MW00844783

Regional Nerve Blocks in Anesthesia and Pain Therapy

Danilo Jankovic • Philip Peng
Editors

Regional Nerve Blocks in Anesthesia and Pain Therapy

Imaging-guided and Traditional Techniques

Fifth Edition

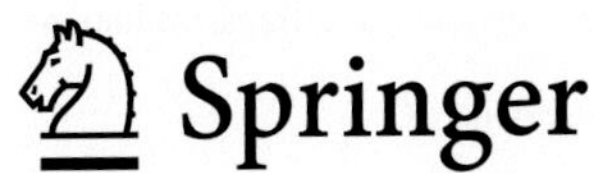
Springer

Editors
Danilo Jankovic
DGS – Cologne – Huerth
Cologne-Hürth
Germany

Philip Peng
Department of Anesthesia and Pain Medicine
Toronto Western Hospital
Toronto, ON, Canada

3rd edition originally published by Wiley-Blackwell, Malden/Oxford/Carlton, 2004

ISBN 978-3-030-88726-1 ISBN 978-3-030-88727-8 (eBook)
https://doi.org/10.1007/978-3-030-88727-8

This Springer imprint is published by the registered company Springer Nature Switzerland AG
The registered company address is: Gewerbestrasse 11, 6330 Cham, Switzerland

This book is dedicated to my wife, Carol, for her continued support, encouragement, and understanding; to my children, Julia and Michael, who fill me with joy and love; and to my sister, Rita, who keeps reminding me to be strong and assertive.
Without them, this book would be impossible.

—Philip Peng

I dedicate this book to my wife, Lydia; to my children Lara and Aleks; and to Julia, Matthias, Lilly, Maximillian, Paul, and Filippa.
Their love, support, and encouragement have made this book possible.

—Danilo Jankovic

Preface

Since the last edition, the literature in both regional anesthesia and pain intervention expands significantly. In the field of regional anesthesia, the increase in interest attributes to the development of a number of fascial plane blocks, as well as the improved understanding of the anatomy and practice from the anatomy publications and systemic reviews. In the field of pain intervention, the application of denervation to different joints, improvement in basic science and technique in neuromodulation, better understanding of the anatomy and pathophysiology of different diseases, and further refinement of some cutting-edge procedures dazzle pain physicians in their practice. Because of this, we feel the need to provide a new edition to embrace these new developments.

What Is New in This Edition?

First, we introduce many new chapters: local anesthetic toxicity, denervation technique for various large joints (hip, knee, shoulder, and sacroiliac joints), neuromodulation (intrathecal drug delivery system, peripheral and spinal cord stimulation), and popular fascial plane blocks (e.g., erector spinae plane block, quadratus lumborum block, iPack blocks). Second, we have re-arranged and organized the large number of chapters, either regional anesthesia or pain therapy, according to the anatomic location. This helps readers to navigate the large number of topics in this new edition. Third, we include both fluoroscopy and ultrasound-guided techniques in various pain intervention procedures

What Is Special About This Textbook?

First, this is the major textbook that comprehensively covers a wide array of regional anesthesia and pain therapy topics, including landmark, ultrasound, and fluoroscopy guidance. Second, the book is contributed by approximately 100 authors, who are the leaders in regional anesthesia and pain therapy across the globe. Third, we made every effort that the overall style of presentation is methodical, practically oriented, thorough, and precise. The description of each block or procedures is broken down into headings: background of the procedures, anatomy, indications and contraindications, techniques, complications and literature review. Lastly, this book contains a generous amount of illustrations and figures, in particular a number of precise anatomical drawings, illustrations, and self-made native anatomical preparations in full color throughout.

The book comprises 76 chapters, organized in 9 parts, covering traditional, ultrasound-guided and fluoroscopy-guided nerve blocks and procedures in anesthesia and interventional pain management. This book is intended for practicing anesthesiologists and all specialties engaged in the field of pain therapy (such as pain specialists, physiatrists, general surgeons, orthopedic surgeons, neurosurgeons, neurologists, and general practitioners).

The start and the finish of this book project coincides with the period of COVID pandemic. During this challenging time, we are indebted to the well-recognized clinicians, academicians, regional anesthesia teams, and pain physicians from around the globe for their support and contribution to this book. We express our sincere thanks to all Springer editorial staff for their expertise and help in editing this book and their constant support and expert assistance.

Cologne-Hürth, Germany Danilo Jankovic
Toronto, ON, Canada Philip Peng

Contents

List of Collaborators

Anne M. Agur Division of Anatomy, Department of Surgery, University of Toronto, Toronto, ON, Canada

Eric Albrecht Department of Anaesthesia, Lausanne University Hospital, Lausanne, Switzerland

Angela Lucia Balocco Department of Anesthesiology, Ziekenhuis Oost-Limburg, Genk, Belgium

Geoff Bellingham Department of Anesthesia and Perioperative Medicine, St. Joseph's Health Care London, Schulich School of Medicine and Dentistry, London, Canada

Thomas Fichtner Bendtsen Department of Anesthesiology, Aarhus University Hospital, Aarhus, Denmark

Anuj Bhatia Anesthesia and Pain Medicine, Toronto Western Hospital, University of Toronto, Toronto, ON, Canada

Sushma Bhatnagar Department of Onco-Anesthesia and Palliative Medicine, AIMS, New Delhi, Delhi, India

Alexandra Bite University of Toronto, Toronto, ON, Canada

Marko Bodor Department of Neurological Surgery, University of California San Francisco, San Francisco, CA, USA

Battista Borghi Anesthesia Research Unit, Instituti Orthopedici Rizzoli, Bologna, Italy

Jens Børglum Department of Anesthesiology and Intensive Care, Zealand University Hospital, Roskilde, Denmark

Department of Clinical Medicine, Faculty of Health and Medical Sciences, University of Copenhagen, Copenhagen, Denmark

Kasha Bornstein Department of Medical Education, University of Miami Medical School, Miami, USA

Hemmo Bosscher Pain Management, Grace Health System/TTU HSC, Lubbock, TX, USA

Matthias R. Braehler Clinical Anesthesia, University of California, San Francisco, CA, USA

Richard Brull Women's College Hospital, University of Toronto, Toronto, ON, Canada

Robert S. Burnham Division of Physical Medicine and Rehabilitation, Faculty of Medicine, University of Alberta, Edmonton, AB, Canada

Central Alberta Pain and Rehabilitation Institute, Lacombe, AB, Canada

Vivo Cura Health, Calgary, AB, Canada

Taylor Burnham Division of Physical Medicine and Rehabilitation, University of Utah, Salt Lake City, UT, USA

Donogh Burns Department of Anesthesiology and Pain Medicine, Toronto Western Hospital, University of Toronto, Toronto, ON, Canada

Michael Catapano Division of Physical Medicine and Rehabilitation, Department of Medicine, University of Toronto, Toronto, ON, Canada

Toronto Rehabilitation Institute, Toronto, ON, Canada

Chin-wern Chan Department of Pain Medicine, Sir Charles Gairdner Hospital, Nedlands, WA, Australia

Vincent Chan Department of Anesthesiology and Pain Medicine, Toronto Western Hospital, University of Toronto, Toronto, ON, Canada

Sara S. K. Cheung University of Alberta, Edmonton, AB, Canada

Department of Anaesthesia, Pamela Youde Nethersole Eastern Hospital, Hong Kong, Hong Kong

Ki Jinn Chin Department of Anesthesiology and Pain Medicine, Toronto Western Hospital, University of Toronto, Toronto, ON, Canada

Niall Cribben Department of Anaesthesia, Critical Care and Pain Management, University Hospital Galway, Galway, Ireland

Miles R. Day Department of Anesthesiology and Pain Management, Texas Tech University Health Sciences Center, Lubbock, TX, USA

James Deering Carolinas Pain Institute and Chronic Pain Research Institute, Winston-Salem, NC, USA

Alessandra Della Porta Department of Medical Education, University of Miami Medical School, Miami, USA

Neel Desai Department of Anaesthesia, Guy's and St Thomas' NHS Foundation Trust, London, UK

Vitaliano Di Grazia Department of Anesthesia and Pain Management, Mount Sinai Hospital, Toronto, ON, Canada

Erica R. Eldon Icahn School of Medicine at Mount Sinai, Rehabilitation and Human Performance, New York, NY, USA

John Paul B. Etheridge Bill Nelems Pain and Research Centre, Kelowna, BC, Canada

Hywel-Gethin Tudur Evans Department of Anesthesiology and Pain Medicine, Toronto Western Hospital, University of Toronto, Toronto, ON, Canada

Guy Feigin Department of Anesthesia and Pain Management, University of Toronto, Toronto Western Hospital, Women's College Hospital, Wasser Pain Management Clinic, Mount Sinai Hospital, Toronto, ON, Canada

Department of Anesthesiology, Critical Care and Pain Management, Meir Medical Center, Kfar-Saba, Israel

Roderick J. Finlayson Bill Nelems Pain and Research Centre, Kelowna, BC, Canada

David Flamer University of Toronto, Toronto, ON, Canada

Mauricio Forero Department of Anesthesia, McMaster University, Hamilton, ON, Canada

Rebecca A. Freedman Icahn School of Medicine at Mount Sinai, Rehabilitation and Human Performance, New York, NY, USA

Laura Girón-Arango Department of Anesthesia, Hospital Pablo Tobón Uribe, Medellín, Colombia

Marina Gitman Department of Anesthesiology, University of Illinois at Chicago, Chicago, IL, USA

Andrew T. Gray Department of Anesthesia and Preoperative Care, University of California San Francisco, San Francisco General Hospital, San Francisco, USA

Paul Gray Department of Anaesthesia, Princess Alexandra Hospital, Woolloongabba, QLD, Australia

Gerbrand Groen Pain Center, University Medical Center Groningen, University of Groningen, Haren, The Netherlands

Amitabh Gulati Department of Anesthesiology and Critical Care, MSKCC, New York, NY, USA

Admir Hadzic Department of Anesthesiology, Ziekenhuis Oost-Limburg, Genk, Belgium

St.Luke's-Roosevelt Hospital Center, College of Physicians and Surgeons, Columbia University, New York, USA

Christian Kruse Hansen Department of Anesthesiology and Intensive Care, Zealand University Hospital, Roskilde, Denmark

Salim M. Hayek Department of Anesthesiology, Division of Pain Medicine, University Hospitals Cleveland Medical Center, Cleveland, OH, USA

Carolina Hernandez-Porras Palliative Care, Instituto Nacional De Cancerologia, Mexico City, Mexico

Louise Hillen P.A., Plymouth, MN, USA

Vivian H. Y. Ip Department of Anesthesiology and Pain Medicine, University of Alberta Hospital, Edmonton, AB, Canada

James M. Jack Guy's and St Thomas' NHS Foundation Trust, London, UK

Danilo Jankovic Pain Management Centre DGS – Cologne – Huerth, Cologne-Hürth, Germany

Leonardo Kapural Carolinas Pain Institute and Chronic Pain Research Institute, Winston-Salem, NC, USA

Manoj Kumar Karmakar Department of Anaesthesia and Intensive Care, The Chinese University of Hong Kong, Prince of Wales Hospital, Shatin, NT, Hong Kong

Michael Kerr Royal Alexandra Hospital, Paisley, Scotland, UK

Jens Kessler Department of Anaesthesiology, University Hospital Division Center for Pain Therapy and Palliative Medicine, Heidelberg, Germany

Michael Seltz Kristensen Department of Anaesthesia, Section 7023, Rigshospitalet, Copenhagen University Hospital, Copenhagen, Denmark

Chandra Kumar Khoo Teck Puat Hospital, Yishun, Singapore

Freelance Consultant Anesthetist, Stockton, TS, UK

Melinda M. Lawrence Department of Anesthesiology, Division of Pain Medicine, University Hospitals Cleveland Medical Center, Cleveland, OH, USA

Danyela Lee Anesthesiology, University of Toronto, Toronto, ON, Canada

Sang Hoon Lee Madiclinic, Jeonju, South Korea

Anam Hospital of Korea University, Seoul, South Korea

Clara Lobo Anesthesiology Department, Hospital das Forças Armadas, Pólo Porto, Portugal

Eldon Loh Department of Physical Medicine and Rehabilitation, Schulich School of Medicine and Dentistry, Western University, London, ON, Canada

Parkwood Institute Research, Lawson Health Research Institute, London, ON, Canada

Parkwood Institute, St. Joseph's Health Care London, London, ON, Canada

Ana M. Lopez Department of Anesthesiology, Ziekenhuis Oost-Limburg, Genk, Belgium

Alan Macfarlane Glasgow Royal Infirmary, University of Glasgow, Glasgow, Scotland, UK

Andre Marques Mansano Department of Interventional Pain Management, Hospital Israelita Albert Einstein, São Paulo, Brazil

Frederik Marynen Section Anesthesiology, Department of Cardiovascular Sciences, KULeuven and University Hospitals Leuven, Leuven, Belgium

Colin J. L. McCartney Department of Anesthesiology and Pain Medicine, The Ottawa Hospital, University of Ottawa, Ottawa, ON, Canada

Jennifer McDonald The Ottawa Hospital, Physical Medicine and Rehabilitation, The Ottawa Hospital Rehabilitation Centre, Ottawa, ON, Canada

John McDonnell Department of Anaesthesia, Critical Care and Pain Management, University Hospital Galway, Galway, Ireland

Wesley Miller Bodor Clinic, Napa, CA, USA

Nimish Mittal Division of Physical Medicine and Rehabilitation, Department of Medicine, University of Toronto, Toronto, ON, Canada

Toronto Rehabilitation Institute, Toronto, ON, Canada

James L. Morgan Department of Anesthesiology and Pain Management, Texas Tech University Health Sciences Center, Lubbock, TX, USA

Farrukh Munshey Department of Anesthesiology and Pain Medicine, University of Toronto, Toronto, ON, Canada

Department of Anesthesia and Pain Medicine, The Hospital for Sick Children, Toronto, ON, Canada

Antoun Nader Acute Pain and Regional Anesthesiology, Northwestern Medicine, Chicago, IL, USA

Tony K. T. Ng Pain Management Unit, Department of Anaesthesia and Operating Theatre Service, Tuen Mun Hospital, Tuen Mun, Hong Kong

Department of Anaesthesiology, LKS Faculty of Medicine, The University of Hong Kong, Pok Fu Lam, Hong Kong

Einar Ottestad Anesthesiology, Perioperative and Pain Medicine, Stanford University School of Medicine, Stanford, CA, USA

Stephanie Pan Department of Anesthesiology, Perioperative and Pain Medicine, Stanford University School of Medicine, Stanford, CA, USA

Amit Pawa Department of Anaesthesia, Guy's and St Thomas' NHS Foundation Trust, London, UK

Philip Peng Department of Anesthesiology and Pain Medicine, Toronto Western Hospital, University of Toronto, Toronto, ON, Canada

Department of Anesthesia and Pain Medicine, Toronto Western Hospital, University of Toronto, Toronto, ON, Canada

Department of Anesthesia and Pain Management, University of Toronto, Toronto Western Hospital, Women's College Hospital, Wasser Pain Management Clinic, Mount Sinai Hospital, Toronto, ON, Canada

Anahi Perlas Anesthesiology and Pain Medicine, University of Toronto, Toronto Western Hospital, University Health Network, Toronto, ON, Canada

Neal Rakesh Department of Anesthesiology and Critical Care, MSKCC, New York, NY, USA

Reva Ramlogan Department of Anesthesiology and Pain Medicine, The Ottawa Hospital, University of Ottawa, Ottawa, ON, Canada

Maria Fernanda Rojas Gomez Cirulaser Andes Clinic, Bogota, Colombia

Vicente Roques Department of Anesthesia and Chronic Pain Treatment, Hospital Universitario Virgen de la Arrixaca, Murcia, Spain

Alexander Sable-Smith Anesthesiology, Perioperative and Pain Medicine, Stanford University School of Medicine, Stanford, CA, USA

Rajendra Sahoo Department of Anesthesia and Pain Management, Kalinga Institute of Medical Sciences, KIIT University, Bhubaneswar, Odisha, India

Piera Santullo DIU Department of Rehabilitation Medicine, Nottingham of University Hospitals, Nottingham, UK

Herman Sehmbi Western University, London, ON, Canada

Ranjith Kumar Sivakumar Department of Anaesthesia and Intensive Care, The Chinese University of Hong Kong, Prince of Wales Hospital, Shatin, NT, Hong Kong

Rakesh V. Sondekoppam Department of Anesthesiology, University of Iowa, Iowa City, IA, USA

David A. Spinner Rehabilitation Mount Sinai, and Human Performance, New York, NY, USA

Kyle Stoffers Department of Physical Medicine and Rehabilitation, University of California Davis, Davis, CA, USA

Agnes R. Stogicza Department of Anesthesiology and Pain Medicine, Saint Magdolna Private Hospital, Budapest, Hungary

Robert Jan Stolker Department of Anesthesiology, Erasmus University Medical Center, Rotterdam, The Netherlands

Katrine Bayer Tanggaard Department of Anesthesiology and Intensive Care, Zealand University Hospital, Roskilde, Denmark

Wendy H. Teoh Private Anaesthesia Practice, Wendy Teoh Pte. Ltd., Singapore, Singapore

Athmaja Thottungal Department of Anaesthesia and Pain Management, Kent and Canterbury Hospital, East Kent Hospitals University NHS Foundation Trust, Canterbury, UK

John Tran Division of Anatomy, Department of Surgery, University of Toronto, Toronto, ON, Canada

Ban C. H. Tsui Department of Anesthesiology, Perioperative Medicine and Pain Medicine, Stanford University, Stanford, CA, USA

Lucille Packard Children's Hospital, Palo Alto, CA, USA

Paul Tumber Department of Anesthesiology and Pain Medicine, University of Toronto, Toronto, ON, Canada

Koen Van Boxem Department of Anesthesiology and Pain Medicine, Maastricht University Medical Centre, Maastricht, Netherlands

Department of Anesthesiology, Critical Care, Urgency Medicine and Multidisciplinary Pain Center, Ziekenhuis Oost-Limburg, Lanaken/Genk, Belgium

Marc Van de Velde Section Anesthesiology, Department of Cardiovascular Sciences, KULeuven and University Hospitals Leuven, Leuven, Belgium

Imré Van Herreweghe Department of Anesthesiology, Ziekenhuis Oost-Limburg, Genk, Belgium

Hans van Suijlekom Department of Anesthesiology, ICU & Pain Therapy, Catharina-ziekenhuis, Eindhoven, The Netherlands

André van Zundert Royal Brisbane and Women's Hospital, Brisbane, QLD, Australia

The University of Queensland & Queensland University of Technology, Brisbane, QLD, Australia

Department of Anaesthesia & Perioperative Medicine, Royal Brisbane & Women's Hospital, Brisbane, QLD, Australia

Jan Van Zundert Department of Anesthesiology and Pain Medicine, Maastricht University Medical Centre, Maastricht, Netherlands

Department of Anesthesiology, Critical Care, Urgency Medicine and Multidisciplinary Pain Center, Ziekenhuis Oost-Limburg, Lanaken/Genk, Belgium

Catherine Vandepitte Department of Anesthesiology, Ziekenhuis Oost-Limburg, Genk, Belgium

Thibaut Vanneste Department of Anesthesiology, Critical Care, Urgency Medicine and Multidisciplinary Pain Center, Ziekenhuis Oost-Limburg, Lanaken/Genk, Belgium

Juan Felipe Vargas Silva Department of Surgery and Image Guided Therapy, Pain Clinic, Hospital Pablo Tobon Uribe, Medellin, Antioquia, Colombia

Department of Surgery, Interventional Radiology and Pain Relief, Hospital Pablo Tobon Uribe, Medellin, Antioquia, Colombia

Sofia Alejandra Velasco Figueroa Pain Management Department, Hospital Zambrano Hellion, TecSalud, San Pedro Garza Garcia, Nuevo Leon, Mexcio, Canada

Juan Venter Bill Nelems Pain and Research Centre, Kelowna, BC, Canada

Barbara Versyck AZ Turnhout, Department of Anesthesia and Intensive Care, Turnhout, Belgium

Department of Anesthesia, Intensive Care and Pain Medicine, Catharina Hospital, Eindhoven, The Netherlands

Ning Nan Wang Anesthesia Department, CIUSSS-du-Nord-de-l'Île-de-Montréal, Montreal, QC, Canada

Guy Weinberg Department of Anesthesiology, University of Illinois at Chicago, Chicago, IL, USA

Arash Yousefi Neurology, Mount Sinai Downtown, New York, NY, USA

Ayden Zarkhah Department of Anesthesiology, University of Illinois at Chicago, Chicago, IL, USA

Zhongxi Zheng Department of Anaesthesia and Surgical Intensive Care, Changi General Hospital, Singapore Health Services, Singapore, Singapore

Anesthesia and Pain Medicine, Toronto Western Hospital, University of Toronto, Toronto, ON, Canada

Xander Zuidema Department of Anesthesiology and Pain Medicine, Maastricht University Medical Centre, Maastricht, Netherlands

Department of Anesthesiology and Pain Management, Diakonessenhuis Utrecht/Zeist, Utrecht, the Netherlands

Jordan Zunder Department of Anesthesiology and Pain Medicine, The Ottawa Hospital, University of Ottawa, Ottawa, ON, Canada

About the Editors

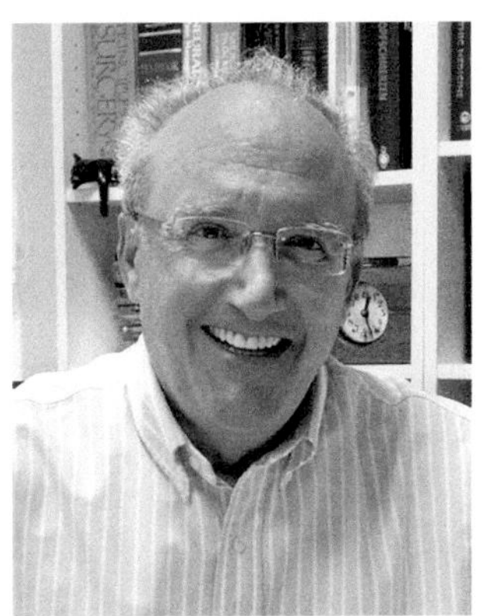

Danilo Jankovic is currently Director of the Regional Pain Management Centre DGS in Cologne-Huerth. Dr. Jankovic's main areas of interest include regional nerve blocks in anesthesia and interventional pain management, regional anesthesia anatomy, treatment of pain by developing new techniques designed and published for the rapid resolution of musculoskeletal pain and dysfunction, medicolegal documentation in regional anesthesia, e.g., Dr. Jankovic is a member of numerous professional associations and has lectured extensively both nationally and internationally.

Dr. Jankovic has been awarded with Rudolf Frey Award 2000 and German Pain Association Award 2007 for his contribution in the field of Regional Anesthesia and Pain Management. Dr. Jankovic has authored the book *Regional Nerve Blocks and Infiltration Therapy* (1st–4th ed.), which has been translated into six languages and awarded "book of the year" 2005 by the Society of Authors and The Royal Society of Medicine in London. He has also contributed many chapters to textbooks edited by colleagues.

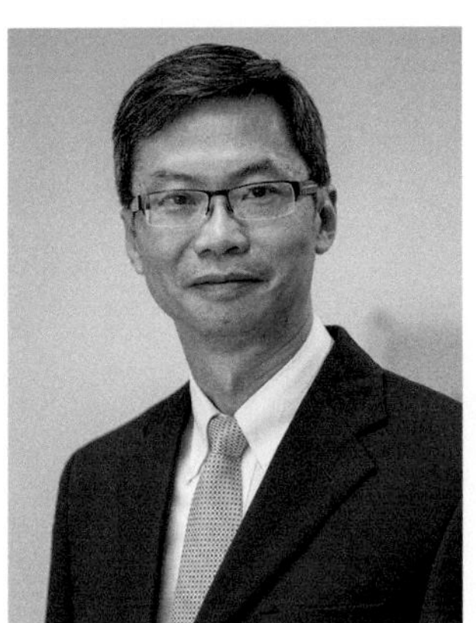

Philip Peng is a Professor in the Department of Anesthesiology and Pain Medicine of the University of Toronto. He has played an important role in the education of pain medicine and established major teaching courses for Pain in Canada such as Canadian Pain Interventional Course and Ultrasound for Pain Medicine Course. The Royal College of Physicians and Surgeons of Canada (RCPSC) honored him with the Founder designation in pain medicine for his role in establishing pain medicine subspecialty in Canada. He is a leader, researcher, educator, and pioneer in the application of ultrasound for pain medicine. His innovative research led to different new procedures in pain intervention, including ultrasound-guided pudendal nerve block and pericapsular nerve group (PENG) block.

He received numerous awards including the prestigious John J Bonica award from American Society of Regional Anesthesia and Pain Medicine and Distinguished Service Award from both the European Society of Regional Anesthesia-Spain Chapter and Canadian Pain Society. He has delivered more than 400 lectures and workshops nationally and internationally. He has edited 8 books and published 240 peer-reviewed publications and book chapters.

Part I

General Consideration

Regional Nerve Block in Anesthesia and Pain Therapy: General Consideration

1

Danilo Jankovic

Contents

D. Jankovic (✉)
Pain Management Centre DGS – Cologne – Huerth, Cologne-Hürth, Germany
e-mail: danilo@jankovic1.de

D. Jankovic, P. Peng (eds.), *Regional Nerve Blocks in Anesthesia and Pain Therapy*,
https://doi.org/10.1007/978-3-030-88727-8_1

Regional Nerve Blocks and Infiltration Therapy in Clinical Practice

General Consideration

Regional anesthesia means the interruption of impulse conduction in the nerves using specific, reversibly acting drugs (local anesthetics). This interruption of impulse conduction can be carried out in every region of the body in which the nerves are accessible for external injection.

The indications for regional anesthesia include:

1. Clinical anesthesia
   Particularly in the fields of traumatology, orthopedics, urology, and gynecology, as well as in large-scale abdominal surgery with continuous procedures for epidural or spinal anesthesia.
2. Obstetrics
   The use of regional anesthesia especially neuraxial anesthesia will be discussed in detail in Chap. 42.
3. Postoperative analgesia
   There is no postoperative analgesia procedure that is more appropriate than regional anesthesia. This field also includes the classic indications for a combination of local anesthetics with opioids or other substances. Optimal patient care can only be achieved using a multimodal approach (effective pain therapy, early mobilization, early enteral nutrition, and emotional and psychological care). Effective pain therapy (e.g., with catheter analgesia procedures) plays a central role here, as it can substantially reduce the perioperative stress response (Fig. 1.1).
4. Pain therapy
   In 1979, a commission set up by the International Association for the Study of Pain (IASP) defined pain as "... an unpleasant sensory and emotional experience, linked to actual or potential tissue damage". Since then, the definition of pain is recently revised. Acute pain is caused by stimulation of pain receptors. This stimulation is transient and sets in motion biologically useful protective mechanisms. Ideally, pain can be relieved by treating

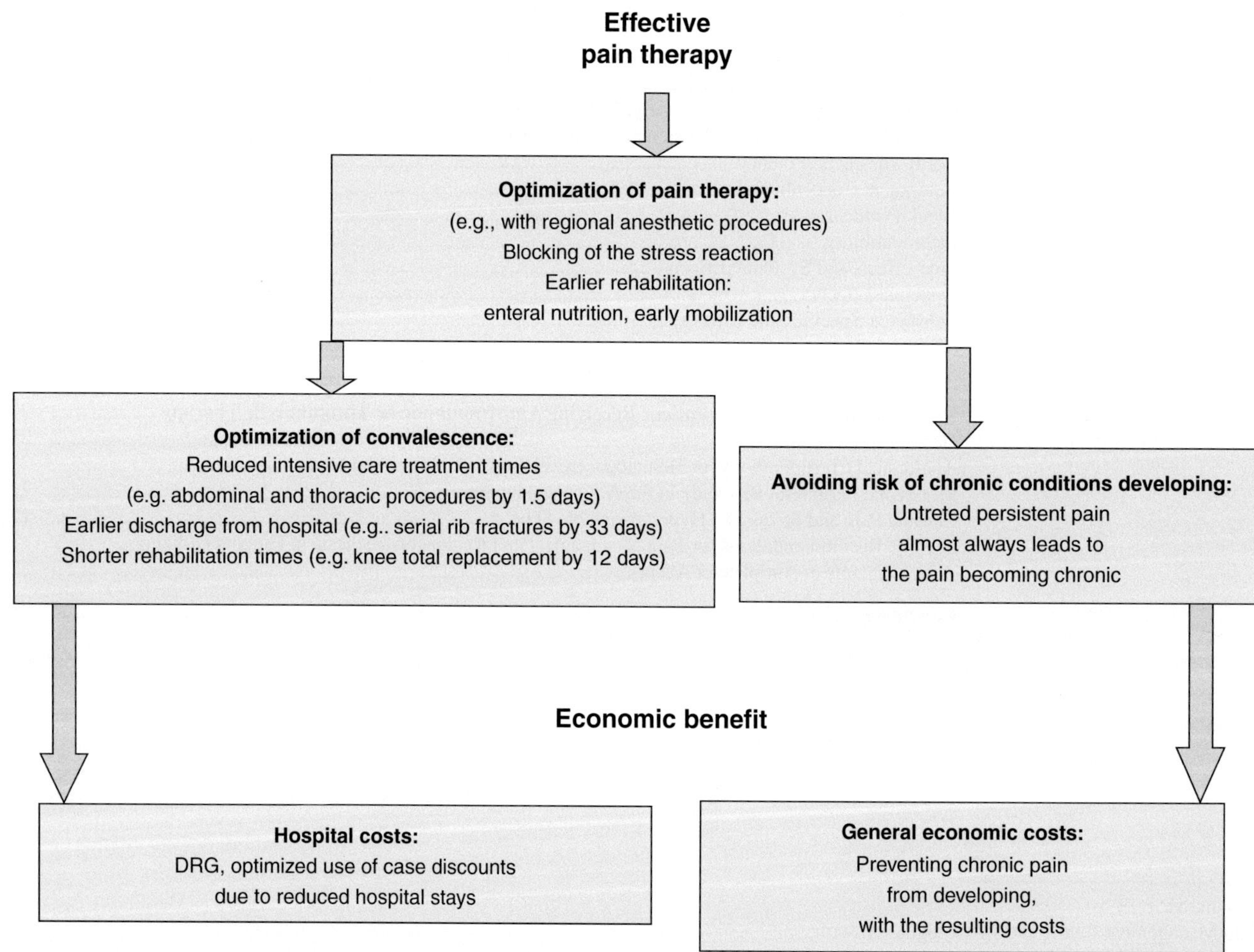

Fig. 1.1 Importance of effective pain therapy as part of a multimodal approach to treatment

the cause. Chronic pain is regarded as a pathological response on the part of the body. The relief of pain should be viewed as a "human right." In this context, there are a significant number of patients who will not obtain effective pain relief without access to potent neural blockade techniques.

It arises due to constant stimulation of nociceptive afferents, or can develop as neuropathic pain after injury or damage to the peripheral nociceptive system. Chronic pain can often lead to alterations in patient's living habits, physical abilities, and personality, and requires a coordinated interdisciplinary approach. This in turn presupposes a clear diagnosis, based on a full general history and pain history, physical examination and functional assessment of the patient's musculature, locomotor apparatus, autonomic nervous system, and neurological and angiological situation.

In addition to medical treatment for pain, nerve blocks have a firmly established place in pain therapy—alongside physical and manual procedures, neurological and neurosurgical methods, physiotherapy and the psychosocial management of patients. In quantitative terms, regional anesthesia procedures play only a minor part in the management of chronic pain, but qualitatively they can produce very good results when used with the correct indications.

Nerve Blocks in Surgery and Pain Therapy

The application of the anesthesiology methods described in the subsequent chapters of this book for temporary interruption of stimulus conduction in a nerve or nerve plexus requires the use of strictly established indications and the implementation of a coordinated therapeutic approach. In principle, these blocks can be administered for surgery, diagnosis, prognosis, and therapy (Table 1.1).

Surgical blocks are administered with high-dose local anesthetics for targeted isolation of a specific body region in order to carry out an operation.

Diagnostic blocks using low-dose local anesthetics are appropriate for the differential diagnosis of pain syndromes. They allow the affected conduction pathways to be recognized and provide evidence regarding the causes of the pain. Diagnostic blocks can also be used to clarify the question of whether the source of the pain is peripheral or central.

Prognostic blocks allow predictions to be made regarding the potential efficacy of a longer-term nerve block, neurolysis or surgical sympathectomy. They should also be used to prepare the patient for the effects of a permanent block.

Therapeutic blocks are used in the treatment of a wide variety of pain conditions. Typical examples of these are post-traumatic and postoperative pain, complex regional pain syndrome (CRPS) types I and II (reflex sympathetic dystrophy and causalgia), joint mobilization, postherpetic neuralgia, and tumor pain.

Table 1.1 Important rules to observe when administering regional anesthesia or therapeutic nerve blocks

Before the block
Patient
1. Preoperative information
– Explain the procedure
– Discuss potential side effects and complications
–Advise the patient about what to do after the procedure
– Document the discussion
2. Determine the patient's neurological status
– Exclude neurological abnormalities
3. Exclude contraindications
4. Avoid premedication in outpatients (particularly in blocks in which there is an increased risk of intravascular injection—e.g., stellate ganglion or superior cervical ganglion)
Anatomy, complications, side effects
1. With rarely used regional blocks, the anatomic and technical aspects should always be studied again beforehand
2. Detailed knowledge of potential complications and side effects of a regional block and how to avoid them
3. Ability to control potential complications and side effects
4. Select the correct block techniques
5. Manual skill and good training on the part of the anesthetist
Preparation
1. Ensure optimal positioning of the patient
2. Always secure intravenous access
3. Check that emergency equipment is complete and fully functioning
4. Added vasopressors are contraindicated in pain therapy
5. Observe sterile precautions
Safety standards when injecting larger doses of local anesthetics
1. Carry out aspiration tests before and during the injection
2. Administer a test dose
3. Inject local anesthetics in incremental doses (several test doses)
4. Maintain verbal contact with the patient
5. Cardiovascular monitoring
6. Keep careful notes of the block

Nerve Blocks and Chronic Pain

A *multimodal treatment approach* to chronic pain is essential for successful treatment. The use of nerve blocks as part of this approach presupposes that the following steps have been taken:

1. Careful analysis of the pain.
2. Correct diagnosis and establishment of the indication.
3. Assessment of the pain chronicity stage.
4. Well-selected patient groups.

Important preconditions for the application of nerve blocks in chronic pain include:

1. A good knowledge of anatomy.
2. Attention to and control of potential side effects and complications.
3. Choice of the correct block techniques.
4. Manual skill and good training on the part of therapist.

The most important tasks facing us include conducting more double-blind, randomized and well-controlled studies on the use of nerve blocks in chronic pain conditions, and developing a consistent standard for carrying out nerve blocks. The answers to two questions need to be found:

1. Selection criteria to identify which patients are suitable for nerve blocks.
2. The number of nerve blocks to be used in the treatment of chronic pain.

Examination and Patient Preparation

Before regional anesthesia, the same type of examination of the patient should be carried out as for general anesthesia. Contraindications must be excluded, as well as neurological abnormalities, and when there are relative contraindications—for example, hemorrhagic diathesis, stable systemic neurological disease or local nerve damage—a careful assessment of the risk-benefit ratio needs to be made.

Particular attention needs to be given to anatomical relationships, palpation of the landmarks and precise localization and marking of the needle insertion point (Table 1.1).

Informed Consent

To ensure cooperation, the patient should be given simple, short information about the aim of the block, its technical performance and possible or probable paresthesias and their significance. The patient should also be informed about potential adverse effects and complications of the block, and outpatients in particular should be familiarized with guidelines on behavior after anesthesia. The patient information session should be documented using a consent form signed by the patient.

*Do not discuss only serious and major risks of the procedure, but also benefits and expected results of the proposed regional anesthetic procedure. The consent process has to be used as a simultaneous education of the patient

Safety Measures

It is important that a number of safety measures are taken to ensure the most suitable regional anesthesia technique is performed for the correct patient. These measures include obtaining patient consent, checking all equipment and drugs, ensuring appropriate monitoring and performance of a correct surgical site check. Once the regional block is performed, it is vital to accurately document the procedure in detail (Table 1.1).

In general, premedication and the administration of sedatives or analgesics should be avoided in outpatient pain therapy. Constant verbal contact should be maintained with the patient during the block, so that potential side effects or complications can be recognized immediately. In addition, any sedation that is not adjusted individually can lead to respiratory and circulatory complications, which may be mistaken for the early symptoms of local anesthetic toxicity.

Documentation of Treatment

The patient history, including investigations at other centers, and diagnostic results should be documented just as carefully as the preparation, implementation, and success of the block.

The checklists and record forms used in our Institution have been adapted for each individual block technique. Samples of record and checklists, for example, stellate ganglion block, neuraxial block, or peripheral nerve block are shown in Figs. 1.2, 1.3, and 1.4.

This comprehensive list has pertinent information including purpose of the block, position and approach, type of local anesthetics used, and complications that might arise. Such standardized recommendations are useful for the purpose of medicolegal documentation and conducting retrospective studies on complications. Paper records are increasingly being replaced with electronic medical record-keeping systems. Legibility and ability to correct errors are advantages to the e-block note. Another useful aspect of regional nerve block documentation is the recording of an ultrasound image or video clip, to be stored in the patient's chart.

Technical Requirements

Carrying out temporary nerve blocks and regional anesthetic procedures in surgery and pain therapy requires the appropriate basic technical equipment and experience in the use of all of the instruments concerned. The conditions for patient positioning, the aseptic conditions required, and the syringes, needle types, and other supplies needed are discussed alongside the individual block techniques described in this book. Complete and properly functioning equipment must be available both for primary care and in case of adverse events and complications, as well as treatment monitoring.

Record and checklist

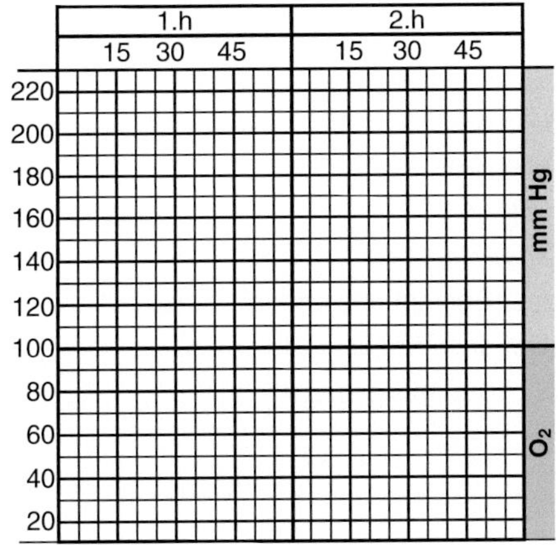

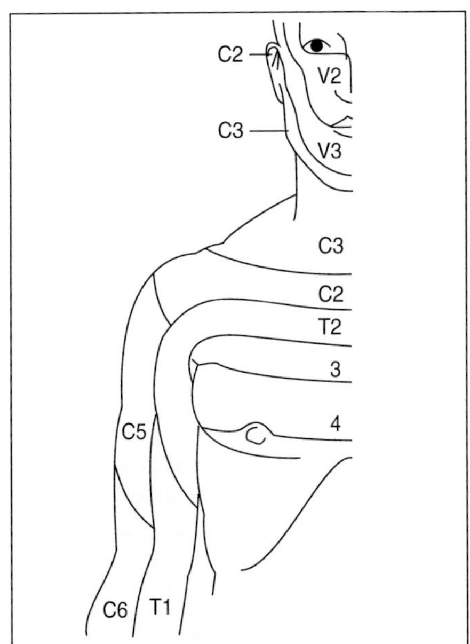

With permission from Danilo Jankovic

Cervicothoracic ganglion (stellate ganglion)

Block no. ☐ Right ☐ Left

Name: ______ Date: ______

Diagnosis: ______

Premedication: ☐ No ☐ Yes ______

Purpose of block: ☐ *Diagnostic* ☐ *Therapeutic*

Needle: ☐ *22 G* ☐ *40 mm long* ☐ *50 mm long*

i.v. access: ☐ *Yes*

Monitoring: ☐ *ECG* ☐ *Pulse oximetry*

Ventilation facilities: ☐ *Yes (equipmet checked)*

Emergency equipment *(drugs)*: ☐ *Checked*

Patient: ☐ *Informed*

Position: ☐ *Supine* ☐ *Neck extended*

Approach: ☐ *Paratracheal* ☐ *C6* ☐ *C7*
☐ *Ultrasound - guided*
☐ *Transducer* ☐ *Linear*
☐ *In plane* ☐ *Out of plane*

Local anesthetic: ____ *ml* ____ *%* ______

Test dose: ____ *ml*

Addition to

Injection solution: ☐ *No* ☐ *Yes* ______

Patient's remarks during injection:

☐ *None* ☐ *Pain* ☐ *Paresthesias* ☐ *Warmth*

Nerve region ______ ______ ______

Objective block effect after 15 min:

☐ *Cold test* ☐ *Temperature measurement right* ____ *°C left* ____ *°C*

Horner's syndrome: ☐ *Yes* ☐ *No*

Segment affected: ☐ *C2* ☐ *C3* ☐ *C4* ☐ *C5* ☐ *T* ___

Monitoring after block: ☐ *< 1 h* ☐ *> 1 h*

Time of discharge ______

Complications: ☐ *None*
☐ *Yes (intravascular, epidural, subarachnoid injection, other)* ______

Side effects: ☐ *None*

☐ *Yes (recurrent laryngeal nerve, phrenic nerve, vagus* ______

Subjective effects of the block: *Duration:* ______

☐ *None* ☐ *Increased pain*

☐ *Reduced pain* ☐ *Relief of pain*

VISUAL ANALOG SCALE

0 10 20 30 40 50 60 70 80 90 100

Special notes:

______

______

______

Fig. 1.2 Checklist and record for cervicothoracic ganglion block. (Courtesy of Danilo Jankovic with permission)

Record and checklist

	1.h			2.h		
	15	30	45	15	30	45

220, 200, 180, 160, 140, 120, 100, 80, 60, 40, 20 — mm Hg — O_2

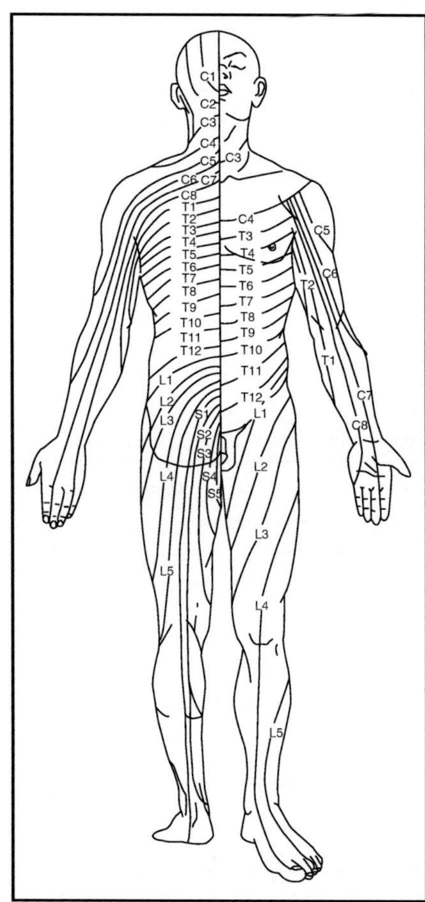

With permission from Danilo Jankovic

Lumbar epidural anesthesia

Name: ____________ Date: ____________

Diagnosis: ____________

Premedication: ☐ No ☐ Yes ____________

Neurological abnormalities: ☐ No ☐ Yes ____________

Purpose of block: ☐ *Surgical* ☐ *Therapeutic* ☐ *Diagnostic*

Needle: ☐ *Tuohy G*___ ☐ *Other* ___

i.v. access, infusion: ☐ *Yes*

Monitoring: ☐ *ECG* ☐ *Pulse oximetry*

Ventilation facilities: ☐ *Yes (equipment checked)*

Emergency equipment (drugs): ☐ *Checked*

Patient: ☐ *Informed*

Position: ☐ *Lateral decubitus* ☐ *Sitting*

Access: ☐ *Median* ☐ *Paramedian*

Injection level: ☐ *L3/L4* ☐ *Other* ________

Injection technique: ☐ *Loss of resistance* ☐ *Other* ________

☐ *Ultrasound guided* ☐ *Transducer* ☐ *Curved* ☐ *Linear*

Approach: ☐ *In plane* ☐ *Out of plane*

Epidural space: ☐ *Identified*

Aspiration test: ☐ *Carried out*

Test dose: ____________ Epinephrine added: ☐ *Yes* ☐ *No*

Check on sensorimotor function after 5 min: ☐ *Carried out*

Abnormalities: ☐ *No* ☐ *Yes*______

Injection:

☐ Local anesthetic: ____________ *mL* ______ *%*
(incremental)

☐ Addition: ____________ *µg/mg*

Patient's remarks during injection:

☐ *None* ☐ *Pain* ☐ *Paresthesias* ☐ *Warmth*

Duration and area: ____________

Objective block effect after 20 min:

☐ *Cold test* ☐ *Temperature measurement before*______ *°C after* ______ *°C*

☐ *Sensory: L*______ *T*______

☐ *Motor*

Complications:

☐ *None* ☐ *Pain*
☐ *Radicular symptoms* ☐ *Vasovagal reactions*
☐ *BP drop* ☐ *Dural puncture*
☐ *Vascular puncture* ☐ *Intravascular injection*
☐ *Massive epidural anesthesia* ☐ *Total spinal anesthesia*
☐ *Subdural spread* ☐ *Respiratory disturbance*
☐ *Drop in body temperature* ☐ *Muscle tremor*
☐ *Bladder emptying disturbances* ☐ *Postdural puncture headache*
☐ *Back pain* ☐ *Neurological complications*

Special notes:

Fig. 1.3 Checklist and record for lumbar epidural anesthesia. (Courtesy of Danilo Jankovic with permission)

Record and checklist

Lumbosacral plexus and individual nerves in the plexus

Block no. ☐ Right ☐ Left

Name: ____________ Date: ____________

Diagnosis: ____________

Premedication: ☐ No ☐ Yes

Neurological abnormalities: ☐ No ☐ Yes ____________

Purpose of block: ☐ Surgical ☐ Diagnostic ☐ Therapeutic

Needle: G____ Length ______ cm ☐ 15° ☐ 30° ☐ Other

i.v. access: ☐ Yes

Monitoring: ☐ ECG ☐ Pulse oximetry

Ventilation facilities: ☐ Yes (equipment checked)

Emergency equipment (drugs): ☐ Checked

Patient: ☐ Informed (behavior after block)

Position: ☐ Prone ☐ Lateral recumbent ☐ Sims-Position ☐ Sitting

Injection: ☐ Inguinal "3-in-one" block ☐ Dorsal psoas compartment block

☐ *Sciatic nerve* ☐ *Femoral nerve* ☐ *Lateral cutaneous nerve of thigh*

☐ *Obturator nerve* ☐ *Ilioinguinal nerve / hypogastric nerve*

Location technique: ☐ Electrostimulation ☐ Other

☐ *Ultrasound- guided* ☐ *Transducer* ☐ *Linear* ☐ *Curved*

Approach: ☐ *In-plane* ☐ *Out of plane*

Plexus (nerve): ☐ *Located* ☐ *Aspiration test* ☐ *Test dose*

Injection:

Local anesthetic: ____________ *mL* ________ *%*

(in incremental doses)

☐ *Inguinal "3-in-one" block* ____ *mL* ☐ *Dorsal psoas compartmt. block* ____ *mL*

☐ *Sciatic nerve* ____ *mL* ☐ *Femoral nerve* ____ *mL* ☐ *Lateral cutaneous nerve of thigh* ____ *mL* ☐ *Obturator nerve* ____ *mL* ☐ *Ilioinguinal nerve/hypogastric nerve* ____ *mL*

☐ Addition to LA ____________ *µg/mg*

	1.h			2.h			
	15	30	45	15	30	45	
220							mm Hg
200							
180							
160							
140							
120							
100							O_2
80							
60							
40							
20							

Patient's remarks during injection:

☐ None ☐ Paresthesias ☐ Warmth ☐ Pain (intraneural position?)

Nerve area: ____________

Objective block effect after 15 min:

☐ Cold test ☐ Temperature measurement before ____°C after ____°C

☐ Sensory ☐ Motor

Monitoring after block: ☐ < 1 h ☐ > 1 h

Time of discharge: ____________ ☐ Sensorimotor function checked

Complications:

☐ None ☐ Intravascular injection ☐ Signs of intoxication

☐ Hematoma ☐ Neurological complications ☐ Other

Subjective effects of the block: Duration: ____________

☐ None ☐ Increased pain ☐ Reduced pain ☐ Relief of pain

VISUAL ANALOG SCALE

0 10 20 30 40 50 60 70 80 90 100

Special notes:

T10 T11 T12 L1 L2 L3 L4 L5

With permission from Danilo Jankovic

Fig. 1.4 Checklist and record for peripheral nerve block. (Courtesy of Danilo Jankovic with permission)

Accessories for Primary Care

Emergency Equipment (Figs. 1.5, 1.6, and 1.7)

- Intubation and ventilation equipment.
- Oxygen source (breathing apparatus).
- Ventilation bag with two masks (large, medium).
- Guedel tubes nos. 3, 4, 5.
- Wendel tubes nos. 26–32.
- Endotracheal tubes nos. 28–36.
- Tube clamp, blocker syringe (10 mL).
- Laryngoscope with batteries (replacement batteries and replacement bulbs), spatula.
- Magill forceps, mouth wedge, 1 tube 2% lidocaine gel.
- Suction device.
- Infusion equipment.
- Two sets of infusion instruments.
- Five plastic indwelling catheters.
- Syringes (2 mL, 5 mL, 10 mL), plaster, gauze bandages.
- Infusion solutions.
- 1 bottle each of Ringer's solution, plasma expander, 8.4% sodium bicarbonate (100 mL).

Defibrillator

- Drugs for emergency treatment.

When blocks are being administered, a sedative (midazolam), a vasopressor (phenylephrine or ephedrine), and a vagolytic (glycopyrrolate) should be available for immediate injection. Lipid emulsion 20% should be available in the presence of local anesthetic systemic toxicity.

Anesthetic Machine

For neuraxial anesthesia, ganglion blocks, intravenous regional anesthesia, and plexus anesthesia, an anesthesia trolley with facilities for intubation is also required (Fig. 1.8).

Monitoring

- Electrocardiogram (ECG).
- Pulse oximeter (Fig. 1.9).

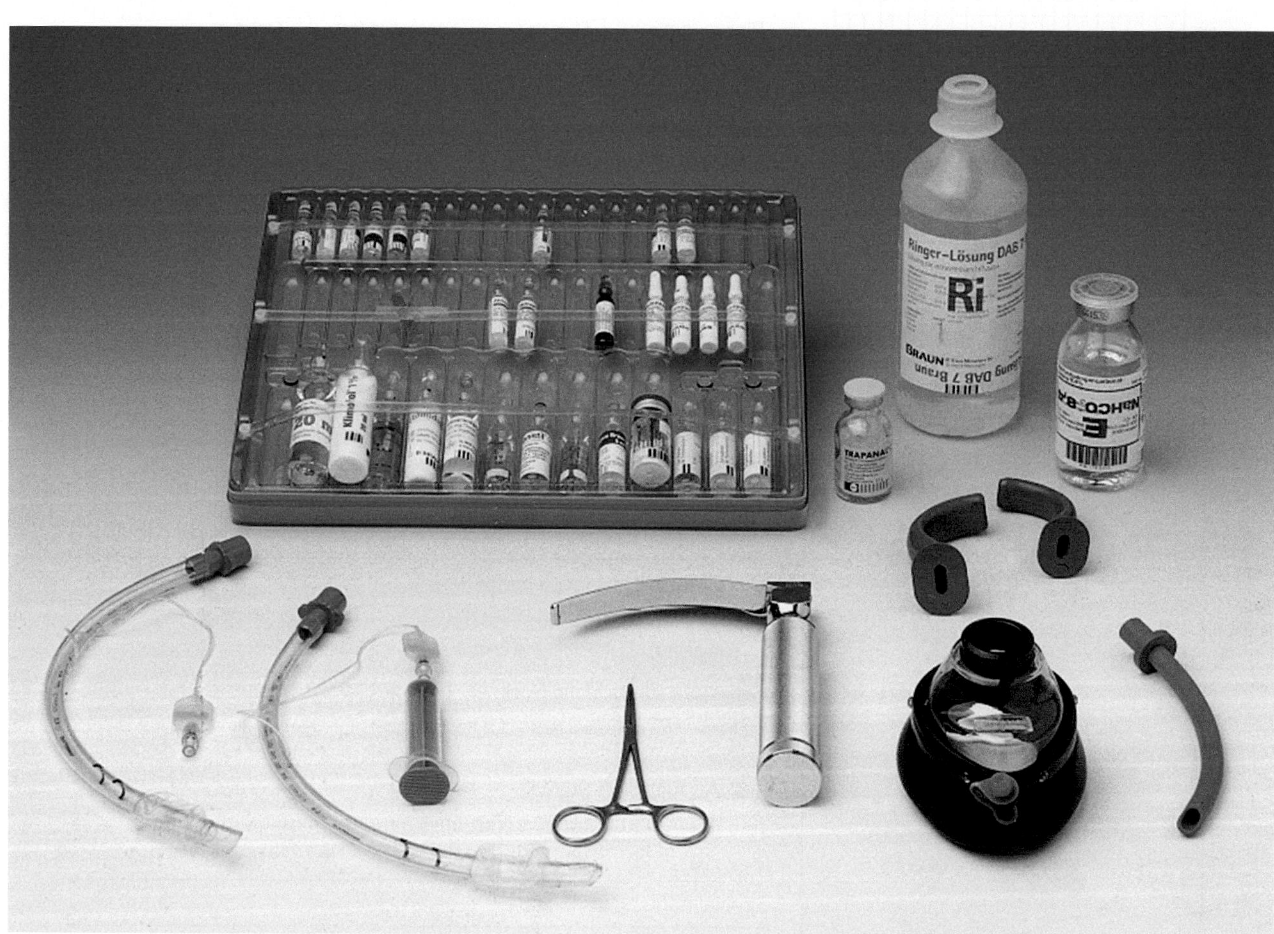

Fig. 1.5 Emergency equipment

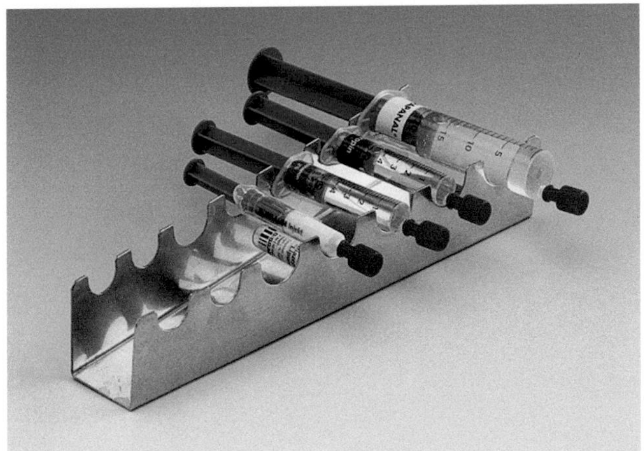

Fig. 1.6 Emergency drugs

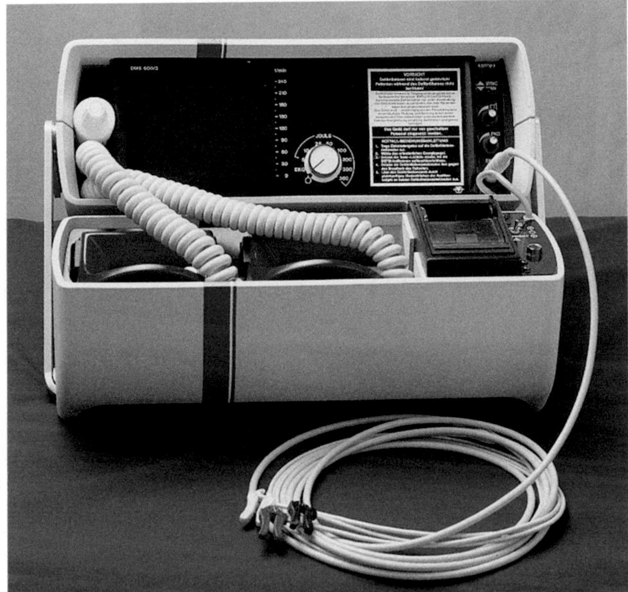

Fig. 1.7 Defibrillator

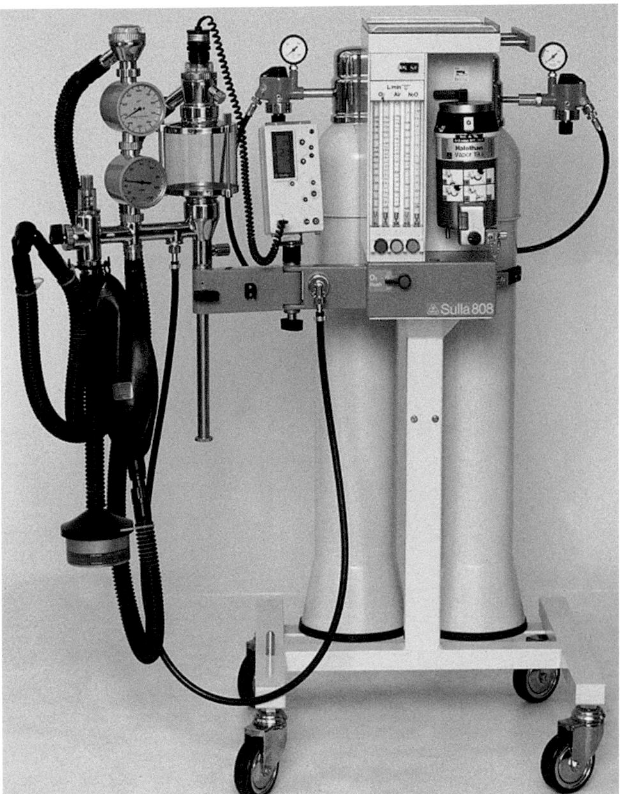

Fig. 1.8 Anesthetic machine

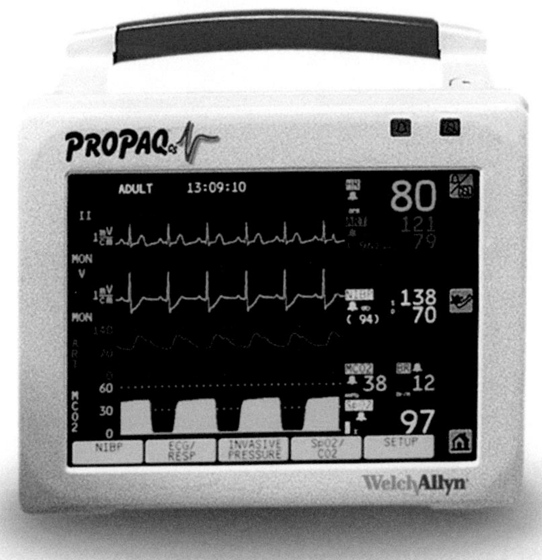

Fig. 1.9 ECG and pulse oximeter

Peripheral Nerve Stimulator

Peripheral nerve stimulation is a valuable aid in clinical practice and has considerable advantages in combination with an atraumatic catheter technique (Fig. 1.10). A full chapter on the electric stimulation for perioperative use will be discussed in Chap. 3.

Ultrasound

In the last two decades, the field of regional anesthesia, and in particular peripheral nerve blockade, has entered an unprecedented renaissance. This renaissance is due primarily to the widespread introduction of ultrasound-guided regional anesthesia (Fig. 1.11). The ability to visualize the anatomy of interest, the needle–nerve relationship, and the spread of the local anesthetic has resulted in significant growth of interest in and use of peripheral, sympathetic, and neuraxial blocks.

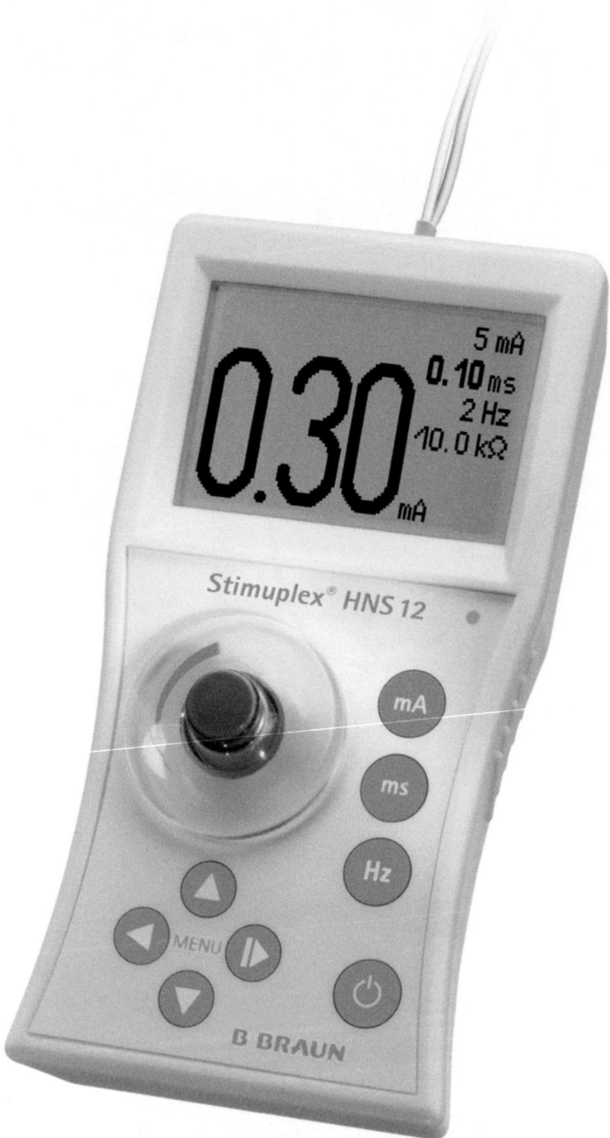

Fig. 1.10 Peripheral nerve stimulator

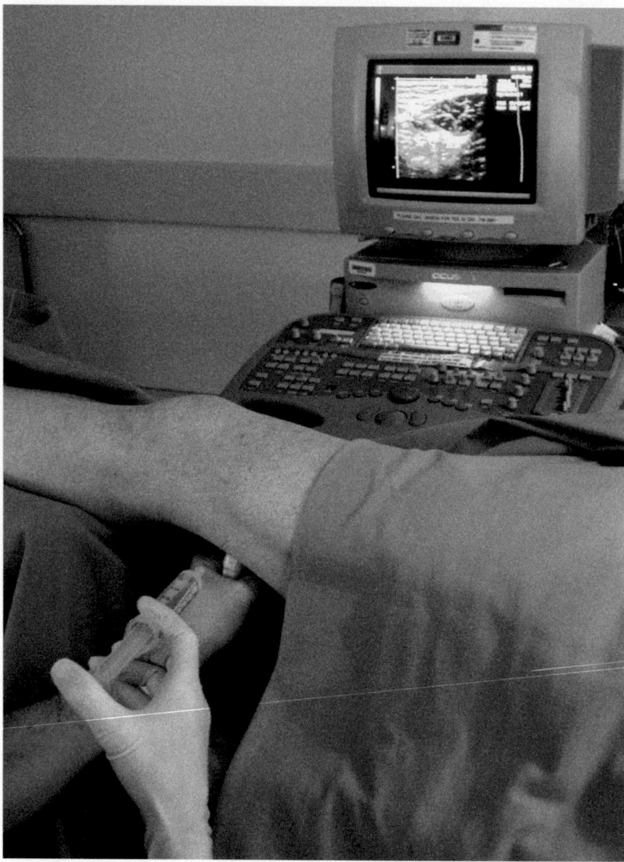

Fig. 1.11 Ultrasound machine

The basic principle of applying ultrasound in regional anesthesia is discussed in detail in Chap. 2.

Use of Local Anesthetic in Regional Anesthesia and Pain Therapy

General Consideration

Local anesthetics produce anesthesia by inhibiting the excitation of nerve endings or by blocking conduction in peripheral nerves. Cocaine, a compound indigenous to the Andes Mountains, West Indies, and Java, was the first anesthetic to be discovered and is the only naturally occurring local anesthetic; all others are synthetically derived. Cocaine was introduced into Europe in the 1800s following its isolation from coca beans. Sigmund Freud, the noted Austrian psychoanalyst, used cocaine on his patients and became addicted through self-experimentation.

Local anesthetics block voltage-gated sodium channels thereby interrupting the initiation and transmission of nerve impulses in axons. Based on this mechanism of action, local anesthetics provide a wide variety of biologic actions, both desirable and unwanted, and have side effects through other mechanisms. Currently available local anesthetics are of two chemical classes: aminoesters and aminoamides. Aminoesters are metabolized primarily by plasma esterases, and aminoamides are metabolized primarily by hepatic cytochrome P450-linked enzymes. The knowledge of their pharmacology is important for safe and optimal use of this group of drugs. The principal systemic toxicities of local anesthetics involve the heart (including atrioventricular conduction block, arrhythmias, myocardial depression, and cardiac arrest) and the brain (including agitation, lethargy, seizures, and generalized central nervous system depression). Local anesthetics are directly toxic to nerve at the concentrations supplied in commercial solutions. Intraneural concentrations during regional anesthesia are generally, but not always, less than a threshold for toxicity because of local vascular removal, and dilutional effects due to spread of solutions through tissues and into nerve. Hence, injection into a constrained tissue space increases the risk for local toxicity. Optimal use of local anesthetics in regional anesthesia requires an understanding of the individual patient's clinical situation, the location, intensity, and duration of regional anesthesia and analgesia required, anatomic factors affecting deposition of drugs near nerves, proper drug selection and dosing, and repeated assessment of clinical effects after administration of a local anesthetic. Local anesthetics are increasingly being used as postoperative infusions and via both local and systemic administration for the management of chronic pain.

Chemical Structure and Physicochemical Properties

All local anesthetics in common clinical use have three characteristic molecular sections in their chemical structure:

An aromatic residue, which basically determines the lipophilic properties of the agent. Substitutions in the aromatic group allow the pKa and lipid solubility of the substance to be influenced.

An intermediate chain, which in local anesthetics of the ester type (Table 1.2) contains a relatively unstable ester bond (CO–O) that can be broken down hydrolytically by pseudocholinesterases. Local anesthetics of the amide type (Table 1.3) are much more stable, since the amide bond (NH–CO) in their intermediate chain cannot be broken down in plasma. The length of the chain between the aromatic residue and the substituted amino group has an influence on the intensity of effect of the local anesthetic. The agent's protein-binding capacity and lipid solubility can be altered by substitution in the intermediate chain.

A substituted amino group, the protonization of which determines the ratio of the cationic to the basic form. Only the free base is capable of penetrating lipoprotein membranes. However, to be able to affect the nerve membrane, the local anesthetic must be available as a cation. The type of amino group substitution affects the distribution coefficient, the plasma protein binding and the intensity and duration of the drug's action.

Clinical Significance of the Physicochemical Properties

Local anesthetics differ with regard to their molecular weight, their lipid and water solubility, pKa, and protein-binding characteristics. These factors in turn have a substantial influence on the potency of the drug's local anesthetic effect on the onset of the effect and on its duration (Tables 1.4a and 1.4b).

Table 1.2 Local anesthetics with an ester bond

Aromatic residue	Intermediate chain	Substit. amino group	Year introduced
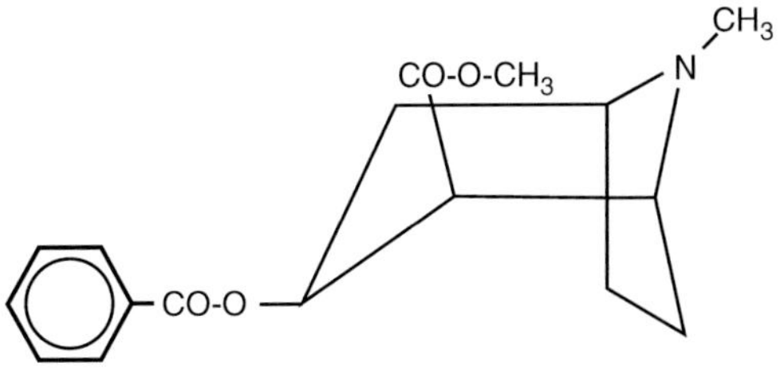 Benzene ring	CO-O (CO-O-CH_3)	N-CH_3	
Cocaine			1884
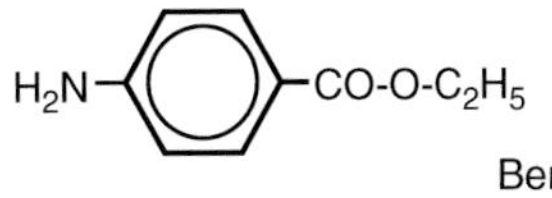 H_2N– benzene ring	CO-O-C_2H_5		
Benzocaine			1900
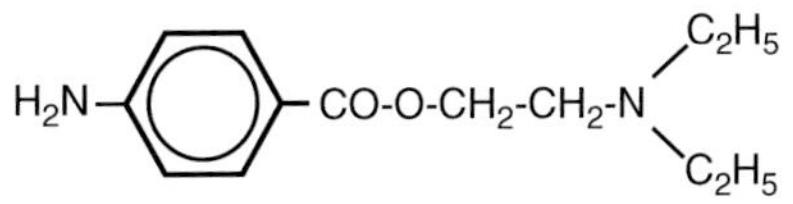 H_2N– benzene ring	CO-O-CH_2-CH_2-	N(C_2H_5)(C_2H_5)	
Procaine			1905
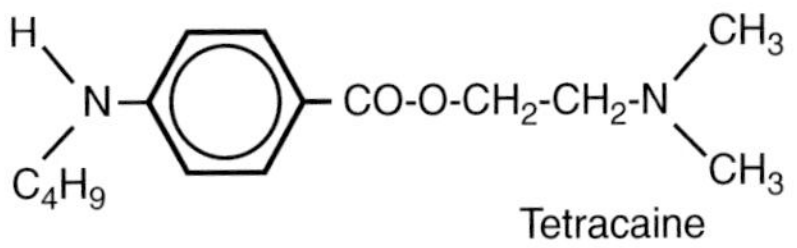 H–N(C_4H_9)– benzene ring	CO-O-CH_2-CH_2-	N(CH_3)(CH_3)	
Tetracaine			1930
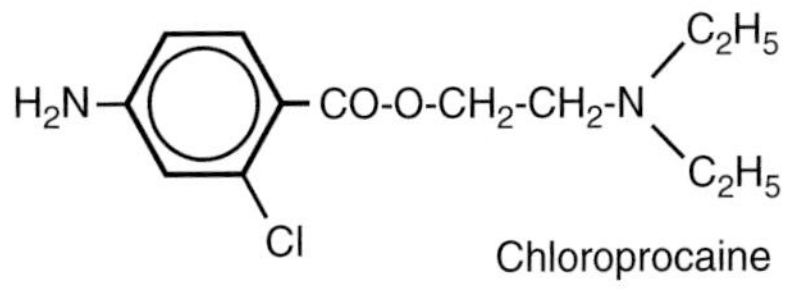 H_2N– benzene ring (Cl)	CO-O-CH_2-CH_2-	N(C_2H_5)(C_2H_5)	
Chloroprocaine			1955

Local Anesthetic Potency

The combined effect of factors such as protein binding, stereoisomeric structure, and lipophilia determine the potency of a local anesthetic agent. To achieve a blocking effect, the local anesthetic has to diffuse across the cell membrane into the interior of the cell (importance of lipophilia for membrane diffusion) so that, from the cytosol (appropriate hydrophilic properties), it can occupy the sodium channel in its then protonated form (Fig. 1.12).

A high degree of lipophilia is associated with good membrane permeation, and a high degree of hydrophilia is associated with good solubility in the cytosol. Local anesthetics therefore have to have both of these properties in a favorable ratio.

However, the clinical distinction that is made in local anesthetics between those of mild potency (procaine), medium

Table 1.3 Local anesthetics with an amide bond

Aromatic residue	Intermediate chain	Substit. amino group	Year introduced
CH_3, CH_3 (benzene ring)	NH-CO-CH_2-N(C_2H_5)(C_2H_5)	Lidocaine	1944
CH_3, CH_3 (benzene ring)	NH-CO (piperidine ring, N-CH_3)	Mepivacaine	1957
CH_3 (benzene ring)	NH-CO-CH(CH_3)-N(C_3H_7)(H)	Prilocaine	1960
CH_3, CH_3 (benzene ring)	NH-CO (piperidine ring, N-C_4H_9)	Bupivacaine	1963
CH_3, CH_3 (benzene ring)	NH-CO-CH(C_2H_5)-N(C_3H_7)(C_2H_5)	Etidocaine	1972
CH_3, S, CO-O CH_3 (thiophene ring)	NH-CO-CH(CH_3)-N(C_3H_7)(H)	Carticaine	1974
CH_3, CH_3 (benzene ring)	NH-CO ····· (H; piperidine ring, N-C_3H_7)	Ropivacaine	1996
CH_3, CH_3 (benzene ring)	NH-CO (piperidine ring, N-C_4H_9)	Levobupivacaine	2000

potency (lidocaine, prilocaine, mepivacaine), and high potency (ropivacaine, bupivacaine, levobupivacaine, etidocaine) does not conform to these correlations in all respects.

The onset of effect in the isolated nerve, at physiological pH, depends on the pKa value of the local anesthetic. The lower this value is, the more local anesthetic base can diffuse toward the membrane receptors, and the shorter the time will

Table 1.4a Physicochemical and pharmacological parameters

Agent	Molecular weight	p*K*a (25°)	Distribution coefficient (lipid/water)	Protein binding (%)	Potency in vitro (isolated nerve)
Procaine	236	8.9	0.02	5.8	1
Lidocaine	220	7.7	2.9	64–70	4
Mepivacaine	234	7.7	0.9	77–80	3–4
Prilocaine	246	7.6	0.8	55	3–4
Bupivacaine	288	8.1	27.5	95	16
Etidocaine	276	7.7	141	95	16
Ropivacaine	274	8.1	9	95	16
Levobupivacaine	288	8.09	27.5	97	16

Table 1.4b Local anesthetic potency and duration of effect

Potency	Structure	Agent
Low	H_2N-(benzene ring)-CO-O-CH_2-CH_2-N(C_2H_5)(C_2H_5)	Procaine
Medium	(benzene ring, CH_3, CH_3)-NH-CO-CH_2-N(C_2H_5)(C_2H_5)	Lidocaine
	(benzene ring, CH_3, CH_3)-NH-CO (piperidine ring, N-CH_3)	Mepivacaine
	(benzene ring, CH_3)-NH-CO-CH(CH_3)-N(C_3H_7)(H)	Prilocaine
High	(benzene ring, CH_3, CH_3)-NH-CO (piperidine ring, N-C_4H_9)	Bupivacaine
	(benzene ring, CH_3, CH_3)-NH-CO (piperidine ring, N-C_4H_9)	Levobupivacaine
	(benzene ring, CH_3, CH_3)-NH-CO-CH(C_2H_5)-N(C_3H_7)(C_2H_5)	Etidocaine
	(benzene ring, CH_3, CH_3)-NH-CO ····· (H; piperidine ring, N-C_3H_7)	Ropivacaine

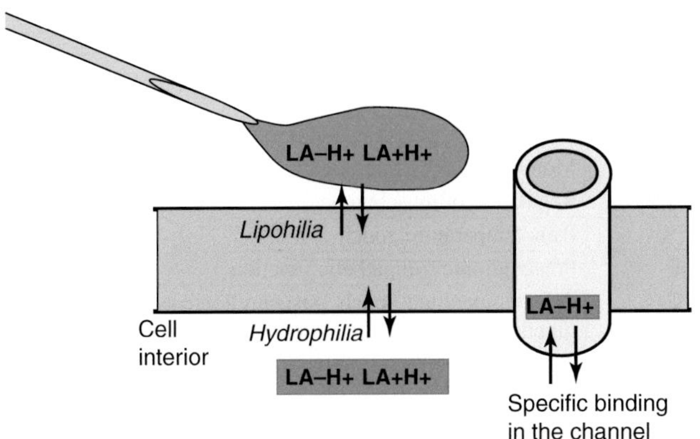

Fig. 1.12 Chemical requirements of a local anesthetic. Local anesthetics must combine lipophilic and hydrophilic properties in a favorable ratio with each other. Hydrophilia = soluble in cytosol, lipophilia = overcoming the cell membrane. (Reprinted with permission from Dr. Danilo Jankovic)

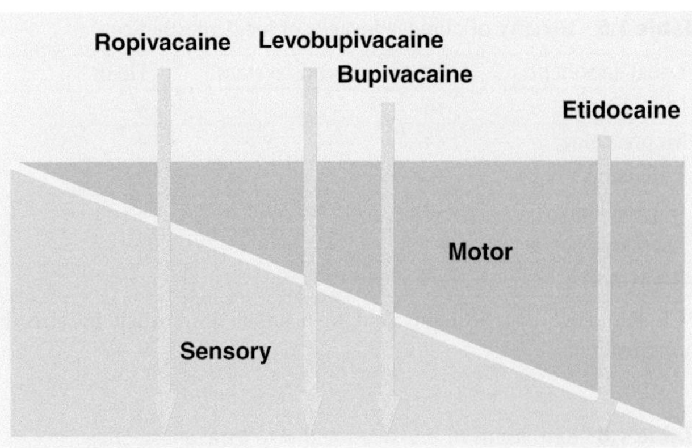

Fig. 1.13 Relative block profile of long-acting local anesthetics

be to the onset of the nerve block. Higher concentrations of local anesthetic accelerate onset.

The duration of effect depends on the dosage and concentration of the local anesthetic, its binding to the membrane receptors (protein-binding capacity), and its reabsorption from the tissue into the blood.

Equipotent Concentrations

Medium-duration local anesthetics have more or less the same clinical potency (except perhaps for lidocaine—due to stronger vasodilation, this local anesthetic is resorbed more readily from the site of action, and this can affect the duration and intensity of the block).

Equipotent concentrations of long-acting local anesthetics cannot be demonstrated in the same way, since the three local anesthetics mentioned have completely different block profiles: etidocaine (highest lipophilic capacity) produces a mainly motor block, ropivacaine has a mainly sensory effect, and bupivacaine has both motor and sensory effects. Anesthetic concentrations of bupivacaine and ropivacaine are equipotent (one to one).

Block Profile

The block profile shows the relation between sensory and motor block (Fig. 1.13). Physicochemical properties determine the block profile. At high anesthetic concentrations—so far as these are toxicologically permissible—the excess quantity of the agent can also block fibers not primarily affected (motor or sensory fibers). On the other hand, the block profile is not altered by low concentrations. A reduced motor block is obtained at the cost of reduced analgesic quality, and this is why opioid supplementation is usually necessary with dilute concentrations of local anesthetic.

Incompatibility

Local anesthetics can precipitate after dilution with alkaline solutions, and should therefore not be diluted with or injected simultaneously with sodium bicarbonate.

Side Effects and Systemic Effects

When assessing the safety and tolerability of a local anesthetic, account needs to be taken not only of its central nervous and cardiovascular effects, but also of its allergenic potential and of toxic degradation products that may form as it is metabolized (Tables 1.5 and 1.6).

Systemic Effects

Adverse systemic effects of local anesthetics can occur when their plasma concentration is high enough to affect organs with membranes that can be irritated.

Toxic plasma levels can be reached as a result of:

- Inadvertent intravascular or intrathecal/epidural injection.
- Overdosing, particularly in areas with good perfusion and correspondingly high resorption.
- Failure to adjust the dosages (mg/kg body weight), particularly in patients with hepatic or renal disease.

The severity of intoxication depends on the absolute plasma level, as well as on the strength of the local anesthetic's effect. While anesthetic dosages of short-acting local anesthetics (prilocaine, mepivacaine, lidocaine) can trigger

Table 1.5 Toxicity of clinical dosages of local anesthetics

Local anesthetic	Central nervous system	Heart
Lidocaine	++	+
Mepivacaine	++	+
Prilocaine	+	+/–
Bupivacaine	+++	++++++[a]
Levobupivacaine	++	++++
Ropivacaine	++(+)	+++

[a]Clinical dose can be equivalent to a lethal dose when incorrectly administered

Table 1.6 Symptoms of intoxication due to local anesthetics

Central nervous system	Cardiovascular system
Stimulation phase, mild intoxication	
Tingling of lips, tongue paresthesias, perioral numbness, ringing in the ears, metallic taste, anxiety, restlessness, trembling, muscle twitching, vomiting	Cardiac palpitation, hypertonia, tachycardia, tachypnea, dry mouth
Stimulation phase, moderately severe intoxication	
Excitation phase, moderate toxicity Speech disturbance, dazed state, sleepiness, confusion, tremor, choreoid movements, tonic-clonic cramp, mydriasis, vomiting, polypnea	Tachycardia, arrhythmia, cyanosis and pallor, nausea and vomiting
Paralytic phase, severe toxicity	
Stupor, coma, irregular breathing, respiratory arrest, flaccidity, vomiting with aspiration, sphincter paralysis, death	Severe cyanosis, bradycardia, drop in blood pressure, primary heart failure, ventricular fibrillation, hyposystole, asystole

clear CNS symptoms in a range extending to generalized cramp, cardiotoxic reactions are also possible with long-acting local anesthetics. In particular, cases of cardiac arrest have been reported with bupivacaine with comparatively small intravascular injections (50 mg; not treatable in half of the cases).

Cardiac symptoms and cardiac arrest can also occur with ropivacaine after inadvertent intravascular injections. However, these can be treated effectively and only occur at higher dosages. The following sequence of increasing systemic toxicity applies to the most frequently used local anesthetics: procaine < prilocaine < mepivacaine < lidocaine < ropivacaine < levobupivacaine < bupivacaine.

CNS toxicity: Central reactions predominate in terms of frequency and clinical significance. The symptoms of these are listed in Table 1.6 in order of severity and toxicity. For speedy and appropriate treatment, it is important to observe and react immediately when even the preconvulsive signs of CNS intoxication are seen—particularly numbness of the tongue and perioral region.

Cardiovascular toxicity: Toxic effects on the cardiovascular system usually occur after the administration of very high doses. They are seen in the form of conduction disturbances in the autonomic cardiac and vascular nerve fibers, depression of cardiac function, and peripheral vasodilation (Tables 1.5 and 1.6).

Table 1.7 Functional distinctions between nerve fibers

Fiber type	Function
^{A}a	Motor, touch, pressure, depth sensation
^{A}|3	Motor, touch, pressure, depth sensation
N Ay	Regulation of muscle tone
^{A}s	Pain, temperature, touch
B	Preganglionic sympathetic function
C	Pain, temperature, touch, postganglionic sympathetic function

A detailed discussion of local anesthetic systemic toxicity (LAST) can be found in Chap. 5 of this book.

Substance-Specific Side Effects

One specific side effect of prilocaine is the increased methemoglobin level caused by the metabolite *o*-toluidine. Clinically, cyanosis, headache, cardiac palpitation and vertigo can be expected at methemoglobin levels of 10–20%, and loss of consciousness, shock and death when the level is 60% or more. This does not call into question the beneficial toxicological properties of prilocaine, since clinically relevant methemoglobinemia can only occur at dosages of more than 600 mg, which is much more than clinically used doses of mepivacaine or lidocaine. A clinically harmful methemoglobin level can be treated within a few minutes by the intravenous administration of 2–4 mg/kg toluidine blue (or alternatively, 1–2 mg/kg methylene blue). Because of this specific side effect, prilocaine is not indicated in patients with congenital or acquired methemoglobinemia, in patients who are anemic or have a history of heart disease, in obstetrics (e.g., for pudendal nerve or paracervical block), or in children under the age of 6 months.

Allergenic Potential

There are no reliable data regarding the frequency of allergic reactions after the administration of local anesthetics. There is no doubt that these are extremely rare, although the symptoms can range from allergic dermatitis to anaphylactic shock. Occasional cases of allergic reactions to ester local anesthetics have been reported, and the preservative substances which the various preparations contain (e.g., parabens) and the antioxidant sodium bisulfide in epinephrine-containing solutions are also under discussion as potential causes. In patients with suspected intolerance of local anesthetics, intracutaneous testing with 20 pL of the agent can be conducted.

When the result is positive, subcutaneous provocation tests at increasing dosages (0.1 mL diluted to 1:10,000, 1:1000, and 1:10; undiluted at 0.1 mL, 0.5 mL, and 1 mL) can be considered. When these tests are being carried out, it is vital to prepare all the necessary safety measures in case of a severe reaction.

Selection of Suitable Substances for Regional Block

When surgical interventions are being carried out under regional anesthesia, priority must go to shutting off both sensory and motor systems, and knowledge of the expected length of the operation is vital to the choice of anesthetic. The onset of effect and the toxicity of the drug used play important parts, but not decisive ones. In the context of pain therapy, in which the fast-conducting A delta fibers and the slow-conducting C fibers (Table 1.7) are the target of the block, toxicity is much more important than the duration of the effect.

In diagnostic and therapeutic blocks, in which there is a risk of intravascular injection—for example, in a stellate ganglion block or superior cervical ganglion block—prilocaine should be selected, as it is the medium-duration local anesthetic with the lowest toxicity (mepivacaine or lidocaine are alternatives) (Tables 1.7 and 1.8).

Bupivacaine has an important role in regional blocks, being a longer-duration local anesthetic that provides high-quality analgesia and an easily controlled motor block. Its anesthetic potency is about four times that of local anesthetics with medium-duration effects (such as prilocaine). When the lower dosage required in pain therapy than in regional anesthesia is taken into account, bupivacaine can be used for practically all pain therapy procedures in spite of its relatively high toxicity.

Ropivacaine is the most recently introduced long-duration local anesthetic in the amino-amide series. The differential block is even more marked than with bupivacaine, and the drug is associated with much lower CNS toxicity and cardiac toxicity. These characteristics make it particularly suitable for regional anesthesia procedures in which higher dosages or concentrations are required. Ropivacaine provides good quality analgesia while largely maintaining motor activity (up to 80% of patients have no measurable motor block on the Bromage scale). At a dosage of 2 mg/mL, the drug is therefore the local anesthetic of choice for epidural obstetric analgesia and for postoperative analgesia (Fig. 1.13). With its pharmacological profile, ropivacaine is the first local anesthetic with primarily analgesic effects, and it is therefore particularly suitable for pain therapy indications.

Every anesthetist and pain therapy physician who uses anesthetic methods for temporary interruption of stimulus conduction in a ganglion, nerve, or neural plexus should be familiar with the properties and potential applications of the following agents.

Short-Acting Local Anesthetics

Cocaine (Table 1.2)

The pioneering work of Koller (1857–1944) on the anesthetic effect of cocaine (10–20%) in the context of ophthalmic surgery was the historical starting point for local and regional anesthesia (11 September, 1884). Cocaine occurs naturally in the leaves of the coca shrub and is ester of benzoic acid. Currently, cocaine is used primarily to provide topical anesthesia of the upper respiratory tract (see Chap. 7; Regional Anesthesia for Airway) and in nasal block of pterygopalatine ganglion (see Chap. 9; Deep Block of Trigeminal Nerve).

Procaine (Novocaine®) (Tables 1.2, 1.4a, and 1.4b)

In 1905, Einhorn in Germany succeeded in synthesizing a new local anesthetic, which he called "procaine." Heinrich Braun introduced procaine into clinical practice the same year, as a 4.5% and 5% solution.

Class of drug: Local anesthetic of the ester type.
Single threshold dose: 500 mg without epinephrine in adults.
LD_{50} (mouse): 52.2–60.0 mg/kg body weight i.v.
Plasma half-life: <0.14 h.
Latency: Medium.
Duration of effect: 0.5–1 h, depending on the area of application and the concentration used.
Metabolism: Procaine is broken down in plasma by pseudocholinesterase into *p*-aminobenzoic acid—a naturally occurring component of folic acid synthesis—and into diethylaminoethanol. The metabolites are excreted in the urine or broken down in the liver.

Table 1.8 Overview of drugs

Drug	Potency	Duration of effect	Toxicity	Half-life	Vdiss
Lidocaine	1 (Ref.)	2 h	1 (Ref.)	96′	91
Mepivacaine	1	2–3 h	1.2	114′	84
Prilocaine	1	2–3 h	0.5	93′	261

Tolerability and control: Procaine is one of the local anesthetics that have the lowest toxicity. Due to its short half-life, procaine is easily controlled.

Clinical uses: It is not so much its local anesthetic potency that predominates in procaine, but rather its muscle-relaxing properties and vasodilatory effect—which are of primary importance in infiltration therapy and trigger point treatment.

In the therapeutic field, very good results can be obtained with superior cervical ganglion block. However, procaine's high allergenic potency in comparison with amide local anesthetics argues against its use.

Dosage: Procaine is administered at concentrations of 0.5–2%. Precise dosages are described in the relevant sections of this book.

2-Chloroprocaine (Table 1.2)

2-Chloroprocaine, an ester local anesthetic, is a chlorinated derivative of procaine and is most rapidly metabolized local anesthetic currently used. Although the potency of chloroprocaine is relatively low, it can be used for epidural anesthesia in large volumes in a 3% solution because of its low systemic toxicity. The duration of action is between 30 and 60 min. This agent enjoyed its greatest popularity for epidural analgesia and anesthesia in obstetrics because of the rapid onset and low systemic toxicity in both mother and fetus. However, frequent injections are needed to provide adequate pain relief in labor, and it is more usual to establish analgesia with chloroprocaine and then change to a longer acting agent such as ropivacaine or bupivacaine.

The use of chloroprocaine declined because of reports of prolonged neurological deficit following accidental subarachnoid injection. This toxicity was ascribed to the sodium metabisulfite used in the past as preservative. However, there are no reports of neurotoxicity with newer preparations of chloroprocaine which contain disodium ethylenediaminetetraacetic acid (EDTA) as the preservative. Nevertheless, these preparations are not recommended for intrathecal administration. However, since then, a number of reports of back pain have appeared. The incidence of back pain appears to be related to the large volume (greater than 40 mL) of drug injected. Chloroprocaine has also proved of value for peripheral nerve blocks and epidural anesthesia when the duration of surgery is not expected to exceed 30–60 min.

Medium-Term Local Anesthetics

Lidocaine (Xylocaine®, Lignocaine) (Tables 1.3, 1.4a, and 1.4b)

Löfgren and Lundqvist in Sweden isolated a new substance in 1943 that was given the working name of "LL 30." It was later renamed "lidocaine." Following extensive pharmacological studies by Goldberg, the first clinical tests in dentistry using lidocaine were carried out in 1947. Thorsten Gordh, the father of Swedish anesthesia, carried out the first investigations of lidocaine in humans.

Class of drug: Lidocaine is a medium-duration local anesthetic of the amide type.

Single threshold dose: 200 mg without epinephrine in adults/70 kg body weight. After injection of a maximum dose, subsequent injections should not be given for 90 min. The second dose must not exceed a maximum of half of the first dose.

LD_{50} (mouse): 31.2–62.2 mg/kg body weight i.v.

Plasma half-life: ca. 1.6 h.

Latency: Fast.

Duration of effect: 1–2 h, depending on the area of application and the concentration used.

Metabolism: Lidocaine is metabolized in hepatic microsomes. Only about 3% of the drug is excreted unchanged via the kidney.

Tolerability and control: Lidocaine is one of the local anesthetics with moderate relative toxicity. It is characterized by a medium-term duration of effect and good distribution characteristics.

Lidocaine causes vasodilation, which may be less than that of procaine. When the medium-duration local anesthetics are compared, the strengths of the associated vasodilatory effects show the following sequence: lidocaine > mepivacaine > prilocaine. Lidocaine is therefore often used with epinephrine.

Clinical uses: Lidocaine is widely used in clinical practice, particularly in neural and segmental therapy. It is also suitable for infiltration anesthesia, for peripheral nerve block, for epidural anesthesia, and for mucosal surface anesthesia (2% gel, Emla®).

Dosage: Lidocaine is mainly administered as a 0.5–1% (1.5)% solution. Specific doses are given in the relevant chapters of this book.

EMLA® Cream

EMLA® (a mixture of 2.5% lidocaine and 2.5% prilocaine) is a topical local anesthetic that penetrates intact skin and reaches an anesthetic depth of up to 5 mm. The onset of effect is approximately 1 h. When the effect takes place, the vessels in the skin show vasoconstriction initially, followed by vasodilation when higher concentrations are reached. This form of administration of this local anesthetic mixture has proved particularly useful in pediatric anesthesia before intravenous access placement, and for minor surgical procedures on the skin surface.

Mepivacaine (Scandicaine®, Meaverine®) (Tables 1.3, 1.4a, and 1.4b)

In 1956, Bo af Ekenstam, a Swedish scientist, developed mepivacaine. It was introduced into clinical practice by K.G. Dhunér in Sweden in 1957.

Class of drug: Mepivacaine is a medium-duration local anesthetic of the amide type.

Single threshold dose without epinephrine in adults (70 kg body weight): 200 mg in the ENT field, 300 mg in other applications.

LD_{50} (mouse): 40.3 ± 3.2 mg/kg body weight i.v.

Plasma half-life: ca. 1.9 h.

Latency: Fast.

Duration of effect: 1–3 h, depending on the area of application and the concentration used.

Metabolism: Mepivacaine is metabolized in the hepatic microsomes.

After intravenous administration, up to 16% of the agent is excreted unchanged via the kidney. Degradation in the liver mainly produces *m*-hydroxymepivacaine and *p*-hydroxymepivacaine. These metabolites are conjugated with glucuronic acid and excreted in the urine. Another metabolite, pipecolylxylidide, collects in bile and passes through the enterohepatic circulation with its degradation products. No 2,6-xylidine is produced when mepivacaine is metabolized, and there is no evidence that either the agent or its metabolites have mutagenic or carcinogenic properties.

Tolerability and control: Mepivacaine is another of the local anesthetics with moderate relative toxicity. It is characterized by a medium-term duration of effect, with good distribution properties and some vasodilatory effect.

Clinical uses: Mepivacaine is the local anesthetic of choice when a medium-duration effect is required for diagnostic and therapeutic blocks in pain therapy—particularly in outpatients. It is suitable for infiltration anesthesia, intravenous regional anesthesia, peripheral nerve block and ganglion block, and for epidural anesthesia. Mepivacaine cannot be recommended in the obstetrics due to its long elimination half-life in the neonate.

Dosage: Mepivacaine is mainly used as a 1% (1.5%) or 0.5% solution. Specific doses are given in the relevant chapters of this book.

Prilocaine (Xylonest®) (Tables 1.3, 1.4a, and 1.4b)

Class of drug: Prilocaine is a medium-duration local anesthetic of the amide type.

Single threshold dose: 400 mg (with or without vasopressor) in adults/70 kg body weight.

LD_{50} (mouse): 62 mg/kg b.w. i.v.

Plasma half-life: ca. 1.5 h.

Latency: Fast.

Duration of effect: 2–3 h, depending on the area of application and the concentration used.

Metabolism: Prilocaine is mainly metabolized in hepatic microsomes, but also in the kidney and lungs. During degradation, the metabolite *ortho*-toluidine is produced. At doses higher than 600 mg, the body's reduction systems may become exhausted. At doses higher than 800 mg, noticeable methemoglobinemia can be expected (see the section on substance-specific side effects). Fast elimination from the blood leads to low systemic toxicity.

Tolerability and control: Among the amide local anesthetics, prilocaine shows the best ratio between anesthetic potency and toxicity. Due to its high distribution volume and marked absorption in the lungs, plasma levels are significantly lower than those of mepivacaine and lidocaine (by a factor of 2–3). It has a medium-term duration of effect.

Clinical uses: Due to its comparatively low toxicity, prilocaine is particularly suitable for regional anesthesia techniques that require a single injection of a large volume or a high anesthetic dosage. The increasing use of prilocaine (2% isobaric solution) for spinal anesthesia is relatively new. Comparative studies in recent years have shown good tolerability, while transient neurological symptoms (TNS; see Chap. 41; Neuraxial Anesthesia and Analgesia for Surgery) were observed more often with lidocaine and mepivacaine. Prilocaine—like other medium-duration agents—is not suitable for continuous blocks. Due to the possibility of raised methemoglobin levels, prilocaine should not be used in anemic patients, children under the age of 6 months, or in obstetrics.

Dosage: Depending on the area of application, a 0.5–2% solution is used. Specific doses are given in the relevant chapters of this book.

Long-Acting Local Anesthetics

Ropivacaine (Naropin®) (Tables 1.3, 1.4a, and 1.4b)

Class of drug: Local anesthetic of the amide type, pure *S*-enantiomer.

Single threshold dose**:** *Anesthesia*: Epidural: 0.5–1%, 200 mg;

Plexus blocks: 0.75%, 300 mg;

Conduction and infiltration anesthesia: 0.5–0.75%, 225 mg;

Injection at myofascial trigger points: 0.2% (1–2 mL per trigger point).

Continuous procedures: 0.2%, up to 14 mL/h. Increased doses may be required during the early postoperative period—up to 0.375%, 10 mL/h (maximum 37.5 mg/h). When it is administered over several days, the resulting concentrations are well below potentially toxic plasma levels.

A dosage of 300 mg should be regarded as a guideline value, as this dosage has been confirmed as tolerable by various pharmacological studies.

LD_{50} (mouse): ca. 11.0–12.0 mg/kg b.w. i.v.

Plasma half-life: ca. 1.8 h.

Duration of effect: Epidural anesthesia ca. 7 h (analgesia); ca. 4 h (motor block), 10 mg/mL.

Plexus anesthesia (brachial plexus, lumbosacral plexus): 9–17 h, 7.5 mg/mL.

Infiltration anesthesia: postoperative analgesia after inguinal herniorrhaphy >7 h (5–23 h), 7.5 mg/mL. Peripheral nerve blocks in pain therapy: 2–6 h (0.2–0.375 mg/mL).

Latency: Medium (decreasing latency at increasing concentrations).

Metabolism: Ropivacaine is metabolized in the liver, mainly through aromatic hydroxylation. Only about 1% of the drug is excreted unchanged in the urine. The main metabolite is 3-hydroxyropivacaine.

Tolerability: Ropivacaine provides relatively low toxicity for a long-term local anesthetic. Compared with bupivacaine, it has a lower arrhythmogenic potential, and the margin between convulsive and lethal doses is wider. Ropivacaine has more favorable receptor kinetics ("fast in, medium out") in cardiac sodium channels, and in comparison with bupivacaine has only slight depressant effects on the energy metabolism of the mitochondria in cardiac muscle cells.

Clinical uses: The first clinical tests were carried out in 1988. Ropivacaine (Naropin®) has been in use since 1996. It is the first local anesthetic with a primary analgetic effect and is therefore of particular interest in pain therapy (postoperative and obstetric, as well as therapeutic blocks).

Ropivacaine is the most comprehensively documented and most widely approved local anesthetic today. It is the most frequently used long-acting local anesthetic throughout the world. It should be noted that it has been approved, with clinical relevance, for use in continuous therapy for acute pain (epidural and peripheral continuous nerve blocks). Approval for administration in children, including continuous epidural administration, was extended to neonates in 2007. It is the first local anesthetic with primarily analgetic effects and is therefore of particular interest for pain therapy (postoperative and obstetric, and therapeutic blocks). In comparison with bupivacaine, it has fewer toxic side effects (CNS and, in particular, cardiac toxicity). High doses are needed before toxic effects develop. CNS symptoms appear well before cardiac symptoms, which in the clinical situation provides time for the local anesthetic injection to be stopped and for early treatment steps to be taken. In an animal model, the chances of successful resuscitation were also found to be better than with bupivacaine (90% vs. 50%). In addition, ropivacaine shows marked differential blocking in epidural analgesia and peripheral blocks. With a good quality of analgesia, up to 80% of patients have no measurable motor block on the Bromage scale. Epidural combinations (e.g., with sufentanil, dosage range 0.5–1 pg/mL) are possible. In view of the increased use of peripheral blocks and infiltrations at painful trigger points, evidence of higher muscular tissue tolerance in comparison with bupivacaine is also of interest. The relatively low toxicity of ropivacaine means that high concentrations can be given (e.g., 10 mg/mL solution for epidural anesthesia)—providing more intense motor block, a higher success rate and better quality analgesia than 0.5% bupivacaine, for example (Tables 1.5 and 1.6).

Dosage: Ropivacaine is administered at concentrations of 2 mg/mL (0.2%), 7.5 mg/mL (0.75%), and 10 mg/mL (1%). Use for continuous epidural infusion has been approved (Naropin® 2 mg/mL polybag, 100 and 200 mL infusion solution). Cumulative daily doses of up to 675 mg (see specialist information) are well tolerated in adults. Precise information on doses is given in the following chapters.

Levobupivacaine (Chirocaine®) (Tables 1.3, 1.4a, and 1.4b)

Class of drug: Local anesthetic of the amide type. A pure *S*-enantiomer of bupivacaine.

Single threshold dose without epinephrine in adults: 150 mg.

LD_{50} (mouse): 10.6 mg/kg b.w.

Plasma half-life: 80 ± 22 min. Plasma protein binding of levobupivacaine in humans has been assessed in vitro, and was more than 97% at concentrations of 0.1–1.0 pg/mL.

Latency: Medium (between ropivacaine and bupivacaine).

Duration of effect: 8–24 h, depending on the area of application and the concentration used.

Metabolism: Levobupivacaine is extensively metabolized, and unaltered levobupivacaine is not found in the urine or feces. 3-Hydroxylevobupivacaine, one of the principal metabolites of levobupivacaine, is excreted via the urine as a glucuronic acid and sulfate ester conjugate. In vitro studies have shown that levobupivacaine is metabolized via CYP3A4 isoforms and CYP1A2 isoforms into desbutyl-levobupivacaine or 3-hydroxylevobupivacaine. The studies showed that the degradation of levobupivacaine and bupivacaine is similar. After intravenous administration of levobupivacaine, the recovery rate within 48 h averaged ca. 95%, quantitatively measurable in urine (71%) and feces (24%). There is evidence of in vivo racemate formation with levobupivacaine.

Tolerability and control: Experimental animal studies have demonstrated a lower risk of CNS and cardiovascular toxicity with levobupivacaine than with bupivacaine. In volunteers, fewer negative inotropic effects were observed after intravenous administration of more than 75 mg levobupivacaine in comparison with bupivacaine. QT interval changes only occurred in a very few cases.

Clinical uses: There is little experience as yet with levobupivacaine in clinical practice. The number of published controlled clinical studies is also comparatively small. Available in vitro, in vivo, and controlled patient studies comparing levobupivacaine and bupivacaine have shown similar potency for neural blocks. After epidural administration of levobupivacaine, the same quality of sensory and motor block as with bupivacaine was seen. However, a significant differential block, as provided by ropivacaine, cannot be expected, as the drug has the same degree of lipophilia as bupivacaine. Levobupivacaine has not been approved for use in Germany.

Dosage: 0.125–0.75%. Precise information on doses is given in the following chapters.

Bupivacaine (Carbostesin®, Marcaine®) (Tables 1.3, 1.4a, and 1.4b)

The first clinical studies of a long-acting local anesthetic, bupivacaine, were carried out in 1965/1966.

Class of drug: Local anesthetic of the amide type.

Single threshold dose: 150 mg without epinephrine in adults.

LD_{50} *(mouse):* 7.8 ± 0.4 mg/kg b.w. i.v.

Plasma half-life: ca. 2.7 h.

Latency: Medium.

Duration of effect: 2.5–20 h, depending on the area of application and the concentration used. A mean duration of effect of 3–6 h can be assumed.

Metabolism: Bupivacaine is broken down in hepatic microsomes at a high rate. The predominant metabolization involves dealkylation to pipecolylxylidide (desbutylbupivacaine). There is no evidence that either the agent or its metabolites have mutagenic or carcinogenic properties.

Tolerability and control: Bupivacaine is one of the local anesthetics that has a high relative toxicity. Its anesthetic potency is about four times greater than that of mepivacaine. It is characterized by a slower onset of effect and by a long duration of effect.

Clinical uses: Bupivacaine is indicated as a long-duration local anesthetic, particularly for regional anesthesia in the surgical field, in postoperative analgesia, and in therapy for various pain conditions.

It is suitable for infiltration anesthesia, peripheral nerve block, ganglion block and plexus block, as well as all forms of neuraxial anesthesia.

The marked cardiac toxicity of bupivacaine has been known since publications dating from the late 1970s, and severe and fatal adverse effects are still reported. Strict observation of safety standards is therefore of fundamental importance for the safe use of this drug at high doses.

Dosage: Depending on the indication, bupivacaine is administered as a 0.125–0.5% solution. A 0.75% solution is still being marketed. Higher concentrations are not required in pain therapy. Specific doses are given in the following chapters.

Tetracaine (Table 1.2)

Tetracaine is a long-acting amino ester. It is significantly more potent and has a longer duration of action than procaine or 2-chloroprocaine. Tetracaine remains a very popular drug for spinal anesthesia in the United States. This drug possesses excellent topical anesthetic properties, and solutions of this agent were commonly used for endotracheal surface anesthesia. Because of its slow onset and high toxicity, tetracaine is rarely used in peripheral nerve blocks.

Regional Anesthesia in the Patient Receiving Antithrombotic or Thrombolytic Therapy

General Consideration

Performing neuraxial anesthesia in patients receiving antithrombotic drugs remains an *individual risk-benefit analysis*. In particular, the patient's individual risk of thromboembolic and ischemic complications as a result of interrupting the anticoagulation must be taken into account. Guidelines on neuraxial anesthesia and anticoagulants aim to assist anesthesiologists to facilitate decisions for or against neuraxial blockades. Compliance with the *substance-specific time interval* allows puncture within lowest anticoagulant blood levels. The current ASRA guidelines for the placement of epidural and spinal catheters *differentiate* between *interventional pain procedures* and *perioperative regional anesthesia* blocks.

Pain-specific procedural guidelines are important because the technical and anatomical considerations for pain interventions are significantly different than for peripheral regional anesthesia. The spectrum of interventional spine and pain procedures is far broader than that for regional anesthesia, with diverse targets and objectives.

Classification of Interventional Pain Procedures According to the Potential Risk of Serious Bleeding is based on the guideline published by American Society of Regional Anesthesia (ASRA) in 2018 (second edition) (Narouze et al.).

Pain procedures vary from minimally invasive procedures with high-risk targets (e.g., spinal cord stimulation trial and implant, intrathecal catheter and pump implant, vertebral augmentation epiduroscopy) to intermediate-risk procedures (e.g., interlaminar ESIs, transforaminal ESIs, cervical facet MBNB and RFA, intradiscal procedures, sympathetic blocks, trigeminal ganglia blocks) and to low-risk peripheral nerve blocks (e.g., peripheral nerve blocks, trigger point injections including piriformis injection, sacroiliac joint injection, peripheral nerve stimulation trial and implant).

It is strongly recommended a *shared assessment, risk stratification*, and *management decision* in conjunction with the treating physician(s) for those patients with higher bleeding risk profiles, *especially when taking concomitant antiplatelet medications*, advanced patient *age*, advanced *liver or renal disease*, or prior *history of abnormal bleeding* exist.

Those important parameters have to be considered before procedure:

- The *degree of invasiveness* (low or intermediate risk or high-risk procedures)
- The *reason* for *anticoagulants utilization*
- *Concomitant* medication
- Significant *spinal abnormalities*
- The *vascular anatomy* surrounding the target area
- The *potential sequelae* associated with *perioperative bleeding*

Anatomical Considerations for Hematoma Development in Spinal and Non-spinal Areas

The risk of formation of *interspinal hematoma* after administration of neuraxial injections is increased in patients who *received anticoagulant therapy* or have a *coagulation disorder, technical difficulties* in the performance of the neuraxial procedures due to anatomic abnormalities of the spine, and *multiple* or *bloody punctures*. Although most cases of *spinal hematoma* have a *multifactorial etiology*, certain anatomical features may pose higher risks secondary to the anatomy and vascular supply of that specific spinal location.

It is important for interventional pain physicians to apply *knowledge of spinal and epidural anatomy* during preprocedural planning. *Other locations* associated with significant undesirable vascularity include the *target ganglia* (cervical, lumbar sympathetic, and celiac plexus). *Radiological imaging* should be reviewed prior to performing *interventional spine and pain procedures* in order to assess for *central* and *foraminal stenosis, disc herniations* that compromise canal diameter, *ligamentum flavum hypertrophy, epidural fibrosis*, and previous surgical *scarring*, which can alter the level of procedural difficulty.

Plexus and Peripheral Blockade in the Anticoagulant Patient

For patients undergoing *peri-neuraxial, deep plexus,* or *deep peripheral* block, ASRA recommends similar guideline as for the neuraxial techniques.

For patients undergoing *neural plexus or peripheral nerve techniques,* ASRA recommends management (performance, catheter maintenance, and catheter removal) based on site compressibility, vascularity, and consequences of bleeding should it occur.

Chronic Pain and Stress as a Hypercoagulable State

Chronic psychosocial stress causes a *hypercoagulable state*, as reflected by increased procoagulant molecules (fibrinogen or coagulation factor VII), reduced fibrinolytic capacity, and increased platelet activity. *Chronic stress* increases many stress hormone levels. Catecholamine and cortisol surges may underlie the hypercoagulability observed with chronic psychological distress. As *chronic pain* frequently coexists with *mental stress*, characterized by a *hypercoagulable state*, *chronic pain patients* may be at increased risk of coronary or cerebrovascular events after discontinuation of protective antiplatelet and anticoagulant medications.

Consider

- *Do not perform* a *neuraxial* or *deep plexus block* in patients on *more than one antiplatelet drug!*
- *Avoid traumatic puncture* (multiple needle and lead insertions-trauma).
- As a rule of thumb, a time interval of *two half-lives* between last (prophylactic) administration and neuraxial puncture is considered as an *adequate safety margin*. In *renal insufficiency* or *"therapeutic" anticoagulation*, the time interval should be *extended* to *four to five half-lives*.

Specific Recommendations for Pain Management and Regional Anesthesia in Patients Utilizing Anticoagulants or Antiplatelet Agents

The following are the recommendations for the management of anticoagulants, antiplatelet agents, and thrombolytic in patients receiving either regional anesthesia or pain management. All those recommendations are based on the two guidelines published by American Society of Regional Anesthesia (ASRA) in 2018 (second edition).

Antiplatelet Medication

Nonsteroidal Anti-inflammatory Drugs (NSAIDs) Including Aspirin

Aspirin

Aspirin is effective at inhibiting platelet activation, platelet aggregation, and thrombosis. Aspirin is rapidly absorbed from the gastrointestinal tract, with peak levels occurring approximately *30 min* following ingestion, resulting in significant platelet inhibition at *1 h*. Aspirin, within *1 h* after ingestion, results in greater than *90%* in thromboxane levels. The *average life span* of a platelet is *7–10 days. Each day*, approximately *10%* of the circulating platelet pool is replaced (at *5–6 days*, approximately *50%*). Zisman et al. demonstrated that in most ASA-treated patients platelet function recovers *4 days* after drug discontinuation.

Non-ASA NSAIDs
Non-steroidal anti-inflammatory drugs inhibit prostaglandin production by inhibiting cyclooxygenase (COX). These drugs may be discontinued without negatively affecting cardiac and cerebral function.

Interventional Pain Management
For *interventional pain high-risk procedures* consideration should be given to discontinue these medications. Each NSAID can be discontinued based on its *specific half-life* (e.g., *discontinuation time = 5 half-lives/h*: Diclofenac, Ketorolac *(1 days)*; Ibuprofen, Indomethacin *(2 days)*; Naproxen, Meloxicam *(4 days)*; Piroxicam *(10 days)*.

Similar to regional anesthesia guidelines, aspirin may be continued when the procedure is low-risk pain procedure (consider concomitant drugs).

If ASA is being taken for *primary prophylaxis*, ASA discontinuation is recommended for high-risk procedures and certain intermediate-risk procedures with heightened risk of perioperative bleeding (e.g., interlaminar cervical ESIs and cervical ganglia) *(6 days*). If ASA is being taken for *secondary prophylaxis*, ASA discontinuation is recommended for high-risk elective pain procedures *(6 days)* and low or intermediate-risk procedures *(4 days)*.

Regional Anesthetic Management
In *perioperative settings, NSAIDs (including Aspirin)* alone appear to represent no added significant risk of the development of spinal hematoma in patients having spinal or epidural anesthesia. There are no specific concerns as to the timing of single injection or catheter techniques in relationship to the dosing of NSAIDs, postoperative monitoring, or the timing of neuraxial catheter removal. Caution is suggested in the performance of neuraxial techniques if the concurrent use of other medications (other antiplatelet agents, oral anticoagulants, unfractionated heparin and low molecular weight heparin) affect clotting mechanisms in the early postoperative period because of the increased risk of bleeding complications. *Careful preoperative assessment* of the patient to identify alterations of health that might contribute to bleeding is crucial (history of easy bruising/excessive bleeding, female sex, and increased age). The evidence suggests that aspirin and non-steroidal anti-inflammatory drugs alone pose only a small increased risk but that in combination with other drugs affecting coagulation, there may be more significant risk.

P2Y12 Inhibitors: Thienopyridine Derivates (Ticlopidine, Clopidogrel, Ticagrelor, Cangrelor)
Thienopyridine, such as ticlopidine and clopidogrel, is a class of selective, irreversible adenosine diphosphate (ADP) receptor/P2Y12 inhibitors used for their antiplatelet activity.

The recommended intervals of discontinuation and resumption of the thienopyridines for regional anesthesia procedures and interventional pain management are based on the two guidelines published by American Society of Regional Anesthesia (ASRA) in 2018 (second edition).

Clopidogrel (Plavix®) (Oral, Irreversible Inhibition)[1]

Regional Anesthetic Management
Discontinuation time: *(5–7 days)*[2]
Restart: *(24 h)*.
Time after puncture/catheter manipulation or removal: *after catheter removal.*

Interventional Pain Management
Discontinuation time:
High- and intermediate-risk procedures: *(7 days)* (footnote 2)
Low-risk procedures: No (risk-benefit assessment)[3]
Restart: *(12–24 h)*.

Ticlopidine (Ticlid®) (Oral, Irreversible Inhibition) (Footnote 1)

Regional Anesthetic Management
Discontinuation time: *(10 days)*.
Restart: *(24 h)*.
Time after puncture/catheter manipulation or removal: *after catheter removal.*

Interventional Pain Management
Discontinuation time: *(10 days)*.
Restart: *(24 h)*.

[1]The antiplatelet effect is not immediate. *Neuraxial catheters* may be maintained for *1–2 days* provided a loading dose of the antiplatelet agent is not administered.

[2]In patients with high risk of thromboembolic events or for trial of SCS: a 5 day discontinuation is recommended (e.g., a "bridge" therapy with low molecular weight heparin). After an intervention, the usual daily dose (75 mg) of clopidogrel can be started 12 h later.

[3]Risk-benefit assessment: higher bleeding risk profiles, concomitant antiplatelet medications, advanced patient age, advanced liver or renal disease, or prior history of abnormal bleeding exist.

Prasugrel (Efient®) (Oral, Irreversible Inhibition)[4]

Regional Anesthetic Management
Discontinuation time: *(7–10 days).*
Restart: *(24 h).*
Time after puncture/catheter manipulation or removal: *(6 h).*

Interventional Pain Management
Discontinuation time:
High- and intermediate-risk procedures: *(7–10 days).*
Low-risk procedures: No (Risk-benefit assessment) (footnote 3)
Restart: *(24 h).*

Ticagrelor (Brilique®) (Oral, Reversible Inhibition) (Footnote 4)

Regional Anesthetic Management
Discontinuation time: *(5–7 days).*
Restart: *(24 h).*
Time after puncture/catheter manipulation or removal: *(6 h).*

Interventional Pain Management
Discontinuation time:
High- and intermediate-risk procedures: *(5 days).*
Low-risk procedures: No (Risk-benefit assessment) (footnote 3)
Restart: *(24 h).*

Cangrelor (Intravenous Direct, Reversible Inhibition; Onset: 2.6–3.3 min; Offset: 60–90 min)

Interventional Pain Management
Discontinuation time:
High- and intermediate-risk procedures: *(3 h).*
Low risk procedures: No (Risk-benefit assessment (footnote 3)).
Restart: *(24 h).*

Older Anticoagulants

Warfarin and Acenocoumarol

The oral anticoagulants exercise their pharmacological action by inhibiting ϒ-carboxylation of the vitamin K-dependent coagulation factors (II, VII, IX, and X) and proteins C and S. Warfarin is difficult to dose, because it has narrow therapeutic index and wide interpatient dosing variability, with genetic factors accounting for a large proportion of the variations in dose requirements. Monitoring of anticoagulation is performed with the INR. In Europe, acenocoumarol is the most commonly used drug in this group, whereas in the United States warfarin is used.

The recommended intervals of discontinuation and resumption of the *older anticoagulants* for regional anesthesia procedures and interventional pain management are based on the two guidelines published by American Society of Regional Anesthesia (ASRA) in 2018 (second edition).

Regional Anesthetic Management

- The anticoagulant therapy must be *stopped (ideally 5 days prior* to the planned procedure), and *INR normalized* prior to initiation of neuraxial block *(INR ≤ 1.4).*
- The performance of neuraxial anesthesia or removal of epidural catheters *within 24 h* of initial warfarin intake is probably safe.
- In patients receiving an initial dose of warfarin *prior to surgery*, the *INR* should be checked *prior to neuraxial block* if the first dose was given *more than 24 h earlier* or a *second dose* of oral anticoagulant has been administered.
- Caution should be used when performing neuraxial techniques in patients recently *discontinued from chronic warfarin therapy*. Consider *increased sensitivity* to warfarin (e.g., age > 65, female sex, weight, liver, cardiac, renal disease).
- ASRA recommends *against the concurrent use of medication* that affects other components of clotting mechanisms (e.g., aspirin, NSAIDs, thienopyridines, UFH, and LMWH).
- *Neurologic testing* should be performed routinely during epidural (neuraxial) analgesia for patients on warfarin therapy.

The *indwelling catheters* may be maintained with caution, based on INR and duration of warfarin therapy. As a thromboprophylaxis with warfarin is initiated, ASRA suggests that *neuraxial catheters be removed* when the *INR is <1.5.* In patients with an INR of >3, ASRA recommends that the warfarin be held or reduced in patients with indwelling neuraxial catheters and the neurologic assessment be continued for at least 24 h following catheter removal.

Interventional Pain Management
Warfarin
Discontinuation time:
High- and intermediate-risk procedures: *(5 days)*; Normal INR (≤1.2).
Low-risk procedures: No (Risk-benefit assessment[5]).
Restart: *(6 h).*

[4]*Neuraxial catheters* should *not be maintained with prasugrel or ticagrelor* because of the *rapid onset*. *Thienopyridine therapy* may be resumed *immediately* after needle placement/ catheter removal, provided a loading dose of the drugs is not administered. If *loading dose* is administered, ASRA suggests a time interval of *6 h* between catheter removal and administration.

[5]Risk-benefit assessment: higher bleeding risk profiles, concomitant antiplatelet medications, advanced patient age, advanced liver or renal disease, or prior history of abnormal bleeding exist.

Acenocoumarol

Discontinuation time:

High- and intermediate-risk procedures *(3 days);* Normal INR (≤1.2);

Low-risk procedures: No (Risk-benefit assessment (footnote 5));

Restart: *(24 h).*

Heparin

Intravenous Unfractionated Heparin (IV UFHs)

Unfractionated heparin inactivates thrombin (factor IIa), factor Xa, and factor IXa. The anticoagulant effect of IV heparin is immediate. Heparin has a *half-life of 1.5–2 h,* and its therapeutic effect *ceases 4–6 h* after its administration.

Subcutaneous Unfractionated Heparin (SC UFHs)

The anticoagulant effect of low-dose, BID subcutaneous heparin (5000 U every 8–12 h) is through heparin-mediated inhibition of activated factor Xa. After subcutaneous injection of heparin, maximum anticoagulation is observed in *40–50* min, which dissipates within *4–6 h.*

Enoxaparin (Lovenox®, Clexane®)

Low-molecular-weight heparins (LMWH)[6] are used for both prophylaxis and treatment of arterial and venous thromboembolism (VTE). The biochemical and pharmacologic properties of LMWH differ from those of UFH. Most relevant are the prolonged half-life and irreversibility with protamine. Anti-factor Xa levels peak 3–5 h after administration. The elimination half-life of LMWH is 3–6 h. LMWH exhibits a dose-dependent antithrombotic effect that is assessed by the anti-factor activity level. The recovery of anti-factor Xa activity after subcutaneous injection of LMWH approaches 100%. The plasma *half-life* of the LMWHs ranges from *2 to 4 h* after an *intravenous* injection and *3 to 6 h* after *subcutaneous* injection.

The recommended intervals of discontinuation and resumption of the *Intravenous Unfractionated Heparin, Subcutaneous Unfractionated Heparin,* and *Enoxaparin (LMWH)* for interventional pain management and regional anesthesia:

Interventional Pain Management

Intravenous Unfractionated Heparin (UFHs)

Discontinuation time:

High-, intermediate- and low-risk procedures: *(6 h); (24 h* especially if it was bloody).

Restart: *minimum* > *(2 h)* after pain procedure.

Subcutaneous Unfractionated Heparin (UFHs)

Discontinuation time:

High-risk procedures: *(24 h)* (INR normalization).

Intermediate-risk procedures: *(6 h)* (BID or TID dosing).

Restart: *(6–8 h);*

Low-risk procedures (No; Risk-benefit assessment); Restart > *(2 h).*

Enoxaparin (LMWH)

Discontinuation time:

High-/intermediate-low risk procedures:

Prophylactic dose (30 mg BID or 40 mg once d.) *(12 h).*

Therapeutic dose (1 mg/kg BID or 1.5 mg/kg once d.) *(24 h).*

Restart:

Low risk: *(4 h).*

High/intermediate risk procedures

Prophylactic dose: (12–24 h). (Laboratory tests: Platelets during treatment for >5 days).

Therapeutic dose: low-risk procedures: *(4 h)*; intermediate/high-risk procedures:*(12–24 h).*

(Laboratory tests: Platelets during treatment for >5 days);

Consider

- *Concomitant drugs* that affect hemostasis (e.g., antiplatelet, NSAIDs, other anticoagulants) should be used with extreme caution in patients on LMWH.

Regional Anesthetic Management

IV Heparin (UHFs) **(for prophylaxis, ≤15,000 IU/and for treatment)**

Discontinuation time: *(4–6 h).*

Time after puncture/catheter manipulation or removal: *(4–6 h).*

Restart: *(1 h).*

(Laboratory tests: Platelets during treatment for >5 days, aPTT, ACT, platelets)

Consider increased risk:

<1 h between the administration of heparin and lumbar puncture, *traumatic needle placement* or *bloody tap.*

Concomitant use of other anticoagulants, avoid neuraxial techniques in patients with *other coagulopathies.*

SC Heparin (UHFs)

- Low dose (e.g., 5000 U BID or TID).
  Discontinuation time: *(4–6 h).*
  Time after puncture/catheter manipulation or removal: *(4–6 h* after last heparin dose); Restart: *(1 h).*

[6] Although the LMWHs constitute a relatively homogenous pharmacological group, the most studied and referenced drug is *Enoxaparin*; there are different commercial preparations on the market that share common characteristics but that also possess different clinical and pharmacological properties and must be regarded as *similar but not equal drugs.*

- Higher dose[7] (e.g., 7500–10,000 U BID or daily dose ≤20,000 U).
  Discontinuation time: *(12 h)*.
  Time after puncture/catheter manipulation or removal: *(12 h)*.
  Restart: *(1 h)*.
  (Laboratory tests: Coagulation status).
- Therapeutic dose(e.g., >10,000 U per dose or >20,000 U total daily dose). Discontinuation time*:(*24 h*)*.
  Time after puncture/catheter manipulation or removal: *(24 h)*.
  Restart: *(1 h)*.
- ASRA guidelines of regional anesthesia considered minidose BID subcutaneous heparin not a contraindication to neuraxial injections.

Enoxaparin (LMWH)
Discontinuation time:

- *Prophylactic dose*[8]: *(12 h)*.
  Time after puncture/catheter manipulation or removal:
  - Twice daily dose*:(>12 h following day)*.
  - Single daily dose: (a) first day*:(>12 h after)*; (b) second day: *(24 h after the first dose)*.
- *Therapeutic dose*[9]: *(24 h)*.
  Time after puncture/catheter manipulation or removal: *(24 h* after non-high-bleeding risk surgery); *(48–72 h* after high-bleeding risk surgery).
  Indwelling neuraxial catheters be removed: *(4 h* prior to the first postoperative dose and *(24 h* after needle/catheter placement*)*.

Consider

- LMWH should not be given ≤*2 h after epidural catheter removal.*
- *Risk-benefit assessment* (risk of thrombosis versus risk of bleeding).
- ASRA recommends *against concomitant antiplatelet or oral anticoagulant medications* that affect hemostasis.
- *The presence of blood during needle/catheter placement* does not necessitate postponement of surgery. *The initiation of LMWH should be delayed for 24 h postoperatively.*
- Routine monitoring of the anti-factor Xa level *is not recommended.*

In patients administered a dose of LMWH *2 h preoperatively* (general surgery patients), ASRA recommends *against neuraxial techniques.*

[7] *The safety of indwelling neuraxial catheters* in patients receiving doses >5000 U or > 15,000 U of UFH/day has not been established. The risk and benefits be assessed on an individual basis (neurologic monitoring).

[8] Enoxaparin 30 mg BID or 40 mg /once d.

[9] *Enoxaparin 1 mg/kg every 12 h;* Dalteparin 120 U/kg every 12 h, 200 U/kg every 12 h; Tanzaparin 175 U/ kg day.

New Anticoagulants

Anti-Factor Xa Agents Fondaparinux (Arixtra®)

Fondaparinux (Arixtra®) is a synthetic anticoagulant that selectively inhibits factor Xa. The drug is *100% bioavailable*, attains *maximum concentration* within *1.7 h* of administration, and has a *half-life of 17–21 h*. Its extended half-life allows *once-daily* dosing. It is usually administered *6 h after surgery.* Fondaparinux is recommended as an antithrombotic agent after major orthopedic surgery and as initial treatment of pulmonary embolism.

The recommended intervals of discontinuation and resumption of fondaparinux for pain management and regional anesthesia management:

Interventional Pain Management

Fondaparinux (1 × 2.5 mg/day)
Discontinuation time:
High-/intermediate-risk procedures: *(4 days)*.
Low-risk (Risk-benefit assessment *(2 days = 2 half-life*, for more conservative approach).

Restart: High-/intermediate-risk procedures: *(24 h);* Low-risk procedures: *(6 h)*.

Regional Anesthetic Management

Fondaparinux (1 × 2.5 mg/day)
Discontinuation time: *(36–42 h)*.
Time after puncture/catheter manipulation or removal: *(6–12 h)*.
(Laboratory tests: Anti-factor Xa (<0.1 U/mL)

- *Based on the sustained and irreversible antithrombotic effect, early postoperative dosing, and the spinal hematoma reported during initial clinical trials, ASRA recommends that until further clinical experience is available performance of neuraxial techniques should occur under conditions used in clinical trials (single needle pass, atraumatic needle placement, avoidance of indwelling neuraxial catheters).*

New (or Direct) Oral Anti-Factor Xa Agents (Dabigatran, Rivaroxaban, Apixaban, Edoxaban)

These drugs are at least as effective anticoagulants as the vitamin K antagonists but seem to be safer in terms of bleeding, have a rapid onset of action and a short half-life, and are devoid of the need for routine laboratory monitoring. Do not require serial coagulation monitoring and are safer, partly because of their short half-lives.

Dabigatran (Pradaxa®)

Dabigatran etexilate is a direct thrombin inhibitor that blocks the interaction of thrombin with different substances. It acts independently of anti-thrombin. Dabigatran is highly dependent (>80%) on renal excretion. The bioavailability after oral dabigatran etexilate is 7.2%, and peak plasma concentrations are attained 1.5–3 h after intake of prodrug. The half-life of dabigatran is 12–17 h (28 h in severe renal disease).

Rivaroxaban (Xarelto®)
Rivaroxaban, a direct factor Xa inhibitor, has a rapid onset of action. Peak plasma concentrations are observed within 2.5–4 h, and maximum inhibition of factor Xa (up to 68%) occurs 3 h after dosing. Factor Xa Inhibition occurs for 12 h or 24–48 h when higher doses are given in the elderly. The half-life of Rivaroxaban is 5.7–9.2 h and can be as long as 13 h in elderly patients secondary to the age-related decline in renal function.

Apixaban (Eliquis®)
Apixaban is rapidly absorbed, attaining peak concentrations in 1–2 h. The half-life of apixaban is 13.5 ± 9.9 h after a single 20 mg dose, and 15.2 ± 8.5 h after a single 5 mg dose, and 11.7 ± 3.3 after multiple 5 mg doses.

Edoxaban (Lixiana®)
Edoxaban is indicated for the prevention of stroke in patients with atrial fibrillation and for treatment of deep venous thrombosis and pulmonary embolism.

Maximum concentration is attained in 1–2 h; it is 60% bioavailable and 50% of the drug is excreted by the kidneys. Its half-life is 8.75–14 h.

The recommended intervals of discontinuation and resumption of new oral anti-coagulants for pain management and regional anesthesia management:

Interventional Pain Management
Dabigatran(Pradaxa®)
Discontinuation time:
High-/intermediate-risk procedures *(4 days);* end-stage of renal disease *(5–6 days);*
Low-risk procedures (Risk-benefit assessment—more conservative approach *(2 days = 2 half-lives).*
Restart: *(24 h); Risk of VTE (12 h).*

Rivaroxaban (Xarelto®)
Discontinuation time:
High-/intermediate-risk procedures: *3 days (65 h).*
Low-risk procedures (Risk-benefit assessment—more conservative approach *(2 days = 2 half-lives).*
Restart: *(24 h); Risk of VTE (12 h).*

Apixaban(Eliquis®)
Discontinuation time:
High-/intermediate-risk procedures: *3 days (75 h).*
Low-risk procedures (Risk-benefit assessment—more conservative approach *(2 days = 2 half-lives).*
Restart: *(24 h); Risk of VTE (12 h).*

Edoxaban(Lixiana®)
Discontinuation time:
High-/intermediate-risk procedures: *3 days (70 h).*
Low-risk procedures (Risk-benefit assessment—more conservative approach *(2 days = 2 half-lives).*
Restart: *(24 h);* Risk of VTE *(12 h).*

Regional Anesthetic Management
Dabigatran: **(110/220 OD[10] 150 mg BID[11])**
Time before puncture/catheter manipulation or removal: *72 h (3 days)–120 h (5 days)*[12]
Time after puncture/catheter manipulation or removal: *(6 h).*
(Laboratory tests: a PTT, ECT, TT)

Consider:

- With *unanticipated administration with indwelling catheter*, dabigatran dosing be held for *34–36 h* or the dTT or ECT assessed before catheter removal.
- *Avoid performance* of neuraxial blocks in patients with *CrCl of <30 mL/min.*
- Age > 65, hypertension, concomitant antiplatelet medication.

Rivaroxaban

- (≤10 mg/day).
  Time before puncture/catheter manipulation or removal: *(22–26 h).*
  Time after puncture/catheter manipulation or removal: *(6 h).*
- (2 × 15 mg/day or 1 × 20 mg/day).
  Time before puncture/catheter manipulation or removal: *44–65 h (3 days).*
  Time after puncture/catheter manipulation or removal: *(6 h).*
  (Laboratory tests: Anti-factor Xa, standardized for specific agent)

Consider

- With *unanticipated administration with indwelling catheter*, ASRA recommends that rivaroxaban dosing be held for 22–26 h before or an anti-factor Xa assay calibrated to rivaroxaban be assessed before the catheter is removed.

Apixaban

- *(2 × 2.5 mg/day).*
  Time before puncture/catheter manipulation or removal: *(26–30 h).*
  Time after puncture/catheter manipulation or removal *(6 h).*

[10]Prophylactic dose for joint replacement.

[11]Risk reduction or treatment for VTE or PE; RA-regional anesthesia procedure including manipulation or removal of catheter.

[12]*72 h (3 days)* (CrCl ≥80 mL/min); *96 h (4 days)* (CrCl 50–79 mL/min); *120 h (5 days)* (CrCl 30–49 mL/min) (ASRA).

- *(2 × 5 mg/day).*
  Time before puncture/catheter manipulation or removal: *40–75 h (3 days).*
  Time after puncture/catheter manipulation or removal *(6 h).*
  (Laboratory: Anti-factor Xa, standardized for specific agent)

Consider

- With *unanticipated administration with indwelling catheter*, ASA recommend that apixaban dosing be held for 26–30 h or an anti-factor Xa assay calibrated to apixaban before the catheter is removed.

Edoxaban

- *(≤30 mg/day).*
  Time before puncture/catheter manipulation or removal: *(20–28 h).*
  Time after puncture/catheter manipulation or removal: *(6–7 h).*
- *(≤60 mg/day).*
  Time before puncture/catheter manipulation or removal: *40–70 h (3 days).*
  Time after puncture/catheter manipulation or removal: *(6–7 h).*

Consider

With *unanticipated administration with indwelling catheter*, ASRA recommends that edoxaban dosing be held for 20–28 h or an anti-factor Xa assay calibrated to edoxaban before the catheter is removed.

Thrombolytic Agents

Thrombolytic agents convert plasminogen and thrombin to plasmin, the enzyme that causes fibrinolysis. Cases of spontaneous spinal hematoma have been reported in patients on thrombolytic therapy. There are also cases of spinal hematoma in patients who had neuraxial procedures and had subsequent thrombolytic therapy.

Recommended Management of Thrombolytic for Interventional Pain Management

- Interventional pain management should *be avoided* in patients who just received fibrinolytic agents.
- If an intervention has to be performed, a *minimum of 48 h* between discontinuation of a thrombolytic agent and a neuraxial injection is probably safe. Longer intervals, that is, *72 h*, should be considered for *high-risk* surgical pain procedures.
- In *emergency situations* wherein a thrombolytic needs to be administered after a spine pain intervention, the *pain service* should preferably be informed.
- If the patient has a neuraxial catheter or SCS lead, the device can be left in place. Fibrinogen levels can be determined and the *device removed after 48 h* or after a minimum of the two half-lives of the drug has elapsed.

Recommended Management of Thrombolytic for Regional Anesthetic Management

- *Avoid performance of neuraxial block* in patients who have received fibrinolytic and thrombolytic drugs. Guidelines detailing original *contraindications* to thrombolytic drugs suggest *avoidance of these drugs for 10 days following puncture* of noncompressible vessels.
- In patients *scheduled* to receive thrombolytic therapy, guidelines suggests that the patient be *queried and medical record reviewed* for a recent history of lumbar puncture, spinal or epidural anesthesia, or ESI to allow appropriate monitoring.
- Data are not available to clearly outline the length of time neuraxial puncture should be avoided after discontinuation of these drugs. However, a *48 h* time interval and documentation of normalization of clotting studies (including fibrinogen) are suggested.
- In those patients *who have received neuraxial blocks* at or near the time of fibrinolytic / thrombolytic therapy, ASRA recommends that *neurological monitoring* should be considered for an appropriate interval.
- There is no definitive recommendation for *removal of neuraxial catheters* in patients who *unexpectedly received* fibrinolytic and thrombolytic therapy during a neuraxial catheter infusion. ASRA recommends the measurement of fibrinogen level.

Conclusion

The management of anticoagulants or antiplatelet agents in the perioperative period is based on their pharmacokinetics and pharmacodynamic profile. Understanding clinical indications for the drugs will make an anesthesiologist more aware of the risks of discontinuation. Several new oral anticoagulants offer oral routes of administration, simple dosing regimen, efficacy with less bleeding risks, reduced requirement for clinically monitoring. Due to safety concerns of bleeding risks, guidelines and recommendations have been designed to reduce patient morbidity/mortality during regional anesthesia. Patient-specific factors and surgery-related issues should be considered to improve patient-oriented outcomes.

Suggested Reading

Ahmed I, Gertner E. Safety of arthrocentesis and joint injection in patients recieving anticoagulation at therapeutic levels. Am J Med. 2012;125:265–9.

Akers WS, Oh JJ, Oestreich JH, et al. Pharmacokinetics and pharmacodynamics of a bolus and infusion of cangreol: a direct, parenteral P2Y12 receptor antagonist. J Clin Pharmacol. 2010;50:27–35.

Albright GA. Cardiac arrest following regional anesthesia with etidocaine or bupivacaine. Anesthesiology. 1978;51:285–7.

Auroy Y, Narchi P, Messiah A, et al. Serious complications related to regional anesthesia: results of a prospective survey in France. Anesthesiology. 1997;87:479–86.

Bara L, Billaud E, Gramond G, et al. Comparative pharmacokinetics of a low molecular weight heparin (PK 10 169) and unfractionated heparin after intravenous and subcutaneous administration. Thromb Res. 1985;39:631–6.

Baranowski AP, De Courcey J, Bonelle E. A trial of intravenous lidocaine on the pain and allodynia of postherpetic neuralgia. J Pain Symptom Manage. 1999;17(6):429–33.

Benedek ICH, Joshi AS, Pieniaszek HJ, King SY, et al. Variability in the pharmacokinetics and pharmacodynamics of low dose aspirin in healthy male volunteers. J Clin Pharmacol. 1995;35:1181–6.

Benzon HT. Regional anesthesia in the anticoagulated patient. In: Hadzic A, editor. Peripheral nerve blocks. 2nd ed. New York: Mc Graw Hill; 2012. p. 107–13.

Benzon HT, Avram J, Green D, et al. New oral anticoagulants and regional anesthesia. Br J Anesth. 2013;111:i96–i113.

Bonica JJ. Biology, pathophysiology, and treatment of acute pain. In: Lipton S, Miles J, editors. Persistent pain, vol. 5. New York: Grune & Stratton; 1985. p. 1–32.

Bonica JJ, Buckley PF. Regional analgesia with local anesthetics. In: Bonica JJ, editor. Management of pain. 2nd ed. Philadelphia: Lea & Febiger; 1990.

Borchard U, Niesel HC. Grundlagen der Pharmakologie der Lokalanästhetika. In: Niesel HC, editor. Regionalanästhesie, Lokalanästhesie, Regionale Schmerztherapie. Stuttgart: Georg Thieme; 1994.

Bradlow BA, Chetty N. Dosage frequencyfor supression of platelet function by low dose aspirin therapy. Thromb Res. 1982;27:99–110.

Braid BP, Scott DB. The systemic absorptionof local analgesic drugs. Br J Anesth. 1965;37:394.

Brandt JT, Payne CD, Wiviott CD, et al. A comparison of prasugrel and clopidogrel loading doses on platelet function: magnitude of platelet inhibition is related to active metabolite formation. Am Heart J. 2007;153:66.e9–e16.

Burch JW, Stanford N, Majerus PW. Inhibition of platelet prostaglandin synthetase by oral aspirin. J Clin Invest. 1978;61:314–9.

Butterworth JF, Strichartz GR. The molecular mechanisms by which local anesthetics produce impulse blockade:a review. Anesthesiology. 1990;72:711–34.

Campbell JN, Raja SN, Cohen RH, Manning D, Khan A, Meyer RA. Peripheral neural mechanisms of nociception. In: Wall PD, Melzack R, editors. Textbook of pain. 2nd ed. Edinburgh: Churchill Livingstone; 1989.

Campion FX. Good medical records can be strongest malpractice defense. In: Grand rounds on medical malpractice. Chicago: American Medical Association; 1990.

Catterall W. Cellular and molecular biology of voltage-gated sodium channels. Physiol Rev. 1992;72:S15–48.

Convay R, O'Shea FD, Cunnane G, et al. Safety of joint and soft tissue injections in patients on warfarin anticoagulation. Clin Rheumatol. 2013;32:1811–24.

Covino BG. Toxicity and systemic effects of local anesthetic agents. In: Stricharzt GR, editor. Handbook of experimental pharmacology, vol. 81. Berlin: Springer; 1987. p. 187–212.

Davies NM, Anderson KE. Clinical pharmacocinetics of naproxen. Clin Pharmacokinet. 1997;32:268–93.

Dawes PJ, O'Keefe L, Adcock S. Informed consent: Using structured interview changes patients attitudes towards informed consent. J Laryngol Otol. 1993;107:775–9.

Devit JH, Rapanos T, Kurreck M, et al. The anesthetic record: accuracy and completeness. Can J Anaesth. 1999;46:122–8.

Devor M. Central changes mediating neuropathic pain. In: Dubner R, Gebhart GF, Bond MR, editors. Proceedings of the Vth world congress on pain. Pain research and clinical management. Amsterdam: Elsevier; 1988. p. 7.

Di Gregorio G, Neal MJ, Rosenquist RW, Weinberg LG. Clinical presentation of local anesthetic systemic toxicity. A review of published cases, 1979 to 2009. Reg Anesth Pain Med. 2010;35:181–7.

Di Nisio M, Middeldrop S, Buller HR. Direct thrombin inhibitors. N Engl J Med. 2005;353:1028–40.

Enders S, Shufelt A, Bogduk N. The risks of continuing or discontinuing anticoagulants for patients undergoing common interventional pain procedures. Pain Med. 2017;18:403–9.

Feldman JM. Do anesthesia information systems increase malpractice exsposure? Result of a survey. Anesth Analg. 2004;99:840–3.

Fields HL, Basbaum AI. Central nervous system mechanisms of pain modulation. In: Wall PD, Melzack R, editors. Textbook of pain. 3rd ed. London: Churchill Livingstone; 1994. p. 243–57.

Frost C, Wang J, Nepal S, et al. Apixaban, an oral, direct factor Xa inhibitor. Xa inhibitor Single dose safety, pharmacokinetics, pharmacodynamics and food effect in healthy subjects. Br J Clin Pharmacol. 2013a;75:476–87.

Frost C, Nepal S, Wang J, et al. Safety pharmacokinetics and pharmacodynamics of multiple oral doses of apixaban, a factor Xa inhibitor, in healthy subjects. Br J Clin Pharmacol. 2013b;76:776–86.

Gadsen J. Local anesthetics: clinical pharmacology and rational selection. In: Hadzic A, editor. Peripheral nerve blocks and anatomy for ultrasound-guided regional anesthesia. New York: McGraw Hill; 2012. p. 30–40.

Gadsen J, Hadzic A, Gandhi K, et al. The effect of mixing 1.5% mepivacaine and 0.5% bupivacaine on duration of analgesia and latency of block onset in ultrasound-guided interscalene block. Anesth Analg. 2011;112:471–6.

Galer BS, Rowbotham MC, Perander J. Topical lidocaine patch relieves postherpetic neuralgia more effectively than a vehicle topical patch: results of an enriched enrollment study. Pain. 1999;80:533–8.

Gammaitoni AR, Alvarez NA, Galer BS. Safety and tolerability of the lidocaine patch 5%, a targeted peripheral analgesic: a review of the literature. J Clin Pharmacol. 2003;43(2):111–7.

Gerancher JC. Documentation of regional anesthesia procedures. In: Hadzic A, editor. Textbook of regional anesthesia and acute pain management. New York: McGraw Hill; 2007. p. 1164–70.

Gerancher JC, Viscusi ER, Liguori GA, et al. Development of standardized peripheral nerve block procedure note form. Reg Anesth Pain Med. 2005;30(1):67–71.

Gogarten W, Vandermeulen E, van Aken H, et al. Regional anaesthesia and antithrombotic agents: recommendations of the European Society of Anaesthesiology. Eur J Anaesthesiol. 2010;27: 999–1015.

Graf BM, Martin E, Bosnjak ZJ, et al. Stereospecific effect of bupivacaine isomers on atrioventricular conduction in the isolated perfused guinea pig heart. Anesthesiology. 1997;86:410–9.

Groban L, Deal DD, Vernon JC, James RL, Butterworth J. Cardiac resuscitation after incremental overdosage with lidocaine, bupivacaine, levobupivacaine, and ropivacaine in anesthetized dogs. Anesth Analg. 2001;92:37–43.

Guay J. The epidural test dose: a Review. Anesth Analg. 2006;102:921–9.

Gurbel PA, Bliden KP, Butler K, et al. Randomized double–blind assessment of the ONSET and OFFSET oft he antiplatelet effects of ticagrelor versus clopidogrell in patients with stable coronary artery disease: the ONSET/OFFSET study. Circulation. 2009;120:2577–85.

Gy L, Endoxaban AG. A focussed review of ist clinical pharmacology. Eur Heart J. 2014;35:1884–5.

Hadzic A, Vloka JD. Equipment and patient monitoring in regional anesthesia. In: Hadzic A, Vloka JD, editors. Peripheral nerve blocks: principles and practice. New York: McGraw-Hill; 2004. p. 29–41.

Hall R, Mazer CD. Antiplatelet drugs: a review of their pharmacology and managemant in the perioperative period. Anesth Analg. 2011;112:292–318.

Hebl JR. The.importance and implications of aseptic tecniques during regional anesthesia. Reg Anesth Pain Med. 2006;31(4):311–23.

Helleberg L. Clinical pharmacocinetic of indometacin. Clin Pharmacokinet. 1981;6:245–58.

Horlocker TT, Heit JA. Low molecular weight heparin: biochemistry, pharmacology, perioperative prophylaxis regimes, and guidelines for regional anesthetic management. Anesth Analg. 1997;85:874–85.

Horlocker TT, Bajwa ZH, Ashraf Z, et al. Risk assessment of hemorrhagic complications associated with nonsteroidal antiinflammatory medications in ambulatory pain clinic patients undergoing epidural steroid injection. Anesth Analg. 2002;95:1691–7.

Horlocker TT, Vandermeulen E, Kopp SL, Gogarten W, Leffert L, Benzon HAT. Regional anesthesia in the patient recieving antithrombotic therapy or thrombolytic therapy: American Society of Regional Anesthesia and Pain Medicine evidence- based guide; 153:line(fourth edition). Reg Anesth Pain Med. 2018;43: 263–309.

Hudson P, Gnanaseakaran S, Knowles M. Improvement of documentation of epidural insertion with the addition of a sticker to the anesthetic chart: an audit circle. Reg Anesth Pain Med. 2008;33:e34.

Jankovic D. New approaches to chronic pain: Nerve blocks in the head. In: Van Zundert A, Rawal N, editors. Highlights in regional anesthesia and pain therapy. XI (Special Edition: World Congress on Regional Anaesthesia and Pain Therapy, Barcelona); 2002. p. 258–69.

Jiang J, Hu Y, Zhang J, et al. Safety, pharmacokinetics and pharmacodynamic of single doses of rivaroxaban- an oral, direct factor Xa inhibitor-in elderly Chinese subjects. Thromb Haemost. 2010;103:234–41.

Jimenez AH, Stubbs ME, Tofler GH, et al. Rapidity and duration of platelet supression by enteric-coated aspirin in healthy young men. Am J Cardiol. 1992;69:258–62.

Kubitza D, Becka M, Wensing G, et al. Safety, pharmacodynamics, and pharmacokinetics of BAY 59-7939-an oral, direct factor Xa inhibitor-after multiple dosing in healthy male subjects. Eur J Clin Pharmacol. 2005;61:873–88.

Laux V, Perzborn E, Kubitza, et al. Preclinical and clinical characteristics of rivaroxaban: a novel, oral direct factor Xa inhibitor. Semin Thromb Hemost. 2007;33:515–23.

Leighton BL, Bauman J, Seltzer J. The effect of a detailed anesthesia consent form on patient recall and anxiety. Anesthesiology. 1987;67:A567.

Levy JH, Faraoni D, Spring JL, et al. Managing new oral anticoagulans in the perioperative and intensive care unit setting. Anesthesiology. 2013;118:1466–74.

Matthews J, Rutter S, Paul R. Standardized peripheral nerve block label can improve documentation. Reg Anesth Pain Med. 2007;32:128.

Matushima N, Lee F, Sato T, et al. Bioavailability and safety of the factor Xa inhibitor edoxaban and the effects of quinidine in healthy subjects. Clin Pharmacolol Drug Dev. 2013;2:358–66.

Meisel A, Roth LH. What we do and do not know about informed consent. JAMA. 1981;246:2473–7.

Meyer RA, Campbell JN, Raja SN. Peripheral neural mechanisms of nociception. In: Wall PD, Melzack R, editors. Textbook of pain. 3rd ed. London: Churchill Livinstone; 1994. p. 13–44.

Mroszczak EJ, Jung D, Yee J, et al. Ketorolac tromethamine pharmacokinetics and metabolsm after intravenous, intramuscular, and oral administration in humans and animals. Pharmacotherapy. 1990;10:33S–9S.

Mulroy MF, Hejtmanek MR. Prevention of local anesthetic systemic toxicity. Reg Anesth Pain Med. 2010;35:177–80.

Narouze S, Benzon HT, Provenzano D, Buvanendran A, De Andres J, Deer T, Rauck R, Huntoon MA. Interventional spine and pain procedures in patients on antiplatelet and anticoagulant medications (second edition): guidelines from the American Society of Regional Anesthesia and Pain Medicine, the European Society of Regional Anaesthesia and Pain Therapy, the American Academy of Pain Medicine, the International Neuromodulation Society, the North American Neuromodulation Society, and the World Institute of Pain. Reg Anesth Pain Med. 2018;43(3):225–62.

Neal JM. McMahon DJ. Equipment. In Brown DL(eds): Regional anesthesia and analgesia. 1. WB Saunders Philadelphia 2005; pp 159-172

Neal MJ, Bernards MC, Butterworth FJ, Di Gregorio G, Drasner K, Hejtmanek M, Mulroy MF, Rosenquist RW, Weinberg GL. ASRA Practice Advisory on local anesthetic systemic toxicity. Reg Anesth Pain Med. 2010;35:152–61.

Olkkola KT, Brunetto AV, Mattila MJ. Pharmacokinetic of oxicam nonsteroidal anti-inflamatory agents. Clin Pharmacokinet. 1994;26:107–20.

Raghavan N, Frost CE, Yu Z, et al. Apixaban metabolism and pharmacokinetic after oral administration to humans. Drug Metab Dispos. 2009;37:74–81.

Rainsford KD. Ibuprofen:pharmacology, efficacy and safety. Inflammopharmacology. 2009;17:275–342.

Raj PP. Guidelines for regional anesthestic technique. In: Hahn MB, Mc Quillan PM, Shepöpck GJ, editors. Regional anesthesia: an atlas of anatomy and techniques. Maryland Heights: Mosby; 1996. p. 21–38.

Reitz S, Haggmark S, Johansson G, et al. Cardiotoxicity of ropivacaine- a new amide local anesthetic agent. Acta Anaesthesiol Scand. 1989;33:93–8.

Ritchie JM, Greengard P. On the mode of action of local anesthetics. Annu Rev Pharmacol. 1966;6:405–30.

Rowbotham MC, Reisner-Keller LA, Fields HL. Both intravenous lidocaine and morphine reduce the pain of postherpetic neuralgia. Neurology. 1991;41:1024–8.

Rowbotham MC, Davies PS, Fields HL. Topical lidocaine gel relieves postherpetic neuralgia. Ann Neurol. 1995;37:246–53.

Rowbotham MC, Davies PS, Galer BS. Multicenter, double-blind, vehicle-controlled trial of long term use of lidocaine patches for postherpetic neuralgia (abstract). In: 8th World congress on pain. IASP Press; 1996a. p. 274.

Rowbotham MC, Davies PS, Verkempinck C. Lidocaine patch: double-blind controlled study of a new treatment method for postherpetic neuralgia. Pain. 1996b;65:39–44.

Ruff RL, Dougherty JH Jr. Complication of lumbar puncture followed by anticoagulation. Stroke. 1981;12:879–81.

Santos AC, Arthur GR, Lehning EJ, et al. Comparative pharmacokinetics of ropivacaine and bupivacaine in nonpregnant and pregnant ewes. Anesth Analg. 1997;85:87–93.

Slaughter S, et al. A comparison of the effect of universal use of gloves and gowns with that of glove use alone on acquisition of vancomycin- resistant enterococci in medical intensive care unit. Ann Intern med. 1996;125(6):448–56.

Small RE. Diclofenac sodium. Clin Pharm. 1989;8:545–58.

Sonksen JR, Kong KL, Holder R. magnitude and time course of impaired primary haemostasis after stopping chronic low back and medium dose aspirin in healthy volunteers. Br J Anesth. 1999;82: 360–5.

Tsui BC, Wagner A, Finucane B. Regional anesthesia in elderly: a clinical guide. Drugs Aging. 2004;21:895–910.

Tucker GT, Mather LE. Pharmacocinetics of local anesthetic agents. Br J Anesth. 1975;47:213–4.

Türc D, Roth W, Busch U. A review oft he clinical pharmacokinetics of meloxicam. Br J Rheumatol. 1996;(35 Suppl 1):13–6.

Vandermeulen EP, van Aken H, Vermylen J. Anticoagulants and spinal-epidural anesthesia. Anesth Analg. 1994;79:1165–77.

Von Känel R, Mills PJ, Fainman C, et al. Effects of psychological stress and psychiatric disorders on blood coagulation and fibrinolysis: a biobehavioral pathway to coronary artery disease? Psychosom Med. 2001;63:531–44.

Warner NS, Moeschler SM, Warner MA, et al. Bleeding complications in patients undergoing celiac plexus block. Reg Anesth Pain Med. 2016;41:488–93.

Warner NS, Bendel MA, Warner MA, et al. Bleeding complications in patients undergoing intrathecal drug delivery system implantation. Pain Med. 2017;18:2422–7.

Waurick K, Riess H, Van Acken H, Kessler P, Gogarten W, Volk T. S1-Leitlinie. Rückenmarksnahe Regionalanästhesien und Thromboembolieprophylaxe/antithrombotische Medikation. Anästh Intensivmed. 2014;55:464–92.

Weinberg LG. Treatment of local anesthetic systemic toxicity (LAST). Reg Anesth Pain Med. 2010;35:188–93.

Weitz JL. Drug therapy: low -molecular-weight heparins. N Engl J Med. 1997;337:688–98.

Weninger E. Pharmakodynamik der Lokalanästhetika. Anästhesiol Intensivmedizin. 1996a;5(37):249–67.

Weninger E. Pharmakodynamik der Lokalanästhetika. Anästhesiol Intensivmedizin. 1996b;5(37):249–67.

Zimmermann M. Physiologie von Nozizeption und Schmerz. In: Zimmermann M, Handwerker HO, editors. Schmerz-Konzepte und ärztliches Handeln. Berlin: Springer; 1984.

Zink W, et al. Bupivacaine but not Ropivacaine induces apoptosis in mammalian skeletal muscle fibers. Poster Discussion, Local Anesthesia and Pain, Basic Science II, ASA: A-971; 2002.

Zisman E, Erport A, Kohanovsky E, et al. Platelet function recovery after cessation of aspirin: preliminary study of volunteers and surgical patients. Eur J Anesthesiol. 2010;27:617–23.

Zwara DA, Nelson JM, Brooker RF, et al. The importance of the postoperative anesthetic visit: do repeated visits improve patient satisfaction or physitian recognition? Anesth Analg. 1996;83: 793–7.

Basics of Ultrasound Imaging

2

Herman Sehmbi and Anahi Perlas

Contents

H. Sehmbi
Western University, London, ON, Canada
e-mail: Herman.Sehmbi@Lhsc.on.ca

A. Perlas (✉)
Anesthesiology and Pain Medicine, University of Toronto, Toronto Western Hospital, University Health Network, Toronto, ON, Canada
e-mail: Anahi.Perlas@Uhn.ca

Basics of Ultrasound Physics

Introduction

Ultrasound-guided regional anesthesia and pain procedures have seen significant strides in technological advances and wide clinical acceptance in the last decade. Ultrasound provides real-time image guidance for regional anesthesia and interventional pain procedures. It is a practical tool as it is portable, moderately priced, and devoid of radiation risks. It

D. Jankovic, P. Peng (eds.), *Regional Nerve Blocks in Anesthesia and Pain Therapy*,
https://doi.org/10.1007/978-3-030-88727-8_2

has been shown to hasten block onset, to improve the success rate, and to be cost-effective. This chapter provides a brief overview of some of the fundamental principles and physics underlying ultrasound technology as well as some of its limitations and pitfalls.

Characteristics of an Ultrasound Wave

An ultrasound wave is a *non-audible sound wave* with frequencies above 20 kHz. It can be characterized by the following basic parameters (Fig. 2.1):

(a) Wavelength (λ): It is the spatial period of the wave, that is, the distance over which the wave's shape repeats. It is determined by measuring the distance between two consecutive corresponding points of the same phase. It is expressed in *meters* (m).
(b) Amplitude (A): It is a measure of the wave's height, that is, maximal particle displacement. It is expressed in *meters* (m).
(c) Period (T): It is the time taken for one complete wave cycle to occur. The unit of a period is *seconds* (s).
(d) Frequency (f): It is the number of completed cycles per second. Thus, it is the inverse of the period (T) of a wave and is measured in *hertz* (Hz). Medical imaging uses high-frequency waves (1–20 MHz).
(e) Velocity (c): It is the speed of propagation of a sound wave through a medium. The velocity (c) of a sound wave is the product of its frequency (f) and wavelength (λ). The unit of velocity is *meters per second* (m/s). The speed of sound in a biological medium is assumed to be constant at 1540 m/s for practical purposes. However, it varies greatly, being as low as 330 m/s in air and as high as 4000 m/s through bone.

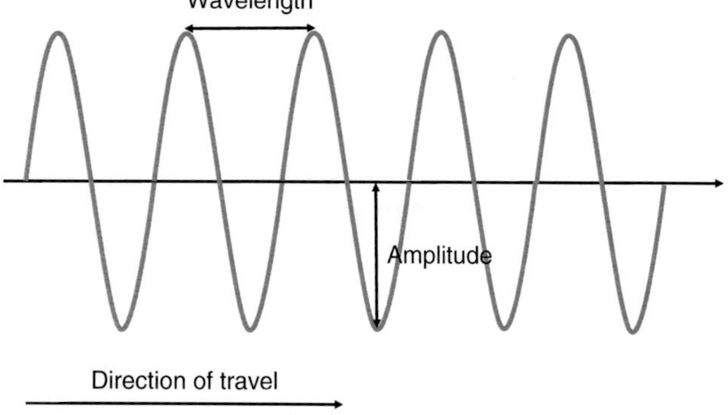

Fig. 2.1 Characteristics of a transverse sound wave. (Reproduced with permission from Dr. Herman Sehmbi)

(f) The energy (E) of a sound wave is proportional to the square of its amplitude (A). This means that as the amplitude of a wave decreases (such as with deeper penetration), the wave's energy reduces drastically. It is measured in *joules* (J).
(g) Power (P): Power of a sound wave is the energy (E) delivered per unit of time (J/t).

Generation of Ultrasound Waves

The piezoelectric crystals (e.g., quartz) in an ultrasound transducer produce a small electrical potential difference across them when compressed. Their ability to convert mechanical energy into electrical energy is termed the *piezoelectric effect* (Fig. 2.2a). This effect is used in image generation when returning ultrasound waves apply mechanical energy to the crystals, generating an electrical signal. The converse, that is, electrical energy across a piezoelectric crystal, causes mechanical distortion of the crystals resulting in their vibration and generation of sound waves termed the *reverse piezoelectric effect* (Fig. 2.2b). This property is utilized to generate ultrasound waves from transducers.

Structure of an Ultrasound Transducer

An ultrasound transducer has *dual functionality*. It is responsible for both the production of ultrasound waves and, after a set period, the reception of waves reflected back from the tissues. This function is called *pulsed ultrasound*. The *pulse repetition frequency* (PRF) is the number of pulses emitted by the transducer per unit of time. The PRF for medical imaging devices ranges from 1 to 10 kHz (Fig. 2.3).

An ultrasound transducer has the following layers (Fig. 2.4):

(a) *Backing material*: It is located behind the piezoelectric element and serves to prevent excessive vibration. As a result, the element generates ultrasound waves with a shorter pulse length, improving axial resolution in images.
(b) *Piezoelectric elements*: They generate ultrasonic waves and images. Piezoelectric ceramic (PZT: lead zirconate titanate) is most used because of its high conversion efficiency.
(c) *The acoustic matching layer* reduces the acoustic impedance mismatch between the transducer and the object, minimizing reflection off the interface. This is usually made up of a resin.

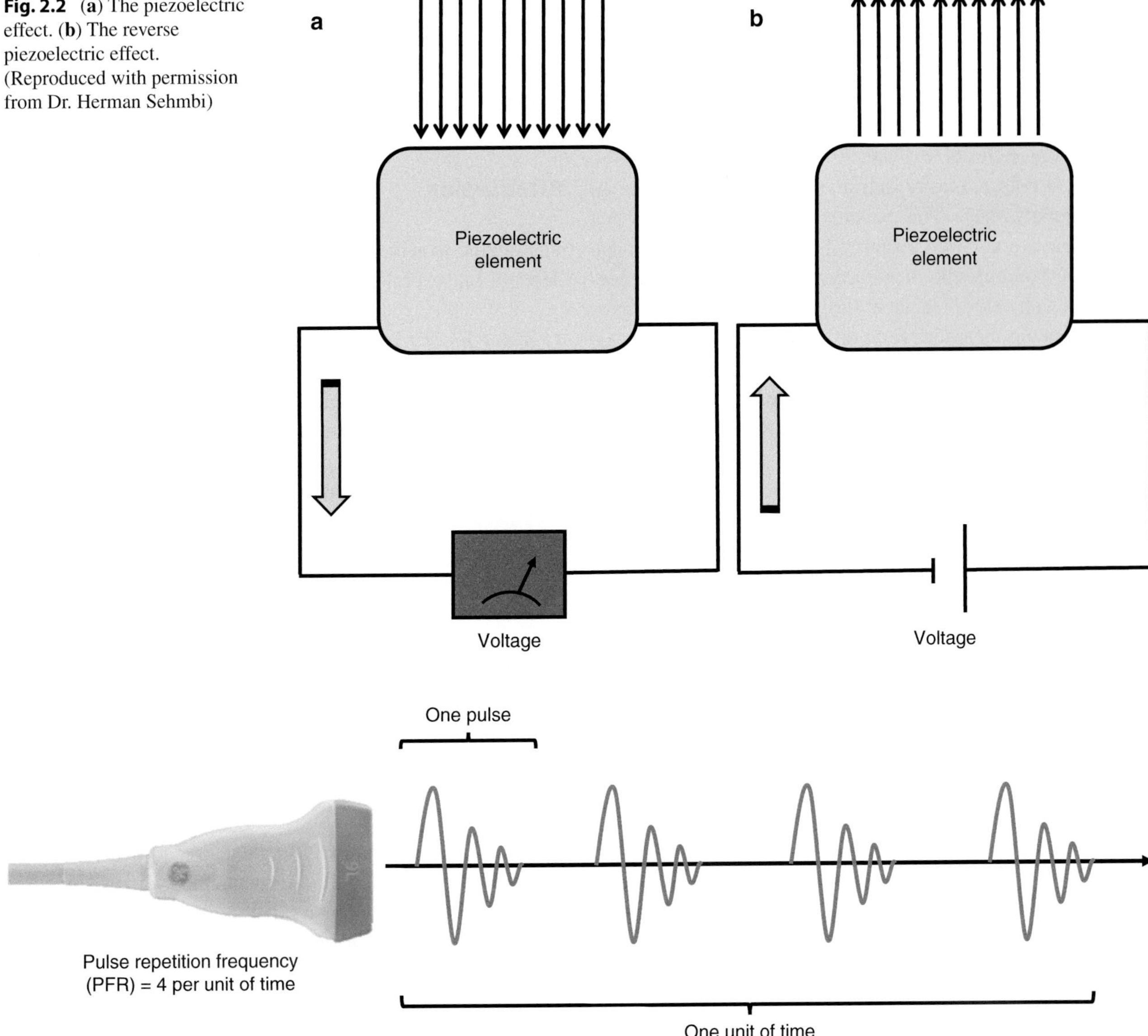

Fig. 2.2 (**a**) The piezoelectric effect. (**b**) The reverse piezoelectric effect. (Reproduced with permission from Dr. Herman Sehmbi)

Fig. 2.3 Pulse repetition frequency. (Reproduced with permission from Dr. Herman Sehmbi)

(d) *Acoustic lens*: The acoustic lens prevents the ultrasonic waves from spreading and focuses them in the slice direction to improve the resolution.

Interaction of Ultrasound with Tissues

The image on the screen of an ultrasound machine results from ultrasound waves' interaction with the tissues being examined. As the ultrasound wave travels through the tissues, it loses amplitude (and hence energy). This reduction in amplitude is called *attenuation*. Attenuation is the summative effect of absorption (conversion of acoustic energy to heat), reflection, and refraction of ultrasound waves.

Absorption

Absorption is the transfer of the ultrasound beam's energy to the medium through which it travels. This results in heat generation and accounts for most of the energy attenuation.

Reflection

When an incident ultrasound pulse encounters an interface of two body tissues with different acoustic impedances, the sound energy is reflected to the transducer. When the ultrasound wave is incident upon objects smaller than its wavelength, it is reflected in multiple directions (*diffuse scattering*).

However, when incident upon smooth structures such as fascial planes, the wave is mostly reflected back to the transducer in a linear manner (*specular reflection*, Fig. 2.5). If the incident angle is near 90°, most of the waves are reflected and get back to the transducer, generating good images. However, with incident angles of less than 90°, an increasing proportion of waves is reflected away from the transducer producing an inferior quality image. This explains why needles inserted at a steep angle are not well visualized on the ultrasound image (Fig. 2.6). Some needle manufacturers have introduced needles with "reflectors" in their design. Many of these have indentations on their surface at different angles which maximize the proportion of waves reflected back to the transducer. This makes such needles more "echogenic."

Refraction

Refraction refers to a change in the wave's direction after reaching an interface of two tissues with different sound transmission speeds. It depends on the *change in velocity* and not due to acoustic impedance differences (Fig. 2.7). Refraction is one of the most frequent causes of artifacts on an ultrasound image.

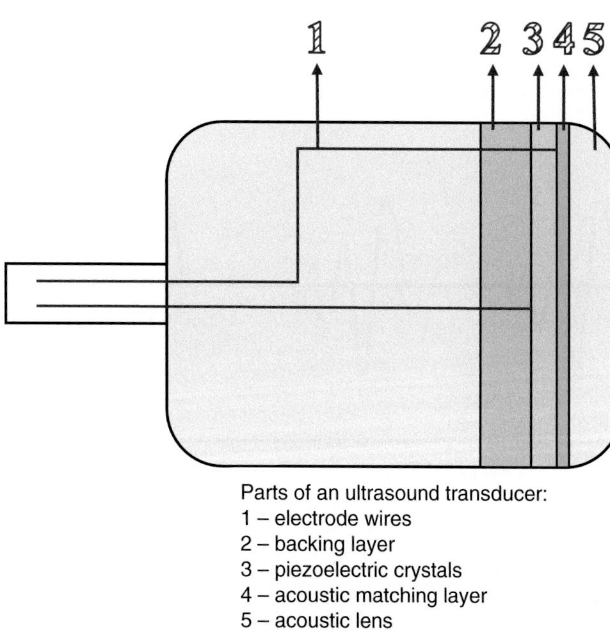

Fig. 2.4 Layers of an ultrasound transducer. (Reproduced with permission from Dr. Herman Sehmbi)

Attenuation

The degree to which a given ultrasound wave is attenuated depends on several factors, such as:

1. The *type of tissue*: Attenuation is greater for denser tissues such as bone and less for fluid mediums such as blood or fluid-containing cysts or cavities.
2. *The frequency* of the ultrasound wave: The degree of attenuation for a given distance unit is greater for higher frequency waves. This explains why higher frequency transducers (commonly up to 13–15 MHz) are mostly used to image superficial structures (up to 5–6 cm deep) while lower frequency (2–5 MHz) transducers are required to image deeper structures (>6–10 cm deep).
3. *Distance traveled*: For any ultrasound wave, the attenuation degree is directly proportional to the distance traveled (Fig. 2.8).

Acoustic Impedance

The *acoustic impedance* (*Z*) is the degree to which medium particles resist change due to mechanical disturbance and is a product of the density (ρ) of the medium and the acoustic velocity (c) of the ultrasound wave. The degree of ultrasound wave reflection (how much gets back to the transducer to form the ultrasound image) depends upon the relative difference in the acoustic impedance (resistance at the interface) between the two tissues (or mediums) across an interface. This is determined by the *reflection coefficient* (*R*). A large difference in acoustic impedance occurs at air/soft tissue and bone/soft tissue interface, causing very high reflection at such sites. This makes the bone cortex appear hyperechoic (white) as there is a drastic **increase** in acoustic impedance from the soft tissues with

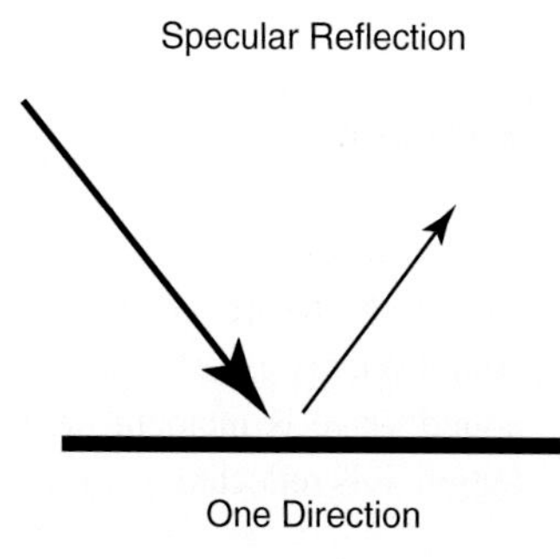

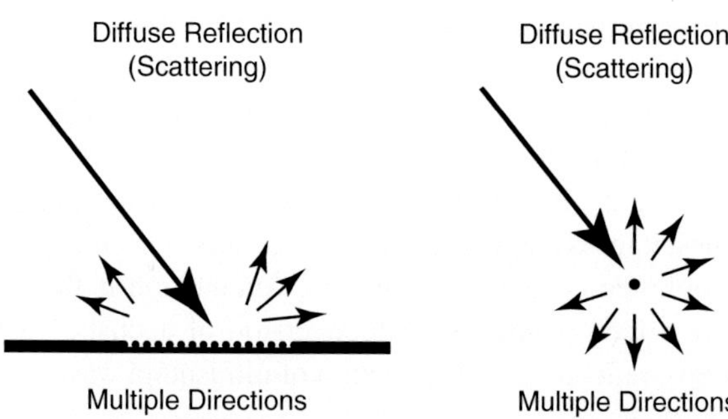

Fig. 2.5 Different types of reflection, including specular and diffuse reflection. (Reproduced with permission from www.usra.ca)

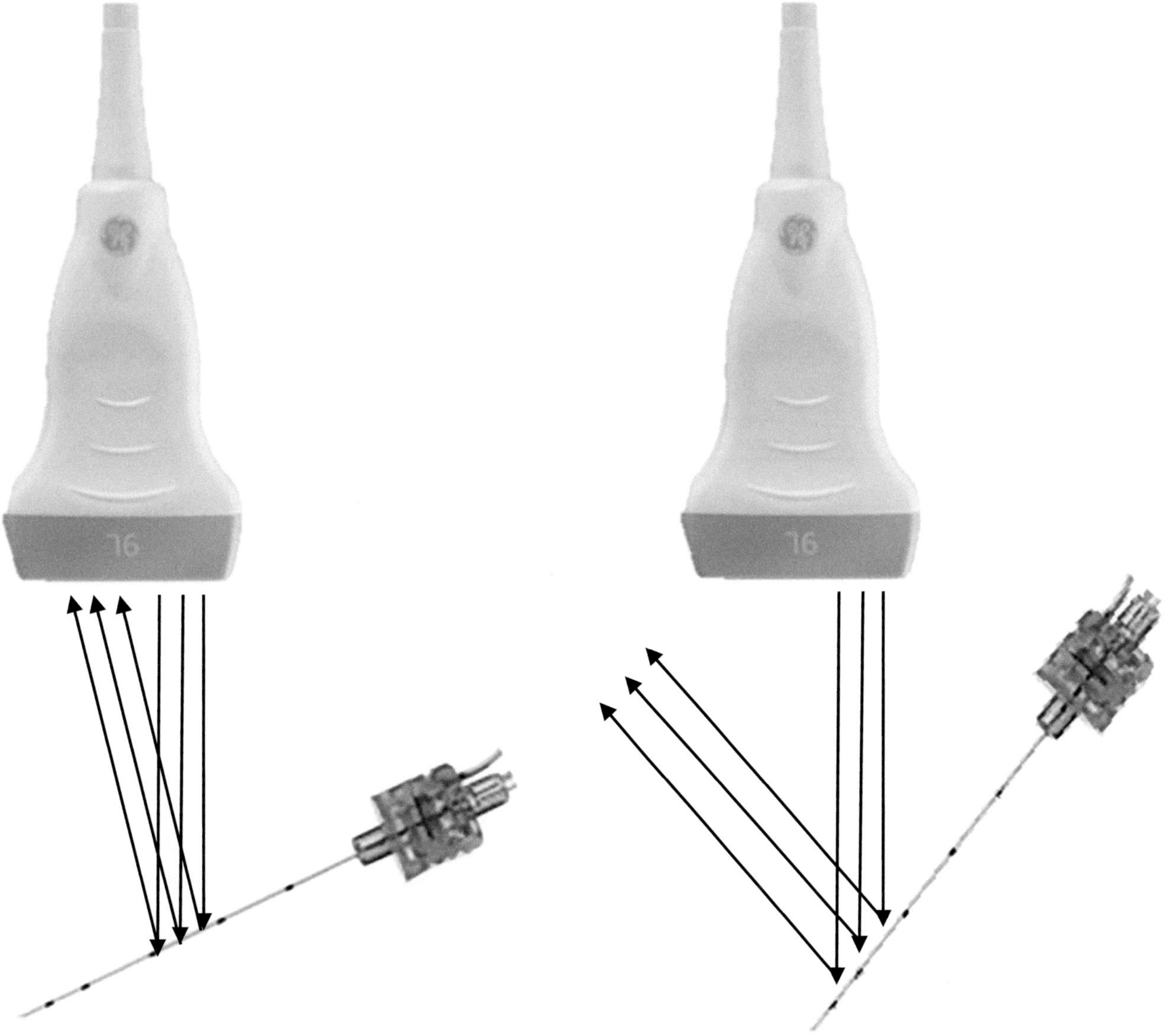

Fig. 2.6 Effect of angle of needle insertion on the acquisition of reflected ultrasound waves. (Reproduced with permission from Dr. Herman Sehmbi)

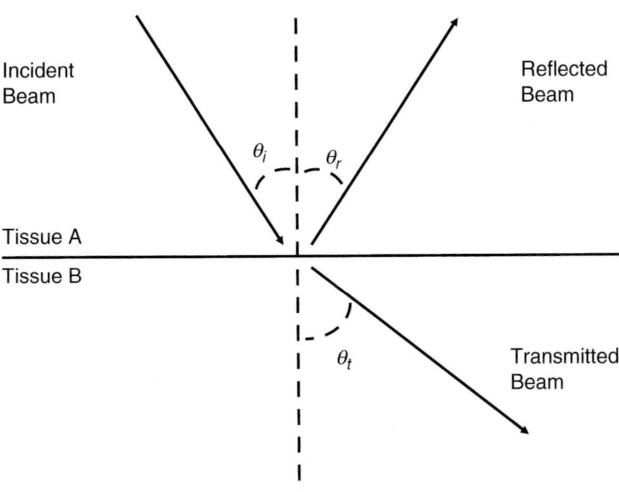

Fig. 2.7 Refraction across two mediums. (Reproduced with permission from Dr. Herman Sehmbi)

relatively low acoustic impedance, to the bone surface with very high acoustic impedance. Similarly, at the pleural surface, there is a high degree of reflection of the ultrasound waves, with the pleural surface appearing hyperechoic. In this latter case, however, the high degree of reflection is due to a drastic *decrease* in acoustic impedance with the soft tissues having a relatively high acoustic impedance compared to the very low acoustic impedance of air. Regardless of the direction of the difference (increase or decrease) in acoustic impedance, the resulting effect is a high degree of reflection with the interface appearing hyperechoic. This phenomenon is also why a gel is needed at the transducer surface to perform "acoustic coupling". In other words, to eliminate the air/soft tissue interface at the skin would result in a high degree of reflection of the ultrasound wave with loss of wave energy available to penetrate the tissues.

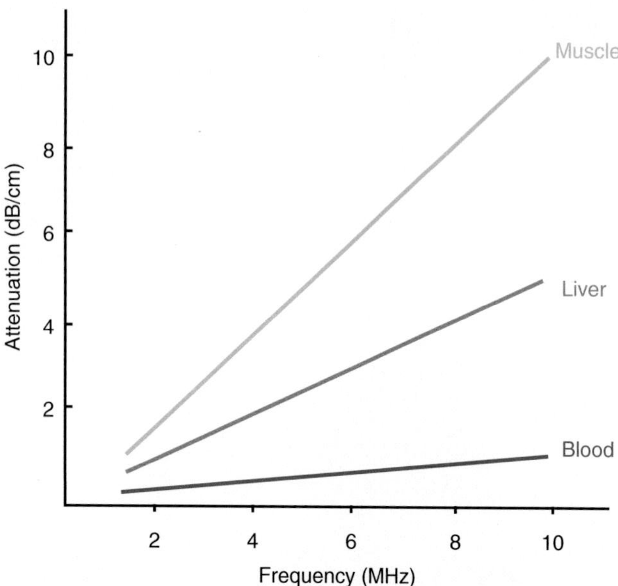

Fig. 2.8 Relationship of attenuation with tissue type and frequency. (Reproduced with permission from www.usra.ca)

Image Acquisition and Processing

The echo signals returning from the tissues reach the crystals and produce an electric current (*piezoelectric effect*). This is then converted to a pixel, with the returning wave's energy being proportional to the pixel dot's brightness on the image. However, the generation of the final image involves these additional processes:

(a) *Amplification (gain):* The amplitude of the returning echo signals is minimal in amplitude to be appropriately displayed on a screen. Hence, it needs amplification. However, amplification adds to "background noise."
(b) *Time gain compensation:* Because the ultrasound waves undergo attenuation, the intensity (and hence brightness) of the returning waves from deeper tissues is much lower than the ones returning from the nearer tissues. This is overcome by preferential enhancement of signals returning from deeper tissues and the so-called time gain compensation. Those echoes returning from similar reflectors are represented by the same grey shade regardless of their depth (Fig. 2.9a, b).
(c) *Analog to digital conversion:* This eliminates external interference and, more importantly, allows for signal processing to improve image quality.
(d) *Post-processing:* This involves techniques such as frame averaging, grey-level transfer curves, edge enhancement, and adaptive image processing to yield the final image on display.

The final image allows structures to be represented according to their brightness or echogenicity as follows:

(a) *Hyperechoic:* Areas with returning echoes of higher energy than their surrounding structures, appearing whiter (such as peripheral nerves and muscle tendons) (Fig. 2.10a).
(b) *Hypoechoic:* Areas with returning echoes of lower energy than their surrounding structures, appearing as dark grey (such as proximally located spinal nerve roots) (Fig. 2.10b).
(c) *Anechoic:* Areas with no returning echoes, appearing as black (such as the fluid within vessels or cysts) (Fig. 2.10c).

Ultrasound Transducer Characteristics

Ultrasound transducers can be classified by their shape. The most used transducers for UGRA and pain procedures are linear array and curved array transducers.

Linear Array Transducer

These have a linear footprint (Fig. 2.11a). They are high-frequency transducers (8–12 MHz) and best reserved for imaging superficial structures (such as the brachial plexus). They provide a square or rectangular field of view (Fig. 2.11b).

Curved Array Transducers

These have a curved footprint (Fig. 2.12a). They are low-frequency transducers (1–5 MHz) and best reserved for imaging deeper structures (such as the sciatic nerve in the gluteal area or neuraxial structures). They provide a sectorial field of view (Fig. 2.12b).

Resolution

The resolution of an ultrasound machine is its ability to distinguish two close objects as separate. In simple terms, it provides clarity to the ultrasound image. Different types of resolution important for a regional anesthesiologist are:

(a) *Axial resolution* is the ultrasound machine's ability to separate two structures lying at different depths, parallel to the ultrasound wave's direction (Fig. 2.13a). The maximum axial resolution of a particular ultrasound

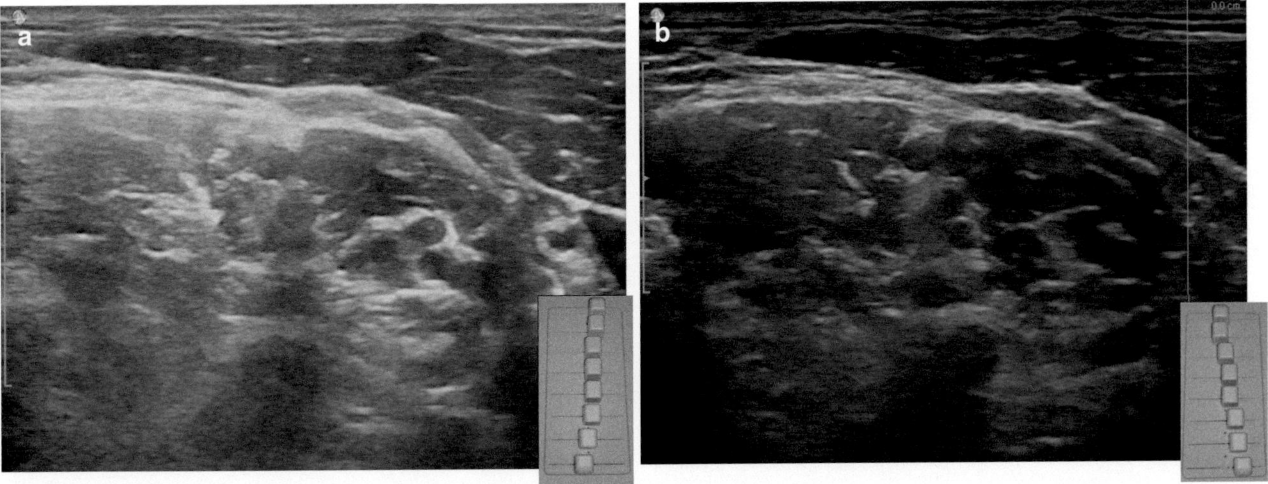

Fig. 2.9 Time gain compensation (**a**) not applied, (**b**) correctly applied. (Reproduced with permission from Dr. Herman Sehmbi)

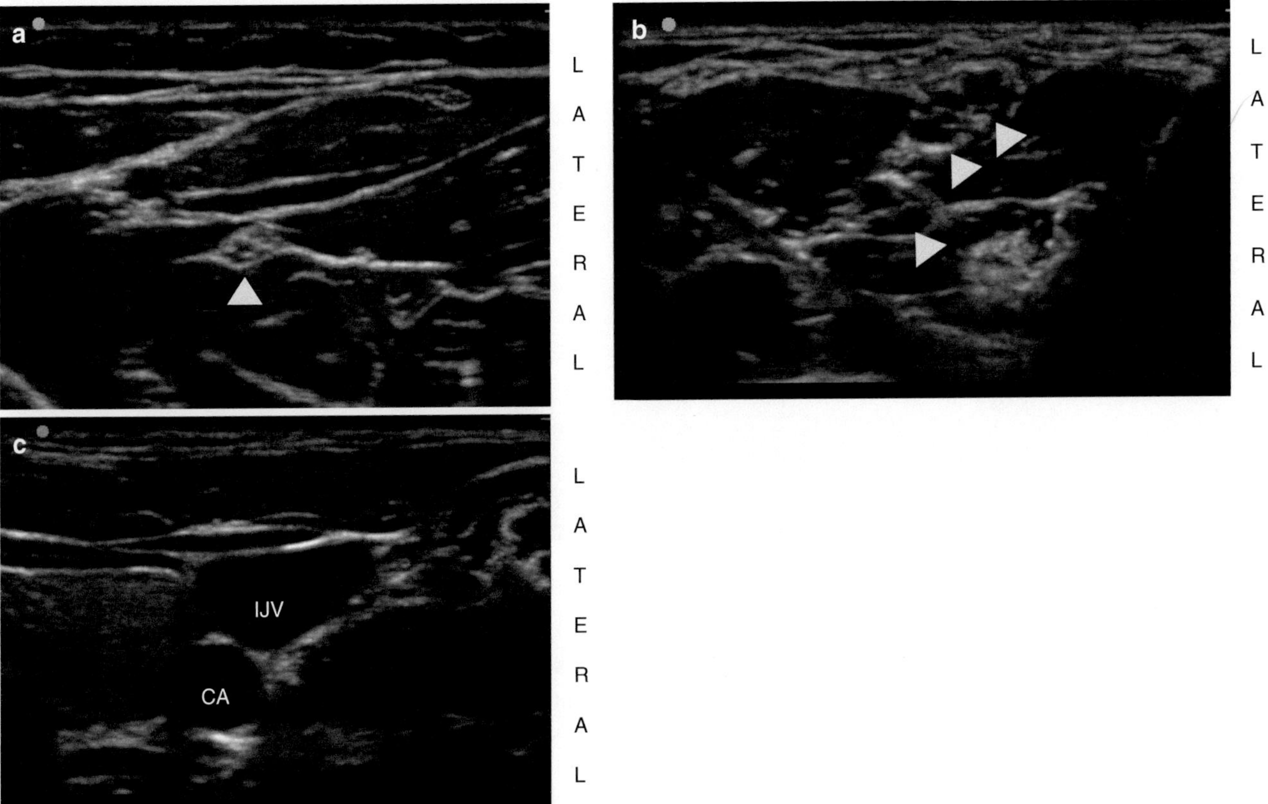

Fig. 2.10 Structures of different echogenicity. (**a**) Hyperechoic peripheral nerves (*yellow arrowhead* = median *n*). (**b**) Hypoechoic cervical nerve roots (*yellow arrowhead* = cervical nerve roots). (**c**) Anechoic vein and artery (*IJV* internal jugular vein and *CA* carotid artery in the neck). (Reproduced with permission from Dr. Herman Sehmbi)

wave is half of its pulse width. Structures that are closer to one another than that distance will be displayed as one. Thus high-frequency transducers (with a shorter pulse width) have a better axial resolution. However, they also have a higher attenuation, resulting in low depth penetration.

(b) *Lateral resolution* is the ultrasound machine's ability to differentiate two separate structures lying at the same depth, on a plane perpendicular to the ultrasound wave's direction (Fig. 2.13b). The lateral resolution of a given ultrasound wave is inversely related to the ultrasound beam's width. Therefore, high-frequency transducers

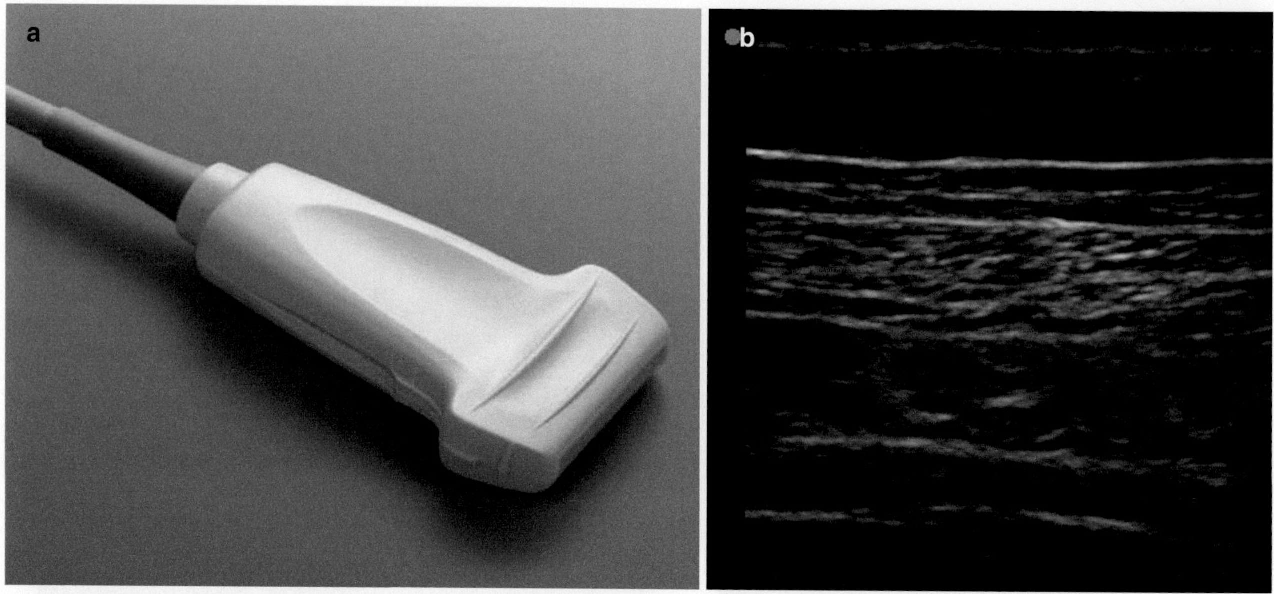

Fig. 2.11 (**a**) A linear array transducer. (**b**) Field of view of a linear transducer. (Reproduced with permission from Dr. Herman Sehmbi)

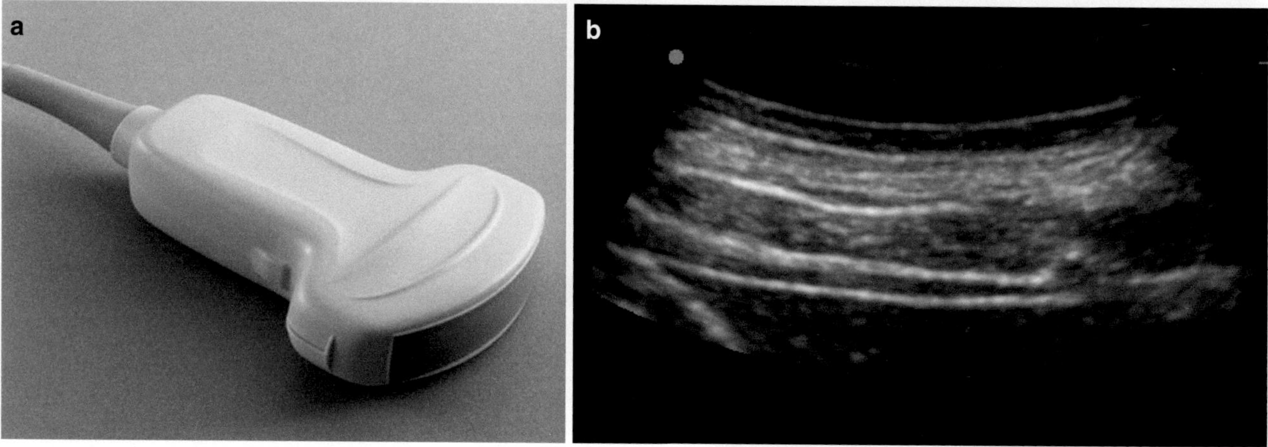

Fig. 2.12 (**a**) A curved array transducer. (**b**) Field of view of a curved array transducer. (Reproduced with permission from Dr. Herman Sehmbi)

(with a lower ultrasound width) also have better lateral resolution compared to lower frequency transducers.

(c) *Temporal resolution* is directly related to the frame rate of the ultrasound machine, and how quickly the ultrasound image can adapt to a moving transducer. Slowing needle manipulation and injection of local anesthetic can compensate for relatively low temporal resolutions, minimizing blur and improving image quality.

Image Optimization

The images generated by an ultrasound machine can be enhanced through appropriate preselection of specific parameters and by post-acquisition optimization techniques. The following steps can be considered to optimize an ultrasound image:

Transducer Selection

Linear transducers are best suited for most superficial nerve blocks (such as the brachial plexus block). In contrast, curvilinear transducers help perform blocks at deeper sites (such as sciatic blocks at the subgluteal region and neuraxial procedures). While smaller footprint transducers (e.g., 25 mm linear transducers) are better suited to pediatric patients and smaller adults, they also provide a narrow field of view (Fig. 2.14). Curvilinear transducers are also available in different footprint sizes.

Frequency

Most transducers are broadband transducers and allow adjustment of their frequency (5–15 MHz). Selecting a higher frequency provides superior lateral resolution at the expense of increased attenuation and lower depth penetration. Lowering the frequency of a given transducer allows

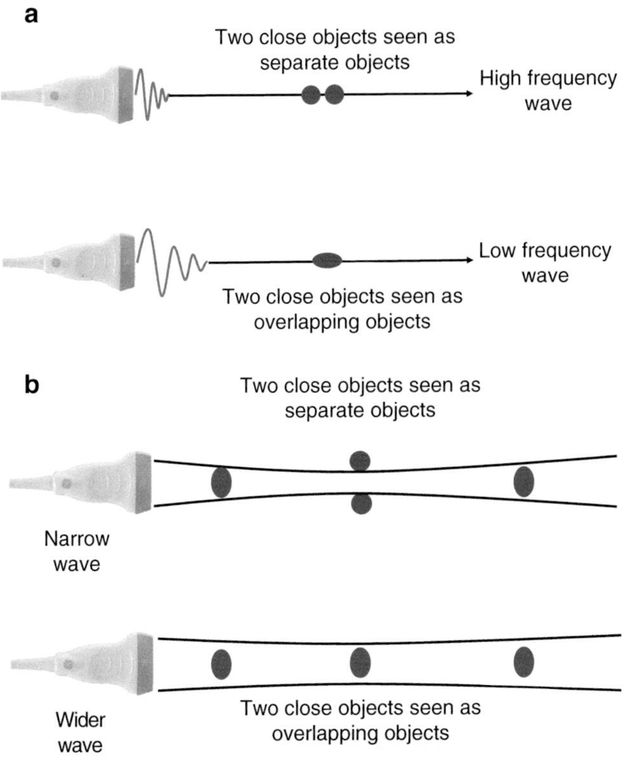

Fig. 2.13 (**a**) The effect of ultrasound frequency on axial resolution. (**b**) The effect of the width of the ultrasound beam on lateral resolution. (Reproduced with permission from Dr. Herman Sehmbi)

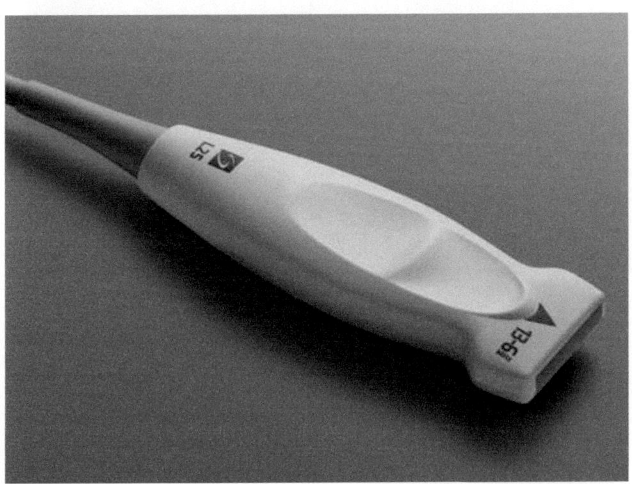

Fig. 2.14 Smaller footprint linear transducer. (Reproduced with permission from Dr. Herman Sehmbi)

better visualization of deeper structures at the cost of axial and lateral resolution (Fig. 2.15).

Default Pre-optimized Modes

Most ultrasound units provide preset modes that can be customized for the user for commonly encountered clinical settings. They represent the most common machine settings (depth, gain, focus, multi-beam, frequency range, frame rate) useful for a specific area.

Gain

The gain setting allows the operator to change the brightness of the image. This happens through amplification (increasing gain) or dampening (decreasing gain) of the returning signals rendering the image more hyperechoic or hypoechoic, respectively. However, it also increases the background noise, resulting in artifacts (Fig. 2.16a–c).

Time Gain Compensation (TGC)

While the signals returning from a superficial target undergo less attenuation, those returning from deeper structures undergo greater attenuation (Fig. 2.17). Therefore, an un-optimized image is generally brighter (representing superficial tissues) at the top than at the bottom (representing deeper tissues). "Time gain compensation" allows for selective amplification of signals at various depths. Thus, increasing the optimization of gain with increasing depth allows for a properly optimized image. Some machines have individual controls for TGC, while others allow adjustment of far/near/overall gain.

Depth

For optimal depth selection, it is usually recommended that the target structure should be placed around the center, or slightly deeper than the center of the screen (Fig. 2.18a). Choosing a greater depth than needed may reduce the target size (Fig. 2.18b), while too shallow a depth may obscure the target altogether (Fig. 2.18c). Optimal depth also optimizes temporal resolution.

Focus

The ultrasound beams do not run exactly parallel to one another. Their trajectory, rather, has an hourglass shape. The narrowest part of this hourglass is where the ultrasound beams have their best lateral resolution. The "focus" of the image can be changed up or down to center this area of best lateral resolution (focal zone) where it is most needed, at the target structure/s. In most ultrasound units, both the number of areas of focus and their depth can be optimized (Fig. 2.19).

Color-Flow Doppler

The "Doppler effect" in medical ultrasound allows for identification and quantification (velocity and direction) of blood flow. The blood cells moving towards the transducer create returning waves of higher frequency while those moving away return lower frequency waves. This is represented as a red (moving towards the transducer) or blue (moving away from the transducer) color spectrum (Fig. 2.20a, b). Color-flow Doppler mode is recommended to identify vascular structures within the intended needle trajectory.

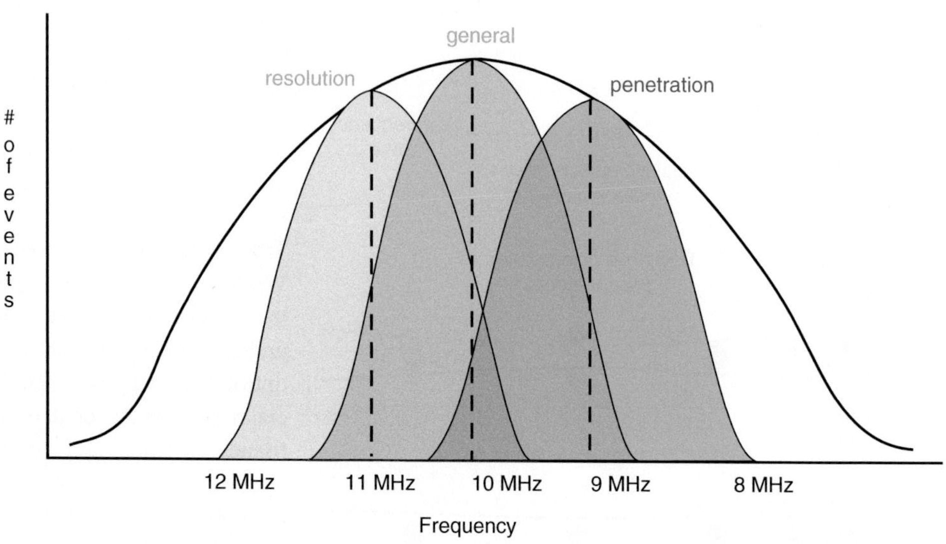

Fig. 2.15 Linear broadband transducers generate higher frequencies. (Reproduced with permission from www.usra.ca)

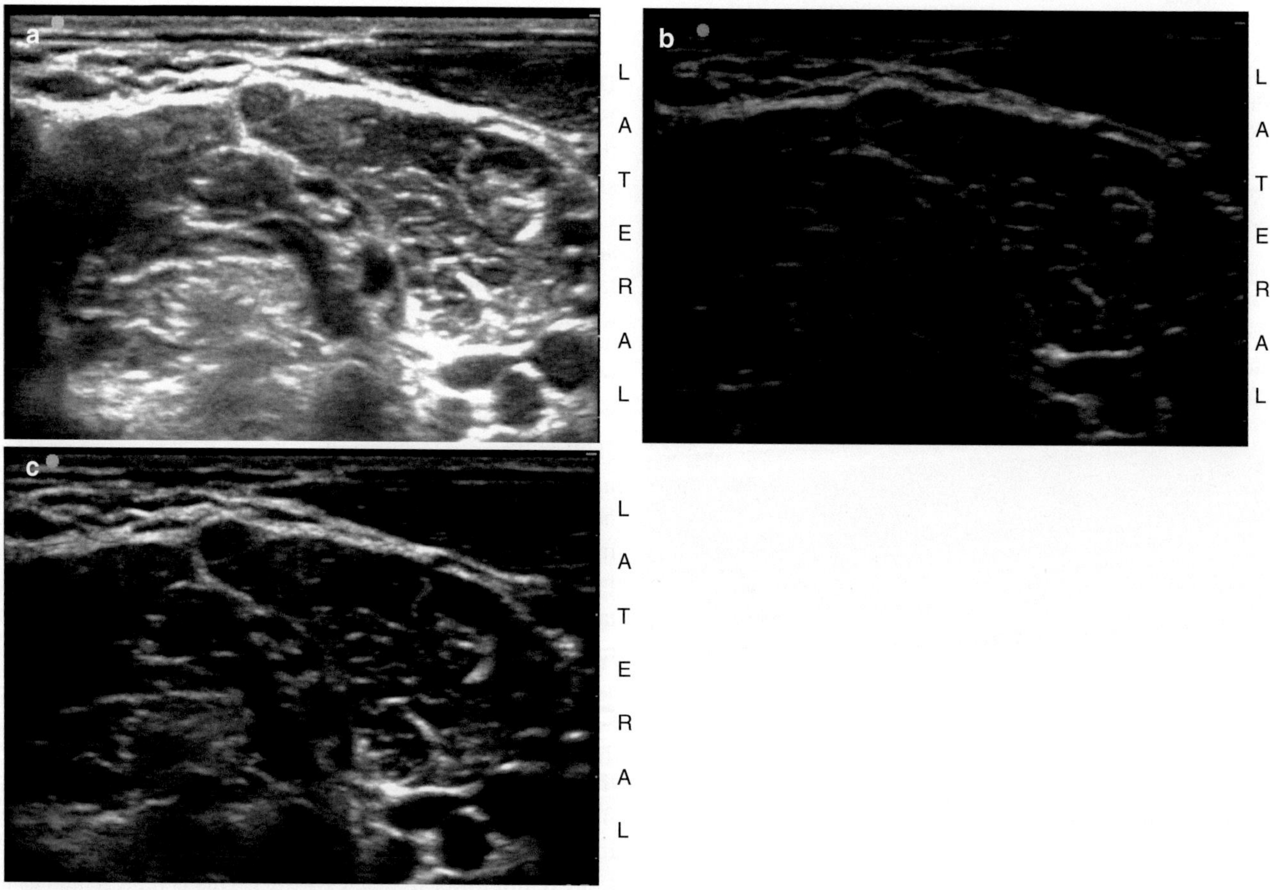

Fig. 2.16 Effects of too high (**a**), too low (**b**), and optimal gain (**c**) settings on the view at interscalene brachial plexus (*SA* subclavian artery, *yellow arrowhead* brachial plexus). (Reproduced with permission from Dr. Herman Sehmbi)

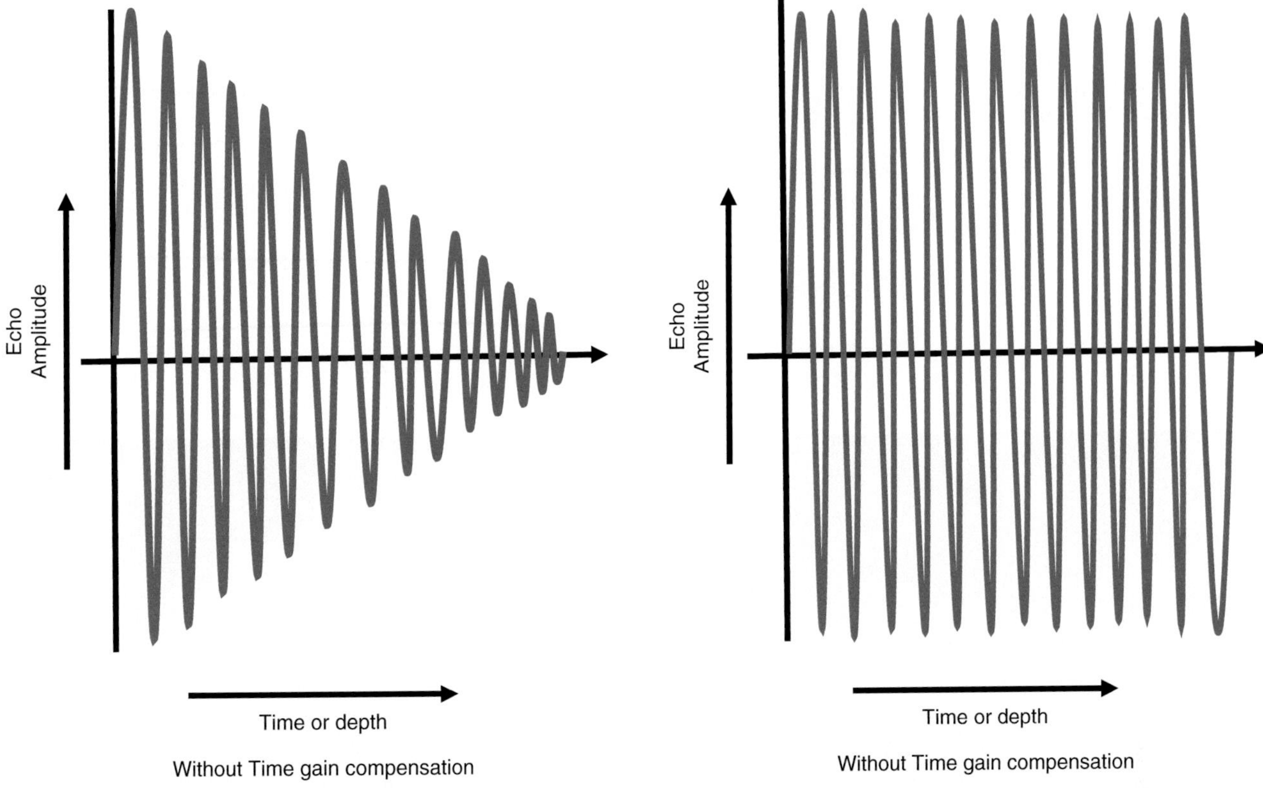

Fig. 2.17 Time gain compensation. (Reproduced with permission from Dr. Herman Sehmbi)

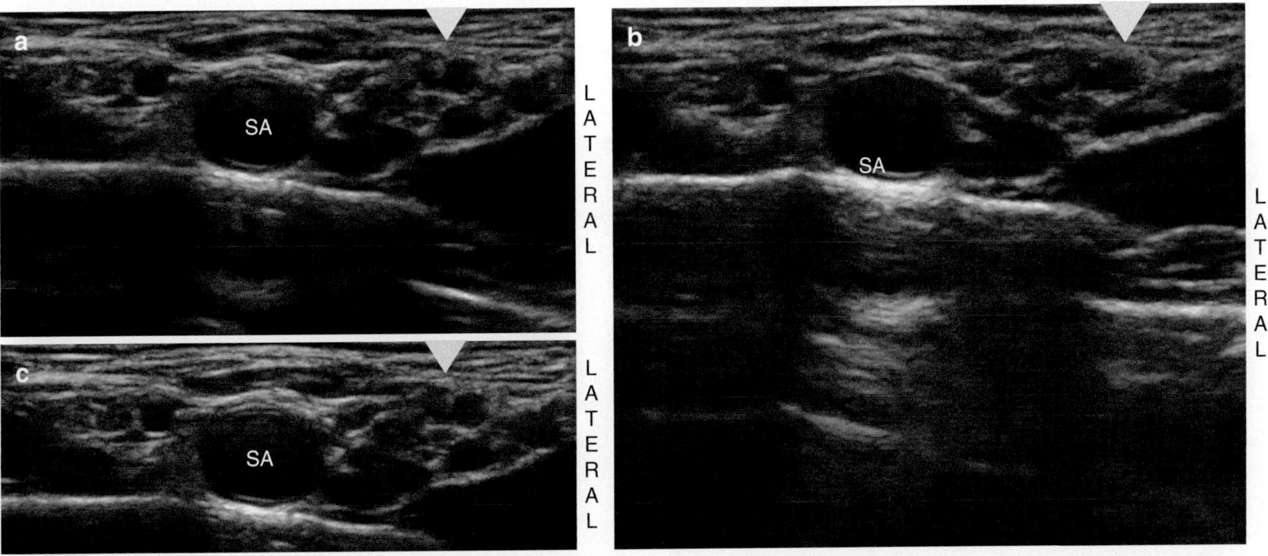

Fig. 2.18 Depth setting in the supraclavicular block (**a**) optimal, (**b**) too deep, and (**c**) too shallow. (Reproduced with permission from Dr. Herman Sehmbi)

Pulse-Wave Doppler

This mode provides flow data from a small preselected area along the ultrasound beam. The displayed pulse wave information is displayed along with generated sound allowing differentiation of arterial from venous pulsation (Fig. 2.21).

Other Optimization Modes

1. *Compound imaging*: This involves capturing multiple images of the tissue under examination, using ultrasound beams that travel in different angles. The combined resulting image has better resolution and reduced artifacts.

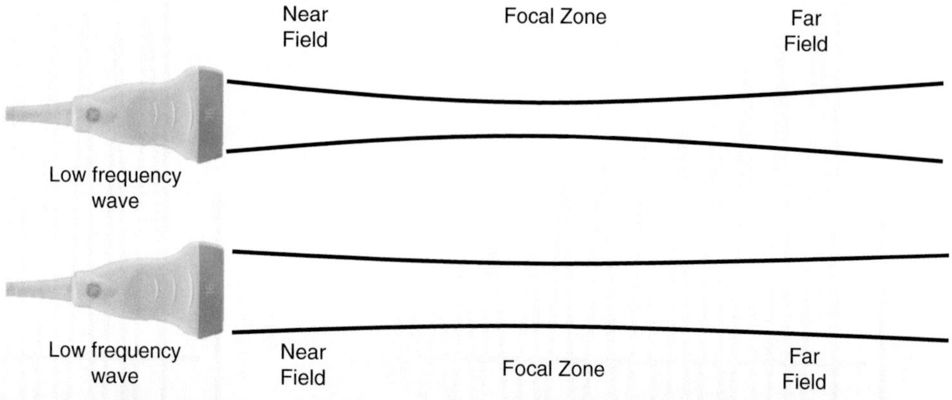

Near
Field
Focal Zone
Far
Field
Low frequency
wave
Low frequency
wave
Near
Field
Focal Zone
Far
Field

Fig. 2.19 Focal zones and the focal length of an ultrasound beam. (Reproduced with permission from Dr. Herman Sehmbi)

a
LATERAL
b
LATERAL

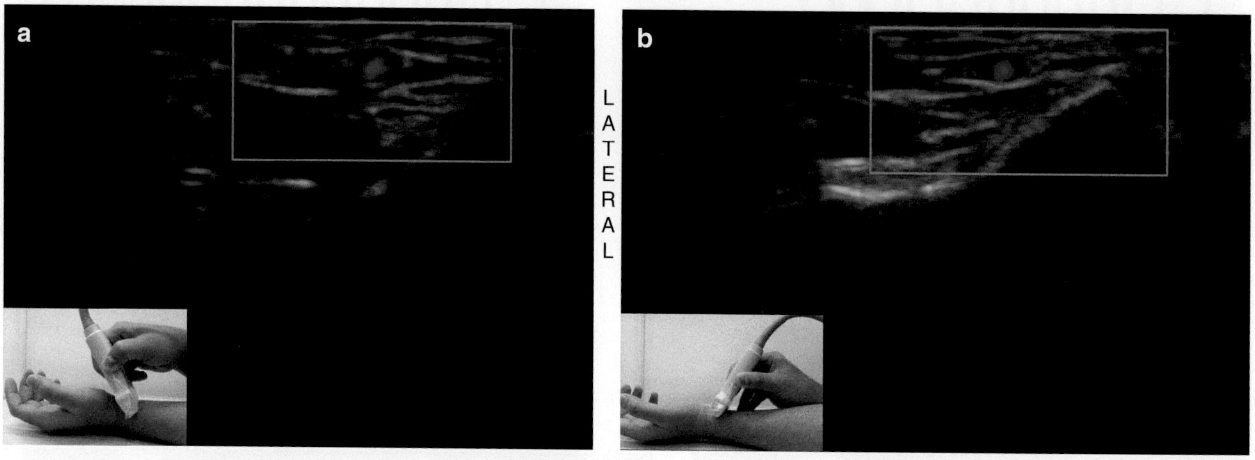

Fig. 2.20 Use of color-flow Doppler for detection of blood flow in radial artery: (**a**) *Red*—towards the transducer; (**b**) *Blue*—away from the transducer. (Reproduced with permission from Dr. Herman Sehmbi)

a
2.7
cm/s
-20
LATERAL
b
2.7
cm/s
-20
LATERAL

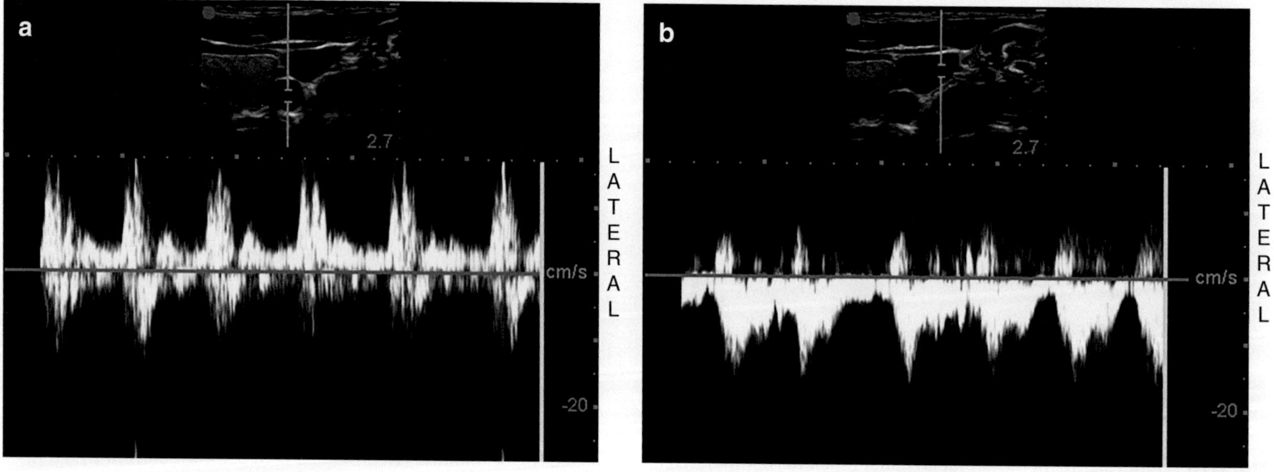

Fig. 2.21 Pulse-wave Doppler shows an arterial (**a**) and a venous waveform (**b**) in the femoral artery and vein, respectively. (Reproduced with permission from Dr. Herman Sehmbi)

2. *Tissue Harmonic imaging*: Echoes are reflected by the examined tissue not only at the original frequency but also at various multiples of the original frequency. Tissue harmonic imaging utilizes these harmonic multiples producing better imaging via reduced scatter and artifacts. However, this may negatively impact needle visibility.

Artifacts

An artifact is an image or a part of an image that does not correspond to any given anatomic structure but is rather the result of the physical properties underlying ultrasound beam generation and capturing. Artifacts are generated because the imaging system makes several *assumptions* about ultrasound propagation in tissue, including assuming a fixed speed of ultrasound wave in tissues, a straight path for the beam's axis, a constant degree of attenuation, and that the pulse returns directly to the transducer. Whenever there is a significant deviation from these assumptions, visible image artifacts are likely to occur.

These artifacts can be classified into *acoustic, anatomic, optical illusions, and electrical noise artifacts*. For a regional anesthesiologist or pain specialist, acoustic and anatomic artifacts are most important. Some of these artifacts are considered below.

Over-Gain and Under-Gain Artifact

Inappropriately low-gain settings can result in a "missing structure" artifact, while a very high gain can obscure existing structures. A correctly applied "time gain compensation" allows appropriate image production and attenuation reduction (Figs. 2.16a–c and 2.17).

Acoustic Shadowing

This occurs when a structure with a high attenuation coefficient lies above a structure with a lower attenuation coefficient. This causes the underlying structure to appear far less echogenic. For example, the tip of a needle can be obscured by an overlying transverse process while performing a paravertebral block.

Posterior Acoustic Enhancement Artifact

This occurs when the ultrasound waves returning from a structure behind a weak attenuator (such as a fluid-containing organ) result in stronger echoes. The reason for this artifact is that the ultrasound unit assumes that attenuation of the ultrasound wave occurs equally across the width of the image for any given depth. Because fluid-filled structures (such as vessels and cysts) are very good conductors of ultrasound waves with little attenuation, the echogenicity of the structures that lie posterior to them will be overcompensated by the ultrasound unit, generating a hyperechoic image (Fig. 2.22).

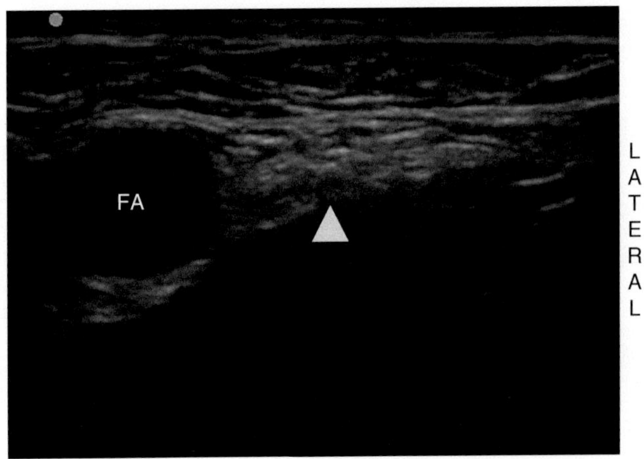

Fig. 2.22 Posterior acoustic enhancement deep to the femoral artery (FA) could be mistaken for the femoral nerve (*yellow arrowhead*), which lies lateral to the artery. (Reproduced with permission from Dr. Herman Sehmbi)

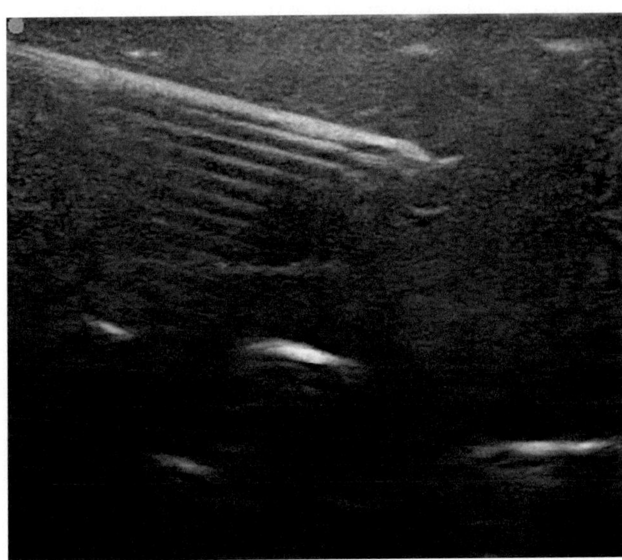

Fig. 2.23 Reverberation artifact with a Tuohy needle. (Reproduced with permission from Dr. Herman Sehmbi)

Lateral Resolution Artifact

Lateral resolution refers to the system's ability to differentiate between two objects lying side by side at the same depth (on a plane perpendicular to the incident beam's direction). Lateral resolution is greatest at the focal zone of the ultrasound beams, where individual ultrasound beams are closest to one another. With beams of lower frequency, two objects that are very close together may appear as one. Choosing an appropriate transducer and frequency will help eliminate this artifact.

Reverberation Artifact

Reverberation occurs when ultrasound contacts a strong specular reflector (such as a needle or the surface of pleura). For a needle, a part of the ultrasound wave is reflected, creating an initial image. The remaining part passes through the shaft to be reflected by the back surface. As this continues, the returning echoes' strength continually decreases, while the time taken to return to the transducer is prolonged. This results in an image of multiple needles of decreasing brightness, a "reverberation artifact" (Fig. 2.23).

Anisotropy

Anisotropy refers to the different appearance of a single structure depending on the angle of the incident ultrasound beams. This occurs because reflection is maximum when the transducer, and the incident waves, is perpendicular to the

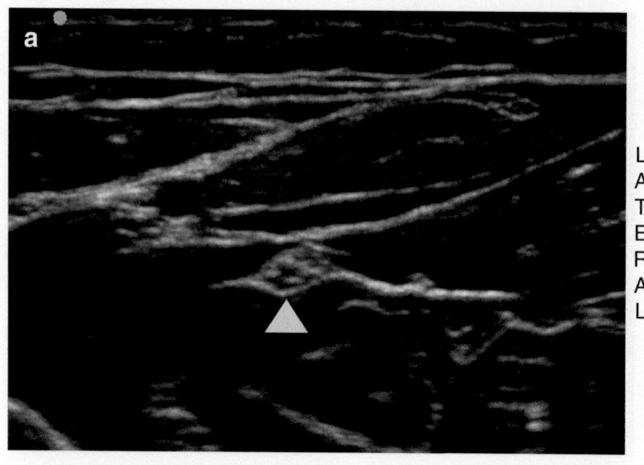

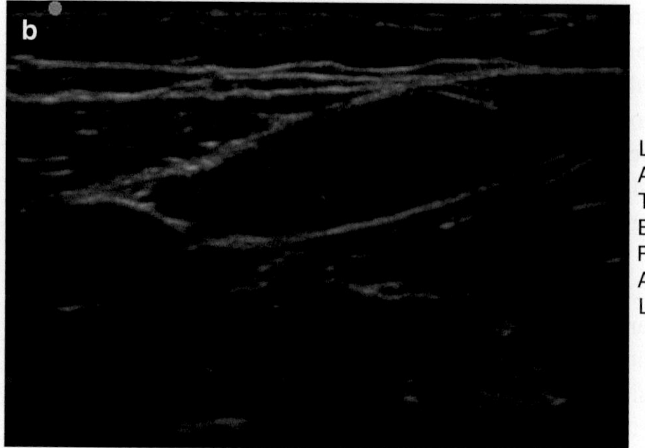

Fig. 2.24 (**a**) Median nerve (*yellow arrowhead*) nerve when the transducer is perpendicular to the nerve. (**b**) Disappearance of the nerve on tilting the transducer. (Reproduced with permission from Dr. Herman Sehmbi)

structure under examination. Any change in this incidence angle dramatically reduces the returning echo, causing the structure to "disappear" out of the image (Fig. 2.24a, b). Manipulation of the transducer (to direct the incident beam perpendicular to the structure of interest) and beam-steering can help address anisotropy.

In conclusion, having a high degree of suspicion, a good knowledge of anatomy and basic ultrasound physics, rotating the transducer from a transverse to a longitudinal view (or vice versa), using appropriate gain, using tissue compression, and observing the structure under examination from another window are a few ways to identify and interpret commonly occurring artifacts correctly.

Practical Approach to Scanning

Procedural Ergonomics

Ergonomics is the study (or science) of the interaction between humans and their working environment. Recent years have witnessed an increasing application of optimal procedural ergonomics in regional anesthesia and pain practice to improve outcomes. Poor ergonomics may not only lead to suboptimal performance of a procedure but may contribute to work-related musculoskeletal discomfort. A sound application of the principles of ergonomics to regional anesthesia include the consideration of the following factors:

Positioning and Care of the Patient

The patient must be placed in a comfortable position for the block. This position may vary with the type of block being performed; for example, the patient may need a supine position for an upper limb block, a prone position for a popliteal block, and a sitting position for a spinal anesthetic. Additionally, the position of the limb may be adjusted to assist the procedure. For example, performing an interscalene block may need a semi-recumbent positioning of the patient with the face turned towards the contralateral side. Similarly, placing a cushion under the lower leg may assist in performing an ankle block.

Positioning of the Physician

Maintaining a good position in reference to the patient helps ensure operator comfort and allows optimal block performance (Fig. 2.25). This includes the following:

(a) Adjusting the *height* of the patient bed to an appropriate level for the operator, ideally working with the elbows flexed at 90°.
(b) Assuming a *good posture* by choosing to stand or sit down (on a chair).
(c) Performing the block from the side being blocked to *avoid reaching over* the patient.

Positioning the Equipment

The ultrasound machine must be placed such that the operator, the target site, and the screen of the ultrasound machine are in a *straight alignment*. Often this is achieved by placing the ultrasound machine on the opposite side to the one that the operator assumes. This allows for a smooth, coordinated scanning and needling, without the need for excessive movements on the operator's part.

Also, the ultrasound machine must be placed sufficiently close to the operator. It can be reached by the operator or

Body Ergonomics

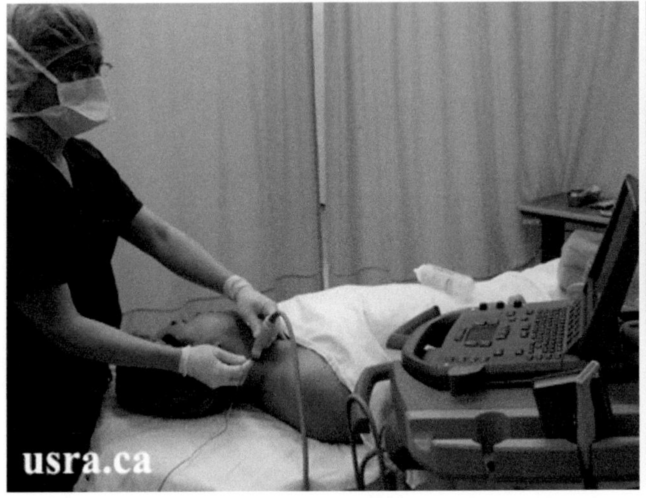

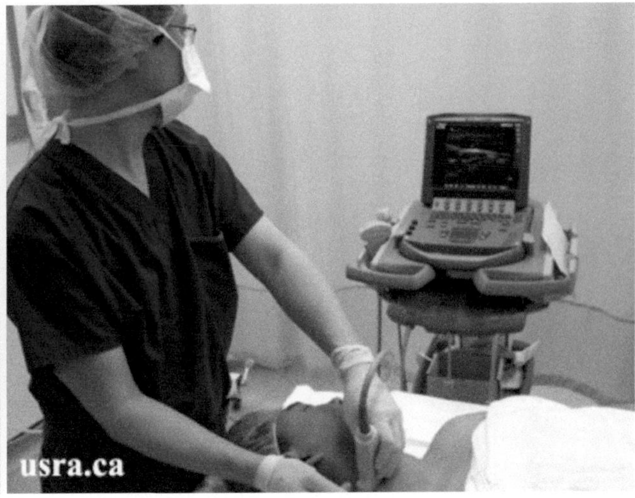

Fig. 2.25 The optimal position of the operator, equipment, and the assistant during an upper limb block. (Reproduced with permission from www.usra.ca)

their assistant if any manipulation of the settings is required. The ultrasound machine must have brake pedals locked to avoid its movement relative to the operator. The screen of the monitoring equipment must be turned to face the operator during the block to allow prompt recognition of any significant change of vital signs.

Position of the Assistant

An assistant may be needed both to operate the ultrasound machine and inject the local anesthetic solution. This may be achieved by standing opposite to the operator and near the ultrasound machine.

Scanning Methodology

Anatomical Planes

While scanning, it is common to refer to the "anatomical plane" of the scan. These include the axial (or transverse) plane, the sagittal plane, and the coronal plane. They are all perpendicular to one another (Fig. 2.26).

(a) The *axial (or transverse) plane* is an imaginary horizontal plane that divides the body into superior and inferior parts.
(b) A *sagittal plane* is an imaginary vertical plane from anterior to posterior that divides the body into left and right halves.
(c) A *coronal plane* is a vertical plane running from right to left that divides the body into ventral and dorsal sections.

Besides, a body part may be scanned obliquely (e.g., "parasagittal oblique" or "transverse oblique" planes).

Transducer Orientation

All ultrasound transducers have an *orientation marker* (Fig. 2.27a). By convention, the orientation marker is placed on the patient's right in a transverse orientation, and cephalad in a longitudinal orientation. The marker is usually placed on the left top corner of the screen on the ultrasound machine (Fig. 2.27b) but can be placed at any corner upon the operator's choice. The orientation of the transducer can be correctly identified by touching one side of the transducer after the gel has been applied and observing the screen for movement. Another way to identify the correct orientation is to move the transducer to one side while scanning and observing the direction of movement of anatomical structures on the screen.

Axis of Scanning

Nerves and vessels may be scanned along their transverse axis, obtaining a cross-sectional view of the structure (Fig. 2.28a) or along their longitudinal axis (Fig. 2.28b). The scans so obtained are commonly referred to as a "transverse scan" and a "longitudinal scan." Transverse scans are commonly used for many ultrasound-guided peripheral nerve blocks, while longitudinal scans are more often used to confirm perineural or intravascular catheter placements.

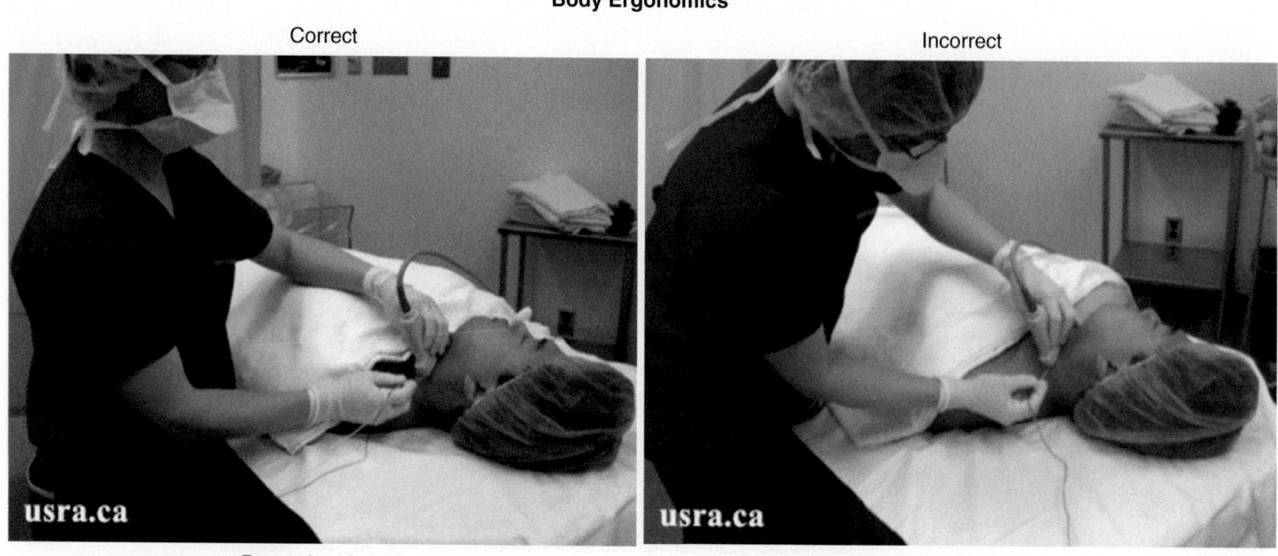

Fig. 2.26 The standard anatomical planes of the body. (Reproduced with permission from www.usra.ca)

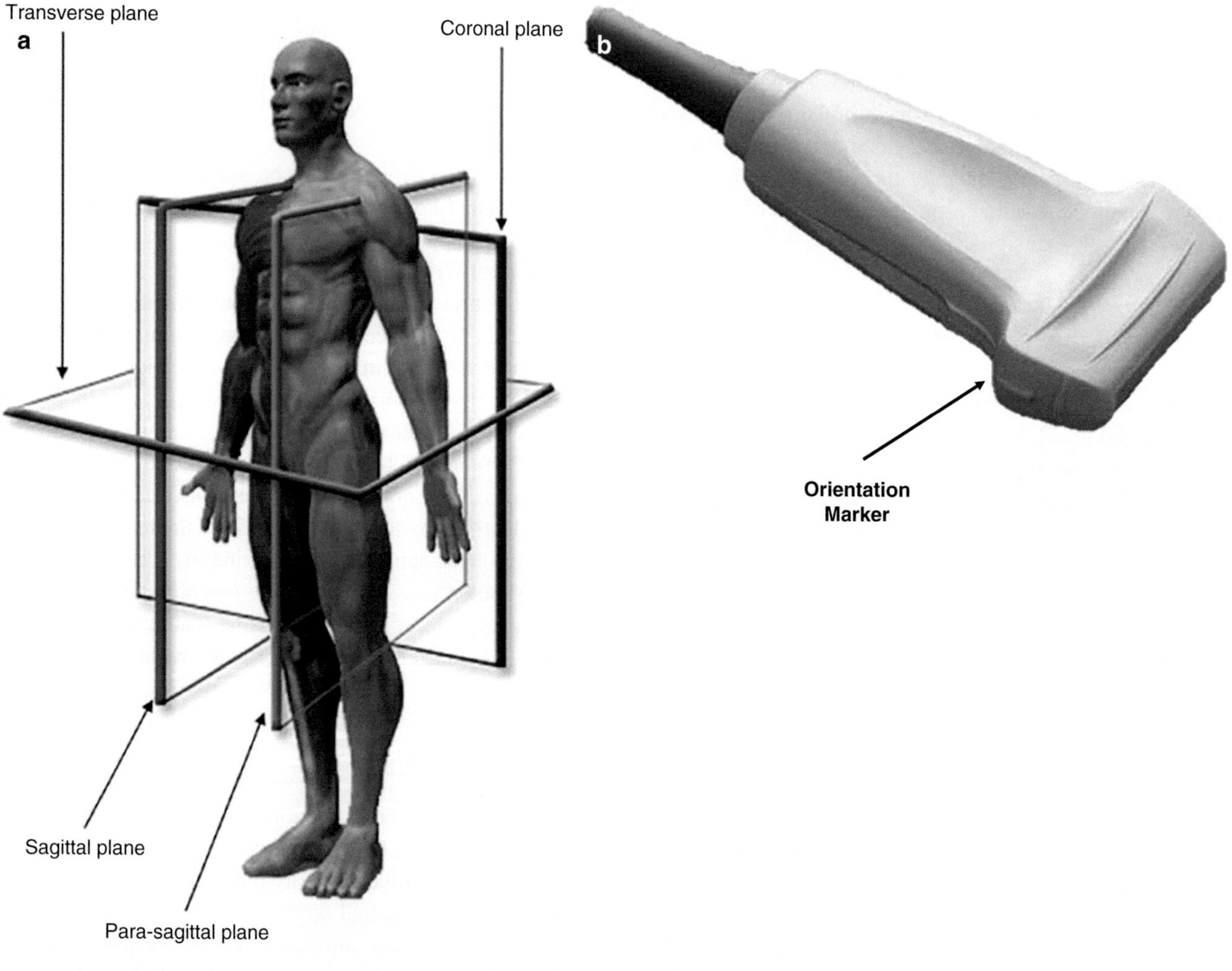

Fig. 2.27 (**a**) Orientation marker on a linear transducer. (**b**) Orientation marker on the top left corner of the ultrasound screen. (Reproduced with permission from Dr. Herman Sehmbi)

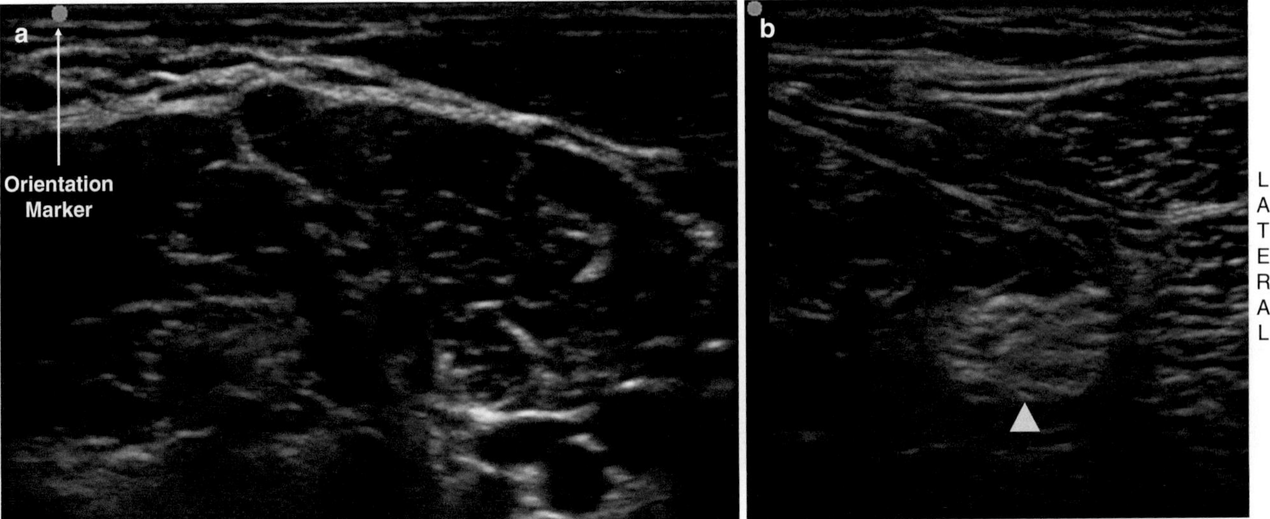

Fig. 2.28 (**a**) Transverse scanning of sciatic nerve at the popliteal fossa. (**b**) Longitudinal scanning of sciatic nerve at the popliteal fossa. (Reproduced with permission from Dr. Herman Sehmbi)

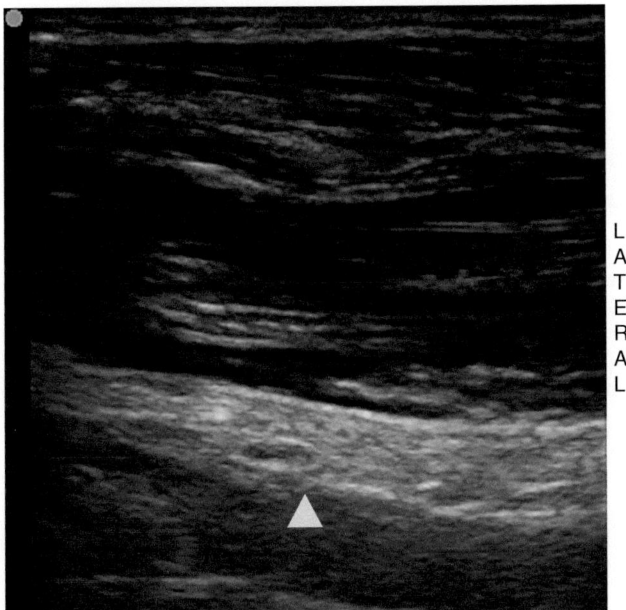

Fig. 2.29 Holding the transducer linear transducer. (Reproduced with permission from Dr. Herman Sehmbi)

Handling the Transducer

(a) *Holding the transducer.*

A linear transducer is usually held between the thumb and the fingers, with the heel of the palm or ulnar aspect of the hand placed on the patient providing stability while scanning (Fig. 2.29). A curvilinear transducer may be held by wrapping fingers around it, supported by the scanning hand's ulnar aspect.

(b) *Transducer movements.*

Obtaining the right image of a structure under examination requires a systemic scanning approach, involving both major and minor movements. These include pressure, alignment, rotation, and tilt (commonly called the PART maneuver).

- *Pressure:* Applying adequate pressure while scanning improves the image quality by shortening the distance between the transducer and the target (Fig. 2.30a). Additionally, it may allow compressing a vein (helping in its identification). One-sided pressure may also allow directing the ultrasound waves at a desired angle. However, excessive pressure may also cause underestimation of the target depth.
- *Alignment (or sliding):* This allows the target structure to be centralized in the image as this provides the best resolution (Fig. 2.30b). Sliding along the long axis also allows us to follow the structure of interest proximally or distally (*scout scan*).
- *Rotation:* Rotating the transducer clockwise or counterclockwise helps identify a correct transverse plane (Fig. 2.30c). Additionally, rotating the transducer from a transverse plane to a longitudinal plane allows a better examination of the target and the best needle trajectory.
- *Tilt:* Tilting the transducer along its vertical axis allows an examination of the target (along its long axis) without the need for sliding the transducer proximally or distally (Fig. 2.30d). Tilting is very useful to track the needle tip.

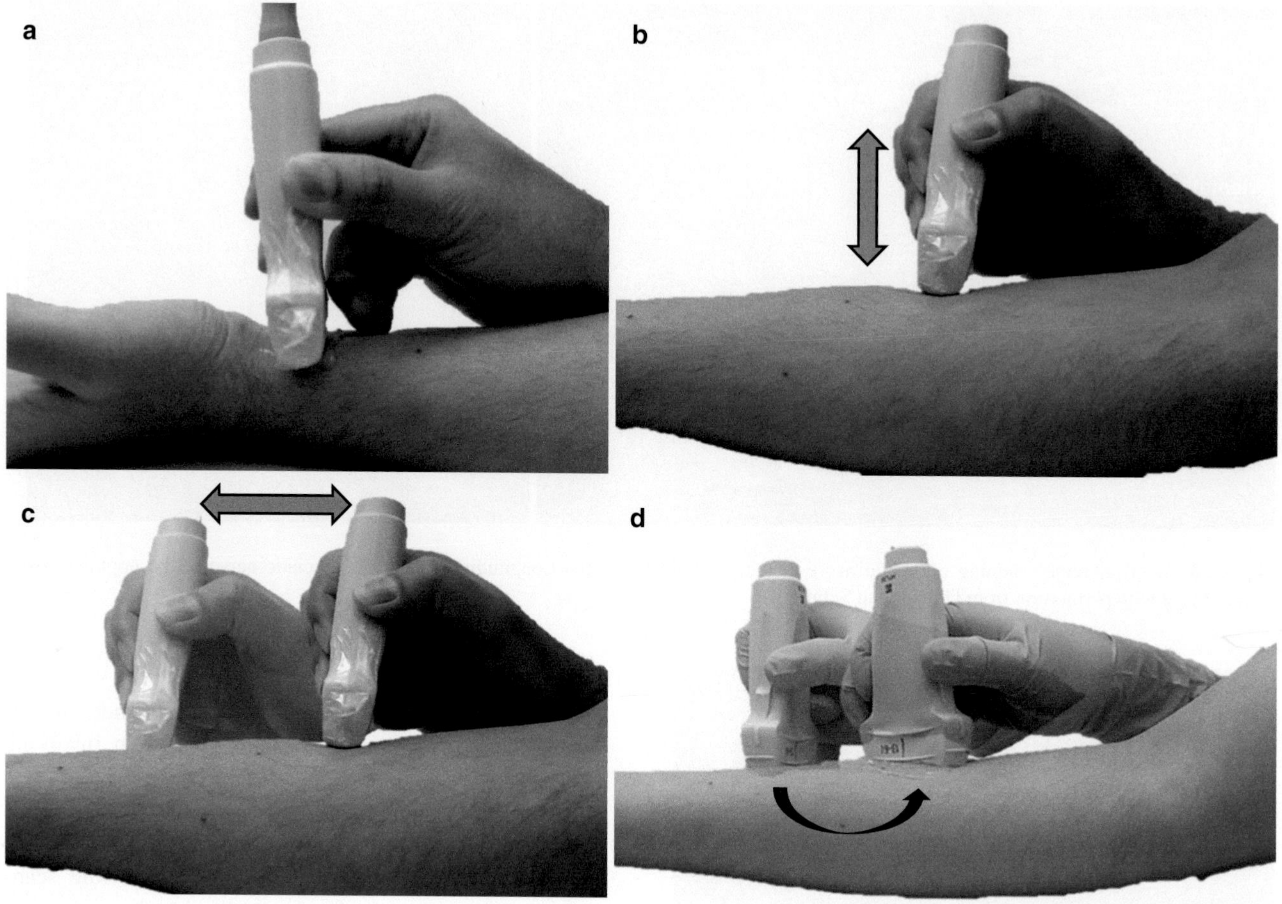

Fig. 2.30 Transducer movements (PART): (**a**) pressure, (**b**) alignment, (**c**) rotation, (**d**) tilt. (Reproduced with permission from Dr. Herman Sehmbi)

Identifying Signposts

Structures that help orient an operator to the underlying anatomy are sometimes referred to as *signposts*. They also provide a starting point for a systematic scan of the target area. For example, the subclavian artery is a vital signpost while scanning for the brachial plexus in the supraclavicular region.

Needling Techniques

Needle Insertion Technique

The "in-plane" and "out-of-plane" needle approaches are most used:

(a) *In-plane needle insertion*: The needle is advanced in the ultrasound beam plane to visualize the needle from the shaft to its tip (Fig. 2.31a). A shallower trajectory will result in better visibility.

(b) *Out-of-plane needle insertion*: here, the needle trajectory is perpendicular to the ultrasound transducer such that the needle tip or its shaft is seen as a hyperechoic dot on the screen (Fig. 2.31b). This approach offers a shorter route to the target structure (nerve or vessel), but it can prove challenging to follow the exact needle tip position in real time, especially for novice users.

In combination with the transverse (short) axis or the longitudinal (long) axis, the following combinations are possible:

(a) Short-axis in-plane needle insertion.
(b) Short-axis out-of-plane needle insertion.
(c) Long-axis in-plane needle insertion.
(d) Long-axis out-of-plane needle insertion.

Short-axis in-plane needling and short-axis out-of-plane needling are commonly used in regional anesthesia. Short-

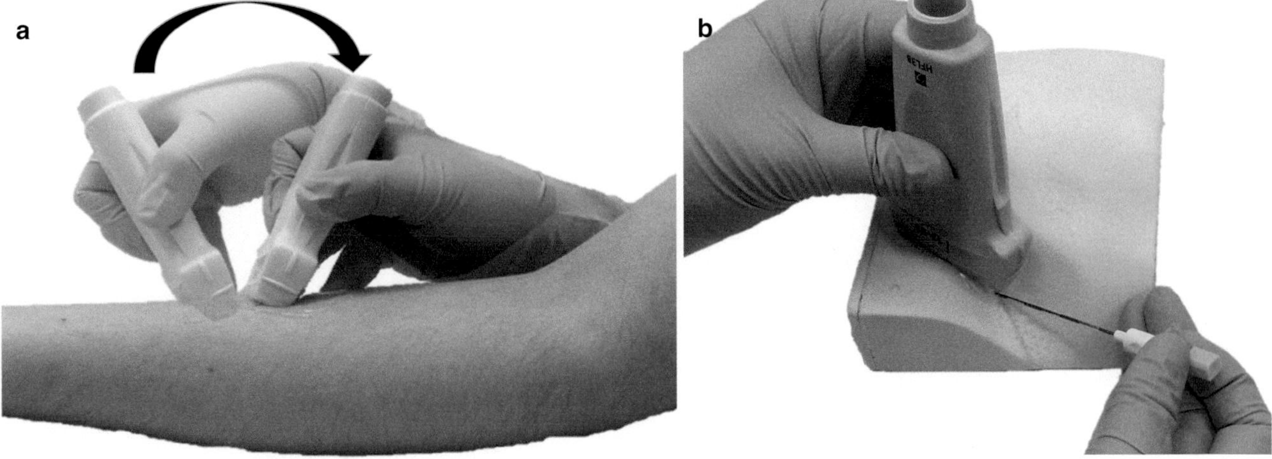

Fig. 2.31 Needling techniques. (**a**) In-plane needle insertion. (**b**) Out-of-plane needle insertion. (Reproduced with permission from Dr. Herman Sehmbi)

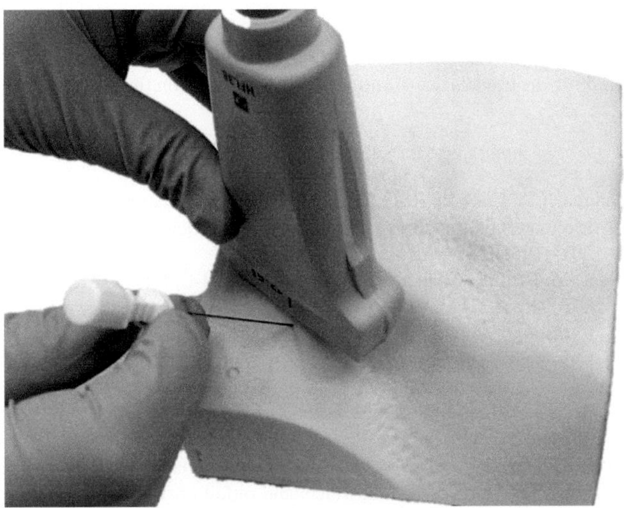

Fig. 2.32 In-plane needle advancement. (Reproduced with permission from Dr. Herman Sehmbi)

axis out-of-plane needling is beneficial while placing perineural catheters. There is no evidence to suggest that one method is better than the other, and it may be prudent to follow the most familiar method.

Needle Advancement

Correct needle advancement techniques allow tracking of needle tip from the point of insertion to the target structure.

(a) *In-plane needling:* Following the needle is easier in in-plane needling. The needle is inserted initially at a shallow angle to allow visualization (Fig. 2.32, point A). It is then redirected deeper towards the target structures, keeping the advancing needle in view always (Fig. 2.32, point B). If the needle is directed slightly obliquely, only a part of it may be visualized. Using *PART maneuver* for transducer manipulation, one can then attempt to visualize the entire needle.

(b) *Out-of-plane needling:* This is more challenging and can be achieved using two methods:

- *Sliding the transducer*: After inserting the needle in an anticipated trajectory, the transducer is first brought closer to the needle until the needle tip is a hyperechoic dot on the screen (Fig. 2.33a, plane A). Then the transducer is moved away from the needle, followed by advancement of the needle till its tip reappears on the screen (Fig. 2.33a, plane B). Using such sliding motions of the transducer, the needle tip can be followed and guided to the target structure.
- *Tilting the transducer*: Here the transducer is kept stationary. The needle is inserted out-of-plane in an anticipated trajectory. The transducer is tilted towards the needle to visualize its tip on the screen (Fig. 2.33b, plane A). Next, the transducer is tilted away from the needle such that the needle tip disappears. The needle is advanced until the tip reappears (Fig. 2.33b, plane B). This motion is repeated until the needle tip approaches the target structure (Fig. 2.33b, plane C). This method may cause difficulty if the underlying structure is quite anisotropic (as a minor tilt may result in a poor image of the structure of interest).

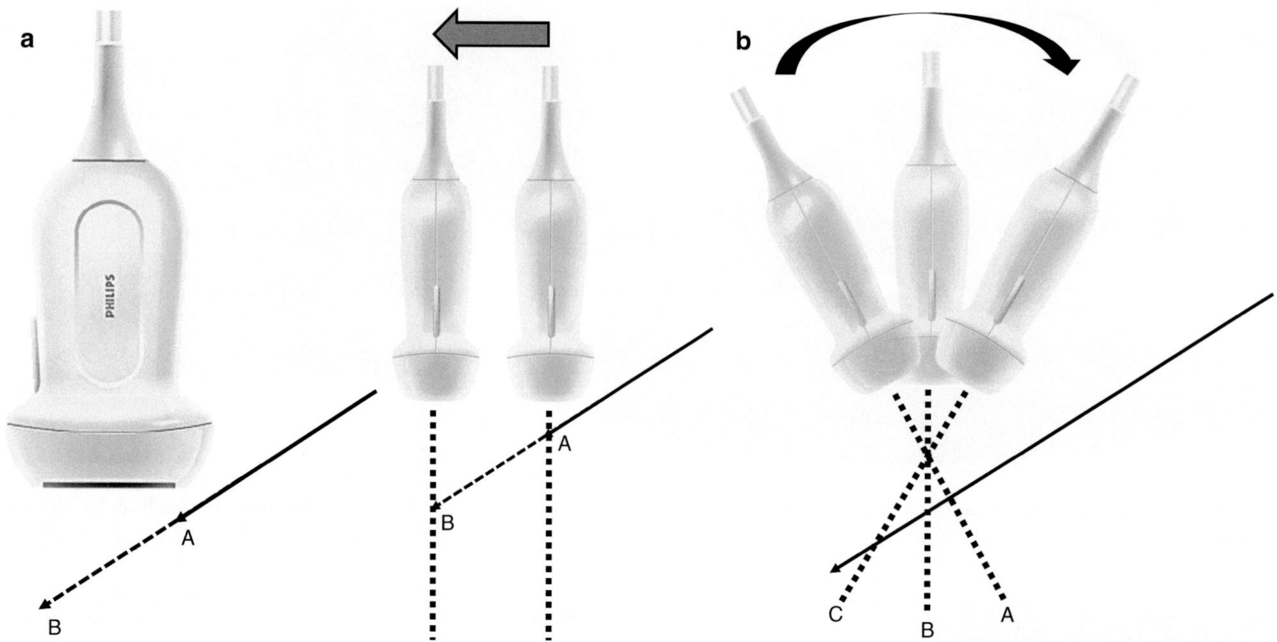

Fig. 2.33 Out-of-plane needle advancement. (**a**) Sliding the transducer. (**b**) Tilting the transducer. (Reproduced with permission from Dr. Herman Sehmbi)

Suggested Reading

Antonakakis JG, Sites B. The 5 most common ultrasound artifacts encountered during ultrasound-guided regional anesthesia. Int Anesthesiol Clin. 2011;49(4):52–66.

Blaivas M, DeBehnke D, Sierzenski PR, Phelan MB. Tissue harmonic imaging improves organ visualization in trauma ultrasound when compared with standard ultrasound mode. Acad Emerg Med. 2002;9(1):48–53.

Brull R, Macfarlane AJR, Tse CCH. Practical knobology for ultrasound-guided regional anesthesia. Reg Anesth Pain Med. 2010;35(2 Suppl):S68–73.

Chin KJ, Perlas A, Chan VWS, Brull R. Needle visualization in ultrasound-guided regional anesthesia: challenges and solutions. Reg Anesth Pain Med. 2008;33(6):532–44.

Chin KJ, Ramlogan R, Arzola C, Singh M, Chan V. The utility of ultrasound imaging in predicting ease of performance of spinal anesthesia in an orthopedic patient population. Reg Anesth Pain Med. 2013;38(1):34–8.

Guo S, Schwab A, McLeod G, Corner G, Cochran S, Eisma R, Soames R. Echogenic regional anaesthesia needles: a comparison study in thiel cadavers. Ultrasound Med Biol. 2012;38(4):702–7.

Ihnatsenka B, Boezaart AP. Ultrasound: basic understanding and learning the language. Int J Shoulder Surg. 2010;4(3):55–62.

Lancée CT, Souquet J, Ohigashi H, Bom N. Transducers in medical ultrasound: part one. ferro-electric ceramics versus polymer piezoelectric materials. Ultrasonics. 1985;23(3):138–42.

Manbachi A, Cobbold RSC. Development and application of piezoelectric materials for ultrasound generation and detection. Ultrasound. 2011;19(4):187–96.

Neal JM, Brull R, Chan VWS, Grant SA, Horn J-L, Liu SS, McCartney CJL, et al. The ASRA evidence-based medicine assessment of ultrasound-guided regional anesthesia and pain medicine: executive summary. Reg Anesth Pain Med. 2010;35(2 Suppl):S1–9.

Reusz G, Sarkany P, Gal J, Csomos A. Needle-related ultrasound artifacts and their importance in anaesthetic practice. Br J Anaesth. 2014;112(5):794–802.

Sites BD, Brull R, Chan VWS, Spence BC, Gallagher J, Beach ML, Sites VR, Hartman GS. Artifacts and pitfall errors associated with ultrasound-guided regional anesthesia. part i: understanding the basic principles of ultrasound physics and machine operations. Reg Anesth Pain Med. 2007;32(5):412–8.

Sites BD, Chan VW, Neal JM, Weller R, Grau T, Koscielniak-Nielsen ZJ, Ivani G. The American Society of Regional Anesthesia and Pain Medicine and the European Society of Regional Anaesthesia and Pain Therapy Joint Committee recommendations for education and training in ultrasound-guided regional anesthesia. Reg Anesth Pain Med. 2009;34(1):40–6.

Stone R, McCloy R. Ergonomics in medicine and surgery. BMJ. 2004;328(7448):1115–8.

Tokumine J, Lefor AT, Yonei A, Kagaya A, Iwasaki K, Fukuda Y. Three-step method for ultrasound-guided central vein catheterization. Br J Anaesth. 2013;110(3):368–73.

Nerve Stimulation and Stimulating Catheter

3

Vivian H. Y. Ip, Rakesh V. Sondekoppam, and Ban C. H. Tsui

Contents

Introduction

Regional anesthesia (RA), historically regarded as an "art" with the success confined to a few gifted individuals, has been transforming into a predictable science in the last three to four decades, due to the availability of better guidance techniques. The introduction of nerve stimulation (NS) was the first step towards that transformation which was followed by the more popular ultrasound (US) guidance. Although a combined US/NS guidance remains popular in some institutions, the perceived advantages of US image guidance, including increased efficacy and "safety" due to the ability to visualize the nerve and surrounding structures, has earned its reputation as the sole monitor for regional anesthesia in many centers, thereby displacing the NS. This is perhaps due to the superior advantages of US guidance such as improved block success, decreased local anesthetic volume, or decrease in the incidence of Local Anesthetic Systemic Toxicity (LAST). This begs the question: what role does neurostimulation play in the current era of regional anesthesia? We hope this chapter will enlighten readers to recognize NS is very much alive both in the performance of RA and in the realm of acute pain management.

V. H. Y. Ip
Department of Anesthesiology and Pain Medicine, University of Alberta Hospital, Edmonton, AB, Canada
e-mail: hip@ualberta.ca

R. V. Sondekoppam
Department of Anesthesiology, University of Iowa, Iowa City, IA, USA
e-mail: rakesh-sondekoppam@uiowa.edu

B. C. H. Tsui (✉)
Department of Anesthesiology, Perioperative Medicine and Pain Medicine, Stanford University, Stanford, CA, USA

Lucille Packard Children's Hospital, Stanford, USA
e-mail: bantsui@stanford.edu

D. Jankovic, P. Peng (eds.), *Regional Nerve Blocks in Anesthesia and Pain Therapy*,
https://doi.org/10.1007/978-3-030-88727-8_3

Background and Basic Principles of Nerve Stimulation

To appreciate the place of nerve stimulation in RA and acute pain medicine, we first need to understand the background and basic principle. Interests in electrophysiology properties of nerve conduction date as early as eighteenth century when Galvani demonstrated "animal electricity" being responsible to induce muscle contraction. In anesthesia practice, nerve stimulators were first used to monitor the depth of neuromuscular blockade, and subsequently to localize the nerves for RA, as NS was thought to be safer and efficacious than landmark-based techniques.

Electrical Principle

An electrical "current" is the flow of charge, and the difference in charge between two surfaces is the "voltage". For the sake of comparison, if we could imagine a tank of water at a height with a hose connected to its bottom, the water in the tank can be thought to represent "charge", the pressure at the end of the hose the "voltage" and the flow of water through the hose is the "current". The main impediment to the flow is represented by the "resistance" to flow. This forms the basis of Ohm's law ($V = IR$) where voltage is the product of current and resistance.

NS exerts its effect by initiating ion flow in nearby neuronal cells causing nerve depolarization. Current and stimulus duration requirements are different for different nerves and depends on rheobase and chronaxie. Rheobase (literally translates into "bottom flow") is the minimum current of indefinite pulse duration producing an action potential when applied to a given nerve (Fig. 3.1). Chronaxie (time value) is the minimum time required for a current intensity double the rheobase to elicit a nerve stimulation. In other words, chronaxie is an indication of the excitability of a neuron (an index of the density of the voltage-gated Na^+ channels) which depends on nerve fiber types and the tissue resistance (electrical impedance). The resulting response of muscle contraction, paresthesia or pain not only depends on nerve type (i.e., motor/mixed vs. sensory, respectively) but more importantly on the amount of energy applied.

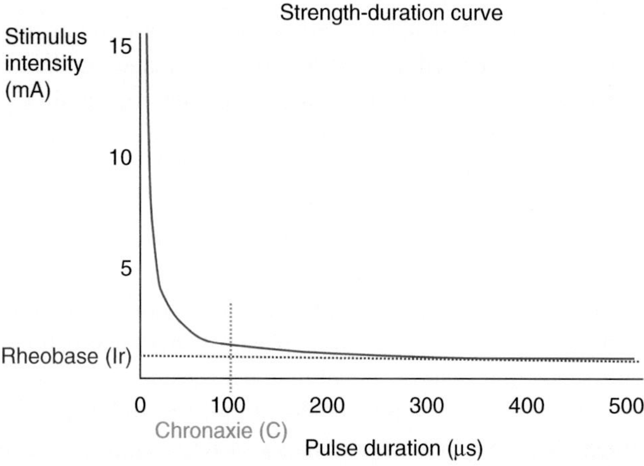

Fig. 3.1 Strength-duration curve showing strength of stimulus against pulse duration in nerve stimulation

This energy (Q) or charge [$Q = I*t$] is a product of the current intensity (I: amplitude) and the duration of stimulus (t). Strength–duration relationship dictates that as the stimulus duration increases, the required amplitude decreases until it reaches the rheobase, while the charge–duration relationship dictates that as the stimulus duration increases, the charge at the end of the electrode increases. Hence, as a trade-off to prevent high charge at the end of the needle or catheter, nerve stimulators are often started using the lowest pulse duration setting to be the closest to the chronaxie of a nerve and then the pulse duration increases if no response ensues.

Whether a set charge stimulates a given nerve is determined by Coulomb's law [$I = k(i/D^2)$] where I = required current, k = Coulomb's constant, i = minimum stimulating current or threshold current for the nerve, and D = distance between the needle and the nerve. For a given nerve, assuming a set threshold current, the required current is inversely proportional to the square of the distance between the nerve and the stimulating electrode. In other words, the closer the needle is to the nerve, the lesser the required current will be.

To overcome the problems of varying tissue resistance, constant current-generating nerve stimulators are utilized in regional anesthesia. Modern nerve stimulators typically produce a square wave pulse of current, with a short pulse width (e.g., 0.2 ms). The nerve stimulators sense the change in current due to a change in tissue resistance and increase or decrease the voltage of the circuit accordingly. This change in resistance is denoted on modern nerve stimulators as electrical impedance (EI).

The Use of Nerve Stimulation in Nerve Localization

Prior to the introduction of ultrasound in regional anesthesia, nerve localization was largely facilitated using nerve stimulation. A high stimulating current of 1–1.5 mA was typically used, and the current slowly reduced to the minimum at which motor response is elicited, usually at a stimulating current of 0.5 mA for most peripheral nerves. More often, this was followed by losing the motor response at lower stimulating currents (0.3 mA or less) to rule out intraneural injections, following which the local anesthetic was administered. Local anesthetic or normal saline test dose was often given after negative aspiration for blood, to note a diminishing or absence of motor response which was reobtained after increasing the stimulating current (Raj Test). It was initially presumed that LA or NS pushing the target nerve away from the needle thereby abolished the motor response elicited by the low current. However, this hypothesis was refuted by studies demonstrating the dissipation of current along the length of the needle by both conducting solutions (local anesthetic or saline) (Fig. 3.2). When dextrose 5% in water (D5W), a non-conducting fluid is used, the elicited motor response is continued or augmented. This response occurs because D5W enables the electric field to be focused on the needle tip. Therefore, when using nerve stimulation, it is important to use D5W when performing the initial injection to confirm correct needle tip position prior to switching the injectate to local anesthesia; otherwise, a higher current threshold is required to obtain a motor response.

Limitations of Nerve Stimulation in Practice

Neurostimulation relies on the physiological response of neural structures to electrical impulse which can be affected by considerable interindividual variation. Moreover, a number of other factors influence the stimulation response, ranging from the characteristic of electrical pulses, surrounding environment (i.e., injectates, tissue, and blood), and the patient's own physiological and pathological states affecting the nervous system.

Stimulating Environmental Factor

Traditional teaching is that in order to ascertain an accurate needle placement in relation to the nerve, motor response should still be present when the stimulating current is reduced between 0.2 and 0.5 mA. *However*, needle nerve contact or intraneural needle placement may not always elicit a motor response or paresthesia, and the same has also been confirmed under US guidance. Briefly, these fallacies can be listed as follows:

- A lack of motor response at higher currents (>0.5 mA) is still possible, despite a complete intraneural needle location. The needle may not come in contact with the motor fibers in the mixed nerve.
- Each nerve has its own threshold current, and it varies along the course of the nerve and the threshold current may also be influenced by the intervening tissue impedances, and subsequently, the resulting motor response.
- Another drawback is the use of nerve stimulator on patients with diabetes or preexisting neuropathy. Studies into their excitability and strength–duration properties have led to

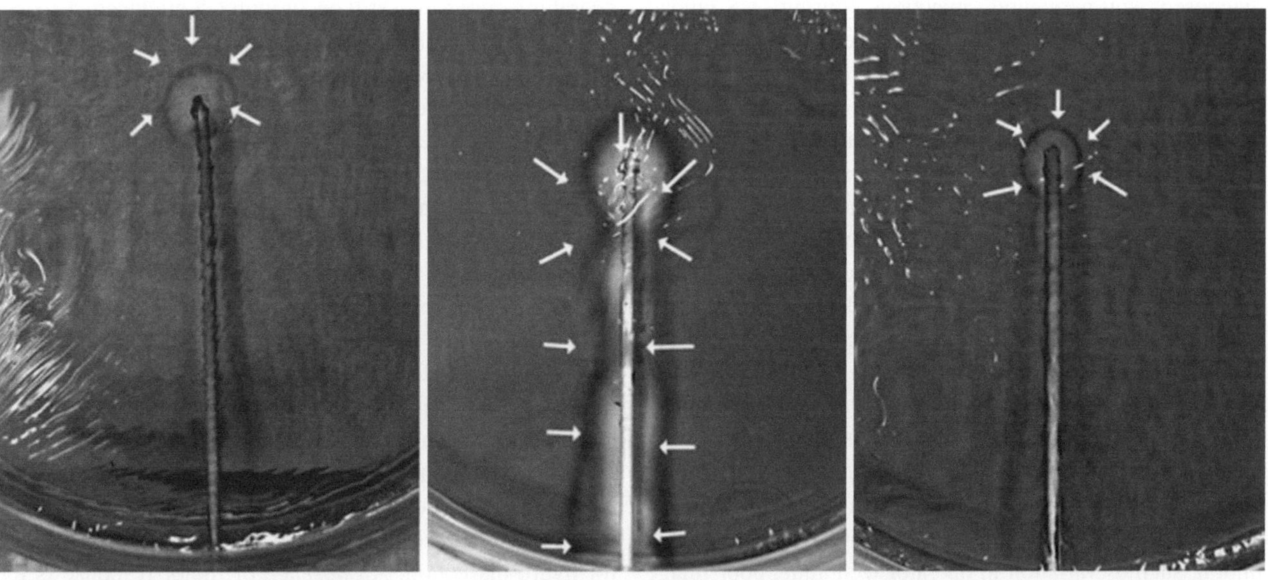

Fig. 3.2 Electrical field after injection of conductive (saline) vs nonconductive (Dextrose 5% in water) injectates with insulated needle. White arrows depict electrical conducting field

conflicting results, with an increased rheobase or its reduction. Although the needle can be in close proximity to the nerve, or even within it, there may not be any visible motor response.

To complicate things further, not all nerve stimulators perform the same, in terms of current output especially at low current output settings. The performance characteristics of 15 nerve stimulators for regional anesthesia have been studied which showed that all nerve stimulators performed well when the current settings were set at 1.0 mA and a standard resistance of 1 or 2 kΩ. The nerve stimulators showed increasing error rates in current outputs at lower current settings of 0.5 and 0.1 mA.

Peripheral Nerve Stimulation in Ultrasound Era

Despite the popularity of peripheral nerve stimulation in regional anesthesia, it was gradually phased out with the introduction of US as imaging technology at the turn of the twenty-first century. The use of US in RA was perceived to reduce procedural time, improve block quality and increase safety. Nonetheless, studies have demonstrated that US resolution is not reliable for visually interpreting the proximity between the needle and nerve. One example is the cadaver study by *Retter* et al. where the incidence of histologically diagnosed sub-perineural injections during US-guided supraclavicular blocks was 24%. While such a high incidence of neurological complications or cadaveric structural integrity is not seen in clinical practice, their findings demonstrate that the lateral resolution of the ultrasound is not high enough to differentiate intra- and extrafascicular injections. Since LA deposition directly around nerve fascicles has been hypothesized to result in cytotoxicity and ischemia, one cannot advocate for intraneural injection even though it may not translate to clinical neurologic deficits. Both animal and human studies suggest that direct needle to nerve contact and intraneural injections be avoided.

Peripheral nerve injuries occur with a similar frequency whether US guidance or PNS is used as the primary nerve localization tool—2 to 4/10,000 blocks. US-guided studies have not demonstrated a significant reduction in the incidence of this event. Several factors may contribute to this finding such as variation in operator technique, poor image resolution, or attempting to inject directly adjacent to a nerve despite a lack of sonographic evidence of tissue expansion with local anesthetic injection represent potentially unsafe regional anesthesia practices. With the use of the nerve stimulator, one may suspect that the needle is intraneural (parafascicular) if a low current threshold (≤0.2 mA) elicit a motor response. Similarly, motor response could be absent with intraneural needle placement at a current intensity of up to 1.7 mA. Therefore, PNS has a low sensitivity but high specificity for direct nerve contact since the ideal minimal threshold current that limits the incidence of intraneural injections yet still provokes a motor response is debatable. Hence, the American Society of Regional Anesthesia (ASRA) Advisory Panel suggests that a current of <0.5 mA which evokes a motor response effectively indicates intraneural needle placement. Other published literature has suggested a lower threshold to illicit concern for intraneural needle placement (closer to 0.2 mA) but that higher thresholds should be considered in certain patient populations (for instance, those with diabetes, multiple sclerosis, and obesity).

Multimodal Monitoring Technique

To reduce the risk of neurological injury, experts advocate the use of multimodal monitoring technique in minimizing intraneural injection during peripheral nerve block (Fig. 3.3). If PNS and US each has its limitations when used independently in RA, would intraneural injection be minimized and neurological injury be reduced with their combined use? Multimodal guidance is employed by some performers of RA as it is noted that nerve contact and intraneural injections may still occur with US guidance. A recent Swiss survey on the practice of RA demonstrates that the dual guidance (US+NS) is still a popular technique. Based on our practice, we suggest the use of multimodal monitoring which includes: US+NS guidance, injection pressure monitoring, impedance measurements, hydro-localization with D5W and patient feedback. A more recent study showed that a high injection pressure combined with low minimal intensity of stimulation during US-guided nerve block might be an alert for the intraneural location of the needle tip.

The technique for using nerve stimulator to avoid nerve-to-needle contact is somewhat different from that for nerve localization. When performing peripheral nerve blocks, US is used to locate the nerve with the current threshold on the nerve stimulator set to 0.2 mA. The insulated nerve block needle is primed with D5W and is used as the initial injectate for hydro-dissection. An *absence* of motor response is the desired outcome and if motor response is present, the needle is withdrawn slightly until no motor response is observed. The spread of the initial injectate is observed in real time under US to confirm the correct needle-tip position and not intraneural or intravascular. Opening pressure monitoring of <15 psi is also used, either in the form of the commercially

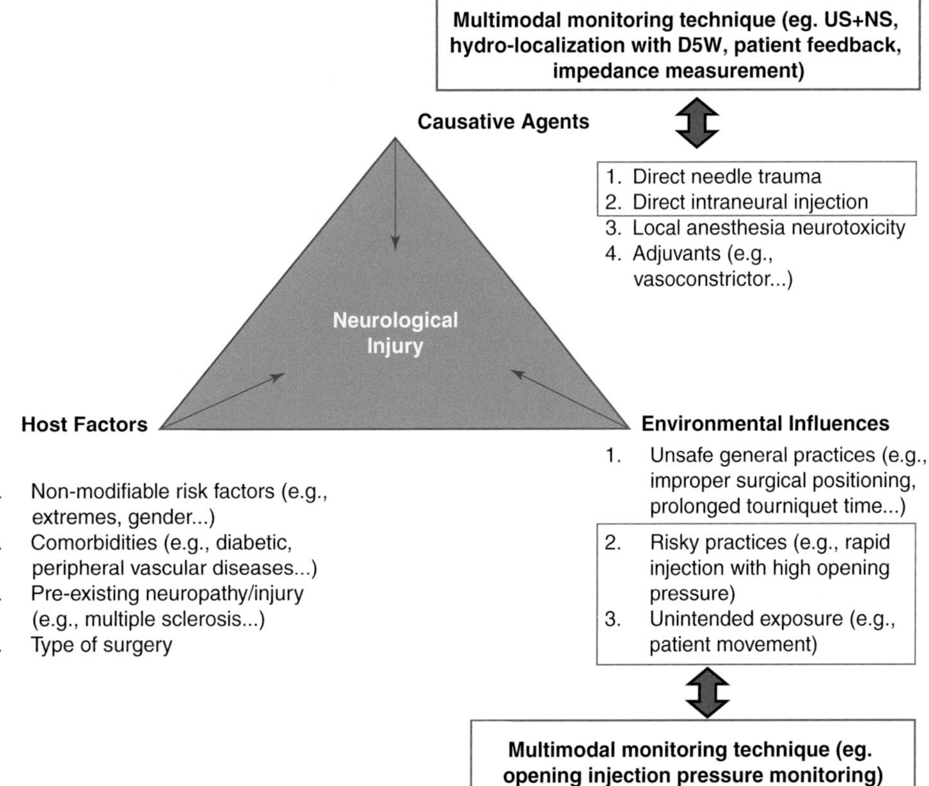

Fig. 3.3 Multimodal monitoring technique

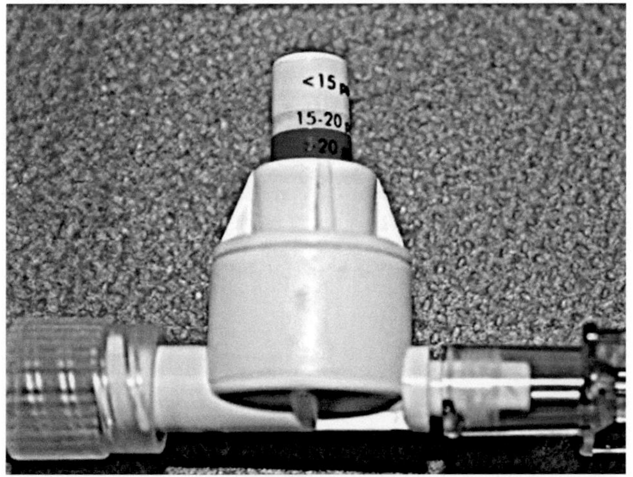

Fig. 3.4 Photo of a commercially available pressure monitoring device (B-smart, Braun, Bethlehem, PA, USA)

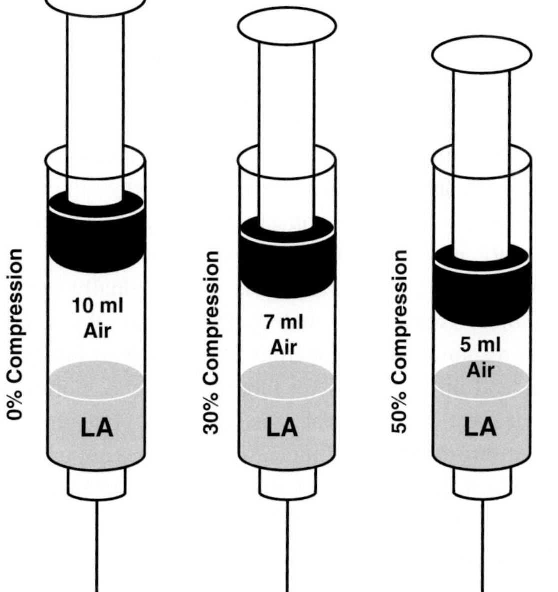

Fig. 3.5 Compressed air injection technique (CAIT) described by Tsui et al. v33 2008: pp 168–173

available pressure monitoring device (Fig. 3.4) or compressed air injection technique (CAIT). The compressed air injection technique (CAIT) applies the principle of Boyle's law when a column of air is aspirated above the column of fluid, and then compressed by ≤50%, the injection pressure is ≤760 mmHg (1 atm or 14.7 psi) (Fig. 3.5). Lastly, insulated nerve block needles should be used, and patients should be awake or minimally sedated for real-time feedback during nerve block performance.

Stimulating Nerve Block Catheters

Peripheral nerve block catheters with metal coil within consist of a wire extension beyond the distal tip (Fig. 3.6) and an injection port for normal saline to be injected. Studies have found that stimulating catheter improves postoperative analgesia when compared to non-stimulating catheter. However, insertion of stimulating catheter may be more technically challenging and require additional helpers. One must note that these studies compare the conventional stimulating peripheral nerve block catheters and newer types of catheter-over-needle stimulating catheters (E Cath Stim, Pajunk, Germany) have been developed with simple, less cumbersome insertion techniques (Fig. 3.7). There are also less likely to meet resistance during catheter advancement, compared to the conventional stimulating catheters.

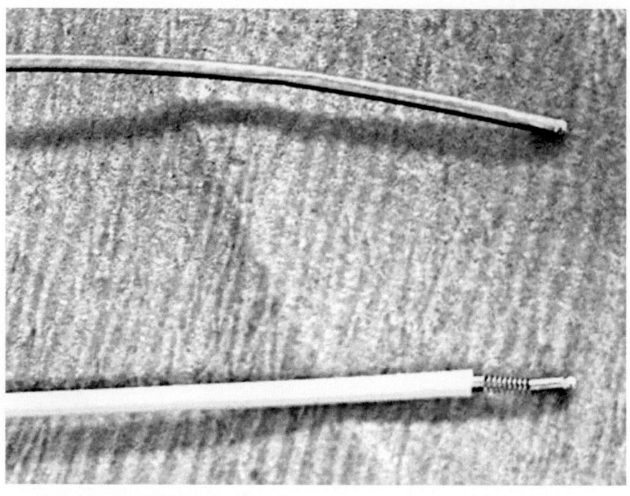

Fig. 3.6 Photo of commercially available stimulating catheters (Stimulong, Pajunk, Germany; Stimu Cath, Arrow, Reading, PA, USA)

Epidural Stimulation Test

For epidural catheters, correct placement can also be confirmed by stimulating the spinal nerves with a catheter that conducts electrical current. In contrast to the stimulating peripheral catheter, in most epidural catheters only the metal reenforced coil within the lumen (i.e., no metal beyond the catheter tip) to reduce air-trapping and to reduce resistance to current flow because of the catheter length. The metal coil is essential to induce electrical pulses, catheter's electrical resistance must remain low by priming the catheter with conducting fluid such as normal saline to overcome resistance when advancing the catheter. The nerve stimulator can be connected to the stimulating epidural catheter using an electrode adapter (Fig. 3.8). The catheter and the adaptor should be primed with normal saline. The cathode lead of the nerve stimulator can be attached to the metal part of the adaptor, and the grounding anode attached to the patient. The nerve stimulator is set to low frequency and pulse width (1 Hz, 0.2 ms). The current intensity is then gradually increased until motor response is noted. The current threshold for motor response can range from 5 to 10 mA in lumbar epidural, and up to 17 mA for thoracic epidural. Following a standard test dose of local anesthetic with epinephrine, the current threshold should increase if the epidural catheter is placed correctly since the current is dispersed by the ionic solution. Other responses to the test dose combined with the use of epidural stimulation test are useful to diagnose the epidural catheter tip position (Table 3.1).

Epidural stimulation test is an important tool for confirmation of correct epidural catheter tip placement, which is more relevant in patients who are noncommunicable such as the pediatric population, patients with language barrier or confusion.

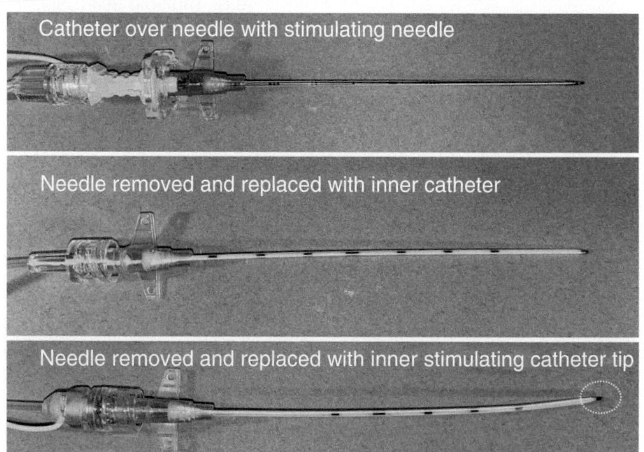

Fig. 3.7 Photo of a catheter over needle with regular tip (E-Cath, Pajunk, Germany) or stimulating tip (E-Cath Stim, Pajunk, Germany)

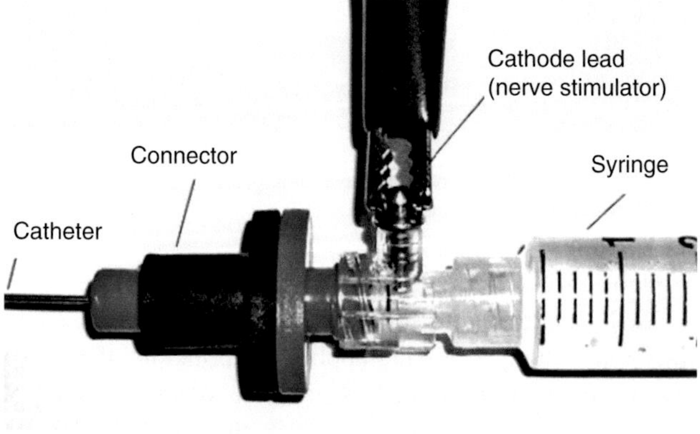

Fig. 3.8 Photo of an ECG electrode adapter (Johans ECG adapter, Arrow, Reading, PA, USA)

Table 3.1 Epidural catheter location determined by standard test dose (lidocaine with 1:200,000 epinephrine) combined with the epidural stimulation test

Catheter location	Test dose	Epidural stimulation test
Subarachnoid	Hypotension/total spinal response	Unilateral/bilateral motor response (1 mA)
Subdural	Unknown	Diffuse motor response in many segments (1 mA)
Epidural space		
Against/Close to spinal nerve root	Narrow unilateral sensory changes	Unilateral motor response (1 mA)
Correct epidural catheter placement	Bilateral sensory changes	Unilateral or bilateral motor response (2–17 mA) Threshold current ↑ after local anesthetic injection
Intravascular	↑ Heart rate/ECG change	Threshold current remains or returns to baseline with positive motor response despite local anesthetic injection
Subcutaneous	No changes	Negative response

Tool for Teaching

Nerve stimulation is underutilized in clinical practice and teaching in the US era. Many trainees may not have the opportunities to elicit motor response with the corresponding peripheral nerve stimulation during their training. For some peripheral nerve blocks, the importance of combining US with NS is not only for multimodal monitoring purpose, but also aid nerve localization. An example would be axillary brachial plexus nerve block, which is an ideal nerve block for teaching trainees since it is a superficial block which makes visualizing and maneuvering the needle less challenging. The trainees can trace the terminal nerves from axillary apex to the elbow and vice versa, learning US transducer handling for image optimization, practicing different probe manipulation techniques such as tilting and rotating. Once the peripheral nerves of the upper limb are identified, motor response can be elicited by gradually increasing the current intensity. This approach enables trainees to appreciate small, incremental needle movement, slick US transducer handling and different motor responses. The use of US and NS are complimentary rather than against each other, even though study has proposed the skills required to perform successful ultrasound-guided axillary brachial plexus block can be learnt faster and lead to a higher final success rate compared to nerve stimulator-guided axillary brachial plexus block.

Furthermore, trainees should learn different techniques to assess the end point of an effective block or epidural placement.

Future Directions

While the drawbacks of NS require consideration in the performance of RA and its role remains as the secondary monitoring device, the basic concepts and the practice of incorporating nerve stimulation during regional techniques may make a resurgence, as increasing number of studies are emerging in support of peripheral nerve stimulation in the management of acute postoperative pain. Hence, combining US with NS may not only become a necessity for the safe and effective performance of RA, but NS may be functioning as a neuromodulatory therapy for acute pain management. Clinically, the main proposed mechanism appears to be based on the "Gate theory" where stimulation of large nerve fibers (Aœ, or Aß) with lower minimum stimulating threshold leads to decreased transmission of A∂ or C fibers responsible for pain perception.

Recently, feasibility studies on using ultrasound-guided peripheral nerve neuromodulation by positioning specialized electrodes near a nerve have demonstrated success in a variety of orthopedic surgeries. However, it is important to note that this technique is still at its infancy and specialized stimulating electrodes and stimulators are required. Despite differences in the utilization of electricity, the application of basic principles of neurostimulation continues.

Challenges of Neuromodulation in Acute Pain Management

At present, specialized equipment and nerve stimulator are required for PNS in acute pain management. The insertion of electrodes is also cumbersome, time-consuming and labor-intensive. More importantly, their effectiveness and safety necessitate careful balance and further research. Recently, peripheral nerve block catheters used in regional anesthetic block have been successfully used for neuromodulation trialing despite having a comparably shorter surface area and may serve as an example to be replicable in the acute pain management.

A Birth of New "Hybrid Regional Technique"

With the accelerating drive for early mobilization, there is a need to explore whether early neuromodulation may be served to bridge the traditional chemical means of local anesthetic with electric means of neuromodulation to smooth the transition in acute pain management. By combining local anesthesia in the acute phase perioperatively, and bridging with early neuromodulation, this novel concept of "hybrid regional technique" may offer patients with the "best of both worlds," as supported by several case reports. In addition, early neuromodulation may prevent priming/sensitization of the nervous system thereby offering better analgesia for patients with preexisting or evolving neuropathic pain. Hence, the hybrid regional anesthesia may serve as an effective strategy to address transitional pain.

Conclusion

Nerve stimulation is anything but being displaced by ultrasound in the twenty-first century. Undoubtedly, its role has changed from facilitating nerve localization to being part of the multimodal monitoring tool to minimize nerve injury in regional anesthesia. It is essential to understand the principle of nerve stimulation to fully appreciate its potential. More importantly, it may be the next game changer as the "hybrid regional technique" to compliment locoregional anesthesia in acute pain medicine.

Suggested Reading

Albrecht E, Chin KJ. Advances in regional anesthesia and acute pain management: a narrative review. Anaesthesia. 2020;75(Suppl 1):e101–10.

Auroy Y, Benhamou D, Bargues L, et al. Major complications of regional anesthesia in France: the SOS regional anesthesia hotline service. Anesthesiology. 2002;97:1274–80.

Barrington MJ, Gledhill SR, Kluger R, et al. A randomized controlled trial of ultrasound versus nerve stimulator guidance for axillary brachial plexus block. Reg Anesth Pain Med. 2016;41(6):671–7. https://doi.org/10.1097/AAP.0000000000000486.

Bigeleisen PE, Groen G, Nizar M. Ultrasound-guided supraclavicular block: what is intraneural? Anesthesiology. 2010;112:251–2.

Birnbaum J, Kip M, Spies CD, et al. The effect of stimulating versus nonstimulating catheters for continuous interscalene plexus blocks in short-term pain management. J Clin Anesth. 2007;19(6):434–9. https://doi.org/10.1016/j.jclinane.2007.03.006.

Cappelleri G, Ambrosoli AL, Gemma M, et al. Intraneural ultrasound-guided sciatic nerve block: minimum effective volume and electrophysiologic effects. Anesthesiology. 2018;129(2):241–8.

Cappelleri G, Ghisi D, Ambrosoli AL, et al. Stimulating versus non-stimulating catheter for lumbar plexus continuous infusion after total hip placement. Minerva Anestesiol. 2019;85(3):236–43. https://doi.org/10.23736/S0375-9393.18.12527-2.

Chan VWS, Brull R, McCartney CJL, Xu D, Abbas S, Shannon P. An ultrasonographic and histological study of intraneural injection and electrical stimulation in pigs. Anesth Analg. 2007;104(5):1281–4. https://doi.org/10.1213/01.ane.0000250915.45247.24.

Choquet O, Noble GB, Abbal B, et al. Subparaneural versus circumferential extraneural injection at the bifurcation level in ultrasound-guided popliteal sciatic nerve blocks: a prospective, randomized, double-blind study. Reg Anesth Pain Med. 2014;39(4):306–11.

Forouzan A, Masoumi K, Motamed H, Gousheh MR, Rohani A. Nerve stimulator versus ultrasound-guided femoral nerve block; a randomized clinical trial. Emergency (Tehran, Iran). 2017;5(1):e54. https://doi.org/10.22037/emergency.v5i1.15782.

Gabriel RA, Ilfeld BM. Percutaneous peripheral nerve stimulation and other alternatives for perineural catheters for postoperative analgesia. Best Pract Res Clin Anaesthesiol. 2019;33(1):37–46. https://doi.org/10.1016/j.bpa.2019.02.002.

Galvani L. Aloysii Galvani De Viribus Electricitatis in Motu Musculari Commentarius. Ex Typographia Instituti Scientiarium. 1791. https://doi.org/10.5479/sil.324681.39088000932442.

Gandhi K, Lindenmuth DM, Hadzic A, et al. The effect of stimulating versus conventional perineural catheters on postoperative analgesia following ultrasound-guided femoral nerve localization. J Clin Anesth. 2011;23(8):626–31. https://doi.org/10.1016/j.jclinane.2001.04.006.

Günter C, Delbeke J, Ortiz-Catalan M. Safety of long-term electrical peripheral nerve stimulation: review of the state of the art. J Neuroeng Rehabil. 2019;16(1):13. https://doi.org/10.1186/s12984-018-0474-8.

Hadzic A, Vloka J, Hadzic N, Thys DM, Santos AC. Nerve stimulators used for peripheral nerve blocks vary in their electrical characteristics. Anesthesiology. 2003;98(4):969–74. https://doi.org/10.1097/00000542-200304000-00026.

Hadzic A, Dilberovic F, Shah S, et al. Combination of intraneural injection and high injection pressure leads to fascicular injury and neurologic deficits in dogs. Reg Anesth Pain Med. 2004;29(5):417–23.

Hara K, Sakura S, Yokokawa N, et al. Incidence and effects of unintentional intraneural injection during ultrasound-guided subgluteal sciatic nerve block. Reg Anesth Pain Med. 2012;37(3):289–93.

Ilfeld BM, Finneran JJ. Cryoneurolysis and percutaneous peripheral nerve stimulation to treat acute pain. Anesthesiology. 2020;133(5): 1127–49. https://doi.org/10.1097/ALN.0000000000003532.

Ip VHY, Ozelsel TJP, Sondekoppam RV, et al. Multimodal monitoring approach: the key to safe performance of peripheral nerve blocks. Br J Anaesth. 2019;123(3):e469–70.

Klein SM, Melton MS, Grill WM, Nielsen KC. Peripheral nerve stimulation in regional anesthesia. Reg Anesth Pain Med. 2012;37(4):383–92. https://doi.org/10.1097/AAP.0b013e3182576647.

Krishnan AV, Kiernan MC, Kiernan M. Altered nerve excitability properties in established diabetic neuropathy. Brain. 2005;128:1178–87. https://doi.org/10.1093/brain/awh476.

Luedi MM, Upadek V, Vogt AP, Steinfeldt T, Eichenberger U, Sauter AR. A Swiss nationwide survey shows that dual guidance is the preferred approach for peripheral nerve blocks. Sci Rep. 2019;9(1):1–8. https://doi.org/10.1038/s41598-019-45700-3.

Luyet C, Schupfer G, Wipfli M, et al. Different learning curves for axillary brachial plexus block: ultrasound guidance versus nerve stimulation. Anesthesiol Res Pract. 2011;2010:309462. https://doi.org/10.1155/2-10/309462.

Mariano ER, Marshall ZJ, Urman RD, et al. Ultrasound and its evolution in perioperative regional anesthesia and analgesia. Best Pract Res Clin Anaesthesiol. 2014;28(1):29–39.

Neal JM. Ultrasound-guided regional anesthesia and patient safety: an evidence-based analysis. Reg Anesth Pain Med. 2010;35:S59–67.

Neal JM, Barrington MJ, Brull R, et al. The second ASRA practice advisory on neurologic complications associated with regional anesthesia and pain medicine. Reg Anesth Pain Med. 2015;40(5):401–30.

Perlas A, Niazi A, McCartney C, Chan V, Xu D, Abbas S. The sensitivity of motor response to nerve stimulation and paresthesia for nerve localization as evaluated by ultrasound. Reg Anesth Pain Med. 2006;31(5):445–50. https://doi.org/10.1016/j.rapm.2006.05.017.

Reddy CG, Flouty OE, Holland MT, Rettenmaier LA, Zanaty M, Elahi F. Novel technique for trialing peripheral nerve stimulation: ultrasonography-guided StimuCath trial. Neurosurg Focus. 2017;42(3):E5. https://doi.org/10.3171/2016.12.FOCUS16475.

Retter S, Szerb J, Kwofie K, et al. Incidence of sub-perineural injection using a targeted intracluster supraclavicular ultrasound-guided approach in cadavers. Br J Anaesth. 2019;122(6):776–81.

Sauter AR, Dodgson MS, Stubhaug A, Cvancarova M, Klaastad O. Ultrasound controlled nerve stimulation in the elbow region: high currents and short distances needed to obtain motor responses. Acta Anaesthesiol Scand. 2007;51(7):942–8. https://doi.org/10.1111/j.1399-6576.2007.01349.x.

Sauter AR, Dodgson MS, Kalvøy H, Grimnes S, Stubhaug A, Klaastad Ø. Current threshold for nerve stimulation depends on electrical impedance of the tissue: a study of ultrasound-guided electrical nerve stimulation of the median nerve. Anesth Analg. 2009;108(4):1338–43. https://doi.org/10.1213/ane.0b013e3181957d84.

Stan TC, Krantz MA, Solomon DL, et al. The incidence of neurovascular complications following axillary brachial plexus block using a transarterial approach: a prospective study of 1000 consecutive patients. Reg Anesth. 1995;20:486–92.

Steinfeldt T, Poeschle S, Nimphius W, et al. Forced needle advancement during needle-nerve contact in a porcine model: histologic outcome. Anesth Analg. 2011;113:417–20.

Tsai TP, Vuckovic I, Dilberovic F, et al. Intensity of the stimulating current may not be a reliable indicator of intraneural needle placement. Reg Anesth Pain Med. 2008;33(3):207–10. https://doi.org/10.1016/j.rapm.2007.12.010.

Tsui BCH, Kropelin B. The electrophysiological effect of dextrose 5% in water on single-shot peripheral nerve stimulation. Anesth Analg. 2005;100(6):1837–9.

Tsui BCH, Wagner A, Finucane A. Electrophysiologic effect of injectates on peripheral nerve stimulation. Reg Anesth Pain Med. 2004;29:189–93.

Tsui BCH, Chan V, Finucane BT, et al. Electrical nerve stimulation. In: Tsui BCH, Chan V, Finucane BT, et al., editors. Atlas of ultrasound and nerve stimulation-guided regional anesthesia. New York: Springer; 2007. p. 9–20.

Tsui BCH, Knezevich MP, Pillay JJ. Reduced injection pressure using a compressed air injection technique (CAIT): an in vitro study. Reg Anesth Pain Med. 2008;33:168–73.

Tsui B, Sondekoppam R, Ip V. Nerve stimulation in regional anesthesia: a game-changer as a 'hybrid regional technique'? Anesthesiology. 2020.

Urmey WF, Stanton J. Inability to consistently elicit a motor response following sensory paresthesia during interscalene block administration. Anesthesiology. 2002;96(3):552–4. https://doi.org/10.1097/00000542-200203000-00008.

Varobieff M, Choquet O, Swisser F. Ultrasound-guided peripheral nerve blocks: an exploratory observational trial. Analg Anesth. 2020; https://doi.org/10.1213/ANE.0000000000005308.

Wiesmann T, Steinfeldt T, Exner M, et al. Intraneural injection of a test dose of local anesthetic in peripheral nerves. Acta Anaesthesiol Scand. 2017;61:91–8.

Yerdelen D, Koç F, Uysal H, Sarica Y. Strength-duration properties in diabetic polyneuropathy. Diabetes Res Clin Pract. 2007;78(1):56–9. https://doi.org/10.1016/j.diabres.2007.03.001.

Serious Complications of Regional Anaesthesia

4

M. Kerr, R. Brull, and A. Macfarlane

Contents

M. Kerr
Royal Alexandra Hospital, Paisley, Scotland, UK
e-mail: michael.kerr@ggc.scot.nhs.uk

R. Brull
Women's College Hospital, University of Toronto, Toronto, ON, Canada
e-mail: richard.brull@uhn.ca

A. Macfarlane (✉)
Glasgow Royal Infirmary, University of Glasgow, Glasgow, Scotland, UK
e-mail: alan.macfarlane@ggc.scot.nhs.uk

D. Jankovic, P. Peng (eds.), *Regional Nerve Blocks in Anesthesia and Pain Therapy*,
https://doi.org/10.1007/978-3-030-88727-8_4

Serious complications of regional anaesthesia are rare. In order to choose the most appropriate anaesthetic technique for an individual, a thorough knowledge of the factors that influence both risk and benefit are essential. The aim of this chapter is to outline the serious complications of both central neuraxial blocks (CNB) and peripheral nerve blocks (PNB), discussing in each case the incidence, presentation, mechanism of injury and factors which may increase or reduce risk. The reference list included is not exhaustive, but rather aims to guide the reader towards contemporary data, detailed management, and landmark studies with reference to each complication.

Central Neuraxial Blockade

Serious complications of CNB may be divided into neurological including post-dural puncture headache, infectious, cardiovascular, respiratory or the consequences of wrong route injection. Adverse effects such as pruritus, urinary retention and back pain, whilst potentially distressing for patients, are not included.

Neurological Complications

Neurological complications of CNB range from temporary paraesthesia to irreversible, catastrophic paraplegia. Calculating the incidence of neurological complications can be challenging as figures vary depending on how robustly the data is collected and how nerve injury is defined. Furthermore, the specific neuraxial technique, the population studied and individual patient risk factors such as pre-existing neurological disease, immunosuppression or altered coagulation are all important. It is therefore difficult to provide accurate figures on an individual patient basis, particularly for rare complications.

In a large national audit of CNB practice in the United Kingdom published in 2009, paraplegia or death was estimated to occur between 0 and 3 per 100,000 CNB procedures. Permanent nerve injuries overall ranged between 1 and 6 per 100,000 depending on 'optimistic' or 'pessimistic' interpretation of the data. This range includes the figure of 1 in 53,000 quoted in a similar national audit of CNB practice in Finland published in 2013. Evidence suggests injury is higher with epidural and CSE compared to spinal or caudal anaesthesia. Furthermore, the risk for each technique appears to be higher in perioperative patients compared to the obstetric, chronic pain and paediatric settings.

The various mechanisms that can lead to neurological injury are discussed below.

Trauma

Direct trauma may occur to either the spinal cord, where symptoms reflect the spinal tract(s) injured, or to the nerve roots forming the cauda equina, which can present as radicular pain with motor involvement. In addition to spinal and epidural needles, skin infiltration needles have also been implicated in trauma to the neuraxis. The true rate of injury attributable to direct trauma appears to be very rare, ranging between 1 in 200,000 and 1 in 1,000,000 in case series. Treatment is generally conservative, and although steroids have been used in other cases of spinal trauma, the associated hyperglycaemia may worsen ischaemic neuronal injury. Steroids should therefore only be used following specialist advice.

Reducing Risk

The spinal cord usually terminates at L1–2 but it can be further caudad. Introducing a needle below this level is therefore the most obvious method of reducing direct spinal cord damage. The safest intervertebral space for spinal anaesthesia is L3–4 and below. Identification of this space using Tuffier's line can be inaccurate, however, with practitioners often inserting the needle one to two interspaces more cephalad than perceived. Where surface anatomy is challenging, identification of vertebral levels using anatomical landmarks can be even more difficult. Both fluoroscopy and ultrasound may be used to assist identify vertebral levels albeit fluoroscopy is a less practical tool. Ultrasound can also be used to determine the midline, as well as estimate the depth from the skin to the epidural or intrathecal space. In the lumbar region particularly, where sonographic windows are better compared to the thoracic region, using ultrasound helps reduce the number of attempts and thus potential trauma.

Unlike spinal anaesthesia, epidural needle or catheter insertion may take place at any vertebral level. Many different methods exist to help identify the epidural space or determine catheter tip position such as loss of resistance, the Tsui test, ultrasound, fluoroscopy or CT epidurography but none can truly prevent the rare complication of spinal cord injury. Anatomical variants such as failure of fusion of the ligamentum flavum may also increase the risk of inadvertent needle advancement.

Below the termination of the spinal cord, particularly when deviating from the midline or if there is inadvertent lateral placement of the spinal needle, a nerve root may be contacted. Paraesthesia during needle advancement does not necessarily relate to injury, but nevertheless it should be considered as potential neural contact and the needle withdrawn and re-positioned. The spinal cord has no sensory receptors, and permanent nerve injury can occur without paraesthesia, as evidenced in cases where a needle has accidentally entered the cord in awake patients. The consensus remains however that neuraxial procedures should not be performed under heavy sedation or general anaesthesia in adults whereby this potential warning sign is lost.

Epidural (or Subdural) Haematoma

An epidural or subdural haematoma from vascular trauma can result in direct compression and subsequent ischaemia of the spinal cord, which must be recognised and acted upon promptly to reduce the risk of permanent damage. The majority of cases present within 24 h of needle insertion or catheter removal. In the 2009 UK national audit, the incidence of epidural haematoma was found to be 1 in 19,500 epidural anaesthetics, but there were no cases of haematoma after 360,000 spinals. The rate of epidural hematoma reported in a recent American series was found to be approximately 1 in every 10,500 epidural anaesthetics. These figures are higher than previous estimates, possibly reflecting increased anticoagulant use. Prolonged motor or sensory deficit, radicular back pain and altered bowel or bladder function mandate urgent radiological imaging to evaluate whether or not surgical management is required. MRI is the modality of choice although CT will identify any potential surgical targets. The best results are generally seen if surgical intervention occurs within 8–12 h, although full recovery has still been reported with surgery up to 56 h. Conservative management appears not to be inferior in patients with mild symptoms that show improvement during diagnosis.

Reducing Risk

The risk of bleeding and a subsequent epidural or subdural haematoma formation are increased by medications that affect coagulation or platelet function, and also in coagulopathic and thrombocytopenic states. Risk also increases with epidural anaesthetics compared to spinals, particularly in non-obstetric, elderly, and female patients. Minimising the number of needle passes is also of theoretical benefit. Practice guidelines recommend when to stop and restart medications in relation to needle insertion, catheter removal and with respect to appropriate haematological parameters. In certain groups of patients, the small increased risk of undertaking CNB outwith these guidelines may be offset by a greater benefit of avoiding general anaesthesia and decisions must be made on an individual patient basis.

Hypoperfusion Ischaemic Cord Injury

Hypotension and the potential for hypoperfusion occurs after neuraxial anaesthesia due to loss of sympathetically mediated vasoconstriction and subsequent reduction in systemic vascular resistance. In the 2009 UK National Audit, four cases of ischaemic cord injury were reported, all occurring in patients receiving thoracic epidurals. However the extent, if any, that CNB-related hypotension contributed to injury is impossible to state, and therefore it is difficult to provide an exact incidence for this complication. The presentation of hypoperfusion-related ischemic injury to the spinal cord largely depends on the location of ischaemia, but back pain and sensorimotor loss are common. Anterior spinal artery syndrome is the commonest presentation, occurring due to lack of collateral blood supply to the singular anterior spinal artery, and it may manifest as paraplegia, and a loss of temperature and pain sensation with intact proprioception/vibration. Imaging, preferably MRI, is required to exclude other causes, and treatment involves supporting normo-high blood pressure. CSF drainage to improve perfusion pressure may also be considered.

Reducing Risk

Factors that increase the risk of hypoperfusion ischaemic injury are listed in Table 4.1. It appears likely that the lower limit of spinal cord autoregulation in the majority of patients is between a MAP of 60–65 mmHg. However, this varies between individuals, and avoiding prolonged hypotension (defined as greater than 20–30% below baseline MAP) is recommended in all patients undergoing neuraxial procedures, but particularly in at risk groups.

Cauda Equina Syndrome

Cauda Equina Syndrome (CES) presents with the constellation of symptoms of altered bladder and bowel function, with sciatic pain and/or variable sensorimotor disturbance. The rate of CES following neuraxial procedures reportedly ranges between 1 in 53,000–94,000. Whilst the majority of cases appear to occur without a definitive understanding of causation, exposure of the lumbosacral nerve roots to prolonged or high concentrations of local anaesthetic (LA) is considered to be a risk, as is spinal stenosis which can limit spread of LA cranially. Spinal stenosis is potentially problematic given it is often undiagnosed but has a prevalence of up to 19% in the over sixties. CES may also occur in cases of

Table 4.1 Factors that increase the risk of spinal ischaemia

Hypertension
Smoking
Atherosclerosis
Hypocapnia
Raised intra-thoracic pressure
Surgical positioning • Hyperlordosis • Extreme lateral flexion • Lithotomy

epidural haematoma and arachnoiditis. Management depends on the cause. Where imaging reveals a correctable lesion such as an epidural haematoma (see above), surgery is indicated. Steroids may be indicated in other cases.

Reducing Risk

Risk can be reduced by considering whether spinal anaesthesia is indicated in patients with known moderate to severe spinal stenosis. In cases of inadequate block following spinal anaesthesia, where a predominantly sacral motor and/or sensory block may indicate pooling of LA, avoiding repeat dosing may be advisable. Small bore intrathecal catheters were withdrawn from North American practice after reports of CES and concerns of consequent local anaesthetic pooling at the thecal sac terminus. Use of intrathecal catheters outwith the field of chronic pain remains relatively uncommon.

Arachnoiditis

Arachnoiditis is a rare meningeal inflammatory process that can be seen after trauma (including back surgery), infection and neuraxial anaesthesia. Causality is difficult to attribute to anaesthesia and delayed presentation after the initial insult ranging from weeks to years further complicates calculating incidence attributable to neuraxial techniques. Only one case of arachnoiditis, following a spinal anaesthetic, was reported in the UK National Audit project of over 700,000 CNB procedures. Other large retrospective reviews of over 750,000 patients reported no cases of arachnoiditis following CNB. Inflammation, fibrosis, adhesion and clumping of nerve roots may occur, reducing CSF and blood flow. Magnetic resonance imaging is diagnostic, and syringomyelia and hydrocephalus may also be present. Treatment options are limited although surgical intervention including shunts have been described. Prognosis is unfortunately poor with permanent disability and pain common.

Reducing Risk

Contamination with the antiseptic chlorhexidine has been implicated in the development of several cases of catastrophic arachnoiditis following obstetrical epidural anaesthesia for labour analgesia. Practice guidelines in the United Kingdom now suggest using 0.5% chlorhexidine rather than 2% for asepsis. Care should also be taken to allow the chlorhexidine solution to fully dry whilst ensuring it also remains separate from the sterile field and instruments.

Transient Neurological Symptoms

Transient Neurological Symptoms (TNS) present as delayed onset gluteal pain radiating into the lower limbs in the absence of other abnormal neurological findings. Symptoms generally start within 24 h, usually are self-limiting, and typically resolve by the fifth day. The frequency of TNS is mostly dependent on the type of LA utilised, with rates of 10–20% reported when using lidocaine. Rates may be similar with 2-chloroprocaine and mepivacaine but appear to be significantly less with other agents. Investigations such as MRI and nerve conduction studies reveal no causative abnormalities. Treatment is simple analgesia including NSAIDs if tolerated.

Reducing Risk

Although TNS has been reported with epidural administration, this is predominantly an issue with intrathecal LA administration. Risk is therefore dependent on the LA utilised as outlined above. A two-orifice needle may reduce risk whereas incidence appears to increase with lithotomy positioning.

Post-dural Puncture Headache

Post-dural puncture headache (PDPH) typically presents with a frontal or, less commonly, occipital headache which is relieved with supine positioning. Photophobia, neck pain, nausea and vomiting, tinnitus and diplopia may all be associated. Rarely cranial nerve palsies, seizures, cerebral venous thrombosis and intracranial haemorrhage can occur. PDPH occurs following approximately 1% of epidural insertions based upon an accidental dural puncture rate of 1.5% and 50–70% of patients subsequently becoming symptomatic. In spinal anaesthesia, where by definition the dura must be punctured, various patient and equipment factors affect the rate which may be as low as 0.2%. Initial management is usually conservative with simple analgesics, hydration and resting in the supine position. Caffeine is of disputed benefit, whilst small studies suggest gabapentin, hydrocortisone and theophylline but not sumatriptan may reduce pain scores. An epidural blood patch performed 24 h after onset of symptoms has been reported to resolve or improve symptoms in over 90% of cases although other evidence suggests only a third of patients may have lasting complete relief, with persistent symptoms present in a considerable proportion even after a second blood patch.

Reducing Risk

Risk of headache following dural puncture is increased with young age, female gender, lower body weight and pre-existing headache. Using cutting needle tips during spinal anaesthesia increases the risk of PDPH by a factor of at least two over atraumatic (pencil point) needles. Recent studies suggest, contrary to previous evidence, that if an atraumatic needle is used, then gauge does not appear to influence risk. With regard to epidural technique, there is still no conclusive evidence to suggest using air or saline to determine loss of resistance is superior in terms of reducing accidental dural puncture and therefore subsequent PDPH.

Infectious Complications

Infectious complications manifest as either abscesses or meningitis. Serious infections following spinal anaesthesia are rare, with documented rates less than 3 in 100,000. Although rates have been reported to increase where an epidural catheter is left in situ, the latest American Society of Anesthesiologists (ASA) Task Force Advisory states that there is no strong evidence to suggest any difference in infectious complications between spinal or epidural techniques, or between continuous catheter or single shot procedures. The estimated incidence of epidural abscess ranges between 1.2 and 8.7 per 100,000 perioperative epidurals with no apparent difference in the risk between thoracic, lumbar or caudal approaches. Meningitis following CNB is reported to occur between 1 and 4 per 100,000 procedures. The most common pathogens identified are streptococcal oral pathogens from the practitioner or staphylococcal skin pathogens from the patient. Abscesses generally present within a week of undergoing CNB, with insidious back pain and pyrexia. Local infection at the injection site may be present whilst motor deficit and other signs of cord compression can occur. Management of abscesses classically involves surgical decompression and prolonged antibiotics, although conservative antibiotic-only therapy may not be inferior in selected patients. Meningitis often presents with fever, photophobia and meningism. Lumbar puncture to isolate the causative pathogen is required, and treatment is antibiotics.

Reducing Risk

Aseptic technique, including adequate skin cleansing with chlorhexidine and the donning of masks and gloves, is important. The risk of infection following CNB is higher in immunocompromised patients. In bacteraemic patients, neuraxial, and particularly spinal, anaesthesia is not an absolute contraindication but serious consideration should be given to the benefit versus risk, and prophylactic antibiotics should be considered. In general, the number of disconnections of epidural catheters should be minimised, filters should be used, and in the case of unwitnessed accidental disconnection and contamination, the catheter should be removed. The duration of neuraxial catheterisation should be minimised with one large retrospective study finding that all abscesses occurred when epidural catheters were left in situ for longer than 72 h.

Cardiovascular Complications

Important cardiovascular complications range from hypotension and bradycardia to cardiovascular collapse. Cardiovascular collapse in the context of CNB may be due to anaphylaxis secondary to either the skin preparation or any drugs used, or alternatively a high or total spinal. The overall rate of cardiovascular collapse reported in the UK national audit project was 0.085 per 10,000 CNB procedures, reflecting six cases of cardiovascular collapse in over 700,000 patients, three of which followed spinal anaesthesia. Sudden cardiac arrest appears to be less likely with an epidural compared to spinal anaesthesia.

Bradycardia can occur if the block reaches sympathetic cardiac accelerator fibres at T1-T5. The reduction in preload can also result in a paradoxical reflex bradycardia mediated by sinus baroreceptors called the Bezold–Jarisch reflex. Associations with severe bradycardia (<40 bpm) include basal heart rate <60 bpm and male gender whilst for moderate bradycardia (40–50 bpm) young age, beta-blocker use and non-emergency surgery may be predictive.

Reducing Risk

Factors associated with hypotension in spinal anaesthesia can be seen in Table 4.2. There is little evidence that either preloading or co-loading with fluid reduces hypotension following spinal anaesthesia. Elderly patients may have a reduction in stroke volume after spinal anaesthesia with block heights of well below T5. Choosing as low a dose of LA as possible to minimise excessive block height is therefore important in this group of patients in particular whilst still ensuring adequate surgical coverage and duration. In fixed cardiac output states such as aortic stenosis where the heart is less able to compensate for the reduced systemic vascular resistance, spinal anaesthesia is relatively contraindicated. Combined spinal epidural anaesthesia may be more cardiovascularly stable in such cases, administering a low-dose spinal anaesthetic combined with epidural volume extension using either saline or LA to gradually extend the block height.

Table 4.2 Association of hypotension with spinal anaesthesia

Patient factors	Technique factors
Hypertension	Block height > T5
Age $\geq$ 40	Baseline systolic BP <120 mmHg
Obesity	Combined spinal and general anaesthesia
Emergency surgery	Interspace at or above L2/3 used
Chronic alcohol use	Phenylephrine added to spinal solution
Hypovolaemia	

Respiratory Complications

Respiratory complications may occur either as a result of neuraxially administered drugs, most commonly opioids, or the effects of a high block. Respiratory depression is centrally mediated, and follows either vascular uptake of neuraxial drug or direct rostral spread within the CSF. The incidence of respiratory depression secondary to neuraxial opioids depends on the route of administration, lipophilicity, and dose utilised.

Spinal bioavailability of opiates increases with decreasing lipid solubility, with hydrophilic agents having a slower onset of action, a longer duration and a higher risk of rostral spread. The peak effect of lipophilic drugs such as fentanyl occurs at 20–30 min, and there is little risk of respiratory depression after 2 h. Hydrophilic morphine conversely has a biphasic profile. Some systemic absorption occurs after 30–40 min with a second peak at 6 h, but there is still a risk of respiratory depression for up to 24 h. With intrathecal morphine doses under 1 mg, the reported incidence of respiratory depression ranges widely, in part due to varying definitions of respiratory depression, the population studied and the nature of surgery. Although higher figures have been reported, many studies report ranges between 0.02 and 3%.

The spread of epidural opioids is also governed by lipid solubility. Compared to lipophilic drugs, epidural morphine reaches the CSF more readily and in higher concentrations, with less being sequestered in epidural fat. Reported rates of respiratory depression after doses of up to 5 mg epidural morphine range from 0.59 to 2.8%.

Respiratory rate and sedation should always be monitored for at least 2 h following the administration of neuraxial lipophilic opioids, and 24 h for hydrophilic opioids. A reduction in oxygen saturation can be a late sign, particularly with supplemental oxygen usage. Treatment with opioid antagonists such as naloxone readily improves respiration.

Dyspnoea may also occur with progressively high levels of neuraxial block, where the intercostal muscles become increasingly affected. Respiratory arrest requiring intubation and ventilation may also occur with a total spinal.

Reducing Risk

Reducing the dose of morphine, or using lipophilic agents, minimises risk. Extra care should be exercised in groups that may be at increased risk such as patients with obstructive sleep apnoea, renal impairment, obese and elderly patients, or those given concurrent parenteral opiates. For many operative procedures, the optimal dose of intrathecal opioid which maximizes analgesia and minimizes the risk of respiratory depression remains unclear. There is good evidence, however, that respiratory depression is reduced with intrathecal morphine at doses below 0.3 mg. Liposomal epidural morphine appears to be more likely to cause respiratory depression compared to parenteral patient-controlled opiates.

Wrong Route of Injection

Inadvertent systemic injection of LA solution is possible during neuraxial techniques but is of more concern with epidurals due to the doses administered. This could either be during insertion, catheter migration intravascularly or wrong route of drug administration. One of the deaths in the UK national audit project was attributed to intravenous injection of LA solution as part of a CSE. Whilst using non-interchangeable connectors (e.g. NRFit) should prevent an epidural infusion being connected to an intravenous infusion, such systems remain no substitute for checking the appropriate drug is administered intrathecally, epidurally or intravenously. Administration of the wrong drug neuraxially, and intrathecally in particular, can be potentially catastrophic.

Peripheral Neuraxial Blockade

Complications of PNB may be divided into those that are generic, and those specific to individual blocks. Generic complications include neurological injury, infection, local anaesthetic toxicity (LAST), anaphylaxis and wrong-sided block. Vessel puncture and bleeding is a generic complication but this is not discussed in detail. Rather, we note that it is linked to both neurological damage and LAST and that whilst haemorrhagic complications may occur with any block, particular care must be taken with blocks targeting deep nerve structures, where manual compression cannot always be easily applied and vessels may be more difficult to visualise when using ultrasound (US) guidance. Complications specific to individual blocks depend on nearby structures but respiratory complications and organ damage are the most serious.

Generic Complications

Neurological

Neurological injury secondary to PNB ranges from transient 'postoperative neurological symptoms' (PONS) to permanent loss of nerve function. PONS appear to be frequent, with an incidence of up to 10% in the initial weeks following surgery. In most cases, however, symptoms resolve, with the rate at

12 months reported to be between 0 and 0.2%. Permanent injury is rare, with the risk believed to be between 1 and 5 per 10,000 PNBs. Calculating the exact incidence can be difficult as figures vary depending upon the definition of nerve injury and the quality of data collection, whilst in some cases it may also be difficult to establish the role of other potential causes of nerve injury such as intraoperative positioning, surgical traction, surgical trauma and tourniquet use. Reassuringly, retrospective data suggests rates of peripheral nerve injury after surgery are similar regardless of whether a PNB was administered or not. It must also be remembered that general anaesthesia is associated with peripheral nerve injuries, most commonly due to positioning.

Presentation depends on the target nerve or plexus involved and the severity of injury. PONS are primarily sensory in nature and typically include pain or paraesthesia although motor deficits are possible. The nature of injury may include one or more of the following: mechanical trauma, toxicity, ischaemic or inflammatory. These are summarised in turn below, followed by a general outline of risk mitigation.

Mechanical Trauma

There are two primary mechanisms whereby mechanical trauma may occur. Direct needle trauma is one possibility, but the more important risk appears to be a pressure-related effect secondary to the injection of LA into neural tissue. Whilst simply touching, and not even penetrating, the epineurium of a peripheral nerve has been shown to cause histological injury in animal models, there are many clinical studies whereby both intentional or inadvertent intraneural injection do not result in clinical injury. The key factor appears to be the precise location of the needle tip during an intraneural injection and any subsequent pressure effect secondary to injection. If the epineurium is penetrated, an intraneural injection may be either extra-/interfascicular (sub-epineural) or intrafascicular (sub-perineural). Intrafascicular injection results in more severe histological injury in animal models, even when saline is used. Injection into the less compliant intrafascicular space generates a higher pressure, and if intraneural pressure exceeds capillary perfusion pressure then nerve ischaemia may occur. Additional injury may occur if the perineurium ruptures due to a high-pressure injection or direct needle trauma.

Toxicity

Animal studies reveal that all local anaesthetics can be neurotoxic at clinical doses. Toxicity-related injury to peripheral nerves is related to LA concentration, duration of exposure and the type of LA, with bupivacaine being the most toxic. Neurotoxicity appears to result from DNA damage and interference with oxidative phosphorylation leading to apoptosis. Schwann cell death and demyelination are also to linked to LA exposure, whilst damage secondary to local ischaemia due to the intrinsic vasoconstrictor properties of some LAs is another possible mechanism. Fascicular contents are protected by the perineurium but if this layer is breached the exposure of axons to higher concentrations of LA can lead to neurotoxicity or inflammation (see below) and subsequent axonal or myelin degeneration.

Local anaesthetic adjuncts or preservatives may also be toxic. Adrenaline reduces blood flow, potentially worsening ischaemia whilst also prolonging exposure to LA by reducing systemic uptake. Dexamethasone displays some in vitro neurotoxicity albeit it is unclear if this is relevant clinically whilst alpha 2 agonists and the partial opiate agonist buprenorphine do not appear to be neurotoxic at clinical concentrations. Midazolam, ketamine and neostigmine appear to be neurotoxic, and given a lack of evidence of effectiveness these should not be used as additives.

Ischaemic

Nerve ischaemia may occur due to either LA or adrenaline-mediated vasoconstriction, or a pressure effect as described above. The use of a tourniquet can also contribute, whilst injury to the vasa nervorum or arterial supply and haemorrhage within the nerve sheath, or extraneural compression by local haematoma are further mechanisms. Haemorrhage and haematoma causing neurological deficit generally have a good prognosis with full recovery over 6–12 months common.

Inflammatory

Non-specific inflammation of peripheral nerves presenting with either sensory or motor involvement can occur after surgery. This post-surgical inflammatory neuropathy can mimic compressive or ischaemic nerve damage in both a focal or diffuse pattern and may occur local or distal to the surgical site. Inflammatory injury has been implicated in persistent phrenic nerve dysfunction after interscalene block for shoulder surgery. Subcutaneous tracking of sonographic gel along the needle path has also been reported to cause local inflammation.

Reducing Risk

Given the rarity of nerve damage there are no randomised studies to guide practice. General principles relate to avoiding intraneural injection and the method of nerve localisation, the choice of needle, and drug and patient selection.

Whilst intentional intraneural injection does not consistently result in injury, and unintentional intraneural injection without subsequent injury may be common, the consensus remains that breach of the epineurium and subsequent intraneural injection should be avoided. No single nerve localisation technique however has conclusively been shown to be superior in terms of avoiding intraneural injection and subsequently reducing nerve injury.

The traditional use of paraesthesia to detect nerves is now an uncommon technique. Paraesthesia during block performance is not always indicative of needle-nerve contact nor does it predict subsequent injury. Nevertheless, guidance in adults remains to perform blocks in awake patients, partly because if this warning sign occurs it may alert practitioners to stop further needle advancement or local anaesthetic injection.

When using peripheral nerve stimulator guidance, a motor response elicited with a stimulating current of <0.2 mA is highly specific for intraneural needle placement. The needle should be withdrawn before injection of LA, preventing pressure-related damage in addition to potential mechanical damage secondary to the intraneural needle tip. Sensitivity is low however as a motor response may not be produced even with intraneural needle placement.

Whilst ultrasound can reliably detect intraneural injection of volumes over 0.5 mL, the resolution makes it difficult to differentiate between intra- and extrafascicular intraneural injections. As with a nerve stimulator, however, the needle tip must already be intraneural to detect such a change; therefore, US does not necessarily prevent mechanical damage.

The pressure required to inject intrafascicularly is greater than that for extrafascicular injection. Subjective assessment of ease of injection is, however, unreliable. Injection pressure monitors can detect needle nerve contact and high injection pressures but there is no clinical data to suggest a reduction in harm. Furthermore, a high-pressure injection is not specific to intrafascicular injections alone. Nevertheless, although unproven it may be that the combination of 'triple monitoring' (i.e. ultrasound to observe for intraneural injection, nerve stimulation to detect possible intraneural needle tip position and pressure monitoring to detect possible high-pressure intrafascicular injection) offers the safest outcome by drawing on the benefits of all three techniques.

The choice of needle is important. Short bevelled (45° angle), 'blunt' needles are less likely to penetrate the epineurium and perineurium compared to a long bevelled (15° angle), sharper needle. However, if a fascicular breach does occur, the damage from a short bevelled needle appears to be worse, and with a longer recovery time. Severity of injury also increases with increasing needle diameter.

Finally, patient-related factors are important. A higher risk of injury theoretically exists in patients with pre-existing neurological impairment due to the 'double-crush' phenomenon. The prevailing theory is that axoplasmic flow is reduced where there is pre-existing disease, increasing the risk of complete cessation of flow and possible nerve injury after a subsequent (double) insult. Despite the 'crush' nomenclature, pre-existing pathology is not limited to compressive injuries and encompasses a vast range of clinical or subclinical neuropathies including metabolic, post-chemotherapy and auto-immune conditions. In diabetic neuropathy, the nerves may be more susceptible to LA due to chronic ischaemia, whilst via a similar mechanism smoking, hypertension and peripheral vascular disease have been proposed to increase risk.

Careful consideration should be given to the risks and benefits of PNB in patients who may be at higher risk of injury. In such circumstances, avoiding vasoconstrictor adjuncts such as adrenaline has been suggested, along with using the lowest concentration of LA possible. Care must also be taken in patients at risk due to coagulopathy or thrombocytopaenia whether due to disease or concomitant medications. The risk here varies depending on whether a PNB is superficial or deep, and guidance to inform practitioners about the timing of stopping anticoagulant medication for the different PNBs should be consulted.

Infectious

Infections relating to PNBs range from localised skin infections to abscesses and systemic sepsis. Incidence of localised infection is difficult to state accurately for single injection blocks although fatal necrotising fasciitis following a single shot axillary block has been reported. Whilst a significant number of continuous infusion perineural catheters may become colonized, the rate of actual infection varies between 0.25 and 3%, with rates generally increasing the longer catheters are left in situ. Abscesses following a continuous technique are rarer, with rates estimated at less than 1%.

Reducing Risk

Diabetes, immunosuppression and male sex are all risk factors for infection with a continuous catheter technique, whilst ICU admission has also been identified as an independent predictor. The duration of the infusion is also important, whereby beyond 48 h the risk of infection appears to increase. Femoral and axillary perineural catheters may also carry greater risk of infection. Catheter sites should be regularly inspected for signs of infection. As well as strict aseptic precautions during insertion, tunnelling the catheter or administering antibiotic prophylaxis may reduce infection.

Local Anaesthetic Systemic Toxicity

Despite advances in treatment, local anaesthetic systemic toxicity (LAST) still remains a potentially fatal complication of PNB. The reported incidence of LAST varies between 0.08 and 0.98 episodes per 1000 blocks. This wide range incorporates both minor and major symptoms of LAST but if restricted to major symptoms (seizure or cardiotoxicity) then the rate reduces to less than 0.37 per 1000 blocks.

Local anaesthetics primarily block axonal Na_V channels, therefore interrupting nerve action potential conduction. Na_V channels however are also abundant in the brain and heart, and if toxic levels of LA occur in these organs then neurological and cardiac symptoms may occur. Some of the consequences of LAST may also result from LA blockade of additional molecular targets such as potassium, calcium and sodium/potassium/ATPase channels as well as a variety of intracellular signalling and metabolic pathways.

Neurological symptoms generally present first, and as LA levels increase there is an initial excitatory phase of sensory or visual changes including a metallic taste and tinnitus, progressing to seizures followed finally by coma and respiratory arrest. Cardiovascular issues typically arise later and include hypotension due to the loss of regulation of peripheral vascular tone and negative inotropic effects. Impairment of conduction pathways can lead to arrhythmias with both brady and re-entrant tachyarrhythmias possible. In severe cases, cardiac arrest occurs. CNS presentation with seizures is more common, either alone or progressing to cardiovascular involvement. Whilst symptoms often occur within minutes of injection suggesting inadvertent intravascular injection, a significant number or presentations may be delayed by up to an hour.

Reducing Risk

The risks of LAST are related to the patient, the technique and the type of LA used. Patient risk factors include those where LA clearance may be impaired, where reduced protein binding occurs therefore increasing the free fraction of LA or where there are less LA storage reservoirs (most importantly muscle). At risk groups therefore include those at extremes of age (<6 months old and elderly), pregnancy, heart failure, renal failure, hepatic failure, pre-existing cardiac conduction defects and those with certain metabolic pathway deficiencies. In these groups, extra caution must therefore be applied and the dose reduced appropriately.

Technique and the type of PNB chosen also influence risk as these determine the dose of LA administered, local vascularity and the surface area for LA absorption all of which influence speed of uptake and peak plasma concentration. Historically, intercostal and interpleural blocks were associated with the highest plasma levels of LA. In some registries, the risk of LAST was higher with paravertebral block compared to upper limb which in turn was higher than lower limb PNB. More recently, fascial plane blocks have been recognised to represent a risk given large volumes of LA are injected into what are often vascular areas, and adding adrenaline has been suggested to reduce absorption. Whilst the addition of adrenaline may also serve as a marker of intravascular injection by increasing heart rate, this is not always reliable. Continuous catheter techniques also increase risk, with reports of presentation days later likely due to tissue uptake and systemic absorption of LA, or accumulation of active metabolites. Using ultrasound reduces the risk of LAST significantly, most likely by minimising vascular puncture and allowing smaller doses/volume of LA to be administered.

The choice of LA also influences risk. Each LA has a cardiotoxic/neurotoxic (CVS/CNS) ratio which is the dose required to cause cardiovascular collapse compared to that to cause seizures. A high ratio means less cardiotoxicity and thus a greater safety margin because CNS symptoms occur further in advance of cardiovascular symptoms, allowing more time to institute treatment. For this reason, levobupivacaine and ropivacaine, which are both single enantiomers, are favoured over bupivacaine. LAST continues to occur and therefore prevention remains important, noting that the traditional mg/kg recommended doses vary amongst texts and countries, and that patient risk factors and the technique of administration are critical.

Anaphylaxis

True anaphylaxis to LA is extremely rare. In one case series of 162 peri-operative reactions referred over 10 years to an allergy clinic none were due to LA. In another series, only two confirmed cases were found from 402 suspected reactions over 20 years. These patients are invariably exposed to several potential allergens and many are found to have a separate, non-LA allergen, most commonly chlorhexidine followed in turn by antibiotics. Allergies to LA additives and preservatives are similarly rare. Ester LAs are thought to be more likely to be allergenic than amides.

Wrong Site Block

The overall incidence of wrong site block has been estimated at 4 per 10,000 blocks. The 'Stop Before You Block' (SBYB) campaign was launched in 2011, but despite this, events continue to occur at the same rate and the impact of SBYB has been called into question. Similar systems exist in Australia and the USA. Contributing factors include distractions, patient positioning, miscommunication as well as delay between performing checks/pauses and the actual block.

Block-Specific Complications

Pneumothorax

Pneumothorax remains a risk in certain brachial plexus block techniques due to the proximity of the lung apex and pleura, particularly supraclavicular and the more medial infraclavicular block approaches. Rates have historically been as high as around 6% following supraclavicular block but whilst it has been suggested that ultrasound should increase safety, cases still exist in the literature. The rate of incidence with ultrasound has been estimated to be between 0.4–0.6 per 1000 blocks for ultrasound-guided supra- and infraclavicular blocks although this may be an underestimate. Other blocks adjacent to the thoracic cavity such as intercostal or paravertebral blocks are a recognised risk. Whilst no case reports of pneumothorax following PECs or serratus anterior plane blocks exist, one has recently been published following the erector spinae plane block.

Reducing Risk

Knowledge of anatomy to guide needle placement during both landmark and US-guided blocks, and meticulous needle tip visualisation either using direct vision or surrogate markers when using US are paramount. However, iatrogenic pneumothoraces have still been reported despite the use of US guidance in experienced hands. Where pneumothorax would be catastrophic (e.g. patients with a contralateral pneumonectomy), serious consideration should be given to risk, benefit and the alternatives to undertaking any block where this is a possibility.

Phrenic Nerve Blockade

Phrenic nerve blockade occurs due to local anaesthetic spread from proximal brachial plexus blocks, especially interscalene blocks. Whilst ultrasound guidance has allowed for smaller volumes of LA to be injected, the incidence of phrenic nerve blockade may still approach 100% for interscalene blocks and 50% for supraclavicular blocks. The resulting hemi-diaphragmatic paralysis reduces FVC and FEV1 volumes by approximately 25% but in the majority of patients this is well-tolerated. A small rise in respiratory rate or mild fall in oxygen saturations can occur which may be managed with supplementary oxygen if necessary until the block resolves. In patients with pre-existing lung pathology or who are severely obese, ipsilateral hemidiaphragmatic paresis must be more carefully considered. Non-invasive ventilation has been used in such patients where the aim has been to avoid general anaesthesia and perform surgery under PNB anaesthesia. Persistent phrenic nerve palsy after interscalene block has been described, possibly due to either inflammation secondary to LA myotoxicity or pressure ischaemia.

Reducing Risk

Using a dose of between 5 and 10 mL retains the post-operative analgesic benefits whilst reducing the incidence of phrenic nerve palsy to approximately 50%. Reducing the concentration of LA, independent of volume, or using ultrasound compared to nerve stimulator guidance also reduces the incidence of phrenic nerve blockade, as does injecting 'extrafascially' slightly further from the nerves (also termed 'periplexus'). Where there is concern about lung function, alternative 'phrenic sparing' analgesic techniques such as suprascapular nerve blocks may be useful though these alone, even in combination with blockade of the axillary nerve, cannot provide complete anaesthesia for shoulder surgery.

Inadvertent Neuraxial Blockade or Spinal Cord Injury

Total spinal blocks have been reported after interscalene, lumbar plexus and paravertebral blocks sometimes resulting in cardiac arrest. Experiments show that proximal flow of LA reaching the spinal cord is possible with high-pressure intrafascicular injections. Alternatively, a needle may inadvertently be placed within the subarachnoid space during a PNB. There are also case reports of catastrophic cervical cord damage after interscalene blocks. Whilst direct visualisation with ultrasound should in theory reduce such complications, it must not be thought of as a panacea.

Inadvertent Organ Damage

Any structure near to, or indeed distal from, a nerve may be punctured with a long enough needle. In abdominal wall blocks, the needle may breach the peritoneum and puncture organs, with case reports of liver and bowel trauma existing as well as haematomas. In studies of the landmark ilioinguinal or TAP block techniques, the incidence of entering the peritoneal cavity has been reported to be as high as 18% in paediatric practice. Direct needle trauma to the renal system has also been reported after both lumbar plexus blocks and TAP blocks. As with all complications, ultrasound will not necessarily eliminate such problems given the element of operator error, although it has been shown to reduce the risk of inadvertent peritoneal puncture during TAP block.

Suggested Reading

Absalom AR, Martinelli G, Scott NB. Spinal cord injury caused by direct damage by local anaesthetic infiltration needle. Br J Anaesth. 2001;87:512–5.

Ahn KS, Kopp SL, Watson JC, Scott KP, Trousdale RT, Hebl JR. Postsurgical inflammatory neuropathy. Reg Anesth Pain Med. 2011;36:403–5.

Alakkad H, Naeeni A, Chan VWS, Abbas S, Oh J, Ami N, Ng J, Gardam M, Brull R. Infection related to ultrasound-guided single-injection peripheral nerve blockade: a decade of experience at Toronto Western hospital. Reg Anesth Pain Med. 2015;40:82–4.

Altermatt FR, Cummings TJ, Auten KM, Baldwin MF, Belknap SW, Reynolds JD. Ultrasonographic appearance of intraneural injections in the porcine model. Reg Anesth Pain Med. 2010;35:203–6.

American Society of Anesthesiologists Task Force on Neuraxial Opioids, Horlocker TT, Burton AW, Connis RT, Hughes SC, Nickinovich DG, Palmer CM, Pollock JE, Rathmell JP, Rosenquist RW, et al. Practice guidelines for the prevention, detection, and management of respiratory depression associated with neuraxial opioid administration. Anesthesiology. 2009;110:218–30.

Anderson TL, Morris JM, Wald JT, Kotsenas AL. Imaging appearance of advanced chronic adhesive arachnoiditis: a retrospective review. AJR Am J Roentgenol. 2017;209:648–55.

Anonymous. Practice advisory for the prevention, diagnosis, and management of infectious complications associated with neuraxial techniques: an updated report by the American Society of Anesthesiologists Task Force on infectious complications associated with neuraxial techniques and the American Society of Regional Anesthesia and Pain Medicine. Anesthesiology. 2017;126:585–601.

Arevalo-Rodriguez I, Muñoz L, Godoy-Casasbuenas N, Ciapponi A, Arevalo JJ, Boogaard S, Roqué I, Figuls M. Needle gauge and tip designs for preventing post-dural puncture headache (PDPH). Cochrane Database Syst Rev. 2017;4:CD010807.

Aromaa U, Lahdensuu M, Cozanitis DA. Severe complications associated with epidural and spinal anaesthesias in Finland 1987-1993. A study based on patient insurance claims [see comment]. Acta Anaesthesiol Scand. 1997;41:445–52.

Auroy Y, Benhamou D, Bargues L, Ecoffey C, Falissard B, Mercier FJ, Bouaziz H, Samii K. Major complications of regional anesthesia in France: the SOS Regional Anesthesia Hotline Service. Anesthesiology. 2002;97:1274–80.

Bai JW, Singh M, Short A, Bozak D, Chung F, Chan VWS, Bhatia A, Perlas A. Intrathecal morphine and pulmonary complications after arthroplasty in patients with obstructive sleep apnea: a retrospective cohort study. Anesthesiology. 2020;132:702–12.

Barrington MJ, Kluger R. Ultrasound guidance reduces the risk of local anesthetic systemic toxicity following peripheral nerve blockade. Reg Anesth Pain Med. 2013;38:289–99.

Barrington MJ, Watts SA, Gledhill SR, Thomas RD, Said SA, Snyder GL, Tay VS, Jamrozik K. Preliminary results of the Australasian Regional Anaesthesia Collaboration: a prospective audit of more than 7000 peripheral nerve and plexus blocks for neurologic and other complications. Reg Anesth Pain Med. 2009;34:534–41.

Basurto Ona X, Osorio D, Bonfill Cosp X. Drug therapy for treating post-dural puncture headache. Cochrane Database Syst Rev. 2015;CD007887

Bateman BT, Mhyre JM, Ehrenfeld J, Kheterpal S, Abbey KR, Argalious M, Berman MF, Jacques PS, Levy W, Loeb RG, et al. The risk and outcomes of epidural hematomas after perioperative and obstetric epidural catheterization: a report from the Multicenter Perioperative Outcomes Group Research Consortium. Anesth Analg. 2013;116:1380–5.

Benson JS. U.S. Food and Drug Administration safety alert: cauda equina syndrome associated with use of small-bore catheters in continuous spinal anesthesia. AANA J. 1992;60:223.

Bogod D. The sting in the tail: antiseptics and the neuraxis revisited. Anaesthesia. 2012;67:1305–9.

Bomberg H, Bayer I, Wagenpfeil S, Kessler P, Wulf H, Standl T, Gottschalk A, Döffert J, Hering W, Birnbaum J, et al. Prolonged catheter use and infection in regional anesthesia: a retrospective registry analysis. Anesthesiology. 2018;128:764–73.

Bos EME, Haumann J, de Quelerij M, Vandertop WP, Kalkman CJ, Hollmann MW, Lirk P. Haematoma and abscess after neuraxial anaesthesia: a review of 647 cases. Br J Anaesth. 2018;120:693–704.

Brull R, Hadzic A, Reina MA, Barrington MJ. Pathophysiology and etiology of nerve injury following peripheral nerve blockade. Reg Anesth Pain Med. 2015;40:479–90.

Buddeberg BS, Bandschapp O, Girard T. Post-dural puncture headache. Minerva Anestesiol. 2019;85:543–53.

Carpenter RL, Caplan RA, Brown DL, Stephenson C, Wu R. Incidence and risk factors for side effects of spinal anesthesia. Anesthesiology. 1992;76:906–16.

Cook TM, Counsell D, Wildsmith JAW, Royal College of Anaesthetists Third National Audit Project. Major complications of central neuraxial block: report on the Third National Audit Project of the Royal College of Anaesthetists. Br J Anaesth. 2009;102:179–90.

Dahan A, Aarts L, Smith TW. Incidence, reversal, and prevention of opioid-induced respiratory depression. Anesthesiology. 2010;112:226–38.

Desai N, Albrecht E, El-Boghdadly K. Perineural adjuncts for peripheral nerve block. BJA Educ. 2019;19:276–82.

Di Gregorio G, Neal JM, Rosenquist RW, Weinberg GL. Clinical presentation of local anesthetic systemic toxicity: a review of published cases, 1979 to 2009. Reg Anesth Pain Med. 2010;35:181–7.

Drummond JC. Blood pressure and the brain: how low can you go? Anesth Analg. 2019;128:759–71.

El-Boghdadly K, Chin KJ, Chan VWS. Phrenic nerve palsy and regional anesthesia for shoulder surgery. Anesthesiology. 2017;127:173–91.

El-Boghdadly K, Pawa A, Chin KJ. Local anesthetic systemic toxicity: current perspectives. Local Reg Anesth. 2018;11:35–44.

Etezadi F, Karimi Yarandi K, Ahangary A, Shokri H, Imani F, Safari S, Khajavi MR. The effect of needle type, duration of surgery and position of the patient on the risk of transient neurologic symptoms. Anesth Pain Med. 2013;2:154–8.

Evron S, Gurstieva V, Ezri T, Gladkov V, Shopin S, Herman A, Sidi A, Weitzman S. Transient neurological symptoms after isobaric subarachnoid anesthesia with 2% lidocaine: the impact of needle type. Anesth Analg. 2007;105:1494–9, table of contents.

Farber SJ, Saheb-Al-Zamani M, Zieske L, Laurido-Soto O, Bery A, Hunter D, Johnson P, Mackinnon SE. Peripheral nerve injury after local anesthetic injection. Anesth Analg. 2013;117:731–9.

Ferré F, Mastantuono J-M, Martin C, Ferrier A, Marty P, Laumonerie P, Bonnevialle N, Minville V. [Hemidiaphragmatic paralysis after ultrasound-guided supraclavicular block: a prospective cohort study]. Rev Bras Anestesiol. 2019;69:580–6.

Forget P, Borovac JA, Thackeray EM, Pace NL. Transient neurological symptoms (TNS) following spinal anaesthesia with lidocaine versus other local anaesthetics in adult surgical patients: a network meta-analysis. Cochrane Database Syst Rev. 2019;12:CD003006.

Fredrickson MJ, Kilfoyle DH. Neurological complication analysis of 1000 ultrasound guided peripheral nerve blocks for elective orthopaedic surgery: a prospective study. Anaesthesia. 2009;64:836–44.

Furness G, Reilly MP, Kuchi S. An evaluation of ultrasound imaging for identification of lumbar intervertebral level: forum. Anaesthesia. 2002;57:277–80.

Gadsden JC, Lindenmuth DM, Hadzic A, Xu D, Somasundarum L, Flisinski KA. Lumbar plexus block using high-pressure injection leads to contralateral and epidural spread. Anesthesiology. 2008;109:683–8.

Gadsden J, Gratenstein K, Hadzic A. Intraneural injection and peripheral nerve injury. Int Anesthesiol Clin. 2010;48:107–15.

Gadsden J, Latmore M, Levine DM, Robinson A. High opening injection pressure is associated with needle-nerve and needle-fascia contact during femoral nerve block. Reg Anesth Pain Med. 2016;41:50–5.

Ganem EM, Vianna PT, Marques M, Castiglia YM, Vane LA. Neurotoxicity of subarachnoid hyperbaric bupivacaine in dogs. Reg Anesth. 1996;21:234–8.

Gehling M, Tryba M. Risks and side-effects of intrathecal morphine combined with spinal anaesthesia: a meta-analysis. Anaesthesia. 2009;64:643–51. https://doi.org/10.1111/j.1365-2044.2008.05817.x.

Gilbar P. Inadvertent intrathecal administration of vincristine: has anything changed? J Oncol Pharm Pract. 2012;18:155–7.

Gitman M, Barrington MJ. Local anesthetic systemic toxicity: a review of recent case reports and registries. Reg Anesth Pain Med. 2018;43:124–30.

Guglielminotti J, Landau R, Li G. Major neurologic complications associated with postdural puncture headache in obstetrics: a retrospective cohort study. Anesth Analg. 2019;129:1328–36.

Guidelines for the Management of Major Regional Analgesia Australian and New Zealand College of Anaesthetists (ANZCA). http://www.anzca.edu.au/documents/ps03-2014-guidelines-for-the-management-of-major-r.pdf. Accessed 3 May 2020.

Hadzic A, Dilberovic F, Shah S, Kulenovic A, Kapur E, Zaciragic A, Cosovic E, Vuckovic I, Divanovic K-A, Mornjakovic Z, et al. Combination of intraneural injection and high injection pressure leads to fascicular injury and neurologic deficits in dogs. Reg Anesth Pain Med. 2004;29:417–23.

Hartmann B, Junger A, Klasen J, Benson M, Jost A, Banzhaf A, Hempelmann G. The incidence and risk factors for hypotension after spinal anesthesia induction: an analysis with automated data collection. Anesth Analg. 2002;94:1521–9.

Hewson DW, Bedforth NM, Hardman JG. Spinal cord injury arising in anaesthesia practice. Anaesthesia. 2018;73(Suppl 1):43–50.

Hofhuizen C, Lemson J, Snoeck M, Scheffer G-J. Spinal anesthesia-induced hypotension is caused by a decrease in stroke volume in elderly patients. Local Reg Anesth. 2019;12:19–26.

Hogan Q. Anatomy of spinal anesthesia: some old and new findings. Reg Anesth Pain Med. 1998;23:340–3. https://doi.org/10.1016/s1098-7339(98)90002-5.

Hopping M, Merry AF, Pandit JJ. Exploring performance of, and attitudes to, stop- and mock-before-you-block in preventing wrong-side blocks. Anaesthesia. 2018;73:421–7. https://doi.org/10.1111/anae.14167.

Horlocker TT, Vandermeuelen E, Kopp SL, Gogarten W, Leffert LR, Benzon HT. Regional anesthesia in the patient receiving antithrombotic or thrombolytic therapy: American Society of Regional Anesthesia and Pain Medicine evidence-based guidelines (fourth edition). Reg Anesth Pain Med. 2018;43:263–309.

Jeng CL, Torrillo TM, Rosenblatt MA. Complications of peripheral nerve blocks. Br J Anaesth. 2010;105(Suppl 1):i97–107.

Karasawa M, Yokouchi K, Kawagishi K, Moriizumi T, Fukushima N. Effects of repeated nerve injuries at different time intervals on functional recovery and nerve innervation. J Clin Neurosci. 2018;48:185–90.

Koning MV, Klimek M, Rijs K, Stolker RJ, Heesen MA. Intrathecal hydrophilic opioids for abdominal surgery: a meta-analysis, meta-regression, and trial sequential analysis. Br J Anaesth. 2020;125:358–72.

Kvisselgaard AD, Krøigaard M, Mosbech HF, Garvey LH. No cases of perioperative allergy to local anaesthetics in the Danish Anaesthesia Allergy Centre. Acta Anaesthesiol Scand. 2017;61:149–55.

Lee JE, George RB, Habib AS. Spinal-induced hypotension: incidence, mechanisms, prophylaxis, and management: summarizing 20 years of research. Best Pract Res Clin Anaesthesiol. 2017;31:57–68.

Lee SI, Sandhu S, Djulbegovic B, Mhaskar RS. Impact of spinal needle type on postdural puncture headache among women undergoing cesarean section surgery under spinal anesthesia: a meta-analysis. J Evid Based Med. 2018;11:136–44.

Lesser JB, Sanborn KV, Valskys R, Kuroda M. Severe bradycardia during spinal and epidural anesthesia recorded by an anesthesia information management system. Anesthesiology. 2003;99:859–66.

Lirk P, Messner H, Deibl M, Mitterschiffthaler G, Colvin J, Steger B, Rieder J, Keller C. Accuracy in estimating the correct intervertebral space level during lumbar, thoracic and cervical epidural anaesthesia. Acta Anaesthesiol Scand. 2004;48:347–9.

Liu H, Tariq R, Liu GL, Yan H, Kaye AD. Inadvertent intrathecal injections and best practice management. Acta Anaesthesiol Scand. 2017;61:11–22.

Macdonald A, Chatrath P, Spector T, Ellis H. Level of termination of the spinal cord and the dural sac: a magnetic resonance study. Clin Anat. 1999;12:149–52.

Management Of Severe Local Anaesthetic Toxicity. Association of Anaesthetists. https://anaesthetists.org/Home/Resources-publications/Guidelines/Management-of-severe-local-anaesthetic-toxicity. Accessed 29 May 2020.

McDermott G, Korba E, Mata U, Jaigirdar M, Narayanan N, Boylan J, Conlon N. Should we stop doing blind transversus abdominis plane blocks? Br J Anaesth. 2012;108:499–502.

McNicol ED, Ferguson MC, Hudcova J. Patient controlled opioid analgesia versus non-patient controlled opioid analgesia for postoperative pain. Cochrane Database Syst Rev. 2015; https://www.cochranelibrary.com/cdsr/doi/10.1002/14651858.CD003348.pub3/abstract

Membership of the Working Party, Campbell JP, Plaat F, Checketts MR, Bogod D, Tighe S, Moriarty A, Koerner R. Safety guideline: skin antisepsis for central neuraxial blockade: Association of Anaesthetists of Great Britain and Ireland Obstetric Anaesthetists' Association Regional Anaesthesia UK Association of Paediatric Anaes. Anaesthesia. 2014;69:1279–86.

Meylan N, Elia N, Lysakowski C, Tramèr MR. Benefit and risk of intrathecal morphine without local anaesthetic in patients undergoing major surgery: meta-analysis of randomized trials. Br J Anaesth. 2009;102:156–67.

Miranda P, Corvetto MA, Altermatt FR, Araneda A, Echevarría GC, Cortínez LI. Levobupivacaine absorption pharmacokinetics with and without epinephrine during TAP block: analysis of doses based on the associated risk of local anaesthetic toxicity. Eur J Clin Pharmacol. 2016;72:1221–7.

Moen V, Dahlgren N, Irestedt L. Severe neurological complications after central neuraxial blockades in Sweden 1990-1999. Anesthesiology. 2004;101:950–9.

Mulroy MF, Weller RS, Liguori GA. A checklist for performing regional nerve blocks. Reg Anesth Pain Med. 2014;39:195–9.

Neal JM. Ultrasound-guided regional anesthesia and patient safety: update of an evidence-based analysis. Reg Anesth Pain Med. 2016;41:195–204.

Neal JM, Bernards CM, Butterworth JF 4th, Di Gregorio G, Drasner K, Hejtmanek MR, Mulroy MF, Rosenquist RW, Weinberg GL. ASRA practice advisory on local anesthetic systemic toxicity. Reg Anesth Pain Med. 2010;35:152–61.

Neal JM, Barrington MJ, Brull R, Hadzic A, Hebl JR, Horlocker TT, Huntoon MA, Kopp SL, Rathmell JP, Watson JC. The second ASRA practice advisory on neurologic complications associated with regional anesthesia and pain medicine: executive summary 2015. Reg Anesth Pain Med. 2015a;40:401–30.

Neal JM, Kopp SL, Pasternak JJ, Lanier WL, Rathmell JP. Anatomy and pathophysiology of spinal cord injury associated with regional anesthesia and pain medicine: 2015 update. Reg Anesth Pain Med. 2015b;40:506–25.

Neal JM, Brull R, Horn J-L, Liu SS, McCartney CJL, Perlas A, Salinas FV, Tsui BC-H. The second American Society of Regional Anesthesia and Pain Medicine evidence-based medicine assessment of ultrasound-guided regional anesthesia: executive summary. Reg Anesth Pain Med. 2016;41:181–94.

Neal JM, Barrington MJ, Fettiplace MR, Gitman M, Memtsoudis SG, Mörwald EE, Rubin DS, Weinberg G. The third American Society of Regional Anesthesia and Pain Medicine practice advisory on local anesthetic systemic toxicity: executive summary 2017. Reg Anesth Pain Med. 2018;43:113–23.

Nseir S, Pronnier P, Soubrier S, Onimus T, Saulnier F, Mathieu D, Durocher A. Fatal streptococcal necrotizing fasciitis as a complication of axillary brachial plexus block. Br J Anaesth. 2004;92:427–9.

Partridge BL. The effects of local anesthetics and epinephrine on rat sciatic nerve blood flow. Anesthesiology. 1991;75:243–50.

Patel S, Robertson B, McConachie I. Catastrophic drug errors involving tranexamic acid administered during spinal anaesthesia. Anaesthesia. 2019;74:904–14. https://doi.org/10.1111/anae.14662.

Perez-Castro R, Patel S, Garavito-Aguilar ZV, Rosenberg A, Recio-Pinto E, Zhang J, Blanck TJJ, Xu F. Cytotoxicity of local anesthetics in human neuronal cells. Anesth Analg. 2009;108:997–1007.

Perlas A, Niazi A, McCartney C, Chan V, Xu D, Abbas S. The sensitivity of motor response to nerve stimulation and paresthesia for nerve localization as evaluated by ultrasound. Reg Anesth Pain Med. 2006;31:445–50.

Perlas A, Lobo G, Lo N, Brull R, Chan VWS, Karkhanis R. Ultrasound-guided supraclavicular block: outcome of 510 consecutive cases. Reg Anesth Pain Med. 2009;34:171–6.

Perlas A, Chaparro LE, Chin KJ. Lumbar neuraxial ultrasound for spinal and epidural anesthesia: a systematic review and meta-analysis. Reg Anesth Pain Med. 2016;41:251–60.

Pitkänen MT, Aromaa U, Cozanitis DA, Förster JG. Serious complications associated with spinal and epidural anaesthesia in Finland from 2000 to 2009. Acta Anaesthesiol Scand. 2013;57:553–64.

Pollock JE, Burkhead D, Neal JM, Liu SS, Friedman A, Stephenson C, Polissar NL. Spinal nerve function in five volunteers experiencing transient neurologic symptoms after lidocaine subarachnoid anesthesia. Anesth Analg. 2000;90:658–65.

Renes SH, Rettig HC, Gielen MJ, Wilder-Smith OH, van Geffen GJ. Ultrasound-guided low-dose interscalene brachial plexus block reduces the incidence of hemidiaphragmatic paresis. Reg Anesth Pain Med. 2009;34:498–502.

Reynolds F. Damage to the conus medullaris following spinal anaesthesia. Anaesthesia. 2001;56:238–47.

Riazi S, Carmichael N, Awad I, Holtby RM, McCartney CJL. Effect of local anaesthetic volume (20 vs 5 ml) on the efficacy and respiratory consequences of ultrasound-guided interscalene brachial plexus block. Br J Anaesth. 2008;101:549–56.

Rigler ML, Drasner K, Krejcie TC, Yelich SJ, Scholnick FT, DeFontes J, Bohner D. Cauda equina syndrome after continuous spinal anesthesia. Anesth Analg. 1991;72:275–81.

Rosero EB, Joshi GP. Nationwide incidence of serious complications of epidural analgesia in the United States. Acta Anaesthesiol Scand. 2016;60:810–20.

Russell R, Laxton C, Lucas DN, Niewiarowski J, Scrutton M, Stocks G. Treatment of obstetric post-dural puncture headache. Part 2: epidural blood patch. Int J Obstet Anesth. 2019;38:104–18.

Safe Anaesthesia Liaison Group. Wrong site blocks during surgery. 2011. https://www.accs.ac.uk/system/files/CSQ-PS-10-wrong-site-block.pdf. Accessed 15 June 2020.

Selander D, Sjöstrand J. Longitudinal spread of intraneurally injected local anesthetics. An experimental study of the initial neural distribution following intraneural injections. Acta Anaesthesiol Scand. 1978;22:622–34.

Shelton C, White S. Anaesthesia for hip fracture repair. BJA Educ. 2020;20:142–9.

Sinha AC, Cheung AT. Spinal cord protection and thoracic aortic surgery. Curr Opin Anaesthesiol. 2010;23:95–102.

Sites BD, Taenzer AH, Herrick MD, Gilloon C, Antonakakis J, Richins J, Beach ML. Incidence of local anesthetic systemic toxicity and postoperative neurologic symptoms associated with 12,668 ultrasound-guided nerve blocks: an analysis from a prospective clinical registry. Reg Anesth Pain Med. 2012;37:478–82.

Steinfeldt T, Werner T, Nimphius W, Wiesmann T, Kill C, Müller H-H, Wulf H, Graf J. Histological analysis after peripheral nerve puncture with pencil-point or Tuohy needletip. Anesth Analg. 2011;112:465–70.

Sultan P, Gutierrez MC, Carvalho B. Neuraxial morphine and respiratory depression: finding the right balance. Drugs. 2011;71:1807–19.

Trautmann A, Goebeler M, Stoevesandt J. Twenty years' experience with anaphylaxis-like reactions to local anesthetics: genuine allergy is rare. J Allergy Clin Immunol Pract. 2018;6:2051–2058.e1.

Tsai TP, Vuckovic I, Dilberovic F, Obhodzas M, Kapur E, Divanovic K-A, Hadzic A. Intensity of the stimulating current may not be a reliable indicator of intraneural needle placement. Reg Anesth Pain Med. 2008;33:207–10.

Tsui BCH, Armstrong K. Can direct spinal cord injury occur without paresthesia? A report of delayed spinal cord injury after epidural placement in an awake patient. Anesth Analg. 2005;101:1212–4, table of contents.

Upton AR, McComas AJ. The double crush in nerve entrapment syndromes. Lancet. 1973;2:359–62.

Weintraud M, Marhofer P, Bösenberg A, Kapral S, Willschke H, Felfernig M, Kettner S. Ilioinguinal/iliohypogastric blocks in children: where do we administer the local anesthetic without direct visualization? Anesth Analg. 2008;106:89–93, table of contents.

Weisman RS, Bhavsar NP, Schuster KA, Gebhard RE. Evaluation of the B-Smart manometer and the CompuFlo computerized injection pump technology for accurate needle-tip injection pressure measurement during peripheral nerve blockade. Reg Anesth Pain Med. 2019;44:86–90.

Werdehausen R, Fazeli S, Braun S, Hermanns H, Essmann F, Hollmann MW, Bauer I, Stevens MF. Apoptosis induction by different local anaesthetics in a neuroblastoma cell line. Br J Anaesth. 2009;103:711–8.

Williams BA, Hough KA, Tsui BYK, Ibinson JW, Gold MS, Gebhart GF. Neurotoxicity of adjuvants used in perineural anesthesia and analgesia in comparison with ropivacaine. Reg Anesth Pain Med. 2011;36:225–30.

Working Party: Association of Anaesthetists of Great Britain & Ireland, Obstetric Anaesthetists' Association, and Regional Anaesthesia UK. Regional anaesthesia and patients with abnormalities of coagulation: the Association of Anaesthetists of Great Britain & Ireland The Obstetric Anaesthetists' Association Regional Anaesthesia UK. Anaesthesia. 2013;68:966–72.

Yajnik M, Kou A, Mudumbai SC, Walters TL, Howard SK, Edward Kim T, Mariano ER. Peripheral nerve blocks are not associated with increased risk of perioperative peripheral nerve injury in a Veterans Affairs inpatient surgical population. Reg Anesth Pain Med. 2019;44:81–5.

Yang S, Abrahams MS, Hurn PD, Grafe MR, Kirsch JR. Local anesthetic Schwann cell toxicity is time and concentration dependent. Reg Anesth Pain Med. 2011;36:444–51.

Zorrilla-Vaca A, Mathur V, Wu CL, Grant MC. The impact of spinal needle selection on postdural puncture headache: a meta-analysis and metaregression of randomized studies. Reg Anesth Pain Med. 2018;43:502–8.

Local Anesthetic Systemic Toxicity

5

Marina Gitman, Kasha Bornstein, Alessandra Della Porta, Ayden Zarkhah, and Guy Weinberg

Contents

Introduction

Optimizing patient safety during regional anesthesia requires awareness of current best practices in managing local anesthetic systemic toxicity (LAST) including how to recognize and treat this potentially life-threatening complication and, optimally, how to prevent it. Like all rare events, there is a tendency to underestimate the likelihood of an occurrence or undervalue its impact on personal practice. However, LAST occurs with sufficient frequency that a busy regionalist can expect to experience an event more than once in the course of a career. Interestingly, as practice changes the clinical presentation, settings, and context of LAST, the range of places it occurs and forms it can take also evolve. As a result, we are continually revising our understanding of the range of patient features and comorbidities that lower the threshold for LAST—identifying such patients is an important step in mitigating the risk. An increasing fraction of published cases involve local anesthetics administered by non-anesthesiologists indicating that it is important for us as consultants with expertise in the topic to educate our colleagues on how best to manage and prevent LAST. Working to increase awareness of the problem outside our specialty will reduce patient risk. In sum, educating ourselves, our colleagues, and others caring for patients at risk for LAST will contribute to improving patient safety overall.

M. Gitman · A. Zarkhah · G. Weinberg (✉)
Department of Anesthesiology, University of Illinois at Chicago, Chicago, IL, USA
e-mail: guyw@uic.edu

K. Bornstein · A. Della Porta
Department of Medical Education, University of Miami Medical School, Miami, USA

D. Jankovic, P. Peng (eds.), *Regional Nerve Blocks in Anesthesia and Pain Therapy*,
https://doi.org/10.1007/978-3-030-88727-8_5

Mechanisms

Local anesthetics are small molecules with both polar and nonpolar features making them at once both hydrophilic and lipophilic. This amphipathic nature renders them able to penetrate cells and interact with (read, alter, or inhibit) a wide range of molecules and pathways. The ability to block voltage-gated sodium channel is responsible for the main clinical benefit of local anesthetics; however, their interaction with systems responsible for a variety of key cellular ionotropic and metabotropic signals as well as energy transduction can also contribute to the pathophysiological effects we recognize clinically as LAST. The specific clinical features of LAST provide a clue in identifying oxidative phosphorylation as one of the most important of the potential "targets of toxicity." The predominance of alterations in central nervous system and cardiac function in the toxidrome of LAST comports with this view given that these tissues are highly intolerant of anaerobic metabolism. When both are seen together, they provide a signature of mitochondrial dysfunction. Bupivacaine, a highly lipophilic local anesthetic that is well-known for its potential to produce cardiac toxicity impairs hydrogen-electron transport, carnitine-dependent fatty acid uptake, adenosine triphosphate (ATP) synthase, and formation of the proton-motive force, four key functions of the inner mitochondrial membrane necessary for ATP synthesis. It is plausible that the resulting depletion of tissue ATP is responsible for the organs specifically targeted in LAST (brain and heart) and the resulting signs and symptoms. This can also explain why LAST is traditionally viewed as resistant to standard resuscitation measures since vasopressor therapy alone does not address underlying tissue toxicity or cellular dysfunction including those related to impaired ATP synthesis.

Incidence

Despite technological advances such as ultrasound-guided regional anesthesia and patient safety efforts in the form of practice guidelines, recent analyses of large administrative databases indicate the incidence of LAST has not substantially changed over the past 20 years from the millennial benchmark of 1 per 1000 nerve blocks reported by Mulroy et al. in 2002. Rubin et al. and Morwald et al. interrogated different databases for surrogate markers of LAST that together included more than 900,000 patients having orthopedic procedures with the benefit of regional anesthesia. These studies each identified a rate of 1.8 LAST events per 1000 nerve blocks. This incidence is likely an underestimation as it does not include other causes of LAST or events that are not captured due to misdiagnosis or recognition failure. Compared with other rare events such as malignant hyperthermia (approximately 1 per 50,000 general anesthetics), one can conclude that while rare, LAST is not so rare that we can let down our collective guard. Currently, the reported mortality rate of LAST is anywhere from 4 to 10% (see Table 5.1).

Table 5.1 Clinical features of LAST described in published, peer-reviewed case reports

Date range of case reports				
Presenting features	10/1979–10/2209 93 cases	03/2010–03/2014 67 cases	01/2014–11/2016 47 cases	12/2016–05/2020 36 cases
Providers	Not reported	Anesthesiologists 65%	Anesthesiologists 49%	Anesthesiologists 50%
Setting	Not reported	Hospital 81% OR 69%	Hospital 80% OR 54%	Hospital 61% OR 68%
Patients	<16 y/o—16% >60 y/o—29%	<16 y/o—30% >60 y/o—20%	<20 y/o—53% >70 y/o—9%	<5 y/o—6% >65 y/o—30%
Route of administration	Neuraxial—33% PNBs—30%	Neuraxial—16% PNBs—23% Field blocks—22%	Neuraxial—13% PNBs—17% Field blocks—17%	Neuraxial—14% PNBs—19% Field blocks—25% Intravenous—11% Airway—17%
Local anesthetic	Bupivacaine—59% Ropicavaine—30%	Bupivacaine—20% Ropicavaine—33% Lidocaine—33%	Bupivacaine—43% Ropicavaine—21% Lidocaine—26%	Bupivacaine—11% Ropicavaine—11% Lidocaine—44% Lidocaine mix—22%
Timing of onset	Within 10 min—83%	Within 10 min—58%	Within 10 min—53%	Within 10 min—53%
Clinical spectrum	CNS only—45% CV only—11% CNS + CV—44% Prodrome—16%	CNS only—50% CV only—14% CNS + CV—36% Prodrome—34%	CNS only—45% CV only—23% CNS + CV—32% Prodrome—17%	CNS only—32% CV only—24% CNS + CV—35% Prodrome—20%
Treatment	Not reported	Lipid emulsion—34% CPR—22%	Lipid emulsion—21% CPR 21%	Lipid emulsion—64% CPR—not reported
Outcomes	Not reported	Death 10%	Death—4.3%	Death 5.6%

PNB peripheral nerve block, *CNS* central nervous system, *CV* cardiovascular

Clinical Context

The varying and evolving context of LAST is best conveyed in collective analyses of cases from October 1979 to May 2020, summarized in four key review articles (Table 5.1). The clinical setting in which LAST occurs is changing in response to more widespread use of local anesthetics, with regard to both location and technique. Although LAST is best recognized in the perioperative setting, where anesthesiology practitioners perform the majority of nerve blocks, the published cases and poison control center reports attest that LAST is a risk wherever and whenever local anesthetics are used. Published case reports of LAST since 2014 indicate that anesthesiology services account for only half of the reported LAST cases, while surgeons, dentists, and emergency medicine physicians account for most of the remaining occurrences. A third of LAST events within the hospital now occur away from the operating room suites, including hospital wards, labor and delivery suites, interventional radiology, intensive care units, echocardiography laboratories, outpatient clinics, and emergency departments (ED). In the ED, local anesthetics are used in routine care, including incision and drainage of abscesses, repair of lacerations, for which field or nerve blocks are used, and more recently, intravenous lidocaine infusion for multimodal analgesia. Whereas the majority of LAST events tend to occur in a hospital setting, the more recent trend indicates an increase in outside settings. A recent review found that 40% of published reports occurred away from the hospital: in standalone surgery centers and clinics, doctors' offices, including dental, pain medicine, urology, and plastic surgery clinics. While tumescent solutions for liposuction are generally considered safe, they commonly carry total lidocaine doses of up to 55 mg/kg, reflecting a potentially high-risk situation for patients with reduced threshold for LAST (see Prevention, below). Notably, several cases reported to United States Poison Control Centers involved self-administration of a local anesthetic at home that resulted in clinical overdose. As clinical use of local anesthetics expands, so too do the range of providers and locations where LAST occurs. Educating non-anesthesiology practitioners about safe use of local anesthetics and management of LAST becomes essential to mitigating LAST-related patient morbidity and mortality.

The majority of LAST events occurs in patients at the extremes of age. Infants less than 6 months and the elderly (older than 65) seem to be at particularly high risk compared to the general population. Review of the published LAST events from before 2010 indicates that the most common routes of administration associated with toxicity were epidural and upper extremity blocks. Review of published cases since then shows that local infiltration (field blocks), topical administration (airway, nasopharyngeal), and intravenous infusions have emerged as common culprits. Another significant change in the clinical pictures of LAST is the choice of anesthetic. The most recent collection of cases shows that the pendulum has swung away from bupivacaine and ropivacaine to lidocaine. Lidocaine, alone or in combination, is now the most commonly (66%) reported agent responsible for LAST. This may be due to more frequent use of this local anesthetic by surgeons and other non-anesthesiologists. Moreover, lidocaine may be erroneously considered as entirely safe, leading to lower levels of vigilance for associated complications. Moreover, many Enhanced Recovery After Surgery (ERAS) protocols now often include continuous lidocaine infusions as part of the perioperative analgesic regimen, and several cases of delayed toxicity have been reported in this setting.

Clinical Presentation

Data from large-scale studies inform us of the incidence of LAST but provide little detail on the clinical presentation of LAST to assist physicians with diagnosis. The traditional, textbook description of local anesthetic systemic toxicity (LAST) begins with a prodrome of tinnitus, metallic taste, or perioral numbness, followed by loss of consciousness, seizures, and possibly complete cardiopulmonary collapse. However, the clinical presentation of LAST is evolving, and so too is our understanding of the range of its potential signs and symptoms. For instance, a progressive delay in the reported time to onset of LAST is observed in published cases. Before 2010, more than 80% of published LAST events occurred within 10 min of drug administration. However, since then roughly half of cases are delayed, presenting more, or much more than 10 min after injection. The increasing use of ultrasound guidance carries a paradox. On the one hand, expert use of ultrasound reduces the risk of LAST caused by direct intravascular injection; however, it is likely also responsible for the relative increase in delayed LAST since this now occurs more often as a result of absorption from the local anesthetic depot. Notably, with continuous intravenous or catheter infusions, symptoms may not appear for many hours or even days. Despite the aforementioned changes, the clinical presentation of LAST still commonly includes central nervous system dysfunction and cardiovascular disturbances, alone or in combination as seen in Table 5.1. The most common CNS presenting feature throughout the last 40 years continues to be seizures.

Prevention

Prevention of local anesthetic systemic toxicity does not reliably hinge on any one specific method but can be improved by combining several safety measures. First is adherence to use of a reasonable local anesthetic dose. Recommended dosing limits of commonly used local anesthetics provide a general guide at best. However, there is no completely "safe" dosing limit that applies to all patients. This is true in part because weight-based dosing does not accurately predict resulting blood levels. Moreover, well-defined groups of patients are at an increased risk for LAST. Patients at the extremes of age, or with small muscle mass (i.e., sarcopenia), and those with preexisting heart disease and patients with metabolic disturbance have a lower-than-normal threshold for developing LAST. An appropriate weight-based dose for a healthy young male patient may produce fatal overdose for a patient at higher risk. Therefore, it is important to be mindful of every patient's comorbidities when selecting the total dose of local anesthetic to be delivered and consider reducing the dose by at least 20% if there are relevant comorbidities or identifying an alternative method of regional anesthesia that uses a smaller total dose (e.g., spinal anesthesia in place of combined nerve blocks for lower extremity surgery, or a digital block for finger surgery in place of brachial plexus block). It is also reasonable to avoid regional anesthesia altogether for patients at extremely high risk of LAST.

The next consideration for preventing LAST is the method of local anesthetic use. Whether performing a field block or peripheral nerve block, local anesthetic should be given in small increments (e.g., 5 mL) with some interval of time (e.g., 30–60 s) between each and aspirating the syringe before each injection to diminish the risk of inadvertent intravascular injection or stacking such injections. Intravascular injection can occur with surprising frequency with certain blocks; it is relatively common with a positive (intravascular) injection occurring in 14–23% of aspirations during inferior alveolar nerve block.

The addition of intravascular markers such as epinephrine (1:200,000 or 5 μg/mL) or fentanyl (especially in parturients) can help detect intravascular injection. With the use of 10–15 μg of epinephrine, an increase in the heart rate of more than 8–10 beats per minute or elevation of the systolic blood pressure by more than 13–15 mmHg can be an early indicator of positive intravascular spread. With fentanyl, intravascular spread should lead to sedation and decreased respiratory rate.

Accurately targeted deposition of the local anesthetic can decrease (but not eliminate) the risk of direct intravascular injection. This was attempted for decades in virtually all plexus and nerve blocks by use of anatomic landmarks with or without nerve stimulation or other endpoints (e.g., paresthesia). The introduction of ultrasound guidance into clinical practice over the last two decades has unquestionably improved the safety and efficacy of regional anesthesia. Ultrasound provides continuous real-time visualization of structures, needle position, and drug deposition and spread. This reduces the likelihood of direct intravascular injection and also allows use of smaller volumes of drug by as much as 50% in some studies; that is, a smaller dose of local anesthetic can be deposited to a precise location near the target nerves without compromising the effectiveness of the block. These two factors contribute to the decreased incidence of local anesthetic toxicity when ultrasound guidance is used for peripheral nerve blocks. Moreover, more precise location of local anesthetic injection leads to longer block thereby reducing the need for redosing; this also should decrease the risk of potential overdose.

Finally, topical application of local anesthetics provides additional challenges for preventing toxicity. First, it is impossible to know with accuracy the dose of gels, pastes, creams, and sprays that are absorbed. Second, these formulations are frequently used for topicalizing extremely vascular areas that permit rapid uptake of the drug (e.g., the airways and naso- or oropharyngeal mucosa), and this can be accelerated when the tissues are inflamed or injured as is often the case. Unlike peripheral nerve blocks, there is no method for targeted and confined deposition and because it is "only topical" there might be less awareness or concern of possible toxicity. Accordingly, extreme caution must be exercised with the use of topical local anesthetics.

Treatment

In 2010, the American Society of Regional Anesthesiologists and Pain Management (ASRA) published the first set of practice guidelines for the management of LAST. These were updated in 2012, 2017, and again in 2020 (Fig. 5.1). Because the pharmacologic management of LAST differs significantly from other causes of hemodynamic collapse and cardiac arrest, ASRA provides specific guidance and a treatment checklist to facilitate high-quality care of LAST. This text summarizes these recommendations and provides insight into the role and mechanism of recommended therapies.

Understanding the cellular sites of local anesthetic toxicity helps explain both the clinical presentation of LAST-associated multi-organ toxicity and the treatment modalities used to counter these toxicologic effects. In brief, rapid treatment of seizures, hypoxia, and hypoventilation are priorities. Equal critical consideration is then given to hemodynamic support and attenuating the underlying toxicity by using lipid emulsion to remove local anesthetic agent from target organs (viz., CNS and heart)—those whose dysfunction underlies the most life-threatening clinical presentations.

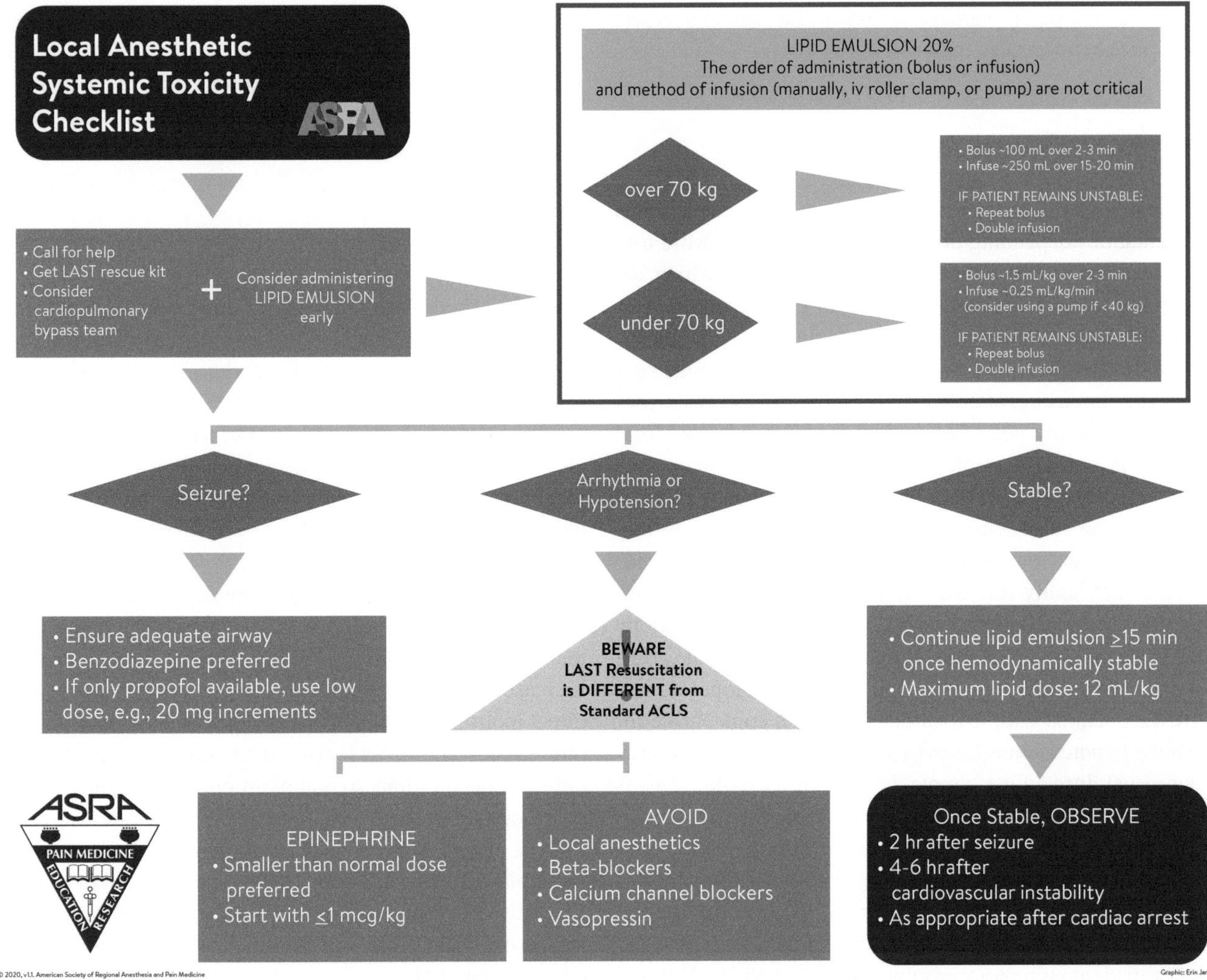

Fig. 5.1 ASRA 2020 checklist for treating LAST. "Copyright 2020 American Society of Regional Anesthesia and Pain Medicine. Used with permission. All rights reserved. Use of this image does not constitute or imply endorsement by ASRA of the website or material on which it appears or the product of service provided"

NOTE: It is important to immediately stop injecting local anesthetic and call for help if signs or symptoms consistent with LAST are observed.

Airway Management

While local anesthetics have no intrinsic effects on pulmonary function, LAST-associated seizures and cardiovascular decompensation both contribute to acute hypoventilation, hypoxemia, and acidosis. Given that both hypoxia and acidosis exacerbate LAST, there is a basis for a life-threatening vicious cycle that can lead to rapid clinical decline. Quick intervention is key to stopping and reversing this process, and airway management is the first step. Ensuring adequate oxygenation and ventilation where patients are unable to maintain their own airway is critical to resuscitation. One hundred percent oxygen supplementation and appropriate ventilation, but not hyperventilation, are needed; placement of advanced airways may also be indicated in these patients. Airway management should also consider other agents in use (opioids, benzodiazepines, paralytics) that contribute to respiratory depression.

Neurologic Support

Local anesthetics can produce a wide array of neurologic findings, including sensory prodromes such as a metallic taste or tinnitus. Neurologic clinical toxicity includes neurological excitation with seizure activity or CNS depression, leading to obtundation and coma. Benzodiazepines are preferred for suppressing seizures. Propofol in very small doses can be considered; however, it is inadequate as a source of lipid and is a potent cardio-depressant that can exacerbate local anesthetic cardiac toxicity.

Cardiovascular Toxicity Management

The cardiovascular system can also have varying clinical presentations depending on the degree of toxicity. Mild toxicity can lead to hypertension and tachycardia, which are often the earliest signs of LAST. With progression, LAST causes conduction disturbances producing either bradycardia or dysrhythmias and contractile depression. Management of dysrhythmias in patients with LAST is distinct from conventional therapy per ACLS guidelines. For instance, local anesthetic anti-arrhythmics are contraindicated since they will aggravate LAST. Beta-blockers and calcium channel blockers are also contraindicated because they further depress cardiac contractility. In severe cases, LAST can produce a sufficiently low cardiac output that requires cardiopulmonary resuscitation. Notably, the mechanism of toxicity has important implications for management of cardiac arrest in the setting of LAST. As opposed to cardiopulmonary arrest associated with myocardial ischemia, epinephrine for treating hypotension is given to patients with LAST at lower-than-usual doses, for example, boluses of <1 μg/kg. This is because standard dosing can directly interfere with lipid resuscitation. Vasopressin and other pure afterload vasopressor agents should be avoided as they may further reduce cardiac output and tissue perfusion. Hypotension and bradycardia can be treated with conventional therapies and are aimed at symptom resolution (i.e., lightheadedness) when present.

Lipid Emulsion

Infusing lipid emulsion (ILE) is one mainstay in the treatment of LAST. The mechanism of action is well understood; although exerting multimodal effects, the main benefit is pharmacokinetic: accelerating the redistribution of local anesthetic. Local anesthetic partitions into the lipid phase of the plasma created by ILE. The lipid then functions as a shuttle carrying local anesthetic to the skeletal muscle, a neutral reservoir and liver/hepatobiliary tract where local anesthetic is excreted. The net effect is to reduce tissue local anesthetic content and toxicity in target organs (brain and heart). Initiation of ILE begins with a bolus of 1.5 mL/kg of 20% lipid emulsion to rapidly establish the bulk lipid phase. This is followed by infusion at a slower rate of 0.25 mL/kg/min to sustain an effective level of lipidemia. Pending the patient's clinical response, additional boluses may be considered but the total lipid dose should not exceed 10–12 mL/kg over 30 min.

For severe LAST that does not respond to these measures, extracorporeal support (e.g., venoarterial ECMO or cardiopulmonary bypass) may be required, and it is therefore important to consider involvement of the necessary personnel or facility early in the treatment sequence.

Mechanism of ILE

Local anesthetics are lipid-soluble and positively charged at physiological pH. Particles comprising the infused lipid emulsion have a negative surface charge and therefore rapidly bind local anesthetic molecules and shuttle them from sensitive organs (brain and heart) to liver and skeletal muscle. This shuttling effect accelerates redistribution of the local anesthetic and directly mitigates the progression of its underlying pharmaco-toxicity.

Cardiovascular improvement with ILE also results from both bulk volume resuscitation provided by the initial bolus and a direct cardiotonic effect of lipid emulsion which increases cardiac output and contributes to the redistribution. Increase in arterial blood pressure results from both the direct inotropic effect and constriction of peripheral vasculature. Local anesthetics also exert vasodilatory effects at higher concentrations so that partitioning and shuttling local anesthetic away from vascular endothelium can also play a role in increasing vascular tone. Finally, ILE attenuates ischemia-reperfusion-injury (IRI) and is thereby cardioprotective for the patient following resuscitation. This is known to result from activation of cyto-protective kinases that attenuate IRI.

Conclusion

Understanding the pathophysiology and treatment of LAST is important for all healthcare providers who use or treat patients that receive local anesthetics. Studies indicate an incidence of local anesthetic systemic toxicity to be about 1.8 events per 1000 nerve blocks with a mortality rate of 4–10%. As clinical context and presentation vary widely and symptom onset can be delayed, the risk of LAST remains present as use of local anesthetics in operative settings and beyond continues to expand. Roughly half of the published cases of LAST occur under an anesthesiologist's care in the perioperative setting. Changes in our practice (lidocaine infusions, extended release local anesthetics, larger volume blocks, office-based surgical procedures, etc.) make for a dynamic situation that warrants continuous reassessment and education. Providers in all areas of the hospital and outpatient community should recognize and be able to appropriately respond to toxicity. Prevention focuses on using the lowest amount of anesthetic possible to achieve the desired effect, markers like epinephrine, and ultrasound guidance whenever possible. Treatment focuses on seizure suppression, airway management, and hemodynamic support as needed and infusing lipid emulsion to reverse underlying tissue toxicity. As local anesthetic use is deployed further under the purview of non-anesthesiology medical practitioners, vigilance to reduce risks and attenuate adverse outcomes are ever more critical to safe use.

Suggested Reading

Abrahams MS, Aziz MF, Fu RF, Horn JL. Ultrasound guidance compared with electrical neurostimulation for peripheral nerve block: a systematic review and meta-analysis of randomized controlled trials. Br J Anaesth. 2009;102(3):408–17.

Barrington MJ, Kluger R. Ultrasound guidance reduces the risk of local anesthetic systemic toxicity following peripheral nerve blockade. Reg Anesth Pain Med. 2013;38(4):289–99.

De Oliveira K, Eipe N. Intravenous lidocaine for acute pain: a single-institution retrospective study. Drugs Real World Outcomes. 2020;7(3):205–12.

Di Gregorio G, Schwartz D, Ripper R, et al. Lipid emulsion is superior to vasopressin in a rodent model of resuscitation from toxin-induced cardiac arrest. Crit Care Med. 2009;37(3):993–9.

Di Gregorio G, Neal JM, Rosenquist RW, Weinberg GL. Clinical presentation of local anesthetic systemic toxicity: a review of published cases, 1979 to 2009. Reg Anesth Pain Med. 2010;35(2):181–7.

Drasner K. Local anesthetic systemic toxicity: a historical perspective. Reg Anesth Pain Med. 2010;35(2):162–6.

Fettiplace MR, Weinberg G. The mechanisms underlying lipid resuscitation therapy. Reg Anesth Pain Med. 2018;43(2):138–49.

Fettiplace MR, Ripper R, Lis K, et al. Rapid cardiotonic effects of lipid emulsion infusion*. Crit Care Med. 2013;41(8):e156–62.

Fettiplace MR, Lis K, Ripper R, et al. Multi-modal contributions to detoxification of acute pharmacotoxicity by a triglyceride microemulsion. J Control Release. 2015;198:62–70.

Gitman M, Barrington MJ. Local anesthetic systemic toxicity: a review of recent case reports and registries. Reg Anesth Pain Med. 2018;43(2):124–30.

Kim DC. Malignant hyperthermia. Korean J Anesthesiol. 2012;63(5):391–401.

Kramer ME, Holtan EE, Ives AL, Wall RT. Perioperative intravenous lidocaine infusion adverse reaction: a case report. A A Pract. 2019;13(3):96–8.

Liu SS, Carpenter RL. Hemodynamic responses to intravascular injection of epinephrine-containing epidural test doses in adults during general anesthesia. Anesthesiology. 1996;84(1):81–7.

Lou PH, Lucchinetti E, Zhang L, et al. The mechanism of Intralipid(R)-mediated cardioprotection complex IV inhibition by the active metabolite, palmitoylcarnitine, generates reactive oxygen species and activates reperfusion injury salvage kinases. PLoS One. 2014;9(1):e87205.

Macfarlane AJR, Gitman M, Bornstein KJ, El-Boghdadly K, Weinberg G. Updates in our understanding of local anaesthetic systemic toxicity: a narrative review. Anaesthesia. 2021;76(Suppl. 1):27–39.

McNaught A, Shastri U, Carmichael N, et al. Ultrasound reduces the minimum effective local anaesthetic volume compared with peripheral nerve stimulation for interscalene block. Br J Anaesth. 2011;106(1):124–30.

Morwald EE, Zubizarreta N, Cozowicz C, Poeran J, Memtsoudis SG. Incidence of local anesthetic systemic toxicity in orthopedic patients receiving peripheral nerve blocks. Reg Anesth Pain Med. 2017;42(4):442–5.

Mosaffa F, Gharaei B, Qoreishi M, et al. Do the concentration and volume of local anesthetics affect the onset and success of infraclavicular anesthesia? Anesth Pain Med. 2015;5(4):e23963.

Mulroy MF. Systemic toxicity and cardiotoxicity from local anesthetics: incidence and preventive measures. Reg Anesth Pain Med. 2002;27(6):556–61.

Mulroy MF, Hejtmanek MR. Prevention of local anesthetic systemic toxicity. Reg Anesth Pain Med. 2010;35(2):177–80.

Neal JM, Barrington MJ, Fettiplace MR, et al. The Third American Society of Regional Anesthesia and Pain Medicine Practice Advisory on Local Anesthetic Systemic Toxicity: executive summary 2017. Reg Anesth Pain Med. 2018;43(2):113–23.

Neal JM, Neal EJ, Weinberg GL. American Society of Regional Anesthesia and Pain Medicine Local Anesthetic Systemic Toxicity checklist: 2020 version. Reg Anesth Pain Med. 2021;46:81.

Ok SH, Hong JM, Lee SH, Sohn JT. Lipid emulsion for treating local anesthetic systemic toxicity. Int J Med Sci. 2018;15(7):713–22.

Rosenberg PH, Veering BT, Urmey WF. Maximum recommended doses of local anesthetics: a multifactorial concept. Reg Anesth Pain Med. 2004;29(6):564–75; discussion 524.

Rubin DS, Matsumoto MM, Weinberg G, Roth S. Local Anesthetic systemic toxicity in total joint arthroplasty: incidence and risk factors in the United States from the national inpatient sample 1998-2013. Reg Anesth Pain Med. 2018;43(2):131–7.

Taghavi Zenouz A, Ebrahimi H, Mahdipour M, Pourshahidi S, Amini P, Vatankhah M. The incidence of intravascular needle entrance during inferior alveolar nerve block injection. J Dent Res Dent Clin Dent Prospects. 2008;2(1):38–41.

Vasques F, Behr AU, Weinberg G, Ori C, Di Gregorio G. A review of local anesthetic systemic toxicity cases since publication of the American Society of Regional Anesthesia recommendations: to whom it may concern. Reg Anesth Pain Med. 2015;40(6):698–705.

Wang QG, Wu C, Xia Y, et al. Epinephrine deteriorates pulmonary gas exchange in a rat model of bupivacaine-induced cardiotoxicity: a threshold dose of epinephrine. Reg Anesth Pain Med. 2017;42(3):342–50.

Weinberg GL. Treatment of local anesthetic systemic toxicity (LAST). Reg Anesth Pain Med. 2010;35(2):188–93.

Weinberg GL, Di Gregorio G, Ripper R, et al. Resuscitation with lipid versus epinephrine in a rat model of bupivacaine overdose. Anesthesiology. 2008;108(5):907–13.

Part II

Nerve Block for Regional Anesthesia and Pain Therapy in Head and Neck Region

Regional Anesthesia in Ophthalmology

6

André van Zundert, Chandra Kumar,
and Danilo Jankovic

Contents

General Consideration

The pioneering work of Carl Koller (1884) on the anesthetic effect of cocaine in the context of ophthalmic surgery was the historical starting point for local and regional anesthesia worldwide. Local/regional anesthesia is commonly used for the majority of ophthalmic surgical procedures. Cataract surgery is the commonest performed surgery and local/regional anesthesia is the norm, but the provision of anesthesia varies worldwide. The exact frequency of the use of a technique is unknown. Patient comfort, safety, and low complication rates are the essentials of local anesthesia. Ophthalmic regional techniques (blocks) provide anesthesia and is usu-

A. van Zundert (✉)
Royal Brisbane and Women's Hospital, Brisbane, QLD, Australia

The University of Queensland & Queensland University of Technology, Brisbane, QLD, Australia

C. Kumar
Khoo Teck Puat Hospital, Yishun, Singapore

Freelance Consultant Anesthetist, Stockton TS, UK

D. Jankovic
Pain Management Centre DGS – Cologne – Huerth, Cologne-Hürth, Germany
e-mail: danilo@jankovic1.de

D. Jankovic, P. Peng (eds.), *Regional Nerve Blocks in Anesthesia and Pain Therapy*,
https://doi.org/10.1007/978-3-030-88727-8_6

ally associated with reduction of eye movements. Ophthalmic regional blocks can be achieved by inserting either a needle or a blunt cannula.

The terminology used for regional orbital blocks is controversial (Kumar). An intraconal (retrobulbar) block involves the injection of a local anesthetic agent into the muscle cone behind the globe formed by four recti muscles and the superior and inferior oblique muscles. An extraconal (peribulbar) block involves the injection of local anesthetic outside the muscle cone. Many studies confirm that there are multiple communications between the two compartments, and it is sometimes difficult to differentiate if the injection is intraconal or extraconal. A combination of intraconal and extraconal blocks is described as combined retro-peribulbar block. In sub-Tenon's block, local anesthetic agent is injected under the Tenon's capsule. This block is also known as parabulbar block, pinpoint anesthesia, and medial episcleral block.

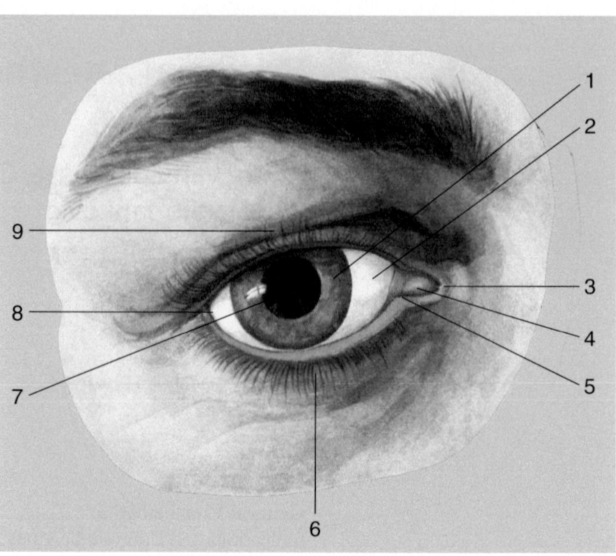

Fig. 6.1 Eyelids and lacrimal apparatus. (*1*) cornea, (*2*) conjunctiva, (*3*) medial angle of the eye, (*4*) lacrimal caruncle, (*5*) lacrimal papilla, (*6*) inferior eyelid, (*7*) pupil, (*8*) lateral angle of the eye, (*9*) superior eyelid. (Reproduced with permission from Danilo Jankovic)

Indications and Contraindications

Both intraocular procedures (cataract extraction, vitrectomy) and extraocular procedures (strabismus surgery, retinal detachment with encircling silicone band) can be carried out under local/regional anesthesia in suitable patients. There are only a few absolute contraindications, such as patient refusal to accept local anesthesia, allergy to local anesthetic agent, local infection, excessive abnormal body movements, severe breathlessness, psychiatric conditions, and in situations where it is difficult to establish a good communication between patients and health-care workers but the list is shrinking and local anesthesia is increasingly used even in the above group.

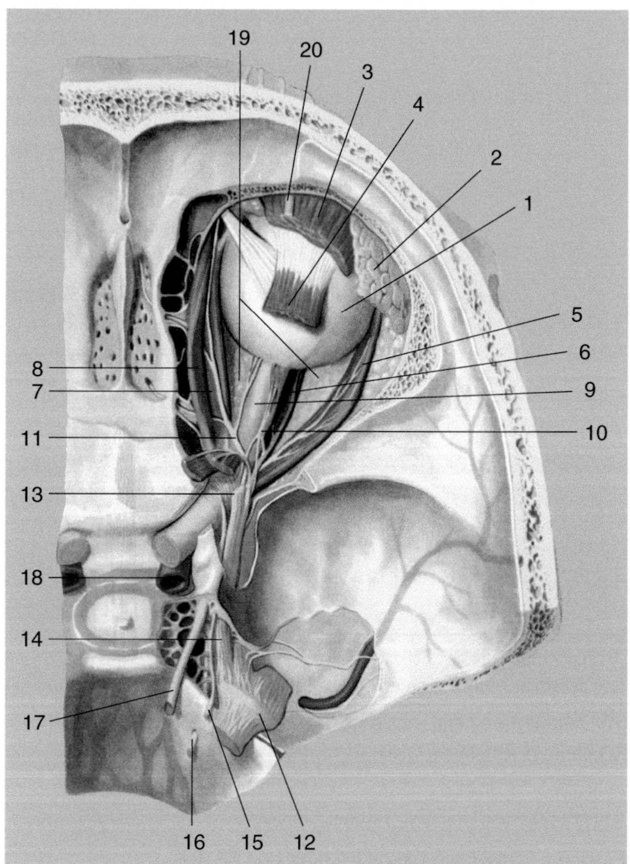

Fig. 6.2 Anatomy of the eye. (*1*) Eyeball, (*2*) lacrimal gland, (*3*) levator palpebrae superioris muscle, (*4*) superior rectus muscle, (*5*) lateral rectus muscle, (*6*) inferior rectus muscle, (*7*) medial rectus muscle, (*8*) superior oblique muscle, (*9*) optic nerve, (*10*) ciliary ganglion, (*11*) nasociliary nerve, (*12*) trigeminal ganglion, (*13*) frontal nerve, (*14*) ophthalmic nerve, (*15*) trochlear nerve, (*16*) abducent nerve, (*17*) oculomotor nerve, (*18*) internal carotid artery, (*19*) retrobulbar fat, (*20*) supraorbital nerve. (Reproduced with permission from Danilo Jankovic)

Functional Orbital Anatomy

The globe or bulbus oculi lies in front of the orbit and is covered by eyelids. The orbit is an irregular four-sided pyramid with its apex pointing posteromedially and its base facing anteriorly (Figs. 6.1, 6.2, and 6.3). The base is formed by the surface of the cornea, the conjunctiva and the lids. The medial wall of orbit is parallel to the sagittal plane, but the lateral wall is angled inwards at 45°. The roof is horizontal but the floor slopes upwards, front to back by 10°. The globe is closer to the roof than the floor of the orbit.

The length of orbit varies from 42 to 54 mm. The globe (7 ml) fills one-fourth of the orbit, and the remainder is filled with fatty tissue, vessels, lacrimal gland, connective tissue, nerves, and extraocular muscles. The transparent cornea lies on the anterior surface of the eyeball (Fig. 6.4). Underneath this lies the crystalline lens, which is located in front of the iris, with its central opening, the pupil. The conjunctiva covers relatively tough sclera.

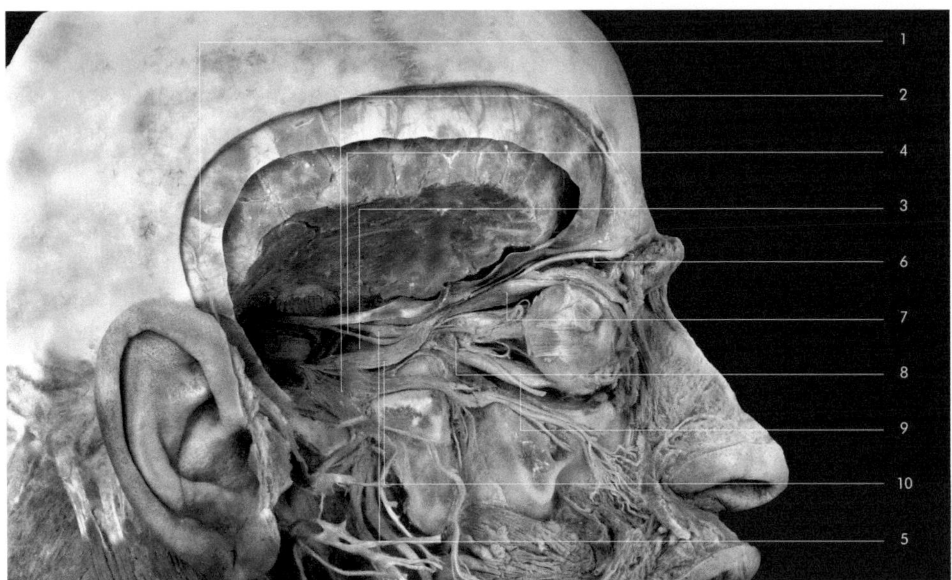

Fig. 6.3 Anatomy. (*1*) Spinal dura mater, (*2*) trigeminal ganglion, (*3*) internal carotid artery, (*4*) trochlear nerve, (*5*) oculomotor nerve, (*6*) supraorbital nerve, (*7*) superior rectus muscle, (*8*) ciliary ganglion, (*9*) inferior rectus muscle, (*10*) ophthalmic nerve. (Reproduced with permission from Danilo Jankovic)

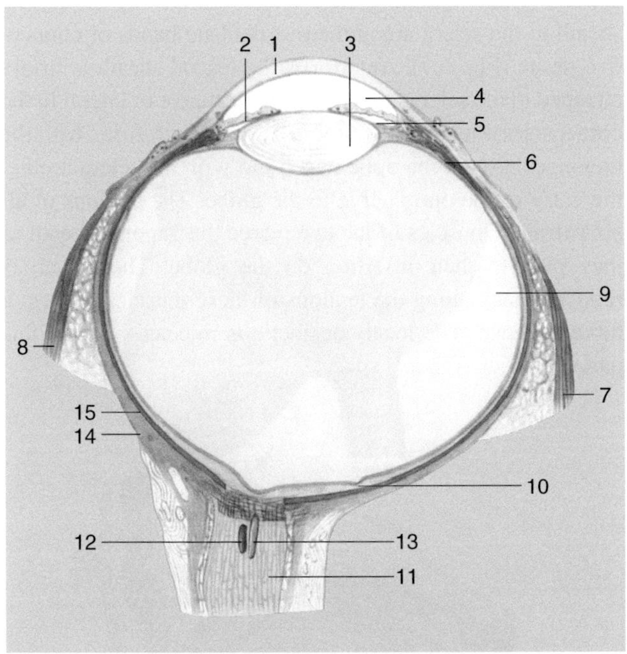

Fig. 6.4 Horizontal section through the eyeball. (*1*) Cornea, (*2*) iris, (*3*) lens, (*4*), anterior chamber of the eyeball, (*5*) posterior chamber of the eyeball, (*6*) ciliary body, (*7*) lateral rectus muscle, (*8*) medial rectus muscle, (*9*) vitreous body, (*10*) central retinal fovea, (*11*) optic nerve, (*12*) central retinal artery, (*13*) central retinal vein, (*14*) sclera, (*15*) chorioid. (Reproduced with permission from Danilo Jankovic)

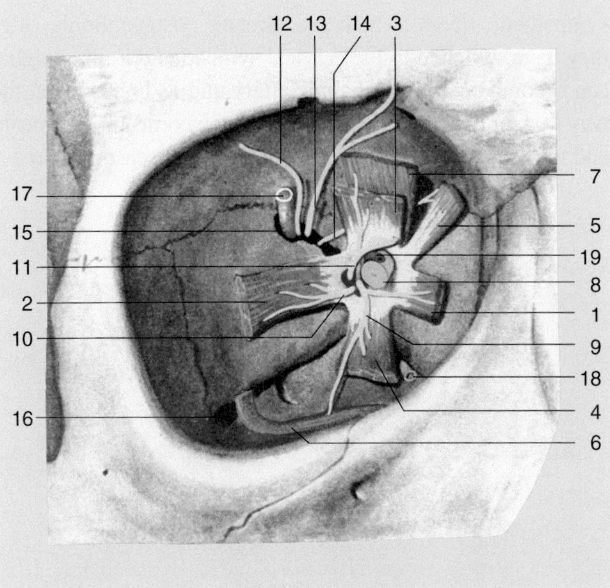

Fig. 6.5 Eye: muscles, nerves, and vessels. (*1*) Medial rectus muscle, (*2*) lateral rectus muscle, (*3*) superior rectus muscle, (*4*) inferior rectus muscle, (*5*) superior oblique muscle, (*6*) inferior oblique muscle, (*7*) levator palpebrae superioris muscle, (*8*) optic nerve, (*9*) oculomotor nerve, (*10*) abducens nerve, (*11*) nasociliary nerve, (*12*) lacrimal nerve, (*13*) frontal nerve, (*14*) trochlear nerve, (*15*) superior orbital fissure, (*16*) inferior orbital fissure, (*17*) superior ophthalmic vein, (*18*) inferior ophthalmic vein, (*19*) ophthalmic artery. (Reproduced with permission from Danilo Jankovic)

The anterior chamber of the eye is bounded by the cornea, the iris and the lens. The posterior chamber of the eye encircles the lens in a ring-like shape and the posterior chamber of the eye contains the vitreous body.

Movements of the globe are made possible by four straight muscles—inferior rectus (oculomotor nerve, CN III), lateral rectus (abducens nerve, CN VI), medial rectus (oculomotor nerve) and superior rectus (oculomotor nerve), and two oblique muscles—superior oblique muscle (trochlear nerve, CN IV) and inferior oblique muscle (oculomotor nerve) (Figs. 6.2, 6.3, and 6.5). The rectus muscles arise from the annulus of Zinn near the apex of the orbit and insert anterior to the equator of the globe thus forming an incomplete cone. Thus, the orbit is divided into two compartments, although not completely separate, an extraconal compartment and an intraconal compartment. Injected local anesthetic agents are easily able to cross the barrier between two compartments by diffusion. Within the annulus and the muscle cone lie the optic nerve (CN II), the oculomotor nerve (CN III containing both superior and inferior branches), the abducent nerve (CN VI), the nasociliary nerve (a branch of CN V), the ciliary ganglion and vessels.

Lacrimal, frontal, and nasociliary branches of the ophthalmic division of the trigeminal nerve provide the sensory supply of the orbit (see Chap. 8; Trigeminal Nerve Anatomy and Peripheral Branches Block). Autonomic fibers run from the ciliary ganglion situated within the cone near to the orbital apex (Figs. 6.2 and 6.3). The ciliary ganglion, a tiny collection of nerve cells, lies in the posterior part of the orbit between the optic nerve and the lateral rectus muscle. The nasociliary nerve and the neural network around the internal carotid artery provide the sensory and sympathetic roots of the ciliary ganglion, but do not always connect to the ciliary ganglion. Their fibers can reach the eye directly via the ciliary nerves. The sympathetic fibers, which are already postganglionic after they have switched to the cervical sympathetic trunk ganglia, can accompany the ophthalmic artery and its branches on the way to their destination. Stimuli from the cornea, iris, choroid and intraocular muscles are conducted in the sensory fibers.

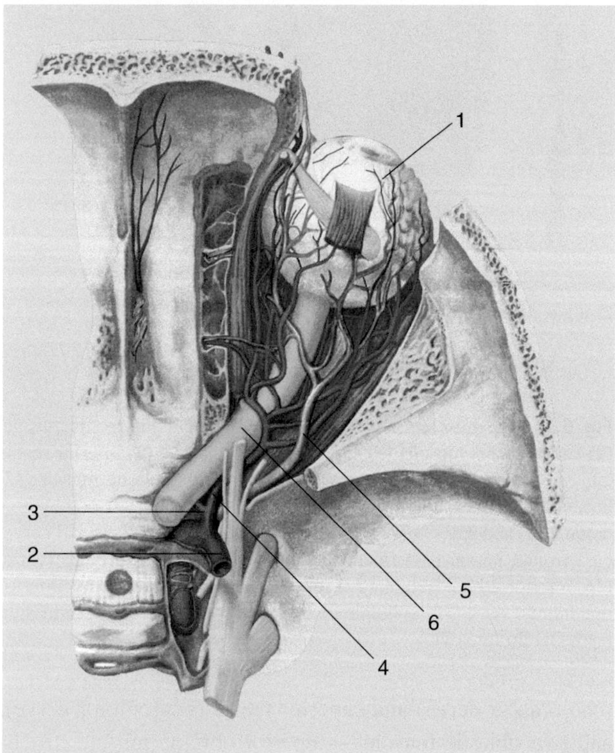

Fig. 6.6 Blood supply in the eye. (*1*) Eyeball, (*2*) internal carotid artery, (*3*) central retinal artery, (*4*) ophthalmic artery, (*5*) superior ophthalmic vein, (*6*) optic nerve. (Reproduced with permission from Danilo Jankovic)

The eye and orbital contents receive their main arterial supply from the ophthalmic artery (Fig. 6.6). The ophthalmic artery is a branch of the internal carotid artery. In the orbital cavity, the artery runs forward for a short distance lateral to the optic nerve and medial to the lateral rectus muscle, the abducens, and oculomotor nerves and the ciliary ganglion. The artery then turns medially and crosses above the optic nerve, accompanied by the nasociliary nerve. The venous blood of the orbit is drained by the superior and inferior ophthalmic veins, which in turn drain into the cavernous sinus. The superior ophthalmic vein crosses the optic nerve with the ophthalmic artery. The veins of the orbit are tortuous and freely anastomose with one another, and they have no valves. These vessels are known to be damaged when a long needle is inserted deep into the apex.

Tenon's capsule (fascial sheath) is a thin membrane that envelops the eyeball and separates it from the orbital fat. The inner surface is smooth and shiny and is separated from the outer surface of the sclera by a potential space, the sub-Tenon's space. Crossing the space and attaching the fascial sheath to the sclera are numerous delicate bands of connective tissue (Fig. 6.7). Anteriorly, the fascial sheath is firmly attached to the sclera about 5–8 mm posterior or lateral to the corneoscleral junction. Posteriorly, the sheath fuses with the meninges around the optic nerve and with the sclera around the entry of the optic nerve to the globe. The tendons of all six extrinsic muscles of the eye pierce the Tenon's sheath as they pass to their insertion on the globe. The sheath is reflected back along the tendons of these muscles to form a tubular sleeve. The local anesthetic is injected beneath this part of the sub-Tenon's space.

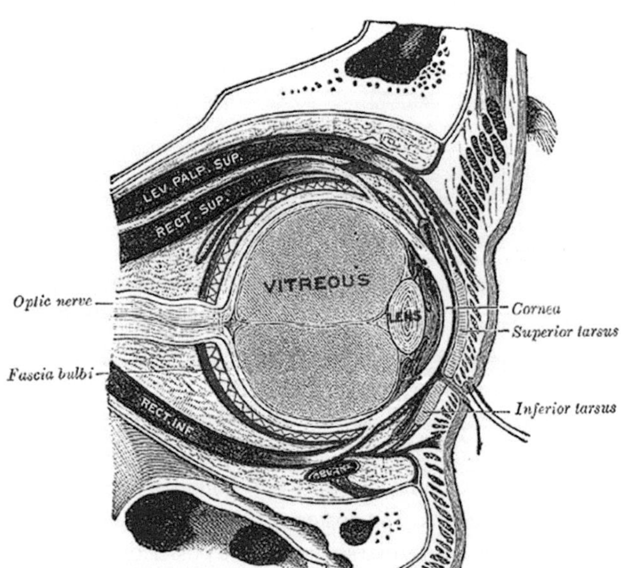

Fig. 6.7 Sub-Tenon's space showing multiple connective tissue bands. (With kind permission from www.bartleby.com)

The average distance between the orbital margin and the ciliary ganglion is approximately 38 mm (range 32–44 mm). If a 38 mm needle is used, it may reach the optic nerve in a large number of patients leading to serious catastrophic events. A needle <31 mm must be used to protect the globe, optic nerve and other major structures behind the globe during both extraconal and intraconal blocks. In cadaver studies, Karampatiakis et al. (1998) found that when a retrobulbar block was carried out with a needle 40 mm long, the needle tip would reach the posterior optic nerve in 100% cases; even with needles 35 mm long, the covering of the optic nerve would be touched.

Average axial length (anteroposterior distance of the globe) of the eye varies from 22 to 24 mm. Eye with axial length >26 mm is more prone to globe damage during needle block. The axial length measurement is made available during cataract surgery by the surgeon. If a patient is scheduled for non-cataract surgery, spherical power of the spectacles may offer some clue. A patient having very thick prescription glasses indicate high myopia. The risk of damage to the globe and optic nerve is also greater when the globe is rotated during injection. Therefore, it is recommended that the globe should be in the neutral gaze during the injection. It is safer to introduce a needle as far lateral as possible below the lateral rectus muscle. If a needle is introduced at the junction of medial 2/3rd and lateral 1/3rd of the inferior orbital rim, there is a possibility of damage to inferior rectus, inferior oblique and inferior braches of the oculomotor nerve.

Functional Orbital Physiology

The physiological pressure (intraocular pressure) in the interior of the eye varies between 10 and 20 mmHg. It is higher in patients with a large diameter eyeball and in the recumbent position. It is higher in the morning than in the evening. It increases during coughing, physical exertions, and vomiting. An increase in the plasma concentration of carbon dioxide and decrease in oxygen concentration increase the intraocular pressure. Intraocular pressure increases after needle technique, and this is due to injected volume of local anesthetic agent behind the globe. There is little or hardly any increase in intraocular pressure after sub-Tenon's block.

Assessment and Preparation of Patients

Most ophthalmic surgical procedures are carried out as outpatient basis. There is debate as to the degree of preoperative assessment and investigation required and they vary worldwide. Routine investigation of patients undergoing cataract surgery under regional anesthesia is not essential because it neither improves the health nor improves the outcome of surgery, but tests can be done to improve the general health of the patient if required. Preoperative testing before cataract surgery was noted to be more frequent and was more strongly associated with provider practice patterns than with patient characteristics.

The preoperative assessment should always include a specific enquiry about bleeding disorders and related drugs. There is an increased risk of hemorrhage, and this requires that a clotting profile is available (and recorded) prior to injection (see later). Patients receiving anticoagulants are advised to continue their medications. Clotting results should be within the recommended therapeutic range. Blood pressure should be controlled in hypertensive patients. Diabetic patients are allowed to take their usual medications, and active control of blood sugar is not necessary and they can continue food and medications as usual on the day of surgery. In the UK, the Joint Royal Colleges Working Party Report recommended that routine laboratory and other investigations are unnecessary and the patients are not fasted and the subject has been reviewed recently. There is no need for antibiotic prophylaxis in patients with valvular heart disease, and surgery is not performed if patient has suffered myocardial infarction during the last 3 months. The presence of a long eye, staphyloma or enophthalmos, the use of faulty technique, a lack of appreciation of risk factors, an uncooperative patient and the use of unnecessarily long needles are some of the contributing causes. Knowledge of axial length measurement is essential. A precise axial length measurement is generally available for intraocular lens diopter power calculation before cataract surgery. If the block is performed for other surgery and the axial length measurement is not known, close attention to the diopter power of patients' spectacles or contact lenses may provide valuable clues to globe dimension (patients usually provide this history).

Preparation Before Ophthalmic Blocks

The patient and the person performing the block must be involved in full discussion of the proposed technique. The anesthetic and surgical procedures are explained to the patients. The (often elderly) patient is placed in a comfortable sitting/semi-sitting position and oxygen is administered via a suitable device (nasal prongs). All monitoring and anesthetic equipment in the operating environments should be fully functional. Blood pressure, oxygen saturation and ECG leads are connected, and baseline recordings are obtained. Insertion of an intravenous line is a prerequisite for needle-based blocks, but its use has been questioned during sub-Tenon's injections. It is not unusual to observe adverse medical events in elderly patients and a working intravenous line could only be a good clinical practice.

Sedation and Analgesia During Ophthalmic Blocks

The use of sedation varies in different parts of the world and may or may not be used. Sedation is used during the block and surgical procedure. Sedation is much more common during topical anesthesia. Selected patients, in whom explanation and reassurance have proved inadequate, may benefit from sedation. There is currently no ideal sedative agent. Short-acting benzodiazepines, opioids and small doses of intravenous anesthetic induction agent (propofol) are favored but the dosage must be minimal. An increased incidence of adverse intraoperative events is anticipated with sedation in elderly. Small IV doses of propofol (0.2–0.5 mg/kg) or midazolam 0.5–1 mg can be administered before the block but there are other drugs and preferences vary. Deep sedation should be avoided during regional anesthesia; the patient should be able to cooperate.

Technique

Conduction Block

Needle-Based Techniques

The Atkinson's or classical retrobulbar block involves insertion of 38 mm long needle through the skin at the junction of medial 2/3rd and lateral 1/3rd of the inferior orbital margin in a rotated eye (upwards and inwards). The needle is directed towards the apex and 2 ml of anesthetic agent of choice (e.g., lidocaine 2%) is injected. A supplemental facial nerve block (seventh nerve block CN VII) is usually used (See below). The classical retrobulbar block has now been superseded by a higher volume modern intraconal (retrobulbar) and extraconal (peribulbar) blocks.

Modern Retrobulbar Block (Intraconal Block)

A needle <31 mm is deliberately directed towards the apex and within the muscle cone (see above) while the globe is in neutral gaze.

Indications

Both intraocular and extraocular surgery may include cataract surgery, viteroretinal surgery, panretinal photocoagulation, trabeculectomy, optic nerve sheath fenestration, delivery of drugs (steroids, neurolytic agents), and sometimes strabismus surgery in willing patients. Retrobulbar block is also performed for the delivery of neurolytic agents for the treatment of chronic orbital pain.

Preparation

See above.

Materials

Equipment such as local anesthetic eye drop, local anesthetic agent, needle and syringe (Fig. 6.8) are essential for needle block. Other materials such as syringe, small needle, oculocompression device, gauge swab, hyaluronidase, epinephrine and balanced salt solution (BSS) may be required.

The short and sharp needles are favored because they reduce the discomfort on insertion but at the expense of a reduced tactile feedback, hence a higher risk of failing to recognize a globe perforation. Conversely, the blunt or dull needles are favored by some because it is believed that blood vessels are pushed rather traumatized and tissue planes could be more accurately defined but these are more likely to cause greater damage when misplaced.

Patient Positioning

The best position for the patient is semi-recumbent position (45°).

Injection Technique

Topical local anesthetic eye drops and antiseptic (5% povidone iodine) are instilled (Fig. 6.9). A dilute local solution is

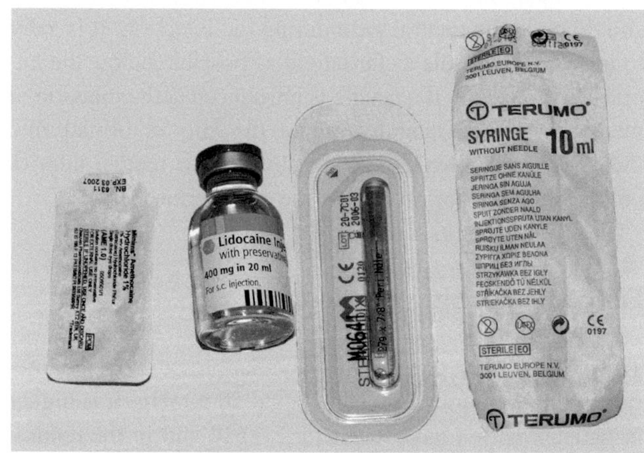

Fig. 6.8 Essential equipment for needle block. (Reproduced with permission from A. van Zundert, Ch. Kumar)

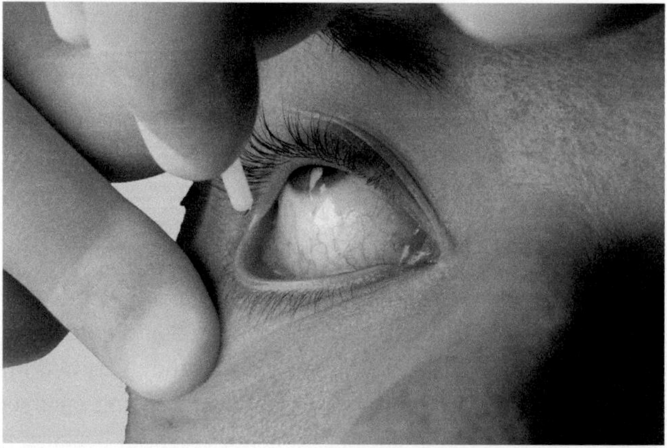

Fig. 6.9 Surface anesthesia. (Reproduced with permission from Danilo Jankovic)

prepared by adding 2 ml of concentrated local anesthetic agent to 13 ml of BSS and is helpful before the main injection of concentrated local anesthetic agent. Of this dilute solution, 1.5–2 ml is injected through the conjunctiva under the inferior tarsal plate in the inferotemporal quadrant. A 27 gauge, 1 cm long needle (Fig. 6.10) is inserted under the inferior tarsal plate through the conjunctiva to deliver dilute local anesthetic.

A 25 gauge or 27 gauge, 31 mm long needle is inserted through the skin or conjunctiva in the main inferotemporal quadrant as far lateral as possible (5 o'clock position on the right eye or 7 o'clock position on the left eye) below the lateral rectus muscle (Fig. 6.11) while the patient's eye is in the neutral gaze position. It is important that the needle hub is visible all the time and that the skin is not indented. The initial direction of the needle is tangential to the globe, then passed below the globe, and once passed the equator as gauged by axial length of the globe, is allowed to go upwards and inwards along the floor of the orbit to enter the central space just behind the globe (Figs. 6.12 and 6.13). The globe is continuously observed during the needle placement. Motility testing of the eye must be carried out before the procedure.

Drugs

Oxybuprocaine HCl 0.4% or tetracaine 1% for surface anesthesia and 4–5 ml of the chosen local anesthetic agent (2% lidocaine, 0.5% bupivacaine) should be prepared.

Optional adjunct agents (hyaluronidase 15 IU/ml, epinephrine 1:200,000), added to the local anesthetic, usually improve diffusion and thus to a faster onset. This provides very good conditions for surgical procedures in the eye.

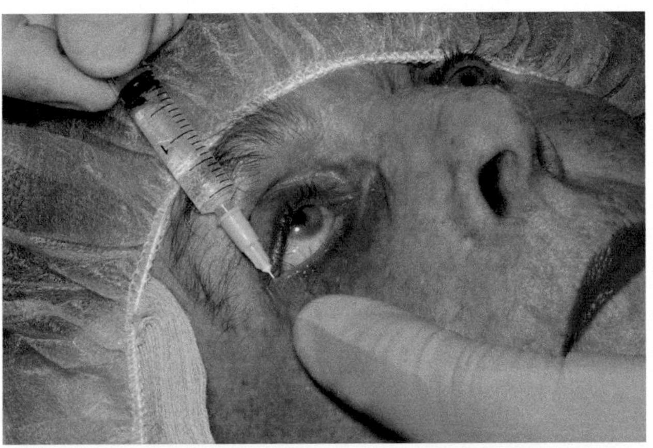

Fig. 6.10 27 gauge, 1 cm long needle inserted under the inferior tarsal plate through the conjunctiva to deliver dilute local anesthetic. (Reproduced with permission from A. van Zundert, Ch. Kumar)

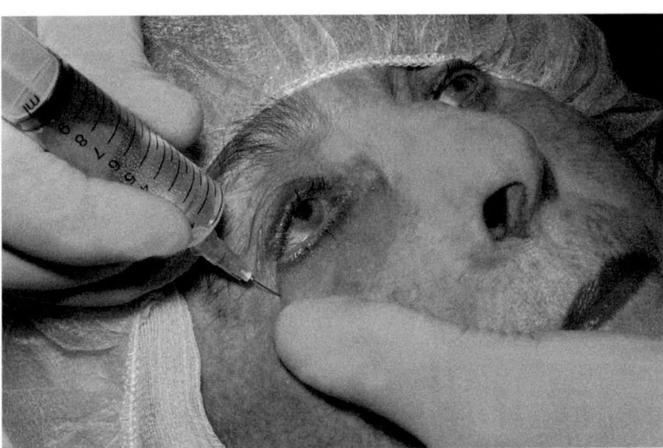

Fig. 6.12 Initial direction of needle (tangential to the globe) during modern retrobulbar block. (Reproduced with permission from A. van Zundert)

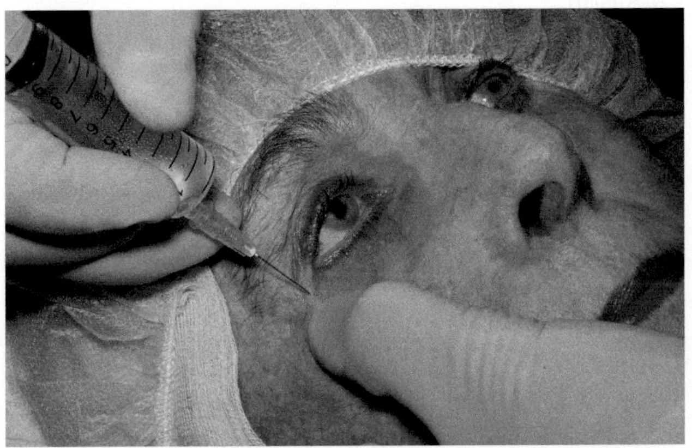

Fig. 6.11 27 gauge, 2 cm long needle is inserted at *the extreme* inferolateral quadrant percutaneously during intended modern retrobulbar block. (Reproduced with permission from A. van Zundert, Ch. Kumar)

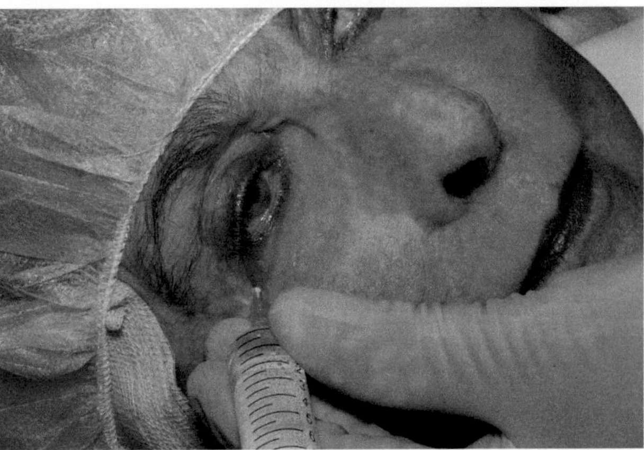

Fig. 6.13 The needle is directed upwards and inwards during modern retrobulbar block. (Reproduced with permission from A. van Zundert, Ch. Kumar)

Akinesia and anesthesia usually follow but they are dose-dependent. If amount injected is small, anesthesia may follow but complete akinesia may not occur. On the other hand, higher volume can generally guarantee anesthesia and akinesia but intraocular pressure rises and other complications such as chemosis may occur. Sometimes, a supplementary injection as a medial peribulbar block is required (see further).

Advantages

Anesthesia and akinesia are very predictable and quick. It is easy to learn the technique provided knowledge of basic sciences relevant to block is achieved.

Disadvantages

There are reports of serious complications of retrobulbar blockade, both sight and life-threatening (see later).

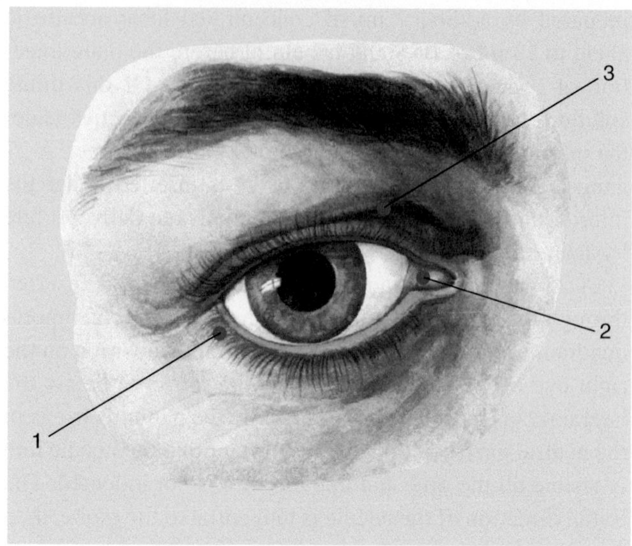

Fig. 6.14 Peribulbar block. Possible approaches: (*1*) inferotemporal, (*2*) medial caruncular, (*3*) superonasal. (Reproduced with permission from Danilo Jankovic)

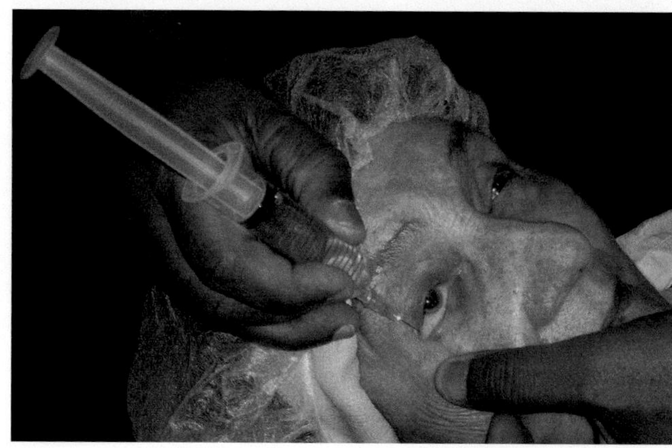

Fig. 6.15 Inferotemporal peribulbar block—a needle inserted through the conjunctiva in the extreme inferotemporal quadrant below the lateral rectus muscle. (Reproduced with permission from A. van Zundert, Ch. Kumar)

Peribulbar Block

Inferotemporal Peribulbar Block

This block is used as a main injection alternative to modern retrobulbar block.

Indications, Preparation, and Materials (See Above)

Patient Positioning

(See above).

Injection Technique

Possible approaches of peribulbar injection are presented in Fig. 6.14.

A 25 G or 27 G, 31 mm long needle is inserted through the conjunctiva or skin as far laterally as possible in the inferotemporal quadrant. Once the needle is under the globe, it is not directed upward and inward, but it is directed along the orbital floor. 4–5 ml of local anesthetic agent of choice is injected. Many patients require a supplementary injection a repeat inferotemporal or usually a medial peribulbar.

Medial Peribulbar Injection (The Medial Canthus or Caruncular Single Injection)

A medial peribulbar block is usually performed to supplement inferotemporal retrobulbar or peribulbar injection, when akinesia or anesthesia is not adequate. A 27 gauge, 2.5 cm long needle is inserted in the blind pit between the caruncle and the medial canthus (Figs. 6.14, 6.15, 6.16, and 6.17) to a depth of 15–20 mm. The needle is inserted at the medial side of caruncle, at the extreme medial side of the palpebral fissure and directed at a 5° angle away from the sagittal plane toward the medial orbital wall. The needle should never be introduced more than 20 mm for the caruncular puncture. A medial peribulbar with a 25G, 31 mm long needle may be used as primary technique in patients with long axial length, which may be associated with higher incidence of staphyloma.

Dosage

Three milliliters of local anesthetic agent of choice is injected if this technique is used as a supplementary injection. However, if this technique is used as a primary injection technique, a volume 6–8 ml may be required.

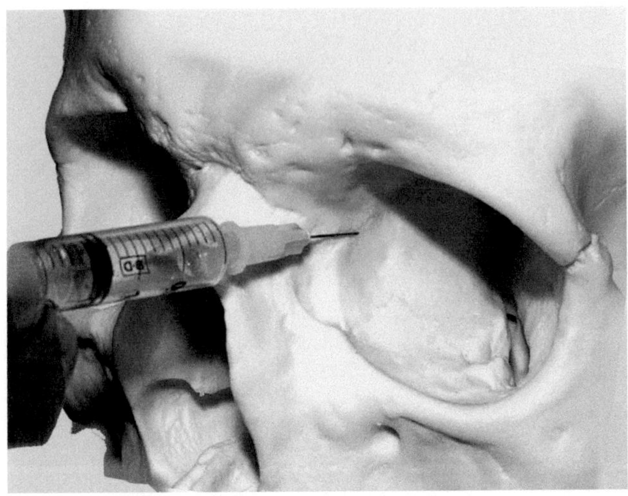

Fig. 6.16 A photography of the skull showing direction of needle during medial (caruncular) peribulbar block. (Reproduced with permission from A. van Zundert, Ch. Kumar)

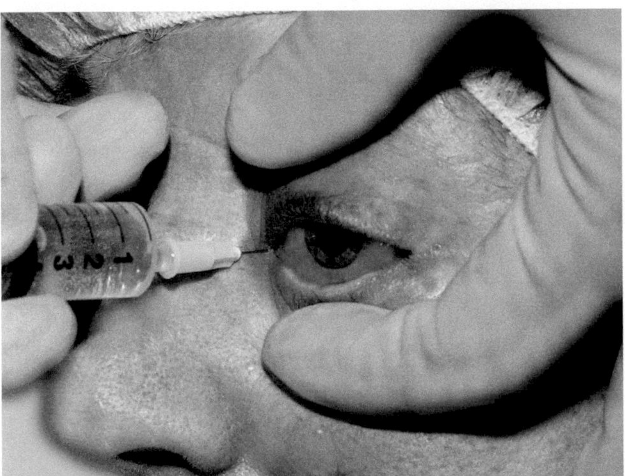

Fig. 6.17 Medial (caruncular) block: 27 gauge 2 cm long needle is inserted between the caruncle and medial canthus during medial peribulbar block. (Reproduced with permission from A. van Zundert)

Advantages of Medial Peribulbar or Caruncular Technique

The medial canthus single-injection peribulbar anesthesia is significantly less painful and required less anesthetic agent than the double-injection peribulbar anesthesia. The diffusion space of anesthetic agents around the globe is segmented by a network of numerous tiny aponeuroses, which may be less dense in the medial canthus region, and this might explain better diffusion and low volume requirement. Further extraconal space in this compartment is relatively large and avascular, and this may reduce the risk of hematoma or intravascular injection.

Disadvantages

Multiple injections may be required during peribulbar block. Caution is required during supplementary injection as the first injection is likely to alter the position of the globe in the orbit.

Complications of Needle-Based Blocks

There are many complications of needle-based blocks, ranging from simple to serious, that have been reported and published. The complications may be limited to the orbit or may be systemic. Orbital complications include failure of the block, corneal abrasion, chemosis, conjunctival hemorrhage, vessel damage leading to retrobulbar hemorrhage, globe perforation, globe penetration, optic or other nerves damage and extraocular muscle damage. Oculocardiac reflex leading to bradycardia or even cardiac arrest due to the vasovagal reflex is observed in younger and frail patients and may be rarely seen both during the block procedure and also intraoperatively. Injury to the extraocular muscles (usually the inferior oblique muscle or inferior rectus muscle) can lead to muscle necrosis, contractions, or disturbances of healing. The systemic complications, such as local anesthetic agent toxicity, brain stem anesthesia and cardiorespiratory arrest, may be due to intravenous or intrathecal injections or the spread or misplacement of drug in the orbit during or immediately after injection.

Sub-Tenon's Block

This block was introduced as a simple, safe and effective alternative to needle blocks. The technique involves gaining access to the sub-Tenon's space, the insertion of a blunt cannula and the administration of local anesthetic agent into the sub-Tenon's space. Injection of local anesthetic into sub-Tenon's space allows spread along the extraocular muscle sheaths, diffusion into the retrobulbar space, spread into the fascial planes around the lids, as well as a direct action on the nerves supplying the globe that pass through this space. The sub-Tenon's space can be accessed from all four quadrants but the inferonasal quadrant is the most commonly reported site of access in the published studies as the placement of cannula in this quadrant allows good fluid distribution superiorly while avoiding the area of access for surgery and damage to the vortex veins.

Indications

Sub-Tenon's block is a versatile and effective technique. Its use has been advocated primarily for cataract surgery but is also effective for viteroretinal surgery, panretinal photocoagulation, trabeculectomy, strabismus surgery, optic nerve sheath fenestration and the delivery of drugs. This technique is also increasingly favored in patients who are on anticoagulants, aspirin and nonsteroidal anti-inflammatory drugs (NSAID).

Materials

Topical local anesthetic agent, povidone iodine (5%), scissors, forceps, local anesthetic agent, blunt sub-Tenon can-

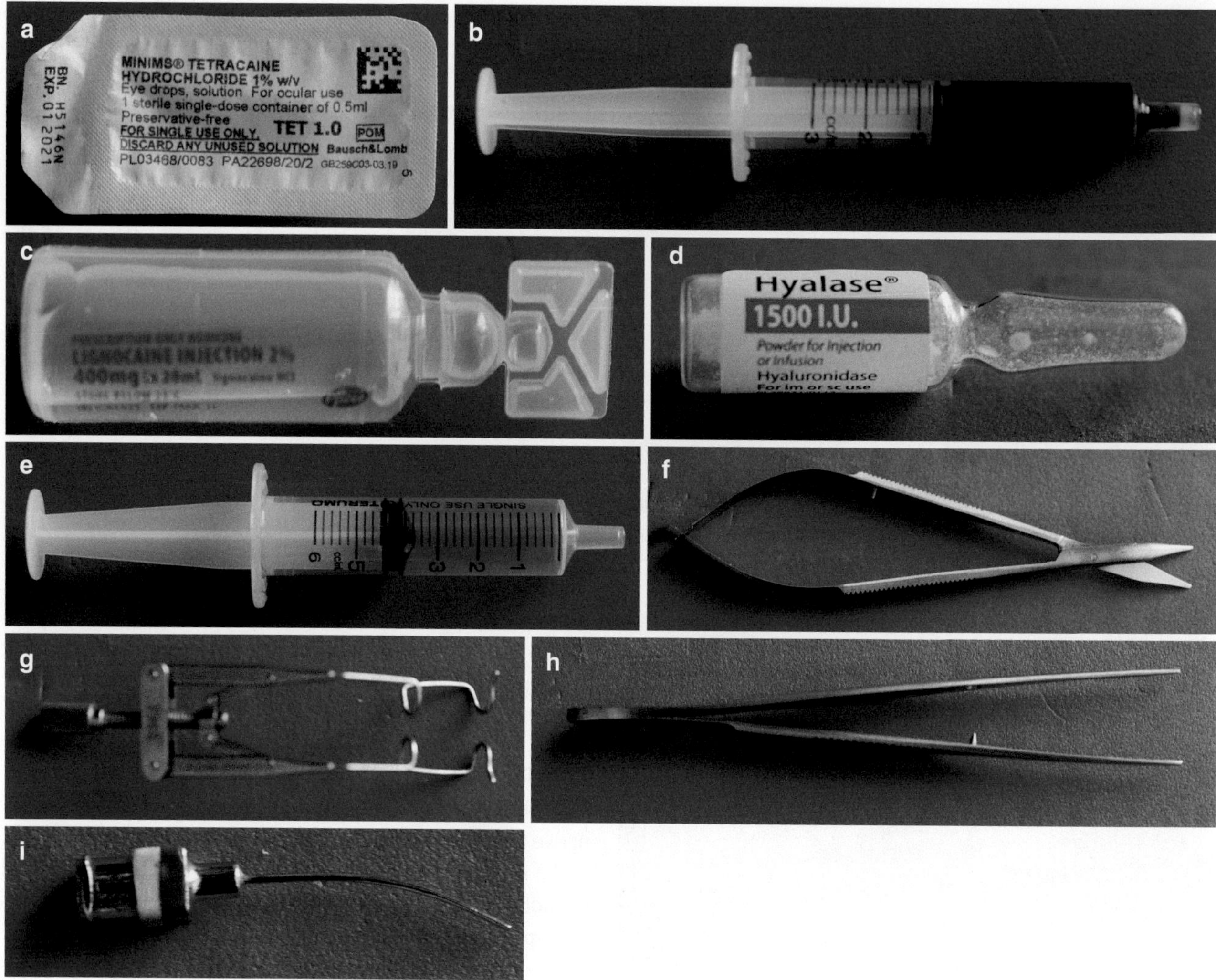

Fig. 6.18 Materials required for a sub-Tenon's block. (**a**) Tetracaine eye drop, (**b**) Povidone iodine 5%, (**c**) Lidocaine, (**d**) Hyaluronidase (**e**) Syringe, (**f**) Westcott scissors, (**g**) Eye speculum, (**h**) Non-toothed forceps, (**i**) sub-Tenon's cannula. (Reproduced with permission from A. van Zundert, Ch. Kumar)

nula and syringe are required (Figs. 6.18, 6.19, and 6.20). Additional materials such as speculum (Clarke or Screw speculum), gloves, cotton buds, hyaluronidase and epinephrine may be helpful.

Preparation

Surface anesthesia and Speculum placement All topical local anesthetic drops have been used but preservative-free topical preparations in single-dose containers (0.4% oxybuprocaine or 1% tetracaine eye drop) are usually preferred but most of them produce stinging on initial application. Surface anesthesia can also be achieved with the application of a cotton bud soaked with topical agent in the area of dissection. The procedure is carried out under sterile conditions, and no-touch technique is advocated as infections are known to occur. Conjunctiva is cleaned with aqueous 5% povidone iodine for 3 min. Some prefer to use a speculum but if not available the lower lid is retracted by an assistant.

Patient Positioning and Injection Technique

Anesthetists can approach from head end or from the side. The patient is positioned supine with comfortable pads and sponges. The patient is asked to look upwards and outwards to allow adequate space for dissection (Fig. 6.21). If sedation is used, dissection can be performed in neutral gaze position. Under sterile conditions, the conjunctiva and Tenon capsule are gripped with non-toothed forceps 5–8 mm away from the limbus (Fig. 6.22a). A small incision is made through these layers (conjunctiva and Tenon capsule) with scissors to expose the white area and a sub-Tenon cannula (2.54 cm curved and blunt) is inserted along the curvature of the globe (Fig. 6.22a, b). It is not unusual to meet a resistance during this procedure especially when Tenon's capsule is not dissected properly or

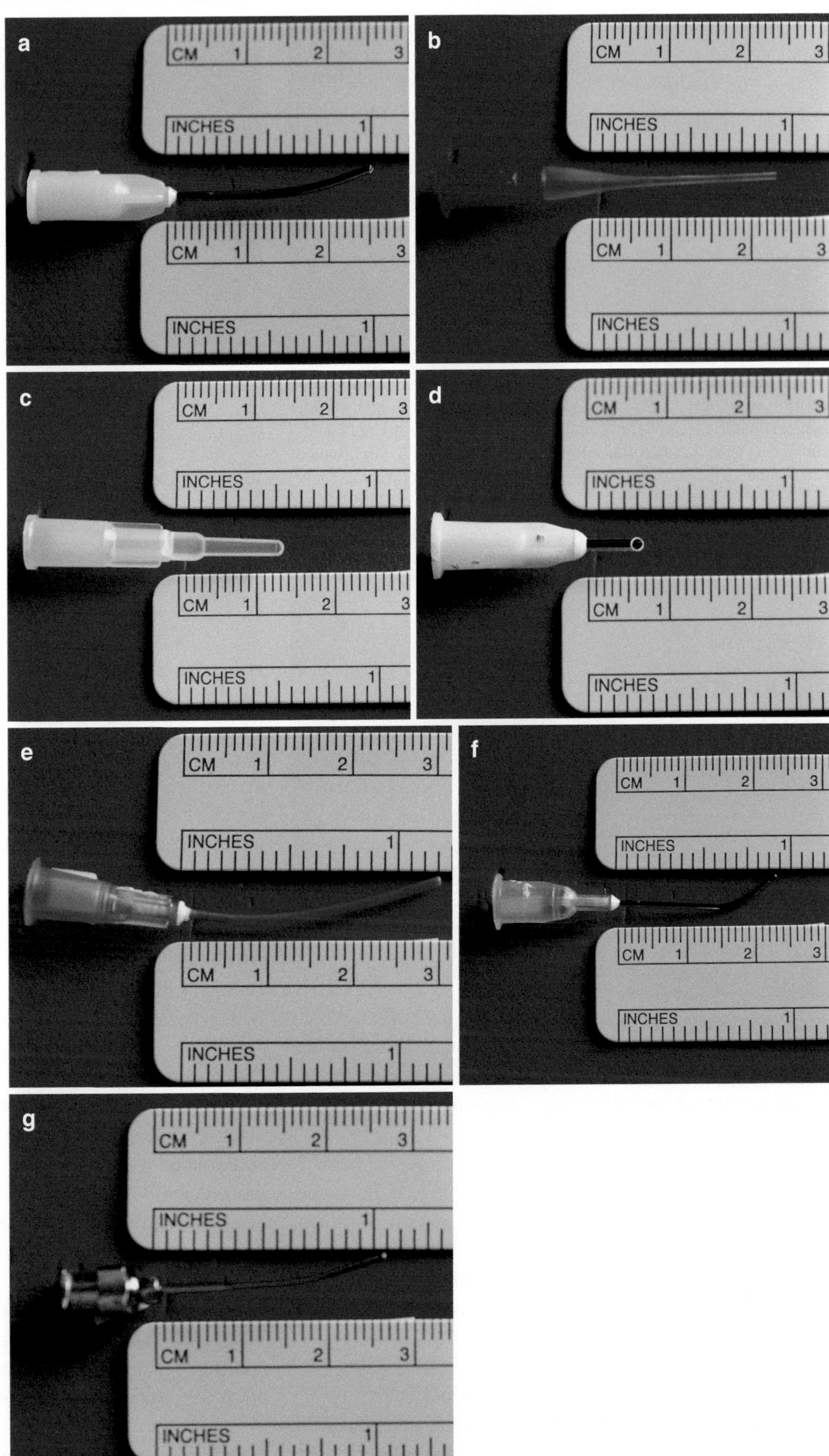

Fig. 6.19 Sub-Tenon's cannulae. (**a**) A standard posterior sub-Tenon's cannula, 19 gauge and 2.54 cm long, metal. (**b**) Mid sub-Tenon's cannula (Kumar Dodds), 21 gauge and 1.8 cm long, plastic. (**c**) Anterior sub-Tenon's cannula (Greenbaum cannula), 14 gauge and 1.2 cm long, plastic. (**d**) Ultra-short cannula, 14 gauge and 0.6 cm long, metal. (**e**) Helica cannula 20.0 mm, curved, internal diameter 1.0 mm (Helica Instruments Ltd. UK). (**f**) Triport sub-Tenon's cannula, 21 gauge, 25.4 cm long (1 in.), angled, curved, metal, disposable cannula. (**g**) Disposable metal sub-Tenon's cannula 21 gauge, 2 cm long. (Reproduced with permission from A. van Zundert, Ch. Kumar)

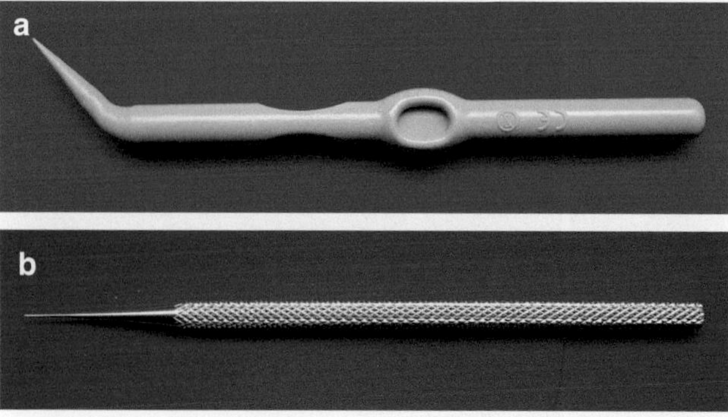

Fig. 6.20 (**a**) Conjunctival probe (angulated and pointed and made of plastic material, CPO-1 Ref. 270, Blink Medical, Birmingham, UK) to perform incisionless sub-Tenon's block. (**b**) Lacrimal dilator (Wilder punctal dilator, Size 1, Serial Number K7-2110) to perform incisionless sub-Tenon's block. (Reproduced with permission from A. van Zundert, Ch. Kumar)

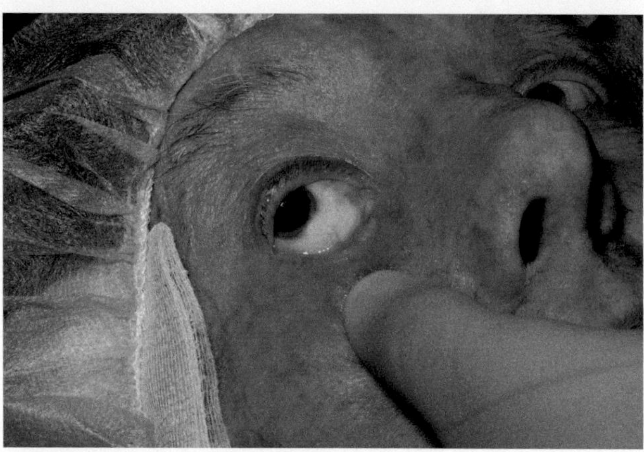

Fig. 6.21 Gaze of the globe (upwards and outwards) during dissection for inferonasal access for sub-Tenon's block. Upwards and outwards rotation helps to expose the area of dissection. (Reproduced with permission from A. van Zundert, Ch. Kumar)

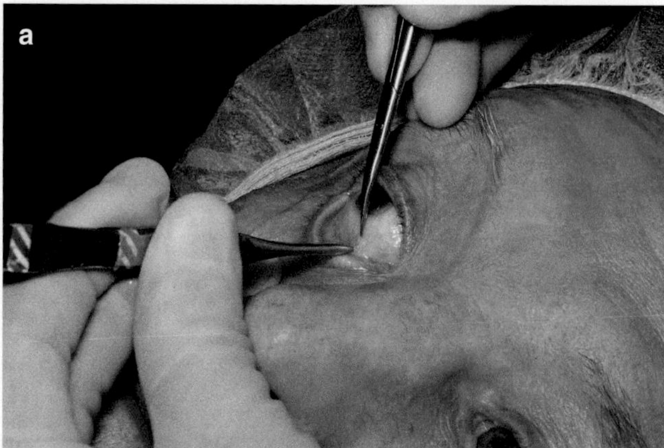

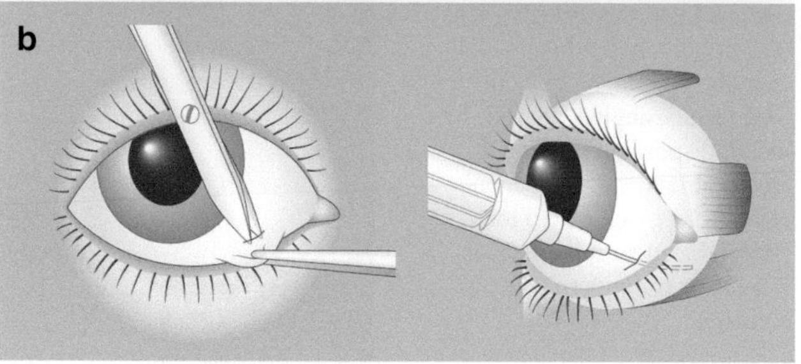

Fig. 6.22 (**a**) Inferonasal dissection for sub-Tenon's block with Wescott scissors and Moorfields forceps. (Reproduced with permission from A. van Zundert, Ch. Kumar). (**b**) Carrying out a sub-Tenon block. (*a*) The conjunctiva and Tenon capsule are opened with Westcott scissors. (*b*) The sub-Tenon cannula is introduced into the posterior sub-Tenon space. (Reproduced with permission from Danilo Jankovic)

the cannula does not advance because resistance is met by tissues (connective tissue bands), the cannula should be repositioned or inserted but force is never applied.

Dosage

3–5 mL of local anesthetic agent of choice (2% lidocaine, 0.5% bupivacaine, 0.5% bupivacaine) is usually sufficient for most surgeries.

The volume can be increased for vitreoretinal surgery. Addition of hyaluronidase and vasoconstrictor with local anesthetic is a subject of debate (see later).

Recent Developments in Sub-Tenon's Block

Sub-Tenon's block has undergone several changes since the technique was popularized in 1992 by Stevens and Greenbaum. These changes include the use of different types of blunt metal cannulae, plastic cannulae, ultrashort cannulae, and "incisionless" approaches using a blunt cannula without dissection or with help of conjunctival probe and lacrimal probe.

Advantages

Advantages include low risk of orbital and systemic complications, safer in anticoagulated patient, suitable in patients with myopic eyes and minimum rise in intraocular pressure.

Disadvantages

The technique is associated with frequent chemosis and conjunctival hemorrhage. Muscle and eyelid akinesia are variable and volume-dependent. It is an invasive and a surgical technique. Asepsis is of paramount importance. The technique could be difficult to learn initially but gets easier with experience. Loss of local anaesthetic during this procedure may occur.

Contraindications of Sub-Tenon's Block

There is hardly any contraindication but absolute contraindications would include patient refusal, inability to cooperate, and infection at the injection site.

Complications of Sub-Tenon's Block

Although sub-Tenon's block was introduced as a very safe technique over the years, a number of complications both minor (see above) and major have been reported.

Major complications, although rare, include orbital and retrobulbar hemorrhage, rectus muscle paresis and trauma, globe perforation, the central spread of local anesthetic, orbital cellulitis and others. Most of these complications have occurred following the use of a 2.54 cm metal cannula but the exact mechanism and their incidence are not known. Smaller or flexible cannulae appear to be safer but the incidence of minor complications increases.

Topical Anesthesia

Topical anesthesia is increasingly used for cataract surgery and preferred by ophthalmic surgeons or nonmedical healthcare professionals. This is not an invasive technique and different considerations apply. There is no sight or life-threatening complications. Readers are advised to consult relevant texts.

Checking Adequacy of Anesthesia

There is no objective method of checking anesthesia. It is anticipated that if akinesia is complete or near complete, anesthesia would accompany. If akinesia is not adequate or surgeon prefers complete akinesia, a repeat injection is considered.

Anticoagulation and Eye Block (See Chap. 1)

There is an increased incidence of subconjunctival and orbital hemorrhage in patients who receive aspirin, nonsteroidal anti-inflammatory drugs, oral anticoagulants, and antiplatelet agents. Clotting profile should be checked and values must be in the therapeutic range. If the patient is receiving warfarin, it should not be stopped. INR must be checked. If INR is higher than 3.5, the injection technique is better avoided. Long needles with sharp tips increase the risk of hemorrhage. Smaller needles and single-shot injections appear to be safer, and the sub-Tenon's technique is apparently safer still.

Local Anesthetic Agents for Ophthalmic Blocks

The ideal agent for ophthalmic block should be safe, painless to inject and produce a rapid onset of dense motor and sensory block, the duration of which must be sufficient for surgery yet not excessively prolonged. A technique based on higher volume can lead to an increased incidence of chemosis. The speed of onset is partially determined by the properties of the anesthetic, but more directly by the proximity to the nerves. All the modern, high-potency local anesthetic agents are suitable for ophthalmic blocks, and numerous studies have shown little difference in the quality of anesthesia, analgesia and akinesia. A complete blockade of nerves may not occur. Many patients reported retained visual sensations (see later). Muscles regain their full activities after a few hours and double vision may be experienced. It is important to inform the patient that while local anesthetic is present, it is important to avoid rubbing the eye.

Role of Vasoconstrictor

Vasoconstrictor (epinephrine) may be mixed with local anesthetic solution to increase the intensity and duration of block and minimize bleeding from small vessels. A concentration 1:200,000 appears to have no systemic effect. However, epinephrine may cause vasoconstriction of the ophthalmic artery, compromising the retinal circulation. The use of epinephrine-containing solutions is avoided in elderly patients suffering from cerebrovascular and cardiovascular diseases. If anesthesia for longer duration is required, an agent which lasts longer, such as bupivacaine, ropivacaine or levobupivacaine, should be used.

Role of Hyaluronidase

Hyaluronidase is an enzyme, which reversibly liquefies the interstitial barrier between cells by depolymerization of hyaluronic acid to a tetrasaccharide, thereby enhancing the diffusion of molecules through tissue planes. It is available as a powder readily soluble in local anaesthetic solution. Hyaluronidase has been shown to improve the effectiveness and the quality of needle as well as sub-Tenon's block, but its use remains controversial. The amount of hyaluronidase used varies from 5 to 150 IU/ml; however, The British National Formulary recommends limiting hyaluronidase to 15 IU/ml for ophthalmic anesthesia. Orbital swelling and allergic reactions can occur. Excellent blocks can be achieved without hyaluronidase, but there are reports of muscle dysfunction when it is not used during needle block. It is generally believed that local anesthetic agents stay in contact with thin muscles for a longer period leading to myotoxicity.

Intraocular Pressure and Ophthalmic Blocks

Rise in intraocular pressure is observed immediately after retrobulbar and peribulbar injections, but no such rise is reported after sub-Tenon's block. Oculocompression devices such as Honan's balloon, McIntyre mercury bag may be necessary to reduce the intraocular pressure. However, when an oculocompression device is used, the pressure should not exceed 25 mmHg and checked intermittently and removed after 5 min.

Retained Visual Sensations During Ophthalmic Blocks

Some patients experience intraoperative visual sensations that include light, colors, movements and instruments during surgery under all forms of local ophthalmic anesthesia. Although the majority of patients feel comfortable with the visual sensations they experience, a small proportion may find the experience unpleasant or frightening. Therefore, patients receiving orbital blocks should receive preoperative advice as this may alleviate an unpleasant experience and sedatives are known to help.

Intraoperative Care

The patient should be comfortable and soft pads are placed under pressure areas. All patients undergoing major eye surgery under local anesthesia are monitored with pulse oximetry, ECG, noninvasive blood pressure measurement and the maintenance of verbal contact. Patients should receive low flow oxygen to prevent hypoxia and rebreathing of carbon dioxide under the drape. ECG and pulse oximetry should be continued. Once the patient is under the drapes, verbal and tactile contacts are maintained.

Advantages and Disadvantages of Different Techniques

There are conflicting reports on the relative effectiveness of akinetic blocks. The evidence indicates that peribulbar and retrobulbar anesthesia produce equally good akinesia and equivalent pain control during cataract surgery. Although there is insufficient evidence in the literature to make a definite statement concerning the relative effectiveness of sub-Tenon's block in producing akinesia when compared with peribulbar or retrobulbar block but, there was moderate evidence that sub-Tenon's block produced better pain control than retrobulbar, peribulbar block and topical anesthesia.

Choosing a Technique

There are numerous studies illustrating the diversity of preference for anesthetic technique by surgeons. The choice of the technique will depend on a balance between the patient's wishes, the operative needs of the surgeon, the skills of the anesthetist and the place where such surgery is being performed. The practice of local anesthesia varies around the world. Although akinesia is not desirable during modern phacoemulsification surgery, other ophthalmic surgeries will require a complete akinesia and anesthesia (viscocanalostomy, vitrectomy). Needles blocks are usually a single shot technique of anesthesia but akinesia depends on the choice of local anesthetic agent and technique used. Sub-Tenon's anesthesia usually provides excellent anesthesia and should the need arise it can be repeated through the initial dissection.

Conclusion

Eye blocks provide excellent anesthesia for ophthalmic surgery and success rates are high. Satisfactory anesthesia and akinesia can be obtained with both needle and cannula blocks. At present, there is no perfect technique. Although rare, orbital injections may cause severe local and systemic complications but much less frequently with sub-Tenon's block. Knowledge of orbital anatomy and training are essential for the practice of safe orbital regional anesthesia.

Akinesia of the Orbicularis Oculi Muscle: Facial Nerve Block

Danilo Jankovic and Chandra M. Kumar

General Consideration

Facial nerve block used to be routinely performed after a low-volume classical retrobulbar block to provide orbicularis akinesia. If the orbicularis muscle is not immobilized, the patient may squeeze the eyelids, which may interfere with surgery and increase intraocular pressure. The orbicularis muscle is supplied by the facial nerve and akinesia can be achieved by blocking the facial nerve by a distal infiltration block of the nerve endings of the facial nerve that provide the motor supply to the orbit. Modern higher volume local anaesthetic agent single injection peribulbar block or double injection techniques provide anesthesia and usually block the terminal branches of the seventh nerve and paralysis of the orbicularis per se is not required. Orbicularis akinesia can also be achieved by injecting local anaesthetic in the inferior fornix, in the lower lid near the lateral canthus, or in the subcutaneous space of the lower or upper lid when withdrawing the retrobulbar needle, making a separate facial nerve block unnecessary.

Indications

1. To produce akinesia of orbicularis muscle after classical retrobulbar block but this block rarely recommended for routine practice.
2. Surgery involving face and eyelid.
3. As a therapeutic procedure for hemifacial spasm and blepharospasm. After a successful nerve block, facial spasm stops immediately.
4. Postherpetic neuralgia.

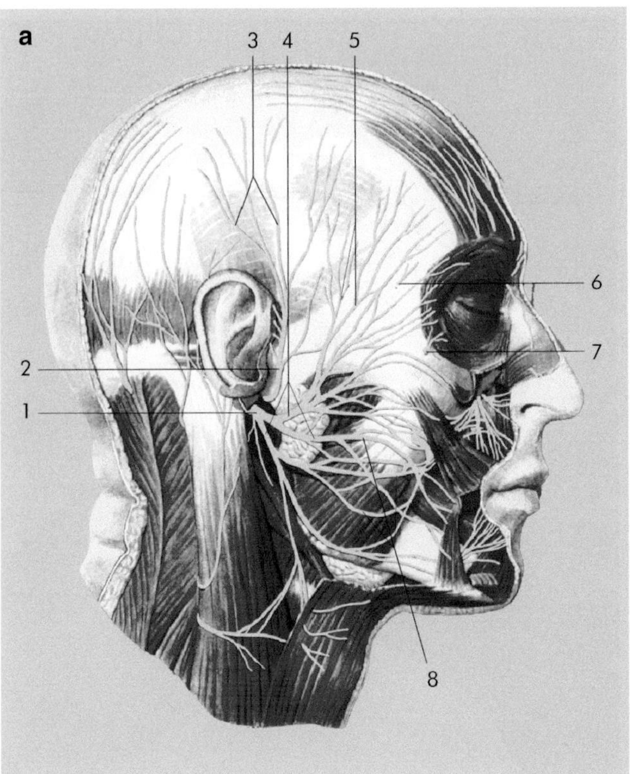

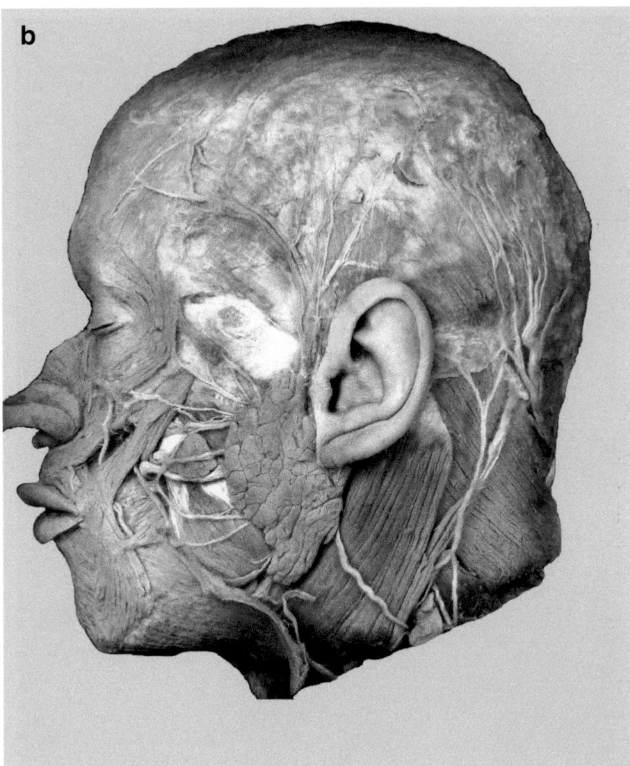

Fig. 6.23 (**a**) Anatomy of the facial nerve. (*1*) Facial nerve, (*2*) auriculotemporal nerve, (*3*) superficial temporal branches, (*4*) parotid plexus, (*5*) temporal branches, (*6*) zygomaticotemporal branch of zygomatic nerve, (*7*) zygomaticofacial branch of zygomatic nerve, (*8*) buccal branches of facial nerve. (Reproduced with permission from Danilo Jankovic). (**b**) Facial nerve. Anatomic specimen. (Reproduced with permission from Danilo Jankovic)

Functional Anatomy (Fig. 6.23a, b)

The seventh cranial nerve carries motor fibers for the muscles of facial expression. The facial nerve emerges from the posterolateral angle of the pons, proceeds laterally to enter the internal auditory meatus, in which it traverses until reaching the medial wall of the epitympanic recess, where it suddenly curves posteriorly and inferiorly, and travels within the facial canal to make its exit from the skull by way of the stylomastoid foramen. While the nerve is within the facial canal, about 0.5 cm above the stylomastoid foramen, it gives rise to the chorda tympani. Blocking the nerve at the stylomastoid foramen, therefore, does not involve the chorda tympani.

Block Techniques

The facial nerve can be blocked using various techniques along its course to the orbit. These locations are topographically related to the facial nerve and its ramifications. These blocks differ in efficacy as well as akinesia of lid.

Van Lint Method (Fig. 6.24)

Blocking the facial nerve to paralyze the orbicularis muscle was first advocated by van Lint in 1914. The injection is carried out temporally from the exterior margin of the eyelid or classically just below it temporally. A 27 gauge, short hypodermic needle 12–17 mm long is initially introduced until bone contact is made. After careful aspiration, the injection is carried out medially and downward and then medially and upward. Fan-shaped injection is carried out as the needle is advanced (dosage, 1.5–2 ml local anesthetic). The van Lint facial nerve block is still commonly used in the original or modified form.

O'Brien Method (Fig. 6.25)

The facial nerve trunk is blocked just above the condylar process of the mandible. It is helpful for the patient to open and close the mouth. After palpation of the condylar process of the mandible, a 27 gauge, short hypodermic needle 12–17 mm long is introduced until bone contact is made, and 1 ml local anesthetic is injected. The needle is then withdrawn, followed by injection first in the caudal direction and then in the cranial direction (dosage, 1.5–2 ml local anesthetic). Due to anatomi-

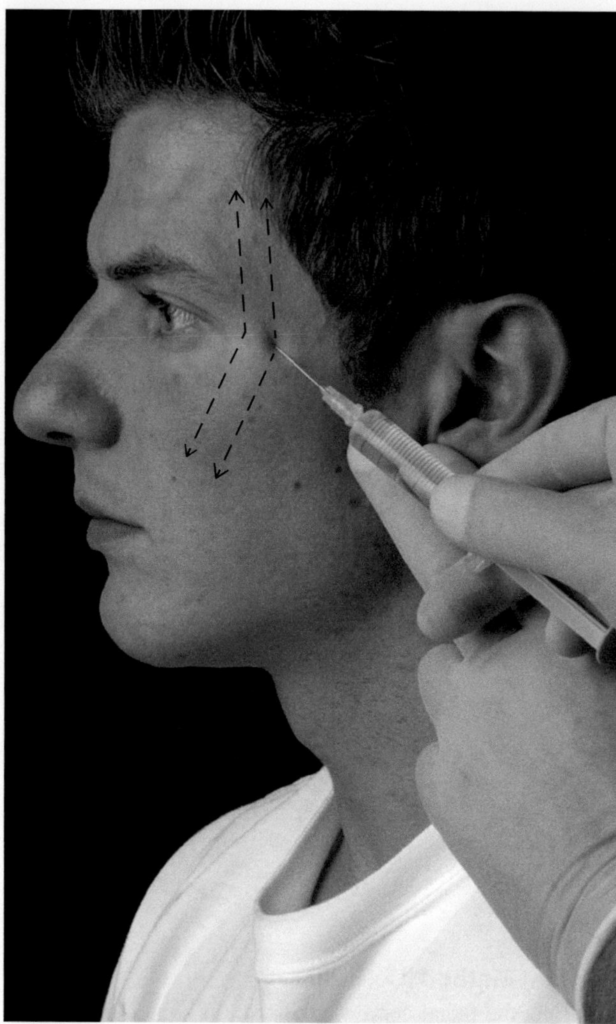

Fig. 6.24 Block for eyelid anesthesia. van Lint method. (Reproduced with permission from Danilo Jankovic)

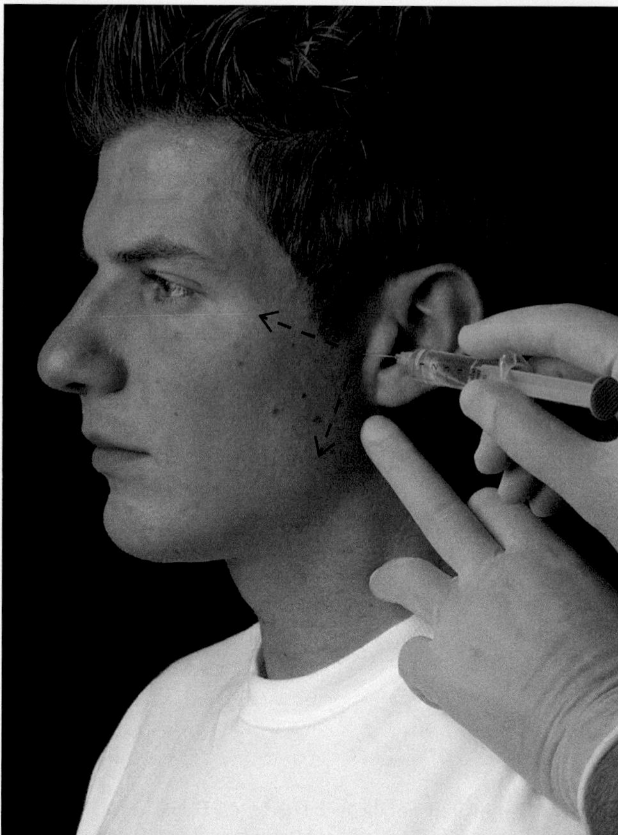

Fig. 6.25 Block for eyelid anesthesia. O'Brien method. (Reproduced with permission from Danilo Jankovic)

cal variations, occasionally the facial nerve is not successfully blocked. This block can be painful at the time of injection. The lower branches of the facial nerve supplying the lips and face are frequently blocked, leading to facial paralysis.

Atkinson Method (Fig. 6.26)

A 27 gauge short hypodermic needle 12–17 mm long is introduced below the exterior angle of the eye at the level of the zygomatic arch and is moved upward and outward (dosage, 2 ml local anaesthetic). This block is usually painful. Firm pressure is then applied over the site of the injection and rarely fails to obtain complete akinesia of the orbicularis.

Nadbath–Rehman Method (Fig. 6.27)

The Nadbath facial nerve block selectively blocks the facial nerve directly underneath the mastoid process as it leaves the skull through the stylomastoid foramen. A 27 gauge short hypodermic needle 12–17 mm long is introduced vertically to a depth of 1–1.5 cm (dosage, 1.5–2 ml local anesthetic). This block is painful.

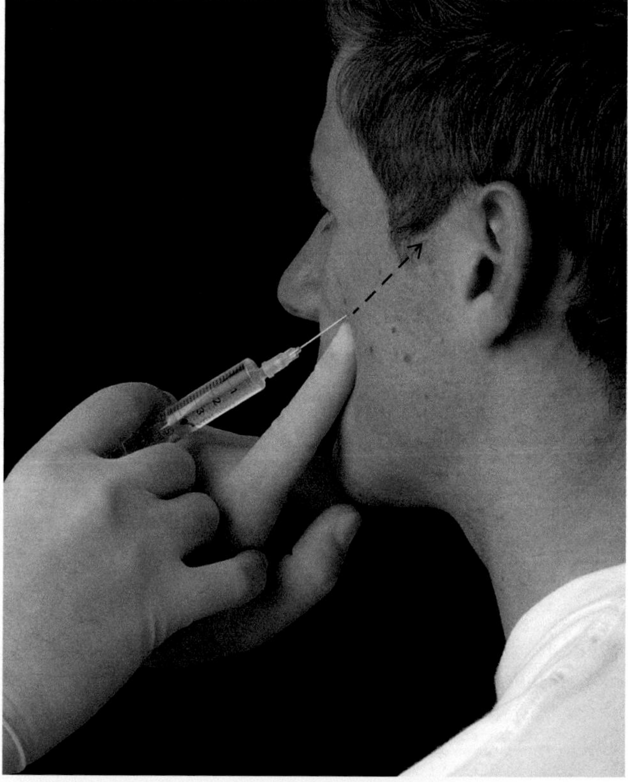

Fig. 6.26 Block for eyelid anesthesia. Atkinson method. (Reproduced with permission from Danilo Jankovic)

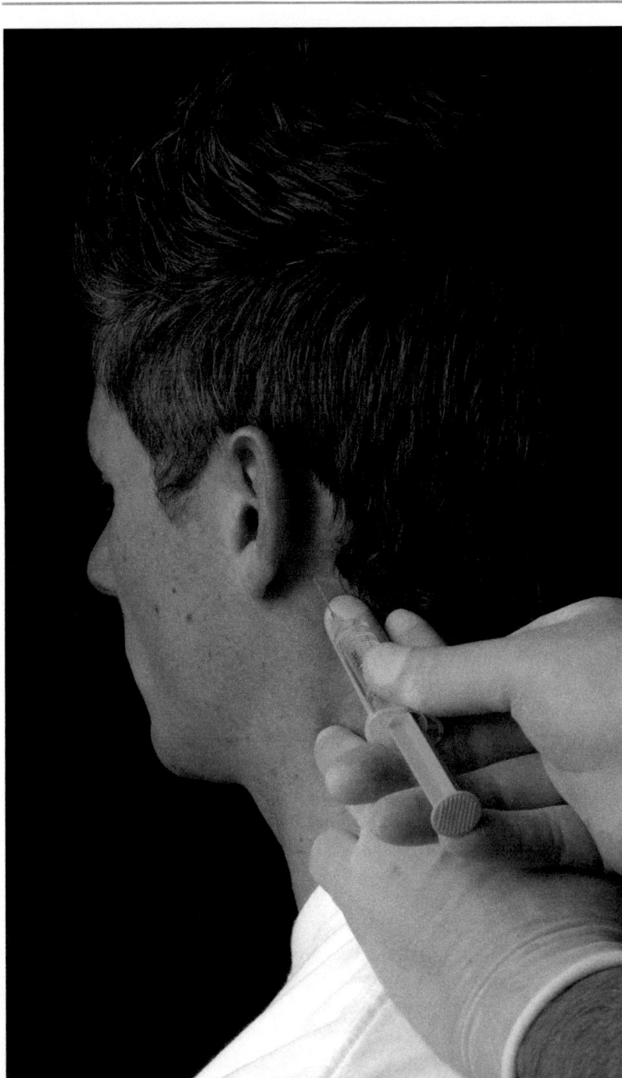

Fig. 6.27 Block for eyelid anesthesia. Nadbath–Rehmann method. (Reproduced with permission from Danilo Jankovic)

Complications

All distal facial nerve blocks are associated with complications. van Lint method sometimes causes eyelid oedema and lid hemorrhage, which may contribute to postoperative ptosis. Vertigo with nystagmus may occur when a local anaesthetic is injected near the stylomastoid foramen. This is the influence of the local anaesthetic infusing into the internal ear. Bleeding in the external auditory canal may occur when the skin of an external auditory canal is damaged with the block needle. Nadbath block is unfortunately associated with more frequent complications compared to other distal facial nerve blocks. These complications include paralysis of the facial nerve, sudden onset of respiratory obstruction and cord paralysis. If a long needle and large volumes of anaesthetic solution are used in thin patients, inadvertent injection of anesthetic solution into the jugular foramen, which lies approximately 10 mm medial to the stylomastoid foramen, has resulted in paralysis of the vagus, glossopharyngeal and spinal accessory nerves causing dysphagia, hoarseness, dysphonia, coughing, unilateral vocal cord paralysis and respiratory distress from pooling of oropharyngeal secretions and laryngospasm.

Prophylaxis: Use of short hypodermic needles, small volumes of local anesthetic solution, and omission of hyaluronidase may reduce the incidence of complications.

Suggested Reading

Regional Anesthesia in Ophthalmology

Allman KG, Theron AD, Byles DB. A new technique of incisionless minimally invasive sub-Tenon's anaesthesia. Anaesthesia. 2008;63:782–3.

Alwitry A, Koshy Z, Browning AC, Kiel W, Holden R. The effect of sub-Tenon's anaesthesia on intraocular pressure. Eye (Lond). 2001;15:733–5.

Benzimra JD, Johnston RL, Jaycock P, Galloway PH, Lambert G, Chung AKK, et al. The Cataract National Dataset electronic multicentre audit of 55,567 operations: antiplatelet and anticoagulant medications. Eye (Lond). 2009;23:10–6.

Chen CL, Lin GA, Bardach NS, Clay TH, Boscardin WJ, Gelb AW, et al. Preoperative medical testing in Medicare patients undergoing cataract surgery. N Engl J Med. 2015;372:1530–8.

Chua A, Chua MJ, Kumar CM. Punctal dilator facilitates insertion of blunt cannula during sub-Tenon's block. Anaesth Intensive Care. 2018;46:239–40.

Deruddre S, Benhamou D. Medial canthus single-injection peribulbar anesthesia: a prospective randomized comparison with classic double-injection peribulbar anesthesia. Reg Anesth Pain Med. 2005;30:255–9.

Greenbaum S. Parabulbar anesthesia. Am J Ophthalmol. 1992;114:776.

Guise P. Sub-Tenon's anesthesia: an update. Local Reg Anesth. 2012;5:35–46.

Guise P, Laurent S. Sub-Tenon's block: the effect of hyaluronidase on speed of onset and block quality. Anaesth Intensive Care. 1999;27:179–81.

Joint Formulary Committee, editor. BNF 79 (British National Formulary) March 2020. 79th Revised edition. Pharmaceutical Press; 2020.

Karampatakis V, Natsis K, Gigis P, Stangos NT. Orbital depth measurements of human skulls in relation to retrobulbar anesthesia. Eur J Ophthalmol. 1998;8:118–20.

Katz J, Feldman MA, Bass EB, Lubomski LH, Tielsch JM, Petty BG, et al. Adverse intraoperative medical events and their association with anesthesia management strategies in cataract surgery. Ophthalmology. 2001;108:1721–6.

Kumar CM. Needle-based blocks for the 21st century ophthalmology. Acta Ophthalmol. 2011;89:5–9.

Kumar CM, Dodds C. A disposable plastic sub-Tenon cannula. Anaesthesia. 2001;56:399–400.

Kumar CM, Dodds C. Ophthalmic regional block. Ann Acad Med Singap. 2006a;35:158–67.

Kumar CM, Dodds C. Sub-Tenon's anesthesia. Ophthalmol Clin North Am. 2006b;19:209–19.

Kumar CM, Dowd TC. Complications of ophthalmic regional blocks: their treatment and prevention. Ophthalmologica. 2006;220:73–82.

Kumar CM, McNeela BJ. Ultrasonic localization of anaesthetic fluid using sub-Tenon's cannulae of three different lengths. Eye (Lond). 2003;17:1003–7.

Kumar CM, Seet E. Stopping antithrombotics during regional anaesthesia and eye surgery: crying wolf? Br J Anaesth. 2017a;118:154–8.

Kumar CM, Seet E. Effective and cost-saving incisionless sub-Tenon's block. Indian J Anaesth. 2017b;61:84–5.

Kumar CM, Dodds C, Fanning GL. Ophthalmic anaesthesia. 1st ed. Netherland: Swets and Zeitlinger; 2002.

Kumar CM, Dowd TC, Dodds C, Boyce R. Orbital swelling following peribulbar and sub-Tenon's anaesthesia. Eye (Lond). 2004;18:418–20.

Kumar CM, Dowd TC, Hawthorne M. Retrobulbar alcohol injection for orbital pain relief under difficult circumstances: a case report. Ann Acad Med Singap. 2006;35:260–5.

Kumar CM, Eid H, Dodds C. Sub-Tenon's anaesthesia: complications and their prevention. Eye (Lond). 2011;25:694–703.

Kumar CM, Eke T, Dodds C, Deane JS, El-Hindy N, Johnston RL, et al. Local anaesthesia for ophthalmic surgery--new guidelines from the Royal College of Anaesthetists and the Royal College of Ophthalmologists. Eye (Lond). 2012;26:897–8.

Kumar CM, Seet E, Eke T, Dhatariya K, Joshi GP. Glycaemic control during cataract surgery under loco-regional anaesthesia: a growing problem and we are none the wiser. Br J Anaesth. 2016;117:687–91.

Kumar CM, Seet E, Eke T, Joshi GP. Hypertension and cataract surgery under loco-regional anaesthesia: not to be ignored? Br J Anaesth. 2017;119:855–9.

Kumar CM, Seet E, Eke T, Irwin MG, Joshi GP. Peri-operative considerations for sedation-analgesia during cataract surgery: a narrative review. Anaesthesia. 2019;74:1601–10.

Malik A, Fletcher EC, Chong V, Dasan J. Local anesthesia for cataract surgery. J Cataract Refract Surg. 2010;36:133–52.

McLure HA, Rubin AP. Review of local anaesthetic agents. Minerva Anestesiol. 2005;71:59–74.

McNeela BJ, Kumar CM. Sub-Tenon's block with an ultrashort cannula. J Cataract Refract Surg. 2004;30:858–62.

Nanji KC, Roberto SA, Morley MG, Bayes J. Preventing adverse events in cataract surgery: recommendations from a Massachusetts Expert Panel. Anesth Analg. 2018;126:1537–47.

Palte HD, Gayer S. Novel technique for minimally invasive sub-Tenon's anesthesia. Reg Anesth Pain Med. 2019;44:131–2.

Riad W, Ahmad N, Kumar CM. Comparison of metal and flexible sub-Tenon cannulas. J Cataract Refract Surg. 2012;38:1398–402.

Roman SJ, Chong Sit DA, Boureau CM, Auclin FX, Ullern MM. Sub-Tenon's anaesthesia: an efficient and safe technique. Br J Ophthalmol. 1997;81:673–6.

Seet E, Kumar CM, Eke T, Joshi GP. Starving patients before cataract surgery under regional anesthesia: needed or not? Anesth Analg. 2018;127:1448–51.

Stevens JD. A new local anesthesia technique for cataract extraction by one quadrant sub-Tenon's infiltration. Br J Ophthalmol. 1992;76:670–4.

Tan CSH, Au Eong K-G, Kumar CM. Visual experiences during cataract surgery: what anaesthesia providers should know. Eur J Anaesthesiol. 2005;22:413–9.

Venkatakrishnan JV, Kumar CM, Ratra V, Viswanathan J, Jeyaraman VA, Ragavendera T. Effect of sedation on visual sensations in patients undergoing cataract surgery under topical anaesthesia: a prospective randomized masked trial. Acta Ophthalmol. 2013;91:247–50.

Vohra SB, Good PA. Altered globe dimensions of axial myopia as risk factors for penetrating ocular injury during peribulbar anaesthesia. Br J Anaesth. 2000;85:242–5.

Winder S, Walker SB, Atta HR. Ultrasonic localization of anesthetic fluid in sub-Tenon's, peribulbar, and retrobulbar techniques. J Cataract Refract Surg. 1999;25:56–9.

Akinesia of the Orbicularis Oculi Muscle: Facial Nerve Block

Atkinson WS. Local anesthesia in ophthalmology. Trans Am Ophthalmol Soc. 1934;32:399–451.

Cofer HF. Cord paralysis after Nadbath facial nerve block. Arch Ophthalmol. 1986;104(3):337.

Eker HE, Yalçın Çok O, Açıl M, Ülger H, Arıboğan A. [Modified van-Lint technique for the management of postherpetic neuralgia: case report]. Agriculture 2011;23(2):84–7.

Feibel RM. Disadvantages of Nadbath facial nerve block. Ophthalmic Surg. 1988;19(8):607.

Kim C, Lee Y-B, Lee H-K, Yoon K-B, Choi R. Facial nerve block for the treatment of facial spasm-a retrospective analysis of 27 patients. Korean J Pain. 1994;7(1):43–8.

Koenig SB, Snyder RW, Kay J. Respiratory distress after a Nadbath block. Ophthalmology. 1988;95(9):1285–7.

Kumar CM. Needle-based blocks for the 21st century ophthalmology. Acta Ophthalmol. 2011 Feb;89(1):5–9.

van Lint A. Paralysie palpebrale temporaire provoquee' par l'ope'ration de la cataracte. Ann Ocul (Paris). 1914;151:420.

Nadbath RP. Rehmani null. Facial nerve block. Am J Ophthalmol. 1963;55:143–6.

Netter FH. Autonomes Nervensystem. Autonome Innervation von Kopf und Hals. In: Kramer G, Hrsg: Farbatlanten der Medizin (Band 5). Nervensystem I: Neuroanatomie und Physiologie. Stuttgart: Thieme; 1987.

O'Brien CS. Akinesia during cataract extraction. Arch Ophthalmol. 1929;1:447.

Rabinowitz L, Livingston M, Schneider H, Hall A. Respiratory obstruction following the Nadbath facial nerve block. Arch Ophthalmol. 1986;104(8):1115.

Sanchez-Capuchino A, Meadows D, Morgan L. Local anaesthesia for eye surgery without a facial nerve block. Anaesthesia. 1993;48(5):428–31.

Schimek F, Fahle M. Techniques of facial nerve block. Br J Ophthalmol. 1995;79(2):166–73.

Schimek F, Steuhl KP, Fahle M, Thiel HJ. [Eyelid akinesia after various techniques of facial nerve block]. Fortschr Ophthalmol. 1990;87(6):696–702.

Shoch D. Complications of the Nadbath facial nerve block. Arch Ophthalmol. 1986;104(8):1114–5.

Wakasugi B. Facial nerve block in the treatment of facial spasm. Arch Otolaryngol. 1972;95(4):356–9.

Wilson CA, Ruiz RS. Respiratory obstruction following the Nadbath facial nerve block. Arch Ophthalmol. 1985;103(10):1454–6.

7 Airway

Michael Seltz Kristensen, Wendy H. Teoh, and Danilo Jankovic

Contents

M. S. Kristensen
Department of Anaesthesia, Section 7023, Rigshospitalet, Copenhagen University Hospital, Copenhagen, Denmark
e-mail: Michael.seltz.kristensen@regionh.dk

W. H. Teoh
Private Anaesthesia Practice, Wendy Teoh Pte. Ltd., Singapore, Singapore

D. Jankovic (✉)
Pain Management Centre DGS – Cologne – Huerth, Cologne-Hürth, Germany
e-mail: danilo@jankovic1.de

Anesthesia of the Airways

General Considerations

Local anesthesia of the upper airway is crucial for awake intubation, a cornerstone approach in patients with predicted difficult airways including patients with airway compromise, trauma to the upper airway, or unstable cervical vertebrae.

Anatomy

Air passes to the pulmonary alveoli via the airways in the nose and nasal cavity, pharynx, larynx, and thus trachea, and bronchial tree, which divides at multiple levels. The upper

D. Jankovic, P. Peng (eds.), *Regional Nerve Blocks in Anesthesia and Pain Therapy*,
https://doi.org/10.1007/978-3-030-88727-8_7

airways are mainly located in the head. The lower airways are located in the neck and chest and include the larynx, trachea, and all the branches of the bronchial tree. The functional anatomy of the airways is illustrated in Figs. 7.1 and 7.2. The *nasal cavity* is divided by the nasal septum into right and left halves. The sensory innervation of the skin of the external nose is provided by the branches of the *ophthalmic nerve* and *maxillary nerve* (Fig. 7.1; cf. Chaps. 6, 8, 9), and the motor innervation of the facial muscles around the nose is from the *facial nerve* (cf. Chap. 6).

Each nasal cavity opens via a posterior choana into the upper level of the *pharynx*, the nasopharynx. The nasopharynx connects with the choanae and is enclosed by the skull base superiorly and by the pharyngeal wall posteriorly. Inferiorly, the soft palate forms the boundary to the middle level of the pharynx (oropharynx). The *larynx* is an air-conducting organ that stretches from the lower pharyngeal space (laryngopharynx) as far as the trachea. In adult males, the larynx is located at the level of the C3–C6 vertebrae (Fig. 7.3), while in women and children, it lies further up. The laryngeal mucosa is innervated as far as the vocal folds by the purely sensory *internal branch* of the *superior laryngeal nerve* and below that by the *recurrent laryngeal nerve*, both are branches of the *vagus nerve*. The inner laryngeal muscles are all supplied by the (*inferior*) *recurrent laryngeal*

Fig. 7.1 Functional anatomy of the airways. (*1*) Trigeminal nerve (V) with the ophthalmic and maxillary nerves. *Dotted red area*: field of sensory olfactory innervation via the olfactory nerve. (*2*) The sensory innervation area of the glossopharyngeal nerve (IX), (*3*) the sensory innervation area of the vagus nerve (X), (*4*) mandible, (*5*) epiglottis, (*6*) trachea, (*7*) esophagus. (With permission from Danilo Jankovic)

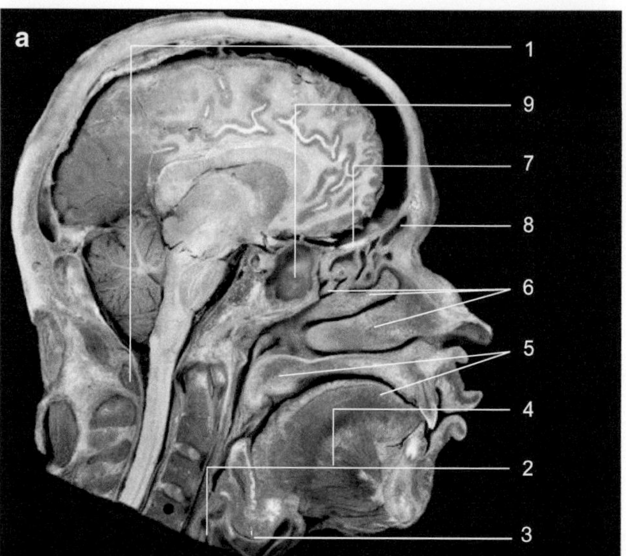

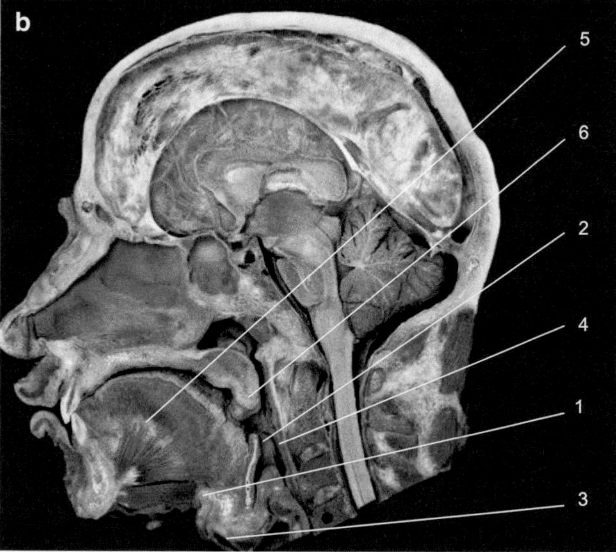

Fig. 7.2 (**a**) Functional anatomy of the airways. Median section through the head. (*1*) Posterior arch of the atlas, (*2*) cricoid cartilage, (*3*) geniohyoid, (*4*) genioglossus, (*5*) soft/hard palate and tongue, (*6*) nasal concha (superior, middle, inferior), (*7*) olfactory tract, (*8*) frontal sinus, (*9*) sphenoid sinus (With permission from Danilo Jankovic). (**b**) Functional anatomy of the airways. Median section through the head. (*1*) Hyoid bone, (*2*) epiglottis, (*3*) thyroid cartilage, (*4*) posterior pharyngeal wall (5) genioglossus, (*6*) uvula. (With permission from Danilo Jankovic)

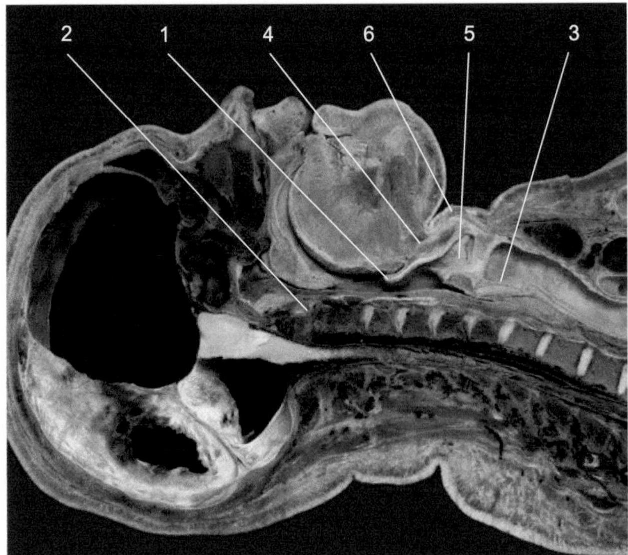

Fig. 7.3 Anatomic specimen. Paramedian sagittal section. In adults, the larynx is located over the C3–C6 vertebrae. (*1*) Epiglottis, (*2*) atlantodental joint, (*3*) trachea, (*4*) hyoid bone, (*5*) laryngeal ventricle, (*6*) thyroid cartilage. (With permission from Danilo Jankovic)

nerve. The only exterior laryngeal muscle, the *cricothyroid*, is innervated by the external branch of the *superior laryngeal nerve* (Fig. 7.4).

The *tongue* is basically a powerful muscle body that is covered with a mucosal layer, the mucosa of the tongue. The lingual mucosa in the anterior (presulcal) part of the tongue receives its sensory innervation from the lingual nerve (a branch of the mandibular nerve; cf. Chap. 8) and (with the exception of the vallate papillae) from the *chorda tympani* (branching from the intermediofacial nerve). The posterior (postsulcal) part of the tongue receives its sensory innervation from the *glossopharyngeal nerve* (with the exception of the epiglottic valleculae, which are supplied from the vagus nerve). The exterior lingual muscles (with the exception of the palatoglossus) are innervated from the *hypoglossal nerve* (Fig. 7.4).

The trachea is 10–12 cm long and stretches from the cricoid to the tracheal bifurcation. The smooth trachealis muscle is innervated from the recurrent laryngeal nerve, which is also responsible for the sensory and secretory innervation.

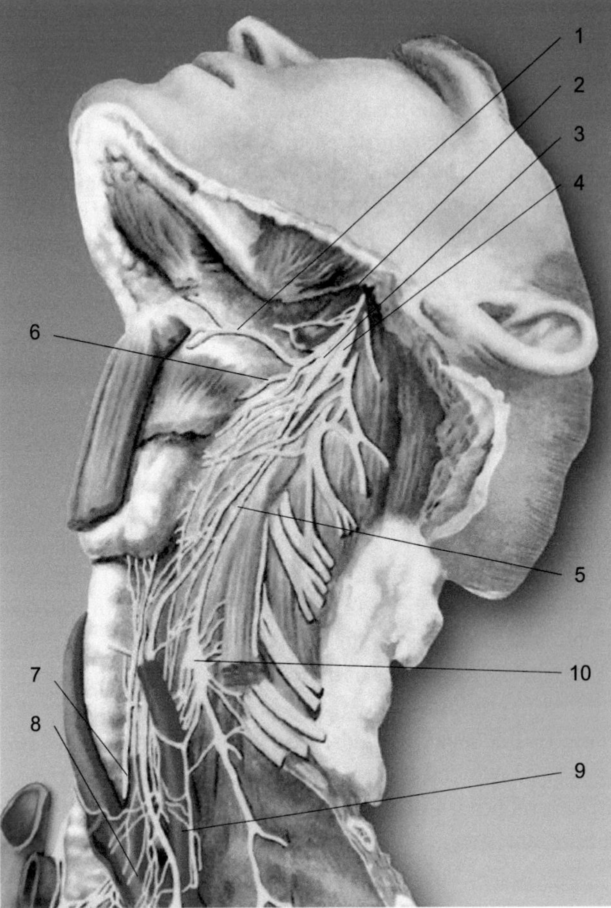

Fig. 7.4 Anatomy. (*1*) Hypoglossal nerve, (*2*) internal carotid artery,(*3*) inferior ganglion of the vagus nerve, (*4*) inferior cervical ganglion, (*5*) vagus nerve, (*6*) superior laryngeal nerve, (*7*) recurrent laryngeal nerve (*8*) aortic arch, (*9*) left subclavian artery, (*10*) cervicothoracic ganglion. (With permission from Danilo Jankovic)

Anesthesia of the Larynx and Trachea for AWAKE Intubation

Various procedures can be used for anesthesia of the laryngeal and tracheal mucosa: spraying and advancement with the fiber endoscope, injection of local anesthetic through the cricothyroid membrane, bilateral blockade of the superior laryngeal nerve, and aerosol inhalation or combinations of the above-mentioned techniques. If local anesthesia is planned for awake intubation, it should be tailored to suit the method of intubation, flexible bronchoscope-guided intubation, videolaryngoscope-guided or other techniques.

Flexible Bronchoscope-Guided Intubation

Awake intubation with flexible bronchoscopy, videolaryngoscopy, or other devices are cornerstone techniques in managing the difficult airway. For indications and concomitant sedation, we refer to new clinically focused literature on the subject. In this chapter, we will focus on the *local anesthesia* part of the procedure.

Local Anesthesia for Flexible Bronchoscopic Intubation

Adequate topical anesthesia of the mucosa in the upper respiratory tract is required for flexible bronchoscopic intubation, in order to subdue coughing, swallowing movements, laryngospasm, and excessive secretion. Lidocaine is usually used for topical anesthesia in the respiratory tract for endoscopic intubation in conscious patients with possible supplement of cocaine for nasal approach.

Lidocaine is administered as a 4% solution for mucosal anesthesia. A 10% pump spray is also used for the oropharynx and nasopharynx. Gargling with a 2% viscous lidocaine solution can also induce oropharyngeal anesthesia. Anesthesia of the nose can be achieved with a 2% gel.

Bleeding in the region of the nasopharynx and mesopharynx can become a severe hindrance to endoscopic intubation. In the nasal procedure, an attempt therefore needs to be made to achieve not only good mucosal anesthesia (with lidocaine spraying) but also bleeding prophylaxis using vasoconstrictive agents. The local anesthetic and vasoconstrictive effects of *cocaine* are therefore advantageous during nasal endoscopic intubation. The synthetic analogs lack cocaine's vasoconstrictive action. Cocaine nose drops (4–10%, 0.5 mL into each nostril) have been found to be very useful in practice. Keep the maximum dosage of cocaine at 100 mg. Alternatively, a mixture of lidocaine (4%) and phenylephrine (1%) at a proportion of 3:1 can be used in the nasal procedure, or lidocaine with adrenaline can be applied. Cocaine should be avoided if there is suspicion of coronary disease. In the oral procedure, pretreatment of the meso pharynx with a lidocaine spray is necessary.

Before anesthesia in the oropharynx, an anti-sialogogue, glycopyrrolate, 5 μg/kg (maximum 400 μg) should be injected to dry out the mucosa. This drug takes time to work and should be administered early, even in advance of the procedure if possible. Oropharyngeal anesthesia is administered with spray shots of 10% lidocaine or by gargling with 2–4 mL of a viscous solution of 2% lidocaine for 30–40 s. Maximum dose of lidocaine spray on the mucosa should be kept below 6 mg/kg. Injecting boluses of 1–2 ml lidocaine 4% via the injection port of the flexible scope allows delivery of the drug precisely where it is wanted; fill the syringe with both the lidocaine and some ml of air in order to flush the drug all the way through the working channel of the flexible scope.

Techniques for Blocking Individual Nerves of the Airway

The following nerve blockades are used in the region of the upper airways:

- Superior laryngeal nerve blockade—above the vocal folds.
- Translaryngeal block—larynx and trachea below the vocal folds.
- Glossopharyngeal nerve blockade—oropharynx.

Vagus Nerve, Superior Laryngeal Nerve, and Recurrent Laryngeal Nerve

Anatomy

The *vagus nerve* (cranial nerve X) not only supplies areas of the head but also descends into the thoracic and abdominal space. It is the largest *parasympathetic nerve* and carries motor fibers (pharyngeal muscles), exteroceptive sensory fibers, visceromotor fibers, viscerosensory fibers, and gustatory fibers. The fibers emerge immediately behind the oliva, combine into a nerve trunk, and exit from the skull through the *jugular foramen.*

The nerve forms the superior ganglion of the vagus nerve (jugular ganglion) within the foramen and after passing through it forms the much larger inferior ganglion of the vagus nerve (nodose ganglion) (Fig. 7.5).

- The *superior ganglion of the vagus nerve* is connected to the *superior cervical ganglion* and also to the *facial nerve, glossopharyngeal nerve*, and *accessory nerve* (Fig. 7.6a, b).
- The *inferior ganglion* of the *vagus nerve* has connections with the cerebral part of the *accessory nerve* and with the *superior cervical ganglion*, the *hypoglossal nerve*, and the loop between the first and second spinal nerves.

In the area of the head, the vagus nerve gives off a *meningeal branch* (for sensory supply to the dura in the posterior cranial fossa) and also an *auricular branch.*

The *vagus nerve* descends along with the *internal carotid artery, common carotid artery*, and *internal jugular vein*, enclosed in a common connective-tissue sheath, down through the neck and passes along with them through the superior thoracic aperture. It gives off four branches in the cervical area:

1. *Pharyngeal branches*. The motor vagus fibers innervate muscles in the soft palate and throat: the muscles of the tonsillar niche, the levator veli palatini, and the constrictor muscles of the pharynx.
2. *Superior laryngeal nerve*. This arises below the inferior ganglion (nodose ganglion) and divides at the level of the hyoid bone into an external branch (the motor branch for the cricothyroid muscle) and an internal branch (the sensory branch for the laryngeal mucosa as far as the vocal folds) (Figs. 7.5 and 7.6a).
3. *Recurrent laryngeal nerve*. This divides in the chest after the vagus nerve has passed over the *aortic arch* on the *left side* and over the *subclavian artery* on the *right side*. Between the trachea and the esophagus, where the nerve gives off the tracheal branches and esophageal branches, it passes to the larynx. Its terminal branch, the *inferior laryngeal nerve*, provides the motor supply for all of the laryngeal muscles except for the cricothyroid and the sensory supply for the laryngeal mucosa below the vocal folds.

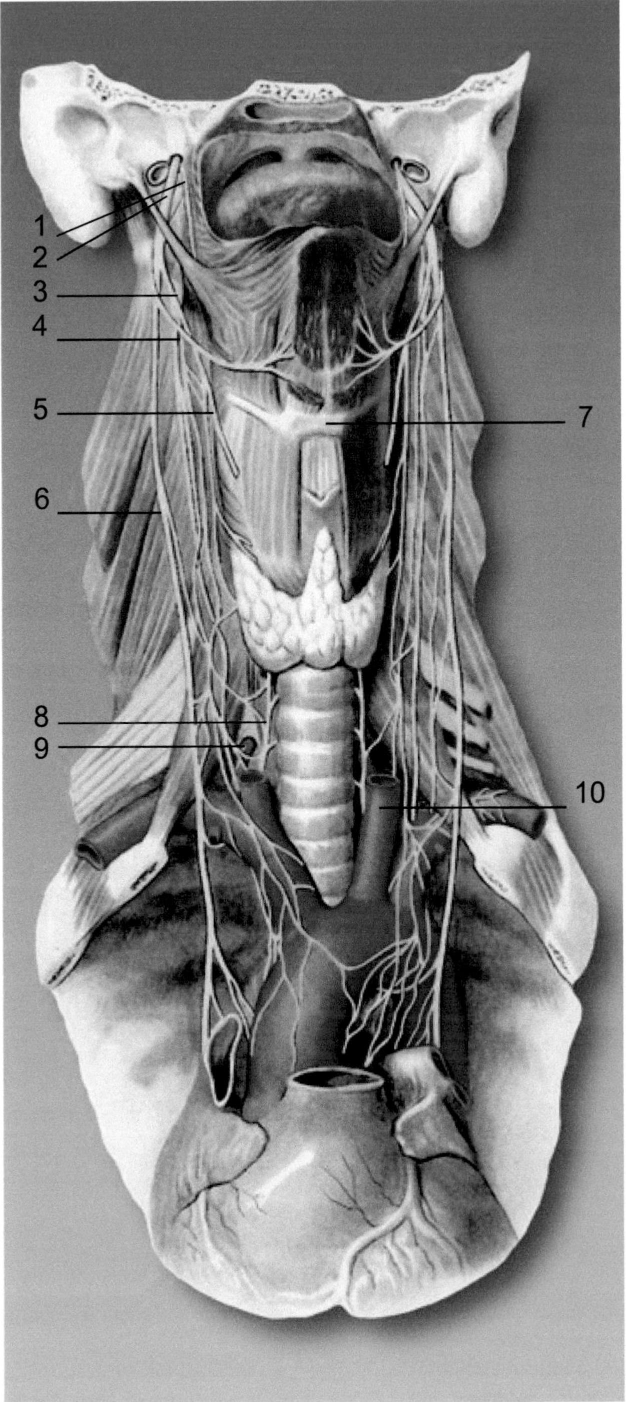

Fig. 7.5 Anatomy. (*1*) Glossopharyngeal nerve, (*2*) inferior ganglion of the vagus nerve, (*3*), superior cervical ganglion, (*4*) hypoglossal nerve, (*5*) superior laryngeal nerve, (*6*) vagus nerve, (*7*) hyoid bone, (*8*) recurrent laryngeal nerve, (*9*) vertebral artery, (*10*) left common carotid artery. (With permission from Danilo Jankovic)

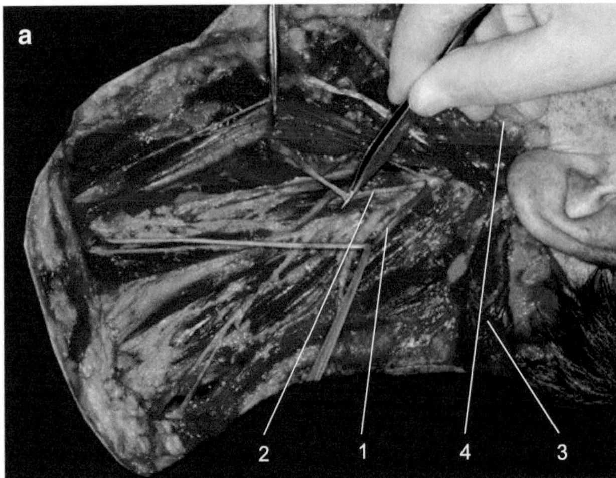

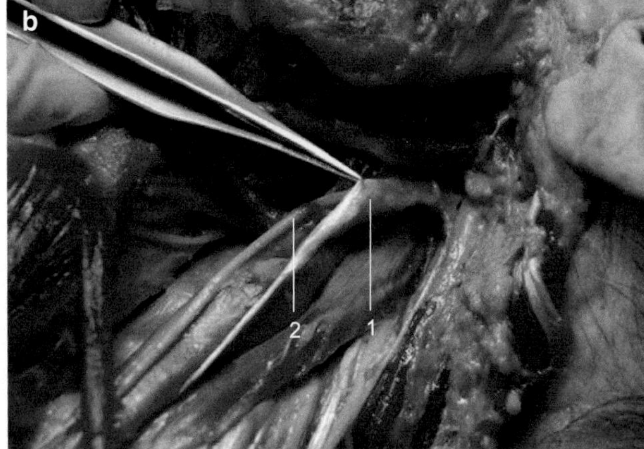

Fig. 7.6 (**a**) Anatomic specimen. (*1*) Division of the vagus nerve. (*2*) Branching of the superior laryngeal nerve, (*3*) sternocleidomastoid (reflected back), (*4*) mandible. (With permission from Danilo Jankovic). (**b**) Anatomic specimen. (*1*) Superior cervical ganglion and (*2*) vagus nerve. (With permission from Danilo Jankovic)

After the inferior ganglion, the two vagus nerves course caudally in each ipsilateral carotid sheath to the superior thoracic aperture. Fibers are exchanged on both sides with the cervical part of the sympathetic nerve, so that from the neck downward, the vagus nerves are actually mixed with parasympathetic and sympathetic nerves (Figs. 7.5 and 7.6).

N.B.

The blockade technique for the vagus nerve is practically identical with that for the glossopharyngeal nerve (see below) and the superior cervical ganglion (cf. Chap. 12).

The present chapter describes blockades of the branches of the vagus nerves (the superior laryngeal nerve and recurrent laryngeal nerve). The use of a vagus nerve blockade as a therapeutic option in the treatment of bronchial asthma has been reported.

Superior Laryngeal Nerve Block

Indications

1. Anesthesia of the airways for intubation of the conscious patient. Superior laryngeal nerve block may be employed as a routine in combination with surface anesthesia but may be especially indicated in the following scenarios: (1) In the contagious setting (e.g., Covid-19 infected patient), in order to diminish coughing during application of local anesthetics (as compared to spraying local anesthetics on the mucosa. (2) In the patient at risk of aspiration (where a SLN block will provide anesthesia to the endolarynx including on the upper surface of the vocal cords but NOT in the trachea itself, this allowing the patient to be able to cough if gastric content should enter the trachea during the intubation. The downside will be some coughing when advancing the tube in the trachea. (3) In the bleeding upper-airway patient where surface anesthesia is unlikely to work and it is also desirable that the patient can cough if blood should enter the trachea. (4) If maximum effect with the minimal amount of local anesthetic is desired.
2. Pain and swallowing symptoms or neuralgia in the innervation area: superior laryngeal neuralgia is characterized by pain in the proximal laryngeal area and hyoid bone, as well as the lateral neck region. Swallowing, coughing, and yawning are reported as triggering factors. The symptoms are usually not accompanied by any major neurological deficits.
3. Laryngoscopy, esophagoscopy, and transtracheal echocardiography.

Contraindications

1. When declined by the patient.
2. Local infections and skin diseases at the injection site.
3. Anticoagulant treatment.
4. Second-degree atrioventricular block.

Procedure

This blockade should be carried out by experienced anesthesiologist or under their supervision.

Preparations

An information discussion with the patient is absolutely necessary.

Check that the emergency equipment is complete and in working order.

Sterile precautions.

Intravenous access, ECG monitoring, ventilation facilities, and pulse oximetry.

Materials

A 25–30 mm-long 23 (25)-G needle.

Patient Positioning

Supine, with slightly extended neck.

Landmarks (Fig. 7.7)

Greater horn of the hyoid bone, thyrohyoid membrane

Injection Technique

This branch of the vagus nerve can be easily blocked at the caudal boundary of the hyoid bone (often easily palpable, even in obese patients) (Fig. 7.7b). The hyoid bone is pushed with the thumb of the left hand toward the side that is to be

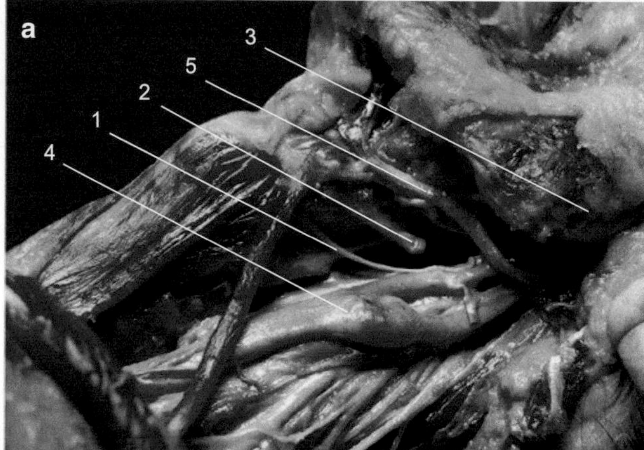

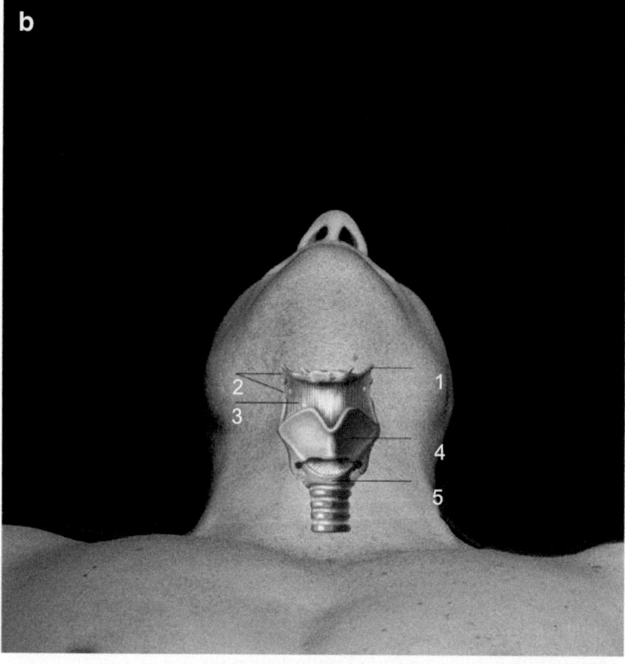

Fig. 7.7 (**a**) Anatomic specimen. (*1*) Superior laryngeal nerve, (*2*) greater horn of the hyoid bone, (*3*) mandible, (*4*) common carotid artery, (*5*) hypoglossal nerve. (With permission from Danilo Jankovic) (**b**) Blockade of the superior laryngeal nerve. Landmarks. (*1*) Greater horn of the hyoid bone, (*2*) thyrohyoid ligament, (*3*) thyrohyoid membrane, (*4*) thyroid cartilage, (*5*) cricoid cartilage. (With permission from Danilo Jankovic)

blocked, to make the greater horn easier to palpate (Fig. 7.8). The short puncture needle is introduced until there is contact with the greater horn and then withdrawn slightly and advanced at a more oblique angle by approximately 2 mm over the caudal edge of the hyoid bone in the direction of the thyrohyoid ligament. Perforation of the thyrohyoid ligament is noted when a loss of resistance occurs. The needle is then located between the thyrohyoid ligament and the laryngeal mucosa and must not be advanced any deeper.

Following aspiration to exclude an intralaryngeal location, 2 mL of local anesthetic is administered. As the needle is being withdrawn, a further 1 mL of local anesthetic is injected into the neighboring tissue.

The *area of anesthesia* covers the caudal region of the epiglottis, the larynx, and the glottis. A higher concentration of the local anesthetic may produce a motor blockade of the cricothyroid.

Complications

1. Laryngeal perforation (intralaryngeal injection).
2. Intravascular injection.

Ultrasound-Guided Superior Laryngeal Nerve Block

The cartilages of the larynx are presented in Fig. 7.9. A high-frequency linear US probe (6–15 MHz) is used.The superior laryngeal nerve (SLN) bifurcates near the pharynx into the external and internal sensory branches. The bilateral SLN block can be used to obtain airway anesthesia, using a percutaneous approach based on anatomic landmarks (greater cornua of the hyoid bone and the thyroid cartilage) (Figs. 7.7 and 7.9). These landmarks may be difficult to locate in some patients. The anatomical study confirmed the presence of a space (named SLN space) containing the internal branch of the superior laryngeal nerve, with hyoid bone superiorly, the thyroid cartilage inferiorly, the thyrohyoid muscle anteriorly, the external carotid artery posteriorly, and the thyrohyoid membrane as the floor (Figs. 7.9 and 7.10). The thyroid cartilage and hyoid bone were identified first, with a probe in a parasagittal plane. The probe was then moved laterally to visualize from the skin to the larynx (Fig. 7.10):

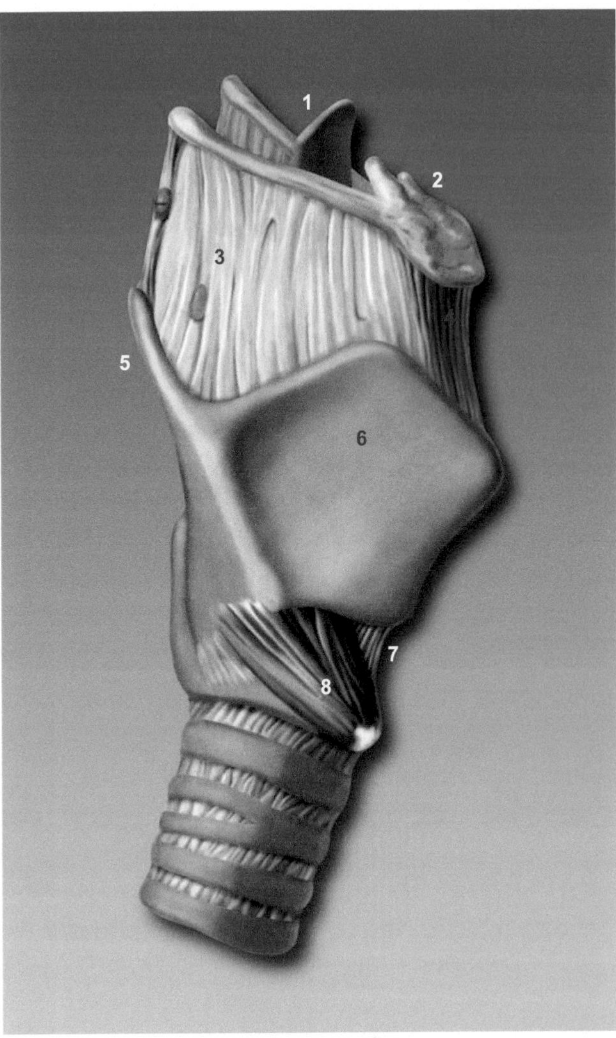

Fig. 7.9 Cartilages of the larynx. (*1*) Epiglottis, (*2*) hyoid bone, (*3*) thyrohyoid membrane, (*4*) thyrohyoid ligament, (*5*) superior horn of thyroid cartilage, (*6*) thyroid cartilage lamina, (*7*) cricothyroid ligament, (*8*) cricothyroid muscle. (With permission from Danilo Jankovic)

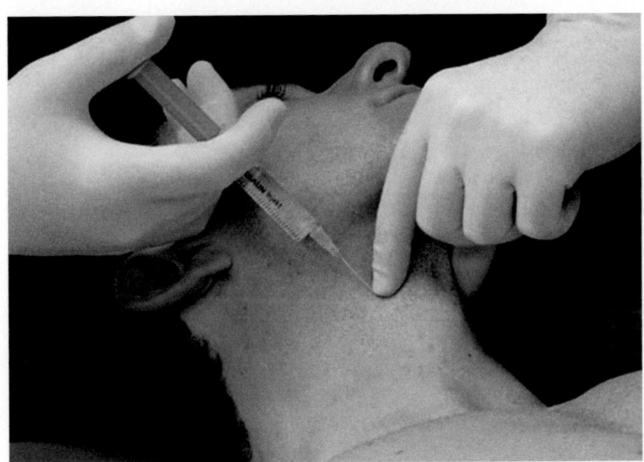

Fig. 7.8 Blockade of the superior laryngeal nerve. The puncture needle is introduced until there is contact with the greater horn of the hyoid bone. (With permission from Danilo Jankovic)

1. Thyrohyoid muscle—large hypoechoic band, inserted on the hyoid bone and passing over the thyroid cartilage (TC) (Fig. 7.10).
2. Thyrohyoid membrane (hyperechoic layer, marking the interface with the hypoechoic pre-epiglottis space) (Fig. 7.10).

The quality of the ultrasound image was rated optimal when all the following were seen: thyrohyoid muscle, pre-epiglottis space, hyoid bone (HB), thyroid cartilage (TC), and thyroid membrane (Fig. 7.10).

As an alternative to in-plane injection, one may use ultrasonography to identify and mark the hyoid bone and the thyroid cartilage and subsequently perform the block.

Injection

In-plane is the preferred technique. The SLN may not be visualized well in ultrasound scan. With a 23-G needle, 2–3 mL of local anesthetics was injected into the surface of the thyrohyoid membrane, anterior to the external carotid artery and posterior to the thyrohyoid muscle under ultrasound guidance (Fig. 7.11). This area correlates with the location of the internal branch of the superior laryngeal nerve.

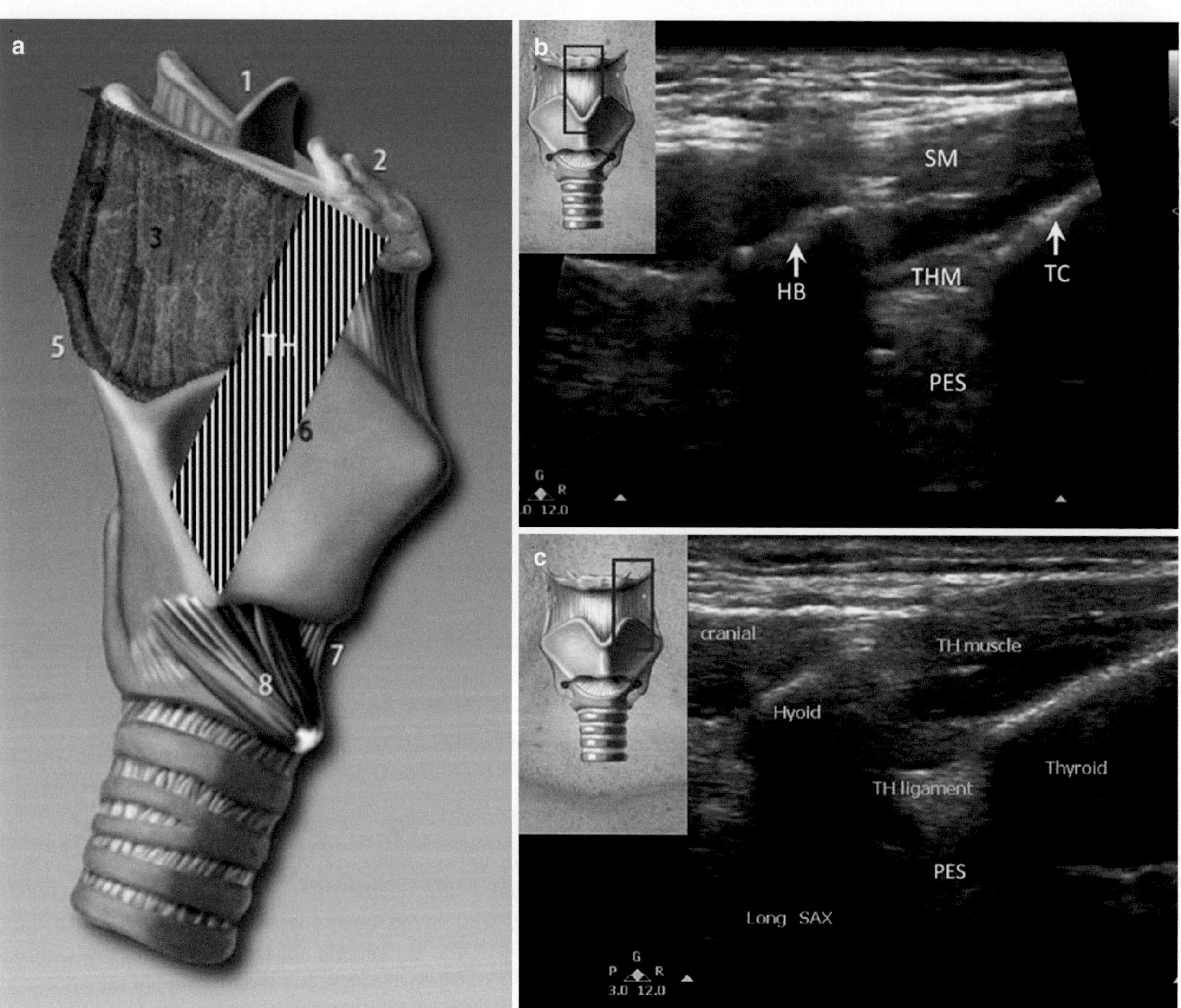

Fig. 7.10 Sonoanatomy of the superior laryngeal nerve. (**a**) The *green* area, the superior laryngeal nerve (SLN) space, is bounded by the hyoid bone superiorly, thyroid cartilage inferiorly, thyrohyoid muscle (black and white striated area) anteriorly, and external carotid artery posteriorly (not shown); (**b**) Sonoanatomy of the anterior aspect of thyrohy oid region. *HB* hyoid bone, *THM* thyrohyoid membrane, *SM* strap muscle, *TC* thyroid cartilage, *PES* pre-epiglottis space (fat). The position of the probe is shown in the inset. (Numbers 1–7: see legend to Fig. 7.9) (**c**) Parasagittal scan of the thyrohyoid region. *TH ligament* (thyrohyoid ligament or membrane), (**d**) Short-axis scan of the thyrohyoid membrane. The superior laryngeal nerve SLA is seen here (*arrows*). In case the nerve is not seen, the location can be approximated by the thyrohyoid (*TH*) muscle anteriorly, external carotid artery (*ECA*) posteriorly, and the thyrohyoid membrane (*arrowheads*) deep to the nerve. *ICA* internal carotid artery. (Reproduced with permission from Peter Cheng)

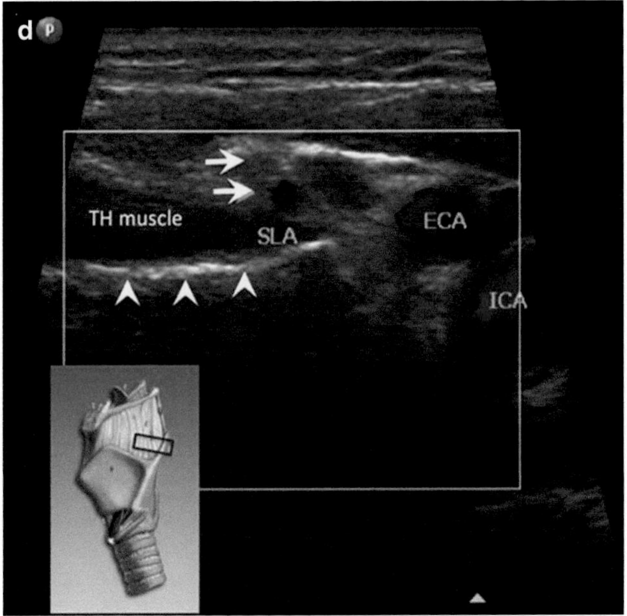

Fig. 7.10 (continued)

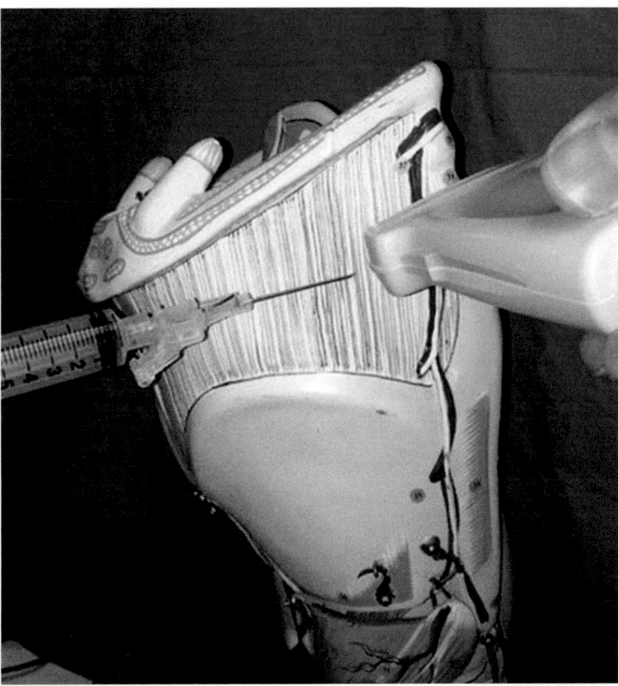

Fig. 7.11 Diagram showing the probe position (similar to Fig. 7.10d) and the direction of the needle insertion for the injection of the internal branch of the superior laryngeal nerve. (Reproduced with permission from Peter Cheng)

Recurrent Laryngeal Nerve Block by Trans-Cricothyroid-Membrane Injection. Palpation Method

Indications

Local anesthesia in the lower pharynx, larynx, and trachea for procedures such as bronchoscopy, esophagoscopy, and endotracheal intubation and for prophylaxis against laryngospasm.

Contraindications

Inability to identify the cricothyroid membrane, overlying malignancy or infection and clinically important coagulopathy.

Procedure Positioning

With extended neck.

Landmarks (Fig. 7.12)

1. Thyroid cartilage.
2. Cricoid cartilage.
3. Median cricothyroid ligament.

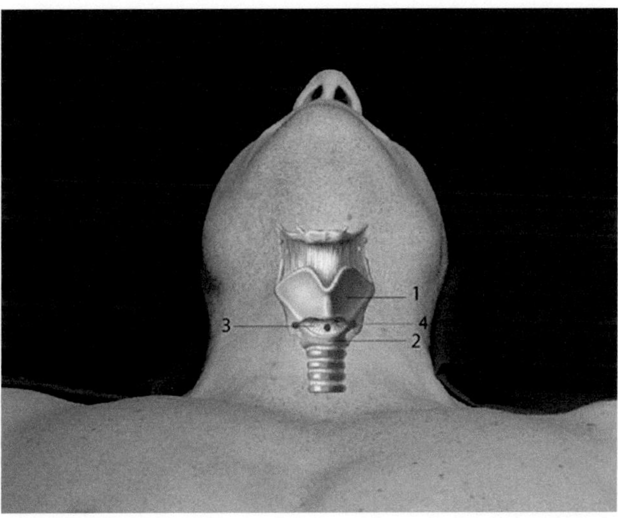

Fig. 7.12 Transtracheal injection. Landmarks. (*1*) Thyroid cartilage (*2*) cricoid cartilage, (*3*) median cricothyroid ligament, (*4*) puncture site (*red*). (With permission from Danilo Jankovic)

Injection Technique

The patient must not swallow, speak, cough, or move. Sedation with fentanyl and midazolam is recommended to prevent heavy coughing attacks.

As the correct identification is often missed, the authors recommended to identify the cricothyroid membrane both from the cranial and from the caudal.

From the caudal end, the hyoid bone and the thyroid cartilage are identified and the groove caudal to the thyroid cartilage represents the cricothyroid membrane and should be marked. Subsequently, the jugular notch is identified and tracheal rings are palpated from the caudal end until the larger cricoid cartilage is identified. The groove cranially to the cricoid cartilage represents the cricothyroid membrane and should be marked. Only if these identifications give the same results, one should rely on the markings; otherwise, if there is discrepancy between these two attempts at identification, one should proceed with ultrasonography.

The anesthetist stands at the patient's head. The puncture is carried out in the *midline* of the neck, as this area has the poorest vascularization. The *cricothyroid membrane* is palpated with the index and *middle fingers* of the left hand (Fig. 7.12).

Vertically to the examination table, a fine 30–40 mm-long 23-G needle with a local anesthetic syringe attached is introduced through the cricothyroid membrane into the lumen of the trachea (Fig. 7.13).

After air has been aspirated (to confirm the intratracheal position), the local anesthetic is rapidly injected into the tracheal lumen. The needle is then quickly removed again. Strong coughing accelerates the spread of the local anesthetic.

Dosage

2–4 mL 2–4% lidocaine. A higher concentration (2–4%) accelerates the onset of effect.

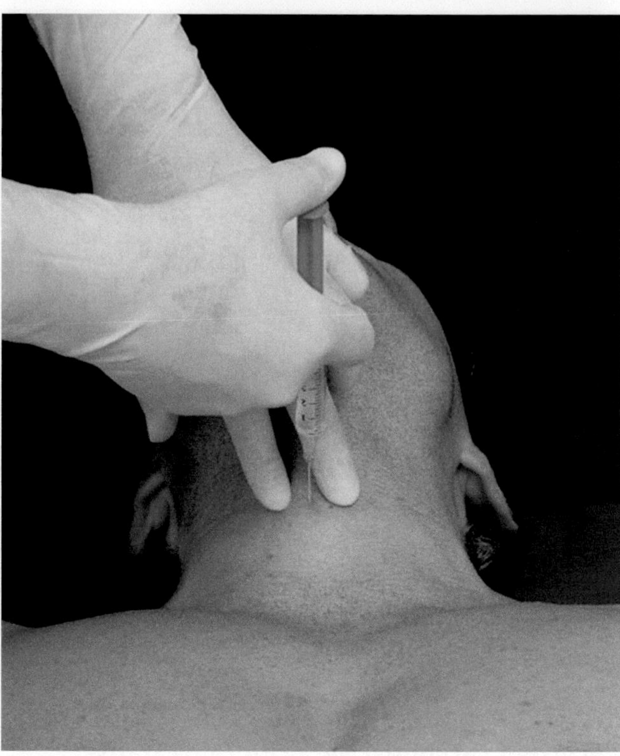

Fig. 7.13 Transtracheal injection. Puncture in the midline of the neck, through the cricothyroid membrane, vertical to the examination table. (With permission from Danilo Jankovic)

N.B.

1. External blockade of the recurrent laryngeal nerve is rarely indicated (e.g., for administering neurolyt ics in carcinoma of the glottis).
2. The recurrent laryngeal nerve lies in a fossa between the esophagus and the trachea and can be blocked underneath the cricoid cartilage. The injection is carried out at the posterolateral edge of the first tra cheal ring.
3. Unintentional blockade of the recurrent laryngeal nerve occurs very often after blockades of the stel late ganglion (cf. Chap. 12 stellate ganglion block).

Complications

1. Intravascular injection, with toxic reactions due to rapid resorption of the (high-dose) local anesthetic.
2. Esophageal perforation.

Recurrent Laryngeal Nerve Block (Transtracheal/Trans-Cricothyroid-Membrane Injection) - Ultrasound Guided

In obese patients and in patients with pathology in the neck, palpation is not reliable for identification of the cricothyroid membrane, whereas ultrasonography has a high success rate and should be trained and applied.

The best documented and proven successful technique is the "string of pearls" approach, Fig. 7.14.

1. The sternal bone is identified by palpation, and the transducer is placed transversely on the patient's neck just cephalad to the suprasternal notch to visualize the trachea (horseshoe-shaped dark structure with a posterior white line) (Fig. 7.14 first panel).
2. The transducer is slid towards the patient's right side (towards the operator), so that the right border of the transducer is positioned midline of the trachea, and the ultrasound image of the tracheal ring is thus truncated into half on the screen (Fig. 7.14 second panel).
3. The right end of the transducer is maintained over the midline of the trachea, **while** the left end is rotated 90° into the sagittal plane resulting in a longitudinal scan of the midline of the trachea. A number of dark (hypoechoic) rings will be seen anterior to the white hyperechoic line (air–tissue border), akin to a "string of pearls". The dark hypoechoic "pearls" are the anterior part of the tracheal rings (Fig. 7.14 third panel).
4. The transducer is kept longitudinally in the midline and slid cephalad until the cricoid cartilage comes into view

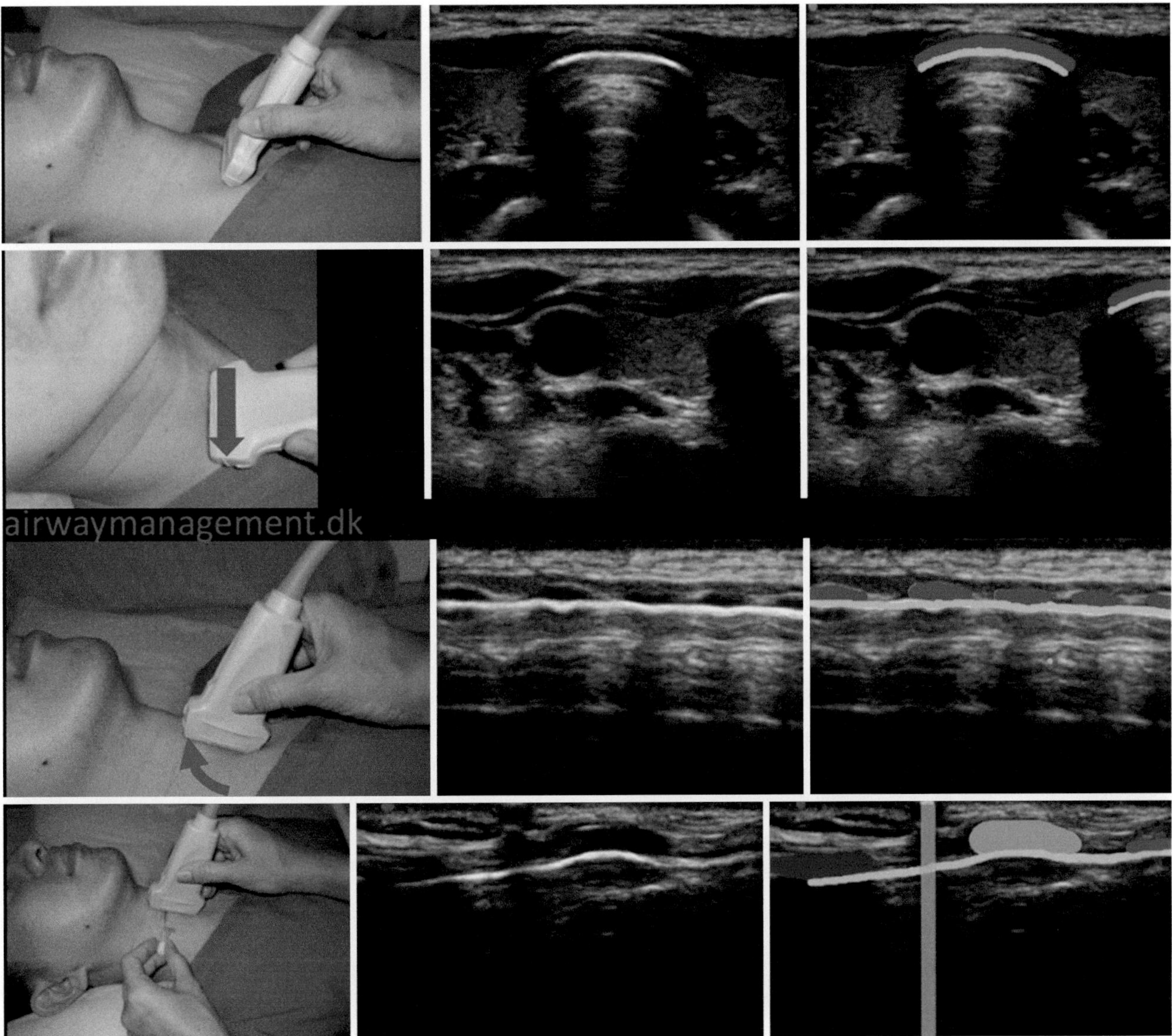

Fig. 7.14 The longitudinal "string of pearls" technique for identifying the cricothyroid membrane, the midline of the airway and the interspaces between tracheal rings. Orange-red = tracheal ring; light blue = the tissue–air border; green = the cricoid cartilage; purple = the distal end of the thyroid cartilage. Yellow = the shadow from the needle slid in between the transducer and the skin. See video at www.airwaymanagement.dk/pearls. (Figure with permission from The Scandinavian Airway Management course "www.airwaymanagement.dk")

(seen as a larger, more elongated and anteriorly placed dark "pearl" compared to the other tracheal rings). Further cephalad, the distal part of the thyroid cartilage can be seen as well (Fig. 7.14 fourth panel). The longitudinal course of the midline of the airway can be marked with a pen.

5. While still holding the transducer, the other hand is used to slide a needle (as a marker, for its ability to cast a shadow in the ultrasound image) between the transducer and the patient's skin until the needle's shadow is seen midway between the caudal border of the thyroid cartilage and the cephalad border of the cricoid cartilage (Fig. 7.14 fourth panel).
6. Now the transducer is removed, and the needle marks the center of the cricothyroid membrane in the transverse plane and this can be marked on the skin with a pen.

The technique is demonstrated on this video: http://airwaymanagement.dk/pearls.

If the neck is too short, or cannot be extended, for the "string of pearls" approach, one can apply the *TACA (Thyroid cartilage, Airline, Cricoid cartilage, Airline) technique* (Fig. 7.15):

1. With the patient's neck extended, estimate where the level of the thyroid cartilage is on the neck and place the

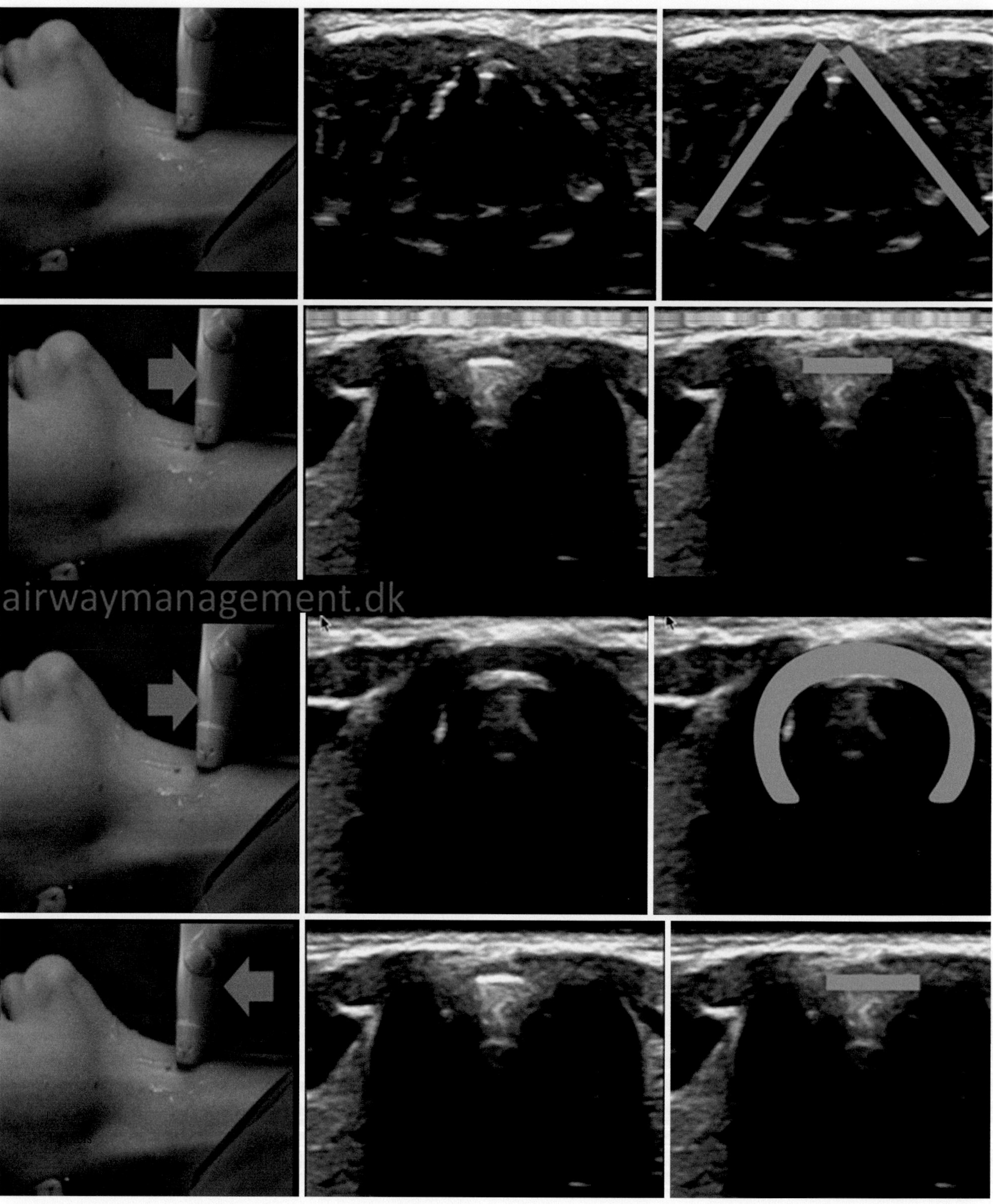

Fig. 7.15 The transverse "TACA (Thyroid-Airline-Cricoid-Airline)" method for identifying the cricothyroid membrane. See the text for details. Blue triangle = Thyroid cartilage, blue horizontal line = the "Airline" = the cricothyroid membrane, Blue "Lying C" = the anterior part of the cricoid cartilage. See video at: www.airwaymanagement.dk/taca. (With permission from The Scandinavian Airway management course "www.airwaymanagement.dk")

ultrasound transducer transversely over it, scanning to identify the thyroid cartilage as a hyperechoic triangular structure (Fig. 7.15 first panel).
2. Move the transducer caudally until the cricothyroid membrane is identified: this is recognizable as a hyperechoic white line resulting from the echo of the air–tissue border of the mucosal lining on the inside of the cricothyroid membrane, often with parallel white lines (reverberation artefacts) below (Fig. 7.15 second panel).
3. Move the transducer further caudally until the cricoid cartilage is identified (a "black lying-"C" with a white lining) (Fig. 7.15 third panel).
4. Finally, move the transducer slightly back cephalad until the center of the cricothyroid membrane is identified (Fig. 7.15 fourth panel).
5. The center can be marked both transversely and sagittal on the skin with a pen. By identifying both the highly characteristic shapes of the thyroid and the cricoid cartilages, both the cephalad and caudal borders of the cricothyroid membrane can be identified.

The technique is demonstrated in this video: http://airwaymanagement.dk/taca.

These techniques can be applied individually or combined, a video demonstrating this is available here: https://airwaymanagement.dk/ultrasound_needle_cricothyrotomy.

Glossopharyngeal Nerve Block

Anatomy

Cranial nerve IX (the glossopharyngeal nerve) is closely related to the vagus nerve (X), both topographically and functionally (Fig. 7.16). It provides the *sensory* innervation for the *middle ear*, for areas of the tongue and *pharynx*, and for *motor muscles* of the pharynx. It contains motor, visceromotor (parasympathetic), viscerosensory, and gustatory fibers.

Behind the oliva, it passes directly above the vagus nerve out of the medulla and exits the skull along with the vagus nerve through the *jugular foramen*. Within the foramen, it forms the *superior ganglion* and after passing through it forms the larger *inferior ganglion* (the *petrosal ganglion*). Lateral to the internal carotid artery and the pharynx, it follows an arching course toward the base of the tongue, where it divides into several terminal branches. The *tympanic nerve* provides the sensory supply for the mucosa of the tympanic cavity and pharyngotympanic (auditory) tube. The secretory fibers pass as the lesser petrosal nerve to the otic ganglion. In addition to connections to the vagus nerve, facial nerve, and sympathetic nerve, the *carotid branch of the glossopharyngeal nerve* is also given off from the inferior ganglion. Also given off are the *pharyngeal branches*, which along with part

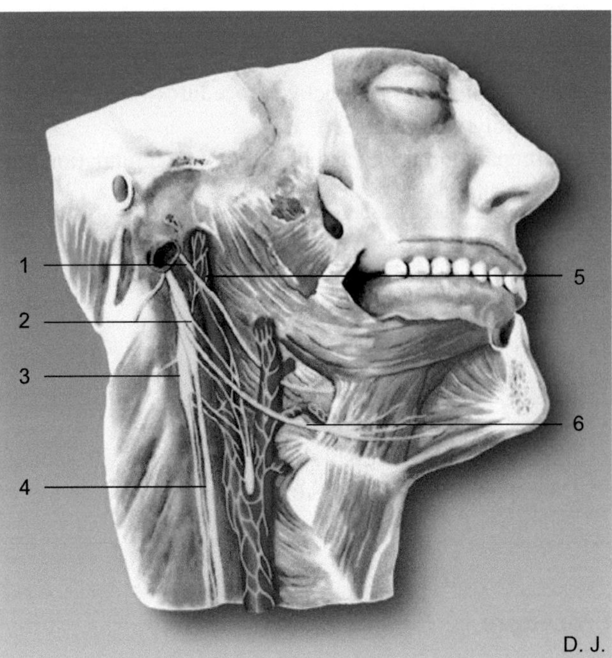

Fig. 7.16 Anatomy. (*1*) Glossopharyngeal nerve, (*2*) inferior ganglion of the vagus nerve, (*3*) superior cervical ganglion, (*4*) vagus nerve, (*5*) internal carotid artery, (*6*) hypoglossal nerve. (With permission from Danilo Jankovic)

of the vagus nerve form the *pharyngeal plexus* and are involved in the sensory and motor supply to the pharynx, the *stylopharyngeal branch* (stylopharyngeus muscle), the *tonsillar branches* (to the tonsils and soft palate), and the *lingual branches* (posterior third of the tongue).

Indications

Diagnostic

- Differential diagnosis of trigeminal neuralgia (anterior two thirds of the tongue) and glossopharyngeal neuralgia (posterior third of the tongue).
- Before neurodestructive procedures.

Therapeutic

- Glossopharyngeal neuralgia. Glossopharyngeal neuralgia is characterized by strictly unilateral, fulminant paroxysms of severe stabbing and burning pain (oropharynx, tonsillar niches, more rarely in the area of the ear—due to co-involvement of the tympanic branch—or mandibular angle). The first report of this clinical picture was by Sicard and Robineau in 1920. In 10–30% of cases, there is simultaneous trigeminal neuralgia. The symptoms are unilateral in 75% of cases. Triggering factors include chewing, speaking, swallowing, coughing, yawning, and cold food and drinks. The glossopharyngeal nerve can sometimes be paralyzed along with the vagus nerve and

accessory nerve due to a tumor or aneurysm in the posterior cranial fossa.
- Tumor pain (neurodestructive procedures—e.g., injection of neurolytic agents).
- As preparation for awake intubation, in conjunction with other techniques.

Contraindications

- When declined by the patient.
- Second-degree atrioventricular block.
- Anticoagulant treatment
- Simultaneous bilateral blockade.
- Contralateral paresis of the glossopharyngeal and adjacent nerves.

Procedure

This blockade should only be carried out by experienced anesthetists or under their supervision.

Preparations

Check that emergency equipment is complete and in working order; sterile precautions; intravenous access; ECG monitoring; ventilation facilities; and pulse oximetry. An information discussion with the patient is absolutely necessary.

Materials

- A 40 mm-long 23-G needle.

Patient Positioning

- Supine, with the head rotated to the contralateral side by approximately 30°.

Landmarks (Fig. 7.17)

- Angle of the mandible.
- Mastoid process.
- Styloid process. The variable anatomy and depth of the styloid process need to be taken into account during the puncture procedure.

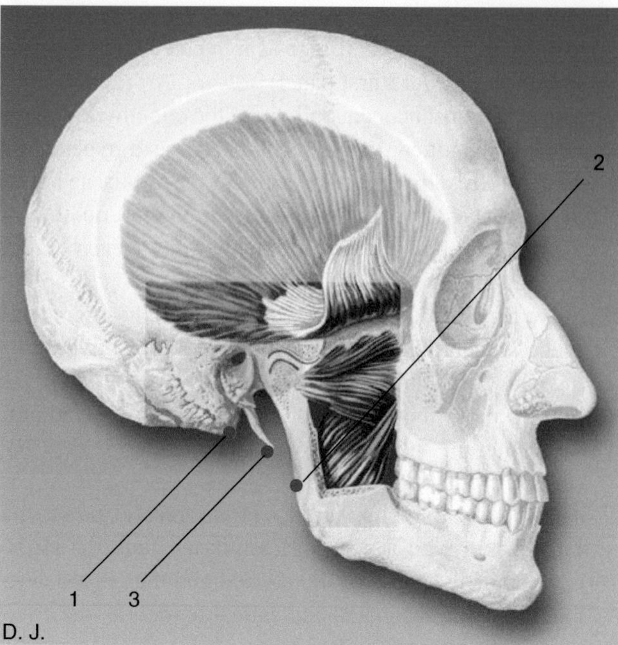

Fig. 7.17 Landmarks. (*1*) Mastoid process, (*2*) angle of the mandible (*3*) styloid process. (With permission from Danilo Jankovic)

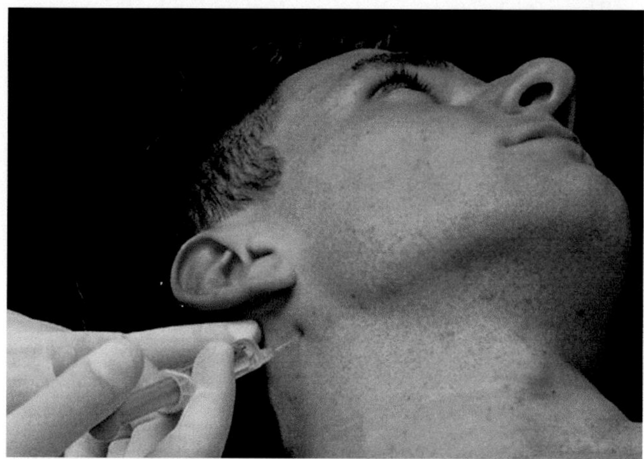

Fig. 7.18 Glossopharyngeal nerve. Injection technique vertical to the skin, toward the styloid process

Injection Technique

Extraoral Access (Lateral Cervical Technique): The needle is introduced at the midpoint between the mastoid tip and the angle of the mandible, vertically to the skin, until there is bone contact with the styloid process (Fig. 7.18). This is usually after approximately 3 cm. The needle is then withdrawn slightly and, after loss of bone contact with the styloid process, is introduced posteriorly at a depth of 0.5–1.0 cm.

After aspiration, fractionated administration of a local anesthetic is carried out.

Intraoral Access

Following topical anesthesia of the tongue, the patient's mouth is opened widely and the posterior tonsillar pillar (palatopharyngeal fold) identified by using a Macintosh laryngoscope blade. In an aseptic manner, the stylet of the 22G spinal needle should be removed from the disposable spinal needle and discarded. Subsequently, utilizing the sterile container that the 22G spinal needle was packed in, the distal 1 cm of the needle is bent to allow more controlled submucosal insertion. The needle tip is inserted submucosally, and following careful aspiration for blood, 2–3 mL of local anesthetic is injected. The block is then repeated on the contralateral side (Fig. 7.19).

Glossopharyngeal Nerve Block, Ultrasonographic Approach

Small retrospective case series of ultrasound-guided external approach to glossopharyngeal nerve blocks have demonstrated its usefulness for treating glossopharyngeal neuralgia, and a cadaver and volunteer study has proved the concept of blockade distally in the parapharyngeal space away from high-risk collateral structures.

Potential Problems

Effects of the Blockade

Globus sensation in the neck, swallowing difficulties, loss of sensation in the pharynx and mucosa, retropharyngeal and tonsillar paresthesias are signs that the glossopharyngeal nerve is blocked. The vagus nerve, which is in the vicinity of the glossopharyngeal nerve, and the superior cervical ganglion and hypoglossal nerve are always anesthetized as well.

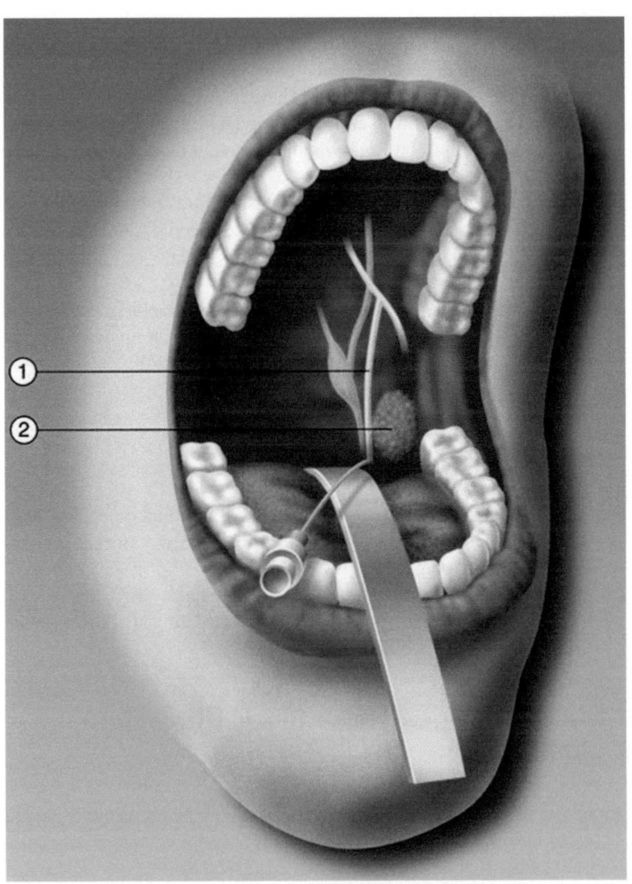

Fig. 7.19 Intraoral glossopharyngeal nerve block. (*1*) Glossopharyngeal nerve, (*2*) palatine tonsil

Dosage

Two to three milliliters of local anesthetic—e.g., procaine 0.5–1.0%, prilocaine 0.5–1.0%, ropivacaine 0.2%, bupivacaine 0.125% (levobupivacaine 0.125%); if appropriate, mixed with 80 mg methylprednisolone.

Complications

- Intravascular injection, with toxic reactions (internal carotid artery, internal jugular vein) (cf. Chap. 12 stellate ganglion).
- Hematoma formation.
- Intraoral approach
- With the intraoral approach, the terminal branches of the glossopharyngeal nerves are closely related to the internal carotid arteries, which lie immediately lateral to the nee dle tips if they are correctly positioned.

Side Effects

Simultaneous anesthetization of the following nerves:

- Vagus nerve (paresis of the vagus nerve is characterized by the collection of saliva in the piriform fossa when there is paresis of the posterior cricoarytenoid muscle—hoarseness, accompanied by nasal vocalization) (Fig. 7.16).
- Hypoglossal nerve (the outstretched tongue deviates toward the paralyzed side) (Fig. 7.16).
- Accessory nerve (weakness in the area of the trapezius) (Fig. 7.20).
- Superior cervical ganglion.

These side effects usually arise after the injection of larger amounts of local anesthetic (cf. Chap. 12).

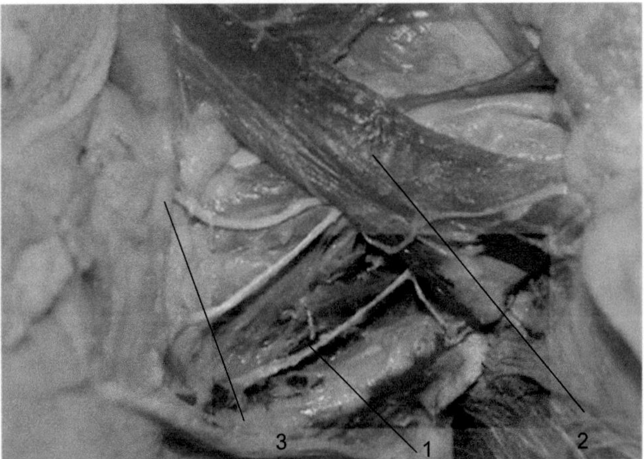

Fig. 7.20 Anatomic specimen. (*1*) Course of the accessory nerve, (*2*) sternocleidomastoid, (*3*) clavicle. (With permission from Danilo Jankovic)

Acknowledgement Peter Cheng, MD is thanked for his substantial contribution to the previous version of the chapter.

Suggested Reading

Ultrasonography in Airway Management

Kristensen MS. Ultrasonography in the management of the airway. Acta Anaesthesiol Scand. 2011;55:1155–73.

Kristensen MS, Teoh WH, Graumann O, Laursen CB. Ultrasonography for clinical decision-making and intervention in airway management: from the mouth to the lungs and pleurae. Insights Imaging. 2014;5:253–79.

Teoh WH, Kristensen MS. Ultrasonography for airway management. In: Cook T, Kristensen MS, editors. Core topics in airway management. Cambridge: Cambridge University Press; 2020. p. 63–71.

Airway Anaesthesia and Awake Intubation in General

Jankovic D. Anästhesie der luftleitenden Wege. In: Jankovic D, editor. Regionalblockaden & Infiltrationstherapie. Berlin: ABW Wissenschaftsverlag; 2007. p. 49–61.

Klock PA, Rai M, Popat M. Tracheal intubation using the flexible optical bronchoscope. In: Cook T, Kristensen MS, editors. Core topics in airway management. Cambridge: Cambridge University Press; 2020. p. 140–52.

Law JA, Heidegger T. Structured planning of airway management. In: Cook T, Kristensen MS, editors. Core topis in airway management. Cambridge: Cambridge University Press; 2020. p. 38–49.

Murphy P. A fiberoptic endoscope used for nasal intubation. Anaesthesia. 1967;22:489.

Ovassapian A. Fiberoptic airway endoscopy in anesthesia and critical care. New York: Raven; 1990.

Rosenstock CV, Hodzovic I. Awake tracheal intubation. In: Cook T, Kristensen MS, editors. Core topics in airway management. Cambridge: Cambridge University Press; 2020. p. 80–6.

Simmons ST, Schleich AR. Airway regional anesthesia for awake fiberoptic intubation. Reg Anesth Pain Med. 2002;27(2):180–92.

Anatomy and Airway Blocks in General

Brown DL. Atlas of regional anesthesia. 3rd ed. Philadelphia: Saunders, Elsevier; 2006.

Gervasio A, Mujahed I, Biasio A, Alessi S. Ultrasound anatomy of the neck: the infrahyoid region. J Ultrasound. 2010;13:85–9.

Jankovic D. Luftleitende Wege-Nervenblockaden. In: Jankovic D, editor. Regionalblockaden & Infiltrationstherapy. 4th ed. Berlin: ABW-Wissenschaftsverlag; 2007. p. 53–6.

Kiray A, Naderi S, Ergur I, Korman E. Surgical anatomy of the internal branch of the superior laryngeal nerve. Eur Spine J. 2006; 15:1320–5.

Lida T, Suzuki A, Kunisawa T, Iwasaki H. Ultrasound-guided superior laryngeal nerve block and translaryngeal block for awake tracheal intubation in a patient with laryngeal abscess. J Anesth. 2013;27:309–10.

Monfared A, Kim D, Jaikumar S, Gorti G, Kam A. Microsurgical anatomy of the superior and recurrent laryngeal nerves. Neurosurgery. 2001;49(4):925–31.

Murphy TM. Somatic blockade of head and neck. In: Cousins MJ, Bridenbaugh PO, editors. Neural blockade. 4th ed. Philadelphia: Lippincott-Raven; 1998.

Paraskevas G, Raikos A, Ioannidis O, Brand-Saberi B. Topographic anatomy of the internal laryngeal nerve: surgical considerations. Head Neck. 2012;34:534–40.

Superior Laryngeal Nerve Block

Ambi US, Arjun BK, Masur S, Endigeri A, Hosalli V, Hulakund SY. Comparison of ultrasound and anatomical landmark-guided technique for superior laryngeal nerve block to aid awake fibreoptic intubation: a prospective randomised clinical study. Indian J Anaesth. 2017;61:463–8.

Barberet G, Henry Y, Tatu L, et al. Ultrasound description of a superior laryngeal nerve space as an anatomical basis for echoguided regional anaesthesia. Br J Anaesth. 2012;109:126–8.

Stockwell M, Lozanoff S, Lang S, Nyssen J. Superior laryngeal nerve block: an anatomical study. Clin Anat. 1995;8:89–95.

Zhipeng L, Meiyi H, Meirong W, et al. Ultrasound-guided internal branch of superior laryngeal nerve block on postoperative sore throat: A randomized controlled trial. PLoS One. 2020;15:e0241834.

Identification of the Trachea/Cricothyroid Membrane for Recurrent Laryngeal Nerve Block

Airwaymanagement_for_Anaesthesiologists. Longitudinal. "String of Pearls" approach to identification of the ricothyroid membrane. http://airwaymanagement.dk/pearls. Accessed 10 Sept 2020.

Airwaymanagement_for_Anaesthesiologists. Transverse "Thyroid-Airline-Cricoid-Airline" approach for identification of the cricothyroid membrane. http://airwaymanagement.dk/taca. Accessed 10 Sept 2020.

Airwaymanagement_for_Anaesthesiologists. Ultrasound guided marking of the cricothyroid membrane and needle cricothyrotomy. https://airwaymanagement.dk/ultrasound_needle_cricothyrotomy. Accessed 8 Sept 2020.

Kristensen MS, Teoh WH, Rudolph SS. Ultrasonographic identification of the cricothyroid membrane: best evidence, techniques, and clinical impact. Br J Anaesth. 2016;117(Suppl 1):i39–48.

Glossopharyngeal Nerve Block

Jankovic D. Nervus glossopharingeus. In: Jankovic D, editor. Regionalblockaden & Infiltrationstherapy. Berlin: ABW-Wissenschaftsverlag; 2007. p. 57–8.

Murphy TM. Somatic blockade of head and neck. In: Cousins MJ, Bridenbaugh PO, editors. Neural blockade. 4th ed. Philadelphia: Lippincott-Raven; 1998.

Glossopharyngeal Nerve Block, Ultrasound Guided

Azman J, Stopar Pintaric T, Cvetko E, Vlassakov K. Ultrasound-guided glossopharyngeal nerve block: a cadaver and a volunteer sonoanatomy study. Reg Anesth Pain Med. 2017;42:252–8.

Liu Q, Zhong Q, Tang G, He G. Ultrasound-guided glossopharyngeal nerve block via the styloid process for glossopharyngeal neuralgia: a retrospective study. J Pain Res. 2019;12:2503–10.

Trigeminal Nerve Anatomy and Peripheral Branches Block

8

Danilo Jankovic and Ban Tsui

Contents

General Consideration

Danilo Jankovic

The trigeminal nerve (CN V) is a nerve responsible for sensation in the face and motor functions such as biting and chewing; it is the most complex of the cranial nerves. Its name ("trigeminal"=tri- or three, and geminus or twin: thrice-twinned) derives from the fact that each of the two nerves (one on each side of the pons) has three major branches. The ophthalmic and maxillary nerves are purely sensory, whereas the mandibular nerve supplies motor as well as sensory (or "cutaneous") functions. Adding to the complexity of this nerve is the fact that autonomic nerve fibers as well as special sensory fibers (taste) are contained within it.

D. Jankovic (✉)
Pain Management Centre DGS – Cologne – Huerth, Cologne-Hürth, Germany
e-mail: danilo@jankovic1.de

B. Tsui
Pediatric Anesthesia and Adult Regional Anesthesia, Stanford University, Palo Alto, USA
e-mail: bantsui@stanford.edu

Functional Anatomy

The trigeminal nerve is the largest cranial nerve and gives origin to three major branches: the *ophthalmic, maxillary,* and *mandibular* nerves (Table 8.1; Figs. 8.1 and 8.2).

The *trigeminal nerve* is attached to the ventrolateral aspect of the *pons* near its upper border and consists of a *larger sensory root* and a much *smaller, medial motor root.*

It transmits *sensory impulses* from most of the face and scalp, parts of the auricle and the external acoustic (auditory) meatus, the nasal and oral cavities, the teeth, the temporomandibular joint, the nasopharynx, and most of the *meninges* in the anterior and middle cranial fossae. It also carries *proprioceptive impulses* from the masticatory and from the extraocular and facial muscles.

D. Jankovic, P. Peng (eds.), *Regional Nerve Blocks in Anesthesia and Pain Therapy*,
https://doi.org/10.1007/978-3-030-88727-8_8

Its *motor root* fibers supply muscles derived from the first branchial (mandibular) arch: the *masticatory muscles*, the *mylohyoid*, the anterior belly of the *digastric*, and the *tensor veli palatini* and *tensor tympani*.

Numerous *parasympathetic* and *sympathetic* fibers join branches of the trigeminal nerve through interconnections with the *oculomotor (III), trochlear (IV), facial (VII), and glossopharyngeal (IX) nerves* and with *sympathetic plexuses* around branches of the *carotid arteries*. From their attachments to the *pons*, the *sensory and motor roots* pass over the superior border of the petrous temporal bone near its apex.

Table 8.1 Trigeminal nerve (CN V) distribution

Trigeminal nerve (CN V)	
Type	Mixed (motor and sensory)
Nuclei	• Motor nucleus of trigeminal nerve
	• Principal sensory nucleus of trigeminal nerve
	• Spinal nucleus of trigeminal nerve
	• Mesencephalic nucleus of trigeminal nerve
Divisions	• Ophthalmic nerve (CN V1)
	• Maxillary nerve (CN V2)
	• Mandibular nerve (CN V3)
Field of innervation	*Motor*: Muscles of mastication, mylohyoid, anterior belly of digastric, tensor tympani muscles
	Sensory: Scalp, face, orbit paranasal sinuses, anterior two-thirds of the tongue

The *sensory root* expands into the semilunar-shaped *trigeminal ganglion (semilunar ganglion, Gasserian ganglion)* (see Chap. 9, Fig. 9.14), which contains *pseudounipolar cells.* The processes of these cells divide into a *peripheral* and *central* part; the former constitutes the majority of sensory fibers in *the ophthalmic and maxillary nerves* and in the *larger part of the mandibular nerve* (Fig. 8.3); the latter coalesces to form the *trigeminal sensory root*, which enters the brainstem and either ends in the principal sensory (pontine) trigeminal nucleus or descends in the *trigeminal spinal tract* to end in the *spinal (inferior) trigeminal nucleus*. The *proprioceptive fibers* are the peripheral processes of unipolar cells located in the *trigeminal mesencephalic nucleus.* They are unique in being the only primary sensory neurons whose cell bodies lie within CNS.

The *motor fibers* originate in the *trigeminal motor nucleus*, which is embedded in the *upper pons* on the medial side of the principal sensory motor nucleus.

The *ophthalmic, maxillary, and mandibular nerves* arise from the convex margin of the trigeminal ganglion; the *small motor root* passes under the ganglion to join the *mandibular nerve.*

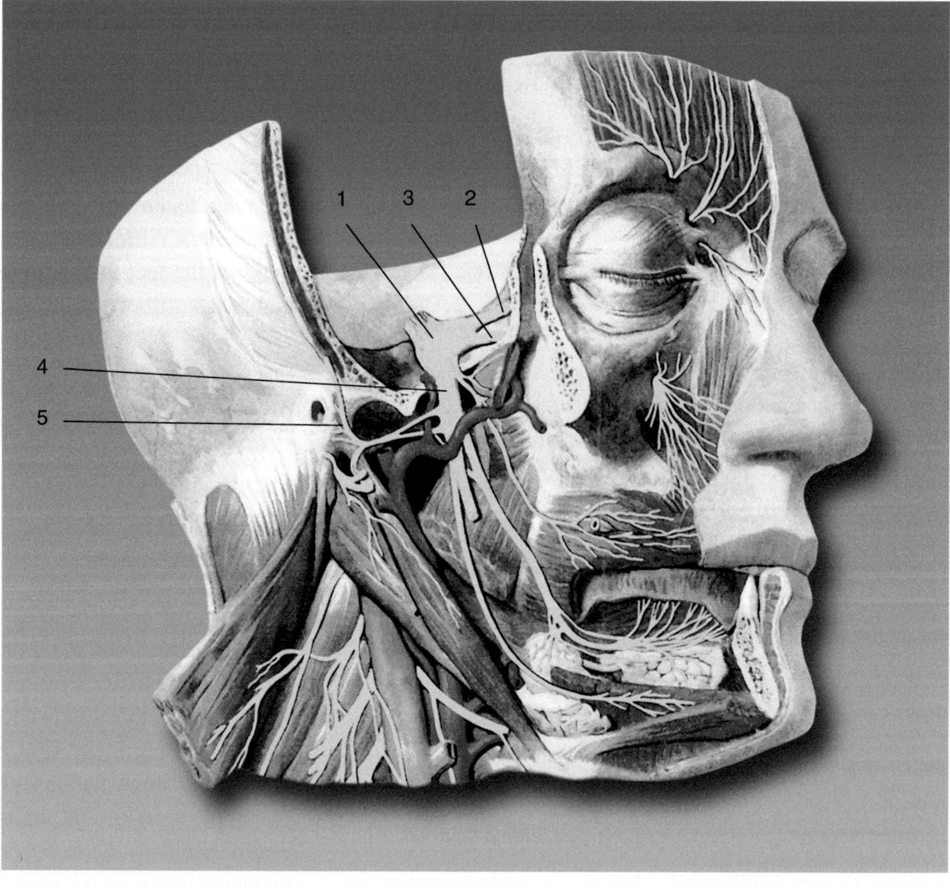

Fig. 8.1 Sensory supply to the face. (*1*) Trigeminal ganglion, (*2*) ophthalmic nerve, (*3*) maxillary nerve, (*4*) mandibular nerve, and (*5*) auriculotemporal nerve. (Reproduced with permission from Danilo Jankovic)

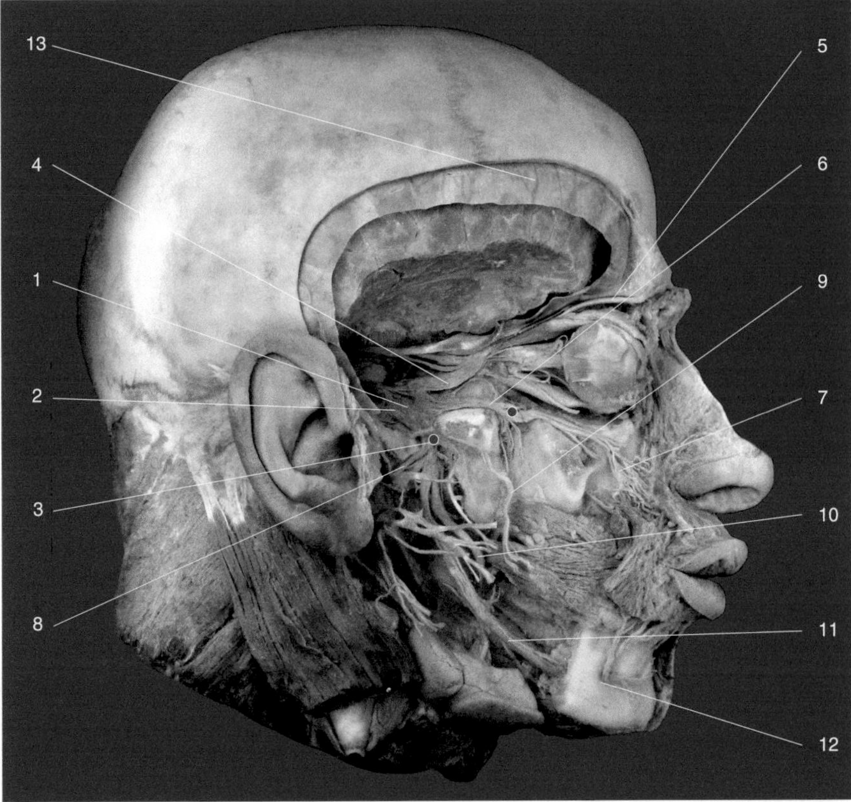

Fig. 8.2 Trigeminal nerve. (*1*) Trigeminal (Gasserian, semilunar) ganglion, (*2*) mandibular nerve in oval foramen, (*3*) mandibular nerve and otic ganglion (red point), (*4*) ophthalmic nerve, (*5*) frontal nerve, (*6*) maxillary nerve and pterygopalatine ganglion, (*7*) infraorbital nerve, (*8*) auriculotemporal nerve, (*9*) buccal nerve, (*10*) lingual nerve, (*11*) alveolar inferior nerve, (*12*) mental nerve, (*13*) dura mater. (Reproduced with permission from Danilo Jankovic)

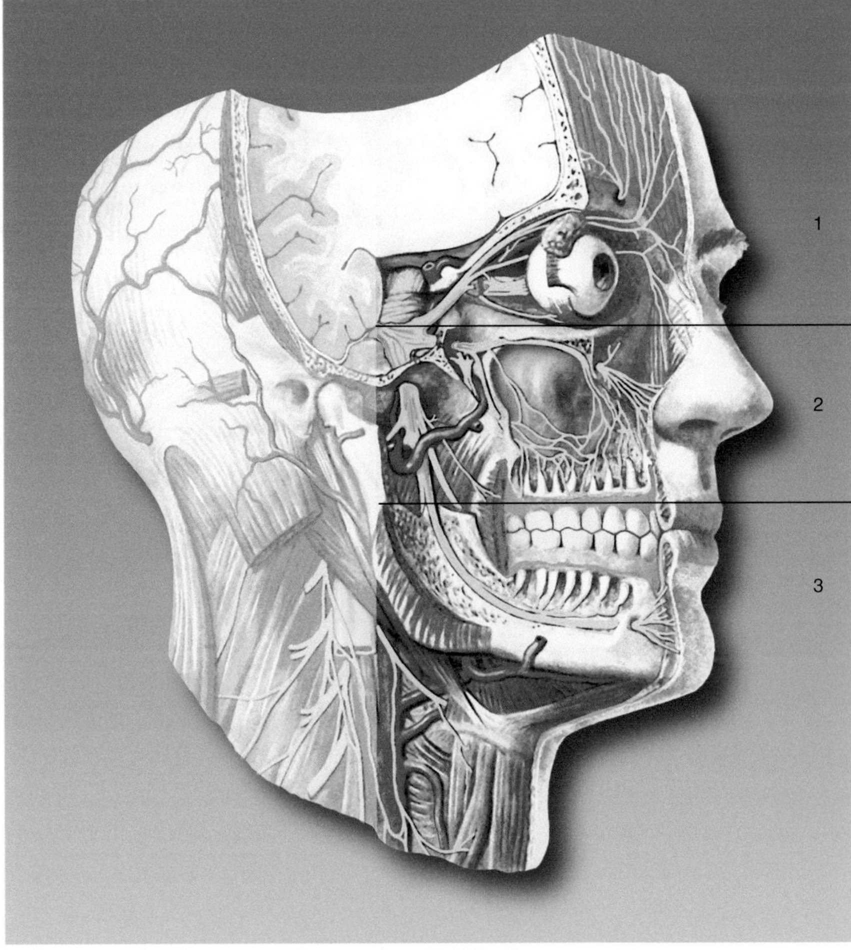

Fig. 8.3 (*1*) Supraorbital and supratrochlear nerves, (*2*) infraorbital nerve, (*3*) mental nerve. (Reproduced with permission from Danilo Jankovic)

Ophthalmic Nerve (Figs. 8.1 and 8.2)

The optic branch is purely *sensory* and passes lateral to the cavernous sinus and abducent nerve to the *superior orbital fissure.* It draws *sympathetic fibers* from the internal carotid plexus and in turn gives off *sensory fibers* to the oculomotor nerve, trochlear nerve, and abducent nerve. Before entering the fissure, the ophthalmic nerve branches into the *lacrimal nerve, nasociliary nerve,* and *frontal nerve.*

The *frontal nerve* runs along the levator palpebrae superioris muscle to behind the center of the orbital cavity. There it divides into the *supraorbital nerve*, which passes to the supraorbital notch, and the *supratrochlear nerve*, which runs in a medial direction toward the trochlea. The branches of the supratrochlear nerve supply the upper eyelid, the root of the nose, and the adjoining skin of the forehead (upper end branch), as well as the skin and conjunctiva of the medial canthus (lower end branch) (Fig. 8.3).

Maxillary Nerve & Pterygopalatine Fossa (PPF) & Pterygopalatine Ganglion (PPG)

The maxillary nerve is larger than the ophthalmic and is also *sensory*. Like the other branches of the trigeminal nerve, it acts as a *vehicle* for the distribution of *sympathetic* and *parasympathetic fibers*. The maxillary nerve gives off a small *meningeal branch* to the *meninges* of the middle cranial fossa before passing forward in the lower part of the lateral wall of the *cavernous sinus* (Figs. 8.1 and 8.2).

It then leaves the skull through the *foramen rotundum* and enters the *(PPF),* where it communicates with corresponding ganglion *(PPG)* (Figs. 8.2 and 8.4), to enter the *orbit* through the *inferior orbital fissure*. Finally, the maxillary nerve traverses the infraorbital groove as the *infraorbital nerve* and emerges on the *face,* where it divides into *inferior palpebral, external,* and *internal nasal* and *superior labial branches,* which supply the *lower eyelid, nasal alae,* and *upper lip* (skin and mucous membrane), respectively (Fig. 8.3).

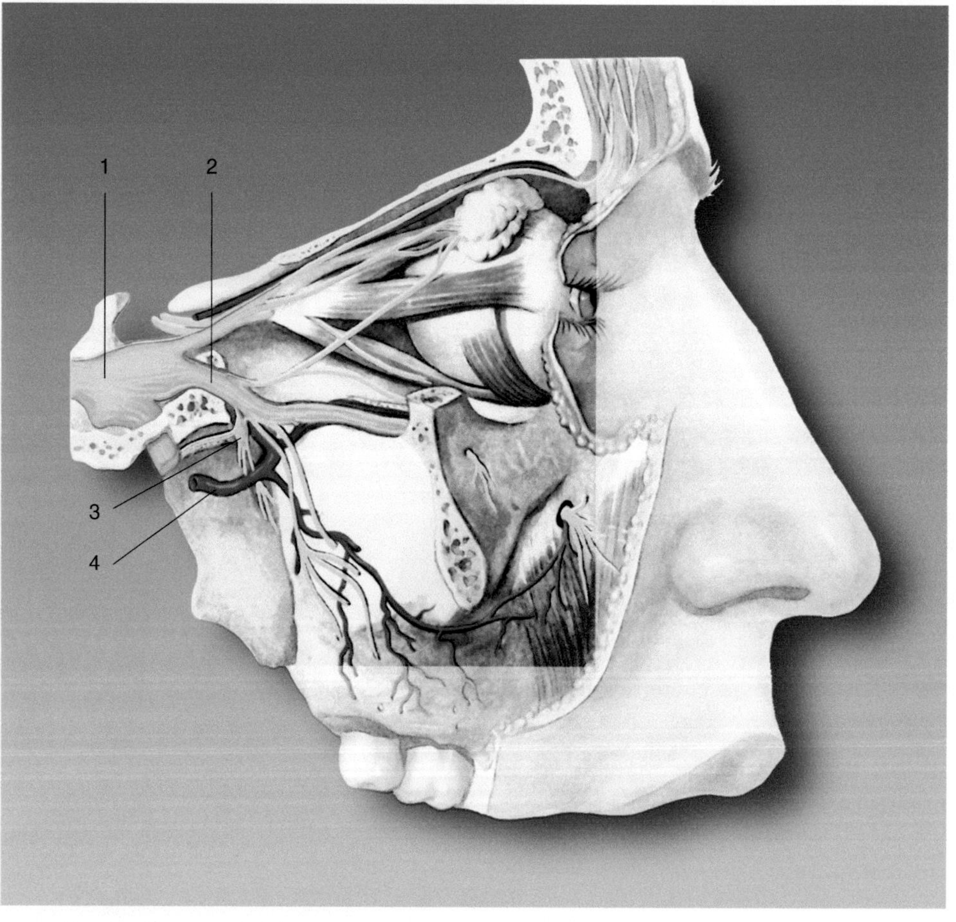

Fig. 8.4 (*1*) Trigeminal ganglion (Gasserian ganglion) and (*2*) pterygopalatine fossa with the maxillary nerve, (*3*) pterygopalatine ganglion, and (*4*) maxillary artery. (Reproduced with permission from Danilo Jankovic)

Anatomy of the Pterygopalatine Fossa (PPF)

The *PPF* is a small, fat-filled space located in the deep face that serves as a *major neurovascular crossroad* between the oral cavity, nasal cavity, nasopharynx, orbit, masticator space, and the middle cranial fossa.

Contents

- The *pterygopalatine ganglion (PPG)* suspended by nerve roots from the *maxillary nerve* (see below) (Figs. 8.2 and 8.4).
- The *maxillary division (V2) of the trigeminal nerve* (purely sensory) and its *branches* (*zygomatic nerve*, *posterior superior alveolar nerve(s)*), the *infraorbital nerve,* and the *Vidian (pterygoid) nerve*. The *PPF* communicates with the *foramen lacerum* via the *Vidian canal* which traverses posterolaterally through the body of the sphenoid bone. The *Vidian canal* contains the *Vidian nerve*, which carries *parasympathetic preganglionic fibers* from the *facial nerve* to the *PPG*. The *postganglionic* fibers from the *PPG* supply the *lacrimal gland* and the mucosa of the *nasal cavity* and *nasopharynx.*
- The terminal third of the *maxillary artery* and *veins,* as well as their associated branches. The *maxillary artery* is one of the major branches of the *external carotid artery*. At the *PPF*, it is located anterior to the *PPG* and gives rise to *six branches* that accompany the branches of the maxillary nerve and the *PPG* (Figs. 8.1, 8.3, 8.4, and 8.5).

Innervation (Figs. 8.1, 8.2, and 8.3)

Branches of the *maxillary nerve* form most of the nerves that enter and exit the *PPF.*

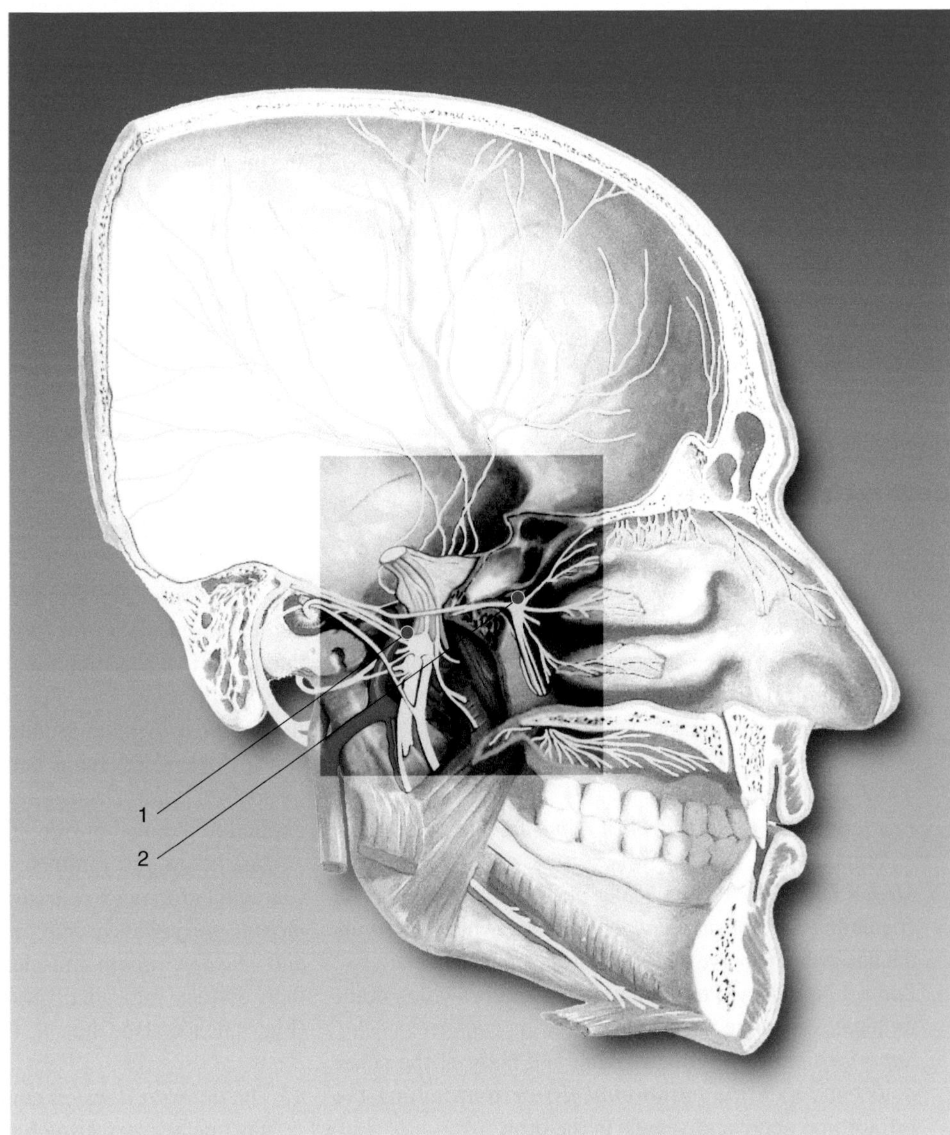

Fig. 8.5 Nerves and ganglia in the vicinity: (*1*) Otic ganglion, (*2*) pterygopalatine ganglion. (Reproduced with permission from Danilo Jankovic)

Maxillary nerve enters the fossa via the *foramen rotundum* and branches as follows:

- *Posterior superior alveolar nerves* (maxillary molar teeth and gingivae)
- *Infraorbital nerve* (maxillary premolars, canines, and incisors and the gingivae and mucosal lining of the maxillary sinus)
- *Zygomatic nerve* (zygomaticotemporal and zygomaticofacial nerves), which supply the skin over the zygomatic arch and the temporal region
- *Pharyngeal nerve* (part of the nasopharynx)
- *Greater and lesser palatine nerves* (roof of the mouth, soft palate, tonsil, and lining membrane of the nasal cavity)

The *ganglionic branches* allow the *maxillary nerve* to communicate with the *PPG*, thus serving as a conduit for *parasympathetic and sympathetic postganglionic* fibers to travel through. Along with the sensory fibers of the maxillary nerve, these fibers (sympathetic and parasympathetic) leave directly either from the *PPG* as orbital, palatine, nasal, and pharyngeal branches or from the maxillary nerve along with its associated branches.

Gateways

The *PPF* serves as a gateway for *seven openings* (foramen rotundum, pterygoid canal, palatovaginal canal, palatine canal, sphenopalatine foramen, inferior orbital fissure, and pterygomaxillary fissure). These openings transmit branches of the *maxillary nerve,* the *pterygopalatine ganglion*, and the *maxillary vessels.*

Boundaries

1. *Anterior.* Superomedial part of the infratemporal surface of maxilla
2. *Posterior.* Root of the pterygoid process and adjoining anterior surface of the greater wing of the sphenoid bone with *openings* for the following structures:
   - *Foramen rotundum* for (V2)
   - *Pterygoid canal* for the nerve of the pterygoid canal (Vidian nerve)
   - *Pharyngeal (palatovaginal) canal* for the pharyngeal branch of V2
3. *Medial boundary.* Perpendicular plate of the palatine bone containing the *sphenopalatine foramen,* which transmits the nasopalatine nerve (V2) and the sphenopalatine artery
4. *Lateral boundary.* Pterygomaxillary fissure, which communicates with the infratemporal fossa
5. *Superior boundary.* Greater wing and body of the sphenoid bone with *the infraorbital fissure* transmitting the infraorbital nerve and vessels in the orbit
6. *Inferior boundary.* Palatine process of the maxilla and the pterygoid process of the sphenoid bone with *the greater and lesser palatine canals and foramina,* which transmit the greater and lesser palatine nerves and vessels

Pterygopalatine Ganglion (PPG)

The *PPG* is the *largest of the four parasympathetic ganglia* located in the head. The pterygopalatine (sphenopalatine) ganglion is triangular in shape; extending to ~5 mm, it is the largest neuronal conglomerate outside of the brain (Figs. 8.2, 8.4, and 8.5).

The *PPG* houses the cell bodies of *parasympathetic postganglionic neurons* and receives *parasympathetic preganglionic fibers* and *sympathetic postganglionic fibers* from the *nerve of the pterygoid canal.* The *nerve of the pterygoid canal* is formed by the union of the *greater petrosal nerve* (branch of the *facial nerve* VII) and the *deep petrosal nerve* (branch of *carotid plexus*); it thus carries *parasympathetic preganglionic fibers* of the *greater petrosal nerve* and *sympathetic postganglionic fibers* of the *deep petrosal nerve.* Once formed, the *nerve of the pterygoid canal* leaves the middle cranial fossa, travels through the *pterygoid canal* via the *foramen lacerum,* and enters the *PPF* to *join the PPG.* Only the *parasympathetic preganglionic fibers* of the *nerve of the pterygoid canal* synapse at the *PPG,* while the *sympathetic postganglionic* fibers travel through it. In addition, the *maxillary nerve is purely sensory* and thus has *no autonomic function;* however, it is used as a *vehicle* by *parasympathetic and sympathetic fibers* to reach their targets.

Mandibular Nerve and Otic Ganglion (Figs. 8.1 and 8.2)

Mandibular Nerve

The mandibular nerve is the largest branch of the trigeminal nerve and consists of a *large sensory root* issuing from the lateral half of the trigeminal ganglion and the entire, *small trigeminal motor root.* The two parts leave the skull through the *foramen ovale* and unite almost immediately to form a short, thick nerve lying between the *lateral pterygoid* and *tensor veli palatini muscles.* A small *otic ganglion* is closely applied to the medial side of the nerve.

Just below the foramen, the mandibular nerve gives off : *meningeal branch (nervus spinosus)* and the nerve to the *medial pterygoid muscle* to supply the *tensor veli palatini* and *tensor tympani* muscles. The *main mandibular nerve* then divides into small *anterior* and large *posterior* parts (Fig. 8.6; see also Chap. 9, Fig. 9.11).

1. The *anterior division* contains *mostly motor fibers,* but it has one *sensory branch (buccal nerve).* The *other motor*

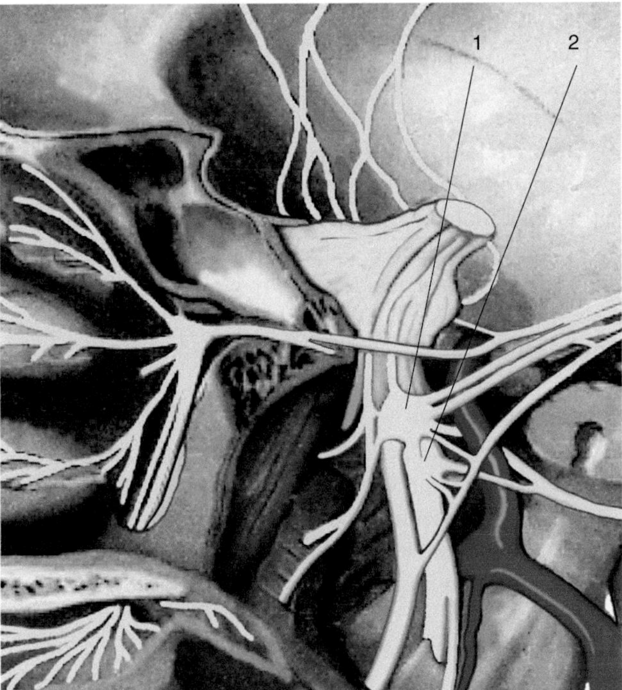

Fig. 8.6 There are close anatomical connections between the otic ganglion (*1*) and the mandibular nerve (*2*). (Reproduced with permission from Danilo Jankovic)

branches are masseteric nerve(s), deep temporal nerves, and nerve to lateral pterygoid muscle.

2. The *posterior division* of the mandibular nerve is *mainly sensory*, but also contains *motor fibers* that are distributed in the mylohyoid branch of the *inferior alveolar nerve*. The most important nerves and areas of the posterior trunk are:
   - The *auriculotemporal nerve* gives branches to the *temporomandibular joint*, the *external acoustic meatus*, and the *tympanic membrane*, to the *skin of the tragus and part of the helix* and *secretomotor and vasomotor fibers* to the *parotid* gland, which reach the nerve through the otic ganglion.
   - The *lingual nerve* carries general sensory fibers from the *anterior two thirds* of the *tongue* and the *floor of the mouth*. It is *joined* near its origin by a branch of the *facial nerve, the chorda tympani*, which conveys special sensory (taste) fibers from the anterior two thirds of the tongue or from the part anterior to the V-shaped sulcus terminalis. The branches communicate with terminal branches of *glossopharyngeal and hypoglossal nerves*.
   - The *inferior alveolar nerve* is mainly sensory, but it does carry *some motor* fibers. Before entering the *mandibular canal*, it gives off its only motor branch, the mylohyoid nerve, which supplies the *mylohyoid muscle* and anterior belly of the *digastric*. The *other branches of the inferior alveolar* nerve are the *mental* nerve (skin and mucosa of the lower lip and chin) and the *inferior dental and gingival rami*, which arise from the nerve as it runs in the mandibular canal.

Otic Ganglion (Figs. 8.2, 8.5, and 8.6)

Located in the *infratemporal fossa, the otic ganglion is the smallest of the four parasympathetic* ganglia found in the head region. The otic ganglion may exist only as a *group of microganglia, medial to the mandibular nerve. It is an oval but flat ganglion and approximately 2 × 1.5 × 0.4 mm in size*. It lies inferomedial to the foramen ovale. Even though the otic ganglion is *topographically* related to *mandibular nerve, functionally*, it is related to the *glossopharyngeal nerve (IX)* and innervates the *parotid gland for salivation*.

The *preganglionic pathway* is usually said to arise from the *glossopharyngeal nerve (IX)* via the *tympanic plexus* and the *lesser petrosal nerve*. However, an additional *preganglionic* pathway runs via the *chorda tympany nerve,* carrying *preganglionic* input from the *facial nerve. Postganglionic* axons leave *the ganglion* mainly via the *auriculotemporal nerve. Otic ganglion neurons are morphologically similar to those of the pterygopalatine ganglion.*

Trigeminal Nerve: Peripheral Branches Block

General Consideration

For superficial trigeminal nerve blocks, the local anesthetic solution should be injected in close proximity to the three terminal superficial branches of the trigeminal nerve divisions: frontal nerve (of the ophthalmic nerve, V1 division); infraorbital nerve (of the maxillary nerve, V2 division); and mental nerve (sensory terminal branch of the mandibular nerve, V3 division). Each nerve is anatomically close to its respective foramen. The supraorbital foramen, infraorbital foramen, and mental foramen lie on a single line running about 2.5 cm lateral to the midfacial line and passing through the pupil (Fig. 8.7).

Block of the Ophthalmic Nerve Branches

Supraorbital and Supratrochlear Nerves

The end branches of these two nerves provide the sensory supply for the skin of the forehead, top of the nose and the skin, and conjunctiva of the medial canthus (Fig. 8.3; see also Chap. 9, Fig. 9.18).

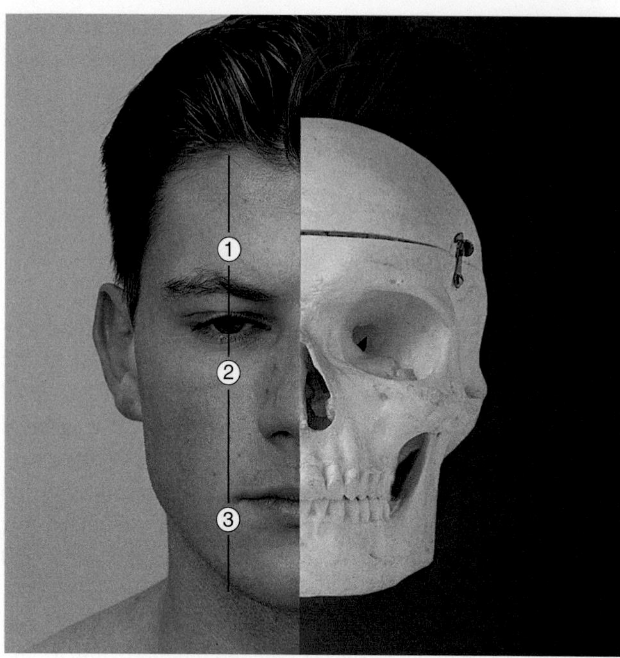

Fig. 8.7 The supraorbital foramen (*1*), infraorbital foramen (*2*), and mental foramen (*3*) lie on a single line running about 2.5 cm lateral to the midfacial line and passing through the pupil. (Reproduced with permission from Danilo Jankovic)

Indications

Diagnostic

- Differential diagnosis of hyperalgesic zones—e.g., the frontal part of the occipitofrontalis muscle

Therapeutic

- Trigeminal neuralgia of the first branch and post-herpetic neuralgia
- Postoperative and posttraumatic pain
- Minor surgical interventions (note higher doses) along the surface of the innervated area—e.g., removal of cysts and atheromas, wound care

Procedure

Preparations

Check that the emergency equipment is complete and in working order. Sterile precautions.

Materials

2-mL syringes, fine 26-G needles (25 mm), disinfectant, swabs for compression

Skin prep

For all blocks

Patient Positioning

Supine

Landmarks

- Supraorbital foramen, upper angle of the orbit
- Supraorbital nerve: palpation of the supraorbital foramen at the orbital margin
- Supratrochlear nerve: palpation of the upper angle of the orbit on the medial side of the root of the nose

Technique

Supraorbital Nerve

After palpation of the supraorbital foramen, a swab is laid on the eyelid to prevent uncontrolled spread of the local anesthetic. The needle is introduced as far as the supraorbital foramen (bone contact), slightly withdrawn, and after aspiration the injection is carried out slowly (Figs. 8.8).

Supratrochlear Nerve

After palpation of the upper angle of the orbit, a swab is laid on the eyelid to prevent uncontrolled spread of the local anesthetic. The needle is introduced at the upper internal angle of the orbit (Fig. 8.9) and minimally withdrawn after bone contact. Slow injection of the local anesthetic follows after careful aspiration.

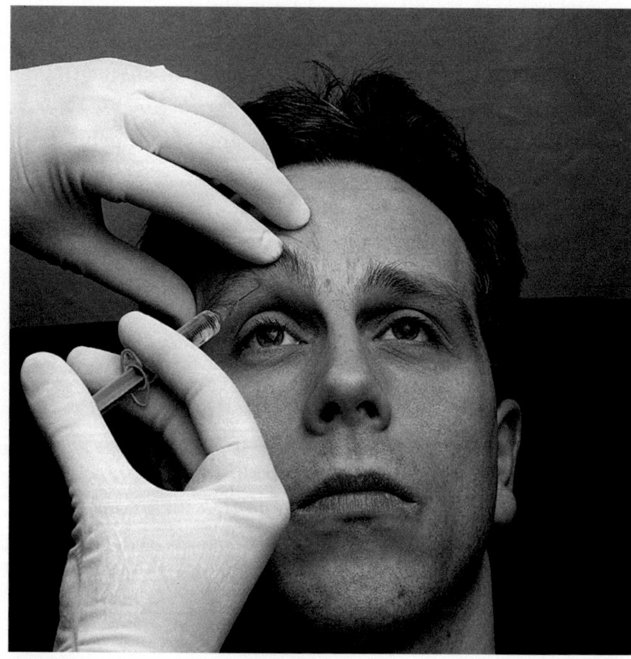

Fig. 8.8 Anesthetizing the supraorbital nerve. (Reproduced with permission from Danilo Jankovic)

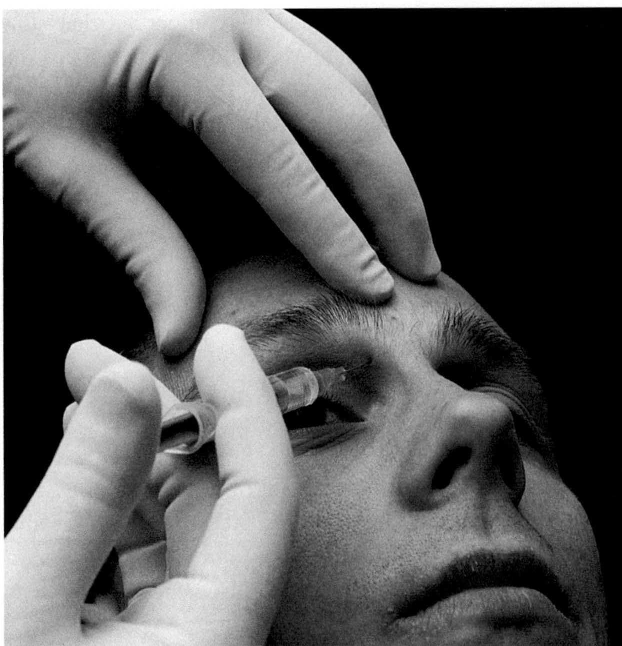

Fig. 8.9 Anesthetizing the supratrochlear nerve. (Reproduced with permission from Danilo Jankovic)

*It is not necessary to elicit paresthesias. Look for bone contact, withdraw the needle slightly, aspirate, and inject.

Dosage

Diagnostic
0.5–1 mL local anesthetic—e.g., 0.5–1% prilocaine, mepivacaine, lidocaine

Therapeutic
0.5–1 mL local anesthetic—e.g., 0.5–0.75% ropivacaine, 0.25–0.5% bupivacaine (levobupivacaine 0.25–0.5%)

Surgical
Up to 5 mL local anesthetic

Shorter procedures: e.g., 1% prilocaine, mepivacaine, lidocaine

Longer procedures: 0.75% ropivacaine, 0.5% bupivacaine (0.5% levobupivacaine)

Side Effects
Possible hematoma formation (prophylactic compression)

After the injection, carry out thorough compression (massaging in) to prevent hematoma formation and to encourage the local anesthetic to spread

Complications
Risk of blood vessel and nerve damage with injections into the foramina and bone channels.

No injections should be made into the supraorbital foramen due to the risk of nerve injury.

Block of the Maxillary Nerve Branches

Infraorbital Nerve
The infraorbital nerve, the end branch of the maxillary nerve, emerges about 1 cm below the middle of the lower orbital margin through the infraorbital foramen (Fig. 8.3; see also Chap. 9; Fig. 9.20).

Indications

Diagnostic
- Differential diagnosis of trigger zones

Therapeutic
- Trigeminal neuralgia in the second branch and postherpetic pain
- Facial pain in the innervation area of the infraorbital nerve, posttraumatic pain, and pain after dental extraction
- Minor surgical procedures on the surface of the area of distribution (note higher dosages)

Procedure

Preparation and Materials (See Supraorbital Block)
Skin Prep

For all blocks

Patient Positioning
Supine

Landmarks
Infraorbital foramen, orbital margin (Figs. 8.3 and 8.7)

Extraoral Injection
Palpation of the infraorbital foramen, about 1 cm below the middle of the lower orbital margin

Intraoral Injection
Palpation of the lower orbital margin

Technique

Extraoral Injection
After palpating the infraorbital foramen, the needle is introduced cranially just below the palpation point until bone contact is made (Fig. 8.10) and then withdrawn slightly.

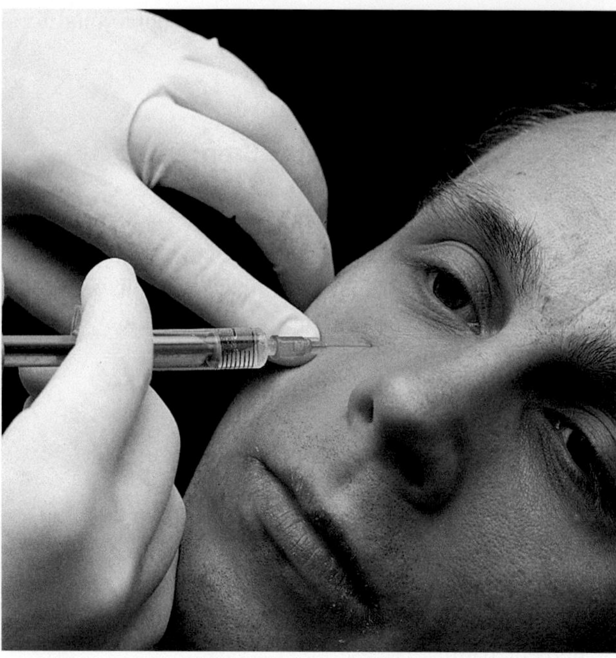

Fig. 8.10 Extraoral technique for blocking the infraorbital nerve. (Reproduced with permission from Danilo Jankovic)

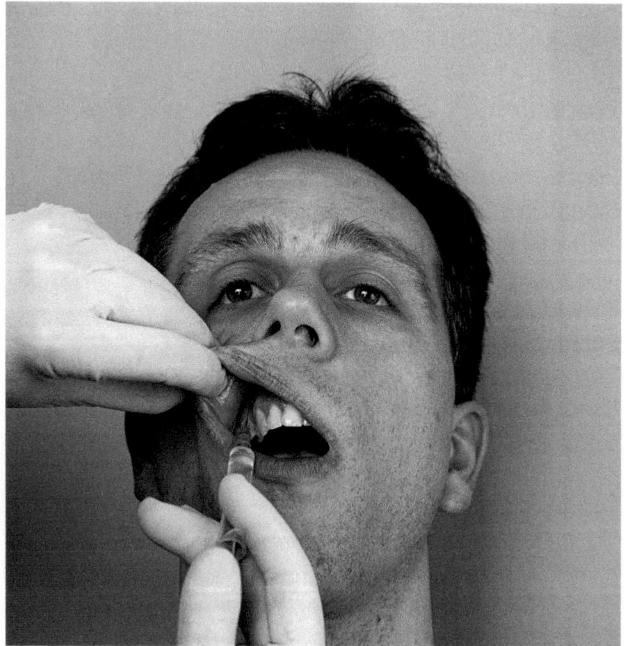

Fig. 8.11 Intraoral technique for blocking the infraorbital nerve. (Reproduced with permission from Danilo Jankovic)

Intraoral Injection

The center of the lower orbital margin is palpated and marked with the middle finger. The upper lip is raised with a spatula or with the thumb and index finger. The needle is introduced above the second premolar tooth toward the infraorbital foramen, until bone contact is made, and then withdrawn slightly (Fig. 8.11).

For both of these techniques, it is important that slow injection of the local anesthetic should only be carried out after careful aspiration. Afterwards, thorough compression should be carried out to prevent hematoma formation and to obtain better distribution of the local anesthetic.

*No injections should be made into the infraorbital canal due to the risk of nerve injury.

Dosages

Diagnostic

0.5–1 mL local anesthetic—e.g., 0.5–1% prilocaine, mepivacaine, lidocaine

Therapeutic (Extraoral Technique)

0.5–1 mL local anesthetic—e.g., 0.5–0.75% ropivacaine, 0.5% bupivacaine (0.5% levobupivacaine)

Surgical

Up to 5 mL local anesthetic extraorally

Shorter procedures: 1% prilocaine, mepivacaine, lidocaine.

Longer procedures: 0.75% ropivacaine, 0.5% bupivacaine (0.5% levobupivacaine)

Intraorally: 2–3 mL local anesthetic

Side Effects

Potential hematoma formation (prophylactic compression).

If the needle is advanced too far, penetration of the orbit can occur.

Symptom: temporary double vision.

Complications

Injection into the bone canal carries a risk of nerve damage.

Block of the Mandibular Nerve Branches

Mental Nerve

The mental nerve, the sensory end branch of the mandibular nerve, emerges from the mental foramen at the level of the second premolar (Figs. 8.3 and 8.12). It provides the sensory supply of the skin and mucosa of the lower lip and chin (see also Chap. 9; Fig. 9.22).

Indications

Diagnostic

- Differential diagnosis of trigger points and hyperalgesic zones

Therapeutic

- Trigeminal neuralgia of the third branch
- Posttraumatic pain and pain in the innervation area of the mental nerve

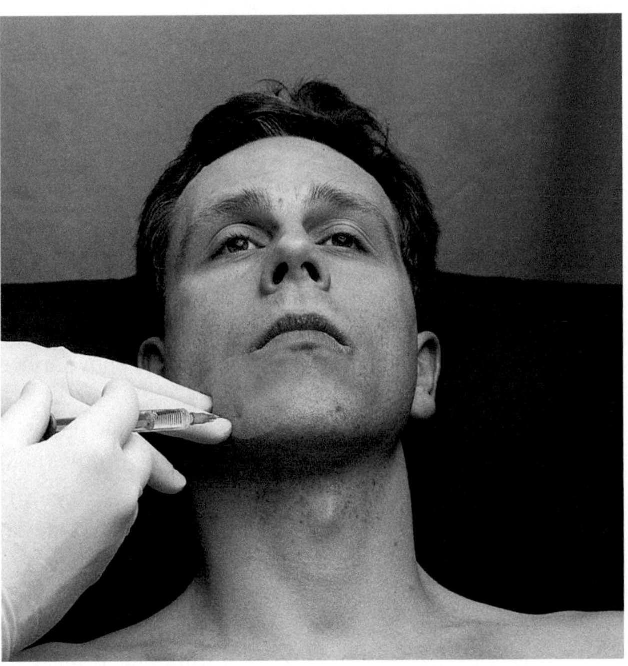

Fig. 8.12 Extraoral technique for blocking the mental nerve. (Reproduced with permission from Danilo Jankovic)

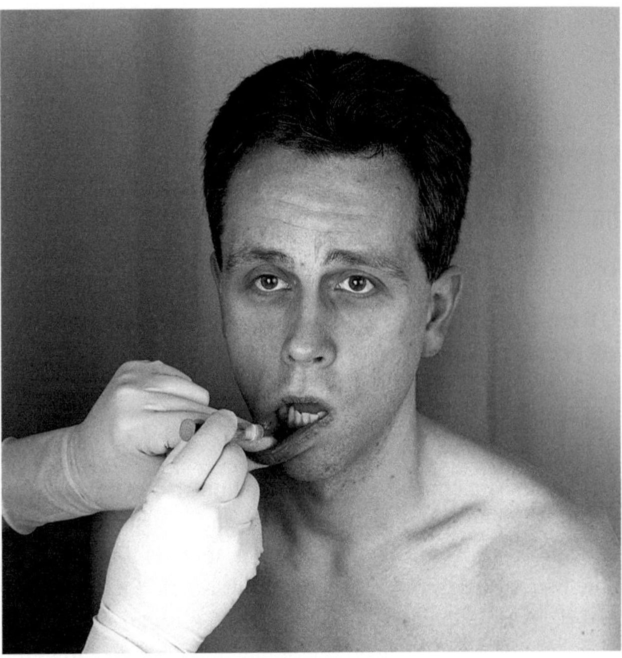

Fig. 8.13 Intraoral technique for blocking the mental nerve (Reproduced with permission from Danilo Jankovic)

- Dental treatment of canine tooth, first premolars and incisors of the lower jaw
- Post-dental extraction pain (intraoral technique)
- Surgical procedures on the surface of the lower lip (note higher dosages)

Procedure

Preparation and Materials (See Supraorbital Nerve Block)

Skin Prep

In all blocks

Patient Positioning

Supine

Landmarks

Mental foramen (Figs. 8.3 and 8.7)

Extraoral and intraoral injection

Palpation of the mental foramen at the level of the second premolar

Technique

- Extraoral Injection

  After palpation of the mental foramen, the needle is inserted about 2.5 cm lateral to the midline until bone contact is made (Fig. 8.12).
- Intraoral Injection

  After palpation of the mental foramen, the lower lip is pressed downward using a spatula. The needle is inserted between the first and second premolars, into the lower reflection of the oral vestibule, in the direction of the neurovascular bundle (Fig. 8.13).

For both of these techniques, it is important that slow injection should only be carried out after careful aspiration. Afterward, thorough compression should be carried out to prevent hematoma formation and to obtain better distribution of the local anesthetic.

Dosage

Diagnostic

0.5–1 mL local anesthetic—e.g., 0.5–1% prilocaine, mepivacaine, lidocaine

Therapeutic (Extraoral Technique)

0.5–1 mL local anesthetic—e.g., 0.5–0.75% ropivacaine, 0.5% bupivacaine (0.5% levobupivacaine)

Surgical

Up to 5 mL local anesthetic *extraorally*

Shorter procedures: 1% prilocaine, mepivacaine, lidocaine

Longer procedures: 0.75% ropivacaine, 0.5% bupivacaine (0.5% levobupivacaine)

Intraorally: 2–3 mL local anesthetic

Side Effects

Potential hematoma formation (prophylactic compression).

Complications

Injections should never be made into the mental canal, due to the risk of nerve injury.

Ultrasound Imaging for Peripheral Branches of Trigeminal Nerve

Ban Tsui

Ultrasound imaging is a common, noninvasive modality to facilitate many regional nerve blocks and to visualize nerves and surrounding soft tissue. However, there is limited available literature describing the use of ultrasound for superficial and deep trigeminal nerve block. This is because the most comprehensive of the deep trigeminal nerve blocks target the central ganglion. Because the ganglion is deep, blockade is often performed under fluoroscopic guidance or computerized tomography.

While blockade of deep structures is inaccessible to ultrasound, superficial branches of the trigeminal nerve (i.e., supraorbital, infraorbital, and mental nerves) are too small to visualize with most common ultrasound machines. In fact, the superficial branches can be performed easily by palpating their respective foramina. Although these bony foramina are usually easy to palpate physically, they can also be identified by observing a disruption or discontinuity within the bony hyperechoic line when imaging with ultrasound, as described below. Due to the superficial nature of these blocks, most experts find it more practical to use ultrasound imaging for landmarking the foramina rather than for real-time guidance.

Scanning Technique

1. As described in previous section, all three foramina are typically located approximately 2.5 cm lateral to the midfacial line passing through the pupil in the sagittal plane on each side of the face.
2. Using a high-frequency linear transducer, the foramina can be identified dynamically by subtle movement of the probe position after placing it in the usual vicinity of the foramina; this technique will allow the user to capture breaks in the linear hyperechogenicity of the bony surface caused by the foramina.
   (a) To locate the supraorbital landmark, the probe is positioned transversely above the roof of the orbital rim and in alignment with the pupil. The bone is scanned slowly in a cephalad-to-caudad direction to identify the supraorbital foramen.
   (b) The infraorbital foramen can be located by scanning in a sagittal plane from medial to lateral along the lower orbital margin or inferior rim of the orbit. This foramen is usually located about 1 cm below the middle of the lower orbital margin.
   (c) The mental foramen can be localized using a transverse plane and scanning in a cephalad direction from the inferior border of the mandible. The nerve typically lies inferior to the outer lip at the level of the second premolar, midway between the upper and lower borders of the mandible.

As shown in Fig. 8.14, the image of the bony surface will change from a definite linear border to a border with a hypoechoic break caused by the foramen during dynamic scanning. It is important to note that the location of each orifice is associated with its respective blood vessels, which can be illuminated using color Doppler. However, the relatively small size of the arteries upon exiting the foramen renders them difficult to identify.

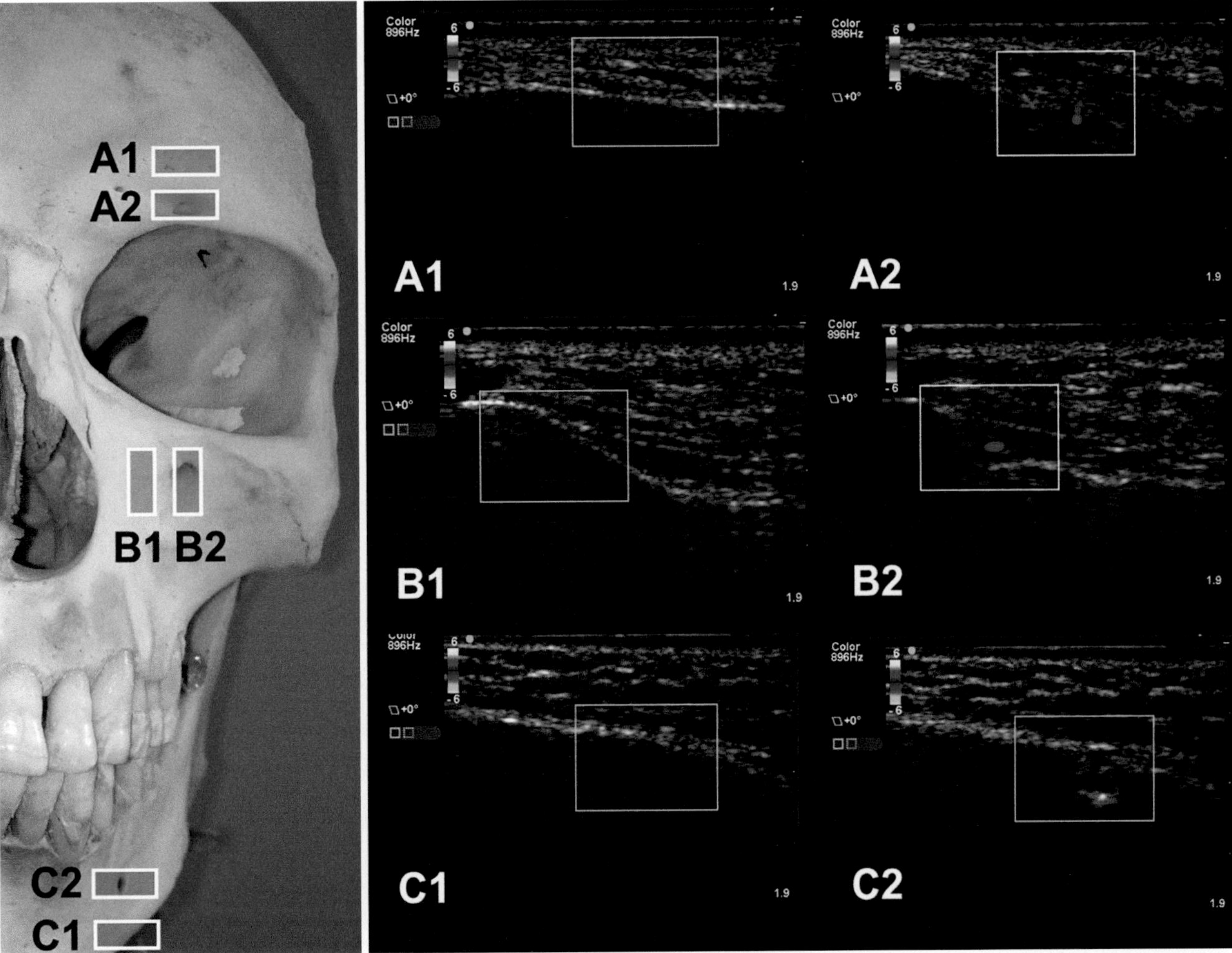

Fig. 8.14 *Left*, ultrasound scanning locations to identify supraorbital *(A1,A2)*, infraorbital *(B1,B2)*,and mental *(C1,C2)* foramina. *A1, B1,* and *C1* represent starting position of probe; *A2, B2,* and *C2* represent position of probe over foramen. *Right*, ultrasound images corresponding to probe positions. Doppler imaging *(far right)* allows identification of supraorbital and infraorbital arteries. (Reproduced with permission from Ban Tsui)

Suggested Reading

Anderson JE. The cranial nerves. Trigeminal nerve. Distribution of the trigeminal nerve. Section 8. In: Grant's atlas of anatomy. 7th ed. Philadelphia: Williams & Wilkins; 1978.

Auberger HG, Niesel HC. Gesichtsschädel: Proximale Leitungsanästhesie im Bereich des N. trigeminus. In: Auberger HG, Niesel HC, editors. Praktische Lokalanästhesie. 4th ed. Stuttgart: Georg Thieme; 1982.

Bonica JJ. Block of cranial nerves. In: Bonica JJ, editor. The management of Pain. 2nd ed. Philadelphia: Lea & Febiger; 1990.

Jenkner FL. Nervenblockaden auf pharmakologischem und auf elektrischem Weg. Wien: Springer; 1980.

Moore KL, Dalley AMR, Agur AMR. Moore clinically oriented anatomy. 7th ed. Philadelphia: Wolters Kluwer Health, Lippincott Williams & Wilkins; 2014. p. 951–4.

Moore DC. Regional block. 4th ed. Springfield: Charles Thomas; 1976.

Murphy TM. Somatic blockade of head and neck. In: Cousins MJ, Bridenbaugh PO, editors. Neural blockade. 2nd ed. Philadelphia: Lippincott; 1988.

Netter FH. Nervous system, part I. Anatomy and physiology. Cranial nerves, section V. Trigeminal nerve (V). The Ciba Collection of Medical Illustrations; 1991. p. 100–2.

Pernkpf E. Atlas der Topographischen und angewandten Anatomie des Menschen. 1.Band Kopf und Hals. 2 Auflage. Urban & Schwarzenberg; 1980. p. 73–5, 150–2.

Petren T. Anatomie des Nervus trigeminus. In: Eriksson E, editor. Atlas der Lokalanästhesie. 2nd ed. Berlin: Springer; 1980.

Raj P, Rawal N. Techniques of regional anesthesia in adults. In: Clinical practice of regional anesthesia. London: Churchill Livingston; 1991. p. 271.

Thiel W. Photograpischer Atlas der Praktischen Anatomie. 5132. Ausgabe. Berlin: Springer; 2003. p. 492–513.

Tsui BC. Ultrasound imaging to localize foramina for superficial trigeminal nerve block. Can J Anesth. 2009;56:704–6.

Tucker J, Flynn J. Head and neck regional blocks. In: Brown D, editor. Regional anesthesia and analgesia. Philadelphia: WB Saunders; 1996. p. 240–53.

Trigeminal Nerve: Deep Block

9

Antoun Nader, Louise Hillen, and Danilo Jankovic

Contents

Ultrasound-Guided Blockade of the Trigeminal Nerve Divisions Through the Pterygopalatine Fossa

General Considerations

Patients presenting with facial pain due to trigeminal neuralgia or atypical facial pain often do not have adequate relief with medical therapy alone. Trigeminal neuralgia is a neuropathic pain syndrome that typically involves the maxillary branch (V2) of the fifth cranial nerve. Twenty-five percent of patients with trigeminal neuralgia are refractory to medical treatment, and 8% may develop tolerance to their pharmacologic regimen. Patients who fail medical management may have the option to undergo surgical or minimally invasive procedures in an attempt to provide pain relief. In patients who are not surgical candidates, have side effects from medical management, or would rather avoid invasive techniques, a trigeminal nerve block under ultrasound guidance is a reasonable alternative. Blockade of the trigeminal nerve may also be an effective diagnostic tool to determine whether further potential treatment options such as radiofrequency ablation or neurolysis with glycerol would be beneficial. The use of trigeminal nerve blocks have also been used to help with acute pain from surgical procedures, such as cleft lip and palate repair. The use of ultrasound guidance allows for real-time visualization of soft tissue and surrounding vasculature and can help to confirm that local anesthetic has spread to the intended target. There are multiple different approaches to ultrasound-guided blockade of the trigeminal divisions through the pterygopalatine

A. Nader (✉)
Acute Pain and Regional Anesthesiology, Northwestern Medicine, Chicago, IL, USA
e-mail: a-nader2@northwestern.edu

L. Hillen
P.A., Plymouth, MN, USA

D. Jankovic
Pain Management Centre DGS – Cologne – Huerth, Cologne-Hürth, Germany
e-mail: danilo@jankovic1.de

D. Jankovic, P. Peng (eds.), *Regional Nerve Blocks in Anesthesia and Pain Therapy*,
https://doi.org/10.1007/978-3-030-88727-8_9

fossa (PPF). The three main approaches include the infrazygomatic anterior-to-posterior in-plane approach, infrazygomatic posterior-to-anterior in-plane approach, and the suprazygomatic out-of-plane approach.

Indication (Patient Selection)

Injection of local anesthetic, steroids, or glycerol at the trigeminal nerve and its branches may be indicated in patients who have failed pharmacological management or surgical interventions or those who are not candidates for surgical procedures or balloon decompression. A block may also be used to decrease facial pain in patients waiting for balloon decompression or surgical intervention for pathologies such as acoustic neuroma or chiari malformation.

Contraindications

Patients should not undergo the nerve block if they have an allergy to local anesthetic, or if they have an active infection or coagulopathy.

Functional Anatomy

(See also Chap. 8, Trigeminal Nerve Anatomy and Peripheral Branches Block)

The trigeminal ganglion (also known as the Gasserian ganglion) is situated within Meckel's cave in the middle cranial fossa. The trigeminal nerve gives rise to three branches: the ophthalmic (V1), maxillary (V2), and mandibular (V3). These branches exit the skull through foramina, the superior orbital fissure, the foramen rotundum, and the foramen ovale, respectively. The foramen rotundum opens into the posterior part of the pterygopalatine fossa (PPF), which is medial to the lateral pterygoid plate. Due to the connection of the PPF and the middle cranial fossa via the foramen rotundum, spread at the upper part of the PPF causes blockade of the trigeminal nerve. Because the space within the PPF is small, placing just 2 ml of contrast results in a retrograde passage in order to reach the middle cranial fossa. The PPF is a pyramidal-shaped space that contains the maxillary nerve (V2), maxillary artery, and sphenopalatine ganglion, and it communicates with the infratemporal fossa via the pterygomaxillary fissure. The boundaries of the PPF are the lateral pterygoid plate posteriorly, the maxillary bone anteriorly, and the orbital apex superiorly. The maxillary artery is tortuous and enters from the infratemporal fossa into the PPF from a posterior-anterior and lateral-medial course. It can be visualized on ultrasound as a deep structure within the PPF. Other contents of the PPF that will be blocked via this approach include the maxillary nerve and the afferent and efferent branches of the sphenopalatine ganglion. The PPF communicates with the foramen rotundum, supraorbital fissure, and vidian canal, which may account for the success of these blocks by way of local anesthetic spreading to the various branches of the trigeminal nerve.

Technique

There are three main approaches to ultrasound-guided trigeminal nerve blocks via the pterygopalatine fossa. The three will be described in detail below.

- Infrazygomatic Posterior-to-Anterior (In-Plane Approach)

  This approach was first described by Nader et al. in a prospective case series involving 15 patients with refractory facial pain. The patient is positioned in the lateral decubitus position with standard ASA monitors applied. The face is prepped and draped in a sterile fashion. The ultrasound is placed below the zygomatic process, superior to the mandibular notch, and anterior to the mandibular condyle (Fig. 9.1a). The zygomatic bone, the lateral pterygoid muscle, the lateral pterygoid plate, and the maxillary bone are identified using ultrasound. The superficial branches of the maxillary artery can be visualized anterior to the mandible using color Doppler (Fig. 9.1c). A 21-gauge 70–100 mm echogenic needle is inserted in-plane parallel to the transducer probe and advanced in a lateral-to-medial and posterior-to-anterior direction toward the pterygopalatine fossa (Fig. 9.1b). The needle will advance in-plane through the lateral pterygoid muscle and stop at the pterygopalatine fissure, typically located 4–5 cm below the surface of the skin and just above the lateral pterygoid plate. While dosing can vary, for the typical adult, 4 ml of 0.25–0.5% bupivacaine with 4 mg (1 ml) of dexamethasone can be injected. The procedure itself typically takes less than 5 min to complete.
- Infrazygomatic Anterior-to-Posterior (In-Plane Approach)

  Kampitak et al. describes an ultrasound technique using a curved probe for a selective maxillary (V2) nerve block using the lateral pterygoid plate (LPP) by way of the PPF. The PPF communicates with the infratemporal fossa via the pterygomaxillary fissure (PMF). The boundary of the PMF, the maxilla, and the lateral pterygoid plate (LPP) are used as anatomical landmarks for orientation during this ultrasound-guided maxillary nerve block. The goal is to find the PMF, which is the narrow gap between the infratemporal surface of the maxilla and the LPP.

  The ultrasound probe is first placed transversely below the zygomatic arch with identification of the maxillary tuberosity and LPP. The patient's mouth should be open to avoid shadowing by the coracoid process and the

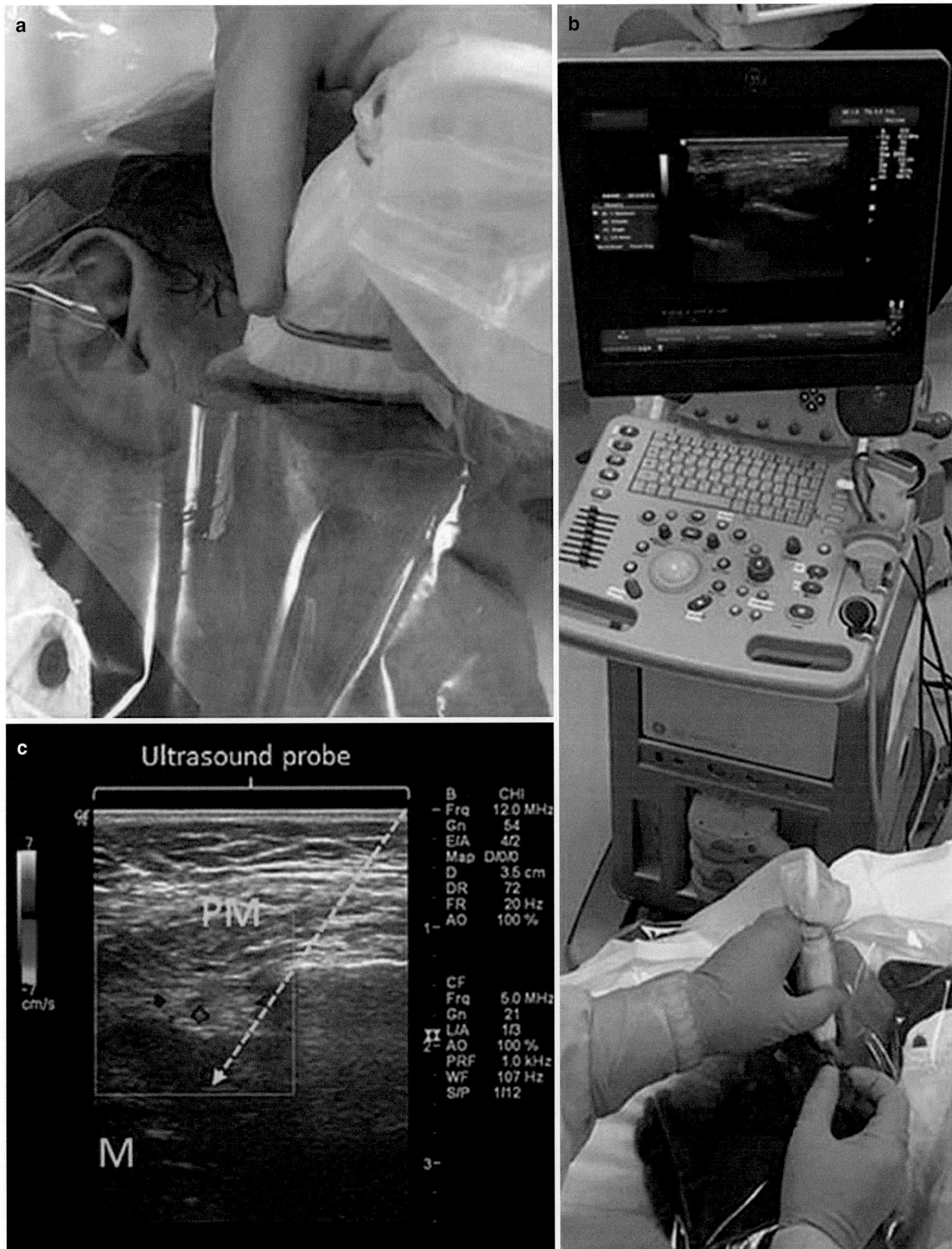

Fig. 9.1 (**a**) The ultrasound probe is positioned below the zygomatic arch with cephalad angulation in order to visualize the target area below the zygoma. (**b**) The needle is placed in-line with the transducer from lateral to medial. (**c**) The ultrasound image is a transverse view. Superficial branches of the maxillary and facial artery can be seen with Doppler. *Dashed line* needle trajectory, *PM* lateral pterygoid muscle, *M* Maxilla. (Reproduced with permission from Nader et al.)

mandible. The probe can be tilted from caudal to cranial direction to observe the boundary between the maxillary tuberosity and the LPP. At the bottom of the PMF, the LPP connects with the MT and appears to be a hyperechoic continuous line. By tilting the probe from caudal to cranial, one will see an interruption in this continuous line between the MT and LPP, which is the PPF or PMF opening. The needle injection point should be the uppermost part of the LPP.

The needle trajectory is anterior-to-posterior and lateral-to-medial, and in-plane with the ultrasound transducer. A 21-gauge 70–100 mm echogenic needle can be used and is advanced through the lateral pterygoid muscle until it contacts the anterior border of the lateral pterygoid plate. The needle is then withdrawn 1–2 mm and redirected medially into the PPF. Typically, just 3 ml of local anesthetic is needed for successful spread into the PPF.

- Suprazygomatic (Out-of-Plane)

  Sola et al. describes a suprazygomatic out-of-plane approach, first utilized in children undergoing cleft palate repair. The ultrasound is placed below the zygomatic process over the maxilla at a 45° angle. A 21-gauge 70–100 mm echogenic needle is inserted perpendicular to the skin at the frontozygomatic angle above the zygomatic process, out-of-plane with the ultrasound. The needle is advanced until, typically around 20 mm in-depth, the needle tip contacts the great wing of the sphenoid (Figs. 9.2c and 9.3). The needle is withdrawn and directed caudally and posteriorly roughly 35–45 mm deep within the PPF. In Sola et al.'s study, 0.15 ml/kg of 0.2% ropivacaine was given, resulting in 70% of spread to the intermediate (anterior) part of the PPF and 22% deep in the PPF.

Complications

Each of the ultrasound-guided approaches has its limitations and potential complications. Both the anterior infrazygomatic and the suprazygomatic approaches involve making contact with the sphenoid bone, which can be particularly uncomfortable in an awake patient. Importantly, the parotid gland, facial nerve, and artery are superficial to the mandibular notch, and are in close proximity to the needle trajectory needed for the posterior infrazygomatic approach. In the suprazygomatic out-of-plane approach, the needle cannot be seen at the entry point and can only be seen once it passes below the zygoma. Without needle visualization at all times, injury to surrounding structures, including neurovascular structures, can occur. With all approaches, puncture of the maxillary artery is of concern. The risk of injury to the artery can be lessened by placing the needle tip beneath the lateral pterygoid muscle at the level of the pterygomaxillary fissure, which causes the muscle to indirectly force the spread of the injectate into the PPF.

The performance of the block may also be limited by patient comfort, and sedation may need to be given to the

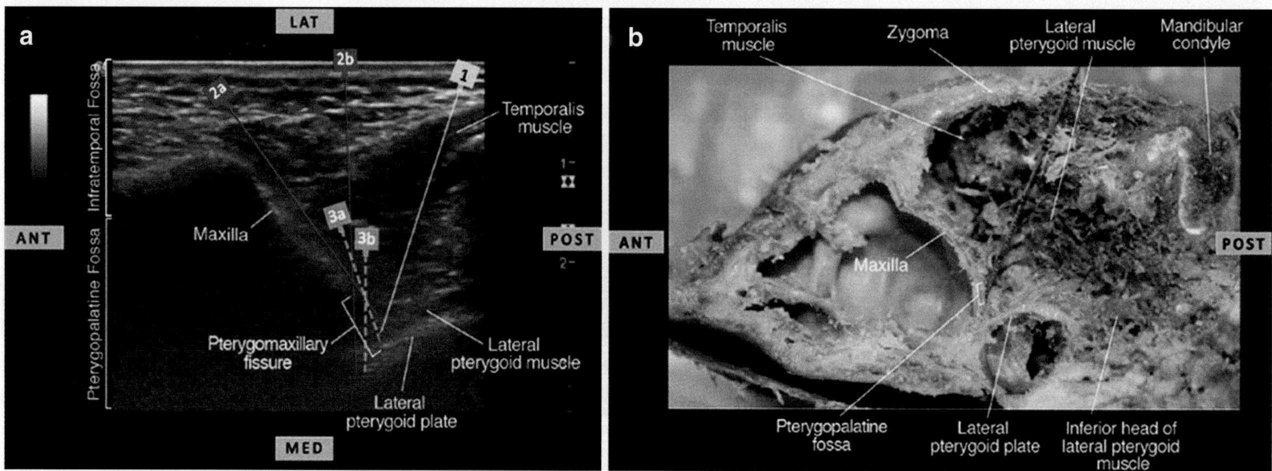

Fig. 9.2 (**a**) An ultrasound image comparing the three main approaches with anatomic landmarks. Yellow needle (1) is the posterior-to-anterior infrazygomatic approach, while the red needle (2) is the anterior infrazygomatic approach, with (2a) being the contact with the lateral pterygoid plate, followed by movement into the pterygopalatine fossa (2b). The blue needle represents the suprazygomatic approach, with (3a) representing the initial contact with the lateral pterygoid plate, followed by redirection towards the pterygopalatine fossa through the fissure (3b). (**b**) is an image of a cadaver skull with a needle demonstrating placement through the pterygoid muscle towards the pterygopalatine fossa. (Reproduced with permission from Nader et al.)

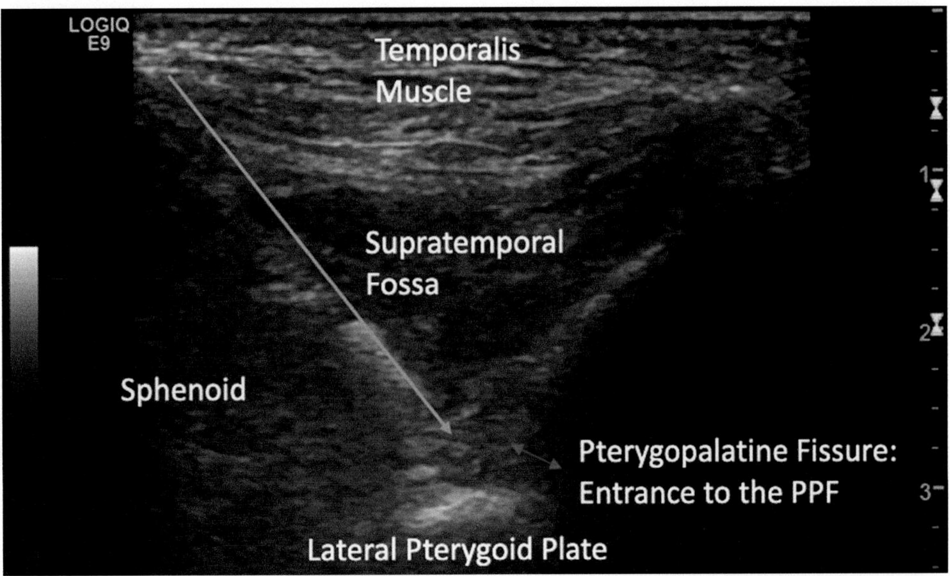

Fig. 9.3 Demonstrates a suprazygomatic approach to maxillary nerve block, with the needle (represented by the gray arrow) directed toward the pterygopalatine fissure, which is the entrance to the PPF. The maxillary nerve rests deep in the PPF

patient in order to tolerate the procedure. Furthermore, the procedure should be completed while monitoring the patient's heart rate, blood pressure, and pulse oximetry, as the procedure may induce an autonomic response of the trigeminal-vagal nerve reflex.

Practical Tips (How to Improve Success and Avoid Complications)

In order to improve the angle of insonation, the transducer probe can be placed closer (just anterior) to the mandibular condyle. Additionally, to avoid the acoustic shadow of the coronoid process, you can ask the subject to slightly open their mouth while directing the transducer probe in a slightly superior direction.

Literature Review

Trigeminal neuralgia is typically a neuropathic chronic pain syndrome that affects the maxillary branch (V2) of the trigeminal nerve. Patients typically describe a unilateral, electric shock-like, sensation that is often provoked by light touch. Medical therapy with antiepileptics drugs (such as carbamazepine) can be ineffective in up to 10% of patients. For refractory trigeminal neuralgia or atypical facial pain, workup by a neurologist to rule out brain tumors, multiple sclerosis, vascular anomalies, or other secondary causes of pain is important. Evidence suggests that vascular compression of the trigeminal nerve root is associated with symptoms in roughly 95% of patients, and microvascular decompression by a neurosurgeon may be helpful in relieving symptoms. While the exact pathophysiology of vascular compression of the trigeminal nerve leading to symptoms is unknown, the "ignition hypothesis" suggests that the neuropathic pain is due to abnormalities or injury of trigeminal afferent neurons in the trigeminal root that leaves the axons hyperexcitable and leads to synchronized electrical activity manifesting as pain.

The traditional approach to maxillary (V2) blockade of the trigeminal nerve was via a landmark approach by entering the PPF and advancing until paresthesia in the V2 distribution was felt by the patient. Alternative non-ultrasound approaches include using fluoroscopic guidance to target the LPP and redirecting off the bone, confirming that the spread of injectate did not spread intravascularly. This approach is limited by the use of bony landmarks that are often difficult to visualize and difficulty avoiding vascular structures. The use of ultrasound guidance for trigeminal nerve block includes better visualization of soft tissues, vasculature, needle placement, and direct observation of injectate spread. A review of the literature supporting each of the different block approaches is included below:

- Infrazygomatic Posterior-to-Anterior (In-Plane Approach)

  Literature supporting the infrazygomatic posterior-to-anterior approach stems largely from a prospective case series from Nader et al. in which 15 patients (14 of which had pain symptoms refractory to medical or surgical treatment) underwent a nerve block using the infrazygomatic posterior-to-anterior approach using 5 ml of 0.25% bupivacaine and steroid. All of the patients achieved complete sensory analgesia to pinprick sensation in the V2 distribution, while 80% achieved complete sensory analgesia in all three distributions of the trigeminal nerve within 15 min of the injection. Two-thirds of the patients reported good or excellent pain relief throughout the duration of the 3-month study. There were no reports of local anesthetic toxicity or new neurologic sequelae. Of the 15 patients, 14 required repeated injections, with three blocks as the median number of injections necessary to provide sustained relief.

- Infrazygomatic Anterior-to-Posterior (In-Plane Approach)

  This approach is intended for targeted maxillary nerve (V2) blockade. The maxillary nerve is a sensory branch of the trigeminal nerve that gives rise to multiple branches, including the palatine, zygomatic, nasopalatine, superior alveolar, and pharyngeal nerves. An alternative approach to a selective V2 nerve blockade via ultrasound includes an entry point within the oral cavity, which can make direct visualization of the block needle very difficult and is associated with serious complications, such as intravascular injection and infraorbital nerve injury. Some would argue that the using the anterior-to-posterior trajectory rather than the posterior-to-anterior approach previously described helps to avoid the needle pathway going through branches of the facial nerve and the parotid gland. Limitations of using this approach may include sparing of the infraorbital nerve, which in dye studies failed to be stained in 20% of cadavers.

- Suprazygomatic (Out-of-Plane Approach)

  The suprazygomatic out-of-plane approach has typically been described in pediatric patients undergoing cleft lip repair. A prospective randomized double-blind study of pediatric patients receiving bilateral suprazygomatic maxillary nerve block for cleft palate repair showed reduced total consumption of morphine at 48 h postoperatively. Furthermore, completing the block was considered easy by the anesthesiologist in 94% of cases with median time to completion at 56 s. This suggests that this allows good visualization of the pterygopalatine fossa and of the local spread. Ultrasound images obtained during this approach showed that 70% of the local anesthetic solution spread into the intermediate part of the pterygopalatine fossa. Additionally, because the maxillary artery is located in the anterior part of the pterygopalatine fossa while the needle trajectory has a more caudal inclination, vascular puncture risk is low.

Conclusion

The use of ultrasound-guided trigeminal nerve blocks provides a safe alternative for patients with trigeminal neuralgia or atypical facial pain who have failed surgical or medical management. This chapter aimed to identify three main techniques in order to achieve trigeminal nerve blockade using ultrasound visualization. Ultrasound use is relatively simple, free of radiation, and generally safe. The use of ultrasound imaging can assist with delineating surrounding bony structures, the PPF, and vascular structures, even though the identification of actual nerves is not possible. Therefore, understanding of anatomical landmarks under ultrasound is important for safe use in clinical practice.

Traditional Techniques

Block of the Main Trunk of Maxillary Nerve and Pterygopalatine Ganglion in the Pterygopalatine Fossa (PPF)

Functional Anatomy

The maxillary nerve emerges from the skull through the round foramen. It connects with the pterygopalatine (sphenopalatine) ganglion (PPG) in the pterygopalatine fossa (PPF) (see Chap. 8; Trigeminal Nerve Anatomy and Peripheral Branches Block, Figs. 8.4 and 8.5). The nerve and ganglion are responsible for sensory and autonomic supply to the central area of the face and head. The PPG, which lies in the PPF, is triangular in shape; extending to ca. 5 mm; it is the largest neuronal conglomerate outside of the brain. The ganglion has three types of nerve fibers and is connected to the trigeminal nerve via sensory fibers. It is linked to the facial nerve, internal carotid plexus, and superior cervical ganglion via sympathetic fibers; the motor fibers have parasympathetic (visceromotor) connections. There is also direct contact between the anterior horn of the spinal cord and the neurohumoral axis (adenohypophysis).

Indications

Diagnostic

1. Differential diagnosis of facial pain.

Therapeutic

1. Trigeminal neuralgia in the second branch, post-herpetic neuralgia.
2. Cluster headache, histamine headache, Sluder's neuralgia
3. Facial pain in the area of supply.
4. Pain in the eye region (iritis, keratitis, corneal ulcer), root of the nose, upper jaw and gums.
5. Postoperative pain in the area of the maxillary sinus and teeth.
6. Pain after dental extraction.

Neural Therapy

1. Allergic coryza.
2. Diseases of the oral mucosa.
3. Localized paresthesias.

Contraindications

Anticoagulant treatment (see Chap. 1), local infection and skin disease.

Procedure

These blocks should only be carried out only with appropriate experience. It is absolutely necessary to have a detailed discussion with the patient before the procedure.

Preparations and Materials

Check that the emergency equipment is complete and in working order. Sterile precautions.

Intravenous access. 22-G needle (4 cm) for the intraoral technique, 23-G needle (5–6 cm) for the extraoral technique. Disinfectant, spatula for the intraoral technique, compresses, cooling element available, emergency drugs.

Intraoral Technique

Patient Positioning and Landmarks

The patient should be sitting, leaning back slightly and with the head tilted back.

Posterior edge of the *upper seventh tooth (second maxillary molar)* (Fig. 9.4).

Technique

Using a 22-G needle (4 cm), the puncture is made medial to the posterior edge of the upper seventh tooth (second maxillary molar) through the greater palatine foramen. The needle is introduced at an angle of about 60°. The vicinity of the ganglion is reached at a depth of 3.5–4 cm. The greater palatine canal is about 3.4 cm long in adults. After careful aspiration at various levels, the local anesthetic is injected (Fig. 9.5).

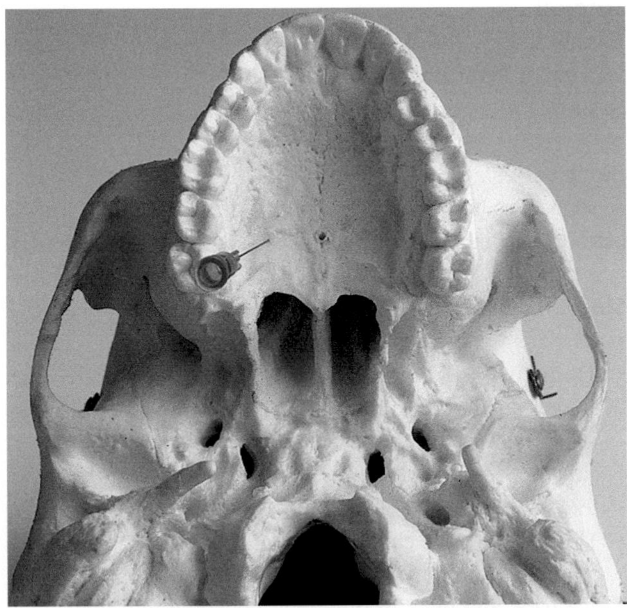

Fig. 9.4 Intraoral technique: orientation. (Reproduced with permission from Danilo Jankovic)

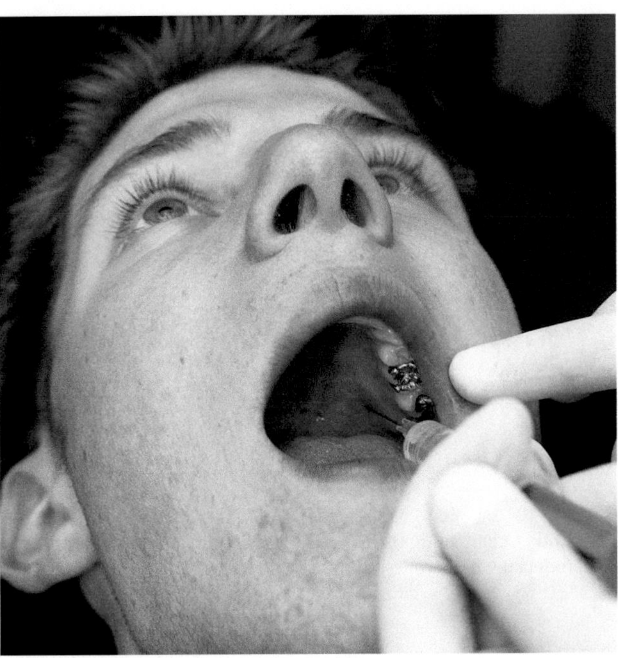

Fig. 9.5 Intraoral block of the pterygopalatine ganglion. (Reproduced with permission from Danilo Jankovic)

Dosage

1–2 ml local anesthetic—e.g., 0.75% ropivacaine, 0.5% bupivacaine (0.5% levobupivacaine).

Extraoral Technique

- Suprazygomatic Technique

  Injection above the zygomatic arch is more comfortable for the patient.

Patient Positioning and Landmarks

Sitting, with face to the side and with the mouth slightly opened. Alternative: supine.

Center of the upper margin of the zygomatic arch.

Technique

A skin injection is made directly above the middle of the zygomatic arch. A 23-G, 5–6 cm long needle is introduced at an angle of ca. 45° in the direction of the pterygopalatine fossa (*contralateral molar teeth*) (Fig. 9.6). After the weak paresthesias have been elicited in the area of the nostril, the upper lip, and the cheek, the needle is withdrawn slightly and aspirated carefully at various levels, and the local anesthetic is administered slowly in several small doses. Repeated aspiration at various levels must be carried out during this procedure.

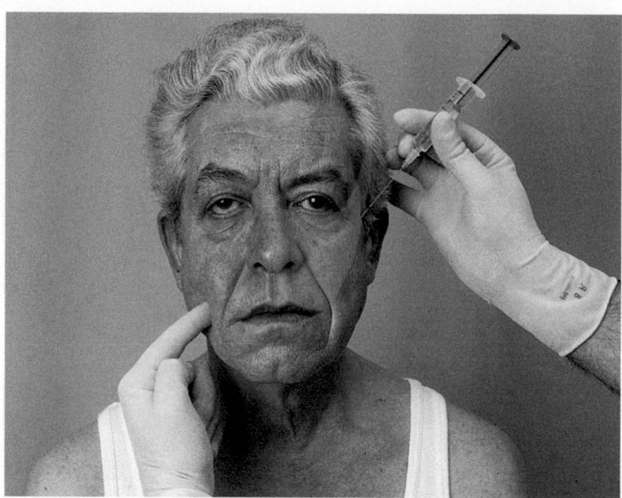

Fig. 9.6 Orientation for injections above the zygomatic arch. (Reproduced with permission from Danilo Jankovic)

Separate blocking of the maxillary nerve and pterygopalatine region is rarely possible with this method.

- Infrazygomatic Technique

Patient Positioning and Landmarks

Supine or sitting, face to the side with the mouth slightly open. *Mandibular fossa.*

Technique

The most important requirement for carrying out this block successfully is accurate location of the mandibular fossa between the condylar and coronoid processes of the mandible. It is helpful for the patient to open and close the mouth. After skin infiltration, a 23-G, 5–6 cm needle is introduced at an angle of 45° in the direction of the back of the eyeball (Fig. 9.7). After ca. 4–4.5 cm, the lateral part of the pterygoid process is reached and the needle is withdrawn slightly and lowered into the pterygopalatine fossa (about 0.5 cm medial to the pterygoid). After the weak paresthesias described above have been elicited and after careful aspiration at various levels, the local anesthetic is carefully injected in several small doses. If pain occurs in the region of the orbit, the procedure should be stopped.

The area supplied by the maxillary nerve is shown in Fig. 9.19.

Dosage

Diagnostic

3 ml local anesthetic—e.g., 0.5% prilocaine, mepivacaine, lidocaine.

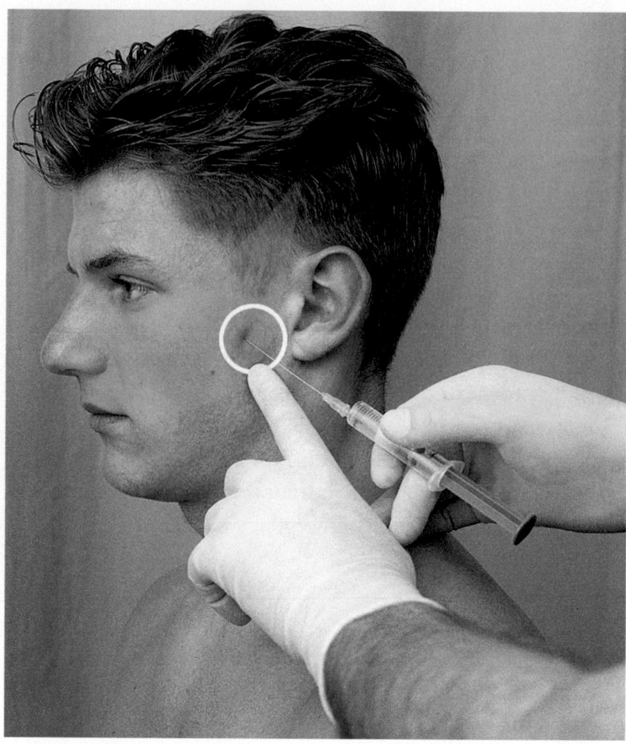

Fig. 9.7 Extraoral technique beneath the zygomatic arch (mandibular fossa). (Reproduced with permission from Danilo Jankovic)

Therapeutic

Extraorally: 3–5 ml local anesthetic—e.g., 0.2–0.5% ropivacaine, 0.25–0.5% bupivacaine (0.25–0.5% levobupivacaine). In acute conditions, with corticosteroids added.

Surgical

Extraorally: 5–7 ml local anesthetic—e.g., 0.5–0.75% ropivacaine, 0.5% bupivacaine (0.5% levobupivacaine), 1% prilocaine, 1% mepivacaine.

Block Series

A sequence of six to eight blocks is recommended for the extraoral technique.

Side Effects

- Transient visual weakness (extremely rare).
- Horner's syndrome, extremely rare and usually with higher doses. There are connections with the superior cervical ganglion via the pterygoid canal, deep petrosal nerve, and greater superficial petrosal nerve (see Chap. 12, Superior Cervical Ganglion Block).
- Hematoma in the cheek or orbital cavity due to blood vessel puncture. Immediate outpatient treatment: alternating ice pack and heparin ointment, depending on the spread

of the hematoma, for ca. 1 h. This can be continued at home, with the patient also taking coated Reparil® tablets (sodium aescinate) if appropriate. Resorption of the hematoma, which is harmless but visually uncomfortable for the patient, occurs within 2 weeks at the most.

Complications

- Intravascular injection (maxillary artery and maxillary vein) (See Chap. 8, Figs. 8.4 and 8.5); Chaps. 1 and 5 (Local Anesthetic Systemic Toxicity)
- Epidural or subarachnoid injection

Both of these complications are extremely rare. Immediate treatment: (See Chap. 41, Neuraxial Blocks: Spinal and Epidural Anesthesia; Complications, p. 604.)

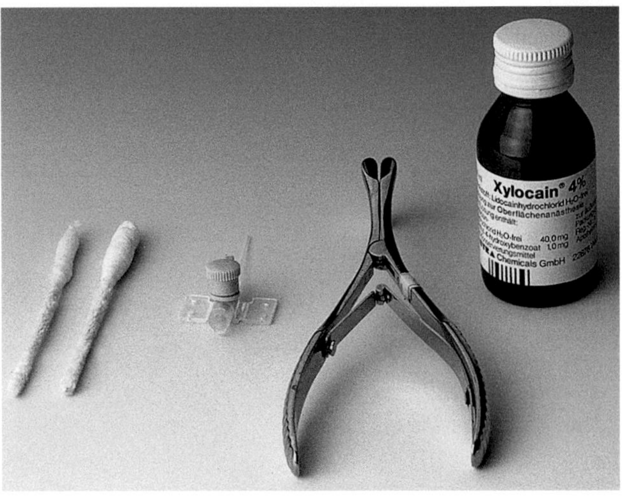

Fig. 9.8 Materials. (Reproduced with permission from Danilo Jankovic)

Nasal Block of the Pterygopalatine Ganglion

Indications

Greenfield Sluder drew attention to the significance of this ganglion as long ago as 1903. In 1918, he described a number of symptoms capable of being treated by injection or topical application of a local anesthetic or cocaine, with the associated anesthesia of the pterygopalatine ganglion: headache; pain in the eyes, mouth, or ears; lumbosacral pain, arthritis, glaucoma, and hypertension. Similar observations were reported by Ruskin, Byrd and Amster. More recent studies have shown that nasal local anesthesia of the ganglion can be used with good success rates in the treatment of:

1. Acute migraine.
2. Acute or chronic cluster headache.
3. Various types of facial neuralgia.
4. Tumor pain in the nasal and pharyngeal area.
5. Post-dural puncture headaches.

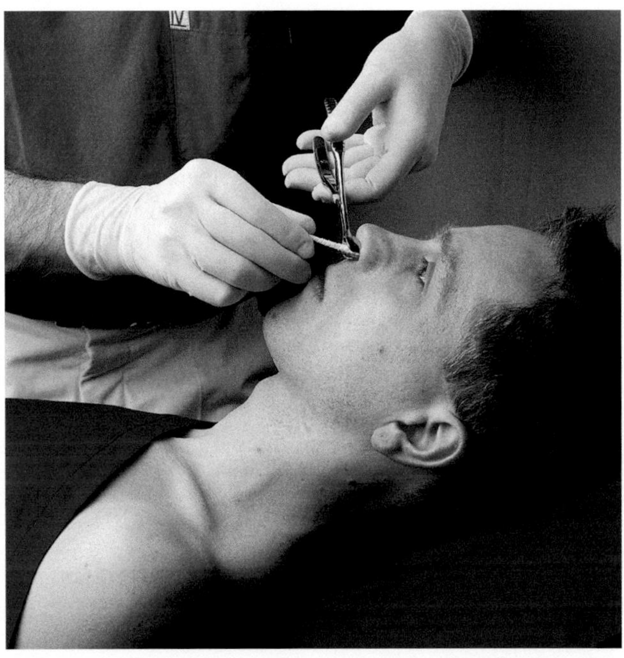

Fig. 9.9 Nasal application. (Reproduced with permission from Danilo Jankovic)

Procedure

Materials (Fig. 9.8)

2 ml syringe, plastic part of a plastic indwelling catheter (for self-administration in tumor pain), nasal speculum, applicators (cotton buds).

Patient Positioning

Supine or sitting, with head tilted back.

Application

An applicator, preferably a cotton bud, soaked in local anesthetic—e.g., 2% lidocaine gel or a 4% aqueous lidocaine solution—is carefully advanced along the inferior nasal concha as far as the posterior wall of the nasopharynx (Fig. 9.9) and left in place for 20–30 min (Fig. 9.10). In patients with cancer pain, the plastic part of a plastic indwelling catheter can be advanced as far as possible into the nasal cavity, and the local anesthetic—e.g., 0.5% bupivacaine—can be instilled with a 2 ml syringe. The block can be carried out bilaterally.

To prevent trauma, the applicator should not be advanced forcefully if resistance is encountered.

Dosage

- Local anesthetics: 2% lidocaine gel, 1.5–2 ml 4% lidocaine (aqueous solution) or 1.5–2 ml 0.5% bupivacaine (0.5% ropivacaine). Disadvantage: the onset of effect is slightly slower.

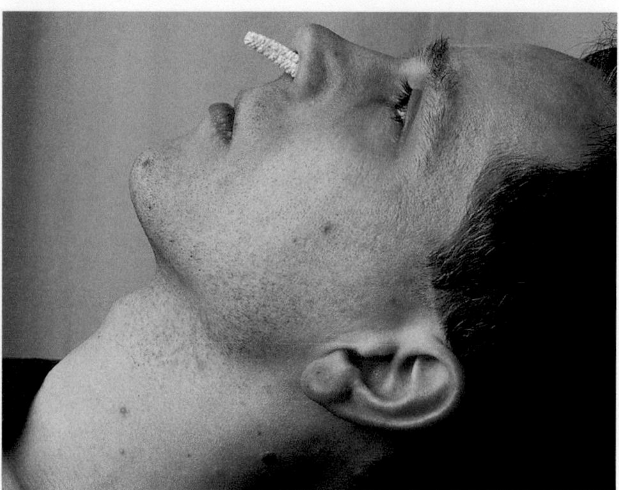

Fig. 9.10 The anesthetic should be allowed 20–30 min to take effect. (Reproduced with permission from Danilo Jankovic)

- 10% cocaine: at a dosage of 0.2–0.4 ml, there is no reason to fear adverse CNS effects. Advantage: very fast onset of effect.

If the recommended doses are used, there is no difference between these substances with regard to effectiveness and resorption.

Block Series

In acute pain, one or two applications are recommended. In chronic conditions, one to three applications can be given over a period of up to 3 weeks. In cancer pain, applications may be indicated three times per day over a longer period.

Side Effects

The method is not very invasive and has minimal side effects. Effects that may occur include: a sense of pressure in the nose, sneezing, short-term lacrimation due to irritation of branches of the lacrimal gland, a bitter taste, and slight numbness in the oral and pharyngeal cavity.

Complications

Very occasionally, toxic effects may occur as a result of absorption of the local anesthetic into very well-vascularized tumor tissue. In long-term treatments, erosions may sometimes lead to spinal absorption of the local anesthetic. To prevent this, periodic rinsing with a physiological saline solution can be carried out.

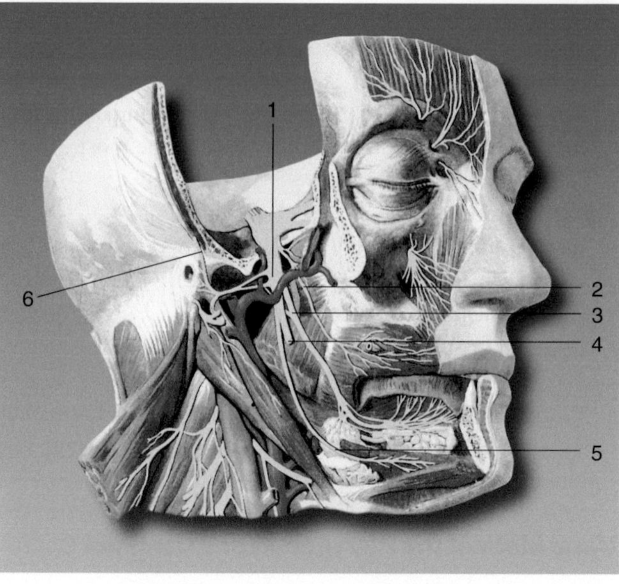

Fig. 9.11 Distribution areas of: (*1*) mandibular nerve; (*2*) buccal nerve; (*3*) lingual nerve; (*4*) inferior alveolar nerve; (*5*) mental nerve; (*6*) auriculotemporal nerve. (Reproduced with permission from Danilo Jankovic)

Block of the Mandibular Nerve and Otic Ganglion in the Infratemporal Fossa

Functional Anatomy

After passing through the oval foramen, the mandibular nerve forms a short, thick nerve trunk, with the otic ganglion lying on the medial side of it. Its most important branches are the buccal nerve, lingual nerve, inferior alveolar nerve, mental nerve, and auriculotemporal nerve (Fig. 9.11). See also Chap. 8; Trigeminal Nerve Anatomy and Peripheral Branches Block.

Indications

Diagnostic

1. Differential diagnosis of trigeminal neuralgia (anterior two-thirds of the tongue) and glossopharyngeal neuralgia (posterior third of the tongue).

Therapeutic

1. Tinnitus (the otic ganglion has connections with the chorda tympani, the nerves of the pterygoid canal, and the medial pterygoid nerve).
2. Trigeminal neuralgia in the third branch.
3. Trismus after dental extraction.

4. Dental surgery and maxillary surgery (higher dosages required).
5. Temporomandibular joint dysfunction syndrome (in collaboration with an orthodontist), if infiltration of the trigger points of the temporalis muscle, lateral pterygoid muscle and masseter muscle is unsuccessful.

Contraindications

Anticoagulant treatment (see Chap. 1), local infection, and skin disease in area of injection.

Procedure

This block should only be carried out only with appropriate experience. It is absolutely necessary to have a detailed discussion with the patient before the procedure.

Preparation and Materials

Check that the emergency equipment is complete and in working order. Sterile precautions.

Intravenous access. 23-G needle (5–6 cm), compresses, cooling element available, emergency drugs.

Patient Positioning and Landmarks

Supine, with face to the side. *Mandibular fossa, zygomatic arch, tragus* (the needle insertion point lies ca. 2 cm laterally (Fig. 9.12).

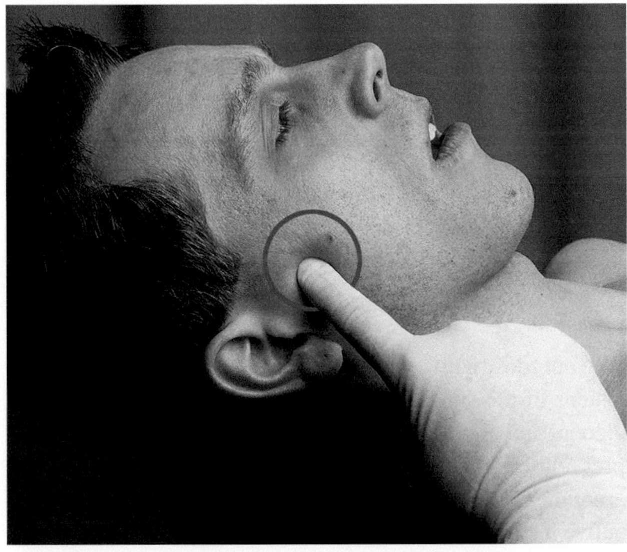

Fig. 9.12 The most important requirement is that the mandibular fossa should be identified precisely. It lies between the condylar process and the coronoid process of the mandible and is easiest to localize when the patient opens and closes his or her mouth. (Reproduced with permission from Danilo Jankovic)

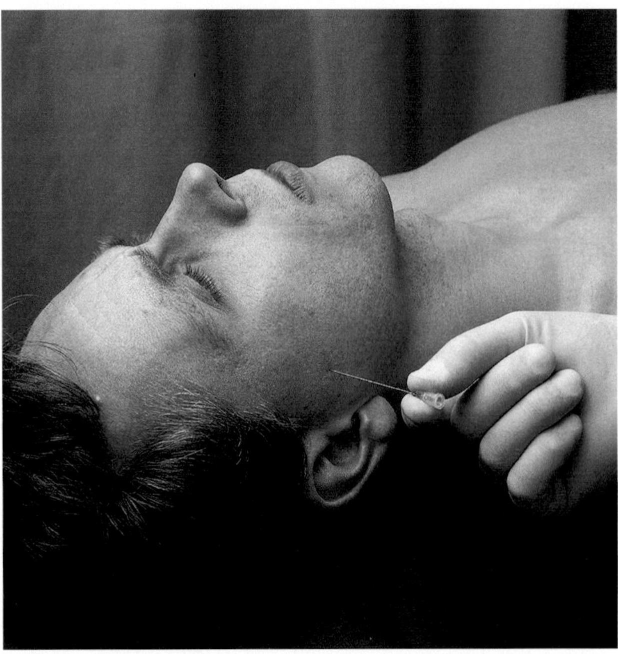

Fig. 9.13 Needle insertion technique: the needle is directed at an angle of 90°. (Reproduced with permission from Danilo Jankovic)

Technique (Fig. 9.13)

Paresthesias in the lower jaw region, lower lip and lower incisors occur when the needle reaches a depth of ca. 4–4.5 cm. After paresthesias have clearly developed, the needle is withdrawn slightly, aspirated carefully at various levels and the local anesthetic is slowly injected in several small doses. Aspiration should be repeated several times at different levels as this is done. There is a delayed onset of the desired effect in the area of the auriculotemporal nerve.

Practical Tips

If contact is made with the pterygoid process when the needle is being introduced, withdraw the needle 0.5–1 cm and redirect dorsally.

Distribution of the Block

The area supplied by the mandibular nerve is shown in Fig. 9.21. The otic ganglion which lies directly under the oval foramen, is always anesthetized along with the nerve. (See Chap. 8, Trigeminal Nerve Anatomy and Peripheral Branches Block, Fig. 8.6),

Dosage

Diagnostic

3 ml local anesthetic—e.g., 5% prilocaine, mepivacaine, lidocaine.

Therapeutic

3–5 ml local anesthetic—e.g., 0.5% ropivacaine, 0.25% bupivacaine (0.25% levobupivacaine). In acute conditions, with corticosteroids added.

Surgical

5–7 ml local anesthetic—e.g., 0.75% ropivacaine, 0.5 bupivacaine (0.5% levobupivacaine), 1% prilocaine, 1% mepivacaine, 1% lidocaine.

Block Series

A series of six to eight blocks is recommended. When there is evidence of symptomatic improvement, further blocks can also be carried out.

Side Effects

- Transient facial paralysis caused by injecting too superficially.
- Hematoma in the cheek due to vascular puncture. These harmless hematomas can take up to 2 weeks to resolve. Immediate treatment: see the section on blocks of the maxillary nerve and pterygopalatine ganglion.

Complications

- Intravascular injection (middle meningeal artery and maxillary artery) (see Chap. 8; Figs. 8.4 and 8.5; Chaps. 1 and 5 Local Anesthetic Systemic Toxicity)
- Epidural or subarachnoid injection. Immediate treatment: see Chap. 41 Neuraxial Blocks: Spinal and Epidural Anesthesia; Complications, p. 604.

Gasserian Ganglion Block (Fluoroscopic or CT-Guided)

Functional Anatomy

The trigeminal ganglion (semilunar ganglion, Gasserian ganglion) lies on the dorsal surface of the petrous bone. The intracranial Gasserian ganglion lies medially in the middle cranial fossa, lateral to the cavernous sinus, internal carotid artery and cranial nerves III–VI, and posterior and superior to the oval foramen, through which the mandibular nerve exits from the intracranial cavity Fig. 9.14; See also Chap. 8, Figs. 8.1 and 8.2). All of these structures can be injured when the ganglion is blocked. The average size of the ganglion is ca. 1–2 cm. Part of the ganglion (the posterior two-thirds) is located within the trigeminal cave (Meckel cavity), a duplication of the dura that encloses the ganglion. The oval foramen is a channel ca. 5 mm long and its largest diameter is ca. 8 mm.

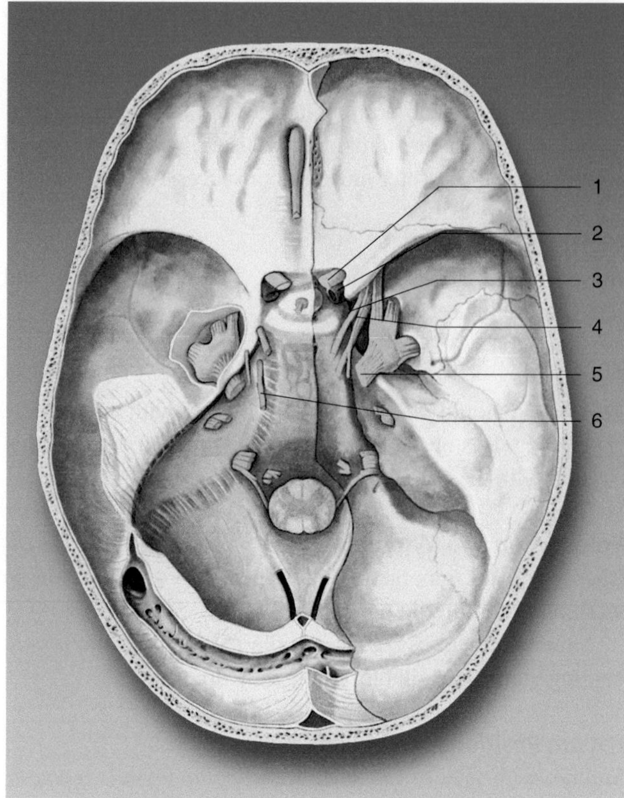

Fig. 9.14 The trigeminal ganglion and the neighboring cranial nerves and internal carotid artery. (*1*) Optic nerve, (*2*) internal carotid artery, (*3*) oculomotor nerve, (*4*) trochlear nerve, (*5*) trigeminal nerve, (*6*) abducent nerve. (Reproduced with permission from Danilo Jankovic)

Indications

1. Local Anesthetics.
   Diagnostic, before neurodestructive procedures.
2. Neurodestructive Procedures.

Neurodestructive methods—particularly radiofrequency lesions of the ganglion, and more rarely glycerol rhizolysis, alcohol injection, corticosteroid injection, or balloon compression of the ganglion—are used in pain conditions that are unbearable and cannot be influenced using other conservative measures:

1. Cancer pain.
2. Trigeminal neuralgia.
3. Cluster headache.

4. Intractable pain in the eye region.
5. Postherpetic neuralgia.

Contraindications

Local infection, sepsis, hemorrhagic diathesis, anticoagulation treatment (see Chap. 1) significantly increased intracranial pressure.

Procedure

This block should only be carried out by highly experienced specialists. A very good knowledge of anatomy, manual skill, radiographic guidance when conducting the procedure, and strictly aseptic conditions are required. It is necessary to have a detailed discussion with the patient before the procedure.

Premedication

This method is painful, and preoperative administration of 0.05 mg fentanyl is therefore recommended.

Preparations

The completeness and functioning of the emergency equipment should be checked. Sterile precautions. Intravenous access, ECG monitoring, ventilation facilities, pulse oximetry.

Materials

Sterile precautions. A fine 22-G spinal needle 8 cm long, 2-ml and 5-ml syringes,

disinfectant, sterile compresses, emergency medication, intubation kit, and cooling element should be ready to hand.

Patient Positioning

Supine; the head is raised with a cushion.

Landmarks (Figs. 9.15a, b)

- Medial edge of the masseter muscle, ca. 3 cm lateral from the angle of the mouth at the level of the second molar tooth.
- Ipsilateral pupil.
- Center of the zygomatic arch and articular tubercle (external acoustic meatus).

Procedure

The following should be noted during puncture:

- The operator should stand on the side on which the block is being carried out.
- Fluoroscopic (or CT) guidance for the puncture is indispensable.
- An intraoral location should be excluded after introduction of the needle (risk of contamination).

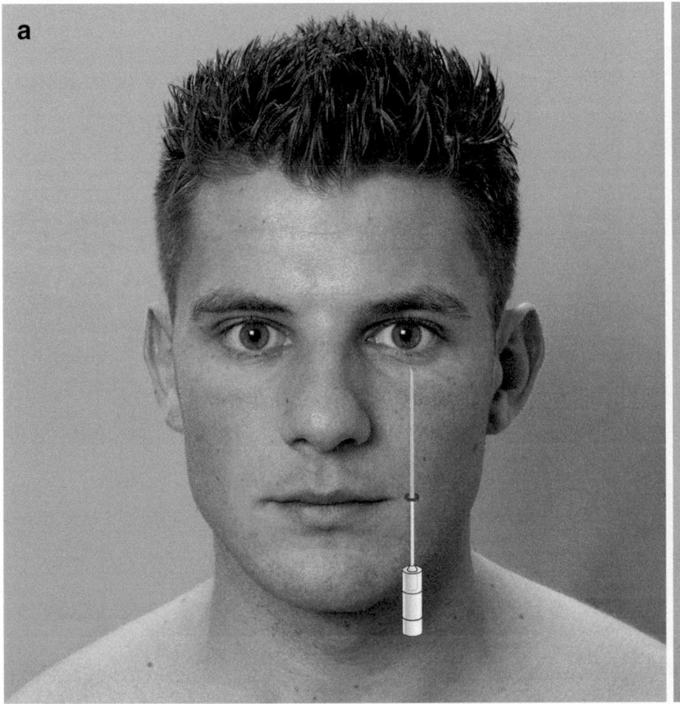

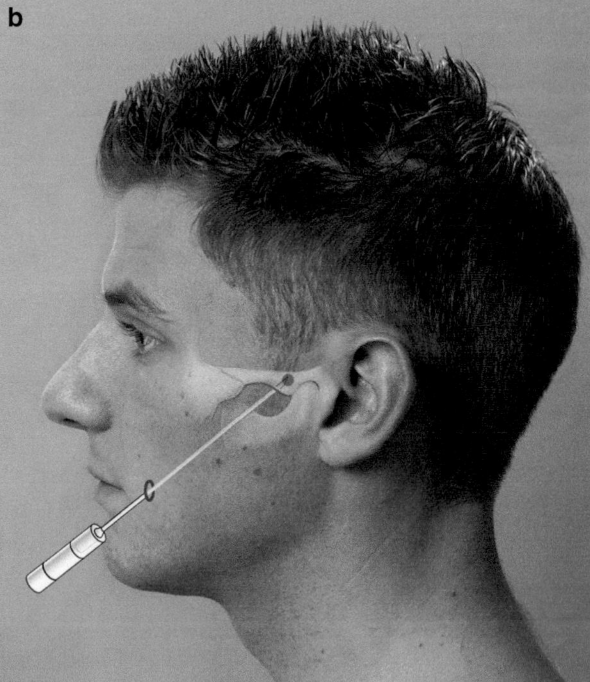

Fig. 9.15 (**a**, **b**) Landmarks: medial edge of the masseter muscle, ipsilateral pupil, center of the zygomatic arch. (Reproduced with permission from Danilo Jankovic)

- There is a risk of perforating the dural cuff (subarachnoid injection).
- Frequent aspiration and fractionated injection of the smallest possible fractions (blood, CSF?).

Technique

Local anesthesia at the needle insertion site is carried out ca. 3 cm from the angle of the mouth (medial edge of the masseter muscle). The patient is asked to gaze straight ahead and focus on a marked point on the wall. The needle should be directed toward the forward-gazing pupil when seen from the front and toward the articular tubercle of the zygomatic arch or external acoustic meatus when viewed from the side (Fig. 9.15a, b).

The needle is then introduced at the level of the second molar tooth, through the previous skin injection in the direction indicated. An intraoral location of the needle must be excluded (risk of contamination). After 4.5–6 cm, bone contact should be made (infratemporal surface of the large wing of the sphenoid bone, directly in front of the upper boundary of the oval foramen; (Fig. 9.16)). The needle is now withdrawn slightly, and the path to the oval foramen ca. 1–1.5 cm away from the first bone contact is probed millimeter by millimeter by advancing and withdrawing the needle. If the tip of the needle is located in the oval foramen, the patient will report pain and paresthesias in the area of distribution of the mandibular nerve (mandible). The needle is now slowly advanced for a further 0.5–1 cm. A small test dose of 0.1–0.2 ml local anesthetic is carefully administered. The remaining dose of 1–1.5 ml is injected in small fractions with constant aspiration. Particular attention should be given to possible subarachnoid or intravascular positioning of the needle. The sensory distribution of the block is shown in Fig. 9.17.

Dosage

1–2 ml local anesthetic—e.g., 1% lidocaine, 0.5–0.75% ropivacaine, or 0.5% bupivacaine.

Complications

1. Subarachnoid injection (total spinal anesthesia)
   Immediate measures: See Chap. 41, Neuraxial Blocks: Spinal and Epidural Anesthesia; Complications, p. 604.
   Important prophylactic measures:
   - Very good knowledge of anatomy
   - Precise execution of the procedure (radiographic guidance)
   - Careful dosage

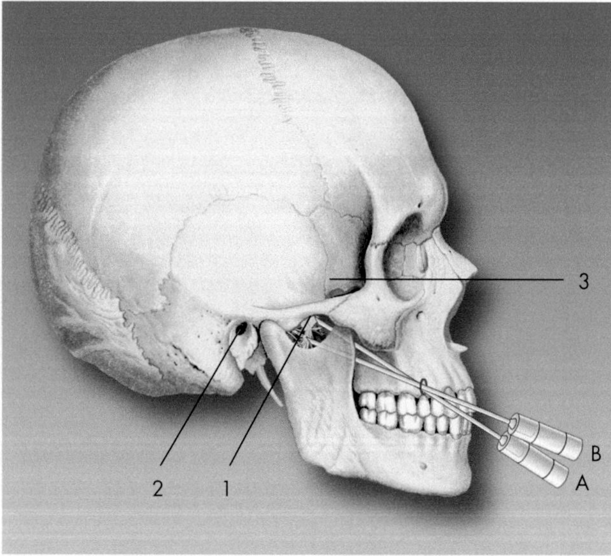

Fig. 9.16 Injection point (level of the second molar tooth). Needle position *A*: bone contact—infratemporal. Needle position *B*: entrance into the oval foramen. (*1*) Zygomatic arch, (*2*) external acoustic pore, (*3*) temporal fossa. (Reproduced with permission from Danilo Jankovic)

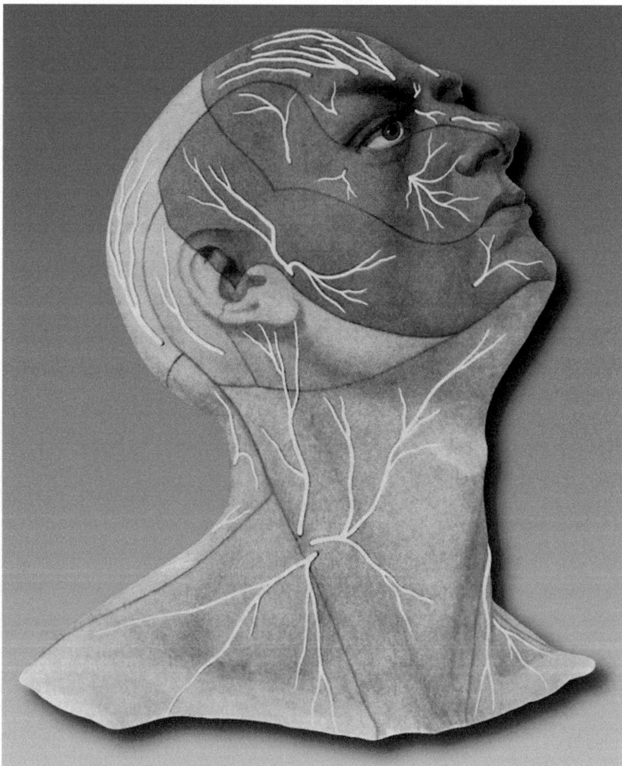

Fig. 9.17 Sensory deficit after blocking of the trigeminal ganglion. (Reproduced with permission from Danilo Jankovic)

- Constant aspiration and injection in the tiniest fractions of 0.1 ml local anesthetic (several test doses)
- No time pressure

2. Intravascular injection.
   Intravascular injection (middle meningeal artery) is always possible (in this highly vascularized region).
3. Hematoma in the cheek or orbit due to vascular puncture.
4. Transient visual weakness or blindness.
   Optic nerve; extremely rare.

Trigeminal Nerve: Comparison of Analgesia Zones

Figures 9.17, 9.18, 9.19, 9.20, 9.21, and 9.22 provide schematic illustrations of the areas supplied by the individual nerves. During blocks, the anesthetic spread may overlap.

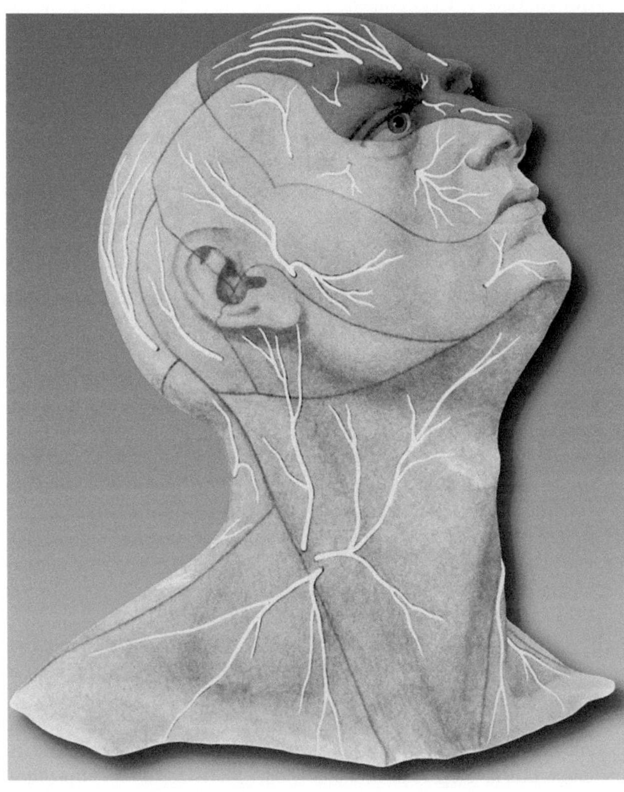

Fig. 9.18 Ophthalmic nerve. (Reproduced with permission from Danilo Jankovic)

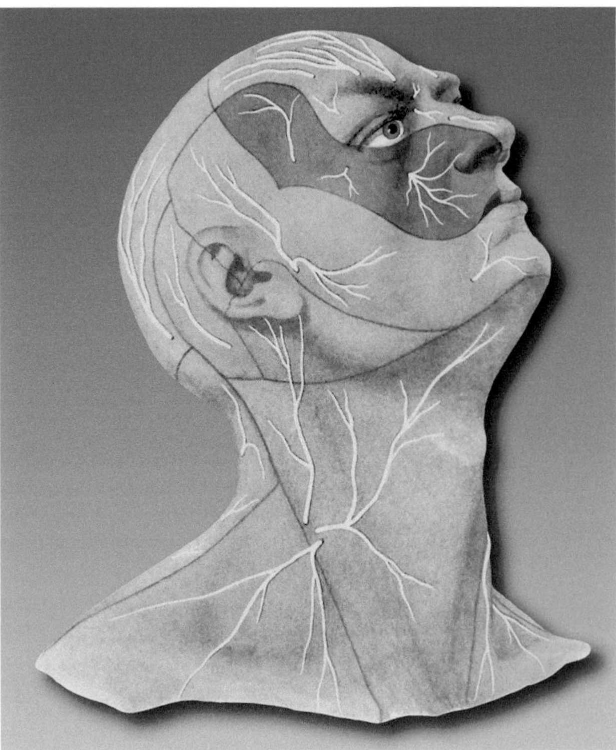

Fig. 9.19 Maxillary nerve. (Reproduced with permission from Danilo Jankovic)

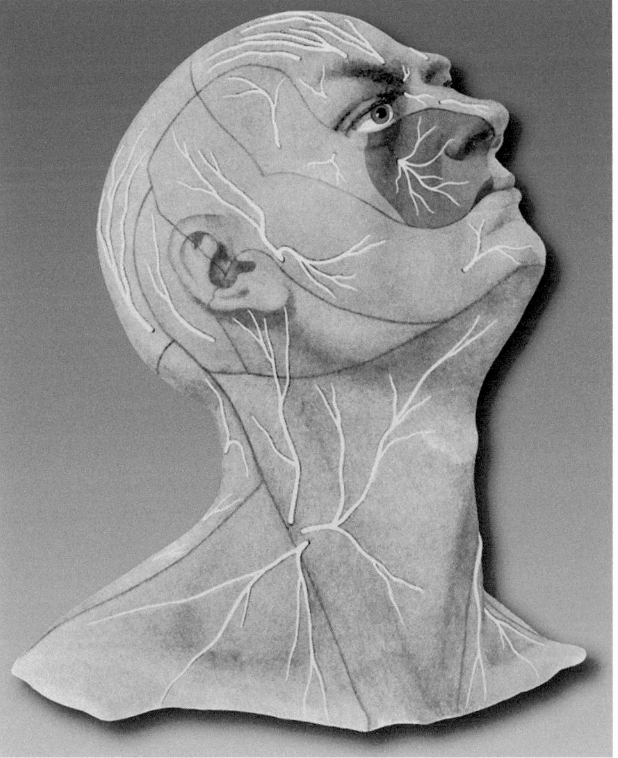

Fig. 9.20 Infraorbital nerve. (Reproduced with permission from Danilo Jankovic)

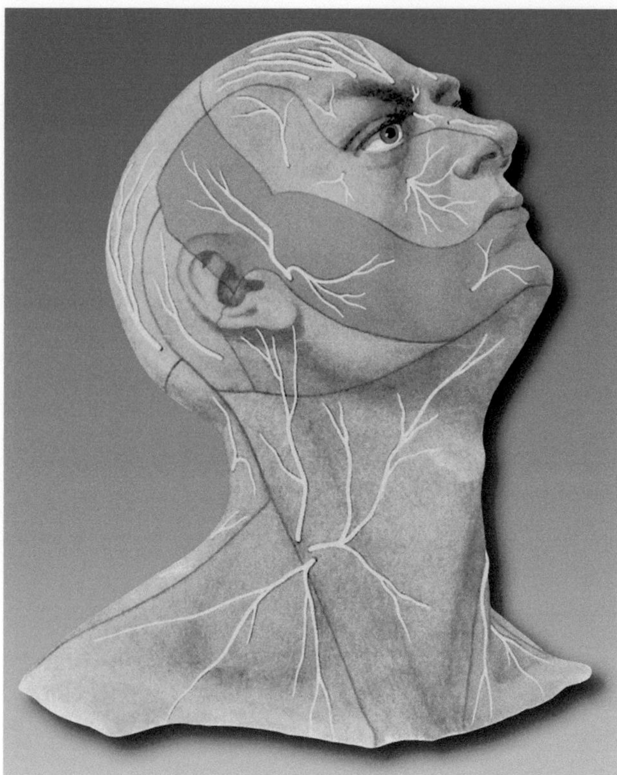

Fig. 9.21 Mandibular nerve. (Reproduced with permission from Danilo Jankovic)

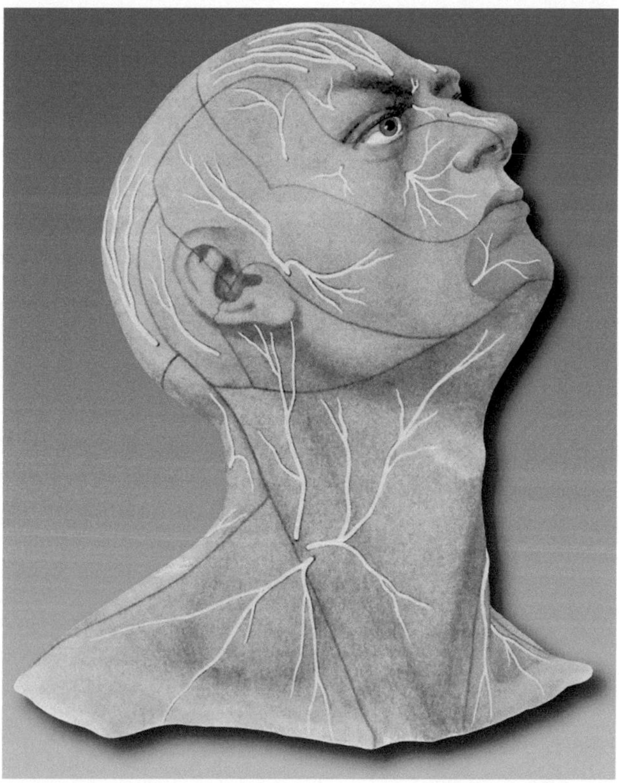

Fig. 9.22 Mental nerve. (Reproduced with permission from Danilo Jankovic)

Suggested Reading

Amster LJ. Sphenopalatine ganglion block for the relief of painful vascular and muscular spasm with special reference to lumbosacral pain. NY State J Med. 1948;48:2475–80.

Anderson JE. The cranial nerves. Trigeminal nerve distribution of the trigeminal nerve. Section 8. In Grant's atlas of anatomy. 7th ed. Wiliams & Wilkins; 1978.

Anugerah A, Nguyen K, Nader A. Technical considerations for approaches to the ultrasound-guided maxillary nerve block via the pterygopalatine fossa: a literature review. Reg Anesth Pain Med. 2020;45(4):301–5.

Auberger HG, Niesel HC. Gesichtsschädel: Proximale Leitungsanästhesie im Bereich des N. trigeminus. In: HG Auberger, HC Niesel (Hrsg) Praktische Lokalanästhesie (4. Auflage) Georg Thieme Verlag, Stuttgart; 1982.

Berger JJ, Pyles ST, Saga-Rumley SA. Does topical anesthesia of the sphenopalatine ganglion with cocaine or lidocaine relieve low back pain? Anesth Analg. 1986;65:700–2.

Bonica JJ. Block of cranial nerves. In: Bonica JJ, editor. The management of pain. 2nd ed. Philadelphia: Lea & Febiger; 1990.

Bovim G, Sand T. Cervicogenic headache, migraine without aura and tension-type headache. Diagnostic blockade of greater occipital and supra-orbital nerves. Pain. 1992;51(1):43–8.

Brown DL. Atlas of regional anesthesia. Trigeminal block. 3rd ed. Amsterdam: Elsevier; 2006. p. 159–79.

Byrd H, Byrd W. Sphenopalatine phenomena: present status of knowledge. Arch Intern Med. 1930;46:1026–38.

Cohen S, Levin D, Mellender S, et al. Topical sphenopalatine ganglion block compared with epidural blood patch for postdural puncture headache management in postpartum patients: a retrospective review. Reg Anesth Pain Med. 2018;43:880–4.

Devogel JC. Cluster headache and sphenopalatine block. Acta Anesth Belg. 1981;32:101–7.

Devor M, Amir R, Rappaport ZH. Pathophysiology of trigeminal neuralgia: the ignition hypothesis. Clin J Pain. 2002;18(1):4–13.

Jenkner FL. Nervenblockaden auf pharmakologischem und auf elektrischem Weg. Wien: Springer; 1980.

Jespersen MS, Jager P, Ægidius KL, et al. Sphenopalatine ganglion block for the treatment of postdural puncture headache: a randomized, blinded, clinical trial. Br J Anesth. 2020;124:739–47.

Kampitak W, Tansatit T, Shibata Y. A cadaveric study of ultrasound-guided maxillary nerve block via the pterygopalatine fossa: a novel technique using the lateral pterygoid plate approach. Reg Anesth Pain Med. 2018;43(6):625–30.

Lebovits AH, Alfred H, Lefkowitz M. Sphenopalatine ganglion block: clinical use in the pain management clinic. Clin J Pain. 1990;6:131–6.

Levin D, Cohen S. Images in anesthesiology: three safe, simple and inexpensive methods to administer the sphenopalatine ganglion block. Reg Anesth Pain Med. 2020;45:880–2. https://doi.org/10.1136/rapm-2020-101765.

Levin D, Cohen S, Kiss G, et al. Reply to DR Araujo, et al. Reg Anesth Pain Med. 2019.

Moore DC. Regional block. 4th ed. Springfield: Charles Thomas; 1976.

Moore KL, Dalley AMR, Agur AMR. Moore clinically oriented anatomy. 7th ed. Philadelphia: Wolters Kluwer Health, Lippincott Williams & Wilkins; 2014. p. 951–4.

Murphy TM. Somatic blockade of head and neck. In: Cousins MJ, Bridenbaugh PO, editors. Neural blockade. 2nd ed. Philadelphia: Lippincott; 1988.

Nader A, Schittek H, Kendall MC. Lateral pterygoid muscle and maxillary artery are key anatomical landmarks for ultrasound-guided trigeminal nerve block. Anesthesiology. 2013;118(4):957.

Nader A, Kendall MC, Vanderby B, Rosenow JM, Bendok BR. Ultrasound-guided trigeminal nerve block via the pterygopalatine fossa: an effective treatment for trigeminal neuralgia and atypical facial pain. Pain Phys. 2013;16:E537.

Netter FH. Nervous system, part I. Anatomy and physiology. Cranial nerves, sectionV. Trigeminal nerve (V). The Ciba collection of medical illustrations. 1991:100–2.

Petren T. Anatomie des Nervus trigeminus. In: Eriksson E (Hrsg.) Atlas der Lokalanästhesie (2. Auflage). Springer, Berlin; 1980.

Prasanna A, Murthy PSN. Sphenopalatine ganglion block and pain of cancer. J Pain. 1993;8(3):125.

Reder M, Hymanson AS, Reder M. Sphenopalatine ganglion block in treatment of acute and chronic pain. In: Hendle NH, Long DM, Wise TN, editors. Diagnosis and treatment of chronic pain. Boston: John Wright; 1982.

Robbins MS, Robertson CE, Kaplan E, et al. The sphenopalatine ganglion: anatomy, pathophysiology, and therapeutic targeting in headache. Headache. 2016;56:240–58.

Rosen S, Shelesnyak MC, Zacharias LR. Naso-genital relationship II. Pseudopregnancy following extirpation of sphenopalatine ganglion in rat. Endocrinology. 1940;27:463–8.

Ruskin SL. The neurologic aspects of nasal sinus infections. Headaches and systemic disturbances of nasal ganglion origin. Arch Otolaryngol. 1929;4(10):337–82.

Ruskin AP. Sphenopalatine (nasal) ganglion: remote effects including psychosomatic symptoms, rage reaction, pain and spasm. Arch Phys Med Rehabil. 1979;60:353–8.

Saade E, Paige GB. Patient administrated sphenopalatine ganglion block. Reg Anesthesia. 1996;21(1):68–70.

Sato J, Saitoh T, Notani K, Fukuda H, Kaneyama K, Segami N. Diagnostic significance of carbamazepine and trigger zones in trigeminal neuralgia. Oral Surg Oral Med Oral Pathol Oral Radiol Endodontol. 2004;97(1):18–22.

Sluder G. Injection of the nasal ganglion and comparison of methods. In: Nasal neurology, headaches and eye disorders. St. Louis: CV Mosby; 1918.

Sola C, Raux O, Savath L, Macq C, Capdevila X, Dadure C. Ultrasound guidance characteristics and efficiency of suprazygomatic maxillary nerve blocks in infants: a descriptive prospective study. Pediatr Anesth. 2012;22(9):841–6.

Tashi S, Purohit BS, Becker M, Mundana P. The pterygopalatine fossa: imaging anatomy, communications, and pathology revisited. Insights Imaging. 2016;7(4):589–99.

Thiel W. Photograpischer Atlas der Praktischen Anatomie. 5132. Ausgabe. Springer; 2003. p. 492–513.

Tsui BC. Ultrasound imaging to localize foramina for superficial trigeminal nerve block. Can J Anesth. 2009;56:704–6.

Waldman SD. Sphenopalatine ganglion block – 80 years later. Reg Anesthesia. 1990;18:274–6.

Zacharias LR. Further studies in naso-genital relationship: anatomical studies of perihypophyseal region in rat. J Comp Neurol. 1941;74:421–45.

Zakrzewska JM, Coakham HB. Microvascular decompression for trigeminal neuralgia: update. Curr Opin Neurol. 2012;25(3):296–301.

Zakrzewska JM, Linskey ME. Trigeminal neuralgia. BMJ [Internet] 2014 [cited 2020 Oct 13];348. http://www.jstor.org/stable/26513978.

Trigeminal and Sphenopalatine Procedures

10

Andre Marques Mansano and Agnes R. Stogicza

Contents

Trigeminal Procedures

General Considerations

Trigeminal neuralgia, characterized by episodes of paroxysmal shock-like facial pain, is considered to be one of the worst types of pain. Hence, it is also known as the "suicide disease." The prevalence varies from 0.03 to 0.3%, occurring more frequently in women and patients over 50–60 years old. Inconsistent data on risk factors include multiple sclerosis, systemic arterial hypertension, diabetes mellitus, and even the presence of migraine.

A. M. Mansano (✉)
Department of Interventional Pain Management, Hospital Israelita Albert Einstein, São Paulo, Brazil

A. R. Stogicza
Anesthesia and Pain Medicine, St Magdolna Private Hospital, Budapest, Hungary

Indication for Trigeminal Nerve Intervention

- Refractory trigeminal neuralgia.
- Refractory facial pain.

Functional Anatomy

The trigeminal ganglion lies in the Meckel's cave, a dural recess extending from the posterior fossa into the posteromedial portion of the middle cranial fossa.

The intracranial Gasserian ganglion lies medially in the middle cranial fossa; lateral to the cavernous sinus, internal carotid artery, and cranial nerves III–VI; and posterior and superior to the oval foramen.

The ganglion gives off three branches: the ophthalmic (V1), maxillary (V2), and mandibular (V3) nerve which exit, respectively, through the superior orbital fissure, foramen rotundum, and foramen ovale (Fig. 10.1). The two medial branches (V1 and V2) are sensory, whereas the most lateral branch (V3) also innervates the masticatory and tympanic muscles.

D. Jankovic, P. Peng (eds.), *Regional Nerve Blocks in Anesthesia and Pain Therapy*,
https://doi.org/10.1007/978-3-030-88727-8_10

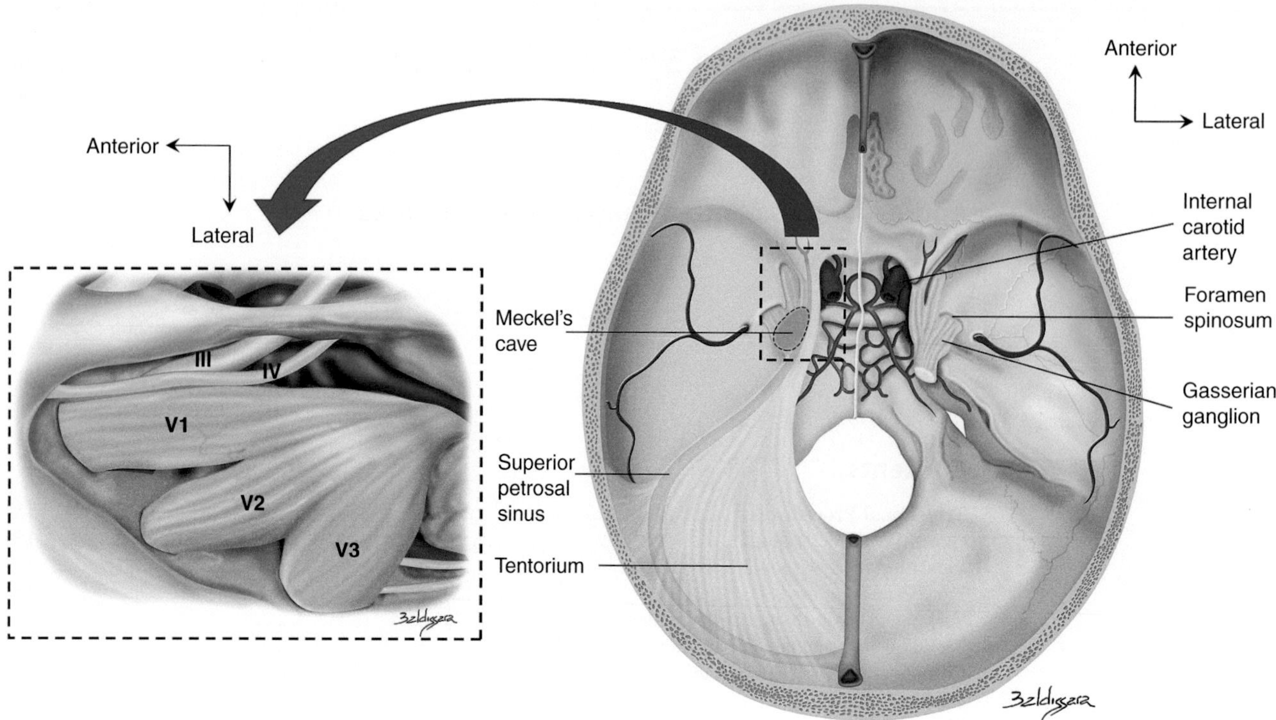

Fig. 10.1 Superior view of skull base showing the Gasserian ganglion and Meckel's cave. The insert showed the trigeminal branches inside the Meckel cave: V1—Ophthalmic nerve; V2—Maxillary nerve; V3—Mandibular nerve. III—Oculomotor nerve; IV—Trochlear nerve (Image courtesy of Dr. Andre Mansano)

The Foramen Ovale

The foramen ovale is particularly important for percutaneous trigeminal procedures as it is relatively easy to visualize with fluoroscopy and serves as an entrance for the Meckel's cave. It is located at the great sphenoid wing and contains the mandibular branch, the meningeal accessory artery, and the minor petrosal nerve.

The Trigeminal Cistern

The trigeminal cistern is an outpocketing of the intrathecal space, reaching out along the trigeminal nerves inside the Meckel's cave. Its length and size varies and it communicates with the lumbar intrathecal space. It is very common to encounter cerebrospinal fluid during trigeminal percutaneous procedures, especially when sharp needles are used. This is acceptable when radiofrequency ablation or balloon compression is performed, but local anesthetics must be used with caution inside the Meckel cave, as it may result in brainstem anesthesia.

Technique: Radiofrequency Trigeminal Ablation

Before treatment, informed consent is required, and all advantages and disadvantages of the procedure should be discussed with the patient. Use of anticoagulants and antiplatelets should be assessed according to the latest guidelines. Currently, percutaneous trigeminal procedures are considered intermediate-risk procedures.

An IV line and standard ASA monitoring are mandatory. The procedure is extremely painful once the needle engages in the Gasserian ganglion, so sedation is usually done with propofol and fentanyl. After needle positioning, the anesthetic is discontinued enabling the patient to communicate with the medical staff during the stimulation phase. The patient is placed in the supine position on a radiolucent table with a pillow/cushion under the shoulders to extend the head. Taping the head is not mandatory but can prevent unintentional movements.

The oval foramen can be found with a submental fluoroscopic view that is accomplished by AP view followed by ipsilateral oblique rotation and subsequent caudal tilt (Figs. 10.2, 10.3, and 10.4). After skin infiltration with local anesthetic and under deep sedation, a radiofrequency needle (20–22G, 2–5 mm active tip) is introduced in a coaxial view to the entrance of the foramen ovale (Fig. 10.5).

The depth of the needle is checked in a true lateral view, which is identified by the lack of double lines at the clivus, overlapping posterior clinoid processes and sellar tubercles. The mandible is highly mobile, so true lateral fluoroscopy view should not be guided by its position (Fig. 10.6a, b). Great care must be taken not to pass the posterior border of the clivus.

Fig. 10.2 AP view of the skull

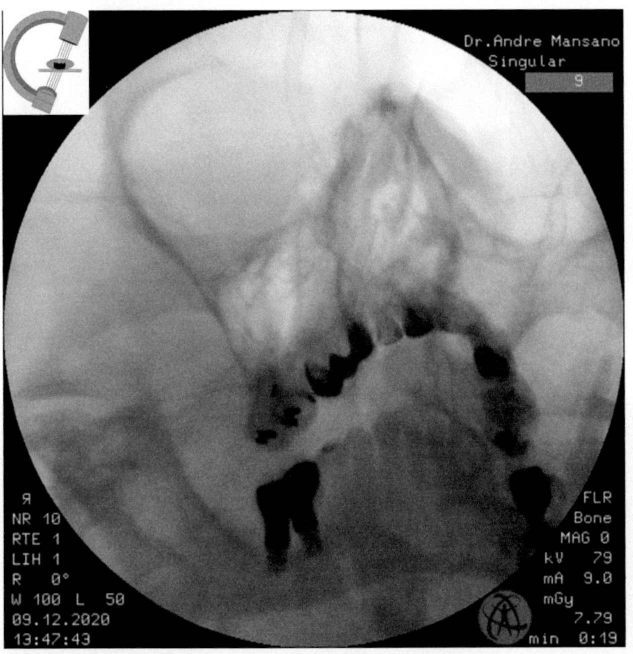

Fig. 10.3 Oblique view toward the side of the procedure

At this point, the stylet is removed and replaced by the electrode. Motor (2 Hz, 1 ms/pulse, 0.1–0.5 V) and sensory (50–100 Hz, 1 ms/pulse, 0.1–0.5 V) stimulations are performed to assure the correct tip location. Motor stimulation provokes masseteric contractions when the active tip is at V3, and sensory stimulation provokes paresthesia over the innervation area of each trigeminal branch. It is very important to wake up the patient before performing sensory stimulation.

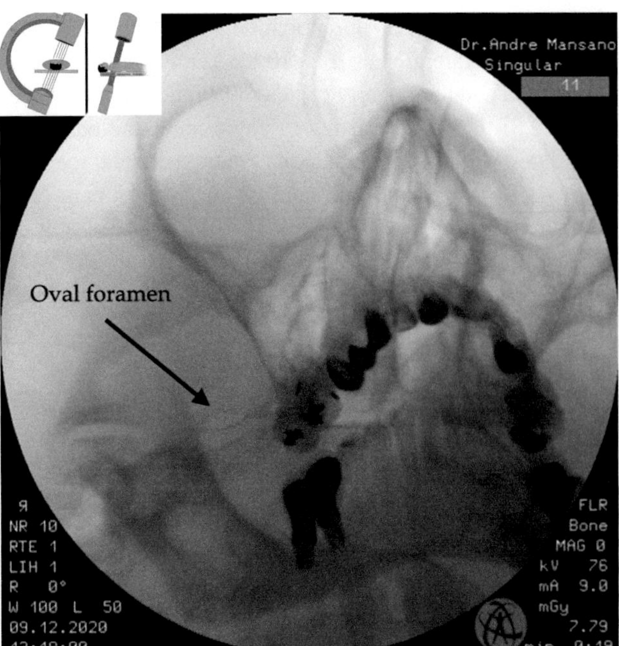

Fig. 10.4 Caudal oblique view. Dark arrow ponting ovale foramen

There is no consensus regarding the optimal temperature of the radiofrequency lesion. The majority of physicians perform sequential lesions starting at 60 °C for 1 min, increasing 5 °C in each lesion, testing the sensibility between them. For this, the patient should be awake between each lesioning and had his/her tactile sensibility assessed, which may be challenging. The concept is to stop increasing the temperature once hypoesthesia is overcome. One study evaluated several temperatures by a Kaplan–Meier estimator and proposed that 75 °C is the optimal temperature balancing between pain relief and occurrence of complications.

Pulsed radiofrequency is also feasible, although less effective than thermal RF. There is also no consensus regarding the best parameters. One frequently used set is 42 °C, 45 V, 5 Hz, 5 ms/pulse, 3–8 min. Some studies suggest that high-voltage PRF is more effective than low voltage, but this may be due to temperature spikes unmeasured by the RF machine.

Technique: Percutaneous Trigeminal Balloon Compression

As indicated in the above section on trigeminal radiofrequency, the first steps of trigeminal balloon compression include informed consent, assessment of anticoagulants/antiplatelets drugs, IV line and ASA monitors and anesthesia. In this approach, general anesthesia is acceptable, as patient feedback is not required.

After skin infiltration with local anesthetic, a 22G spinal needle is introduced to allow deeper tissue anesthesia. A 14G needle is then introduced inside the Meckel's cave, through a coaxial approach, using the oval foramen as the entrance point (Fig. 10.7). The appropriate depth of the needle must be checked in lateral view (Fig. 10.8). At this point, the stylet is removed and the Fogarty catheter (4 French) is introduced (Fig. 10.8). Under lateral fluoroscopic view, the balloon is insufflated with sterile nonionic contrast media for 60 s (Fig. 10.9). Pear shape is related to longer term pain relief compared with other shapes (Fig. 10.10).

Complications of Thermal Radiofrequency and Balloon Compression Techniques

Complications are quite common with both techniques and are summarized in the graphic below (Fig. 10.11).

Practical Tips

The skin entry is usually about 2 cm lateral from the angle of the mouth. If the planned entry point is far from this, the fluoroscopy setup must be rechecked (submental view).

One of the concerns about percutaneous trigeminal procedures is the penetration of the oral mucosa, carrying bacteria to the Meckel's cave, leading to meningitis. Some physicians prefer to put a finger in the patient's mouth to check for potential mucosa penetration. Moving the skin entry slightly more lateral also helps to avoid this problem.

The maxillary and mandibular divisions are very easy to reach. Choosing the entry point in the middle of the oval foramen will access V3 right at the foramen ovale entrance and V2 once the needle is advanced slightly. The ophthalmic

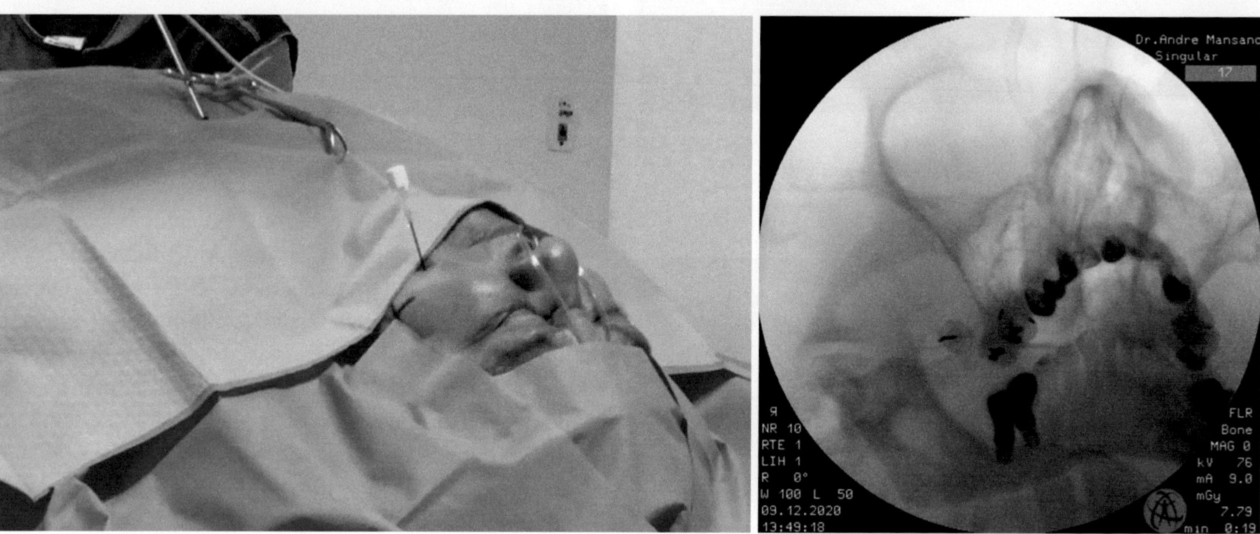

Fig. 10.5 RF needle in coaxial position

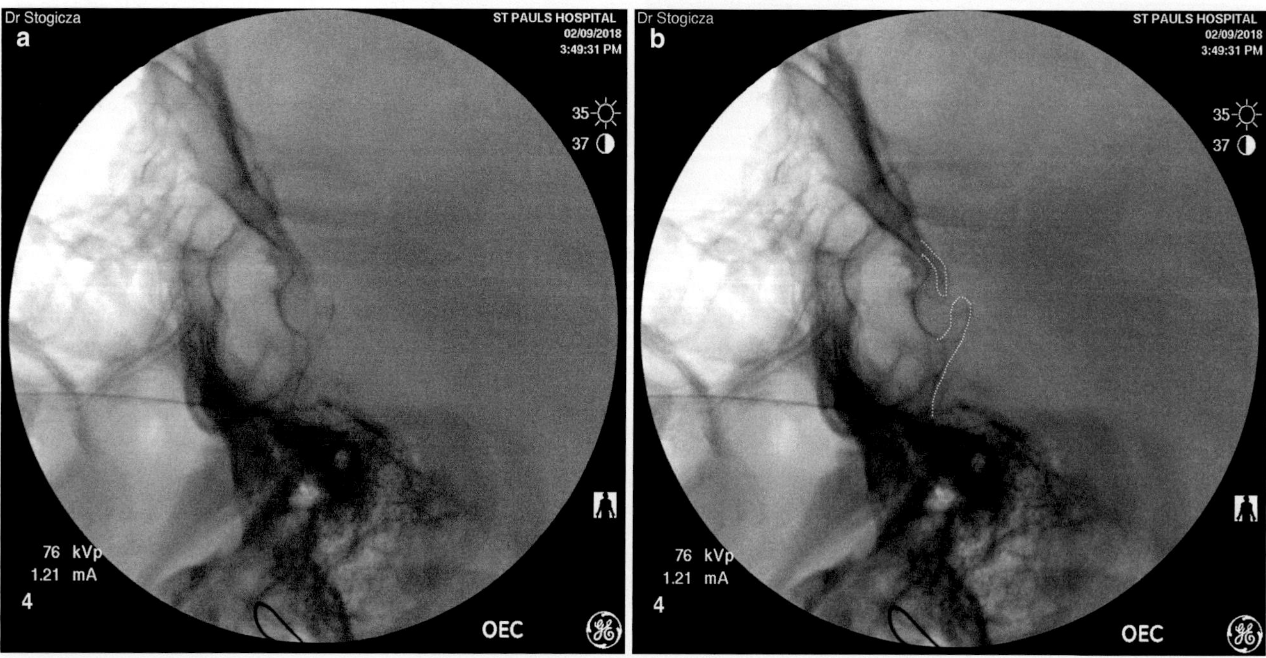

Fig. 10.6 (**a**) RF needle inside de Meckle cave - lateral view. (**b**) Orange line - turcica sella; Yellow line. Posterior border of the clivus

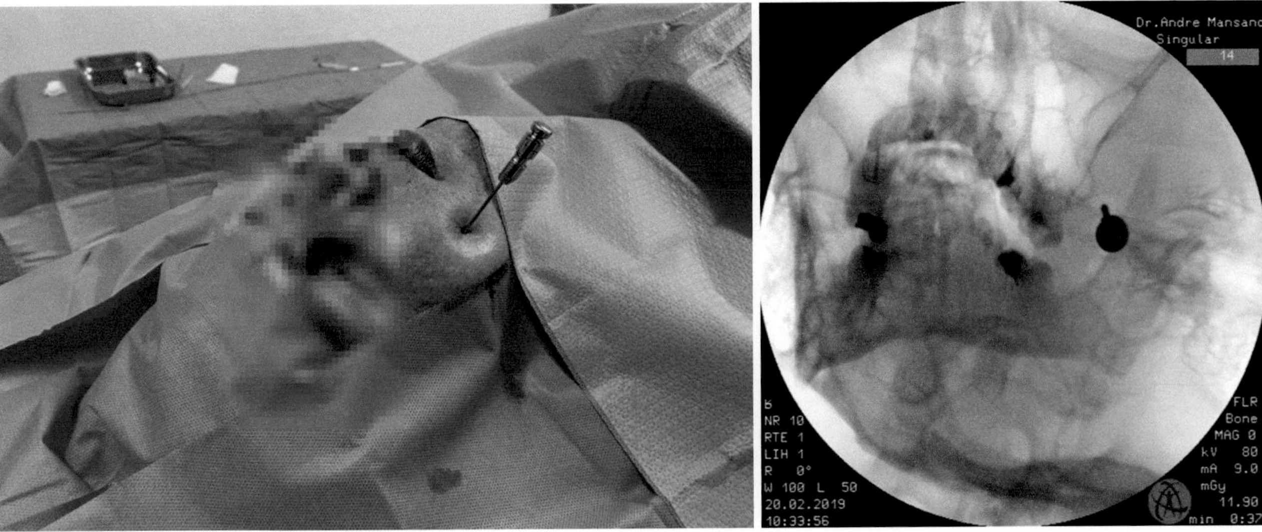

Fig. 10.7 14G needle in coaxial view, inside the Meckle cave

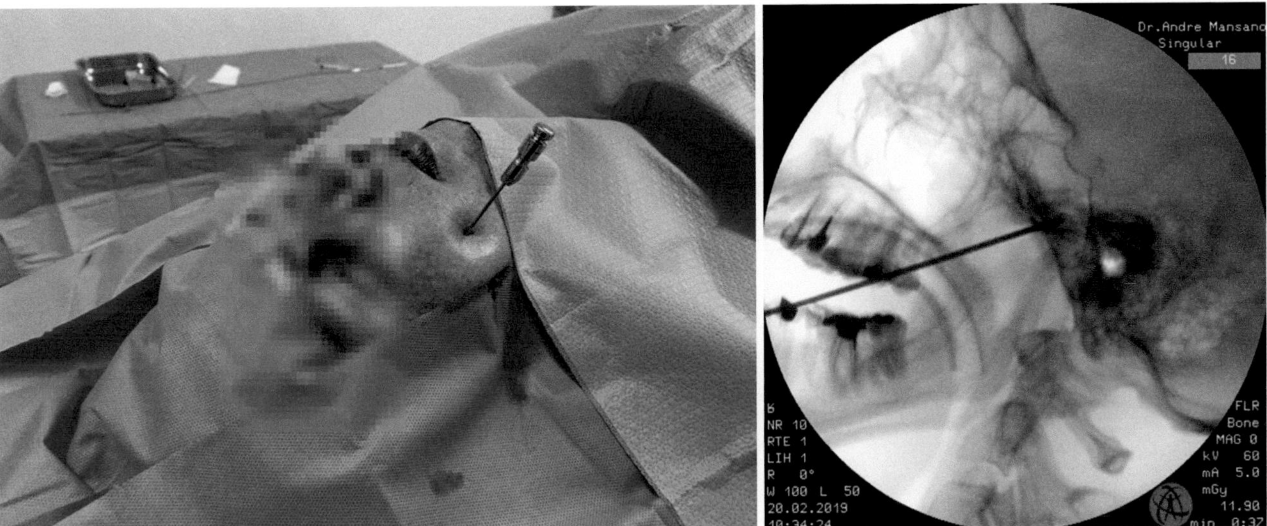

Fig. 10.8 14G needle in coaxial view, inside the Meckle cave - Lateral view

division is located more medial and deeper inside the Meckel cave. Moving the skin entry slightly more lateral and inferior will allow access to V1, located more medial and superior (deeper in the Meckel's cave) (Fig. 10.12).

Literature Review

There is limited evidence available for percutaneous trigeminal procedures as there is no high-quality RCT available. The largest, although uncontrolled study, is from Kanpolat who evaluated 1600 patients, who underwent radiofrequency ablation of the Gasserian ganglion with a long-term follow-up, who showed a 97.6% initial success rate and a recurrence rate of 47.4% and 59% in 10 and 20 years, respectively.

Thermal radiofrequency is superior to pulsed radiofrequency, although it has a higher complication rate. There are some retrospective studies suggesting that combining pulsed and thermal radiofrequency can increase the success rate and decrease complications.

Percutaneous balloon compression efficacy is 96% with a recurrence rate of 31% in 3 years. One recent study showed no superiority of balloon compression over thermal radiofrequency (Fig. 10.13).

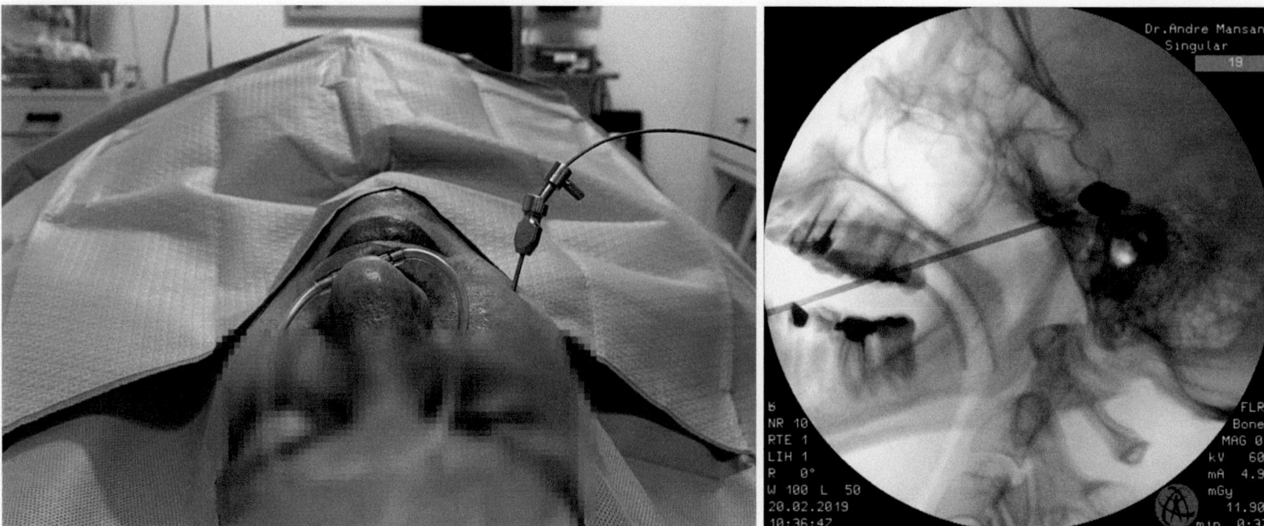

Fig. 10.9 4F Fogarty catheter throught the needle. Pear shaped balloon

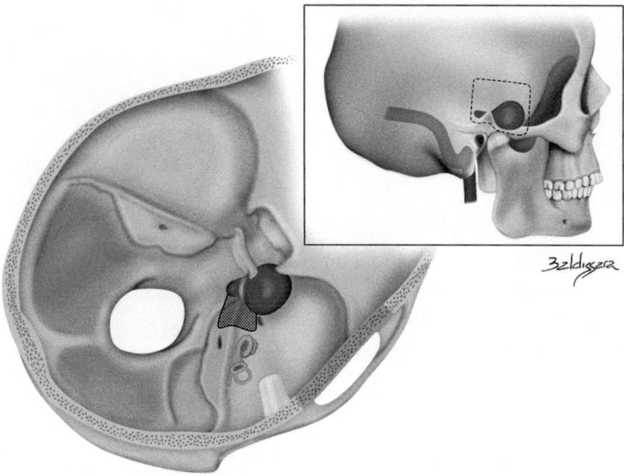

Fig. 10.10 Cartoon drawing of a pear shaped baloon

Sphenopalatine Procedures

General Considerations

The sphenopalatine ganglion (SPG), also known as pterygopalatine ganglion, Meckel ganglion, or sphenomaxillary ganglion, regulates vascular tone of cerebral vessels and has been implicated in several kinds of facial pain and headaches.

Indication

- Sphenopalatine neuralgia (Sluder's neuralgia).
- Cluster headache.
- Side-locked migraine.
- Facial postherpetic neuralgia.
- Persistent idiopathic facial pain.

Functional Anatomy

SPG has somatosensorial, sympathetic, and parasympathetic fibers with multiple connections with facial, trigeminal nerve and sympathetic chain. Sphenopalatine parasympathetic innervation comes from the intermediate nerve, also called "Wrisberg nerve," through the great petrosal nerve. It promotes vasodilation and/or secretion of the soft palate, tonsils, uvula, floor of the mouth, superior lips/gums, pharynx, and lacrimal glands. SPG sympathetic innervation comes from the internal carotid plexus though the deep petrosal nerve (Fig. 10.14). The deep petrosal nerve joins with the superficial petrosal nerve to form the vidian nerve that enters the SPG fossa.

The SPG lies inside the sphenopalatine fossa, which is bounded anteriorly by the maxilla, posteriorly by the pterygoid process, medially by the perpendicular plate of the palatine bone, and inferiorly by the palatine bone.

Technique

Intranasal

This technique is very simple although has low specificity. The rationale is delivering local anesthetic posterior to the posterior conchae (Fig. 10.15) through soaked gauze or cotton swab or even with specific instillation devices. (Please refer to Samer Narouze's recent daring discourse on RAPM

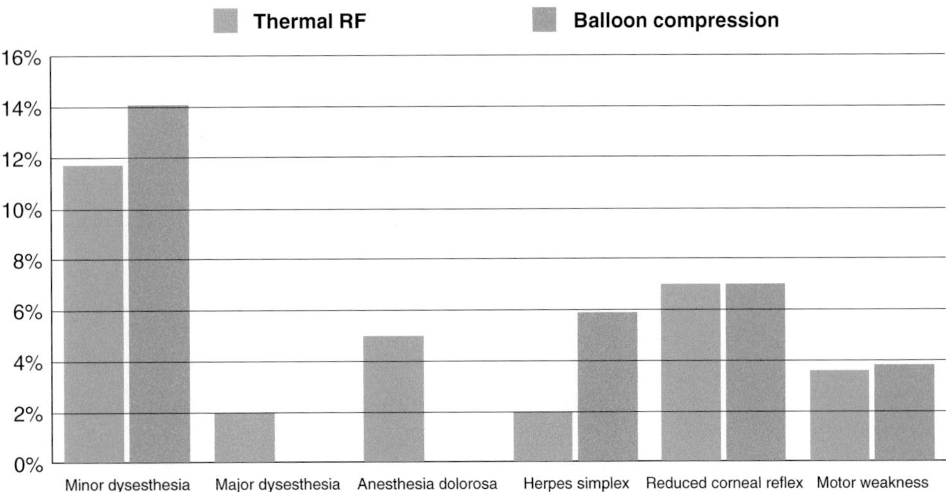

Fig. 10.11 RF and balloon compression complication rates

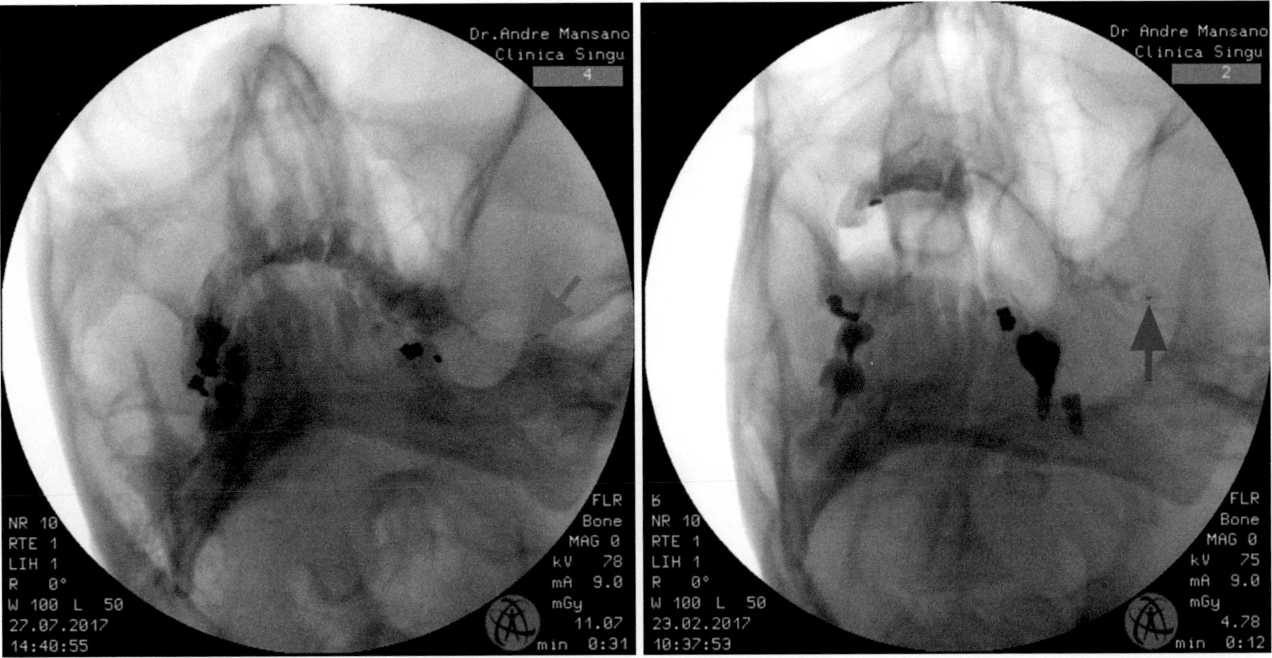

Fig. 10.12 Green arrow poiting Ramus of mandible. Blue arrow pointing oval foramen with a 30G needle marking the the needle entry point

"Topical intranasal lidocaine is not a sphenopalatine ganglion block".)

Fluoroscopic-Guided Infrazygomatic Classical Technique

Before treatment, informed consent is required, and all advantages and disadvantages of the procedure should be discussed with the patient. Use of anticoagulants and antiplatelets should be assessed according to the latest guidelines (Table 10.1). Currently, percutaneous sphenopalatine procedures are considered intermediate-risk procedure. An IV line and ASA standard monitors are mandatory. The patient should be placed in the supine position on a radiolucent. Taping the head is not mandatory but can prevent unintentional movements.

Before the procedure, we draw a line under the zygoma to allow a better entry point. The SPG fossa can be found with a lateral fluoroscopic view. It is important to superimpose both sphenopalatine fossae (Fig. 10.16). After skin infiltration with local anesthetic, a spinal or radiofrequency needle (20–22G, 2–5 mm active tip) is introduced under the zygoma (Fig. 10.17) toward the superior posterior aspect of the SPG fossa. The depth of the needle is checked in an AP view (Fig. 10.18).

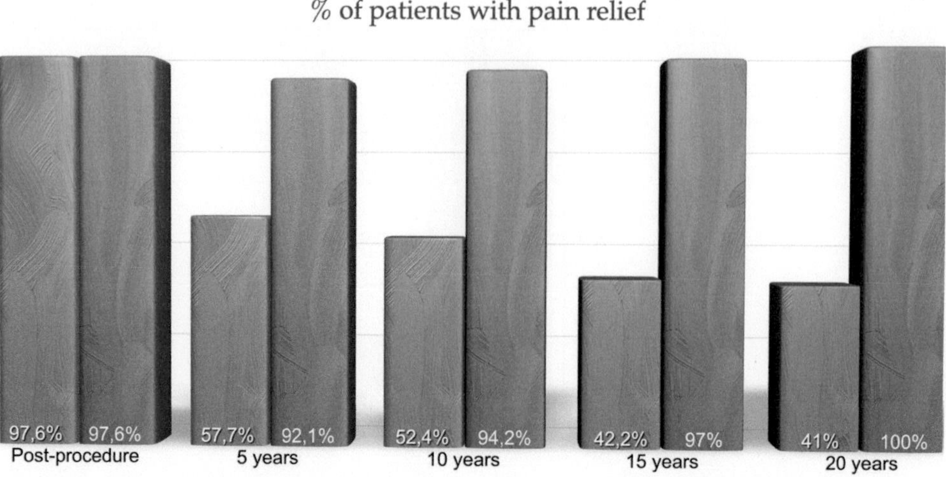

Fig. 10.13 Trigeminal radiofrequency outcomes. Follow up: 20 years

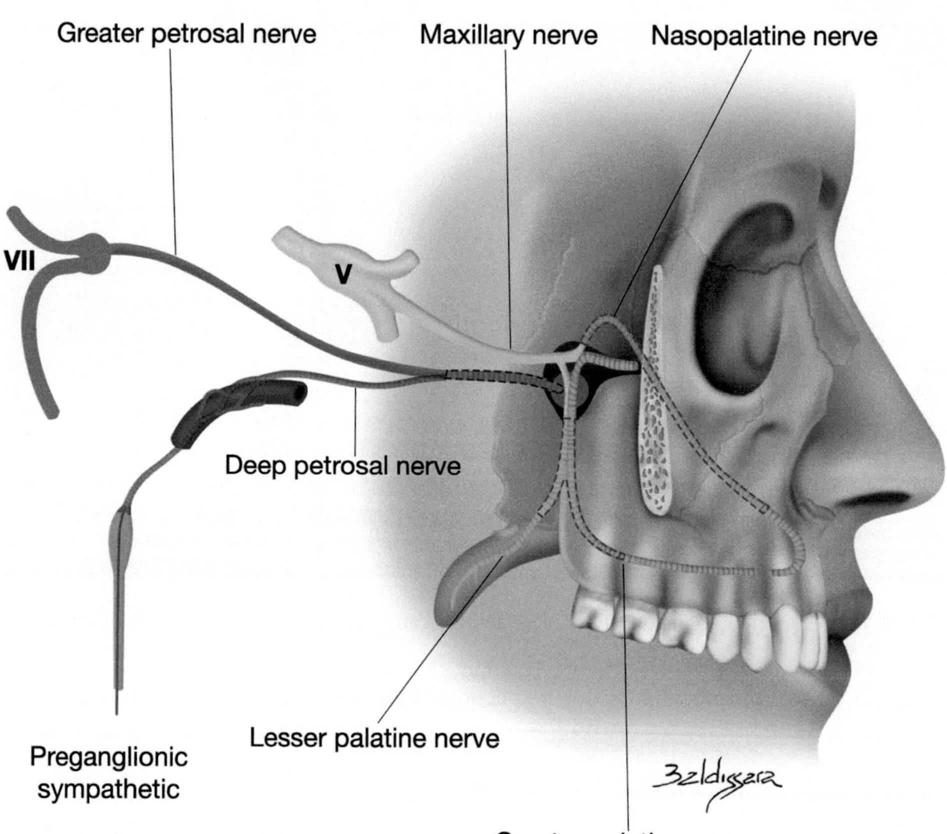

Fig. 10.14 SPG sitted inside the SPG fossa and it's somatic and autonomic relationships

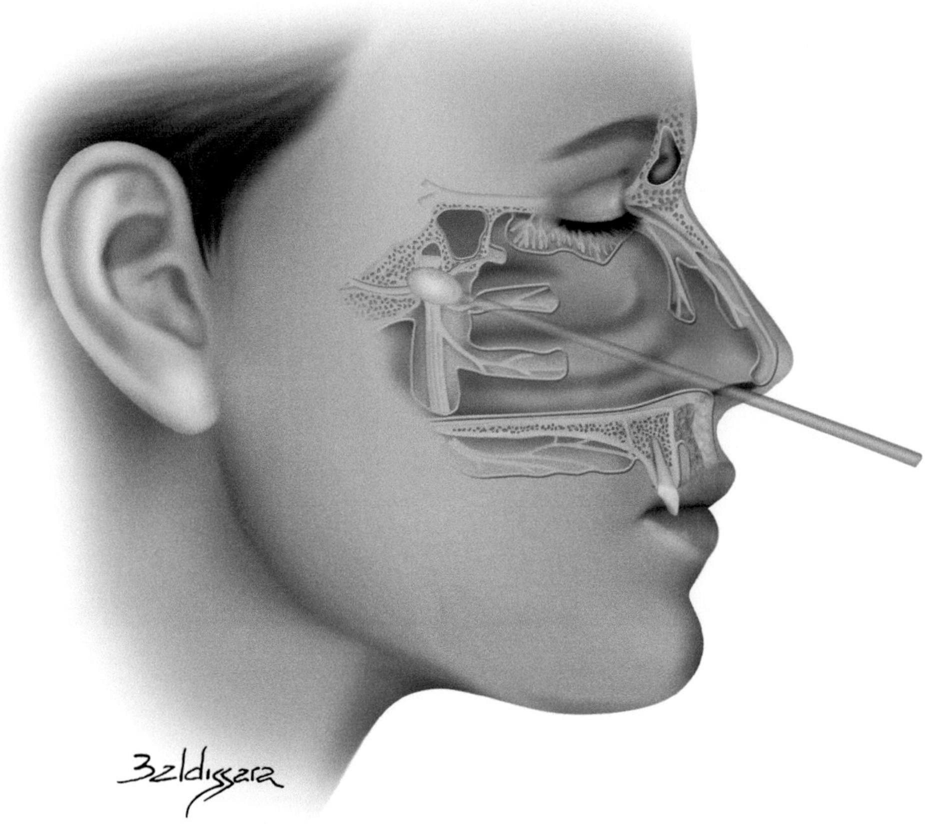

Fig. 10.15 Cartoon drawing - Intranasal SPG block technique

Table 10.1 Most common anticoagulants and antiplatelets drugs and their need of withdrawal prior to trigeminal and sphenopalatine percutaneous procedures

Drug	When to stop	When to restart
Aspirin primary prophylaxis	Shared assessment and risk stratification	24 h
Aspirin secondary prophylaxis	No	24 h
Clopidrogrel	7 days	12–24 h
Warfarin	5 days INR ≤ 1.2	6 h
Dabigatran Pradaxa®	4 days 5–6 days (impaired renal function)	24 h
Rivaroxaban Xarelto®	3 days	24 h
Apixaban Eliquis®	3 days	24 h
IV heparin	6 h	2 h
Subcutaneous heparin	6 h	2 h
Enoxaparin (prophylatic)	12 h	12–24 h
Enoxaparin (therapeutic)	24 h	12–24 h

At this point, the stylet is removed and replaced by the electrode. Sensory stimulation (50–100 Hz, 1 ms/pulse, 0.1–0.5 V) is done to properly assure the correct tip location (the patient must feel paresthesia at the base of the nose). Thermal or pulsed radiofrequency are both options although the literature supporting either is scarce.

Fluoroscopic-Guided Infrazygomatic, Coaxial Technique

The patient is placed in lateral decubitus with the affected side up. The C-arm is initially positioned to provide a lateral view (Fig. 10.19), and the ideal visualization and alignment of the pterygopalatine fossa is accomplished with tiny

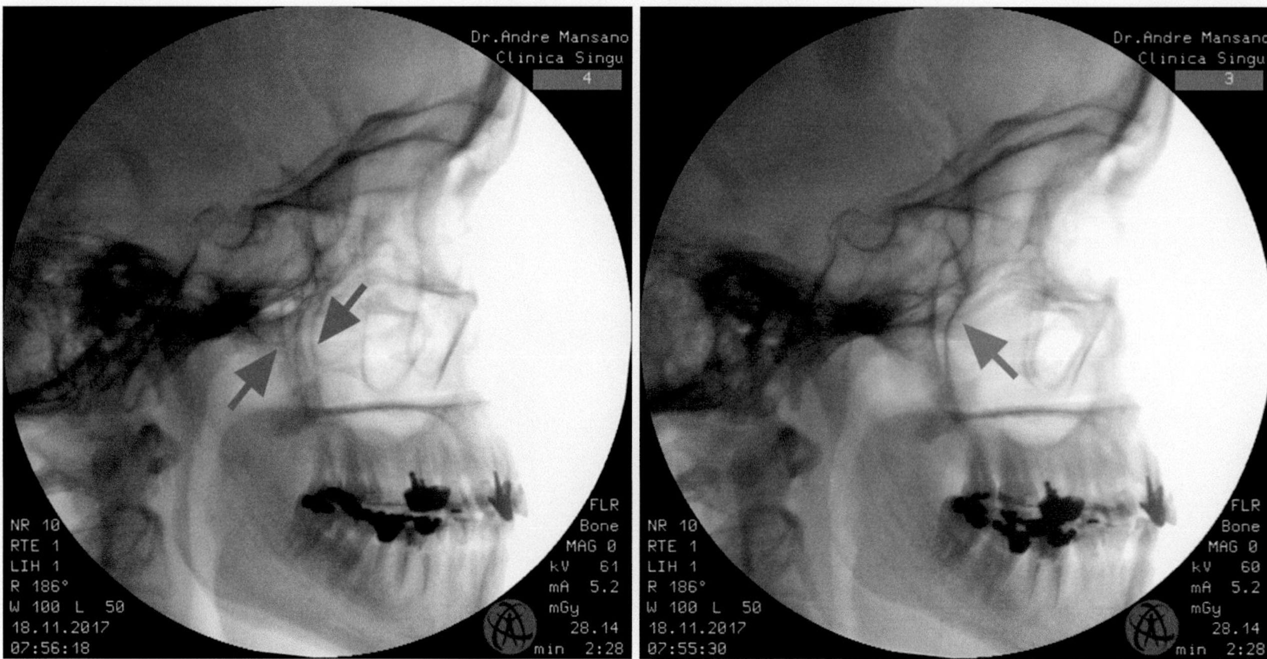

Fig. 10.16 Left picture - Misaligned SPG fossa; Right picture - Aligned SPG fossa

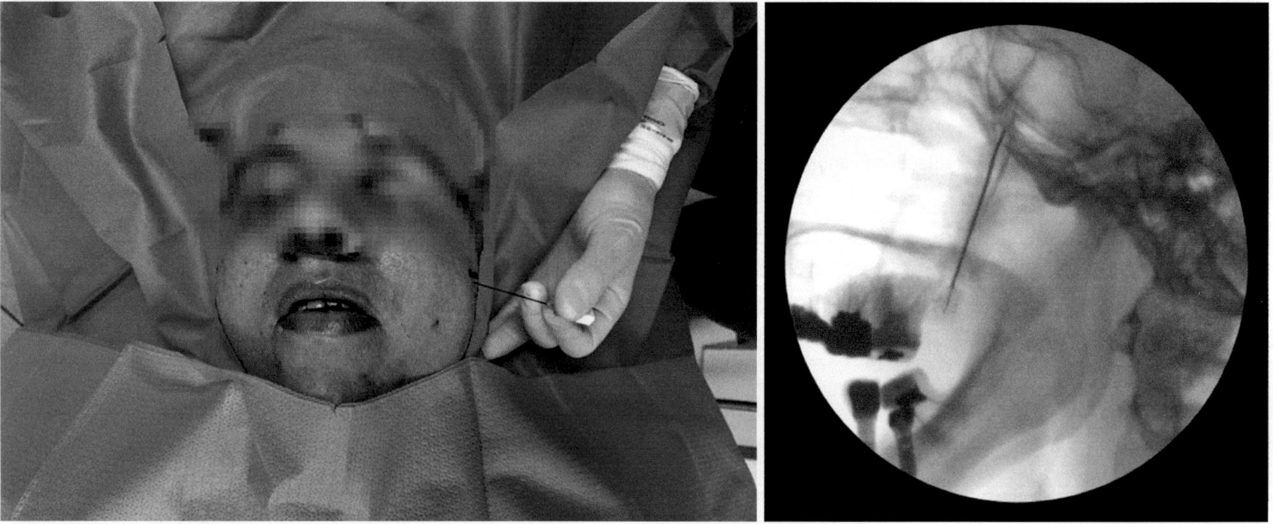

Fig. 10.17 22G needle in place - Conventional lateral tecnhique

oblique movements of the C-arm (rather than moving the patient's head).

After palpation, a 30-gauge, 1.5 cm needle is placed under the zygoma (Figs. 10.20, 10.21, and 10.22), and the C-arm is caudally tilted (Fig. 10.23) until this needle projection reaches the superior aspect of the pterygopalatine fossa (Fig. 10.24). A 22G spinal needle is inserted in a coaxial view, under the zygoma (Figs. 10.25 and 10.26) until the needle touched the palatine bone. The C-arm is then returned to the initial lateral view and then to an AP view to confirm the ideal position of the needle lateral to the nasal wall at the middle turbinate level (Fig. 10.27).

Complications: Sphenopalatine Procedures

Complications are infrequent, but include epistaxis, maxillary artery injury, facial, palatine or superior alveolar nerve lesions, bradycardia, parotid injury, hematoma, hypoesthesia, diplopia and infection.

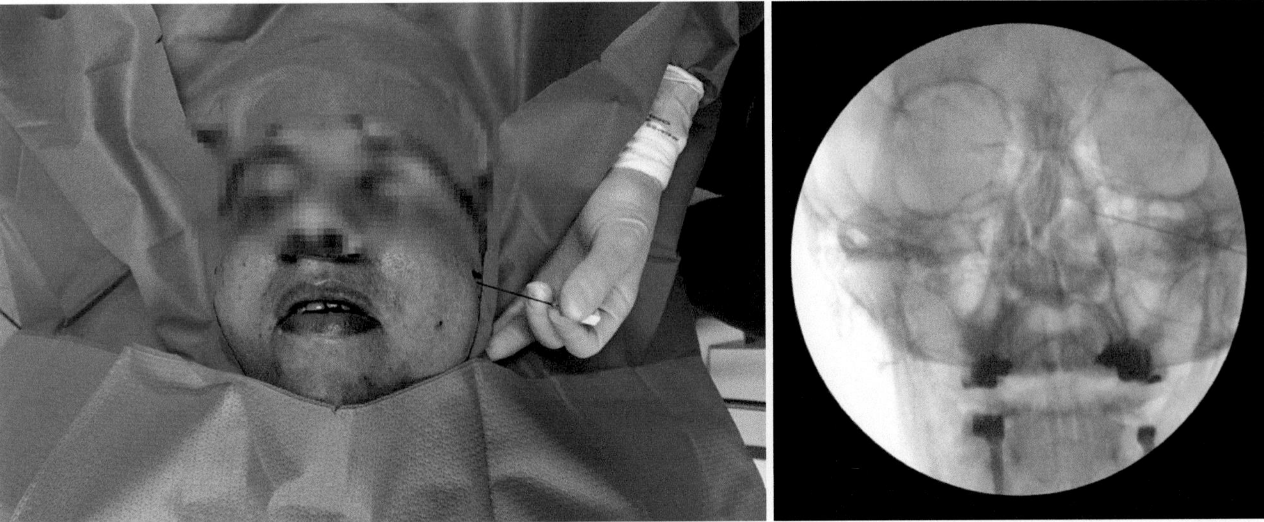

Fig. 10.18 22G needle in place - Conventional lateral tecnhique. AP view

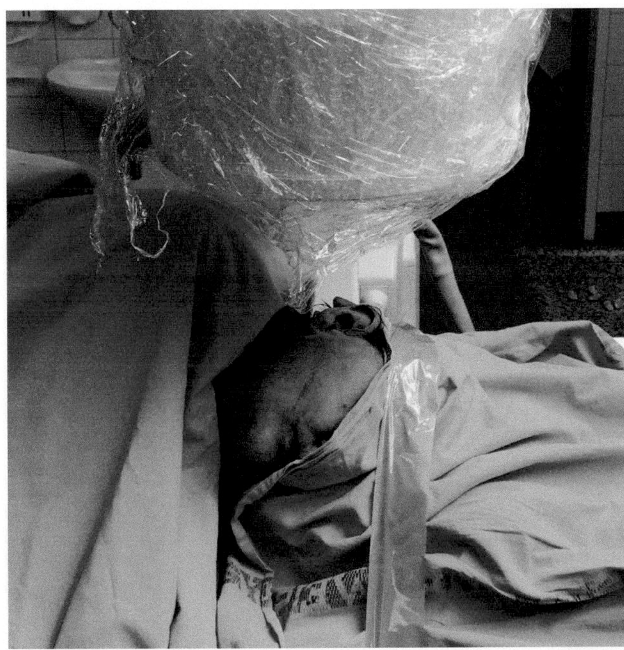

Fig. 10.19 Cadaver specime in lateral position. C-Arm showing lateral view

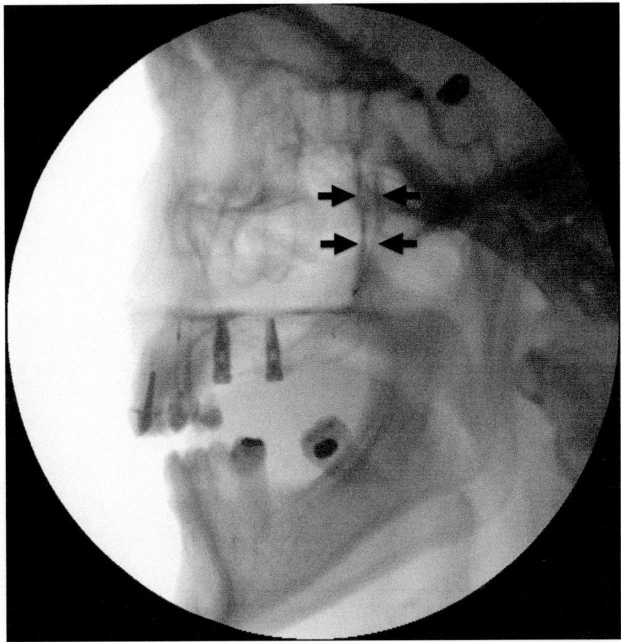

Fig. 10.20 Black arrows showing SPG fossa

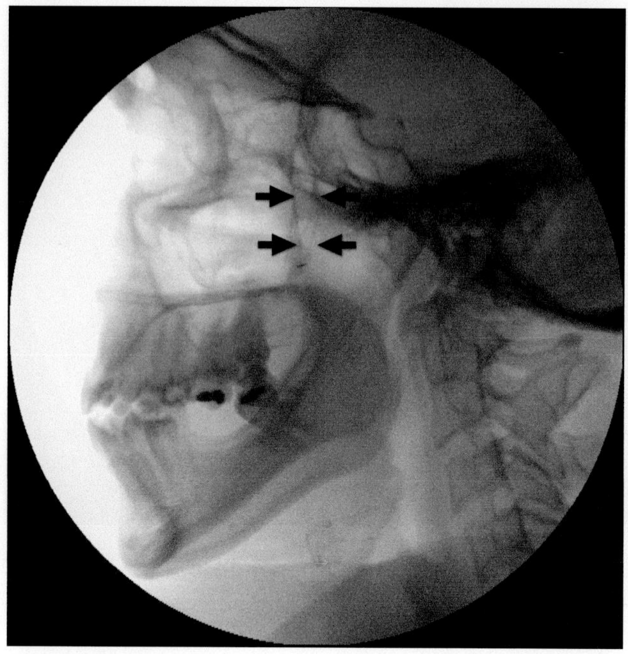

Fig. 10.21 Black arrows showing SPG fossa. 30G needle marking the entry point at the inferiore aspect of the SPG fossa

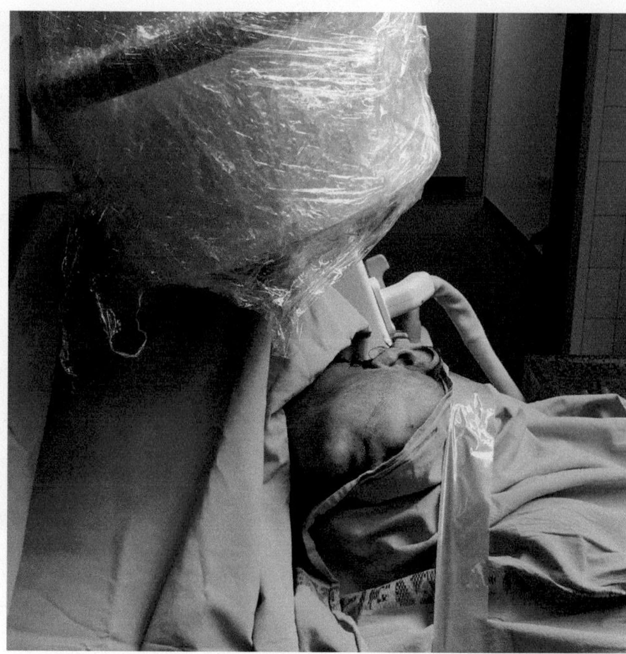

Fig. 10.23 C-arm tilted caudally

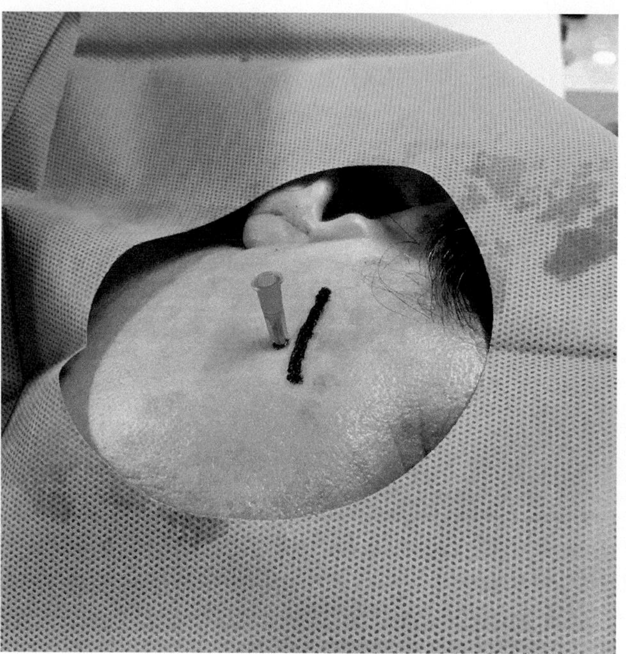

Fig. 10.22 27G needle marking the entry point bellow the maxilla

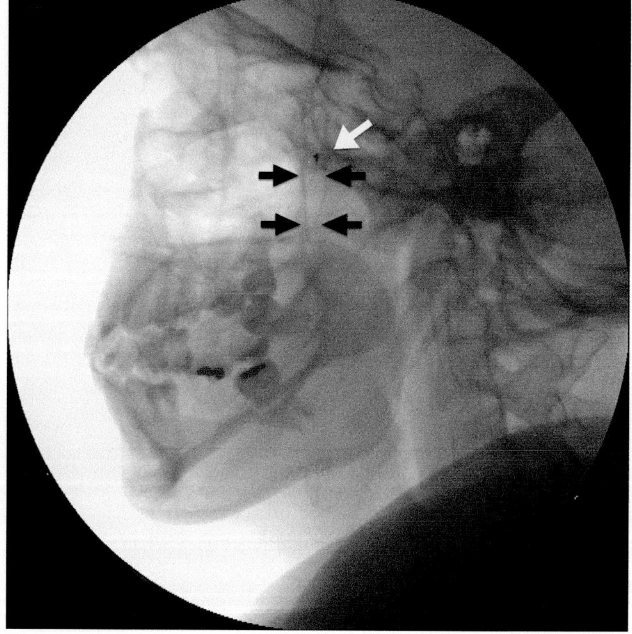

Fig. 10.24 Fluoroscopic view after tilting the C-arm caudally. The 30-gauge needle projection is in thesuperior aspect of the pterygopalatine fossa

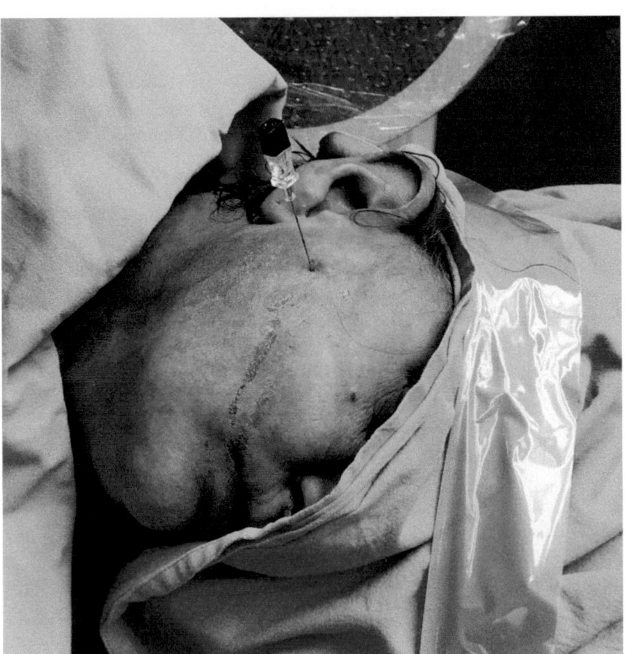

Fig. 10.25 22G needle inserted in a coaxial view

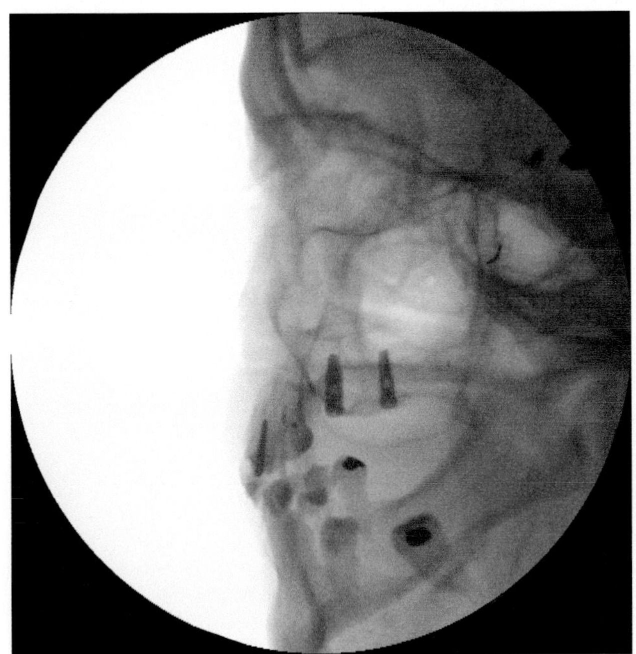

Fig. 10.26 22G needle inserted in a coaxial view till it touches the bone

Literature

Unfortunately, the literature is scarce regarding SPG procedures. Racz et al. evaluated the efficacy of SPG pulsed radiofrequency in 30 patients with facial pain, showing good

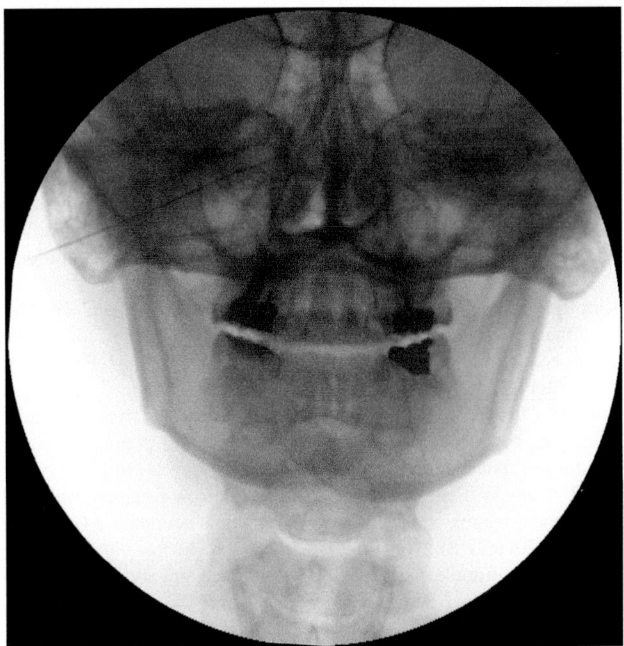

Fig. 10.27 AP view showing the needle lateral to the middle turbinate level

results in more than 80% of patients. In another study, Kapural showed a 50% decrease in pain frequency and intensity in patients with chronic recalcitrant cluster headache. A retrospective series using chemical neurolysis (alcohol) in patients with orofacial pain also supported its efficacy.

Suggested Reading

Bayer E, Racz GB, Miles D, Heavner J. Sphenopalatine ganglion pulsed radiofrequency treatment in 30 patients suffering from chronic face and head pain. Pain Pract. 2005;5(3):223–7.

Brown JA, McDaniel MD, Weaver MT. Percutaneous trigeminal nerve compression for treatment of trigeminal neuralgia: results in 50 patients. Neurosurgery. 1993;32(4):570–3.

Cheng JS, Lim DA, Chang EF, Barbaro NM. A review of percutaneous treatments for trigeminal neuralgia. Neurosurgery. 2014;10(Suppl 1):25–33; discussion 33.

Ding Y, Li H, Hong T, Zhu Y, Yao P, Zhou G. Combination of pulsed radiofrequency with continuous radiofrequency thermocoagulation at low temperature improves efficacy and safety in V2/V3 primary trigeminal neuralgia. Pain Phys. 2018;21(5):E545.

Emril DR, Ho K-Y. Treatment of trigeminal neuralgia: role of radiofrequency ablation. J Pain Res. 2010;3:249–54.

Erdine S, Ozyalcin NS, Cimen A, Celik M, Talu GK, Disci R. Comparison of pulsed radiofrequency with conventional radiofrequency in the treatment of idiopathic trigeminal neuralgia. Eur J Pain. 2007;11(3):309–13.

Fang L, Tao W, Jingjing L, Nan J. Comparison of high-voltage- with standard-voltage pulsed radiofrequency of Gasserian ganglion in the treatment of idiopathic trigeminal neuralgia. Pain Pract. 2015;15(7):595–603.

Kanpolat Y, Savas A, Bekar A, Berk C. Percutaneous controlled radiofrequency trigeminal rhizotomy for the treatment of idiopathic trigeminal neuralgia: 25-year experience with 1,600 patients. Neurosurgery. 2001;48(3):524–32; discussion 532-4.

Kastler A, Cadel G, Comte A, Gory G, Piccand V, Tavernier L, et al. Alcohol percutaneous neurolysis of the sphenopalatine ganglion in the management of refractory cranio-facial pain. Neuroradiology. 2014;56(7):589–96.

Katusic S, Williams DB, Beard M, Bergstralh EJ, Kurland LT. Epidemiology and clinical features of idiopathic trigeminal neuralgia and glossopharyngeal neuralgia: similarities and differences, Rochester, Minnesota, 1945-1984. Neuroepidemiology. 1991;10(5–6):276–81.

Kim JH, Yu HY, Park SY, Lee SC, Kim YC. Pulsed and conventional radiofrequency treatment: which is effective for dental procedure-related symptomatic trigeminal neuralgia? Pain Med. 2013;14(3):430–5.

Lin KH, Chen YT, Fuh JL, Wang SJ. Increased risk of trigeminal neuralgia in patients with migraine: a nationwide population-based study. Cephalalgia. 2016;36(13):1218–27.

Liu P, Zhong W, Liao C, Liu M, Zhang W. Narrow foramen ovale and rotundum: a role in the etiology of trigeminal neuralgia. J Craniofac Surg. 2016;27(8):2168–70.

Manzoni GC, Torelli P. Epidemiology of typical and atypical craniofacial neuralgias. Neurol Sci. 2005;26(S2):s65–7.

Narouze S, Kapural L, Casanova J, Mekhail N. Sphenopalatine ganglion radiofrequency ablation for the management of chronic cluster headache. Headache. 2009;49(4):571–7.

Narouze S, Benzon HT, Provenzano D, Buvanendran A, De Andres J, Deer T, et al. Interventional Spine and Pain Procedures in Patients on Antiplatelet and Anticoagulant Medications (Second Edition): Guidelines from the American Society of Regional Anesthesia and Pain Medicine, the European Society of Regional Anaesthesia and Pain Therapy, the American Academy of Pain Medicine, the International Neuromodulation Society, the North American Neuromodulation Society, and the World Institute of Pain. Reg Anesth Pain Med. 2018;43:225–62.

Neto HS, Fukuda CY, Duarte KP, da Silva VA, de Lima Rodrigues AL, Geront RG, et al. Balloon compression versus radiofrequency for primary trigeminal neuralgia: a randomized, controlled trial. Pain. 2021;162:919.

Reinard K, Nerenz DR, Basheer A, Tahir R, Jelsema T, Schultz L, et al. Racial disparities in the diagnosis and management of trigeminal neuralgia. J Neurosurg. 2017;126(2):368–74.

Sabanci PA, Batay F, Civelek E, Al Mefty O, Husain M, Abdulrauf SI, et al. Meckel's cave. World Neurosurg. 2011;76:335–41.

Somesh MS, Sridevi HB, Prabhu LV, Swamy MSG, Krishnamurthy AK, Murlimanju BV, et al. A morphometric study of foramen ovale. Turk Neurosurg. 2011;21(3):378–83.

Tang Y-Z, Yang L-Q, Yue J-N, Wang X-P, He L-L, Ni J-X. The optimal radiofrequency temperature in radiofrequency thermocoagulation for idiopathic trigeminal neuralgia: a cohort study. Medicine (Baltimore). 2016;95(28):e4103.

Van Kleef M, Van Genderen WE, Narouze S, Nurmikko TJ, Van Zundert J, Geurts JW, et al. 1. Trigeminal neuralgia. Pain Pract. 2009;9:252–9.

Wu H, Zhou J, Chen J, Gu Y, Shi L, Ni H. Therapeutic efficacy and safety of radiofrequency ablation for the treatment of trigeminal neuralgia: A systematic review and meta-analysis. J Pain Res. 2019;12:423–41.

Xu Z, Zhang P, Long L, He H, Zhang J, Sun S. Diabetes mellitus in classical trigeminal neuralgia: a predisposing factor for its development. Clin Neurol Neurosurg. 2016;151:70–2.

Zhao WX, Wang Q, He MW, Yang LQ, Wu BS, Ni JX. Radiofrequency thermocoagulation combined with pulsed radiofrequency helps relieve postoperative complications of trigeminal neuralgia. Genet Mol Res. 2015;14(3):7616–23.

Occipital Nerve Block

11

Vitaliano Di Grazia and Philip Peng

Contents

General Consideration

Greater and lesser occipital nerve blocks are widely and effectively used in the management of primary and secondary headaches. Literature has reported improvement in pain associated with occipital neuralgia, cervicogenic headache, and cluster headache. The reported efficacy of this treatment is considered to be related to the role played by the sensory inputs from the occipital nerves in the functional neural network known as the trigeminocervical complex: inputs from the occipital segments converge with the nuclei of the trigeminal nociceptive system and then connect further to the thalamus and cortex. Therefore, the occipital nerve block would modulate central nociceptive pathway and reduce central sensitization.

The use of ultrasound to perform this procedure has proven to enhance its efficacy and reduce risks compared to the traditional landmark-based approach.

Indication/Patient Selection

Occipital nerve blocks are carried out for prognostic, diagnostic, and therapeutic purposes in patients with primary and secondary headaches. The occipital nerve block plays a diagnostic role in the diagnosis of occipital neuralgia and cervicogenic headache. It is commonly performed therapeutically for occipital neuralgia.

The International Headache Society defines occipital neuralgia as a paroxysmal jabbing pain in the distribution of the occipital nerves sometimes accompanied by dimin-

V. Di Grazia (✉)
Department of Anesthesia and Pain Management, Mount Sinai Hospital, Toronto, ON, Canada
e-mail: vitaliano.digrazia@one-mail.on.ca

P. Peng
Department of Anesthesia and Pain Medicine, Toronto Western Hospital, University of Toronto, Toronto, ON, Canada
e-mail: philip.peng@uhn.ca

D. Jankovic, P. Peng (eds.), *Regional Nerve Blocks in Anesthesia and Pain Therapy*,
https://doi.org/10.1007/978-3-030-88727-8_11

ished sensation or dysesthesia in the affected area. For the other types of headaches, the nerve block can be considered in patient's failure to respond to conservative management.

Anatomy

The greater occipital nerve (GON) arises from the dorsal ramus of the second spinal nerve (C2) and to a lesser extent from the dorsal ramus of the third spinal nerve. It contributes to the sensory innervation of the major portion of the posterior scalp as far anterior as the vertex of the skull.

In order to appreciate the course of the occipital nerves and recognize them on ultrasound scanning, it is important to visualize the several muscle layers of the upper posterior neck (Fig. 11.1). The greater occipital nerve emerges below the lower border of the obliquus capitis inferior muscle (OCIM), and passes cranially superficial to this muscle across the roof of the suboccipital triangle. It then turns dorsally to pierce the semispinalis capitis, after which it runs a short distance rostrally and laterally, lying deep to the trapezius muscle. The GON becomes subcutaneous slightly inferior to the superior nuchal line. At this point, the GON is immediately medial to the occipital artery

Laterally, the greater occipital nerve communicates with the lesser occipital nerve (LON).

The LON is composed of branches from the ventral ramus of the second and third cervical nerves and ascends toward the occiput by running parallel to the posterior border of the sternocleidomastoid muscle, becoming the most cranial part of the superficial cervical plexus. Near the scalp, it perforates the deep fascia and continues superiorly over the occiput, where it is located lateral to and in the same fascial plane as the greater occipital nerve (Fig. 11.2). The LON supplies the skin over the posterolateral portion of the scalp and above the ear.

Technique for Greater Occipital Nerve

Distal Approach at the Nuchal Line

The key landmark is the superior nuchal line and occipital artery. It can be performed with both landmark and ultrasound guidance with the patient in the sitting position and head tilted forward resting on a soft surface.

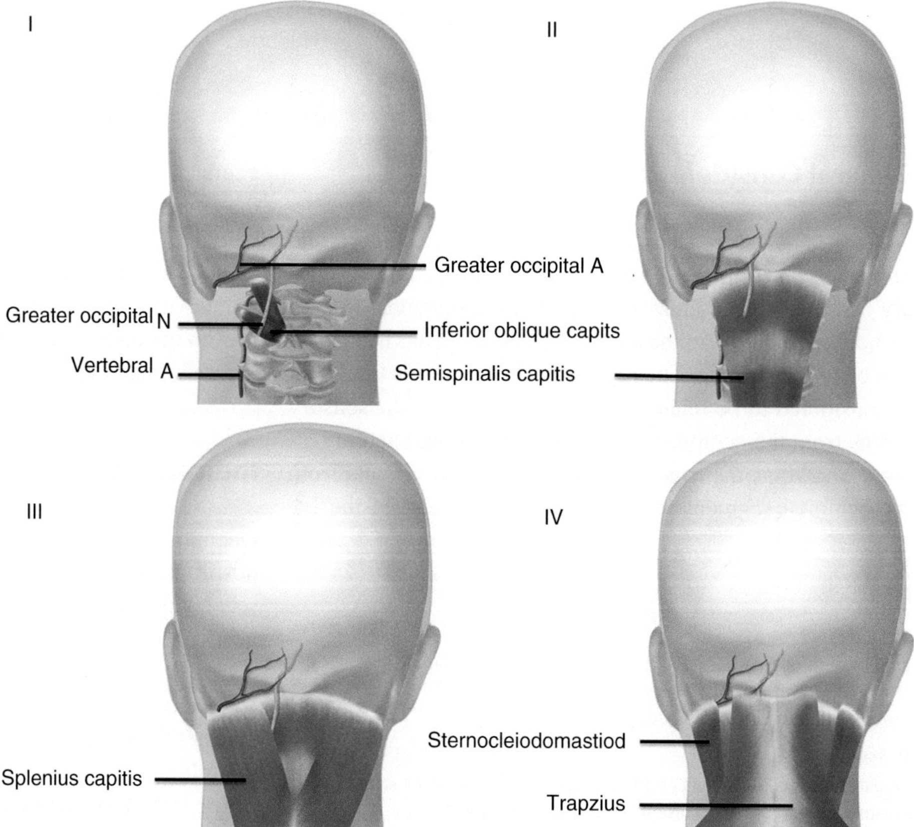

Fig. 11.1 Fours layers of muscles relevant to the greater occipital nerve. N and A – nerve and artery. Reprinted with permission from Philip Peng Educational Series

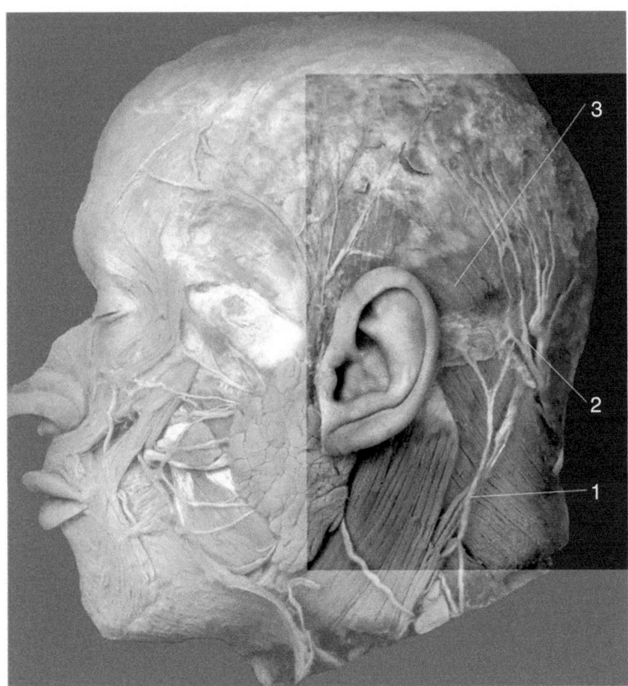

Fig. 11.2 (1) Lesser occipital nerve, (2) greater occipital nerve, (3) occipitalis muscle. Reprinted with permission from Dr. Danilo Jankovic

For landmark-guided technique, the needle is inserted about 2.5 cm from the midline, directly medial to the easily palpable occipital artery (Fig. 11.3). If the artery is not palpable, the needle is inserted lateral to the lateral border of the trapezius at the superior nuchal line. A 25-gauge 1.5-inch needle is advanced at a slightly cranial angle until bone contact is made, and the depth should not exceed more than 1cm. After minimal withdrawal and aspiration, 1 to 1.5 mL of local anesthetic is administered for diagnostic purpose, and for therapeutic block, a small amount of steroid (Depo-Medrol 10–20 mg) is added.

For ultrasound technique, a linear ultrasound probe is covered in sterile dressing and positioned transversally over the superior nuchal line (Fig. 11.4a) and moved laterally until the greater occipital artery can be visualized (Fig. 11.4b). The GON is not commonly visualized as it is divided into small branches. An in-plane technique can be used and a 25-G 1.5-inch needle can be inserted to anesthetize the skin and then advanced into the fascial plane containing the greater occipital artery, greater occipital nerve, and more laterally the lesser occipital nerve. Therapeutic medication containing local anesthetic and steroid can be injected into this fascial plane.

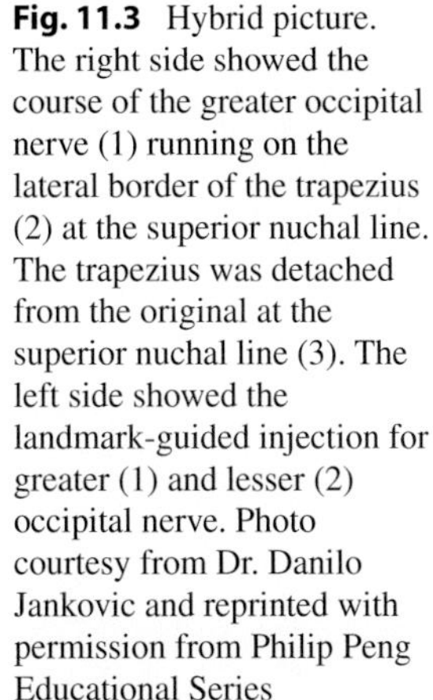

Fig. 11.3 Hybrid picture. The right side showed the course of the greater occipital nerve (1) running on the lateral border of the trapezius (2) at the superior nuchal line. The trapezius was detached from the original at the superior nuchal line (3). The left side showed the landmark-guided injection for greater (1) and lesser (2) occipital nerve. Photo courtesy from Dr. Danilo Jankovic and reprinted with permission from Philip Peng Educational Series

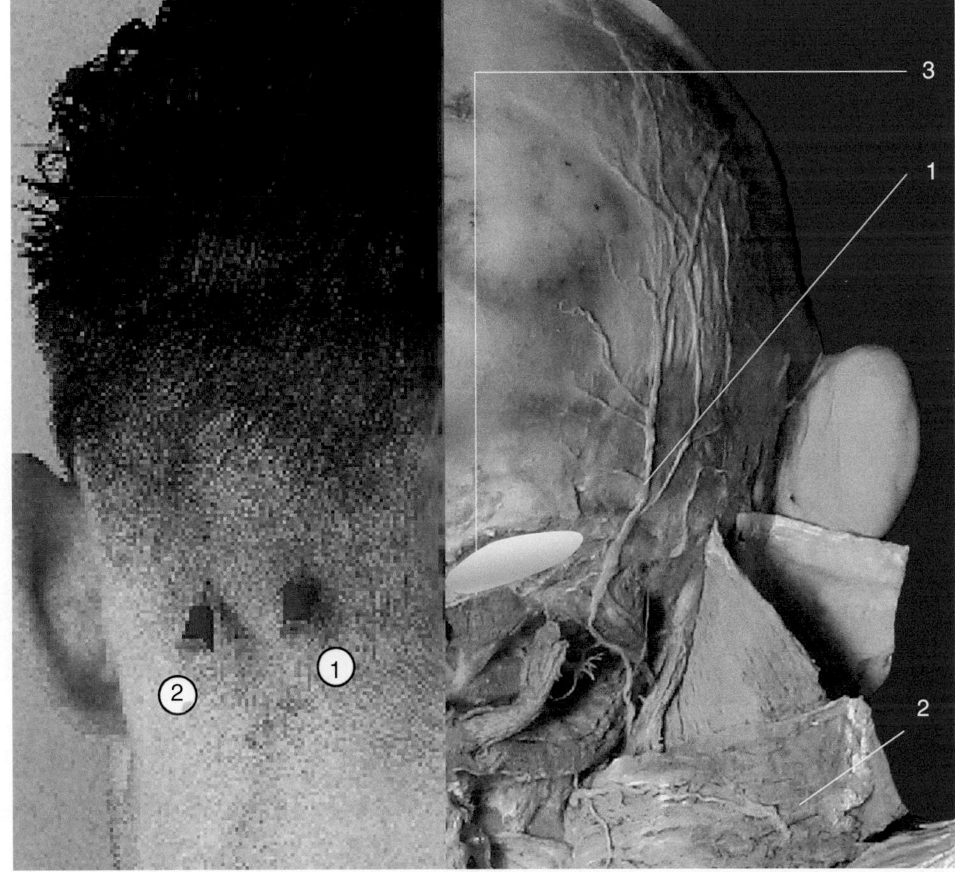

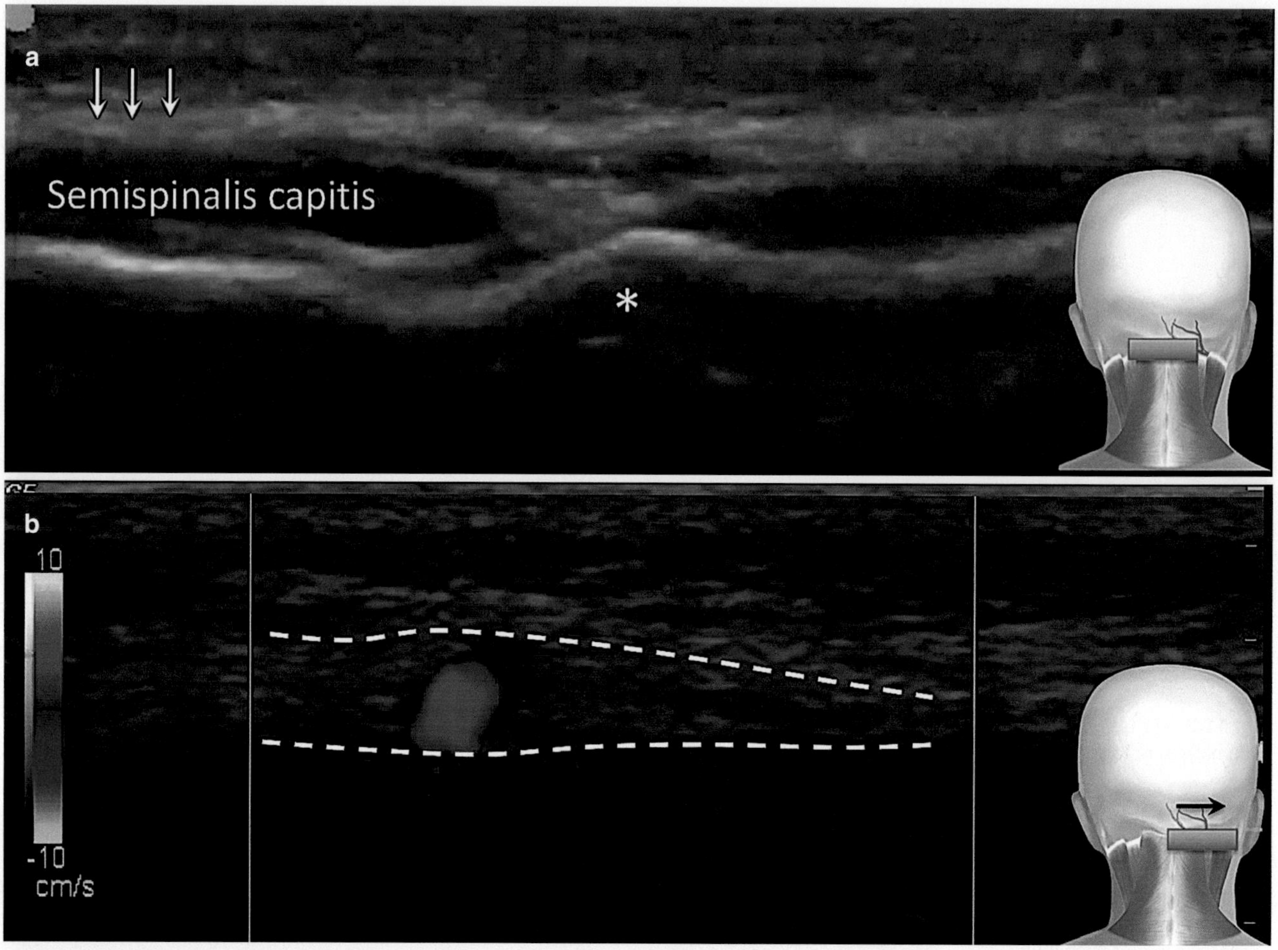

Fig. 11.4 (**a**) Sonogram shows the occipital protuberance (*). The arrows indicates the fascia. (**b**) Sonogram shows the occipital artery. The dotted line shows the fascial layer that the occipital artery and nerve reside. Reprinted with permission from Philip Peng Educational Series

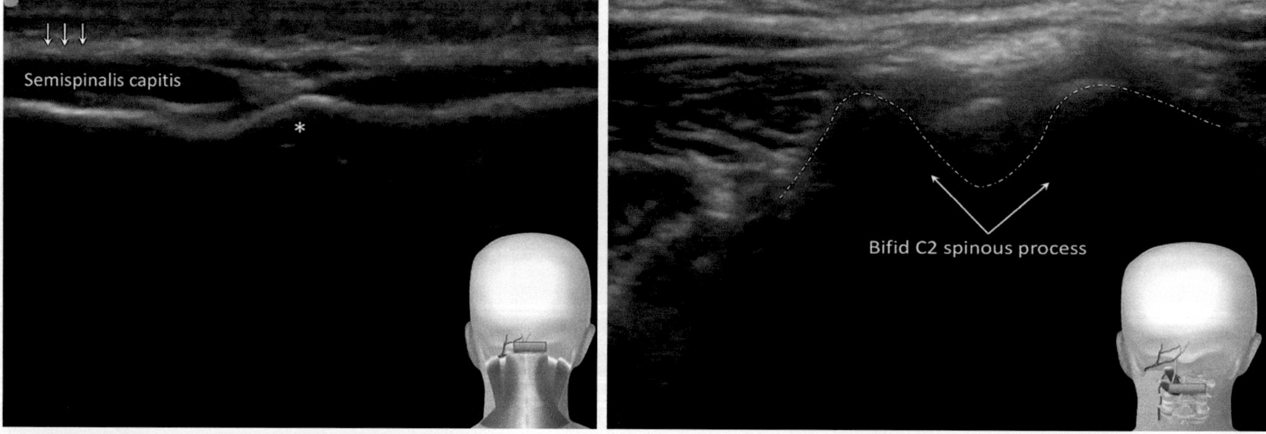

Fig. 11.5 Steps by steps of scanning for greater occipital at C2 level. Starting from occipital protuberance (left) and the probe move in caudal direction to reveal the bifid C2 spinous process. Reprinted with permission from Philip Peng Educational Series

Proximal Approach at C2

This approach aims at the nerve when it emerges below the lower border of the OCIM. Because it is deep, ultrasound should be used for guidance. Patient is positioned prone and the posterior aspect of the neck is prepped and draped in a sterile fashion. A high-frequency linear probe (12–18MH) is used and covered in sterile dressing.

The probe is positioned in a transverse orientation over the occipital protuberance and moved caudally to visualize the bifid C2 spinous process (Fig. 11.5). Then the probe is moved laterally and the lateral edge of the probe directed obliquely to the mastoid process. The C2 lamina appears boat-shaped and the obliquus capitis inferior and the semispinalis capitis visualized (Fig. 11.6). Doppler scan on the lateral side reveals the vertebral artery and the dorsal root ganglion (Fig. 11.7).

After anesthetizing the skin, a 25-G 1.5-inch needle is inserted in plane lateral to medial direction toward to greater occipital nerve, which is located in the plane separating the obliquus capitis inferior and the semispinalis capitis muscles. Needle tip position is then confirmed through hydrodissection with normal saline (Fig. 11.8). After negative aspiration, the therapeutic medication (3 ml of local anesthetic and steroid) can be injected. Injection in this fascial plane results in analgesia in the distribution of greater and lesser occipital nerve.

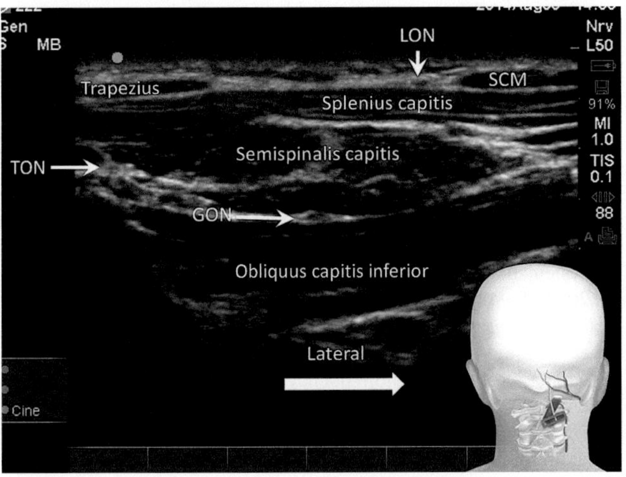

Fig. 11.6 With the medial side of the probe on the spinous process of C2 and the lateral side on the lateral mass of C1, the occipital nerves are revealed in one scan. GON, greater occipital nerve; LON, lesser occipital nerve; TON, third occipital nerve. Reprinted with permission from Philip Peng Educational Series

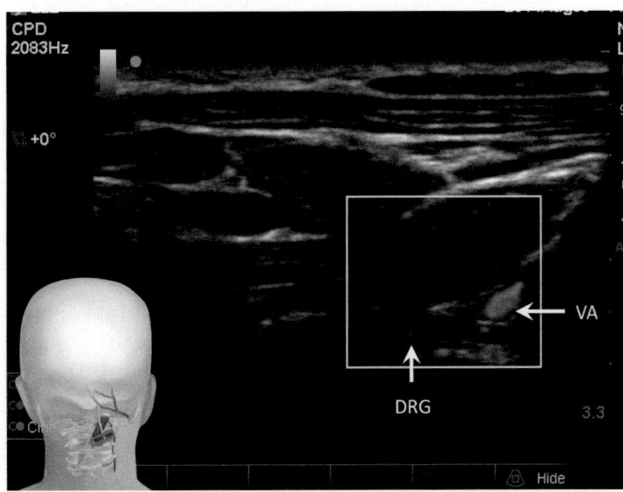

Fig. 11.7 Moving the ultrasound probe slightly laterally in Fig. 11.6, the vertebral artery (VA) and the dorsal root ganglion (DRG) of C2 are revealed. Reprinted with permission from Philip Peng Educational Series

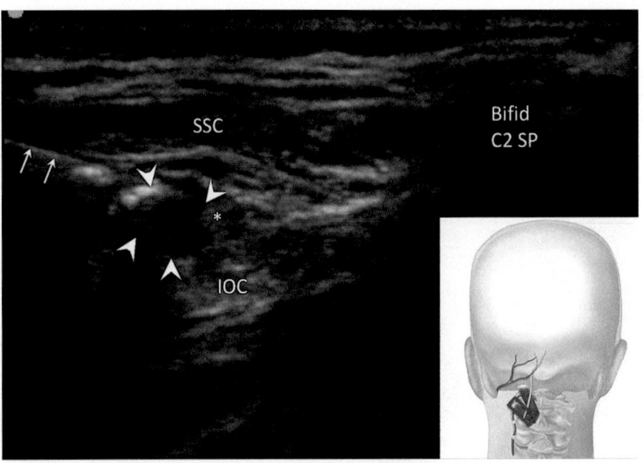

Fig. 11.8 Injection of the greater occipital nerve at Ca. The needle is indicated with arrows and the injectate with arrowheads. *SSC* semisplenius capitis, *IOC* obliquus inferior capitis; *SP* spinal process. Reprinted with permission from Philip Peng Educational Series

Technique for Lesser Occipital Nerve

The key landmark is the posterior border of the sternocleidomastoid muscle, caudal to the mastoid. The probe is moved cranially and caudally along the posterior border of sternocleidomastoid (SCM) until a nerve structure is identified (Fig. 11.9). Alternatively, it can be performed as landmark-guided technique (Fig. 11.3) when the medial border of sternocleidomastoid is traced to the superior nuchal line. In general, 1 mL of injectate is required for this nerve.

Complication

Although the most common complication is vasovagal syndrome, other complications can occur such as intravascular injection, hematoma, intramuscular injection, worsening of symptoms, and spread of local anesthetic to the brain stem (extremely rare). Infection, bleeding, nerve damage, and allergic reactions must be always taken into account, as per any procedures performed.

Practical Tips

- When performing landmark-guided technique for greater occipital nerve, the clinician should be cognizant about the superficial position of the superior nuchal line. If the needle is inserted more than 1 cm with no bony contact, the needle may be placed too caudally and should be redi-

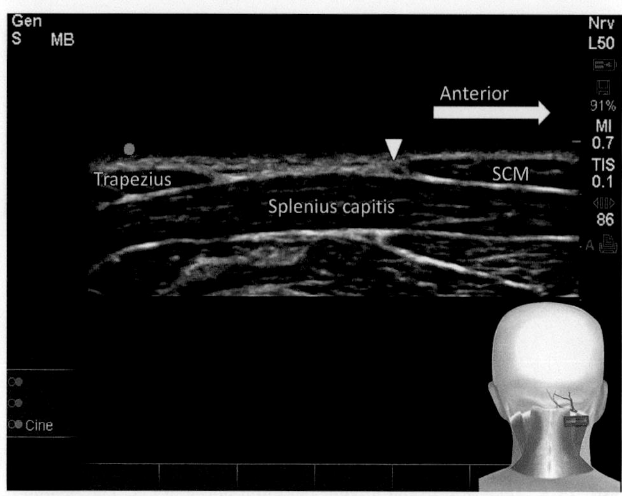

Fig. 11.9 Scanning the posterior border of sternocleidomastoid close to the nuchal line revealed the highest branch of the superficial cervical plexus, the lessor occipital nerve (arrowhead). Reprinted with permission from Philip Peng Educational Series

rected slightly in cephalad position. If this correction is not performed, the needle may end up in the spinal cord through the space between the occiput and C1.

- A block is successful if it creates absence of light-touch sensation in the dermatome of GON.
- The target area in the proximal approach is not far from the vertebral artery and epidural space; constant visualization of the needle and injectate is mandatory.
- Proximal approach might be the technique of preference for patients with occipital neuralgia, since nerve entrapment is often in proximal location.
- When performing the proximal approach, the GON is usually 3–4 cm from the midline. Quite commonly, another nerve appears in the same plane but much closer to the midline. It is the third occipital nerve.
- The angle of mandible approximates C3 level. Thus, a simpler way to find the bifid C2 spinous process is to put the transducer in midline at this level and scan in cephalad direction to search for the bifid spinous process.

Literature Review

Several studies have evaluated the efficacy of the greater occipital nerve block in different types of headache. Tobin and Flitman performed a literature review and concluded that occipital nerve block is an effective treatment for cervicogenic headache, cluster headache, and occipital neuralgia.

The choice of a distal versus a proximal approach has been a matter of debate for years. A multicenter, prospective, randomized control trial compared accuracy, effectiveness, and safety of proximal and distal techniques in patients with chronic migraines in 2019. Results demonstrate that both distal and proximal techniques can provide a short-term improvement in headache intensity, reduction in number of headache days per week, and an improvement in sleep interruption. The proximal GON technique may confer more sustained analgesic benefit compared with the distal approach in patients with chronic migraine headaches.

Consistently, trials in scientific literature showed efficacy that lasted beyond the duration of action of local anesthetics and steroids. Some small studies of pulsed radiofrequency treatment of GON have demonstrated better and longer-lasting pain relief comparing to steroid injection in patients with occipital neuralgia, migraine, or cervicogenic headache.

Suggested Reading

Ashkenazi A, Blumenfeld A, Napchan U, Narouze S, Grosberg B, Nett R, De Palma T, Rosenthal B, Tepper S, Lipton RB. Peripheral nerve blocks and trigger point injections in headache management – a systematic review and suggestions for future research. Headache. 2010;50:943–52.

Cohen SP, Peterlin BL, Fulton L, Neely ET, Kurihara C, Gupta A, et al. Randomized, double-blind, comparative-effectiveness study comparing pulsed radiofrequency to steroid injections for occipital neuralgia or migraine with occipital nerve tenderness. Pain. 2015;156(12):2585–94.

Curatolo M. Greater occipital nerve. In: Peng P, editor. Ultrasound for pain medicine intervention: a practical guide, peripheral structures, Philip Peng Educational Series, vol. 1. California: iBook, Apple Inc.; 2013. p. 13.

Ducic I, Hartmann EC, Larson EE. Indications and outcomes for surgical treatment of patients with chronic migraine headaches caused by occipital neuralgia. Plast Reconstr Surg. 2009;123(5):1453–61.

Flamer D, Alakkad H, Soneji N, Tumber P, Peng P, Kara J, Hoydonckx Y, Bhatia A. Comparison of two ultrasound-guided techniques for greater occipital nerve injections in chronic migraine: a double blind, randomized, controlled trial. Reg Anesth Pain Med. 2019;44(5):595–603.

Gille O, Lavignolle B, Vital JM. Vital: Surgical treatment of greater occipital neuralgia by neurolysis of the greater occipital nerve and sectioning of the inferior oblique muscle. Spine. 2004;29(7):828–32.

Greher M, Moriggl B, Curatolo M, Kirchmair L, Eichenberger U. Sonographic visualization and ultrasound-guided blockade of the greater occipital nerve: a comparison of two selective techniques confirmed by anatomical dissection. Br J Anaesthesia. 2010;104:637–42.

Jankovic D. Occipital nerves. In: Jankovic D, editor. Regional nerve blocks and infiltration therapy. Malden: Blackwell; 2004. p. 30–2.

Jurgens TP, Muller P, Seedorf H, Regelsberger J, May A. Occipital nerve block is effective in craniofacial neuralgias but not in idiopathic persistent facial pain. J Headache Pain. 2012;13:199–213.

Klinger M, Villani F, Klinger F, Gaetani P, Rodriguez Y, Baena R, Levi D. Anatomical variations of the occipital nerves: implications for the treatment of chronic headaches. Plast Reconstr Surg. 2009;124(5):1727–8.

Lauretti G, Correa S, Mattos A. Efficacy of the greater occipital nerve block for cervicogenic headache: comparing classical and subcompartmental techniques. Pain Pract. 2015;15:654–61.

Ploveran EJ, Kowacs PA, Tatsui CE, Lange MC, Ribas LC, Wernek LC. Referred pain after painful stimulation of the greater occipital nerve in humans: evidence of convergence of cervical afferents on trigeminal nuclei. Cephalalgia. 2001;21:107–9.

Tobin J, Flitman S. Occipital nerve blocks: when and what inject? Headache. 2009;49(10):1521–33.

Tubbs RS, Mortzavi MM, Loukas M, et al. Anatomical study of the third occipital nerve and its potential role in occipital headache/neck pain following midline dissections of the craniocervical junction. J Neurosurg Spine. 2011;15(1):71–5.

Tubbs RS, Salter EG, Wellons JC, et al. Landmarks for the identification of the cutaneous nerves of the occiput and nuchal regions. Clin Anat. 2007;20(3):235–8.

Cervical Sympathetic Chain and Superior Cervical Ganglion Block

12

Paul Tumber and Danilo Jankovic

Contents

P. Tumber (✉)
Department of Anesthesiology and Pain Medicine, University of Toronto, Toronto, ON, Canada
e-mail: paul.tumber@uhn.ca

D. Jankovic
Pain Management Centre DGS – Cologne – Huerth, Cologne-Hurth, Germany
e-mail: danilo@jankovic1.de

D. Jankovic, P. Peng (eds.), *Regional Nerve Blocks in Anesthesia and Pain Therapy*,
https://doi.org/10.1007/978-3-030-88727-8_12

General Considerations: Stellate Ganglion Block

Concurrent with the advent of ultrasound guidance technology, the stellate ganglion block (SGB) has become a sympatholytic procedure that can now be safely performed without the need for fluoroscopy or blind palpation techniques. The initial description of using ultrasound to directly visualize the spread of local anesthesia in the neck for an SGB was by Kapral and colleagues in 1995, and this was refined and validated by Gofeld and colleagues in 2009. The volume required to perform an SGB has been reduced from 10–15 cc to 4–5 cc, and with the refinement offered by a proper ultrasound technique, there has been an associated reduction in undesirable complications such as life-threatening hematoma.

Indications

The cervical sympathetic nervous system is involved with a myriad of structures, including viscera, sweat glands, and blood vessels, and the innervation extends to the eyes, face, brain, head and neck, heart, and upper extremity (Fig.12.1). Therefore, there is a corresponding range of indications and case reports highlighting the potential benefits of a SGB, although the effects may only be short-lived and may require repeat injections.

Painful medical conditions involving the head, neck, or upper extremity

- Sympathetically mediated pain/complex regional pain syndromes.
- Acute herpes zoster or post-herpetic neuralgia.
- Phantom limb pain.
- Headache (e.g., cluster, migraine, atypical facial pain).
- Intractable angina pectoris.
- Joint stiffness.
- Post-stroke pain (contralateral block).

Non-painful medical conditions

- Raynaud's.
- Hyperhidrosis.
- Lymphedema after breast amputation.
- Traumatic cerebral edema.
- Post-traumatic stress disorder.
- Vascular conditions (obliterative vascular disease, cerebral vasospasm).
- Cardiac conditions (refractory ventricular arrhythmias).
- Postmenopausal flushing.
- Ménierè's disease, sudden sensorineural hearing loss, and tinnitus.
- Positive effect on the immune system.

Contraindications

Anticoagulation treatment, contralateral paresis of the phrenic nerve or recurrent laryngeal nerve, glaucoma, severe emphysema, and simultaneous bilateral block.

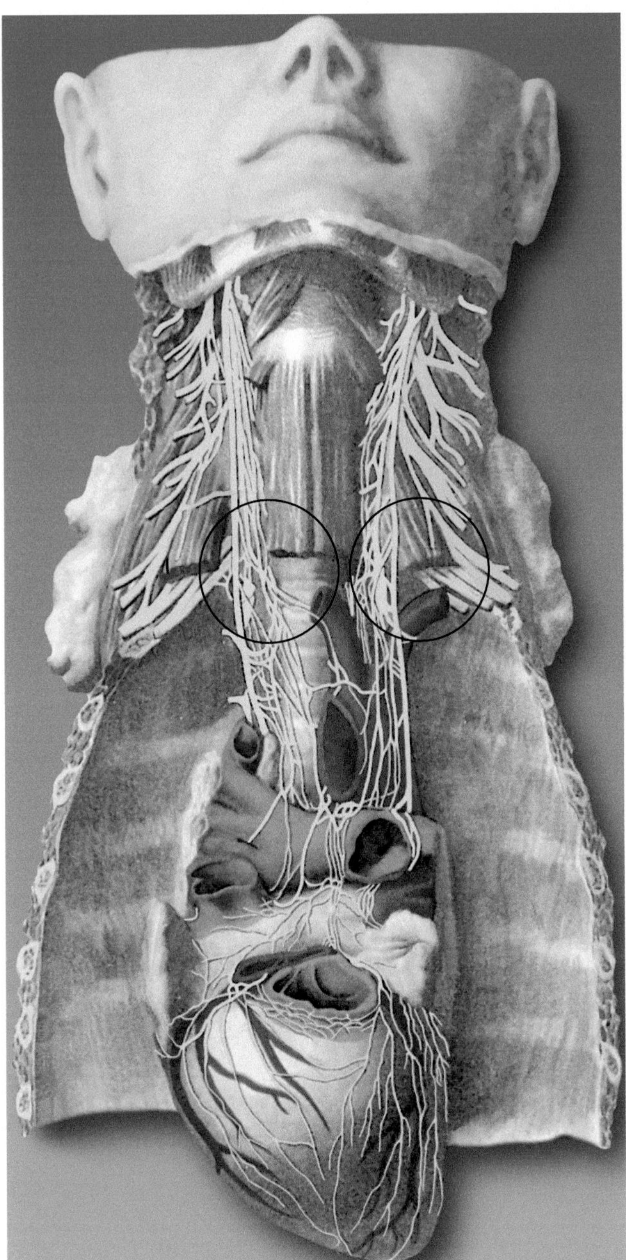

Fig. 12.1 Fibers from the gray rami communicantes *(circles)* supply the heart, esophagus, airways, and thymus (Reproduced with permission from Danilo Jankovic)

Functional Anatomy

Sympathetic nerve cell bodies exist in the first few thoracic segments and send preganglionic sympathetic nerve fibers that ascend through the paravertebral cervical sympathetic chain. These nerve fibers synapse in the superior, middle, and inferior cervical ganglions. In approximately 80% of the population, there is a fusion of the inferior cervical ganglion with the first thoracic ganglion, and this structure is termed the cervicothoracic ganglion but is more commonly known as the stellate ganglion. The size and development of the STG are subject to considerable variation. Average sizes of between 25 mm (15–50 mm) × 3–10 mm × 5 mm have been reported. This average corresponds to the superior cervical ganglion size and is much more voluminous than the middle cervical ganglion. Some authors have only been able to identify it in 38% of individuals studied (Fig. 12.2). The stellate ganglion is situated in the region of the lower part of C7 extending to the T1 transverse process. The STG is deep to the prevertebral fascia, is often just anterior or superior to the neck of the first rib, and is closely located medial or posterior to the vertebral artery in proximity to the dome of the pleura (Fig. 12.3). Some practitioners attempted to block the STG at the C7-T1 region, but several serious complications are possible at this level, and thus it has considered safer to block the cervical sympathetic ganglia and chain at the C6 level instead. The middle cervical ganglion is variable in location and size, although it is the smallest of the three cervical sympathetic ganglia and is likely blocked at the C6 level although this has not been rigorously studied. Performance of a STB at the C6 level relies on a planar spread of the local anesthesia between the prevertebral fascia layer and the surface of the longus colli muscle in order to block the stellate ganglion (Figs. 12.4, 12.5, and 12.6). It is also judicious to choose C6 as the level for the injection as the vertebral artery becomes protected from potential needle injury as it dives into the bony foramen transversarium in at least 90% of subjects (Fig. 12.7).

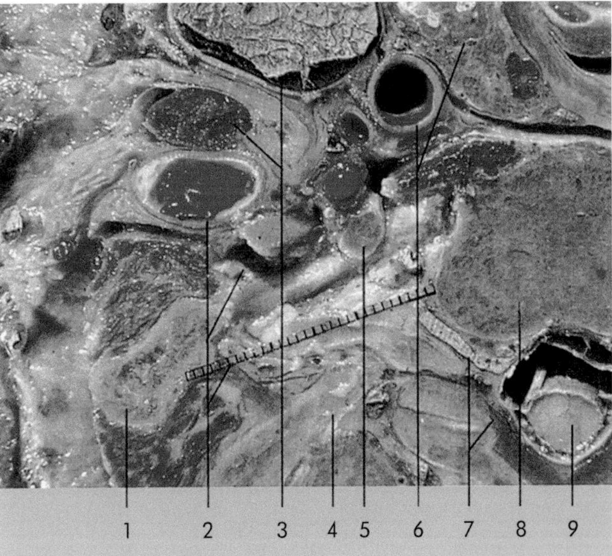

Fig. 12.2 The immediate vicinity of the ganglion (transverse section). *(1)* First rib, *(2)* subclavian artery and scalenus anterior muscle, *(3)* jugular vein, *(4)* second rib, *(5)* cervicothoracic ganglion, *(6)* common carotid artery and thyroid gland, *(7)* T2 intervertebral artery and zygapophyseal joint, *(8)* T2 vertebral body, *(9)* spinal medulla. The average size of the cervicothoracic ganglion is 25 mm × 3–10 mm × 5 mm (Reproduced with permission from Danilo Jankovic)

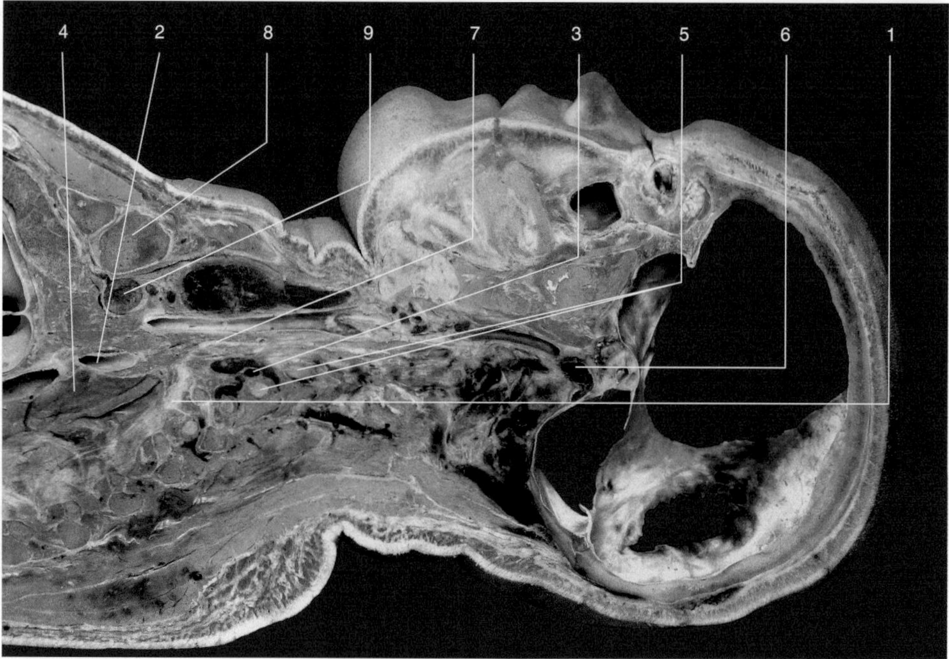

Fig. 12.3 Paramedian sagittal dissection (head and thorax): *(1)* Stellate ganglion, *(2)* the subclavian artery, *(3)* the vertebral artery, *(4)* pleura, *(5)* the brachial plexus, *(6)* the carotid artery, *(7)* the vagus nerve, *(8)* clavicle, *(9)* V. brachiocephalica (Reproduced with permission from Danilo Jankovic)

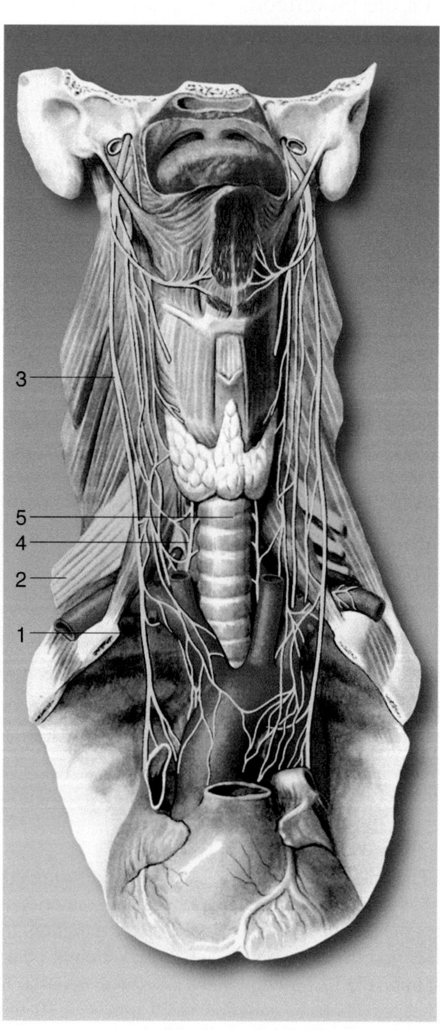

Fig. 12.4 The immediate vicinity of the stellate ganglion: *(1)* pleura, *(2)* brachial plexus, *(3)* vagus nerve, *(4)* recurrent laryngeal nerve, *(5)* trachea (Reproduced with permission from Danilo Jankovic)

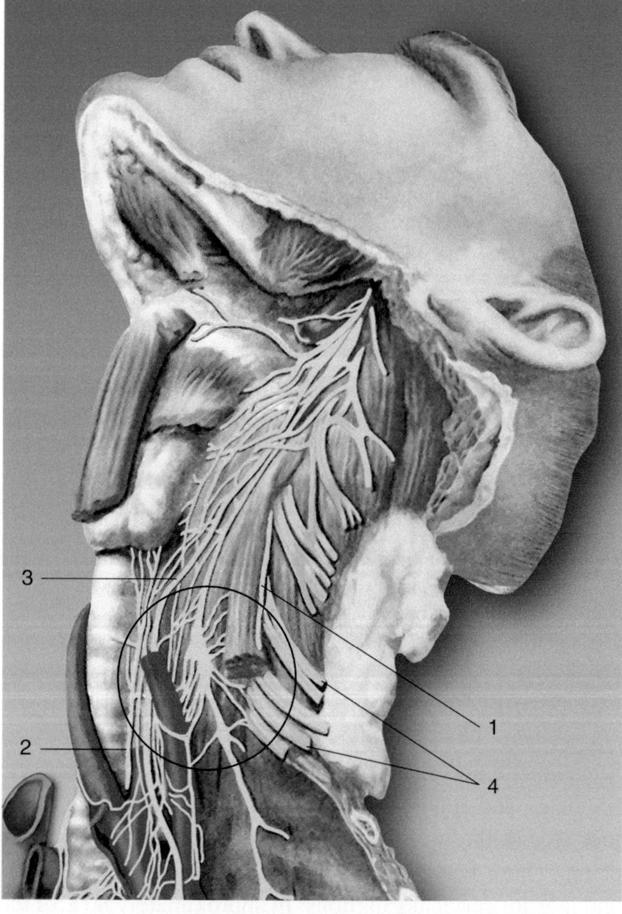

Fig. 12.5 Close anatomical connections in the ganglion trunk include those to *(1)* the phrenic nerve, *(2)* the recurrent laryngeal nerve, *(3)* the vagus nerve, and *(4)* the brachial plexus (Reproduced with permission from Danilo Jankovic)

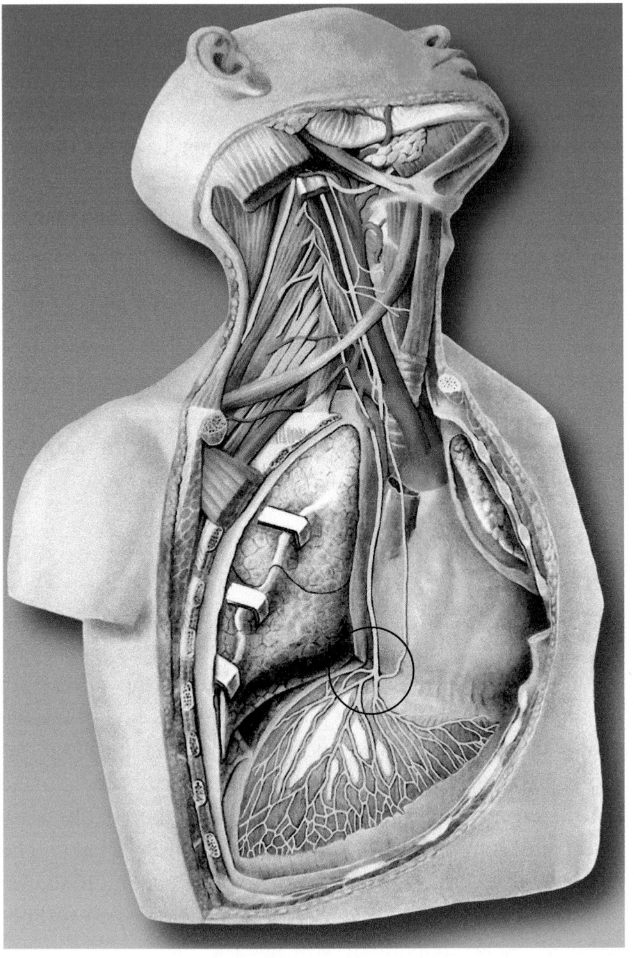

Fig. 12.6 Course of the phrenic nerve (*circle* shows the end position of the phrenic nerve). (Reproduced with permission from Danilo Jankovic)

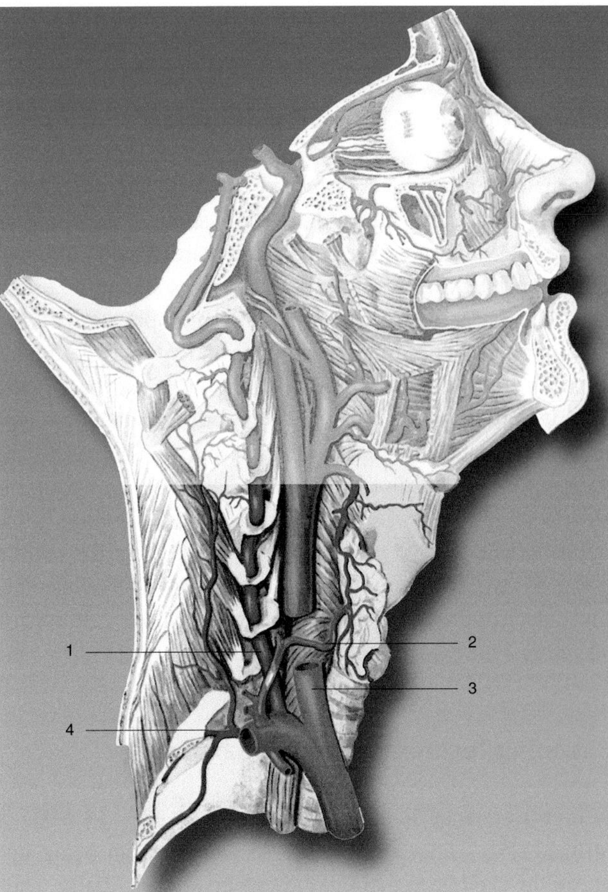

Fig. 12.7 Risk of intravascular injection into *(1)* the vertebral artery, *(2)* the inferior thyroid artery, *(3)* the carotid artery, and *(4)* the first intercostal artery (Reproduced with permission from Danilo Jankovic)

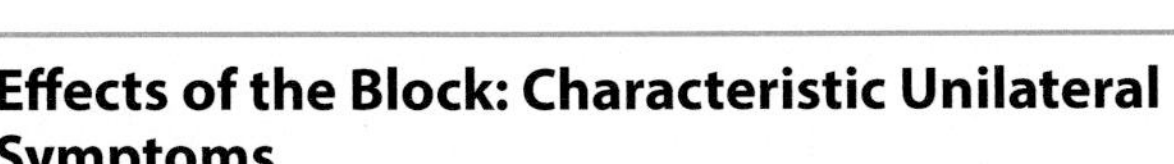

Effects of the Block: Characteristic Unilateral Symptoms

Block of the STG can denervate sympathetic supply to the head, neck, and upper extremity. A successful block is demonstrated most commonly by an ipsilateral Horner's syndrome (Fig. 12.8) and an increased skin temperature of at least 1° Celsius. Other techniques to confirm a successful block include the observation of an abolished skin resistance response and increased skin blood flow. It is possible to completely block the STG in some individuals, but there may still be sympathetic innervation maintained to the upper extremity. Such a situation may occur if there is anomalous sympathetic innervation via gray rami communicantes from the second thoracic sympathetic ganglia that pass directly to the upper limb via a second thoracic nerve that joins the first thoracic spinal nerve and ultimately onto the brachial plexus. These anomalous pathways are known as the Kuntz nerves and maybe a reason for a partial or failed effect of an STGB on the upper extremity.

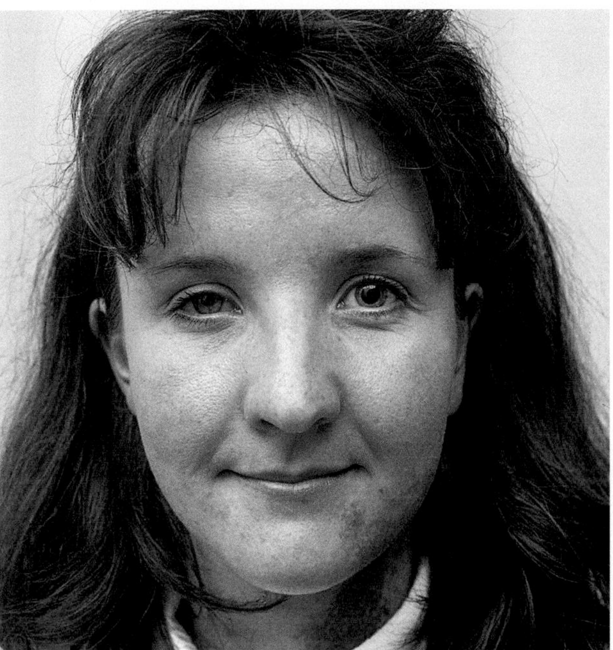

Fig. 12.8 Horner's syndrome: Note ptosis, miosis, anhidrosis, and unilateral conjunctival engorgement. (Reproduced with permission from Danilo Jankovic)

Procedure for Ultrasound-Guided Stellate Ganglion Block

Preparation and Patient Positioning

The patient should be fasted as per standard anesthesia guidelines and have standard monitors applied, including an automated blood pressure cuff, electrocardiogram, and continuous pulse oximeter. Intravenous access should be established in order to treat any potential complication. Light sedation may be necessary to help the patient relax their neck muscles and shoulder, and a slight head up or reverse Trendelenburg position may help to reduce venous congestion and reduce the size of the internal jugular vein. The patient can be placed supine or turned slightly away from the side to be blocked with a wedge. The head is turned to the opposite side to help increase the distance from the carotid artery to the C6 anterior tubercle, and this can be adjusted to find the optimal position under real-time ultrasound scanning.

Scanning Technique and Sonoanatomy

A high-frequency linear ultrasound probe of 6–13 MHz is utilized (Fig. 12.9a, b). Transverse scanning can begin just above the clavicle to identify the carotid artery initially. Then deep and lateral to this can be visualized the pulsatile vertebral artery and C7 nerve root, lateral to which is the C7 posterior tubercle. The vertebral artery can then be tracked cephalad as the transducer maintains a transverse orientation, and it will disappear as it enters the C6 transverse process in 90% of individuals, whereas in the remainder, the vertebral artery will enter the bony canal at C5. The level of C6 is confirmed by the presence of a prominent anterior tubercle and a smaller posterior one, whereas at C5 the two tubercles are similar in size. At the C6 level, the longus colli muscle can be seen deep to the carotid artery and carotid sheath (which also contains the vagus nerve and internal jugular vein). Superficial and lateral to the longus colli may be seen a smaller muscle which may be the longus capitis muscle. The needle tip's target will be a plane deep to the prevertebral fascia between the longus capitis and longus colli muscles. The middle cervical ganglion or cervical sympathetic chain may be seen in some individuals immediately overlying the longus colli muscle.

Technique

Typically, the needle is directed from lateral to medial, and an in-plane approach is used to visualize the needle tip throughout the procedure. Once the target is identified, the probe should be adjusted such that the lateral end of the probe just overlies the US image of the anterior tubercle and not the corresponding foramen. This way, the needle has a direct and short path to the target from the probe's lateral end and can bypass the neurovascular structures lateral to the C6 anterior tubercle. A 25-gauge, 1.5-inch needle often suffices although some individuals will need a 25G or 22G spinal needle (3.5 inch) to reach the target. Before needle placement, a color Doppler scan should rule out the presence of

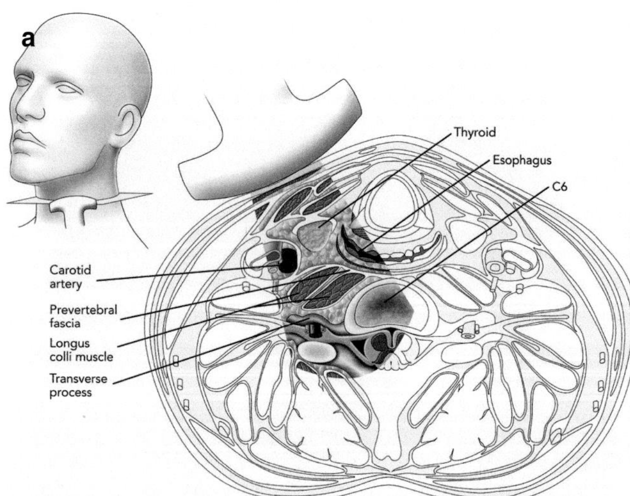

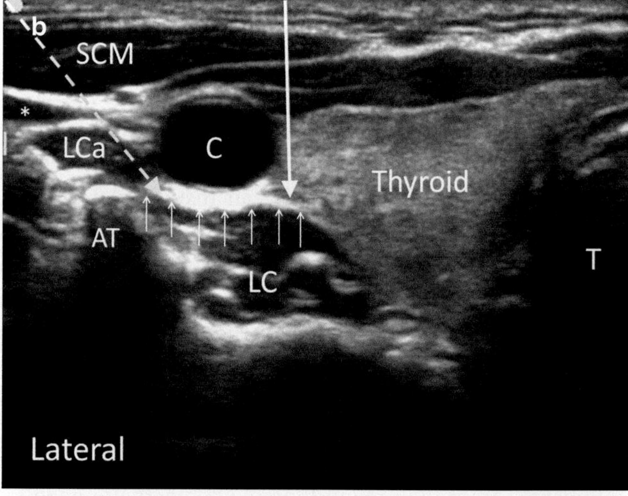

Fig. 12.9 (**a**) Cross section of the neck at the sixth cervical vertebral level correlating with the ultrasonographic image. (**b**) Ultrasonographic image of neck at C6. *C6* sixth cervical vertebra, *C* carotid artery, *, internal jugular vein (compressed), *SCM* sternocleidomastoid muscle, *LC* longus colli muscle, *LCa* longus capitis muscle, *T* airway, *AT* anterior tubercle. The prevertebral fascia is marked by small solid arrows. The needle paths of anterior and lateral approach are marked by long solid and dotted arrow, respectively. (Reproduced with permission from Philip Peng Educational Series)

any arteries such as the transverse inferior thyroid or smaller ascending cervical arteries that may be in the path of the needle (Figs. 12.10 and 12.11). Occasionally, a more medial out-of-plane approach may be necessary and care should be taken to visualize the needle tip as best possible as it may traverse vessels and the thyroid gland itself. In all cases, hydrodissection with small amounts of normal saline should be employed before any local anesthesia injection. Once the needle is in position, negative aspiration is confirmed.

A test dose of 0.5 mL of the local anesthetic may then be injected to confirm proper spread and lack of any immediate adverse response. A final volume of 4–5 mL is adequate to elicit a STGB, and bupivacaine 0.25–0.5% is often used (Fig. 12.12). An ipsilateral Horner's syndrome should develop within a few minutes, and the patient should be observed for a minimum of 30 minutes after the procedure to ensure a lack of any undesirable adverse effects such as a recurrent laryngeal nerve palsy.

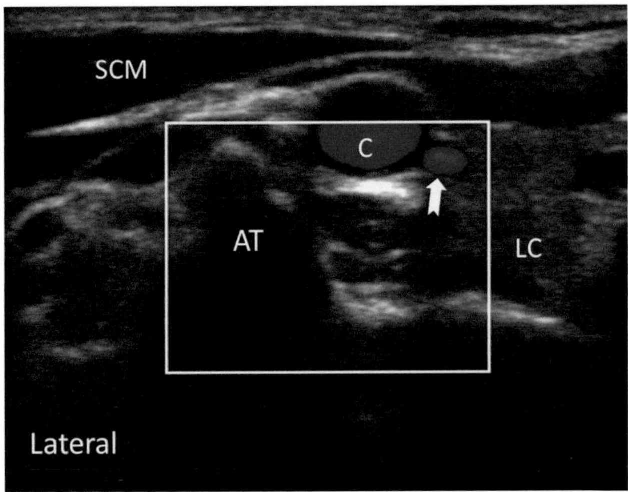

Fig. 12.10 Ultrasonographic image of neck at C6 level on the right side showing a vessel in the short axis (bold arrows). LC, longus colli muscle; C, carotid artery; SCM, sternocleidomastoid muscle; AT, anterior tubercle. (Reproduced with permission from Philip Peng Educational Series)

Dosage

Local anesthetic (e.g., 0.2–0.375–0.5 ropivacaine, 0.25–0.5% bupivacaine (0.25–0.5% levobupivacaine), or 1% prilocaine, 1% lidocaine, 1% mepivacaine).

- "Low dose" for indications in the head region (cerebrofacial effects): 2 mL (for traditional technique: 2–3 mL)
- "Medium-high dose" for indications in the shoulder and arm region: 4–5 mL (for traditional blind technique: 8–10 mL)

In acute intractable pain (e.g., postzosteric neuralgia), low dose of local anesthetic could be combined with steroids, opioids, or clonidine in mixture.

Block Series

If the clinical picture being treated does not show temporary improvement after the second block, there is no point in performing series of treatments. Otherwise, for all indications mentioned, a series of six to ten blocks can be carried out typically 5–7 days apart. In difficult cases (e.g., herpes zoster ophthalmicus), further blocks can also be carried out when there is a visible trend toward improvement.

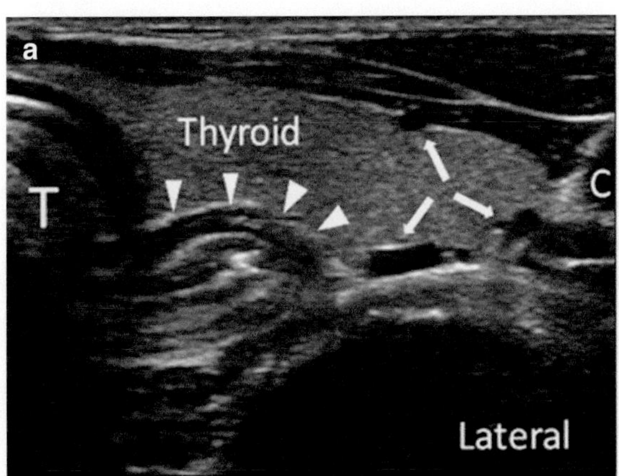

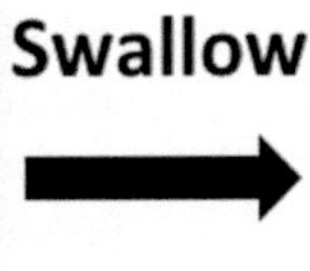

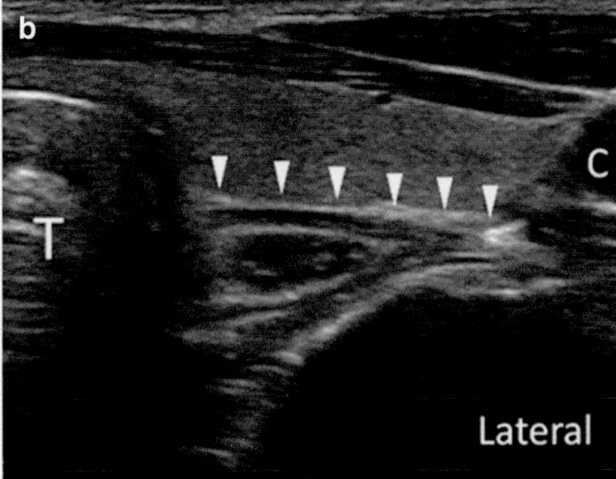

Fig. 12.11 (**a**, **b**) Ultrasonographic image of the neck at C7 level showing the variation of position of the esophagus with swallowing. (**a**) Before swallowing, the esophagus (arrow heads) was seen covering half of the distance between the trachea (T) and carotid artery (C); (**b**) During swallowing, the esophagus moved laterally toward the carotid artery, virtually covering the whole area between the trachea and carotid artery. Note that the bold arrows showed the presence of three vessels in the pre-swallow scan. Swallowing action was evident by the increased in hyperechogenic shadow in the trachea. (Reproduced with permission from Philip Peng Educational Series)

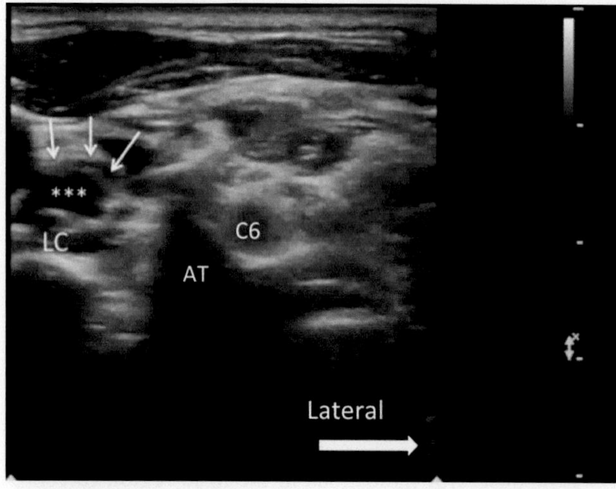

Fig. 12.12 Ultrasonographic image of the neck at C6 level showing the local anesthetic spread within the prevertebral fascia following the injection. *C6* C6 nerve root, *AT* anterior tubercle of C6, *LC* longus colli muscle, *arrows* prevertebral fascia; *** local anesthetic. (Reproduced with permission from Philip Peng Educational Series)

Side Effects

- Partial block of the following nerves :
  - *Phrenic nerve* (ipsilateral phrenic nerve palsy and hemidiaphragm paralysis), main symptom: dyspnea with normal auscultation findings (Fig. 12.6).
  - *Vagus nerve*, main symptom: tachycardia and hypertension (Fig. 12.4).
  - *Recurrent laryngeal nerve*, main symptom: foreign body sensation in the throat and hoarseness. It should be noted here that in ca. 43% of individuals, anastomoses with the cervicothoracic ganglion are found (Figs. 12.4 and 12.5).
  - *Brachial plexus*: a partial brachial plexus block may occur if the local anesthetic spreads into the area of the roots of C6–T1 (Fig. 12.5).
- Hematoma formation (may occur in the neck but is rarely dangerous when proper ultrasound techniques are employed). Carotid puncture in a patient with atherosclerosis can lead to cerebrovascular ischemia or stroke.
- Persistent coughing.
- Locked-in syndrome.
- Bradycardia.

Complications

Intravascular Injection

Leading to seizure, coma, and cardiovascular collapse as it is recognized that even small amounts of local anesthesia injected in arteries in the neck can lead to disastrous effects (see Chap. 5, "Local Anesthetic Systemic Toxicity"). In particular, there is a risk of injection into the vertebral artery (the diameter of which is ca. 0.3 mm larger on the left side than on the right). More rarely, there is a risk of puncturing the carotid artery, the inferior thyroid artery, or the first intercostal artery (Fig. 12.7).

Epidural or Subarachnoid Injection

(See Chap. 41, Neuraxial Blocks: Spinal and Epidural Anesthesia; Complications, p.604). There is a risk of perforating the dural membrane if the needle is inserted incorrectly toward the nerve root. Cerebrospinal fluid (CSF) pressure is very low in the cervical area and it is almost impossible to aspirate CSF. High epidural anesthesia or high spinal anesthesia is extremely rare. It can lead to bradycardia, hypotension, and possibly to respiratory arrest and loss of consciousness. The first signs are heaviness in the limbs, sweating, dyspnea, apprehension, and anxiety.

Pneumothorax (Figs. 12.3 and 12.6)

The incidence of this complication is low. If it occurs at all, it usually produces a small pneumothorax that resolves spontaneously. If there is suspicion of a pneumothorax, a chest radiograph is required after 4–6 h.

- Esophageal perforation or tracheal perforation (extremely rare)
- Cardiac arrest

Practical Tips

Patients should be forewarned about the expected development of a Horner's syndrome as a sign of a successful block and the expected warmth that develops in the upper extremity if it is cold beforehand. Patients should understand beforehand the challenge posed by the STGB and that it is not unusual to have some degree of hoarseness, dysphagia, and foreign body sensation for hours after the block. When performing the US-guided block, it is easy to apply enough pressure with the transducer to occlude the internal jugular vein, so the pressure should be minimal at first to help identify this structure, and then more pressure is applied as it improves visualization of the target. It may be necessary for the needle to traverse the IJ vein and this does not normally cause a problem. In some patients, it may be helpful to angle the probe with the medial end more caudad than the lateral end of the probe as this may help improve the visualization of a clear trajectory from lateral to medial and assist in avoiding the carotid artery contents. Inject only a small amount of lidocaine to anesthetize the skin before needle placement as the lidocaine may cause undesirable numbness on the side of the neck by blocking branches of the superficial cervical plexus. If the correct subfascial plane is not easy to visualize, then one can deliberately advance the needle into the longus colli muscle. Then an injection of small 0.5 mL aliquots with slow withdrawal of the needle tip will allow visualization of the change in the spread seen from the typical intramuscular injection pattern to the anticipated planar spread pattern seen just under the prevertebral fascia (the injectate should envelope the longus colli muscle in an inverted U shape).

Literature Review

There are various case reports of STGB being therapeutic for several painful and non-painful conditions involving the upper extremity, head, neck, and heart. Typically, local anesthesia is employed, but there have been reports of using pulsed radiofrequency of the stellate ganglion. There is also a report of using long-acting liposomal bupivacaine to try and prolong the benefit from a STGB as well as placing a catheter for continuous infiltration of local anesthesia. In current practice, a stellate ganglion block is commonly performed with US guidance at the C6 level, and it blocks a length of the cervical sympathetic chain from about C4 to the first thoracic vertebral level. Ultrasound has the added benefit of being a portable technique that allows one to avoid radiation exposure. The use of US guidance allows for identifying important structures relevant to the successful blockade of the cervical sympathetic chain. It is critical to maintain real-time visualization of the needle as it advances toward the target in addition to using hydrodissection with normal saline before active drug administration. There is still a need for more research to support many of the reported indications for stellate ganglion blockade.

Traditional Approach for SGB (Paratracheal Anterior Technique)

The injection can be made at the level of C6 or C7. The transverse process of the sixth cervical vertebra is easily palpated at the level of the cricoid; the distance from the pleura is greater and there is less danger of puncturing the vertebral artery. Block at the level of C7 can extend as far as T3, with a reduced dose of local anesthetic. However, the likelihood of injuring the pleura or puncturing the vertebral artery is greater here (Fig. 12.13). For palpation of the site between the larynx and the sternocleidomastoid muscle, a cushion is placed under the shoulder blades and the head is tilted back. The index and middle fingers are moved between the trachea and sternocleidomastoid muscle to locate the pulse in the common carotid artery. This is displaced laterally together with the medial margin of the sternocleidomastoid muscle. After skin infiltration, a 22-gauge, 3–5-cm needle with injection tube (depending on patient's anatomy) is introduced vertical to the skin at this point and advanced until bone contact is made with the transverse process (2–4 cm). After bone contact, the needle is withdrawn about 1–2 mm, and with careful aspiration at various levels, an initial test dose of 0.5–1 mL of the local anesthetic is injected (Fig. 12.14). After approximately 1 min, slow injection of the remaining dose can be injected in small portions. Two effects of the block need to be distinguished: after 1–2 min, Horner's syndrome develops due to cerebral facial spread. This can be achieved with a low dose of the local anesthetic. Complete block, including the shoulder and arm region, requires a higher dose, and the local anesthetic needs to spread as far as T4.

Practical Tips

If there is no bone contact or paresthesias in the brachial plexus are elicited, the needle must be withdrawn and corrected medially. If the transverse process is still not reached, the needle's direction should be carefully corrected caudally or cranially. A single test dose by no means guarantees correct positioning of the needle. The remaining dose must never be injected quickly and carelessly. It must be adminis-

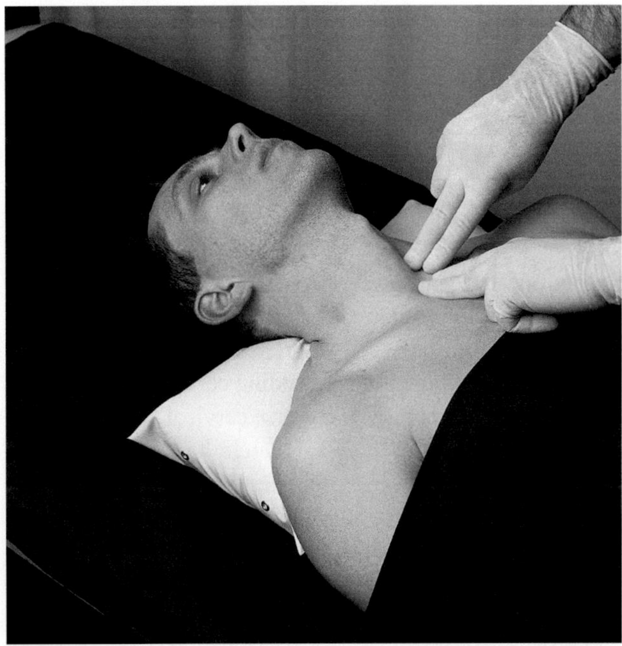

Fig. 12.13 Two-finger method of locating the level of C7 (Reproduced with permission from Danilo Jankovic)

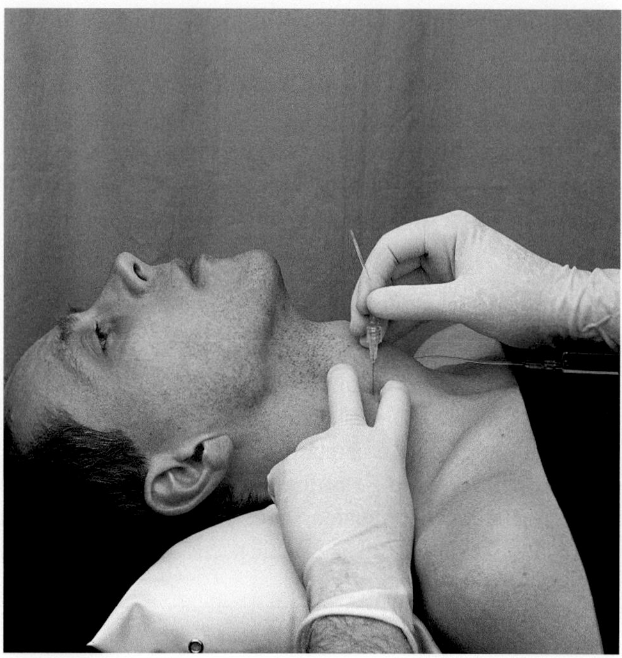

Fig. 12.14 The immobile needle with injection tube is introduced vertical to the skin and advanced until bone contact is made with the transverse process. After bone contact, the needle is withdrawn ca. 1–2 mm. The injection is carried out after aspiration in various levels. (Reproduced with permission from Danilo Jankovic)

tered slowly in small quantities (several test doses) with constant aspiration.

Disadvantages and Limitations of Non-ultrasound-Guided Approaches

Possible consequences of non-ultrasound-guided approaches are as follows:

- Potential for penetration of vascular structures and intravascular injection:

  Retropharyngeal and cervicomediastinal hematomas after SGB have been reported despite negative aspiration tests, causing severe airway compromise. Possibility of other arteries of risk (e.g., the ascending cervical branch of the inferior thyroid artery, transverse cervical artery) that traverse over the C6 anterior tubercle has also been mentioned. Narouze and Siegenthaler found that the vertebral or other arteries were located in the needle path for traditional approach for SGB in over 28% of subjects, while Bhatia and colleagues reported that major vessel was observed in up to 29 and 43% of patients at the C6 and C7 levels, respectively. It was also noted that the vertebral artery was outside the foramen transversarium in 7% of subjects at the C6 level.

- Potential for penetration of the esophagus, pleura, lateral lobes of the thyroid gland, and cervical nerve roots:

  The recent studies have indicated that the *esophagus* is frequently located in the needle path of SGB performed using traditional approaches. The esophagus was located along the needle path in 37–50% and 65–74% of subjects at the C6 and C7 levels, respectively, in these studies. *Pneumothorax* is also a potential complication with anatomic landmark- or fluoroscopy-guided techniques, primarily if a SGB is performed at the C7 level. Finally, a needle traversing through the *thyroid gland* can result in a hematoma, and exiting *cervical nerve roots* can also be traumatized during SGB.

Conclusion

In addition to the risk of potential complications with traditional approaches for SGB, *precision in the deposition of the injectate and adequacy of its spread to the first and second thoracic vertebral levels* are vital considerations for ensuring efficacy. The location of CST is in the loose connective tissues of the prevertebral fascia. However, traditional approaches rely on contact with bony landmarks (transverse processes of C6 or C7) followed by the needle's withdrawal by a few millimeters and then injection. The spread of injectate seen with these approaches has been anterior to the prevertebral fascia and in most patients' paratracheal space, without much caudal spread In contrast a subfascial injection results in a more caudal spread, a higher rate of sympathetic block of the upper limbs, and a lower incidence of blockade of the vagus or recurrent laryngeal nerve.

General Considerations: Superior Cervical Ganglion Block

The SCG is the largest of the three cervical sympathetic ganglia. Selective block of this ganglia can be therapeutic for a variety of craniofacial conditions, and the block may now be performed with ultrasonography whereas in the past a blind intraoral or fluoroscopic/CT approach was required. Most of the evidence reported about this selective block is limited to case series or retrospective analysis. More research is needed to determine the optimal technique and volume of local anesthesia to use and understand its role versus a standard cervical sympathetic ganglion block performed at the C6 level. This does not appear to be a common block, and there are no active research trials underway according to Clinical Trials.gov.

Indications

The areas of application are partly identical to those for the stellate block, but due to its marked cerebro-facial effects, the superior cervical ganglion block (SCGB) is particularly suitable in situations where there was pain or dysfunction involving the head and face, such as:

- Migraine,
- Cluster headache, headaches of cervical origin,
- Neuropathic pain of the head/neck region,
- Cerebral vasospasm and microvascular ischemia,
- Central post-stroke syndrome (contralateral block!),
- Peripheral facial paralysis facial pain,
- Vertigo (of vertebral origin),
- Tinnitus,
- Trigeminal neuralgia in the 1st and 2nd branches*,
- Acute herpes zoster or post-herpetic neuralgias (otic, ophthalmic)*,
- Glossopharyngeal neuralgia,
- Hyperhidrosis in the head region,
- Asthma, allergic coryza,
- Depression (S.below)

* SCGB in combination with pterygopalatine ganglion block may be useful (Coauthors clinical experience over many years) (See. Chaps. 8 and 9)

Contraindications

(See above, SGB)

Functional Anatomy (Figs. 12.15, 12.16, 12.17, and 12.18)

The SCG is usually formed by the fusion of the upper four cervical paravertebral sympathetic ganglia and contains the preganglionic sympathetic nerve fibers that synapse with postganglionic sympathetic fibers that travel widely to the head and neck. Rami communicants connect the SCG with structures such as the carotid arteries, the pharyngeal plexus of CN IX (glossopharyngeal) and CN X (vagus) (Figs. 12.15, 12.16, and 12.17) the eye, tympanic and choroid plexus, lacrimal gland, salivary glands, thyroid and pineal gland. The widest part is often noted to be at the C2-3 level, and it often assumes a vertical fusiform shape but may also appear flattened. In cadavers, it may be an average length of 26.6 mm (14–43 mm), 7.2 mm in width and 3.4 mm in depth.

In a cadaveric study of 30 subjects, the SCG was reliably located just above the carotid artery bifurcation. The SCG lies in a plication of the deep cervical fascia, separate from the sheath that encloses the carotid artery, vagus nerve and internal jugular vein. An MRI study confirms that the SCG is usually located medial to the internal carotid sheath and superficial to the longus capitis muscle at the level of C2.

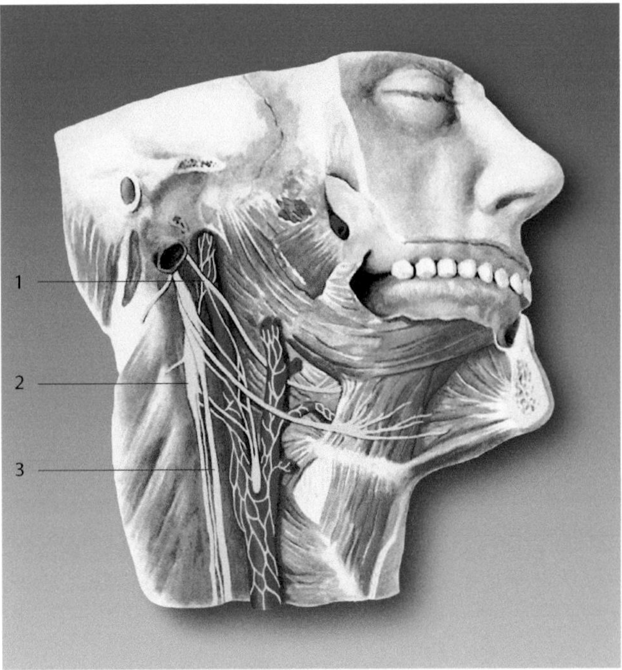

Fig. 12.15 Topographic position of the superior cervical ganglion. The widest part is often to be at the C2-3 level (carotid artery bifurcation). (1) glossopharyngeal nerve, (2) superior cervical ganglion, (3) vagus nerve. (Reproduced with permission from Danilo Jankovic)

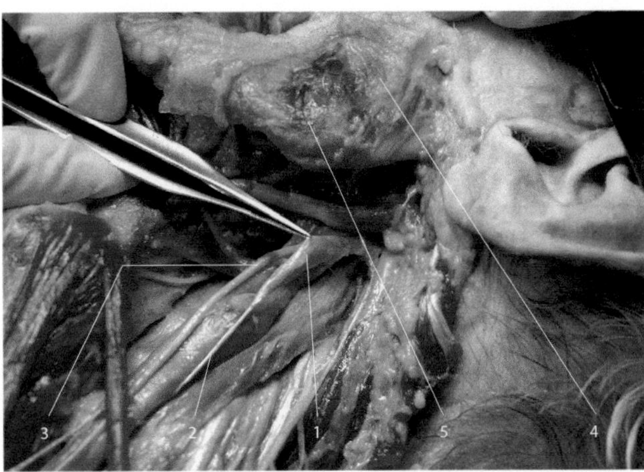

Fig. 12.16 The superior cervical ganglion has an average size of: 26.6 mm (14–43 mm) × 7.2 mm × 3.4 mm. *(1)* Superior cervical ganglion above the carotid artery bifurcation *(2)* sympathetic trunk, *(3)* vagus nerve with inferior vagal ganglion, *(4)* masseter muscle, *(5)* angle of the mandible. Hypoglossal nerve-underneath of angulus mandible. (Reproduced with permission from Danilo Jankovic)

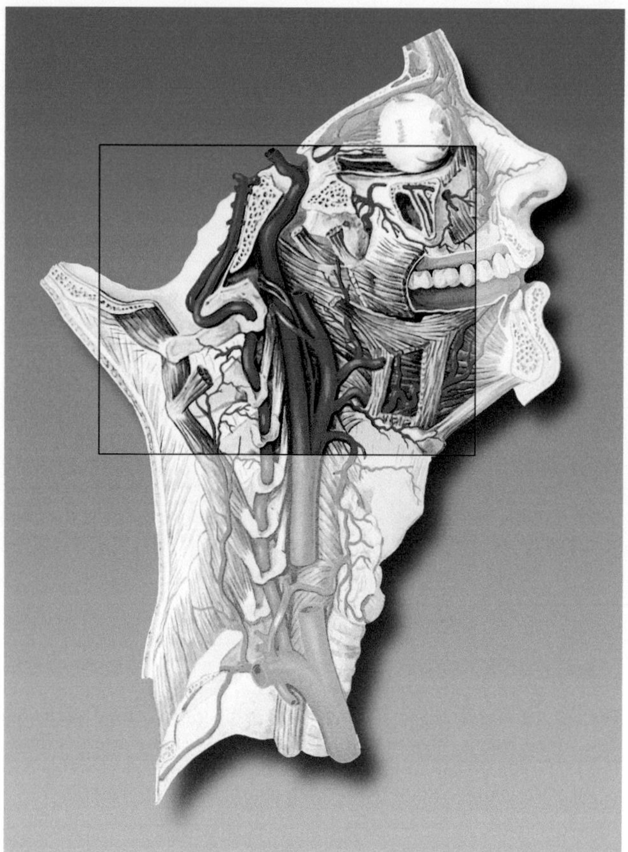

Fig. 12.17 Arteries in the immediate vicinity of the ganglion. Course of the vertebral artery and internal carotid artery bifurcation (risk of intra-arterial injection) (Reproduced with permission from Danilo Jankovic)

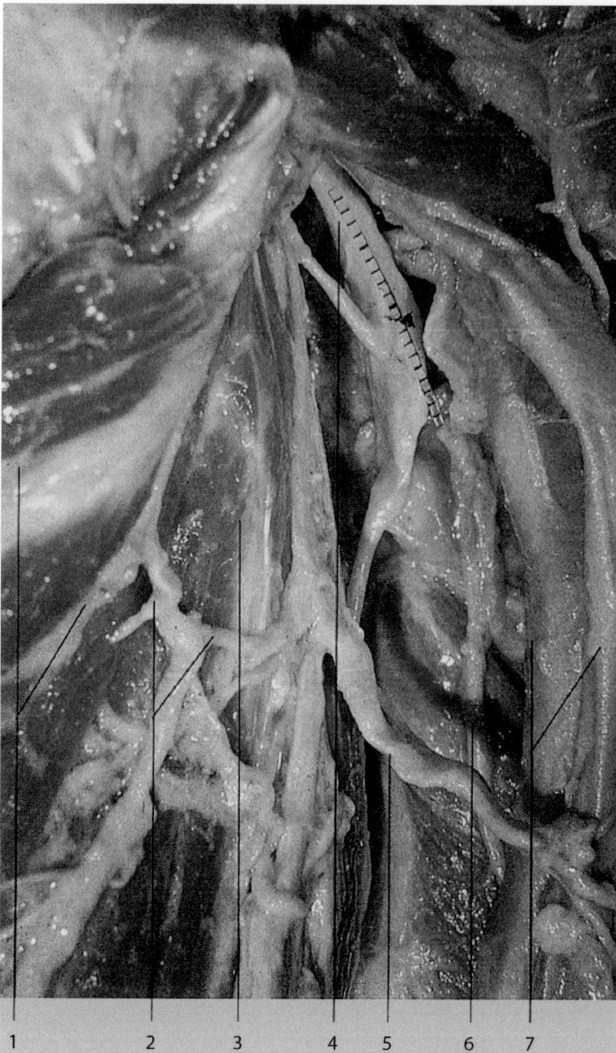

Fig. 12.18 Immediate vicinity of the superior cervical ganglion: (1) *sternocleidomastoid* muscle, repositioned dorsally, and the accessory nerve, (2) anastomosis between the C2 vertebral branch and CN XII, (3) scalenus medius muscle, (4) superior cervical ganglion, (5) hypoglossal nerve, (6) external branch of the superior laryngeal nerve, (7) neurovascular fascicle, repositioned anteriorly (Reproduced with permission from Danilo Jankovic)

Procedure for Ultrasound-Guided Superior Cervical Ganglion Block

Siegenthaler and colleagues first described how to block the SCG using ultrasonography in 2013, utilizing a cadaveric model to confirm the accuracy of the approach. Subsequently, there has been a case report using US guidance to block the SCG by pulsed RF ablation to treat refractory migraine and another case report using local anesthesia to improve recovery from abducens nerve palsy caused by microvascular ischemia.

Patient Positioning

The patient is placed supine, and the head is rotated in a slightly contralateral direction.

Scanning Technique and Sonoanatomy

A short length US probe is ideal for minimizing contact with the jaw medially, and the head may need to be extended to help improve imaging. A high-frequency linear ultrasound probe is placed transverse across the neck in order first to identify the C6 transverse process (Fig. 12.19a). After that, the probe is translated cephalad to count the cephalad transverse processes and arrive at the C3 level (Fig. 12.19b,c).

Injection Technique

Attention is drawn to visualize the start of the *bifurcation of the common carotid artery* (Figs. 12.16, 12.17, and 12.19d). At this point, the SCG may be visualized superficial to the longus capitis muscle and deep to the carotid artery and sheath. It is recommended to advance the 25G to 22G needle

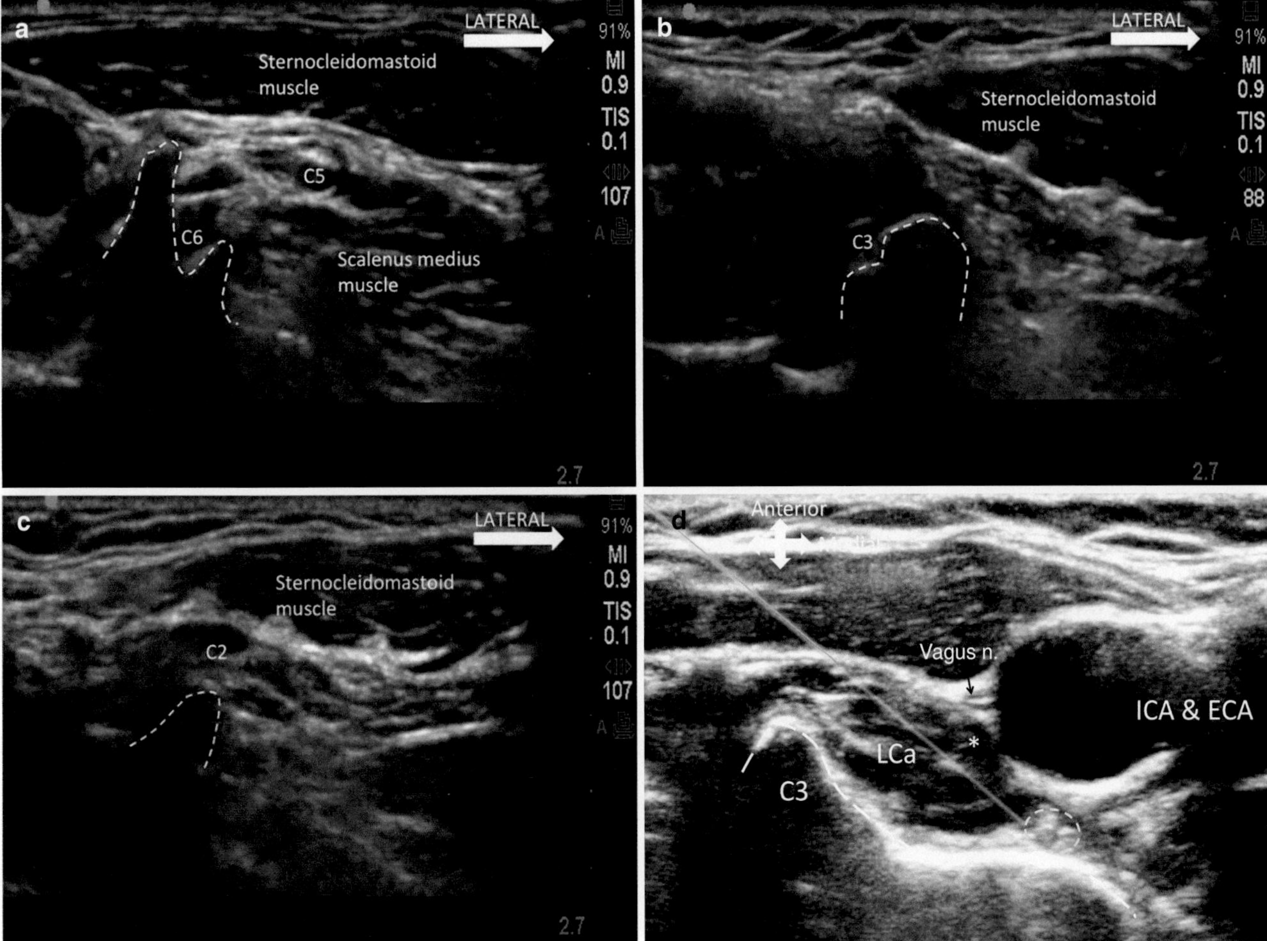

Fig. 12.19 (**a**) Sonogram showing the transverse process of C6. Note the prominent anterior tubercle of C6. (Reproduced with permission from Philip Peng Education Series). (**b**) Sonogram of C3. Note the discrepancy in the shape of anterior and posterior tubercle. (Reproduced with permission from Philip Peng Education Series). (**c**) Sonogram of C2. Note the prominence of the posterior tubercle. (Reproduced with permission from Philip Peng Education Series). (**d**) Sonogram of C3. Carotid bifurcation, vagus nerve, longus capitis muscle. Needle path and target for hydrodissection. (Reproduced with permission from Paul Tumber)

from lateral to medial in-plane with the US transducer and hydrodissect with small aliquots of normal saline until the needle tip is in position. After that one author injected 5mL of 0.2% ropivacaine to elicit an SCG block. Further research is necessary to determine the ideal or minimal volume required as the transoral route may only require 1mL of volume according to a cadaver study Whereas Wisco and colleagues(2010)' report indicated a maximum of 2.5 mL should suffice by the US or CT guided approach.

Effects of the Block

Characteristic signs of a successful block are radiation and a warm sensation in the area of the back of the head, ear, eyes, and corner of the mouth and the ipsilateral half of the face (Figs. 12.23 and 12.24). Conjunctival injection, increased tear production, and ipsilateral nasal congestion are equally characteristic, as is Horner's syndrome – which is by no means restricted to stellate block, but occurs in all blocks of the sympathetic cervical trunk.

Dosage

2.5–5 mL local anesthetic (e.g. 0.2% ropivacaine, 0.125–0.25% bupivacaine/ levobupivacaine, 0.5–1% procaine, 0. 5–1% lidocaine, 0. 5–1% mepivacaine).

In acute intractable pain (e.g. postzosteric neuralgia), low dose of local anesthetics could be combined with steroids, opioids, or clonidine in mixture.

Block Series

(See above, SGB)

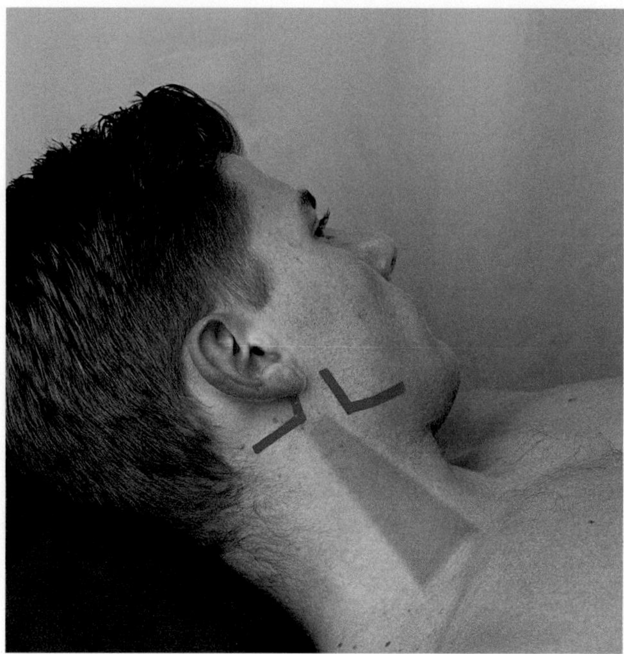

Fig. 12.20 Landmarks for locating the needle insertion position. Angle of the mandible, mastoid, medial margin of the sternocleidomastoid muscle (Reproduced with permission from Danilo Jankovic)

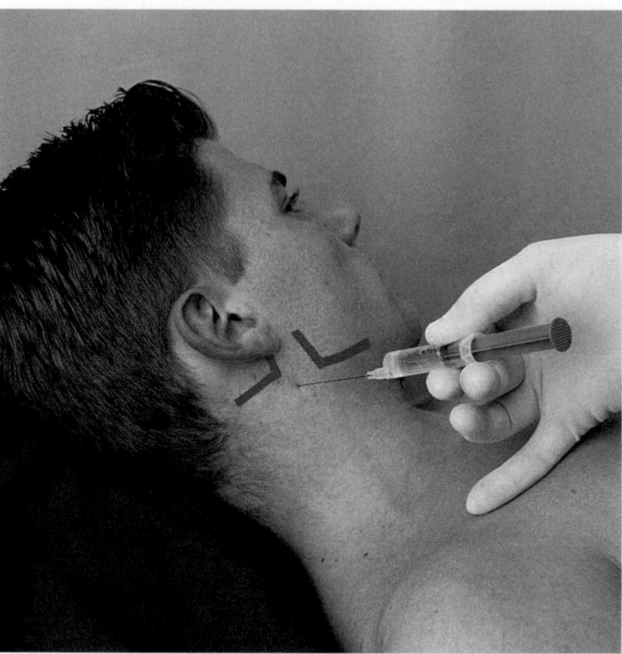

Fig. 12.22 Craniodorsal puncture in the direction of the *contralateral mastoid*. No injection without prior bone contact! (Reproduced with permission from Danilo Jankovic)

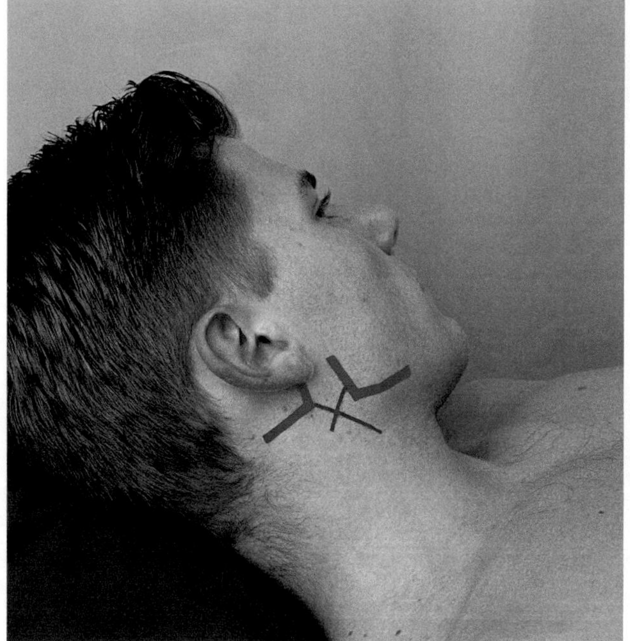

Fig. 12.21 Marking the injection site (Reproduced with permission from Danilo Jankovic)

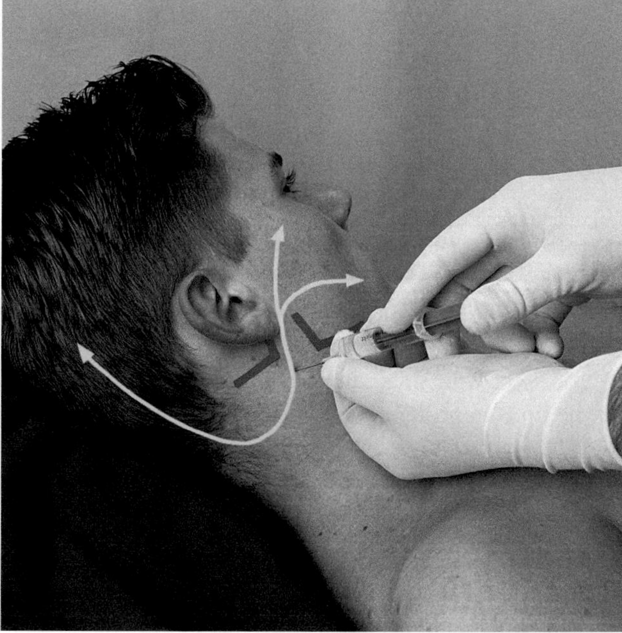

Fig. 12.23 Characteristic directions of radiation during the injection (Reproduced with permission from Danilo Jankovic)

Side Effects and Complications

(See above, SGB)

This is a potentially hazardous block to perform via blind or transoral techniques as there several structures (nerves and vessels) in the vicinity of the SCG. The side effects and complications are mostly the same as by SGB except for a reduced risk of pneumothorax, esophageal perforation, or tracheal perforation. When giving consent, the patient must be informed about all the potential risks.

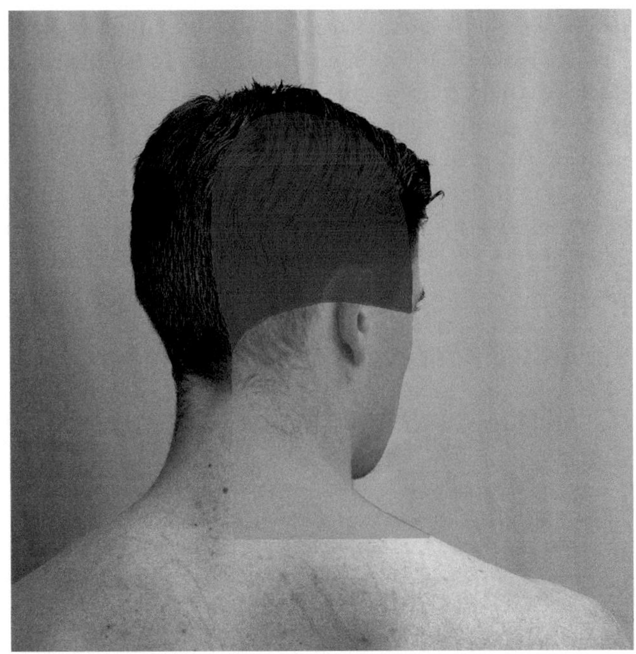

Fig. 12.24 Distribution of the block (Reproduced with permission from Danilo Jankovic)

Side Effects

Partial blockade of the phrenic nerve can lead to shortness of breath; the recurrent laryngeal nerve leading to hoarse voice; vagus nerve (CN X) block leading to tachycardia and hypertension; glossopharyngeal nerve (CN IX) leading to paresis of the pharyngeal muscles and numbness in the posterior third of the tongue; hypoglossal nerve (CN XII)- motor nerve of tongue muscles may be anesthetized (Figs. 12.15, 12.16, and 12.17); cervical plexus spread leading to anesthesia along C2-3 dermatomes especially (See above SGB).

Complications

A vascular puncture can lead to a hematoma, and a carotid puncture in a patient with atherosclerosis can lead to cerebrovascular ischemia or stroke. If the needle tip is not visualized correctly on ultrasound, intravascular injection of small volumes of local anesthesia can lead to local anesthetic systemic toxicity (See Chap. 5), and epidural or spinal anesthesia can result if the needle is placed too deep to the intended target. (See above, SGB).

Practical Tips

If available, it is helpful to review an MRI scan of the patient before attempting this block. Particular attention is drawn to the location of the SCG in relation to the *common carotid artery bifurcation* (Fig. 12.19d) as this is readily visualized using ultrasonography. The *location of the C3 transverse process* (Fig. 12.19b) *and longus capitis muscle* are also crucial landmarks. One should consider the presence of lymph nodes that may mimic the appearance of the SCG. It would be prudent to ensure negative aspiration through the needle and then inject a small test dose of 0.5 mL and wait a minute to assure the absence of any undesirable side effects. After the procedure, the patient should be kept with the head elevated to maintain comfort in the event of any recurrent laryngeal nerve blockade, and the patient should be monitored for at least 30 min to ensure there is no adverse spread of the local anesthesia or hematoma. As ultrasound technology continues to improve, this is a block that will become more familiar.

Traditional Approach for SCG (Lateral Extraoral Technique)

An experienced regional anesthetist should only carry out this block. The patient should have a full explanation of the procedure before it is performed. The patient should be fasted as per standard anesthesia guidelines (See above SGB).

Patient Positioning and Landmarks

The patient is placed supine, and the head is turned about 30–40° to the opposite side. Landmarks for locating the needle are: mastoid process, angle of the mandible, medial margin of the sternocleidomastoid muscle (Figs. 12.20 and 12.21).

Injection Technique

After skin infiltration, a 4–5 cm 23-G long needle is introduced in the direction of the *contralateral mastoid* at a *craniodorsal angle of about 20°*(Fig. 12.22). In normal anatomy, bone contact is made mostly at about 3.5–4 cm, and careful aspiration is carried out at various levels after the needle has been minimally withdrawn. Only then can a test dose of 0.5 mL of the local anesthetic be administered. After about 1 min, slow injection of the remaining dose can be carried out. The patient's upper body is then raised.

Dosage

4–5 mL local anesthetic-e.g., 0.5–1% procaine, 0.5–1% lidocaine, and 0.5–1% prilocaine, 0.2% ropivacaine and 0.125% bupivacaine (levobupivacaine) Side Effects and complications (see above).

Practical Tips

Most complications arise when the local anesthetic is administered without prior bone contact. A single test dose by no means guarantees the correct positioning of the needle. The remaining dose must never be injected quickly or carelessly. It must be administered slowly in small quantities (several test doses) with repeated aspiration. Bilateral block of the superior cervical ganglion is contraindicated, since bilateral paralysis of the recurrent laryngeal nerve or phrenic nerve is life-threatening. Due to the potential complications, the patient must be monitored after the injection has been carried out—for at least 30 min after procaine administration and at least 60 min after administration of ropivacaine or bupivacaine.

Disadvantages

Possible consequences of non-ultrasound-guided approaches (See above, SGB).

Superior Cervical Ganglion Blocks in Pain Therapy or as an Option in Depressive Conditions

In the coauthor's clinical experience over many years with the superior cervical ganglion block (10–12 on average per series), there have been surprisingly good results in a large number of patients. These observations principally concern patients with pain-associated depression in chronic pain (especially in various types of headache, migraines, facial pain, post-nucleotomy pain, fibromyalgia, etc.). In the superior cervical ganglion block, the volume of 5 mL of local anesthetic (e.g. 1% procaine) covers neighboring nerves such as the vagus nerve, for example. The superior cervical ganglion is often barely distinguishable from the vagus nerve. Left-sided vagus stimulation with an implantable electrode has been successfully used since 1938 to treat various neurological diseases such as epilepsy, treatment- resistant depression, anxiety states, sleep disturbances, and other conditions. Dysfunction of the autonomic nervous system is almost always present as an accompanying symptom of depression The long-term analgetic effect of vagus stimulation was demonstrated in a study by Kirchner 2001. Like the anti-epileptic and antidepressive action of vagus stimulation, this is probably due to neurobiochemical effects. For example, patients receiving vagus stimulation show a significant increase in norepinephrine and serotonin levels and a significant decrease in proalgetic excitatory amino acids such as aspartate and glutamate. The same group of authors reported marked symptomatic improvement during vagus stimulation in a patient with chronic tension headaches. In this context, answers will have to be found in the future to the following questions: What role does the superior cervical ganglion play in this? Is the functioning of the superior cervical ganglion more important than that of the vagus nerve? It should not be forgotten that the superior cervical ganglion is the last station where information from the body can be modulated before entering the CNS.

Suggested Reading

General Considerations: Stellate Ganglion Block

Alino J, Kosatka D, Mclean B, et al. Efficacy of stellate ganglion block in the treatment of anxiety symptoms from combat-related post traumatic stress disorder: a case series. Mil Med. 2013;178:e473–6.

Alshuraim FM, Flamer D. Cervical sympathetic trunk. In: Peng P, et al., editors. Ultrasound for interventional pain management. Cham: Springer Nature; 2019. p. 43–50.

Atez Y, Asik I, Özgencil E, Açar HI, Yağmurlu B, Tekdemir I. Evaluation of the longus colli muscle in relation to stellate ganglion block. Reg Anesth Pain Med. 2009;34(3):219–23. https://doi.org/10.1097/AAP.0b013e3181a32a02.

Baig S, Moon JY, Shankar H. Review of sympathetic blocks: Anatomy, sonoanatomy, evidence, and techniques. Reg Anesth Pain Med. 2017;42(3):377–91. https://doi.org/10.1097/AAP.0000000000000591.

Bhatia A, Flamer D, Peng PW. Evaluation of sonoanatomy relevant to performing stellate ganglion blocks using anterior and lateral simulated approaches: an observational study. Can J Anaesth. 2012;59:1040–7.

Bhatia A, Peng PWH. Stellate Ganglion Block. In: Jankovic D, Peng P, editors. Regional nerve blocks in anesthesia and pain therapy: traditional and ultrasound-guided techniques. Cham: Springer International Publishing; 2015. p. 189–201.

Chan C-w, Chalhiadis G. A case of sympathetically mediated headache treated with stellate ganglion blockade. Pain Med. 2010;11(8):1294–8.

Christie JM, Martinez CR. Computerized axial tomography to define the distribution of solution after stellate ganglion nerve block. J Clin Anesth. 1995;7:306–11.

Colding A. The effect of regional sympathetic blocks in the treatment of herpes zoster. Acta Anesth Scand. 1969;13:133–41.

Dan K, Higa K, Noda B. Nerve block for herpetic pain. In: Fields HL, et al., editors. Advances in pain research and therapy, vol. 9. New York: Raven Press. 1985.

Dobias M, Michalek P, Neuzil P, et al. Interventional treatment of pain in refractory angina. A review. Biomed Pap Med Fac Univ Palacky Olomouc Czech Repub. 2014;158:518–27.

Dukes RR, Leroy AA. Transient locked- in syndrome after vascular injection during stellate ganglion block. Reg Anesth. 1993;18:378–80.

Elias M. Cervical sympathetic and stellate ganglion blocks. Pain Physician. 2000;3:294–304.

Ferrillo M. Treatment of complex regional pain syndrome with stellate ganglion local anesthetic blockade: a case report of one patient' experiences with traditional bupivacaine HCL and liposome bupivacaine. Clin Case Rep. 2016;4(9):861–5.

Fine PG, Ashburn MA. Effect of stellate ganglion block with fentanyl on postherpetic neuralgia with a sympathetic component. Anesth Analg. 1998;67:897–9.

Floyd JB Jr. Traumatic cerebral edema relieved by stellate ganglion anesthesia. South Med J. 1987;80:1328.

Franklin AD, Llobet JR, Sobey CM, Daniels JM, Kannankeril PJ. Stellate ganglion catheter effective for treatment of ventricular tachycardia storm in a pediatric patient on extracorpo-real membrane oxygenation. A A Pract. 2019;13(7):245–9. https://doi.org/10.1213/xaa./0000000000001036.

Fudim M, Qadri YJ, Waldron NH, et al. Stellate ganglion blockade for the treatment of refractory ventricular arrhythmias. JACC Clin Electrophysiol. 2020;6(5):562–71. https://doi.org/10.1016/j.jacep.2019.12.017.

Ganz H, Klein H. Verläufe und Spätergebnisse beim Hörsturz. HNO. 1968;16(11):334–9.

Gautam D, Rangalakshmi LNU, Anagha MV. Stellate ganglion block for treatment of patient with Raynaud's syndrome. J Recent Adv Pain. 2019;5(3):90–1.

Goel V, Patwardhan AM, Ibrahim M, Howe CL, Schultz DM, Shankar H. Complications associated with stellate ganglion nerve block: A systematic review. Reg Anesth Pain Med. 2019;44(6):669–78. https://doi.org/10.1136/rapm-2018-100127.

Gofeld M, Bhatia A, Abbas S, Ganapathy S, Johnson M. Development and validation of a new technique for ultrasound-guided stellate ganglion block. Reg Anesth Pain Med. 2009;34:475–9.

Goto F, Fujita T, Kitani Y, et al. Hyperbaric oxygen and stellate ganglion blocks for idiopathic sudden hearing loss. Acta Otorionolaring. 1979;88:335–42.

Gross D. Therapeutische Lokalanästhesie des Halsgrenzstranges. In: Gross D, editor. Therapeutische Lokalanästhesie. Stuttgart: Hippokrates; 1972.

Guirguis M, Abdelmalak J, Jusino E, Hansen MR, Girgis GE. Stellate ganglion block for the treatment of hot flashes in patients with breast cancer: a literature review. Ochsner J. 2015;15(2):162–9.

Haug O, Draper WL, Haug SA. Stellate ganglion blocks for idiopathic sensorineural hearing loss. Arch Otorinolaring. 1976;102(1):5–8.

Heinig B, Koch A, Wollina U. Palmar hyperhidrosis treated by noninvasive ultrasound stellate ganglion block. Wien Med Wochenschr. 2018;168(9-10):250–3.

Higa K, Hirata K, Hirota K, Nitahara K, Shono S. Retropharyngeal hematoma after stellate ganglion block. Anesthesiology. 2006;105:1238–45.

Hogan Q, Erickson S, Haddox D, et al. The spread of solution during stellate ganglion block. Regional Anesthesia. 1992;17:78–83.

Jadon A, Jain P, Agrawal A. Efficacy of stellate ganglion block in the management of CRPS-not otherwise specified. Indian J Pain. 2016;30:171–5.

Jain V, Rath GP, Dash HH, Bithal PK, Chouhan RS, Suri A. Stellate ganglion block for treatment of cerebral vasospasm in patients with aneurysmal subarachnoid hemorrhage - a preliminary study. J Anaesthesiol Clin Pharmacol. 2011;27(4):516–21. https://doi.org/10.4103/0970-9185.86598.

Jankovic D. Postherpetic neuralgia treated with stellate ganglion block. In: Jankovic D, editor. Regional nerve blocks & infiltration therapy. 3rd ed. Oxford: Blackwell; 2004. p. 59–68.

Jankovic D. Ganglion cervicothoracicum (stellatum). In: Jankovic D, editor. Regionalblockaden & Infiltrationstherapie. Oxford: Blackwell; 2008. p. 109–20.

Jung G, Kim BS, Shin KB, Park KB, Kim SY, Song SO. The optimal volume of 0.2% ropivacaine required for an ultrasound-guided stellate ganglion block. Korean J Anesthesiol. 2011;60(3):179184. https://doi.org/10.4097/kjae.2011.60.3.179.

Kapral S, Krafft P, Gosch M, Fleischmann M, Weinstabl C. Ultrasound imaging for stellate ganglion block: direct visualization of puncture site and local anesthetic spread. A pilot study. Reg Anesth. 1995;20:323–8.

Khan M, Ahmed I. Role of stellate ganglion block in post CABG sympathetically mediated chest pain. J Pak Med Assoc. 2007;57:470.

Kim ED, Yoo WJ, Kim YN, Park HJ. Ultrasound-guided pulsed radiofrequency treatment of the cervical sympathetic chain for complex regional pain syndrome: A retrospective observational study. Med (United States). 2017;96(1):1–5. https://doi.org/10.1097/MD.0000000000005856.

Kimm J, Hahck SP, Soo Young C, et al. The effect of stellate ganglion block on intractable Lymphedema after breast cancer surgery. Korean J Pain. 2015;28(1):61–3.

Kyung Im Lim. Stellate ganglion block for the preventive effect on the attacks of cluster headache: a case report. Korean J Anesthesiol. 1998;35(6):1205–9.

Lang J. Klinische Anatomie der Halswirbelsäule. New York: Thieme, Stuttgart; 1991.

Lang J. Einige Befunde zur Anatomie des Halssympathikus. Med Orth Tech. 1992;112:194–200.

Lee YY, Park HS, Lee YS, et al. The effect of stellate ganglion block on breast cancer-related infectious lymphedema. Korean J Hosp Palliate Care. 2018;21(4):158–62.

Lemonica L, Trentin L. Raynaud's syndrome: two treatment techniques in comparison. Reg Anesth Pain Med. 1993;18(S1):46.

Lipov EG, Navaie M, Brown PR, et al. Stellate ganglion block improves refractory post-traumatic stress disorder and associated memory dysfunction: a case report and systematic literature review. Mil Med. 2013;178:e260–4.

Liu Q, Zhong Q, Tang G, Ye L. Ultrasound-guided stellate ganglion block for central post-stroke pain: a case report and review. J Pain Res. 2020;13:461–4. https://doi.org/10.2147/JPR.S236812.

Makharita MY, Amr YM, Bayoumy Y. Effect of early stellate ganglion blockade for facial pain from acute herpes zoster and incidence of postherpetic neuralgia. Pain Physician. 2012;15:467–74.

Matsuoka H, Tokutomi Y, Muteki T, Yokojama MM. Influence of stellate ganglion block on the immune system. Masui J Anesthes. 1985;34(7):917–23.

Mays KS, North WC, Schnapp M. Stallate ganglion blocks with morphine in sympathetic type pain. J Neurol Neurosurg Psychiat. 1981;44:189–90.

Melis M, Zawawi K, Al-Badawi E, a l. Complex regional pain syndrome in the head and neck: a review of the literature. J Orofac Pain. 2002;16:93–104.

Miligan NS, Nash TP. Treatment of postherpetic neuralgia.A review of 77 consecutive cases. Pain. 1985;23:381–6.

Nabil MKA. Does sympathetic ganglion block prevent postherpetic neuralgia? Reg Anesth. 1995;20(3):227–3.

Narouze S. Beware of the "serpentine" inferior thyroid artery while performing stellate ganglion block. Anesth Analg. 2009;109:289–90.

Naveira FA, Morales A. Treatment of persistent cough after stellate ganglion block. Reg Anesth. 1993;18:312–4.

Okuda Y, Urabe K, Kitajima T. Retropharyngeal or cervicomediastinal haematomas following stellate ganglion block. Eur J Anaesthesiol. 2003;20:757–9.

Olson ER, Ivy HB. Stellate block for trigeminal zoster. J Clin Neuro Ophth. 1981;1(1):53–5.

Park DY, Kang S, Kang HJ, Choi JK, Do Kim J, Yoon JS. Impact of neck position on the probability of common carotid artery puncture during ultrasound-guided stellate ganglion block. PM R. 2019;11(5):463–9. https://doi.org/10.1016/j.pmrj.2018.08.376.

Park JH, Min YS, Chun SM, et al. Effects of stellate ganglion block on breast cancer-related lymphedema: comparison of various injectates. Pain Physician. 2015;18(1):93–9.

Park KH, Lee CK, Lee JD, Park MK, Lee BD. Combination therapy with systemic steroids, an antiviral agent, anticoagulants, and stellate ganglion block for treatment of sudden sensorineural hearing loss. Korean J Audiol. 2012;16(2):71–4. https://doi.org/10.7874/kja.2012.16.2.71.

Qureshi AI, Waqas MA, Jadhav V, Saleem MA, Campbell J, Wallery SS. Long acting liposomal bupivacaine for percutaneous sympathetic stellate ganglion blockade: a technical note. J Vasc Interv Neurol. 2017;9(5):49–53.

Rastogi S, Tripathi S. Cardiac arrest following stellate ganglion block performed under ultrasound guidance. Anesthesia. 2010;65:104.

Salvaggio I, Aduci E, Dell'Aquila L, et al. Facial pain: a possible therapy with stellate ganglion block. Pain Med. 2008;9:958–62.

Sankstone A, Cornbleet T. Facial hyperhidrosis interruption with stellate ganglion block. JAMA. 1962;179:571.

Sekhri NK, Parikh S, Foo RM. Radiofrequency Ablation of the Stellate Ganglion for Management of Acute Digital Ischemia: A Case Report. A A Pract. 2018;11(7):189–92. https://doi.org/10.1213/XAA.0000000000000869.

Seung DY, Sang SJ, Hee-Sang K, et al. Efficacy of ultrasonography guided stellate ganglion blockade in the stroke patients with complex regional pain syndrome. Ann Rehabil Med. 2012;36(5):633–9.

Shibata Y, Fujiwara Y, Komatsu T. A new approach of ultrasound-guided stellate ganglion block. Anesth Analg. 2007;105:550–1.

Siegenthaler A, Mlekusch S, Schliessbach J, Curatolo M, Eichenberger U. Ultrasound imaging to estimate risk of esophageal and vascular puncture after conventional stellate ganglion block. Reg Anesth Pain Med. 2012;37:224–7.

Summers MR, Nevin RL. Stellate ganglion block in the treatment of post-traumatic stress disorder: a review of historical and recent literature. Pain Pract. 2017;17(4):546–53. https://doi.org/10.1111/papr.12503.

Takanami I, Abiko T, Koizumi S. Life-threatening airway obstruction due to retropharyngeal and cervicomediastinal hematomas following stellate ganglion block. Thorac Cardiovasc Surg. 2009;57:311–2.

Tenicella R, Lovasik D, Eaglstein W. Treatment of herpes zoster with sympathetic blocks. Clin J Pain. 1985;1:63–7.

Umeda S, Hasihida T, Kakita T. Clinical application of stellate ganglion morphine infiltration for chronic pain relief. Masui Jap J Anesthesiol. 1982;31:1403–6.

Van Gastel P, Kallewaard JW, Van der Zanden M, et al. Stellate-ganglion block as a treatment for severe menopausal flushing. Climacteric. 2013;16:41–7.

Waldman SD, Waldman K. Reflex sympathetic dystrophy of the face and neck: report of 6 patients treated with stellate ganglion block. Reg Anesth. 1987;12:15–175.

Wassef MR. Phantom pain with probable reflex sympathetic dystrophy: efficacy of fentanyl infiltration of the stellate ganglion. Reg Anesth. 1997;22(3):287–90.

Wei K, Feldmann R, Brascher AK. Ultrasound guided stellate ganglion blocks combined with pharmacological and occupational therapy in complex regional pain syndrome (CRPS): A pilot Case series Ad Interim. Pain Med. 2014;15(12):2120–7.

Winnie AP, Hartwell PW. Relationship between time of treatment of acute herpes zoster with sympathetic blockade and prevention of postherpetic neuralgia: Clinical support For a new theory of the mechanism by which sympathetic blockade provides therapeutic benefit. Reg Anesth. 1993;18:277–82.

Wittwer ED, Radosevich MA, Ritter M, Cha YM. Stellate ganglion blockade for refractory ventricular arrhythmias: implications of ultrasound-guided technique and review of the evidence. J Cardiothorac Vasc Anesth. 2020;34(8):2245–52. https://doi.org/10.1053/j.jvca.2019.12.015.

Won JC, Chung JY, Ok Young S, et al. Comparison of effectiveness of stellate ganglion block between chronic tension headache and chronic migraine patients. Koren. J Anesth. 2006;51(2):201–6.

Yucel I, Demiraran Y, Ozturan K, et al. Complex regional pain syndrome type I: efficacy of stellate ganglion blockade. J Orthop Traumatol. 2009;10(4):179–83.

General Considerations: Superior Cervical Ganglion Block

Amar AP, Heck CN, Levy ML, et al. An institutional experience with cervical vagus nerve trunk stimulation for medically refractory epilepsy: Rationale,technique and outcome. Neurosurgery. 1998;43:1265–80.

Ben-Menacham E, Manon-Espaillat R, Ristanovic R, et al. Vagus nerve stimulation for treatment of partial seizures: a controlled study of effect on seizures. Epilepsia. 1994;35:616–26.

Carcamo CR. Pulsed radiofrequency of superior cervical sympathetic ganglion for treatment of refractory migraine. Pain Med (United States). 2017;18(8):1598–600. https://doi.org/10.1093/pm/pnw301.

Descomps H, Dorgeuille C. Traitement de l'asthme par l'infiltration anesthesique retro-stylienne. Results Sur 564 cas. Fr Med Chir Thorac. 1963 Apr;17:285–95.

Feigl G, Rosmarin W, Likar R. Blockade des ganglion cervicale superius des truncus sympathicus. Ursachen für fehlblockaden Schmerz. 2006;20(4):277–84. https://doi.org/10.1007/s00482-005-0435-6.

Glassmann AH. Depression, cardiac death and the central nervous system. Neuropsychobiology. 1998;37:80–3.

Gross D. Therapeutische Lokalanästhesie des Halsgrenzstranges. In: Gross D, editor. Therapeutische Lokalanästhesie. Stuttgart: Hippokrates; 1972.

Gutierrez S, Iwanaga J, Pekala P, et al. The pharyngeal plexus: an anatomical review for better understanding postoperative dysphagia. Neurosurg Rev. 2020;1-2 https://doi.org/10.1007/s10143-020-01303-514.

Harder HJ. Die Behandlung der Migraine Blanche und Ophthalmique mit Blockaden des Ganglion cervicale superius. Reg Anaesth. 1981;4:1–9.

Jankovic D, Peng P. Regional nerve blocks in Anesthesia and pain therapy. Reg Nerve Blocks Anesth Pain Ther. 2015; https://doi.org/10.1007/978-3-319-05131-4.

Jenkner FL. Blockade des Ganglion cervicale superius. In: Jenkner FL, editor. Nervenblockaden auf pharmakologischem und auf elektrischem Weg. Wien: Springer; 1980.

Kirchner A, Birklein F, Stefan H, Handwerker HO. Vagusstimulation – Eine Behandlungsoption für chronische Schmerzen? Schmerz. 2001;15:272–7.

Koning HM, Dyrbye BA, van Hemert FJ. Percutaneous radiofrequency lesion of the superior cervical sympathetic ganglion in patients with tinnitus. Pain Pract. 2016;16(8):994–1000. https://doi.org/10.1111/papr.12348.

Lang J. Klinische Anatomie der Halswirbelsäule. Stuttgart-New York: Thieme; 1991.

Lang J. Einige Befunde zur Anatomie des Halssympathikus. Med Orth Techn. 1992;112:194–200.

Moon S, Ko M, Kim S, Kim H, Oh D. Superior cervical sympathetic ganglion block under ultrasound guidance promotes recovery of abducens nerve palsy caused by microvascular ischemia. Scand J Pain. 2019;20(1):211–4. https://doi.org/10.1515/sjpain-2019-0096.

Murphy TM. Somatic blockade of head and neck. In: Cousins MJ, Bridenbaugh PO, editors. Neural Blockade. 4th ed. Philadelphia: Lippincot-Raven; 1998.

Olfson M, Marcus S, Sackeim HA, et al. Use of ECT for the inpatient treatment of reccurent major depression. Am J Psychiatry. 1998;155:22–9.

Rosenbaum JF, Heninger G. Vagus nerve stimulation for treatment-resistant depression. Biol Psychiatry. 2000;47:273.

Rush AJ, George MS, Sackeim HA, et al. Vagus nerve stimulation (VNS) for treatment-resistant depressions: a multicenter study. Biol Psychiatry. 2000;47:277–86.

Siegenthaler A, Haug M, Eichenberger U, Suter MR, Moriggl B. Block of the superior cervical ganglion, description of a novel ultrasound-guided technique in human cadavers. Pain Med (United States). 2013;14(5):646–9. https://doi.org/10.1111/pme.12061.

Treggiari MM, Romand JA, Martin JB, Reverdin A, Rüfenacht DA, De Tribolet N. Cervical sympathetic block to reverse delayed ischemic neurological deficits after aneurysmal subarachnoid hemorrhage. Stroke. 2003;34(4):961–6. https://doi.org/10.1161/01.STR.0000060893.72098.80.

Vaugh BV, D'Cruz OF. Effect of vagal nerve stimulation on sleep (abstract). Epilepsia. 1999;40:137.

Wisco JJ, Stark ME, Rahman S. Localization of the superior cervical ganglion for targeted anesthetic blockade. Clin Anat. 2010;23(8):1039.

Wisco JJ, Stark ME, Safir I, Rahman S. A heat map of superior cervical ganglion location relative to the common carotid artery bifurcation. Anesth Analg. 2012;114(2):462–5. https://doi.org/10.1213/ANE.0b013e31823b676d.

Yokota H, Mukai H, Hattori S, Yamada K, Anzai Y, Uno T. MR imaging of the superior cervical ganglion and inferior ganglion of the vagus nerve: structures that can mimic pathologic retropharyngeal lymph nodes. Am J Neuroradiol. 2018;39(1):170–6. https://doi.org/10.3174/ajnr.A5434.

Cervical Plexus Block

13

Danilo Jankovic and Philip Peng

Contents

Introduction

The cervical plexus, superficial and deep, was used by anesthesiologists for a variety of superficial surgery in the neck, including thyroid and carotid endarterectomy. Traditionally, it is performed by landmark guidance, but ultrasound-guided technique has been described.

Anatomy

The anterior branches of the four upper cervical spinal nerves (C1 to C4) form the cervical plexus (Fig. 13.1), which is covered by the sternocleidomastoid muscle. The branches of the cervical plexus carry motor, sensory, proprioceptive, and autonomous fibers and divide into superficial cutaneous branches penetrating the cervical fascia and deeper muscular branches that mainly innervate the joints and muscles. The cutaneous branches of the cervical plexus are the lesser occipital nerve, great auricular nerve, transverse cervical (colli) nerve, and supraclavicular nerves (Fig. 13.2). The lesser occipital nerve (from C2 and C3) passes on the splenius capitis muscle to its insertion area, where it fans out into several branches and supplies the skin on the upper side of the neck and upper part of the auricle and the adjoining skin of the scalp. The largest plexus branch is usually the great auricular nerve (from C2 and C3), which passes upward behind the external jugular vein and divides into a posterior and an anterior end branch. The posterior branch supplies the skin lying behind the ear and the medial and lateral surfaces of the lower part of the auricle. The anterior branch supplies the skin in the lower posterior part of the face and the concave surface of the auricle. The transverse cervical nerve (from C2 and C3) passes almost horizontally over the external surface of the sternocleidomastoid muscle in an anterior direction toward the hyoid bone, divides into superior and inferior branches, and supplies the skin over the anterolateral side of the neck between the mandible and the sternum. The common trunk of the supraclavicular nerves (from C3 and C4) appears at

D. Jankovic (✉)
Pain Management Centre DGS – Cologne – Huerth, Cologne-Hürth, Germany
e-mail: danilo@jankovic1.de

P. Peng
Department of Anesthesia and Pain Medicine, University of Toronto Toronto Western Hospital, Toronto, ON, Canada
e-mail: philip.peng@uhn.ca

D. Jankovic, P. Peng (eds.), *Regional Nerve Blocks in Anesthesia and Pain Therapy*,
https://doi.org/10.1007/978-3-030-88727-8_13

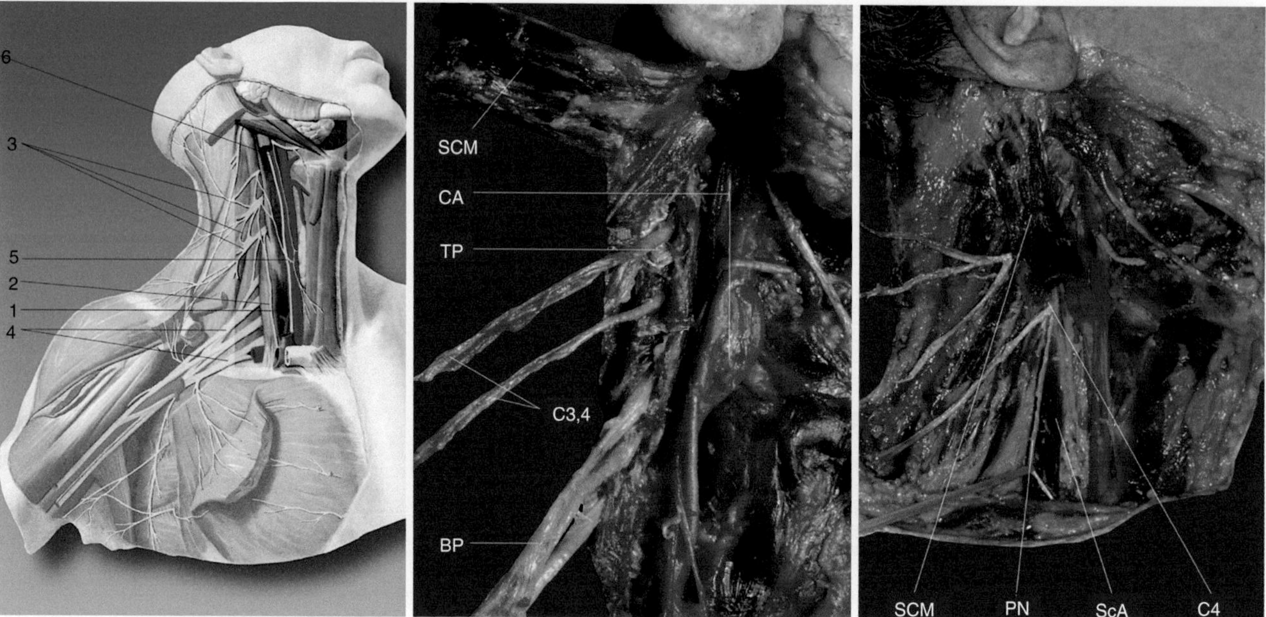

Fig. 13.1 Left. Schematic diagram. (1) Phrenic nerve, (2) scalenus anterior, (3) cervical plexus (C3, C4), (4) brachial plexus, (5) vagus nerve, (6) internal carotid artery. Middle. Dissection showing *SCM* sternocleidomastoid muscle (cut), *CA* common carotid artery, *C3,4* deep cervical plexus from C3 to C4, *BP* trunks of the brachial plexus, *TP* sulcus of transverse process. Right. Dissection showing *PN* phrenic nerve, *ScA* scalenus anterior, *C3* deep cervical plexus from C3. (Reproduced with permission from Danilo Jankovic)

the posterior margin of the sternocleidomastoid muscle, just below the transverse cervical nerve, passes downward, and divides into anterior, medial, and posterior supraclavicular nerve branches. The areas supplied by the supraclavicular nerves include the skin over the caudal part of the neck and the skin above the shoulders and the lateral upper chest, as well as the skin covering the anterior part of the deltoid muscle and occupying the acromial region.

The muscular branches of the cervical plexus include segmentally arranged nerve branches supplying the deeper anterior neck muscles (the rectus capitis anterior and lateralis, longus colli, longus capitis and intertransverse, scalenus anterior and medius, and levator scapulae), as well as the inferior descending cervical nerve, the trapezius branch, and the phrenic nerve. The inferior descending cervical nerve (from C2 and C4) gives off several fibers to the carotid and jugular neural plexus and joins with the superior descending cervical nerve to form the ansa cervicalis. The area supplied includes the sternothyroid muscle, sternocleidomastoid muscle, thyrohyoid muscle, geniohyoid muscle, and omohyoid muscle.

The trapezius branch appears at the surface just below the accessory nerve and passes to the trapezius muscle. The phrenic nerve (from C4 and C3/5) is the motor nerve for the diaphragm, but it also contains sensory and sympathetic fibers that supply the fibrous pericardium, mediastinal pleura, and the central part of the diaphragmatic pleura as the nerve courses through the thorax. Connections have been described between the phrenic nerve (left or right branch) or the phrenic plexus and the following structures: inferior and middle cervical ganglion, subclavian plexus, pulmonary plexus, inferior vena cava, esophagogastric junction, cardiac end of the stomach, hepatic portal, and suprarenal cortex.

Indications

Superficial cervical plexus

1. Superficial procedure for submandibular, post-auricular, and lower neck area
2. Combined with deep cervical plexus block for surgical procedures listed below
3. Isolated nerve (supraclavicular nerve) block adjunct to brachial plexus block for shoulder surgery

Deep cervical plexus

1. Diagnostic block for localization and differentiation of various types of neuralgia. However, with current advance of investigational methods (magnetic resonance image and electrophysiological studies) and image-guided nerve block, this indication is growing out of favor.

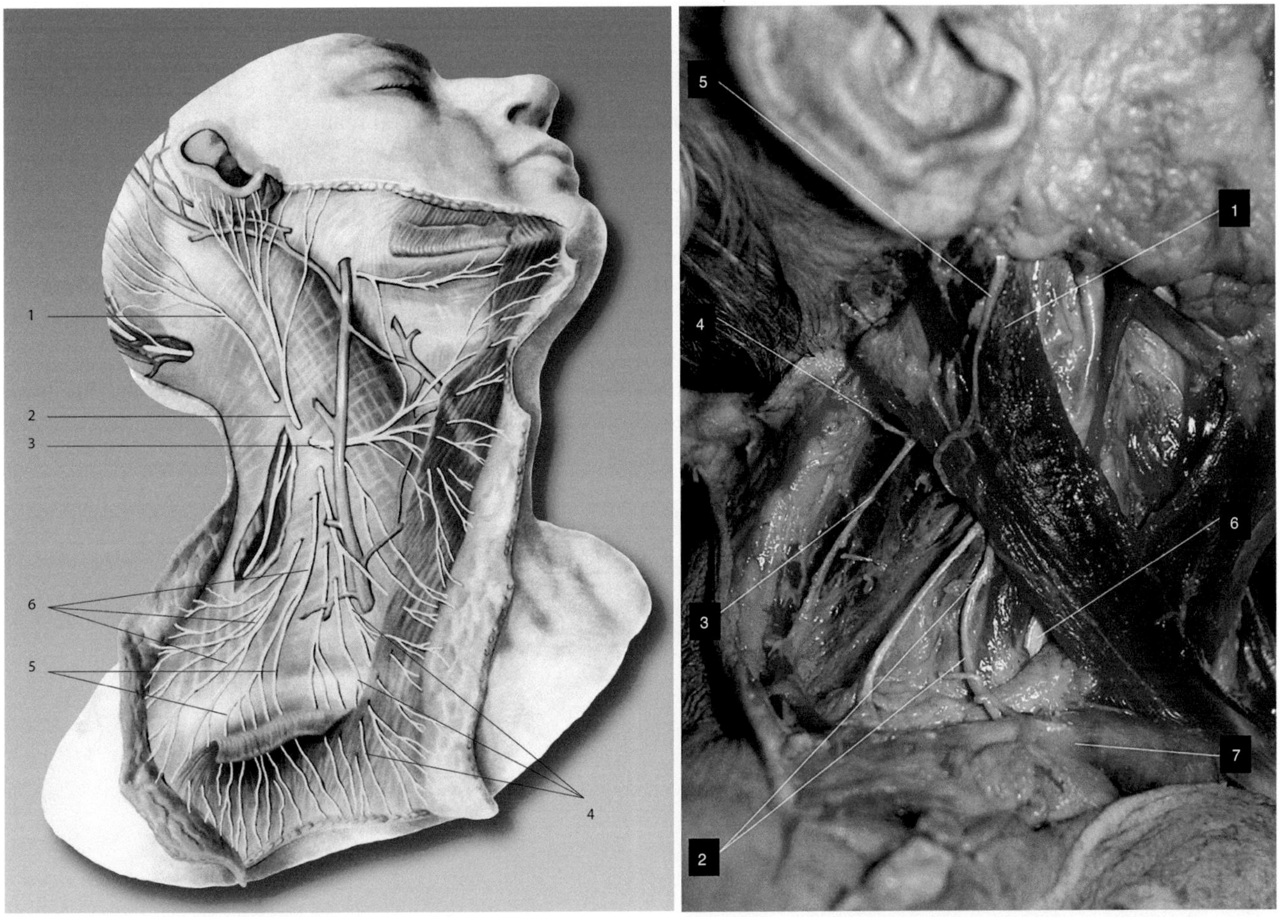

Fig. 13.2 Superficial cervical plexus. Left. Anatomy drawing. (1) Lesser occipital nerve, (2) great auricular nerve, (3) transverse cervical (colli) nerve, (4) medial supraclavicular nerves, (5) intermediate supraclavicular nerves, (6) lateral supraclavicular nerves. Right. Dissection. (1) Sternocleidomastoid muscle, (2) supraclavicular branches of the superficial plexus, (3) accessory nerve, (4) lesser occipital nerve, (5) great auricular nerve, (6) brachial plexus, (7) clavicle (Reproduced with permission from Danilo Jankovic)

2. Some physicians use this block for management of postherpetic neuralgia, torticollis, and occipital and cervicogenic headache.

Procedure

Superficial Cervical Plexus Block: Landmark-Guided

The landmark is the midpoint of the posterior edge of the sternocleidomastoid muscle between the mastoid process and the clavicular head. Once this landmark is palpated, a 25 gauge needle is inserted at the midpoint of the posterior margin with a fanlike injection into the superficial cervical plexus. Five to eight mL of local anesthetic is sufficient (Fig. 13.3).

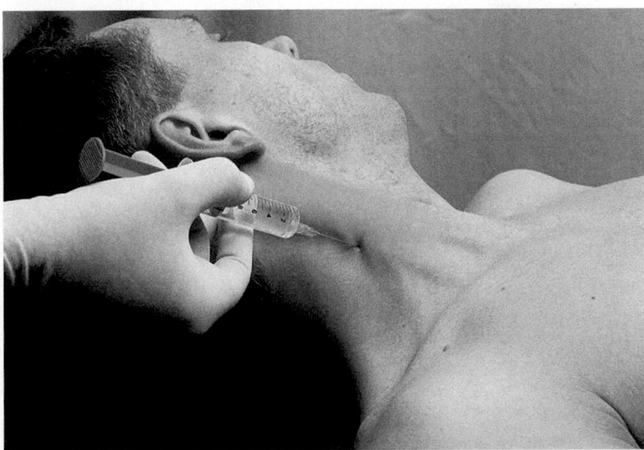

Fig. 13.3 Superficial cervical plexus block (Reproduced with permission from Danilo Jankovic)

Superficial Cervical Plexus Block: Ultrasound-Guided

With ultrasound, the typical morphology of cervical transverse processes from C2 to C7 can be easily revealed (Fig. 13.4a–d). At the level of C4 or C5, the superficial cervical plexus can be seen deep to the sternocleidomastoid muscle (Fig. 13.5). Both in-plane and out-of-plane approaches can be performed and a total of 5 mL of local anesthetic will be sufficient.

For the clavicle, blockade of the supraclavicular nerve of the superficial plexus is possible. The anatomical landmark is the supraclavicular area 2–3 cm above the clavicle, posterior to the sternocleidomastoid muscle superficial to the deep cervical investing fascia (Fig. 13.6). The nerve usually appears as a single nerve trunk before it branches into medial, intermediate, and lateral branches and is in intimate relation to the external jugular vein. To inject this nerve, only 2 mL of local anesthetic is sufficient.

Deep Cervical Plexus Block: Landmark-Guided

This block should only be carried out by experienced anesthetists with standard anesthesia monitoring and the presence of emergency equipment. It is absolutely necessary to

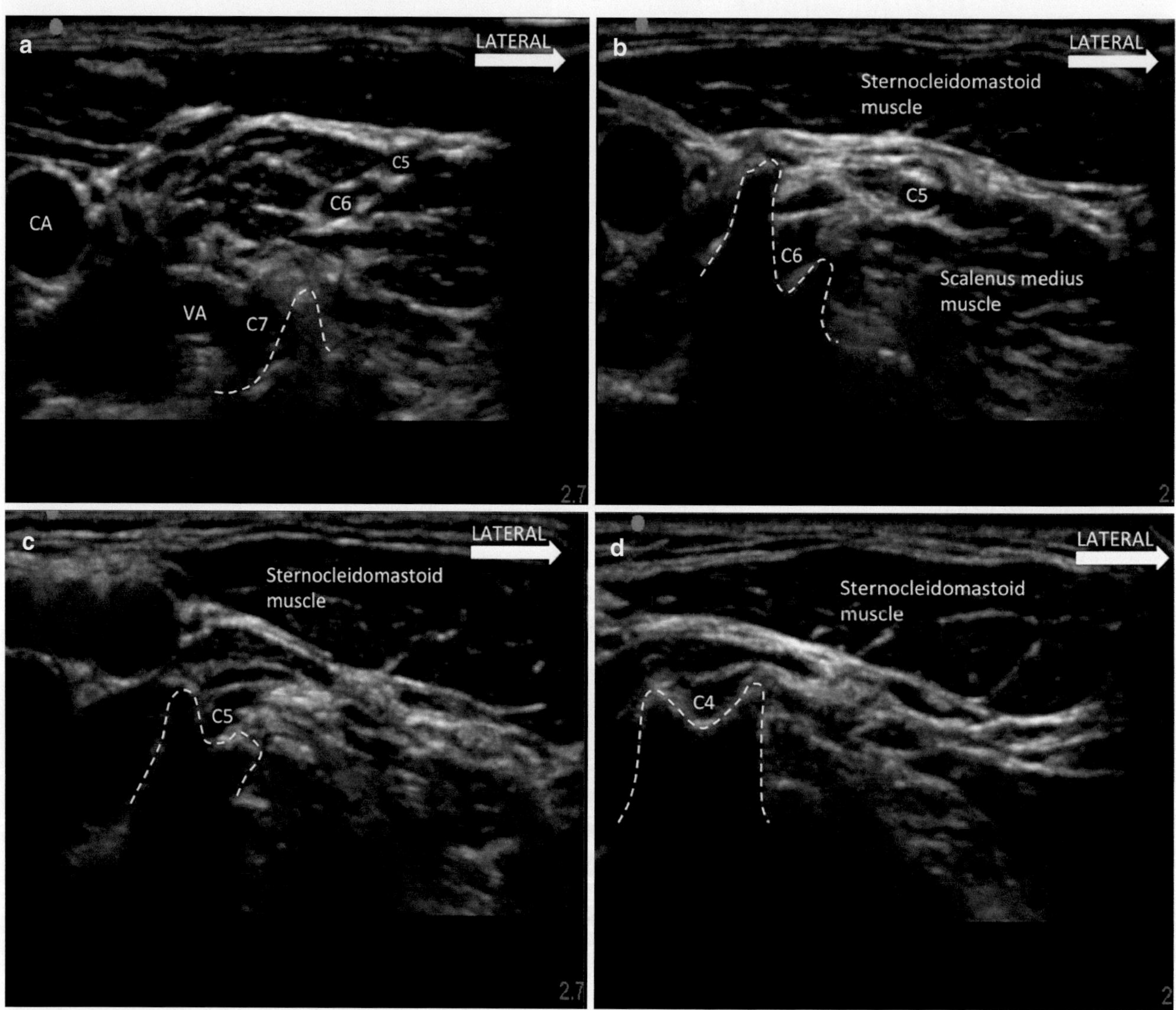

Fig. 13.4 (**a**) Sonogram showing transverse process of C7. Note that only the posterior tubercle is seen as the anterior tubercle is usually vestigial. The nerve roots of C5 to C7 is seen aligned in the interscalene groove. *VA* Vertebral artery, *CA* carotid artery. (**b**) Sonogram showing the transverse process of C6. Note the prominent anterior tubercle of C6. (**c**) Sonogram showing C5. Note the anterior and posterior tubercles are similar in size, in contrast to that in C6. (**c**) Sonogram of C4. Note the morphology is similar to C5 but the tubercles are usually closer together than that of C5 (Reproduced with permission from Philip Peng)

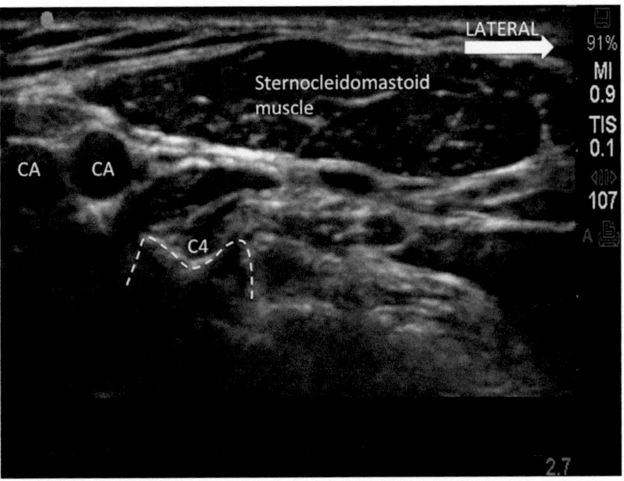

Fig. 13.5 Sonogram of the superficial cervical plexus (shaded with purple color) at the level of C4. Multiple nerves in short axis are seen sequestered in this space deep to the sternocleidomastoid muscle. *CA* carotid artery, which bifurcates into internal and external carotid arteries (Reproduced with permission from Philip Peng)

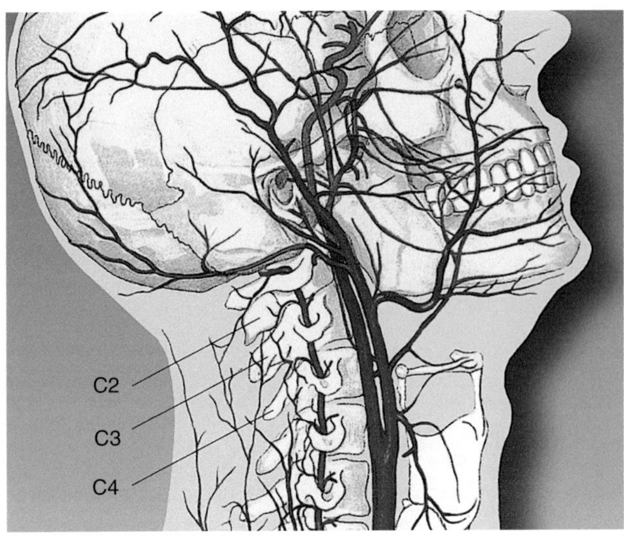

Fig. 13.7 Landmarks: transverse processes of C2 to C4 (Reproduced with permission from Danilo Jankovic)

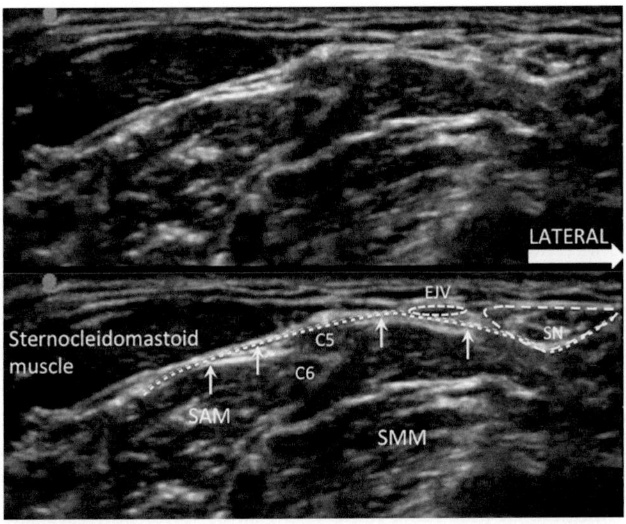

Fig. 13.6 Sonogram of the supraclavicular nerve (SN). The top picture is the unlabeled version of the bottom picture. Note the investing layer of the deep cervical fascia (dotted line indicated by arrows). The SN is superficial to this layer and is in close proximity with external jugular vein (EJV). *SAM* scalenus anterior muscle, *SMM* scalenus medius muscle. (Reproduced with permission from Philip Peng)

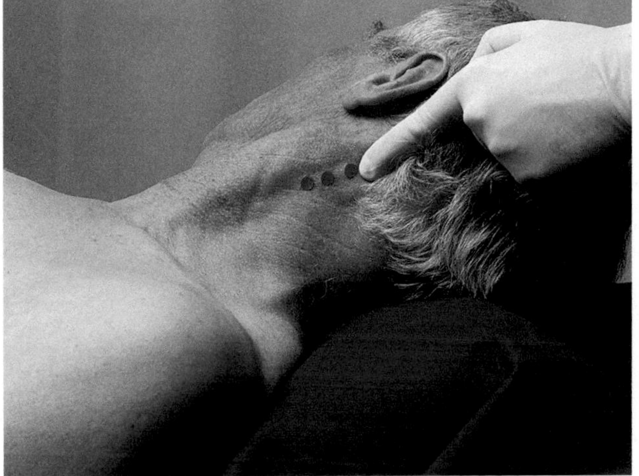

Fig. 13.8 Marking the guiding lines (Reproduced with permission from Danilo Jankovic)

have a detailed discussion with the patient before the procedure. The procedure is performed under sterile condition with patient placed in supine position, and the head tilted slightly backward and turned about 45° to the opposite side.

The transverse process of C6 and the caudal tip of the mastoid process are located. A line is drawn from the mastoid process along the posterior edge of the sternocleidomastoid muscle to the level of C6. The transverse process of C2 is palpated and marked on the skin. This lies about 1.5 cm caudal to the mastoid process and about 0.5–1 cm dorsal to the marked line. The transverse processes of C3, C4, and C5 are also palpated and marked (Figs. 13.7 and 13.8). The distances between them are each ca. 1.5 cm, and like C2 they lie about 0.5–1 cm dorsal to the marked line.

The aim is to block the anterior branches of the cervical plexus in the groove of the transverse process. After thorough skin prep, skin infiltration is carried out at the marked areas of C2, C3, and C4, and the needles are introduced (Fig. 13.9). Standing on the side of the injection, the clinician directs the needles perpendicular to the skin in the sequence C2 to C4, and advanced medially slightly caudal (ca. 30°) to contact the "gutters" in the superior surface of the transverse processes. In normal anatomy, the distance from the transverse processes to the skin varies between 1.5 and 3.5 cm. After clear bone contact and minimal withdrawal

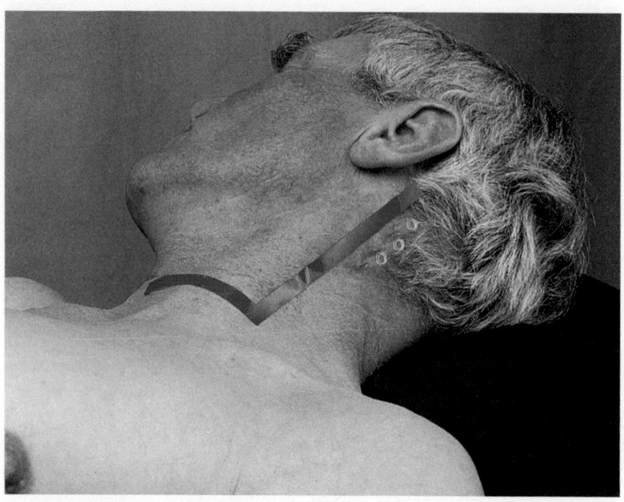

Fig. 13.9 Needle insertion in the area of the transverse processes of C2, C3, and C4

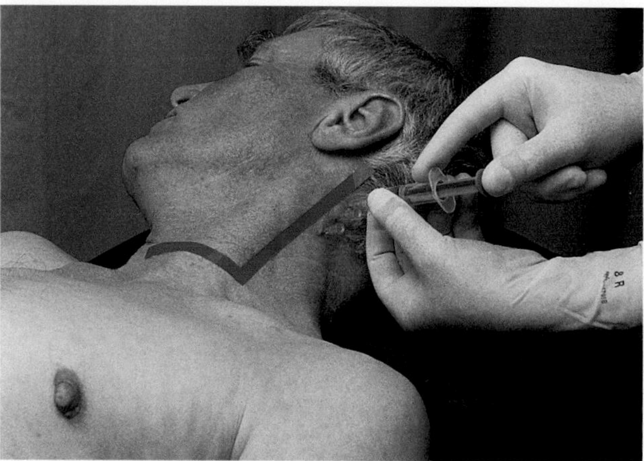

Fig. 13.10 Injection after aspiration (Reproduced with permission from Danilo Jankovic)

of the needle, careful aspiration needs to be carried out at various levels (Fig. 13.10). At each level, 2 mL local anesthetic (e.g., 1% prilocaine, mepivacaine, lidocaine) is administered for diagnostic purpose and 3 mL local anesthetic (e.g., 0.2–0.375% ropivacaine, 0.125–0.25% bupivacaine, 0.125–0.25% levobupivacaine) per segment for therapeutic purpose.

If the local anesthetic spreads in the direction of the superior cervical ganglion and/or the cervicothoracic ganglion, Horner's syndrome may develop (see chapter "Stellate Ganglion Block"). If there is improvement after two treatment sessions, a series of 8–12 therapeutic blocks is indicated.

It is important to note that this block is contraindicated in patient with grade 2 atrioventricular (AV) block, anticoagulant treatment, and contralateral paresis of the phrenic nerve or recurrent laryngeal nerve. Furthermore, this procedure should not be performed simultaneously on both sides.

Complication

The superficial cervical plexus is usually well tolerated due to the superficial location and the local volume of injectate.

With the deep location of the deep cervical plexus, the local anesthetic may spill to various nerves resulting in adverse effects.

- Phrenic nerve, main symptom: unilateral paralysis of diaphragmatic movement
- Recurrent laryngeal nerve, main symptoms: hoarseness and foreign body sensation in the throat
- Glossopharyngeal nerve, main symptoms: numbness in the final third of the tongue and paralysis of the pharyngeal muscles
- Vagus nerve, main symptoms: tachycardia and hypertension
- Partial block of the upper part of the brachial plexus

Because of this, the patient should be informed of these possible side effects in obtaining consent and be monitored for 60 min after the procedure.

The other possible complications are intravascular injection. There is always a risk of intravascular injection due to the rich vascular supply in this area. Particular attention should be given to avoiding puncture of the vertebral artery. Toxic reactions may occur after intravascular administration of local anesthetics, and the symptoms and treatment of these are outlined in Chap. 5. Another possibility is

epidural or subarachnoid injection when the needle slides along the transverse process and enters an intervertebral foramen. In that case, there is a risk of dural puncture and subarachnoid injection of local anesthetic. This can lead to a high spinal or high epidural block. The clinical picture and management of this complication is covered in other chapters.

Practical Tips

- The tip of the needle must reach the groove of the transverse process in order to ensure good anesthesia. Note that caudal direction is essential to avoid penetration of an intervertebral foramen, with possible injection into epidural space or dural sleeve.
- An injection should never be carried out without definite bone contact. The local anesthetic must be slowly administered in small amounts (several test doses) and with repeated aspiration.

Literature Review

Superficial, with or without deep, cervical plexus block can be used to provide analgesia for a variety of superficial surgery in head and neck region. It is popular in thyroid surgery and can be performed by anesthesiologist preoperatively or by surgeon during the operation. Systematic review supported the analgesic efficacy with a reduction in analgesic requirement, improvement of pain scores, increase in time for first analgesic, and reduction of hospital stay with no significant change in incidence of postoperative nausea and vomiting. There is no advantage of performing this under ultrasound because of the consistent location deep to the sternocleidomastoid muscle. It is effective in reducing the pain in insertion of the vascular access.

Carotid endarterectomy can be performed with regional block alone. In the past, anesthesiologist combined superficial and deep cervical plexus block. When comparing superficial with deep cervical plexus blocks for carotid endarterectomy, addition of deep cervical plexus block did not show any advantage. Performing the superficial plexus block alone becomes a more favorable approach because of the ease of procedure and lower risk of complication. However, the largest randomized trial comparing general anesthesia and local anesthesia did not show a difference in the major outcome: 30-day stroke or mortality rate.

Suggested Reading

Aunac S, Carlier M, Singelyn F, De Kock M. the analgesic efficacy of bilateral combined superficial and deep cervical plexus block administered before thyroid surgery under general anesthesia. Anesth Analg. 2002;95:746–50.

Benzon HT, Raja SN, Borsook D, Molloy RE, Strichartz G. Essentials of pain medicine and regional anesthesia. Philadelphia: Churchill Livingstone; 1999.

Brull SJ. Superficial cervical plexus block for pulmonary artery catheter insertion. Crit Care Med. 1992;20:1362–3.

Davies MJ, Silbert BS, Scott DA, Cook RJ, Mooney PH, Blyth C. Superficial and deep cervical plexus block for carotid artery surgery: A prospective study of 1000 blocks. Reg. Anesthesia. 1997;22(5):442–6.

GALA Trial Collaborative Group. General anaesthesia versus local anaesthesia for carotid surgery (GALA): a multicentre, randomised controlled trial. Lancet. 2008;372:2132–42.

Guay J. Regional anesthesia for carotid surgery. Curr Opin Anaesthesiol. 2008;21:638–44.

Harbaugh RE, Pikus HJ. Carotid endarterectomy with regional anesthesia. Neurosurgery. 2001;49:642–5.

Jankovic D. Deep and superficial plexus block. In: Jankovic, editor. Regional nerve blocks& infiltrattion therapy. Berlin: Blackwell Scientists; 2007. p. 129–36.

Johnson TR. Transient ischaemic attack during deep cervical plexus block.Br. J Anesth. 1999;83:965–7.

Mayhew D, Sahgal N, Khirwadar R, Hunter JM, Banerjee A. Analgesic efficacy of bilateral superficial cervical plexus block for thyroid surgery: meta-analysis and systematic review. BJA. 2018;120:241–51.

Papavasiliou AK, Magnadottir HB, Gonda T, et al. Clinical outcomes after carotid endarterectomy: Comparison of the use of regional and general anesthetics. J Neurosurg. 2000;92:291–6.

Sandeman DJ, Griffiths MJ, Lennox AF. Ultrasound guided deep cervical plexus block. Anaesth Intensive Care. 2006;34:240–4.

Soeding P, Eizenberg N. Review article: anatomical considerations for ultrasound guidance for regional anesthesia of the neck and upper limb. Can J Anaesth. 2009;56:518–33.

Stoneburner JM, Nishanian GP, Cukingnan RA, et al. Carotid endarterectomy using regional anesthesia: a benchmark for stenting. Am Surg. 2002;68:1120–3.

Stoneham MD, Knighton JD. Regional anaesthesia for carotid endarterectomy. Br J Anaesth. 1999;82:910–9.

Stoneham MD, Wakefield TW. Acute respiratory distress after deep cervical plexus block. J Cardiothorac Vasc Anesth. 1988;12:197–8.

Tran DQ, Dugani S, Finlayson RJ. A randomized comparison between ultrasound-guided and landmark-based superficial cervical plexus block. Reg Anesth Pain Med. 2010;35(6):539–43.

Usui Y, Kobayashi T, Kakinuma H, et al. An anatomical basis for blocking of the deep cervical plexus and cervical sympathetic tract using an ultrasound-guided technique. Anesth Analg. 2010;110:964–8.

Vaniyapong T, Chongruksut W, Rerkasem K. Local versus general anaesthesia for carotid endarterectomy. Cochrane Database Syst Rev. 2013;19:12.

Weiss A, Isselhorst C, Gahlen J, et al. Acute respiratory failure after deep cervical plexus block for carotid endarterectomy as a result of bilateral recurrent laryngeal nerve paralysis. Acta Anaesthesool scand. 2005;49:715–9.

Cervical Interlaminar Epidural (CIE) Block

14

Paul Gray, Jan van Zundert, and André van Zundert

Contents

General Considerations

Cervical interlaminar epidural (CIE) block was first described by Dogliotti in 1933. It has demonstrated to be of benefit in managing chronic radicular pain at this level secondary to a number of pathologies including disc herniation. It should be reserved for the experienced interventionist, as the complications can be devastating and permanent. Patients should be carefully selected and provided with informed consent with respect to proposed advantages and potential adverse effects and complications.

P. Gray
Department of Anaesthesia, Princess Alexandra Hospital, Woolloongabba, QLD, Australia

J. van Zundert
Department Anesthesiology, Critical Care, Urgency Medicine and Multidisciplinary Pain Center, Ziekenhuis Oost-Limburg, Genk, Belgium

Department of Anesthesiology and Pain Medicine, Maastricht University Medical Centre, Maastricht, The Netherlands
e-mail: jan.vanzundert@zol.be

A. van Zundert (✉)
Department of Anaesthesia and Perioperative Medicine, Royal Brisbane and Women's Hospital, Brisbane, QLD, Australia

Indications

The cervical interlaminar epidural block may be used for both surgical anaesthesia and analgesia as well as for persistent pain states. The possible surgical indications include upper limb surgery, neck surgery and breast surgery. However, the large majority of indications for CIE is in the management of persistent pain states and is usually restricted to the treatment of radicular pain originating from the cervical spine. Radicular pain, a condition due to a compressed or irritated nerve in the cervical spine, is usually characterised by pain and numbness, tingling or weakness along the course of that nerve. Several studies provide evidence of moderate quality that interlaminar corticosteroid administration in combination with conservative treatment gives a greater pain reduction than conservative treatment or epidural corticosteroid alone.

Contraindications

Contraindications can be considered from a spectrum of relative to absolute. Systemic or local infection at the site of insertion can increase the risk of seeding bacteria into the

D. Jankovic, P. Peng (eds.), *Regional Nerve Blocks in Anesthesia and Pain Therapy*,
https://doi.org/10.1007/978-3-030-88727-8_14

epidural space which could result in an epidural infection, and this must be taken into account when considering the risk-to-benefit ratio of the procedure. Hereditary, acquired or induced coagulopathies are absolute contraindications as they increase the chances of epidural haematoma, which can have catastrophic consequences such as paralysis or death. Current therapy with anticoagulant or antiplatelet medication must be ceased prior to the procedure with the clinician deciding upon the need for bridging therapy based on the individual patient circumstances (see Chap. 1). Aspirin or other non-steroidal anti-inflammatory drug therapy does not seem to increase the risk of epidural haematoma and can be continued. Special caution must be exercised when considering this procedure in patients on the newer factor Xa inhibitors (e.g. rivaroxaban) or direct thrombin inhibitors (dabigatran) as studies are lacking with regard to the optimal time period to withhold these medications. At our institution, in patients with normal hepatic function, we recommend withholding rivaroxaban for at least 3 days and dabigatran for 5 days. More detailed information on these newer agents is available from the ASRA guidelines (see Chap. 1). Previous surgery of the cervical spine, particularly posteriorly, is a relative contraindication as the epidural space may be very thin if not obliterated increasing the risk of dural puncture and spinal cord injury. In this situation, the interventionist can consider accessing the space at a level below the surgical site and feeding a catheter up to the desired level of blockade. Severe spinal canal stenosis, reduced neck flexion and ankylosing spondylitis are also relative contraindications as successfully accessing the epidural space may be significantly reduced.

Finally, caution should be exercised in those patients with a background of severe cardiovascular or respiratory disease.

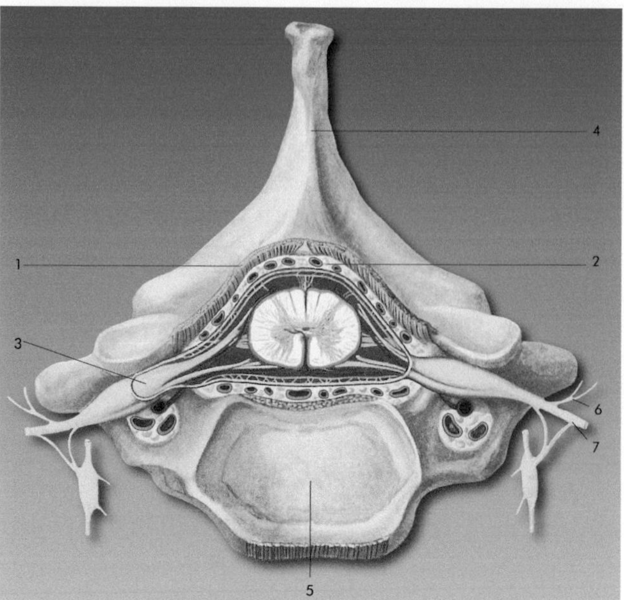

Fig. 14.1 Cross section of epidural space: *(1)* Ligamentum flavum, *(2)* epidural space with venous plexus, *(3)* spinal ganglion, *(4)* spinous process, *(5)* body of vertebra, *(6)* dorsal branch of spinal nerve, *(7)* ventral branch of spinal nerve (Reproduced with permission from the Danilo Jankovic)

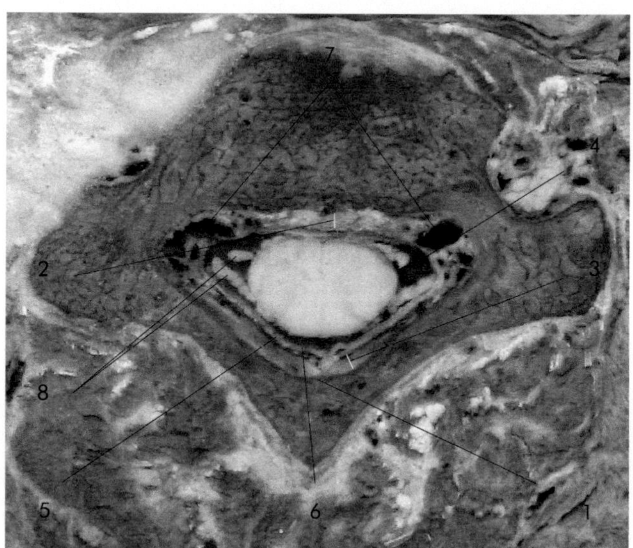

Fig. 14.2 Cross section at the level of the C6: *(1)* Ligamentum flavum, *(2)* anterior epidural space, *(3)* posterior epidural space, *(4)* subarachnoid space with the spinal cord, *(5)* spinal dura mater, *(6)* spinal pia mater, *(7)* epidural veins, *(8)* anterior and posterior spinal nerve roots (Reproduced with permission from Danilo Jankovic)

Functional Anatomy

An understanding of the anatomical differences at the cervical level will aid in performing the interlaminar epidural block as it allows the interventionist to visualise the cervical spine in a three-dimensional manner and make informed choices of how best to acquire images and direct the needle under fluoroscopic or CT guidance (Figs. 14.1 and 14.2). Vertebra prominens (C7) is the most prominent of all the cervical spinous processes and aids in determining the level for injection. At the lower cervical spine, the spinous processes are quite horizontal in a similar way to the lumbar spinous processes and in contrast to the mid-thoracic region where the spinous processes are inclined (Fig. 14.3). Therefore, with flexion of the cervico-thoracic junction, there is usually good separation of the spinous processes allowing access to the epidural space. The distance to the epidural space in the cervical region is similar to that in the lumbar region. It is influenced by the weight and neck size of the patient. The ligamentum flavum is relatively thin when compared to the thoracic and lumbar regions resulting in a more subtle loss-of-resistance when the advancing needle penetrates the ligament and enters the epidural space. Moreover, there is evidence that for many patients, the ligamentum flavum fails to fuse in the midline at the cervical level with the added risk that the endpoint of

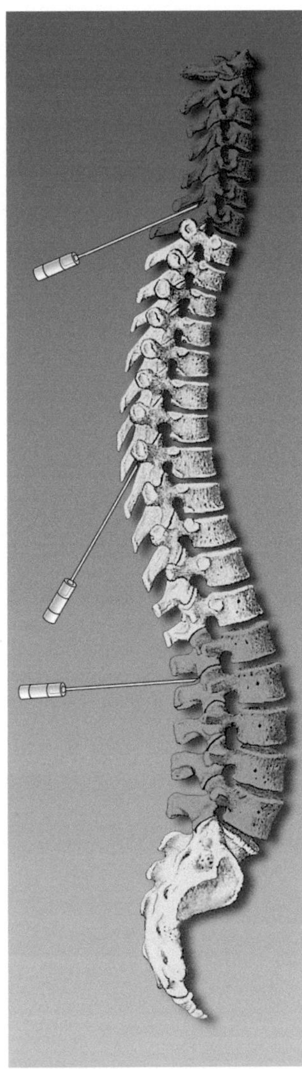

Fig. 14.3 Cervical, thoracic and lumbar spine (Reproduced with permission from Danilo Jankovic)

loss-of-resistance will be difficult to determine. The approximate anterior-posterior width of the epidural space is 1.5–2.0 mm at C7 but increases to 3.0–4.0 mm on flexion of the neck. This compares to 5.0–6.0 mm in the lumbar region. The joining of the periosteal and spinal dura at the foramen magnum forms the superior boundary of the cervical epidural space, and therefore an epidural injection should not enter the cranium. Epidural veins are concentrated in the anterolateral aspect of the epidural space. However, a blood tap is still possible with a posterior midline approach to the epidural space (see Chap. 40, "Neuraxial Anatomy and Sonoanatomy").

Technique

Informed consent for cervical interlaminar epidural block must be obtained prior to the procedure. This should include a discussion of the potential advantages and risks both

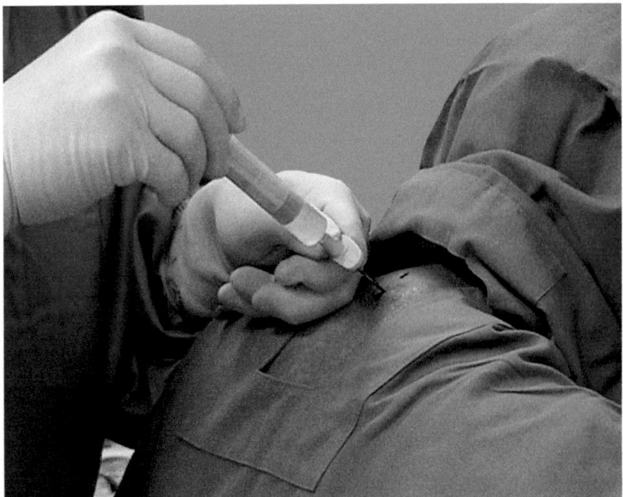

Fig. 14.4 Patient positioning for the sitting approach to the cervical epidural interlaminar block using loss-of-resistance to saline. (Reproduced with permission from Paul Gray)

general and specific to the patient. The cervical epidural interlaminar block should be reserved for the experienced interventionist who is proficient in epidural blockade at the lumbar level. Intravenous access should be established, and the block performed in an area where staff, drugs and equipment are available for resuscitation. Regular monitoring of blood pressure and continuous pulse oximetry should occur during and for 60 minutes following the procedure. The block can be performed in the sitting (Fig. 14.4), prone or lateral recumbent positions, with a supportive nurse stabilising the patient. Pre-syncope and syncope may occur when the block is performed in the sitting position with the added risk of misplacement of the needle. This risk could be reduced with intravenous loading with a crystalloid or colloid solution and doses of a vasopressor as needed. Due to this risk, the prone position is preferred. The use of fluoroscopy is recommended to aid with needle direction.

Position of the neck is extremely important with MRI studies demonstrating that when the cervical spine is in the extended position, there is the tendency for the ligamentum flavum to buckle toward the spinal cord and reduce the epidural space. Moreover, the epidural space width increases significantly on flexion of the cervical spine. For this reason, the patient is positioned with the cervical spine flexed as this maximises the distance between the ligamentum flavum and the dura compared with the extended position. This flexion is achieved in the prone position through the patient having two pillows under their chest with the forehead resting on a rolled towel (Fig. 14.5).

The technique should be performed with full sterile technique using mask, sterile gloves and gown by the interventionalist. Due to the ligamentum flavum being thinner at the cervical region, the loss-of-resistance may be more reliably detected with the use of a 16-gauge Tuohy needle rather than an 18-gauge.

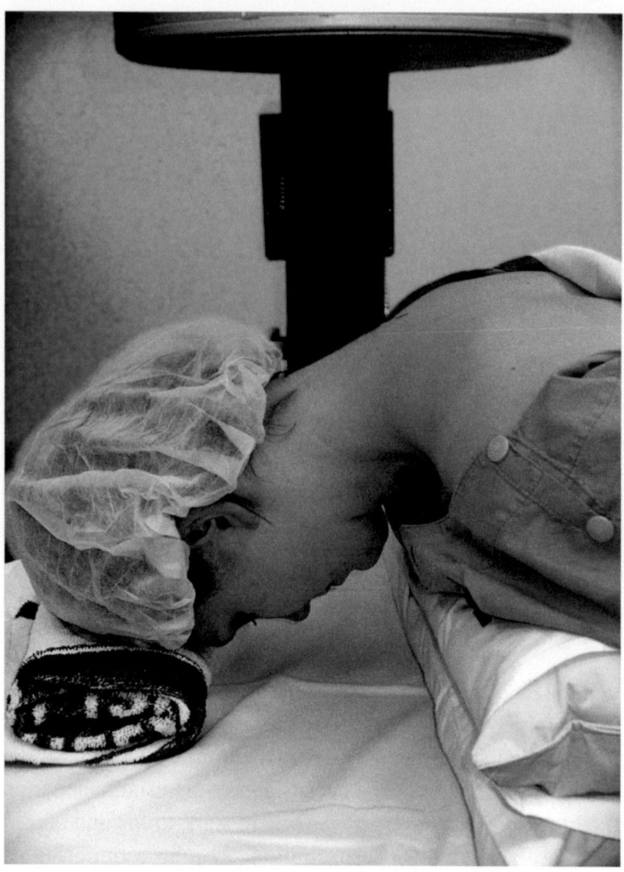

Fig. 14.5 Patient positioning for the preferred prone approach. Pillows under the chest achieve good flexion of the cervical spine while still allowing for a clear face to support breathing. Fluoroscopy can be easily performed with this position. (Reproduced with permission from Paul Gray)

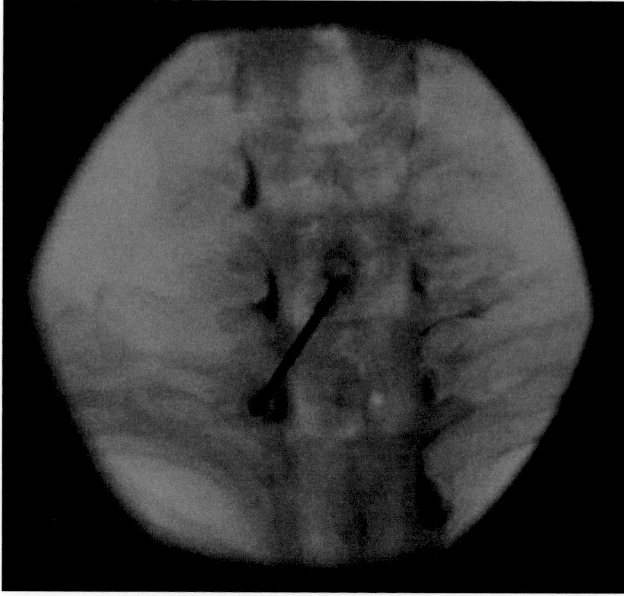

Fig. 14.6 Epidurogram of the cervical epidural space with a small volume of contrast solution. The epidural Tuohy needle is in position at the C7/T1 interspace. (Reproduced with permission from Paul Gray)

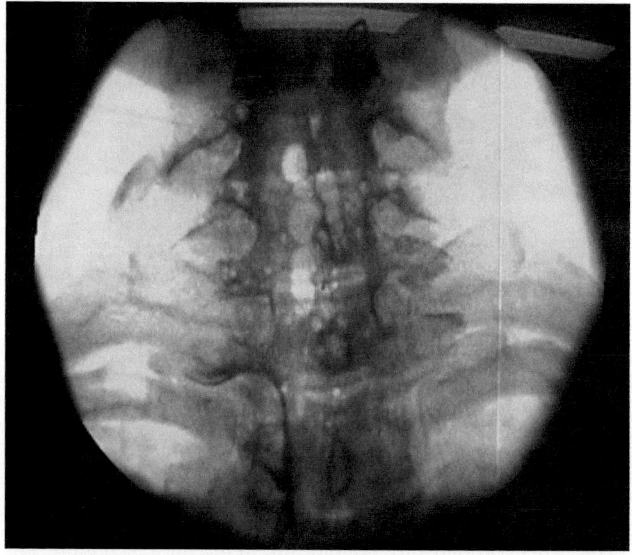

Fig. 14.7 Epidurogram of the cervical epidural space following a larger volume of contrast solution. Loss-of-resistance to air was used in this case with the bubbles of air visible in the epidural space following injection of the contrast solution. (Reproduced with permission from Paul Gray)

The cervical interlaminar epidural block is most commonly accessed between the C6/C7 and C7/T1 interspace. After clear identification of the interlaminar space, a local anaesthetic is used to numb the trajectory of the Tuohy needle.

Using loss-of-resistance with saline in the epidural syringe is recommended as using loss-of-resistance to air can rarely result in pneumocephalus in the event of a dural puncture. With the spinous processes being quite vertical in the prone patient, the direction of the needle should be perpendicular to the skin and therefore perpendicular to the floor. The right-handed interventionist would stand on the patient's left side when in the prone position.

A small volume (1–2 ml) of radio-opaque contrast approved for epidural use can be injected to confirm the placement within the epidural space. Figure 14.6 demonstrates an epidurogram with a smaller volume of contrast solution, whereas Fig. 14.7 shows the normal appearance of an epidurogram with a larger volume of contrast.

The injectate usually consists of a combination of glucocorticoid (dexamethasone 4–8 mg, triamcinolone 20–40 mg or methylprednisolone 40 mg) and low concentration local anaesthetic (ropivacaine 0.2% or lidocaine 1%). A 2 ml injection of contrast at C6–C7 or C7–T1 will spread laterally and cranially up to approximately C3. Considering the narrow epidural margin at the cervical level it is theoretically possible that injection of higher volumes increases the risk for dural puncture. Therefore, a volume of max 3 ml slowly injected is recommended. A recent RCT comparing low-dose lidocaine to saline as the diluent in cervical epidural corticosteroid injection demonstrated no difference in myotomal weakness or immediate meaningful pain relief.

If a longer-term unilateral block is required, an epidural catheter can be directed to the desired side by rotating the epidural needle 45 degrees to that side and gently introducing the catheter. This position can again be confirmed with 1–2 mL of radio-opaque solution.

Complications

Injury to the spinal cord at the level of the cervical interlaminar epidural block or brain can be devastating and may include localised neurological injury, paraplegia, quadriplegia or death. This injury may occur via epidural haematoma, drug error, epidural infection, intravascular injection or direct trauma from the advancing epidural needle. The use of particulate steroid likely adds to the risk of injury due to the embolic effect with inadvertent intravascular injection.

Inadvertent injections may occur into an epidural vein resulting in local anaesthetic toxicity or injection into the subarachnoid space resulting in high (or even total) spinal anaesthesia, hence the importance of conducting the block in an environment where resuscitation can be performed.

More common adverse effects include those from the injected local anaesthetic including hypotension secondary to the blocking of cardiac sympathetic fibres plus peripheral vasodilatation. This can be managed with supplemental oxygen, increased intravenous fluids, vasopressors and atropine for the management of bradycardia and hypotension.

A mild reduction of respiratory function may be seen due to the effect of local anaesthetic on the phrenic nerve (C3–C5) and therefore the contractility of the diaphragm.

The deposit of glucocorticoid steroids may be beneficial but may cause systemic effects including temporary disruption of the hypothalamus-pituitary-adrenal axis, prolonged menses in women for one or two menstrual cycles or poorly controlled blood sugar levels in diabetics.

Practical Tips

As the use of loss-of-resistance alone has been shown to have a high false positive rate, injecting a small volume of radio-opaque solution approved for epidural use can be used to help confirm the position of the needle.

On loss-of-resistance, careful aspiration of the needle should be performed as venous tap and dural puncture is generally only detected on aspiration of the needle. This is especially the case in the prone position due to the 10 cm of vertical height of the epidural needle.

The use of a contralateral oblique view at 50 ° to the anterior-posterior may allow better view of the tip of the epidural needle to reduce the risk of advancing the needle too far with subsequent dural puncture or spinal cord injury.

In patients with diabetes, it may be prudent to reduce the dose of steroid by 50% to minimise the disruption of blood sugar control.

Sedation should be avoided but if administered, only in small doses. Excessive sedation can result in sudden movement of the patient if they become disorientated adding to the risk of needle misplacement. The procedure can usually be performed with minimal discomfort using local anaesthetic infiltration of the skin prior to introducing the Tuohy needle.

Literature Review

Cervical interlaminar epidural steroid administration for the treatment of subacute radicular pain was tested in eight RCTs and various observational studies. The evidence is of moderate quality mainly due to the heterogeneity of the study methodology and lack of a true placebo comparison. Cervical interlaminar epidural steroid administration provides pain relief up at 3-month follow-up. Reported cases of severe neurological injury using the interlaminar technique are rare and significantly less when compared to transforaminal injections at the same level. The transforaminal risk is such that it has been suggested this approach be abandoned.

A case series of 394 patients undergoing carotid surgery received a cervical interlaminar epidural block for surgical anaesthesia and analgesia. The authors described two inadvertent dural punctures and six blood taps. Of the six venous taps, five were only detected on aspiration and one detected when the patient had a seizure following the injection of local anaesthetic. Three patients developed respiratory failure requiring ventilation. However, all of these patients had pre-existing chronic obstructive airways disease and the dose used in this study was a generous 15 ml of 0.5% bupivacaine. It is also important to note that it is difficult to completely block the phrenic nerve. A cervical epidural injection of 15 ml of 2% lidocaine at C7/T1 resulted in a 12–16% reduction in FVC and FEV1 but no change to maximum inspiratory pressure or SpO_2.

In conclusion, cervical interlaminar epidural block has indications in surgical anaesthesia and especially in chronic pain therapy. However, meticulous attention to the technique and careful selection of the drugs injected into the epidural space are warranted while the patient is kept under monitoring for at least 1-hour post puncture. Complications do occur and question the validity of epidural injections of steroids, highlighting potential disadvantages. Further research is needed, to define the exact role of cervical interlaminar epidural block in chronic pain medicine.

Suggested Reading

Ahsan SN, Faridi S. Cervical epidural anesthesia for sub-total thyroidectomy in a patient with aortic incompetence. J Pak Med Assoc. 1998;48(9):281–3.

Bao C, Bao S. Hemorrhagic infarction of cerebellum and brainstem due to cervical epidural steroid injection - case report and review of the literature. Acad Forensic Pathol. 2018;8(4):952–6. https://doi.org/10.1177/1925362118821494.

Bonnet F, Szekely B, Abhay K, Touboul C, Boico O, Saada M. Baroreceptor control after cervical epidural anesthesia in patients undergoing carotid artery surgery. J Cardiothorac Anesth. 1989;3(4):418–24. https://doi.org/10.1016/s0888-6296(89)97411-5.

Buchheit T, Crews JC. Lateral cervical epidural catheter placement for continuous unilateral upper extremity analgesia and sympathetic block. Reg Anesth Pain Med. 2000;25(3):313–7. https://doi.org/10.1016/s1098-7339(00)90019-1.

Cohen SP, Hayek S, Semenov Y, Pasquina PF, White RL, Veizi E, et al. Epidural steroid injections, conservative treatment, or combination treatment for cervical radicular pain: a multicenter, randomized, comparative-effectiveness study. Anesthesiology. 2014;121(5):1045–55. https://doi.org/10.1097/ALN.0000000000000409.

Dogliotti AM. Segmental peridural spinal anesthesia. Am J Surg. 1933;20(1):107–18.

Epstein NE. Major risks and complications of cervical epidural steroid injections: an updated review. Surg Neurol Int. 2018;9:86. https://doi.org/10.4103/sni.sni_85_18.

Gill JS, Aner M, Nagda JV, Keel JC, Simopoulos TT. Contralateral oblique view is superior to lateral view for interlaminar cervical and cervicothoracic epidural access. Pain Med. 2015;16(1):68–80. https://doi.org/10.1111/pme.12557.

Han KR, Kim C, Park SK, Kim JS. Distance to the adult cervical epidural space. Reg Anesth Pain Med. 2003;28(2):95–7.

Horlocker TT, Vandermeuelen E, Kopp SL, Gogarten W, Leffert LR, Benzon HT. Regional anesthesia in the patient receiving antithrombotic or thrombolytic therapy: American Society of Regional Anesthesia and Pain Medicine evidence-based guidelines (fourth edition). Reg Anesth Pain Med. 2018;43(3):263–309. https://doi.org/10.1097/AAP.0000000000000763.

House LM, Barrette K, Mattie R, McCormick ZL. Cervical epidural steroid injection: techniques and evidence. Phys Med Rehabil Clin N Am. 2018;29(1):1–17. https://doi.org/10.1016/j.pmr.2017.08.001.

Huygen F, Kallewaard JW, van Tulder M, Van Boxem K, Vissers K, van Kleef M, et al. "Evidence-based interventional pain medicine according to clinical diagnoses": update 2018. Pain Pract. 2019;19(6):664–75. https://doi.org/10.1111/papr.12786.

Kim YD, Ham HD, Moon HS, Kim SH. Delayed Pneumocephalus following fluoroscopy guided cervical Interlaminar epidural steroid injection: a rare complication and anatomical considerations. J Korean Neurosurg Soc. 2015;57(5):376–8. https://doi.org/10.3340/jkns.2015.57.5.376.

Landers MH. Spinal cord injury during attempted cervical Interlaminar epidural injection of steroids. Pain Med. 2018;19(4):652–7. https://doi.org/10.1093/pm/pnx081.

Lirk P, Kolbitsch C, Putz G, Colvin J, Colvin HP, Lorenz I, et al. Cervical and high thoracic ligamentum flavum frequently fails to fuse in the midline. Anesthesiology. 2003;99(6):1387–90. https://doi.org/10.1097/00000542-200312000-00023.

Manchikanti L, Cash KA, Pampati V, Wargo BW, Malla Y. A randomized, double-blind, active control trial of fluoroscopic cervical interlaminar epidural injections in chronic pain of cervical disc herniation: results of a 2-year follow-up. Pain Physician. 2013;16(5):465–78.

Manchikanti L, Falco FJ, Diwan S, Hirsch JA, Smith HS. Cervical radicular pain: the role of interlaminar and transforaminal epidural injections. Curr Pain Headache Rep. 2014;18(1):389. https://doi.org/10.1007/s11916-013-0389-9.

McCormick ZL, Burnham T, Cunningham S, Kendall RW, Bougie D, Teramoto M, et al. Effect of low-dose lidocaine on objective upper extremity strength and immediate pain relief following cervical interlaminar epidural injections: a double-blinded randomized controlled trial. Reg Anesth Pain Med. 2020;45(10):767–73. https://doi.org/10.1136/rapm-2020-101598.

Narouze S, Benzon HT, Provenzano D, Buvanendran A, De Andres J, Deer T, et al. Interventional spine and pain procedures in patients on antiplatelet and anticoagulant medications (second edition): guidelines from the American Society of Regional Anesthesia and Pain Medicine, the European Society of Regional Anaesthesia and Pain Therapy, the American Academy of pain medicine, the international neuromodulation society, the north American neuromodulation society, and the world Institute of Pain. Reg Anesth Pain Med. 2018;43(3):225–62. https://doi.org/10.1097/AAP.0000000000000700.

Nystrom UM, Nystrom NA. Continuous cervical epidural anesthesia in reconstructive hand surgery. J Hand Surg Am. 1997;22(5):906–12. https://doi.org/10.1016/s0363-5023(97)80089-5.

Simopoulos T, Peeters-Asdourian C. Pneumocephalus after cervical epidural steroid injection. Anesth Analg. 2001;92(6):1576–7. https://doi.org/10.1097/00000539-200106000-00045.

Singh AP, Tewari M, Singh DK, Shukla HS. Cervical epidural anesthesia: a safe alternative to general anesthesia for patients undergoing cancer breast surgery. World J Surg. 2006;30(11):2043–7; discussion 8-9. https://doi.org/10.1007/s00268-006-0117-2.

Stevens RA, Frey K, Sheikh T, Kao TC, Mikat-Stevens M, Morales M. Time course of the effects of cervical epidural anesthesia on pulmonary function. Reg Anesth Pain Med. 1998;23(1):20–4. https://doi.org/10.1016/s1098-7339(98)90106-7.

Stojanovic MP, Vu TN, Caneris O, Slezak J, Cohen SP, Sang CN. The role of fluoroscopy in cervical epidural steroid injections: an analysis of contrast dispersal patterns. Spine. 2002;27(5):509–14.

Trentman TL, Rosenfeld DM, Seamans DP, Hentz JG, Stanek JP. Vasovagal reactions and other complications of cervical vs. lumbar translaminar epidural steroid injections. Pain Pract. 2009;9(1):59–64. https://doi.org/10.1111/j.1533-2500.2008.00242.x.

Van Boxem K, Rijsdijk M, Hans G, de Jong J, Kallewaard JW, Vissers K, et al. Safe use of epidural corticosteroid injections: recommendations of the WIP Benelux work group. Pain Pract. 2019;19(1):61–92. https://doi.org/10.1111/papr.12709.

Van Zundert J, Huntoon M, Patijn J, Lataster A, Mekhail N, van Kleef M, et al. 4. Cervical radicular pain. Pain Pract. 2010;10(1):1–17. https://doi.org/10.1111/j.1533-2500.2009.00319.x.

Young WF. Cervical spondylotic myelopathy: a common cause of spinal cord dysfunction in older persons. Am Fam Physician. 2000;62(5):1064–1070, 1073.

Cervical Medial Branch Blocks and Radiofrequency Ablation

15

Roderick J. Finlayson, John Paul B. Etheridge, and Juan Venter

Contents

Abbreviations

AP	Articular pillars
CMBBs	Cervical medial branch blocks
LA	Local anesthetic
SSC	semispinalis capitis muscle
TON	Third occipital nerve
TP	transverse process
US	ultrasound
USG	ultrasound-guided

Considerations

Cervical medial branch blocks and radiofrequency ablations are commonly employed for the diagnosis and management of facet-related pain. The latter constitutes the most important cause of axial neck pain and has been implicated in 40% of all cases. In addition, the upper cervical joints can also cause cervicogenic headaches, an often-debilitating condition representing up to 20% of chronic headaches. Well-defined pain referral patterns for each joint can help operators select the appropriate injection level. Fluoroscopy has long been the imaging standard for spinal procedures, as it allows operators to reliably define bony structures while remaining impervious to the depth of overlying tissue. Nonetheless, several anatomic features unique to the neck offer an ideal canvas for ultrasound guidance (USG). For instance, cervical targets are relatively shallow (usually ≤3 cm under the skin surface): this falls within the range of high-resolution linear array probes. Another particularity of the cervical spine stems from the large number of critical soft tissue structures (blood vessels, nerves) in close proximity to the needle path. Unlike fluoroscopy, USG allows the operator to visualize and avoid these structures during needle insertion, which may reduce complication rates related to vascular breach. This chapter will review techniques based on both the imaging modalities, which can often be combined for optimal effect.

R. J. Finlayson (✉) · J. P. B. Etheridge · J. Venter
Bill Nelems Pain and Research Centre, Kelowna, BC, Canada

D. Jankovic, P. Peng (eds.), *Regional Nerve Blocks in Anesthesia and Pain Therapy*,
https://doi.org/10.1007/978-3-030-88727-8_15

Patient Selection

Eligible patients will typically have had neck pain for at least 3 months and not responded to conservative therapies. Levels to be treated are determined by known pain referral patterns (Fig. 15.1), and specific joints are blocked by targeting the medial branch above and below (i.e., the C5 and C6 nerves for the C5/C6 joint), while the TON is anesthetized for the C2/C3 joint. Although clinical trials examining the effect of cervical medial branch radiofrequency ablation have selected only patients with complete (100%) relief of the affected segment following controlled diagnostic blocks, such stringent criteria are often not followed in clinical practice. As this may result in more modest post-procedural pain relief, the clinical significance of any pain reduction following a diagnostic block should be carefully considered before proceeding with an ablation.

Functional Anatomy

Each zygapophyseal joint is innervated by the medial branch above and below it, except for the C2/C3 level, which is solely innervated by the third occipital nerve. The later originates from C3 spinal nerve in the C2/C3 foramen and curves posteriorly through the intertransverse space where it divides into several smaller branches, in addition to a larger superficial branch (the third occipital nerve), which crosses the C3 articular pillar at or below the C2/C3 facet joint. Whereas from C4 to C7, the posterior ramus divides into a lateral and medial branch as it crosses the transverse process. The medial branch then courses posteriorly, following the contour of the articular pillar (typically 1–2 mm lateral to the periosteal surface), and sends articular branches to the adjacent joints from the posterior aspect of the articular pillar (Fig. 15.2). In contrast to other segments where medial

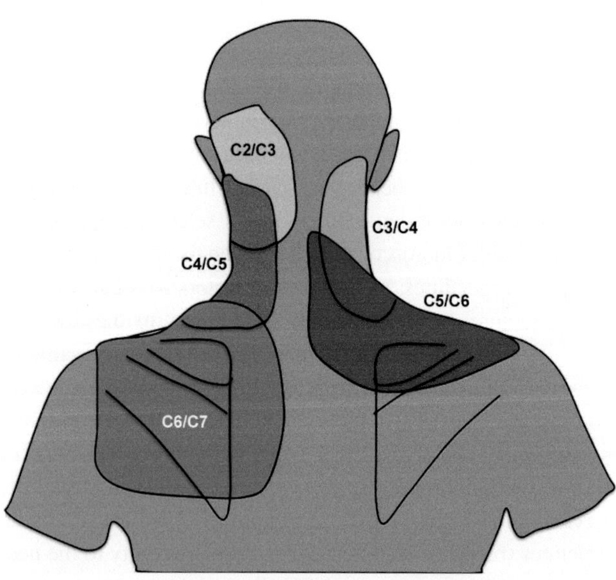

Fig. 15.1 Segmental pain referral patterns for cervical zygapophyseal joints. (Adapted from Dwyer A, Aprill C, Bogduk N. Cervical zygapophyseal joint pain patterns: a study in normal volunteers. *Spine* 1990;15:453–457. Reproduced with permission from Philip Peng Educational Series)

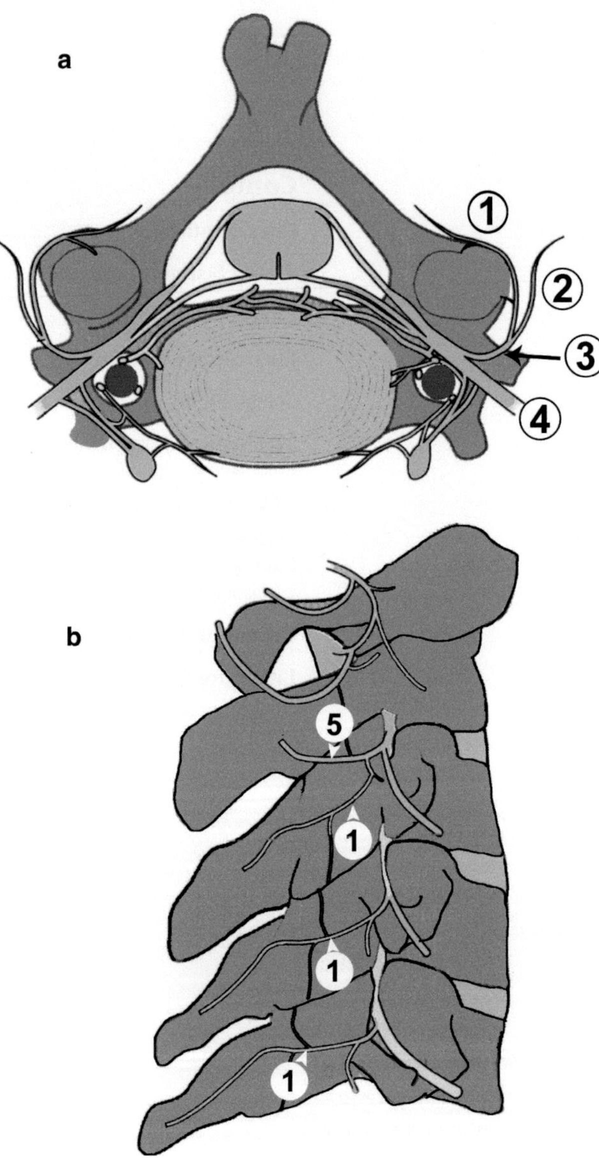

Fig. 15.2 (**a**) Transverse view of a C5 vertebra demonstrating the spinal nerve anatomy. Medial branch of posterior ramus (1); lateral branch of posterior ramus (2); posterior primary ramus (3); anterior ramus (4). (**b**) Lateral view of a cervical spine model demonstrating the course of the cervical medial branches. A cervical medial branch traverses the articular pillar, supplying the zygapophyseal joint above and below (1); The C2/C3 joint is unique as it is innervated solely by the third occipital nerve (5), which emerges from the posterior ramus along with the medial branch of C3. The latter innervates the C3/C4 joint with the C4 medial branch. (Reproduced with permission from Philip Peng Educational Series)

branches course near the centroid of the articular pillar, at C7 the nerve crosses the superior articular process, or less commonly, the root of the transverse process. Whereas all medial branches innervate segments of the posterior neck muscles (multifidus and interspinalis), the third occipital nerve is unique in providing cutaneous sensory innervation to a suboccipital patch of skin.

Although fluoroscopy and ultrasound provide different imaging perspectives, an understanding of bony anatomy is critical for the performance of techniques using either modality.

Fluoroscopic Anatomy

Lateral and anteroposterior views and their bony correlates are illustrated in Fig. 15.3. Additional views used during radiofrequency ablation procedures, including oblique and pillar view, are also presented (Fig. 15.4).

Sonoanatomy

Coronal (long axis) scan: This view is used for level confirmation in both the upper and the lower cervical spines. In the long axis, the AP appears as a series of peaks (zygapophyseal joints lines) and valleys (convex shapes of the APs) (Fig. 15.5). Above the C2-C3 joint, the slope of the inferior articular process of C2 creates a characteristic drop-off with the vertebral artery visible immediately cephalad to it (Fig. 15.6). In the lower cervical spine, the TP of C7, which can be found anterior to the AP, provides a reference for needle positioning (Fig. 15.7).

Transverse (short axis) scan: This view is used for needle placement. The targets are the C2–C3 zygapophyseal joint (TON) and the centroid aspect of the AP (C3–C6 medial branches, MB). The latter appears as a distinctive flat hyperechoic line that can be appreciated when moving the probe in a cephalo-caudal direction (Fig. 15.8). It can be differentiated from the joint line, which is rounded and less echogenic (Fig. 15.9). The tendinous insertions of the SSC (semispinalis capitis) can be identified just above the AP; their importance lies in the fact that they confine the injectate to the periosteal plane, thus ensuring a successful block with small volumes of local anesthetic. A useful landmark in the lower cervical spine is the narrow TP of C7, which has no anterior tubercle: this permits its differentiation from the TPs of other cervical levels and the wider square shape of the more posterior T1 TP (Fig. 15.10).

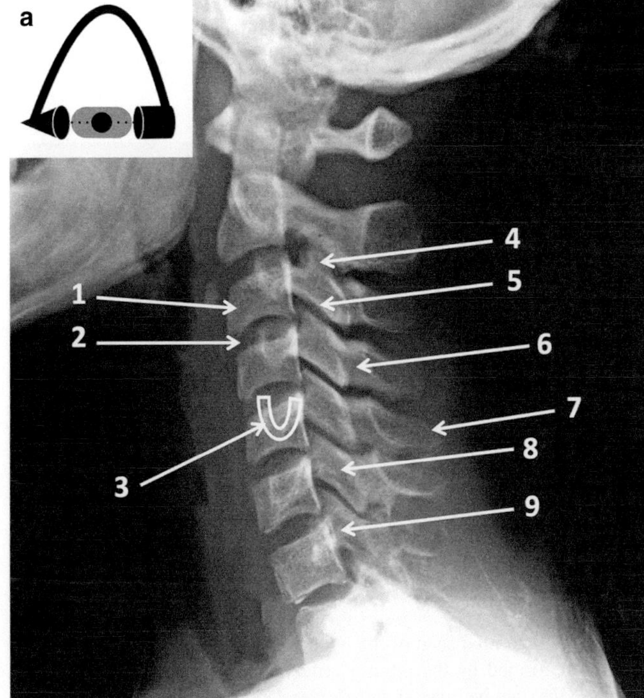

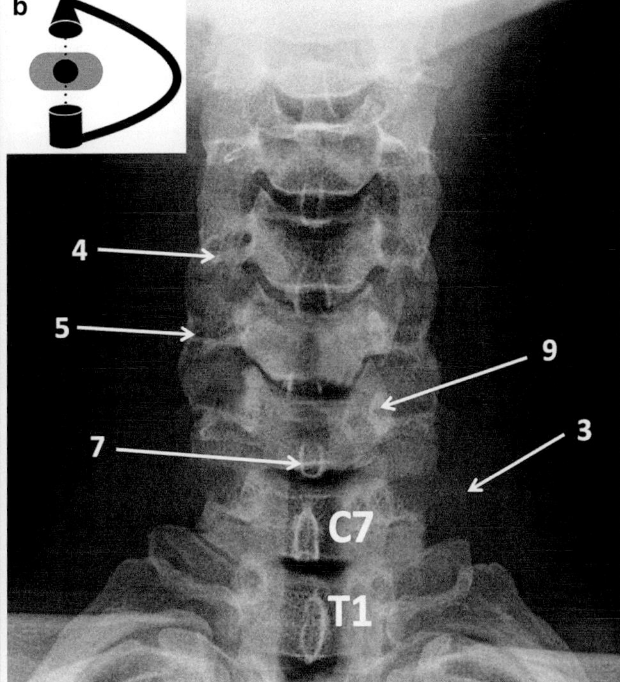

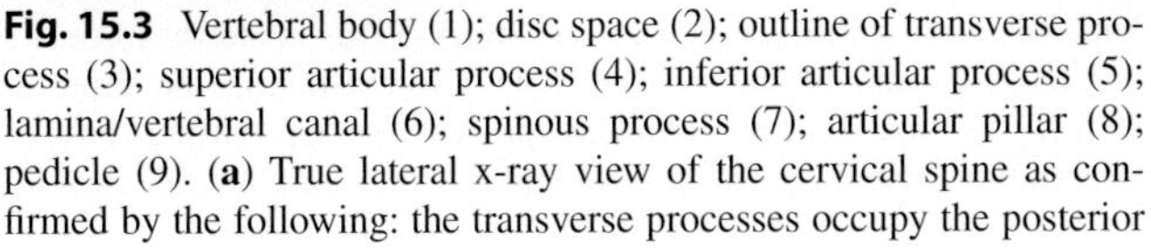

Fig. 15.3 Vertebral body (1); disc space (2); outline of transverse process (3); superior articular process (4); inferior articular process (5); lamina/vertebral canal (6); spinous process (7); articular pillar (8); pedicle (9). (**a**) True lateral x-ray view of the cervical spine as confirmed by the following: the transverse processes occupy the posterior superior quadrant of their vertebral body; the disc spaces are clear; half the vertebral canal can be seen between the articular pillar and bases of the spinous processes; the articular pillars of both sides are superimposed. (**b**) Anteroposterior view of the cervical spine. (Reproduced with permission from Philip Peng Educational Series)

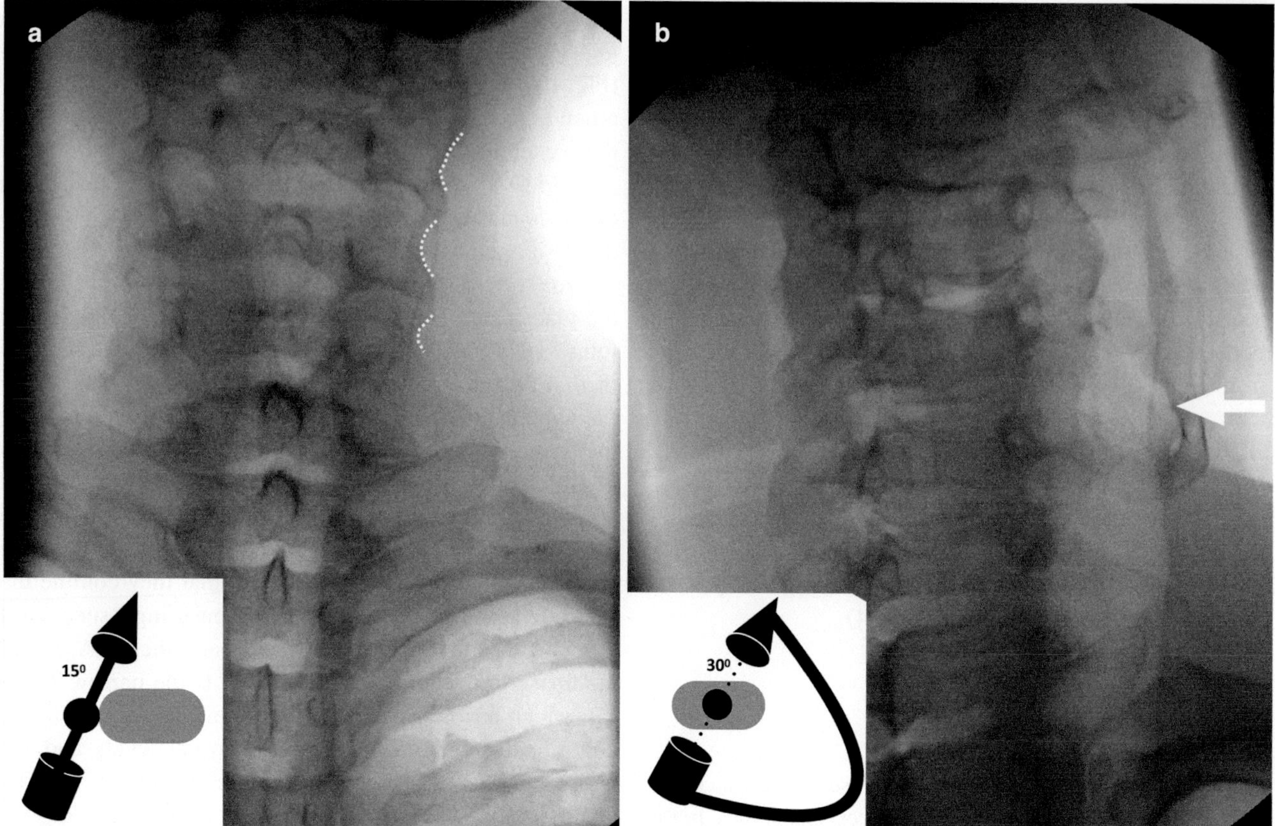

Fig. 15.4 (**a**) Pillar or declined anteroposterior view of the cervical spine in which the c-arm head has been inclined 15° caudally (left lower inset), allowing the articular pillar contours to be visualized (white dashed lines). This view is used for parasagittal cannula placements. (**b**) 30° ipsilateral oblique view, the targeted side is indicated by the white arrow. This view is used for oblique cannula placements. Because the contours of the articular pillars are not readily visualized in this view, the use of a finder needle is generally required for accurate placement. (Reproduced with permission from Philip Peng Educational Series)

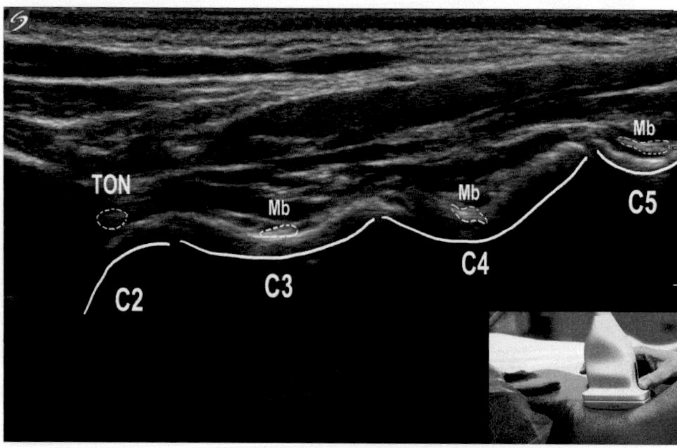

Fig. 15.5 Coronal scan of the cervical spine demonstrating the articular pillars of C4, C5, and C6, as well as the inferior articular process of C2. This view is used for level and needle position confirmation. The medial branches (mb) of C3, C4, and C5 can be seen, as well as the third occipital nerve (TON). (Reproduced with permission from Philip Peng Educational Series)

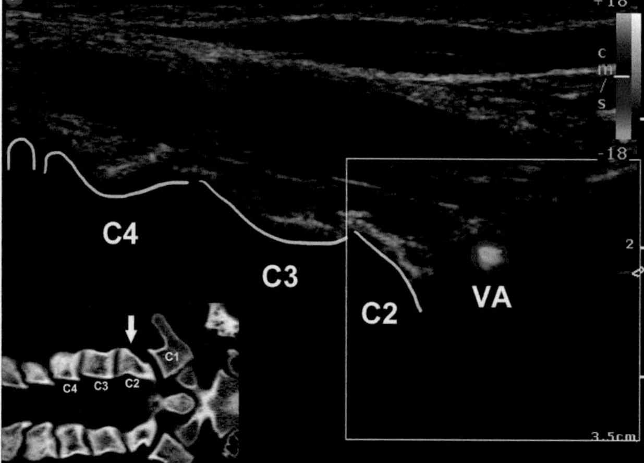

Fig. 15.6 Coronal scan of the upper cervical spine demonstrating the drop-off formed by the inferior articular process of C2; the vertebral artery (VA) can be imaged with duplex Doppler immediately cephalad. This view facilitates identification of the C2/C3 joint which is used as a landmark during third occipital nerve blocks. The left lower inset is a coronal CT scan of the cervical spine demonstrating the drop-off formed by the inferior articular process of C2 (white arrow). (Reproduced with permission from Philip Peng Educational Series)

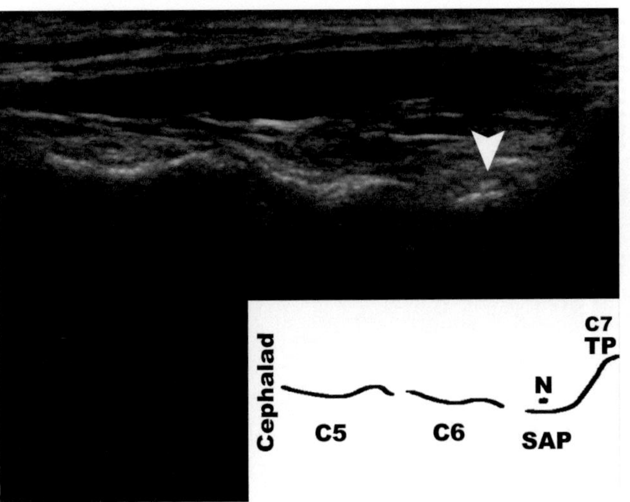

Fig. 15.7 Coronal scan of the lower cervical spine demonstrating the transverse process of C7 (C7 TP); superior articular process of C7 (SAP); articular pillar of (C5) and (C6). This view is used to confirm needle (N) positioning for blocks of the lower cervical medial branches. (Reproduced with permission from Philip Peng Educational Series)

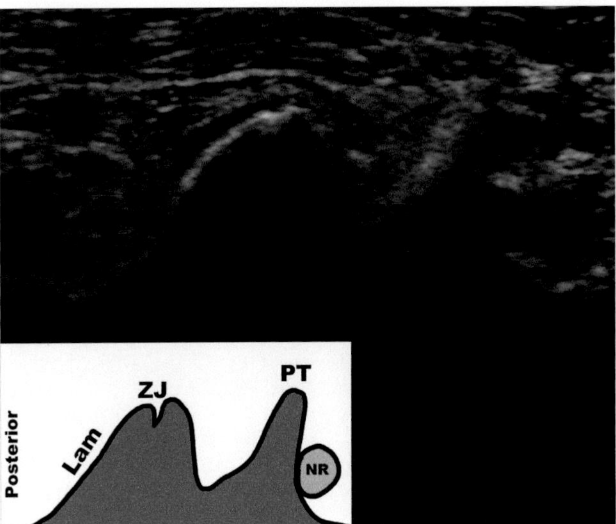

Fig. 15.9 Transverse scan at the level of the C5/C6 zygapophyseal joint (ZJ). When moving the probe in a cephalo-caudal direction, the joints, which are rounded and hypoechoic, can be differentiated from the flatter and hyperechoic articular pillars. *Lam* lamina, *PT* posterior tubercle, *NR* nerve root. (Reproduced with permission from Philip Peng Educational Series)

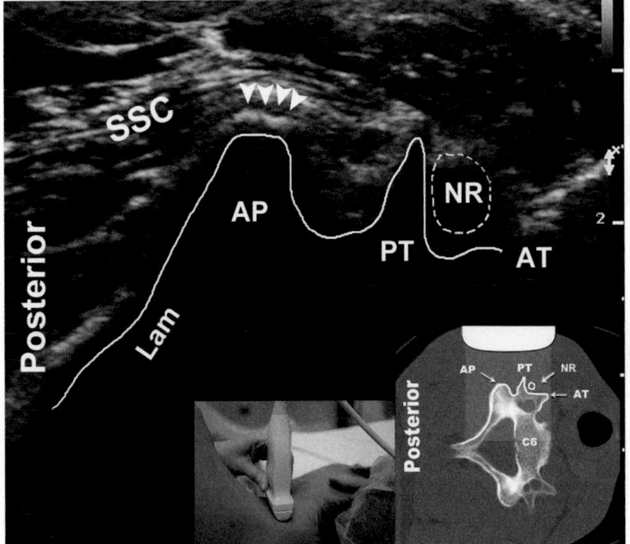

Fig. 15.8 Transverse scan of the cervical spine at the level of C6. The centroid of the articular pillar (AP) forms a distinct flat hyperechoic line and constitutes the target for cervical medial branch blocks (arrows). The (SSC) inserts on the posterior tubercle of the transverse process (PT) and courses over the AP. Further anterior, the nerve root (NR) and anterior tubercle (AT) can be seen. A CT overlay of the same bony landmarks is depicted in the right lower inset. When performing a cervical medial branch block, the injectate should be deposited along the periosteum of the AP, beneath the SSC. (Reproduced with permission from Philip Peng Educational Series)

Technique: Medial Branch Block

Common supplies include a 2.5-in., 22- or 25-gauge block needle and a local anesthetic (lidocaine or bupivacaine). In addition, a radiocontrast agent is required if fluoroscopic imaging is used. Volumes used for diagnostic blocks are 0.3 mL (MB C3-C6), 0.6 mL (MB C7), and 0.9 mL (TON). Steroids appear to have limited value when added to local anesthetics for cervical medial branch blocks (CMBB), and the use of particulate steroids should be avoided in the cervical spine.

Fluoroscopy

While a posterior parasagittal approach has been described, this section will review the more commonly used lateral approach, which is performed with the patient in a supine or lateral decubitus position. The acquisition and maintenance of a true lateral view are critical for the safe conduct of this procedure, and frequent adjustments of the c-arm may be required to compensate for patient movement or rotation of the cervical spine (Fig. 15.3a). In addition, needles should be inserted parallel to the x-ray beam in the lateral view and advanced cautiously in small increments, with frequent reevaluation of their position using a biplanar imaging technique (lateral and anteroposterior views) to avoid misdirection. As an additional precaution, 0.3 mL of contrast agent is usually injected before the LA to excluded intravascular or aberrant spread. In contrast to other levels, where a single point is targeted at the centroid of the AP, the C7 and TON (C2/C3) levels require multiple injections (Fig. 15.11). Indeed, for the TON, three injections of 0.3 mL are performed around the C2/C3 joint to ensure coverage of the nerve and the resulting caudal spread over the C3 AP

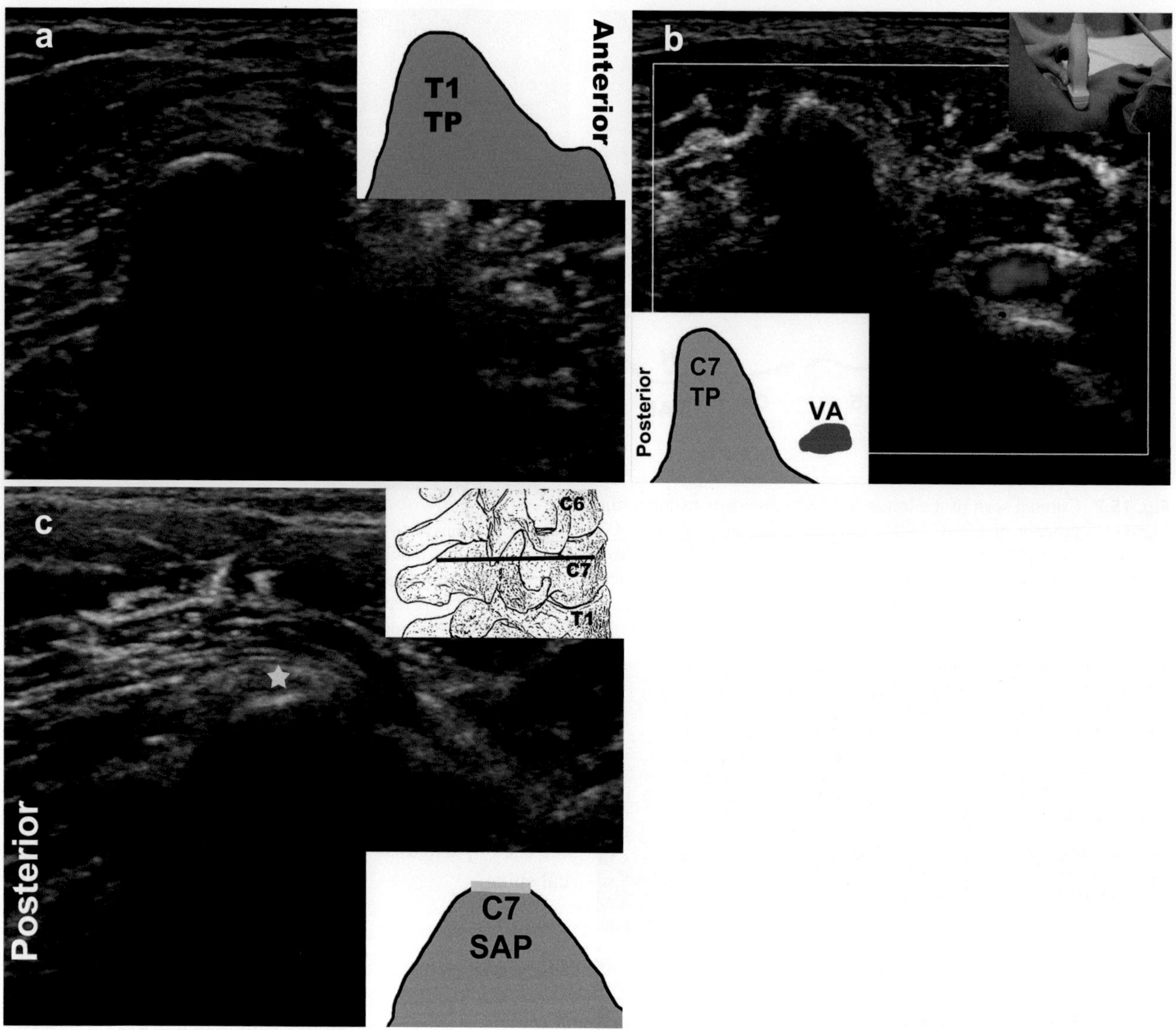

Fig. 15.10 Transverse scan of the lower neck. (**a**) The T1 transverse process (T1 TP) can be recognized because of its typical wide and square contour. Further confirmation can be obtained by tilting the probe caudally and imaging the pleura. (**b**) When scanning cephalad in a transverse plane from T1, the C7 transverse process (C7 TP) can be found anterior to that of T1. Visualizing this posterior to anterior translation is a reliable way to identify the C7 TP, which can be differentiated from that of C6 (depicted in Fig. 15.8) because it lacks an anterior tubercle. The vertebral artery (VA) can be imaged anterior to the C7 TP. (**c**) The C7 superior articular process (C7 SAP) is targeted when performing C7 medial branch blocks (white star). It can be found immediately cephalad to the C7 transverse process and appears as a small hyperechoic line. The right upper inset shows the scan line on a model spine. (Reproduced with permission from Philip Peng Educational Series)

obviates the need to separately target the C3 MB. While only one point on the superior articular process is targeted for the C7 level, two injections of 0.3 mL are performed (on the periosteum and 3 mm lateral) to ensure spread over the proximal transverse process (Fig. 15.12).

Ultrasound

1. *TON, C3, C4 medial branches*: The neck is first scanned in the coronal plane along the posterior edge of the AP in order to identify the drop-off at the C2-C3 level (Figs. 15.5 and 15.6). The probe is then rotated to a transverse plane, and the C2-C3 zygapophyseal joint identified for the TON block (Fig. 15.13). From this point, the probe is moved caudally to the target points on the C3 and C4 APs.
2. *C5, C6 medial branches*: The base of the neck is scanned in the transverse plane and the TP of T1 identified. As the probe is moved cephalad from this point, the more anterior TP of C7 is localized (Fig. 15.10b), followed by the targets on the AP of C6 and C5 (Fig. 15.8).

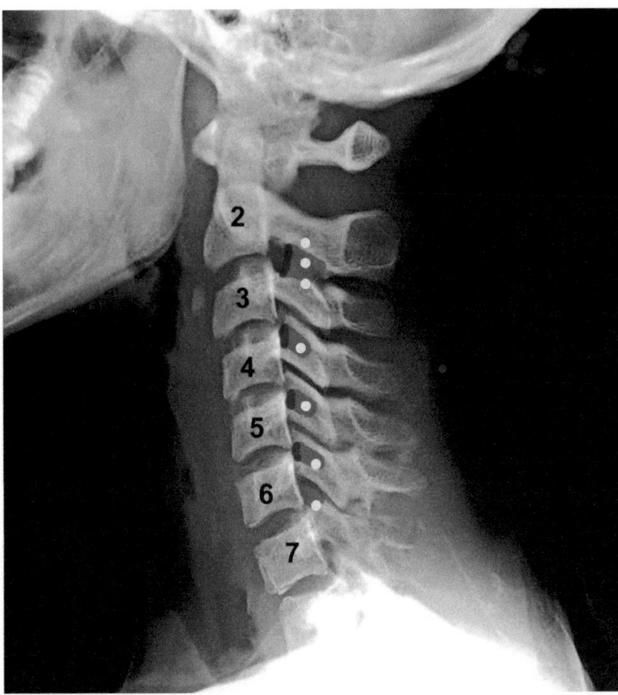

Fig. 15.11 Lateral x-ray view of the cervical spine demonstration of the targets for third occipital and cervical medial branch block (yellow dots). In addition, the target zone for radiofrequency ablation is represented for the parasagittal (red) and oblique (blue) cannula placements. Vertebral bodies are numbered to reflect their respective levels. (Reproduced with permission from Philip Peng Educational Series)

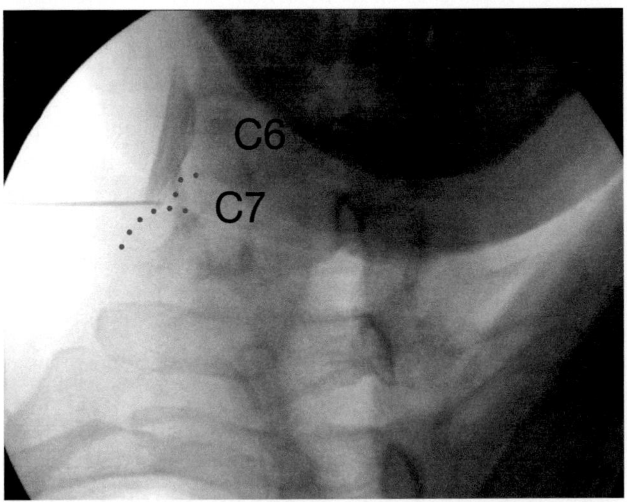

Fig. 15.12 Anteroposterior fluoroscopic view taken during a C7 medial branch block demonstrating contrast spread over the proximal C7 transverse process and superior articular process, as well as the articular pillar of C6. A needle can be seen adjacent to the superior articular process and cephalad to the transverse process (both outlined by red dots). (Reproduced with permission from Philip Peng Educational Series)

3. *C7 medial branch*: The base of the neck is scanned in the transverse plane and the TP of T1 identified. As the probe is moved cephalad from this point, the more anterior TP of C7 is localized (Fig. 15.10). The superior articular process of C7 can be imaged cephalad to the TP of C7 (Fig. 15.10c).

Needle placement after target level has been identified: Once the target has been identified in the transverse plane, pressure on the probe is reduced and the color Doppler mode engaged to detect potential blood vessels in the needle path. A posterolateral in-plane approach is used and the needle advanced until contact with the periosteum (Fig. 15.13). The probe is then rotated to obtain a coronal scan and the needle confirmed to be in the middle of the targeted AP (Fig. 15.7). Returning to a transverse view, local anesthetic (LA) is then injected under real-time visualization; if necessary, the position of the needle tip is adjusted to obtain an LA spread under the semispinalis capitis muscle that covers the anteroposterior diameter of the AP or joint (TON) (Fig. 15.14). Local anesthetic spread can also be visualized in the coronal plane, and this view can be useful when confirming coverage of the different cervical levels (Fig. 15.15). When performing a TONB, needle placement can be further refined by placing the tip next to the nerve as it can often be imaged near the C2–C3 joint in the coronal plane (Fig. 15.5). The C7 MB, because of its variable anatomy, requires two injections, with half the volume deposited on the superior articular process of C7 and the remainder 3 mm lateral to it.

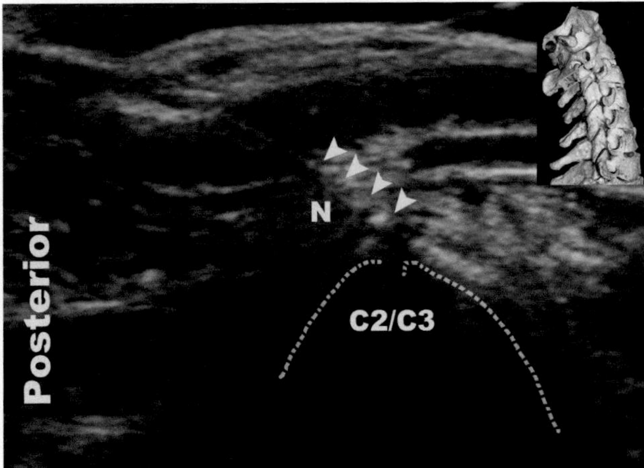

Fig. 15.13 Transverse scan of the upper neck demonstrating a needle (N) outlined by arrows, which has been placed on the (C2/C3) zygapophyseal joint using an in-plane technique and a posterolateral approach during the performance of a third occipital nerve block. The right upper inset shows the scan line on a model spine. (Reproduced with permission from Philip Peng Educational Series)

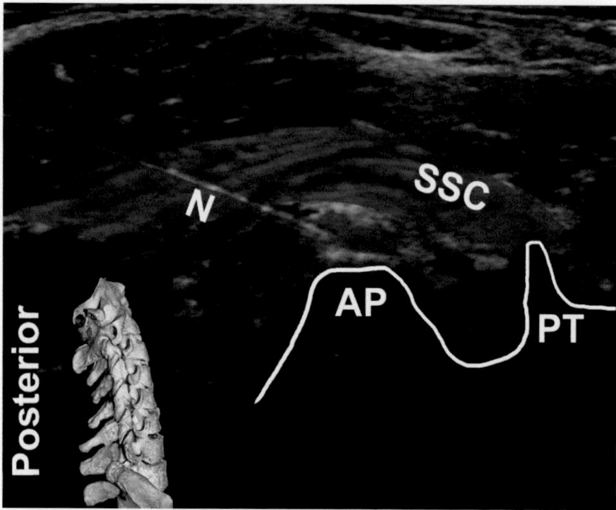

Fig. 15.14 Transverse scan of the lower neck demonstrating a needle (N) that has been placed on the C6 articular pillar (AP) using an in-plane technique and a posterolateral approach during the performance of a C6 medial branch block. The injectate (blue outline) can be seen spreading under the semispinalis capitis muscle (SSC, red highlight). Posterior tubercle (PT); left lower inset illustrates the scan line on a model spine. (Reproduced with permission from Philip Peng Educational Series)

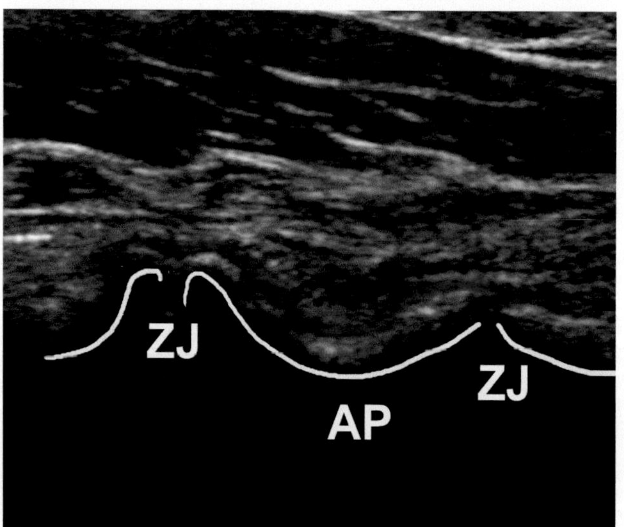

Fig. 15.15 Coronal scan of a C4 articular pillar (AP) illustrating the cephalocaudal spread of local anesthetic (blue highlight) along the periosteum and under the semispinalis capitis muscle following an ultrasound-guided medial branch block; zygapophyseal joint (ZJ). (Reproduced with permission from Philip Peng Educational Series)

Technique: Cervical Medial Branch Radiofrequency Ablation

Common supplies include a temperature-controlled radiofrequency lesion generator and a compatible probe/cannula set. Whereas cannula length (50 or 100 mm) is determined by patient body habitus, an active tip of 5 mm generally provides an adequate lesion for most individuals while minimizing unnecessary damage to posterior soft tissue structures. In addition, lesioning times of 90–120 s at 80–90 °C are commonly used.

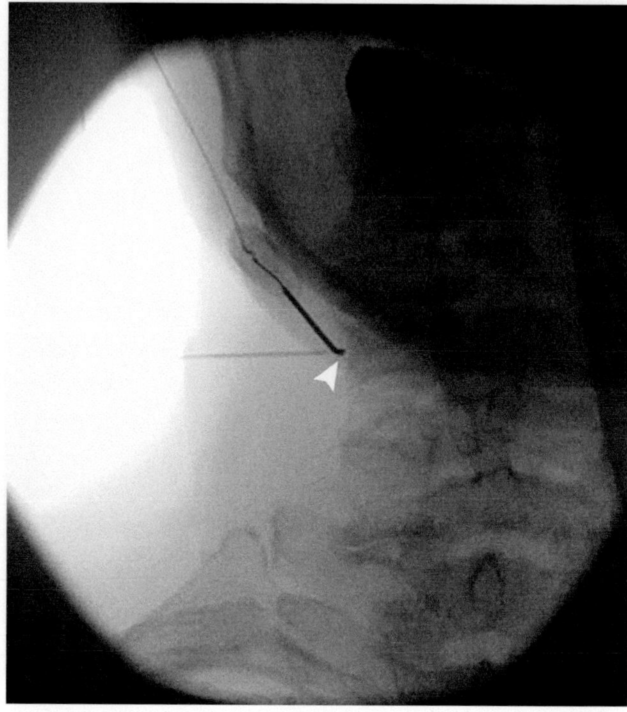

Fig. 15.16 Anteroposterior fluoroscopic view of the cervical spine demonstrating a finder needle that was previously inserted using a lateral view to facilitate the placement of a radiofrequency cannula on the C5 articular pillar (arrow). (Reproduced with permission from Philip Peng Educational Scries)

A pre-procedural medial branch block should be performed to provide anesthesia at the targeted levels using 1 mL of local anesthetic and 2 mg of dexamethasone per segment. When inserted using a lateral approach, block needles can be left in situ and serve as finder needles to facilitate level recognition in anteroposterior fluoroscopic views (Fig. 15.16).

Fluoroscopy

Effective radiofrequency ablation requires targeting a sufficiently long portion of the targeted nerve to produce long-lasting pain relief. To this aim, a two-step lesioning process involving oblique and parasagittal cannula positioning has traditionally been advocated, as it follows the curve of the medial branch around the AP (Fig. 15.17a). In order to maximize the contact with the medial branches, parasagittal passes are performed in a pillar or declined view, a modification of the standard anteroposterior approach which aligns the cannula with the natural cephalocaudal inclination of the

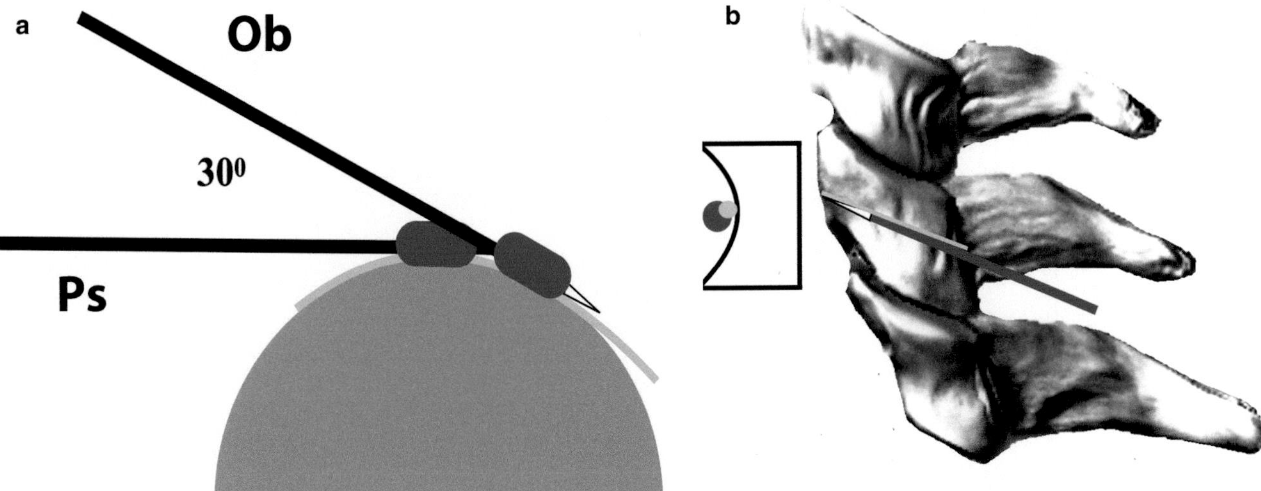

Fig. 15.17 Cervical medial branch radiofrequency ablation techniques are influenced by the bony contours of the articular pillars and zygapophyseal joints. (**a**) Both parasagittal (Ps) and 30° oblique (Ob) cannula placements are performed to maximize the length of the medial branch lesioned. (**b**) Parasagittal cannula placements are performed using a pillar view (Fig. 15.4), which aligns the insertion angle to match that of the zygapophyseal joints. In contrast, cannula placed in the 30° oblique view does not require a similar cephalocaudal angulation, as it targets the anterior aspect of the articular pillar and thus less likely to be deflected by the raised surface of the joint. (Reproduced with permission from Philip Peng Educational Series)

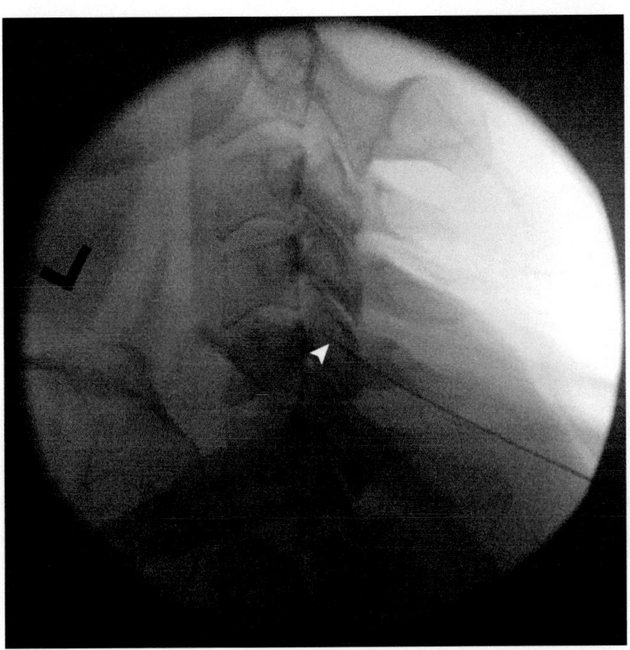

Fig. 15.18 Lateral fluoroscopic view illustrating a parasagittal radiofrequency cannula placement on the articular pillar of C5 (arrow). (Reproduced with permission from Philip Peng Educational Series)

facet joints (Figs. 15.17b and 15.18). In contrast, oblique placements target the anterior portion of the AP and are therefore less likely to be deflected laterally by the raised joint contours. As such, they can be performed in a standard oblique view. Radiofrequency ablation targets are represented in Fig. 15.11, and the number of lesions required per level depends on cannula width, as well as patient-related factors such AP length. In addition, there are level-specific considerations, such as the TON, which generally requires six lesions (three each in oblique and parasagittal) to cover the length of superior articular process of C3 (Fig. 15.19), and C4 and C5 where at least two lesions should be considered because of the 20% incidence of double medial branches at those levels.

Ultrasound

Ultrasound imaging can be used as adjunct to fluoroscopy or as a standalone modality for cervical medial branch radiofrequency ablation procedures. When used in an assistive role, US can help refine cannula positioning by providing a two-dimensional view of bony surface anatomy, which can be useful in patients with altered anatomy caused by degenerative changes. In addition, when significant vascular structures are visualized in proximity to a targeted site, potentially affecting the safety and efficacy of a planned lesion, an operator may decide to modify or abandon the intervention for that level. When using US as a primary imaging modality, two different strategies have been described. The first relies on identifying target nerves in a coronal scan and then positioning a cannula next to it using a transverse view. Unfortunately, because medial branches cannot always be identified, particularly in the lower

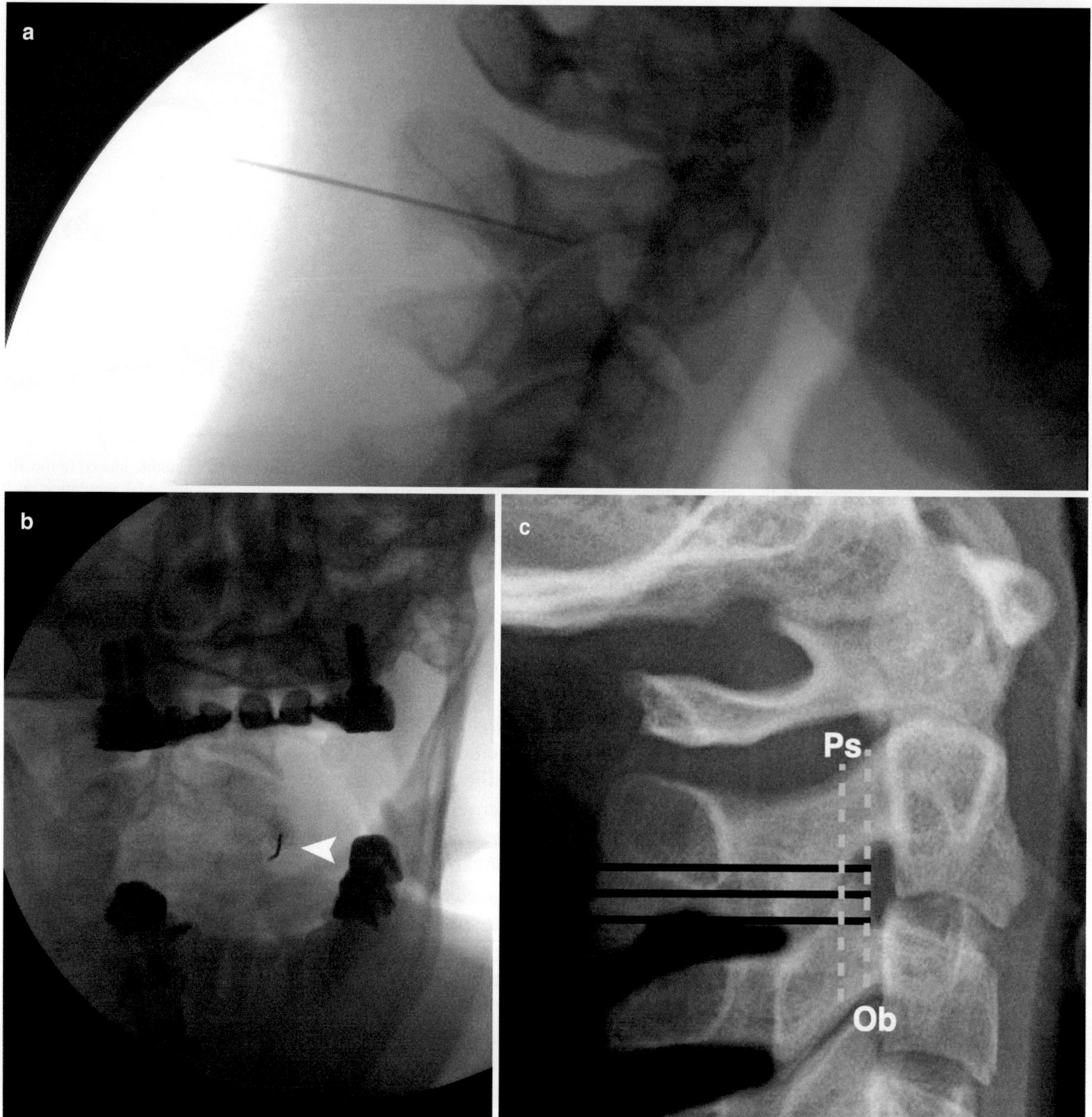

Fig. 15.19 Radiofrequency ablation of the third occipital nerve. (**a**) Lateral fluoroscopic view of the upper cervical spine demonstrating a parasagittal radiofrequency cannula placement at the upper target point for third occipital nerve ablation. (**b**) Anteroposterior open-mouth view of the cannula placement illustrated in (**a**). (**c**) The three transverse cannula placements (black lines) targeting the superior articular process of C3 for radiofrequency ablation of the third occipital nerve are shown. Final cannula tip positions for the parasagittal (Ps) and oblique (Ob) passes are also illustrated (broken white lines). (Reproduced with permission from Philip Peng Educational Series)

cervical spine and in the presence of degenerative changes, this strategy may not be reliable. The second strategy uses bony landmarks and a bi-planar USG technique to produce a lesion pattern similar to that of the fluoroscopic technique (Fig. 15.20). Indeed, by visualizing the contours of the articular pillars, operators can adjust insertion angles to optimize periosteal contact. While nerve roots are readily imaged, smaller structures such as lateral branches can be more difficult to identify. However, unintended damage to the latter can be avoided by ensuring that cannula tips remains 3 mm behind the posterior tubercle of the transverse process.

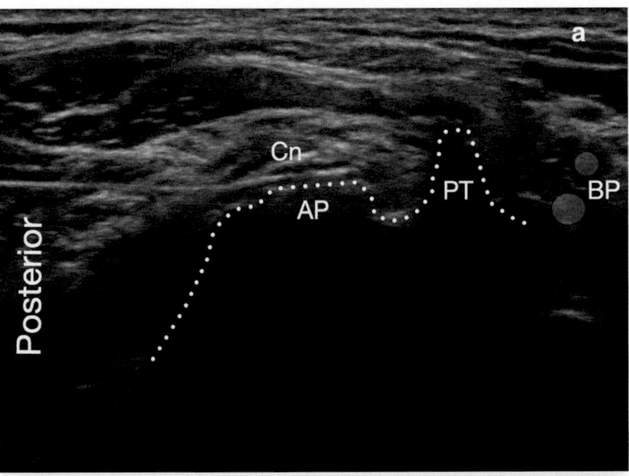

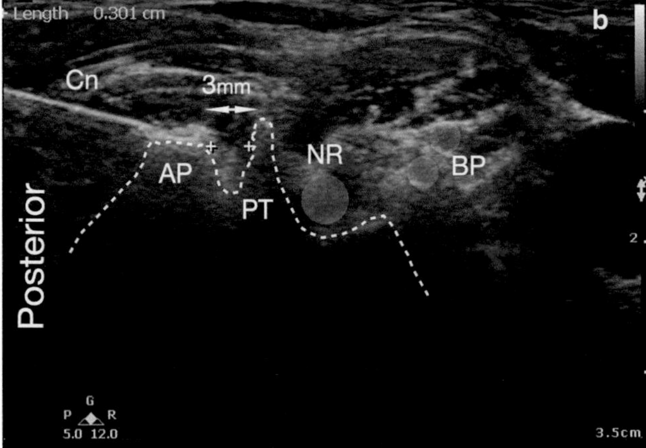

Fig. 15.20 (**a**) A conventional radiofrequency cannula (Cn) has been placed on a C5 articular pillar (AP) using an in-plane ultrasound-guided technique. The posterior tubercle (PT) and brachial plexus (BP) can be visualized anteriorly. (**b**) A deployment multi-tined radiofrequency cannula (Cn) has been placed on a C6 articular pillar (AP) using a posterolateral approach and in-plane technique. The distal tine has been placed 3 mm behind the posterior tubercle (PT) to minimize the possibility of unintentional lesioning of the lateral branch. The nerve root of C6 (NR) and brachial plexus (BP) can be seen anteriorly. (Reproduced with permission from Philip Peng Educational Series)

Ultrasound image quality is significantly affected by the presence of air, which can be introduced to the target area by needle or cannula insertions, as well as tissue degassing caused by the lesioning process. Therefore, technologies that minimize the number of lesions required can be particularly useful in the context of ultrasound guidance. One such recent innovation is the multi-tined deployment cannula, which creates a large lesion adjacent to the periosteum that is less affected by approach angles and bony contours than conventional cannula. These valuable characteristics could thus form the basis of a simplified ultrasound technique involving an approach similar to that used for medial branch blocks (Fig. 15.20b).

Complications and Safety Considerations

- Rare reports in the scientific and medicolegal literature indicate that cervical medial branch procedures can be associated with serious neurological complications when improper technique is used. In contrast, transient minor side effects (segmental skin numbness and dysesthesia) are common, affecting 20–30% of patients undergoing C4–C7 lesions and 55–95% of those undergoing TON procedures, which carry the additional risk of transient ataxia.
- Injections of local anesthetic around the cervical spine carry the risk of accidental intravascular or intrathecal spread, which can sometimes result in life-threatening complications. Fortunately, most patients will make a full recovery with timely treatment and therefore resuscitation capability should be available when performing these procedures. Furthermore, injections of particulate steroids carry the additional risk of causing vascular events affecting the anterior spinal cord (radicular artery) or posterior circulation (vertebral artery) and should therefore be eschewed in favor of dexamethasone.
- Vertebral arteries can frequently be found in proximity to the cannula path when targeting the TON at C2/C3, particularly in older age groups where patients are more likely to present arterial loops that course caudally toward the joint. A pre-procedural ultrasound scan can help identify this potentially dangerous situation.
- The use of precautionary motor stimulation prior to lesioning is controversial and its value in preventing unintended lesioning of the lateral branches or nerve roots is uncertain. Therefore, lesions should not be performed if imaging cannot confirm a safe cannula position.

Literature Review

The use of radiofrequency ablation to treat cervical pain is supported by two randomized controlled trials and several cohort studies. These suggest that approximately 63% of patients selected with dual comparative blocks (100% relief required for inclusion) will present complete pain relief at 6 months. While cervical medial branch blocks are used primarily as a diagnostic tool, they can also have a therapeutic effect. Indeed, one randomized controlled trial found that patients selected with dual comparative blocks achieved 50% relief for an average of 14 weeks following CMBB with bupivacaine. In addition, the authors found no advantage to the addition of steroids.

An emerging body of literature supports the use of ultrasound imaging for CMMBs. Compared to fluoroscopy, the latter provides similar accuracy but reduces performance time and the number of required needle passes. In addition, USG CMBBs are associated with the same short- and long-term clinical effects (pain reduction, improved functional status) as their fluoroscopy-guided counterparts. Although several trials have reported a lower incidence of vascular breach in patients assigned to ultrasound guidance, further prospective studies involving larger numbers of patients are required to determine whether US can reduce procedural complications. While there are several proof of concept studies examining the use of USG for radiofrequency ablation, no randomized controlled trials have been published.

Suggested Reading

Elgueta MF, Jimenez JO, Wang NN, Lara AP, Chankowsky J, Charghi R, Tran DQ, Finlayson RJ. Anatomical variations of the vertebral artery in the upper cervical spine: clinical relevance for procedures targeting the C1/C2 and C2/C3 joints. Reg Anesth Pain Med. 2018;43:367–71.

Finlayson RJ, Etheridge JP, Vieira L, Gupta G, Tran DQH. A randomized comparison between ultrasound- and fluoroscopy-guided third occipital nerve block. Reg Anesth Pain Med. 2013;38:212–7.

Finlayson RJ, Etheridge JP, Tiyaprasertkul W, Nelems B, Tran DQH. A prospective validation of bi-planar ultrasound imaging for C5-C6 medial branch blocks. Reg Anesth Pain Med. 2014;39:160–3.

Finlayson RJ, Etheridge JP, Tiyaprasertkul W, Nelems B, Tran DQH. A randomized comparison between ultrasound- and fluoroscopy-guided C7 medial branch blocks. Reg Anesth Pain Med. 2015;40:52–7.

Finlayson RJ, Thonnagith A, Elgueta MF, Perez J, Etheridge JP, Tran DQH. Ultrasound-guided cervical medial branch radiofrequency neurotomy: can multitined deployment cannulae be the solution? Reg Anesth Pain Med. 2017;42:45–51.

Kweon TD, Kim JY, Lee HY, Kim MH, Lee YW. Anatomical analysis of medial branches of dorsal rami of cervical nerves for radiofrequency thermocoagulation. Reg Anesth Pain Med. 2014;39:465–71.

Lord SM, Barnsley L, Wallis BJ, McDonald GJ, Bogduk N. Percutaneous radiofrequency neurotomy for chronic cervical zygapophyseal joint pain. N Engl J Med. 1996;335:1721–6.

Manchikanti L, Singh V, Falco FJ, Cash KM, Fellows B. Cervical medial branch blocks for chronic cervical facet joint pain: a randomized, double-blind, controlled trial with one-year follow-up. Spine. 2008;33:1813–20.

Siegenthaler A, Eichenberger U, Curatolo M. A shortened radiofrequency denervation procedure for cervical zygapophysial joint pain based on ultrasound localization of the nerves. Pain Med. 2011;12:1703–9.

Radiofrequency Treatment Adjacent to the Cervical Dorsal Root Ganglion

16

Xander Zuidema, Thibaut Vanneste, Koen Van Boxem, and Jan Van Zundert

Contents

General Considerations

Neck pain was ranked ninth as the leading cause of years lived with disability. Its prevalence is increasing faster than low back pain. Besides degenerative neck pain, mainly originating from the cervical facet joints, cervical radicular pain is a frequent cause of neck pain.

X. Zuidema
Department of Anesthesiology and Pain Medicine, Maastricht University Medical Centre, Maastricht, Netherlands

Department of Anesthesiology and Pain Management, Diakonessenhuis Utrecht/Zeist, Utrecht, the Netherlands
e-mail: xander.zuidema@mumc.nl

T. Vanneste
Department of Anesthesiology, Critical Care, Urgency Medicine and Multidisciplinary Pain Center, Ziekenhuis Oost-Limburg, Lanaken/Genk, Belgium

K. Van Boxem · J. Van Zundert (✉)
Department of Anesthesiology and Pain Medicine, Maastricht University Medical Centre, Maastricht, Netherlands

Department of Anesthesiology, Critical Care, Urgency Medicine and Multidisciplinary Pain Center, Ziekenhuis Oost-Limburg, Lanaken/Genk, Belgium
e-mail: jan.vanzundert@zol.be

Cervical radicular pain is pain perceived in the arm, shooting or electric in quality, caused by irritation or injury of a cervical spinal nerve root. It affects approximately 1 in 1000 adults annually. There may be confusion between cervical radicular pain and cervical radiculopathy. The latter is a condition with an objective loss of sensory and/or motor function. Radicular pain and radiculopathy are therefore not synonymous, although they are frequently used interchangeably in the literature. The former is a symptom caused by ectopic impulse generation. Radiculopathy also includes neurological signs. The two conditions may coexist and share the same etiologies: foraminal stenosis, intervertebral disc herniation, and radiculitis due to arteritis, infection, or inflammatory exudates. The two conditions can be part of a continuum, and radiculopathy may follow radicular pain as the underlying disease progresses.

In patients with cervical radicular pain, the symptoms and signs are related to dysfunction of cervical spinal nerve roots and should be attributed to the distribution of the affected

D. Jankovic, P. Peng (eds.), *Regional Nerve Blocks in Anesthesia and Pain Therapy*, https://doi.org/10.1007/978-3-030-88727-8_16

nerve root. This distribution was verified in clinical experiments, where radicular pain was elicited in the characteristic distributions by mechanical stimulation of cervical spinal nerves with a needle under fluoroscopic control. Bogduk summarized the distributions as follows: pain from C4 is restricted to the neck and suprascapular regions. Pain from C5 extends into the upper arm, while pain from C6 and C7 extends from the neck and shoulder into the forearm and hand. In both instances, the pain covers the lateral border of the upper limb, but that of C7 extends more onto the dorsal aspect. Pain from successive spinal nerves overlaps considerably, and no particular region of the upper limb is characteristic of any particular segment. Somatic referred pain from the zygapophyseal joint or from the cervical intervertebral disc can have similar distributions as radicular pain, when the pain is perceived in the proximal upper limb. However, when pain is distributed in the forearm or hand, it is far more likely to be radicular in origin. Nevertheless, radicular pain should not be restricted to a dermatome, and might be perceived in any of the structures innervated by the affected nerve, because cervical spinal nerves are also distributed to deep structures, such as muscles, joints, and ligaments as well as the skin.

A variety of treatment modalities for cervical radicular pain have been described, but the optimal treatment approach remains unclear. In clinical practice, treatment is often started with conservative measures. When conservative treatment fails to provide satisfactory outcome, epidural steroid administration, pulsed radiofrequency, or surgery may be considered as part of a multidisciplinary approach.

Indication and Patient Selection

As with other types of spinal pain, if cervical radicular pain is not resolved spontaneously within 3 months, vertebral column infections and cancer (e.g., Pancoast tumor) should be ruled out before further symptomatic treatment is offered. Somatic referred pain and shoulder pathology should also be excluded, because their clinical presentation may be similar to radicular pain. Neurological examination of patients with cervical radicular pain includes sensory, motor, and reflex evaluation. Five different clinical tests have been reported as useful for the diagnosis of cervical radicular pain: the neck compression test or Spurling test, shoulder abduction test, Valsalva maneuver, axial manual traction test, and Elvey's upper limb tension test. The validity of these three tests in radicular pain, Spurling, axial manual traction, and shoulder abduction test, has been investigated in the diagnosis of root compression in cervical disc disease. All tests had a high specificity (81–100%) but a low sensitivity (26–50%) for the validity parameters. Additionally, Spurling test has also been validated in a controlled trial using electromyography as reference, with comparable results (sensitivity of 30%; specificity of 93%). Despite low sensitivity, the three investigated tests are considered valuable aid in the clinical diagnosis of a patient with neck and arm pain.

Besides, diagnosis of cervical radicular pain and radiculopathy requires a complete medical history, clinical diagnosis using standardized test methods of physical examination, imaging techniques, electrophysiological investigation, and determination of the symptomatic level by means of diagnostic selective nerve root blocks. Nevertheless, the discrepancy found in clinical practice between symptoms and pathology identified with imaging techniques and electrophysiological testing remains striking. Moreover, recent research on genetically determined differences in sensitivity to pain highlights the problem of inter-individual variability, which is often observed in clinical practice where pain symptoms and treatment effects vary among patients with similar clinical conditions.

Functional Anatomy

The cervical spinal vertebrae can be divided in two segments: the upper spine (C1–C2) and the lower spine (C3–C7). It accommodates the spinal cord. At each segment, the nerve root arises from the spinal cord and divides into the ventral and dorsal root. The ventral root carries motor signals and the dorsal root sends sensory signals to the brain. Both nerve roots merge in the spinal foramen and become the spinal nerves. There are eight spinal nerves and each nerve exits cranially to its corresponding vertebrae, except C8, which exits caudally to C7 (Fig. 16.1).

The dorsal root ganglion (DRG) is oval and proportional in size to its related root. These ganglia are located just distal to the intervertebral foramina, immediately lateral to the perforation of the dura mater by the nerve roots. The first cervical ganglion lies on the vertebral arch of the atlas, and the second cervical ganglion is located behind the lateral atlantoaxial joint.

Technique

Prior to performing a radiofrequency (RF) procedure, confirmation of the involved level is sought by means of a prognostic block.

Prognostic Block

After the clinical diagnosis of cervical radicular pain is made, the segmental level that appears to be involved should be confirmed by a diagnostic block.

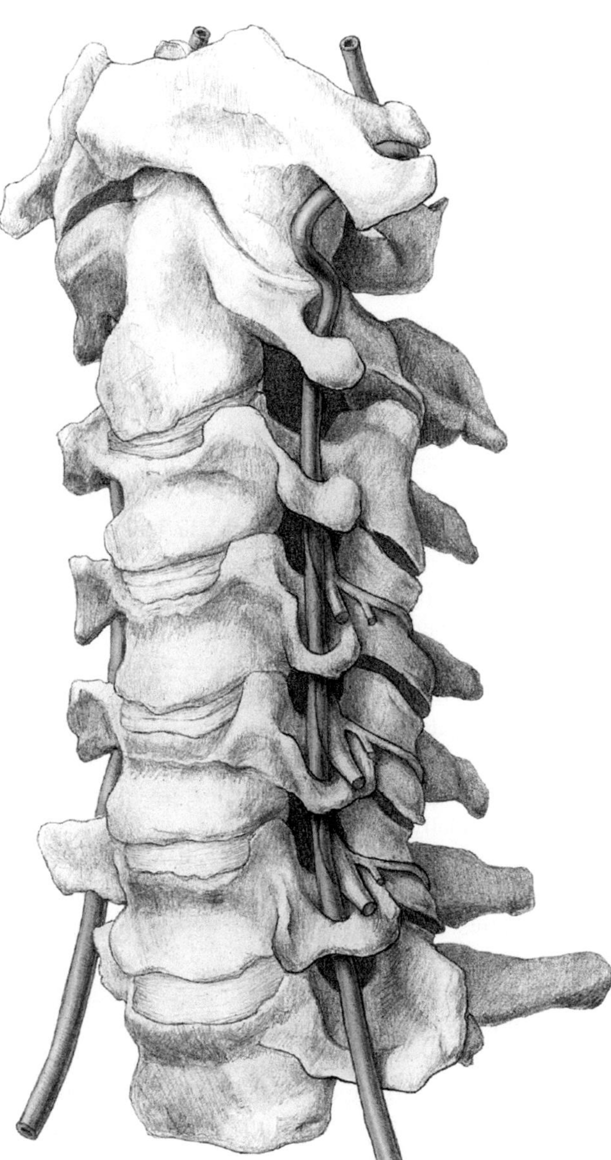

Fig. 16.1 Anatomy of the cervical spine

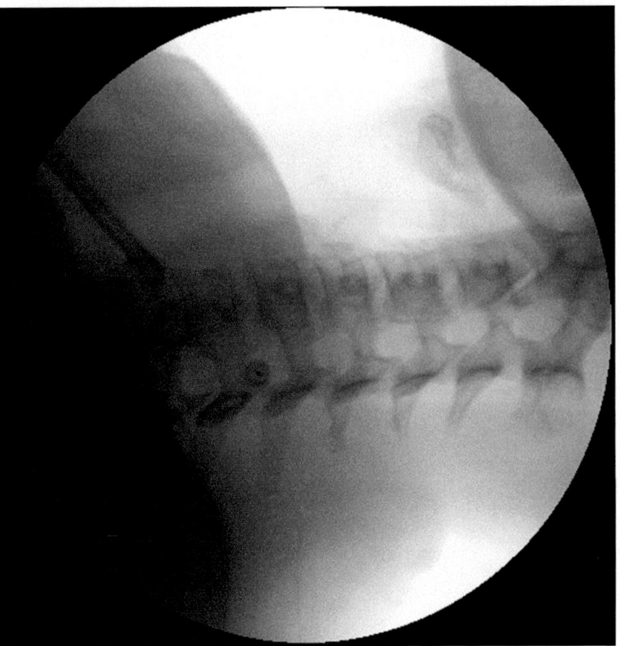

Fig. 16.2 X-ray detection with the C-arm in the lateral oblique position. The needle in the posterior caudal quadrant of the neuroforamen

The patient is placed in supine position on a translucent operation table. The C-arm of the fluoroscope is placed such that the beam is parallel to the axis of the intervertebral foramen. The axis points 25–35° oblique and 10° caudally. In this way, the entry point is determined by the projection of a metal ruler over the caudal and posterior part of the intervertebral foramen. A 60 mm 24G neuroradiography needle is introduced parallel to the beam (tunnel view). Then the beam direction is changed to the anteroposterior position, and the introducer needle is further introduced until the tip is projected just laterally to the facet column. When the segmental nerve is identified using 0.4 mL iohexol contrast dye, 0.5–1.0 mL lidocaine is slowly injected around the nerve. Overflow into the epidural space is avoided by "real-time" observation of the radio-opaque mixture.

Pain relief is assessed within 30 min following the procedure. A diagnostic block is considered positive if it results in a minimum of 50% pain reduction, as measured on the visual analogue scale (VAS) within 30 min.

Radiofrequency Treatment

The technique used for the radiofrequency (RF) intervention is similar to the one for performing prognostic nerve block. The C-arm of the fluoroscopy unit is positioned with the beam parallel to the axis of the intervertebral foramen (25–35° anteriorly and 10° caudally). The entry point is located by projecting a metal ruler over the caudal and posterior part of the foramen—"tunnel view." In practice, this dot should lie directly over the dorsal portion of the intervertebral foramen at the transition between the middle and most caudal third.

A 22 G radiofrequency cannula (54 mm with 4 mm active tip) is introduced coaxial to the beam, and, if necessary, the position is corrected in the superficial subcutaneous layers until the cannula was projected on the screen as a single dot (Fig. 16.2). This position is chosen to avoid possible penetration of the vertebral artery, which runs anterior to the ventral part of the foramen. The fluoroscope is then adjusted to the anterior-posterior view, and the cannula is inserted further until the tip projects over the middle of the facetal column (Fig. 16.3).

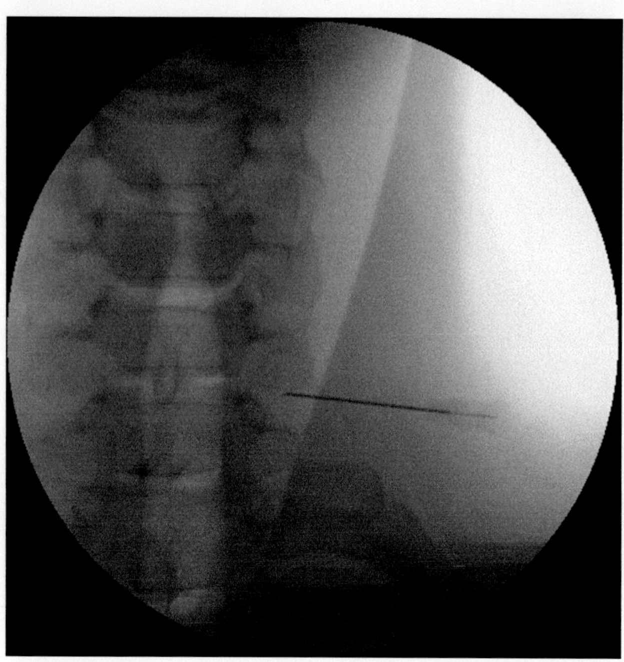

Fig. 16.3 Cervical DRG procedure: needle is in the middle of the facetal column

The stylet of the cannula is then replaced by the RF probe. After checking the impedance, which indicates a normal closed electrical circuit, stimulation is started at a frequency of 50 Hz to obtain a sensory stimulation threshold. A paresthesia is elicited along the tested cervical nerve root at less than 0.5 V. Motor stimulation is performed at a frequency of 2 Hz. Muscle contractions should not occur below a voltage of 1.5 × the sensory threshold.

The treatment can be performed using either conventional radiofrequency or pulsed radiofrequency current.

Conventional radiofrequency current is applied to slowly increase the temperature to 67 °C at the electrode tip. This temperature is maintained for 60 s. The PRF current is applied during 120 s from the lesion generator as described by Sluijter et al. With the use of PRF, the output is set at 45 V so that the temperature at the electrode tip does not exceed 42 °C.

Side Effects and Complications

The most frequently reported side effect with conventional radiofrequency treatment is a vague burning sensation in the treated dermatome. This pain usually subsides spontaneously 6 weeks after treatment. Also, hypoesthesia may be observed in the treated dermatome. Though rarely occurring, the most troublesome complication of conventional radiofrequency treatment is the deafferentation pain.

No side effects and complications of pulsed radiofrequency treatment adjacent to the cervical DRG have been reported in the literature.

Practical Tips

To obtain a good tunnel view, the entry point is located by projecting a metal ruler over the caudal and posterior part of the foramen

Real-time contrast injection is obligatory for correct needle placement for the prognostic block

Literature Review

Chronic cervical radicular pain is a complex syndrome that has a high impact on patients' quality of life. An integrated approach involving psychological counseling, physical therapy, cognitive behavioral treatment, and symptomatic management of the pain is recommended. The multidisciplinary evaluation also aims at providing guidance for the selection of any treatment. In this chapter, we focus on conventional or pulsed RF treatment.

The efficacy of RF treatment adjacent to the cervical DRG has been illustrated in two randomized clinical trials. Van Kleef et al. demonstrated a significant reduction in pain 8 weeks after RF at 67 °C compared to sham treatment. Additionally, Slappendel et al. found that treatment with RF at 40 °C was equally effective as treatment at 67 °C. According to two systematic reviews, there is currently limited evidence that radiofrequency treatment of the dorsal root ganglion is more effective than placebo in chronic cervical radicular pain.

Recently, PRF was introduced in clinical practice as a non- or minimal neurodestructive modification of conventional RF heat lesions. A clinical audit on the use of PRF treatment adjacent to the cervical DRG showed a positive outcome in 72% of the patients after 8 weeks and in 33% after 1 year. In the first randomized controlled trial (RCT) on PRF adjacent to the cervical DRG in patients with chronic cervical radicular pain, the PRF group showed a significantly better outcome with regard to the global perceived effect (>50% improvement) and VAS (20-point pain reduction) at 3-month follow-up. The need for pain medication was significantly reduced in the PRF group after 6 months. No complications were observed during the study period.

Two additional case series with a total of 43 patients suggested that more than 60% of patients benefited in terms of more than 50% pain relief or treatment success after 6 months with no serious adverse effects reported. This relief appears to be sustained at 1-year follow-up (12 of 21 patients).

The updated guidelines for evidence-based interventional pain medicine give the recommendations listed in Table 16.1 for the different treatment options for cervical radicular pain.

Table 16.1 Level of evidence and recommendation for the intervention of cervical radicular pain

Description	Strength of recommendation	Level of evidence
Interlaminar epidural corticosteroid administration could be used in addition to conservative treatment in patients with cervical radicular pain	Weak	Moderate
Transforaminal epidural preservative-free dexamethasone could be considered for the treatment of subacute cervical radicular pain	Very weak	Very low
Pulsed radiofrequency treatment adjacent to the cervical spinal ganglion (DRG) should be used for the treatment of patients with cervical radicular pain	Moderate	Moderate
Radiofrequency treatment adjacent to the cervical spinal ganglion (DRG) could be used for the treatment of patients with cervical radicular pain	Weak	Moderate
Spinal cord stimulation for cervical radicular pain could be considered for the treatment of patients with cervical radicular pain	Very weak	Not graded

Conclusions

Cervical radicular pain may be refractory to pharmacological treatment and rehabilitation. Before offering symptomatic treatment, infection and cancer (e.g., Pancoast tumor) should be excluded. After careful neurological examination and ruling out shoulder pathology, the causative level should be confirmed by means of a prognostic block. Epidural corticosteroid administration, by intralaminar or transforaminal route, may be a treatment option. There is, however, no comparison between both techniques, though the transforaminal administration route has gained in interest because it is supposed to deliver the drug as close as possible to the inflammatory nerve root. Recently, published case reports on serious adverse events after transforaminal steroid administration at the cervical level urge for a cautious use of this treatment. Surgical techniques for decompression with or without anterior interbody fusion are often performed to reduce the pain and disability, but are associated with a small but definite risk. A randomized controlled trial indicates that a multidisciplinary treatment with cognitive behavioral therapy and psychological interventions are preferred over surgery. Systematic reviews showed that there is little evidence for better efficacy of surgery compared to cognitive behavioral treatment, justifying the higher risk of complications from surgical option.

The available evidence on RF treatment adjacent to the cervical DRG suggests pain relief and improved patient satisfaction. The evidence on PRF adjacent to the cervical DRG indicates potentially similar clinical results. The perceived better safety of the latter technique justifies trying this minimal invasive procedure prior to other interventional treatment options.

Suggested Reading

Bland J. Cervical spine syndromes. J Muscoloskel Med. 1986;3:23–41.

Bogduk N. Medical management of acute cervical radicular pain: and evidence-based approach. 1st ed. Newcastle: The Newcastle Bone and Joint Institute; 1999.

Choi GS, Ahn SH, Cho YW, Lee DG. Long-term effect of pulsed radiofrequency on chronic cervical radicular pain refractory to repeated transforaminal epidural steroid injections. Pain Med. 2012;13:368–75.

Daffner SD, Hilibrand AS, Hanscom BS, Brislin BT, Vaccaro AR, Albert TJ. Impact of neck and arm pain on overall health status. Spine. 2003;28:2030–5.

Date E, Gray L. Electrodiagnostic evidence for cervical radiculopathy and suprascapular neuropathy in shoulder pain. Electromyogr Clin Neurophysiol. 1996;36:333–9.

Davidson RI, Dunn EJ, Metzmaker JN. The shoulder abduction test in the diagnosis of radicular pain in cervical extradural compressive monoradiculopathies. Spine. 1981;6:441–6.

Devereaux MW. Neck and low back pain. Med Clin North Am. 2003;87:643–62.

Dwyer A, Aprill C, Bogduk N. Cervical zygapophysial joint pain patterns. I/ A study in normal volunteers. Spine. 1990;15:453–7.

Elvey R. The investigation of arm pain: signs and adverse responses to the physical examination of the brachial plexus and related tissues. In: Boyling J, Palastanga N, editors. Grieve's modern manual therapy. New York: Churchill Livingstone; 1994. p. 557–85.

Fager CA. Identification and management of radiculopathy. Neurosurg Clin N Am. 1993;4:1–12.

Ford DJ, Pither C, Raj PP. Comparison of insulated and uninsulated needles for locating peripheral nerves with a peripheral nerve stimulator. Anesth Analg. 1984;63:925–8.

Fouyas IP, Statham PF, Sandercock PA. Cochrane review on the role of surgery in cervical spondylotic radiculomyelopathy. Spine. 2002;27:736–47.

G. B. D., Disease I, Incidence, Prevalence, Collaborators. Global, regional, and national incidence, prevalence, and years lived with disability for 354 diseases and injuries for 195 countries and territories, 1990-2017: a systematic analysis for the Global Burden of Disease Study 2017. Lancet. 2018;392:1789–858.

Geurts J, van Wijk RM, Stolker R, Groen GJ. Efficacy of radiofrequency procedures for the treatment of spinal pain: a systematic review of randomized clinical trials. Reg Anesth Pain Med. 2001;26:394–400.

Hession WG, Stanczak JD, Davis KW, Choi JJ. Epidural steroid injections. Semin Roentgenol. 2004;39:7–23.

Huygen F, Kallewaard JW, van Tulder M, et al. "Evidence-based interventional pain medicine according to clinical diagnoses": update 2018. Pain Pract. 2019;19:664–75.

Jacobs W, Anderson P, Limbeek J, Willems P, Pavlov P. Single or double-level anterior interbody fusion techniques for cervical degenerative disc disease. Cochrane Database Syst Rev. 2004;CD004958

Johnson GM. The sensory and sympathetic nerve supply within the cervical spine: review of recent observations. Man Ther. 2004;9:71–6.

Kerns RD, Habib S. A critical review of the pain readiness to change model. J Pain. 2004;5:357–67.

Merskey H, Bogduk N. Classification of chronic pain: descriptions of chronic pain syndromes and definitions of pain terms. 2nd ed. Seattle: IASP Press; 1994.

Mogil JS. The genetic mediation of individual differences in sensitivity to pain and its inhibition. Proc Natl Acad Sci U S A. 1999;96:7744–51.

Mogil JS, Wilson SG, Bon K, et al. Heritability of nociception II. 'Types' of nociception revealed by genetic correlation analysis. Pain. 1999;80:83–93.

Niemisto L, Kalso E, Malmivaara A, Seitsalo S, Hurri H. Radiofrequency denervation for neck and back pain. A systematic review of randomized controlled trials. Cochrane Database Syst Rev. 2003;CD004058

Persson LC, Lilja A. Pain, coping, emotional state and physical function in patients with chronic radicular neck pain. A comparison between patients treated with surgery, physiotherapy or neck collar—a blinded, prospective randomized study. Disabil Rehabil. 2001;23:325–35.

Radhakrishnan K, Litchy WJ, O'Fallon WM, Kurland LT. Epidemiology of cervical radiculopathy. A population-based study from Rochester, Minnesota, 1976 through 1990. Brain. 1994;117(Pt 2):325–35.

Rathmell JP, Aprill C, Bogduk N. Cervical transforaminal injection of steroids. Anesthesiology. 2004;100:1595–600.

Rothstein J, Roy S, Wolf S. The rehabilitation specialist's handbook. Philadelphia, PA: FA Davis; 1991.

Rowlingson JC. Epidural steroids: do they have a place in pain management? Barcelona: V. Permanyer Publications; 1996.

Saal JS, Saal JA, Yurth EF. Nonoperative management of herniated cervical intervertebral disc with radiculopathy. Spine. 1996;21:1877–83.

Schellhas KP, Smith MD, Gundry CR, Pollei SR. Cervical discogenic pain. Prospective correlation of magnetic resonance imaging and discography in asymptomatic subjects and pain sufferers. Spine. 1996;21:300–11; discussion 311–302.

Slappendel R, Crul BJ, Braak GJ, et al. The efficacy of radiofrequency lesioning of the cervical spinal dorsal root ganglion in a double blinded randomized study: no difference between 40 degrees C and 67 degrees C treatments. Pain. 1997;73:159–63.

Sluijter ME, Cosman ER, Rittman IIWB, van Kleef M. The effects of pulsed radiofrequency field applied to the dorsal root ganglion—a preliminary report. Pain Clin. 1998;11:109–17.

Spurling R, Scoville W. Lateral rupture of the cervical intervertebral discs: a common cause of shoulder and arm pain. Surg Gynecol Obstet. 1944;78:350–8.

Tong HC, Haig AJ, Yamakawa K. The Spurling test and cervical radiculopathy. Spine. 2002;27:156–9.

van Kleef M, Spaans F, Dingemans W, Barendse GAM, Floor E, Sluijter ME. Effects and side effects of a percutaneous thermal lesion of the dorsal root ganglion in patients with cervical pain syndrome. Pain. 1993;52:49–53.

van Kleef M, Liem L, Lousberg R, Barendse G, Kessels F, Sluijter M. Radiofrequency lesion adjacent to the dorsal root ganglion for cervicobrachial pain: a prospective double blind randomized study. Neurosurgery. 1996;38:1127–31; discussion 1131–1122.

Van Zundert J, Raj P, Erdine S, van Kleef M. Application of radiofrequency treatment in practical pain management: state of the art. Pain Pract. 2002;2:269–78.

Van Zundert J, Lamé IE, de Louw A, et al. Percutaneous pulsed radiofrequency treatment of the cervical dorsal root ganglion in the treatment of chronic cervical pain syndromes: a clinical audit. Neuromodulation. 2003;6:6–14.

Van Zundert J, Patijn J, Kessels A, Lame I, van Suijlekom H, van Kleef M. Pulsed radiofrequency adjacent to the cervical dorsal root ganglion in chronic cervical radicular pain: a double blind sham controlled randomized clinical trial. Pain. 2006;127(1–2):173–82.

Viikari-Juntura E, Porras M, Laasonen EM. Validity of clinical tests in the diagnosis of root compression in cervical disc disease. Spine. 1989;14:253–7.

Wainner RS, Gill H. Diagnosis and nonoperative management of cervical radiculopathy. J Orthop Sports Phys Ther. 2000;30:728–44.

Yoon YM, Han SR, Lee SJ, Choi CY, Sohn MJ, Lee CH. The efficacy of pulsed radiofrequency treatment of cervical radicular pain patients. Korean J Spine. 2014;11:109–12.

Part III

Nerve Block for Regional Anesthesia and Pain Therapy for Shoulder

Suprascapular Nerve Block

17

Chin-wern Chan and Philip Peng

Contents

Introduction

The suprascapular nerve (SSN) is the major sensory nerve of the shoulder. It provides sensory innervation to the posterior and superior aspects of the shoulder joint. Due to its consistent course through the suprascapular notch, the suprascapular nerve is an accessible target for neural blockade.

There have been numerous variations and refinements in the technique of suprascapular nerve block (SSNB) since its introduction. Techniques based on anatomical landmarks and radiological guidance have been described in the literature. The more recent implementation of ultrasound guidance has attempted to improve the accuracy of SSNB while reducing complications.

Indication (Patient Selection)

Blockade of the suprascapular nerve has been performed to assist in the diagnosis of suprascapular neuropathy, as well as in the management of acute and chronic shoulder pain. There has been a resurgence of interest in the role of suprascapular nerve block for shoulder surgery due to its ability to spare the phrenic nerve. In chronic pain management, there is also an increased interest in suprascapular nerve intervention in the management of various types of shoulder pain. These interventions include perineural injection, radiofrequency (ablation or pulsed) treatment, cryotherapy, and neuromodulation.

C.-w. Chan (✉)
Department of Pain Medicine, Sir Charles Gairdner Hospital, Nedlands, WA, Australia

P. Peng
Department of Anesthesia and Pain Medicine, University of Toronto, Toronto Western Hospital, Toronto, ON, Canada
e-mail: philip.peng@uhn.ca

D. Jankovic, P. Peng (eds.), *Regional Nerve Blocks in Anesthesia and Pain Therapy*,
https://doi.org/10.1007/978-3-030-88727-8_17

Anatomy of the Suprascapular Nerve

The SSN is a large peripheral nerve possessing both motor and sensory fibers. It originates from the ventral rami of the fifth and sixth cervical nerve roots with a variable contribution from the fourth cervical nerve root. Following its formation, the nerve emerges from the lateral aspect of the upper trunk of the brachial plexus. It then travels through the posterior triangle of the neck, courses deep to the trapezius and omohyoid muscles, and enters the supraspinous fossa via the suprascapular notch underneath the superior transverse scapular ligament (STSL) (Fig. 17.1). In the majority of cases, the suprascapular artery runs above (78.3%) the STSL.

Shortly after passing through the suprascapular notch, the SSN emits two branches: one is the motor nerve for the supraspinatus muscle and the other is known as the superior articular branch. The latter nerve is sensory and supplies the coracoclavicular and coracohumeral ligaments, the acromioclavicular joint, the glenohumeral joint (posterior and superior aspects), and the subacromial bursa. For readers who are interested in the details of these articular branches, please refer to the Chap. 22 on shoulder denervation. The main trunk then exits the suprascapular fossa by curving around the lateral border of the scapula spine through a fibro-osseous tunnel formed by the spinoglenoid ligament and the spine of the scapula, and terminates in motor branches to the infraspinatus muscle (Fig. 17.2).

The anatomy of the suprascapular notch is important for several reasons. The nerve is susceptible to injury and impingement at the level of the notch as it passes beneath the STSL. This site represents an attractive region for SSN blockade as the nerve has not divided yet. The variable shape of the notch has been described and has been categorized into different types (Fig. 17.3). In the adult, the most common type is a u-shaped or semicircular notch (Type 1 and 2 in Fig. 17.3). The notch is absent or converted into a foramen by the ossified STSL in 15% of the specimens.

Technique of Localizing the Suprascapular Nerve

Traditionally, suprascapular nerve blockade has been performed via use of anatomical landmarks (blind techniques). Subsequently, the use of imaging guidance to more accurately guide needle placement has been described.

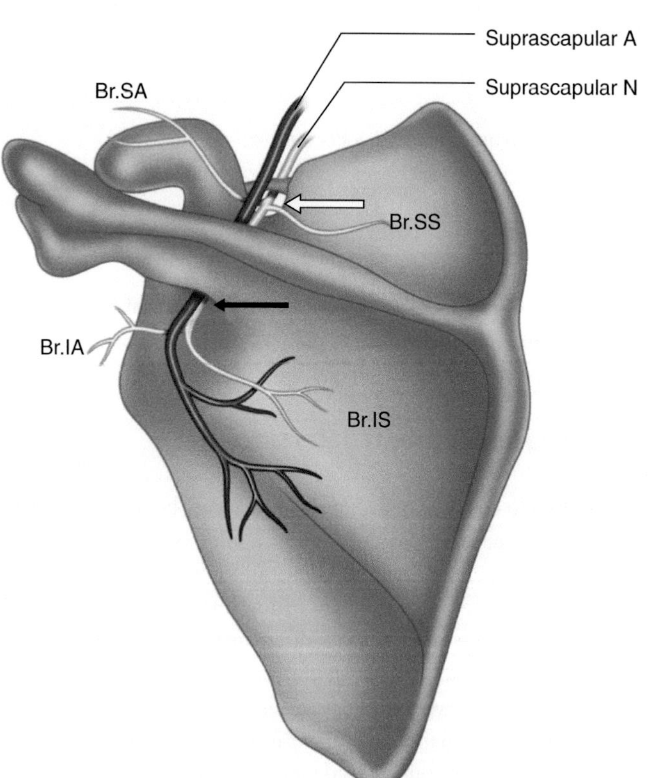

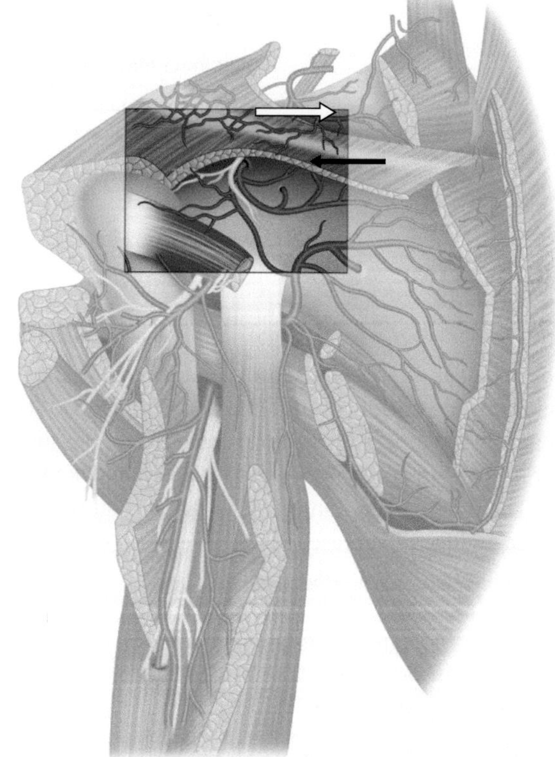

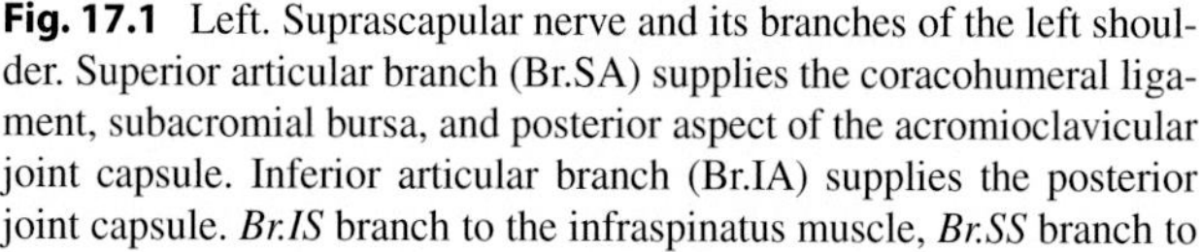

Fig. 17.1 Left. Suprascapular nerve and its branches of the left shoulder. Superior articular branch (Br.SA) supplies the coracohumeral ligament, subacromial bursa, and posterior aspect of the acromioclavicular joint capsule. Inferior articular branch (Br.IA) supplies the posterior joint capsule. *Br.IS* branch to the infraspinatus muscle, *Br.SS* branch to the supraspinatus muscle. Right. Anatomy drawing based on dissection. The course of suprascapular nerve is highlighted. The suprascapular notch and spinoglenoid notches are indicated by open and solid arrows, respectively. (Reproduced with permission from Philip Peng Educational Series and Dr. Danilo Jankovic)

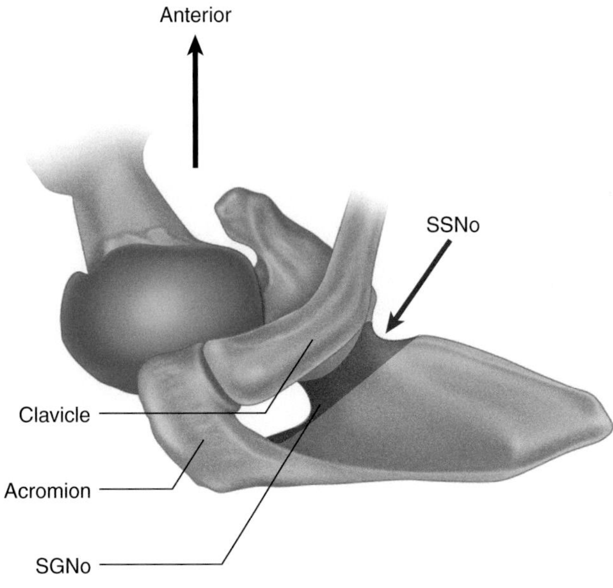

Fig. 17.2 Superior view of the left shoulder. The course of the suprascapular nerve (shaded) enters the suprascapular fossa through the suprascapular notch (SSNo) and then enters the infrascapular fossa through the spinoglenoid notch (SGNo). The clavicle and coracoid processes are also displayed in the diagram. (Reproduced with permission from Philip Peng Education Series)

Blind Techniques

Various landmark approaches have been described and can be grouped into posterior, superior, and lateral approaches. Only the superior approach will be described here which can be performed with the patient in the sitting or lateral positions. In general, the needle is directed to the lateral half of the floor of the suprascapular fossa because the supraspinatus muscle is attached to the medial half. A 1.5-in. needle is usually sufficient to reach the floor of the scapular fossa. Potential advantages of this approach include ease of access, no reference to the notch, and extremely low risk of pneumothorax

Image-Guided Techniques for SSNB

Techniques using imaging guidance such as fluoroscopy, computed tomography (CT), and more recently ultrasound have been described.

Fluoroscopic Imaging

For the fluoroscopic technique, the patient is placed in the prone position. A C-arm is then used to identify the notch

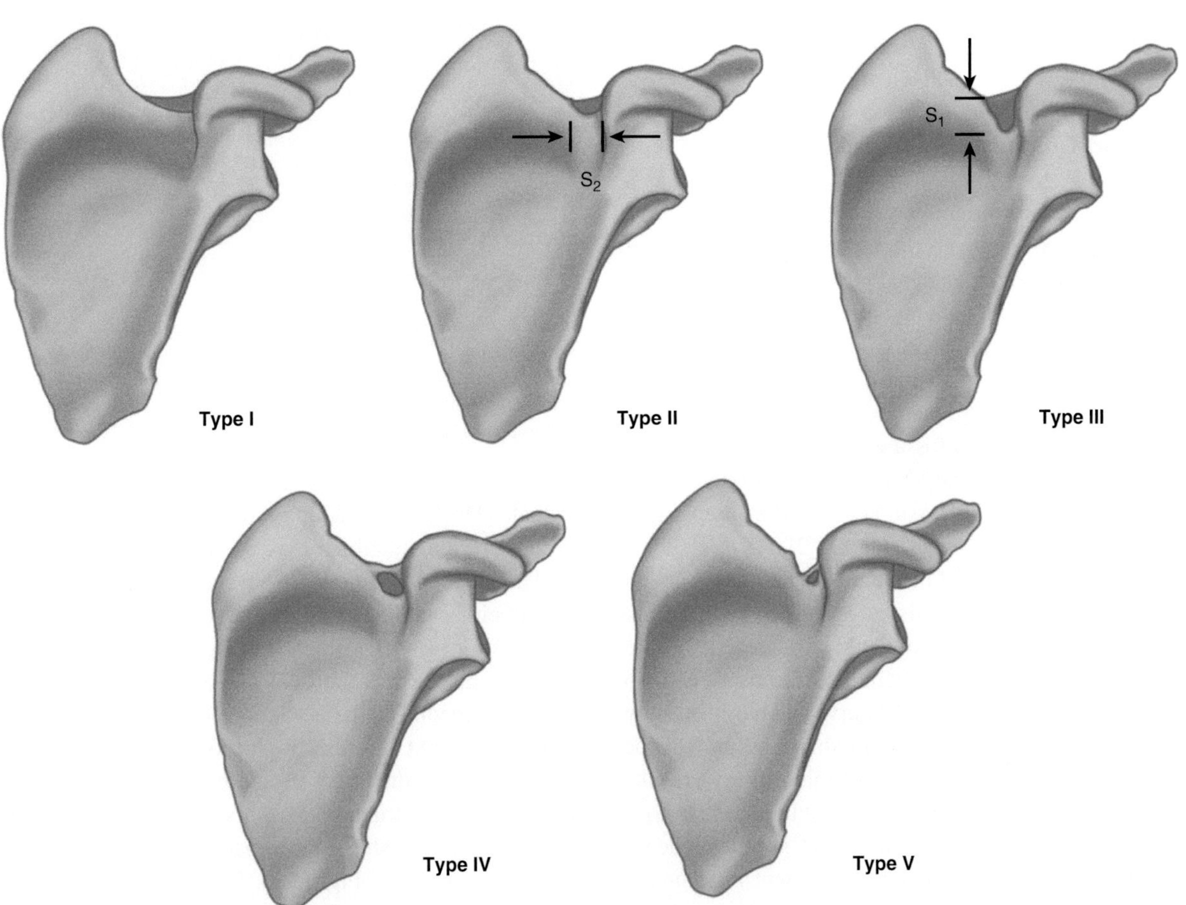

Fig. 17.3 Variation of morphology of the suprascapular notch. Type I indicates no notch (8.3%); type II, notch with greater transverse diameter, S2 (41.85%); type III, notch with greater vertical diameter, S1 (41.85%); type IV, bony foramen (7.3%); type V, notch with bony foramen (0.7%). (Reproduced with permission from Philip Peng Educational Series)

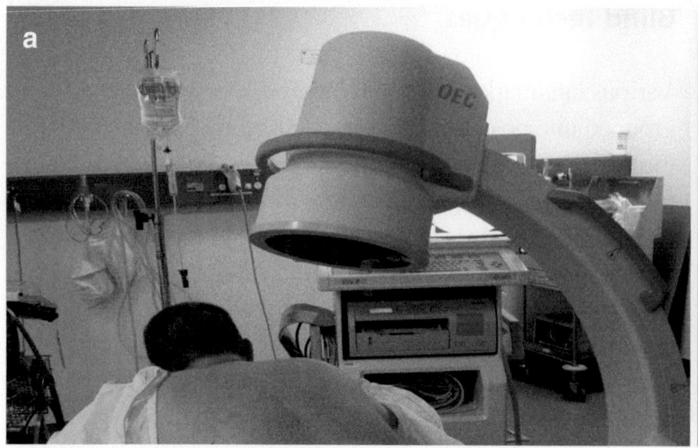

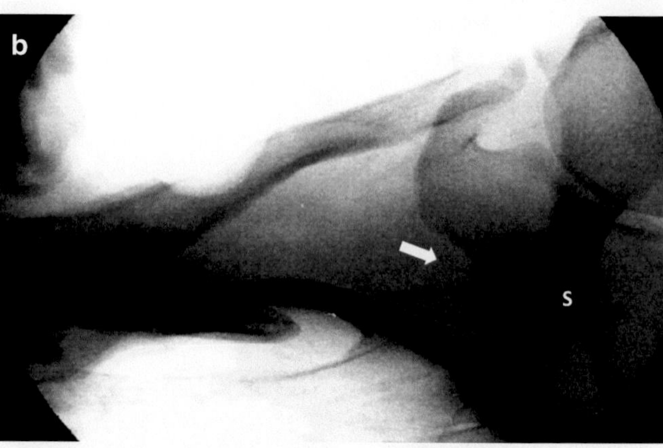

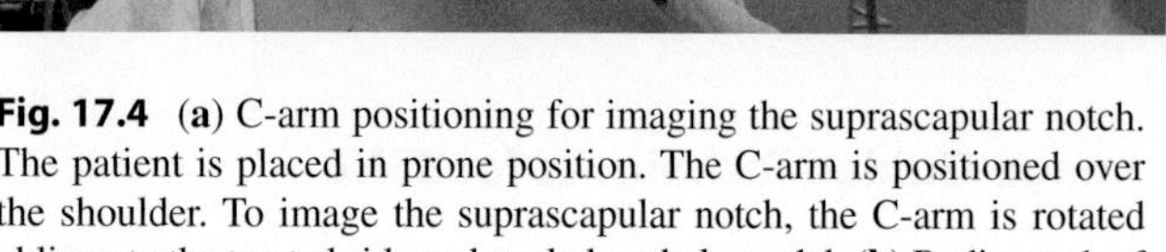

Fig. 17.4 (**a**) C-arm positioning for imaging the suprascapular notch. The patient is placed in prone position. The C-arm is positioned over the shoulder. To image the suprascapular notch, the C-arm is rotated oblique to the treated side and angled cephalocaudal. (**b**) Radiograph of the right suprascapular notch. White arrow points to the suprascapular notch. S indicates spine of scapula. (Reproduced with permission from Philip Peng Educational Series)

(Fig. 17.4). The suprascapular notch will be seen superior to the spine of the scapula, medial to the coracoid process, and lateral to the rib margins. To obtain an optimal image, the C-arm will often need to be obliquely angled away from the side of the proposed block and in the cephalo-caudad orientation. Visualization of the suprascapular notch is further improved when the ipsilateral arm is placed above the shoulder ("arm up" position) compared to when the affected arm is placed by the side ("arm down position").

Ultrasound-Guided Suprascapular Nerve Blockade

Both anterior and posterior approaches have been described. The anterior approach targets the suprascapular nerve shortly after it branches from the brachial plexus (in the supraclavicular area) underneath the omohyoid muscle. The major limitation of this approach is the proximity to the brachial plexus (median 8 mm; range 4–15 mm). For the purpose of this chapter, the more widely practiced technique of US-guided SSNB at the suprascapular fossa will be described.

The ideal site to perform SSNB with ultrasound is at the floor of the suprascapular fossa, between the suprascapular notch and spinoglenoid notch (Fig. 17.2). At this site, the SSN runs along the floor of the suprascapular fossa covered by the fascia of supraspinatus in a natural compartment, which will contain the spread of the local anesthetic or injectate. Applying an ultrasound-guided injection technique approximated the needle tip to the nerve and has been shown to achieve a complete block with a reduced volume of local anesthetic. A small volume (5 ml) of injectate will result in adequate flooding of the nerve with minimal spread to the brachial plexus. Furthermore, this target is independent of the suprascapular notch, which can be absent in some individuals. The risk of pneumothorax is substantially reduced because of the direction of the needle.

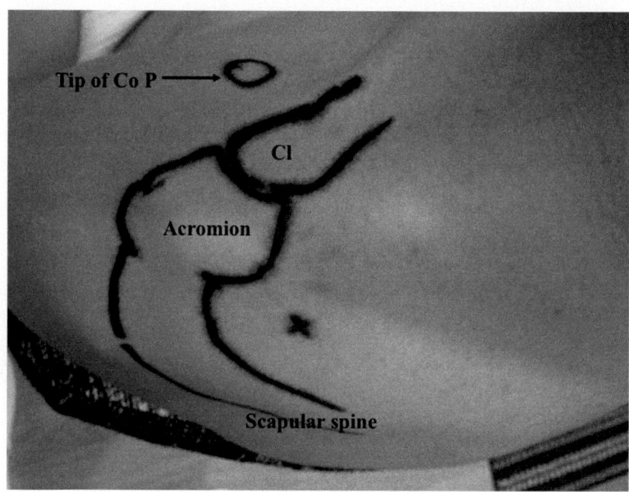

Fig. 17.5 Surface anatomy demonstrating landmarks for the lateral approach to SSNB. The x marks the site known as Nevasier portal, which is determined but the soft spot just medial to acromion. The o represents the coracoid process. (Reproduced with permission from Philip Peng Education Series)

The ultrasound-guided SSNB may be performed with the patient either in the sitting, lateral or prone position. A high-frequency (7–13 Hz) linear ultrasound probe is used. The probe is placed in a coronal plane over the suprascapular fossa just medial to the acromion (also called Nevasier portal) with a slight anterior tilt placed on the probe to improve visualization of the target structures (Fig. 17.5). In this view, the identifiable structures (from superficial to deep) are the trapezius muscle, the supraspinatus muscle, and the suprascapular fossa floor (Fig. 17.6). The suprascapular nerve and

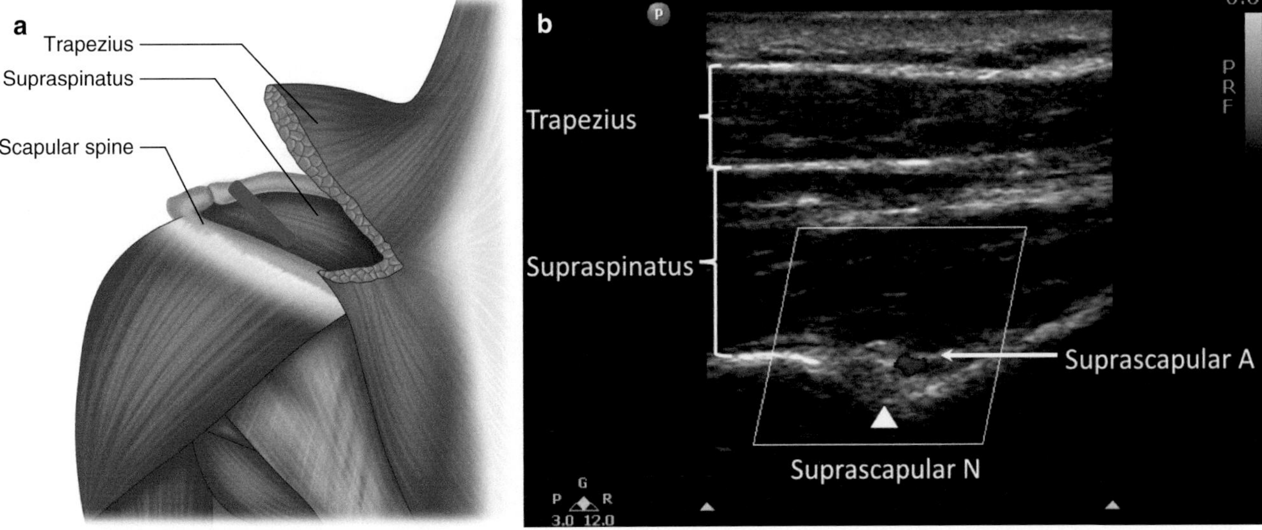

Fig. 17.6 (**a**) Ultrasound probe (blue rectangle) placed in a coronal plane over the suprascapular fossa with a slight anteromedial tilt. The trapezius muscle was removed to show the underlying supraspinatus muscle. (**b**) Ultrasonographic image of the suprascapular nerve on the floor of the scapular spine between suprascapular notch and spinoglenoid notch. Both suprascapular nerve and artery run underneath the fascia of supraspinatus muscle. Suprascapular artery and nerve are indicated with arrow and bold arrowhead, respectively. (Reproduced with permission from Philip Peng Education Series)

artery are commonly seen on the floor running underneath the supraspinatus muscle layer (Fig. 17.6).

SSNB is performed by passing a 22-gauge 3-in. needle in an in-plane approach from medial to lateral. For treatment of chronic shoulder pain, injectable steroid (methylprednisolone) usually is added to the local anesthetic solution. However, the value of this practice has been questioned by a double-blinded study demonstrating that the addition of methylprednisolone fails to confer any benefit.

In summary, various approaches have been described for the blockade of SSN. Disadvantages of the approach using the notch as a landmark are the potential absence of the notch in some individuals and the potential risk of pneumothorax. The superior approach may negate these disadvantages. On limited evidence, these studies would suggest ultrasound is useful in approximating the block needle in the vicinity of the SSN and thereby increasing efficacy and reducing complications of SSNB. The majority of recent studies utilizing US-guided SSNB for acute and chronic shoulder pain management may reflect this.

SSNB achieved with radiofrequency or cryolesion provides a long-lasting effect that can endure for up to 18 months. Furthermore, one of these studies demonstrated a significant reduction in pain, improvement in function, and a reduction in analgesic medication (81% of study patients) following pulsed RF of the SSN.

The use of chemical neurolysis for SSNB has mainly been in the form of case reports. Injection of phenol causes protein coagulation and necrosis when applied directly to the nerve, thereby alleviating pain. A larger study involved 16 patients with shoulder pain secondary to rheumatoid arthritis. These patients received SSNB with prilocaine (4 ml) and 6% aqueous phenol (4 ml) with significant reduction in pain and improved shoulder range of motion at 13-week follow-up.

Complications

SSNB is a safe procedure with a generally low rate of complications (Table 17.1).

One large study retrospectively analyzed 1005 SSNBs performed by multiple clinicians in multiple centers over a 6-year period. There were no major complications reported. There were only six minor adverse events which included transient dizziness (n = 3), transient arm weakness (n = 2), and facial flushing (n = 1). Several systematic reviews confirm the safety of SSNB with negligible reports of complications. The possible complications are pneumothorax (<1%), intravascular injection, residual motor weakness, local trauma, and vasovagal response of the patient.

Literature Review

Suprascapular Nerve Block for Acute Pain

The studies investigating the efficacy of SSNB in acute pain states are summarized in Table 17.2.

It is now well established that SSNB is highly effective in the control of postoperative pain following open and

Table 17.1 Complications of suprascapular nerve block and rhizotomy

Study authors	Type of study	No of patients	Clinical indication for SSNB or SSN rhizotomy	Complications reported (numbers)
Shanahan et al. (2012)	O (multicenter study 2003–2009)	1005	Chronic shoulder pain	6 side effects: Transient dizziness (3) Transient arm weakness (2) Facial flushing (1)
[a]Eyigor et al. (2010)	R	50	Chronic shoulder pain	No complications reported
Gorthi et al. (2010)	R,C	50	Chronic shoulder pain	US group—no complications; blind technique: arterial puncture (2), direct nerve injury (1)
Martinez-Barenys et al. (2010)	R	74	Ipsilateral shoulder pain post-thoracotomy	No complications reported
Saha et al. (2010)	O	178	Ipsilateral shoulder pain post-thoracotomy	No complications reported
Mitra et al. (2009)	O	28	Adhesive capsulitis	No complications reported
[a]Liliang et al. (2009)	O	11	Chronic shoulder pain	Puncture wound pain for 1 week (1)
[a]Kane et al. (2008)	O	12	Painful cuff tear arthropathy in patients unfit for surgery	No complications reported
Checucci et al. (2008)	O	20	Patients undergoing arthroscopic procedures for rotator cuff disease	No complications reported
Jerosch et al. (2008)	R	260	Arthroscopic and shoulder surgery	No complications reported
Price DJ (2007)	O	40	Arthroscopic and open shoulder surgery	No complications reported from SSNB
Di Lorenzo et al. (2006)	R	40	Rotator cuff tendinitis	No major complications
Taskaynata et al. (2005)	R	60	Chronic shoulder pain	No complications reported
Singelyn et al. (2004)	R, C	120	Arthroscopic shoulder surgery	No complications reported
Shanahan et al. (2004)	R, SB	67	Degenerative joint or rotator cuff disease	No complications reported
Schneider-Kolsky et al. (2004)	O	40	Chronic shoulder pain	No complications reported
Neal et al. (2003)	R, DB, C	50	Acromioplasty, rotator cuff repair, or combination of both	No complications reported
Shanahan et al. (2003)	R, DB, C	83	Shoulder pain from rheumatoid arthritis and/or degenerative disease of the shoulder	Minor bruising (1)
Tan et al. (2002)	R, DB, C	44	Ipsilateral shoulder pain post-thoracotomy	No complications reported
Karatas and Meray (2002)	R, SB	41	Adhesive capsulitis	No complications reported
Dahan et al. (2000)	R, DB, C	34	Frozen shoulder	No major complications reported
Jones and Chattopadhyay (1999)	R	30	Frozen shoulder	No major complications reported
Lewis (1999)	O	16	Rheumatoid or osteoarthritis of shoulder	No complications reported
Ritchie et al. (1997)	R, DB, C	50	Arthroscopic shoulder surgery	No complications
Dangoisse et al. (1994)	O	12	Frozen shoulder (6 patients), others (6 patients)	Sensation of heaviness in arm (1), numbness, and aching shoulder (1)
Gado and Emery (1993)	R, DB	26	Rheumatoid arthritis	No complications reported
Vecchio et al. (1993)	R, C	28	Rotator cuff tendinitis	Mild aching in the injection area (16)
Wassef (1992)	O	9	Frozen shoulder	No complications reported
Emery et al. (1989)	R, DB, C	17	Rheumatoid arthritis	No complications reported
[a]Brown et al. (1988)	O	22	Rheumatoid arthritis	Impaired abduction (1)

C placebo-controlled, *DB* double-blinded, *O* observational, *R* randomized, *No* number, *SSNB* suprascapular nerve (SSN) block, *US* ultrasound
[a] Rhizotomy study

Table 17.2 Suprascapular nerve block for acute pain control

Study authors	Type of acute pain	Study design	Number of participants	Results	Conclusions
SSNB as the only form of regional anesthesia					
Cho et al. (2020)	Acute postoperative shoulder surgery pain	Systematic review comparison of SSNB vs no block (control)	700 patients	SSNB was statistically superior in analgesia and reducing opioid consumption in the first 24 h SSNB reduced odds of nausea SSNB improved patient satisfaction	In acute post shoulder surgical pain, SSNB provides improved analgesia, improved patient satisfaction, reduced opioid consumption, and reduced odds of nausea compared to placebo
Koga et al. (2019)	Arthroscopic surgery: Rotator cuff repair	Retrospective comparison	97 patients SSNB (33 patients) ISBPB (52 patients) Glenohumeral injection (control) 12 patients)	VAS pain scores reduced in SSNB group at 1 and 6 h vs control No significant differences in pain scores between the SSNB and ISBPB groups at all time points	No significant differences in VAS pain scores at all times between SSNB and ISBPB following arthroscopic rotator cuff repair
Kay et al. (2018)	Arthroscopic shoulder surgery: mixed	Systematic review comparison of SSNB vs ISB vs no block	1382 patients (14 RCT)	Pain control superior in SSNB vs control group (no block) at 6 h post-surgery SSNB inferior to ISBPB for first hour after surgery	SSNB was only inferior to ISBPB for first hour after surgery; beyond the first hour, SSNB provided analgesia similar to ISBPB
Auyong et al. (2018)	Arthroscopic shoulder surgery: mixed	Randomized, double-blind, noninferiority trial	189 patients randomized ISB Supraclavicular block SSNB	Mean pain score difference between SSNB and ISBPB (0.1) $P = 0.012$ for noninferiority Supraclavicular vs ISBPB (0.4) $P = 0.088$ for noninferiority Similar opioid consumption between all groups Better preservation of vital capacity in the SSNB and supraclavicular groups compared to ISBPB	SSNB provides noninferior analgesia to ISBPB SSNB provides superior preservation of pulmonary function compared to ISBPB
Hussain et al. (2017)	Shoulder Surgery	Meta-analysis Comparison of SSNB vs ISBPB	1152 patients (16 studies)	Area under the curve pain scores less in ISBPB group only for the first 24 h ISBPB reduced opioid consumption in recovery room compared to SSNB After 24 h, no difference in pain scores between groups SSNB reduced odds of block-related and respiratory complications	No clinically meaningful difference between SSNB and ISBPB Reduced potential for side effects and complications from SSNB

(continued)

Table 17.2 (continued)

Study authors	Type of acute pain	Study design	Number of participants	Results	Conclusions
Auyong et al. (2017)	Total shoulder arthroplasty	RCT Comparison of continuous ISB vs supraclavicular block (SCV) vs SSNB	75 patients, 25 patients each treatment arm	Pain scores at 24 h ISBPB = 2.2, SCV = 1.6, SSNB = 2.6 (no significant difference) Opioid consumption not significantly different Lung function Vital capacity reduction ISBPB—991 ml SCV—803 ml SSNB—464 ml	In patients where there is concern about lung function, continuous SSNB via catheter would be preferable compared to ISBPB for preservation of lung function
Chang et al. (2016)	Acute postoperative shoulder pain: Shoulder surgery Laparoscopic surgery Thoracotomy	Systematic review comparison of SSNB vs placebo Outcomes Pain scale Nausea (odds ratio)	681 patients (7 RCT, 2 comparative studies)	SSNB significant reduction in pain compared to placebo for shoulder surgery group SSNB did not provide significant reduction in pain in non-shoulder surgery group Odds ratio of SSNB compared with placebo 0.2	SSNB provides significant reduction in acute pain post shoulder surgery *but not* in patients post-thoracotomy or laparotomy SSNB significantly reduces nausea post shoulder surgery compared to placebo
Dhir et al. (2016)	Arthroscopic shoulder surgery: mixed	RCT Comparison of analgesic efficacy of combined SSNB and axillary nerve block vs ISBPB	60 patients Pain scores recorded at 6 h, 24 h, 7 days after surgery	ISBPB better mean static pain scores (ISBPB 1.8 vs combined block 5.45) in the recovery room At 24 h, combined block has superior pain score of 3.92 vs ISBPB 6.35	ISBPB provided superior analgesia in the immediate postoperative period 1 h Beyond 24 h, there was no significant difference
Jerosch et al. (2008)	Arthroscopic shoulder surgery: mixed	Prospective, non-randomized study. Comparison of 2 consecutive cohorts	260 patients. Received SSNB = 130. No nerve block = 130.	No difference in baseline VAS scores. Postoperatively, significant reduction in VAS scores at 24, 48, and 72 h in the SSNB group. No complications of SSNB	SSNB is effective in reducing postoperative shoulder pain in arthroscopic shoulder surgery. SSNB is associated with minimal complications
Singelyn et al. (2004)	Arthroscopic shoulder acromioplasty	Prospective, randomized, blinded study	120 patients randomized to 4 treatment groups: SSNB = 30 IALA = 30 ISBPB = 30 Control (no regional analgesia) = 30	No significant difference in pain scores between control and IALA groups. SSNB and ISBPB reported significantly less pain than the other 2 groups. The ISBPB group had significantly less pain on movement than the SSNB group. Only the ISBPB group recorded significantly less morphine consumption and higher satisfaction	ISBPB is the most efficient regional technique for arthroscopic shoulder acromioplasty. SSNB improves analgesia for arthroscopic acromioplasty but is less efficient than ISBPB. When ISBPB is contraindicated, SSNB is a clinically appropriate alternative

Table 17.2 (continued)

Study authors	Type of acute pain	Study design	Number of participants	Results	Conclusions
Ritchie et al. (1997)	Arthroscopic shoulder surgery	Randomized, double-blind, placebo-controlled study	50 patients randomized to: Placebo = 25 SSNB = 25	VAS significantly lower in SSNB group at 120 and 180 min. VPS score significantly lower in SSNB group at 120, 180, and 240 min. Significantly reduced morphine consumption (SSNB group) on the day of surgery. Significantly less nausea and vomiting in SSNB group. Reduced stay in ambulatory surgical unit	SSNB is an effective regional anesthetic technique for arthroscopic shoulder surgery in terms of improved analgesia, reduced opioid requirements, and less nausea and vomiting
Martinez-Barenys et al. (2010)	Ipsilateral post-thoracotomy shoulder pain	Randomized, single-blinded study	74 patients First group: phrenic group (PNI) received 10 ml 2% lidocaine into perinephric fat pad prior to closure = 37 Second group: SSNB with 10 ml 0.5% bupivacaine at completion of surgery = 37	Shoulder pain intensity was significantly lower in the PNI group compared with the SSNB group	Shoulder pain post-thoracotomy does not appear to arise from the shoulder joint. This study suggests that pain arises from diaphragmatic irritation. Therefore, routine preemptive blockade of the suprascapular nerve is not recommended
Saha et al. (2010)	Ipsilateral post-thoracotomy shoulder pain	Retrospective case review of post-thoracotomy patients	178 patients post-thoracotomy. New onset shoulder pain post-thoracotomy = 92 (51%). 34 patients (27%) with localizing signs suggestive of musculoskeletal origin underwent SSNB	29 of 34 patients reported satisfactory pain relief following SSNB	In patients with post-thoracotomy shoulder pain and whom have localizing signs suggestive of musculoskeletal origin, SSNB is an effective treatment. However, SSNB is not the treatment per se for post-thoracotomy shoulder pain as the musculoskeletal system is responsible for less than one third of cases
Tan et al. (2002)	Ipsilateral post-thoracotomy shoulder pain	Double-blinded, randomized, placebo-controlled study	44 patients who had undergone thoracotomy under general anesthesia and mid-thoracic epidural. 30 patients experienced shoulder pain within 2 h post-surgery and were randomized to: SSNB with 10 ml 0.5% bupivacaine = 15 Control: SSNB with 10 ml 0.9% saline = 15	No significant decrease in VAS or VRS in patients receiving SSNB with bupivacaine	SSNB not effective for ipsilateral shoulder pain post-thoracotomy

(continued)

Table 17.2 (continued)

Study authors	Type of acute pain	Study design	Number of participants	Results	Conclusions
SSNB in combination with another regional technique					
Lee et al. (2014)	Ambulatory arthroscopic shoulder surgery	Prospective randomized controlled trial	42 patients 21 patients received US-guided SSNB and axillary nerve block 21 patients received US-guided SSNB alone	Addition of US-guided axillary nerve block to SSNB resulted in reduced pain scores (VAS) in the first 24 h post-surgery, compared to SSNB alone	Axillary nerve block improves analgesic efficacy of SSNB for ambulatory arthroscopic shoulder surgery
Checucci et al. (2008)	Arthroscopic shoulder surgery	Case series	20 consecutive patients Each patient received a SSNB and an axillary nerve block as the sole anesthetic for the operation, with midazolam sedation	All patients were able to have surgery under the combination block. No patients required opioids, analgesics, or general anesthesia. Postoperative pain control was effective with negligible use of nonopiate analgesics. No opiate analgesic was required postoperatively	SSNB in combination with axillary nerve block is sufficient for arthroscopic shoulder surgery
Price (2007)	Shoulder surgery: arthroscopic and open. Postoperative analgesia in patients who had ISBPB failure	Retrospective case series	40 patients with ISBPB failure received combined SSNB and axillary nerve block	57% of cases required no morphine in PACU. 83% of cases required no morphine overnight. Complications: radial nerve blockade which resolved (2/70 cases)	If ISBPB fails, combined SSNB and axillary nerve block is effective in providing postoperative analgesia for shoulder surgery
Neal et al. (2003)	Ambulatory nonarthroscopic shoulder surgery	Prospective randomized study	50 patients SSNB and ISBPB-general anesthesia = 25 Sham injection and ISBPB-general anesthesia = 25	Addition of SSNB significantly delayed the time to first significant report of pain. However, addition of SSNB did not improve PACU measures, 24 h assessment of pain, supplemental analgesic use, or QOL measures	SSNB combined with ISBPB does not significantly improve outcomes in ambulatory nonarthroscopic shoulder surgery

IALA intra-articular local anesthetic, *ISBPB* interscalene brachial plexus block, *PACU* post-anesthesia care unit, *PNI* phrenic nerve infiltration, *QOL* quality of life, *SSNB* suprascapular nerve block, *VAS* visual analog scale, *VPS* verbal pain scale, *VRS* verbal rating scale

arthroscopic shoulder surgery (Table 17.2). SSNB provides significantly improved pain control post arthroscopic shoulder surgery compared to analgesia with no nerve block (i.e., no regional technique) at 1 and 6 h postoperatively. Comparing SSNB vs placebo for both arthroscopic and open shoulder surgeries, SSNB was significantly associated with lower pain scores and reduced nausea. SSNB also allows good control of severe postoperative pain at rest and with movement in the early postoperative period, resulting in a significant reduction in analgesic dose and demand, discharge time, and the incidence of nausea.

Historically, interscalene brachial plexus block (ISB) is the usual regional technique employed for analgesia during and after shoulder surgery. Blockade of the brachial plexus provides more complete analgesia of the shoulder joint. One systematic review has been performed comparing SSNB and ISB for shoulder surgery. This review found that the analgesia provided by SSNB provides noninferior analgesia for arthroscopic shoulder surgery compared to ISB except in the initial stay in the recovery room where ISB produced superior analgesia. To improve the success rate of SSNB, a combined technique with axillary nerve block has been used to provide increased coverage of the shoulder joint for arthroscopic rotator cuff procedures. A subsequent randomized controlled trial compared the effects of the combined US-guided axillary nerve and SSN blocks with SSNB alone for arthroscopic rotator cuff repairs. This study found that the combination block (axillary and SSN block) resulted in superior analgesia in the immediate postoperative period.

In addition to the management of acute pain associated with shoulder surgery, several studies have assessed SSNB for control of shoulder pain post-thoracotomy. One of these studies demonstrating that SSNB was beneficial in post-thoracotomy patients only when those with shoulder pain and localizing signs suggestive of musculoskeletal pain. If selected in this manner, then this study found that 85.3% of selected patients obtained satisfactory pain relief post SSNB. Nevertheless, in a more extensive systematic review encompassing nine studies (including seven RCT), it was found that SSNB did not significantly reduce postoperative shoulder pain in patients undergoing laparoscopic surgery or thoracotomy. Therefore, in the current climate, SSNB would only be recommended in post-thoracotomy patients with shoulder pain suggestive of musculoskeletal origin which is refractory to oral analgesia and physical therapy.

Diagnostic Block for Suprascapular Neuropathy

Suprascapular neuropathy is believed to be the cause in 1–2% of patients with shoulder pain. The possibility of suprascapular neuropathy is suggested by posterior shoulder pain, a history of trauma or traction to the suprascapular nerve, and weakness and atrophy of the muscles (supraspinatus, infraspinatus) supplied by the suprascapular nerve. Neuropathy of the SSN can be caused by traction or compression of the nerve at the spinoglenoid region or the suprascapular notch. The causes of traction or compression include trauma, repetitive use, and space occupying lesions. The differential diagnosis is broad. The diagnosis is often made based on clinical, investigative parameters (electrophysiologic and imaging studies) and exclusion of other pathologies, mainly rotator cuff pathology, cervical radiculopathy, and brachial plexopathy. The optimal management of suprascapular neuropathy has not been determined. Studies have reported good to excellent results in either nonsurgical management or surgical management.

Due to the difficulty in differentiating suprascapular neuropathy from other shoulder pathologies, SSNB can be performed to aid in the diagnosis. A diagnosis of SSNB is often based on clinical history and examination findings together with electrodiagnostic studies and MRI. In cases where the diagnosis is uncertain after electrodiagnostic studies, SSNB may be helpful. The test is positive if the pain is completely relieved.

SSNB for Chronic Shoulder Pain

Chronic Shoulder Pain (General)

SSNB has gained popularity in the treatment of chronic shoulder pain from a number of causes. The relevant studies are summarized in Table 17.3. While conclusions can be difficult due to the heterogenous nature of chronic shoulder pain (e.g., multiple etiologies, variable treatments prior to and in association with SSNB), SSNB has been shown to be an effective and safe therapeutic modality in reducing chronic shoulder pain but more importantly improving function. One meta-analysis (11 RCT) found that SSNB was superior to placebo injection (SMD = 0.75; 95% CI 0.35–1.1.4) and superior to physical therapy (SMD = 0.70; 95% CI 0.40–1.00) for pain relief at 12 weeks.

The efficacy of ultrasound-guided SSNB was compared to the landmark-based technique. In this study, patients with chronic nonspecific shoulder pain were randomized with 25 patients in each group. The investigators found that initially both groups improved in terms of pain relief. However, the analgesic effect was better sustained at 1 month in the ultrasound-guided group compared to the control group. Furthermore, while there were no complications in the ultrasound group, the control group recorded two cases of arterial puncture and three cases of direct nerve injury with neurological deficit. The most common pathologies individually studied are chronic pain from rheumatoid arthritis or osteoarthritis, adhesive capsulitis (frozen shoulder), and persistent rotator cuff lesions.

Shoulder Joint Arthritis: Rheumatoid Arthritis and Osteoarthritis

A number of studies have assessed the efficacy of SSNB for the pain and disability in patients with osteoarthritis and rheumatoid arthritis.

Local corticosteroid injection and gentle mobilization may improve rheumatoid shoulder in the early stages of disease. However, when glenohumeral damage is advanced, this treatment option is not as effective. Two randomized controlled trials have been published demonstrating the efficacy of SSNB in shoulder joint arthritis. One is a randomized controlled trial comparing the efficacy of intra-articular steroid injection with SSNB in patients with long-standing rheumatoid arthritis (average 17 years). SSNB provided prolonged pain relief (3 months) and superior improvement in shoulder movement. Another study consisted of a double-blind placebo-controlled RCT of patients suffering from rheumatoid shoulder. A total of 108 shoulders were randomized, to receive an injection of 10 ml of bupivacaine 0.5% and 40 mg methylprednisolone into the suprascapular fossa or a placebo injection of 5 ml of normal saline. SSNB was performed using surface anatomical landmarks as described by Dangoisse et al. At 3-month follow up, the active injection (local anesthetic and steroid) group recorded significantly superior pain reduction (VAS) and functional improvement (Shoulder Pain and Disability Index [SPADI], SF-36 scales) compared to the placebo group. A notable finding was that 67% of the patients receiving the active injection improved by at least 10 points on the SPADI which is a significant clinical improvement. The only adverse effects were minor

Table 17.3 Suprascapular nerve block for chronic pain conditions

Study authors	Type of chronic pain	Study design	Number of participants	Results	Conclusions
Terlemez et al. (2020)	Hemiplegic shoulder pain	Randomized controlled study	34 stroke patients Placebo (local anesthetic into trapezius) Local SSNB (local anesthetic suprascapular notch) Local and steroid SSNB (local anesthetic and steroid SSN)	Reduced VAS in all three injections Local anesthetic and local anesthetic plus steroid reduced pain significantly more than placebo group	SSNB facilitates pain relief and rehabilitation
Shanahan et al. (2020)	Shoulder pain in motor neurone disease	Case series	27 patients with motor neurone disease and shoulder pain; 10 patients had bilateral shoulder pain Total 37 shoulders Pain measured by pain scale (out of 100)	Significant reductions in pain over 3-month follow-up Baseline (58.4) Week 12 (30.4) $P = 0.001$	SSNB effective therapeutic modality in shoulder pain in patients with MND
Aydin et al. (2019)	Painful hemiplegic shoulder	Case control US-guided SSNB vs no SSNB	42 patients with hemiplegic shoulder pain: 21 patients no SSNB 21 patients SSNB	At 3-month follow-up, the SSNB group had significant reduction in pain and improved shoulder joint range of motion compared to the control group (no change from baseline scores)	US-guided SSNB is safe and effective compared to conservative (no nerve block) management of hemiplegic shoulder pain
Sencan et al. (2019)	Effects of fluoroscopy-guided intra-articular injection, suprascapular nerve block, and combination therapy in hemiplegic shoulder pain	Double-blind randomized clinical study	30 patients with hemiplegic shoulder pain SSNB treatment = 10 IAI treatment = 10 Combination (SSNB and IAI) = 10	Significant decrease in VAS and increased ROM in all groups post intervention Only internal rotation was significantly greater in combined treatment group	SSNB and IAI are effective in reducing pin and improving function in hemiplegic shoulder pain
Coory et al. (2019)	Symptomatic rotator cuff tears	Double-blinded randomized controlled trial SSNB vs SAB injection	42 shoulders with symptomatic partial and full-thickness rotator cuff tears SSNB treatment = 21 shoulders SAB treatment = 22 shoulders	At 12-week follow-up, SSNB group recorded significantly greater improvements in pain (as measured by VAS) Function (as measured by Constant-Murley [CM] score)	SSNB superior to SAB injection for pain and function at 12 weeks
Jung et al. (2019)	Adhesive capsulitis	Retrospective cohort study Comparison of SSNB and intra-articular injection (IAI) compared to IAI only	102 patients SSNB + IAI = 48 patients IAI only = 54 patients	Both groups recorded significant improvements in pain and function SSNB + IAI group recorded significantly greater improvement than IAI only group in FVAS and American Shoulder and Elbow Surgeons (ASES) functional scores	Treatment efficacy for adhesive capsulitis is significantly improved when SSNB is combined with IAI

Table 17.3 (continued)

Study authors	Type of chronic pain	Study design	Number of participants	Results	Conclusions
Sir and Eksert (2019)	Chronic shoulder pain—partial rotator cuff tear	Retrospective study Effects of pulsed radiofrequency SSNB for partial rotator cuff tears	31 patients Pain (NRS) Function (SPADI)	Baseline NRS 7.32 SPADI 69.0 At 6 months post SSNB PRF NRS 3.2 (significant pain reduction) SPADI 33.9 (significant functional improvement)	Pulsed radiofrequency lesion reduces pain and improves function in patients with partial rotator cuff tear
Ergonenc et al. (2018)	Chronic shoulder pain: adhesive capsulitis, rotator cuff syndrome, impingement syndrome shoulder	Case series Efficacy of pulsed radiofrequency rhizotomy of the SSN following a positive (50% reduction pain) response from diagnostic SSNB	74 patients	70 of 74 patients had a greater than 50% reduction pain following diagnostic SSNB In the patients (n = 70) who proceeded with PRF SSNB, significant reduction in pain (VAS) improvement in function (Shoulder Pain and Disability Index) SPADI was demonstrated up to 6 months post procedure	Longer-term efficacy of PRF SSN in chronic shoulder pain of multiple etiologies
Okur et al. (2017)	Breast cancer survivors with limited shoulder motion	Case series	18 patients following breast cancer surgery with limited shoulder motion, pain, and difficulty positioning the upper extremity for radiation therapy	Significant reductions in pain severity 10 days post SSNB Improved ranges of shoulder abduction, flexion, and external rotation post SSNB	Initial study demonstrating that SSNB may be a promising treatment for shoulder pain and shoulder dysfunction post breast cancer surgery
Mortada et al. (2017)	Adhesive capsulitis in diabetic patients	Comparative trial Single SSNB vs multiple sequential SSNB (9)	96 patients Group 1: single SSNB Group 2: 9 sequential SSNB	Both groups recorded significant reduction in pain and improvement in function at 3-week, 4-month review The group undergoing multiple SSNB recorded significantly greater improvement than the single SSN B group	Multiple SSNB provides superior clinical response than single SSNB
Kurt et al. (2016)	Chronic intractable shoulder pain	Case study Percutaneous lead placement for the SSN for intractable shoulder pain following cervical stenosis surgery	1 patient underwent trial and then permanent lead placement for SSN	9-month follow-up—excellent pain relief	Preliminary study suggestive of the SSN being a target for peripheral neuromodulation for intractable shoulder pain
Chang et al. (2016)	Chronic shoulder pain	Meta-analysis SSNB vs physical therapy vs placebo vs intra-articular injections for chronic shoulder pain	591 patients (11 RCT)	SSNB provided superior pain relief at 12 weeks post intervention compared to physical therapy and placebo. SSNB provided similar analgesia as joint injection US-guided SSNB better effectiveness than landmark or fluoroscopy-guided SSNB	SSNB is superior to physical therapy and placebo for chronic shoulder pain SSNB is of similar efficacy as shoulder joint injection

(continued)

Table 17.3 (continued)

Study authors	Type of chronic pain	Study design	Number of participants	Results	Conclusions
Klc et al. (2015)	Adhesive capsulitis	Randomized controlled trial SSNB vs physical therapy only	41 patients Control group (physical therapy alone) = 22 Intervention group SSNB = 19	Pain severity, general activity, and enjoyment of life significantly superior in the SSNB group	SSNB reduces pain severity and improves functional status compared to physical therapy alone for management of adhesive capsulitis
Chang et al. (2015)	Malignancy associated shoulder pain	Case series US-guided radiofrequency lesioning of the SSN for malignancy associated shoulder pain	6 patients undergoing ablative radiofrequency lesioning of the suprascapular nerve	Substantial reduction in pain	Potential treatment option for shoulder pain associated with malignancy
Dorn et al. (2015)	Chronic shoulder pain	Case series	20 patients SSNB with ropivacaine 0.5 ml Assessed 60 min and 24 h post block Constant-Murley score and numerical rating scales	SSNB improved both CMS and pain scores within the follow-up period	SSNB improves pain and shoulder function in patients suffering from chronic shoulder pain
Wu et al. (2014)	Adhesive capsulitis	Prospective, randomized, controlled study	42 patients Control group: physical therapy alone = 21 Intervention group: PRF applied to SSN via US guidance and physical therapy = 21	12-week follow-up The intervention group (PRF to SSN and physical therapy) demonstrated significantly shorter time to onset of significant pain relief, reduction in VAS, and improvement in SPADI compared to the control group (physical therapy alone)	PRF to the SSN combined with physical therapy is superior (reduction in pain and disability) to physical therapy alone in patients suffering from adhesive capsulitis
Jeon et al. (2014)	Hemiplegic shoulder pain	Comparative clinical trial	30 patients SSNB = 10 Intra-articular injection of corticosteroid = 10 Combination (SSNB followed by intra-articular corticosteroid) = 10	Reduction in VAS and improvement in ROM over observed period in all groups No statistically significant difference between the groups.	Both SSNB and intra-articular steroid injection alone and in combination improve pain and function over time for hemiplegic shoulder pain. However, neither type of injection was demonstrated to be superior to the other
Jang et al. (2013)	Chronic intractable shoulder pain >6 months Heterogeneous etiology: adhesive capsulitis, rotator cuff tear, mixed etiology	Case series	11 patients underwent SSN PRF following favorable response (pain improvement >50%) following diagnostic SSNB	Significant reduction in pain (VAS) and significant improvement in shoulder function (OSS) at 6- and 9-month follow-up	PRF SSN results in long-term improvement (greater than 9 months) in shoulder pain and function in patients with intractable shoulder pain

Table 17.3 (continued)

Study authors	Type of chronic pain	Study design	Number of participants	Results	Conclusions
Adey-Wakeling et al. (2013)	Hemiplegic shoulder pain	Randomized controlled trial	64 stroke patients randomized to SSNB or placebo injection	Patients who received SSNB recorded significantly superior pain reduction (VAS) compared to placebo at 1, 4, and 12 weeks post intervention No significant differences in function (Modified Rankin Scale, Croft Disability Index) or quality of life (EuroQol Health Questionnaire) were demonstrated.	SSNB provides sustained pain reduction in patients with hemiplegic shoulder pain but does not result in improved quality of life
Shabat et al. (2013)	Chronic headache attributable to lower cervical nerve roots (C5, C6)	Case series	69 patients undergoing PRF SSN for shoulder pain with concomitant chronic headache attributed to lower cervical nerve roots (C5, C6)	At 12 months, 45% of patients reported greater than 30% reduction in chronic headache pain	PRF SSN may provide analgesia for patients suffering from chronic headache secondary to lower cervical nerve root (C5, C6) irritation
Gofeld et al. (2013)	Chronic shoulder pain >3 months Heterogeneous etiology: adhesive capsulitis, tendinosis, arthritis, rotator cuff, or capsular tears	Randomized double-blind active placebo-controlled study	22 patients SSNB with lidocaine alone = 10 PRF applied to SSN = 12	Reduction in pain (NRS); improvement in function (SPADI) over 6-month follow-up for PRF SSN No significant difference between lidocaine and PRF SSN groups High dropout rate in both treatment arms (50% for lidocaine group; 33% for PRF SSN group)	Study suggests efficacy of PRF SSN for chronic shoulder pain. Study limited by high dropout rate resulting in study being underpowered
Simopoulos et al. (2012)	Chronic shoulder pain >12 months Heterogeneous etiology	Retrospective case series	6 patients whom had failed conservative management, SSNB with steroid, PRF SSN, and considered unfit for surgery These patients underwent continuous radiofrequency lesion of the SSN (80° for 60 s)	Significant reduction in pain (NRS); functional improvement as measured by ROM	This small study demonstrates that continuous radiofrequency lesioning of the SSN may be an effective treatment for chronic intractable shoulder pain

(continued)

Table 17.3 (continued)

Study authors	Type of chronic pain	Study design	Number of participants	Results	Conclusions
Eyigor et al. (2010)	Chronic shoulder pain >3 months Heterogeneous etiology	Single-blinded, randomized, comparative clinical trial Outcome measures: Pain scores using VAS at rest and movement Range of motion (ROM) of shoulder joint Shoulder Pain and Disability Index (SPADI) Short Form 36 Beck Depression Inventory Medication requirements Complications	50 patients Intra-articular injection of corticosteroid = 25 PRF applied to the SSN = 25	Improvements in pain, ROM of shoulder joint, and quality of life in both groups In the SSN PRF group, improvement lasted for 12 weeks in VAS, ROM, and SPADI Pain reduction was superior in the intra-articular group compared to the SSN PRF group	Both intra-articular steroids and AAN PRF reduced pain and improved function. Intra-articular steroids showed a greater reduction in pain throughout the study period
Gorthi et al. (2010)	Chronic shoulder pain	Prospective randomized comparative study	50 patients SSNB under US guidance (treatment group) = 25 SSNB blind technique (control group) = 25	Both groups recorded significantly reduced pain (VAS) and improved function (CSS) post procedure The SSNB US group showed significantly superior VAS and CSS scores compared to the control group	Performing SSNB under US guidance results in greater efficacy of block in terms of pain and shoulder function measures. In addition, US reduces the risk of vascular and neurological complications
Mitra et al. (2009)	Adhesive capsulitis	Retrospective chart review over 3 years	28 consecutive patients Received SSNB as part of a protocol for adhesive capsulitis management The protocol also included intra-articular steroid, volume dilation of the joint, and finally manipulation of the shoulder	After protocol, patients demonstrated significant improvements in ROM being flexion and abduction	SSNB as part of a multimodal therapy protocol improves shoulder function
Liliang et al. (2009)	Chronic shoulder pain for 3 months	Prospective case series	11 patients, total of 13 shoulder joints Treatment: PRF of the SSN	Significant pain relief in 10/13 joints at 1 month. And 9/13 shoulders at 6 months. Decreased SPADI scores at 6 months and 9 out of 11 patients reduced their analgesic medication	SSN PRF reduces shoulder pain and disability in a range of shoulder pathologies. Furthermore, patient's analgesic consumption is reduced
Di Lorenzo et al. (2006)	Rotator cuff tendinitis	Prospective, randomized, cross-over investigation	40 patients Treatment: SSNB and standard rehabilitation treatment Control: standard rehabilitation treatment alone	The SSNB group reported significantly less pain at rest, activity, and with rehabilitation exercises compared to the control group	SSNB and standard rehabilitation for rotator cuff tendinitis is superior to standard rehabilitation alone for pain control and functional improvement

Table 17.3 (continued)

Study authors	Type of chronic pain	Study design	Number of participants	Results	Conclusions
Taskaynata MA et al. (2005)	Chronic shoulder pain	Prospective randomized study	60 patients Intra-articular steroid injection = 30 SSNB = 30	Significant improvement in pain and ROM in both groups compared to baseline at 1 week and 1 month No significant difference between the two treatments Complications in the intra-articular steroid group No complications in the SSNB group	Both intra-articular steroids and SSNB are effective for managing shoulder pain and improving shoulder function. SSNB is safe with negligible risk of complications
Shanahan EM et al. (2004)	Chronic shoulder pain due to degenerative joint/ rotator cuff disease	Randomized, single blind	67 patients 77 shoulder randomized Group 1: SSNB via anatomical landmark approach Group 2: SSNB via CT guidance	Significant improvements in pain scores and disability in both groups No significant differences between the two groups No significant complications in either group No significant adverse events in either group	Clinically, there is no significant difference between SSNB performed via anatomical landmarks or CT guidance in terms of efficacy and complication rate
Schneider-Kolsky et al. (2004)	Chronic shoulder pain, range of pathology	Case series	40 consecutive patients. Treated with CT-guided SSNB	Significant reduction in pain and disability at both short-term and long-term follow-up. At long term (greater than 3 weeks), 29% of patients had sustained analgesia and reduced disability	CT-guided SSNB provides effective short-term pain relief in chronic shoulder pain
Shanahan et al. (2003)	Chronic shoulder pain due to rheumatoid arthritis and/or degenerative disease	Randomized, double-blind, placebo-controlled trial	83 patients, 108 shoulders studied in total Treatment group: SSNB: 56 Control/placebo group: 52	Treatment group compared to placebo: Significant reduction in pain in the treatment group at 12-week follow-up Modest but significant reduction in shoulder disability at 12 weeks in treatment group No difference in quality of life measures (SF36) between the 2 groups	SSNB is more effective than placebo in reducing pain and disability at 3-month follow-up for chronic shoulder pain of degenerative causes. However, it does not significantly improve quality of life compared to placebo
Karatas and Meray (2002)	Adhesive capsulitis (frozen shoulder)	Single-blinded, randomized comparative clinical trial	41 patients randomized into two groups: Group A: SSNB via anatomical landmarks Group B: near-nerve EMG-guided technique	In both groups, improvements in pain scores and ROM scores from baseline were significant VAS scores were significantly lowered in the EMG group compared to the blind technique at 60 min	EMG-guided SSNB provides more rapid analgesia that the blind approach in immediate post block time

(continued)

Table 17.3 (continued)

Study authors	Type of chronic pain	Study design	Number of participants	Results	Conclusions
Dahan et al. (2000)	Frozen shoulder (adhesive capsulitis)	Double-blind randomized controlled trial	34 patients randomized into two groups: Treatment: 3 SSNB at 7-day intervals with 10 cc bupivacaine 0.5% each block. Control: same as treatment group except 10 cc of normal saline used for SSNB	Significant reduction in pain in the treatment group (64%) compared to the control group (13%) at 1 month Nonsignificant improvement in shoulder function in treatment group. No improvement in shoulder ROM	Repeated SSNB with local anesthetic alone reduces pain compared to placebo but does not improve shoulder function or shoulder ROM
Jones and Chattopadhyay (1999)	Frozen shoulder (adhesive capsulitis)	Randomized trial of 30 patients	30 patients randomized First group: single SSNB Second group: course of intra-articular injections	SSNB produced a faster and more complete reduction in pain and restoration of ROM than intra-articular steroid	SSNB is superior to intra-articular steroid injection for pain reduction and improvements in shoulder ROM
Lewis RN (1999)	Chronic shoulder pain due to rheumatoid or osteoarthritis	Case series	16 patients Treated with combined SSNB and ACNb (4 ml 1% prilocaine and 4 ml 6% aqueous phenol)	Significant reduction in pain intensity (69%) and improvement in ROM (36–67%) over mean follow-up of 13 weeks	The combined SSNB and ACNb with local anesthetic and phenol provides pain relief and improvement in shoulder ROM
Gado and Emery (1993)	Chronic shoulder pain due to rheumatoid arthritis	Double-blind comparative study	29 patients (58 shoulders) First group: SSNB with local anesthetic (bupivacaine) alone Second Group: SSNB with local anesthetic and steroid	Both groups recorded significant improvements in pain, stiffness, and ROM up to 3 months Steroid did not improve outcomes. In fact, the bupivacaine alone group responded better	SSNB is effective for reducing shoulder pain and improving function. But the addition of steroid does not seem to confer added benefit
Vecchio et al. (1993)	Chronic shoulder pain due to rotator cuff lesions, tendinitis, and tears	Randomized clinical controlled trial	28 patients Divided into tendinitis and tears Tendinitis 15 – Active injection = 10 – Placebo injection = 5 Tears – Active injection = 5 – Placebo injection = 8	Tendinitis group: Significant improvement in night pain up to 12 weeks, movement pain significantly improved at 1 week but no difference at later follow-up, no difference to placebo in rest pain. Improvement in ROM only till 4 weeks Tear group: Significant improvement in night pain up to 12 weeks, significant improvement in movement pain till 12 weeks, no difference to placebo in rest pain. Only active abduction improved till 4 weeks; other ROM parameters showed no difference to placebo	SSNB improves the pain of rotator cuff pathology for at least 3-month period. While there is an improvement in shoulder function, this is only short term

Table 17.3 (continued)

Study authors	Type of chronic pain	Study design	Number of participants	Results	Conclusions
Emery et al. (1989)	Chronic shoulder pain due to rheumatoid arthritis	Randomized study	17 patients with bilateral shoulder rheumatoid arthritis 34 shoulders in total In each patient: one shoulder: SSNB and sham intra-articular injection Second shoulder: intra-articular steroid and sham SSNB	Compared with intra-articular steroids, SSNB resulted in longer duration of pain relief and improvement in pain index and range of movement.	
Brown et al. (1988)	Chronic shoulder pain due to glenohumeral arthritis not suitable for and had been receiving conservative medical management	Pilot study Consecutive case series	22 patients, 26 shoulders treated with RF heat lesion of the SSN	Analgesia: 7 produced no relief, 10 obtained good pain relief Duration: 9 produced good relief for 3 months, 14 produced relief for 6 months, and 9 produced relief for more than 7 months Three in last group had 18 months of pain relief	SSNB PRF can provide variable duration pain relief in patients with advanced glenohumeral arthritis who are not suitable for surgery

ACNb articular branches of the circumflex nerve, *CSS* Constant Shoulder Score, *CT* computed tomography, *EMG* electromyography, *IAI* intra-articular injection, *OSS* Oxford Shoulder Score, *MPQ* McGill-Melzack Pain Questionnaire, *NRS* numerical rating scale, *PRF* pulsed radiofrequency, *ROM* range of motion, *SF-36* Short Form 36 Health Survey, *SPADI* Shoulder Pain and Disability Index, *SSN* suprascapular nerve, *SSNB* suprascapular nerve block, *VAS* visual analog scale, *US* ultrasound

including chest wall tenderness in one subject which resolved and minor bruising in another.

Similarly, SSNB provided significantly better analgesia and superior movement in patients with long-standing rheumatoid arthritis who were unresponsive to intra-articular injection of steroid. Interestingly, supplementation of the local anesthetic solution with steroid conferred no additional benefit.

Adhesive Capsulitis (Frozen Shoulder)

As adhesive capsulitis is relatively common, the utility of SSNB in its management has been extensively studied. It is important to note that the studies have generally assessed the efficacy of SSNB compared to conventional therapies, e.g., physical therapy. This is understandable as the mainstay of therapy for adhesive capsulitis is physical therapy.

An RCT focused on the additive effect of SSNB to physical therapy for adhesive capsulitis. Forty-one patients with adhesive capsulitis were randomly assigned to physical therapy alone (control group) vs physical therapy combined with SSNB (injection group). SSNB was performed with prilocaine and triamcinolone steroid. Effects were measured by the brief pain inventory and the constant score. Physical therapy alone significantly reduced pain (~50%) and reduced pain interference. The addition of SSNB reduced pain (>60%) and interference significantly more than physical therapy alone. The Constant score improved by 70% in the injection group and by 54.5% in the physical therapy only group. In this study, patients who had received a subacromial bursa injection in the past 3 months were excluded. Thus, the study focused on the effects of SSNB as the only regional treatment modality.

A subsequent study chose to assess the effects of SSNB in combination with an intra-articular corticosteroid injection on adhesive capsulitis. This retrospective review had more extensive follow-up and a more homogeneous population mainly suffering from adhesive capsulitis than other studies and allows the clinician and assessment of the longer-term effects of SSNB. In this cohort, 48 patients had only an intra-articular injection performed and 54 patients underwent combined SSNB and IAI. Both groups improved relative to baseline in pain (VAS) and shoulder function as measured by the Shoulder Pain and Disability Index. However, there was no significant difference between the IAI and combined injection (SSNB plus IAI) groups.

In the above studies, a single shot SSNB was performed. In clinical practice, often SSNB is repeated for chronic shoulder conditions. Mortada et al. investigated the role of repeated SSNB and found that patients who received multiple SSNB (nine SSNBs) recorded significant greater pain reduction and functional improvement than patients who received only one SSNB.

To provide more sustained analgesia, the beneficial effects of pulsed radiofrequency treatment of the suprascapular nerve for adhesive capsulitis were demonstrated in a RCT. One half of the studied population underwent physical therapy alone ($n = 21$). The other half of the study population underwent physical therapy combined with SSNB via pulsed RF treatment ($n = 21$). The group of patients undergoing the combination therapy (physical therapy and pulsed RF treatment) recorded significantly faster and greater analgesia, improved range of movement, and less disability than the group undergoing physical therapy alone. This difference was evident to the 12-week follow-up period.

Persistent Rotator Cuff Lesions

Rotator cuff tendinitis is a common cause of shoulder pain in adults and may result in considerable morbidity. Many patients respond to conservative management, including avoiding activities likely to aggravate the lesion, use of nonsteroidal anti-inflammatory drugs, local injection of steroid, and physiotherapy. However, significant symptoms may persist: in one retrospective, long-term follow-up study, symptoms of severe shoulder pain persisted in approximately 26% of patients after a mean duration of 12 months following the first presentation of pain.

In this subset of patients with persistent symptoms, SSNB has been demonstrated to provide effective pain relief and improved range of motion. Although the therapeutic effect is temporary (4–12 weeks), it can be simply repeated in outpatient settings with minimal risk of complications. This block is also an effective way to control pain in patients awaiting surgery.

Historically, subacromial bursa injections have been performed in the management of rotator cuff tears. Suprascapular nerve block has now been performed to alleviate the pain of rotator cuff tears. In most clinical cases, patients with a diagnosed rotator cuff tear would have undergone a subacromial bursa injection prior to being selected for a SSNB. This has made it difficult in the past to evaluate the efficacy of SSNB compared to SAB injection. In a double-blinded randomized controlled trial, 43 shoulders with confirmed symptomatic rotator cuff tears were treated with either SSNB or SAB injections. Efficacy was determined by measurement of pain by the visual analog scale and shoulder function by the modified Constant-Murley score. At 12-week follow-up, the SSNB group had a significantly higher CM score than the SAB group (57.6 [SD, 10] vs 44.6 [SD, 16]; P =0.023) and greater improvement from the baseline CM score (23.4 [SD, 17.5] vs 7.8 [SD, 16.5]; $P = 0.014$). At 12 weeks, the visual analog score was significantly better in the SSNB group than in the SAB group (9.9 [SD, 3.3] vs 7.3 [SD, 4.3]; $P = 0.03$). While there were no complications in either the SSNB or SAB group, it is important to note that SAB steroid has a theoretical risk of weakening and potential rupture of tendons.

After pulsed radiofrequency lesioning of the SSN, a significant reduction in pain (VAS) and improvement in shoulder function (Constant and Oxford shoulder scores) were reported, lasting till 3-month follow up. These results are similar to those of Liliang et al., who in addition to improvement in pain and function also demonstrated a reduction in medication requirements in their study group. However, both injection and RF trials did not include a placebo control group, and further investigation is required to confirm the efficacy of the neural blockade or ablation technique in the management of rotator cuff tendinitis.

The timing of when to perform pulsed radiofrequency lesioning of the SSN for rotator cuff tears has not been clearly defined. One retrospective study suggests that whose symptoms do not improve after 3 months of conservative medical management, pulsed radiofrequency lesion of the SSN is an appropriate option. In this study, 31 patients underwent US-guided PRF SSN. At 6 months pain (NRS 7.32 prior to treatment; 3.22 6 months posttreatment; $P < 0.001$) and function (SPADI 68.96 prior to treatment; 33.93 6 months posttreatment $P < 0.001$) showed significant improvements.

Other Chronic Nonmalignant Pain States Responsive to SSNB

SSNB has been found to reduce chronic hemiplegic shoulder pain. One study documented the effectiveness of ultrasound-guided SSNB for pain reduction and functional improvement in hemiplegic shoulder pain. However, the investigators could not determine if ultrasound-guided SSNB was superior to landmark-based SSNB. The most extensive study to date randomized patients to compare placebo vs local anesthetic only SSNB vs local anesthetic and steroid SSNB. Their findings (reduced pain and improved shoulder range of movement in local anesthetic and steroid SSNB) support the utility of SSNB (with or without steroid) to facilitate rehabilitation in painful hemiplegic shoulder pain.

Malignant Pain

There are very few reports assessing the use of SSNB in the management of malignant shoulder pain. Theoretically, SSNB should be considered due to its success in reducing shoulder pain regardless of etiology and its low complication rate. One study has demonstrated this. In a range of malignancies (non-small cell lung cancer, prostate cancer, hepatocellular cancer, breast cancer, colon cancer) with humeral metastases or brachial plexus involvement, a radiofrequency lesion of the SSN was performed. This followed confirmation of a diagnostic SSNB with local anesthesia only. At settings of 80° for 75 s, all patients reported reduction in pain (mean VAS prior to SSN lesion = 7.3 ± 0.5; mean VAS post SSN lesion = 2.0 =/− 0.9; $P = 0.03$). There were no complications and no patients experienced recurrence of shoulder pain. The choice of supraclavicular block was chosen in this setting as this can be performed in the sitting/supine position unlike the posterior approach SSNB. Many patients with extensive malignancy find the prone position uncomfortable due to pain but also respiratory distress. While the numbers in this study are low, this study demonstrates the potential efficacy of SSNB in the management of refractory shoulder pain in malignancy.

In summary, SSNB is effective for short-term pain relief and improvement in shoulder function in a variety of painful shoulder conditions. The main causes of shoulder pain studied were arthritic conditions, rotator cuff lesions, and adhesive capsulitis. The data suggests that SSNB is useful for pain reduction but more importantly functional improvement. Furthermore, SSNB should be considered after 3 months of conservative management if significant pain and disability persist. For patients with short-term analgesia following a single shot SSNB, serial SSNB or pulsed radiofrequency to the SSN provides more sustained analgesia and functional improvement.

Summary and Conclusion

On review of the literature discussed above, the uses of SSNB and pulsed radiofrequency lesioning of the SSN can be summarized in Table 17.4.

There have been many described techniques by which to perform SSNB. While the radiologically guided techniques

Table 17.4 Summary of evidence on suprascapular nerve block and rhizotomy

Studied uses of SSNB	Level of evidence
SSNB is non-inferior to ISBPB for shoulder surgery	I
SSNB is not effective for reducing all cases of ipsilateral shoulder pain post-thoracotomy	I
SSNB does not improve outcomes in ambulatory nonarthroscopic shoulder surgery when added to ISB	I
SSNB reduces hemiplegic shoulder pain	I
SSNB is effective for postoperative pain control for shoulder arthroscopic surgery and reduces opioid requirements and nausea and vomiting	II-1
SSNB is effective for providing short-term (3 months) analgesia and improving function for chronic shoulder pain due to degenerative pathology or rotator cuff lesions	II-1
PRF of the SSN can provide longer lasting analgesia and improved shoulder function than single SSNB	II-2
SSNB combined with axillary nerve block is sufficient for arthroscopic shoulder surgery	II-3

ISB interscalene brachial plexus block, *PRF* pulsed radiofrequency, *SSN* suprascapular nerve, *SSNB* suprascapular nerve block
Based on Quality of Evidence Gradings as recommended by the US Preventive Services Task Force (Appendix)

(fluoroscopic, ultrasound guided) have grown in popularity, a knowledge of surface anatomical landmarks are still recommended. SSNB is a safe regional technique with a very low rate of complications.

While ISB provides the best form of regional anesthesia for shoulder surgery, SSNB is an appropriate alternative particularly for arthroscopic surgery. Combining axillary nerve block with SSNB improves the analgesic effect. The placement of a catheter to provide continuous SSNB shows similar analgesic efficacy to ISB. Importantly, in this setting, SSNB results in significantly less respiratory functional impairment, making SSNB a safer choice in patients with respiratory morbidity.

The studies mentioned in this chapter demonstrate efficacy of SSNB in chronic shoulder pain. While the efficacy of SSNB compared to other modalities has been proven, it should be emphasized that the role of SSNB remains as one component of a multidisciplinary pain management program with physical therapy a core requirement. Compared to SAB injection, the ease of repeating SSNB safely and the adoption of radiofrequency lesioning make SSNB a more attractive option. Furthermore, the theoretical risk of weakening or potential rupturing of tendon by peritendinous injection of steroids makes SSNB a safer regional technique for chronic shoulder pain.

Investigators have now focused on specific shoulder pathologies to assess efficacy of SSNB in different states. However, in many patients, it is likely that multiple pathologies (e.g., combined osteoarthritis and rotator cuff tears) will be present concomitantly. It is reassuring that SSNB has proven to be efficacious across a broad range of musculoskeletal shoulder conditions. The early data on SSNB for non-musculoskeletal conditions (e.g., malignancy, neuropathic shoulder pain) reflect the potential promise of SSNB in alleviating shoulder pain regardless of the causative pathology.

Appendix: Quality of Evidence Grading as recommended by US Preventive Services Task Force

Level of evidence	Description
I	Evidence from at least one properly designed randomized controlled trial
II-1	Evidence obtained from well-designed controlled trials without randomization
II-2	Evidence obtained from well-designed cohort or case-control analytic studies, preferable from more than one center or research group
II-3	Evidence obtained from multiple time series with or without the intervention
III	Opinions of respected authorities, based on clinical experience, descriptive studies, or reports of expert committees

Suggested Reading

Adey-Wakeling Z, Crotty M, Shanahan EM. Suprascapular nerve block for shoulder pain in the first year after stroke: a randomized controlled trial. Stroke. 2013;44:3136–41.

Aiello I, Serra G, Traina GC, Tugnoli V. Entrapment of the suprascapular nerve at the spinoglenoid notch. Ann Neurol. 1982;12:314–6.

Ajmani ML. The cutaneous branch of the human suprascapular nerve. J Anat. 1994;185:439–42.

Alon M, Weiss S, Fishel B, Dekel S. Bilateral suprascapular nerve entrapment syndrome due to an anomalous transverse scapular ligament. Clin Orthop. 1988;234:31–3.

Antoniadis G, Richter HP, Rath S, Braun V, Moese G. Suprascapular nerve entrapment: experience with 28 cases. J Neurosurg. 1996;85:1020–5.

Aszmann OC, Dellon AL, Birely BT, et al. Innervation of the human shoulder joint and its implications for surgery. Clin Orthop Relat Res. 1996;330:202–7.

Auyong DB, Yuan SC, Choi DS, Pahang JA, Slee AE, Hanson NA. A double-blind randomized comparison of continuous interscalene, supraclavicular, and suprascapular blocks for total shoulder arthroplasty. Reg Anesth Pain Med. 2017;42(3):302–9. https://doi.org/10.1097/AAP.0000000000000578. PMID: 28272290

Auyong DB, Hanson NA, Joseph RS, Schmidt BE, Slee AE, Yuan SC. Comparison of anterior suprascapular, supraclavicular, and interscalene nerve block approaches for major outpatient arthroscopic shoulder surgery: a randomized, double-blind, noninferiority trial. Anesthesiology. 2018;129(1):47–57. https://doi.org/10.1097/ALN.0000000000002208. PMID: 29634491

Aydın T, Şen Eİ, Yardımcı MY, Kesiktaş FN, Öneş K, Paker N. Efficacy of ultrasound-guided suprascapular nerve block treatment in patients with painful hemiplegic shoulder. Neurol Sci. 2019;40(5):985–91. https://doi.org/10.1007/s10072-019-03749-y. Epub 2019 Feb 9. PMID: 30739273

Barber FA. Suprascapular nerve block for shoulder arthroscopy. Arthroscopy. 2005;21:1015.

Bennett DL, Cronin AM, Palmer WE, Kattapuram SV, Huang AJ. Optimization and standardization of technique for fluoroscopically guided suprascapular nerve blocks. AJR Am J Roentgenol. 2014;202:576–84.

Bigliani LU, Morrison DS. Miscellaneous degenerative disorders of the shoulder. In: Dee R, Mango E, Hurst LC, editors. Principles of orthopedic practice. New York: McGraw-Hill; 1989.

Bigliani LU, Dalsey RM, McCann PD, April EW. An anatomical study of the suprascapular nerve. Arthroscopy. 1990;6:301–5.

Bonica JJ. Management of pain. Pittsburgh: Lean and Febiger; 1953.

Borgeat A, Pershak H, Bird P, et al. Patient-controlled interscalene analgesia with ropivacaine 0.2% versus patient controlled intravenous analgesia after major shoulder surgery: effects on diaphragmatic and respiratory function. Anesthesiology. 2000;92:102–8.

Breen TW, Haigh JD. Continuous suprascapular nerve block for analgesia of scapular fracture. Can J Anaesth. 1990;37:786–8.

Brown DE, James DC, Roy S. Pain relief by suprascapular nerve block in glenohumeral arthritis. Scan J Rheumatol. 1988;17:411–5.

Brown AR, Weiss R, Greenerg C, et al. Interscalene block for shoulder arthroscopy: a comparison with general anesthesia. Arthroscopy. 1993;9:295–300.

Callahan JD, Scully TB, Shapiro SA, Worth RM. Suprascapular nerve entrapment: a series of 27 cases. J Neurosurg. 1991;74:893–6.

Chan CW, Peng PW. Suprascapular nerve block: a narrative review. Reg Anesth Pain Med. 2011;36(4):358–73. https://doi.org/10.1097/AAP.0b013e3182204ec0. PMID: 21654552

Chang KV, Hung CY, Wang TG, Yang RS, Sun WZ, Lin CP. Ultrasound-guided proximal suprascapular nerve block with radiofrequency lesioning for patients with malignancy-associated recalcitrant shoulder pain. J Ultrasound Med. 2015;34(11):2099–105. https://doi.org/10.7863/ultra.14.12042. Epub 2015 Oct 9. PMID: 26453125

Chang KV, Hung CY, Wu WT, Han DS, Yang RS, Lin CP. Comparison of the effectiveness of suprascapular nerve block with physical therapy, placebo, and intra-articular injection in management of chronic shoulder pain: a meta-analysis of randomized controlled trials. Arch Phys Med Rehabil. 2016a;97(8):1366–80. https://doi.org/10.1016/j.apmr.2015.11.009. Epub 2015 Dec 14. PMID: 26701762

Chang KV, Wu WT, Hung CY, Han DS, Yang RS, Chang CH, Lin CP. Comparative effectiveness of suprascapular nerve block in the relief of acute post-operative shoulder pain: a systematic review and meta-analysis. Pain Physician. 2016b;19(7):445–56. PMID: 27676661

Chard MD, Satelle LM, Hazleman BL. The long term outcome of rotator cuff tendinitis—a review study. Br J Rheumatol. 1988;27:385–9.

Checcucci G, Allegra A, Bigazzi P, Gianesello L, Ceruso M, Gritti G. A new technique for regional anesthesia for arthroscopic shoulder surgery based on a suprascapular nerve block and an axillary nerve block: an evaluation of the first results. Arthroscopy. 2008;24:689–96.

Cho N, Kang RS, McCartney CJL, Pawa A, Costache I, Rose P, Abdallah FW. Analgesic benefits and clinical role of the posterior suprascapular nerve block in shoulder surgery: a systematic review, meta-analysis and trial sequential analysis. Anaesthesia. 2020;75(3):386–94. https://doi.org/10.1111/anae.14858. Epub 2019 Oct 3. PMID: 31583679

Cohen SB, Dines DM, Moorman CT. Familial calcification of the superior transverse scapular ligament causing neuropathy. Clin Orthop. 1997;334:131–5.

Coory JA, Parr AF, Wilkinson MP, Gupta A. Efficacy of suprascapular nerve block compared with subacromial injection: a randomized controlled trial in patients with rotator cuff tears. J Shoulder Elbow Surg. 2019;28(3):430–6. https://doi.org/10.1016/j.jse.2018.11.051. Epub 2019 Jan 14. PMID: 30651194

Cummins CA, Messer TM, Nuber GW. Current concepts review suprascapular nerve entrapment. J Bone Joint Surg. 2000;82:415–24.

D'Alessio J, Rosenblum M, Shea K, Freitas D. A retrospective comparison of interscalene and general anesthesia for ambulatory surgery shoulder arthroscopy. Reg Anesth. 1995;20:62–8.

Dahan TH, Fortin L, Pelletier M, Petit M, Vadeboncoeur R, Suissa S. Double blind randomized clinical trial examining the efficacy of bupivacaine suprascapular nerve blocks in frozen shoulder. J Rheumatol. 2000;27:1464–9.

Dangoisse MJ, Wilson DJ, Glynn CJ. MRI and clinical study of an easy and safe technique of suprascapular nerve blockade. Acta Anaesth Belg. 1994;45:49–54.

Dhir S, Sondekoppam RV, Sharma R, Ganapathy S, Athwal GS. A comparison of combined suprascapular and axillary nerve blocks to interscalene nerve block for analgesia in arthroscopic shoulder surgery: an equivalence study. Reg Anesth Pain Med. 2016;41(5):564–71. https://doi.org/10.1097/AAP.0000000000000436. PMID: 27380105

Di Lorenzo L, Pappagallo M, Gimigliano R, Palmieri E, Saviano E, Bello A, Forte A, Deblasio E, Trombetti C. Pain relief in early rehabilitation of rotator cuff tendinitis: any role for indirect suprascapular nerve block? Eura Medicophys. 2006;42:195–204.

Dorn C, Rumpold-Seitlinger G, Farzi S, Auer J, Bornemann-Cimenti H. The effect of the modified lateral suprascapular block on shoulder function in patients with chronic shoulder pain. Anesth Pain Med. 2015;5(6):e31640. https://doi.org/10.5812/aapm.31640. PMID: 26705528; PMCID: PMC4688809

Drez D Jr. Suprascapular neuropathy in the differential diagnosis of rotator cuff injuries. Am J Sports Med. 1976;4:43–5.

Elsharkawy HA, Abd-Elsayed AA, Cummings KC 3rd, Soliman LM. Analgesic efficacy and technique of ultrasound-guided suprascapular nerve catheters after shoulder arthroscopy. Ochsner J. 2014;14:259–63.

Emery P, Bowman S, Wedderburn L, Grahame R. Suprascapular nerve block for chronic shoulder pain in rheumatoid arthritis. BMJ. 1989;299:1079–80.

Ergonenc T, Beyaz SG. Effects of ultrasound-guided suprascapular nerve pulsed radiofrequency on chronic shoulder pain. Med Ultrason. 2018;20(4):461–6. https://doi.org/10.11152/mu-1543. PMID: 30534653

Eyigor C, Eyigor S, Korkmaz OK, Uyar M. Intra-articular corticosteroid injections versus pulsed radiofrequency in painful shoulder: a prospective, randomized, single-blinded study. Clin J Pain. 2010;26:386–92.

Ferré F, Pommier M, Laumonerie P, Ferrier A, Menut R, Bosch L, Balech V, Bonnevialle N, Minville V. Hemidiaphragmatic paralysis following ultrasound-guided anterior vs. posterior suprascapular nerve block: a double-blind, randomised control trial. Anaesthesia. 2020;75(4):499–508. https://doi.org/10.1111/anae.14978. Epub 2020 Jan 26. PMID: 31984478

Fiegl GC, Anderhuber F, Dorn C, Pipam W, Rosmarin W, Likar R. Modified lateral block of the suprascapular nerve: a safe approach and how much to inject? A morphological study. Reg Anesth Pain Med. 2007;32:488–94.

Fiegl GC, Dorn C, Likar R. What local anesthetic volume should be used for suprascapular nerve block? Reg Anesth Pain Med. 2008;33:571–3.

Gado K, Emery P. Modified suprascapular nerve block with bupivacaine alone effectively controls chronic shoulder pain in patients with rheumatoid arthritis. Ann Rheum Dis. 1993;52:215–8.

Gofeld M. Ultrasonography in pain medicine: a critical review. Pain Pract. 2008;8:226–40.

Gofeld M, Restrepo-Garces CE, Theodore BR, Faclier G. Pulsed radiofrequency of suprascapular nerve for chronic shoulder pain: a randomized double-blind active placebo-controlled study. Pain Pract. 2013;13:96–103.

Gordh T. Suprascapular nerve block. In: Eriksson E, editor. Illustrated handbook in local anesthesia. 2nd ed. Copenhagen: Munkgaard; 1979.

Gorthi V, Moon YL, Kang JH. The effectiveness of ultrasonography-guided suprascapular nerve block for perishoulder pain. Orthopedics. 2010;16:238–41.

Granirer LW. A simple technique for suprascapular nerve block. NY State J Med. 1951;51:1048.

Green S, Buchbinder R, Forbes A, Bellamy N. A standardized protocol for measurement of range of movement of the shoulder using the Plurimeter-V inclinometer and assessment of its intrarater and interrater variability. Arthritis Care Res. 1998;11:43–51.

Grey RG. The natural history of 'idiopathic' frozen shoulder. J Bone Joint Surg. 1978;60:564–5.

Hackworth RJ. A new and simplified approach to target the suprascapular nerve with ultrasound. J Clin Anesth. 2013;25:347–8.

Harmon D, Hearty C. Ultrasound-guided suprascapular nerve block technique. Pain Physician. 2007;10:743–6.

Hayes JMW, Cats A. Rheumatoid arthritis-management: end stage and complication. In: Dieppe PA, Klippel JH, editors. Rheumatology. London: Mosby; 1994.

Hussain N, Goldar G, Ragina N, Banfield L, Laffey JG, Abdallah FW. Suprascapular and interscalene nerve block for shoulder surgery: a systematic review and meta-analysis. Anesthesiology. 2017;127(6):998–1013. https://doi.org/10.1097/ALN.0000000000001894. PMID: 28968280

Ilfeld BM, Finneran JJ 4th, Gabriel RA, Said ET, Nguyen PL, Abramson WB, Khatibi B, Sztain JF, Swisher MW, Jaeger P, Covey DC, Meunier MJ, Hentzen ER, Robertson CM. Ultrasound-guided percutaneous peripheral nerve stimulation: neuromodulation of the suprascapular nerve and brachial plexus for postoperative analgesia following ambulatory rotator cuff repair. A proof-of-concept study. Reg Anesth Pain Med. 2019; https://doi.org/10.1136/rapm-2018-100121. PMID: 30770421

Inouye Y. Conduction along the articular branch of the suprascapular nerve. Acta Neurol Scand. 1978;58:230–40.

Jang JS, Choi HJ, Kang SH, Yang JS, Lee JJ, Hwang SM. Effect of pulsed radiofrequency neuromodulation on clinical improvements in the patients of chronic intractable shoulder pain. J Korean Neurosurg Soc. 2013;54:507–10.

Jayson MIV. Frozen shoulder: adhesive capsulitis. BMJ. 1981;283:1005–6.

Jeon WH, Park GW, Jeong HJ, Sim YJ. The comparison of effects of suprascapular nerve block, intra-articular steroid injection, and a combination therapy on hemiplegic shoulder pain: pilot study. Ann Rehabil Med. 2014;38(2):167–73.

Jerosch J, Saad M, Greig M, Filler T. Suprascapular nerve block as a method of preemptive pain control in shoulder surgery. Knee Surg Sports Traumatol Arthrosc. 2008;16:602–7.

Jones DS, Chattopadhyay C. Suprascapular nerve block for the treatment of frozen shoulder in primary care: a randomized trial. Br J Gen Pract. 1999;49:39–41.

Jung TW, Lee SY, Min SK, Lee SM, Yoo JC. Does combining a suprascapular nerve block with an intra-articular corticosteroid injection have an additive effect in the treatment of adhesive capsulitis? A comparison of functional outcomes after short-term and minimum 1-year follow-up. Orthop J Sports Med. 2019;7(7):2325967119859277. https://doi.org/10.1177/2325967119859277. PMID: 31384617; PMCID: PMC6651672

Kane TPC, Rogers P, Hazelgrove J, Wimsey S, Harper GD. Pulsed radiofrequency applied to the suprascapular nerve in painful tear arthroscopy. J Shoulder Elbow Surg. 2008;17:436–40.

Karatas GK, Meray L. Suprascapular nerve block for pain relief in adhesive capsulitis: a comparison of two different techniques. Arch Phys Med Rehabil. 2002;83:593–7.

Katz J. Atlas of regional anesthesia. 2nd ed. Norwalk: Appleton-Century-Crofts; 1994.

Kay J, Memon M, Hu T, Simunovic N, Duong A, Paul J, Athwal G, Ayeni OR. Suprascapular nerve blockade for postoperative pain control after arthroscopic shoulder surgery: a systematic review and meta-analysis. Orthop J Sports Med. 2018;6(12):2325967118815859. https://doi.org/10.1177/2325967118815859. PMID: 30627589; PMCID: PMC6311591

Klç Z, Filiz MB, Çakr T, Toraman NF. Addition of suprascapular nerve block to a physical therapy program produces an extra benefit to adhesive capsulitis: a randomized controlled trial. Am J Phys Med Rehabil. 2015;94(10 Suppl 1):912–20. https://doi.org/10.1097/PHM.0000000000000336. PMID: 26203643

Koga R, Funakoshi T, Yamamoto Y, Kusano H. Suprascapular nerve block versus interscalene block for analgesia after arthroscopic rotator cuff repair. J Orthop. 2019;19:28–30. https://doi.org/10.1016/j.jor.2019.11.013. PMID: 32021031; PMCID: PMC6994801

Laumonerie P, Blasco L, Tibbo ME, Panagiotis K, Fernandes O, Lauwers F, Bonnevialle N, Mansat P, Ohl X. Ultrasound-guided versus landmark-based approach to the distal suprascapular nerve block: a comparative cadaveric study. Arthroscopy. 2019;35(8):2274–81. https://doi.org/10.1016/j.arthro.2019.02.050. Epub 2019 Jul 23. PMID: 31350084

Lee HY, Chung IH, Sir WS, et al. Variations of the ventral rami of the brachial plexus. J Korean Med Sci. 1992;7:19–24.

Lee JJ, Kim DY, Jwang JT, Lee SS, Hwang SM, Kim GH, Jo YG. Effect of ultrasonographically guided axillary nerve block combined with suprascapular nerve block in arthroscopic rotator cuff repair: a randomized controlled trial. Arthroscopy; 2014

Lewis RN. The use of combined suprascapular and circumflex (articular branches) nerve blocks in the management of chronic arthritis of the shoulder joint. Eur J Anaesthesiol. 1999;16:37–41.

Liliang PC, Lu K, Liang CL, Tsai YD, Hsieh CH, Chen HJ. Pulsed radiofrequency lesioning of the suprascapular nerve for chronic shoulder pain. Pain Med. 2009;10:70–5.

Martin SD, Warren RF, Martin TL, Kennedy K, O'Brien SJ, Wickiewicz TL. Suprascapular neuropathy: results of non-operative treatment. J Bone Joint Surg Am. 1997;79:1159–65.

Martinez-Barenys C, Busquets J, de Castro PE, Garcia-Guasch R, Perez J, Fernandez E, Mesa MA. Randomized double-blind comparison of phrenic nerve infiltration and suprascapular nerve block for ipsilateral shoulder pain after thoracic surgery. Eur J Cardiothorac Surg; 2010.

McGrath B, Elgendy H, Chung F, Kamming D, Curti B, King S. Thirty percent of patients have moderate to severe pain 24 hr after ambulatory surgery: a survey of 5703 patients. Can J Anesth. 2004;51:886–91.

Mestdagh H, Drizenko A, Ghestem P. Anatomical basis of suprascapular nerve syndrome. Anat Clin. 1981;3:67–71.

Meyer-Witting M, Foster JMG. Suprascapular nerve block in the management of cancer pain. Anaesthesia. 1992;47:626.

Mitra R, Harris A, Umphrey C, Smuck M, Fredericson M. Adhesive capsulitis: a new management protocol to improve passive range of movement. PM & R. 2009;1:1064–9.

Moore DC. Block of the suprascapular nerve. In: Moore DC, editor. Regional block. 4th ed. Springfield, IL: Charles C Thomas Co; 1979.

Mortada MA, Ezzeldin N, Abbas SF, Ammar HA, Salama NA. Multiple versus single ultrasound guided suprascapular nerve block in treatment of frozen shoulder in diabetic patients. J Back Musculoskelet Rehabil. 2017;30(3):537–42. https://doi.org/10.3233/BMR-150322. PMID: 27858673

Natsis K, Totlis T, Tsikaras P, Appell HJ, Skandalakis P, Koebke J. Proposal for classification of the suprascapular notch: a study on 423 dried scapulas. Clin Anat. 2007;20:135–9.

Neal JM, McDonald SB, Larkin KL, Polissar NL. Suprascapular nerve block prolongs analgesia after nonarthroscopic shoulder surgery but does not improve outcome. Anesth Analg. 2003;96:982–6.

Neuts A, Stessel B, Wouters PF, Dierickx C, Cools W, Ory JP, Dubois J, Jamaer L, Arijs I, Schoorens D. Selective suprascapular and axillary nerve block versus interscalene plexus block for pain control after arthroscopic shoulder surgery: a noninferiority randomized parallel-controlled clinical trial. Reg Anesth Pain Med. 2018;43(7):738–44. https://doi.org/10.1097/AAP.0000000000000777. PMID: 29659438

Neviaser TJ. Arthroscopy of the shoulder. Orthop Clin North Am. 1987;18:361–72.

Ogino T, Minami A, Kato H, Hara R, Suzuki K. Entrapment neuropathy of the suprascapular nerve by a ganglion: a report of three cases. J Bone Joint Surg Am. 1991;73:141–7.

Okur SC, Ozyemisci-Taskiran O, Pekindogan Y, Mert M, Caglar NS. Ultrasound-guided block of the suprascapular nerve in breast cancer survivors with limited shoulder motion—case series. Pain Physician. 2017;20(2):E233–9. PMID: 28158160

Ozer Y, Grossman JA, Gilbert A. Anatomic observations on the suprascapular nerve. Hand Clin. 1995;11:539–44.

Parris WC. Suprascapular nerve block: a safer technique. Anesthesiology. 1990;72:580–1.

Peng PW, Wiley MJ, Liang J, Bellingham GA. Ultrasound-guided suprascapular nerve block: a correlation with fluoroscopic and cadaveric findings. Can J Anaesth. 2010;57(2):143–8. https://doi.org/10.1007/s12630-009-9234-3. Epub 2010 Jan 6. PMID: 20052627

Petersson CJ. Painful shoulders in patients with rheumatoid arthritis. Scand J Rheumatol. 1986;15:275–9.

Piasecki DP, Romeo AA, Bach BR, Nicholson GP. Suprascapular neuropathy. J Am Acad Orthop Surg. 2009;17:665–76.

Polguj M, Sibinski M, Grzegorzewski A, Grzelak P, Majos A, Topol M. Variation in morphology of suprascapular notch as a factor of suprascapular nerve entrapment. Int Orthop. 2013;37:2185–92.

Post M. Diagnosis and treatment of suprascapular nerve entrapment. Clin Orthop Relat Res. 1999;223:92–100.

Price DJ. The shoulder block: a new alternative to interscalene brachial plexus blockade for the control of postoperative shoulder pain. Anaesth Intensive Care. 2007;35:575–81.

Rengacharry SS, Neff JP, Singer PA, Brackett CE. Suprascapular entrapment neuropathy: a clinical, anatomical and comparative study. Part 1: clinical study. Neurosurgery. 1979;5:441–6.

Riazi S, Carmichael N, Awad I, Holtby RM, McCartney CJ. Effect of local anaesthetic volume (20 vs 5 ml) on the efficacy and respiratory consequences of ultrasound-guided interscalene brachial plexus block. Br J Anaesth. 2008;101:549–56.

Ridsall JE, Sharwood-Smith GH. Suprascapular nerve block. New indications and a safer technique. Anaesthesia. 1992;47:626.

Ritchie ED, Tong D, Chung F, Norris AM, Miniaci A, Vairavanathan SD. Suprascapular nerve block for postoperative pain relief in arthroscopic shoulder surgery: a new modality? Anesth Analg. 1997;84:1306–12.

Rose DL, Kelly CR. Suprascapular nerve block in shoulder pain. J Kansas Med Soc. 1969;70:135–6.

Saha S, Brish EL, Lowry AM, Boddu K. In select patients, ipsilateral post-thoracotomy shoulder pain relieved by suprascapular nerve block. Am J Ther; 2010.

Schneider-Kolsky ME, Pike J, Connell DA. CT-guided suprascapular nerve blocks: a pilot study. Skeletal Radiol. 2004;33:277–82.

Sencan S, Celenlioglu AE, Karadag-Saygı E, Midi İ, Gunduz OH. Effects of fluoroscopy-guıded intraartıcular injectıon, suprascapular nerve block, and combınatıon therapy ın hemıplegıc shoulder paın: a prospective double-blınd, randomızed clınıcal study. Neurol Sci. 2019;40(5):939–46. https://doi.org/10.1007/s10072-019-03733-6. Epub 2019 Jan 28. PMID: 30690679

Shabat S, Leitner J, Folman Y. Pulsed radiofrequency for the suprascapular nerve for patients with chronic headache. J Neurosurg Anesthesiol. 2013;25:340–3.

Shah RV, Racz GB. Pulsed mode radiofrequency lesioning of the suprascapular nerve for the treatment of chronic shoulder pain. Pain Physician. 2003;6:503–6.

Shanahan EM, Ahern M, Smith M, Wetherall M, Bresnihan B, Fitzgerald O. Suprascapular nerve block (using bupivacaine and methylprednisolone acetate) in chronic shoulder pain. Ann Rheum Dis. 2003;62:400–6.

Shanahan EM, Smith MD, Wetherall M, Loft CW, Slavotinek J, Fitzgerald O, Ahern MJ. Suprascapular nerve block in chronic shoulder pain: are the radiologists better? Ann Rheum Dis. 2004;63:1035–40.

Shanahan EM, Shanahan KR, Hill CL, Ahern MJ, Smith MD. Safety and acceptability of suprascapular nerve block in rheumatology patients. Clin Rheumatol. 2012;31:145–9.

Shanahan EM, Glaezter K, Gill T, Hill C, Graf S, Allcroft P. A case series of suprascapular nerve block (with an historical comparator) for shoulder pain in motor neurone disease. Palliat Med. 2020;34(8):1127–33. https://doi.org/10.1177/0269216320929553. Epub 2020 May 29. PMID: 32469625

Siegenthaler A, Morrigl B, Mlekusch S, Schliessbach J, Haug M, Curatolo M, Eichenberger U. Ultrasound-guided suprascapular nerve block, description of a novel supraclavicular approach. Reg Anesth Pain Med. 2012;37:325–8.

Simopoulos TT, Nagda J, Aner MM. Percutaneous radiofrequency lesioning of the suprascapular nerve for the management of chronic shoulder pain: a case series. J Pain Res. 2012;5:91–7.

Singelyn FJ, Lhotel L, Fabre B. Pain relief after arthroscopic shoulder surgery: a comparison of intraarticular analgesia, suprascapular nerve block, and interscalene brachial plexus block. Anesth Analg. 2004;99:589–92.

Sinha P, Sarkar B, Goswami S, Ray Karmakar P, Dasgupta SR, Basu S. Effectiveness of combination of ultrasonography-guided pulsed radiofrequency neuromodulation with steroid at the suprascapular nerve in chronic shoulder pain. Pain Pract. 2020;20(1):16–23. https://doi.org/10.1111/papr.12820. Epub 2019 Aug 24. PMID: 31310702

Sir E, Eksert S. Ultrasound-guided pulsed radiofrequency neuromodulation of the suprascapular nerve in partial rotator cuff tears. Turk J Med Sci. 2019;49(5):1524–8. https://doi.org/10.3906/sag-1906-132. PMID: 31651124; PMCID: PMC7018394

Tan N, Agnew NM, Scawn ND, Pennefather SH, Chester M, Russell GN. Suprascapular nerve block for ipsilateral shoulder pain after thoracic epidural analgesia: a double-blind comparison of 0.5% bupivacaine and 0.9% saline. Anesth Analg. 2002;94:199–202.

Taskaynata MA, Yilmaz B, Ozgul A, Yazicioglu K, Kalyon TA. Suprascapular nerve block versus steroid injection for non-specific shoulder pain. Tohoku J Exp Med. 2005;205:19–25.

Terlemez R, Çiftçi S, Topaloglu M, Dogu B, Yilmaz F, Kuran B. Suprascapular nerve block in hemiplegic shoulder pain: comparison of the effectiveness of placebo, local anesthetic, and corticosteroid injections-a randomized controlled study. Neurol Sci. 2020;41(11):3243–7. https://doi.org/10.1007/s10072-020-04362-0. Epub 2020 May 10. PMID: 32388647

US Preventive Services Task Force. Guide to clinical preventive services: report of the US Preventive Services Task force. Pennsylvania, PA: Diane Publishing Co; 1989.

Vastamaki M, Gorannson H. Suprascapular nerve entrapment. Clin Orthop. 1993;297:135–43.

Vecchio PC, Adebajo AO, Hazleman BL. Suprascapular nerve block for persistent rotator cuff lesions. J Rheumatol. 1993;20:453–5.

Voster W, Lange CPE, Briet RJP, et al. The sensory branch distribution of the suprascapular nerve: an anatomic study. J Shoulder Elbow Surg. 2008;17:500–2.

Walsworth MK, Mills JT, Michener LA. Diagnosing suprascapular neuropathy in patients with shoulder dysfunction: a report of 5 cases. Phys Ther. 2004;84:359–72.

Warner JP, Krushell RJ, Masquelet A, Gerber C. Anatomy and relationships of the suprascapular nerve: anatomical constraints to mobilization of the supraspinatus and intraspinatus muscles in the management of massive rotator-cuff tears. J Bone Joint Surg. 1992;74-A:36–45.

Wassef MR. Suprascapular nerve block. A new approach for the management of frozen shoulder. Anaesthesia. 1992;47:120–4.

Wertheim HM, Rovenstein EA. Suprascapular nerve block. Anesthesiology. 1941;2:541–5.

Wu YT, Ho CW, Chen YL, Li TY, Lee KC, Chen LC. Ultrasound-guided pulsed radiofrequency stimulation of the suprascapular nerve for adhesive capsulitis: a prospective, randomized, controlled trial. Anesth Analg; 2014

Yucesoy C, Akkaya T, Ozel O, et al. Ultrasonographic evaluation and morphometric measurements of the suprascapular notch. Surg Radiol Anat. 2009;31:409–14.

Axillary Nerve Blockade

18

Maria Fernanda Rojas Gomez and Philip Peng

Contents

General Consideration

The innervation of the shoulder is complex and variable, involving multiple nerves which share interconnections with overlapped territories. Therefore, the blockade of a single nerve may not be sufficient to achieve analgesia of shoulder joint or surrounding structures (Fig. 18.1).

Current literature supports the significant contribution of axillary nerve to the total innervation of the shoulder (Fig. 18.1). There is an emerging interest of the phrenic nerve sparing regional anesthesia blockade of the shoulder especially in patients at high risk of respiratory complications. One popular option is the blockade of the axillary nerve in conjunction with suprascapular nerve. In addition, axillary nerve is also one of the targets for shoulder denervation procedure. This chapter summarized the anatomy, sonoanatomy, and technical approaches of the blockade. As the use of axillary nerve block in chronic shoulder pain is covered in another chapter, this chapter focuses on the role of axillary in the perioperative management.

M. F. Rojas Gomez (✉)
Cirulaser Andes Clinic, Bogota, Colombia

P. Peng
Department of Anesthesia and Pain Medicine, Toronto Western Hospital, University of Toronto, Toronto, ON, Canada
e-mail: philip.peng@uhn.ca

Indications

1. Regional Anesthesia

   Axillary nerve block is considered in conjunction with other nerves, mainly suprascapular nerve (others are superficial cervical plexus and lateral pectoral nerve), for perioperative pain control of shoulder surgery, especially in patient with poor respiratory reserve.
2. Chronic Pain

   It is the target for denervation or neuromodulation for chronic shoulder pain.

Functional Anatomy

Both the radial nerve and the axillary nerve are terminal branches of the posterior cord of the brachial plexus (Fig. 18.2). The origin of the axillary is from C5 and C6.

D. Jankovic, P. Peng (eds.), *Regional Nerve Blocks in Anesthesia and Pain Therapy*,
https://doi.org/10.1007/978-3-030-88727-8_18

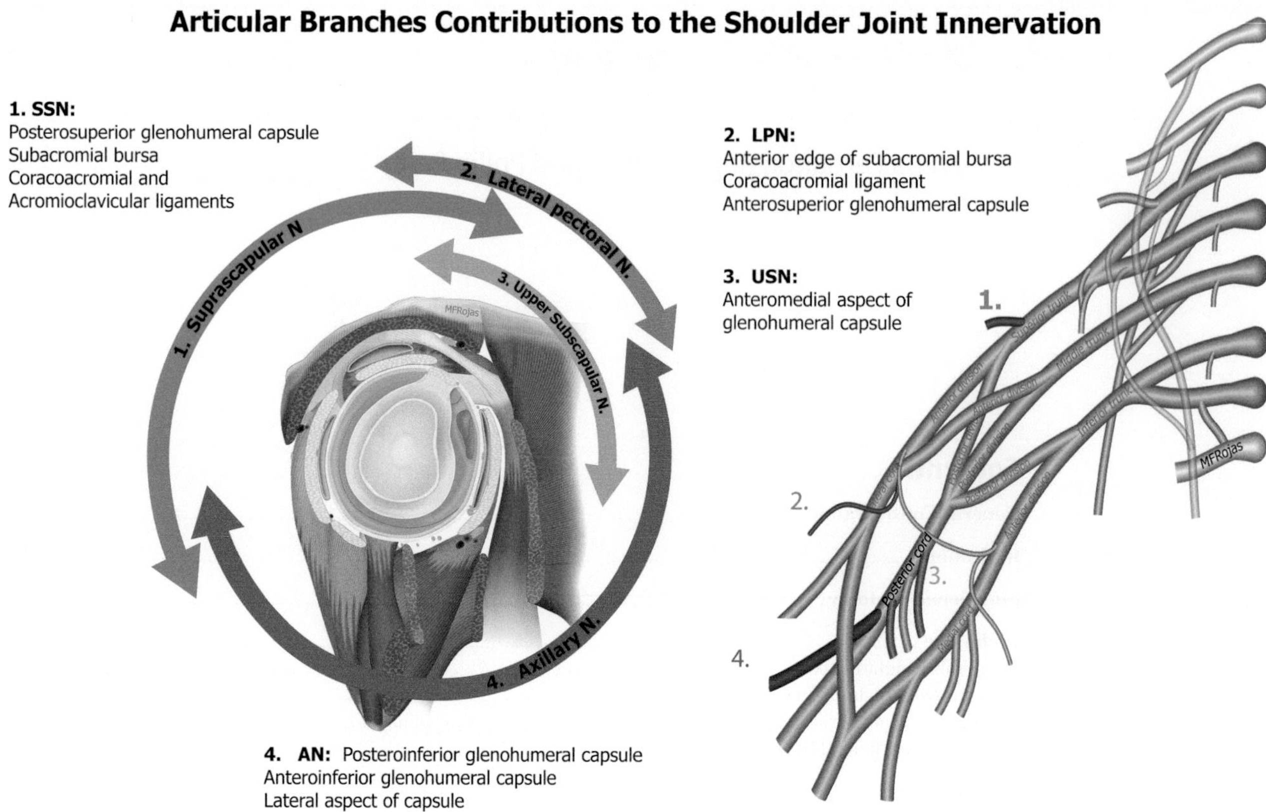

Fig. 18.1 Contribution of articular branches to the shoulder. *LPN* lateral pectoral nerve, *USN* upper subscapular nerve. (Reproduced with courtesy of Dr. Maria Fernanda Rojas)

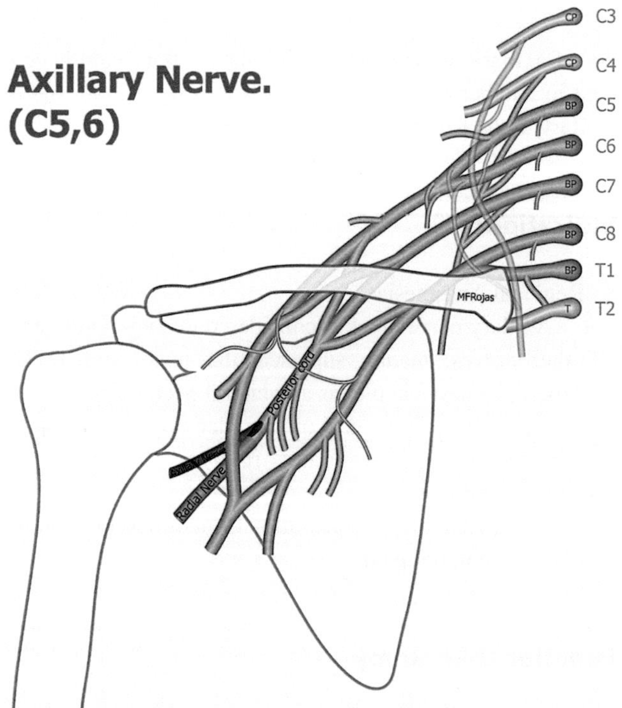

Fig. 18.2 Radial and axillary nerve. Both are branches from the posterior cord. (Reproduced with courtesy of Dr. Maria Fernanda Rojas)

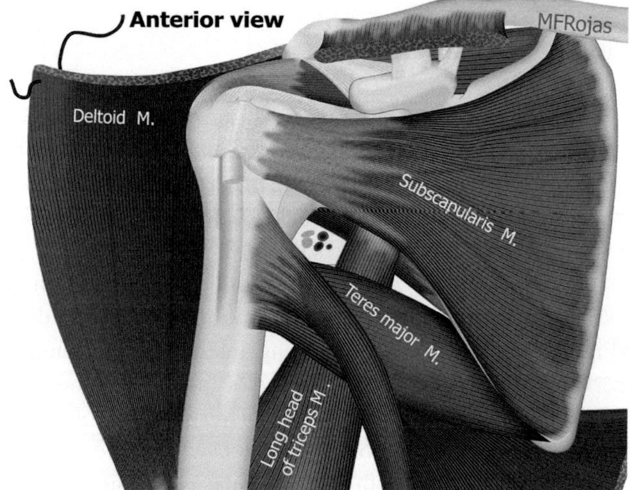

Fig. 18.3 Anterior view of quadrilateral space. The neurovascular bundle (axillary nerve: yellow; posterior humeral circumflex artery and vein in red and blue, respectively) is seen passing through the anterior quadrilateral space (yellow). The boundaries are subscapularis superiorly, teres major inferiorly, humerus laterally, and long head of triceps medially. (Reproduced with courtesy of Dr. Maria Fernanda Rojas)

Emerging from the posterior cord, the axillary nerve runs between the pectoralis minor and serratus anterior medial to the musculocutaneous nerve and descends inferolaterally superficial to the subscapularis muscle. At the caudal border of subscapularis, it passes into the quadrilateral space accompanied by the posterior circumflex humeral artery (Fig. 18.3).

The quadrilateral space (of Velpeau) or quadrangular space or foramen humerotricipital is an intermuscular space through which the axillary nerve and posterior circumflex humeral vessels (artery and vein) pass through backward to encircle the surgical neck of the humerus. It is bounded above by subscapularis and teres minor, below by teres major, medially by long head of triceps, and laterally surgical neck of humerus (Fig. 18.4).

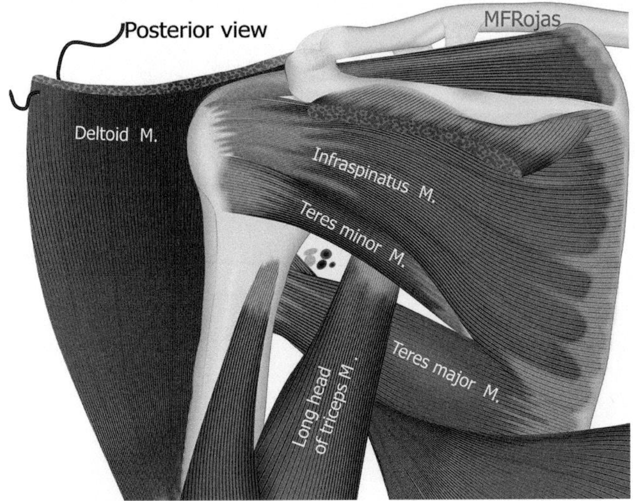

Fig. 18.4 Posterior view of quadrilateral space. The neurovascular bundle (axillary nerve: yellow; posterior humeral circumflex artery and vein in red and blue, respectively) is seen passing through the posterior quadrilateral space (yellow). The boundaries are teres minor superiorly, teres major inferiorly, humerus laterally, and long head of triceps medially. (Reproduced with courtesy of Dr. Maria Fernanda Rojas)

Prior to entering the quadrilateral space, the axillary nerve gives off articular branches to the anteroinferior glenohumeral joint that courses along the inferior border of the musculotendinous junction of the subscapularis muscle (Fig. 18.5). As the axillary nerve passes through the quadrilateral space, it divides into anterior and posterior divisions. The posterior division innervates the posterior deltoid and teres minor and provides a branch that courses superiorly deep to the teres minor to innervate the posteroinferior glenohumeral joint (Fig. 18.5). It terminates as a cutaneous branch supplying the sensation to the skin over the deltoid area. The anterior division of axillary nerve, after wrapping laterally around the surgical neck of the humerus with the posterior circumflex humeral artery, provides motor supply to anterior and middle deltoid but inconsistently supplies articular branches to the lateral humerus and subacromial bursa.

According to Duperc et al., they proposed to divide the course of axillary nerve into five segments: (1) from its origin to the inferior border of the subscapularis muscle (ramifications in this segment are not frequent), (2) from the lower border of the subscapularis to the long head of the triceps, (3) from the long head of the triceps to the surgical neck of the humerus, (4) from humerus to the entrance to the deltoid muscle, and (5) its intramuscular course in the deltoid (Figs. 18.5 and 18.6).

From the perspective of intervention, there are four targets at which the axillary nerve or the relevant branches can

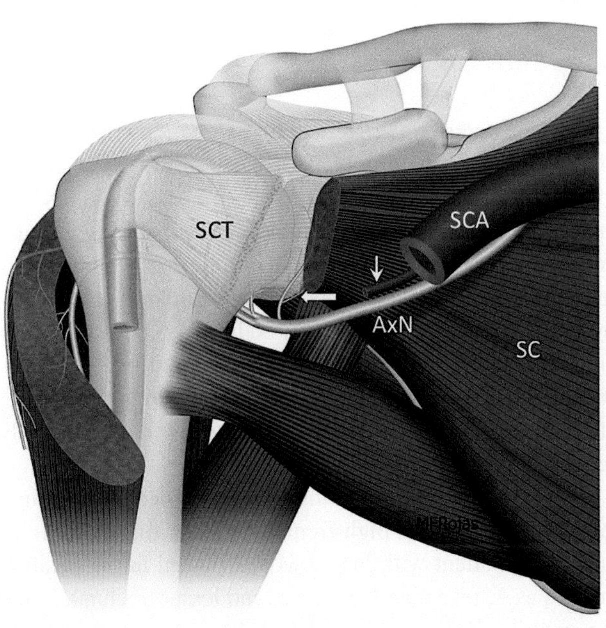

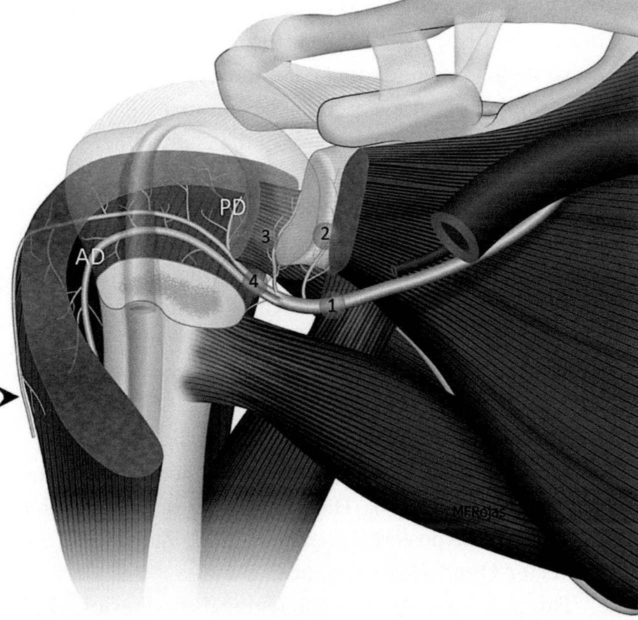

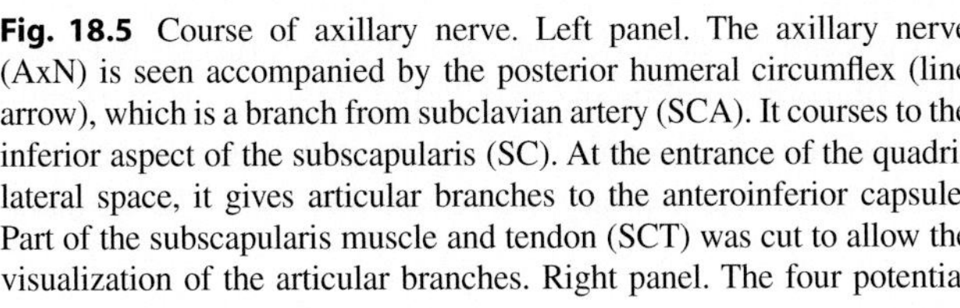

Fig. 18.5 Course of axillary nerve. Left panel. The axillary nerve (AxN) is seen accompanied by the posterior humeral circumflex (line arrow), which is a branch from subclavian artery (SCA). It courses to the inferior aspect of the subscapularis (SC). At the entrance of the quadrilateral space, it gives articular branches to the anteroinferior capsule. Part of the subscapularis muscle and tendon (SCT) was cut to allow the visualization of the articular branches. Right panel. The four potential sites for intervention. (1) Anterior quadrilateral space, (2) deep subscapularis space, (3) deep teres minor space, (4) posterior quadrilateral space. The subscapularis and teres minor muscles were cut to allow the visualization of the articular branches. The humeral head was faded to allow the visualization of the anterior and posterior division (AD and PD, respectively). Arrowhead: upper lateral cutaneous nerve of the arm. (Reproduced with courtesy of Dr. Maria Fernanda Rojas)

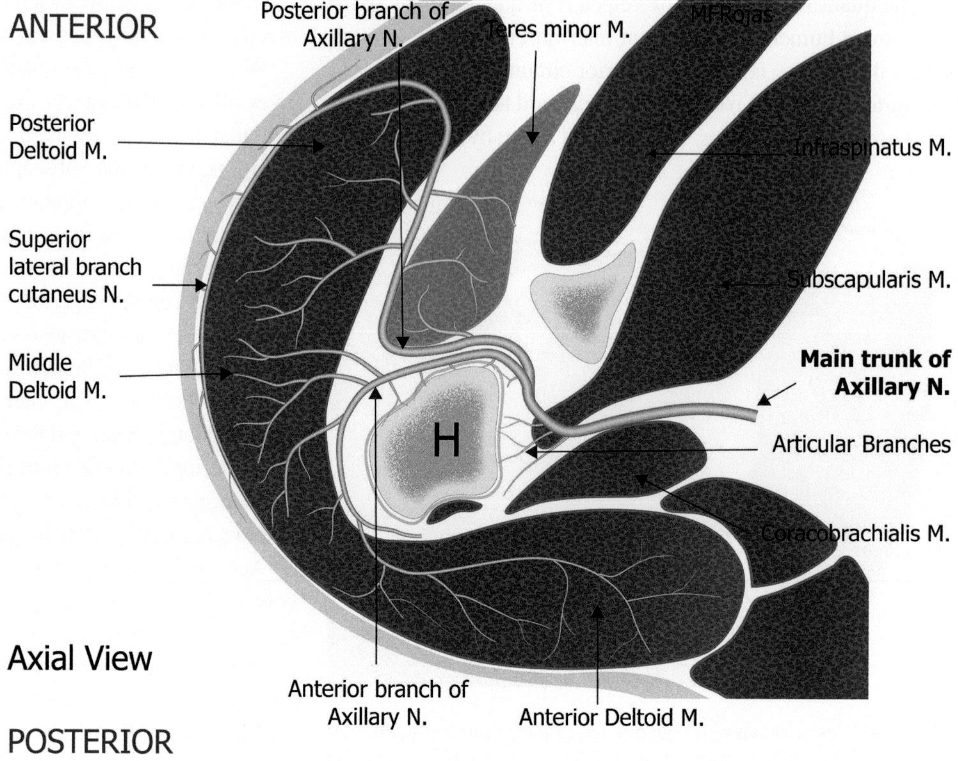

Fig. 18.6 Schematic diagram of the branches of axillary nerve. Note that the branches are not all in the same axial plane. (Reproduced with courtesy of Dr. Maria Fernanda Rojas)

be targeted. To understand the anatomy and sonoanatomy of those four targets, the readers should be familiar with the bony structures of the shoulder (Fig. 18.7).

1. **Deep Subscapularis Space**
   This is the space between the subscapularis and anterior glenoid (Fig. 18.8). The articular branches from the nerve to subscapularis innervate the upper anterior capsule, while the articular branches from axillary nerve cover the anteroinferior capsule of the glenohumeral joint (Fig. 18.8).
2. **Anterior Quadrilateral Space**
   This is the space between subscapularis, long head of triceps, humerus, and teres major, where the axillary nerve enters with posterior circumflex humeral vessels (Figs. 18.3 and 18.5). Blockade at this nerve will block all the branches of axillary nerve (sensory, motor, and articular branches).
3. **Deep Teres Minor Space**
   This is the space between the teres minor and humerus (Figs. 18.5 and 18.9). The space houses the articular branches to the posterior glenohumeral joint capsule.
4. **Posterior Quadrilateral Space**
   This space is well-known to regional anesthesiologists as the target for axillary nerve block. The boundaries are similar to the anterior quadrilateral space except the upper border is teres minor instead. Blockade at this space covers the motor branches to the deltoid and the sensory branches to the skin over the deltoid area (Figs. 18.4 and 18.5). Whether the blockade in this area will cover the articular branches is unknown.

Technique

Deep Subscapularis Space

This space between the subscapularis and the upper half of glenoid contains the articular branches of the nerve to subscapularis, while the space between the subscapularis and inferior half of glenoid contains the anterior articular branches of the axillary nerve. To direct the needle to this space, both ultrasound and fluoroscopy guidance can be considered, but in patient with high body mass index (BMI) or thick chest wall, fluoroscopy is the preferred imaging technique. The fluoroscopy technique is described in the chapter of shoulder denervation. The ultrasound technique is briefly described here.

The patient is put in a sitting position with the upper limb in external rotation. A high-frequency linear transducer (curvilinear in patient with high BMI) is placed in the position marked as A, revealing the greater and lesser trochanters and the anterior deltoid (Fig. 18.10). Moving the transducer medially and caudally as shown in position B, the coracoid process can be seen. Moving the transducer further in caudal direction with a subtle medial tilt, the anterior part of glenoid can be identified, and it is where the anterior articular branches of the axillary nerve are located. The articular

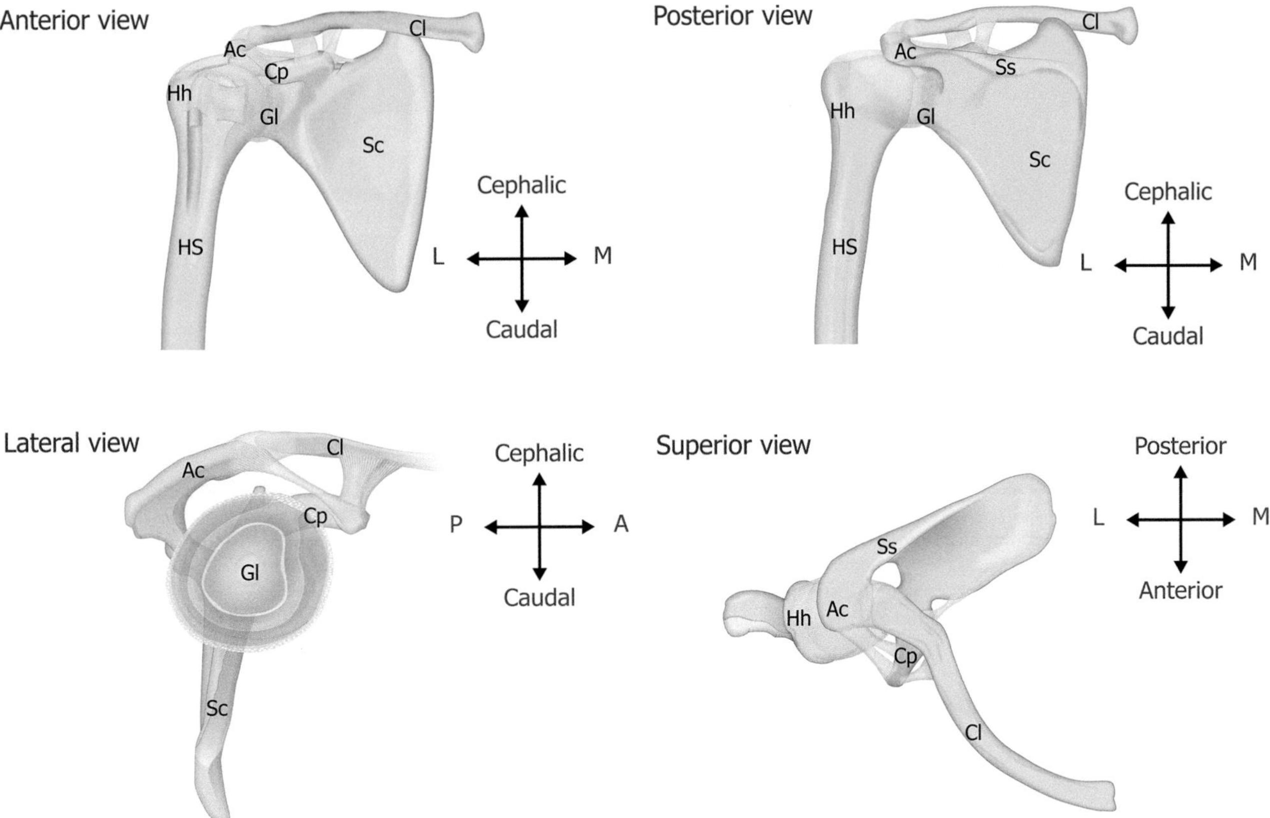

Fig. 18.7 Bony structures of the shoulder girdle. *Ac* acromion, *Hh* humerus head, *HS* humerus shaft, *Cp* coracoid process, *Gl* glenoid, *Sc* scapula, *Cl* clavicle, *Ss* scapular spine. (Reproduced with courtesy of Dr. Maria Fernanda Rojas)

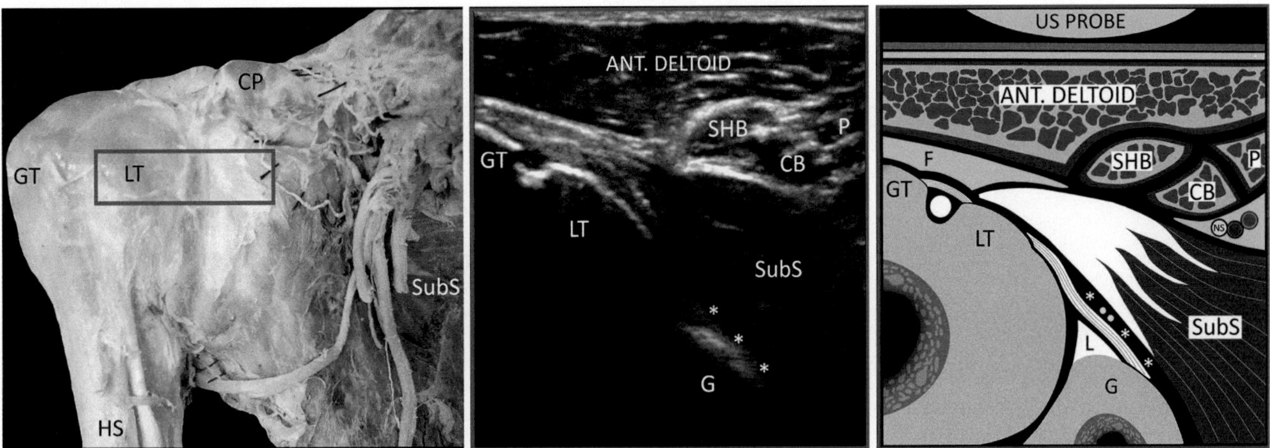

Fig. 18.8 Left panel: anatomic dissection, ultrasonography, and schematic diagram of the deep subscapularis space. The red rectangle depicts the position of the ultrasound probe for the sonographic image of this space. *GT* greater tuberosity, *LT* lesser tuberosity, *SubS* subscapularis, *SHB* short head of biceps, *CB* coracobrachialis, *P* pectoralis minor, *CP* coracoid process, *HS* humerus shaft, *G* glenoid, *L* labrum. (Reprinted with permission from Philip Peng educational series)

branches come out from the main trunk of the axillary nerve before its entrance in the quadrilateral space. A 22-G 3.5-in. needle is inserted out-of-plane until bony contact with the glenoid. Before the needle insertion, a quick scan in the region with Doppler is advisable to scout the vessels (anterior circumflex humeral artery or its branch).

Anterior Quadrilateral Space

The axillary enters into this space on the inferior border of the subscapularis. From there the nerve courses deep and runs around the neck of humerus. Because of this course, the nerve is difficult to be visualized at the entry. However,

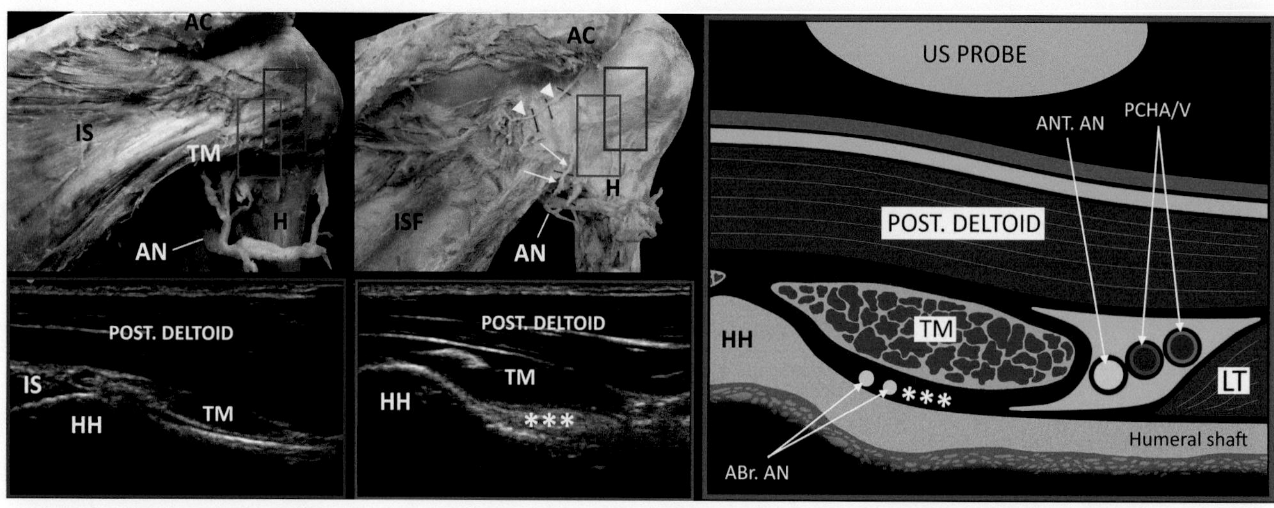

Fig. 18.9 Anatomic dissection, ultrasonography, and schematic diagram of the deep teres minor space (***). The red and blue rectangles depict the position of the ultrasound probe for the sonographic image of this space. *IS* infraspinatus, *TM* teres minor, *HH* humeral head, *AbrAN* articular branches to the axillary nerve, *PCHA/V* posterior circumflex humeral artery and vein. (Reprinted with permission from Philip Peng educational series)

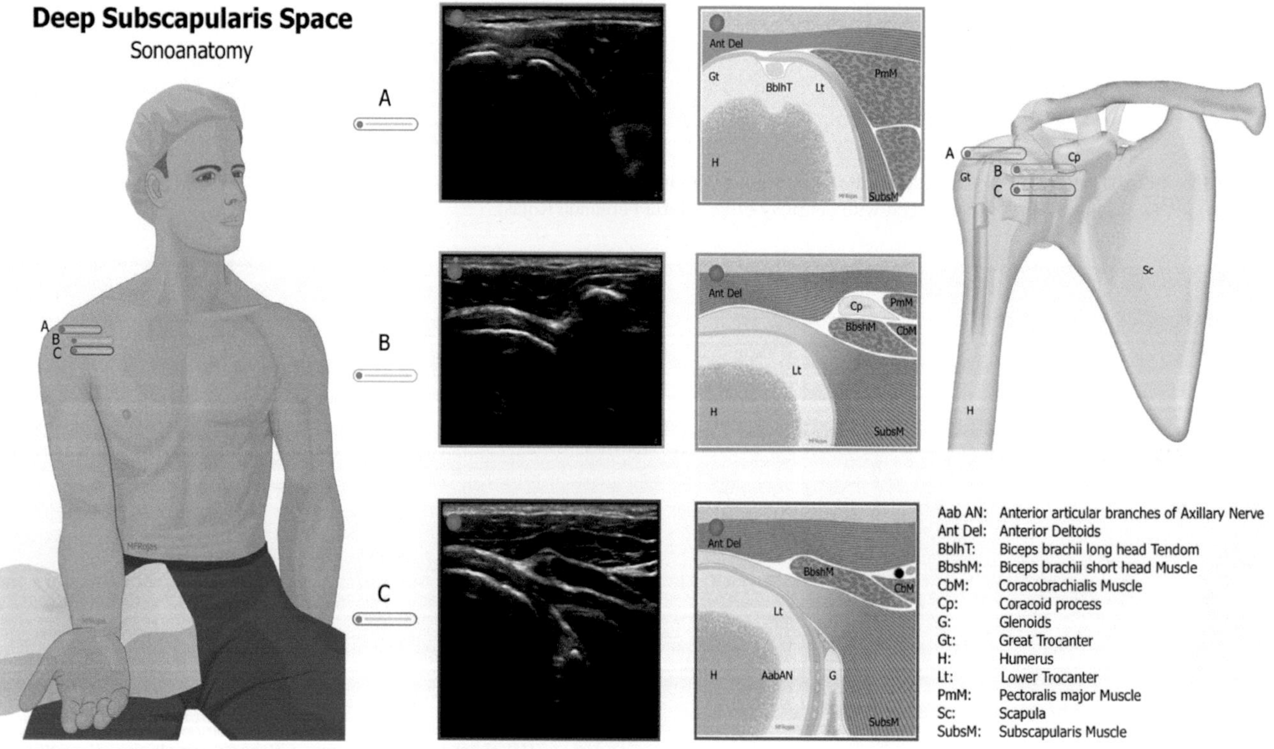

Fig. 18.10 Scanning technique for deep subscapularis space. In the left and right panels, the three different positions of the probe (A to C) are illustrated. In the middle panel, the anatomy and sonoanatomy corresponding to scanning position A to C are shown. (Reproduced with courtesy of Dr. Maria Fernanda Rojas)

before its entrance, the nerve lies on the inferior part of subscapularis, and it is the window that the nerve can be recognized in the ultrasound scanning (Fig. 18.11). At this site, the nerve carries all the sensory branches including the articular branches, making it a suitable target for providing analgesia with suprascapular nerve blockade in shoulder surgery when there is a high risk of performing more proximal blocks.

With the patient in a supine position with the arm abducted (90° or more), the ultrasound probe is initially placed over the posterior axillary fold (Fig. 18.11). Here, two muscles can be seen: teres major and latissimus dorsi. The tendon of the latissimus dorsi wraps around the lower border of the teres major and is inserted into the floor of the bicipital groove with the teres major forming the "conjoint tendon,"

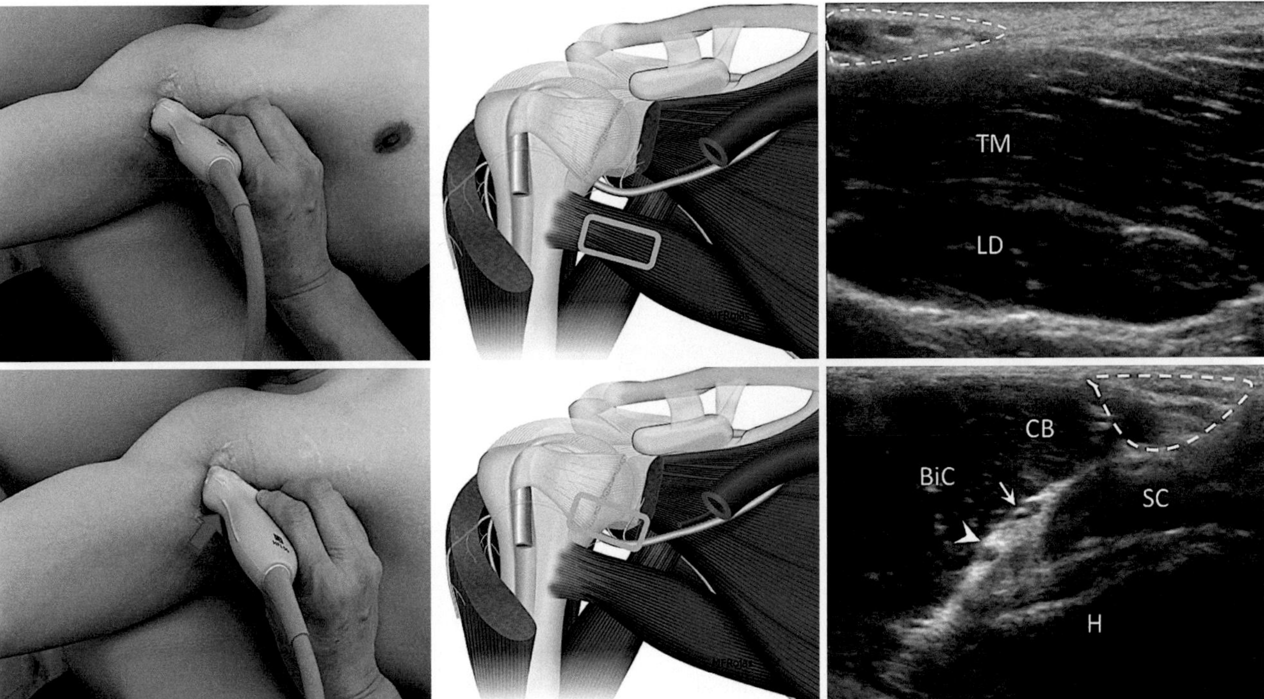

Fig. 18.11 Scanning technique for the anterior quadrilateral space. The left panel showed the position of the transducer in the model. Left upper: the initial probe position is over the posterior axillary fold. Left lower: the probe is then tilted towards the apex of axilla. The middle panel showed the position of transducer (orange rectangle) in the anatomic figure. The right panel shows the sonography. Right upper: the two muscles of posterior axillary fold, teres major (TM) and latissimus dorsi (LM). The brachial plexus can be seen in the left upper corner (dotted line). Right lower: axillary nerve (arrowhead) and the accompanied posterior circumflex humeral artery (arrow) is seen between the subscapularis (SC) and flexor muscles, biceps (BiC) and coracobrachialis (CB). (Reprinted with permission from Philip Peng educational series)

termed commonly in anesthesiology literature. Tilting the probe deep towards the apex of axilla and moving slightly in cephalad direction, the subscapularis can be seen over the humeral head. Superficial to this muscle, the axillary nerve is seen accompanied by posterior circumflex humeral artery. A 50 mm 22-G needle is inserted in-plane toward the nerve. Nerve stimulation can be used for confirmation of the nerve.

Because of the proximity of the radial nerve on the medial side, a small volume of local anesthetic (3 mL of 0.25% bupivacaine) is required to block this nerve.

Deep Teres Minor Space

This is the space deep to the teres minor where the articular branches from the posterior division of the axillary nerve can be located. The patient can be in either sitting or lateral decubitus position, with the arm slightly abducted, and the transducer is placed in the position A of the diagram (Fig. 18.12). Here, the acoustic shadow of the humeral head, the posterior deltoid, the infraspinatus, and the teres minor muscles is identified. The transducer is slided caudally and medially toward the medial edge of humerus, beyond which the hyperechoic shadow of humerus will be lost. The reason to slide the transducer to the most medial part of humerus is to avoid the tendinous attachment of the teres minor, at which the potential space is obliterated with tendon attachment. At this space, a 50 mm 22-G needle is inserted either in-plane or out-of-plane toward the space. Upon hydrodissection, 3–5 mL of local anesthetic is administered.

Posterior Quadrilateral Space

At this space, the target is anterior and posterior divisions of the nerve after the departure of the posterior articular branches (Fig. 18.12). It is commonly described in the anesthesia literature as a space between the teres minor and triceps on the posterior surface of the humerus, where the axillary nerve is accompanied by the posterior circumflex artery. At this site, the articular branches already leave the posterior division and run deep to the teres minor. However, local anesthetic injected at this site may spread to the articular branches deep to the teres minor. A 50 mm 22-G needle is inserted in plane toward this target. Alternatively, the transducer is slided in medial direction until the hyperechoic shadow of humerus disappears. The axillary nerve can be targeted just inferior to the teres minor (Fig. 18.12).

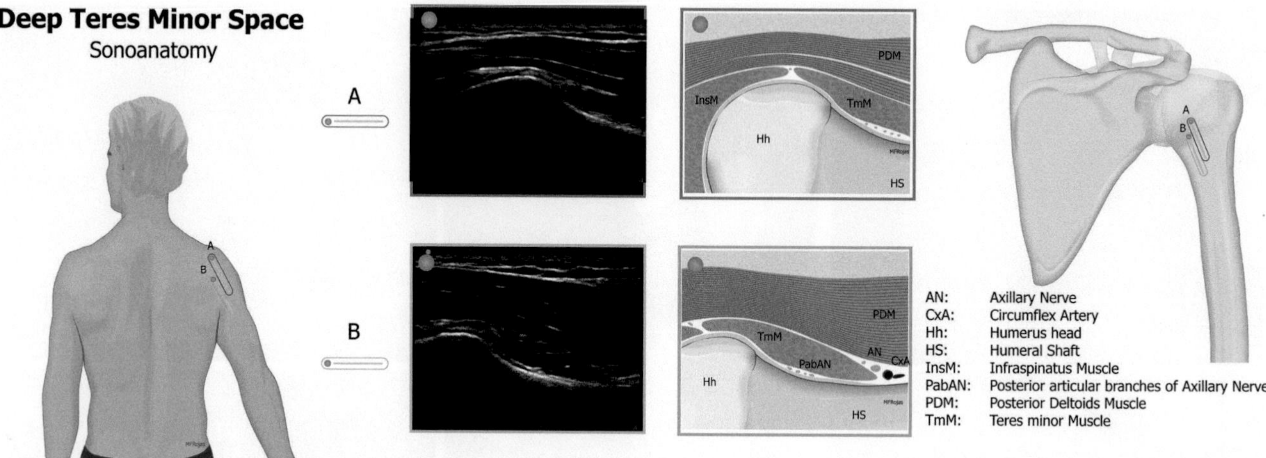

Fig. 18.12 Scanning technique for the deep teres minor space and posterior quadrilateral space. (Reproduced with courtesy of Dr. Maria Fernanda Rojas)

Complications

The axillary nerve block is an advanced regional anesthesia procedure, especially the anterior quadrilateral approach. The vicinity to vessels increases the potential for hematoma. Neurological injury can happen with this advanced block. The local anesthetic administered in the anterior quadrilateral space can spill to the radial nerve and results in inadvertent motor blockade.

Literature Review

Interscalene block is the recommended regional anesthesia technique for the perioperative pain control following shoulder surgery. However, the incidence of phrenic nerve block and the hemi-diaphragmatic paralysis is concerning. With the local anesthetic solution administered 20 mL or more, the incidence of transient phrenic nerve palsy is as high as 100% with landmark- or paresthesia-guided interscalene block. This will be translated to 27% reduction in forced vital capacity, which can be quite detrimental to patients with poor respiratory reserve secondary to pulmonary pathology or preexisting hemi-diaphragmatic paralysis. Various strategies were developed to minimize the phrenic nerve palsy from the interscalene block, such as small local anesthetic volume (5 mL), dilute local anesthetic concentration, or injection point 4 mm lateral to the brachial plexus. Although these strategies have been shown to reduce the incidence of phrenic nerve block, the incidence was still higher than 20%.

Therefore, investigators explored the possibility of blocking the suprascapular nerve with or without the axillary nerve block. A systematic review addressing this question revealed that the interscalene block reduced the postoperative pain but not opioid consumption in the recovery room. Yet, the superiority in pain score did not go beyond to the 24-h postoperative period. Overall, the pain control was better in the interscalene group as evident by the area under the curve of pain score in 24-h interval, but the difference is not clinically important (1.1 cm/h). A couple of issues need to be noted in this review. All the comparative studies were arthroscopic surgery. It is generally believed that the interscalene block should be considered for more painful procedure (open procedure or joint replacement surgery). Also, the role of addition of axillary nerve block was unclear. It was only examined once in a small randomized controlled study in which Lee and colleagues demonstrated the addition of axillary nerve block to the suprascapular nerve block provided superior pain control and satisfaction in the first 24 h. The target of their needle was the posterior quadrilateral space and the volume of injectate ranged from 10 to 15 mL. Although no formal spread study has examined the extent of dispersion of the local anesthetic, the high volume of local anesthetic is likely to spread deep to the articular branches of the shoulder.

Suggested Reading

Aliste J, Bravo D, Fernández D, et al. A randomized comparison between interscalene and small-volume supraclavicular blocks for arthroscopic shoulder surgery. Reg Anesth Pain Med. 2018;43:590–5.

Aszmann OC, Dellon AL, Birely BT, et al. Innervation of the human shoulder joint and its implications for surgery. Clin Orthop Relat Res. 1996;330:202–7.

Dhir S, Sondekoppam RV, Sharma R, et al. A comparison of combined suprascapular and axillary nerve blocks to interscalene nerve block for analgesia in arthroscopic shoulder surgery: an equivalence study. Reg Anesth Pain Med. 2016;41:564–71.

Duparc R, Bocquet G, Simonet J, Freger P. Anatomical basis of the variable aspects of injuries of the axillary nerve (excluding the terminal branches in the deltoid). Surg Radiol Anat. 1997;19:127–32.

Eckmann MS, Bickelhaupt B, Fehl J, et al. Cadaveric study of the articular branches of the shoulder joint. Reg Anesth Pain Med. 2017;42:564–70.

Eckmann MS, Lai BK, Uribe MA, et al. Thermal radiofrequency ablation of the articular branch of the lateral pectoral nerve: a case report and novel technique. A A Pract. 2019;13:415–9.

El-Boghdadly K, Chin KJ, Chan VWS. Phrenic nerve palsy and regional anesthesia for shoulder surgery: anatomical, physiologic, and clinical considerations. Anesthesiology. 2017;127(1):173–91.

Feigl G, Aichner E, Mattersberger C, Zahn PK, Avila Gonzalez C, Litz R. Ultrasound guided anterior approach to the axillary and intercostobrachial nerves in the axillary fossa: an anatomical investigation. Br J Anaesth. 2018;121:883–9.

Hussain N, Goldar G, Ragina N, Banfield L, Laffey JG, Abdallah FW. Suprascapular and interscalene nerve block for shoulder surgery: a systematic review and meta-analysis. Anesthesiology. 2017;127(6):998–1013.

Laumonerie P, Dalmas Y, Tibbo ME, et al. Sensory innervation of the human shoulder joint: the three bridges to break. J Shoulder Elbow Surg. 2020;29:e499–507.

Nam Y-S, Panchal K, Kim I-B, et al. Anatomical study of the articular branch of the lateral pectoral nerve to the shoulder joint. Knee Surg Sports Traumatol Arthrosc. 2016;24:3820–7.

Neuts A, Stessel B, Wouters PF, et al. Selective suprascapular and axillary nerve block versus interscalene plexus block for pain control after arthroscopic shoulder surgery: a noninferiority randomized parallel-controlled clinical trial. Reg Anesth Pain Med. 2018;43:738–44.

Pitombo PF, Barros RM, Matos MA, Modolo NS. Selective suprascapular and axillary nerve block provides adequate analgesia and minimal motor block. Comparison with interscalene block. Rev Bras Anestesiol. 2013;63:45–51.

Tran J, Peng PWH, Agur AMR. Anatomical study of the innervation of glenohumeral and acromioclavicular joint capsules: implications for image-guided intervention. Reg Anesth Pain Med. 2019a;44:452–8.

Tran J, Peng P, Agur A. Evaluation of suprascapular nerve radiofrequency ablation protocols: 3D cadaveric needle placement study. Reg Anesth Pain Med. 2019b;44:1021–5.

Tran J, Peng P, Agur A, Mittal N. Diagnostic block and radiofrequency ablation of the acromial branches of the lateral pectoral and suprascapular nerves for shoulder pain: a 3D cadaveric study. Reg Anesth Pain Med. 2021;46(4):305–12.

Regional Block for Pain Therapy in Shoulder

19

Jennifer McDonald and Philip Peng

Contents

J. McDonald (✉)
The Ottawa Hospital, Physical Medicine and Rehabilitation, The Ottawa Hospital Rehabilitation Centre, Ottawa, ON, Canada

P. Peng
Department of Anesthesiology and Pain Medicine, Toronto Western Hospital, University of Toronto, Toronto, ON, Canada
e-mail: philip.peng@uhn.ca

General Consideration

Shoulder pain is an ubiquitous complaint in both general and pain practices. Encouragingly, it often improves with conservative management strategies, including activity modification, physical therapy, and medications. When required,

D. Jankovic, P. Peng (eds.), *Regional Nerve Blocks in Anesthesia and Pain Therapy*,
https://doi.org/10.1007/978-3-030-88727-8_19

injections can be helpful for both diagnosis and management of shoulder pain.

The shoulder consult can be formidable due to the multiple potential pain generators. One of the more challenging aspects of ultrasound-guided shoulder injections is choosing the appropriate patient and anatomical target. In this chapter, we will review the relevant functional anatomy, appropriate patient selection, and specific interventional techniques to target the primary shoulder pain generators.

If the pain generator is in doubt, or if the injection is not providing the expected benefit, seeking the opinion of a musculoskeletal medicine specialist for diagnostic clarification is recommended. In addition, clinical findings suggestive of acute trauma, marked weakness, instability, or significant mechanical symptoms (i.e., locking) should trigger a referral for diagnostic clarification and to rule out the need for surgical management.

Some patients with chronic shoulder pain present with associated periscapular myofascial pain and/or referred pain and sensory complaints down the arm. These shoulder pain patients can be mistakenly triaged as having cervical spine-mediated pain. It can be very enlightening to screen the shoulder joint during cervical spine pain consult to ensure there is no hidden contributing shoulder pathology.

Functional Anatomy

The glenohumeral (GH) joint is a synovial ball-and-socket joint consisting of the humeral head and shallow glenoid fossa. The latter is deepened by a fibrocartilaginous rim, the glenoid labrum (Fig. 19.1). Because only one-third of the humeral head is covered by the glenoid cavity, it confers the shoulder inherent instability, making it susceptible to subluxation and dislocation. The surrounding ligamentous structures are instrumental in stabilizing the joint.

The four rotator cuff muscles, which create a tight layer of tendons around the GH joint, also play an important role in joint stabilization (Fig. 19.2). The rotator cuff helps to keep the humeral head centered on the glenoid during arm elevation. The subacromial subdeltoid (SASD) bursa lies beneath the deltoid muscle and coracoacromial arch (acromion, coracoacromial ligament, and coracoid) and covers the deeper rotator cuff tendons. The SASD bursa, which is the largest bursa in the body, allows the rotator cuff tendons to glide smoothly under the deltoid muscle and arch.

The long head of biceps (LHB) tendon originates at the supraglenoid tubercle and superior labrum. The intra-articular, extra-synovial proximal tendon travels over the anterosuperior humeral head. It then takes a sharp turn to exit the joint within the bicipital groove, covered by the transverse humeral ligament and accompanied by the ascending branch of the anterior circumflex artery (Fig. 19.3a, b). The synovial membrane lines the deep surface of the capsule and the outer surface of the biceps tendon. As one of the three main synovial recesses, the biceps tendon sheath extends along the extra-articular portion of the LHB tendon.

The rotator interval is a triangular space defined superiorly by the anterior supraspinatus fibers, inferiorly by the lateral subscapularis fibers, and medially, at its base, by the coracoid process (Fig. 19.3a, b). The rotator interval contains the CHL, SGHL, and LHB tendon and sheath and rotator interval joint capsule.

The acromioclavicular (AC) joint, located at the superior aspect of the shoulder complex, is a small diarthrodial joint between the concave medial end of the acromion and the convex lateral end of the clavicle (Fig. 19.4). A wedge-shaped fibrocartilaginous disc separates the articular surfaces of the joint. The movement of this joint is limited to primarily rotation and translation in the anterior–posterior and the superior–inferior planes. The AC joint is stabilized by both static and dynamic stabilizers. The static stabilizers include the acromioclavicular ligaments, the coracoclavicular ligaments (trapezoid and conoid), and the coracoacromial ligament. The inferior surface of the AC joint is in direct contact with the subacromial bursa and supraspinatus muscle and may play a role in the development of the impingement syndrome.

Indication (Patient Selection)

LHB Tendon

The extra-articular LHB tendon sheath can be targeted for injection in cases of primary biceps tendinopathy, which refers to a spectrum of pathology ranging from inflammatory tendinitis and tenosynovitis to degenerative tendinosis. It is important to note that isolated biceps tendon pathology is rare. A circumferential effusion within the biceps tendon sheath is often joint fluid tracking down from the GH joint, thus considering a GH joint pain generator from intra-articular pathology. LHB tendinopathy and/or instability is often associated with other shoulder pathology, especially superior labral tears and anterosuperior rotator cuff tears in the region of the rotator interval.

Rotator Interval

Frozen shoulder or adhesive capsulitis is characterized by marked progressive pain and stiffness and most often impacts

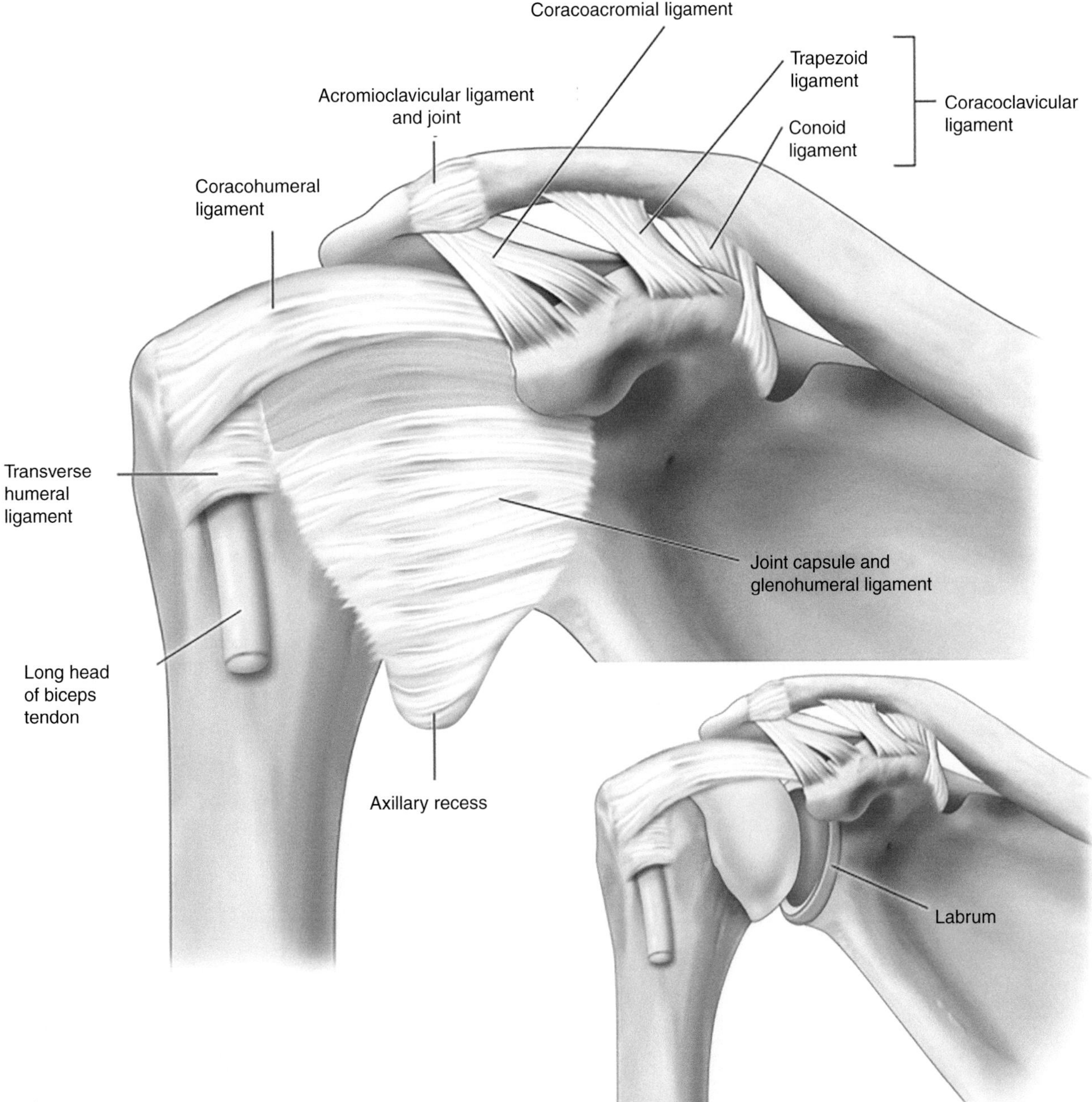

Fig. 19.1 The GH joint capsule and surrounding ligaments are pictured. The coracohumeral ligament (CHL) is a thick fibrous band originating from the coracoid process and inserting on the greater and lesser tuberosities of the humerus. The superior glenohumeral ligament (SGHL) is outlined in green. The inset picture shows the joint's articular surface, glenoid, and labrum. (Figure reproduced with permission from Philip Peng Educational Series)

middle-aged adults. It is thought to be related to inflammation and thickening of the rotator interval structures. Injecting the intra-articular portion of the biceps tendon sheath within the rotator interval allows the interventionalist to access the GH joint indirectly through this synovial recess. At the same time, the anterior capsule is distended through a relatively large volume injection.

GH Joint

The main indication for posterior GH joint injection is glenohumeral osteoarthritis and nonsurgical labral pathology. GH arthropathy is characterized by progressive and irreversible articular destruction and frequent involvement of the surrounding soft tissues. Primary

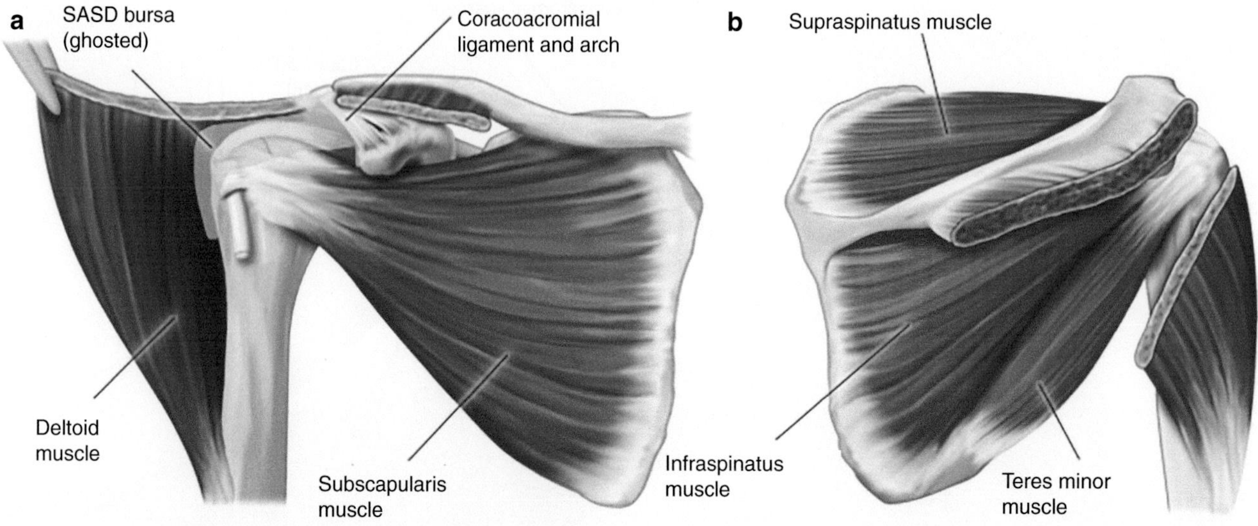

Fig. 19.2 The four rotator cuff muscles are pictured. The supraspinatus passes under the coracoacromial arch (outlined in yellow). The SASD bursa (ghosted) is a synovium-lined potential space deep to the coracoacromial arch and deltoid muscle. (**a**) Anterior view of the rotator cuff muscles with anterior deltoid muscle reflected away. (**b**) Posterior view of the rotator cuff muscles with posterior deltoid muscle partially resected. (Figure reproduced with permission from Philip Peng Educational Series)

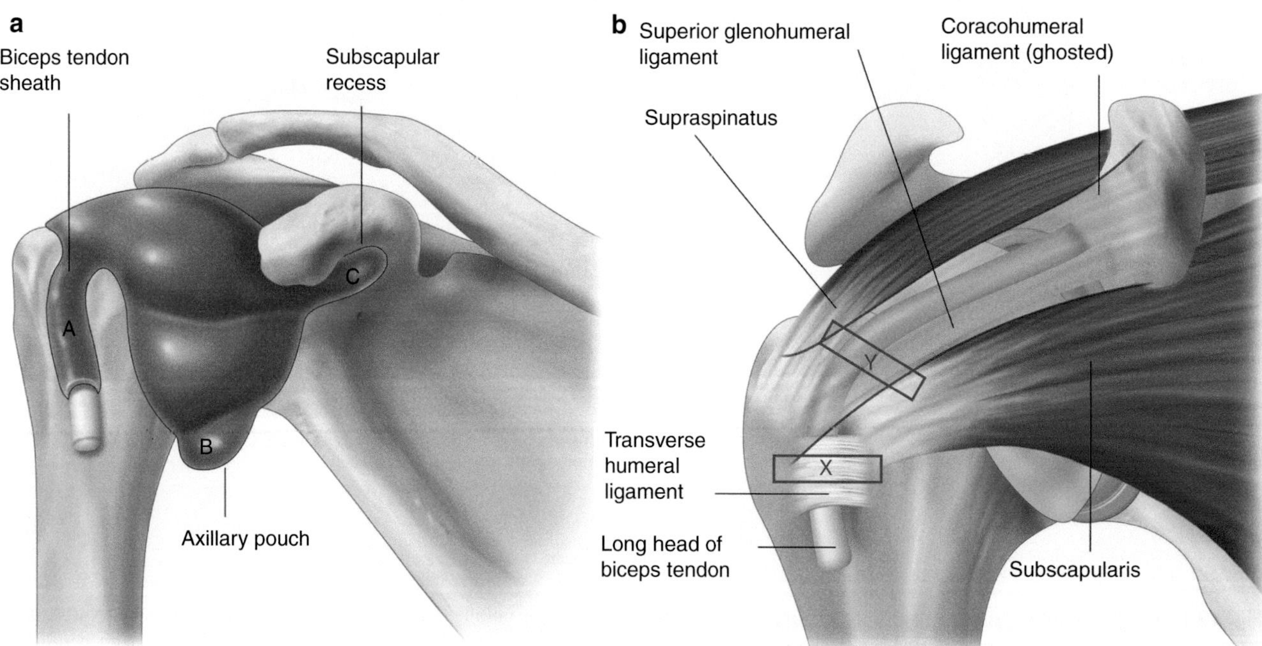

Fig. 19.3 The joint capsule (not pictured) extends from the medial glenoid cavity and base of the coracoid process to the anatomic neck of the humerus. (**a**) The three main synovial membrane recesses are pictured: A, the biceps tendon sheath; B, the axillary pouch; C, the subscapular recess. (**b**) Diagram of the rotator interval (outlined in yellow) with its complex anatomical relationships. Slices x and y mark ultrasound scanning positions applicable to Fig. 19.6. (Figure reproduced with permission from Philip Peng Educational Series)

osteoarthritis is uncommon and most of the causes of chondral damage are secondary to trauma, instability (from associated rotator cuff or labral pathology), post-surgical arthrosis, avascular necrosis, and inflammatory arthropathy. Chronic rotator cuff tears often lead to a high-riding humerus with suboptimal shoulder stability and biomechanics, which eventually results in advanced GH joint OA (rotator cuff arthropathy). Isolated labral pathology is often seen in younger individuals post trauma, and there can be associated shoulder stiffness, locking, and/or instability depending on the location and degree of labral disruption.

SASD Bursa

The SASD bursa is a common injection target in patients with subacromial impingement. Subacromial impingement occurs when the superior aspect of the humeral head and rotator cuff tendons impinge on the undersurface of the coracoacromial arch. The clinical finding of subacromial impingement is often seen together with the clinical diagnoses of rotator cuff pathology, SASD bursitis, and/or abnormal coracoacromial arch anatomy.

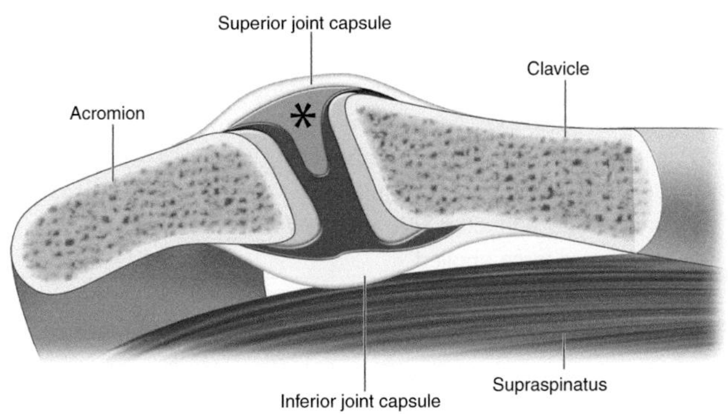

Fig. 19.4 The acromioclavicular joint is pictured. (Figure reproduced with permission from Philip Peng Educational Series)

AC Joint

The AC joint injection can be used as a diagnostic and/or therapeutic block. It is commonly used as a diagnostic test to localize the source of pain when AC joint injury is suspected. The main therapeutic indication for AC joint injection is arthritis (post-traumatic and osteoarthritis) of this joint.

History and Physical Examination

The clinical history (Table 19.1) and physical exam (Table 19.2) are important parts of the shoulder pain consult and provide clues about the primary pain generator. Pain with sleeping, especially when lying on the ipsilateral shoulder, is common and is a nonspecific finding. A simplified algorithm is also provided to assist the pain physician in interpreting the physical examination findings (Fig. 19.5). Palpation is omitted from the algorithm because tenderness of various structures, especially the LHB tendon, is common and nonspecific. The exception is palpation of the AC joint. AC joint tenderness worse on the affected side and that reproduces the patient's typical pain often supports a diagnosis of AC joint pathology. If marked stiffness and pain is apparent on range of motion examination in a middle-aged adult, the diagnosis of frozen shoulder is likely. In this case, the remaining exam can be abbreviated, as most of the provocative maneuvers will be painful and nonspecific.

Table 19.1 Clinical history

DIAGNOSIS	AGE	FUNCTIONAL COMPLAINTS	PAIN LOCATION
LHB tendon pathology	Variable	Marked pain +/- clicking/popping with shoulder movement	Anterior shoulder, referral to anterior upper arm
Labral pathology	Young to middle age	Associated stiffness or instability	Shoulder girdle, variable referral
Frozen shoulder	Middle age	Progressive marked pain/stiffness, difficulty reaching for seat belt	Shoulder girdle, often referred down the arm
RTC pathology/ bursitis	Middle to advanced age	Pain and limitation with overhead activities	Referral to lateral upper arm/deltoid
AC joint OA	Middle to advanced age	Pain and limitation with overhead activities and reaching behind	Superior shoulder, variable referral
GH joint OA	Middle to advanced age	Pain and limitation in all directions, difficulty reaching for seat belt	Shoulder girdle, variable referral

Reproduced with permission from Philip Peng and Jennifer McDonald

Table 19.2 Physical examination

ACTIVE ROM	*Note available range, location of pain, compare side to side*
Abduction	Raise arms towards the ears
Adduction and Internal rotation	Reach behind the back (Apley's scratch test) Note the long finger position relative to the scapula
External rotation	Arms adducted against the trunk, elbows flexed 90°, externally rotate arms
PASSIVE ROM	***Note available range, location of pain, presence of crepitus***
Abduction	Stabilize the scapula (firm downward pressure) to isolate GH joint abduction, raise the arm away from the side
External rotation	Arm fixed against the trunk with elbow flexed 90°, externally rotate the arm
ROTATOR CUFF STRENGTH	***Tested in isometric fashion, note any pain and/or weakness***
Infraspinatus	Arm adducted against the trunk with elbow flexed 90°, patient resists examiner's external force to arms (tries to maintain neutral rotation)
SPECIAL TESTS	***If pain is elicited, note ifreproduces the patient's typical pain***
Cross body adduction	Arm flexed 90°, horizontally adducted, pain localizes over AC joint
Speed's	Arm flexed 90°, elbow extended and forearm supinated (palm up), downward force applied, pain localizesover the bicipital groove
Empty can	Arm flexed 90° in scapular plane (relatively abducted), internally rotated (thumb pointing down), downward force applied
O'Brien's	Arm flexed 90°, horizontally adducted 15°, internally rotated (thumb pointing down), downward force applied

Reproduced with permission from Philip Peng and Jennifer McDonald

Radiographs

A normal shoulder x-ray to rule out early osteoarthritis or bony pathology can help differentiate GH joint osteoarthritis from frozen shoulder. X-ray imaging of the AC joint can also rule in/out AC joint osteoarthritis as a potentially contributing pain generator.

Sonoanatomy

Starting with the patient supine and arm supinated, the LHB tendon at the bicipital groove can be identified in transverse view using a Linear 5–13 MHz ultrasound probe. Starting at Fig. 19.3 position "x," the greater and lesser tuberosities (GT and LT, respectively) of the humerus, LHB tendon within bicipital groove, and overlying transverse humeral ligament (THL) can be visualized (Fig. 19.6a). The target for LHB peritendinous injection (marked by a star) is the biceps tendon sheath, which is a synovial recess of the GH joint. The tendon is accompanied by the ascending branch of the anterior circumflex humeral artery. The THL is an extension of the subscapularis tendon, and disruption of the THL with associated biceps tendon instability often accompanies subscapularis tears.

Translating the probe just cephalad and rotating slightly to remain perpendicular to the LHB tendon, the probe reaches Fig. 19.3 slice "y." The humeral head is now convex in shape and the LHB synovial recess is visible surrounding the oval hyperechoic LHB tendon (Fig. 19.6b). The CHL overlies the LHB tendon. The star marks the target for indirect GH joint injection via the rotator interval.

From the rotator interval, moving medially and rotating the probe, the CHL can be followed to its origin at the coracoid process of the scapula (Fig. 19.6c). The underlying LHB tendon and subscapularis muscle are visible. Externally rotating the shoulder will bring more of the subscapularis into view and tighten the CHL.

Moving the patient to a seated, modified Crass position (arm supinated and extended, as if the hand is in the back pocket), the rotator cuff tendons can be studied in more detail. Starting with the rotator interval view (Fig. 19.6b), the probe is centered on the LHB tendon and then carefully rotated so that the biceps tendon appears as elongated as possible. The LHB tendon will have a typical fibrillar pattern when viewed in the long axis (Fig. 19.7a). From here,

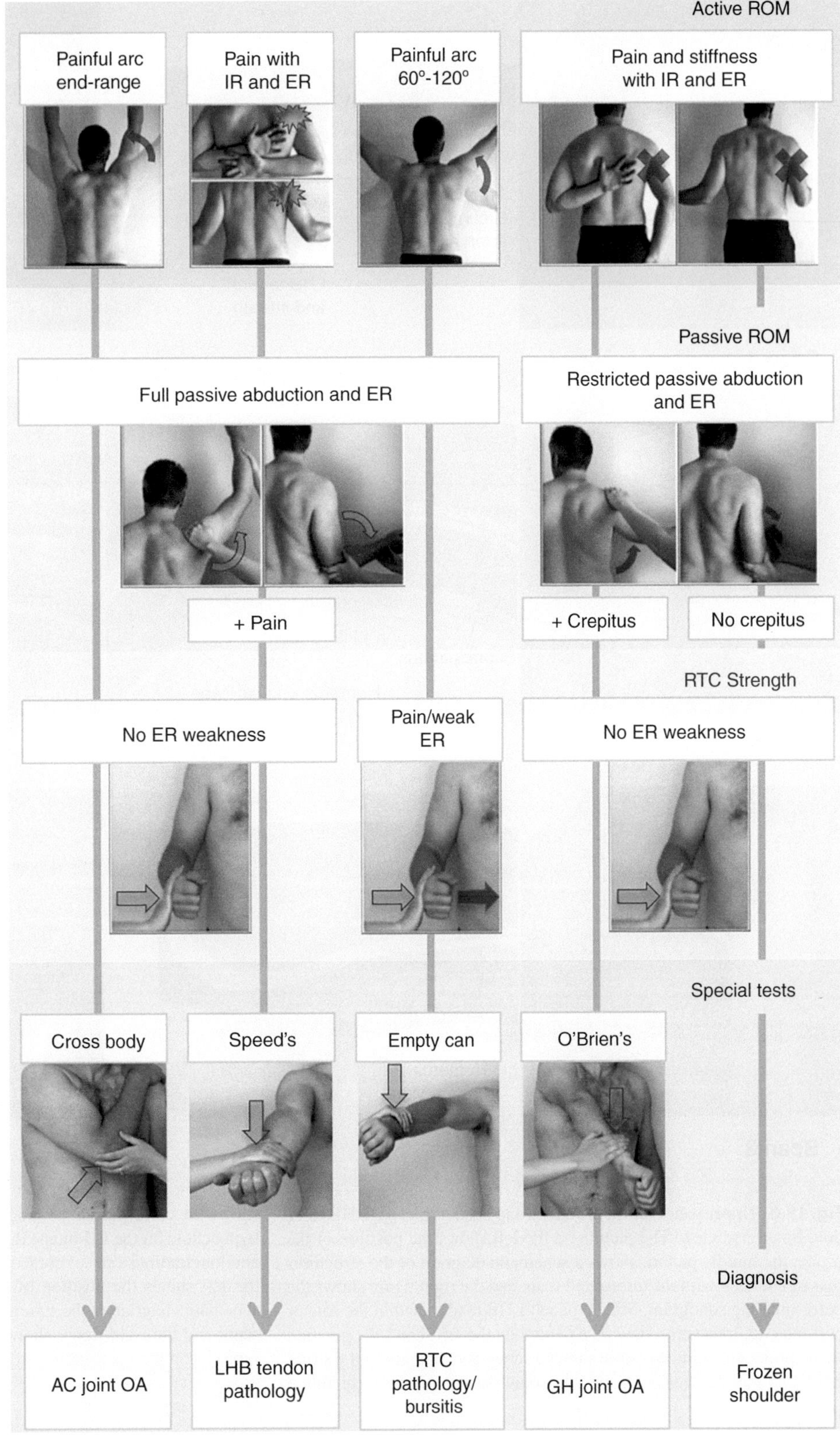

Fig. 19.5 A simplified algorithm of shoulder physical examination. *ROM* range of motion, *RTC* rotator cuff, *ER* external rotation, *IR* internal rotation, *OA* osteoarthritis. (Reproduced with permission from Dr. J McDonald)

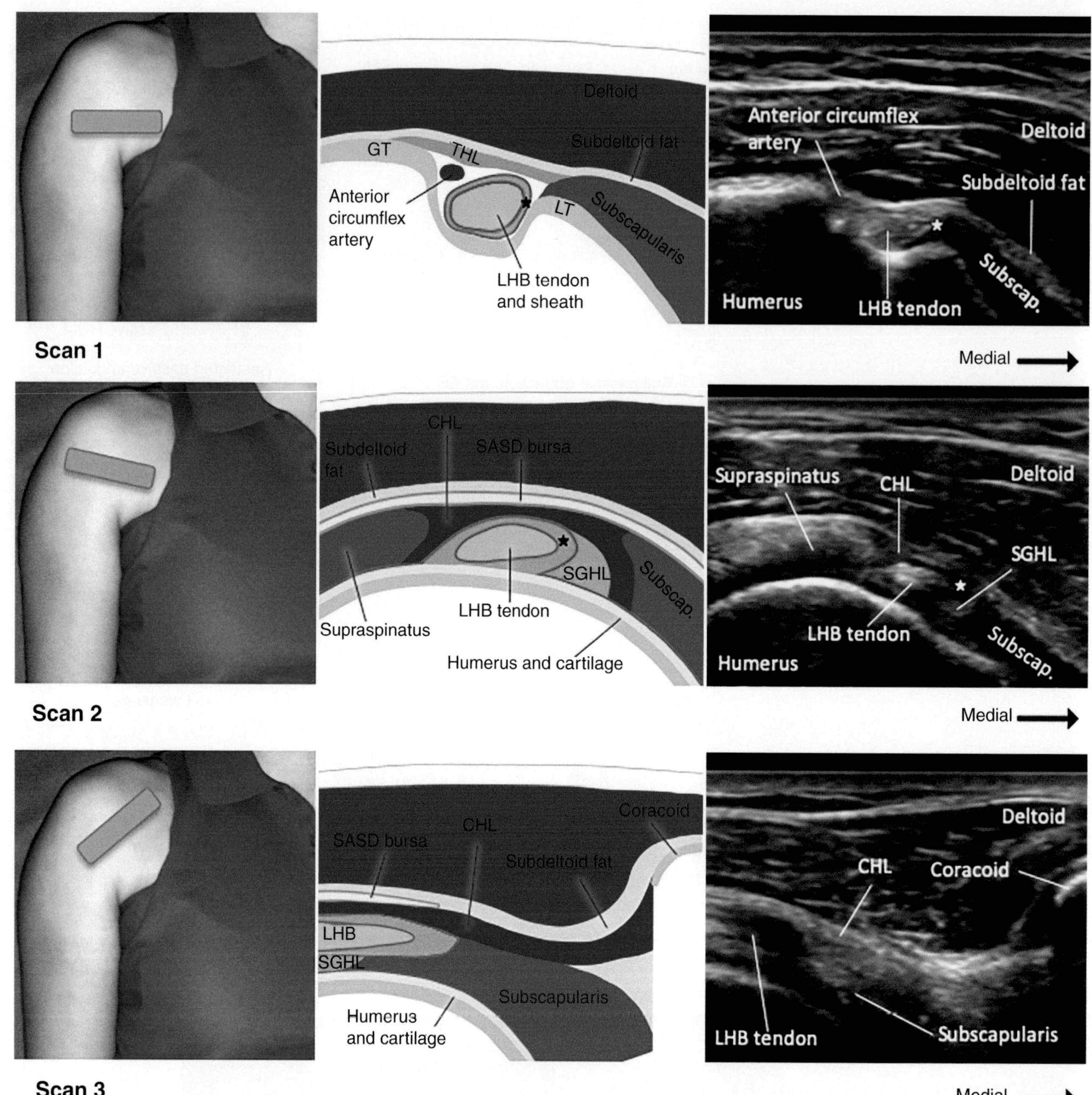

Fig. 19.6 Upper panel: Extra-articular long head of biceps (LHB) tendon, transverse view. The picture on the left shows the position of the probe; the middle picture shows a schematic diagram of the structures that can be seen with the ultrasound scan; and the right figure shows the corresponding sonogram. Middle panel: LHB tendon within the rotator cuff interval, transverse view. The picture on the left shows the position of the probe; the middle picture shows a schematic diagram of the structures that can be seen with the ultrasound scan; and the right figure shows the corresponding sonogram. The subscapularis tendon appears hypoechoic on the US image due to anisotropy. Lower panel: Coracoid and longitudinal view of coracohumeral ligament (CHL) The picture on the left shows the position of the probe; the middle picture shows a schematic diagram of the structures that can be seen with the ultrasound scan; and the right figure shows the corresponding sonogram. (Figure reproduced with permission from Jennifer McDonald)

the probe is translated just lateral to bring the supraspinatus tendon into view (Fig. 19.7b). The supraspinatus tendon inserts onto the beak-shaped greater tuberosity (GT). Note the hypoechoic hyaline cartilage along the humeral head. The SASD bursa can be identified as a thin hypoechoic line flanked by the hyperechoic supraspinatus tendon and subdeltoid fat. When bursitis is present, this bursal space will be fluid-filled with thickening of the peribursal fat. The star marks the target for SASD bursa injection.

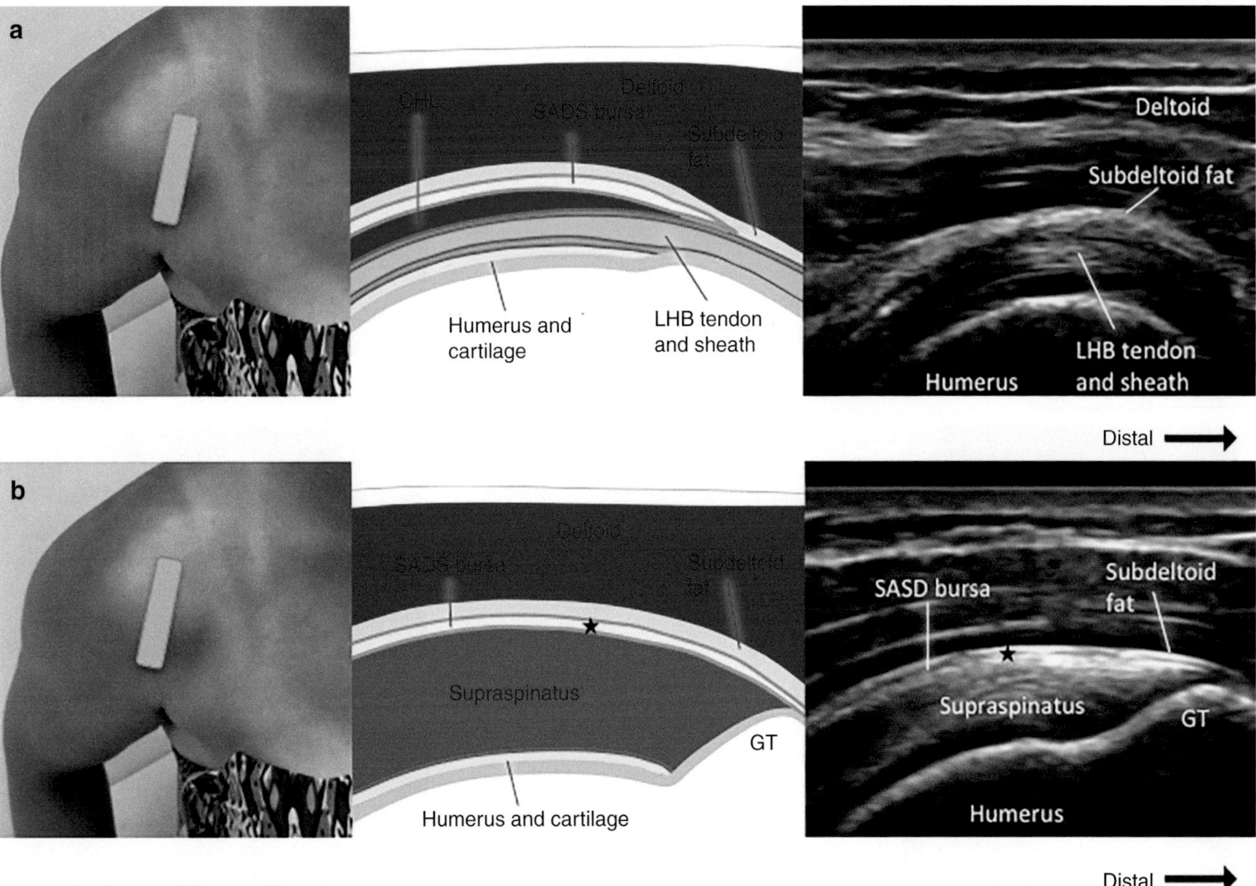

Fig. 19.7 (**a**) Long head of biceps (LHB) tendon, longitudinal view. Starting with the rotator interval view (Fig. 19.6b), the probe is centered on the LHB tendon and then carefully rotated so that the biceps tendon appears as elongated as possible. The LHB tendon will have a typical fibrillar pattern when viewed in the long axis. (**b**) Supraspinatus tendon longitudinal view, obtained by moving the probe in lateral direction. (Figure reproduced with permission from Jennifer McDonald)

Next, with the patient seated with their arm at their side, the AC joint is located by palpating along the concave lateral third of the clavicle to its lateral edge where it articulates with the acromion. The linear probe is centered over the joint in the coronal plane. The superior joint capsule and intra-articular wedge-shaped fibrocartilaginous disk can be seen (Fig. 19.8a). The SASD bursa and supraspinatus tendon lie immediately inferior to the joint. The star marks the target for AC joint injection using an out-of-plane approach. To locate the AC joint in short-axis view, to allow in-plane injection, the probe is rotated 90° and translated laterally over the acromion. The superficial bony acromion is visualized in the sagittal plane (Fig. 19.8b). The probe is then translated medially past the AC joint space to the superficial bony clavicle in short-axis (Fig. 19.8c). Moving back toward the acromion, the AC joint is found when the bone shadows of the clavicle and acromion are not visible and the superficial capsule of the AC joint and underlying bursa and supraspinatus tendon come into view (Fig. 19.8d). The star marks the target for AC joint injection using an in-plane approach.

Finally, with the patient lying on their side with the ipsilateral shoulder facing up and arm touching the contralateral shoulder, the posterior GH joint can be viewed (Fig. 19.9). The acromion can be palpated and followed medially to become the spine of the scapula. A linear US probe (Curvilinear, 2–6 MHz, if large body mass) is placed parallel and directly inferior to the spine of the scapula. The fibers of the infraspinatus muscle can be seen overlying the humeral head and glenoid. The hypoechoic hyaline cartilage can be seen along the surface of the humeral head and hyperechoic triangular labrum. Just medial to the glenoid, the bony spinoglenoid notch cradles the suprascapular nerve and artery. Paralabral cysts can occasionally be seen extending into this notch compressing on the distal suprascapular nerve. If not decompressed through US-guided aspiration or surgical management, they can lead to chronic infraspinatus muscle denervation and external rotation weakness. The star marks the target for posterior intra-articular GH joint injection.

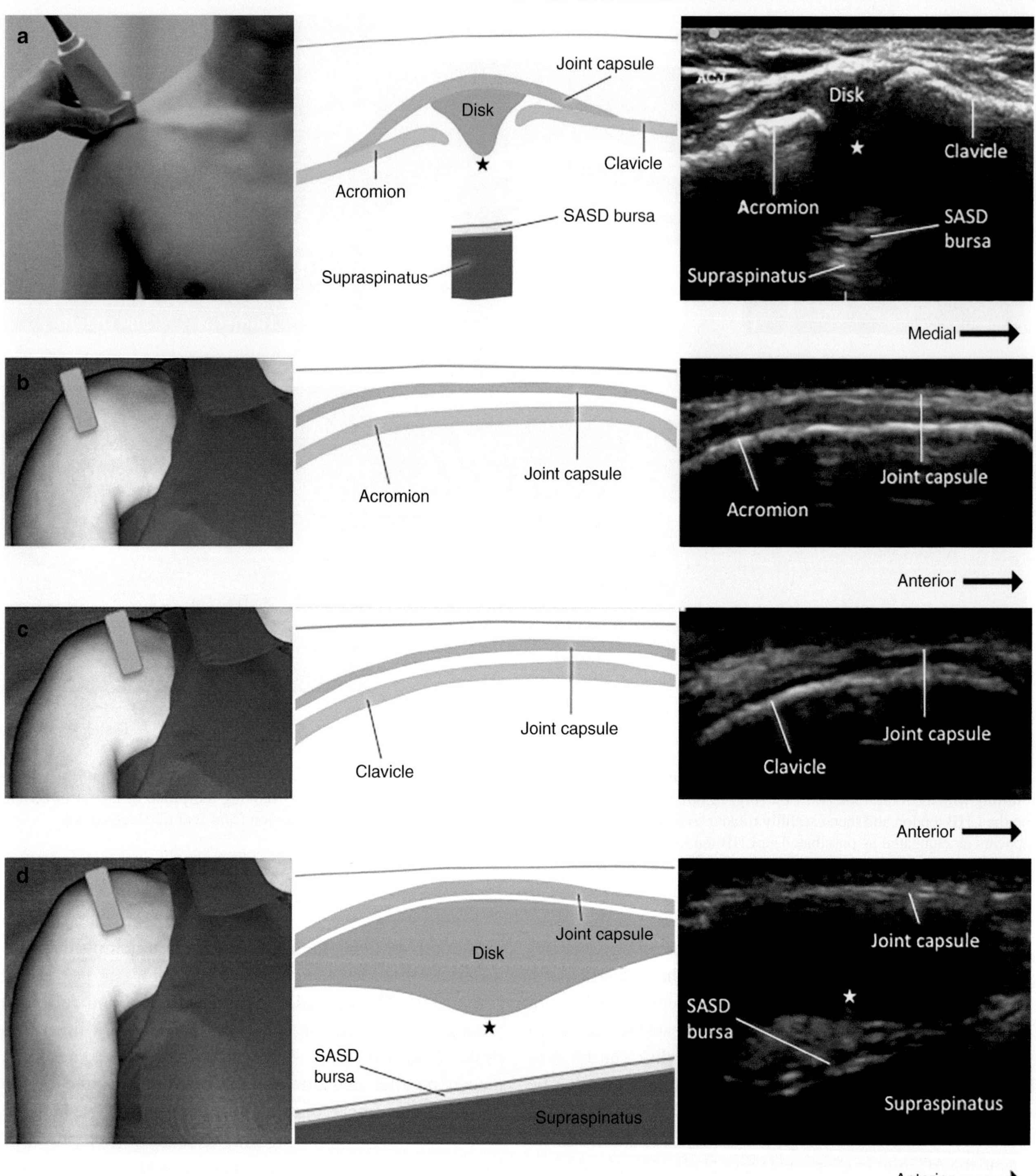

Fig. 19.8 (**a**) Acromioclavicular (AC) joint, coronal plane. (**b**) Acromion, sagittal plane. (**c**) Clavicle, sagittal plane. (**d**) AC joint, short-axis view. In each panel, the picture on the left shows the position of the probe; the middle picture shows a schematic diagram of the structures that can be seen with the ultrasound scan; and the right figure shows the corresponding sonogram. Star indicates the AC joint. (Figure reproduced with permission from Philip Peng Educational Series and Jennifer McDonald)

Ultrasound-Guided Injection Technique

Long Head of Biceps Tendon Sheath Injection

Using a linear high-frequency probe, a 1.5-in. 25-G needle is inserted out-of-plane with 2–3 mL of a mixture of local anesthetic with steroid (0.25% bupivacaine and 20 mg Depo-Medrol). The needle tip is positioned medial to the hyperechoic biceps tendon deep to the transverse humeral ligament (Fig. 19.10). The anterior circumflex artery, just lateral to the tendon, should be visualized using color Doppler

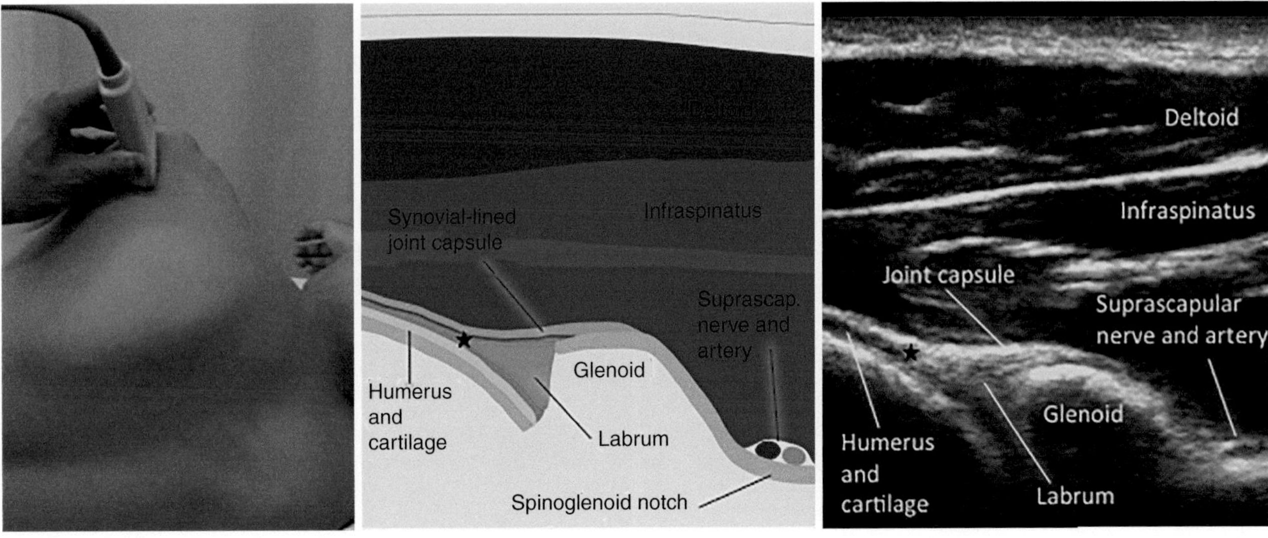

Fig. 19.9 Infraspinatus view of the glenohumeral joint. The picture on the left shows the position of the probe; the middle picture shows a schematic diagram of the structures that can be seen with the ultrasound scan; and the right figure shows the corresponding sonogram. (Figure reproduced with permission from Philip Peng Educational Series and Jennifer McDonald)

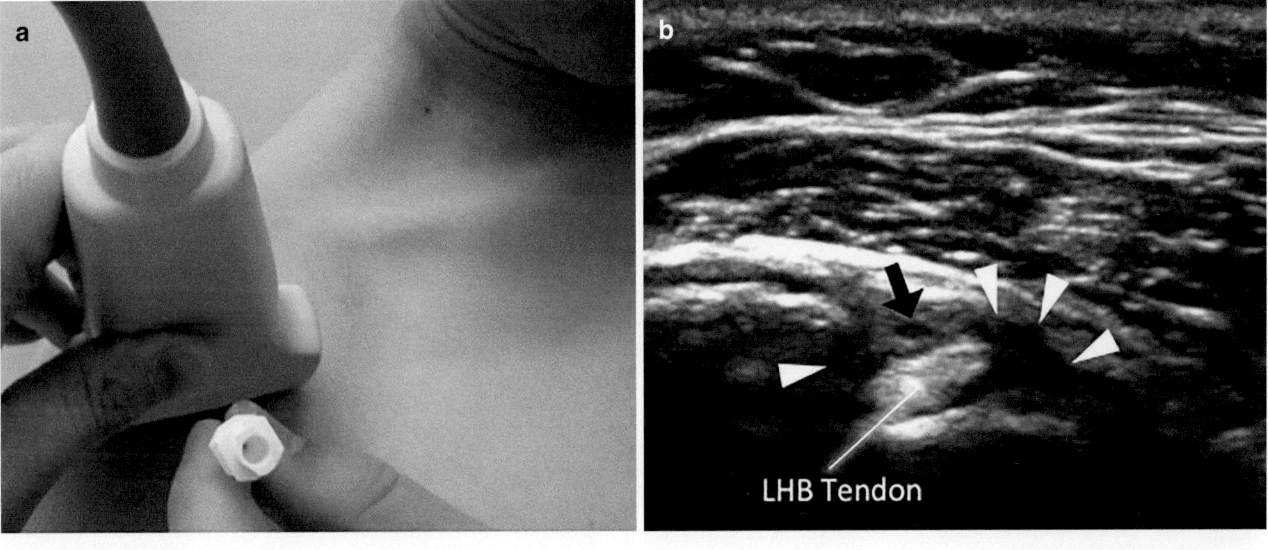

Fig. 19.10 Biceps tendon sheath injection. (**a**) Correct position of ultrasound probe and needle for out-of-plane technique. (**b**) Corresponding US image post-injection. Black arrow marks the anterior circumflex artery. White arrowheads outline the local anesthetic within the biceps tendon sheath. (Figure reproduced with permission from Philip Peng Educational Series)

and avoided. Appropriate spread in a peritendinous fashion should be observed.

Rotator Interval Injection

The anterior GH joint can be targeted through the rotator interval. This approach is commonly used for the treatment of adhesive capsulitis. Using a linear high-frequency probe, a 22-G 2-in. needle is inserted in-plane from the medial aspect of the probe or out-of-plane in caudal to cephalad direction. The target site is the intra-articular portion of the LHB tendon sheath just deep to the CHL (Fig. 19.11). The fluid will fill the synovial recess, which is continuous with the GH joint, and distend the rotator interval capsule. For capsular distension, 10 mL of a mixture of local anesthetic with steroid (0.5–1% lidocaine and 40–80 mg Depo-Medrol) is injected. A recent study looks at direct infiltration of the CHL for cases of early frozen shoulder (without capsular distension or intra-articular injection). In this case, the target

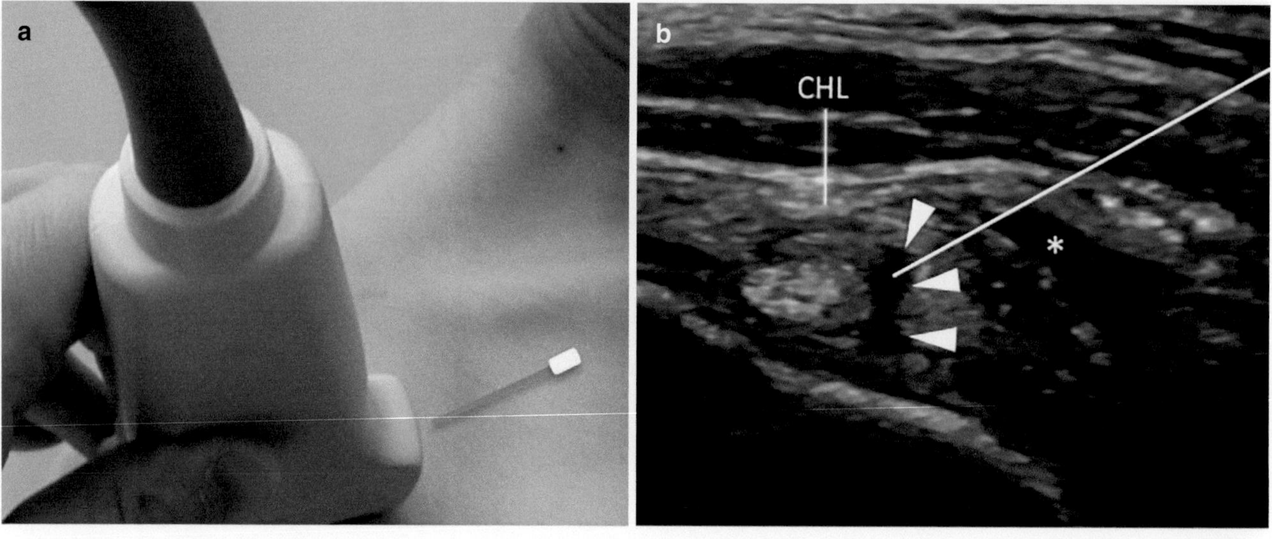

Fig. 19.11 Rotator interval injection. (**a**) Correct position of ultrasound probe and needle for in-plane technique. (**b**) Corresponding US image post-injection. The white line marks the needle trajectory and white arrowheads outline the local anesthetic within the synovial recess. Some injectate commonly leaks back into the subdeltoid bursal space (marked by asterisk) due to the high pressure. (Figure reproduced with permission from Philip Peng Educational Series)

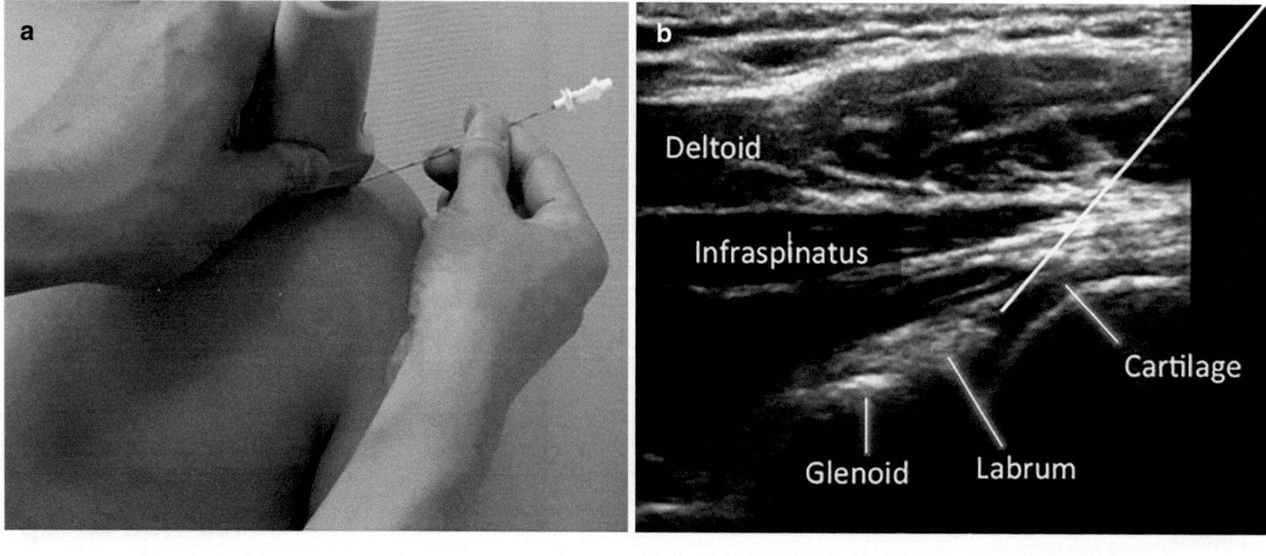

Fig. 19.12 Posterior GH joint injection. (**a**) Correct position of ultrasound probe and needle for in-plane technique. (**b**) Corresponding US image. The white line marks the needle trajectory. (Figure reproduced with permission from Philip Peng Educational Series)

would be the CHL and 2–3 mL total volume with 40 mg Depo-Medrol is suggested.

Posterior GH Joint Injection

For the posterior GH joint approach, the target is the joint space between the free edge of the labrum and the cartilage. The patient is positioned lateral decubitus with the target shoulder facing up and the ipsilateral arm touching the contralateral shoulder. Using a linear high-frequency probe, a 22-G 3.5-in. spinal needle is inserted in-plane in a lateral-to-medial direction (Fig. 19.12). The needle tip is positioned adjacent to the triangular labrum, just deep to the joint capsule. The injectate volume is 4–5 mL of a mixture of local anesthetic with steroid (1% lidocaine and 40 mg Depo-Medrol). A successful

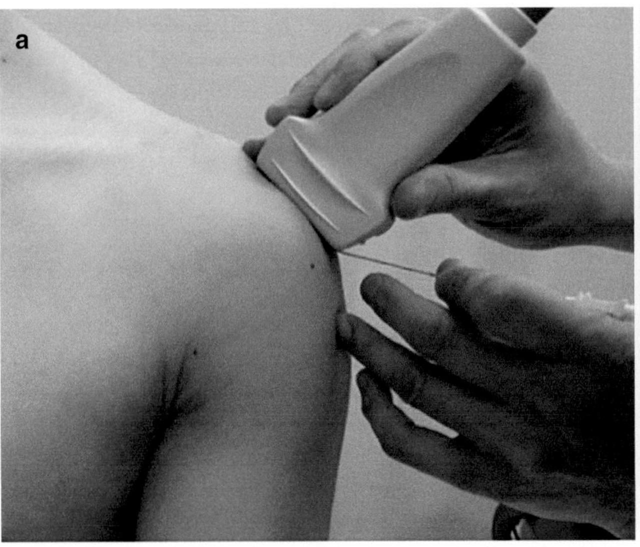

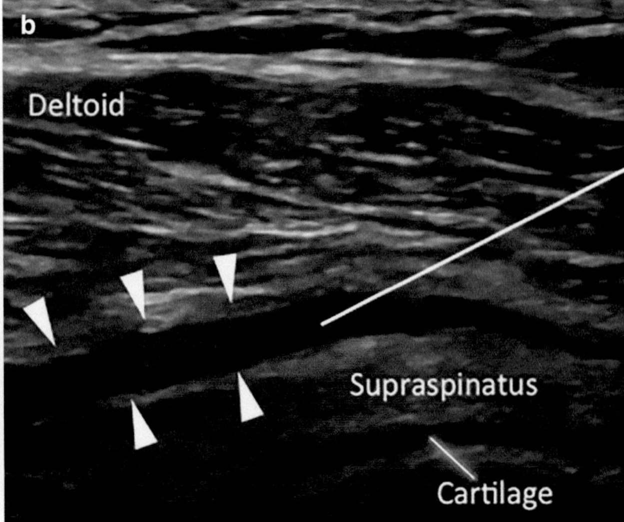

Fig. 19.13 SASD bursa injection. (**a**) Correct position of ultrasound probe and needle for in-plane technique. (**b**) Corresponding US image post-injection. The white line marks the needle trajectory. The white arrowheads outline the local anesthetic within the SASD bursal space. (Figure reproduced with permission from Philip Peng Educational Series)

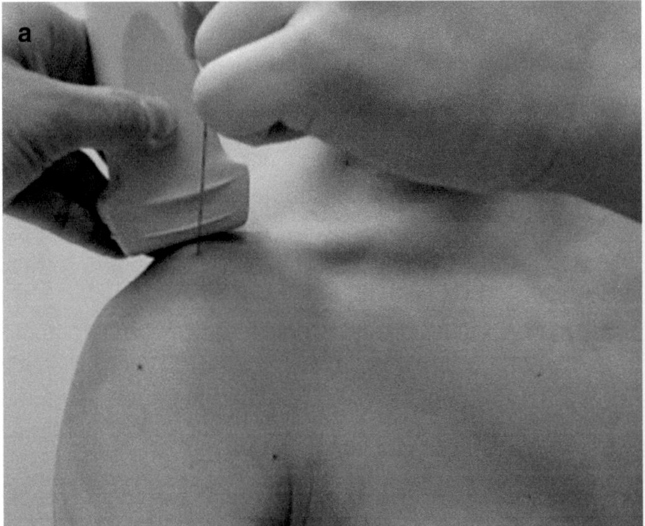

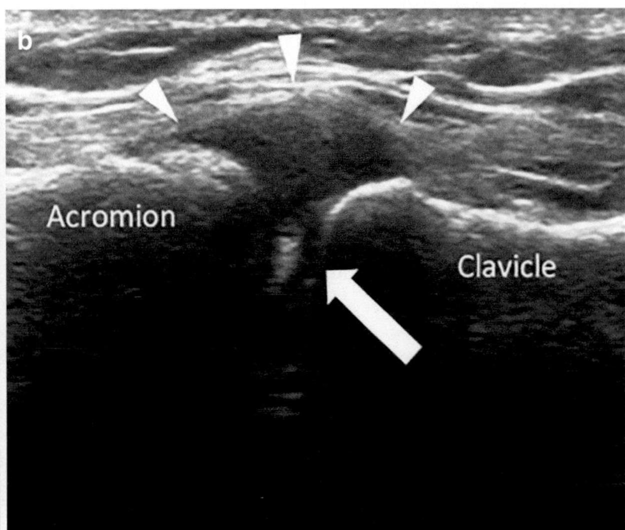

Fig. 19.14 AC joint injection. (**a**) Correct position of ultrasound probe and needle for out-of-plane technique. (**b**) Corresponding US image with out-of-plane needle (solid arrow) and superior joint capsule (white arrowheads) highlighted. (Figure reproduced with permission from Philip Peng Educational Series)

injection will result in transient capsular distension and medial spread of the medication into the joint.

Subacromial Subdeltoid (SASD) Bursa Injection

The target is the subdeltoid portion of the SASD bursa, which lies just deep to the subdeltoid fat and is continuous with the subacromial bursa (Fig. 19.13). Using a linear high-frequency probe, a 25-G 1.5-in. needle or 22-G 2-in. needle is inserted in-plane. The injected volume is 4–5 mL of local anesthetic with steroid (0.25% bupivacaine and 40 mg Depo-Medrol). The fluid will be seen spreading along the bursal space with no resistance to injection.

AC Joint Injection

The target for AC joint injection is just deep to the AC joint capsule (Fig. 19.14). Out-of-plane technique is often used for this superficial structure. A linear high-frequency probe is used and a 25G 1″ or 1.5″ needle is inserted. 1 mL total volume is injected deep to AC joint capsule with a mixture of local anesthetic and steroid (2% lidocaine and 20 mg Depo-Medrol).

Complications

Possible complications to shoulder joint injections are highlighted below:

- Lack of benefit or post-injection pain flare
- Allergy to the injectate
- Infection
  - Includes superficial cellulitis, soft-tissue infection, septic arthritis, and postoperative infection (if steroid injection is administered shortly prior to a planned shoulder surgery)
- Vasovagal reaction
- Steroid-specific systemic side effects
  - Transient blood sugar elevation
  - Transient blood pressure elevation
  - Facial flushing
  - Cataracts
  - Psychosis
- Steroid-specific local side effects
  - Fat atrophy and skin atrophy/depigmentation
  - Muscle atrophy
  - Bone necrosis
  - Tendon rupture/degeneration (risk factors include repeated peritendinous injections, intratendinous injection, and/or early return to full loading of the tendon post-injection)
- Musculoskeletal trauma
  - Needle trauma to the smooth hypoechoic hyaline cartilage lining the humeral head
  - Needle trauma to the posterior labrum during posterior GH joint injections
  - Needle trauma to the discoid meniscus of the AC joint
  - Trauma to the rotator cuff and/or long head of biceps tendon during SASD bursa, biceps tendon sheath, and rotator interval injections
- Vascular trauma
  - Damage to the anterior circumflex humeral artery during extra-articular biceps tendon sheath injection could in theory lead to avascular necrosis of the humeral head.
- Nerve trauma
  - If the needle tip is lost during advancement, the brachial plexus, suprascapular nerve, axillary nerve, or lateral pectoral nerve could be injured.

Practical Tips

LHB Tendon Sheath Injection

1. Before targeting the biceps tendon, consider rotator cuff pathology or GH joint pathology with an effusion tracking down the biceps tendon sheath.
2. Doppler examination is helpful to localize (and avoid) the anterior circumflex humeral artery and to assess for increased vascularity (aka hyperemia), representing inflammation.
3. Intratendinous injection should be avoided. If the tendon begins to swell or resistance is encountered, stop the injection and redirect the needle tip to the tendon sheath.
4. Recommend relative rest for 1–2 weeks (i.e., no heavy lifting) to avoid LHB tendon rupture post-procedure.

Rotator Interval Injection for Adhesive Capsulitis

1. High resistance will be encountered during the injection of the frozen shoulder due to thickening of the CHL and surrounding structures. Thus, proper localization of the needle tip is critical to avoid intratendinous injection, which will also provide high resistance.
2. There is often significant anisotropy of the tendinous structures within the rotator interval. Dynamic subtle probe tilting during the procedure may allow for better visualization of the target site, needle tip and bordering tendons.
3. If a sudden loss of resistance is encountered, the needle tip has likely slipped out into the subdeltoid bursal space. Stop the injection and redirect the needle tip to the correct target site.
4. A home stretching routine, with a focus on passive range of motion of the GH joint, is recommended once the pain starts to subside (approx. 3–7 days post-procedure).

Posterior GH Joint Injection

1. In order to clear the humeral head and access the narrow target, the needle trajectory can be quite steep. To improve needle visualization, a curvilinear probe can

be used and heeled in toward the needle. Gel can be heaped under the toe of the probe to improve contact with the skin.
2. If resistance is encountered during the injection, turn the bevel 90° or withdraw the needle slightly.
3. The hypoechoic hyaline cartilage lining the humeral head can be mistaken for fluid within the joint space. The cartilage should be avoided during needle placement.

SASD Bursa Injection for Subacromial Impingement

1. Correct needle location within the bursal space is confirmed by rapid expansion of the bursa with small volume (0.5 mL) hydrodissection.
2. Partial rotator cuff tears are common incidental findings on shoulder US and MRI in healthy adults. Thus, sonographic evidence of an RTC tear does not guarantee this as the primary pain generator.

AC Joint Injection

1. Since the joint space is narrow, one way to facilitate an easier entry is to put the needle shaft on the skin as a marker to the joint space. Once the joint space is located, the needle is then retracted and inserted into the joint.
2. The AC joint is very shallow. The needle tip should be inserted no more than 1 cm deep. If the needle is too deep, the injectate will be deposited within the underlying subacromial bursa or supraspinatus tendon.
3. AC joint pathology often mimics other pain generators of the shoulder and the examination can be nonspecific. Repeating provocative examination maneuvers post-injection with local anesthetic can be very helpful to rule the AC joint in or out as the primary pain generator.

Literature Review

Long Head of Biceps Tendon Sheath Injection

The target site for biceps tendon disease is the tendon sheath with avoidance of intratendinous injection. As mentioned above, isolated biceps tendon pathology is rare, and the biceps tendon sheath is actually continuous with the GH joint space. Not surprisingly, Gofeld et al. were able to show intra-articular extension of the injectate with distal biceps tendon sheath injection in a recent cadaveric study. Hashiuchi et al., comparing blind injection to US-guided technique, revealed accurate biceps tendon sheath placement on CT confirmation in all of the US-guided injections but only two-thirds of the blind injections.

Rotator Interval Injection

Given the presence of inflammation and thickening in the region of the rotator interval in individuals with frozen shoulder, many have theorized that a steroid injection targeting the rotator interval would be more beneficial than other injection techniques. In a cadaveric study, Majdalani et al. showed that the CHL could be accurately targeted within the rotator interval under US guidance. A recent RCT by Elnady et al. showed that US-guided anterior capsule hydrodistension via the rotator interval was more effective than the conventional posterior GH joint hydrodistension approach. At 3-month follow-up, the rotator interval treatment arm had statistically significant improvements in pain, range of motion, and function on the shoulder pain and disability index scale when compared to the posterior approach. Another RCT by Sun et al. randomized patients with primary frozen shoulder in the freezing stage to three injection groups: rotator interval (CHL infiltration), posterior intra-articular joint, and subacromial bursa. The rotator interval injection group yielded better effects in terms of improvement in pain, passive ROM, and function.

A systematic review by Xiao et al. concluded that corticosteroid injections demonstrate short-term efficacy in frozen shoulder. Another systematic review by Catapano et al., which identified six RCTs comparing capsular distension plus corticosteroid to corticosteroid alone, revealed significant variability with respect to injection approach and method of distension. Two studies demonstrated clinically and statistically significant improvement in both ROM and pain at 3 months. However, more studies with better anatomical approaches and images guidance are needed to better understand benefit of capsular distension.

Glenohumeral Joint Injection

The accuracy of blind GH joint injection ranges from 27 to 100% in the literature. This is compared to an accuracy rate of 87–100% with US guidance. Comparison studies of US versus fluoroscopically guided GH joint injections by experienced radiologists revealed 100% accuracy in both groups, but less time and patient discomfort in the US group. There is no evidence to support or refute the use of GH joint steroid injections in the treatment of GH joint osteoarthritis. The American Academy of Orthopaedic Surgeons 2011 guidelines on the treatment of GH osteoarthritis were unable to recommend for or against steroid injections and recommended the use of hyaluronic acid (HA) injections as an option, citing weak evidence.

Many surgeons will wait 6–12 months between an intra-articular steroid injection and shoulder arthroplasty for the treatment of advanced osteoarthritis because of the theoretical risk of infection. Bhattacharjee et al. found a significant increase in post shoulder arthroscopy infections in patient who received a shoulder injection within 2 weeks before surgery, compared with no injections in the 6-month preoperative period.

SASD Bursa Injection

A systematic review by Koester et al. studying SASD bursa steroid injections for treatment of rotator cuff disease concluded that there was little evidence to support efficacy. None of the studies reviewed used US-guided technique. A systematic review by Cook et al. concluded that corticosteroid injections have a short-term benefit (up to 8 weeks) over local anesthetic injections in management of rotator cuff disease.

Landmark-based injections in the SASD bursa are often inaccurate. There was no observed benefit beyond 8 weeks. Comparing ultrasound-guided to landmark-guided technique, several RCTs (Bhayana, Akbari) have found no significant difference in outcomes.

AC Joint Injection

The accuracy of ultrasound-guided AC joint injection is significantly better than blind injection. The therapeutic role of AC joint injection is unclear as RCTs are lacking.

Suggested Reading

Akbari N, Ozen S, Şenlikçi HB, Haberal M, Çetin N. Ultrasound-guided versus blind subacromial corticosteroid and local anesthetic injection in the treatment of subacromial impingement syndrome: a randomized study of efficacy. Jt Dis Relat Surg. 2020;31(1):115–22.

Bhattacharjee S, Lee W, Lee MJ, Shi LL. Preoperative corticosteroid joint injections within 2 weeks of shoulder arthroscopies increase postoperative infection risk. J Shoulder Elbow Surg. 2019;28(11):2098–102.

Bhayana H, Mishra P, Tandon A, Pankaj A, Pandey R, Malhotra R. Ultrasound guided versus landmark guided corticosteroid injection in patients with rotator cuff syndrome: randomised controlled trial. J Clin Orthop Trauma. 2018;9(Suppl 1):S80–5.

Catapano M, Mittal N, Adamich J, Kumbhare D, Sangha H. Hydrodilatation with corticosteroid for the treatment of adhesive capsulitis: a systematic review. PM R. 2018;10(6):623–35.

Cook T, Lowe CM, Maybury M, Lewis JS. Are corticosteroid injections more beneficial than anaesthetic injections alone in the management of rotator cuff-related shoulder pain? A systematic review. Brit J Sport Med. 2018;52(8):497.

Elnady B, Rageh EM, Hussein MS, Abu-Zaid MH, Desouky DE-S, Ekhouly T, et al. In shoulder adhesive capsulitis, ultrasound-guided anterior hydrodilatation in rotator interval is more effective than posterior approach: a randomized controlled study. Clin Rheumatol. 2020;39(12):3805–14.

Gofeld M, Hurdle MF, Agur A. Biceps tendon sheath injection: an anatomical conundrum. Pain Med. 2018;20(1):138–42.

Hashiuchi T, Sakurai G, Morimoto M, Komei T, Takakura Y, Tanaka Y. Accuracy of the biceps tendon sheath injection: ultrasound-guided or unguided injection? A randomized controlled trial. J Shoulder Elbow Surg. 2011;20(7):1069–73.

Koester MC, Dunn WR, Kuhn JE, Spindler KP. The efficacy of subacromial corticosteroid injection in the treatment of rotator cuff disease: a systematic review. J Am Acad Orthop Surg. 2007;15(1):3–11.

Majdalani C, Boudier-Revéret M, Pape J, Brismée J, Michaud J, Luong DH, et al. Accuracy of two ultrasound-guided coracohumeral ligament injection approaches: a cadaveric study. PM R. 2019;11(9):989–95.

Peng PWH, Cheng P. Ultrasound-guided interventional procedures in pain medicine. Reg Anesth Pain Med. 2011;36(6):592–605.

Rutten MJCM, Collins JMP, Maresch BJ, Smeets JHJM, Janssen CMM, Kiemeney LALM, et al. Glenohumeral joint injection: a comparative study of ultrasound and fluoroscopically guided techniques before MR arthrography. Eur Radiol. 2009;19(3):722–30.

Sabeti-Aschraf M, Lemmerhofer B, Lang S, Schmidt M, Funovics PT, Ziai P, et al. Ultrasound guidance improves the accuracy of the acromioclavicular joint infiltration: a prospective randomized study. Knee Surg Sports Traumatol Arthrosc. 2011;19(2):292–5.

Sun Y, Liu S, Chen S, Chen J. The effect of corticosteroid injection into rotator interval for early frozen shoulder: a randomized controlled trial. Am J Sports Med. 2018;46(3):663–70.

Xiao RC, Walley KC, DeAngelis JP, Ramappa AJ. Corticosteroid injections for adhesive capsulitis. Clin J Sport Med. 2017;27(3):308–20.

Rotator Muscles and Subscapular Nerve Injection

20

Danilo Jankovic

Contents

D. Jankovic (✉)
Pain Management Centre DGS – Cologne – Huerth,
Cologne-Hürth, Germany
e-mail: danilo@jankovic1.de

D. Jankovic, P. Peng (eds.), *Regional Nerve Blocks in Anesthesia and Pain Therapy*,
https://doi.org/10.1007/978-3-030-88727-8_20

General Consideration

A "frozen shoulder" may be a common stage of many disorders affecting the shoulder or an independent, idiopathic condition. The etiology of a frozen shoulder is complex. The numerous concepts are evident when the diagnostic labels applied to this condition are reviewed. It appears that many tissues, mainly synovial, are involved in the ultimate frozen shoulder. Current clinical nomenclature uses three categories of frozen shoulder: idiopathic frozen shoulder, adhesive capsulitis, and subacromial fibrosis. Additional proposal etiologies of the frozen shoulder include acromioclavicular joint irritation, entrapment of the suprascapular nerve, prolonged immobilization of the upper extremity, cervical radiculopathy, hemiplegia, myocardial infarction, bicipital tendonitis, and muscle spasm. There are several references in the literature that assume frozen shoulder to be an algoneurodystrophic process. Recent publications have pointed out similarities with Dupuytren's contracture. Many other synonyms are used in the literature: periarthritis or periarticular arthritis, pericapsulitis, scapulocostal syndrome, calcified tendinitis of the rotator cuff, degenerative tendinitis of the rotator cuff, and acromioclavicular arthritis. Mc Laughlin (1944) stressed the importance of the subscapularis muscle in the etiology of the frozen shoulder.

Clinical Evaluation

Clinical Presentation

This scenario develops insidiously, beginning with pain and tenderness usually over the deltoid insertional area in the upper outer humerus. Motion aggravates the pain, and gradually a limitation of both active and passive motions develops. What at first hampers daily activities gradually interferes with sleep.

The usual stages of evolution are pain, gradual restriction of motion, and ultimately marked limitation without pain. The last stage is stiff, useless, but painless shoulder which hurts only when forcefully moved to ensure or to determine limitation. The condition widely claimed to be a frozen shoulder still remains an enigma as to the exact origin, tissue involvement, causative mechanism, and the ideal forms of prevention and treatment.

Imaging Modalities

X-ray evaluation may reveal no specific diagnostic findings other than some osteopenia or cystic changes in the lateral aspect of the humerus. An arthrogram depicts the presence and degree of adhesive capsulitis. An MRI may rule out other abnormalities but is not specifically diagnostic of adhesive capsulitis with regard to the exact tissues involved or the severity of involvement.

Management of Frozen Shoulder

Treatment for the frozen shoulder varies widely with experienced clinicians. Started early with a frequent intensity—before there is significant adhesion—active physical therapy is more applicable and is advocated by most clinicians who are studying and treating this condition. Pain relief is achieved by local ice, heat, ultrasound application, TENS application, oral NSAIDs, electroacupuncture , oral and local corticosteroids, oral analgesic medication, and shock waves. Mobilization and gentle manipulation may be also advisable in the early stage. Rhythmic stabilization exercises have also proven to be of value. Some of the nerve blocks, e.g., suprascapular or subscapular nerve block, have been recently recommended.

Subscapular Nerve Block and Subscapularis Muscle Trigger Point Infiltration

Introduction

With irritation of subscapularis muscle trigger points, adjacent nerves produce pain both during movement and at rest, resulting in pain radiating to the scapula, posterior deltoid muscle, elbow, and/or dorsal wrist. The pain usually worsens at night. The usual scenario restricts arm abduction and external rotation, reducing movement in all directions, ending in a stiff, frozen shoulder. A common finding is that the subscapularis muscle trigger point plays a key role in the development of a frozen shoulder. The subscapular nerve block and subscapularis trigger point infiltration could be very valuable in producing pain relief in the affected shoulder. Shortly after each block, intensive, physical therapy could be successfully performed. We injected routinely 10–15 mL of a local anesthetic solution with or without the addition of a corticosteroid. The total volume guarantees adequate spread of the corticosteroids. The mechanisms by which corticosteroids have been suggested to modify pain include reduced prostaglandin synthesis, a week local anesthetic action, a change activity in the dorsal horn cells, and reduced ectopic discharge from neuromata. Corticosteroids have also been shown to induce a reversible block of normal C-fibers in animal model.

Functional Anatomy of the Fossa Subscapularis

The subscapularis muscle (the most important internal rotator muscle of the arm—it also acts as an adductor when the arm is raised or flexed, and together with the rotator cuff, keeps the head of the humerus pressed into the glenoid fossa) is located at the anterior surface of the subscapularis fossa. The anatomical insertions of the subscapular muscle are medial to the interior surface of the scapula and lateral to the lesser tubercle on the anterior surface of the humerus (Figs. 20.1, 20.2, and 20.3).

The subscapular nerves consist of two or three nerves emerging from various parts of the brachial plexus for the subscapular, teres major, and latissimus dorsi muscles. The longest and most important of these is the thoracodorsal nerve, which runs along the axillary border of the scapula and supplies the latissimus dorsi muscle.

The superior subscapular nerve emerges from C5 and C6 (C7) and enters the subscapular muscle. The medial subscapular nerve (C5–6) arises from the posterior secondary trunks and supplies the lateral lower part of the subscapular muscle and teres major muscle. The inferior subscapular nerve (thoracodorsal nerve) is the largest in this group. It arises from the posterior secondary branches or from the axillary nerve, or more rarely from the radial nerve, and passes along the lateral edge of the scapula to the latissimus dorsi muscle.

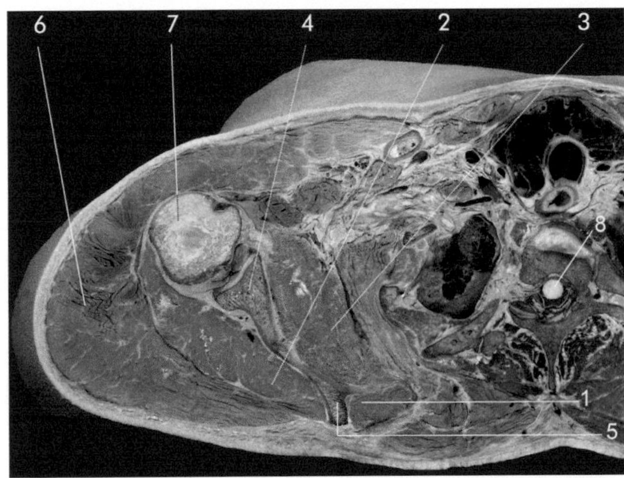

Fig. 20.1 Transverse section at the level of T2–T3. Rotator cuff muscles and neighboring muscles. *(1)* Supraspinatus muscle, *(2)* infraspinatus muscle, *(3)* subscapularis muscle, *(4, 5)* scapula, *(6)* deltoid muscle, *(7)* greater tubercle of the humerus, *(8)* spinal cord. (Reproduced with permission from Danilo Jankovic)

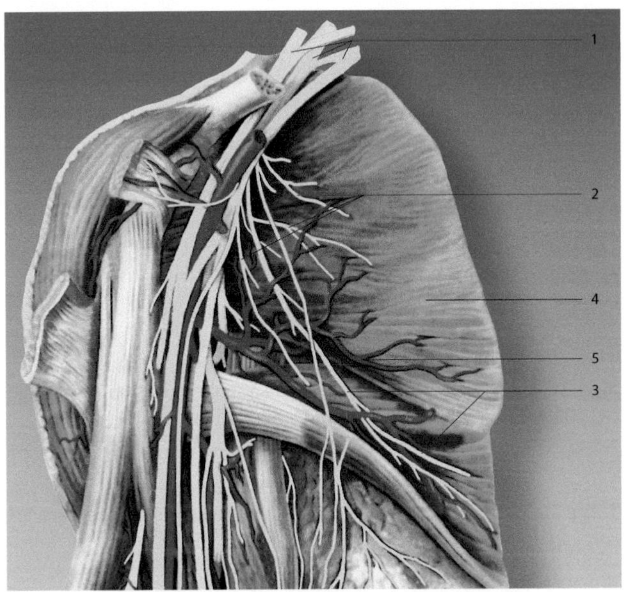

Fig. 20.2 Anatomy (anterior view): *(1)* cords of the brachial plexus, *(2)* subscapular nerve, *(3)* thoracodorsal nerve, *(4)* subscapular muscle, *(5)* circumflex scapular artery. (Reproduced with permission from Danilo Jankovic)

Innervation and Function

Table 20.1.

Indications

Indications for a subscapular nerve block and subscapularis trigger point infiltration are presented in Table 20.2.

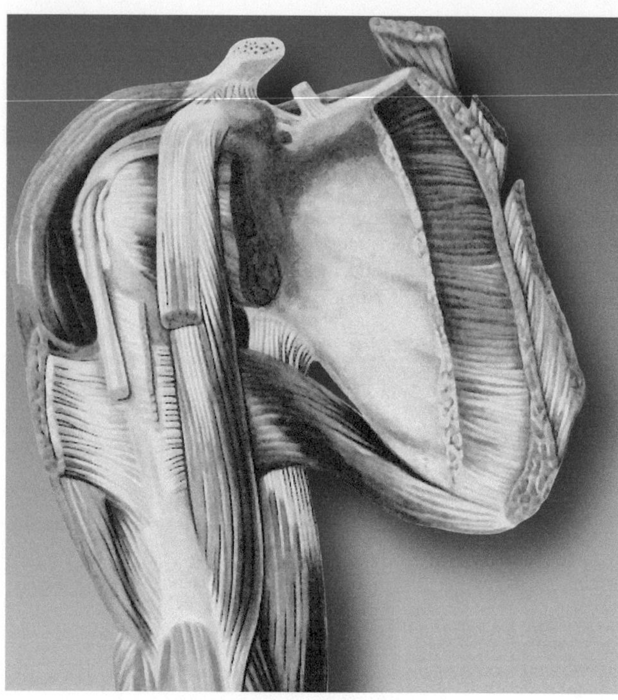

Fig. 20.3 Anatomy. Subscapular fossa and subscapular muscle. (Reproduced with permission from Danilo Jankovic)

Procedure

Preparations

Check that the emergency equipment is complete and in working order, sterile precautions and intravenous access. Prior information for the patient is an absolute necessity.

Materials

Fine 25-mm-long 26-G needle for local anesthesia, 70-mm-long 20-G needle (with the needle shaft angled by about 20°), local anesthetic, disinfectant, swabs, and 2- mL and 10-mL syringes.

Technique

Patient Position

Sitting, with the neck comfortably tilted and the shoulders relaxed.

Location (Fig. 20.4)

1. The patient's arm is pulled back, so that the contours of the scapula are easily recognized. The center of the medial border of the scapula is marked as the injection point.
2. Acromion.

Skin prep, local anesthesia, drawing up the local anesthetic, testing the injection needle for patency.

Table 20.1 Rotator cuff muscle (dark blue) and neighboring muscles: innervation and function

Muscle	Innervation	Function
Supraspinatus	Suprascapular nerve (C5**; superior trunk*)	Abducts the upper arm and pulls the head of the upper arm into the glenoid cavity
Infraspinatus	Suprascapular nerve (C5, C6**; superior trunk*)	External rotation of the arm; stabilizes the head of the humerus in the glenoid cavity
Teres minor	Axillary nerve (C5, C6**; posterior fascicle*)	Almost identical to the infraspinatus muscle
Subscapularis	Subscapular nerve (C5, C6**; posterior fascicle*)	Internal rotation and adduction of the upper arm in the shoulder
Teres major	Inferior subscapular nerve (C5, C6**; posterior fascicle*)	Supports adduction, internal rotation, and extension of the upper arm from a bent position
Deltoid	Axillary nerve (C5, C6**; posterior fascicle*)	Helps the supraspinatus muscle to abduct the upper arm in the shoulder
Latissimus dorsi	Thoracodorsal nerve (C6–C8**; posterior fascicle*)	Adduction and internal rotation of the arm; strong downward movement of the scapula
Coracobrachialis	Musculocutaneous nerve (C5, C6**; lateral fascicle*)	Actions are to assist flexion and adduction of the arm at the shoulder

*Brachial plexus
** Spinal nerves

Table 20.2 Indications for subscapular nerve block and subscapularis trigger point

Infiltration
Diagnostic: in painful conditions of the shoulder girdle/joint
Therapeutic: in the following situations (in combination with physiotherapy):
Frozen shoulder syndrome
Rheumatism
Diabetes
Post-trauma neuralgia
Postherpetic neuralgia
Post-hemiplegia neuralgia
Ankylosing spondylitis

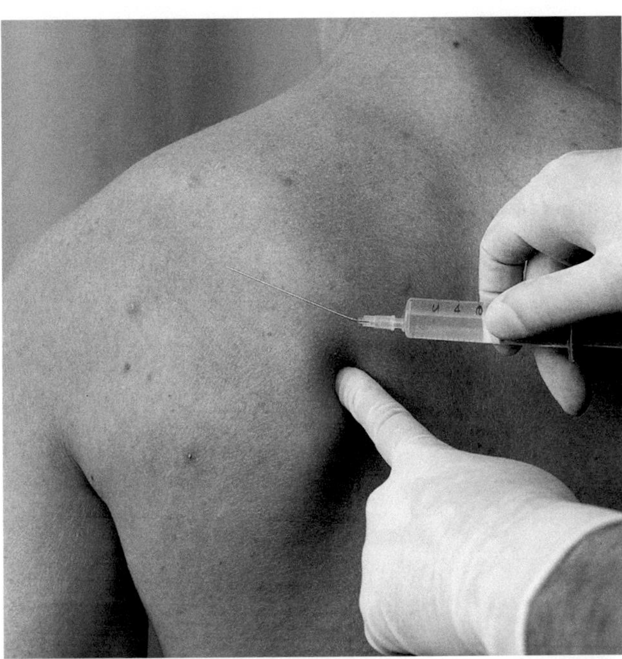

Fig. 20.4 Location. Marking the injection site (center of the medial border of the scapula). (Reproduced with permission from Danilo Jankovic)

Practical Tips

1. Before the injection, the shaft of the injection needle should be bent by about 20°.
2. Targeted paresthesias are not elicited.
3. During the injection, observe the skin for possible subcutaneous spread of the local anesthetic.

Technique

1. Introduce the 20° angled needle into the center of the medial border of the scapula, in the direction of the acromion (Figs. 20.5 and 20.6a, b).

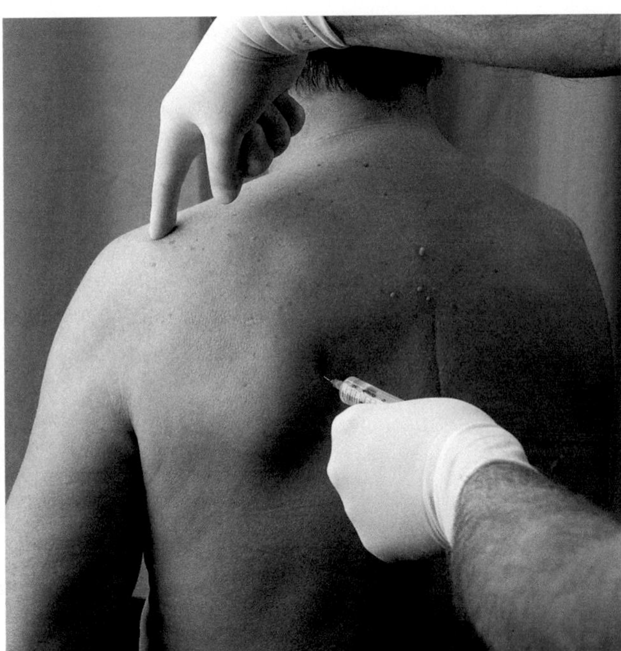

Fig. 20.5 Introducing the needle in the direction of the acromion. (Reproduced with permission from Danilo Jankovic)

2. The needle is introduced subscapularly parallel to the skin surface between the anterior surface of the scapula (costal surface) and the posterior thoracic wall (ribs), into the subscapular fossa. If the needle meets the edge of the ribs, it is withdrawn as far as the subcutaneous tissue and reintroduced.
3. At a depth of 4 cm, then 5 cm, and finally 6 cm—depending on the anatomy—a total of 10–15-mL local anesthetic is then injected after prior aspiration (Figs. 20.5 and 20.6a).

The signs of a successful injection are spread extending into the shoulder joint, upper arm, and often as far as the wrist, corresponding to the radiation pattern of the trigger points of the subscapular muscle (Fig. 20.7a, b).

Dosage

Diagnostic

5-mL local anesthetic—e.g., 1% prilocaine or 1% mepivacaine.

Therapeutic

10–15-mL local anesthetic—e.g., 0.5–0.75% ropivacaine and 0.25–0.5% bupivacaine (0.25–0.5% levobupivacaine). In acute pain, the addition of 40 mg triamcinolone has proved useful.

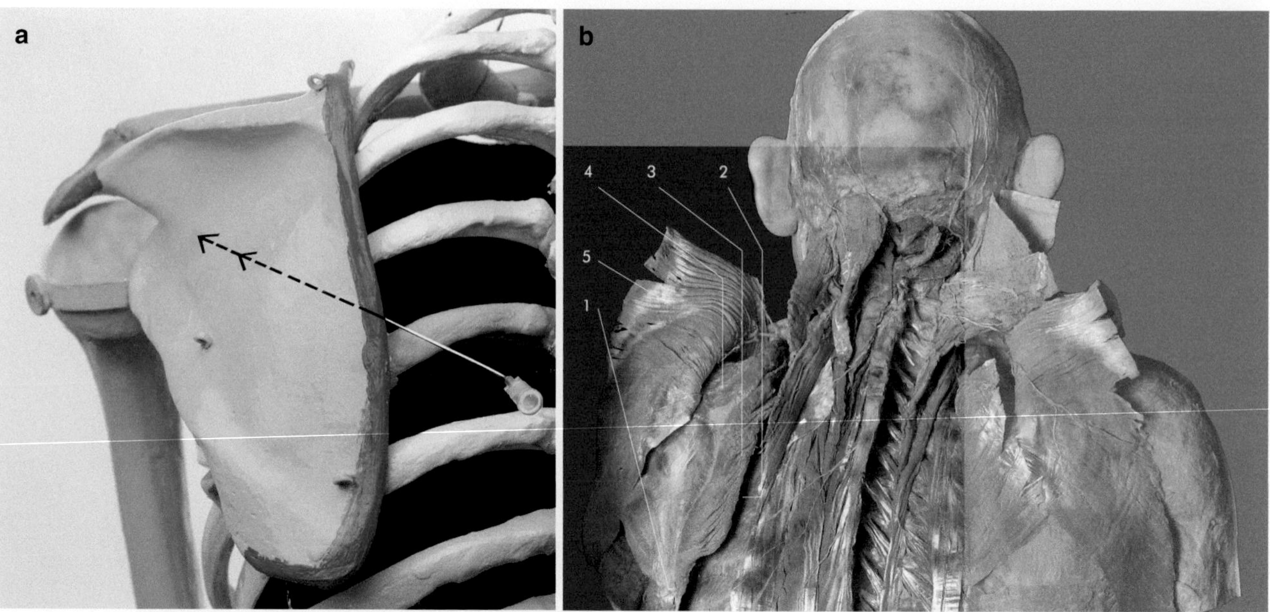

Fig. 20.6 (**a**) Introducing the needle in the direction of the acromion (skeletal model). (Reproduced with permission from Danilo Jankovic). (**b**) *(1)* Inferior angle of the scapula, *(2)* medial border of the scapula with subscapularis muscle inside, *(3)* rhomboideus major muscle, *(4)* infraspinatus muscle, *(5)* trapezius muscle. (Reproduced with permission from Danilo Jankovic)

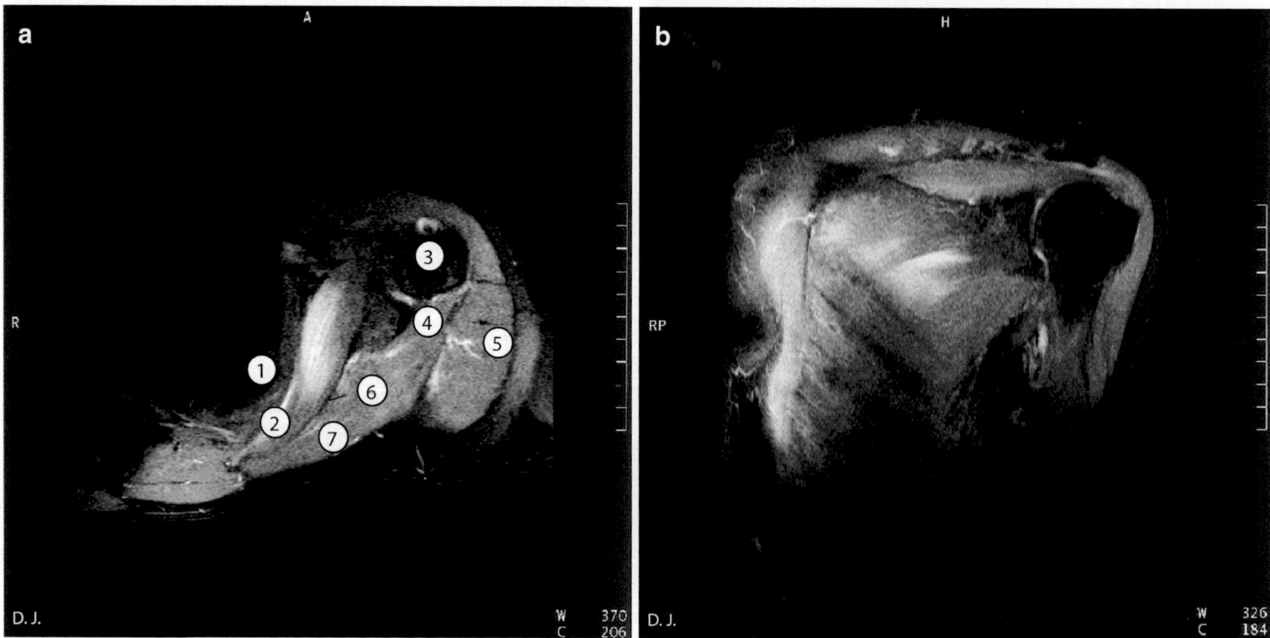

Fig. 20.7 Magnetic resonance images 10 min after injection of 10-mL ropivacaine, without radiographic contrast medium, into the subscapular fossa. (**a**) Axial (crosssection). (**b**) Paracoronal. *(1)* Thorax wall, *(2)* subscapular muscle and subscapular fossa, *(3)* head of the humerus, *(4)* teres minor muscle, *(5)* deltoid muscle, *(6)* scapula, *(7)* infraspinatus muscle. (Reproduced with permission from Danilo Jankovic)

Table 20.3 Shoulder–arm region: blocking techniques in pain therapy

Indications				
		Acute and chronic pain conditions		
		Target area		
Surgical	Postoperative pain therapy	Shoulder	Shoulder–arm	Mobilization of the shoulder
Interscalene[a]	Interscalene[b]	Subscapular nerves	Interscalene	Interscalene
+++++	+++++	+++++	+++++	+++++
Dosage: 20–25 mL 0.75% ropivacaine or 0.5% bupivacaine (0.5% levobupivacaine)	20–25 mL 0.375–0.5% ropivacaine or 0.25% bupivacaine (0.25% levobupivacaine)	10–15 mL 0.5–0.75% ropivacaine or 0.25% bupivacaine (0.25% levobupivacaine)	10–15 mL 0.375–0.5% ropivacaine or 0.25% bupivacaine (0.25% levobupivacaine)	20–25 mL 0.375–0.5% ropivacaine or 0.25% bupivacaine (0.25% levobupivacaine)
	Subscapular nerves[b]	Interscalene	Stellate ganglion	Subscapular nerves[c]
	++	+++	++	++
	15 mL 0.5–0.75% ropivacaine or 0.25–0.375% bupivacaine (0.25–0.375% levobupivacaine)	10–15 mL 0.375–0.5% ropivacaine or 0.25% bupivacaine (0.25% levobupivacaine)	10–15 mL 0.375% ropivacaine or 0.25% bupivacaine (0.25% levobupivacaine)	10–15 mL 0.5–0.75% ropivacaine or 0.25% bupivacaine (0.25% levobupivacaine)

Comparison of interscalene block of the brachial plexus, blocks of the subscapular and suprascapular nerves, and blocks of the stellate ganglion
+++++ Best method
++++ Very suitable method
+++ Suitable method
++ Method suitable with some qualifications
+ Less suitable method
[a] Usually in combination with basic general anesthesia. This provides excellent pain relief
[b] In severe pain, a combination of the two techniques is possible
[c] Usually in combination with a suprascapular nerve block: 8–10 mL 0.5–0.75% ropivacaine or 0.25% bupivacaine (0.25% levobupivacaine)

A combination of the subscapular and suprascapular nerve blocks is possible and often desirable (Table 20.3).

Block Series

In all indications, a series of six to eight blocks is useful if an improvement trend is seen after the first and second treatments.

Side Effects

If the dosage is too high, transient weakness may occur in the shoulder and upper arm. Outpatients should be informed about this. A partial block of the intercostal nerves is possible due to spread of the local anesthetic, and is often desirable.

Complications

- There is a potential risk of pneumothorax (unlikely if the correct technique is observed).
- Intravascular injection.

Author could not observe any side effects or possible complications after injection of local anesthetic with corticosteroid.

Supraspinatus Muscle

Functional Anatomy

The anatomical insertions are medial to the supraspinous fossa and lateral to the greater tubercle of the humerus (Fig. 20.8).

Innervation and Function (See Table 20.1)

Myotatic Unit

This covers the middle part of the deltoid muscle and the upper part of the trapezius muscle, as synergists for abduction.

Trigger Points

The two trigger points (TrPs) in the supraspinatus muscle are located deep in the supraspinous fossa of the scapulae, underneath the relatively thick part of the trapezius

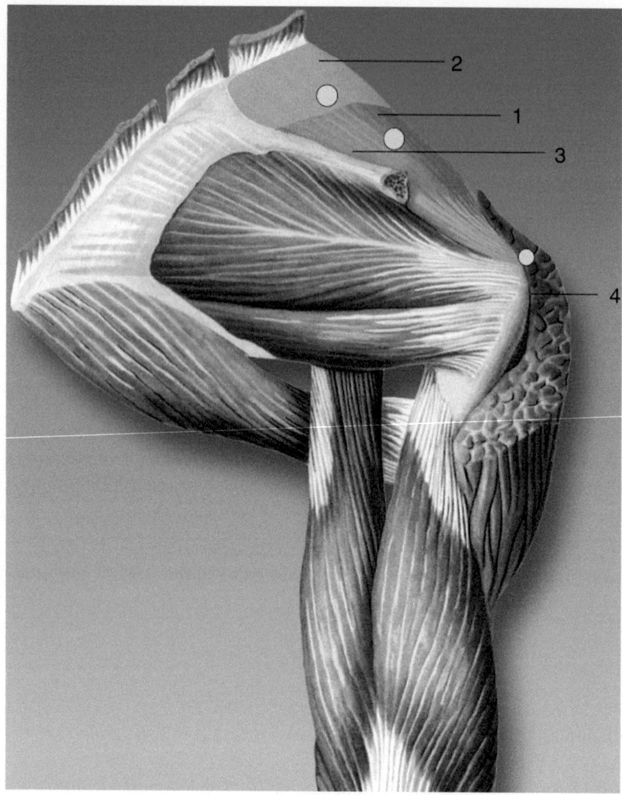

Fig. 20.8 Supraspinatus muscle. Anatomic insertions and myofascial trigger points (yellow circles); adapted from Travell and Simons. *(1)* Infraspinatus muscle, *(2)* supraspinous fascia, *(3)* spine of the scapula, *(4)* greater tuberosity of the humerus. (Reproduced with permission from Danilo Jankovic)

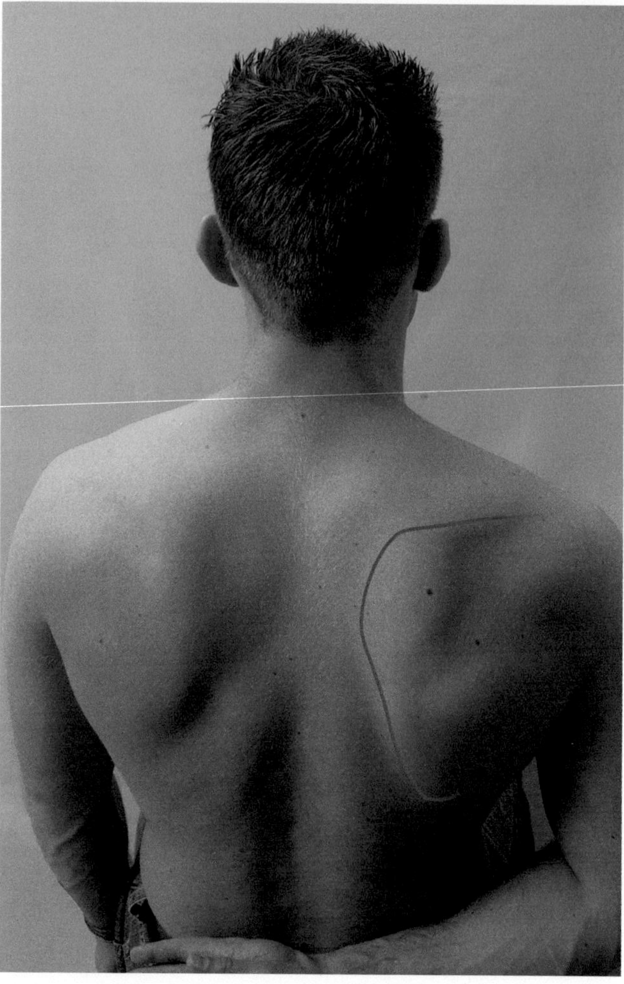

Fig. 20.9 Supraspinatus muscle. Positioning for trigger point injection ("hand behind the back" position). (Reproduced with permission from Danilo Jankovic)

muscle. The medial TrP lies directly above the spine of the scapula, lateral to the medial border of the scapula. The lateral TrP can be palpated medial to the acromion. A third TrP may be located in the tendon of the muscle at its lateral insertion on the joint capsule and the greater tuberosity (Fig. 20.8).

Symptoms

Pain in the middle deltoid region, sometimes radiating to the upper and lower arm, particularly in the area of the lateral epicondyle.

Procedure

Materials

Sterile precautions, 23-G needle 30 mm long, 2-mL and 5-mL syringes, and local anesthetic.

Technique

The lower arm of the seated patient is placed behind the back at waist level ("hand behind the back") (Fig. 20.9). After palpation, injection into the medial TrP is carried out in the direction of the suprascapular notch (Fig. 20.10). After careful aspiration, injection of the local anesthetic follows. The lateral TrP is sought directly medial to the acromion. The muscle's insertion point at the greater tubercle of the humerus requires perpendicular puncture until bone contact is made (Fig. 20.11).

Dosage

1–2-mL local anesthetic—e.g., 0.2–0.375% ropivacaine.

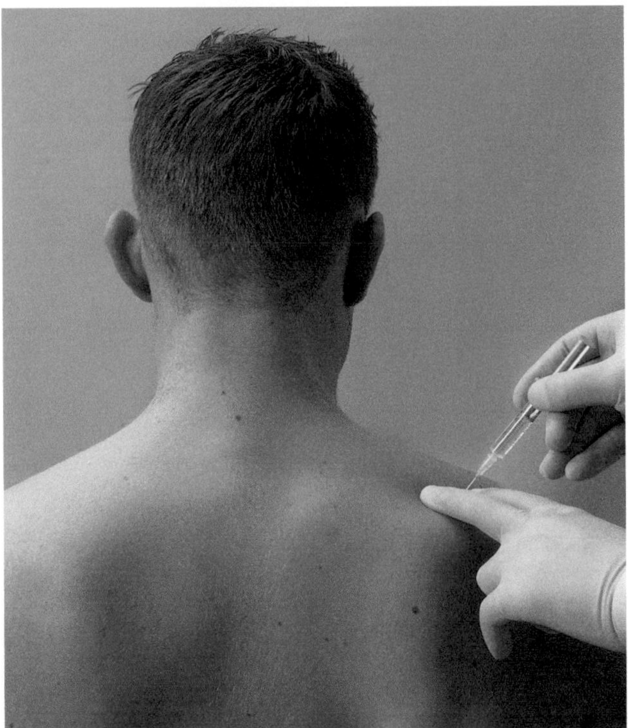

Fig. 20.10 Supraspinatus muscle. Injection into the medial trigger point in the direction of the suprascapular notch. (Reproduced with permission from Danilo Jankovic)

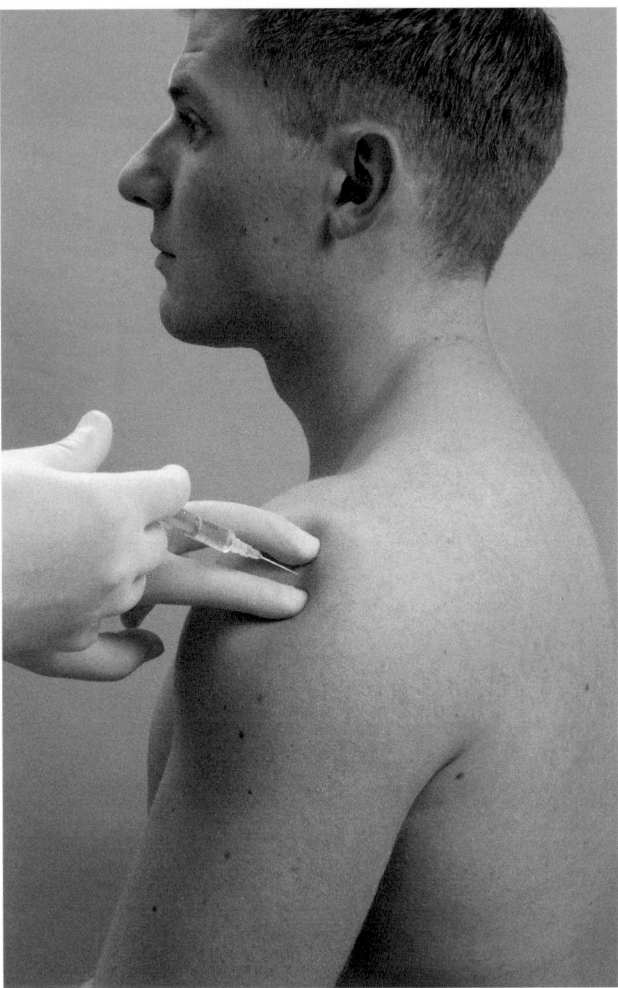

Fig. 20.11 Supraspinatus muscle. Infiltration of the insertion site at the greater tubercle of the humerus. (Reproduced with permission from Danilo Jankovic)

Complications

Pneumothorax must be regarded as a potential complication when injecting into the medial TrP of the supraspinatus muscle.

Infraspinatus Muscle

Functional Anatomy

The anatomic insertions are located medial to the infraspinous fossa of the scapula and lateral to the greater tuberosity of the humerus (Figs. 20.12 and 20.13).

Innervation and Function (See Table 20.1)

Myotatic Unit

With the exception of external rotation of the arm, the infraspinatus muscle acts synergistically with the teres minor muscle (with almost identical function) and the posterior part of the deltoid muscle.

Trigger Points

Two active trigger points (medial and lateral) can be located approximately 2 cm below the spine of the scapula, and sometimes there is also another possible trigger point slightly caudally (Fig. 20.12).

Symptoms

The symptoms consist of referred pain when sleeping in the lateral position and an inability to reach the rear trouser pockets or bra fastener, or to comb the hair or brush the teeth.

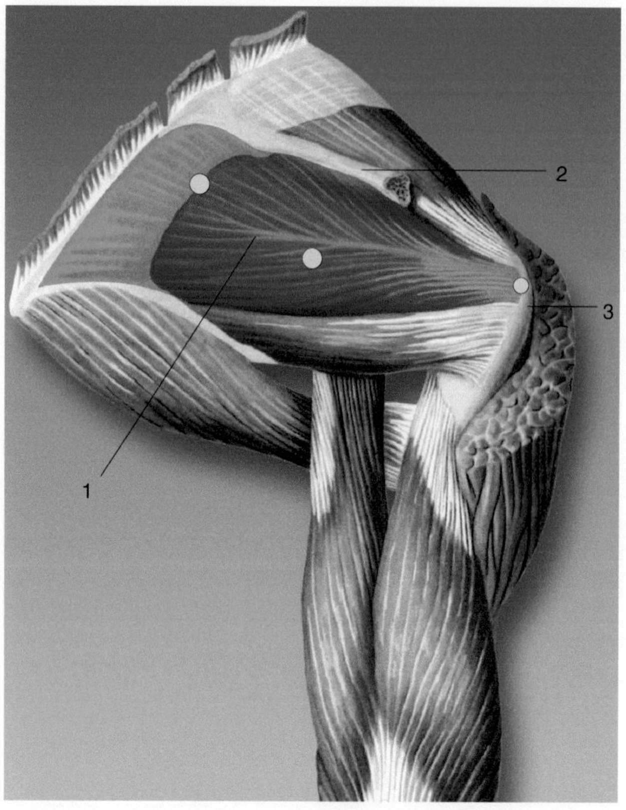

Fig. 20.12 Infraspinatus muscle. Anatomic insertions and myofascial trigger points *(yellow circles)*; adapted from Travell and Simons. *(1)* Infraspinatus muscle, *(2)* spine of the scapula, *(3)* greater tuberosity of the humerus. (Reproduced with permission from Danilo Jankovic)

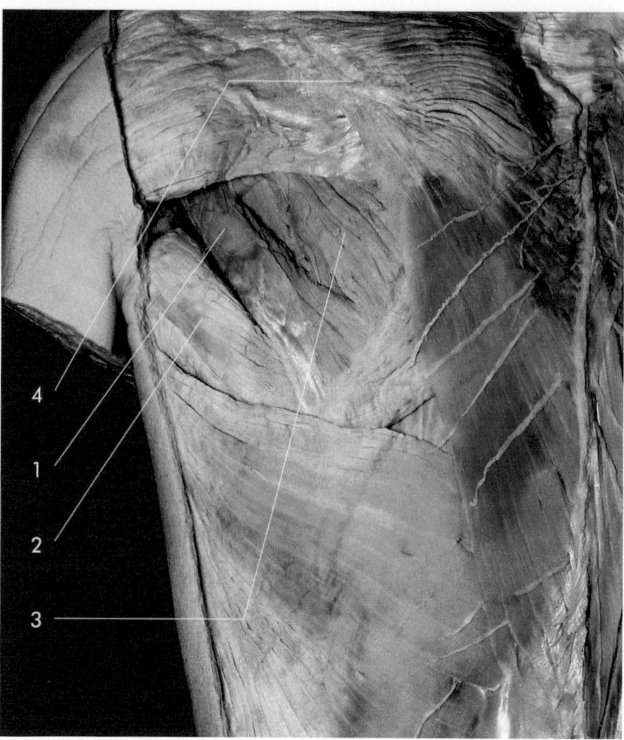

Fig. 20.13 *(1)* Teres minor muscle, *(2)* teres major muscle, *(3)* infraspinatus muscle, *(4)* spine of the scapula. (Reproduced with permission from Danilo Jankovic)

Procedure

Materials

Sterile precautions, 23-G needle 30 mm long, 2-mL and 5-mL syringes, and local anesthetic.

Technique

The patient lies on the side that is not being treated. The arm is bent to 90° and the elbow is laid on a cushion. The contour of the scapula has to be clearly defined.

After careful disinfection and palpation of the trigger point (TrP), the needle is slowly introduced in the direction of the TrP. During injection into the medial TrP, the left middle finger is pressed against the caudal edge of the spine of the scapula. During injection into the lateral TrP, the left ring finger presses against the caudal edge of the spine of the scapula (Figs. 20.14 and 20.15).

The puncture has to be carried out sensitively, as the scapula bones (part of the infraspinous fossa) sometimes offer very little resistance (resembling a fibrous membrane, so that there is a risk of pneumothorax). The insertion site of the muscle into the greater tuberosity of the humerus requires a perpendicular position to be maintained until bone contact is made (Fig. 20.16).

Dosage

1–2-mL local anesthetic—e.g., 0.2–0.375% ropivacaine.

Complications

- Pneumothorax is a potential complication.
- Infection.

Teres Minor Muscle

Functional Anatomy

The muscle's anatomic insertions are located directly alongside and caudal to those of the infraspinatus muscle (Figs. 20.13 and 20.17).

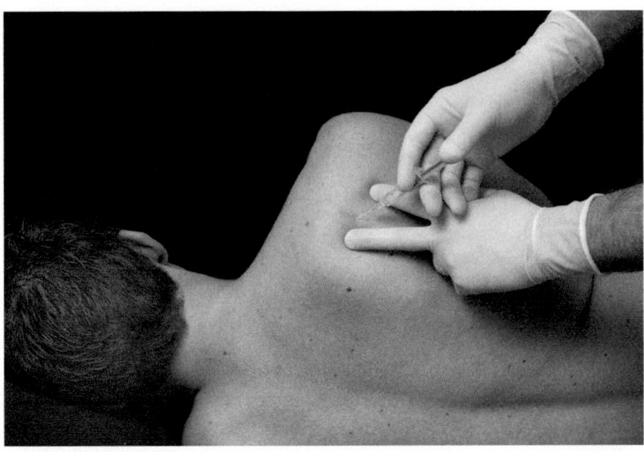

Fig. 20.14 Infraspinatus muscle. Injection into the medial trigger point in the direction of the caudal edge of the spine of the scapula. (Reproduced with permission from Danilo Jankovic)

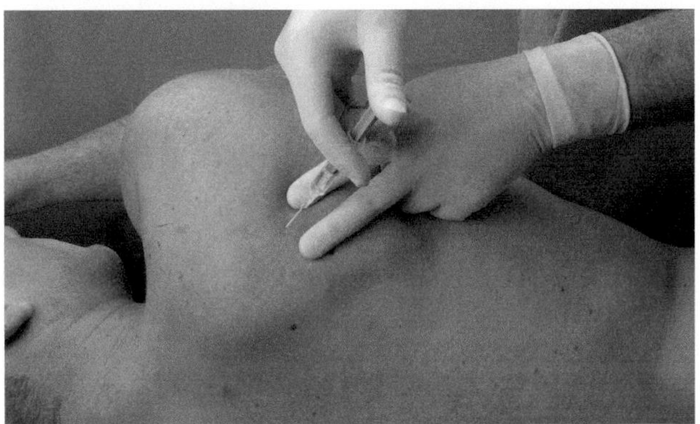

Fig. 20.15 Infraspinatus muscle. Injection into the caudal trigger point. (Reproduced with permission from Danilo Jankovic)

Fig. 20.16 Infraspinatus muscle. Infiltration of the insertion site on the greater tuberosity of the humerus. (Reproduced with permission from Danilo Jankovic)

Innervation and Function (See Table 20.1)

Myotatic Unit

The teres minor muscle acts synergistically with the infraspinatus muscle.

Trigger Points

The teres minor muscle is one of the most rarely affected muscles in the rotator cuff (only involved in 7% of cases). The trigger point usually lies in the center of the muscle (Figs. 20.13 and 20.17). The teres minor muscle is located above the teres major muscle.

Symptoms

Pain in the posterior deltoid area.

Procedure

Materials

Sterile precautions, 23-G needle 30 mm long, 2-mL and 5-mL syringes, and local anesthetic.

Technique

The arm is bent to 90°. The contour of the scapula has to be clearly defined (Fig. 20.18). The TrPs are sought between the teres major and infraspinatus muscles, near the lateral edge of the scapula. The index and middle fingers fix the TrP. The 30-mm needle is directed toward the scapula (Fig. 20.19).

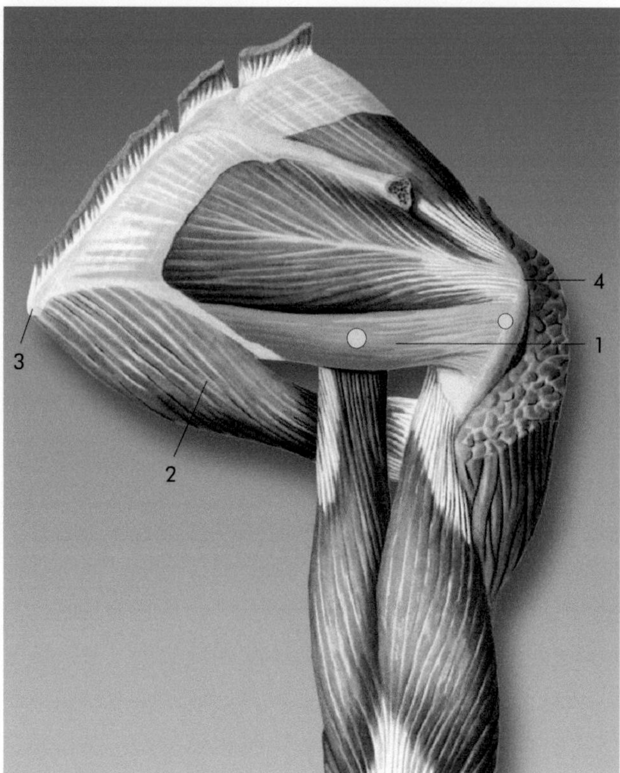

Fig. 20.17 Teres minor muscle. Anatomic insertions and myofascial trigger points *(yellow circles)*; adapted from Travell and Simons. *(1)* Teres minor muscle, *(2)* teres major muscle, *(3)* inferior angle of the scapula, *(4)* greater tuberosity of the humerus. (Reproduced with permission from Danilo Jankovic)

The insertion site of the muscle on the greater tuberosity of the humerus requires a perpendicular needle direction until bone contact is made (Fig. 20.20).

Dosage

2-mL local anesthetic—e.g., 0.2–0.375% ropivacaine.

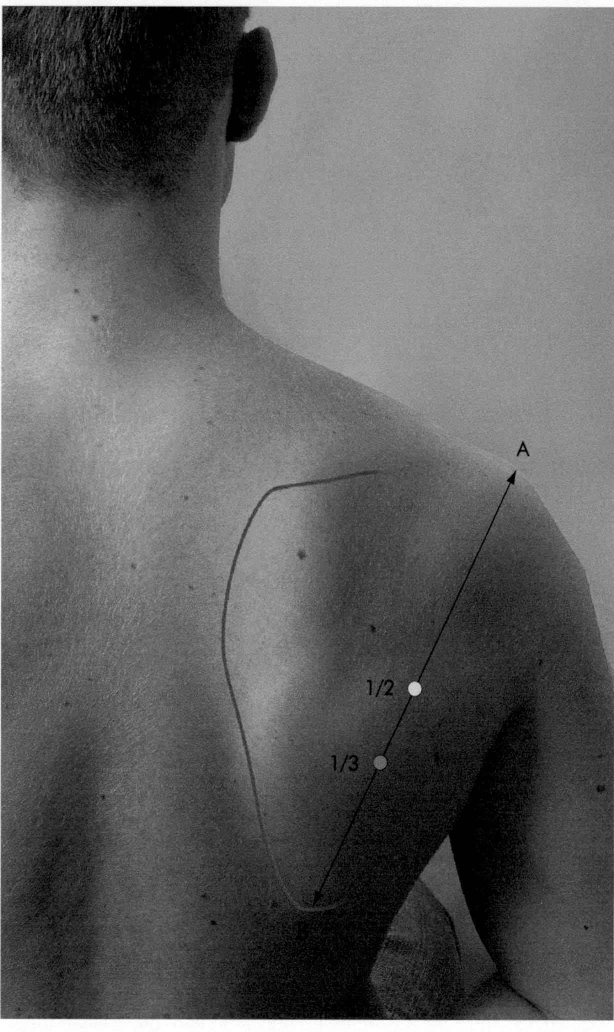

Fig. 20.18 Teres minor muscle *(yellow)* and teres major muscle *(green)*. Landmarks for trigger point injection. A-Acromion, B-inferior angle of the scapula. (Reproduced with permission from Danilo Jankovic)

Complications

Pneumothorax is a potential complication.

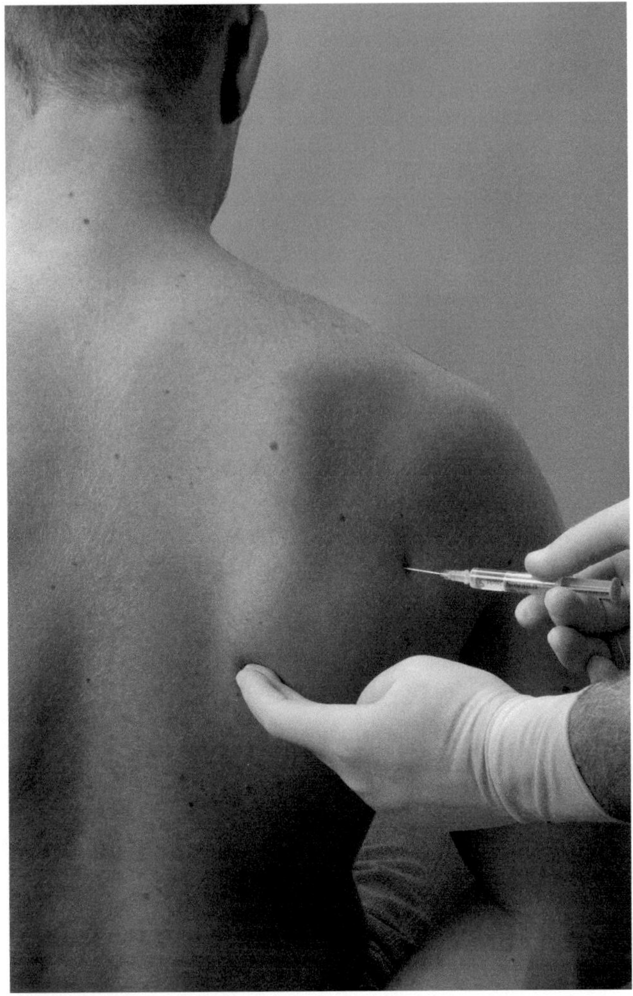

Fig. 20.19 Teres minor muscle. The needle is directed toward the scapula. (Reproduced with permission from Danilo Jankovic)

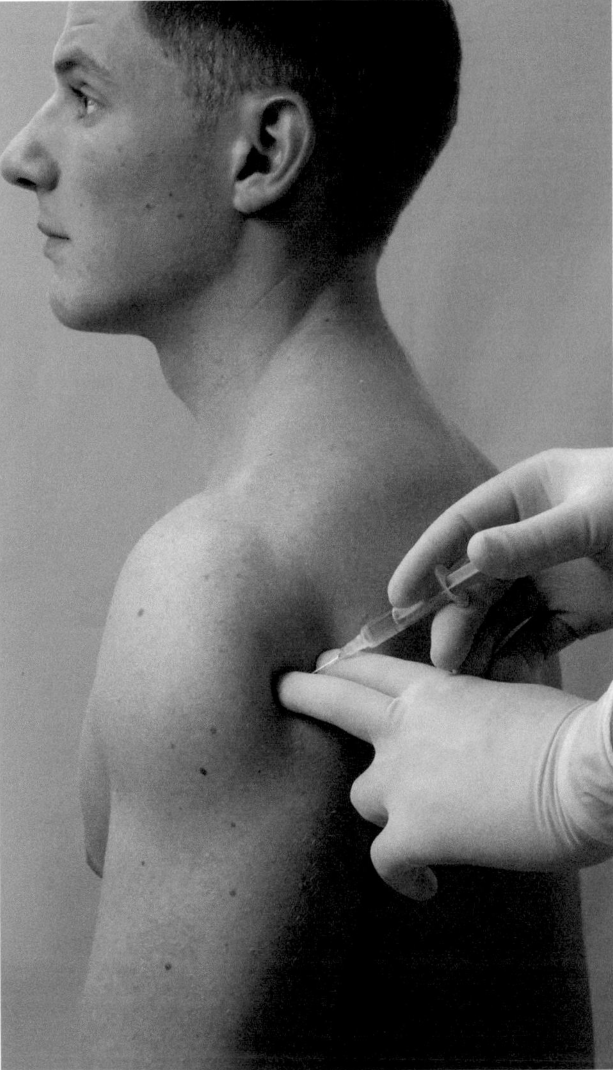

Fig. 20.20 Teres minor muscle. Injection at the insertion point of the greater tuberosity of the humerus. (Reproduced with permission from Danilo Jankovic)

Suggested Reading

Abram S, O'Conor T. complications associated with epidural steroid injections. Reg Anesth. 1996;21:149–61.

Batemann JE. The shoulder and neck. Philadelphia: W. B. Saunders; 1991. p. 134, 145–6, 149, 284–90

Cailliet R. Soft tissue pain and disability. Philadelphia: FA. Davis; 1977. p. 161–2.

Cailliet R. Shoulder pain. 3rd ed. Philadelphia: Davis Company; 1991. p. 105–23, 193–226

Chen CH, Chen TW, Weng MC, et al. The effect of electroacupuncture on shoulder subluxation for stroke patients. Kaoshiung J Med Sci. 2000;16:525–32.

Dahan TH, Fortin L, Pelletier M, et al. Double blind randomized clinical trial examining the efficacy of bupivacaine suprascapular nerve blocks in frozen shoulder. J Rheumatol. 2000;27: 1329–31.

Devor M, Govin-Lippman R, Raber P. Corticosteroids suppress ectopic neural discharge originating in experimental neuromas. Pain. 1985;22:127–37.

Dursun E, Dursun N, Ural CE, Cakci A. Glenohumeral joint subluxation and reflex sympathetic dystrophy in hemiplegic patients. Arch Phys Med Rehabil. 2000;81(7):944–6.

Ekelund A. New knowledge of the mysterious "frozen shoulder". Surgical treatment can accelerate the recovery in more serious cases. Lakartidningen. 1998;95(48):5472–4.

Gray H. In: Goss M, editor. Anatomy of human body. American edition 29. Lea & Febiger; 1973. p. 455–6.

Hall ED. Acute effects of intravenous glucocorticoids on cat spinal motor neuron electrical properties. Brain Res. 1982;240:186–90.

Hecht JS. Subscapular nerve block in the painful hemiplegic shoulder. Arch Phys Med Rehabil. 1992;73(11):1036–9.

Jankovic D. Subscapular nerve block & subscapularis trigger point infiltration. In: Jankovic D, editor. Regional nerve blocks & infiltration therapy. 3rd ed. Oxford: Blackwell Scientists; 2004. p. 128–32.

Jankovic D, van Zundert A. The frozen shoulder syndrome. Description of a new technique and five case reports using the subscapular nerve block and subscapularis trigger point infiltration. Acta Anaesth Belgica. 2006;57:137–43.

Johansson A, Hao J, Sjölund B. Local corticosteroid application block transmission in normal nociceptive C-fibers. Acta Anesthesiol Scand. 1990;34:335–8.

Kopell HP, Thompson WL. Pain and the frozen shoulder. Surg Gynecol Obstet. 1959;109:92–6.

Mackinnon SE, Hudson AR, Gentili F, et al. Peripheral nerve injection injury with steroid agents. Plast Reconst Surg. 1982;69:482–9.

Mc Laughlin HL. Lesions of the musculotendinous cuff of the shoulder. J Bone Joint Surg. 1944;26:31.

Muller LP, Muller LA, Happ J, Kerschbaumer F. Frozen shoulder: a sympathetic dystrophy? Arch Orthop Trauma Surg. 2000;120(1–2):84–7.

Netter FH. Nervengeflechte und periphere Nerven. In: Krämer G, editor. Farbatlanten der Medizin (Band 5). Nervensystem I: Neuroanatomie und Physiologie. Stuttgart: Georg Thieme Verlag; 1987.

Ontjes DA. Adrenal corticosteroids, corticotrophin releasing hormone, adrenocorticotropin and anti-adrenal drugs. In: Munson PL, editor. Principles of pharmacology. Chapman & Hall; 1995. p. 764–5.

Pinedo S, de la Villa FM. Complications in the hemiplegic patients in the first year after the stroke. Rev neurol. 2001;32:206–9.

Reichmister JP, Friedmann SL. Long-term functional results after manipulation of the frozen shoulder. Md Med J. 1999;48:7–11.

Seeman PM. Membrane stabilization by drugs: tranquilizers, steroids and anesthetics. Int Rev Neuro Biol. 1996;9:145–221.

Travell JG, Simons DG. Myofascial pain and dysfunction. The trigger point manual, vol. 1. Baltimore: Williams & Wilkins; 1983.

21 Calcific Tendinitis Intervention

Sang Hoon Lee

Contents

General Considerations

Calcific tendinosis or calcific tendinopathy in the rotator cuff (also referred to as calcifying tendinitis) is caused by the deposition of loosely bonded carbonate apatite crystals in the tendon. Most calcium deposits remain in the silent stage and can be detected on radiographs in 7.5–20% of asymptomatic adults. However, these deposits can become symptomatic, causing acute or chronic pain. The ultrasound imaging is more sensitive than radiography to detect smaller calcific particles. Using this modality in patients with shoulder pain, the prevalence of calcium deposition can be as high as 29%. Symptomatic calcification has been reported most commonly in the supraspinatus tendon, especially in the critical zone, i.e., approximately 1 cm proximal to its insertion. It does not imply that calcification is created in the critical zone for the first time, as described later.

Conservative physical and pharmacological treatment, with or without subacromial subdeltoid steroid injection, can effectively relieve pain in most of the symptomatic calcification. However, a high probability of spontaneous rupture has been reported in some patients with extensive calcifications, resulting in delaminated rotator cuff tear. Delamination is negatively associated with tendon healing. In this situation, early decompression of calcium is logical to salvage tendons.

Calcific tendonitis can be managed with minimally invasive treatments such as (1) barbotage (repeated alternating injection and aspiration of fluid with a syringe, lavage, and aspiration) and (2) fenestration (creating a new opening in calcium deposit by repeated needling procedure to stimulate natural absorption). Dense, hard calcification has less chance of causing symptoms than soft calcification. The stiff calcium deposit can exhibit different degrees of hardness and flexibility compared with neighboring healthy tendon fibers. The shear stress between the calcification and neighboring tendon layers plays a role in its pathogenesis of splitting and delamination tear between superficial and deep components. A delaminated rotator cuff tear is a form of degeneration within the tendon; it generally refers to a horizontal tear occurring between rotator cuff layers. Edge fraying or cleavage greater than or equal to 5 mm was the definition reported by MacDougal and Tod Hunter. Lee defined delaminated tear as the linear pooling of contrast within the long axis of the tendon radiologically.

S. H. Lee (✉)
Madiclinic, Jeonju, South Korea

Anam Hospital of Korea University, Seoul, South Korea

D. Jankovic, P. Peng (eds.), *Regional Nerve Blocks in Anesthesia and Pain Therapy*,
https://doi.org/10.1007/978-3-030-88727-8_21

Chronic degenerative change within the tendon might, therefore, be related to the development of delamination. In these cases, pain arises from the nociceptors of tears with inflammation. Platelet-rich plasma (PRP) treatment may be helpful to these painful conditions.

Patient Selection

The pathogenesis of calcific tendinosis remains elusive. Reactive and dystrophic calcifications are a widely accepted hypothesis. Theoretically, the dystrophic calcification occurs in degenerative tissue and does not heal spontaneously. The reactive calcific tendinosis occurs in healthy tissue, presumed as a cell-mediated process, and is a self-limiting disease. In terms of reactive calcific tendinosis, Uhthoff and Loehr described three distinct stages in the disease process: the pre-calcific, calcific, and post-calcific steps (Fig. 21.1).

It is difficult to differentiate between reactive and dystrophic calcifications and their natural course. But there are some common natural courses of calcifications, no matter how it originated.

The tiny nodular calcium spots are being created in the rotator cuff tendon insertional area and grow larger proximally (Fig. 21.2). Microscopically, calcium crystals are deposited primarily in matrix vesicles in the insertional area. These crystals become coalesce and form large foci of calcifications. Calcium vesicles are separated by chondrocytes and fibrocartilaginous tissue septa from the normal tissue. This theory is well established in calcification of the atherosclerotic calcification wall as well.

Under normal conditions, calcium cavities are well encapsulated without clinical symptoms. The capsule of calcific vesicles may have a chance to be ruptured by external force or daily activities of any size. Broken walls release the chemical substance (calcium) to the environment and induce intense chemical inflammation and pain. If calcific vesicles would rupture in a smaller size, it doesn't generate severe pain and would heal without damaging neighboring healthy tendon fibers. However, if calcium grows enough to be detected with image modalities, it can induce intense pain and harm the adjacent healthy tendon fiber. In general, calcium deposit bigger than 1 cm in diameter is likely to be symptomatic and bears a worse prognosis. Some investigators correlate the morphology of the deposit on ultrasound with symptoms.

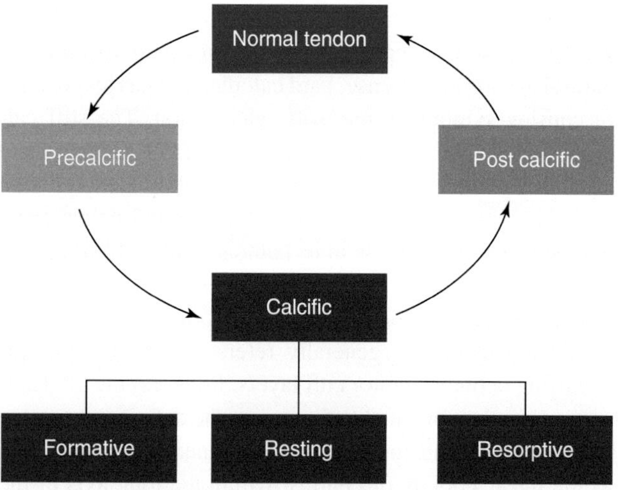

Fig. 21.1 The different phases of calcification. (Reprinted with permission from Philip Peng Educational Series)

Chiou et al. classified calcific depositions into four shapes: an arc shape (echogenic arc with shadowing), a fragmented or punctate shape (at least two separated echogenic spots or plaques, with or without shadowing), a nodular shape (echogenic nodule without shadowing), and a cystic shape (a bold echogenic wall with an anechoic area, weak internal echoes, or layering content). They emphasized the differences between well-defined calcifications with strong shadowing and those with faint or absent shadowing.

These imaging appearances differ significantly with patient symptoms and correlates with the physical consistency of the calcium. The cystic and nodular shapes correlated with patients with severe symptoms.

Physical appearance is different between radiography and ultrasound. On radiography, dense molecules reveal as discrete and radio-opaque like hard calcium deposit. On ultrasonography, dense molecules prevent echo transmission and cast echo shadowing. The solid calcifications tend to be well-circumscribed and discrete in radiographic appearance and often produce significant acoustic shadowing in ultrasound scan (Fig. 21.3). Solid calcification has less chance of capsular rupture and clinical symptoms. All the solid calcifications are not doomed to turn into soft calcification, but a few solid calcifications can be transformed into soft calcium. Most of the typical solid calcification causes impingement syndrome or delamination tear. It is not easy to aspirate the calcifications at this state because the calcifications are quite solid and chalklike. The most typical indication of lavage at this stage is calcification over 1 cm in diameter.

The soft or semiliquid calcium appears ill-defined or well-defined. Still, the opacity is homogeneous and less dense over the hard calcific phase on radiographs, producing little or no acoustic shadowing by ultrasonography (Fig. 21.4). Leaking of calcium into the normal tendon or shedding of calcium crystals into the adjacent subacromial bursa may result in severe acute pain and a restricted range of motion. When aspirated, these calcified deposits typically are soft with a toothpaste-like consistency. This stage is the most common indication for ultrasound-guided intervention.

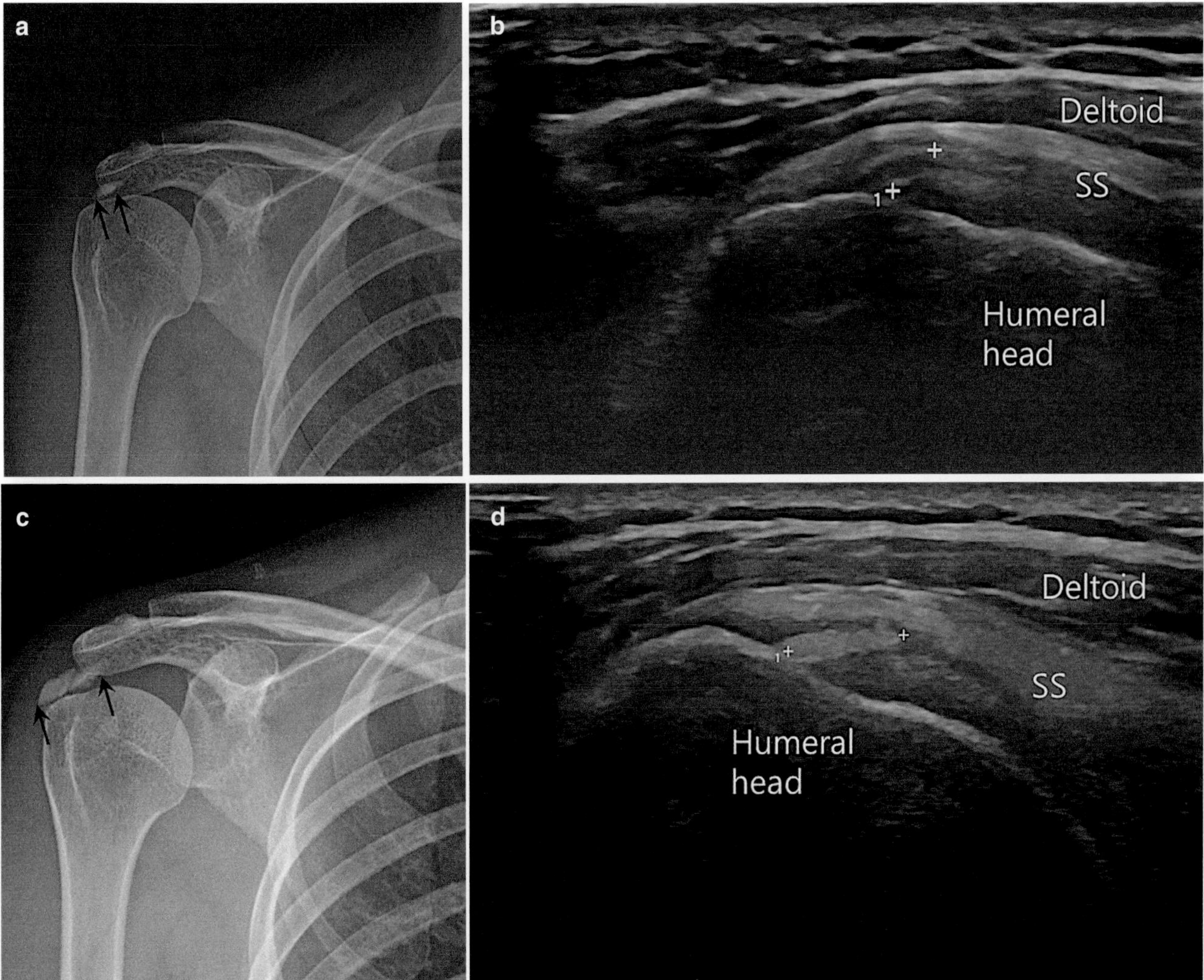

Fig. 21.2 Growing calcification. The small nodular cystic calcium (**a**, **b**) increase is larger proximally (**c**, **d**) by 2-year follow-up check. Calcification (C-1) in (**a**) and (**b**) shows 3.5 mm in long diameter, while in (**c**) (C-1) and (**d**) shows 7 mm in long diameter. Note the secondary calcification(C-2) was formed in another area. (Reprinted with permission from Dr. Sang Hoon Lee)

Some doctors believe that the soft calcification absorbs spontaneously by the self-healing process and does not consider the harmful effect. But most of the calcium results in rupture with the remaining residual space in the tendon and split the tendon fiber (Fig. 21.5). The more enormous calcium proceeds, the larger defect or intrasubstance delamination tear results. Consequently, more extensive calcium has a worse prognosis than the smaller one and has a higher chance of tendon rupture. Therefore, early successful drainage is the best way to minimize subsequent tendon failure. Successful aspiration may not be possible in cases when the calcifications appear already ruptured.

Sometimes multiple and fragmented calcifications can cause painful shoulders. There are several assumptions about the pain in these cases. Concomitant delamination tear would be one of the theories. In these cases, subsequent platelet-rich plasma (PRP) treatment should be performed following the fenestration. These calcifications can be ground gently with the needle tip by rotating the syringe by the fenestration technique.

Fenestration means the surgical creation of a new opening in a body part. For calcific tendinosis, a new window can be made by repeated needling procedure to stimulate natural absorption. This mechanical perturbation of the deposit is hypothesized to stimulate cell-mediated resorption. There is evidence in the surgical literature to support that calcific deposits need not be removed completely to achieve successful outcomes.

There are patients who remain symptomatic even after a successful barbotage or fenestration procedures. Concomitant delamination tear or sequelae intrasubstance tear would be one of the explanations. In some cases, concomitant adhesive capsulitis could be the major contributor to the symptom

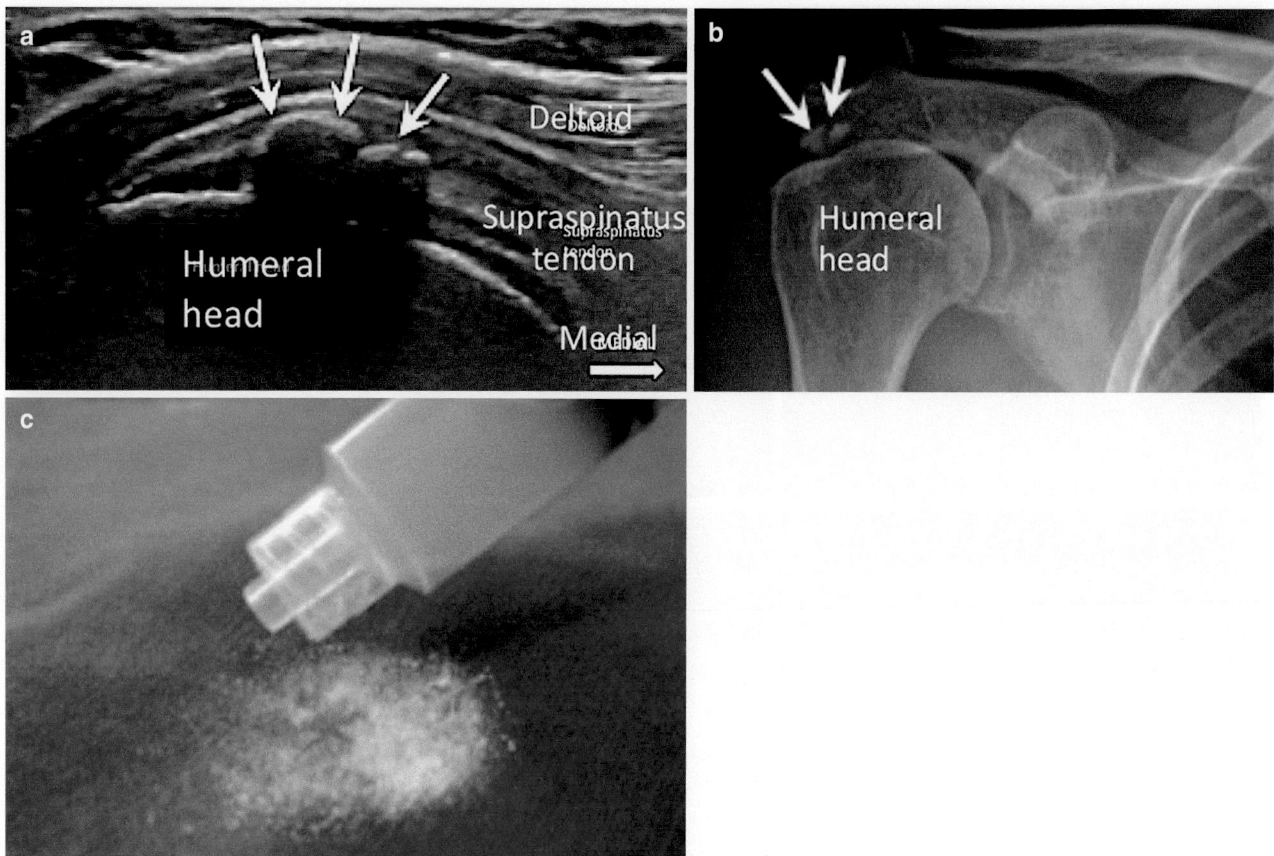

Fig. 21.3 Hard calcific phase: Sonographic (**a**), radiographic image (**b**), and aspirated specimen (**c**). The arrows indicate the calcification. Note the anechoic shadow cast by the calcium in 1A. (Reprinted with permission from Philip Peng Educational Series)

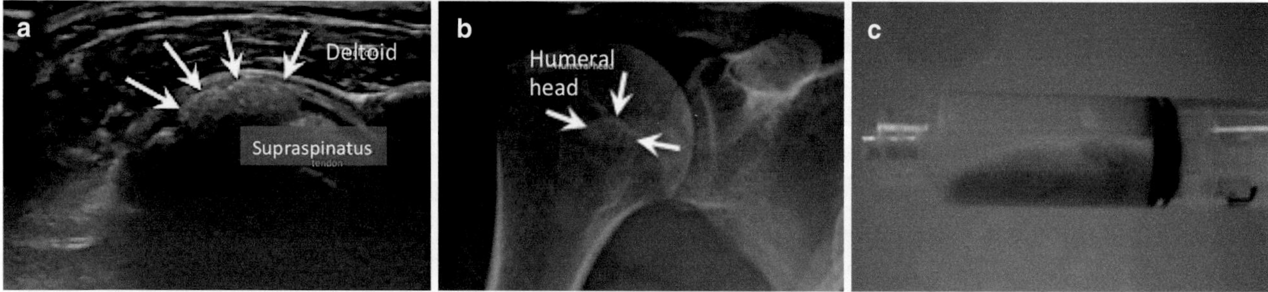

Fig. 21.4 Soft calcific phase: Sonographic (**a**), radiographic image (**b**), and aspirated specimen (**c**). The arrows indicate the calcification. Note the minimal echogenic shadow cast by the calcium in 2A. (Reprinted with permission from Philip Peng Educational Series)

irrespective of the findings of the calcifications in the tendon. The calcification could be only an innocent bystander, not the cause of the pain.

In summary:

1. Small nodular calcifications have less chance of symptoms than large, irregular, extensive calcification.
2. Well-encapsulated calcification has less chance of symptom than irregular, spiculated calcification.
3. Calcium deposit bigger than 1 cm in diameter is likely to be symptomatic.
4. The cystic- and nodular-shaped calcification has a higher chance of symptom than the arc shape and fragmented or punctate form.
5. Well-circumscribed and discrete in radiographic appearance and significant acoustic shadowing in the ultrasound scan has a less probability of being symptomatic.
6. Homogeneous and less dense on radiographs and little or no acoustic shadowing by ultrasonography has a high probability of pain.
7. The more enormous calcium proceeds, the larger defect or intrasubstance delamination tear results.

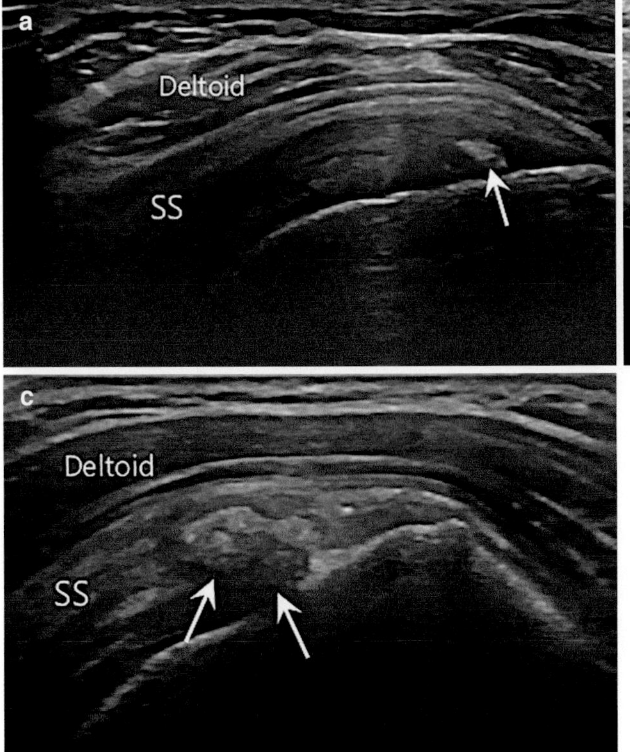

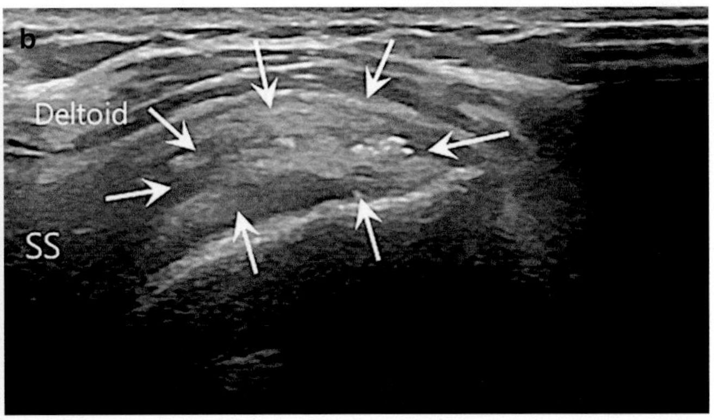

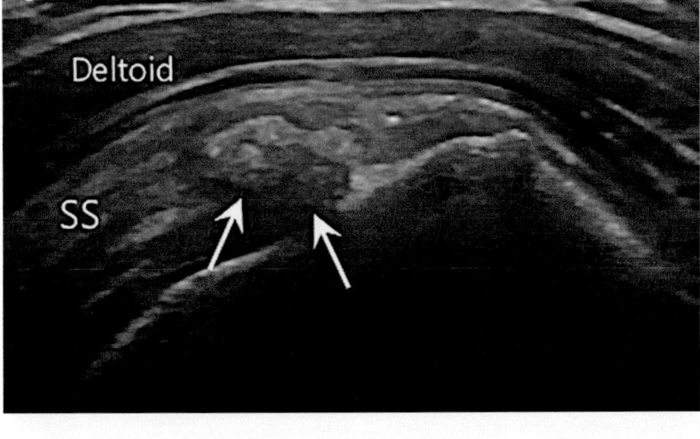

Fig. 21.5 Ultrasound images showing change of calcification configuration during follow-up. (**a**). Initial nodular calcification in supraspinatus tendon; (**b**). Rupture of previous calcification and scattered calcification with the swollen degenerated tendon; (**c**). The large calcification remains a large defect. SS-supraspinatus; arrows-calcification. (Reprinted with permission from Dr. Sang Hoon Lee)

8. More extensive calcium has a worse prognosis than the smaller one and has a higher chance of tendon rupture.
9. Concomitant delamination tear or sequelae intrasubstance tear accounts for the persistence of symptom even after a successful barbotage or fenestration procedures.
10. Concomitant adhesive capsulitis could be the major contributor to the symptom irrespective of the findings of the calcifications in the tendon.

Techniques

In preparing for the procedure, the needles and the drugs needed to be prepared are summarized in Table 21.1.

Needle/syringes
• 26G 1.5-in. needle for local anesthetic infiltration
• 18G 1.5-in. needle for calcium barbotage
• 24G 3.5-in. needle for removal of calcium plug obstructing the 18G needle lumen or fragmentation of the hard calcium before lavage (used as stylet)
• 5 ml lock syringes X5
Drugs
• 3 ml 1% lidocaine for irrigation(fill 3 ml of lidocaine in each 5 ml syringe)
• 3 ml lidocaine with 1 ml dexamethasone after barbotage process

Table 21.1 The needles and the drugs needed to be prepared

Needles			
Diameter	Length	Number	Purpose
26G	1.5 in.	1	Local anesthetic infiltration
18G	1.5 in.	1	Calcium barbotage
24G	3.5 in.	1	For removal of calcium plug obstructing the 18G needle lumen or fragmentation of the hard calcium before lavage (used as stylet)
Syringes			
5 ml Luer lock syringe		5	Local anesthetic infiltration and irrigation
Drugs			
1% lidocaine	3 ml	4	Local anesthetic infiltration and irrigation
Dexamethasone	1 ml	1	Reduce inflammation after barbotage process

The patient lie down supine. The position of the arms depends on the location of the lesion: humerus in external rotation for subscapular lesion, internal rotation for anterior supraspinatus lesion, or arm sling position (put a hand on the abdomen) for posterior supraspinatus lesion. If the calcification is localized in the infraspinatus, the patient's body position will be in oblique supine or lateral decubitus position. All procedure requires the use of a high-frequency probe, and the needle will be inserted in-plane.

One Needle Barbotage Technique (Fig. 21.6)

The first step is to identify the symptomatic calcification through careful physical examination and a full ultrasound scanning. The transducer is then placed along the long axis of the calcium cavity, putting the calcium deposit in the center of the scan image. Then, under the ultrasound guidance, infiltrate local anesthetics in the skin to the subdeltoid bursal space.

Following skin infiltration with a local anesthetic, a 18G needle is advanced until its tip is placed in the calcification center. It will be easy to understand that calcium crystals are deposited in the vesicle encircled by a capsule. With this technique, the operator put in fluid to mix liquid and calcium particles to be aspirated. Therefore, the resolution of calcium particles relies on the optimal increase of the vesicle's hydrostatic pressure. Any unnecessary hole or crack causes leaking the pressure, which is the most common reason for a lavage's technical failure. One should avoid repositioning or adjusting the needle once inserting it in the calcium cavity. Therefore, one should keep in mind that there is only one

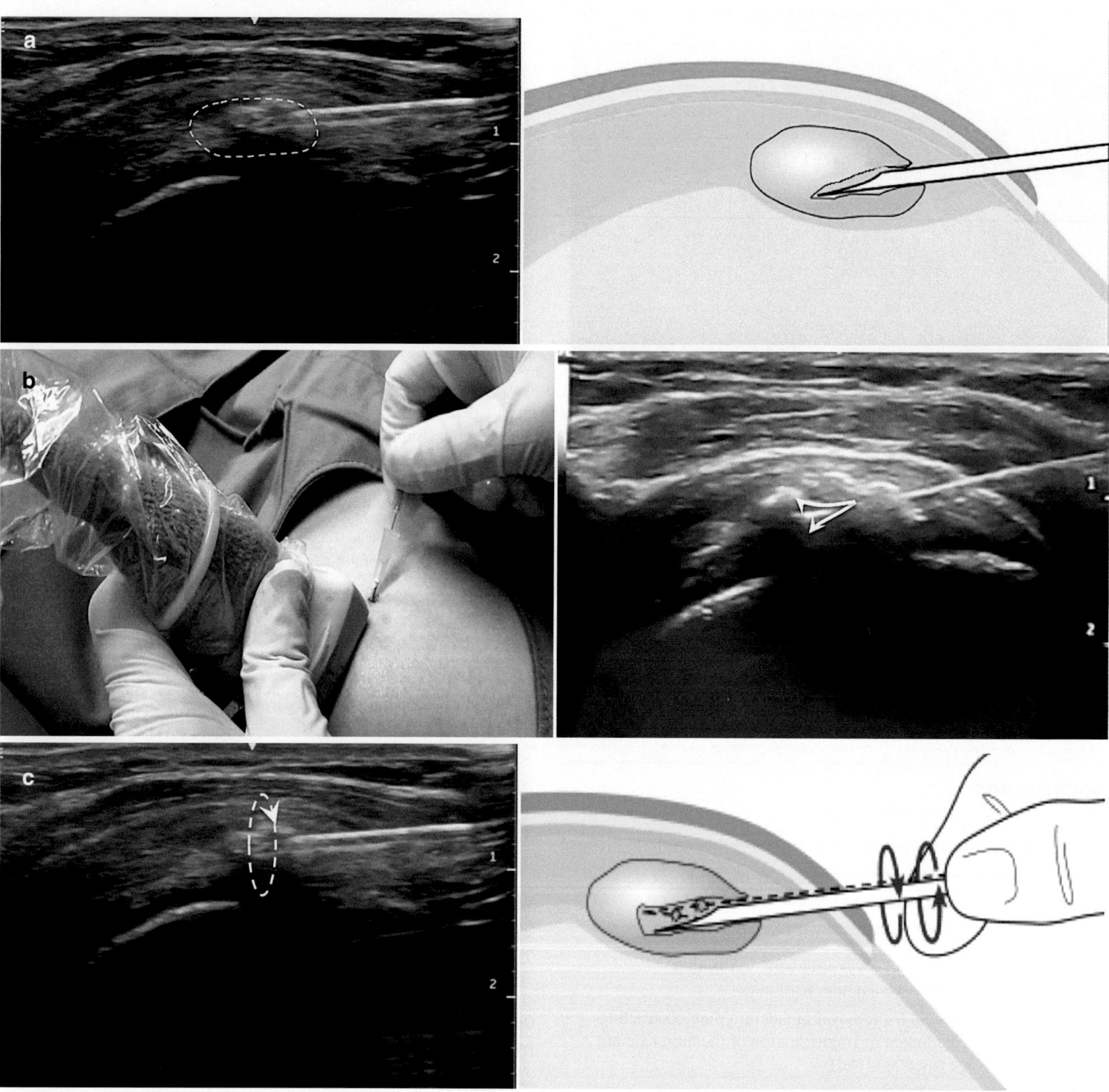

Fig. 21.6 One needle barbotage technique. (**a**) Needle insertion into the center of calcium with an in-plane method. (**b**) Removal of the calcium plug obstructing the needle lumen using 6-cm-long 24G stylet needle. (**c**) Fenestration with rotation of 18G needle. (**d**) Pumping the needle to hydrodissection the calcium. (**e**) Relieve the pressure of the needle to evacuate calcium. (**f**) Subacromial bursa injection of steroid. (Reprinted with permission from Philip Peng Educational Series)

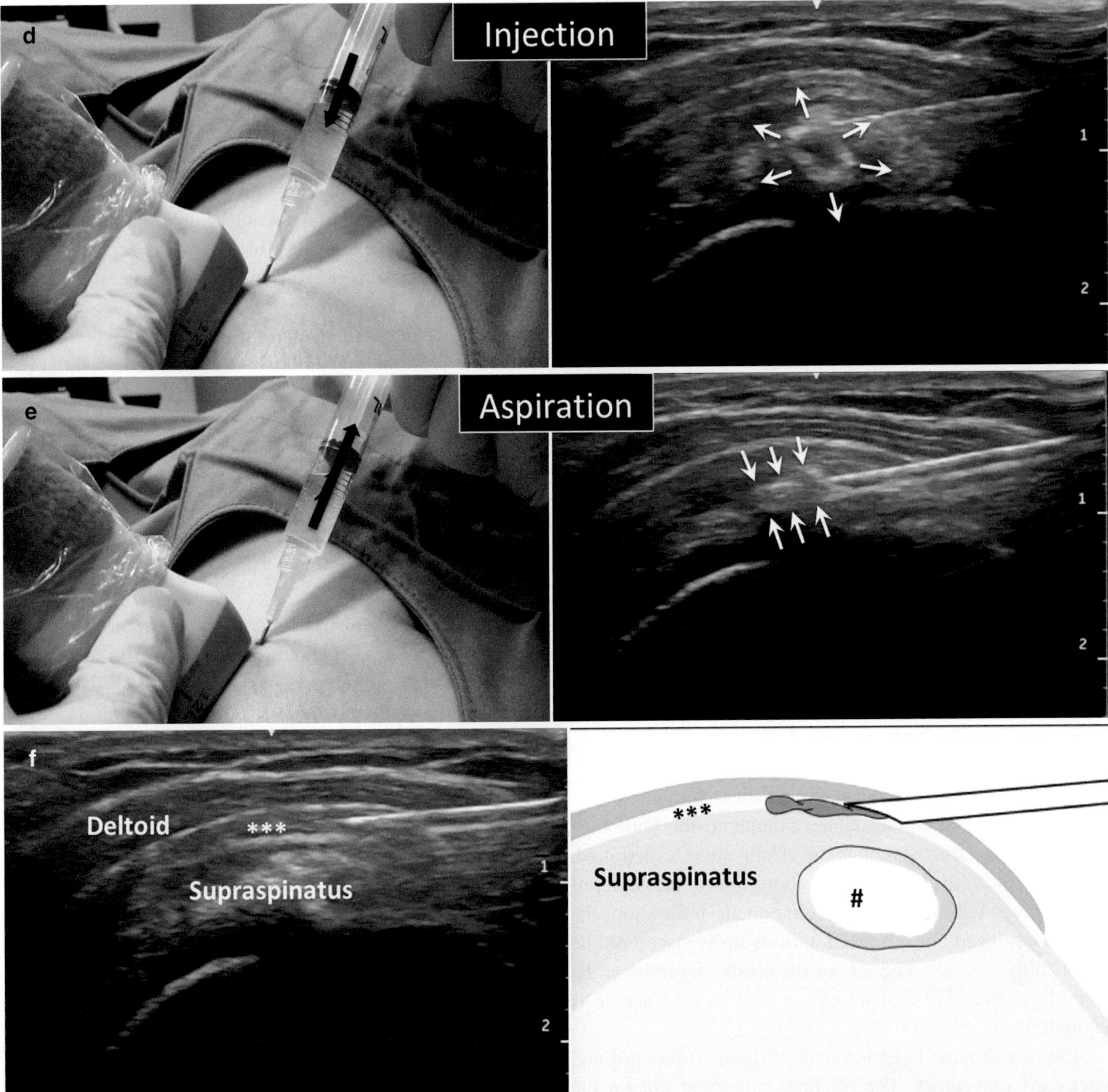

Fig. 21.6 (continued)

chance to insert the needle, so unnecessary penetration of the capsular wall leads to a leak of injecting fluid. The operator should hold tight the lavaging 18G needle inside the capsule.

Usually, calcium plug obstructs the 18G needle lumen during the initial needle insertional process. Removal of the calcium plug with a smaller bore-long needle is an essential step for the irrigation process. A 6-cm-long 24G stylet needle is chosen.

After slightly bending the distal tip of the 6-cm-long 24G stylet needle, insert and pass this stylet needle into the previously positioned lavaging 18G needle until the needle enters the center of the calcium. This process removes the calcium plug obstructing the needle lumen. If the distal tip is bent too much, it will not be easily inserted into the 18G needle. This 6 cm needle is advanced further and rotated to fragment or soften the hard calcium. This maneuver helps the initial hydrostatic irrigation process.

The next step is putting in a fluid to mix liquid and calcium particles to be aspirated. Following the withdrawal of 6 cm 24G stylet needle, a 5 ml syringe prefilled with 3 ml of lidocaine 1% is attached to the 18G needle. Lidocaine instead of saline is chosen because it can relieve pain during the procedure. The initial step is critical. The plunger should be pushed very gently to avoid rupture of the calcium capsule. The premature disruption of the calcium capsule before enough mixing liquid and calcium particles is the most common cause of this single needle technique's technical failure. The plunger should be pushed very slow, progressively aiming to mix liquid and calcium particle resolution. Do not aspirate the plunger by active force but passively "let go" of motion. This slow and low-pressure injection, followed by the passive release of pressure on the plunger, is repeated several times. If successful, lidocaine and calcium fragments will begin to evacuate into the syringe and appear as white particles.

If this initial barbotage steps proceed well, the operator can actively increase the force to the plunger to evacuate more calcium vigorously. If the lavaging fluid becomes turbid, change the lidocaine-filled new syringe. Please continue barbotage until the white calcium particle in the syringe cannot be seen. Withdraw the needle slowly until it reaches the subacromial bursa and stays put the needle tip in the subacromial bursal space. Infiltrate injectant mixture of 1 ml 2% lidocaine and 1 ml of dexamethasone in the subdeltoid bursal space. This steroid will mitigate the risk of post-procedural bursitis.

Fenestration Technique (Fig. 21.6)

Fenestration is usually indicated in a patient with symptomatic multiple solid calcifications. Similar to the barbotage procedure, the target symptomatic calcification is identified, and a transducer is placed along the long axis of the center of calcification. Following the local anesthetic infiltration, the fenestration needle is advanced until its tip is placed on the calcification surface. The size of the needle depends on the size of calcium. For a small one, a 25G or 26G needle is enough.

The calcification is fenestrated by repeated forward and backward movement. The rotating movement allows the needle bevel as a shovel excavating the solid calcium (Fig. 21.7). Continue digging the calcium until the calcification is felt soft and crepitation is diminished.

The needle is slowly withdrawn until it reaches the subacromial bursa and an injectant mixture of 1 ml 2% lidocaine and 1 ml of dexamethasone into the subacromial bursal space. This steroid will decrease the post-procedural pain.

Complications

There are no significant complications related to the procedure. But calcific tendinosis may have other concomitant pathologies, such as secondary adhesive capsulitis, delamination tear, rotator cuff tear, greater tubercular osteolysis, and ossifying tendinitis. While evaluating calcific tendinosis, physical examination and thorough ultrasound examination is vital to rule out associated pathologies because the misjudged diagnosis can lead to an unsatisfactory outcome.

The only expected complication related to the procedure is the technical failure of decompression of the calcium. The calcification wall can be perforated or ruptured iatrogenically before successful lavage, which is the most common cause of technical failure.

A perforated capsule cannot contain hydrostatic pressure inside the calcium, and an intact capsule is an essential part of successful drainage. Post-procedural pain is usually minimal. However, excessive hydrodistension could overstretch the calcium cavity and harm the adjacent normal tendon causing post-procedural pain.

Practical Tips

1. Thorough assessment is crucial to determine the calcification as a cause of shoulder pain. Sometimes calcification could be an innocent bystander.
2. Preoperative ultrasound evaluation is important: calcium size, density, shape, and designing needle approach pathway.
3. While inserting the needle, the target should be the center of the calcium cavity.
4. Do not relocate or adjust the needle after one needle passed the calcification capsule.
5. The initial step of barbotage is critical. Push the plunger very gently to avoid calcium capsular rupture, which is the most common cause of technical failure.
6. Subacromial bursal injection of steroid is essential in minimizing the post-procedural bursitis.
7. Following treatment, the patient is advised to avoid heavy lifting and overhead movement for about 2 weeks. For post-procedure pain, a cold compress is applied over the shoulder. Prescribe analgesics, including a combination of acetaminophen and nonsteroidal anti-inflammatory drugs.

Literature Review

Calcific tendinosis is usually known as a self-limited disease in which the calcification is resorbed after a period of worsening pain. The resolution of calcification correlated well with clinical improvement of symptoms. However, in many patients, the condition can lead to chronic pain and functional impairment. Various causes of pain have been

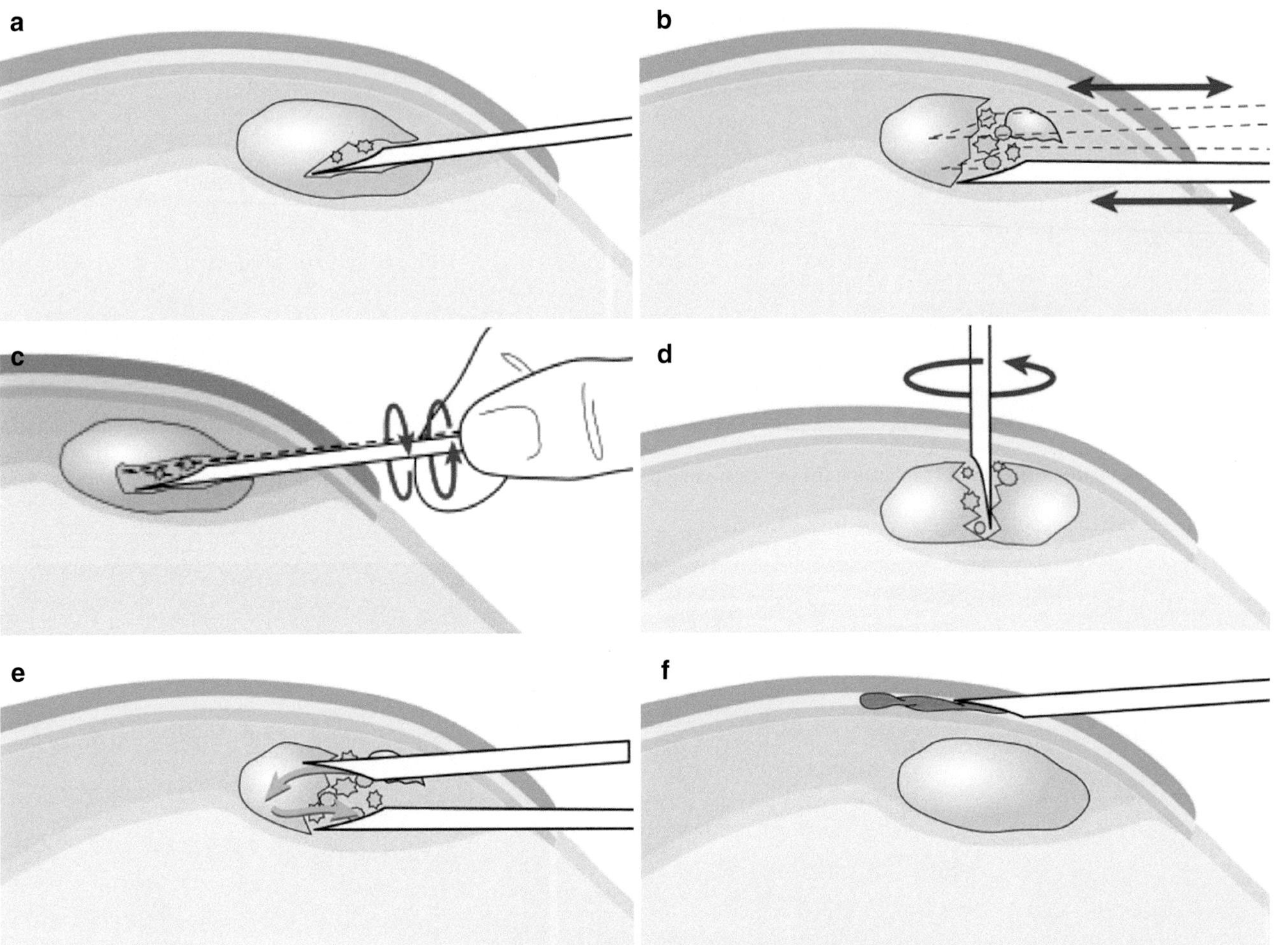

Fig. 21.7 Schematic drawing of the penetration in the calcium deposition in supraspinatus (pink color). (**a**) Needle insertion into the center of calcium with an in-plane method. (**b**) Fenestration with backward and forward movement. (**c**) Fenestration with rotation. (**d**) Fenestration out-of-plane. (**e**) Fenestration with two needles. (**f**) Subacromial bursa injection of steroid. (Reprinted with permission from Philip Peng Educational Series)

postulated, and multiple strategies have been devised to relieve the symptoms.

In terms of the hard calcific phase, there is no conclusive evidence to support the use of intralesional steroid injection, acetic acid iontophoresis, or pulsed ultrasound therapy.

Extracorporeal shockwave lithotripsy uses acoustic waves to fragment calcium deposits, and substantial or complete clinical improvement has been reported in 66–91% of patients with chronic calcific tendinosis. However, it also has a less favorable effect on hard calcific phase and large calcification over 15 mm in diameter.

Image-guided needle irrigation and aspiration (barbotage) of rotator cuff calcific tendinosis is an effective minimally invasive technique and was first described three decades ago. Del Cura and colleagues reported that 91% of patients experienced a significant or complete improvement in range of motion, pain, and disability when aspiration was performed under ultrasound guidance. Given the potential risks of surgery, percutaneous calcium aspiration should be considered after medical therapy failure.

Successful aspiration may not be possible when the calcification appears striated or spiculated because it represents a previous calcification rupture (Fig. 21.8). When attempting to remove numerous, diffuse, small (<5 mm) calcifications, clinical outcomes are only fair to poor, even when treated surgically. If the pain is associated with the multiple small, scattered calcifications, these calcifications may be a degenerative form of calcification or a feature of the tendinosis. Therefore, chronic degenerative change within the tendon might be related to the development of delamination (Fig. 21.9). In these cases, pain arises from the nociceptors of tears with inflammation. PRP treatment may be helpful to these painful conditions.

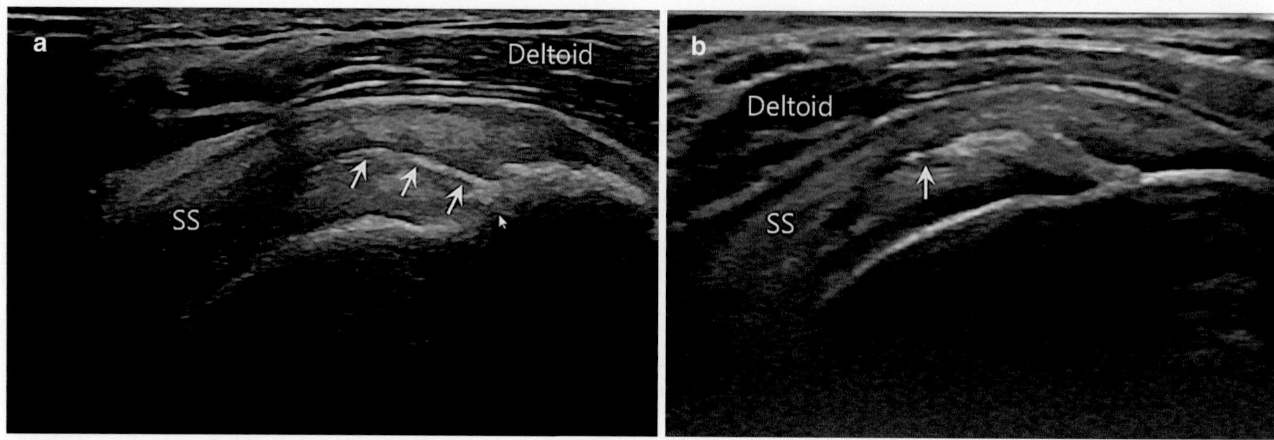

Fig. 21.8 Striation (**a**) or spiculated calcification (**b**) suggestive of a previously ruptured calcification. (Reprinted with permission from Dr. Sang Hoon Lee)

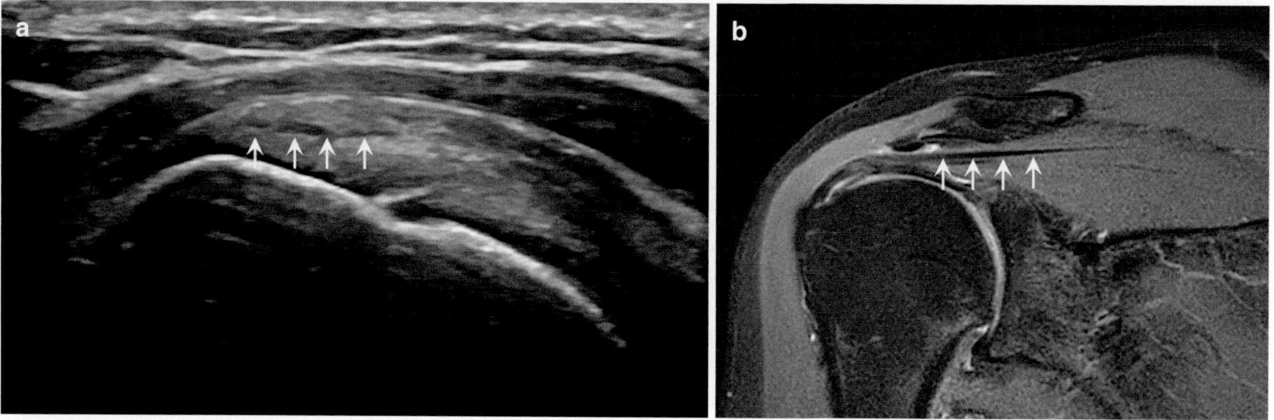

Fig. 21.9 Correlation of supraspinatus tendon between ultrasound (**a**) with MRI (**b**); both show delamination tear of the tendon (arrows) in the site of calcification inside the supraspinatus tendon. (Reprinted with permission from Dr. Sang Hoon Lee)

Suggested Reading

Chiou HJ, Chou YH, Wu JJ, Hsu CC, Huang DY, Chang CY. Evaluation of calcific tendonitis of the rotator cuff: role of color Doppler ultrasonography. J Ultrasound Med. 2002;21:289–95.

Choe W-Y, Want C-J, et al. Prognostic factors for the outcome of extracorporeal shockwave therapy for calcific tendinitis of the shoulder. Bone Joint J. 2017:1643–50.

Ciccone CD. Does acetic acid iontophoresis accelerate the resorption of calcium deposits in calcific tendinitis of the shoulder? Phys Ther. 2003;83:68–74.

Comfort TH, Arafiles RP. Barbotage of the shoulder with image-intensified fluoroscopic control of needle placement for calcific tendinitis. Clin Ortho Relat Res. 1978:171–8.

Cooper G, Lutz GE, Adler RS. Ultrasound-guided aspiration of symptomatic rotator cuff calcific tendonitis. Am J Phys Med Rehab. 2005;84:81.

del Cura JL, Torre I, Zabala R, Legorburu A. Sonographically guided percutaneous needle lavage in calcific tendinitis of the shoulder: short- and long-term results. AJR. 2007;189:W128–34.

Farin PU, Jaroma H, Soimakallio S. Rotator cuff calcifications: treatment with US-guided technique. Radiology. 1995;195:841–3.

Farin PU, Rasanen H, Jaroma H, Harju A. Rotator cuff calcifications. treatment with ultrasound-guided percutaneous needle aspiration and lavage. Skeletal Radiol. 1996;25:551–4.

Farr S, Sevelda F, Mader P, Graf A, Petje G, Sabeti-Aschraf M. Extracorporeal shockwave therapy in calcifying tendinitis of the shoulder. Knee Surg Sport Tr A. 2011;19:2085–9.

Gerdesmeyer L, Wagenpfeil S, Haake M, et al. Extracorporeal shock wave therapy for the treatment of chronic calcifying tendonitis of the rotator cuff: a randomized controlled trial. JAMA. 2003;290:2573–80.

Giacomoni P, Siliotto R. Echo-guided percutaneous treatment of chronic calcific tendinitis of the shoulder. La Radiologia Medica. 1999;98:386–90.

Gosens T, Hofstee DJ. Calcifying tendinitis of the shoulder: advances in imaging and management. Curr Rheumatol Rep. 2009;11:129–34.

Hamada J, Ono W, Tamai K, Saotome K, Hoshino T. Analysis of calcium deposits in calcific periarthritis. J Rheumatol. 2001;28:809–13.

Hsu CJ, Wang DY, Tseng KF, Fong YC, Hsu HC, Jim YF. Extracorporeal shock wave therapy for calcifying tendinitis of the shoulder. J Shoulder Elbow Surg. 2008;17:55–9.

Hurt G, Baker CL Jr. Calcific tendinitis of the shoulder. Orthop Clin of N Am. 2003;34:567–75.

Iwashita S, Hashiguchi H, Okubo A, Yoneda M, Takai S. Characteristics of the patients with delaminated rotator cuff tear. SICOT J. 2018;4:28.

Kim J-H, Jung S-H. Delaminated rotator cuff tear: concurrent concept and treatment. Clin Shoulder Elbow. 2019;22(3):159–70.

Lee KS, Rosas HG. Musculoskeletal ultrasound: how to treat calcific tendinitis of the rotator cuff by ultrasound-guided single-needle lavage technique. AJR. 2010;195:638.

Lin JT, Adler RS, Bracilovic A, Cooper G, Sofka C, Lutz GE. Clinical outcomes of ultrasound-guided aspiration and lavage in calcific tendinosis of the shoulder. HSS J. 2007;3:99–105.

Louis LJ. Musculoskeletal ultrasound intervention: principles and advances. Radiol Clin N Am. 2008;46:515–33.

Maier M, Schmidt-Ramsin J, Glaser C, Kunz A, Kuchenhoff H, Tischer T. Intra- and interobserver reliability of classification scores in calcific tendinitis using plain radiographs and CT scans. Acta Orthop Belg. 2008;74:590–5.

McKendry RJ, Uhthoff HK, Sarkar K, Hyslop PS. Calcifying tendinitis of the shoulder: prognostic value of clinical, histologic, and radiologic features in 57 surgically treated cases. J Rheumatol. 1982;9:75–80.

Minamizaki T, Nakao Y, et al. The matrix vesicle cargo miR-125b accumulates in the bone matrix, inhibiting bone resorption in mice. Commun Biol. 2020;3(1):30.

Ottenheijm RPG, vant Klooster IGM, et al. Ultrasound-diagnosed disorders in shoulder patients in daily general practice: a retrospective observational study. BMC Fam Pract. 2014;15:115.

Sarkar K, Uhthoff HK. Ultrastructural localization of calcium in calcifying tendinitis. Arch Pathol Lab Med. 1978;102:266–9.

Speed CA, Hazleman BL. Calcific tendinitis of the shoulder. N Engl J Med. 1999;340:1582–4.

Speed CA, Richards C, Nichols D, et al. Extracorporeal shockwave therapy for tendonitis of the rotator cuff. A double-blind, randomised, controlled trial. J Bone Joint Surg (B). 2002;84:509–12.

Uhthoff HK, Loehr JW. Calcific tendinopathy of the rotator cuff: pathogenesis, diagnosis, and management. J Am Acad Ortho Surg. 1997;5:183–91.

Walz DM, Miller TT, Chen S, Hofman J. MR imaging of delamination tears of the rotator cuff tendons. Skeletal Radiol. 2007;36(5):411–6.

Yoo JC, Koh KH, Park WH, Park JC, Kim SM, Yoon YC. The outcome of ultrasound-guided needle decompression and steroid injection in calcific tendinitis. J Shoulder Elbow Surg. 2010;19:596–600.

Zazzeroni L, Faggioli G, Pasquinelli G. The Mechanisms of arterial calcification: the role of matrix vesicles. Eur J Vasc Endovasc Surg. 2018:1–8.

22 Shoulder Denervation

John Tran and Philip Peng

Contents

General Consideration

With a prevalence of 18–26%, shoulder pain is the third most common musculoskeletal complaint and the leading cause of nontraumatic pain in the upper limb. It encompasses a constellation of pain conditions including rotator cuff tendinopathy, degenerative tears and impingement, glenohumeral and acromioclavicular joint osteoarthritis, adhesive capsulitis, and labral tears. Pain and the associated decrease in range of motion impact negatively on the quality of life leading to substantial economic and healthcare burdens.

J. Tran
Division of Anatomy, Department of Surgery, University of Toronto, Toronto, ON, Canada
e-mail: johnjt.tran@utoronto.ca

P. Peng (✉)
Department of Anesthesia and Pain Medicine, University of Toronto Toronto Western Hospital, Toronto, ON, Canada
e-mail: philip.peng@uhn.ca

Although the initial management of various shoulder pain is conservative measures such as pharmacologic treatment and physiotherapy, patients with moderate to severe symptoms suffer severe disability and are usually less responsive to conservative treatment. Operative management is often offered if other options fail; however, surgical options do not always provide pain relief. Unlike the hip and knee, the outcome of shoulder surgery is not as promising. The risks of persistent pain following shoulder arthroplasty and subacromial surgery are 22% and 20%, respectively. Various shoulder injections, such as intra-articular or bursa injections, are available, but the effects are short term and the efficacy decreases with advanced disease.

Similar to the facet joints of the spine, and recently hip and knee joints, one approach for pain management is to

D. Jankovic, P. Peng (eds.), *Regional Nerve Blocks in Anesthesia and Pain Therapy*,
https://doi.org/10.1007/978-3-030-88727-8_22

partially denervate the shoulder joint. In the past, the main target has been the entire suprascapular nerve at the suprascapular notch. A recent publication from Tran et al., documenting the course of articular branches supplying the shoulder joint, has laid out an anatomical road map for defining alternative ablation target sites for the suprascapular nerve and other articular branches (Fig. 22.1). This provides the opportunity to develop more selective targets for shoulder denervation procedures with function-preserving implications.

Indication (Patient Selection)

A thorough assessment is important in determining the pathology to be managed. The pathologies can be rotator cuff disease, glenohumeral or acromioclavicular joint and are summarized in Table 22.1. In addition, the assessment allows both clinician and the patient to appreciate the baseline range of movement and strength. This is important in the patient selection process as the denervation procedure may impact the motor function of rotator cuff muscles.

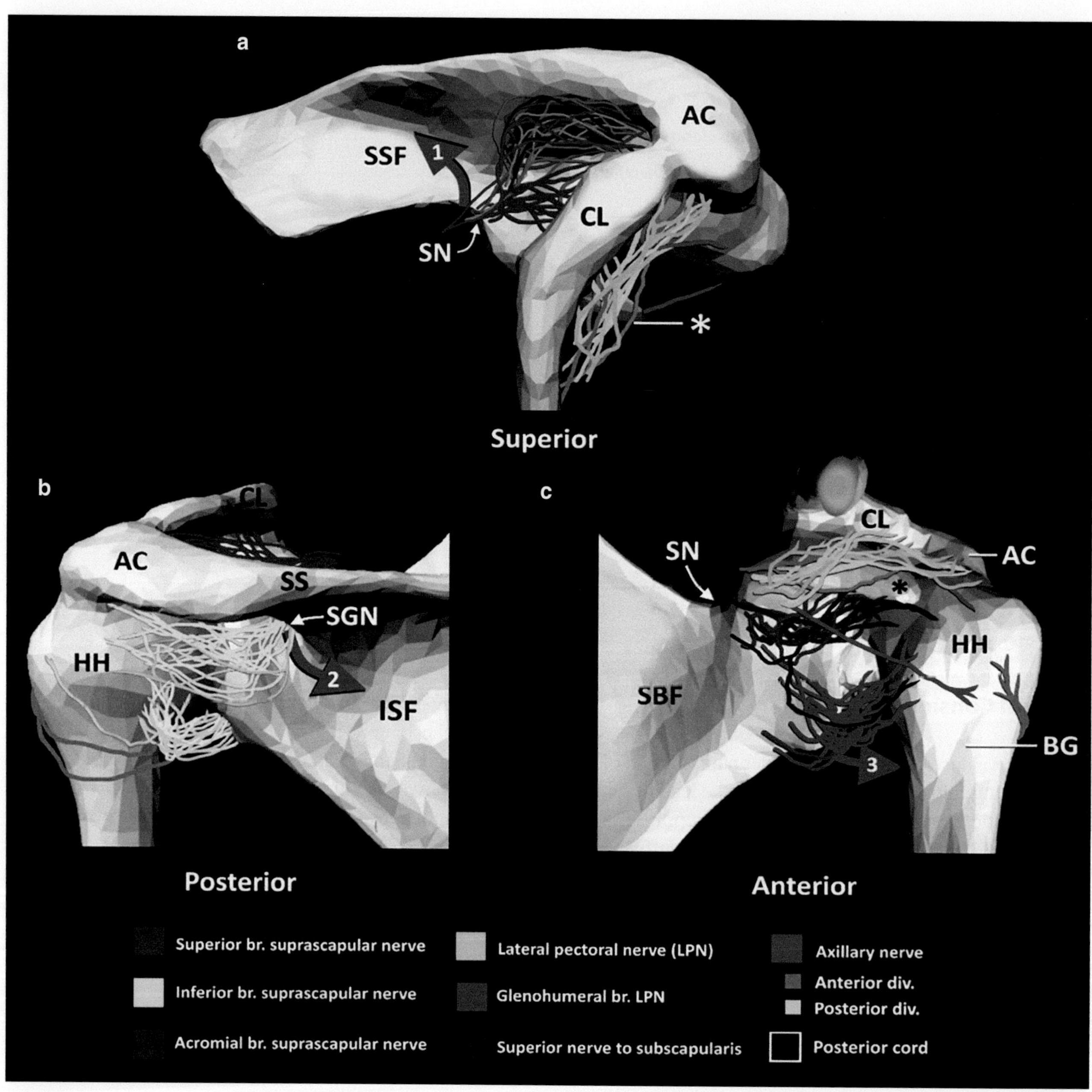

Fig. 22.1 Frequency map of innervation of glenohumeral and acromioclavicular joints. Numbered arrows in Figure **a**–**c** indicate course of (1) medial trunk of suprascapular nerve (SSN), (2) motor branches of SSN supplying infraspinatus, (3) anterior and posterior divisions (div) of AN. *AC* indicates acromion process, *BG* bicipital groove, *CL* clavicle, *CP* coracoid process, *HH* humeral head, *ISF* infraspinous fossa, *SBF* subscapular fossa, *SGN* spinoglenoid notch, *SN* suprascapular notch, *SS* spine of scapula, *SSF* suprascapular fossa, and *, coracoid process. Reproduced with permission from Philip Peng Educational Series

Table 22.1 Targets of articular branches corresponding to the shoulder pathology

Pathology	Nerve(s) to be denervated
Rotator cuff disease	SSN ± LPN-ab
Glenohumeral joint disease	SSN, NSc, ax-ab ± ax-pb ± LPN-ab
Acromioclavicular joint disease	SSN-ab, LPN-ab

SSN suprascapular nerve, *NSc* nerve to subscapularis, *Ax-ab* axillary nerve anterior branch, *Ax-pb* axillary nerve posterior branch, *SSN-ab* suprascapular nerve acromial branch, *LPN-ab* lateral pectoral nerve acromial branch

The two rotator cuff muscles innervated by the suprascapular nerve are supraspinatus and infraspinatus. A detailed pre-procedure examination and radiologic evaluation is important. The impact of loss of motor function from supraspinatus is minimal if there is a complete tear of the supraspinatus or the abduction is predominately from scapulothoracic movement (minimal or absence of glenohumeral movement). The impact of the loss of motor function from infraspinatus is minimal if there is a complete tear of infraspinatus or the external rotation is well compensated by other muscles (serratus anterior, latissimus dorsi, posterior deltoid, and teres minor).

If the baseline function of the rotator cuff is well preserved, the patient should be warned about the potential risk of decrease motor strength in the consent.

Functional Anatomy

The shoulder consists of the glenohumeral, sternoclavicular, and acromioclavicular joints. Clinically, pain from the sternoclavicular joint is rare. Previous cadaveric studies have elucidated the nerve supply to these joints. The glenohumeral joint has been reported to receive innervation from the suprascapular, lateral pectoral, subscapular, and axillary nerves, whereas the acromioclavicular joint is mainly supplied by articular branches of the suprascapular and lateral pectoral nerves. It has also been reported that these four nerves supply innervation to the surrounding bursae and ligaments (coracoclavicular, coracoacromial, and coracohumeral) of the shoulder. The course of articular nerves, supplying joints and bursae, relative to bony and soft tissue landmarks, is important to successfully perform shoulder procedures to manage joint pain and will be described below.

Suprascapular Nerve

The suprascapular nerve originates from the superior trunk of the brachial plexus and courses posterolaterally to the suprascapular notch where it passes deep to the suprascapular ligament to enter the supraspinous fossa (Fig. 22.2). The first branch of the suprascapular nerve, the acromial branch, originates just proximal or at the suprascapular notch. The acromial branch of suprascapular nerve continues deep to the suprascapular ligament and courses laterally along the posterior surface of the coracoid process. The nerve continues in a superolateral direction to emerge anterior to the supraspinatus where it supplies articular branches to the coracoclavicular and coracohumeral ligaments, as well as the subacromial bursa. The acromial branch of suprascapular nerve terminates as articular branches innervating the acromioclavicular joint. After passing through the suprascapular notch, the suprascapular nerve bifurcates into medial and lateral trunks deep to the supraspinatus. The medial trunk mainly supplies innervation to the supraspinatus, whereas the lateral trunk courses along the floor of the supraspinous fossa to reach the spinoglenoid notch. Along its course, deep to the supraspinatus, the lateral trunk gives off articular branches which course posterolaterally to supply the posterosuperior glenohumeral joint, as well as the subacromial bursa. The lateral trunk of suprascapular nerve continues inferiorly to enter the infraspinous fossa. Within the infraspinous fossa, the lateral trunk supplies muscular branches to the infraspinatus as well as articular branches that course laterally to the posterosuperior glenohumeral joint capsule located deep to the tendon of the infraspinatus.

Lateral Pectoral Nerve

The lateral pectoral nerve has its origin from the lateral cord of the brachial plexus and supply muscular branches that innervate the pectoralis muscles. The lateral pectoral nerve also supplies an acromial branch which courses laterally along the superior surface of the coracoid process, just anterior to the coracoclavicular ligament, in a neurovascular bundle with its corresponding vessels (Figs. 22.3 and 22.4). The acromial branch of lateral pectoral nerve continues laterally along the coracoacromial ligament to terminate in the acromioclavicular joint. Prior to terminating in the acromioclavicular joint, the acromial branch of lateral pectoral nerve supplies branches to the coracoclavicular and coracoacromial ligaments as well as the subacromial bursa.

Subscapular Nerves

The subscapular nerves originate from the posterior cord of the brachial plexus and innervate the subscapularis muscle. The most superior subscapular nerve provides an articular nerve that courses superolaterally to reach the superior border of the musculotendinous junction of the subscapularis (Fig. 22.4). At this location, the nerve continues laterally by coursing between the inferior surface of the coracoid process and superior border of the subscapularis musculotendinous junction to supply the subcoracoid bursa and innervate the

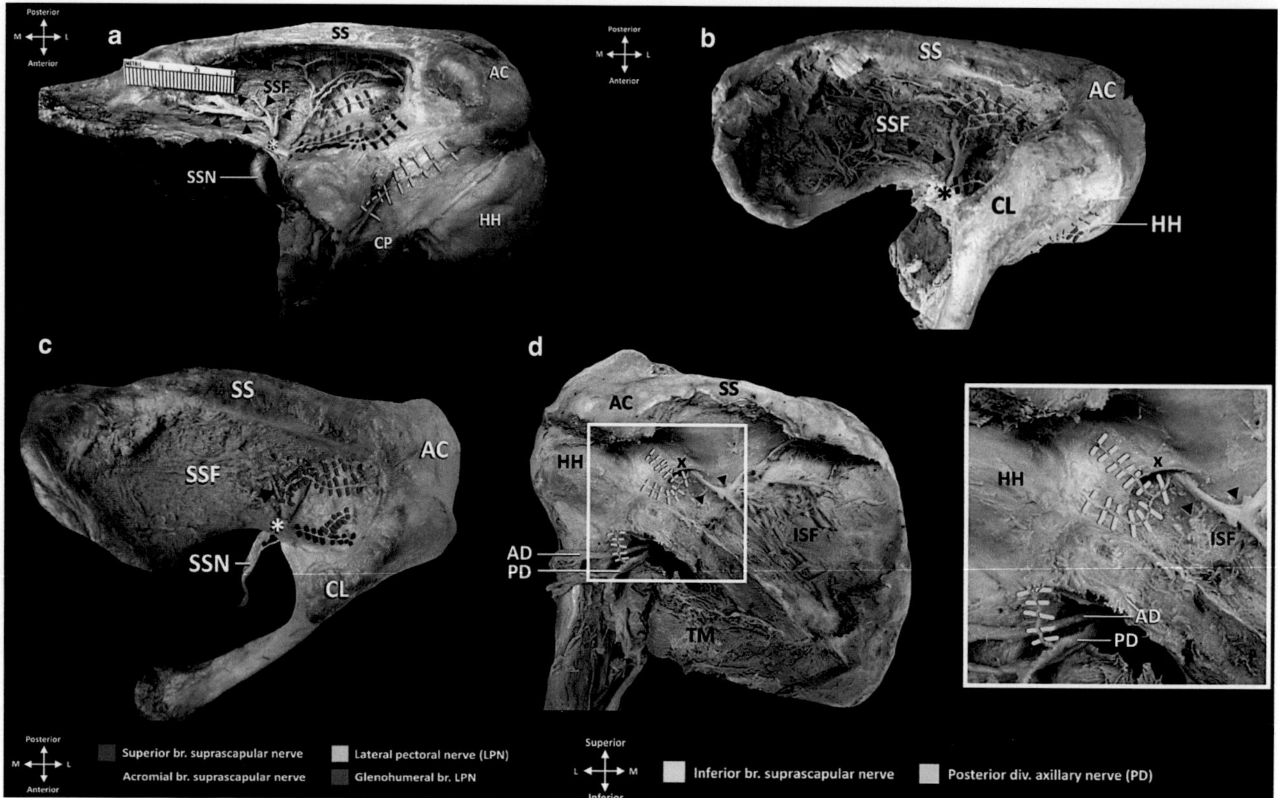

Fig. 22.2 Innervation of acromioclavicular joint (ACJ) and posterosuperior quadrant of glenohumeral joint (GHJ). (**a**) and (**b**). Articular branches to GHJ originating from the lateral trunk of suprascapular nerve (SSN) and acromial branch (br) of SSN and lateral pectoral nerve (LPN) to ACJ. Note the clavicle has been disarticulated and removed in (**a** . (**c**) . SSN articular branches to GHJ and ACJ. Articular branches to GHJ originate from bifurcation of SSN into medial and lateral trunks and acromial branches to ACJ from SSN. (**b**). Inferior branch (br) of SSN and posterior division (div) of AN. Note infraspinatus and teres minor have been removed. *AC* indicates acromion process, *AD* anterior division of axillary nerve, *HH* humeral head, *ISF* infraspinous fossa, *LHT* long head of triceps brachii, *SS* spine of scapula, *TM* teres major; black arrowheads, motor branches of SSN supplying infraspinatus; and x, spinoglenoid ligament. *AC* indicates acromion process, *CL* clavicle, *CP* coracoid process, *HH* humeral head, *SS* spine of scapula, *SSF* suprascapular fossa, *SSN* main trunk of suprascapular nerve; black arrowheads, medial trunk of SSN; and *, transverse scapular ligament. Reprinted with permission from Philip Peng Education Series

anterosuperior glenohumeral joint deep to the tendon of the subscapularis.

Axillary Nerve

The axillary nerve is a terminal branch of the posterior cord. The nerve courses in an inferolateral direction along the surface of the subscapularis to reach its inferior border where it continues posteriorly through the quadrangular space (Figs. 22.3 and 22.4). Prior to entering the quadrangular space, the axillary nerve gives off one to two branches that course along the inferior border of the musculotendinous junction of the subscapularis muscle. These articular branches course superiorly, deep to the tendon of the subscapularis, to supply the anteroinferior glenohumeral joint. As the axillary nerve passes through the quadrangular space, it divides into anterior and posterior divisions. The posterior division which innervates the posterior deltoid and teres minor also provides a branch that courses superiorly deep to the teres minor to innervate the posteroinferior glenohumeral joint. The anterior division of axillary nerve, after wrapping laterally around the surgical neck of the humerus, with the posterior circumflex humeral artery, inconsistently supplies articular branches to the lateral humerus and subacromial bursa.

Target-Specific Anatomy

From a clinical perspective, the clinician should be cognizant about what targets to denervate based on the clinical presentation. If the patient presents with rotator cuff disease, suprascapular nerve is the major target, although lateral pectoral and axillary nerve both contribute to a minor extent. If the patient presents with pain from acromioclavicular joint, both acromial branches of lateral pectoral and suprascapular nerves will be the target. If the patient has symptomatic

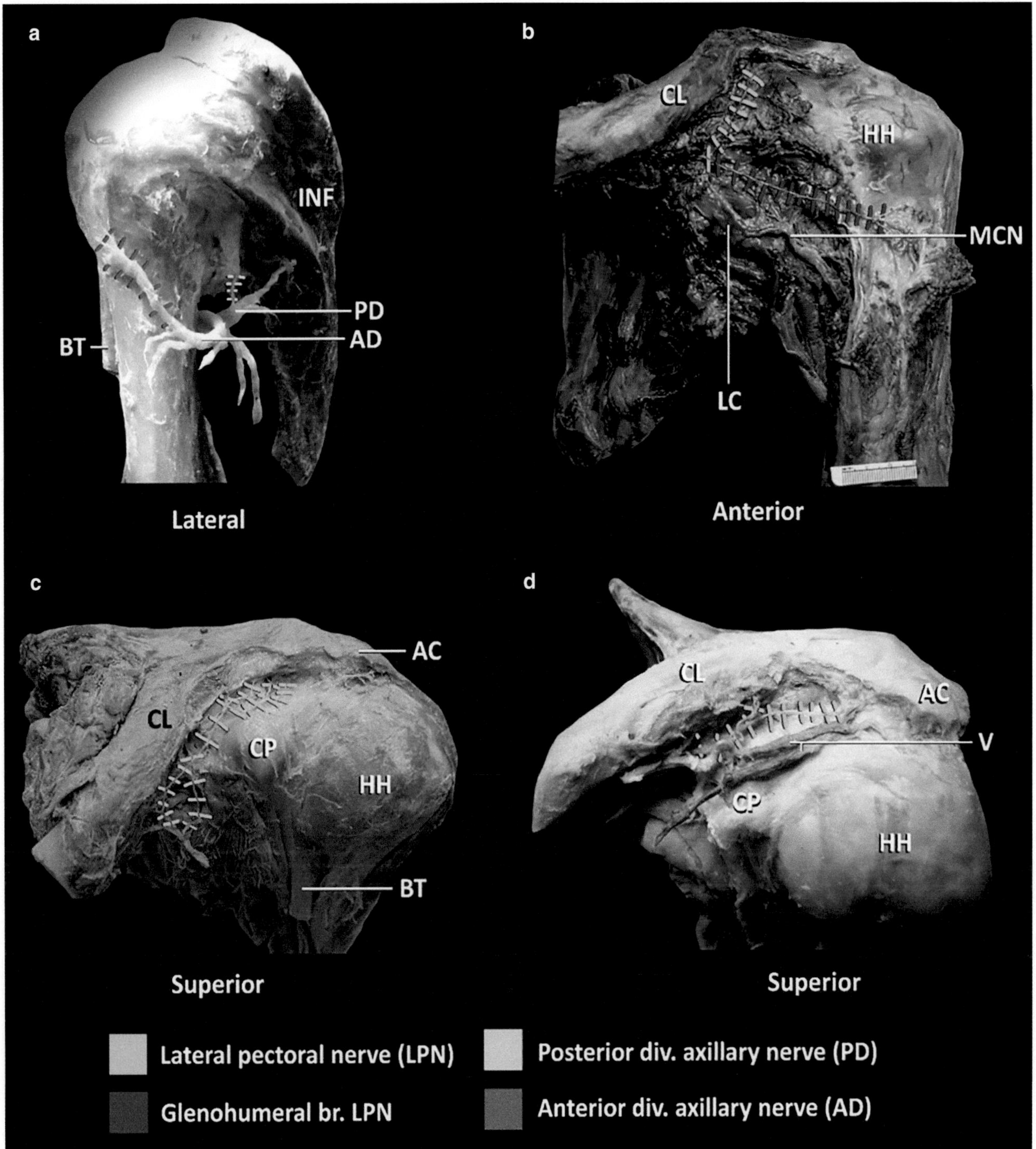

Fig. 22.3 Course of articular branches of anterior division of axillary nerve (AN) and lateral pectoral nerve (LPN). (**a**) and (**b**). Innervation of acromioclavicular joint (ACJ) and posteroinferior/anteroinferior quadrants of glenohumeral joint (GHJ). (**c**) and (**d**). Innervation of ACJ by LPN. *AC* acromion process, *BT* tendon of long head of biceps brachii, *CL* clavicle, *CP* coracoid process, *HH* humeral head, *INF* infraspinatus, *LC* lateral cord, *MCN* musculocutaneous nerve, *V* acromial branches of thoraco-acromial artery and vein. Reprinted with permission from Philip Peng Education Series

glenohumeral joint arthritis, more nerves should be considered for denervation. Suprascapular nerve supplies the superior and posterosuperior joint capsule, while anterior capsule is innervated by nerve to subscapularis, anterior branch of axillary nerve and acromial branch of lateral pectoral nerve. One may consider denervation of the posterior branches of the axillary nerve. At the present time, the literature is scant in this target-orientated denervation.

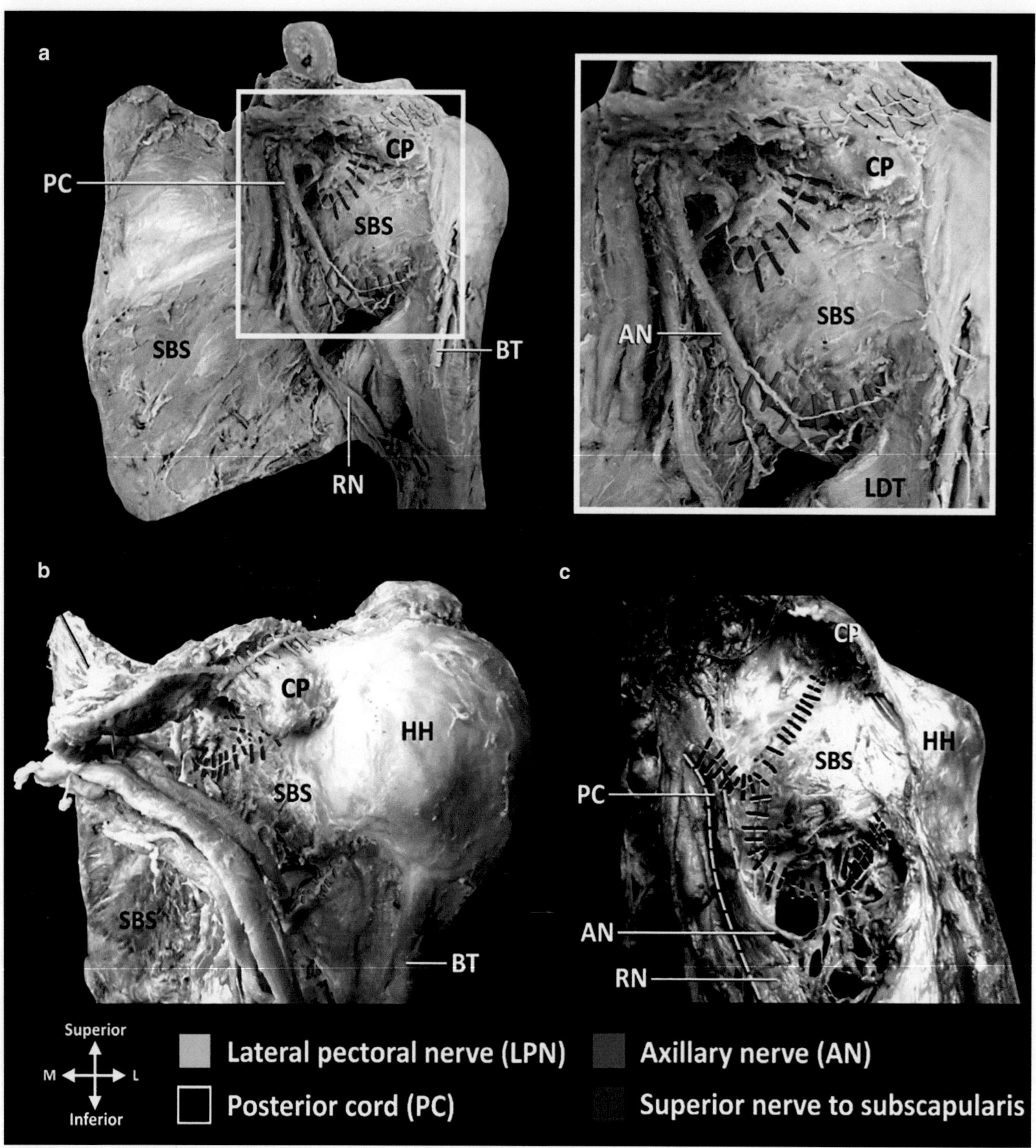

Fig. 22.4 Innervation of acromioclavicular joint (ACJ) and anterior glenohumeral joint (GHJ) capsule. (**a**) and (**b**). Superior nerve to subscapularis and axillary nerve innervate GHJ and lateral pectoral nerve the ACJ. Inset photo is enlargement of area in white box in (**a**). (**c**) Articular branches from posterior cord innervating the GHJ. Yellow dash lines outline the posterior cord and its bifurcation into axillary (AN) and radial (RN) nerves. *BT* indicates tendon of long head of biceps brachii, *CP* coracoid process, *HH* humeral head, *LDT* tendon of latissimus dorsi, and *SBS* subscapularis. Reprinted with permission from Philip Peng Education Series

In addition, the literature also describes the distribution of nociceptor and mechanoreceptors in the shoulder. Subacromial bursa has the highest density of the nociceptor. The superior capsules (both anterior and posterior) are more densely innervated with both mechanoreceptors and nociceptors. In such patients, targeting the suprascapular nerve and acromial branch of lateral pectoral nerve should be considered as they innervate the subacromial bursa.

Technique

From the literature, the denervation technique focused on the suprascapular nerve, which is a mixed motor and sensory nerve. Because of this, most of the publication described the use of pulsed radiofrequency technique. With the current new understanding of the innervation of the shoulder, a few techniques have been proposed but clinical trials are lacking. The techniques below are based on anatomical data and future clinical trials are required to prove analgesic efficacy and safety.

Suprascapular Nerve Midpoint Denervation

Because branches supplying the subacromial bursa and superior capsule originate from the lateral trunk of the suprascapular nerve (Fig. 22.5), the midpoint between the

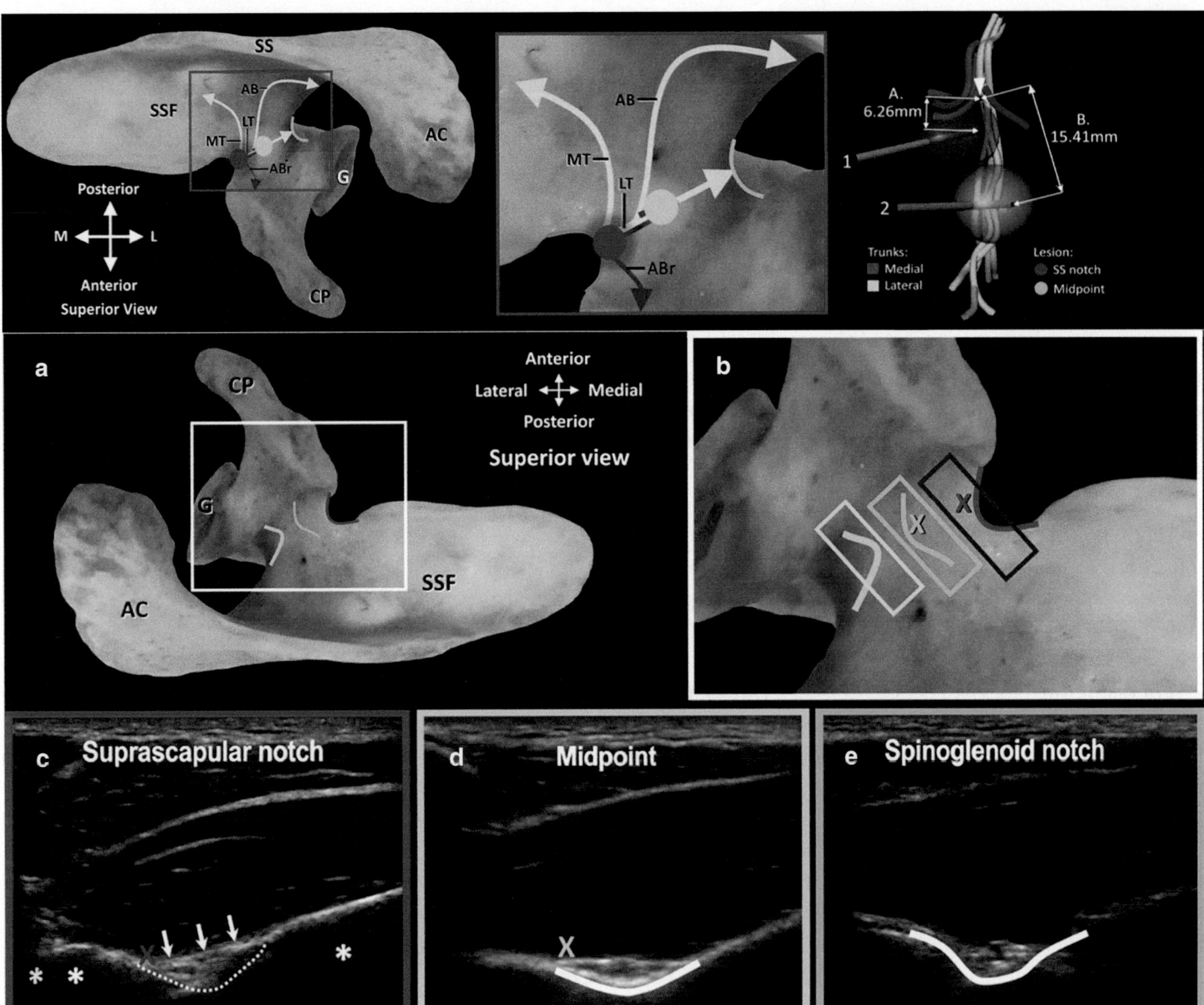

Fig. 22.5 Top panel. Schematic display of two possible lesions on the suprascapular nerve (SSN): one at the suprascapular (SS) notch (red) and the other the midpoint (green) of a line between the suprascapular (light blue curve) and spinoglenoid (green curve) notches. As the SSN enters the suprascapular notch, it gives out two branches: medial trunk (MT) which is the motor branch to supraspinatus and the acromial branch (ABr) which supplies the acromioclavicular joint and subacromial bursa. From the lateral trunk (LT), the articular branch (AB) is the first articular branch from LT of SSN. *AC* acromion process, *CP* coracoid process, *G* glenoid fossa, *SS* spine of scapula, *SSF* supraspinous fossa. The right diagram showed the two hypothetical lesions and the distance measurements from needle tips (1 and 2). A lesion in the midpoint is 15.41 mm from the medial trunk and is a safe distance from the motor branch of the supraspinatus. Middle panel. (**a**) Methodology for landmarking radiofrequency needle placement. (**a**) Localization of needle placement at suprascapular notch (red curve), spinoglenoid notch (turquoise curve), and midpoint between the notches (green curve). (**b**) The ultrasound probe position corresponding to the sonographic pictures in the low panel. Low panel. (**c**) Sonography of suprascapular notch. Note the bony contour of the notch (dotted line) is not as hyperechoic as the adjacent scapular bone, which cast an anechoic shadow (*). The suprascapular ligament is hyperechoic as outlined by white arrows. (**d**) Sonogram of floor of the scapular fossa midpoint between the notches. (**e**) Sonogram of spinoglenoid notch. Note the contour of the bony floor is steeper than that of the floor of scapular fossa midpoint between the notches. *AC* acromion, *CP* coracoid process, *G* glenoid fossa, *SSF* supraspinous fossa, *X* radiofrequency needle placement targets. Reprinted with permission from Philip Peng educational series

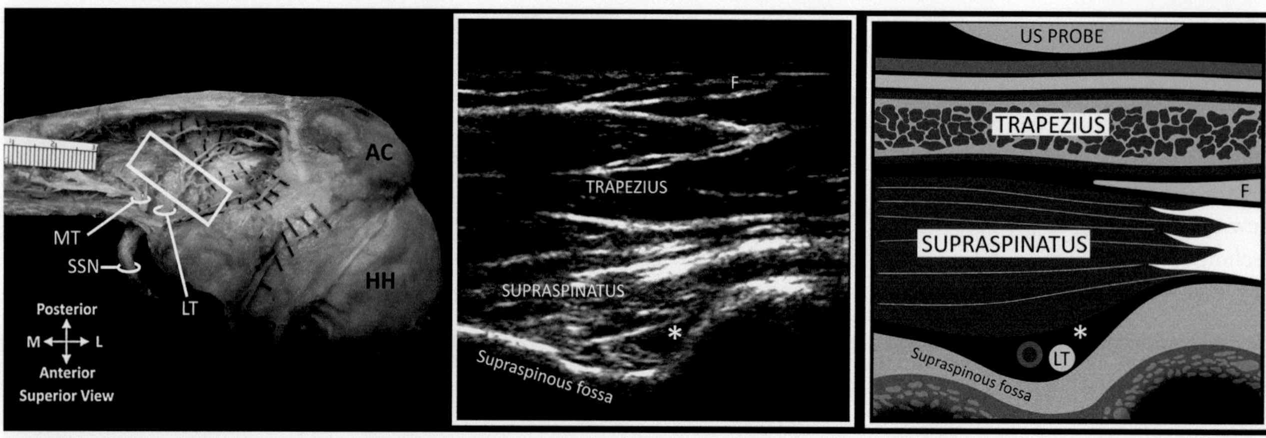

Fig. 22.6 Anatomic dissection, ultrasonography, and schematic diagram of midpoint suprascapular nerve (SSN) target. The white rectangle depicts the position of probe for the sonographic image. *MT* medial trunk, *LT* lateral trunk, *F* adipose tissue. Reprinted with permission from Philip Peng educational series

suprascapular and spinoglenoid notches is an ideal technique to selectively target the lateral trunk of suprascapular nerve.

Under sterile technique and with the patient on the lateral position (the shoulder for procedure on the non-dependent side), the suprascapular nerve in the supraspinatus fossa is scanned methodologically. The orientation of the suprascapular nerve is estimated by a line joining the coracoid process and acromion. The ultrasound probe is placed in short axis to this line. By moving the probe in anterior and posterior direction, the suprascapular and spinoglenoid notch are revealed (Fig. 22.6). The midpoint between the two notches will be the target.

For diagnostic block, a 22-gauge 3.5-inch Quincke needle is inserted out-of-plane or in-plane into the fascia space between the supraspinatus and floor of the supraspinous fossa followed by the administration of 1–2 mL of local anesthetic.

For radiofrequency procedure, the authors recommend out-of-plane technique to minimize the needle trauma. Because of the angle of the needle to the nerve, the authors prefer a Trident needle (Diros® Markham, Canada) or Cooled radiofrequency system so the lesion size can cover the nerve on the floor of the fossa. Motor testing is important. The optimal response is the exclusive stimulation of the infraspinatus without supraspinatus. The clinician should put the hand on both muscles above and below the spine of scapula to detect the muscle contraction. If there is contraction of supraspinatus, the needle can be repositioned in a more distal location. If the infraspinatus contraction is not strong, the needle can be repositioned in a medial-lateral fashion toward the suprascapular nerve.

The target suprascapular nerve is much bigger than the usual articular branches for radiofrequency lesioning. The authors suggest increasing the setting of radiofrequency with longer duration and higher temperature. In the author's experience, it may take more than one radiofrequency lesioning to achieve a long-lasting effect.

Suprascapular Nerve Acromial Branch Denervation

The lesion created by the above midpoint ablation does not cover the acromial branch of the suprascapular nerve (Fig. 22.5). Because this acromial branch supplies the ligaments, subacromial bursa, and posterior aspect of the acromioclavicular joint, patients with pain in this area may benefit from a separate lesion.

The suprascapular notch can be scanned as described in Fig. 22.5. Out-of-plane needle inserted is performed and the direction of the needle is toward the base of the coracoid process (Figs. 22.7 and 22.8).

Lateral Pectoral Nerve Acromial Branch Denervation

This is the terminal sensory branch of the lateral pectoral nerve. The nerve is accompanied by the acromial branch of the thoraco-acromial vessels in the space between the clavicle and coracoid process (Fig. 22.9). Here, the neurovascular bundle is between the anterior deltoid and coracoclavicular ligament (trapezoid).

With a linear high-frequency probe and the patient in supine position, the initial placement is in short axis of clavicle close to the glenohumeral joint. The probe is pivoted until the appearance of the coracoid process (Figs. 22.9 and

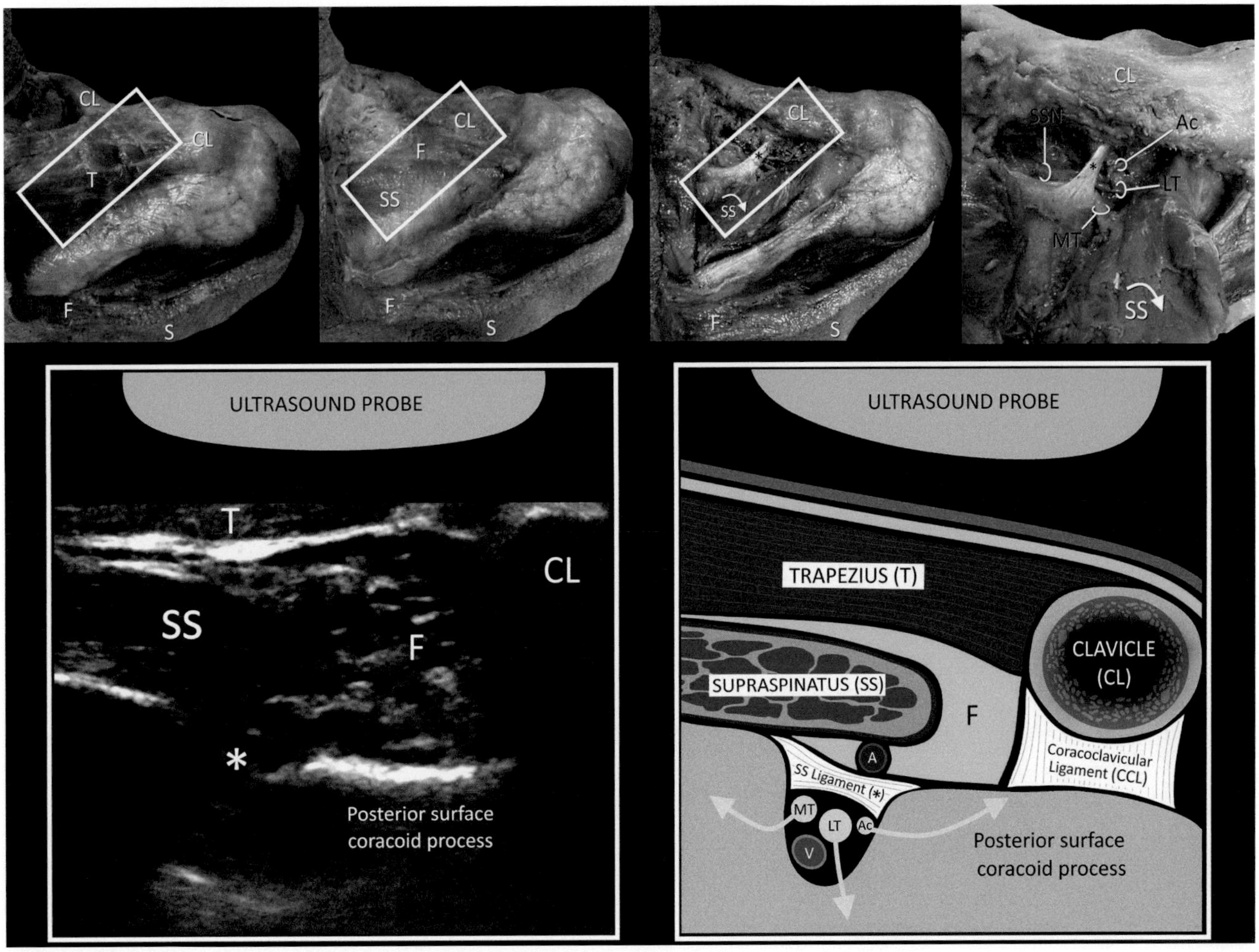

Fig. 22.7 Anatomic dissection, ultrasonography, and schematic diagram of the acromial branch of suprascapular nerve (SSN). The white rectangle depicts the position of probe for the sonographic image. *MT* medial trunk, *LT* lateral trunk, *F* adipose tissue, *SS* supraspinatus, *CL* clavicle, *Ac* acromion, *T* trapezius. Reprinted with permission from Philip Peng educational series

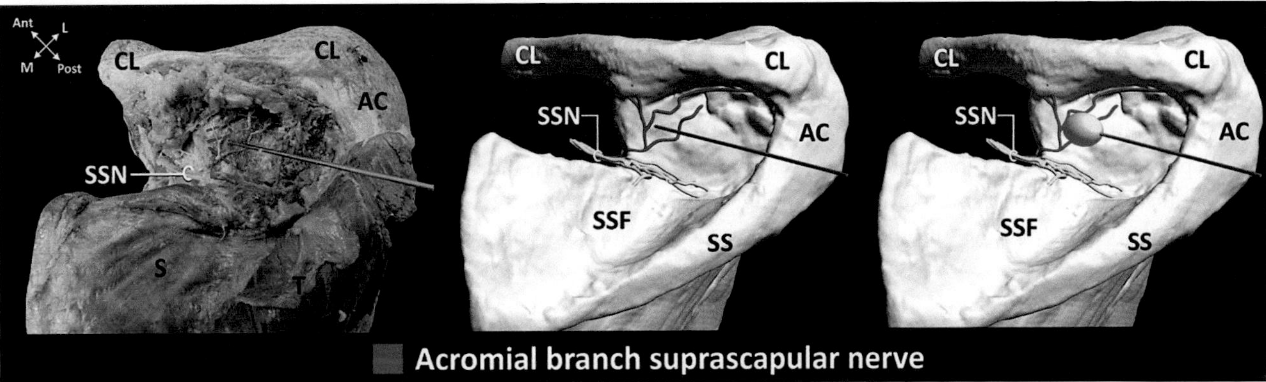

Fig. 22.8 The needle target for the acromial branch of suprascapular nerve (SSN) in the cadaveric specimen. The right two diagrams are the digitalized images of the specimen, and the orange color lesion is the simulated lesion at the base of the coracoid process. *CL* clavicle, *Ac* acromion, *SS* scapular spine, *SSF* suprascapular fossa. Reprinted with permission from Philip Peng educational series

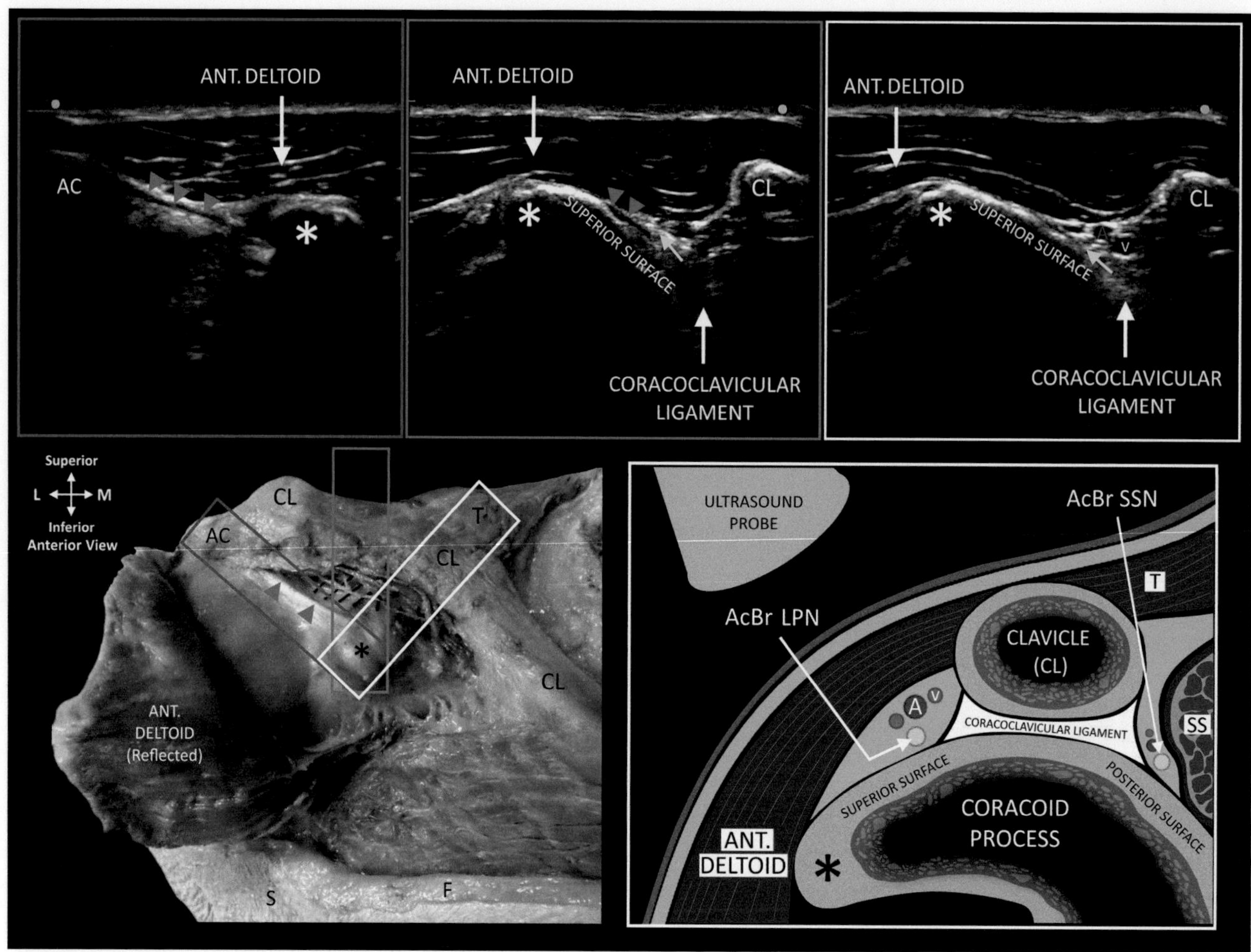

Fig. 22.9 Anatomic dissection, ultrasonography, and schematic diagram of the acromial branch of the lateral pectoral nerve (AcBr LPN). Green, blue, and white rectangles show the positions of the ultrasound probe for the images in the corresponding boxes in the top panel. *CL* clavicle, *Ac* acromion, *SS* supraspinatus, *A&V* suprascapular artery and vein, blue arrowheads, coracoacromial ligament; yellow arrow, acromial branch of the lateral pectoral nerve; *T* trapezius; *, tip of coracoid process. Reprinted with permission from Philip Peng educational series

22.10). With proper positioning, a three-layered display of structures should be seen. The lateral pectoral nerve articular branch is just caudal to the acromial artery. The needle can be inserted either in-plane or out-of-plane. Because of the small space, 0.5 to 1 mL of local anesthetic is sufficient for the diagnostic block. For radiofrequency lesioning, the setting is similar to the lesioning of other articular branches in hip and knee.

Deep Subscapular Space (Nerve to Subscapularis and Anterior Branch of Axillary Nerve)

Both the articular branches from subscapularis and anterior branch of axillary nerves can be found in the fascia plane deep to the subscapularis. On the glenoid side, there is a fascia plane, deep subscapular space (Fig. 22.11). On the humeral side, the subscapularis tendon-bone interface will be easily hydrodissected as the subscapularis inserts onto the facet on the medial side of the lesser tubercle.

This procedure should be performed with imaging, i.e., fluoroscopy and/or ultrasound. With the patient in supine position, the glenoid process is seen deep to the subscapularis in ultrasound and anteroposterior view of the glenohumeral joint. For diagnostic block, the needle is inserted through the subscapularis on the glenoid, and a volume of 2 mL of local anesthetic is administered. For the radiofrequency, the authors suggest a bipolar lesion with one needle on the upper half and another needle on the lower half of the glenoid (Fig. 22.12).

Posterior Division of the Axillary Nerve

The posterior division of the axillary nerve sends articular branches that ascend deep to the teres minor to reach the

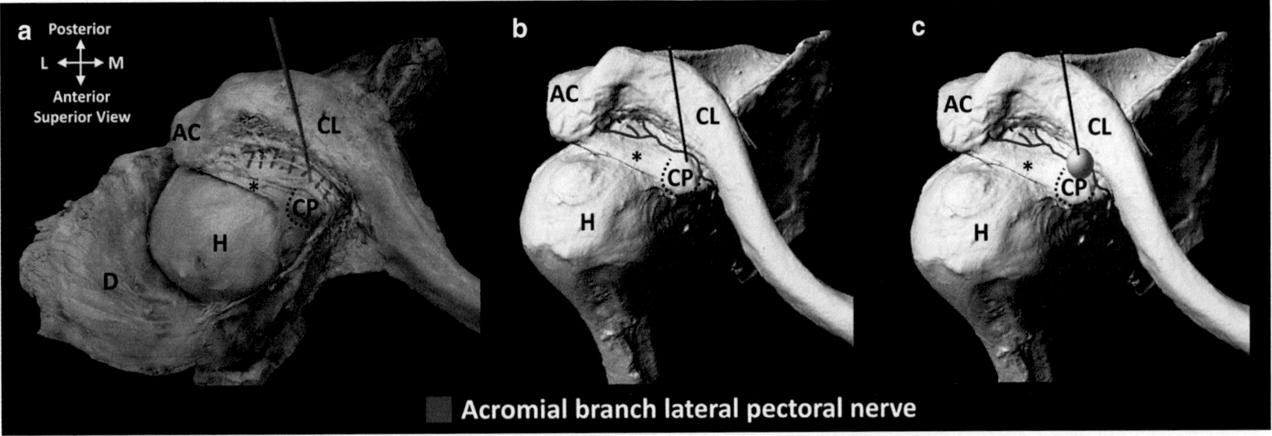

Fig. 22.10 The needle target for the acromial branch of the lateral pectoral nerve in the cadaveric specimen (**a**). The right two diagrams (**b**, **c**) are the digitalized images of the specimen, and the orange color lesion is the simulated lesion at the tip of the coracoid process. *CL* clavicle, *Ac* acromion, *CP* coracoid process, *H* humeral head. Reprinted with permission from Philip Peng educational series

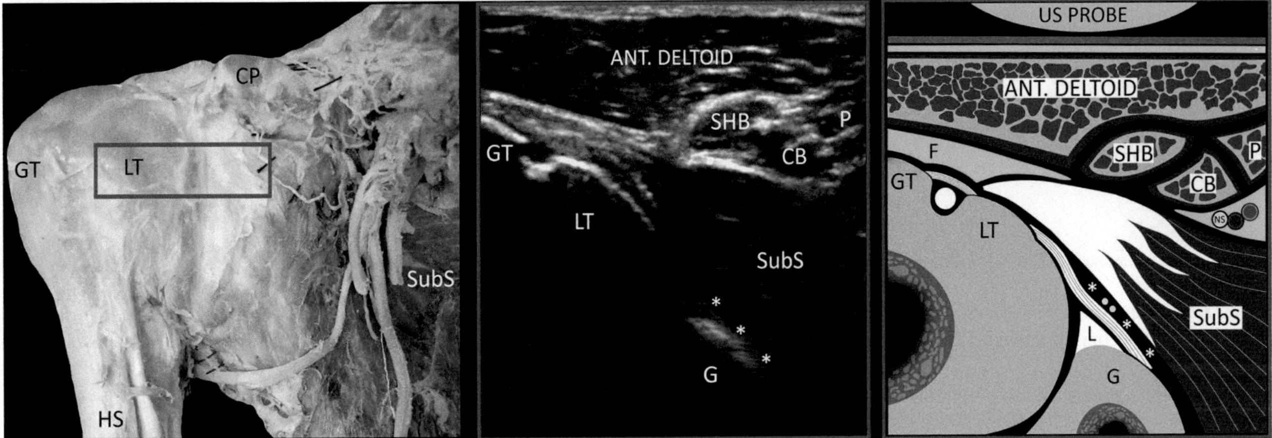

Fig. 22.11 Anatomic dissection, ultrasonography, and schematic diagram of the deep subscapularis space. The red rectangle depicts the position of the ultrasound probe for the sonographic image of this space. *GT* greater tuberosity, *LT* lesser tuberosity, *SubS* subscapularis, *SHB* short head of biceps, *CB* coracobrachialis, *P* pectoralis minor, *CP* coracoid process, *HS* humerus shaft, *G* glenoid, *L* labrum. Reprinted with permission from Philip Peng educational series

posteroinferior glenohumeral joint capsule at the exit of the quadrangular space. The plane (deep teres minor plane) lies between the teres minor and the humeral head (Fig. 22.13).

With the patient placed in lateral position, the initial scan is performed by placing the probe long axis on the humeral head. The infraspinatus and teres minor attach to a different facet of the posterior aspect of greater tubercle. A ridge between the two facets helps to differentiate the two muscles. Because the muscle is adherent to the bone, the plane deep to the teres minor is not well defined. The probe is moved in the medial direction following the teres minor muscle on the medial edge of the humerus. The plane between the teres minor and humerus is the target for diagnostic block and radiofrequency ablation for articular branches originating from the posterior division of axillary nerve (Fig. 22.13). The authors prefer in-plane technique to approach this deep space. For diagnostic block, 1 mL of local anesthetic is enough to allow a thorough spread in this space. For radiofrequency lesion, Trident needle is preferred because of the angle of the needle to the articular branches.

Complications

Review of the literature does not show any serious adverse effects reported from pulsed or radiofrequency ablative procedures. Most studies reported bruises, local discomfort, and pain after the procedure which resolved without treatment. One study reported transient pain and tingling at the site of needle insertion. Radiofrequency ablation of the suprascapular nerve was not associated with worsening of motor function. This likely reflects patient selection who already had

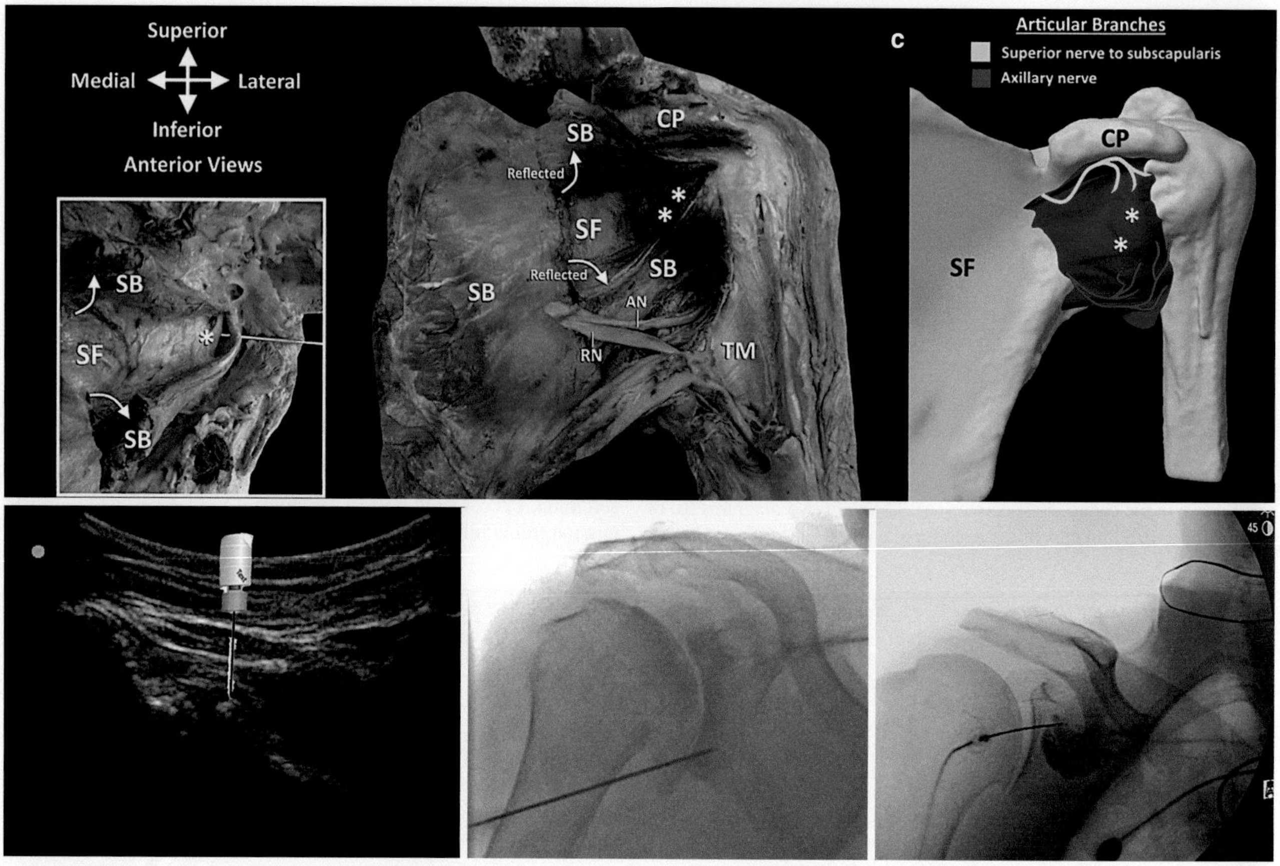

Fig. 22.12 Top panel. The needle target for the deep subscapularis space (DSS). Injection of methylene blue in this space shows the spread of in the anterior capsule (**) and scapular fossa (SF) in the DSS, which was revealed by reflecting the subscapularis (SB). The schematic diagram shows the coverage of the superior nerve to subscapularis and the articular branches from the anterior axillary nerve (AN). *CP* coracoid process. Low panel. Needle position at the glenoid in ultrasound and fluoroscopy images. Reprinted with permission from Philip Peng educational series

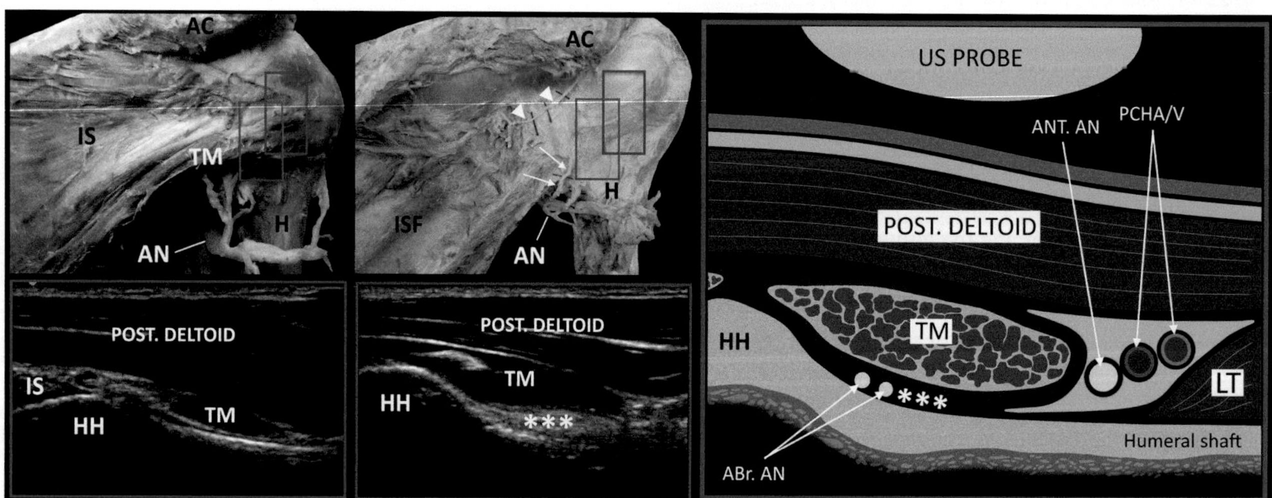

Fig. 22.13 Anatomic dissection, ultrasonography, and schematic diagram of the deep teres minor space (***). The red and blue rectangles depict the position of the ultrasound probe for the sonographic image of this space. *IS* infraspinatus, *TM* teres minor, *HH* humeral head; articular branches to the axillary nerve (AbrAN), *PCHA/V* posterior circumflex humeral artery and vein. Reprinted with permission from Philip Peng educational series

compromised rotator cuff function prior to ablation. Interestingly, in one case report, suprascapular nerve ablation improved the range of movement, which reflected that the pre-procedure decrease range of movement was related to pain.

With the suggestion of new target sites, the deep subscapularis and teres minor planes are both osseous-muscle plane void of important structures and potentially represent a safe area for denervation. However, when targeting the deep subscapularis plane, the practitioner needs to be cognizant of the needle trajectory as the brachial plexus lies in close proximity, and caution is paramount in avoiding those structures.

Practical Tips

In scanning the supraspinous fossa, one needs to remember that the suprascapular nerve runs in an anteromedial to posterolateral direction from the suprascapular notch to the spinoglenoid notch. Thus, the movement of the probe, when tracing the suprascapular nerve, should be in an anteromedial to posterolateral direction. Once the needle is inserted at the midpoint between the suprascapular and spinoglenoid notches, motor stimulation is important. Strong motor response of infraspinatus but absence of muscle twitch of supraspinatus is the ideal end point.

After insertion of the needle at the target in both deep subscapularis and teres minor planes, rotation of the needle along its long axis will enhance piercing of the muscles' underlying fascia to ensure the needle tip is in the right plane.

Literature Review

As of December 31, 2019, there are 42 studies (1018 patients) published on the radiofrequency procedures of the shoulder. Of those publications, there are comparative studies (8), prospective case series (11), retrospective case series (6), and case reports (8). Most studies (36/42) described the use of pulsed radiofrequency lesion (pRF). The targets for the radiofrequency procedures are mainly the suprascapular nerve, with 29 studies describing the nerve as the sole target. The other targets are the axillary nerve, the lower subscapular nerve, the lateral pectoral nerve, cervical nerve roots, and the nerve endings on the surface and in the intra-articular region of the glenohumeral joint or subacromial bursa. Fluoroscopy was the most commonly used modality for guiding these procedures with the suprascapular notch identified as the landmark to target the suprascapular nerve. More recent literature described the use of ultrasound-guided technique, and the target of the suprascapular nerve was at the supraspinous fossa deep to the supraspinatus.

Most studies measure the analgesic and functional outcomes. The duration of follow-up ranged between 1 week and 2 years. Most publications that evaluated pain intensity reported a mean reduction of more than 50% with a few exceptions, and the duration of pain relief ranged from a few days to over 2 years. A meta-analysis of the seven randomized controlled trials (all on pRF lesioning) found no significant reduction in mean pain scores in patients receiving pRF compared with conventional medical treatment at 3 months after the interventions. For the six studies using radiofrequency ablation on the suprascapular nerve, there was no reports on motor functioning deterioration as the patients selected were those with minimal or no range of movement at the shoulder joint. With the new proposed targets for radiofrequency ablation, it represents a new era in the treatment of refractory shoulder pain.

Suggested Reading

Akita K, Kawashima T, Shimokawa T, Sato K, Sato T. Cutaneous nerve to the subacromial region originating from the lateral pectoral nerve. Ann Anat. 2002;184:15–9.

Andrews JR. Diagnosis and treatment of chronic painful shoulder: review of nonsurgical interventions. Arthrosc J Arthrosc Relat Surg. 2005;21:333–47.

Aszmann OC, Dellon AL, Birely BT, McFarland EG. Innervation of the human shoulder joint and its implications for surgery. Clin Orthop Relat Res. 1996;330:202–7.

Chang KV, Hung CY, Wang TG, Yang RS, Sun WZ, Lin CP. Ultrasound-guided proximal suprascapular nerve block with radiofrequency lesioning for patients with malignancy-associated recalcitrant shoulder pain. J Ultrasound Med. 2015;34:2099–105.

Ebraheim NA, Whitehead JL, Alla SR, et al. The suprascapular nerve and its articular branch to the acromioclavicular joint: an anatomic study. J Shoulder Elb Surg. 2011;20:e13–7.

Eckmann M, Bickelhaupt B, Fehl J, et al. Cadaveric study of the articular branches of the shoulder joint. Reg Anesth Pain Med. 2017;42:564–70.

Gelber PE, Reina F, Monllau JC, Yema P, Rodriguez A, Caceres E. Innervation patterns of the inferior glenohumeral ligament: anatomical and biomechanical relevance. Clin Anat. 2006;19:304–11.

Ketola S, Lehtinen J, Rousi T, Nissinen M, Huhtala H, Arnala I. Which patients do not recover from shoulder impingement syndrome, either with operative treatment or with nonoperative treatment? Subgroup analysis involving 140 patients at 2 and 5 years in a randomized study. Bone Joint Res. 2013;2:132–9.

Laumonerie P, Blasco L, Tibbo M, et al. Distal suprascapular nerve block—do it yourself: cadaveric feasibility study. J Shoulder Elb Surg. 2019;28:1291–7.

Laumonerie P, Dalmas Y, Tibbo ME, et al. The sensory innervation of human shoulder: the three bridges to break. J Shoulder Elbow Surg. 2020; https://doi.org/10.1016/j.jse.2020.07.017.

Linaker CH, Walker-Bone K. Shoulder disorders and occupation. Best Pract Res Clin Rheumatol. 2015;29:405–23.

Luedke C, Kissenberth MJ, Tolan SJ, Hawkins RJ, Tokish JM. Outcomes of anatomic total shoulder arthroplasty with B2 Glenoids. A Systematic Review. JBJS Rev. 2018;6(4):e7.

Nam YS, Panchal K, Kim IB, Ji JH, Park MG, Park SR. Anatomical study of the articular branch of the lateral pectoral nerve to the shoulder joint. Knee Surg Sports Traumatol Arthrosc. 2016;24:3820–7.

Nasu H, Nimura A, Yamaguchi K, Akita K. Distribution of the axillary nerve to the subacromial bursa and the area around the long head of the biceps tendon. Knee Surg Sports Traumatol Arthrosc. 2015;23:2651–7.

Roberson TA, Bentley JC, Griscom JT, et al. Outcomes of total shoulder arthroplasty in patients younger than 65 years: a systematic review. J Shoulder Elb Surg. 2017;26(1298–1306):10.

Singh JA, Sperling J, Buchbinder R, McMaker K. Surgery for shoulder osteoarthritis: a Cochrane systematic review. J Rheumatol. 2011;38:598–605.

Tran J, Peng P, Agur A. Anatomical study of the innervation of glenohumeral and acromioclavicular joint capsules: implications for image-guided intervention. Reg Anesth Pain Med. 2019b;44:452–8.

Tran J, Peng P, Agur A. Evaluation of suprascapular nerve radiofrequency ablation protocols: 3D cadaveric needle placement study. Regional anesthesia and pain medicine. Reg Anesth Pain Med. 2019c;44:1021–5.

Tran J, Peng PWH, Agur AMR. Anatomical study of the innervation of glenohumeral and acromioclavicular joint capsules: implications for image-guided intervention. Reg Anesth Pain Med. 2019a;44:452–8.

Vorster W, Lange CP, Briët RJ, et al. The sensory branch distribution of the suprascapular nerve: an anatomic study. J Shoulder Elb Surg. 2008;17:500–2.

Wu YT, Ho CW, Chen YL, Li TY, Lee KC, Chen LC. Ultrasound-guided pulsed radiofrequency stimulation of the suprascapular nerve for adhesive capsulitis: a prospective, randomized, controlled trial. Anesth Analg. 2014;119:686–92.

Yoo JC, Rhee YG, Shin SJ, et al. Subscapularis tendon tear classification based on 3-dimensional anatomic footprint: a cadaveric and prospective clinical observational study. Arthroscopy. 2015;31:19–28.

Part IV

Nerve Block for Regional Anesthesia and Pain Therapy for Upper Limb

Brachial Plexus Anatomy

23

Danilo Jankovic and Philip Peng

Contents

General Consideration

The regional anesthesia blockade of the brachial plexus is classically divided into four approaches: interscalene, supraclavicular, infraclavicular, and axillary approaches, initially described and popularized by Winnie, Kulenkampff, Raj, and Hirschel, respectively. The premise of these approaches is based on the "belief" that the nerves in the plexus are contained within a defined perivascular and perineural space in the course from the transverse process to the axilla. Thus, a single injection of local anesthetic into this confined space will result in spread to the various trunks and nerves. The understanding of the anatomy in this region evolves over the last few decades and this assumption is proven to be oversimplified. For example, there is no evidence of a substantial sheath on cryomicrotome sections of the supraclavicular region. Several investigators had challenged the concept of a tubular axillary sheath and proposed that the sheath is a multi-compartmental structure formed by thin layers of fibrous tissue surrounding the plexus extending inward to create discrete fascial septae. Nerves are thus enmeshed in this tissue rather than lying separate and distinct. As a result, individual fascial compartments are created for each nerve with defined anatomic limit for that neural structure. These compartments functionally limit the circumferential spread of injectate, thereby requiring separate injections into each compartment for maximal nerve blockade. However, proximal connections between compartments have been identified, which may account for the success of single injection techniques. Certain clinical observations may be interpreted as support or counter-support for the existence of a functional tubular sheath. The clinical significance of these septa

D. Jankovic (✉)
Pain Management Centre DGS – Cologne – Huerth, Cologne-Hürth, Germany
e-mail: danilo@jankovic1.de

P. Peng
Department of Anesthesia and Pain Medicine, University of Toronto Toronto Western Hospital, Toronto, ON, Canada
e-mail: philip.peng@uhn.ca

D. Jankovic, P. Peng (eds.), *Regional Nerve Blocks in Anesthesia and Pain Therapy*,
https://doi.org/10.1007/978-3-030-88727-8_23

remains *controversial*, and it makes sense to inject local anesthetic in divided doses at several locations within the sheath.

Functional Anatomy

Along its course from proximal to distal, the brachial plexus passes through four distinct topographical areas: interscalene gap, posterior triangle of the neck (lateral cervical supraclavicular region), infraclavicular fossa, and axillary fossa.

Interscalene Gap

This is a very narrow area bounded ventrally by the anterior and dorsally by the middle scalene muscles (Fig. 23.1). It continues to the epidural space laterally, is filled by loose fat and connective tissue, and accommodates the ventral rami of the spinal nerves C5 to T1. In this way, local anesthetic may spread into the epidural space during plexus blockade via the interscalene route. Each ventral ramus is surrounded by the epineural sheath, which contains mostly fatty tissue. The tissue around the ventral rami is filled with fat and loose connective tissue without a sheath (Fig. 23.1). The *prevertebral fascia* covers both the local nerve structures and the paravertebral muscles (longus colli muscle and scalene muscles); overall, it covers the brachial plexus and the subclavian artery and the phrenic nerve. Originated in the C4 segment, phrenic nerve takes a convex course passing the C5 ventral ramus at a short distance and still covered by the prevertebral fascia. It crosses the anterior surface of the scalenus anterior muscle and enters the superior thoracic aperture in front of the subclavian artery (Figs. 23.1 and 23.2a, b). Caudally, the interscalene gap widens, and the nerve structures closely approach the subclavian artery and the body of the first rib in this anatomical region (Figs. 23.1, and 23.5a, b). Within the interscalene gap, there are two anatomically distinct spaces: laterally the prevertebral space and medially the scalenovertebral triangle (bounded laterally by the anterior scalene muscle and medially by the longus colli muscle). The latter connects prevertebral space to a ventrally located space with-

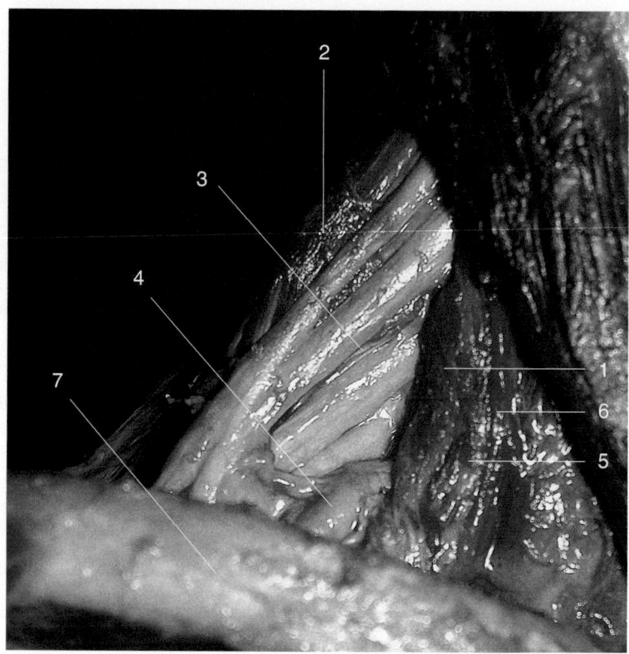

Fig. 23.1 Interscalene region. *(1)* Scalenus anterior muscle, *(2)* scalenus medius muscle, *(3)* trunks of the brachial plexus with subclavian artery, covered by prevertebral fascia *(4)* proximal supraclavicular plexus with connective tissue *(5)* phrenic nerve, *(6)* ascending cervical artery, *(7)* clavicle. (Reproduced with permission from Danilo Jankovic)

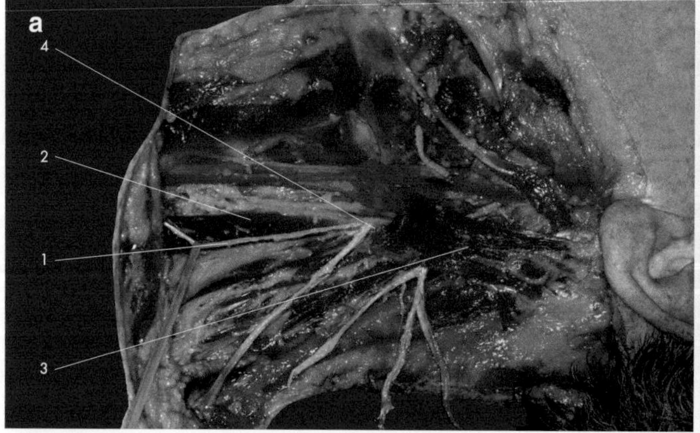

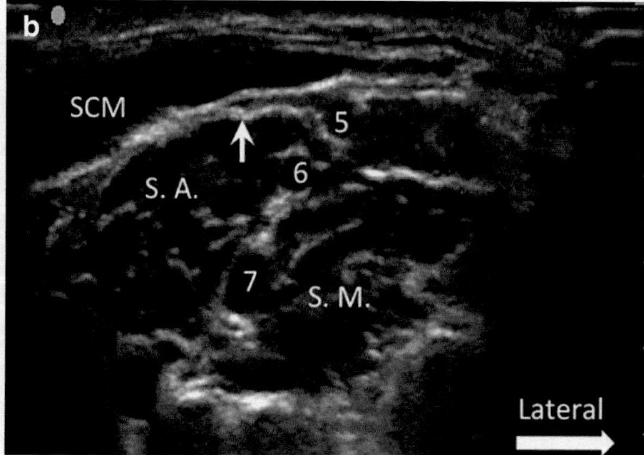

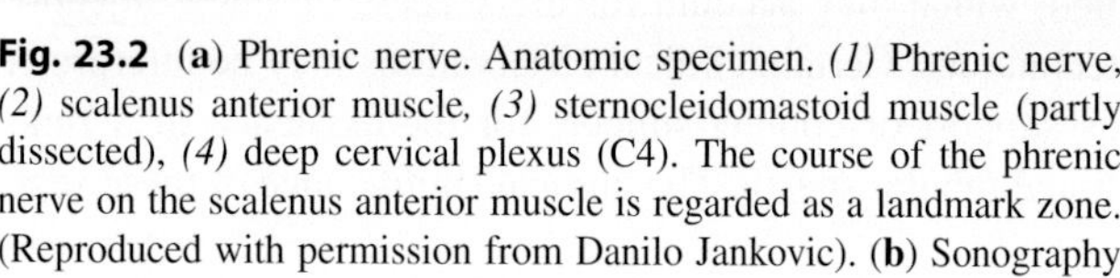

Fig. 23.2 (**a**) Phrenic nerve. Anatomic specimen. *(1)* Phrenic nerve, *(2)* scalenus anterior muscle, *(3)* sternocleidomastoid muscle (partly dissected), *(4)* deep cervical plexus (C4). The course of the phrenic nerve on the scalenus anterior muscle is regarded as a landmark zone. (Reproduced with permission from Danilo Jankovic). (**b**) Sonography of the phrenic nerve. The nerve is small and is usually hypoechoic (arrow). *SCM* sternocleidomastoid muscle, *SA* scalenus anterior muscle, *SM* scalenus medius muscle. Cervical nerve roots 5–7 are numbered accordingly as 5–7. (Reproduced with permission from Philip Peng Educational Series)

out the prevertebral fascia. This spatial connection allows the potential spread of injectate in medial direction inside a space filled with loose connective tissue when a large volume of local anesthetic is administered in the interscalene gap. Thus, it may lead to undesired blockade of neural structures such as the recurrent laryngeal nerve, the cervical sympathetic chain, or autonomic innervation systems of the heart (Fig. 23.3).

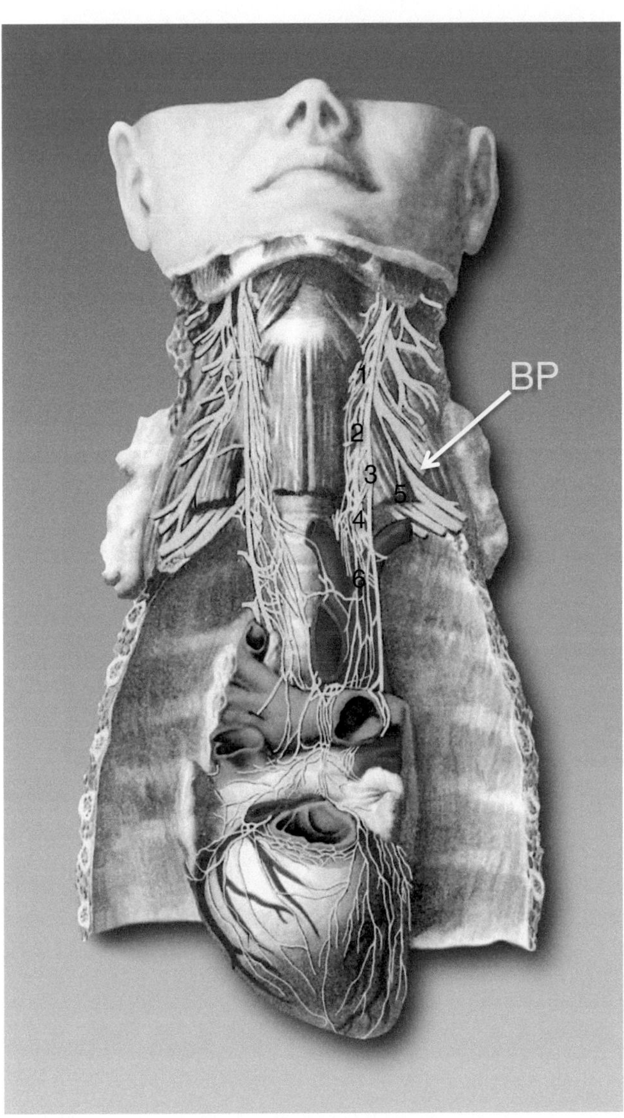

Fig. 23.3 Any large volumes of local anesthetic might spread in medial directions inside a space filled with loose connective tissue, thus potentially leading to blockade of the recurrent laryngeal nerve, the cervical sympathetic chain, or autonomic innervation systems of the heart. *(BP)* brachial plexus, *(1)* N. cardiacus cervicalis superior, *(2)* truncus sympathicus, *(3)* N. vagus, *(4)* ganglion cervicothoracicum, *(5)* N. phrenicus, *(6)* N. cardiacus cervicalis inferior. (Reproduced with permission from Danilo Jankovic)

Sonoanatomy of the Interscalene Gap

With ultrasound, the typical morphology of the interscalene gap can be easily revealed (Fig. 23.4a–f) (see chapter on brachial plexus above the clavicle).

Posterior Triangle of the Neck (Lateral Cervical Supraclavicular Region)

The supraclavicular area is where the ventral rami of the brachial plexus merge into *trunks,* the ventral branches of C5/C6 continuing as superior, C7 as middle, and C8/T1 as inferior trunk (Figs. 23.5a and 23.11).

Boundaries (Fig. 23.5b)

The posterior triangle of the neck (or lateral cervical supraclavicular region) has the following boundaries:

- Apex: union of sternocleidomastoid and trapezius muscles at the superior nuchal line of the occipital bone.
- Anterior: posterior border of the sternocleidomastoid muscle.
- Posterior: anterior border of the trapezius muscle.
- Inferior: middle one third of the clavicle.
- Roof: investing layer of the deep cervical fascia.
- Floor (from superior to inferior): M. semispinalis capitis, M. splenius capitis, M. levator scapulae, M. scalenus posterior.

The posterior triangle is crossed, about 2.5 cm above the clavicle, by the inferior belly of the omohyoid muscle, which divides the space into two triangles: an upper or occipital triangle and a lower or subclavian triangle (or supraclavicular triangle) (Fig. 23.5a). Nerves and plexuses of this region are spinal accessory nerve (CN XI), branches of cervical plexus, roots and trunks of brachial plexus, and phrenic nerve (Figs. 23.2, and 23.5a). The nerve structures have a mediocaudal position in this region, still covered by the *prevertebral fascia*, which fuse with the fascia of the subclavius muscle at the level of the clavicle. The long thoracic and the dorsal scapular nerves form two branches descending directly from the ventral rami of C5 to C7 and enter the region of the posterior triangle after piercing the middle scalene muscle (Fig. 23.4d–e). The trunks are highly relevant for their topographical relationship to the subclavian artery (see below). Two more branches emerge from the brachial plexus almost at the level of the clavicle: the suprascapular and the subclavian nerves (Fig. 23.5c). At the level of the clavicle or slightly underneath,

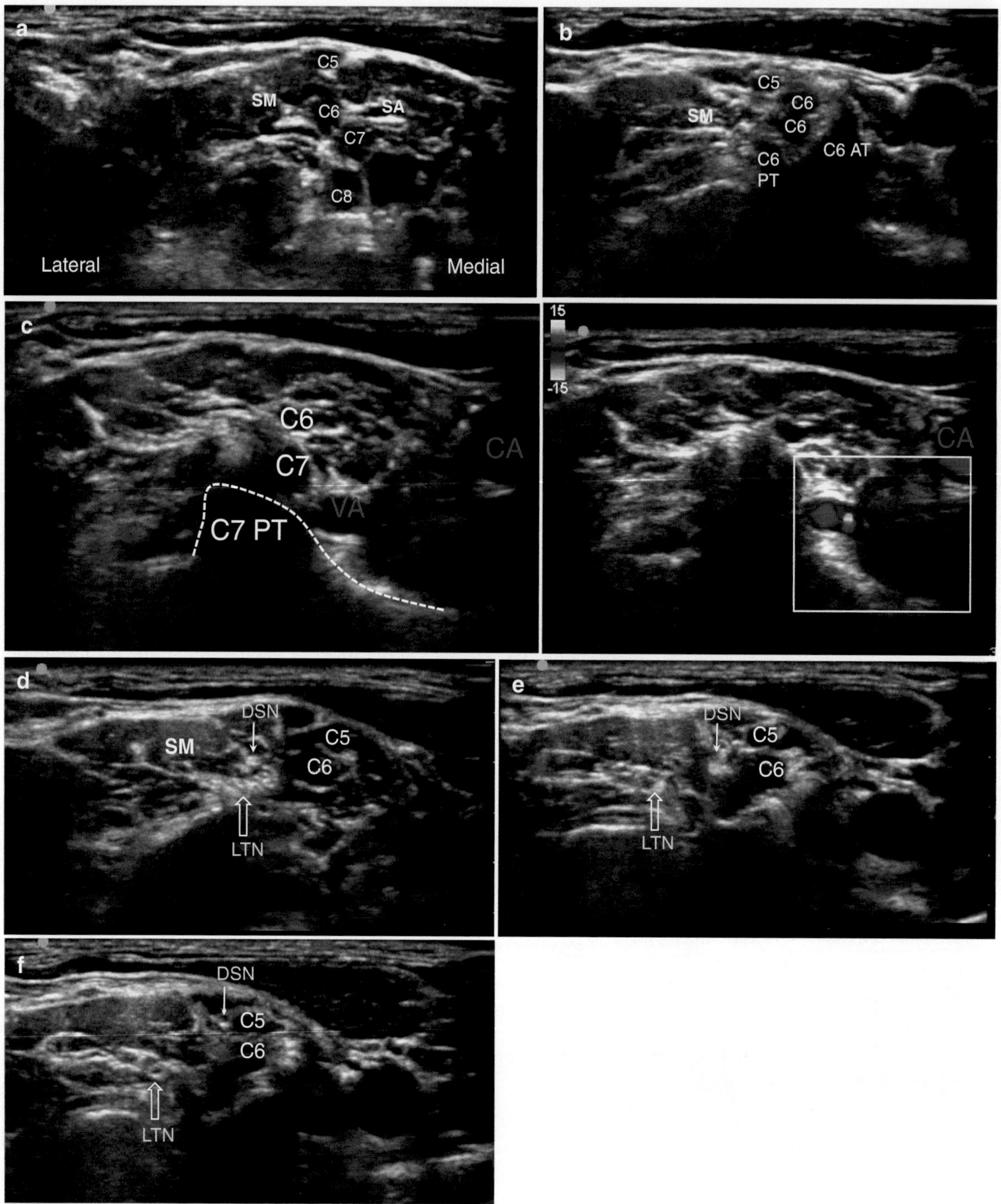

Fig. 23.4 (**a**) Typical ultrasound image of the interscalene gap with C5 to C8. *SM* scalene medius muscle, *SA* scalene anterior muscle. (Reproduced with permission from Philip Peng Education Series). (**b**) Sonogram of the interscalene gap with special angle to show the C6 (bifid) coming out from anterior and posterior tubercle of C6. *SM* scalenus medius muscle, *AT* anterior tubercle, *PT* posterior tubercle. (Reproduced with permission from Philip Peng Education Series). (**c**) Sonogram of the interscalene gap with special angle to show the C7 coming from C7 transverse process with the posterior tubercle shown. The vertebral artery is shown in Doppler. *P* posterior tubercle, *VA* vertebral artery, *CA* carotid artery. (Reproduced with permission from Philip Peng Education Series). (**d**) Sonogram of the dorsal scapular nerve *(DSN)* and long thoracic nerve *(LTN)*. Line arrow shows the dorsal scapular nerve embedded inside scalenus medius muscle *(SM)*. The long thoracic nerve (bold arrow) is embedded in the tendinous part of the muscle. *(SM)* scalenus medius muscle. (Reproduced with permission from Philip Peng Education Series). (**e**) Sonogram of the dorsal scapular nerve *(DSN)* and long thoracic nerve *(LTN)*. Tracing the dorsal scapular nerve (line arrow) in superior direction and it is approaching the C5. The long thoracic nerve is also seen within the tendinous part of the muscle. (Reproduced with permission from Philip Peng Education Series). (**f**) Sonogram of the dorsal scapular nerve *(DSN)* and long thoracic nerve *(LTN)*. By tracing more proximally and superiorly, the dorsal scapular nerve is seen going back to the C5 where it originates. (Reproduced with permission from Philip Peng Education Series)

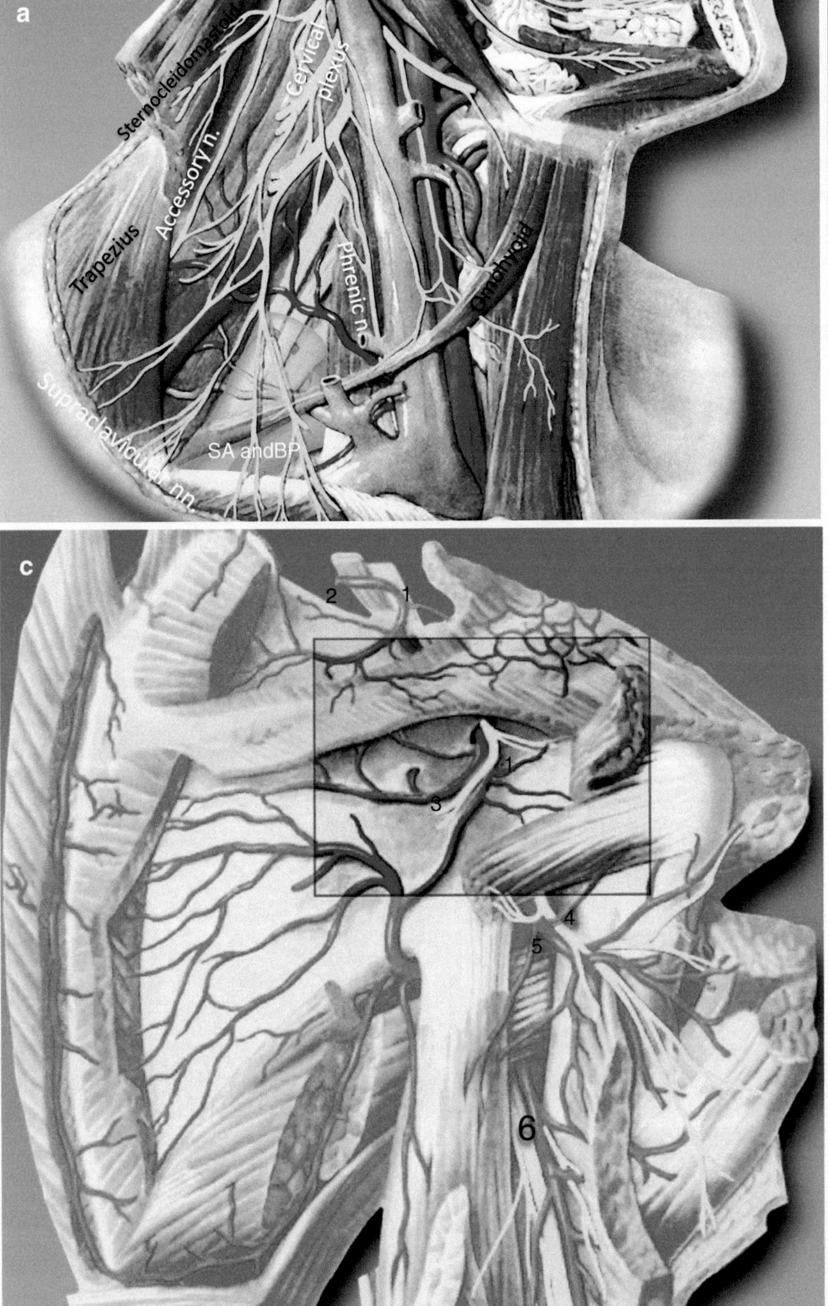

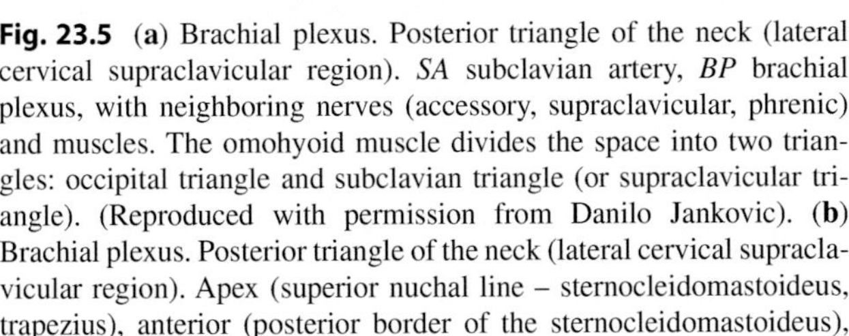

Fig. 23.5 (**a**) Brachial plexus. Posterior triangle of the neck (lateral cervical supraclavicular region). *SA* subclavian artery, *BP* brachial plexus, with neighboring nerves (accessory, supraclavicular, phrenic) and muscles. The omohyoid muscle divides the space into two triangles: occipital triangle and subclavian triangle (or supraclavicular triangle). (Reproduced with permission from Danilo Jankovic). (**b**) Brachial plexus. Posterior triangle of the neck (lateral cervical supraclavicular region). Apex (superior nuchal line – sternocleidomastoideus, trapezius), anterior (posterior border of the sternocleidomastoideus), posterior (anterior border of the trapezius), inferior (middle one third of the clavicle), roof (investing layer of the deep cervical fascia), floor (from superior to inferior: semispinalis capitis, splenius capitis, levator scapulae, scalenus posterior). (Reproduced with permission from Danilo Jankovic). (**c**) The suprascapular nerve originates from the ventral rami of the fifth and sixth cervical nerve roots. *(1)* Suprascapular nerve, *(2)* omohyoid muscle, *(3)* suprascapular a., *(4)* axillary n., *(5)* circumflex humeral a., *(6)* radial n. and profunda brachii a. (Reproduced with permission from Danilo Jankovic)

the trunks continue to split into a lateral, medial, and posterior cord. Supraclavicular nerves (Fig. 23.5a; see chapter on cervical plexus) originating mainly from the C4 ventral ramus extend caudally deep to the prevertebral fascia and pierce the fascia approximately 2 cm inferior to where the greater auricular nerve winds around the sternocleidomastoid muscle dividing into the medial, lateral, and intermediate branches. On approaching the clavicle, the supraclavicular nerves pierce the superficial fascia to innervate the skin of the pectoral region over the greater pectoral muscle and partially extending to the level of mamilla.

Sonoanatomy

Sonoanatomy of the lateral cervical supraclavicular region is presented in Fig. 23.6a–e (see chapter on brachial plexus above the clavicle).

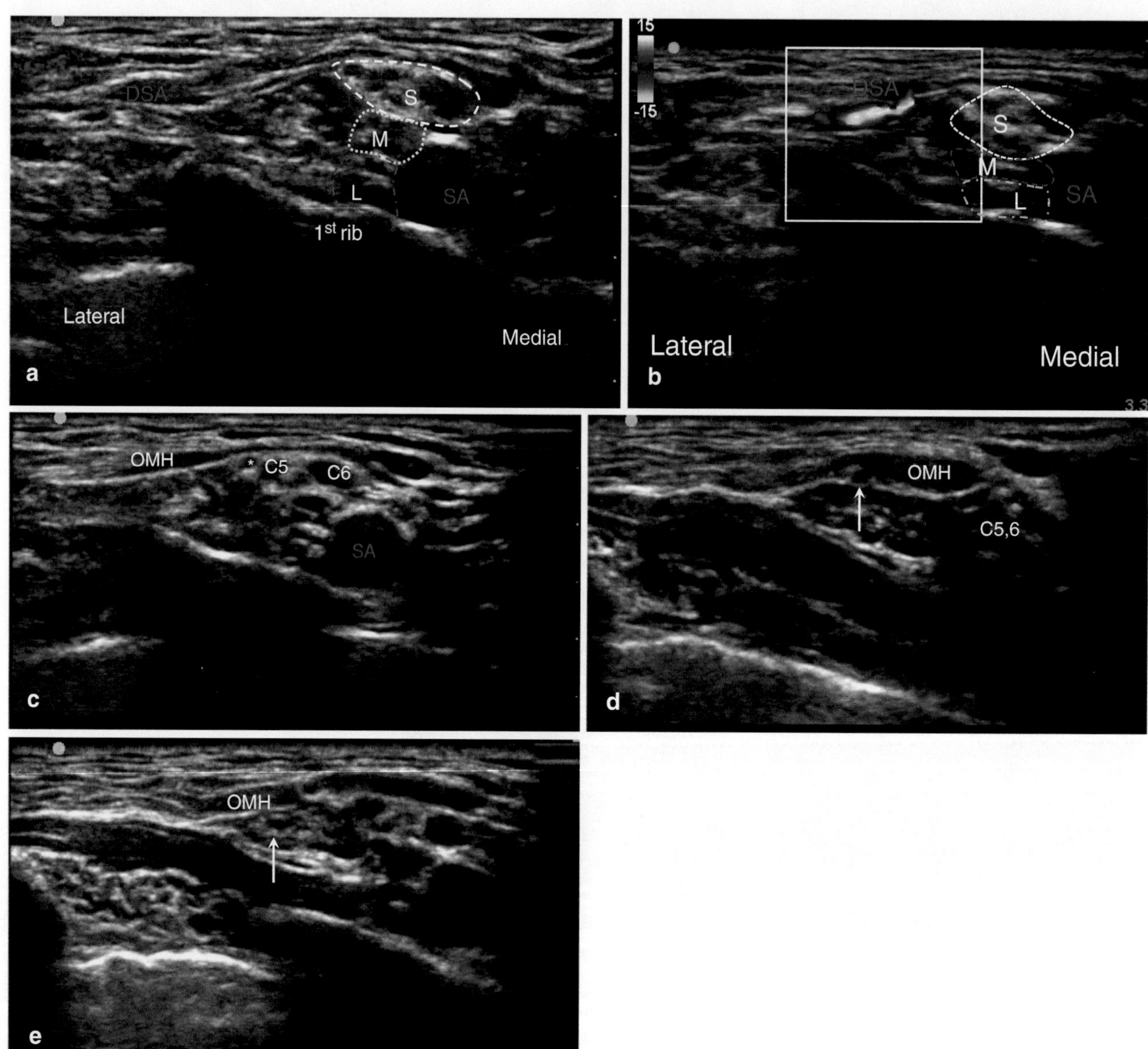

Fig. 23.6 (**a**) The three-trunk arrangement of the brachial plexus in the supraclavicular region. *(SA)* subclavian artery, *(DSA)* dorsal scapular artery. (Reproduced with permission from Philip Peng Education Series). (**b**) Doppler scan to show the dorsal scapular artery *(DSA)* in the supraclavicular region. (Reproduced with permission from Philip Peng Education Series). (**c**) A detailed look of the superior trunk, which is composed of C5, C6 ventral rami and suprascapular nerve *(*)*. *(OMH)* inferior belly of omohyoid muscle, *(SA)* subclavian artery. (Reproduced with permission from Philip Peng Education Series). (**d**) Suprascapular nerve (arrow) is seen moving to the deep surface of omohyoid muscle *(OMH)*. (Reproduced with permission from Philip Peng Education Series). (**e**) Suprascapular nerve (arrow) leaves the superior trunk and is seen moving to the deep surface of omohyoid muscle. *(OMH)* omohyoid muscle. (Reproduced with permission from Philip Peng Education Series)

Infraclavicular Fossa (Mohrenheim's Fossa)

The infraclavicular fossa is situated immediately below the clavicle and is bounded by the clavicle, the deltoid muscle, the pectoralis major, the upper part of the thorax, and the medioclavicular line (Figs. 23.7, 23.12, 23.14). The clavipectoral fascia, continuing the prevertebral fascia laterally with connections to the fascia of the subclavius muscle, divides this space into a superficial and a deep layer. It is pierced by the cephalic vein, which drains the subclavian vein and is the most lateral structure of this deep layer of the infraclavicular fossa. It is important to appreciate that the orientation of the cords around the axillary artery varies with distance from the clavicle. As the brachial plexus emerges from under the clavicle, the cords are bunched together on the superior (cephalad) aspect of artery. As the neurovascular bundle travels more distally, the cords gradually separate out and "spiral" around the axillary artery to eventually adopt the classically described position of lateral, posterior, and medial to the artery (Fig. 23.8). This arrangement is best appreciated when scanning the infraclavicular area with the arm abducted at the shoulder.

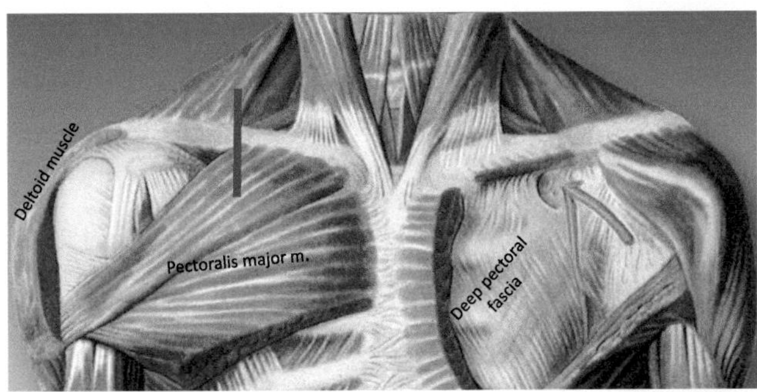

Fig. 23.7 Infraclavicular fossa (Mohrenheim's fossa): bounded by the clavicle, the deltoid muscle, the pectoralis major, the upper part of the thorax, and the medioclavicular line (red). (Reproduced with permission from Danilo Jankovic)

Axillary Fossa

The overall 3D shape of the axilla looks slightly like a pyramid, whose apex is coracoid process and whose base is the superficial axillary fascia, the latter being a cribriform structure pierced by the intercostobrachial nerve (Fig. 23.9a–b).

Borders of the Axillary Fossa (Fig. 23.9c)

- Apex (axillary inlet) is formed by the lateral border of the first rib, superior border of scapula, and posterior border of the clavicle.
- Lateral wall is formed by intertubercular groove of the humerus.
- Medial wall consists of the serratus anterior muscle and the thoracic wall (ribs and intercostal muscles).

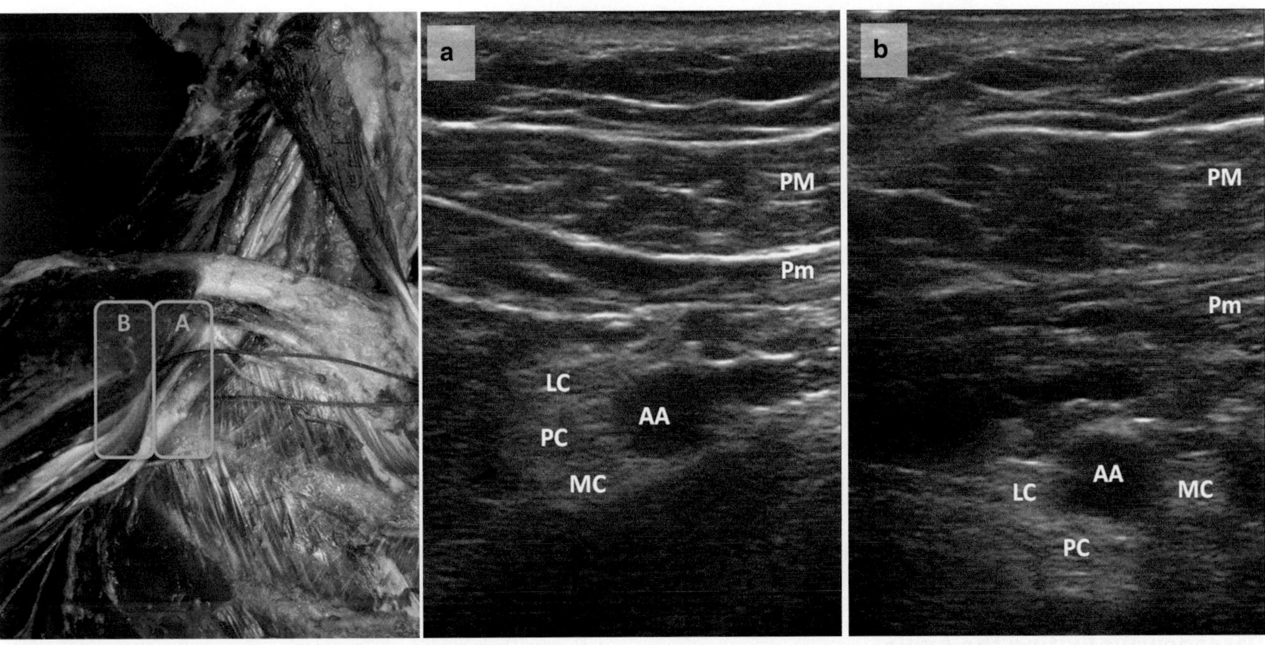

Fig. 23.8 Illustration of the variation in distribution of brachial plexus cords around the axillary artery *(AA)* depending on whether the probe is placed more medially *(position A)* or laterally *(position B)*. In *position A* (sonogram a), the cords are clustered around the cephalad aspect of the artery and are often not distinguishable from each other. This view is usually only obtainable if the arm is abducted at the shoulder so that the clavicle moves up out of the way. In *position B* (sonogram b), the cords start to spread out around the artery. The lateral cord *(LC)* remains at the cephalad aspect of the artery, but the posterior cord *(PC)* and medial cord *(MC)* move into their classically described positions relative to the artery. *(PM)* pectoralis major, *(Pm)* pectoralis minor. (Reproduced with permission from Danilo Jankovic)

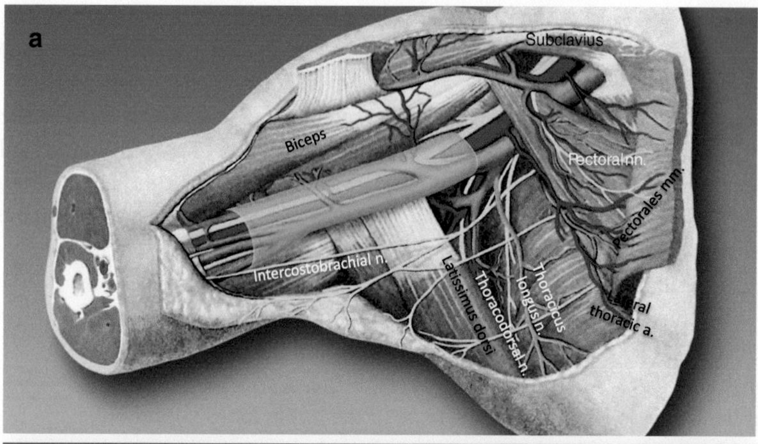

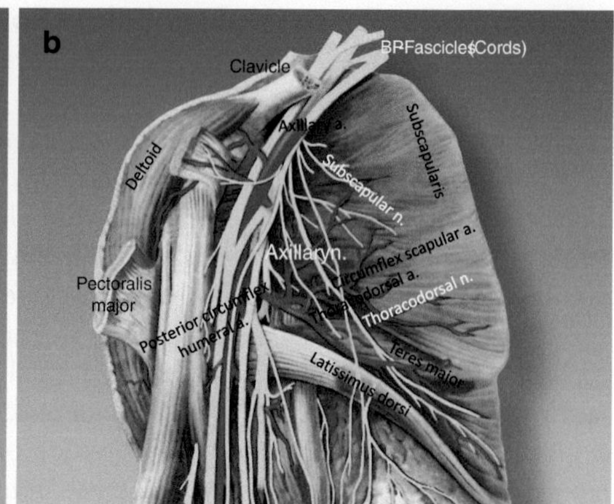

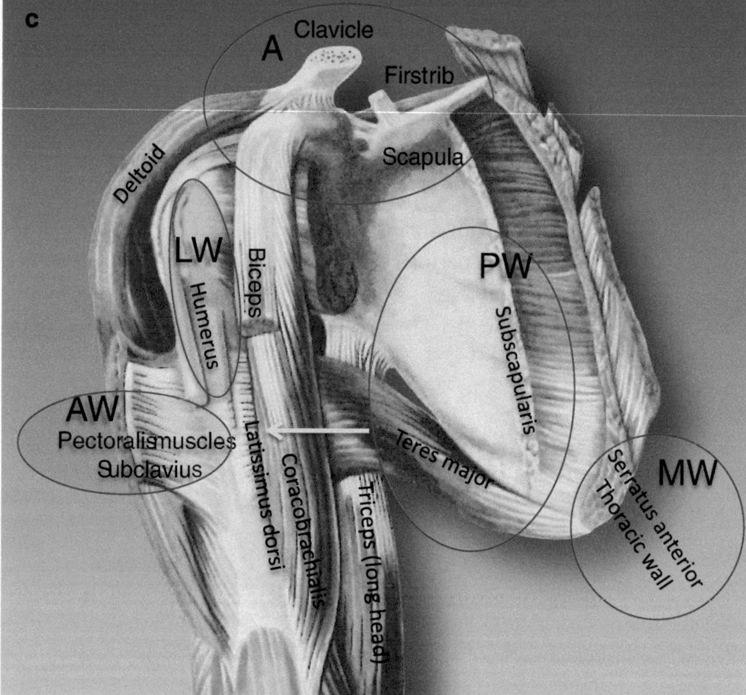

Fig. 23.9 (**a**) Axillary fossa. Distal neurovascular sheath with lateral cord and musculocutaneous, median, ulnar, intercostobrachial, thoracodorsal, thoracicus longus, and pectoral nerves and axillary artery. (Reproduced with permission from Danilo Jankovic). (**b**) Brachial plexus. Anterior view. Fascicles (cords) *(BP)* extending to axillary region. Neighboring nerves (subscapular, thoracodorsal), muscles (subscapularis, teres major, latissimus dorsi, pectoralis minor, deltoid), and vessels (axillary a., posterior circumflex humeral a., circumflex scapular a., thoracodorsal a.). (Reproduced with permission from Danilo Jankovic). (**c**) Borders of the axillary fossa: *A* apex, clavicle, first rib, scapula, *LW* lateral wall, intertubercular groove of the humerus, *MW* medial wall, serratus anterior, ribs, intercostal muscles, *AW* anterior wall, pectoralis muscles, subclavius, *PW* posterior wall, subscapularis, teres major, latissimus dorsi. (Reproduced with permission from Danilo Jankovic)

- Anterior wall contains the pectoralis major and the underlying pectoralis minor and the subclavius muscles.
- Posterior wall is formed by the subscapularis, teres major, and latissimus dorsi muscles.

Passageways Exiting the Axilla

There are three main routes by which structures leave the axilla:

- The main route of exit is immediately inferiorly and laterally, into the upper limb. The majority of contents of the axilla region leave by this way.
- Another pathway is via the quadrangular and triangular spaces. The quadrangular or quadrilateral space is bordered by humerus laterally, long head of triceps medially, subscapularis and teres minor superiorly, and teres major inferiorly. Structures passing through this space include the axillary nerve and posterior circumflex humeral artery (a branch of the axillary artery). The radial nerve exits the triangular space into the spiral groove of the posterior compartment of the arm.
- The last passageway is the clavipectoral triangle, which is an opening in the anterior wall of the axilla. It is bounded by the pectoralis major, deltoid, and clavicle. The cephalic

vein enters the axilla via this triangle, while the medial and lateral pectoral nerves leave.

- Nerve structures enter the axillary fossa underneath the deep axillary fascia, which is the continuation of the clavipectoral fascia. The major neurovascular structures are located in what is known as the "deep axillary space" which is a continuation of the deep layer of the infraclavicular fossa, underlying the clavipectoral and prevertebral fasciae in the posterior triangle of neck.

Sonoanatomy

Sonoanatomy of the axillary fossa is presented in Fig. 23.10a–b (see chapter on brachial plexus below the clavicle).

Brachial Plexus: Trunks, Divisions, and Cords

The brachial plexus arises from the union of the spinal nerve roots of C5, C6, C7, C8, and T1, and it often also contains fine fibers from the fourth cervical nerve and second thoracic nerve.

After they have left their intervertebral foramina, the roots of the plexus appear in the interscalene groove between the scalenus anterior and scalenus medius muscles, and they join together there to form the *primary cords or trunks* (Fig. 23.11). The upper roots (C5, C6) form the *superior trunk*, the roots of C7 continue as the *middle trunk*, and the *inferior trunk* arises from the roots of C8 and T1 (Fig. 23.6a–c). After passing through the interscalene groove, the primary cords of the plexus, lying close together, move toward the first rib (Figs.23.1 and 23.6a). The suprascapular nerve and subclavian nerve already branch off from the superior trunk here, in the posterior triangle of the neck above the clavicle (Figs. 23.5c, 23.6d–e and 23.11).

The dorsal scapular nerve arises from the brachial plexus, usually from the plexus root (anterior/ventral ramus) of the cervical nerve C5 (Fig. 23.4d–f). Once the nerve leaves C5, it commonly pierces the middle scalene muscle, and continues deep to levator scapulae and the rhomboids. The long thoracic nerve arises from the anterior rami of the C5, C6, and C7 cervical spinal nerve. The root from C7 may occasionally be absent. The roots from

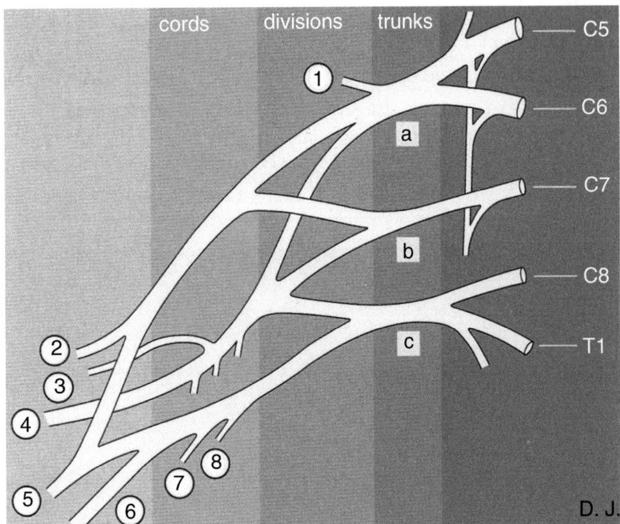

Fig. 23.11 Trunks: (**a**) superior trunk, (**b**) medial trunk, (**c**) inferior trunk, divisions and cords of the brachial plexus. *(1)* Suprascapular nerve, *(2)* musculocutaneous nerve, *(3)* axillary nerve, *(4)* radial nerve, *(5)* median nerve, *(6)* ulnar nerve, *(7)* medial antebrachial cutaneous nerve, *(8)* medial brachial cutaneous nerve (Reproduced with permission from Danilo Jankovic)

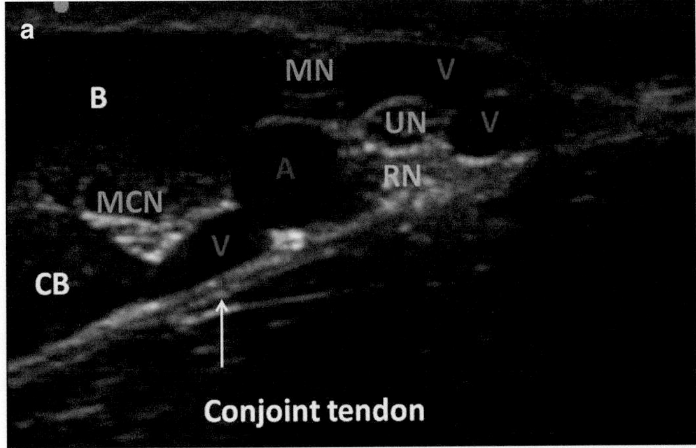

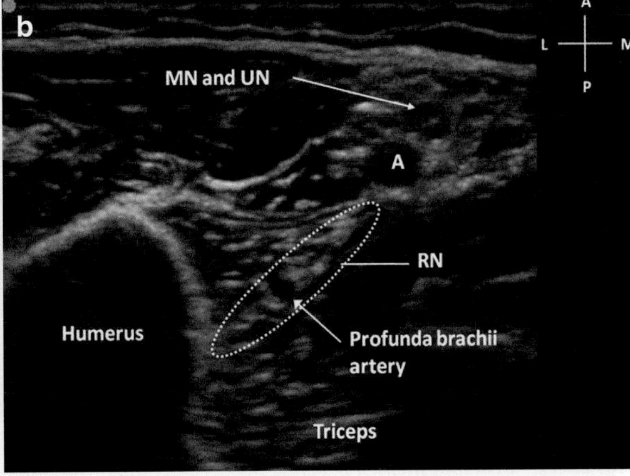

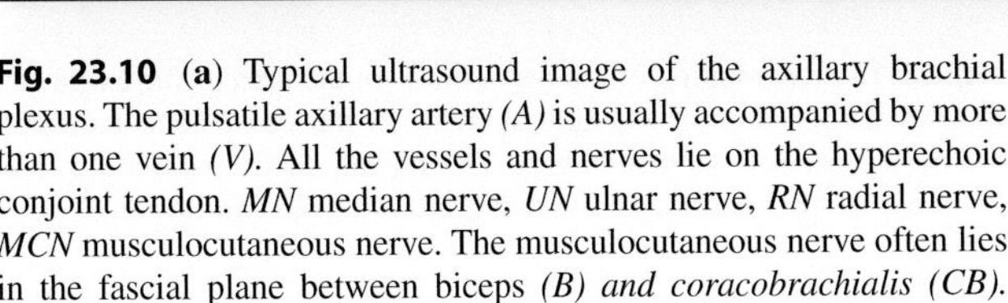

Fig. 23.10 (**a**) Typical ultrasound image of the axillary brachial plexus. The pulsatile axillary artery *(A)* is usually accompanied by more than one vein *(V)*. All the vessels and nerves lie on the hyperechoic conjoint tendon. *MN* median nerve, *UN* ulnar nerve, *RN* radial nerve, *MCN* musculocutaneous nerve. The musculocutaneous nerve often lies in the fascial plane between biceps *(B) and coracobrachialis (CB).* (Image courtesy of KJ Chin MPC). (**b**) Distal to the conjoint tendon zone, the radial nerve runs posterolaterally in a fascial plane between the long and medial heads of the triceps toward the humerus. It is accompanied by the profunda brachii artery *(A artery, MN* median nerve, *RN* radial nerve, *UN* ulnar nerve. (Image courtesy of KJ Chin MCP)

C5 and C6 pierce through the scalene medius, while C7 root passes in front of the muscle (Fig. 23.4d–f). When crossing the first rib, the trunks of the plexus lie dorsolateral to the subclavian artery and are enclosed along with the artery by a *connective tissue*. The plexus runs through under the middle of the clavicle, following the course of the subclavian artery, into the tip of the axilla (Fig. 23.12). As it does so, each of the primary cords divides into the *anterior (ventral) divisions and posterior (dorsal) divisions*. These supply the ventral flexor muscles and the dorsal extensor muscles of the upper extremity. In the axilla itself, the nerve cords regroup and separate into the individual nerves (Fig. 23.13).

The *ventral branches* of the superior and middle trunk combine to form the *lateral cord* (*fasciculus lateralis*, C5, C6, C7; (Figs. 23.14, 23.15, and 23.19)).

The following nerves emerge from this:

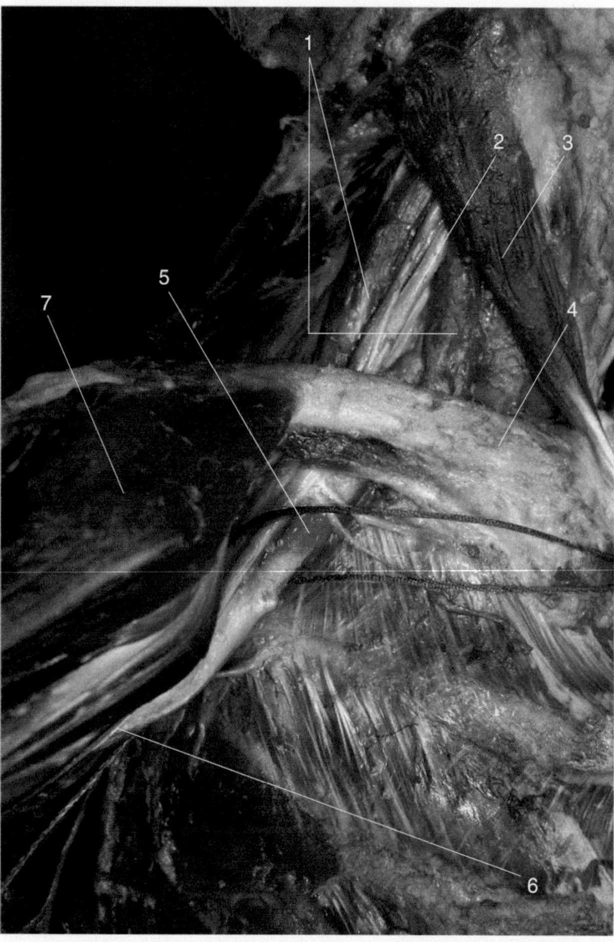

Fig. 23.12 **Brachial plexus.** Brachial plexus extending from interscalene to subclavian and axillary region. Pectoralis muscle separated. *(1)* Middle and anterior scalene muscles, *(2)* trunks of the brachial plexus, *(3)* sternocleidomastoid muscle, *(4)* clavicle, *(5)* infraclavicular region, *(6)* axillary part of the brachial plexus, *(7)* deltoid muscle. (Reproduced with permission from Danilo Jankovic)

- Musculocutaneous nerve (Figs.23.11, 23.13, 23.15, and 23.19).
- Median nerve (lateral root) (Figs. 23.11, 23.13, 23.15, and 23.19).
- Lateral pectoral nerve (Fig. 23.9a).

All of the *dorsal branches* of the three trunks form the *posterior cord* (*fasciculus posterior*, C5–8, T1). The end branches of this are the:

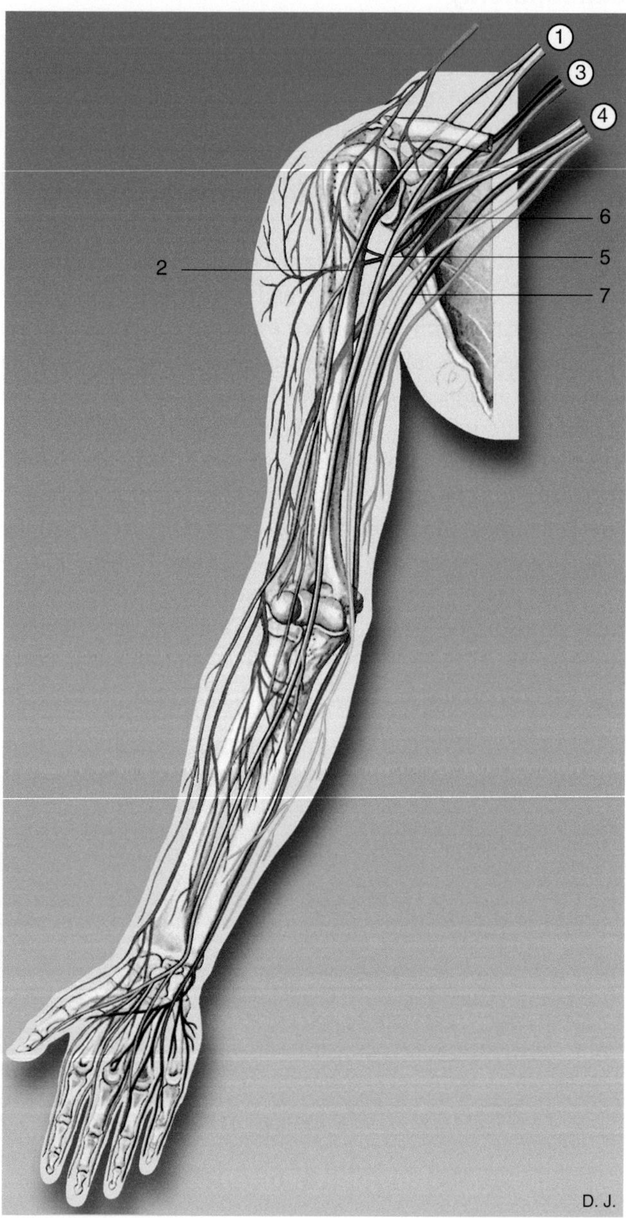

Fig. 23.13 Regrouping of the nerve cords in the area of the axilla and their distal distribution. *(1)* Lateral cord, *(2)* musculocutaneous nerve, *(3)* posterior cord, *(4)* medial cord, *(5)* median nerve, *(6)* radial nerve, *(7)* ulnar nerve. (Reproduced with permission from Danilo Jankovic)

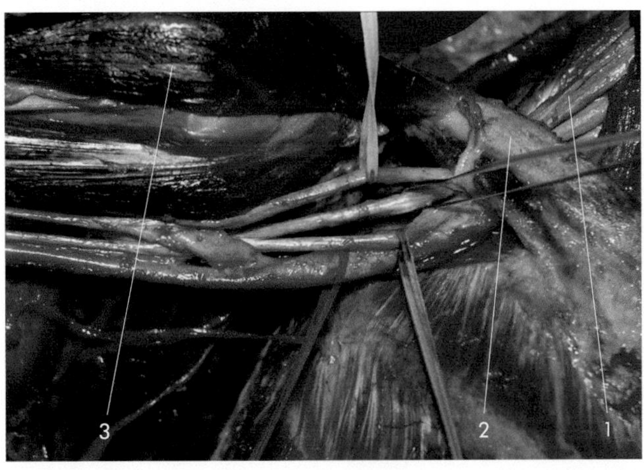

Fig. 23.14 Fascicles (cords) of the brachial plexus. Lateral cord *(white)*, posterior cord *(blue)*, medial cord *(green)*, axillary artery *(red)*. *(1)* Trunks of the brachial plexus above the clavicle *(2)*, deltoid muscle *(3)*. Pectoralis major muscle separated. (Reproduced with permission from Danilo Jankovic)

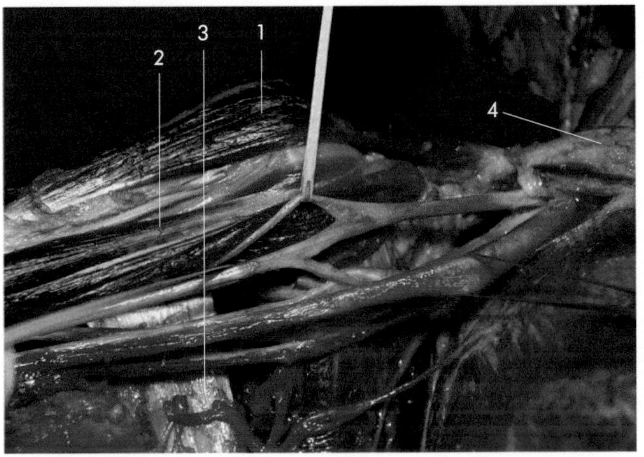

Fig. 23.15 Musculocutaneous nerve *(yellow)*, median nerve *(green)*, and axillary artery *(red)*. *(1)* Deltoid muscle, *(2)* biceps brachii muscle and coracobrachialis muscle, *(3)* latissimus dorsi muscle, *(4)* clavicle (Reproduced with permission from Danilo Jankovic)

- Radial nerve (Figs.23.11, 23.13, 23.16, and 23.19).
- Axillary nerve (Figs. 23.9b, 23.11, and 23.16).
- Thoracodorsal nerve (Figs. 23.9a, b, and 23.17).
- Inferior subscapular nerve (Fig. 23.9b).
- Superior subscapular nerve (Fig. 23.9b).

The *ventral branches of the inferior trunk* continue as the *medial cord* (*fasciculus medialis*, C8, T1). The following nerves emerge from this:

- Ulnar nerve (Figs. 23.11, 23.13, 23.18, and 23.19).
- Median nerve (medial root) (Figs.23.11, 23.13, 23.15, and23.19).
- Medial pectoral nerve (Fig. 23.9a).
- Medial antebrachial cutaneous nerve (Figs. 23.11 and 23.13).
- Medial brachial cutaneous nerve (Figs. 23.11 and 23.13).

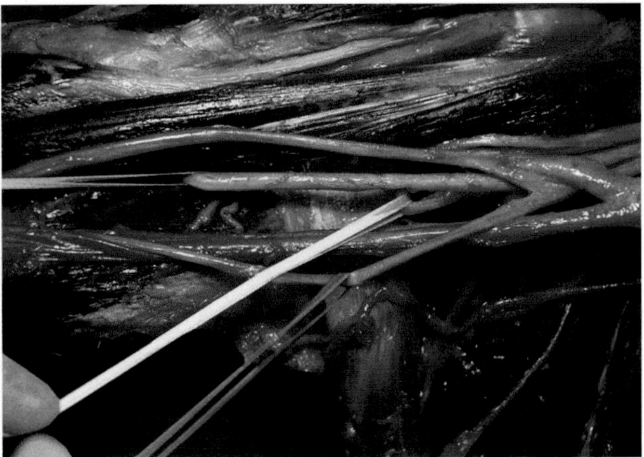

Fig. 23.16 Radial nerve *(green)* and axillary nerve *(yellow)*. (Reproduced with permission from Danilo Jankovic)

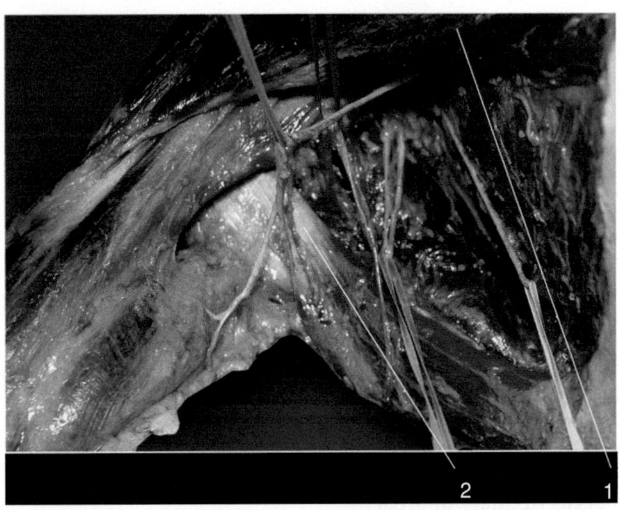

Fig. 23.17 Thoracodorsal nerve *(green)*, thoracicus longus nerve *(yellow)*, intercostobrachial nerve *(blue)*, thoracodorsal artery *(red)*. *(1)* Pectoralis major muscle, *(2)* latissimus dorsi muscle. (Reproduced with permission from Danilo Jankovic)

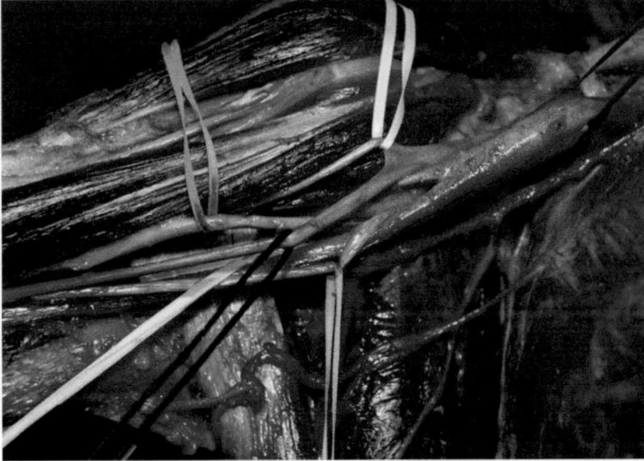

Fig. 23.18 Ulnar nerve *(light blue)*, median nerve *(dark blue)*, axillary nerve *(yellow)*, radial nerve *(green)*, musculocutaneous nerve *(white)*, axillary artery *(red)*. *(1)* Deltoid muscle, *(2)* latissimus dorsi muscle, *(3)* axillary vein. (Reproduced with permission from Danilo Jankovic)

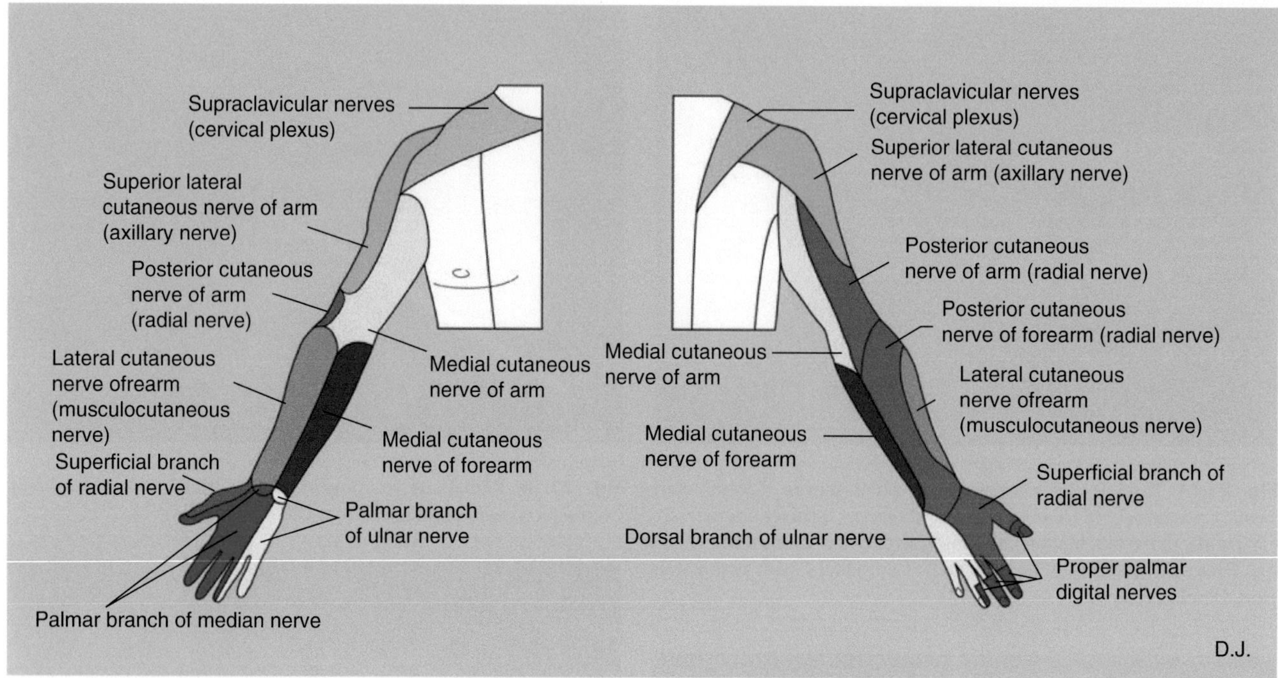

Fig. 23.19 Brachial plexus, cutaneous innervation. (Reproduced with permission from Danilo Jankovic)

Regional anesthesia performed *above the clavicle* will block either the ventral rami of the spinal nerves or, where the trunks have formed, any branched-off terminal nerves like the long thoracic nerve or the dorsal scapular nerve. Techniques performed *below the clavicle* will mainly block fascicles (infraclavicular approach) or any of the terminal nerves (axillary approach).

Suggested Reading

Albrecht E, Bathory I, Fournier N. Reduced hemidiaphragmatic paresis with extrafascial compared with intrafascial tip placement for continuous interscalene brachial plexus block: a randomized, controlled, double-blind trial. Br J Anaesth. 2017;118:586–92.

Albrecht E, Kirkham KR, Tafé P. The maximum effective needle-to-nerve distance for ultrasound-guided interscalene –block: an exploratory study. Reg Anesth Pain Med. 2014;39:56–60.

Benumof JL. Permanent loss of cervical spinal cord function associated with interscalene block performed under general anesthesia. Anesthesiology. 2000;93:1541–4.

Blanchard J, Ramamurthy S. Brachial plexus. In: Benumof LD, editor. Clinical procedures in anesthesia and intensive care. Philadelphia: Lippincott; 1992.

Cornisch PB, Greenfield LJ. Brachial plexus anatomy. Reg Anesth. 1997;22:106–7.

De Jong RH. Axillary block of the brachial plexus. Anesthesiology. 1961;22:215–25.

De Jong RH. Modified axillary block. Anesthesiology. 1965;26:615.

Duton RP, Eckhardt WF, Sunder N. Total spinal anesthesia after interscalene blockade of the brachial plexus. Anesthesiology. 1994;80:939–41.

Feigl G, Hammer GP, Litz R. The intercarotid or alar fascia, other cervical fascias, and their adjacent spaces-a plea for clarification of cervical fascia and spaces terminology. J Anat. 2020b; https://doi.org/10.1111/joa.13175.

Feigl GC, Dreu M. Important structures to be known for a safe ultrasound guided supraclavicular plexus block. Reg Anesth Pain Med. 2010;35:317–8.

Feigl GC, Litz RJ, Marhofer P. Anatomy of brachial plexus and its implications for daily clinical practice: regional anesthesia is applied anatomy. Reg Anesth Pain Med. 2020a;45:620–7.

Feigl GC, Pixner T. The cleidoatlanticus muscle: a potential pitfall for the practice of ultrasound guided interscalene brachial plexus block. Surg Radio Anat. 2011a;33:823–5.

Feigl GC, Pixner T. Combination of variations of the interscalene gap as a pitfall for ultrasound guided brachial plexus block. Reg Anesth Pain Med. 2011b;36:523–4.

Feigl GG. Fascia and spaces on the neck: myth and reality. Medical Fluminensis. 2015;51(4):430–9.

Franco CD, Rahman A, Voronov G. Gross anatomy of the brachial plexus sheath inhuman cadavers. Reg Anesth Pain Med. 2008;33:64–9.

Franco CD, Williams JM. Ultrasound-Guided Interscalene Block. Reevaluation of the "stoplight" sign and clinical implications. Reg Anesth Pain Med. 2016;41:452–9.

Gosling JA, Harris PF, Whitmore I, Willan PLT. Fotoatlas Anatomie. Präparate, Zeichnungen und Text. München: Urban and Fischer; 2005. p. 72–9.

Grodinsky M, Holyoke EA. The fasciae and fascial spaces of the head, neck and adjacent regions. Am J Anat. 1938;63:637–408.

Hickey R, Rogers J, Hoffman J, Ramamurthy S. Comparison of the clinical efficacy of three perivascular techniques for axillary brachial plexus block. Reg Anesth. 1993;18:335–8.

Hirschel G. Anästhesierung des Plexus brachialis bei Operationen an der oberen Extremität. Münchn MedWschr. 1911;58:1555–6.

Hogan QH, Ericson SJ. MR imaging of the stellate ganglion. Normal appearanceAm J Roentgen. 1992;158:655–9.

Kahle W. Taschenatlas der Anatomie.Band 3. Nervensystem und Sinnesorgane. New York: ThiemeStuttgart; 2001.

Kulenkampf D. Die Anästhesierung des Plexus brachialis. Dtsch med Wschr. 1912;38:1878–80.

Maga J, Missair A, Visan A. Comparison of outside versus inside brachial plexus sheath injection for ultrasound guided interscalene nerve blocks. J Ultrasound Med. 2016;35:279–85.

Neal J, Gerancher JC, Hebl J, Ilfeld B, et al. Upper extremity regional anesthesia Essentials of Our Current Understanding, 2008. RAPM. 2009;34(2):134–71.

Netter FH. Nerve plexuses and peripheral nerves. In Netter FH: nervous system. (volume 1): neuroanatomy and physiology. In: The Ciba Collection of Medical Illustrations. Basel: Ciba-Geigy; 1991.

Palhais N, Brull R, Kern C. Extrafascial injection for interscalene brachial plexus block reduces respiratory complications compared with a conventional intrafascial injection: a randomized, controlled ,double –blind trial. Br J Anaest. 2016;116:531–7.

Pertridge BL, Benirschke F. Functional anatomy of the brachial plexus sheath: implications for anesthesia. Anesthesiology. 1987;66:743–7.

Raj PP, Montgomery SJ, Nettles D, Jenkins MT. Infraclavicular brachial plexus block – a new approach. Anesth Analg. 1973;52:897–904.

Rohen JW, Yokochi C, Lütjen-Drecoll E. Anatomie des Menschen. Fotografischer Atlas. New York: Schattauer Stuttgart; 2002. p. 396–401.

Rorie DK. The brachial plexus sheath. Anat Rec. 1974;187:451.

Thompson GE, Rorie DK. Functional anatomy of the brachial plexus sheaths. Anesthesiology. 1983;59:117–22.

Winnie AP. Interscalene brachial plexus block. Anesth Analg. 1970;49:455–66.

Winnie AP, Collins V, J. The subclavian perivascular technique of brachial plexus anesthesia. Anesthesiology. 1964;25:353–63.

Winnie AP, Radonjic R, Akkineni SR, Durrani Z. Factors influencing distribution of local anesthetics injected into the brachial plexus sheath. Anesth Analg. 1979;58:225–34.

Brachial Plexus Block Above the Clavicle

24

Neel Desai, Eric Albrecht, and Danilo Jankovic

Contents

In 1884, Hall first reported on the direct application of cocaine to the brachial plexus after its surgical exposure, with ensuing blockade of this network of nerves that provides the motor, sensory, and sympathetic innervation of the upper limb. Not surprisingly, it was only once the percutaneous approaches to the brachial plexus were developed that the analgesic and anesthetic utility of these techniques were realized. Initially, landmark and paresthesia followed by neurostimulation methods were established. More recently, the introduction of ultrasound-guided techniques has been associated with benefits such as a decreased number of needle passes, increased rates of block success in some trials, less time to onset of sensory and motor blockade, longer duration of analgesia, and reduced patient discomfort. In this chapter, we will review the brachial plexus blocks above the clavicle, namely interscalene and supraclavicular block.

N. Desai
Department of Anaesthesia, Guy's and St Thomas' NHS Foundation Trust, London, UK
e-mail: Neel.Desai@gstt.nhs.uk

E. Albrecht (✉)
Department of Anaesthesia, Lausanne University Hospital, Lausanne, Switzerland
e-mail: eric.albrecht@chuv.ch

D. Jankovic
Pain Management Centre DGS – Cologne – Huerth, Cologne-Hürth, Germany
e-mail: danilo@jankovic1.de

Interscalene Block

General Consideration

Interscalene block is performed at the level of the distal roots and proximal trunks of the brachial plexus. If local anesthetic is injected in the interscalene groove, that is between the anterior and middle scalene muscles, then it blocks the higher nerve roots of the brachial plexus such as C5 and C6, and tends to spread in a proximal and superficial fashion to block the supraclavicular nerve of the cervical plexus. Importantly, the physical distance of the C5 and C6 nerve roots to the lower nerve roots such as T8 and T1 leads to an increased likelihood of incomplete blockade of the inferior trunk of the brachial plexus.

D. Jankovic, P. Peng (eds.), *Regional Nerve Blocks in Anesthesia and Pain Therapy*,
https://doi.org/10.1007/978-3-030-88727-8_24

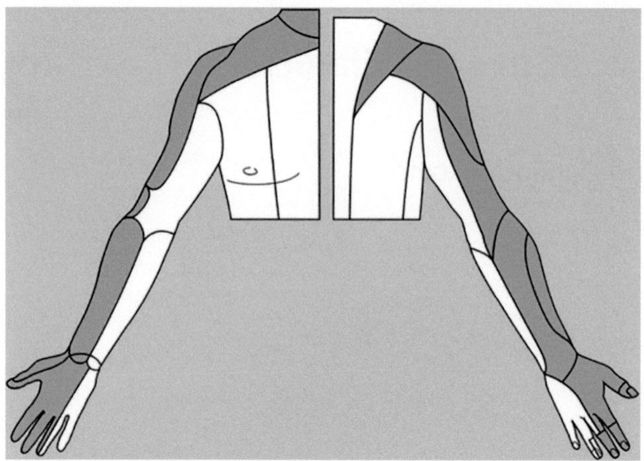

Fig. 24.1 Expected distribution of anesthesia following interscalene block. Reprinted with permission from Danilo Jankovic

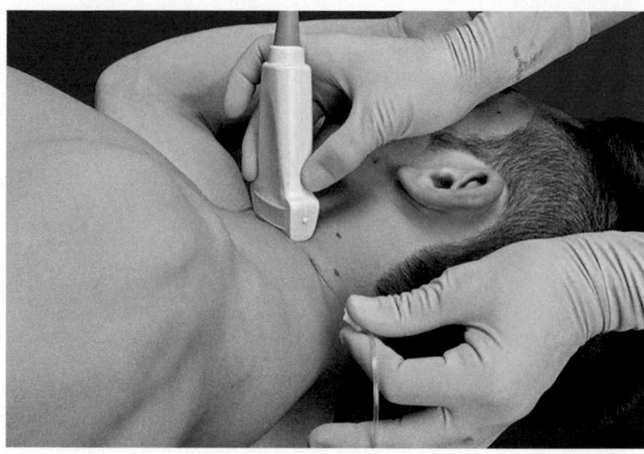

Fig. 24.2 Demonstration of the patient position for the interscalene and supraclavicular block and point of needle insertion for the supraclavicular block

Indication

Interscalene block is indicated for surgical procedures on the shoulder, proximal humerus, and the lateral two thirds of the clavicle. It is not advocated for surgery of the arm or forearm because of the increased risk of incomplete blockade of the inferior trunk or ulnar nerve (Fig. 24.1). Absolute contraindications are as follows: patient refusal, local infection, allergy to local anesthetic, contralateral pneumonectomy or pneumothorax, contralateral paresis of the phrenic or recurrent laryngeal nerve, and contralateral interscalene block. Relative contraindications include coagulopathy, previous neurological deficit of the ipsilateral arm, and reduced pulmonary reserve. In all cases, the balanced view of risks and benefits of the selected brachial plexus block technique should be discussed with the patient and the surgeon.

Technique: Ultrasound-Guided

Preparation, Patient Positioning and Regional Anesthesia Equipment

Before performing the interscalene block, the patient must have functional intravenous access and full monitoring applied, including the electrocardiogram, noninvasive blood pressure monitor, and the pulse oximeter. It is best to position the patient in either a semi-sitting position, in which the head is slightly turned with the pillow moved toward the contralateral side, or a semi-sitting and lateral position, with the pillow shifted toward the contralateral side in order to expose the neck (Fig. 24.2). In both of these positions, the ipsilateral arm of the patient should lie alongside the body.

To optimize the ergonomics, the operator and ultrasound machine should be positioned on the ipsilateral and contralateral side of the block, respectively. In this manner, the operator will have a simultaneous view of the needle, ultrasound probe, and the monitor of the ultrasound machine. In terms of selection of equipment, we recommend a linear and high-frequency ultrasound probe with the depth of field set at approximately 3 cm to start with, and a 50-mm 22-G short beveled regional block needle. For a single shot interscalene block, a hat and mask with sterile gloves should be worn and skin asepsis maintained, and for continuous interscalene block, a hat and mask with sterile gown and gloves should be worn with full aseptic technique.

Sonoanatomy

To find the nerve roots between the anterior and middle scalene muscles in the interscalene groove, the brachial plexus can be located with either a medial-to-lateral approach or a trace back method from the supraclavicular fossa. In the medial-to-lateral approach, the ultrasound probe is placed in a transverse orientation at the level of the cricoid cartilage and, in the preliminary scan, the sternocleidomastoid muscle, internal jugular vein, and the carotid artery are identified (Fig. 24.3). Lateral and posterior movement of the ultrasound probe will subsequently reveal the linear arrangement of the nerve roots between the anterior and middle scalene muscles deep to the tapering posterior border of the sternocleidomastoid muscle. In the trace back method from the supraclavicular fossa, which is the preferred method of the authors, the ultrasound probe is placed in a transverse orientation immediately proximal and parallel to the midpoint of the clavicle with caudad tilt. In the preliminary scan, the subclavian artery and three trunks of the brachial plexus, with the appearance of a "bunch of grapes," are identified (Fig. 24.4). Cephalad movement of the ultrasound probe, following the superior trunk of the brachial plexus, will then show its transition back to the nerve roots, with the appearance of a "string of pearls" or "traffic lights," positioned

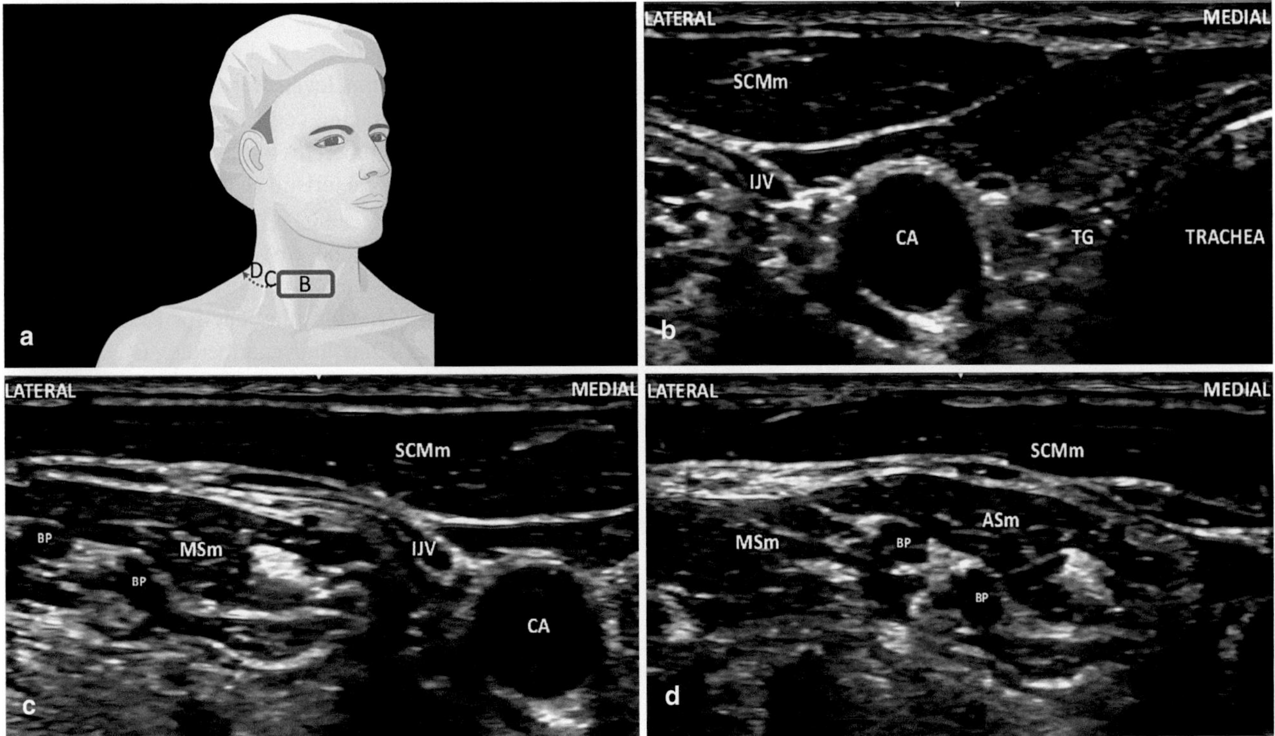

Fig. 24.3 Illustration of the position of the ultrasound probe for the interscalene block (**a**), and, as it is moved from medial-to-lateral to localize the cervical nerve roots, the consecutive sonographic images (**b–d**) are obtained. *ASm* anterior scalene muscle, *BP* brachial plexus, *CA* carotid artery, *IJV* internal jugular vein, *MSm* middle scalene muscle, *SCMm* sternocleidomastoid muscle, *TG* thyroid gland. Reproduced with permission from Philip Peng Educational Series

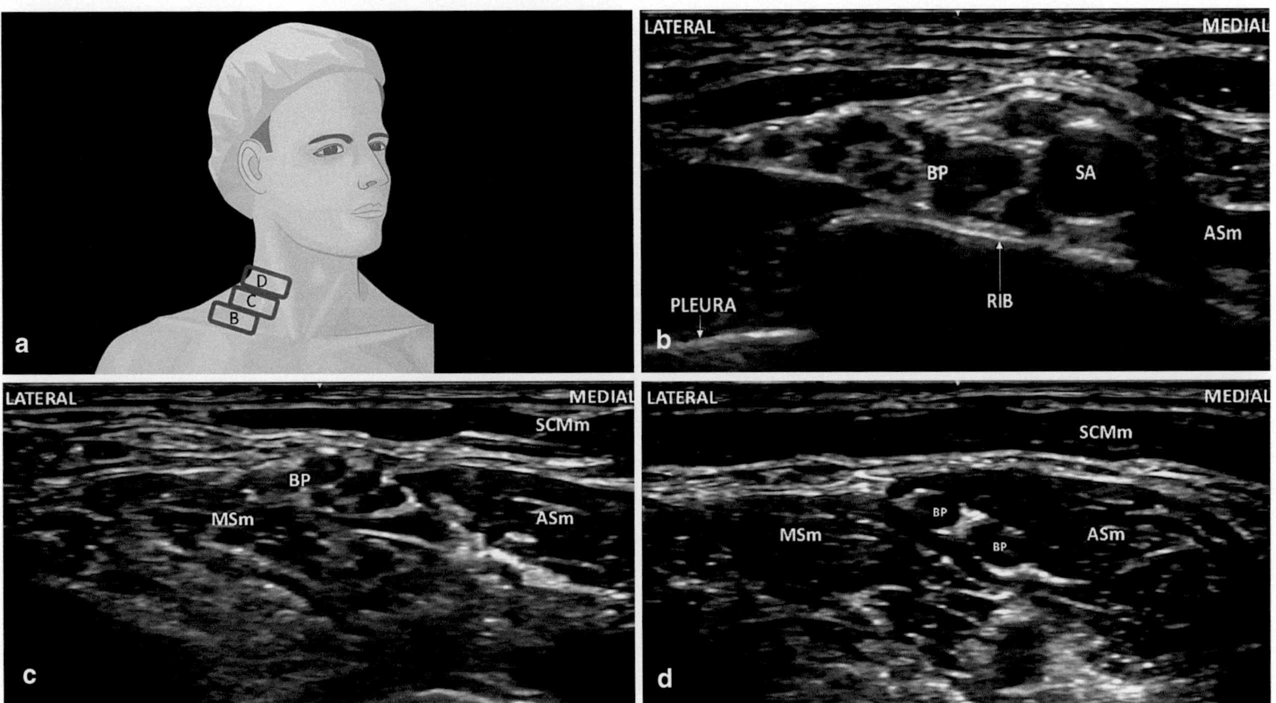

Fig. 24.4 Illustration of the position of the ultrasound probe for the interscalene block (**a**), and, as it is traced cephalad from the supraclavicular fossa to localize the cervical nerve roots, the sequential sonographic images (**b–d**) are obtained. *ASm* anterior scalene muscle, *BP* brachial plexus, *MSm* middle scalene muscle, *SA* subclavian artery, *SCMm* sternocleidomastoid muscle. Reproduced with permission from Philip Peng Educational Series

between the anterior and middle scalene muscles. Caudad tilt of the ultrasound probe should result in the ultrasound beam interacting with the nerve roots at a perpendicular angle, optimizing the image on the monitor of the ultrasound machine. Interestingly, this ultrasound method tends to be performed at a more caudad level compared to the landmark technique. It is likely a reflection, at least in part, of the improved visualization of the scalene muscles on ultrasound as they course distally, owing to the increasing number of muscle fibers joining from the transverse processes of the lower cervical vertebra.

On the interscalene view of the brachial plexus, the nerve roots appear on ultrasound as hypoechoic circular or oval structures, and their low echogenicity is a reflection of the relatively high ratio of neural to nonneural tissue contained within them. Cadaveric studies of the brachial plexus have uncovered the anatomical correlation of the ultrasonographic "traffic lights" sign. From cephalad to caudad, it is composed of the C5 root, the upper fascicle of C6 root, and the lower fascicle of C6 root. The C7 root forms the middle trunk of the brachial plexus, explaining its relatively greater physical separation from the C6 root in comparison to the C5 root. The C8 and T1 roots are deeper and more caudad and so are difficult to visualize at this level. Nerve roots can be identified on ultrasound by tracing cephalad to the point of their emergence between the tubercles of the transverse processes, and recognizing the characteristic shapes of their respective transverse processes (Fig. 24.5). The transverse processes of C5 and C6 have anterior and posterior tubercles, while the transverse process of C7 has only a posterior tubercle but not an anterior tubercle. Of note, the anterior tubercle of C6, often referred to as Chassaignac tubercle, is particularly prominent. Medial to the C7 root at the level of its transverse process, the vertebral artery can be identified prior to its entry into the foramen transversarium of the C6 transverse process.

Importantly, several nerves and blood vessels are present in this anatomical area. If not recognized, they can be at risk of iatrogenic injury should they be in the path of the needle or result in the inadvertent intravascular injection of local anesthetic. The phrenic nerve is located as a hypoechoic structure on the anterior border of the anterior scalene mus-

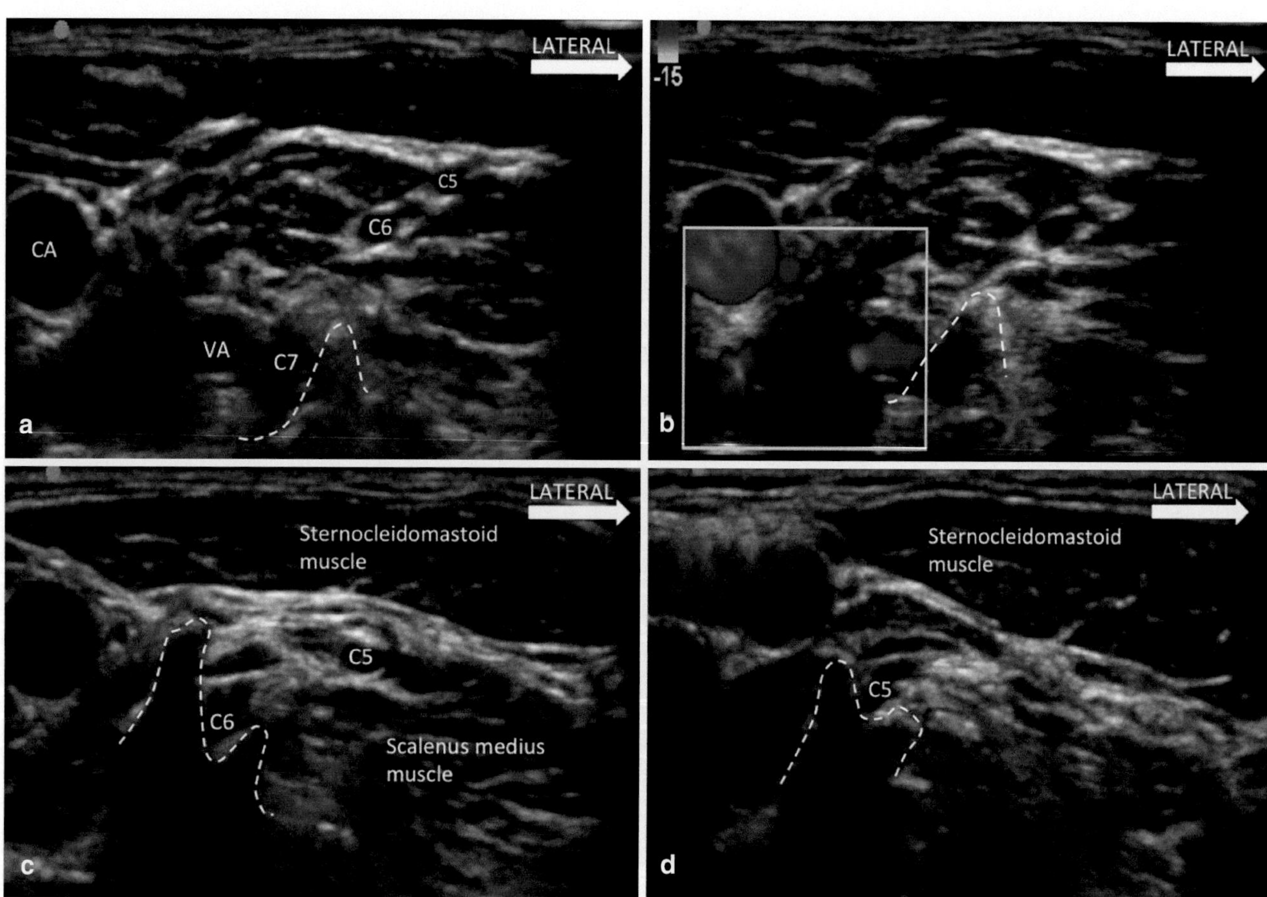

Fig. 24.5 C5, C6, and C7 nerve roots and the characteristic shapes of their respective transverse processes. (**a**) C7. Note the absence of the anterior tubercle. (**b**) C7 with Doppler scan. (**c**) C6. Note the prominence of the anterior tubercle. (**d**) C5. Note the size of anterior and posterior tubercle is similar. *CA* carotid artery, *VA* vertebral artery. Reproduced with permission from Philip Peng Educational Series

cle deep to the sternocleidomastoid muscle (Fig. 24.6). The dorsal scapular nerve and the long thoracic nerve, both hyperechoic in nature, pass through the middle scalene muscle (Fig. 24.7). Of importance, the dorsal scapular nerve is located in the superior portion of the middle scalene muscle and is in the trajectory of the needle for the lateral-to-medial approach. The long thoracic nerve is normally in the inferior portion and close to the tendinous part of the middle scalene muscle, further away from the path of the needle. Blood vessels such as the inferior thyroid, transverse cervical, and the suprascapular arteries, which are all branches of the thyrocervical trunk of the subclavian artery, can be identified with the use of color Doppler.

Single Shot Injection

Once the optimal ultrasound image has been obtained and the structures of interest have been recognized, the needle can be inserted either with an in-plane or out-of-plane approach, the former in a lateral-to-medial or medial-to-lateral direction. It is the preference of the authors that the needle be placed in-plane from lateral-to-medial in order to avoid injury to the phrenic nerve (Fig. 24.8). The dorsal scapular and the long thoracic nerves must be looked for in the middle scalene muscle with this approach to avoid inadvertent neural injury. The needle should be directed through the prevertebral fascia, when a fascial click may be appreciated, to one of three locations: deep to the C6

Fig. 24.6 Identification of the phrenic nerve on the anterior border of the anterior scalene muscle at the level of the interscalene block. *ASm* anterior scalene muscle, *BP* brachial plexus, *MSm* middle scalene muscle, *PHn* phrenic nerve, *SCMm* sternocleidomastoid muscle, *SCP*, superficial cervical plexus. Reproduced with permission from Philip Peng Educational Series

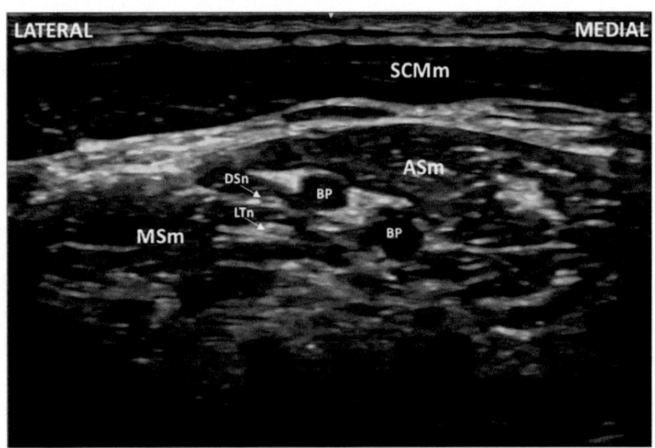

Fig. 24.7 Identification of the dorsal scapular and the long thoracic nerve in the middle scalene muscle at the level of the interscalene block. *ASm* anterior scalene muscle, *BP* brachial plexus, *DSn* dorsal scapular nerve, *LTn* long thoracic nerve, *MSm* middle scalene muscle, *SCMm* sternocleidomastoid muscle. Reprinted with permission from Neel Desai and Eric Albrecht

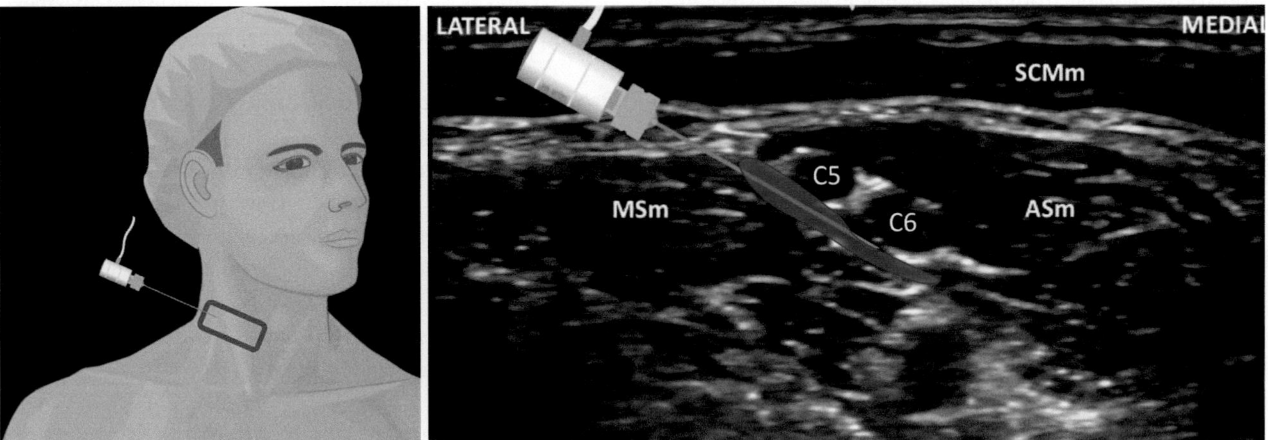

Fig. 24.8 Needle insertion technique for the interscalene block. The left panel demonstrates the direction of needle insertion from lateral-to-medial. The right panel shows the spread of local anesthetic injectate lateral to the C5 and C6 nerve roots. *ASm* anterior scalene muscle, *MSm* middle scalene muscle, *SCMm* sternocleidomastoid muscle. Reprinted with permission from Neel Desai and Eric Albrecht

root, in between the C5 and C6 roots, or superficial to the C5 root. Our recommendation is to place the tip of the needle deep to the C6 root in the first instance and, following negative aspiration, observe the spread of local anesthetic around the brachial plexus at the time of injection. Distal and proximal scanning with the ultrasound probe subsequent to the injection of local anesthetic can evaluate its spread. If the local anesthetic spreads in a suboptimal fashion, including into the middle scalene muscle, then the needle should be redirected, but its tip must never be placed between the fascicles of a nerve root as intraneural injection can otherwise occur. Further, the spread of local anesthetic just outside the fascia of the plexus and on one side of the nerve roots is sufficient for blockade, although its duration is inferior to circumferential and intraplexus spread. Occasionally, the C5 and C6 roots can course separately or together through the anterior scalene muscle, in which case tracing their trajectory can inform optimal placement of the needle. Should identification of the underlying anatomy be difficult, then ultrasound with concomitant nerve stimulation, seeking stimulation of the deltoid or biceps muscles, may be considered.

Superior trunk block remains an attractive alternative to interscalene block. It involves the more caudad injection of local anesthetic to the superior trunk of the brachial plexus once the C5 and C6 roots have united and prior to the leaving of the suprascapular nerve (Fig. 24.8). Its potential advantages include the identification of the C5 and C6 roots as part of the preliminary scan, even if anatomical variation is present, facilitates their blockade at the level of the superior trunk; path of the needle does not need to pass through the middle scalene muscle, and therefore the risk of injury to the dorsal scapular and long thoracic nerve is obviated; the presence of a connective tissue sheath provides protection to the nerves from needle contact; and the potential reduction of phrenic nerve involvement and hemidiaphragmatic paresis.

Surgical anesthesia can be achieved with interscalene block subsequent to only 5 ml of 0.75% ropivacaine, but the failure rate associated with this may be as high as 25%. It is less likely that such a decreased volume of local anesthetic will have the capacity to diffuse to and inhibit the supraclavicular nerve. Moreover, in everyday clinical practice and outside the context of trials, the success rate of these regional techniques with lower volumes of local anesthetic is probably reduced. Given this, within the limits of the maximum recommended dose of local anesthetic, we suggest that between 10 and 20 ml of long-acting local anesthetic such as 0.5% bupivacaine/levobupivacaine or 0.75% ropivacaine should be administered in interscalene block, with the lower and higher range of this dose for analgesia and anesthesia, respectively.

Continuous Catheter Technique

Continuous catheters to extend the benefits of single shot interscalene block involve the in-plane or out-of-plane insertion of a needle similar to the single shot technique. It is the recommendation of the authors that the needle be directed through the prevertebral fascia to the level of the C5 and C6 roots, with the tip of the needle remaining lateral to and outside the fascia of the plexus. Following the injection of local anesthetic to open up the space and verify its appropriate spread, the needle should be maintained in its position while a catheter is inserted up to a maximum of 1–2 cm into this perineural space. It is possible to localize the perineural catheter on ultrasound by either visualizing its trajectory on insertion or injecting local anesthetic or air through it.

Technique: Landmark-Based

Percutaneous access to the brachial plexus was described in the early 1900s. In 1925, Etienne reported the successful blockade of the brachial plexus by inserting a needle at the level of the cricothyroid membrane, halfway between the lateral border of the sternocleidomastoid muscle and anterior border of the trapezius muscle after a single injection through the area around the scalene muscles. This approach is most likely the first clinically useful interscalene block technique. Winnie's approach was further modified, in line with numerous developments in regional anesthesia, e.g., by the placement of a perineural catheter. An interscalene block relies on the spread of local anesthetic solution within the interscalene groove to accomplish blockade of the brachial plexus. This block involves injecting local anesthetic around the trunks of the brachial plexus between the anterior and middle scalene muscles at the level of the cricoid cartilage. The interscalene brachial plexus block is an effective analgesic and anesthesia technique for shoulder and proximal humeral surgery.

Preparation, Patient Positioning, and Regional Anesthesia Equipment

The monitoring and patient position is similar to that with ultrasound-guided technique. However, peripheral nerve stimulator is required and the block needle is 50-mm 22-G short-bevel insulated stimulating atraumatic needle with "immobile needle" injection lead. For continuous technique with catheter insertion, a 50-mm 22-G stimulating atraumatic needle with catheter will be used.

Landmark-Guided Approach with Nerve Stimulator

The landmark is sternocleidomastoid muscle, interscalene groove between the scalenus anterior and scalenus medius muscles, transverse process (C6), and external jugular vein (Figs. 24.9a, b). To locate the injection site, the patient's

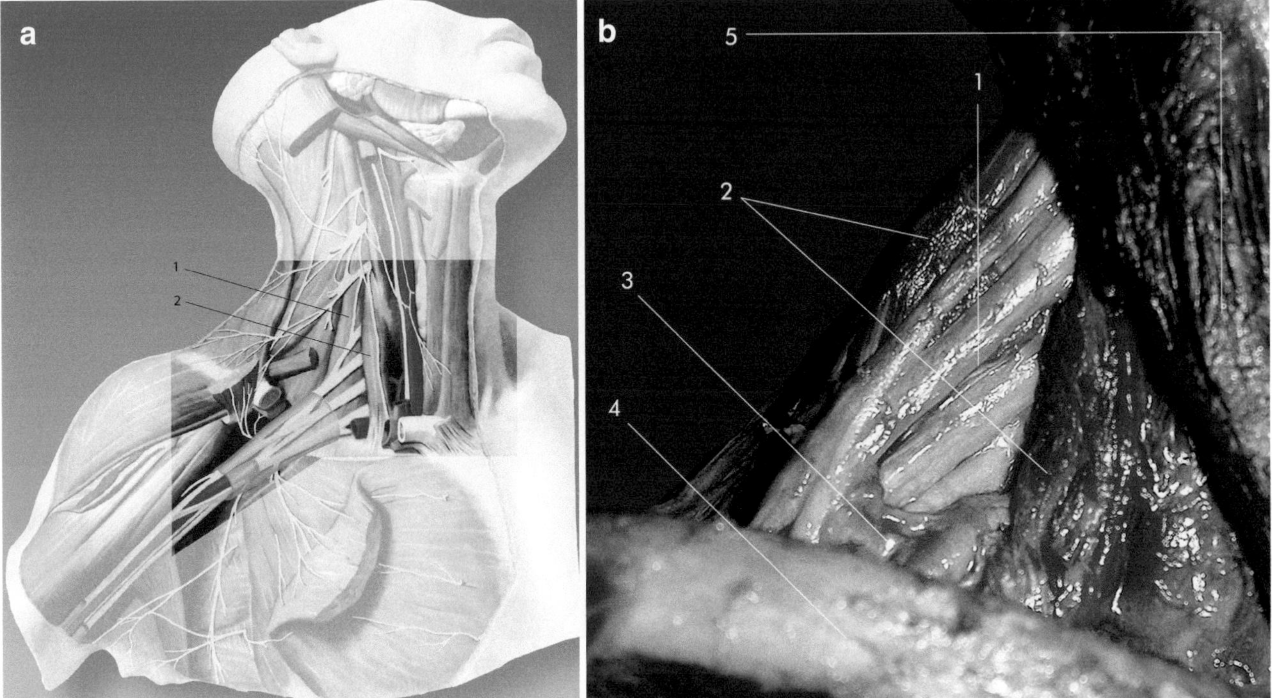

Fig. 24.9 (**a**) The interscalene groove. Scalenus medius muscle *(1)* and scalenus anterior muscle *(2)*. Injection of the local anesthetic into the proximal neurovascular sheath of the brachial plexus. The plexus is located in a kind of "sandwich" between the scalenus anterior muscle and scalenus medius muscle, covered by prevertebral fascia. (Reproduced with permission from Danilo Jankovic). (**b**) *(1)* Trunks of the brachial plexus with subclavian artery, *(2)* middle and anterior scalene muscles, *(3)* proximal supraclavicular plexus sheath, *(4)* clavicle, *(5)* sternocleidomastoid muscle (Reproduced with permission from Danilo Jankovic)

arm is drawn in the direction of the knee (Fig. 24.10). The patient is asked to turn the head to the opposite side and to lift it slightly (ca. 20°), so that the posterior edge of the sternocleidomastoid muscle becomes evident (Fig. 24.11). The transverse process (C6) is palpated at the lateral edge of the sternocleidomastoid muscle. For confirmation and guidance, the pulsation of the subclavian artery (at the lower end of the interscalene groove) and the upper edge of the clavicle can also be palpated and their distance from the injection site can be estimated (Fig. 24.12). Posterior to the sternocleidomastoid muscle, the scalenus anterior muscle is palpated. The interscalene groove between the scalenus anterior and scalenus medius muscles is felt with "rolling fingers" and located (Fig. 24.13). The injection site in the interscalene groove lies at the level of the cricoid, opposite the transverse process of C6 (Chassaignac's tubercle). The external jugular vein often crosses the level of the cricoid cartilage here (Fig. 24.14). When there are anatomical difficulties, it is helpful for the patient to inhale deeply or to try and blow out the cheeks. The scalene muscles then tense up and the interscalene groove becomes more easily palpable.

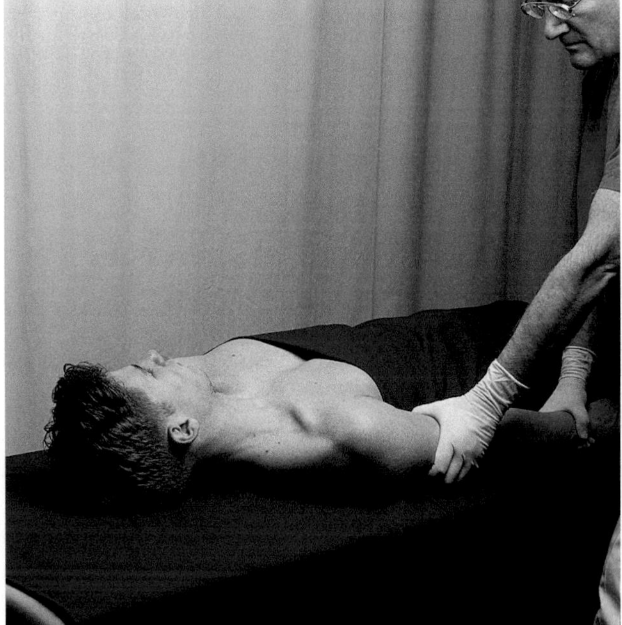

Fig. 24.10 Drawing the arm toward the knee (with permission from Danilo Jankovic)

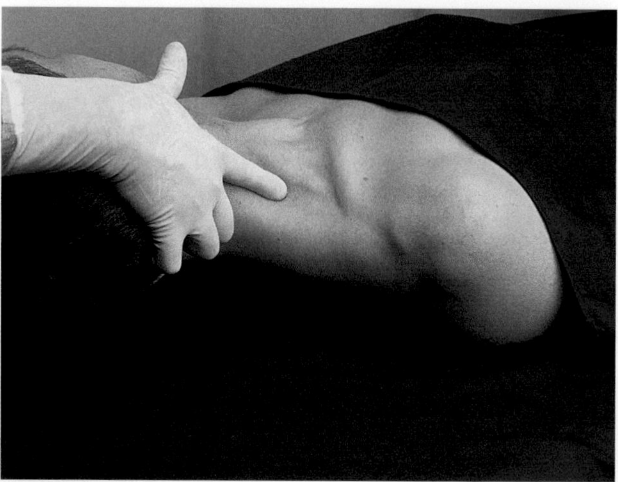

Fig. 24.11 Turning the head to the opposite side and raising it slightly (Reproduced with permission from Danilo Jankovic)

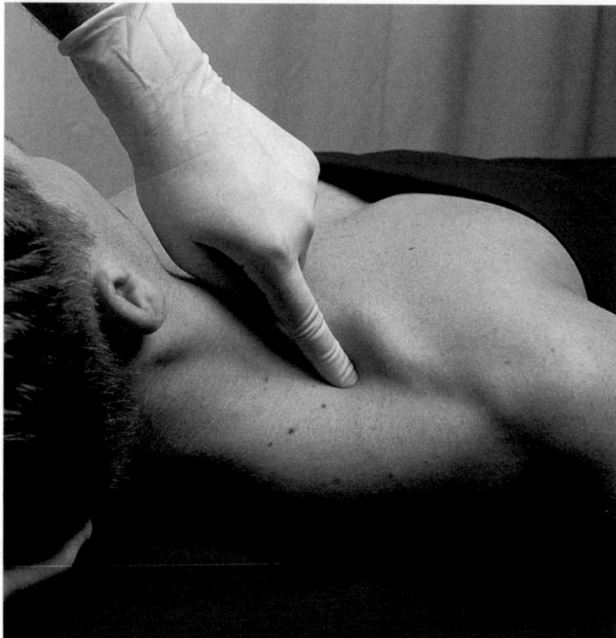

Fig. 24.12 Palpating the clavicle and subclavian artery (Reproduced with permission from Danilo Jankovic)

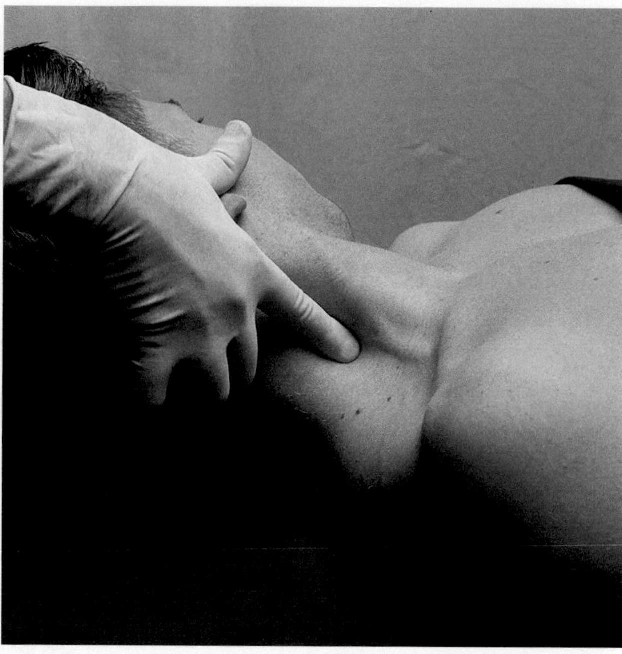

Fig. 24.13 Palpating the interscalene groove with "rolling" fingers (Reproduced with permission from Danilo Jankovic)

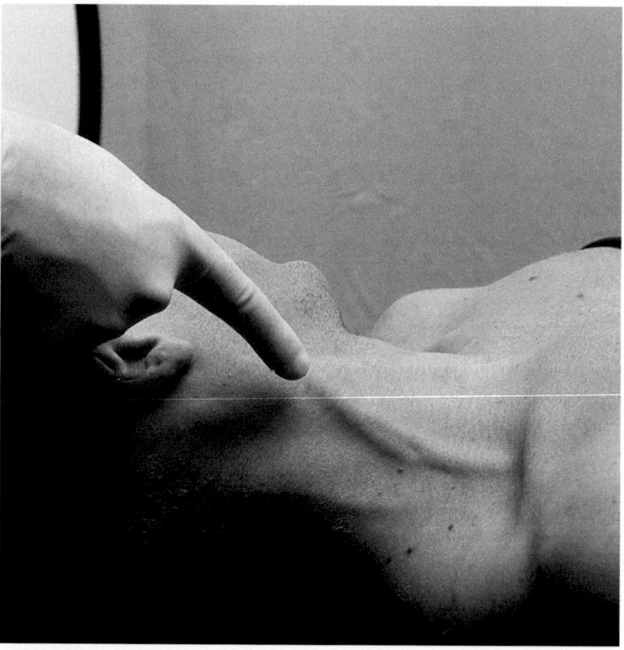

Fig. 24.14 Position of the external jugular vein (Reproduced with permission from Danilo Jankovic)

After identification of the interscalene groove, the block needle is introduced at an angle of 30° caudally and slightly laterally, in the direction of the transition from the middle to the lateral third of the clavicle (Fig. 24.15). A stimulation current of 1–2 mA and 2 Hz is selected with a stimulus duration of 0.1 ms. After a motor response from the relevant musculature (twitching in the biceps brachii muscle and/or deltoid muscle) indicative of C5 or C6, the stimulation current is reduced to 0.2–0.3 mA. Slight twitching suggests that the stimulation needle is in the immediate vicinity of the nerve. Local anesthetic is injected or in the case of a continuous catheter technique, a catheter is advanced approximately 3 cm beyond the end of the cannula or needle (Fig. 24.16). After removal of the cannula or needle, fixation of the catheter, and placement of a bacterial filter, and after careful aspiration and injection of a test dose, the bolus administration of the local anesthetic follows.

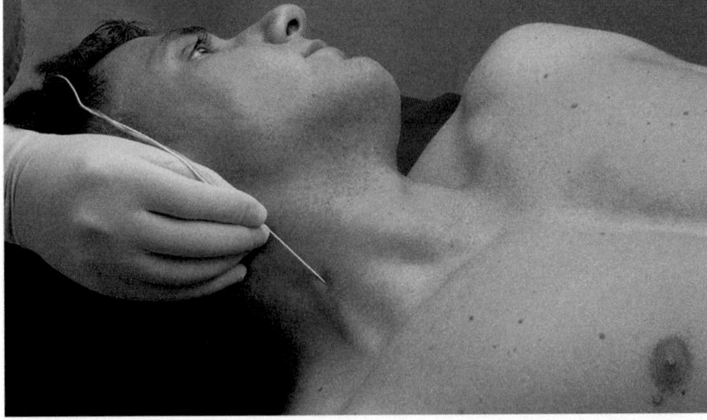

Fig. 24.15 Introducing the puncture needle at an angle of ca. 30° to the skin, caudally and laterally in the direction of the transition from the middle to the lateral third of the clavicle (Reproduced with permission from Danilo Jankovic)

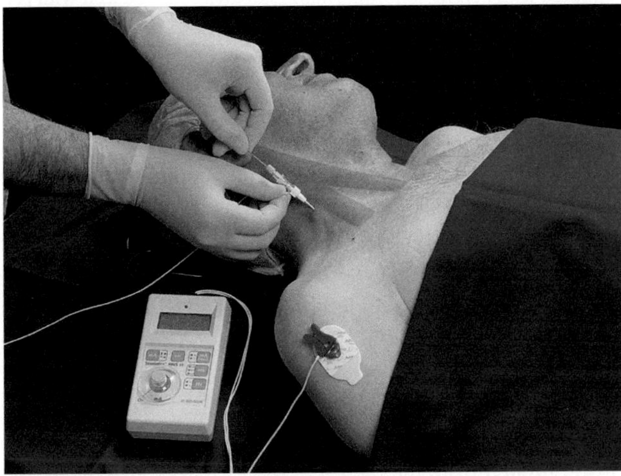

Fig. 24.16 Interscalene block (continuous technique). Introducing the catheter through a Tuohy needle (Reproduced with permission from Danilo Jankovic)

Practical Tips for Landmark-Guided Technique

The needle should never been advanced beyond 2.5 cm to avoid the risk of mechanical complications (cervical cord injury, pneumothorax, vascular puncture).

Intraneural positioning of the needle should be excluded. Never inject when resistance (high pressure) to injection of local anesthetic is met (intrafascicular needle placement). If the patient reports severe pain during the injection, the injection should be stopped at once and the needle should be withdrawn.

Local anesthetic should not be injected when a motor response is obtained at the current intensity < 0.2 mA because this is associated with intraneural needle placement.

If the motor response is elevation of scapula, the needle is most likely in the scalenus medius where the needle is stimulating the dorsal scapular nerve. The needle should be moved in the anterior direction.

Supraclavicular Block

General Consideration

Supraclavicular block is performed at the level of the distal trunks and proximal divisions of the brachial plexus. It has previously been referred to as the spinal of the arm due to its reported capacity to provide complete and reliable anesthesia with a short latency, probably a reflection of the dense arrangement of the brachial plexus at the supraclavicular level. Evidence to date, however, does not confirm this with a meta-analysis demonstrating axillary, infraclavicular, and supraclavicular block to be associated with similar onset times and success rates.

Indication

Supraclavicular block is indicated for surgical procedures on the arm, elbow, forearm, and hand (Fig. 24.17). It is not the brachial plexus block of choice for surgery of the shoulder as the supraclavicular branches of the cervical plexus are even further away for local anesthetic to diffuse to and inhibit, and the suprascapular nerve may have already left the brachial plexus (Fig. 24.18). Absolute and relative contraindications are similar to those relevant to the interscalene block. In all cases, the balanced view of risks and benefits of the selected brachial plexus block technique should be discussed with the patient and the surgeon.

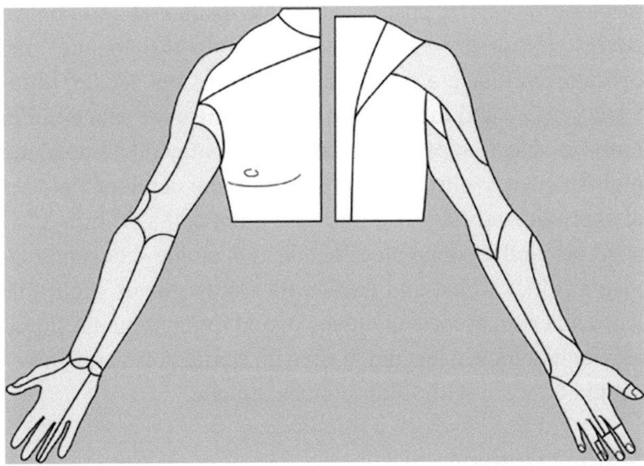

Fig. 24.17 Expected distribution of anesthesia subsequent to supraclavicular block. Reprinted with permission from Danilo Jankovic

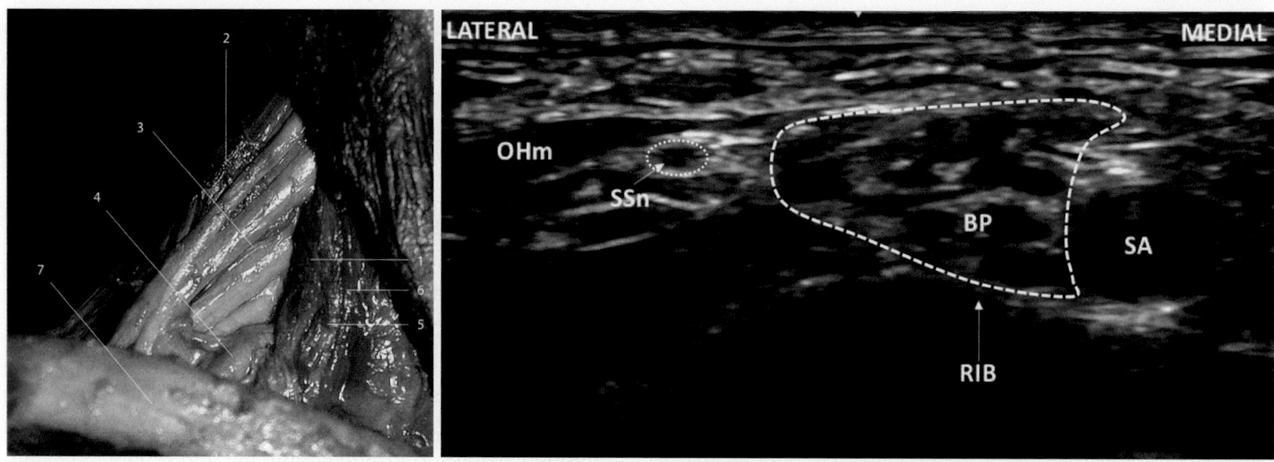

Fig. 24.18 Left panel. Anatomical dissection of the brachial plexus trunk. (1) Anterior scalene muscle, (2) middle scalene muscle, (3) trunks of the brachial plexus and subclavian artery, (4) proximal supraclavicular plexus sheath, (5) phrenic nerve, (6) ascending cervical artery, (7) clavicle. Right panel. Corresponding sonographic image of this supraclavicular region. Supraclavicular nerve is visualized deep to the omohyoid muscle and lateral to the brachial plexus at the level of the supraclavicular block. *BP* brachial plexus, *OHm* omohyoid muscle, *SA* subclavian artery, *SSn* suprascapular nerve. Anatomical dissection reprinted with permission from Danilo Jankovic. Reproduced with permission from Philip Peng Educational Series

Technique

Preparation, Patient Positioning, and Regional Anesthesia Equipment

Before performing the supraclavicular block, the patient must have functional intravenous access and full monitoring applied, including the electrocardiogram, noninvasive blood pressure monitor and the pulse oximeter, and should have functional intravenous access. It is best to position the patient in either a semi-sitting or supine position, in which the head is slightly turned with the pillow moved toward the contralateral side to expose the neck, and the ipsilateral arm is placed alongside the body (Fig. 24.2).

To optimize the ergonomics, the operator and ultrasound machine should be positioned on the ipsilateral and contralateral side of the block, respectively. In this manner, the operator will have a simultaneous view of the needle, ultrasound probe, and the monitor of the ultrasound machine. In terms of selection of equipment, we recommend a linear and high-frequency ultrasound probe, with the depth of field set at approximately 3 to 4 cm to start with, and a 50-mm 22-G short beveled regional block needle. For single shot supraclavicular block, a hat and mask with sterile gloves should be worn and skin asepsis maintained, and for continuous supraclavicular block, a hat and mask with sterile gown and gloves should be worn with full aseptic technique.

Sonoanatomy

To find the distal trunks and proximal divisions in the supraclavicular fossa, the ultrasound probe is placed in a transverse orientation immediately proximal and parallel to the midpoint of the clavicle with caudad tilt, similar to the initial position of the trace back method relevant to the interscalene block. In the preliminary scan, from medial-to-lateral, the subclavian vein, insertion of anterior scalene muscle, subclavian artery, and posterolateral brachial plexus, with the appearance of a "bunch of grapes," and the insertion of middle scalene muscle are identified (Fig. 24.19). Caudad tilt and parasagittal rotation of the ultrasound probe should be adjusted until the first rib, rather than the pleura, is located deep to the subclavian artery and brachial plexus as a bony backstop to subserve safety on needling. The first rib can be differentiated from the pleura as the former is visualized as a discontinuous and hyperechoic line with an underlying acoustic shadow, and the latter as a hyperechoic line that shimmers with the parietal and visceral pleura sliding over one another in respiration.

On the supraclavicular view of the brachial plexus, the distal trunks and proximal divisions appear on ultrasound as hypoechoic circular or oval structures surrounded by fascia. It is often possible to distinguish between the superior, middle, and the inferior trunks. Lateral and superficial to the subclavian artery is the superior trunk, composed of the C5 and C6 roots, and in the corner pocket between the subclavian artery and first rib is the inferior trunk, made up of the C8 and T1 roots. The middle trunk, composed of just the C7 root, is located between the superior and inferior trunks. It is the position of the inferior trunk in this corner pocket which is responsible for the increased vulnerability of the ulnar nerve to incomplete blockade and sparing. The components of the brachial plexus at the supraclavicular level can sometimes be separated by a blood vessel such as the dorsal scapular artery, itself a branch of the thyrocervical trunk or subclavian artery, transverse cervical artery, and the supra-

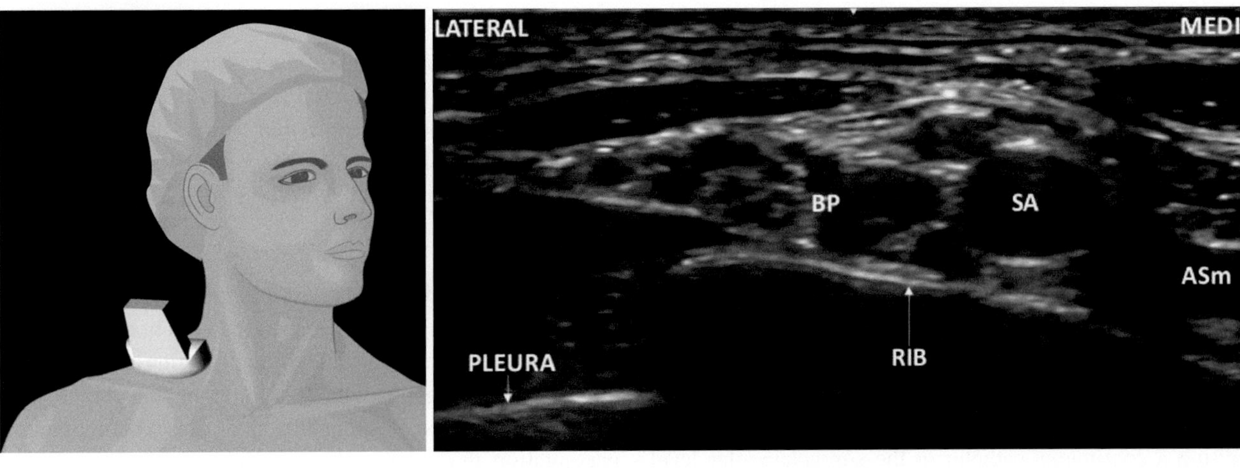

Fig. 24.19 The left panel demonstrates the position of the ultrasound probe for the supraclavicular block, and the right panel shows the corresponding sonographic image in the supraclavicular region. *BP* brachial plexus, *SA* subclavian artery. Reproduced with permission from Philip Peng Educational Series

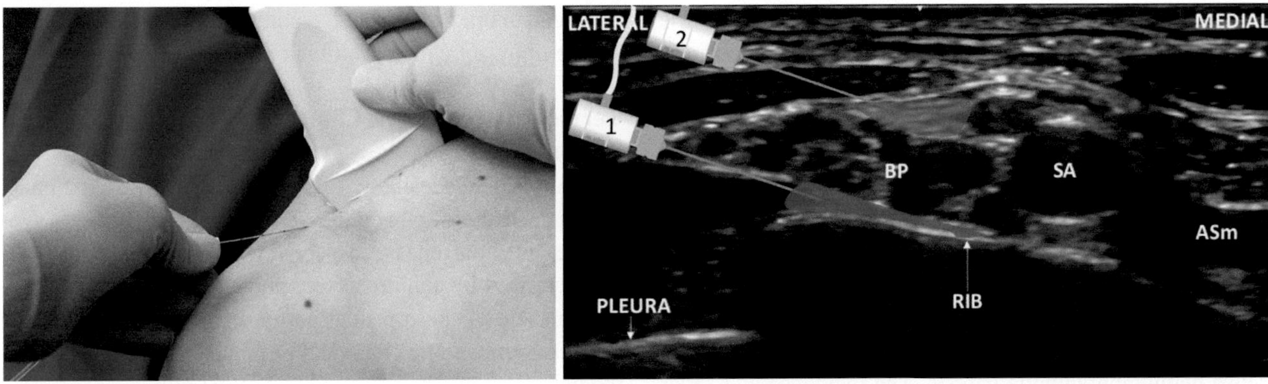

Fig. 24.20 Needle insertion technique for the supraclavicular block. The left panel demonstrates the point of needle insertion. The right panel shows the spread of local anesthetic injectate with the initial insertion of the needle (1) and the insertion of this needle inside the brachial plexus sheath (2). *BP* brachial plexus, *SA* subclavian artery. Reproduced with permission from Philip Peng Educational Series

scapular artery. It is important to identify these before needle insertion with the use of color Doppler.

Single Shot Injection

Once the optimal ultrasound image has been obtained and the structures of interest have been recognized, the needle can be inserted in-plane, either from lateral-to-medial (Fig. 24.20) or medial-to-lateral. It is the preference of the authors that the needle be placed in-plane from lateral-to-medial to facilitate ease of access to the corner pocket. In the approach of the needle toward the elements of the brachial plexus, hydrodissection can lead to the creation of space for its passage and the separation of neural structures. Our recommendation is to first place the tip of the needle in the corner pocket and inject local anesthetic between the brachial plexus, first rib, and the subclavian artery, hence lifting the brachial plexus and subclavian artery. Distal and proximal scanning with the ultrasound probe subsequent to the injection of local anesthetic can evaluate its spread. The needle can then be redirected to the superficial part of the brachial plexus where further local anesthetic can be injected. Compared to a single injection, multiple injections have not been consistently associated with a decrease in the time to onset or an increase in the success rate of the block in randomized controlled trials, and these relationships have not been confirmed on meta-analysis. Further, the procedural time is shorter with a single injection, and the risk of nerve injury may be higher with multiple injections. Relative to an extrafascial injection of local anesthetic, subfascial injection has been associated with a reduced time to onset of the block and the prolongation of the duration of analgesia, albeit with a higher rate of paresthesia. Should identification of the underlying anatomy be difficult, then ultrasound with concomitant nerve stimulation, seeking contraction of the biceps or triceps muscles for surgery proximal to the elbow and stimulation of the hand muscles for surgery distal to the elbow, may be considered.

Surgical anesthesia can be achieved with a minimum effective volume of 32 ml of 1.5% lidocaine and 1:200,000 adrenaline or 15 ml of 1.5% mepivacaine in 90% of patients. In our experience, within the limits of the maximum recommended dose of local anesthetic, we suggest that between 15 and 20 ml of 0.25% bupivacaine/levobupivacaine or 0.2–0.5% ropivacaine and 20–30 ml of 0.5% bupivacaine/levobupivacaine or 0.75% ropivacaine for perioperative analgesia and surgical anesthesia, respectively, should be administered in supraclavicular block.

Continuous Catheter Technique

Similar to continuous interscalene block, the process of inserting a continuous catheter at the supraclavicular level involves the placement of the needle, catheter insertion, and the securement of the catheter. It is the recommendation of the authors that the needle be inserted from lateral-to-medial and placed in the corner pocket. Following the injection of local anesthetic to open up the subfascial space and verify its appropriate spread, the needle should be maintained in its position while a catheter is inserted up to a maximum of 1–2 cm into this perineural space.

Complications

Hemidiaphragmatic Paresis

Given the proximity of the brachial plexus to the C3–5 nerve roots and phrenic nerve, its blockade above the clavicle can cause hemidiaphragmatic paresis. The incidence and severity of this complication differ with the exact site of regional block. Interscalene block is associated with an incidence of hemidiaphragmatic paresis of up to 100%. It can manifest as mild dyspnea and lead to decreases in measures of pulmonary function such as forced vital capacity by 25–30%. Supraclavicular block, in contrast, is related to an incidence of hemidiaphragmatic paresis in the range of 50%. It has not been reported to result in respiratory symptoms or changes in measures of spirometric function to the same extent as that for interscalene block. Strategies to lower the risk of hemidiaphragmatic paresis in interscalene block include reducing the concentration and/or volume of local anesthetic to 0.125% bupivacaine or 5 ml, respectively, and injecting the local anesthetic lateral to the brachial plexus in an extrafascial fashion. None of these techniques, however, decrease the risk of hemidiaphragmatic paresis below 20%, and hence brachial plexus blocks superior to the clavicle are not recommended in patients who are not able to tolerate a 30% reduction in respiratory function.

Pneumothorax

Pneumothorax can develop following interscalene and supraclavicular block at a historical rate of 0.2% and 0.5–6.1%, respectively. If pneumothorax does occur, then patients are not likely to report symptoms until 6–12 h later at which point they may have mild symptoms such as pleuritic chest pain.

Bradycardic and Hypotensive Events

Interscalene block has been associated with bradycardic and hypotensive events in awake patients having shoulder surgery in the sitting position. It is thought that the Bezold-Jarisch reflex is responsible for this hemodynamic presentation that occurs an hour or so following regional blockade in 17–24% of patients. Decreased venous return, owing to the redistribution of blood volume to the legs while sitting, and increased contraction of the therefore relatively empty heart, secondary to increased sympathetic stimulation, lead to bradycardia and hypotension. It can be prevented with prophylactic metoprolol but not glycopyrrolate.

Cervical Sympathetic Chain and Recurrent Laryngeal Nerve

Spread of local anesthetic to the cervical sympathetic chain and/or recurrent laryngeal nerve can result in Horner's syndrome and hoarseness, respectively. Horner's syndrome is characterized by anhidrosis, enophthalmos, miosis, and ptosis. In view of the transient nature of the inhibition of the cervical sympathetic chain and/or recurrent laryngeal nerve, the patient should be educated and reassured.

Suggested Reading

Albrecht E, Mermoud J, Fournier N, Kern C, Kirkham KR. A systematic review of ultrasound-guided methods for brachial plexus blockade. Anaesthesia [Internet]. 2016; [cited 2020 Aug 18];71:213–27. Available from: https://pubmed.ncbi.nlm.nih.gov/26670119/

Allesio JG, Rosenblum M, Shea K, Freitas D. A retrospective comparison of interscalene block and general anesthesia for ambulatory surgery and shoulder arthroscopy. Reg Anesthesia. 1995;20(1):62–8.

Arab SA, Alharbi MK, Nada EMS, Alrefai DA, Mowafi HA. Ultrasound-guided supraclavicular brachial plexus block: single versus triple injection technique for upper limb arteriovenous access surgery. Anesth Analg [Internet]. 2014; [cited 2020 Aug 19];118:1120–5. Available from: https://pubmed.ncbi.nlm.nih.gov/24686046/

Barutell C, Vidal F, Raich M, Montero A. A neurological complication following interscalene brachial plexus block. Anesthesia. 1980;35:365–7.

Blanchard J, Ramamurthy S. Brachial plexus. In: Benumof LJ, editor. Clinical procedures in anesthesia and intensive care. Philadelphia: Lippincott-Raven; 1992.

Borgeat A, Ekatodramis G, Kalberer F, Benz C. Acute and nonacute complications associated with interscalene block and shoulder surgery: a prospective study. Anesthesiology [Internet]. 2001; [cited 2020 Aug 20];95:875–80. Available from: https://pubmed.ncbi.nlm.nih.gov/11605927/

Bridenbaugh DL. The upper extremity: Somatic blockade. In: Cousins MJ, Bridenbaugh DL, editors. Neural Blockade. 2nd ed. Philadelphia: Lippincott-Raven; 1988.

Brown DL, Cahill DR, Bridenbaugh LD. Supraclavicular nerve block: anatomic analysis of a method to prevent pneumothorax. Anesth Analg [Internet]. 1993; [cited 2020 Aug 18];76:530–4. Available from: https://pubmed.ncbi.nlm.nih.gov/8452261/

Burckett-St Laurent D, Chan V, Chin KJ. Refining the ultrasound-guided interscalene brachial plexus block: the superior trunk approach. Can J Anaesth [Internet]. 2014; [cited 2020 Aug 17];61:1098–102. Available from: https://pubmed.ncbi.nlm.nih.gov/25208976/

D'Alessio JG, Weller RS, Rosenblum M. Activation of the Bezold-Jarisch reflex in the sitting position for shoulder arthroscopy using interscalene block. Anesth Analg. 1995; [cited 2020 Aug 20];80:1158–62. Available from: https://pubmed.ncbi.nlm.nih.gov/7762845/

Durrani Z, Winnie AP. Brainstem toxicity with reversible locked-in syndrome after interscalene brachial plexus block. Anesth Analg. 1991;72:249–52.

Etienne J. Regional Anesthesia: Its application in the surgical treatment of cancer of the breast (French). Faculte` de Me`decin de Paris; 1925.

Franco CD, Williams JM. Ultrasound-guided interscalene block: reevaluation of the stoplight sign and clinical implications. Reg Anesth Pain Med [Internet]. 2016; [cited 2020 Aug 17];41:452–9. Available from: https://rapm.bmj.com/content/41/4/452

Gautier P, Vandepitte C, Ramquet C, Decoopman M, Xu D, Hadzic A. The minimum effective anesthetic volume of 0.75% ropivacaine in ultrasound-guided interscalene brachial plexus block. Anesth Analg [Internet]. 2011; [cited 2020 Aug 17];113:951–5. Available from: https://pubmed.ncbi.nlm.nih.gov/21821517/

Gentili ME, Le foulon-Gourves M, Mamelle JC. Acute respiratory failure following interscalene block: Complications of combined general and regional anesthesia. Reg Anesthesia. 1994;19(4):292–3.

Gologorsky E, Leanza RF. Contralateral anesthesia following interscalene block. Anestn Analg. 1992;75:311–2.

Haasio J, Tuominen MK, Rosenberg PH. Continuous interscalene brachial plexus block during and after shoulder surgery. Ann Chir Gynaecol. 1990;79:103–7.

Hall R. Hydrochlorate of cocaine. N Engl J Med. 1884;40:643–6.

Hanson NA, Auyong DB. Systematic ultrasound identification of the dorsal scapular and long thoracic nerves during interscalene block. Reg Anesth Pain Med. 2013; [cited 2020 Aug 17];38:54–7. Available from: https://pubmed.ncbi.nlm.nih.gov/23080352/

Kahn RL, Hargett MJ. Beta-adrenergic blockers and vasovagal episodes during shoulder surgery in the sitting position under interscalene block. Anesth Analg [Internet]. 1999; [cited 2020 Aug 20];88:378–81. Available from: https://pubmed.ncbi.nlm.nih.gov/9972760/

Kardash K, Schools A, Concepcion M. Effects of brachial plexus fentanyl on supraclavicular block. Reg Anesthesia. 1995;20(4):311–5.

Kessler J, Schafhalter-Zoppoth I, Gray AT. An ultrasound study of the phrenic nerve in the posterior cervical triangle: implications for the interscalene brachial plexus block. Reg Anesthsia Pain Med [Internet]. 2008; [cited 2020 Aug 17];33:545–50. Available from: https://pubmed.ncbi.nlm.nih.gov/19258969/

Kumar A, Battit GE, Froese AB, Long MC. Bilateral cervical and thoracic epidural blockade complicating interscalene brachial plexus block:Report of two cases. Anesthesiology. 1971;35:650–2.

Lanz E, Theiss D, Jankovic D. The extent of blockade following various techniques of brachial plexus block. Anesth Analg. 1983;62:55–8.

Liguori GA, Kahn RL, Gordon J, Gordon MA, Urban MK. The use of metoprolol and glycopyrrolate to prevent hypotensive/bradycardic events during shoulder arthroscopy in the sitting position under interscalene block. Anesth Analg [Internet]. 1998; [cited 2020 Aug 20];87:1320–5. Available from: https://pubmed.ncbi.nlm.nih.gov/9842820/

Löfström B, Wennberg A, Widen L. Late disturbances in nerve function after block with local anesthetic agents. Acta Anesth Scand. 1966;10:111–22.

Lombard TP, Couper JL. Bilateral spread of analgesia following interscalene brachial plexus block. Anesthesiology. 1983;58:472–3.

Lu I-C, Hsu H-T, Soo L-Y, Lu DV, Chen T-I, Wang J-J, et al. Ultrasound examination for the optimal head position for interscalene brachial plexus block. Acta Anaesthesiol Taiwanica [Internet]. 2007; [cited 2020 Aug 19];45:73–8. Available from: https://pubmed.ncbi.nlm.nih.gov/17694682/

Mak PHK, Irwin MG, Ooi CGC, Chow BFM. Incidence of diaphragmatic paralysis following supraclavicular brachial plexus block and its effect on pulmonary function. Anaesthesia. 2001; [cited 2020 Aug 20];56:352–6. Available from: https://pubmed.ncbi.nlm.nih.gov/11284823/

Martinoli C, Bianchi S, Santacroce E, Pugliese F, Graif M, Derchi LE. Brachial plexus sonography: a technique for assessing the root level. Am J Roentgenol [Internet]. 2002; [cited 2020 Aug 17];179:699–702. Available from: https://pubmed.ncbi.nlm.nih.gov/12185049/

Meier G, Bauereis C, Heinrich C. Der interskalenäre Plexuskatheter zur Anästhesie und postoperativen Schmerztherapie. Anaesthesist. 1997;46:715–9.

Moayeri N, Bigeleisen PE, Groen GJ. Quantitative architecture of the brachial plexus and surrounding compartments, and their possible significance for plexus blocks. Anesthesiology [Internet]. 2008; [cited 2020 Aug 18];108:299–304. Available from: https://pubmed.ncbi.nlm.nih.gov/18212575/

Muhly WT, Orebaugh SL. Sonoanatomy of the vasculature at the supraclavicular and interscalene regions relevant for brachial plexus block. Acta Anaesthesiol Scand [Internet]. Acta Anaesthesiol Scand. 2011; [cited 2020 Aug 17];55:1247–53. Available from: https://pubmed.ncbi.nlm.nih.gov/22092130/

Neal JM, Gerancher JC, Hebl JR, Ilfeld BM, McCartney CJL, Franco CD, et al. Upper extremity regional anesthesia. Essentials of our current understanding, 2008. Reg Anesth Pain Med [Internet]. 2009; [cited 2020 Aug 17];34:134–70. Available from: /pmc/articles/PMC2779737/?report=abstract

Neal JM, Moore JM, Kopacz DJ, Liu SS, Kramer DJ, Plorde JJ. Quantitative analysis of respiratory, motor, and sensory function after supraclavicular block. Anesth Analg [Internet]. 1998; [cited 2020 Aug 20];86:1239–44. Available from: https://pubmed.ncbi.nlm.nih.gov/9620512/

Neil RS. Postoperative analgesia following brachial plexus block. Br J Anaesth. 1978;50:379–82.

Palhais N, Brull R, Kern C, Jacot-Guillarmod A, Charmoy A, Farron A, et al. Extrafascial injection for interscalene brachial plexus block reduces respiratory complications compared with a conventional intrafascial injection: a randomized, controlled, double-blind trial. Br J Anaesth. 2016;116:531–7.

Pere P. The effect of continuous interscalene brachial plexus block with 0,125% bupivacaine plus fentanyl on diaphragmatic motility and ventilatory function. Reg Anesth. 1993;18:93–7.

Pippa P, Cominelli E, Marinelli C, Aito S. Brachial plexus block using the posterior approach. Eur J Anaesth. 1990;7:411–20.

Poeck K. Therapie der peripheren Nervenschädigungen. In: Poeck K, editor. Neurologie. 9th ed. New York: Springer; 1994.

Ross S, Scarborough CD. Total spinal anesthesia following brachial plexus block. Anesthesiology. 1973;39:458.

Roy M, Nadeau MJ, Côté D, Levesque S, Dion N, Nicole PC, et al. Comparison of a single- or double-Injection technique for ultrasound-guided supraclavicular block: a prospective, randomized, blinded controlled study. Reg Anesth Pain Med. 2012; [cited 2020 Aug 19];37:55–9. Available from: https://pubmed.ncbi.nlm.nih.gov/22030724/

Rucci FS, Pippa P, Barbagli R, Doni L. How many interscalenic blocks are there? A comparison between the lateral and posterior approach. Eur J Anesth. 1993;10:303–7.

Selander D, Dhuner KG, Lundborg G. Peripheral nerve injury due to injection needles used for regional anesthesia. Acta Anesth Scand. 1977;21:182–8.

Siler JN, Liff PI, Davis JF. A new complication of interscalene brachial plexus block. Anesthesiology. 1973;38(6):590–1.

Silverstein WB, Moin U, Saiyed MD, Brown AR. Interscalene block with a nerve stimulator: A deltoid motor response is a satisfactory endpoint for successful block. Reg Anesth Pain Med. 2000;25(4):356–9.

Sivashanmugam T, Ray S, Ravishankar M, Jaya V, Selvam E, Karmakar MK. Randomized comparison of extrafascial versus subfascial injection of local anesthetic during ultrasound-guided supraclavicular brachial plexus block. Reg Anesth Pain Med [Internet]. 2015; [cited 2020 Aug 19];40:337–43. Available from: https://pubmed.ncbi.nlm.nih.gov/26066385/

Song JG, Jeon DG, Kang BJ, Park KK. Minimum effective volume of mepivacaine for ultrasound-guided supraclavicular block. Korean J Anesthesiol [Internet]. 2013; [cited 2020 Aug 19];65:37–41. Available from: /pmc/articles/PMC3726844/?report=abstract

Spence BC, Beach ML, Gallagher JD, Sites BD. Ultrasound-guided interscalene blocks: understanding where to inject the local anaesthetic. Anaesthesia. 2011; [cited 2020 Aug 17];66:509–14. Available from: https://pubmed.ncbi.nlm.nih.gov/21568985/

Tetzlaff JE, Yoon HJ, Brems J. Interscalene brachial plexus block for shoulder surgery. Reg. Anesthesia. 1994;19(5):339–43.

Tetzlaff JE, Yoon HJ, Dilger J, Brems J. Subdural anesthesia as a complication of an interscalene brachial plexus block. Reg. Anesthesia. 1994;19(5):357–9.

Thiagarajah S, Lear E, Azar I, Salzer J, Zeiligson E. Bronchospasm following interscalene brachial plexus block. Anesthesiology. 1984;61:759–61.

Tran DQH, Bertini P, Zaouter C, Muñoz L, Finlayson RJ. A prospective, randomized comparison between single-and double-injection ultrasound-guided infraclavicular brachial plexus block. Reg Anesth Pain Med. 2010; [cited 2020 Aug 19];35:16–21. Available from: https://pubmed.ncbi.nlm.nih.gov/20048654/

Tran DQH, Dugani S, Correa JA, Dyachenko A, Alsenosy N, Finlayson RJ. Minimum effective volume of lidocaine for ultrasound-guided supraclavicular block. Reg Anesth Pain Med. 2011; [cited 2020 Aug 19];36:466–9. Available from: https://pubmed.ncbi.nlm.nih.gov/21857275/

Tran DQH, Elgueta MF, Aliste J, Finlayson RJ. Diaphragm-sparing nerve blocks for shoulder surgery. Reg Anesth Pain Med [Internet]. 2017; [cited 2020 Aug 20];42:32–8. Available from: https://pubmed.ncbi.nlm.nih.gov/27941477/

Urban MK, Urquhart B. Evaluation of brachial plexus anesthesia for upper extremity surgery. Reg Anesth. 1994;19(3):175–82.

Urmey WF. Interscalene Block. The truth about twitches. Reg Anesth and Pain Med. 2000;25(4):340–2.

Urmey WF, Gloeggler PJ. Pulmonary function changes during interscalene brachial plexus block: effects of decreasing local anesthetic injection volume. Reg Anesth [Internet]. 1993; [cited 2020 Aug 20];18:244–9. Available from: https://pubmed.ncbi.nlm.nih.gov/8398959/

Urmey WF, Gloeggler PJ. Pulmonary function changes during interscalene brachial plexus block. Effects of decreasing local anesthetic injection volume. Reg Anesth. 1993;18:244–9.

Urmey WF, McDonald M. Hemidiaphragmatic paresis during interscalene brachial plexus block: effects on pulmonary function and chest wall mechanics. Anesth Analg. 1992; [cited 2020 Aug 20];74:357. Available from: https://pubmed.ncbi.nlm.nih.gov/1539813/

Urmey WF, Talts KH, Sharrock NE. One hundred percent incidence of hemidiaphragmatic paresis associated with interscalene brachial plexus anesthesia as diagnosed by ultrasonography. Anesth Analg. 1991; [cited 2020 Aug 20];72:498–503. Available from: https://pubmed.ncbi.nlm.nih.gov/2006740/

Urmey WF, Talts KH, Sharrock NE. One hundred percent incidence of hemidiafragmatic paresis associated with interscalene brachial plexus anesthesias diagnosed by ultrasonography. Anesth Analg. 1991;72:498–503.

Viel EJ, Eledjam JJ, de la Coussage JE, D'Athis F. Brachial plexus block with opioids for postoperative pain relief: Comparison between buprenorphine and morphine. Reg Anesthesia. 1989;14:274–8.

Vranken JH, van der Vegt MH, Zuurmond WA, Pij AJ, Dzoljic M. Continuous brachial plexus block at the cervical level using a posterior approach in the management of neuropathic cancer pain. Reg Anesth and Pain Med. 2001;26(6):572–5.

Winchell SW, Wolf R. The incidence of neuropathy following upper extremity nerve blocks. Reg. Anesthesia. 1985;10:12–5

Brachial Plexus Below the Clavicle

25

Ki Jinn Chin

Contents

Infraclavicular Brachial Plexus Block

Introduction

The infraclavicular brachial plexus block was described as early as 1917, but was overshadowed in the early part of the twentieth century by the axillary and supraclavicular approaches. Refinements in the technique by Wilson and by Kilka led to a deserved increase in popularity in the mid-1990s, and ultrasound guidance has established it as a highly effective, simple, and safe technique for providing anesthesia of the upper limb below the shoulder.

Indications and Contraindications

It provides anesthesia or analgesia of the elbow, forearm, and hand. It may be performed as either a single-shot or continuous catheter technique.

The contraindications are summarized in Table 25.1.

K. J. Chin (✉)
Department of Anesthesiology and Pain Medicine, Toronto Western Hospital, University of Toronto, Toronto, ON, Canada
e-mail: kijinn.chin@uhn.ca

D. Jankovic, P. Peng (eds.), *Regional Nerve Blocks in Anesthesia and Pain Therapy*,
https://doi.org/10.1007/978-3-030-88727-8_25

Table 25.1 Contraindications to performing an infraclavicular brachial plexus block

Absolute

- There are no absolute contraindications specific to this block. Generic contraindications such as patient refusal, allergy to local anesthetics, and local infection at the site of injection apply as usual.

Relative

- Coagulopathy – The neurovascular bundle and associated vessels lie relatively deep, under the pectoralis muscles, and may therefore be less easy to compress in the event of vascular puncture. However, the likelihood of a clinically significant hematoma in most patients is low.
- Distorted surface anatomy, e.g., from clavicular fracture, prior surgery, etc.
- Foreign bodies in the infraclavicular area, e.g., subclavian central venous lines, pacemaker or other battery packs, etc.

Table 25.2 Advantages and disadvantages of the infraclavicular brachial plexus block versus other approaches

Advantages compared to other brachial plexus block techniques

1. Both surface landmark-guided and ultrasound-guided techniques are associated with high block success rates.
2. The infraclavicular block is a safe block. It carries minimal risk of adverse effects associated with injections administered more proximally in the root of the neck, e.g., phrenic nerve palsy and Horner's syndrome. Pneumothorax has been described with more medial surface landmark-guided approaches (i.e., the vertical infraclavicular block), but we consider the risk to be minimal with other approaches where needle insertion occurs lateral to the thoracic cage.
3. The neurostimulation-guided technique utilizes simple surface anatomical landmarks and a straightforward needle approach.
4. The endpoint for injection in the ultrasound-guided technique (local anesthetic spread posterior to the artery) is simple and easily recognized.
5. There is evidence that tourniquet application may be tolerated better, which is attributed to local anesthetic spread to the intercostobrachial nerve .
6. The infraclavicular block may be performed with the arm in any position (adducted or abducted at the shoulder).
7. Nerve catheters are easily fixed in this location and do not interfere with patient movement.

Disadvantages compared to other brachial plexus block techniques

1. The brachial plexus in the ultrasound-guided infraclavicular block is usually at least 3–4 cm deep in most adults, and a relatively steep needle trajectory is required to reach it. However, this is not usually an issue with modern ultrasound equipment and sufficient experience with ultrasound-guided regional anesthesia in general.
2. Needle insertion through the pectoral muscles can be uncomfortable for the patient.
3. Nerve catheter placement is usually perpendicular to the plexus, rather than parallel to it. This may make advancement of the catheter more difficult and limit the length of catheter that can be advanced into the brachial plexus sheath, which in turn may increase the risk of dislodgement. However, this is true of most of the other brachial plexus approaches.

The advantages and disadvantages of infraclavicular approach compared with other brachial plexus block techniques are summarized in Table 25.2.

Functional Anatomy

The infraclavicular-axillary region can be visualized as a pyramidal space. The apex of the pyramid is formed medially by the confluence of the clavicle, scapula, and first rib; the base is the skin and subcutaneous tissue of the armpit. The posterior wall is formed by the scapula and its associated muscles; the anterior wall by the pectoralis major and minor. The humerus, together with the converging muscles and tendons of the anterior and posterior walls that insert into it, constitutes the lateral wall. The bony thoracic cage, and overlying serratus anterior muscle, forms the medial wall. The contents of this space are the axillary artery and vein, the brachial plexus, lymph nodes, and loose areolar tissue. Of note, the intercostobrachial nerve runs along the inferior aspect of the brachial plexus sheath in the infraclavicular-axillary fossa and is often blocked by anesthetic spread following infraclavicular injection (Fig. 25.1).

The coracoid process of the scapula and the clavicle are the chief bony landmarks. The coracoid process lies superior and lateral to the course of the brachial plexus.

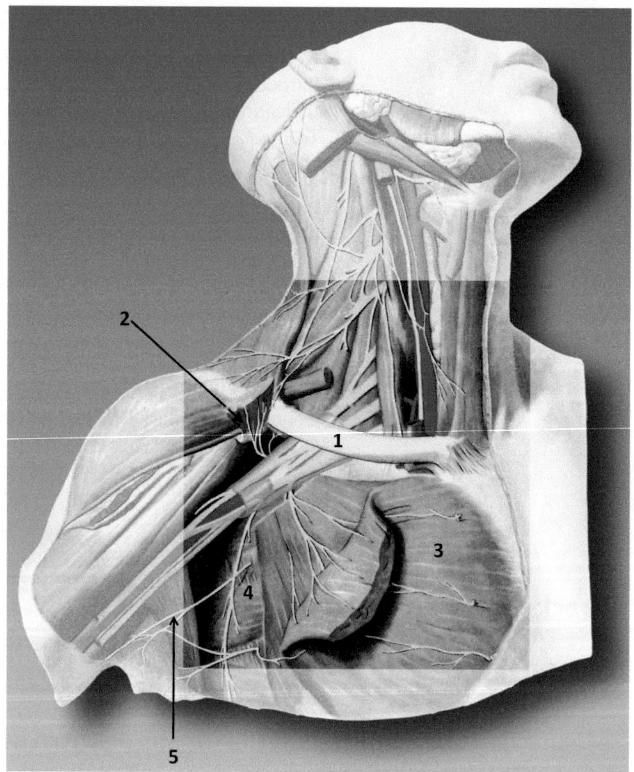

Fig. 25.1 Anatomy of the infraclavicular area. Note that the brachial plexus passes under the approximate midpoint of the clavicle, and then deep to pectoralis major and minor muscle, medial and inferior to the coracoid process. Legend: (1) clavicle, (2) coracoid process and pectoralis minor (cut and reflected), (3) pectoralis major (cut and reflected), (4) thoracic cage, (5) intercostobrachial nerve. Reprinted with permission from Dr. Danilo Jankovic

The brachial plexus runs in a line between the base of the interscalene groove and the axilla, and knowing this is helpful when trying to mentally visualize the location of the brachial plexus. Note that the direction in which this line runs will differ depending on whether the arm is adducted or abducted (Figs. 25.2 and 25.3).

It is important to appreciate that the orientation of the cords around the axillary artery varies with distance from the clavicle. As the brachial plexus emerges from under the clavicle, the cords are bunched together on the superior (cephalad) aspect of the artery. As the neurovascular bundle travels more distally, the cords gradually separate out and "spiral" around the axillary artery to eventually adopt the classically described position of lateral, posterior, and medial to the artery (Fig. 25.4). This arrangement is best appreciated when scanning the infraclavicular area with the arm abducted at the shoulder.

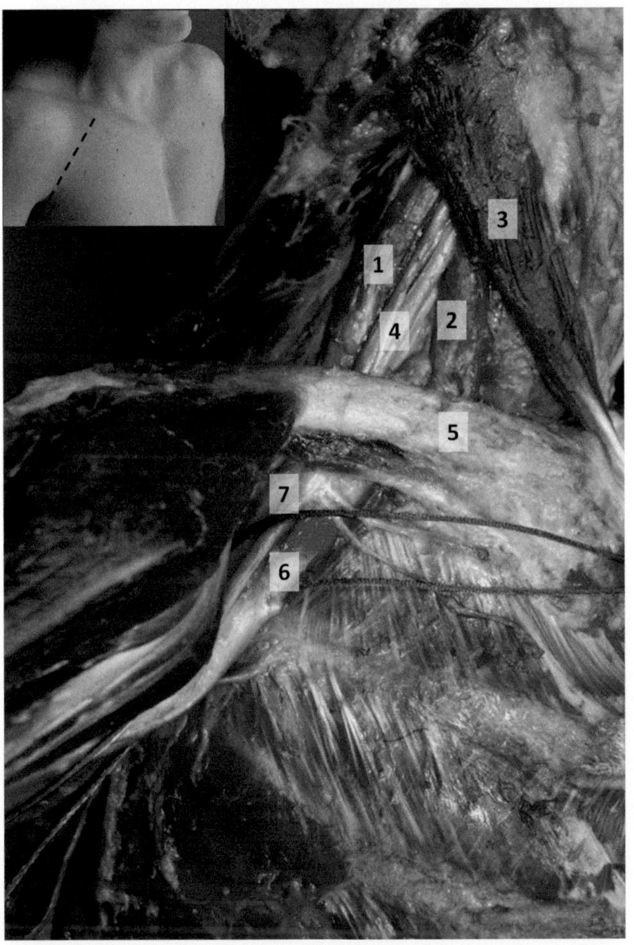

Fig. 25.2 The course of the infraclavicular brachial plexus with arm adducted at the shoulder. The neurovascular bundle is encircled by the blue suture. Note that all the cords of the brachial plexus are clustered superolateral to the axillary artery in the medial portion of the infraclavicular fossa. Legend: (1) middle scalene muscle, (2) anterior scalene muscle, (3) sternocleidomastoid muscle, (4) trunks of the brachial plexus, (5) clavicle, (6) axillary artery, (7) cords of brachial plexus. Reprinted with permission from Dr. Danilo Jankovic

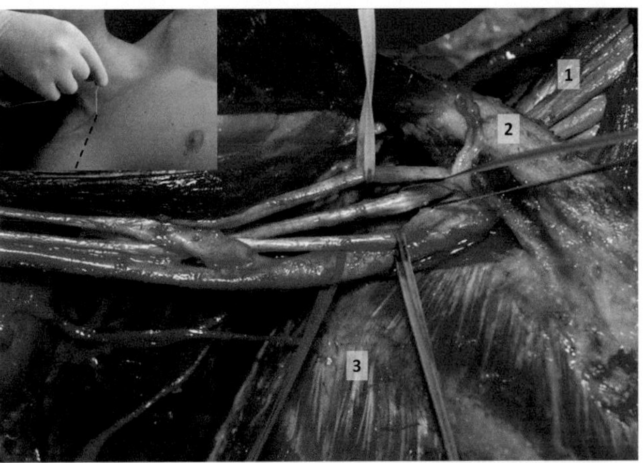

Fig. 25.3 Course of the infraclavicular brachial plexus with the arm abducted at the shoulder. Note that all the cords of the brachial plexus are clustered superolateral to the axillary artery in the medial portion of the infraclavicular fossa. Lateral cord (white), posterior cord (blue), medial cord (green), axillary artery (red). Note the relationship between the brachial plexus and the thoracic cage, which determines the relative risk of pneumothorax with more medial versus lateral approaches. Legend: (1) trunks of the brachial plexus, (2) clavicle, (3) thoracic cage of ribs and intercostal muscles. Reprinted with permission from Dr. Danilo Jankovic

There is a fascial sheath around the neurovascular bundle that contains and directs the spread of local anesthetic. There is usually a fascial septum that separates the lateral cord from posterior and medial cord; piercing this septum is necessary to achieve the U-shaped local anesthetic spread posterior to the artery that is associated with block success (Fig. 25.5). This also explains why obtaining a posterior cord motor response in the landmark-guided approach carries the highest success rates.

Technique: Surface Landmark, Neurostimulation-Guided Approach—Single-Shot

Before the procedure, the preparation of the equipment and patient is summarized in Table 25.3.

Several slightly different surface landmark-guided techniques have been described, all of which use neurostimulation as the endpoint for nerve localization and injection. We recommend one of two techniques:

1. The coracoid (Wilson) approach.
2. The vertical infraclavicular plexus (VIP) approach.

The patient is placed supine with the operative arm adducted, and if possible flexed at the elbow and placed on the patient's abdomen to facilitate observation of motor responses. It is recommended that the operator stand at the head of the patient, on the side to be blocked, as this makes it easier to observe and avoid inadvertent medial direction of the needle. However, the operator may also stand on the side of the patient if preferred.

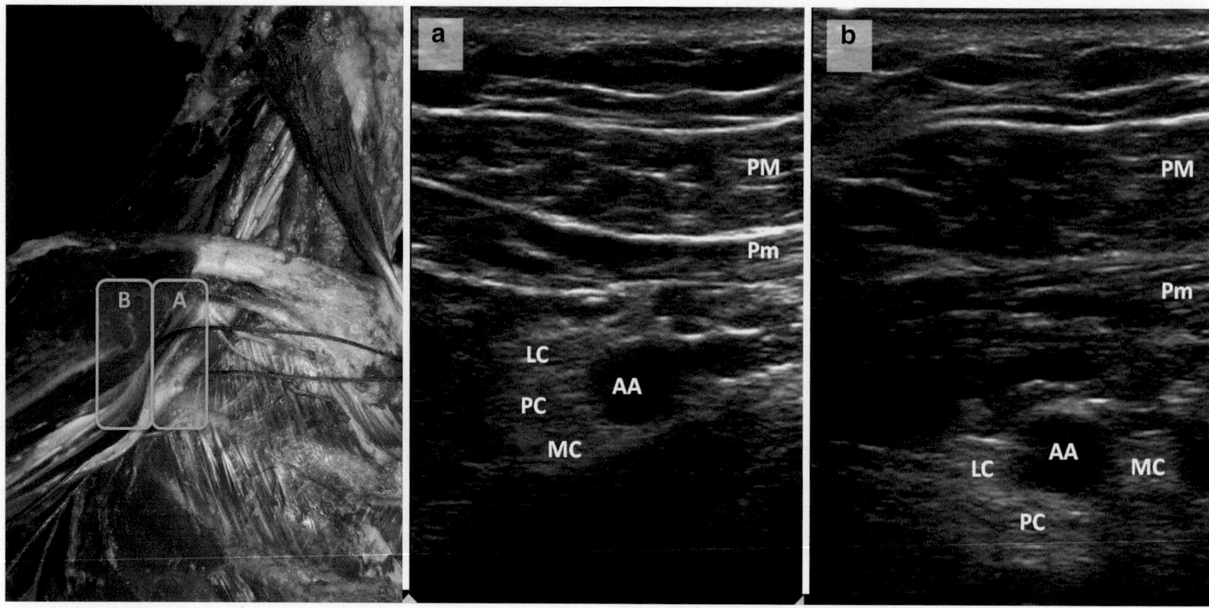

Fig. 25.4 Illustration of the variation in distribution of brachial plexus cords around the axillary artery (AA) depending on whether the probe is placed more medially (*position A*) or laterally (*position B*). In position A (*sonogram a*), the cords are clustered around the cephalad aspect of the artery and are often not distinguishable from each other. This view is usually only obtainable if the arm is abducted at the shoulder so that the clavicle moves up out of the way. In position B (*sonogram b*), the cords start to spread out around the artery. The lateral cord (LC) remains at the cephalad aspect of the artery, but the posterior cord (PC) and medial cord (MC) move into their classically described positions relative to the artery. Legend: *PM* pectoralis major, *Pm* pectoralis minor

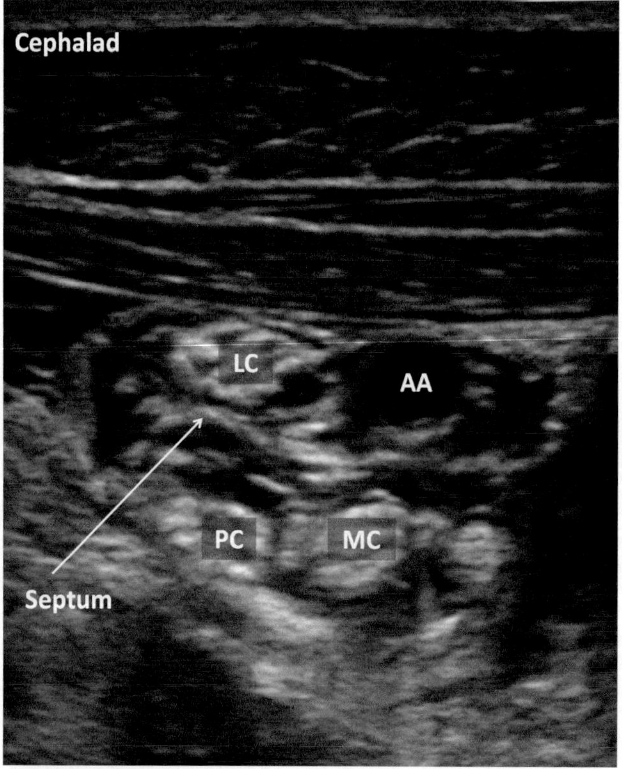

Fig. 25.5 Post-injection ultrasound image of the infraclavicular brachial plexus, illustrating the septum that separates the lateral cord (LC) from the posterior (PC) and medial (MC) cords. Our preference is therefore for a dual-injection technique, but there can be communication between the two compartments, and a single-injection technique posterior/deep to the artery (AA) may also suffice. (Image courtesy of Dr. Ki Jinn Chin)

Table 25.3 Preparation for a surface landmark, neurostimulation-guided infraclavicular brachial plexus block

Required supplies and equipment

- Disinfectant solution and swabs for skin preparation.
- Sterile gloves and drapes.
- Short-beveled 22G block needle with extension tubing.
  - A 50 mm needle is suitable in slimmer patients, but an 80 mm needle may be necessary in patients with a thick chest wall.
- Local anesthetic of choice in 10 ml or 20 ml syringes.
- Peripheral nerve stimulator.
- Lidocaine 1–2% in 3 ml syringe with a 25–27G hypodermic needle for skin infiltration (at operator's discretion).
- Equipment and supplies for managing life-threatening acute complications, including lipid emulsion for local anesthetic systemic toxicity.
- Drugs for intravenous sedation during the block (at operator's discretion).

Preparation of patient

- Obtain informed consent for the block.
- Explain expected clinical course including care of the insensate limb and managing the transition to systemic analgesia.
- Establish intravenous access, supplemental oxygen delivery, and standard monitors (ECG, noninvasive blood pressure, pulse oximetry).
- Perform a time-out to confirm patient identity and site and side of surgery.

Landmark-Guided Infraclavicular Block: Coracoid (Wilson) Approach

The coracoid process is palpated and marked. The site of needle insertion is the point 2 cm inferior and 2 cm medial to the coracoid process (Fig. 25.6).

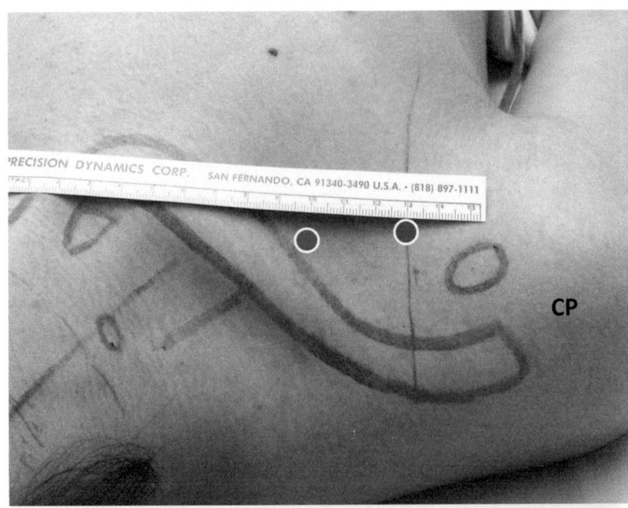

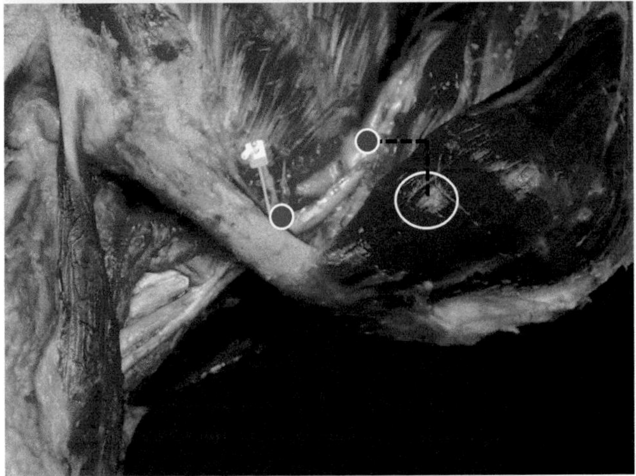

Fig. 25.6 Surface landmarks for the vertical infraclavicular plexus (VIP) approach and the coracoid (Wilson) approach to the infraclavicular block, illustrated in a volunteer and a cadaver. In the VIP approach, the needle insertion site (blue circle) is immediately inferior to the clavicle at its midpoint. In the coracoid approach, the needle insertion site (red circle) is located 2 cm medial and inferior to the coracoid process (CP). In both approaches, the needle is advanced perpendicular to the skin surface. Note that in the coracoid approach, the needle trajectory usually lies lateral to the thoracic cage. The green line indicates the interscalene groove and location of the brachial plexus. Reprinted with permission from Dr. Danilo Jankovic

Needle Insertion and Injection Technique

- Disinfect the skin, drape the area appropriately, prime the block needle and tubing with local anesthetic solution, and attach a nerve stimulator at an initial current setting of 0.5–0.8 mA, pulse duration of 0.1–0.3 msec, and frequency of 1–2 Hz. This lower initial current setting is recommended to reduce patient discomfort during needle passage through the pectoral muscles.
- Infiltrate the needle insertion site with local anesthetic. Fixing the skin over the skin insertion point with the second and third fingers of the nondominant hand, insert a 50–80 mm block needle at a 90° angle to the skin in a strict parasagittal plane. Medial angulation must be avoided to prevent pleural puncture.
- The pectoral muscles will initially be observed to twitch due to local stimulation as the needle passes through it. Once this twitch disappears, the nerve stimulator current may be turned up to 1 mA or more for nerve localization.
- Advance the needle slowly and steadily until a distal motor response in the wrist or hand (first to third fingers) is obtained at a current threshold of 0.3–0.5 mA.
- The ideal motor response, associated with the highest block success rate, is a posterior cord response of wrist or finger extension. A medial cord response may also be accepted. If elbow, wrist, or finger flexion is obtained (lateral cord), the needle should be advanced a little deeper, and may need to be redirected slightly more inferiorly or deeper.
- If no motor response is obtained despite inserting the needle to a depth of 4–5 cm in the average adult patient, or if bone is contacted (scapula), the needle should be withdrawn to the skin and redirected slightly more inferiorly or superiorly in the same parasagittal plane.
- Once an appropriate distal motor response has been obtained, incremental injection of local anesthetic is performed with intermittent aspiration to exclude intravascular injection.

Landmark-Guided Infraclavicular Block: Vertical Infraclavicular Plexus (VIP) Approach

The following surface landmarks are palpated and marked: the suprasternal notch and the anterior acromion. Precise location of the anterior acromion is very important, and it can be distinguished from the mobile humeral head by passive movement of the upper arm. The midpoint of the line between the suprasternal notch and anterior acromion is identified and marked – this is the needle insertion point, immediately inferior to the clavicle (Fig. 25.6).

Needle Insertion and Injection Technique

- Disinfect the skin, drape the area appropriately, prime the block needle and tubing with local anesthetic solution, and attach a nerve stimulator at an initial current setting of 1–2 mA, pulse duration of 0.1–0.3 msec, and frequency of 1–2 Hz.
- Infiltrate the skin insertion point with local anesthetic and advance the block needle at a 90° angle to the skin in a strict parasagittal plane (Fig. 25.7).
- Advance the needle slowly and steadily until a distal motor response in the wrist or hand (first to third fingers) is obtained at a current threshold of 0.3–0.5 mA.
- A posterior or medial cord response is preferred to a lateral cord response.

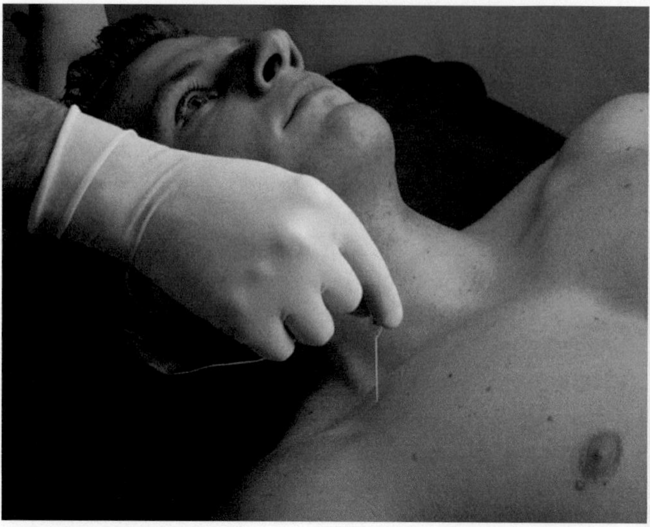

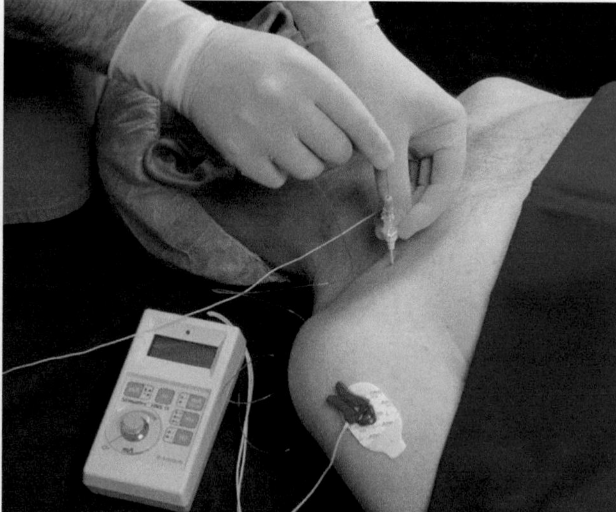

Fig. 25.7 The vertical infraclavicular plexus (VIP) approach to infraclavicular block, using a single-shot block needle (left) and a continuous peripheral nerve block catheter set (right). Note the needle trajectory perpendicular to the skin without any medial angulation. Reprinted with permission from Dr. Danilo Jankovic

- Medial angulation must be avoided to prevent puncture of the subclavian vessels. If blood is aspirated, it signifies that puncture has occurred and the needle should be redirected or reinserted more laterally.
- The plexus lies at a depth of 3–4 cm in the average adult patient. Caution should be exercised if this depth is reached without any motor response, as further insertion increases the risk of a pneumothorax. Contact with bone signals contact with the first rib and this depth should not be exceeded on subsequent passes.
- Once an appropriate distal motor response has been obtained, incremental injection of local anesthetic is performed with intermittent aspiration to exclude intravascular injection.

Technique: Landmark-Guided Continuous Nerve Block Technique

This is identical to the single-shot technique except that a peripheral nerve block catheter kit is used instead (Fig. 25.7). Either of the above approaches may be used, depending on operator preference and expertise.

The introducer needle is advanced as described above until the desired motor response is obtained. If a stimulating catheter is being used, 5–10 ml of 5% dextrose solution can be injected through the introducer needle to distend the paraneural sheath. This should also result in augmentation of the motor response. Injection of other solutions will abolish the motor response.

The catheter is then advanced approximately 3 cm beyond the tip of the introducer needle, looking to maintain a motor response at current thresholds of at least 0.3 mA and up to 0.8–1 mA. As the angle of insertion is at right angles to the course of the plexus, some resistance can be expected when advancing the catheter. This may be improved by the injection of 5–10 ml of fluid as described above. The needle is then withdrawn and the catheter fixed in place in the usual manner.

Technique: Ultrasound-Guided Approach—Single-Shot

Before the procedure, the preparation of the equipment and patient is summarized in Table 25.4.

Scanning Technique

The patient is placed supine. While it is also possible to perform the block with the arm adducted at the shoulder, it is recommended that the arm be abducted if possible. This moves the clavicle superiorly and out of the way of the ultrasound probe and block the needle, which makes the block much easier to perform. The brachial plexus also moves into a more superficial location and is easier to visualize as a result.

It is recommended that the operator stand on the side of the patient to be blocked, either at the head of the patient or at the patient's side depending on operator preference. The ultrasound machine should be positioned in the operator's direct line of sight, i.e., toward the foot of the bed on the same side or on the opposite side of the patient, depending on whether the operator is standing at the head or at the side of the patient, respectively.

Table 25.4 Preparation for an ultrasound-guided infraclavicular brachial plexus block

Required supplies and equipment
- Disinfectant solution and swabs for skin preparation.
- Sterile gloves and drapes.
- Short-beveled 22G block needle with extension tubing.
  - An 80 mm needle is recommended in all adult patients.
  - An echogenic needle helps in needle localization.
- Local anesthetic of choice in 10 ml or 20 ml syringes.
- Lidocaine 1–2% in 3 ml syringe with a 25–27G hypodermic needle for skin infiltration (at operator's discretion).
- Ultrasound machine with high-frequency linear-array probe. A low-frequency curved-array probe may sometimes offer better image quality in patients with a thick chest wall.
- Equipment and supplies for managing life-threatening acute complications, including lipid emulsion for local anesthetic systemic toxicity.
- Drugs for intravenous sedation during the block (at operator's discretion).

Preparation of patient
- Obtain informed consent for the block.
- Explain expected clinical course including care of the insensate limb and managing the transition to systemic analgesia.
- Establish intravenous access, supplemental oxygen delivery, and standard monitors (ECG, noninvasive blood pressure, pulse oximetry).
- Perform a time-out to confirm patient identity and site and side of surgery.

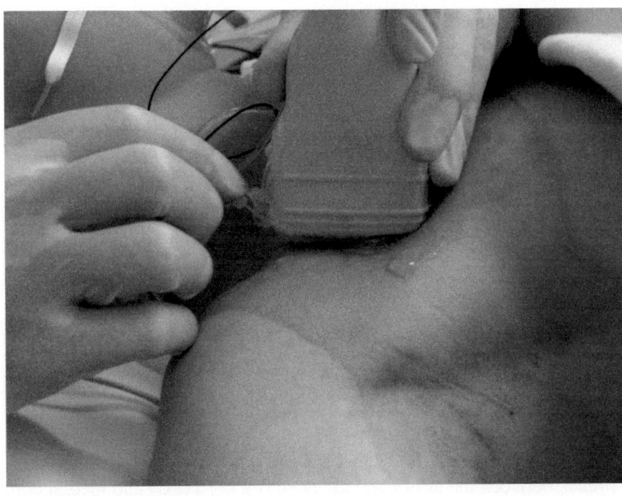

Fig. 25.8 Ultrasound-guided infraclavicular block. The probe is placed in a parasagittal plane, and the needle is advanced in a cephalad-to-caudad direction. Abduction of the shoulder moves the clavicle superiorly, which increases the available space for needle insertion cephalad to the probe. (Image courtesy of Dr. Ki Jinn Chin)

The suggested initial ultrasound settings include a depth of 4 cm, and a frequency in the middle of the probe's range to allow for the relatively greater penetration that is required. Gain, focus, and depth are subsequently adjusted as needed to optimize the image. The probe is placed inferior to the clavicle, in a parasagittal plane perpendicular to the line of the brachial plexus (Fig. 25.8). The chief landmark is the axillary artery, which is easily identified as a round hypoechoic pulsatile structure, deep to the pectoralis major and minor muscles. The lateral cord is visible as a hyperechoic structure immediately superior to the artery and just deep to pectoralis minor. The posterior and medial cords are not usually distinct from each other but appear as a large hyperechoic complex structure posterior to the axillary artery (Fig. 25.4).

The position of the cords in relation to the artery varies depending on where the neurovascular bundle is imaged along its course. More proximally (medially), the cords are grouped together along the superior aspect of the artery, and the plexus has a similar appearance to the first rib view that is used in the supraclavicular plexus block. More distally (laterally), the posterior and medial cords move into a location posterior to the artery, with the medial cord eventually taking up position between the axillary artery and vein (Fig. 25.4).

The operator should scan along the course of the neurovascular bundle to identify the plane in which the plexus is most readily visualized, and ideally where all the cords are bunched close together rather than spread out around the artery. The thoracic cage and pleura are visible in more medial probe positions, but usually lie 1–2 cm deep to the neurovascular bundle, and are therefore at little risk of inadvertent puncture. There are pectoral vessels running between the pectoralis major and minor muscles which should be identified to ensure that they do not lie in the path of the selected needle trajectory.

Needle Insertion and Injection Technique

The needle is advanced using an in-plane approach toward the superior aspect of the lateral cord, aiming to pass at a tangent to its surface, rather than directly at it (Fig. 25.9a). The needle is advanced slowly and carefully through the pectoral muscles until the deep fascia of pectoralis minor has been pierced, which is usually signaled by a tactile pop. At this point, a test injection of 0.5 ml is made – if the needle tip is in the correct location, there will be visible fluid expansion next to the lateral cord, which has the added effect of pushing it out of the needle's path (Fig. 25.9b).

The needle is advanced deeper, aiming to place the tip at the posterior (6 o'clock) aspect of the artery. A test injection at the correct location will create visible fluid spread immediately posterior or deep to the artery (the "double bubble" sign). A total of 20–30 ml of local anesthetic is injected at this point, to create a U-shaped pattern of spread between the posterior aspect of the artery and the plexus (Fig. 25.9c). The needle is then slowly withdrawn until the tip once again lies adjacent to the lateral cord, at which point another 5–10ml of local anesthetic is injected to produce spread in this compartment (Fig. 25.9d).

Note that there is no statistically significant difference between the efficacy of single-injection techniques posterior

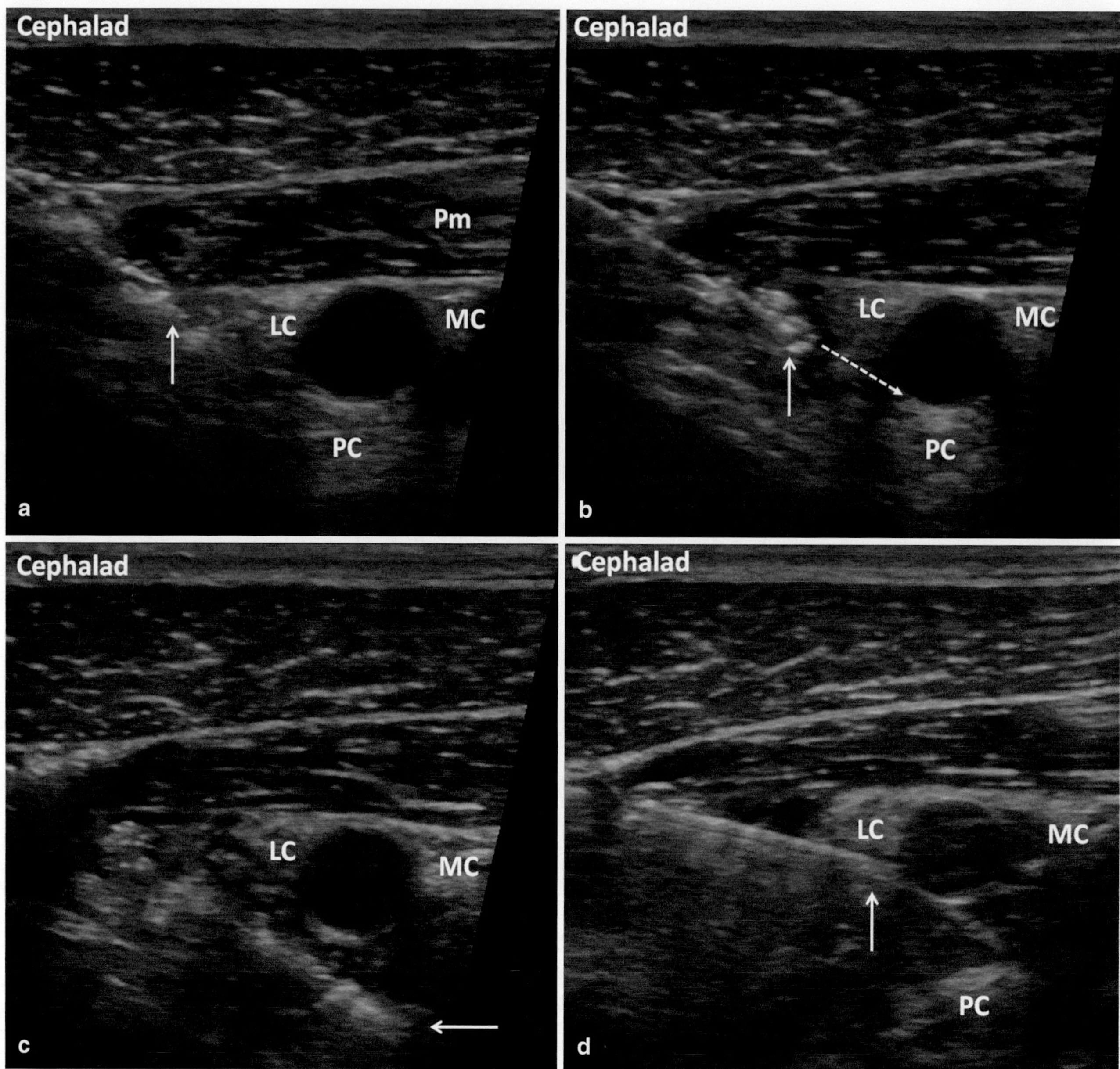

Fig. 25.9 Typical performance of an ultrasound-guided infraclavicular block. (**a**) The needle tip (arrow) pierces the deep fascia of pectoralis minor (Pm), just lateral to the lateral cord (LC). (**b**) 0.5–1 ml of fluid is injected to confirm that the needle tip is in the correct compartment and to push aside the lateral cord so that the needle can reach the posterior aspect of the artery (dotted arrow indicates trajectory). (**c**) Injection at the posterior aspect of the artery creates a pocket of local anesthetic that spreads between the artery and the posterior cord (PC) and medial cord (MC) – the "double bubble" sign. (**d**) In the dual-injection technique, after injection of 20–30 ml posterior to the artery, the needle tip is withdrawn back into the compartment of the lateral cord where a further 5–10 ml is injected. (Image courtesy of Dr. Ki Jinn Chin)

to the artery and the dual-injection technique described above, or even a triple-injection technique. However, the authors consider that a dual-injection technique does not add significant complexity and in clinical practice, may further improve the already high success rates.

Ultrasound-Guided Continuous Nerve Block Technique

This is identical to the single-shot technique except that a peripheral nerve block catheter kit is used instead.

The introducer needle is advanced as described above until the needle tip is located at the posterior aspect of the artery and injection produces the "double bubble" sign of fluid spread immediately adjacent to the artery. It is recommended that 5–10 ml of fluid be injected in this location to create a "pocket" into which the catheter can be advanced. If a stimulating catheter is being used to confirm tip location, 5% dextrose solution should be used to preserve the motor response.

The catheter is advanced approximately not more than 3 cm beyond the tip of the introducer needle. If neurostimulation is used, an appropriate motor response should be sought at current thresholds of at least 0.3 mA and up to 0.8–1 mA. Catheter tip position may also be confirmed by (1) attempting to visualize the catheter tip – this is aided by making small jiggling movements of the catheter, (2) rapid injection of 3–5 ml of fluid which should produce visible expansion posterior to the artery, and (3) injection of agitated saline to produce a color Doppler signal adjacent to the artery. The needle is then withdrawn and the catheter fixed in place in the usual manner.

Local Anesthetic Dosages

Single-Shot Block

- A volume of 30–40 ml (0.4–0.5 ml/kg) is generally recommended.
- The choice of local anesthetic and concentration depends on the desired speed of onset and duration. Commonly used local anesthetics include:
  - A 1:1 mixture of an intermediate-acting local anesthetic (e.g., 2% mepivacaine or lidocaine) and a long-acting local anesthetic (e.g., 0.5% bupivacaine), which will have a faster onset than bupivacaine alone and a longer duration than lidocaine alone
  - 0.25%–0.5% bupivacaine
  - 0.5%–0.75% ropivacaine.
- Epinephrine may be added in a concentration of 25 mcg/ml as a marker of intravascular injection and to reduce systemic vascular absorption.

Continuous Infraclavicular Plexus Block

- 0.2–0.4% ropivacaine at 4–8 ml/h
- 0.125%–0.25% bupivacaine at 4–8 ml/h
- PCA boluses of 2–5 ml may be added if this function is available on the infusion pump
- Both infusion rates and bolus volumes should be titrated to achieve the optimal balance between adequate analgesia and an excessively dense sensory and motor block

Complications and Adverse Effects

In general, the infraclavicular block is an extremely safe technique. The following adverse events have been reported, but all are uncommon.

1. Vascular Puncture
   - This is the most commonly reported complication in the literature.
   - Axillary vein puncture is more likely than arterial puncture in the neurostimulation-guided approach as the brachial plexus cords envelop and protect the axillary artery.
   - Arterial puncture should be avoidable with careful needle handling in the ultrasound-guided approach as it is difficult to puncture the thick elastic arterial wall with a short-beveled block needle.
   - The main concern is that this area can be difficult to compress, and coagulopathy is therefore a relative contraindication to the infraclavicular block. However, no significant complications arising as a result of vascular puncture have been reported to date.
2. Pneumothorax
   - The only published reports of pneumothorax following a surface landmark-guided approach are with the vertical infraclavicular plexus approach, which is more medial than the coracoid approach.
   - Although pneumothorax has been reported following ultrasound-guided infraclavicular block, it is extremely unlikely if proper technique is observed, given the distance between the plexus and the pleura in most patients. An out-of-plane approach and advancement of the needle in a medial direction may increase risk.
3. Phrenic Nerve Palsy and Horner's Syndrome
   - Both of these complications are unlikely, as they require spread of local anesthetic cephalad into the neck.
   - They have however been reported more commonly with the vertical infraclavicular plexus block, which as previously mentioned, targets the plexus in a more proximal/medial location.

Retroclavicular Brachial Plexus Block

Introduction

The retroclavicular brachial plexus is an alternative ultrasound-guided approach to the infraclavicular brachial plexus that was first described in 2007 by Hebbard and Royse, and later in

2015 by Beh et al. (who both called it a posterior ultrasound-guided infraclavicular brachial plexus block). It has since been investigated by others, and compared with other approaches to the brachial plexus. There are both advantages and limitations to the technique, and appeals to some practitioners, but not to others. Reports of faster block performance time or fewer needle passes are related to operator familiarity and preference, and are not inherent in the technique.

Indications

It is indicated when anesthesia or analgesia of the elbow, forearm, and hand is required. The contraindications are summarized in Table 25.5.

The advantages and disadvantages of this retroclavicular approach compared with other brachial plexus block techniques are summarized in Table 25.6.

Table 25.5 Contraindications to performing a retroclavicular brachial plexus block

Absolute
- There are no absolute contraindications specific to this block. Generic contraindications such as patient refusal, allergy to local anesthetics, and local infection at the site of injection apply as usual.

Relative
- Coagulopathy – This is of particular concern as there is a risk of trauma to vessels in the supraclavicular fossa that are not visualized during the first phase of needle insertion.
- A crowded or "full" supraclavicular fossa, due to variations in patient anatomy, which can make it difficult to negotiate a path under the clavicle.

Table 25.6 Advantages and disadvantages of the retroclavicular brachial plexus block versus other approaches

Advantages compared to other brachial plexus block techniques
- Versus conventional infraclavicular brachial plexus block technique.
  - Easier needle visibility (when alignment is achieved), due to needle being perpendicular to ultrasound beam.
  - The arm does not have to be abducted at the shoulder.
- Versus supraclavicular brachial plexus block technique.
  - Lower risk of phrenic nerve palsy.

Disadvantages compared to other brachial plexus block techniques
- Distorted clavicular anatomy, and a short neck with a "full" supraclavicular fossa, can hinder needle insertion.
- Can be associated with more pain due to manipulation and clavicular contact during the "blind" phase of needle insertion past the clavicle.
- The clavicle can hinder attempts at needle tip repositioning and alterations in trajectory.
- There is a risk of damage to non-visualized structures in the supraclavicular fossa, e.g., suprascapular nerve and associated arteries, during the "blind" phase of needle insertion past the clavicle.
- It can be difficult to pass the lateral cord and reach the posterior aspect of the artery without needle contact and elicitation of paresthesia (with the attendant risk of mechanical trauma).
- Few material advantages, apart from better needle visualization, have been demonstrated in the literature when compared to the conventional infraclavicular technique.

Table 25.7 Preparation for performing an ultrasound-guided retroclavicular brachial plexus block

Required supplies and equipment
- Disinfectant solution and swabs for skin preparation.
- Sterile gloves and drapes.
- Short-beveled 22G block needle with extension tubing.
  - An 80 mm needle is recommended in all adult patients.
  - An echogenic needle helps in needle localization.
- Local anesthetic of choice in 10 ml or 20 ml syringes.
- Lidocaine 1–2% in 3 ml syringe with a 25–27G hypodermic needle for skin infiltration (at operator's discretion).
- Ultrasound machine with high-frequency linear-array probe.
- Equipment and supplies for managing life-threatening acute complications, including lipid emulsion for local anesthetic systemic toxicity.
- Drugs for intravenous sedation during the block (at operator's discretion).

Preparation of patient
- Obtain informed consent for the block.
- Explain expected clinical course including care of the insensate limb and managing the transition to systemic analgesia.
- Establish intravenous access, supplemental oxygen delivery, and standard monitors (ECG, noninvasive blood pressure, pulse oximetry).
- Perform a time-out to confirm patient identity and site and side of surgery.

Technique

The equipment and preparation of patient is summarized in Table 25.7.

Scanning Technique

The patient is placed supine with the arm adducted at the shoulder. It may help to gently pull down on the shoulder to maximize the area of the supraclavicular fossa (i.e., the shoulder should not be in a "shrugged" position). It is recommended that the operator stand at the head of the patient. The ultrasound machine should be positioned in the operator's direct line of sight, i.e., toward the foot of the bed on the same side.

The suggested initial ultrasound settings include a depth of 4 cm, and a frequency in the middle of the probe's range to allow for the relatively greater penetration that is required. Gain, focus, and depth are subsequently adjusted as needed to optimize the image. The probe is placed inferior to the clavicle, in a parasagittal plane perpendicular to the line of the brachial plexus (Fig. 25.10). The landmarks are similar as described for the conventional infraclavicular approach (see above). These include the axillary artery, the lateral cord, and the posterior and medial cords (which are not usually distinct from each other but appear as a large hyperechoic complex structure posterior to the axillary artery) (Fig. 25.4).

Needle Insertion and Injection Technique

The needle is inserted an appropriate distance (approximately 2 cm in the adult) superior to the clavicle, in line with the ultrasound probe (Fig. 25.10). The needle should not

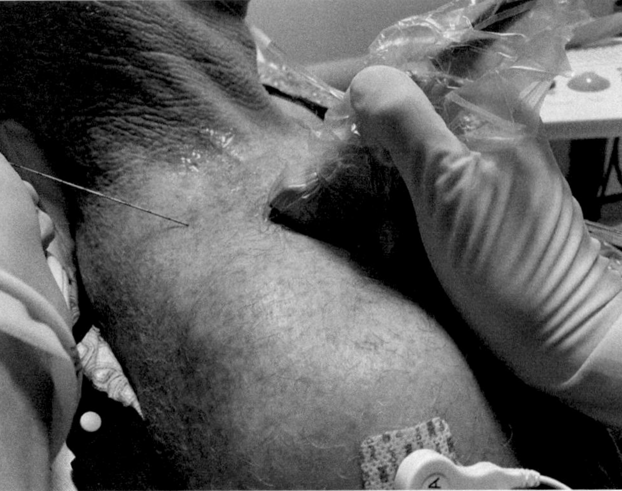

Fig. 25.10 The arm is adducted at the shoulder and depressed slightly. The ultrasound probe is placed inferior to the clavicle to obtain a view of the plexus. The needle is inserted a good distance away from the clavicle in the supraclavicular fossa, in line with the ultrasound probe, so as to be able to pass under the clavicle in a flat trajectory without needing to angle it downward. (Images courtesy of Dr. Jeffrey Gadsden)

need to be angled steeply to avoid the inferior aspect of the clavicle, as the desired trajectory is a flat one. Note that subsequent attempts at readjustments to needle trajectory can be impeded by the clavicle.

Uppal et al. have recommended estimating the distance that the needle will have to travel from the insertion point, superior to the clavicle, to the point where it will enter the field of the ultrasound beam. The needle is held along its shaft at this length during the initial phase of insertion to ensure that this is not exceeded during the attempts to locate and visualize the needle, which will minimize the risk of damage to the neurovascular bundle or pleura. The needle is advanced slowly under the clavicle until it is seen within the ultrasound beam. Complaints of shoulder pain from the patient may signify contact with the suprascapular nerve, and the needle tip should be repositioned accordingly.

The needle is advanced to place the tip at the posterior (6 o'clock) aspect of the artery. A test injection at the correct location will create visible fluid spread immediately posterior or deep to the artery (the "double bubble" sign). A total of 20–30 ml of local anesthetic is injected at this point, to create a U-shaped pattern of spread between the posterior aspect of the artery and the plexus (Fig. 25.11).

Axillary Brachial Plexus Block

Introduction

The axillary brachial plexus block has a long history as a popular technique for providing regional anesthesia at and below the elbow. The surface landmarks (chiefly the axillary artery pulsation) are easily ascertained, and there is no risk of pneumothorax. A variety of landmark-guided approaches have been described, including elicitation of paresthesia, trans-arterial injection, and single- and multiple-injection neurostimulation techniques. The main issues with the landmark-guided approaches were variable efficacy and the risk of intravascular injection of local anesthetic. The advent of ultrasound guidance has effectively addressed these concerns. It is at least as effective as the supraclavicular and infraclavicular blocks, if not more so because of the ability to individually target the four main terminal nerves of the arm. The shallow depth of the brachial plexus in this location allows excellent visualization of both nerves and needle. Inadvertent intraneural and intravascular injections remain the only significant risks, but both are easily avoided with ultrasonographic visualization.

Indications and Contraindications

It is indicated when anesthesia or analgesia of the elbow, forearm and hand is required (Fig. 25.12). It may be performed as either a single-shot or continuous catheter technique; however, it can be more difficult to maintain hygiene of the catheter insertion site compared to other brachial plexus approaches.

The contraindications are summarized in Table 25.8.

The advantages and disadvantages of axillary approach compared with other brachial plexus block techniques are summarized in Table 25.9.

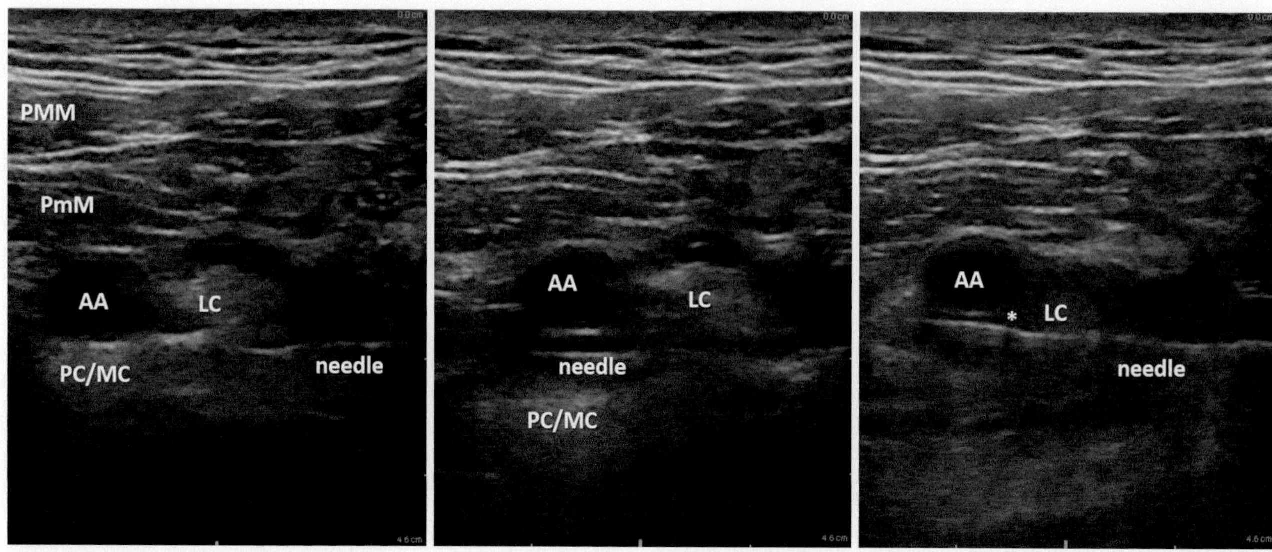

Fig. 25.11 From left to right: the needle is advanced under the lateral cord (LC), toward the posterior aspect of the axillary artery (AA), and superficial to the posterior and medial cords (PC/MC). Correct needle tip location is indicated by hydrolocation and fluid spread under the artery that pushes the posterior and medial cords downward. Further injection will spread to all elements of the plexus. Lateral cord coverage can be ensured by injecting at the 5 o'clock aspect of the artery (asterisk). (Images courtesy of Dr. Jeffrey Gadsden)

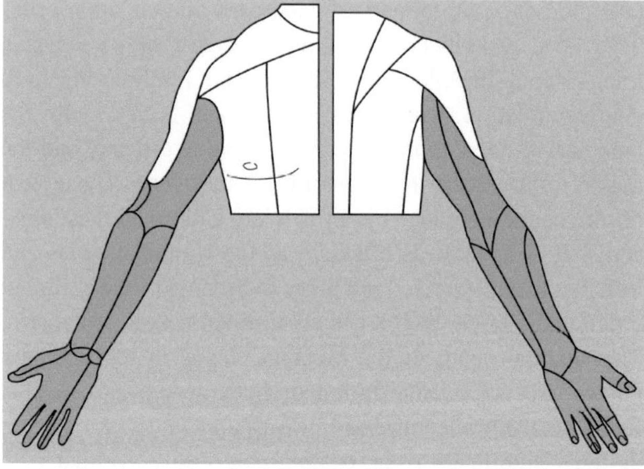

Fig. 25.12 Typical distribution of anesthesia and analgesia following successful axillary plexus blockade. Reprinted with permission from Dr. Danilo Jankovic

Table 25.8 Contraindications to performing an axillary brachial plexus block

Absolute
- Inability to abduct the arm at the shoulder and access the injection site.
- Generic contraindications such as patient refusal, allergy to local anesthetics, and local infection at the site of injection apply as usual.

Relative
- Previous axillary node clearance.
- Congenital or acquired vascular malformations in the upper arm or axilla (e.g., arteriovenous fistula), although the ultrasound-guided approach may still be feasible in skilled hands.

Table 25.9 Advantages and disadvantages of axillary brachial plexus block versus other approaches

Advantages compared to other brachial plexus block techniques
1. The ultrasound-guided technique is a highly efficacious technique, with block success rates as high as 97.5% reported.
2. It is a superficial site that is easily compressible and carries a low risk of compressive injury to surrounding structures by hematoma formation. This makes it a viable option in coagulopathic patients, particularly if ultrasound guidance is used.
3. There is no risk of pneumothorax, or of adverse effects associated with injections administered more proximally in the root of the neck, e.g., phrenic nerve palsy and Horner's syndrome.
4. Adequate ultrasound images can be obtained even in very obese patients.

Disadvantages compared to other brachial plexus block techniques
1. The axillary block can only be performed with the arm abducted (and ideally externally rotated) at the shoulder.
2. The landmark-guided techniques of axillary block have relatively poor block success rates, especially if single-injection techniques are used. Multiple-injection techniques are complex and require good understanding of anatomy as well as dexterity with needle and nerve stimulator.

Functional Anatomy

At the level of the axillary block, the cords of the brachial plexus have divided into the major terminal nerves: the median nerve, ulnar nerve, radial nerve, musculocutaneous nerve, and medial brachial and antebrachial cutaneous nerves (Fig. 25.13). These last two nerves are not usually sought out separately as they lie close to the ulnar nerve and are readily anesthetized with it.

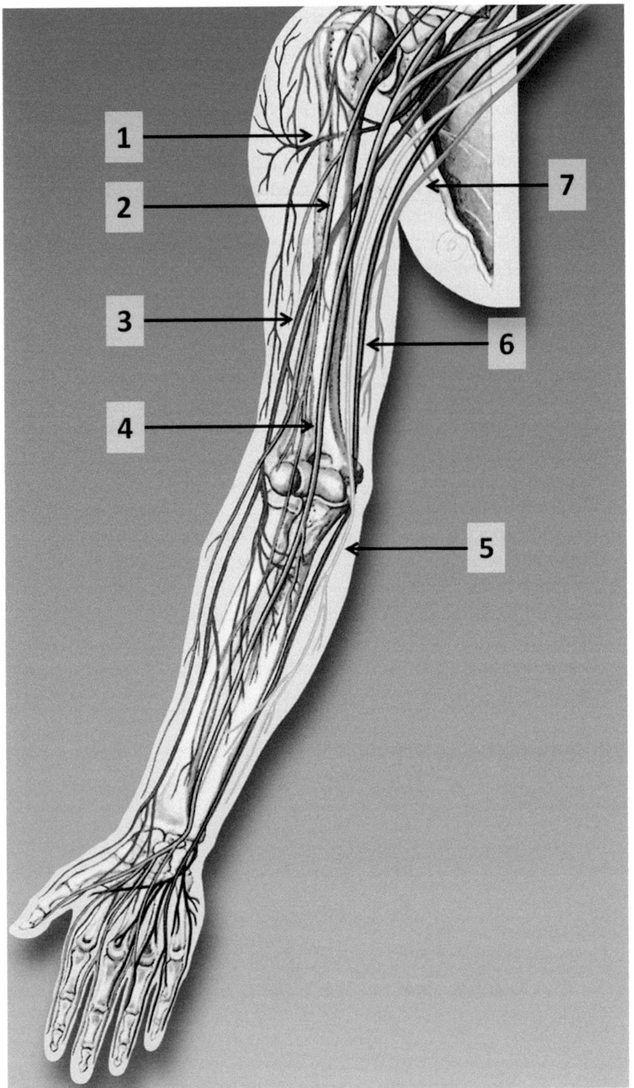

Fig. 25.13 Major terminal branches of the brachial plexus in the axillary region. (1) Axillary nerve, (2) musculocutaneous nerve, (3) radial nerve, (4) median nerve, (5) medial antebrachial cutaneous nerve, (6) ulnar nerve, (7) medial brachial cutaneous nerve. Reprinted with permission from Dr. Danilo Jankovic

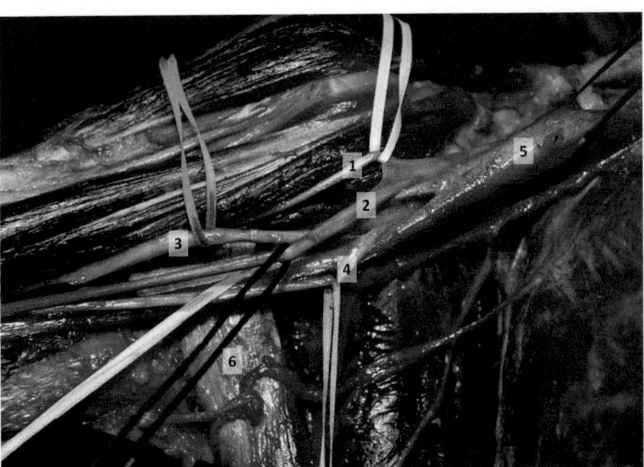

Fig. 25.14 Cadaveric dissection of the axillary brachial plexus. The musculocutaneous nerve (1) (white) and median nerve (2) (dark blue) originate from the lateral cord. The radial nerve (3) (green) and ulnar nerve (4) (light blue) run posterior and medial to the axillary artery (5), but have been displaced here for visibility. Note the conjoint tendon (6) of teres major and latissimus dorsi which inserts onto the humerus posterior to the axillary neurovascular bundle. Reprinted with permission from Dr. Danilo Jankovic

The nerves are distributed around the axillary artery, together with one or more accompanying axillary veins, and together they constitute the neurovascular bundle (Fig. 25.14). The median nerve is most commonly located in the anterolateral quadrant, the ulnar nerve in the anteromedial quadrant, and the radial nerve in the posteromedial quadrant around the artery (Fig. 25.15). However, these nerves are highly mobile, and on ultrasound, their position can be observed to vary significantly with the pressure exerted through the probe. The musculocutaneous nerve starts in a location adjacent to the median nerve in the posterolateral quadrant around the artery, but then courses out laterally in the fascial plane between biceps and coracobrachialis muscle. Its exact location in any given subject is highly variable and depends on how proximally or distally it takes off from the lateral cord; this is the main reason for the high failure rate with single-injection landmark-guided approaches.

A fascial sheath surrounds the brachial plexus in this location, but is subdivided by thinner septae into compartments that contain the median, ulnar, and radial nerves. These are most evident during ultrasound-guided perineural block. While large-volume injection in a single location close to the artery may traverse these septae, they are nevertheless likely to be another reason for the poor efficacy of the single-injection landmark-guided techniques.

The most important landmark in the ultrasound-guided approach, apart from the axillary artery, is the conjoint tendon of teres major and latissimus dorsi (Figs. 25.14 and 25.15). This inserts onto the proximal humerus and forms a "floor" on which the artery and all the associated nerves lie. In particular, the radial nerve can always be visualized lying superficial to the conjoint tendon on ultrasound. Distal to the lateral edge of the conjoint tendon, the radial nerve rapidly courses posteriorly and away from the axillary artery, descending between the heads of the triceps muscle to lie in the spiral groove of the humerus. Ultrasound-guided axillary nerve blocks performed where the conjoint tendon cannot be visualized therefore carry a significant risk of failure to block the radial nerve.

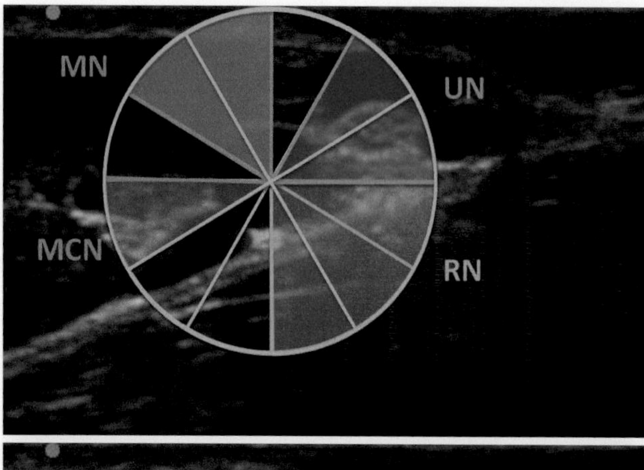

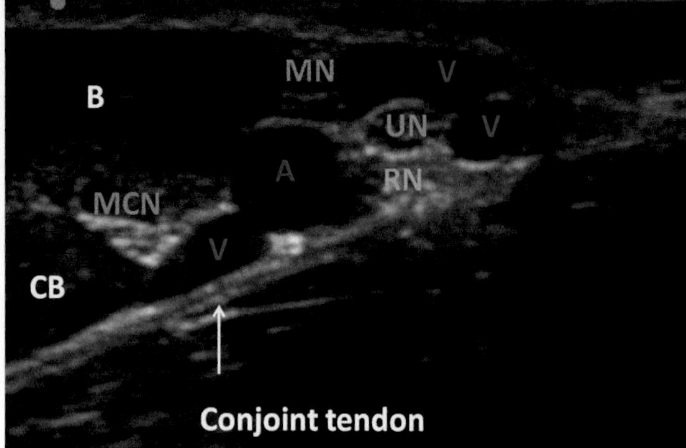

Fig. 25.15 Typical ultrasound image of the axillary brachial plexus. The pulsatile axillary artery (A) is usually accompanied by more than one vein (V). All the vessels and nerves lie on the hyperechoic conjoint tendon. The most common location of the median nerve (MN), ulnar nerve (UN), radial nerve (RN), and musculocutaneous nerve (MCN) in relation to the artery is illustrated in the top image. The musculocutaneous nerve often lies in the fascial plane between biceps (B) and coracobrachialis (CB). (Image courtesy of Dr. Ki Jinn Chin)

Technique: Surface Landmark-Guided Approach – Single-Shot

The equipment and preparation of patient is summarized in Table 25.10.

Scanning Technique

The patient is placed supine with the arm externally rotated and abducted to 90 degrees at the shoulder, with the elbow flexed (Fig. 25.16). Abduction beyond 90 degrees should be avoided, as it makes arterial palpation more difficult and may impair distribution of the local anesthetic. The operator stands on the side of the patient to be blocked.

The main surface landmark is the axillary artery, which is palpated as proximally as possible under the lateral edge of the pectoralis major muscle (Fig. 25.17). This increases the efficacy of the block for two reasons: (1) there is a higher likelihood that the musculocutaneous nerve will be close enough to the plexus for local anesthetic spread to reach it and (2) the plexus is targeted where it lies on the conjoint tendon, which is an important boundary for containing and directing local anesthetic spread, especially around the radial nerve. The median nerve is expected to lie superior and ante-

Table 25.10 Preparation for performance of a surface landmark-guided axillary brachial plexus block

Required supplies and equipment
• Disinfectant solution and swabs for skin preparation.
• Sterile gloves and drapes.
• Short-beveled 22G, 50 mm block needle with extension tubing. – Note that a sharp hypodermic needle may be preferred in the transarterial approach.
• Local anesthetic of choice in 10 ml or 20 ml syringes.
• Peripheral nerve stimulator (optional, depending on approach).
• Lidocaine 1–2% in 3 ml syringe with a 25–27G hypodermic needle for skin infiltration (at operator's discretion).
• Equipment and supplies for managing life-threatening acute complications, including lipid emulsion for local anesthetic systemic toxicity.
• Drugs for intravenous sedation during the block (at operator's discretion).
Preparation of patient
• Obtain informed consent for the block.
• Explain expected clinical course including care of the insensate limb and managing the transition to systemic analgesia.
• Establish intravenous access, supplemental oxygen delivery, and standard monitors (ECG, noninvasive blood pressure, pulse oximetry).
• Perform a time-out to confirm patient identity and site and side of surgery.

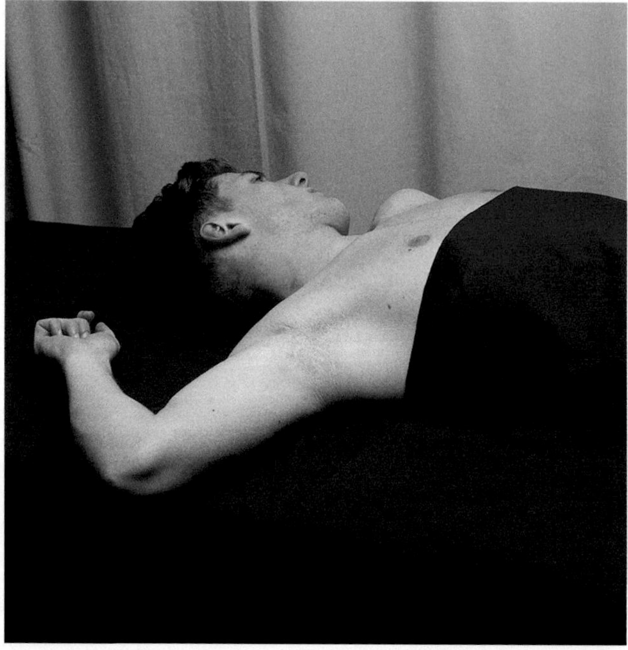

Fig. 25.16 Patient positioning for the axillary block. The patient is supine with the arm externally rotated and abducted to 90° at the shoulder. The shoulder should not be abducted more than 90°, as it makes arterial palpation more difficult, distorts the ultrasonographic view, and may impair distribution of the local anesthetic. Reprinted with permission from Dr. Danilo Jankovic

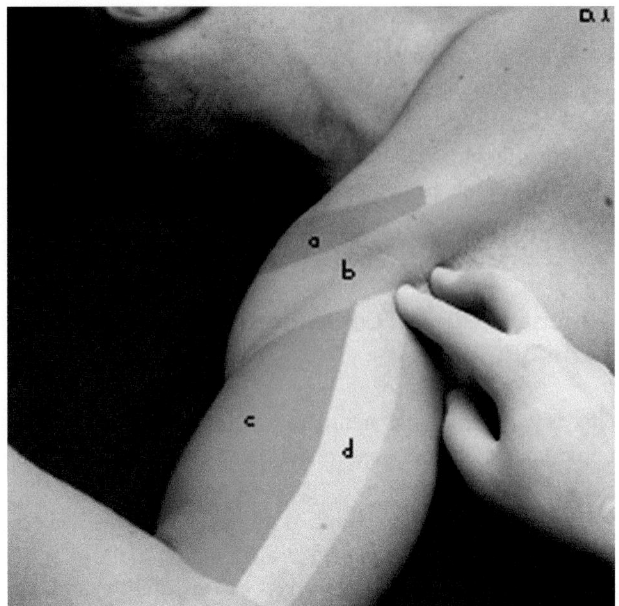

Fig. 25.17 Palpation of the axillary artery. This is done with two fingers (usually the second and third fingers), so that the skin and artery may be fixed in position between them. Palpation should be performed as proximal as possible. (a = deltoid muscle, b = pectoralis major muscle, c = biceps muscle, d = coracobrachialis muscle) Reprinted with permission from Dr. Danilo Jankovic

rior (superficial) to the artery, the ulnar nerve lies inferior and posterior, and the radial nerve lies posterior (deep) to the artery.

Needle Insertion and Injection Technique

A variety of methods of nerve localization have been described, including the elicitation of paresthesia and seeking a fascial click to indicate entry into the fascial sheath. These are primarily of historical interest and will not be described further here. The two methods that will be described are:

1. Transarterial injection technique.
2. Neurostimulation-guided technique.

Transarterial Double-Injection Technique

Before the procedure, the skin is disinfected, the procedure area is draped appropriately, and the block needle and tubing are primed with local anesthetic solution. The second and third fingers of the nondominant hand are placed on either side of the artery to anchor it in position. The block needle is advanced at a 90° angle to the skin to puncture the artery, as evidenced by pulsatile backflow of bright-red blood into the tubing (Fig. 25.18). The needle is advanced further until blood can no longer be aspirated, signaling that the needle tip is now posterior (deep) to the artery. Fractionated injection of half of the total dose of local anesthetic is performed at this location.

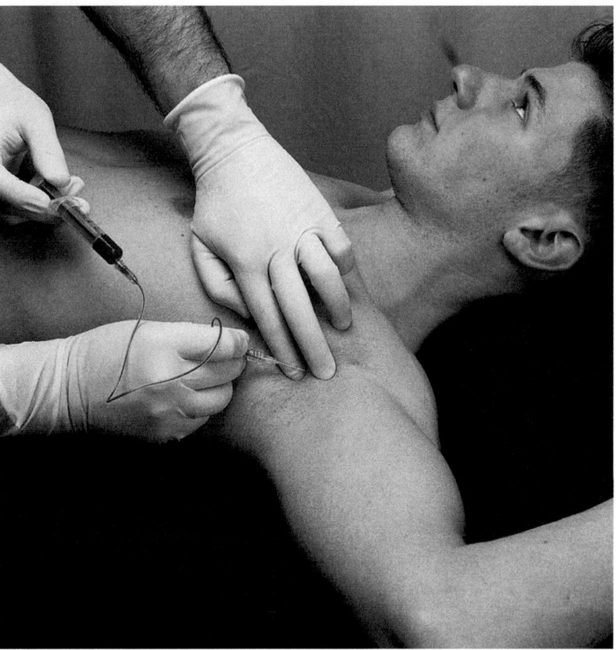

Fig. 25.18 Performance of the transarterial axillary block. The artery is fixed firmly between the fingers of the nondominant hand. The operator advances the block needle, while an assistant aspirates to confirm that the artery has been pierced. The needle is advanced further until blood can no longer be aspirated, signaling that the needle tip is now posterior to the artery. Half the volume of local anesthetic is injected in this location (in fractionated doses). The needle tip is withdrawn; blood is again aspirated as the needle tip reenters the arterial lumen, and ceases as the tip exits the lumen to lie anterior to the artery, at which time the remaining half of local anesthetic is injected (again in fractionated doses). Reprinted with permission from Dr. Danilo Jankovic

The needle is then withdrawn slowly until the needle tip is lying just superficial to the artery, signaled again first by resumption, and then cessation of pulsatile blood flow. The remaining volume of local anesthetic is injected in this location. The primary concerns with the transarterial approach are (1) an increased risk of intravascular injection and local anesthetic systemic toxicity and (2) hematoma formation. Nevertheless, it is an effective technique that does not require additional equipment (nerve stimulator or ultrasound machine).

Neurostimulation-Guided Technique

Before the procedure, the skin is disinfected, the procedure area is draped appropriately, and the block needle and tubing are primed with local anesthetic solution. A nerve stimulator is set at an initial current setting of 1–1.5 mA, pulse duration of 0.1–0.3 msec, and frequency of 1–2 Hz. The second and third fingers of the nondominant hand are placed on either side of the artery to anchor it in position (Fig. 25.19). The skin insertion site is infiltrated with local anesthetic if desired. The block needle is inserted at a 45° angle to the skin in a proximal direction, aiming for the anterolateral

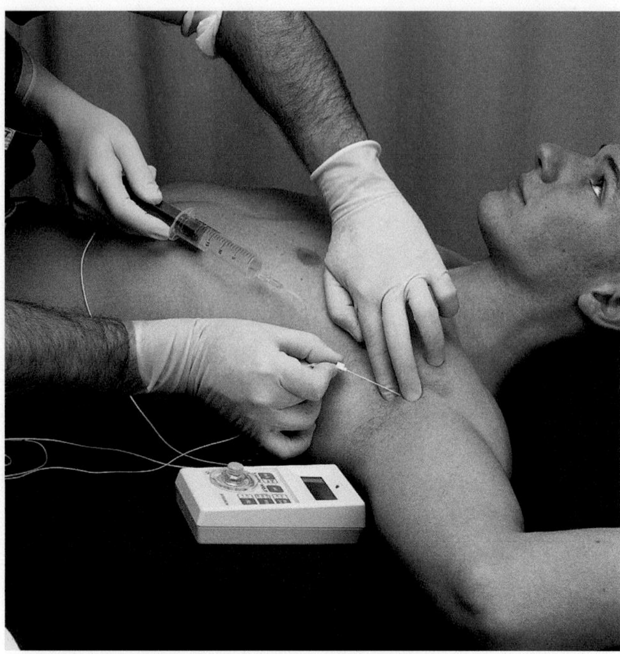

Fig. 25.19 Performance of the neurostimulation-guided axillary brachial plexus block. The artery is fixed firmly between the fingers of the nondominant hand. The operator advances the block needle, while an assistant adjusts the nerve stimulator as required. The operator redirects the needle around the artery to locate one or all of the median, ulnar, radial, and musculocutaneous nerves, depending on whether a single- or multiple-injection technique is employed. Reprinted with permission from Dr. Danilo Jankovic

aspect of the artery where the median nerve is expected to lie. Once a median nerve response is located at a current threshold of 0.3–0.5 mA, 5–8 mL of local anesthetic is injected. The needle is withdrawn from the skin and redirected to the anteromedial aspect of the artery, where the ulnar nerve is expected to lie. The radial nerve lies deeper on the posteromedial aspect of the artery. Finally, the musculocutaneous nerve is sought by redirecting the needle lateral to the arterial pulsation, in the groove between biceps and coracobrachialis. Once an appropriate motor response is obtained at a current threshold of 0.3–0.5 mA, 5–8 mL of local anesthetic is injected at each location.

Variations of the multiple-injection technique have been described, ranging from a single-injection on a motor response from median, ulnar, or radial nerves to a double-injection. It is probably most effective to perform the single injection posterior to the artery, i.e., on a radial nerve response. Double injections should be performed anterior and posterior to the artery, i.e., median or ulnar + radial. Larger volumes (40–50 ml) of local anesthetic are recommended to try and ensure adequate spread. The musculocutaneous nerve is usually sought out separately.

It is recommended that the second and third fingers of the nondominant hand which are palpating the artery also be used to exert pressure distal to the site of injection, which promotes cephalad spread and increases the effectiveness of the block, particularly if the musculocutaneous nerve is not separately sought and injected. Compression and massage of the axilla for 3–5 minutes after completion of injection has also been recommended for the same reason. If paresthesias are obtained, the needle should be withdrawn very slightly to avoid intraneural injection.

Landmark-Guided Continuous Nerve Block Technique

This is similar to the neurostimulation-guided single-shot technique except that a peripheral nerve block catheter kit is used instead.

The patient is positioned as described above, and the introducer needle is advanced at a 45° angle to the skin in a proximal direction, aiming to pass just medial to the artery (Fig. 25.20a-c). Ideally, a radial nerve response is sought as this indicates that the needle tip is posterior to the artery. If a stimulating catheter is being used, 5–10 ml of 5% dextrose solution can be injected through the introducer needle to distend the paraneural sheath. This should also result in augmentation of the motor response. Injection of other solutions will abolish the motor response.

The catheter is then advanced 3–5 cm beyond the tip of the introducer needle, looking to maintain a brachial plexus motor response at current thresholds of at least 0.3 mA and up to 0.8–1 mA. The needle is then withdrawn and the catheter fixed in place in the usual manner.

Technique: Ultrasound-Guided Approach: Single-Shot

The equipment and preparation of patient is summarized in Table 25.11.

Scanning Technique

The patient is placed supine with the arm externally rotated and abducted to 90 degrees at the shoulder, with the elbow flexed. Abduction beyond 90 degrees should be avoided, as it alters the sonoanatomy and can make image recognition more difficult. It is recommended that the operator stand on the side of the patient to be blocked, either at the head of the patient or at the patient's side depending on operator preference. The ultrasound machine should be positioned in the operator's direct line of sight, i.e., toward the foot of the bed on the same side or on the opposite side of the patient, depending on whether the operator is standing at the head or at the side of the patient, respectively.

The transducer is oriented perpendicular to the axis of the brachial plexus and axillary artery to image the neurovascu-

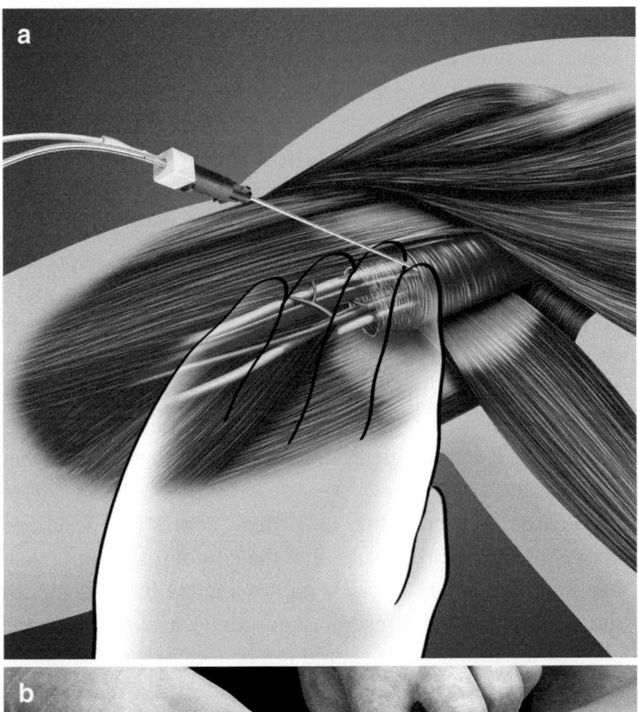

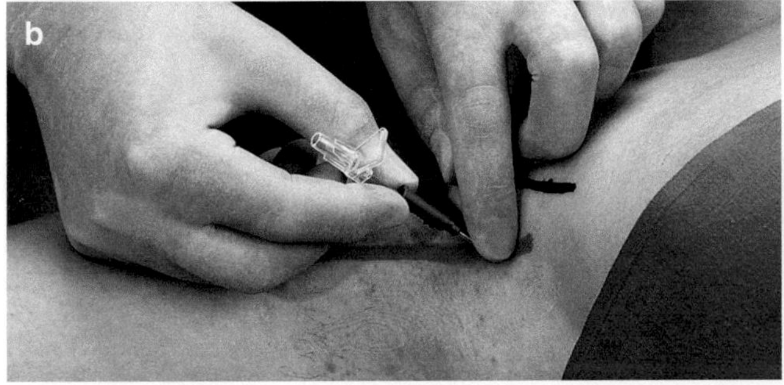

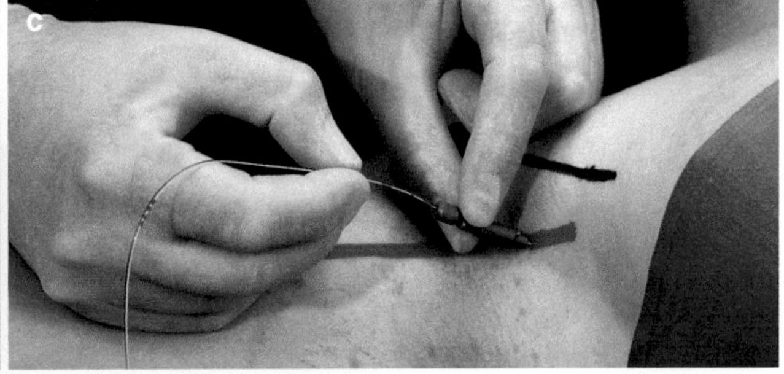

Fig. 25.20 Continuous axillary brachial plexus blockade. **a**. Schematic illustration of the needle approach. The needle tip is placed within the brachial plexus sheath. **b**. In this particular model of continuous peripheral nerve catheter (Contiplex ® D or Contiplex®Tuohy continuous set, e.g., B. Braun Melsungen), an introducer cannula is first inserted into the brachial plexus sheath over the needle. **c**. The nerve catheter is then threaded through the introducer cannula. Reprinted with permission from Dr. Danilo Jankovic

lar bundle in cross section. It is essential that the transducer is placed as high up (proximal) in the axilla as possible. The conjoint tendon of the latissimus dorsi and teres major is identified as a sloping hyperechoic line on ultrasound (Fig. 25.15). The entire neurovascular bundle will be visible superficial (anterior) to it.

The veins in the axillary neurovascular bundle are revealed by varying the downward pressure of the transducer in a "bouncing" motion to alternately expand and compress the veins. This helps to minimize the risk of inadvertent puncture, and often helps delineate the nerves, which might otherwise appear as a single hyperechoic mass.

The median, ulnar, and radial nerves lie in characteristic locations around the artery (Fig. 25.15) and are readily identified with experience. Their identity can further be confirmed by using a "traceback" approach of scanning distally along the arm and observing the characteristic course that each nerve takes. The median and ulnar nerves both lie very close to the axillary artery in the axilla. More distally, the ulnar nerve diverges in a medial direction away from the artery, while the median nerve remains adjacent to the artery. Because of its subcutaneous location, the ulnar nerve can be difficult to distinguish from pockets of adipose tissue on a static image, but is easily recognizable on dynamic scanning.

The radial nerve is always found sandwiched between the axillary artery and the conjoint tendon. Its appearance in this location, as a hyperechoic structure with indistinct margins, resembles that of a "cotton wool ball." Its identity may be further confirmed by scanning distally and observing the nerve descend in a fascial plane between the long and medial heads of the triceps muscle toward the posteromedial aspect of the humerus (Fig. 25.21). The location of the musculocutaneous nerve is highly variable. In general, the nerve lies lateral to the axillary artery and by scanning in a proximal-distal direction, can be observed to "slide" in a lateral-medial

Table 25.11 Preparation for performance of an ultrasound-guided axillary brachial plexus block

Required supplies and equipment • Disinfectant solution and swabs for skin preparation. • Sterile gloves and drapes. • Short-beveled 22G block needle with extension tubing. – An 80 mm needle is recommended in all adult patients. – An echogenic needle helps in needle localization. • Local anesthetic of choice in 10 ml or 20 ml syringes. • Lidocaine 1–2% in 3 ml syringe with a 25–27G hypodermic needle for skin infiltration (at operator's discretion). • Ultrasound machine with high-frequency linear-array probe. • Peripheral nerve stimulator (optional). • Equipment and supplies for managing life-threatening acute complications, including lipid emulsion for local anesthetic systemic toxicity. • Drugs for intravenous sedation during the block (at operator's discretion).
Preparation of patient • Obtain informed consent for the block. • Explain expected clinical course including care of the insensate limb and managing the transition to systemic analgesia. • Establish intravenous access, supplemental oxygen delivery, and standard monitors (ECG, noninvasive blood pressure, pulse oximetry). • Perform a time-out to confirm patient identity and site and side of surgery.

direction in the fascial plane between the biceps and coracobrachialis muscles. Its cross-sectional shape varies from triangular to elliptical, depending on its location.

Needle Insertion and Injection Technique

Different methods of performing the axillary block have been described, including using an out-of-plane (OOP) needle approach instead of an in-plane (IP) approach, approaching from both the lateral and medial sides of the probe, and a perivascular technique in which the aim is to deposit local anesthetic in a circumferential pattern around the artery rather than targeting individual nerves (perineural technique). The in-plane perineural approach is described here as we believe it affords greater precision, and therefore greater efficacy and safety.

Having identified the individual nerves as described above, place the probe such that the conjoint tendon is visible, and the axillary artery is approximately in the center of the screen. The block needle is inserted close to the lateral edge of the probe – this should not be too far away from the plexus or else it creates a longer needle track and hinders needle redirection.

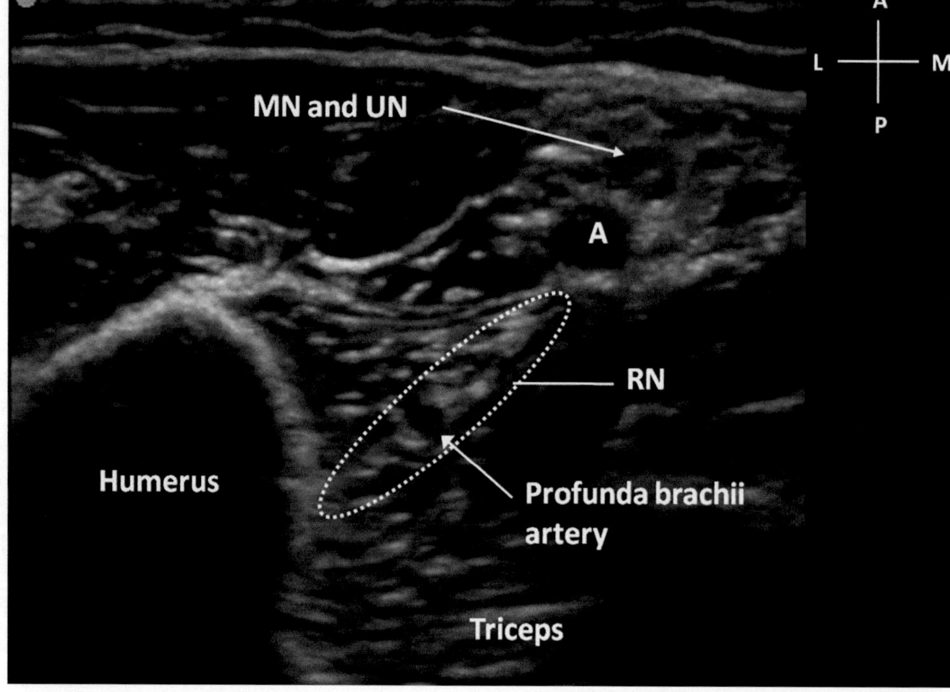

Fig. 25.21 Distal to the conjoint tendon zone, the radial nerve runs posterolaterally in a fascial plane between the long and medial heads of the triceps toward the humerus. It is accompanied by the profunda brachii artery. (*A* artery, MN median nerve, *RN* radial nerve, *UN* ulnar nerve) (Image courtesy of Dr. Ki Jinn Chin)

The block needle is advanced to place the tip onto the conjoint tendon just where it meets the axillary artery (Fig. 25.22). A 0.5 ml bolus of local anesthetic is injected which will hydrodissect the artery and radial nerve off the conjoint tendon. The needle may be advanced a little further under the artery, but does not need to be advanced beyond its 6 o'clock aspect. Injection of 5–8 ml of local anesthetic here will be seen to spread under and around the radial nerve.

The needle is now withdrawn until the tip lies in the subcutaneous layer. It is then readvanced in a shallow trajectory toward the median nerve, aiming to pierce its investing fascia at a tangent to the surface of the nerve so as to avoid accidental transfixion of the nerve. Penetration of the fascia is signaled by a tactile "pop," whereupon local anesthetic is injected in 0.5–1 mL boluses to surround the median nerve and to hydrodissect a safe passage toward the ulnar nerve (Fig. 25.23). A total of 5–8 mL of local anesthetic is injected around the median nerve – note that this can be done before advancing toward the ulnar nerve, or it can be done after injection around the ulnar nerve as the needle is being withdrawn (the author's preference).

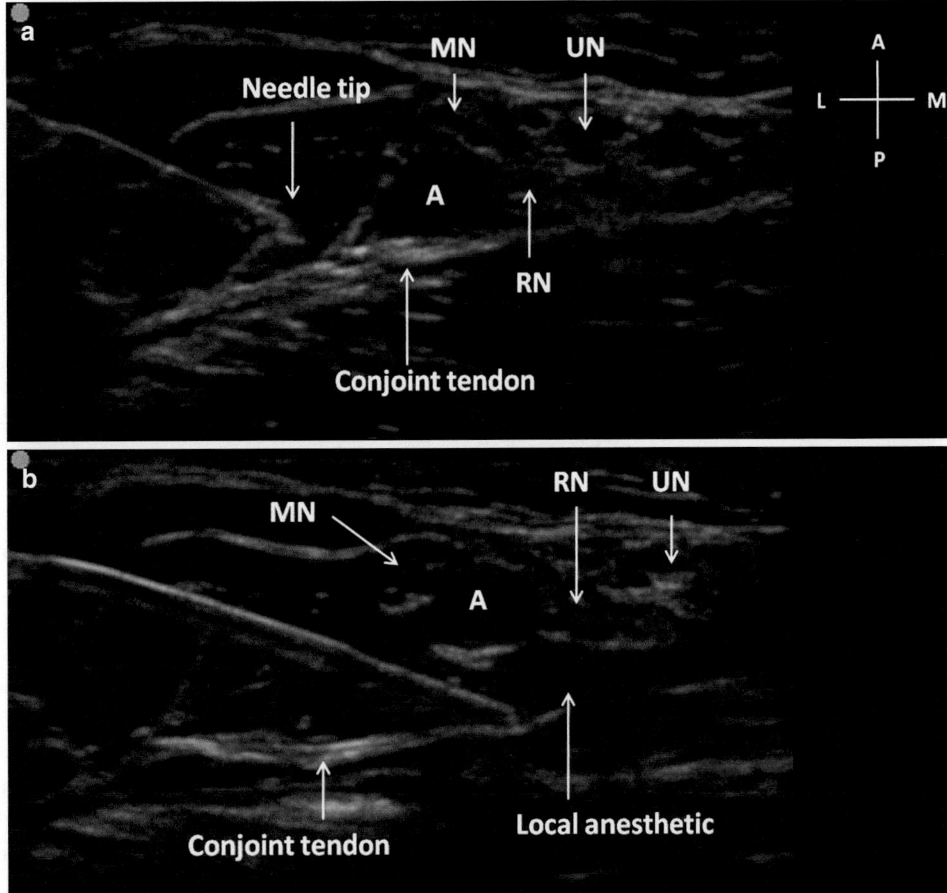

Fig. 25.22 **a**. The needle tip is advanced toward the posterolateral junction of the axillary artery (A) and the conjoint tendon. **b**. Injection at this point causes local anesthetic to spread anterior to the conjoint tendon and under (posterior to) the radial nerve, lifting it up. (*A* artery, *MN* median nerve, *RN* radial nerve, *UN* ulnar nerve) (Image courtesy of Dr. Ki Jinn Chin)

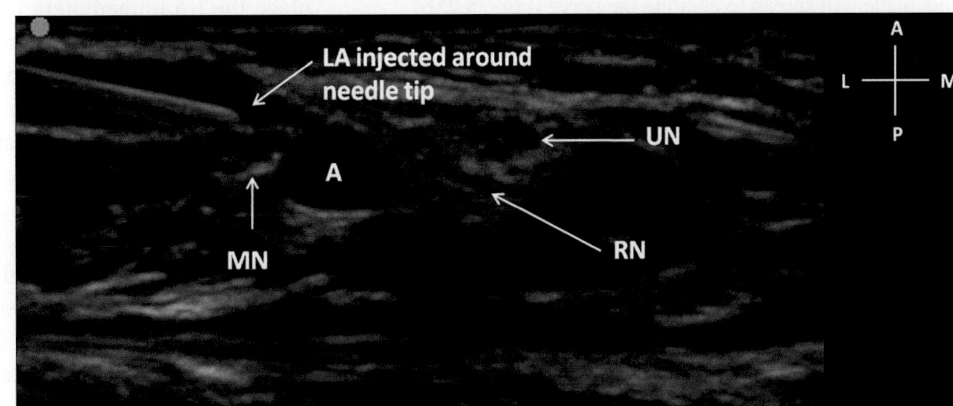

Fig. 25.23 The needle is advanced at a tangent to the median nerve in order to pierce its enveloping fascia without transfixing the nerve. Local anesthetic is injected here to surround the nerve and to hydrodissect a safe passage toward to the ulnar nerve. (*A* artery, *MN* median nerve, *RN* radial nerve, *UN* ulnar nerve) (Image courtesy of Dr. Ki Jinn Chin)

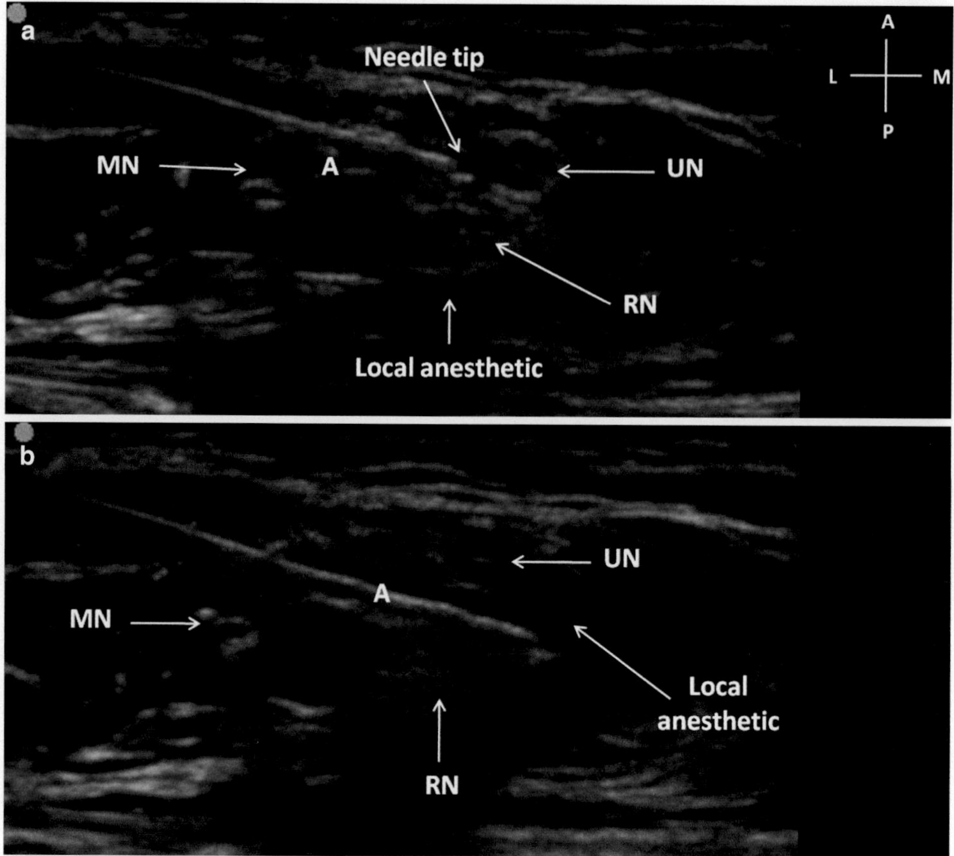

Fig. 25.24 **a**. The needle is advanced over the axillary artery (A) toward the ulnar nerve (UN) at a tangent to its surface. **b**. Injection here surrounds the ulnar nerve (UN) and also often spreads superficial to the radial nerve (RN). (*MN* median nerve) (Image courtesy of Dr. Ki Jinn Chin)

The needle is advanced further into the anteromedial quadrant of the neurovascular bundle and adjacent to the ulnar nerve (Fig. 25.24). Injection of 0.5–1 mL boluses of local anesthetic, up to a total of 5–8 mL, in this area will surround the ulnar nerve and usually delineate it clearly.

Depending on how far lateral the musculocutaneous nerve lies from the axillary artery, the needle may need to be withdrawn and reinserted through a second skin puncture. The nerve lies in the fascial plane between the biceps and coracobrachialis muscles. Once again the needle should be advanced to contact the nerve at a tangent to its surface and pierce this fascial plane (Fig. 25.25a). Three to five mL of local anesthetic injected in this plane will spread to encircle the nerve (Fig. 25.25b).

The endpoint for injection is adequate spread of local anesthetic around the individual nerves. Excessive needle repositioning and contact with the nerves is not recommended. Each nerve has its own fascial compartment which directs and contains local anesthetic spread around the nerve. Although neurostimulation can be used as an additional confirmation of nerve identification, the operator must be aware that needle-nerve contact can occur even in the absence of a motor response at commonly accepted current thresholds. Aggressive needling merely to provoke a motor response at low current thresholds should be avoided.

Ultrasound-Guided Continuous Nerve Block Technique

This is not a commonly used site for long-term catheter placement as it is difficult to maintain adequate hygiene of the insertion site. The nerves are spread out around the artery which can limit the effectiveness of continuous local anesthetic infusion without intermittent boluses.

Patient positioning and pre-scanning are performed in a similar manner to the single-shot technique. If an in-plane approach is selected, the introducer needle should be advanced from the lateral side of the probe, aiming to place the tip immediately posterior to the axillary artery. 5–10 ml of fluid should be injected here to produce a perivascular pocket of fluid into which the catheter should be advanced, usually not more than 3 cm beyond the tip of the needle. If an out-of-plane approach is selected, the introducer needle is advanced at a 45–60° angle to the skin in a proximal direction, aiming to reach the posteromedial aspect of the artery, i.e., placing the needle tip between the artery and radial nerve. Injection of 0.5–1 mL boluses of fluid should be used to confirm needle tip position during advancement as well as to hydrodissect a safe path and avoid needle-nerve trauma. 5–10 ml of fluid is

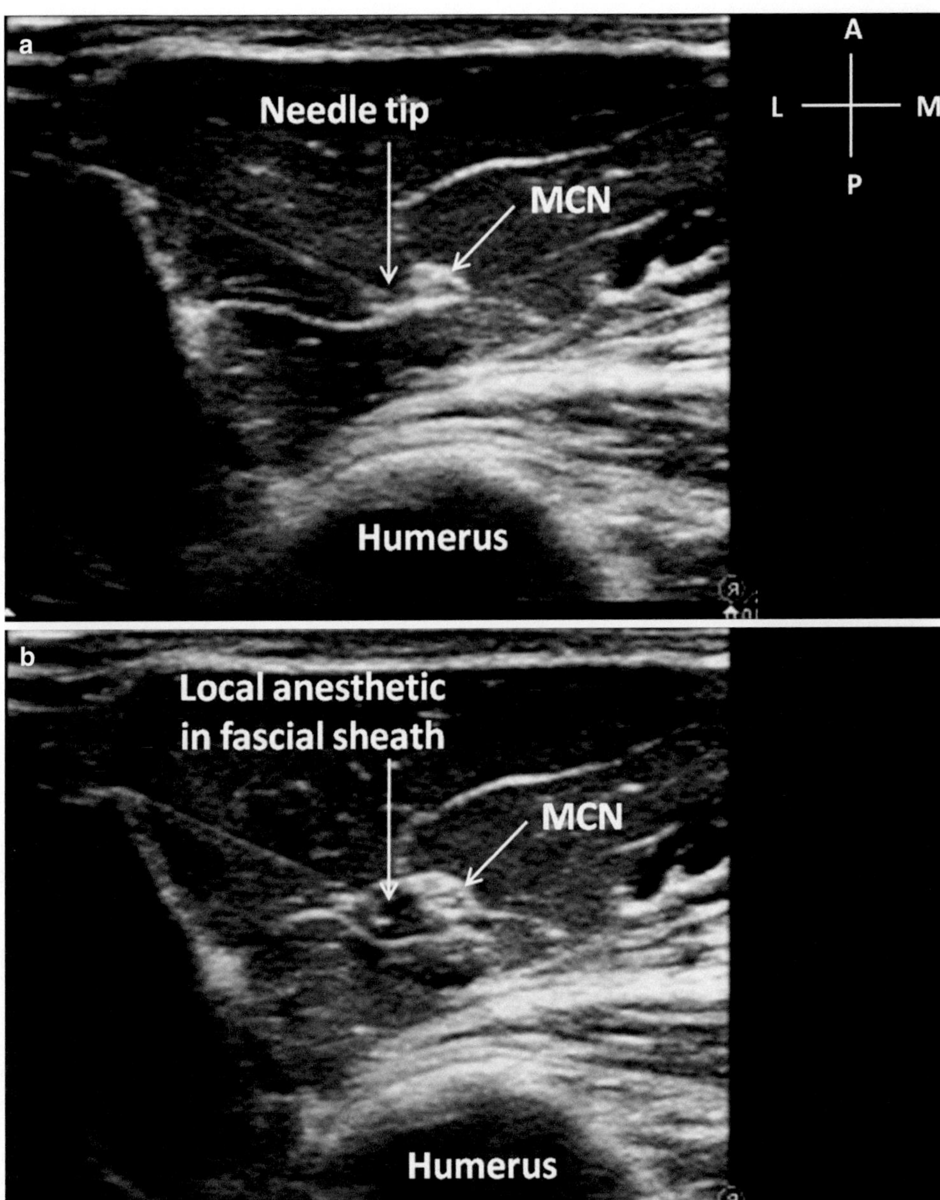

Fig. 25.25 a. The musculocutaneous nerve (MCN) is approached at a tangent, the aim being to enter the enveloping fascia without piercing the nerve.
b. Injection with the needle tip within the fascial sheath will surround the nerve with local anesthetic

injected in the final needle position to create a fluid pocket; the catheter is advanced 3–5 cm beyond the needle tip to travel in a proximal direction parallel to the plexus.

Local Anesthetic Dosages

Single-Shot Block

- A volume of 40–50 ml (0.5–0.6 ml/kg) is generally recommended for the landmark-guided techniques of axillary nerve blockade, but lower volumes of 25–40 ml can be used in the ultrasound-guided approach as long as adequate local anesthetic spread is observed.
- The choice of local anesthetic and concentration depends on the desired speed of onset and duration. Commonly used local anesthetics include:
  - A 1:1 mixture of an intermediate-acting local anesthetic (e.g., 2% mepivacaine or lidocaine) and a long-acting local anesthetic (e.g., 0.5% bupivacaine), which will have a faster onset than bupivacaine alone and a longer duration than lidocaine alone.
  - 0.25%–0.5% bupivacaine
  - 0.5%–0.75% ropivacaine
- Epinephrine in a concentration of 25–50 mcg/ml should always be added when performing an axillary block as a marker of intravascular injection and to reduce systemic vascular absorption.

Continuous Axillary Brachial Plexus Block

- 0.2–0.4% ropivacaine at 4–8 ml/h.
- 0.125%–0.25% bupivacaine at 4–8 ml/h.
- PCA boluses of 2–5 ml may be added if this function is available on the infusion pump.
- Both infusion rates and bolus volumes should be titrated to achieve the optimal balance between adequate analgesia and an excessively dense sensory and motor block.

Complications and Adverse Effects

- The axillary plexus block is a safe technique compared to other brachial plexus blocks as there are no vital structures in the vicinity.
- The main complications relate (1) to inadvertent intravascular injection and local anesthetic systemic toxicity and (2) nerve injury.
- The risk of local anesthetic systemic toxicity can be minimized by taking appropriate precautions, including (1) the addition of epinephrine to local anesthetic and (2) fractionated injections with intermittent *gentle* negative aspiration. If ultrasound guidance is being used, fluid spread must always be observed with injection. If this is not seen, the needle tip must be assumed to be intravascular until proven otherwise, and repositioning must be undertaken before further injection.
- The risk of needle-nerve injury can be minimized by avoiding paresthesia and respecting patient's complaints of pain or discomfort on injection during a surface landmark-guided technique. If ultrasound guidance is used, individual nerves should be clearly visualized and identified, and needle-nerve contact kept to a minimum.

Suggested Reading

Infraclavicular Brachial Plexus Block

Auyong DB, Gonzales J, Benonis JG. The Houdini clavicle: arm abduction and needle insertion site adjustment improves needle visibility for the infraclavicular nerve block. Reg Anesth Pain Med. 2010;35:403–4.

Bigeleisen P, Wilson M. A comparison of two techniques for ultrasound guided infraclavicular block. Br J Anaesth. 2006;96:502–7.

Chin KJ, Alakkad H, Adhikary SD, Singh M. Infraclavicular brachial plexus block for regional anaesthesia of the lower arm. Cochrane Database Syst Rev. 2013;8:CD005487.

Fredrickson MJ, Wolstencroft P, Kejriwal R, Yoon A, Boland MR, Chinchanwala S. Single versus triple injection ultrasound-guided infraclavicular block: confirmation of the effectiveness of the single injection technique. Anesth Analg. 2010;111:1325–7.

Gauss A, Tugtekin I, Georgieff M, Dinse-Lambracht A, Keipke D, Gorsewski G. Incidence of clinically symptomatic pneumothorax in ultrasound-guided infraclavicular and supraclavicular brachial plexus block. Anaesthesia. 2014;69:327–36.

Ilfeld BM, Le LT, Ramjohn J, Loland VJ, Wadhwa AN, Gerancher JC, Renehan EM, Sessler DI, Shuster JJ, Theriaque DW, Maldonado RC, Mariano ER. PAINfRETM investigators: the effects of local anesthetic concentration and dose on continuous infraclavicular nerve blocks: a multicenter, randomized, observer-masked, controlled study. Anesth Analg. 2009;108:345–50.

Kilka HG, Geiger P, Mehrkens HH. Infraclavicular vertical brachial plexus blockade. A new method for anesthesia of the upper extremity. An anatomical and clinical study. Anaesthesist. 1995;44:339–44.

Minville V, Fourcade O, Bourdet B, Doherty M, Chassery C, Pourrut J-C, Gris C, Eychennes B, Colombani A, Samii K, Bouaziz H. The optimal motor response for infraclavicular brachial plexus block. Anesth Analg. 2007;104:448–51.

Rodríguez J, Taboada M, Oliveira J, Ulloa B, Bárcena M, Alvarez J. Single stimulation of the posterior cord is superior to dual nerve stimulation in a coracoid block. Acta Anaesthesiol Scand. 2010;54:241–5.

Sharma D, Srivastava N, Pawar S, Garg R, Nagpal VK. Infraclavicular brachial plexus block: comparison of posterior cord stimulation with lateral or medial cord stimulation, a prospective double blinded study. Saudi J Anaesth. 2013;7:134–7.

The Infraclavicular Brachial Plexus Block. https://youtu.be/zEsDMPCpZKY

Tran DQH, Bertini P, Zaouter C, Muñoz L, Finlayson RJ. A prospective, randomized comparison between single- and double-injection ultrasound-guided infraclavicular brachial plexus block. Reg Anesth Pain Med. 2010;35:16–21.

Tran DQH, Charghi R, Finlayson RJ. The "double bubble" sign for successful infraclavicular brachial plexus blockade. Anesth Analg. 2006;103:1048–9.

Wilson JL, Brown DL, Wong GY, Ehman RL, Cahill DR. Infraclavicular brachial plexus block: parasagittal anatomy important to the coracoid technique. Anesth Analg. 1998;87:870–3.

Retroclavicular Brachial Plexus Block

Beh ZY, Hasan MS, Lai HY. Ultrasound-guided Retroclavicular block (aka posterior approach Infraclavicular block): anatomical variation of the clavicle limits block feasibility. Reg Anesth Pain Med. 2016;41(5):658–9. https://doi.org/10.1097/AAP.0000000000000456.

Beh ZY, Hasan MS, Lai HY, Kassim NM, Md Zin SR, Chin KF. Posterior parasagittal in-plane ultrasound-guided infraclavicular brachial plexus block-a case series. BMC Anesthesiol. 2015;21(15):105. https://doi.org/10.1186/s12871-015-0090-0.

Blanco AFG, Laferrière-Langlois P, Jessop D, D'Aragon F, Sansoucy Y, Albert N, Tétreault P, Echave P. Retroclavicular vs Infraclavicular block for brachial plexus anesthesia: a multi-centric randomized trial. BMC Anesthesiol. 2019;19(1):193. https://doi.org/10.1186/s12871-019-0868-6.

Charbonneau J, Fréchette Y, Sansoucy Y, Echave P. The ultrasound-guided Retroclavicular block: a prospective feasibility study. Reg Anesth Pain Med. 2015;40(5):605–9. https://doi.org/10.1097/AAP.0000000000000284.

Georgiadis PL, Vlassakov KV, Patton ME, Lirk PB, Janfaza DR, Zeballos JL, Quaye AN, Patel V, Schreiber KL. Ultrasound-guided supraclavicular vs. retroclavicular block of the brachial plexus: comparison of ipsilateral diaphragmatic function: a randomised clinical trial. Eur J Anaesthesiol. 2021;38(1):64–72. https://doi.org/10.1097/EJA.0000000000001305.

Grape S, Pawa A, Weber E, Albrecht E. Retroclavicular vs supraclavicular brachial plexus block for distal upper limb surgery: a randomised, controlled, single-blinded trial. Br J Anaesth. 2019;122(4):518–24. https://doi.org/10.1016/j.bja.2018.12.022.

Hebbard P, Royse C. Ultrasound guided posterior approach to the infraclavicular brachial plexus. Anaesthesia. 2007;62(5):539. https://doi.org/10.1111/j.1365-2044.2007.05066.x.

Sancheti SF, Uppal V, Sandeski R, Kwofie MK, Szerb JJ. A cadaver study investigating structures encountered by the needle during a Retroclavicular approach to Infraclavicular brachial plexus block. Reg Anesth Pain Med. 2018;43(7):752–5. https://doi.org/10.1097/AAP.0000000000000826.

Sutton EM, Bullock WM, Gadsden J. The Retroclavicular brachial plexus block: additional advantages. Reg Anesth Pain Med. 2015;40(6):733–4. https://doi.org/10.1097/AAP.0000000000000318.

Uppal V, Kalagara HKP, Sondekoppam RV. Tips and tricks to improve the safety of the retroclavicular brachial plexus block. Am J Emerg Med. 2018;36(6):1107–8. https://doi.org/10.1016/j.ajem.2017.09.056.

Axillary Brachial Plexus Block

Ultrasound-Guided Axillary Brachial Plexus Block – The Simple Guide. https://youtu.be/HLgHSrnaLFo

Bernucci F, Gonzalez AP, Finlayson RJ, Tran DQH. A prospective, randomized comparison between perivascular and perineural ultrasound-guided axillary brachial plexus block. Reg Anesth Pain Med. 2012;37:473–7.

Bloc S, Mercadal L, Dessieux T, Garnier T, Estebe J-P, Le Naoures A, Komly B, Leclerc P, Morel B, Ecoffey C, Dhonneur G. The learning process of the hydrolocalization technique performed during ultrasound-guided regional anesthesia. Acta Anaesthesiol Scand. 2010;54:421–5.

Chin KJ, Alakkad H, Cubillos JE. Single double or multiple-injection techniques for non-ultrasound guided axillary brachial plexus block in adults undergoing surgery of the lower arm. Cochrane Database Syst Rev. 2013;8:CD003842.

Cho S, Kim YJ, Kim J-H, Baik H-J. Double-injection perivascular ultrasound-guided axillary brachial plexus block according to needle positioning: 12 versus 6 o'clock position of the axillary artery. Korean J Anesthesiol. 2014;66:112–9.

Tran DQH, Russo G, Muñoz L, Zaouter C, Finlayson RJ. A prospective, randomized comparison between ultrasound-guided supraclavicular, infraclavicular, and axillary brachial plexus blocks. Reg Anesth Pain Med. 2009;34:366–71.

Intravenous Regional Anesthesia (IVRA)

26

Danilo Jankovic

Contents

General Consideration

The injection of local anesthetics into a vein in an exsanguinated extremity was first described by German surgeon August Bier in 1908. Originally, anesthesia was obtained by the intravenous injection of procaine in a previously exsanguinated vascular space, isolated from the rest of the circulation by two Esmarch bandages used as tourniquet. In 1963, Holmes reintroduced the Bier block with the novel use of lidocaine. It caused anesthesia and a motor block. It is a widely accepted technique well suited for brief minor surgeries such as wrist or hand ganglionectomy, carpal tunnel release, Dupuytren's contractures, etc. IVRA is a simple, effective anesthetic technique with a reported success rate of 96–100%. IVRA is safe but not entirely without the risk of complications. IVRA has been used for many years to empirically treat CRPS with a wide variety of substances, including guanethidine, lidocaine, bretylium, clonidine, droperidol, ketanserin, or reserpine.

D. Jankovic (✉)
Pain Management Centre DGS – Cologne – Huerth, Cologne-Hürth, Germany
e-mail: danilo@jankovic1.de

Indications

Outpatient surgical procedures with a maximum length of 1 h in the forearm or hand (standard application) and in the lower leg and foot (more rarely; Figs. 26.1, 26.2, and 26.3). The only significant difference in IVRA for the upper and lower extremities is that the IVRA technique

D. Jankovic, P. Peng (eds.), *Regional Nerve Blocks in Anesthesia and Pain Therapy*,
https://doi.org/10.1007/978-3-030-88727-8_26

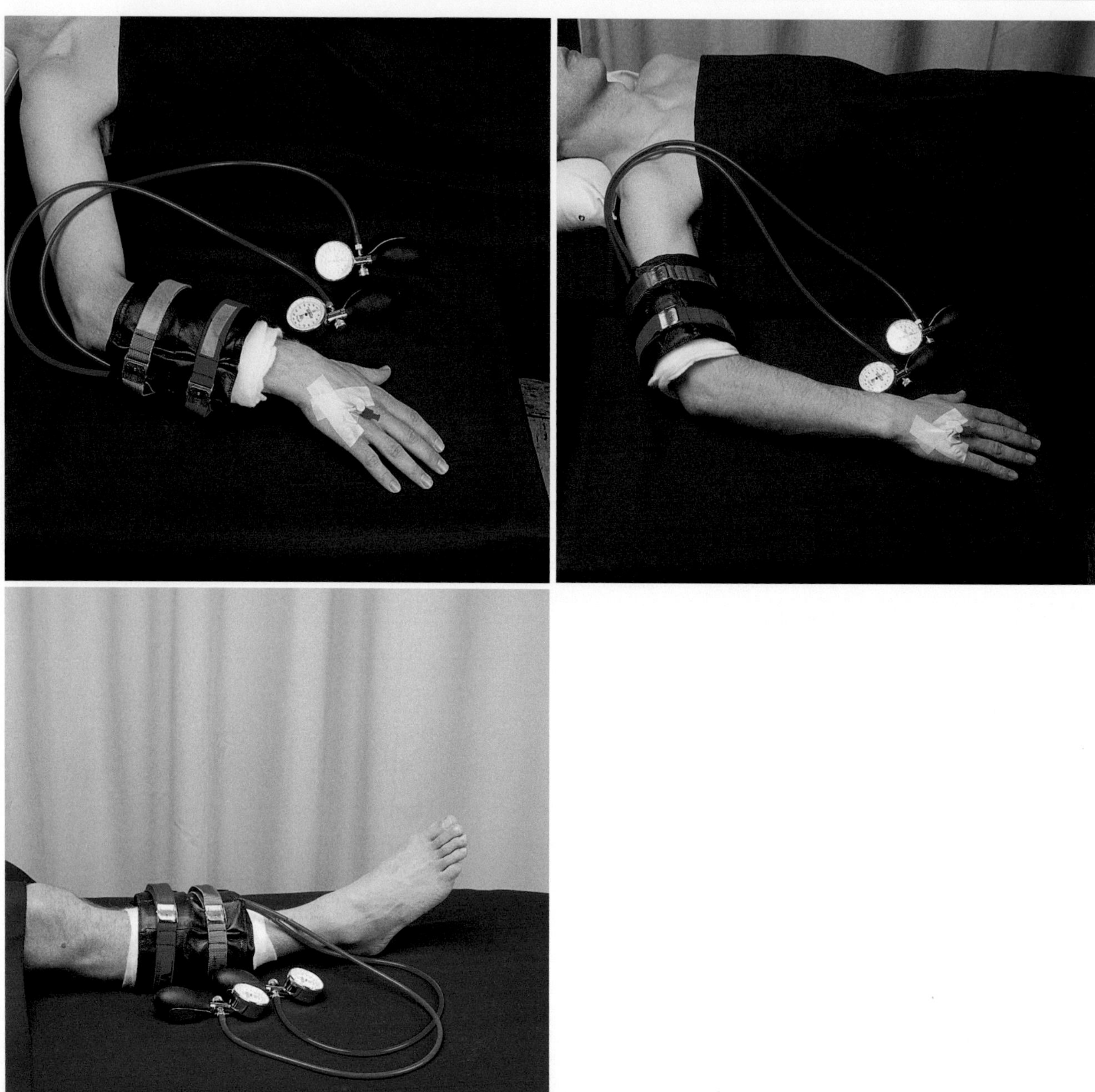

Figs. 26.1, 26.2, and 26.3 Areas of application of intravenous regional anesthesia. (Reproduced with permission from Danilo Jankovic)

for the lower extremity requires relatively larger volumes of local anesthetic solutions by virtue of the obvious size disparity between upper and lower extremities. This is necessary to more completely fill the larger vascular compartment of the lower extremity from the distally placed intravenous cannula to the proximal tourniquet (100 mL vs. 50 mL).

Contraindications

- Patient refusal
- Local infection in the area to be anesthetized
- Local nerve damage
- Peripheral vascular diseases

- Severe decompensated hypovolemia, shock
- Certain cardiovascular diseases
- Hypertonia, bradycardia, second-degree AV block, any history of a tendency to syncope
- Musculoskeletal diseases

Advantages

- Simple technique
- No specific anatomical expertise is needed
- Wide safety margins and very high success rate
- Fast onset of effect (5–10 min)
- The need for supplemental medication is ordinarily minimal
- The technique is particularly suitable for short procedures in an ambulatory surgery center
- Controllable spread of the anesthesia (below the tourniquet cuff)
- Fast return of sensation
- No risk of infection
- The major cause of failure of the technique or serious adverse effects is a technical error
- The incidence of adverse reactions is low (1.6%) and consists of minor events (e.g., transient dizziness, tinnitus, dysphoria, facial tingling, or bradycardia).

Disadvantages

- Tourniquet cuff is needed
- Limited operating time (<1 h)
- Procedures in the upper arm are not possible
- Tourniquet pain during the procedure
- Nerve damage due to the tourniquet cuff
- Does not provide a blood-free operating area
- Insufficient postoperative analgesia due to fast recovery from the anesthesia

Procedure

This block should only be carried out when full anesthetic facilities are available. Full prior information for the patient is mandatory.

Preparations

Check that the appropriate emergency equipment is present and in working order. Sterile precautions. Two intravenous access points (in the healthy extremity as well as the one being operated on), BP and ECG monitoring, pulse oximetry, anesthesia machine. Patient preparation is the same as for general anesthesia.

Materials (Fig. 26.4)

20-mL and 50-mL syringes, saline, cotton wool padding, pneumatic tourniquet (double-lumen), Esmarch bandage, local anesthetic, disinfectant, pneumatic tourniquet device (Fig. 26.5).

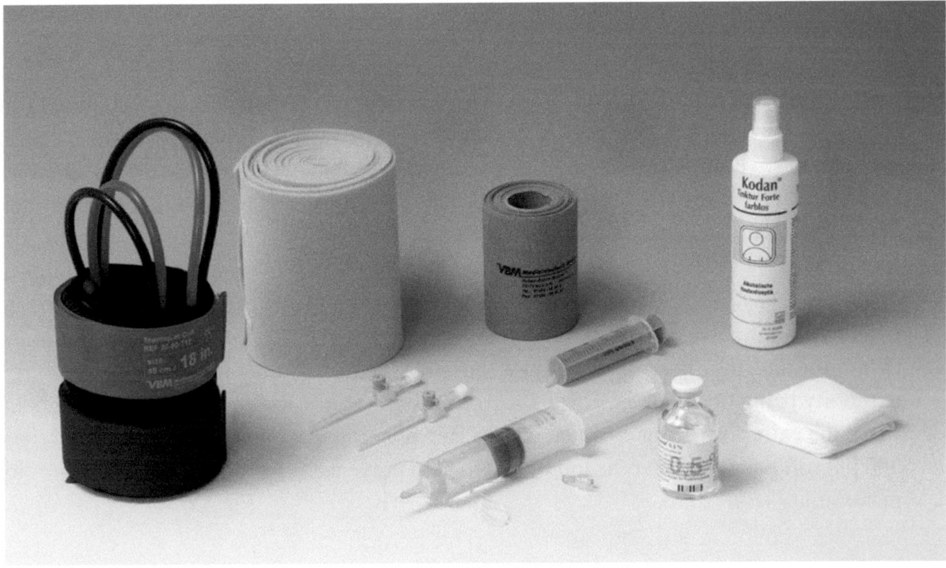

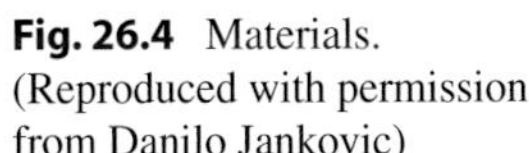
Fig. 26.4 Materials. (Reproduced with permission from Danilo Jankovic)

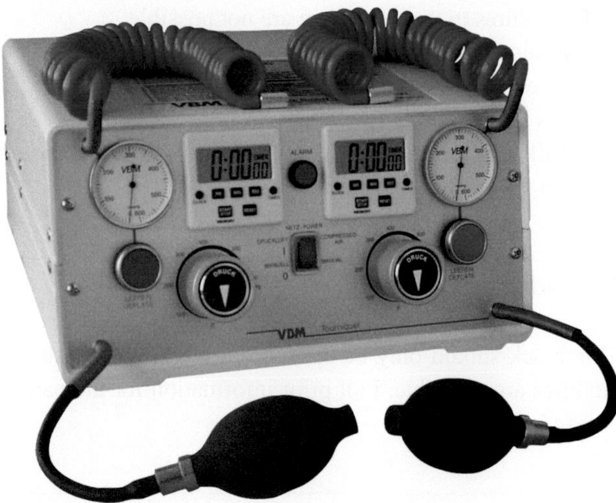

Fig. 26.5 Pneumatic tourniquet device. (Reproduced with permission from Danilo Jankovic)

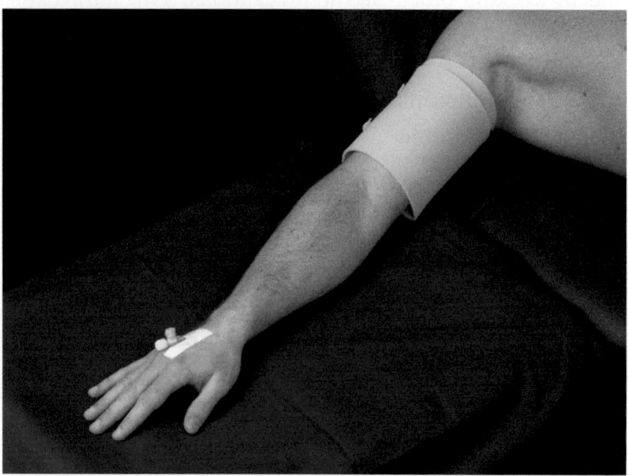

Fig. 26.6 Padding of the tourniquet area, intravenous access. (Reproduced with permission from Danilo Jankovic)

Patient Positioning

Supine, with the extremity free.

Technique

1. Insert two intravenous catheters – one in a healthy extremity and the other as distally as possible in the extremity being operated on.
2. Place the extremity being operated on in a free position, and put soft padding under the tourniquet to help prevent nerve injury (Fig. 26.6).

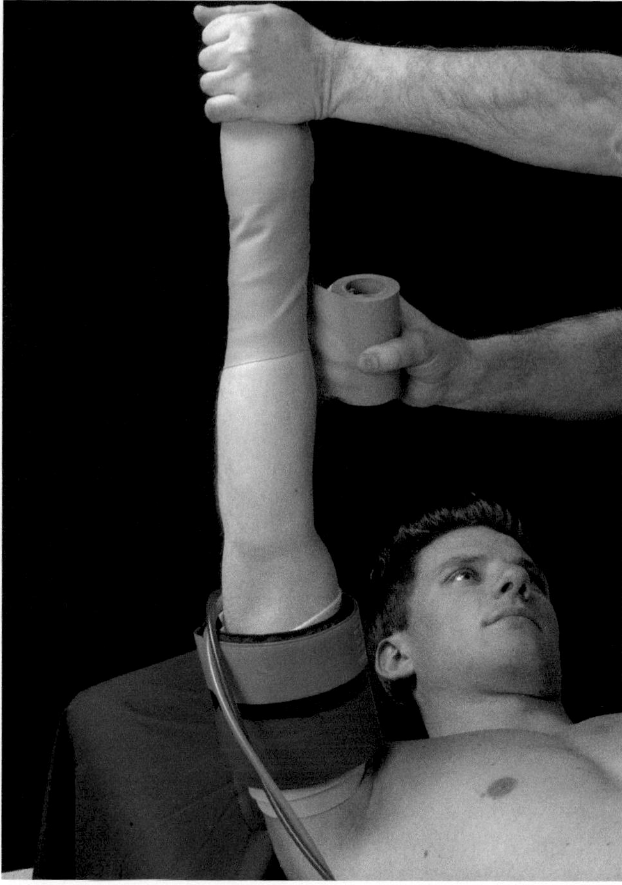

Fig. 26.7 Wrapping with an Esmarch bandage. (Reproduced with permission from Danilo Jankovic)

3. Position the double-lumen tourniquet.
4. Elevate and massage the limb for a few minutes, and then wrap it completely with an Esmarch bandage (Fig. 26.7).
5. Inflate the proximal cuff: the pressure in the cuff has to be ca. 80–100 mmHg higher than the patient's systolic blood pressure. The pressure that should be used depends on the thickness of the muscles being compressed. A pulse oximeter is used to document changes in, and cessation of, the pulse ("pulse occlusion pressure") and the disappearance of the pulse in the radial artery. The "pulse occlusion pressure" can be used to determine the optimal pressure in the proximal cuff (Fig. 26.8).
6. Remove the bandage and place the extremity in a horizontal position.
7. Slowly inject the local anesthetic (20 mL/min; Fig. 26.9).

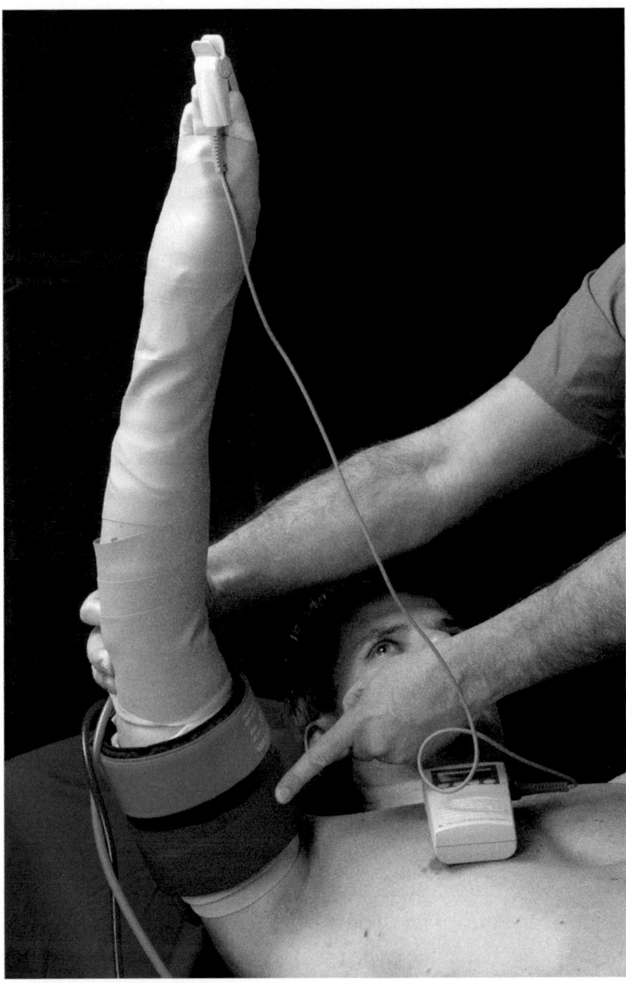

Fig. 26.8 Inflation of the tourniquet. (Reproduced with permission from Danilo Jankovic)

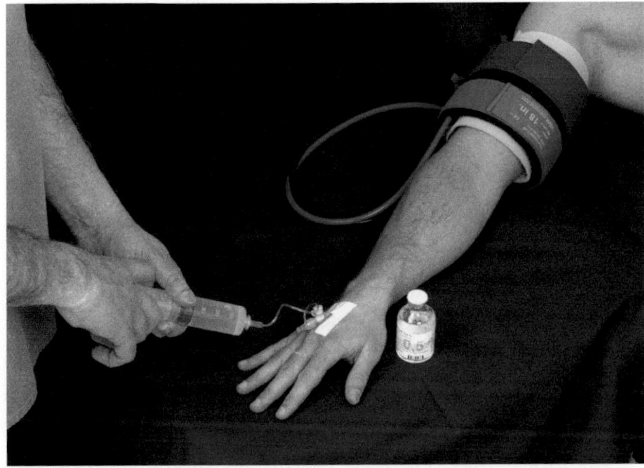

Fig. 26.9 Injection of the local anesthetic. (Reproduced with permission from Danilo Jankovic)

8. Perform stroking massage of the extremity (this improves the spread of the local anesthetic), and remove the catheters.
9. Good analgesia and muscle relaxation develop after ca. 5–10 min.
10. Inflate the distal cuff, which is now in the analgesic area, so that the cuff is better tolerated. Deflate the proximal cuff. After the anesthetic effect has been tested, the operation can begin.

Dosage

Local anesthetics

40–50 mL local anesthetic, e.g.:

- Prilocaine 0.5%, 3–4 mg/kg body weight.

Among the amide local anesthetics, prilocaine provides the best ratio between anesthetic potency and toxicity and should be regarded as the agent of choice for intravenous regional anesthesia (see Chap. 1).

- Lidocaine 0.5%, 1.5–3 mg/kg b.w.
- Ropivacaine 0.2% (0.250.375%), (1.2 mg–1.8 mg/kg).

*The most common local anesthetics for IVRA are lidocaine (United States) and prilocaine (Europe). Ropivacaine use results in similar onset times and tourniquet tolerance as with lidocaine (prilocaine) but increased time to recovery of sensory and motor function and improved postoperative analgesia. Cardiotoxicity is still possible with ropivacaine, and its widespread use for IVRA is limited by this potential.

IVRA adjuncts to local anesthetic agents:

- Opioids (tramadol 50–100 mg, morphine 1–6 mg, meperidine 100 mg, fentanyl 50–200 μg, sufentanil 25 μg)
- Clonidine 1 μg/kg
- Ketamine 0.3–0.5 mg/kg
- Muscle relaxants (atracurium 2 mg, pancuronium 0.5 mg, mivacurium 0.6 mg, and cisatracurium 0.01 mg/kg)
- Nonsteroidal anti-inflammatory drugs: ketorolac (20–30 mg – the optimal dose has not been established)
- Dexmedetomidine (0.5–1 μg /kg)
- Dexamethasone 8 mg

Complications

- Systemic toxic reactions can occur if the local anesthetic enters the circulation due to the release of the tourniquet cuff (see Chap. 5). Prophylaxis: intermittent opening of the tourniquet, maintaining verbal contact with the patient, avoiding strong premedication.

  *Have intralipid readily available

- Toxic effects on the cardiovascular system only occur after very high doses of local anesthetic and become apparent as a drop in blood pressure, bradycardia, circulatory collapse, and cardiac arrest. This type of complication rarely occurs in intravenous regional anesthesia.
- Nerve damage due to the cuff pressure.
- Petechiae or other skin discoloration and hypertension with tourniquet inflation.
- Thrombophlebitis.

Practical Tips

- Minimum tourniquet time is 15–20 min after injection of the local anesthetic. The tourniquet must not be released during this period (risk of toxic reactions!).
- Tourniquet pressure must be monitored continuously.
- After completion of the procedure: intermittent deflation over a period of 10 min, with complete inflation in between (Fig. 26.10).
- Only local anesthetics that contain no vasoconstrictors may be used!

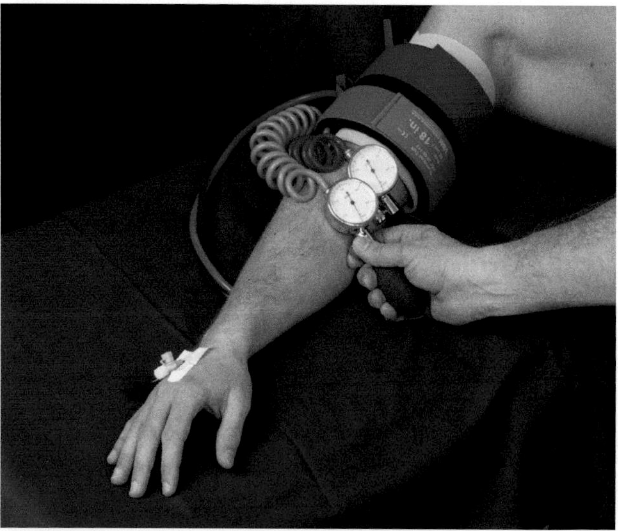

Fig. 26.10 Intermittent deflation of the cuff over a period of 10 min. (Reproduced with permission from Danilo Jankovic)

Literature Review

There are a few limitations associated with IVRA: local anesthetic systemic toxicity, delayed onset of action, poor muscle relaxation, tourniquet pain, and minimal postoperative analgesia. Various adjuncts added to LA have been investigated in an attempt to improve the quality of IVRA, including opioids, muscle relaxants, nonsteroidal anti-inflammatory drugs, clonidine, dexmedetomidine, ketamine, dexamethason, potassium, and alkalizing agents.

Local anesthetic lidocaine and *ropivacaine* were the most common LA agents evaluated. Overall, there were no significant differences in the onset of sensory block between lidocaine, prilocaine, and ropivacaine. Five studies evaluated offset of sensory block with the use of ropivacaine compared to lidocaine and prilocaine. All five studies found recovery to be prolonged when ropivacaine was used.

Opioids – morphine, meperidine, and fentanyl (as a sole adjunct) – do not demonstrate clinically significant benefits as adjuncts, or their side effects preclude their clinical use. Sufentanil data is limited but appears to provide faster onset of sensory block, and not demonstrate postdeflation analgesia. Tramadol provides faster onset of sensory block and improves tourniquet tolerance but lacks consistent postoperative benefits with an increased risk of minor side effects. The *combination* of *fentanyl* with a *muscle relaxant* can achieve an equivalent quality of IVRA with a 50% reduction in LA dose, but at the expense of a potentially slower sensory block.

Muscle relaxants (pancuronium, atracurium, mivacurium, and cisatracurium) improve the quality of motor block but at the expense of delayed motor recovery.

The use of *nonsteroidal anti-inflammatory drugs* (NSAIDs) as adjunct for IVRA has been widely studied. A review of Choice and Peng in 2002 summarized the state of literature at that time, with ketorolac shown to reduce postoperative pain after IVRA. However, the subsequent retraction of several articles published regarding NSAIDs and acute pain has clouded the picture (Schafer 2009). Recent studies have indirectly addressed that question by investigating the use of additional adjuvants. Two of those studies have associated ketorolac with postoperative pain and analgesic requirements when added to IVRA solution compared with lidocaine alone but did not include a systemic administration control group.

Clonidine may increase tourniquet tolerance time and modestly reduce postoperative pain scores, but sedation and hypotension after tourniquet release are significant adverse effects (Choice Peng 2002, Alayurt Memis 2004).

Dexmedetomidine is more selective for alpha-2 receptors than clonidine, which accounts for its preferential sedative over hemodynamic effects. At doses of 0.5–1 μg/kg added to lidocaine, dexmedetomidine improves postoperative analgesia and may shorten sensory block onset time. Importantly, hemodynamic changes (bradycardia, hypotension) may still occur with dexmedetomidine but seem less severe than with clonidine.

Dexamethasone in a dose of 8 mg added to plain lidocaine 3 mg/kg shortens block onset and improves postoperative analgesia in some small studies, and this effect may be manifested by the addition of other additives as ketorolac.

The addition of *ketamine* to the block solution improves postoperative and intraoperative analgesic requirements; however, this effect seems to be no different than with systemic administration. The addition of *potassium* confers no advantages, and changing the temperature of the injectate does not affect the quality of the block, although warmer solutions are less painful on injection.

Suggested Readings

Abdel-Ghaffar HS, Kalefa MA, Imbaby AS. Efficacy of ketamine as an adjunct to lidocaine in intravenous regional anesthesia. Reg Anesth Pain Med. 2014;39(5):418–22.

Akram M, Farooqi FM, et al. Role of addition of dexamethasone and ketorolac to lignocaine intravenous regional anesthesia (Bier's block) to improve tourniquet tolerance and post-operative analgesia in hand and forearm surgery. J Pak Med Assoc. 2015;65(11 supp 3):S128–S31.

Alayurt S, Memis D, Pamukcu Z. The addition of sufentanil, tramadol, or clonidine to lignocaine for intravenous regional anesthesia. Anaesth Intensive Care. 2004;32(1):22–7.

Asik I, Kocum AI, Goktug A. Comparison of ropivacaine 0.2% and 0.25% with lidocaine 0.5% for intravenous regional anesthesia. J Clin Anesth. 2009;21(6):401–7.

Aujla KS, Gupta R, Singh J. Plain lignocaine versus mixture of lignocaine, fentanyl and pancuronium for intravenous regional anesthesia. J Anaesth Clin Pharmacol. 2009;25(3):301–4.

Brown E, McGriff JT, Malinowski RW. Intravenous regional anesthesia (Bier Block): review of 20 years experience. Can J Anesth. 1989;36(3):307.

Chan VW, Weisbrod MJ, Kaszas Z, et al. Comparison of ropivacaine and lidocaine for intravenous regional anesthesia in volunteers: a preliminary study on anesthetic efficacy and blood level. Anesthesiology. 1999;90(6):1602–8.

Chiao FB, Chen J, Lesser JB, et al. Single-cuff forearm tourniquet in intravenous regional anesthesia results in less pain and fewer sedation requirements than upper arm tourniquet. Br J Anaesth. 2013;111(2):271–5.

Choyce A, Peng P. A systematic review of adjuncts for intravenous regional anesthesia for surgical procedures. Can J Anesth. 2002;49(1):32–45.

Erciyes N, Akturk G, Solak M. Morphine/prilocaine combination for intravenous regional anesthesia. Acta Anaesthes Scand. 1995;39:845–6.

Erciyes N, Aktürk G, Solak M, et al. Morphine/prilocaine combination for intravenous regional anesthesia. Acta Anaesthesiol Scand. 1995;39(6):845–6.

Flamer D, Peng PWH. Intravenous regional anesthesia: a review of common local anesthetic options and the use of opioids and muscle relaxants and adjuncts. Local Reg Anesth. 2011;4(1):57–76.

Gentili M, Bernard JM, Bonnet F. Adding clonidine to lidocaine for intravenous regional anesthesia prevents tourniquet pain. Anesth Analg. 1999;88(6):1327–30.

Gorgias N, Maidatsi P, Kyriakidis, et al. Clonidine versus Ketamine to prevent tourniquet pain during intravenous anesthesia with lidocaine. Reg Anesth and Pain Med. 2001;26(6):512–7.

Guay J. Adverse events associated with intravenous regional anesthesia (Bier block): a systematic review of complications. J Clin Anesth. 2009;21(8):585–94.

Gupta A, Björnsson A, Sjöberg F, et al. Lack of peripheral analgesic effect of low- dose morphine during intravenous regional anesthesia. Reg Anesth. 1993;18(4):250–3.

Hadzic A, Vloka JD, Kuroda MM, Koorn R, Birnbach DJ. The practice of peripheral nerve blocks in the United States: a national survey. Reg Anesth Pain Med. 1998;23:241–6.

Hannington-Kiff J. Intravenous regional sympathetic block with guanethidine. Lancet. 1974;I:1010–20.

Hannington-Kiff J. Antisympathetic drugs in limbs. In: Wall PD, Melzack R, editors. Textbook of pain. London: Churchill Livingstone; 1984.

Hartmannsgruber MW, Silverman DG, Halaszynski TM. Comparison of ropivacaine 0.2% and lidocaine 0.5% for intravenous regional anesthesia in volunteers. Anesth Analg. 1999;89(3):727–31.

Hassani E, Mahoori A, Aghdashi MM. Evaluating the quality of intravenous regional anesthesia following adding dexamethasone to lidocaine. Saudi J Anesth. 2015;9(4):418–21.

Hilgenhurst G. The Bier block after 80 years: a historical review. Reg Anesth. 1990;15:2.

Holmes C. Intravenous regional nerve blockade. In: Cousins MJ, Bridenbaugh DL, editors. Neural blockade. 3rd ed. New York: Lippincott-Raven; 1998. p. 395–409.

Ismail O, El-Bahnasawe N, Badran A. Clinical efficacy of ropivacaine 0.2% for intravenous regional anaesthesia. Eg J Anaesth. 2004;20(2):165–9.

Jankovic D. Intravenous regional anesthesia. In: Jankovic D, editor. Regional nerve blocks & infiltration therapy. Berlin: Blackwell Scientists; 2004. p. 164–8.

Kumar K, Railton C, Tawfic Q. Tourniquet application during anesthesia: what we need to know? J Anaesthesiol Clin Pharmacol. 2016;32(4):424.

Langlois G, Estebe JP, Gentili ME, et al. The addition of tramadol to lidocaine does not reduce tourniquet and postoperative pain during iv regional anesthesia. Can J Anesth. 2002;49(2):165–8.

Löser B, Petzoldt M, Löser A, et al. Intravenous Regional Anesthesia: A historical Overview and Clinical Review. J Anesth Hist. 2019 Jul;5(3):99–108.

de May JC. Bier's block. Anesthesia. 1997;52:713.

McKeown DW, Scott DB. Influence of the addition of potassium to 0.5% prilocaine solution during I.V. regional anesthesia. Br J Anaesth. 1988;43(5):362–4.

Mickhael H, Hussanin A. Effect of Addition of Cisatracurium and Ketorolac to Lidocaine for Local Intravenous Anaesthesia. Eg J Anaesth. 2009;25(2):139–45.

Peng P, Coleman MM, McCartney CJ. Comparison of anesthetic effect between 0.375% ropivacaine versus 0.5% lidocaine in forearm intravenous regional anesthesia. Reg Anesth Pain Med. 2002;27(6):595–9.

Perlas A, Peng PW, Plaza MB, et al. Forearm rescue cuff improves tourniquet tolerance during intravenous regional anesthesia. Reg Anesth Pain Med. 2003;28(2):98–102.

Pitkänen MT. Intravenous regional anesthesia. In: Rosenberg P, editor. Local and regional anesthesia. BMJ Books; 2000. p. 55–6.

Prasad SB, Anjan T. Intravenous regional anesthesia (IVRA): Addition of atracurium or ketorolac to lignocaine- a prospective randomised double blind study. J Anaesth Clin Pharmacol. 2010;26(2):203–7.

Ramadhyani U, Park JL, Carollo DS, et al. Dexmedetomidine: clinical application as an adjunct for intravenous regional anesthesia. Anesthesiol Clin. 2010;28(4):709–22.

Sardesai SP, Patil KN, Sarkar A. Comparison of clonidine and dexmedetomidine as adjuncts to intravenous regional anesthesia. Indian J Anesth. 2015;59(11):733–8.

Schafer SL. Notice of retraction. Anesth Analg. 2009;108(4):1350.

Siddiqui AK, Mowafi HA, Al-Ghamdi A, et al. Tramadol as an adjuvant to intravenous regional anesthesia with lignocaine. Saudi Med J. 2008;29(8):1151–5.

Simgen WLA. Intravenöse Regionalanästhesie. In: Hörster W, Zenz M, Niesel HC, Kreuscher H, Redaktion. Regionalanästhesie. Stuttgart: Gustav Fischer; 1989. p. 82–5.

Tan SM, Pay LL, Chan ST. Intravenous regional anesthesia using lignocaine and tramadol. Ann Acad Med Singap. 2001;30(5):516–9.

Viscomi CM, Friend A, Parker C, et al. Ketamine as an adjuvant in lidocaine intravenous regional anesthesia. Reg Anesth Pain Med. 2009;34(2):130–3.

Wahren KL, Gordh T, Torebjörk E. Effects of regional intravenous guanethidine in patients with neuralgia in the hand, a follow up study over a decade. Pain. 1995;62:379–85.

Armstrong P, Power I, Wildsmith JA. Addition of fentanyl to prilocaine for intravenous regional anesthesia. Anaesthesia. 1991;46:278–80.

Peripheral Nerve Block Around the Elbow or Forearm

27

Clara Lobo and Philip Peng

Contents

General Considerations

Distal upper limb blocks are simple and very effective techniques aiming at the peripheral nerves of the brachial plexus at the elbow and wrist level for a variety of procedures involving the hand and fingers. These peripheral nerve blocks are easy to perform, devoid of major systemic complications, and should be part of basic armamentarium for every anesthesiologist. The easily identified nerves under ultrasound guidance are radial, median, and ulnar. Its blockade may prove to be extremely useful in supplementing a failed or incomplete proximal brachial plexus block. Distally, these nerves are predominantly sensory, so its use in combination with a proximal brachial plexus block can reduce onset time and increase block consistency. Another advantage is that their blockade with long-acting local anesthetics, in combination with a short-acting brachial plexus block, can prolong analgesia with limited motor block avoiding the

C. Lobo (✉)
Anesthesiology Department, Hospital das Forças Armadas, Pólo Porto, Portugal

P. Peng
Department of Anesthesiology and Pain Medicine, Toronto Western Hospital, University of Toronto, Toronto, ON, Canada
e-mail: philip.peng@uhn.ca

D. Jankovic, P. Peng (eds.), *Regional Nerve Blocks in Anesthesia and Pain Therapy*,
https://doi.org/10.1007/978-3-030-88727-8_27

immobilization of the whole limb for several hours. In a study comparing the combination of general anesthesia with elbow block versus axillary plexus block favored the first with an improved retention of motor function, a similar analgesia, and an enhanced patient satisfaction.

Before selecting the blockade of individual nerves at the elbow or wrist levels, several facts must be remembered:

1. The innervation of each individual nerve is variable and overlaps are very common (Fig. 27.1). The exception is the motor and sensory innervation of the fifth metacarpal bone and fifth finger, which is consistently covered by the ulnar nerve. The wide, varying distribution and overlapping of ulnar, median, and radial nerves necessitate that either two out of three or all must be anesthetized to produce adequate analgesia for most procedures. The anesthesiologist must be aware of the superficial and deep innervation of these nerves as well as the possible deviation from the description of textbook.
2. The use of tourniquet is very common, and the best place to put it on the upper extremity is above the elbow. Therefore, the elbow and wrist blocks will not be suitable in this situation.
3. Cutaneous infiltration is often necessary, unless you block the involved cutaneous branches separately (see below), namely, the medial antebrachial cutaneous nerve of the forearm and the intercostobrachial nerve that might contribute to the proximal innervation of the forearm.
4. Muscle relaxation might not be adequate. For example, in case of tendinous rupture on the hand, a wrist block will only produce sensory blockage, and the muscles that control the tendon on the forearm are not blocked, making it impossible to recover and suture the retracted tendon. Yet, these types of block can be an advantage in procedures when the surgeon wants to assess the movement of fingers, e.g., after a tendon release.
5. Be aware to not exceed maximal dose of local anesthetic. The blockade of each individual nerve should not require more than 5 mL of local anesthetic solution.

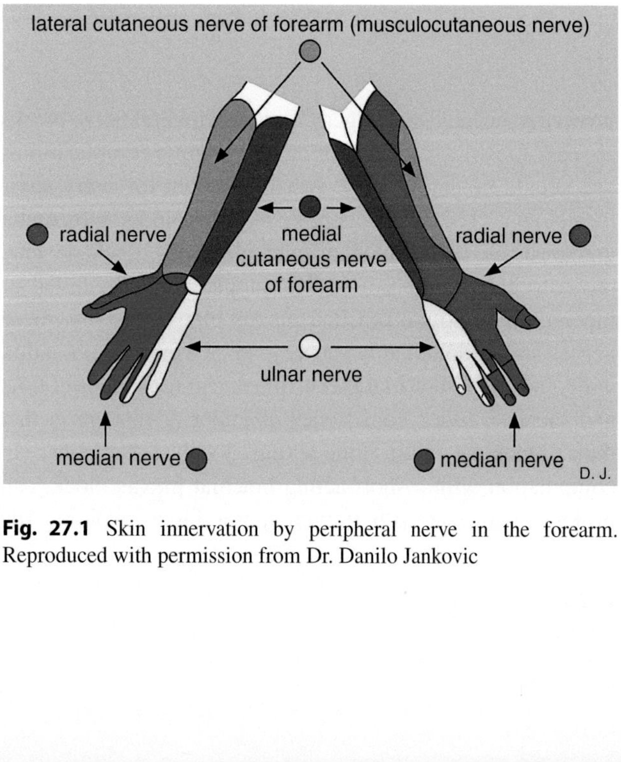

Fig. 27.1 Skin innervation by peripheral nerve in the forearm. Reproduced with permission from Dr. Danilo Jankovic

Indications

Main indications are:

1. Forearm, hand, wrist, and finger interventions (surgery or trauma)
2. Supplementation of incomplete or failed brachial plexus block
3. Prolongation of distal upper limb analgesia
4. Individual nerve block might be a useful tool for diagnostic purposes and localize pain problems.

Functional Anatomy

Innervation of the forearm, wrist, and hand is shared by the radial, median, and ulnar nerves. However, the lateral cutaneous nerve of the forearm (a branch of the musculocutaneous nerve) supplies the lateral aspect of the forearm and wrist and must be blocked separately if the lateral aspect of the forearm or/and wrist is included in the procedure. The sensory innervation of the medial aspect of the forearm is covered by the medial cutaneous nerve of the forearm (Fig. 27.1).

The brachial plexus (BP) is a neuronal network of ventral rami of C5–T1 roots, with possible contributions from C4 or T1 (Fig. 27.2).

Median Nerve

The anterior divisions of the medial and lateral cords of the BP originate the median nerve (contains fibers from all five BP nerve roots: C5–T1). This nerve is in very close relation to axillary artery and brachial artery along its course (Fig. 27.3). At the elbow level, the median nerve (MN) is very superficial and lies medial to the brachial artery, which in turn lies on the medial side of the biceps brachii tendon posterior to the bicipital aponeurosis, medial to the brachialis muscle (Fig. 27.4). The MN separates from the artery and lies deep to the pronator teres muscle and the flexor digitorum superficialis (FDS) as it reaches the forearm. Distal to the ulnar fossa, the MN originates from the anterior interosseous nerve that supplies all flexor muscles of the anterior compartment of the forearm, except the flexor carpi ulnaris. At the mid-forearm level, the MN lies in the plane between the FDS and flexor digitorum profundus (FDP) (Fig. 27.5).

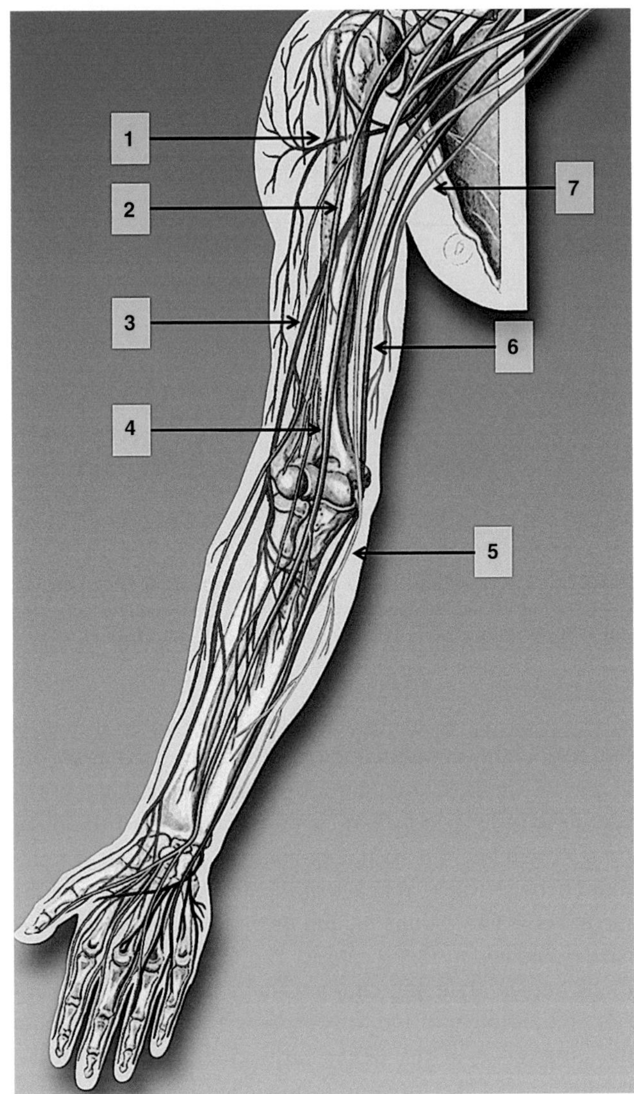

Fig. 27.2 Major terminal branches of the brachial plexus in the axillary region (1). Axillary nerve, (2) musculocutaneous nerve, (3) radial nerve, (4) median nerve, (5) medial antebrachial cutaneous nerve, (6) ulnar nerve, (7) medial brachial cutaneous nerve. Reproduced with permission from Danilo Jankovic

At the wrist level, the MN lies lateral to the FDS and beneath the palmaris longus tendon and continues under the flexor retinaculum to enter the hand, inside the carpal tunnel. It is fairly common to find an absence of palmaris longus muscle (and tendon). In this case, the median nerve is located between the FDS and the flexor carpi radialis tendons. The sensory supply of the MN is through the palmar cutaneous and palmar digital cutaneous branches. Three fingerbreadths proximal to the wrist, the medial nerve gives rise to a palmar cutaneous branch to the thenar eminence.

Hence, a single injection to achieve a complete sensory-motor block of the median nerve is possible by blocking it proximal to the elbow. A sensory block of the median nerve territory of the hand is possible by approaching it at the forearm.

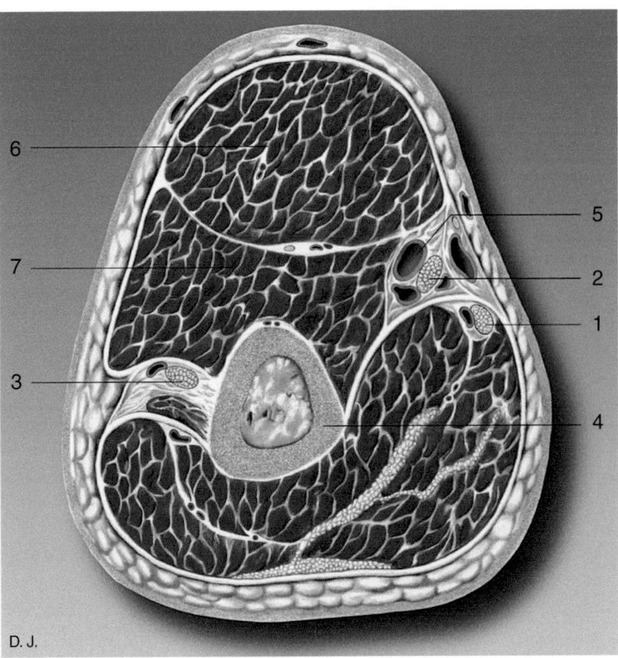

Fig. 27.3 Cross-section view at distal third of the humerus (1). Ulnar nerve, (2) median nerve, (3) radial nerve, (4) humerus, (5) brachial artery, (6) biceps brachii muscle, (7) brachialis muscle. Reproduced with permission from Danilo Jankovic

Radial Nerve

The radial nerve (C5–T1) is the largest branch of the brachial plexus and the terminal branch of the posterior cord (Fig. 27.2). The radial nerve (RN) runs in the posterior aspect of the arm, from medial to lateral between the medial and lateral heads of the triceps muscle, in the radial or spiral groove (Fig. 27.3). It pierces the lateral intermuscular septum, approximately 7 cm above the lateral epicondyle of the humerus, and passes between the brachioradialis (BRM) and the brachialis muscles (BM) to the anterior aspect of the lateral epicondyle and elbow joint capsule, where it divides into deep branch and superficial branch (sensory). The deep branch surrounds the neck of the radius and descends between the two layers of the supinator muscle in the "radial tunnel" or "arcade of Frohse" and enters the posterior compartment of the forearm as the posterior interosseous nerve, often accompanied by the recurrent branch of the radial artery. The superficial branch of the RN has no branches for the forearm, runs under the BRM and on the supinator and pronator teres muscles, and descends close and lateral to the radial artery in the mid-forearm, after which it abandons the artery and travels along the medial side of the BRM (Fig. 27.5). About 7–8 cm proximal to the wrist, it crosses under the tendon of the BRM and reaches the extensor side of the forearm. At the level of the wrist, the RN divides into several peripheral branches.

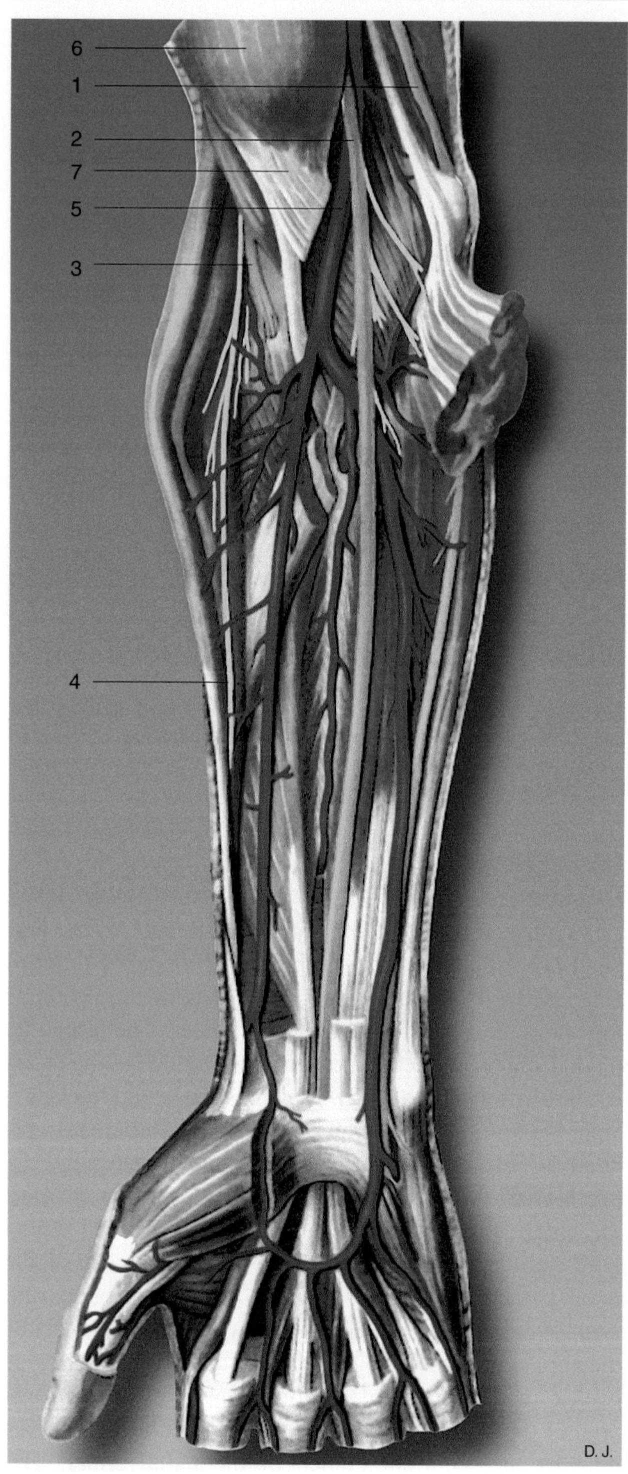

Fig. 27.4 Anatomy of the forearm (1). Ulnar nerve, (2) median nerve, (3) deep branch of the radial nerve (posterior interosseous nerve), (4) superficial branch of the radial nerve, (5) brachial artery, (6) biceps brachii muscle, (7) bicipital aponeurosis. Reproduced with permission from Danilo Jankovic

Ulnar Nerve

The ulnar nerve (UN) originates from the medial cord of the BP (C8–T1, occasionally C7) and can be easily identified medial to the brachial artery in the arm up to about the insertion of the coracobrachialis muscle, where it pierces the medial intermuscular septum to enter the posterior aspect of the arm, lying anterior to the medial head of triceps (Figs. 27.2 and 27.3). It then runs toward the ulnar tunnel bound by the medial epicondyle, the Osborne reticulum between the two heads of the flexor carpi ulnaris, the medial collateral ligament, and the olecranon. The nerve is easily palpated at this location. The UN winds around the medial epicondyle in the ulnar groove and enters the anterior compartment of the forearm between the humeral and the ulnar head of the flexor carpi ulnaris muscle on the medial side of the forearm, sandwiched between the FDS and FDP (Fig. 27.5).

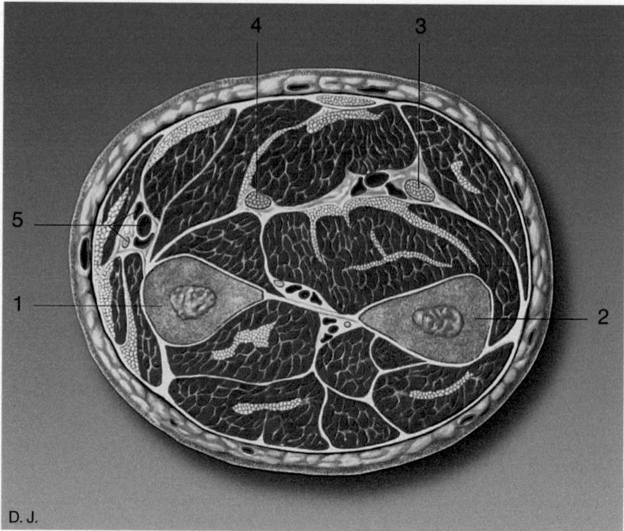

Fig. 27.5 Cross-section view at the mid-forearm (1). Radius, (2) ulna, (3) ulnar nerve, (4) median nerve, (5) radial artery, radial vein, and radial nerve. Reproduced with permission from Danilo Jankovic

In the medial distal third of the forearm, about three fingerbreadths proximal to the wrist, the UN divides into a dorsal branch (sensory to the dorsal surface of the hand and fingers), a small palmar cutaneous branch to the hypothenar eminence, and a mixed branch—the palmar branch. The latter runs superficially between the tendons of the flexor carpi ulnaris and FDS. In the distal forearm, the ulnar artery lies directly radially, alongside the nerve as it enters the hand superficial to the flexor retinaculum.

The UN contributes to the sensory and motor innervation of the forearm and hand. The motor innervation of the flexor carpi ulnaris and medial part of the FDP muscles branches from the ulnar nerve below the elbow crease. Sensory innervation is dependent on the terminal superficial nerve and palmar and dorsal cutaneous branches, which emerge at the mid forearm level. So, for both motor and sensory blockades, the nerve must be blocked proximal to the medial epicondyle. For sensory blockade only, it might be blocked at the forearm or wrist level.

Lateral Cutaneous Nerve of the Forearm

The lateral cutaneous nerve of the forearm (LCNF) is the terminal branch of the musculocutaneous nerve (C5–C7). At the lateral distal one-third aspect of the arm, the musculocutaneous nerve pierces the deep fascia to continue as the LCNF and is consistently in the fascia plane between the biceps brachii and BM. At the elbow level, it lies medial to the cephalic vein where it divides into anterior and posterior branches.

In order to block the sensory musculocutaneous contribution to the forearm, one must block the LCNF proximal to the elbow.

Technique

All nerves are very superficial and easily identified under ultrasound guidance. High-frequency (6–15 MHz) linear ultrasound probe and short-bevel insulated needles should be preferentially used. However, many practitioners use small-gauge long-bevel needles. Peripheral nerve stimulation (settings: 0.3–0.5 mA, 100 ms, 2 Hz) and pressure monitoring are optional. During injection, the practitioner should pay particular attention to the spread of the injectate in order to avoid intravascular injection (absence of spread) or intraneural injection (nerve expansion). The injectate is administered by three separate syringes of 5 mL with the selected local anesthetic solution.

The patient lies in the supine position. For the ulnar and median nerve blocks, the arm is supinated and abducted for elbow and wrist blocks. For the radial nerve block at the elbow, the arm can be flexed at the elbow with the hand over the abdomen, allowing a better technical performance. Alternatively, the radial nerve can be blocked with the arm supine when the target is just proximal to the elbow. Disinfection rules should be followed as for any regional anesthesia technique.

Elbow Block

Medial Nerve Block

The transducer is placed at the elbow crease over the medial epicondyle. In this position, the sonography will show a cross-section view of the brachial artery (using color Doppler). The MN is a hyperechoic oval-shape honeycomb structure, in close proximity of the brachial artery, normally on its medial side. A scan distal to the elbow crease shows the MN detaching from the artery and running deep to the humeral head of the pronator teres muscle and the FDS as it reaches the mid-forearm (Figs. 27.4 and 27.6).

Blocking the nerve distal to the elbow joint may miss the anterior interosseous nerve. The ultrasound probe is placed just proximal to the elbow. The needle is inserted in plane from medial to lateral (preferred direction to avoid the artery) or out of plane (Fig. 27.6). A total volume of 5 mL of local anesthetic is adequate.

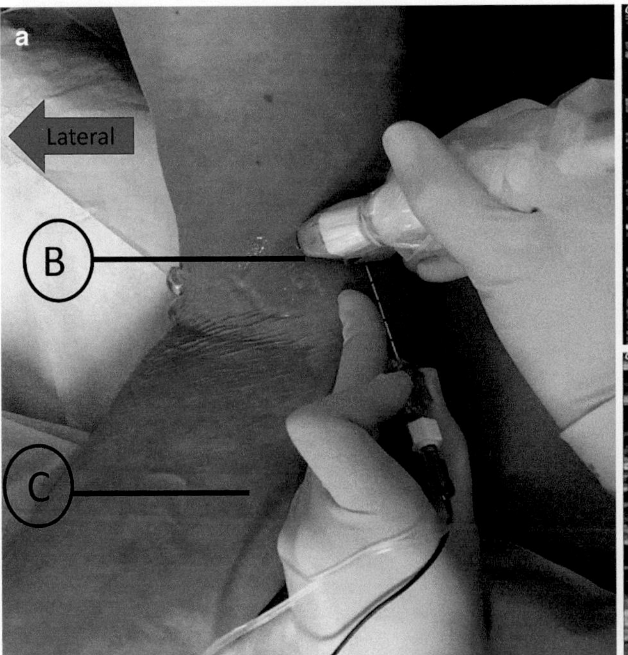

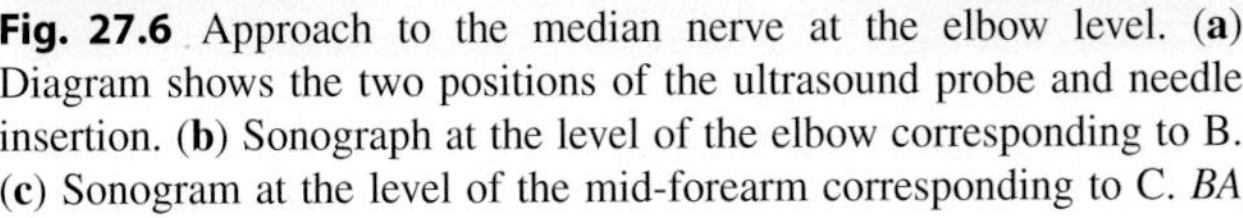

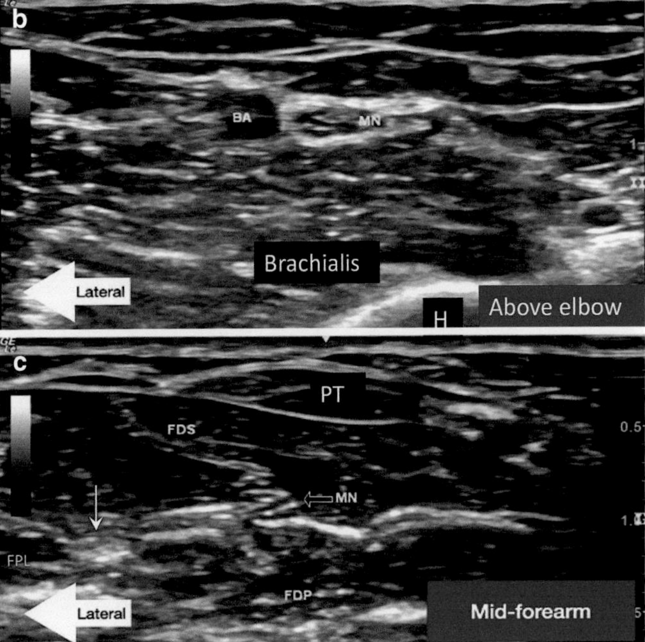

Fig. 27.6 Approach to the median nerve at the elbow level. (**a**) Diagram shows the two positions of the ultrasound probe and needle insertion. (**b**) Sonograph at the level of the elbow corresponding to B. (**c**) Sonogram at the level of the mid-forearm corresponding to C. *BA* brachial artery, *MN* median nerve, *H* humerus, *FDS* flexor digitorum superficialis, *FDP* flexor digitorum profundus, *FDP* flexor digitorum pollicis, *line arrow* anterior interosseous nerve. Reproduced with permission from Philip Peng Educational Series

Radial Nerve Block

The transducer is placed at the lateral aspect of the arm above the lateral epicondyle. The radial nerve courses between the BRM and BM. A needle is inserted in plane from medial to lateral direction (Fig. 27.7). If using the nerve stimulator, proximity to the nerve will cause extension of the wrist and fingers. After negative aspiration, 4–5 mL of local anesthetic is injected.

Ulnar Nerve Block

The UN is very superficial on the medial aspect of the arm, especially above the elbow crease. With the arm with external rotation, a transducer is placed proximal to the medial epicondyle, and the needle can be in plane or out of plane (Fig. 27.8). The nerve stimulator will cause flexion and external rotation of the wrist and fifth finger. Avoid injecting the local anesthetic at the ulnar groove, where the nerve is more vulnerable to injury.

Alternatively, the UN can be blocked distal to the elbow. Using the same arm position, the transducer is placed over the anteromedial aspect of the forearm, and the ulnar artery is identified lateral to the UN. Once identified, the probe is moved proximally to search for the location where the artery is further away from the nerve and where the UN is found lateral to the flexor carpi ulnaris between the FDS and FDP (Fig. 27.9). The needle can be inserted in plane or out of plane. Up to 5 mL of local anesthetic should be enough.

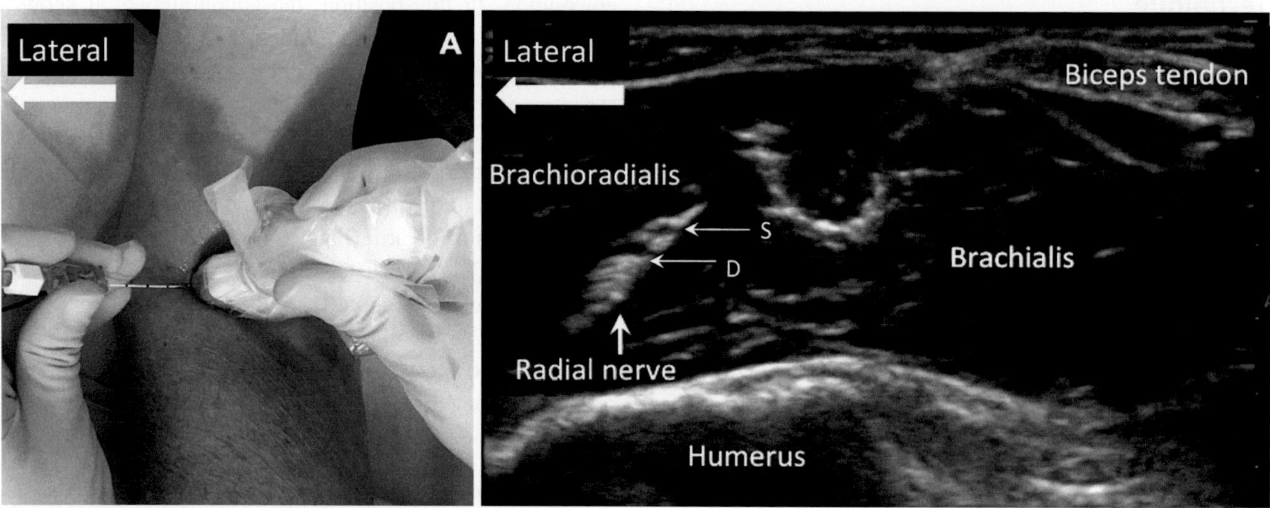

Fig. 27.7 Approach to the radial nerve at the elbow level. Left panel: the position of the probe and needle insertion. Right panel: Sonogram showing the superficial (S) and deep (D) branches of the radial nerve. Reproduced with permission from Philip Peng Educational Series

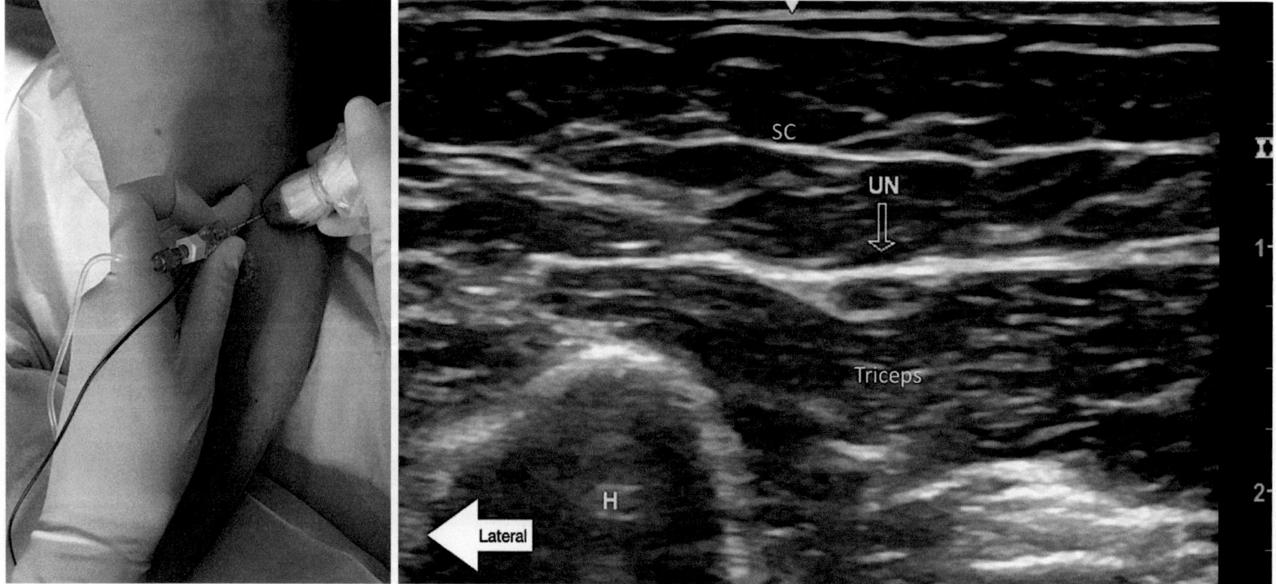

Fig. 27.8 Approach to the ulnar nerve at the elbow. Left panel: the position of the probe and needle insertion. Right panel: sonogram of the ulna nerve at the same level. *UN* ulnar nerve, *H* humerus, *SC* subcutaneous tissue. Reproduced with permission from Philip Peng Educational Series

Lateral Cutaneous Nerve of the Forearm

The transducer is placed at the lower third at the lateral aspect of the arm. The fascial plane between the brachialis and biceps brachii muscles is carefully defined as the nerve is within this plane. The small size, anisotropy of the nerve, and compartment where it is located can make it difficult to identify (Fig. 27.10). A total volume of 3 mL of local anesthetic is appropriate.

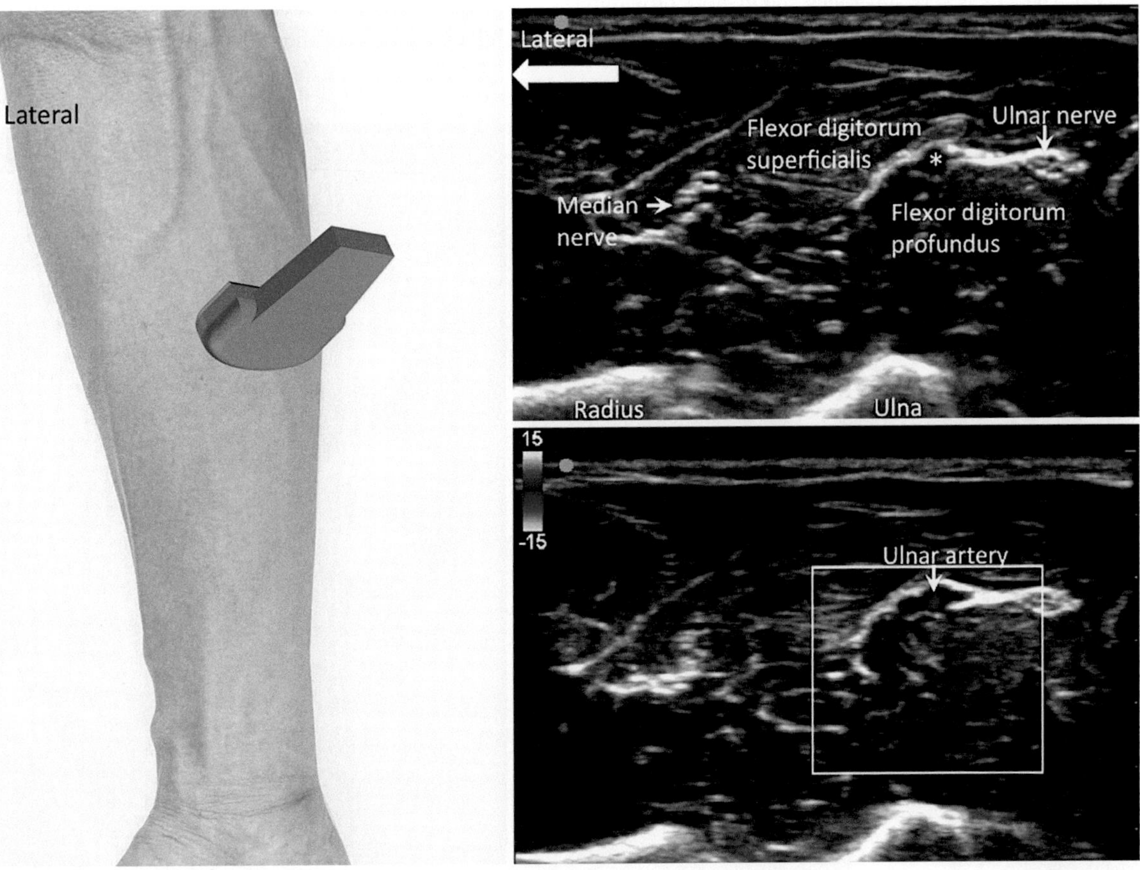

Fig. 27.9 Approach to the ulnar nerve distal to the elbow. Left panel: the position of the probe. Right panel: sonogram of the ulna nerve at the same level (upper) and the Doppler scan (lower). * ulnar artery. Reproduced with permission from Philip Peng Educational Series

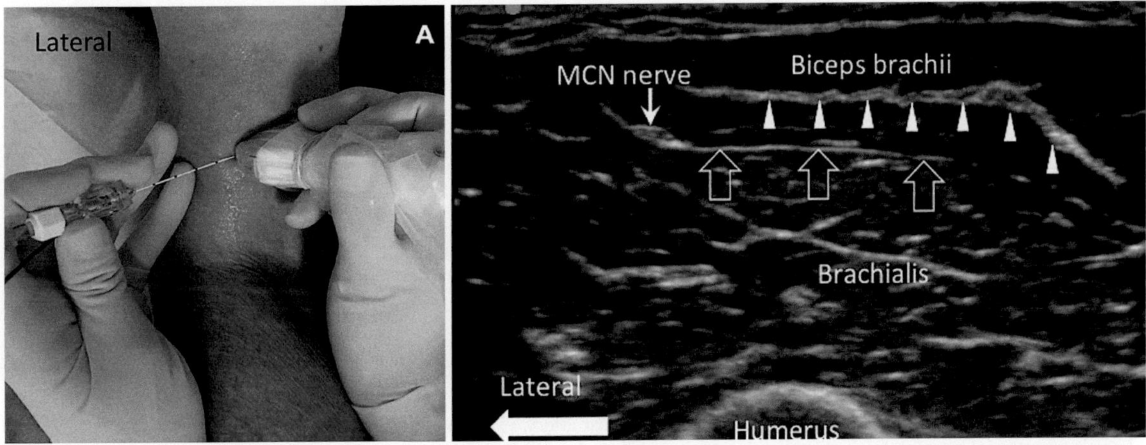

Fig. 27.10 Approach to the lateral cutaneous nerve of the forearm (LCNF) at the elbow level. Left panel: the position of the probe and needle insertion. Right panel: sonogram showing the lateral cutaneous branch of forearm (MCN). Bold arrows, fascial plane between brachialis and biceps brachii; arrowheads, tendon of biceps brachii. Reproduced with permission from Philip Peng Educational Series

Blocks at the Wrist

Median Nerve

The transducer is placed over the palmar crease which is just proximal to the flexor retinaculum of the carpal tunnel (Fig. 27.11a). The MN is very superficial and in close proximity of the FDS, FDP, and flexor pollicis longus (FPL) tendons. At this location, it is easy to confuse the MN with those tendons. Several methods have been described to help identify the MN correctly:

1. Sliding the probe proximally until the tendons disappear (become muscles) and only the nerve remains.
2. Flex the thumb to help identify the FPL. The MN is always on the 2 o'clock position of the left hand and 10 o'clock position of the right hand.

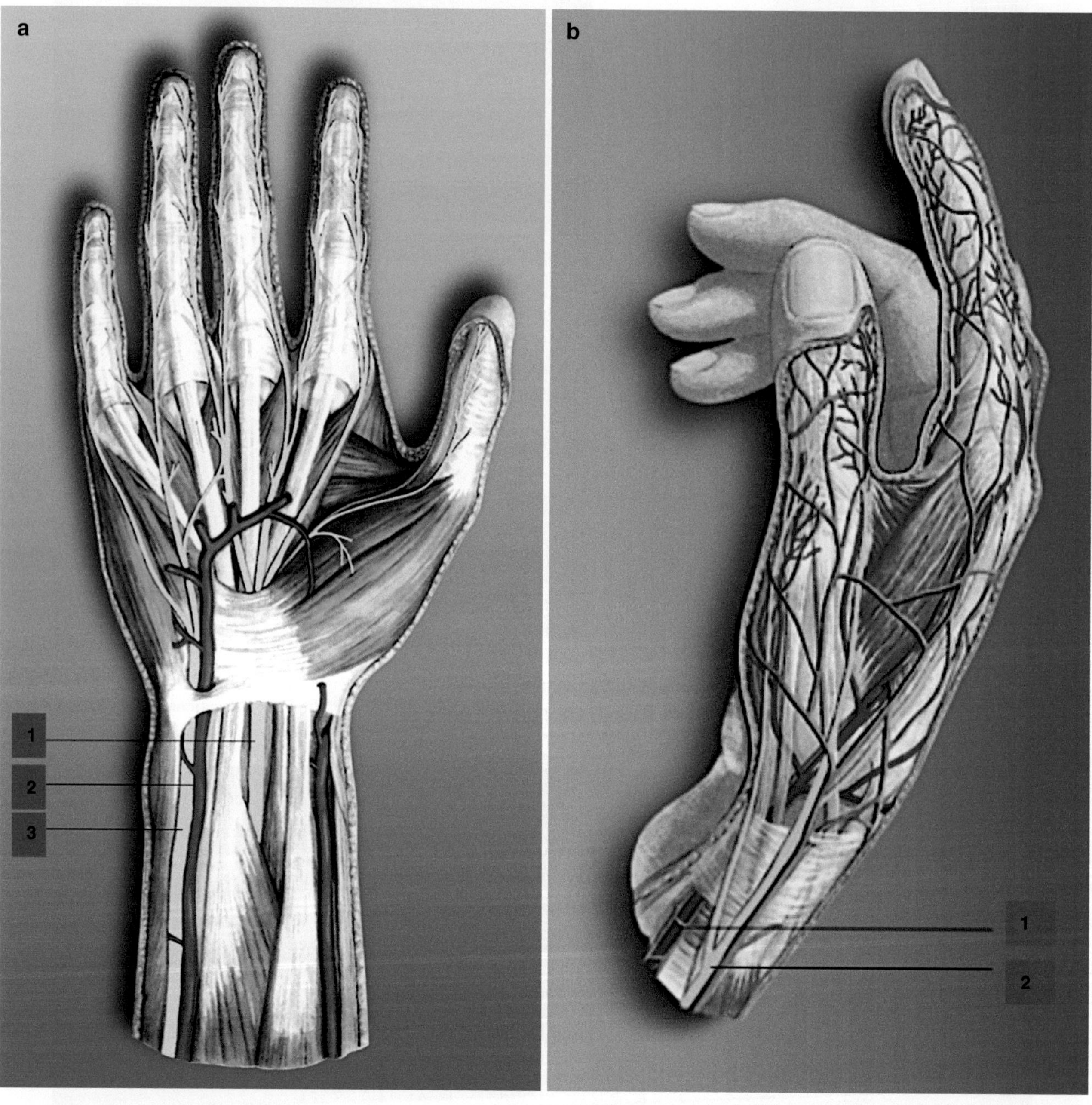

Fig. 27.11 (**a**) Anatomy of hand volar side. (1) Median nerve, (2) ulnar artery, (3) ulnar nerve. (**b**) Anatomy of hand-radial side (1) Radial artery, (2) radial nerve (superficial branch). Reproduced with permission from Danilo Jankovic

3. Tilting the ultrasound probe, the MN will stand out as the tendon is more anisotropic than nerve (Fig. 27.12).

It's easier to use an out-of-plane approach (Fig. 27.13). Three to 5 mL of local anesthetic is enough.

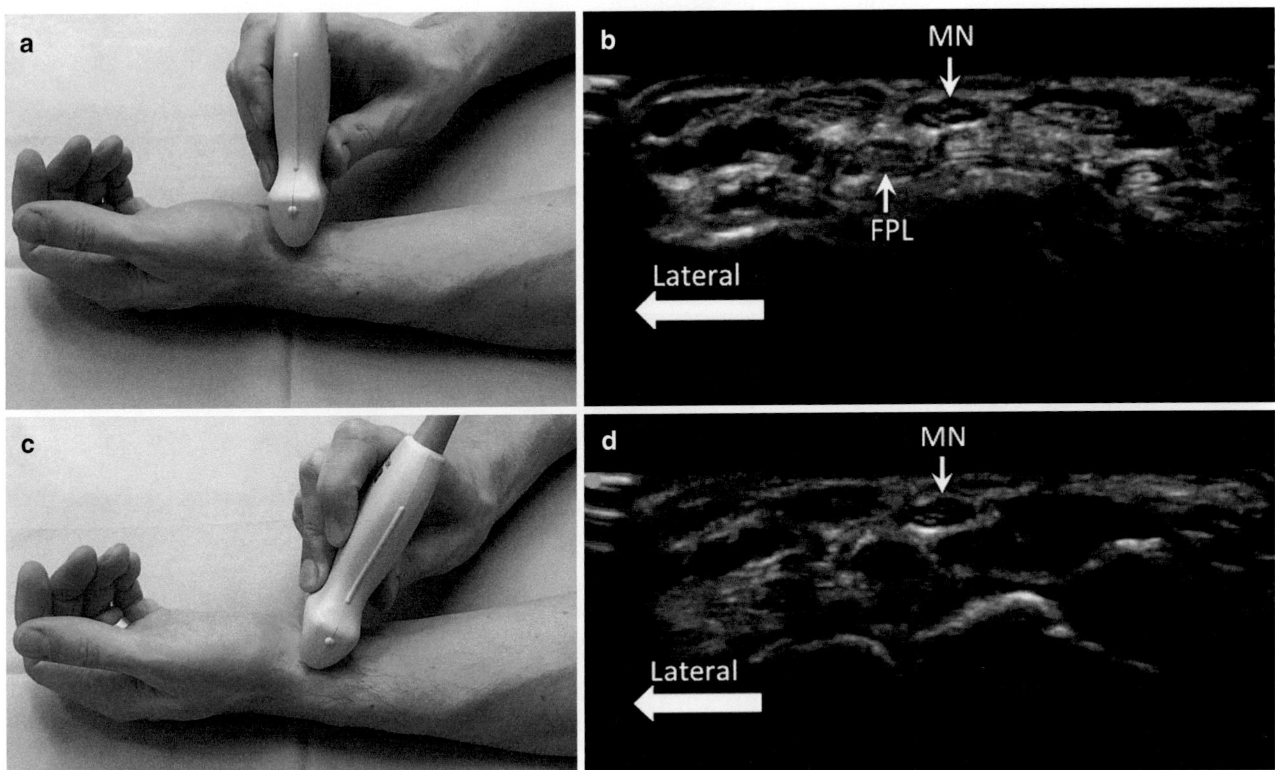

Fig. 27.12 Comparing anisotropy between tendons and median nerve (MN). (**a**, **b**) The tendons and MN look the same at the wrist level. (**c**, **d**) However, on tilting the ultrasound probe, the tendons look hypoechoic, but the echogenicity of MN still remains. *FPL* flexor pollicis longus. Reproduced with permission from Philip Peng Educational Series

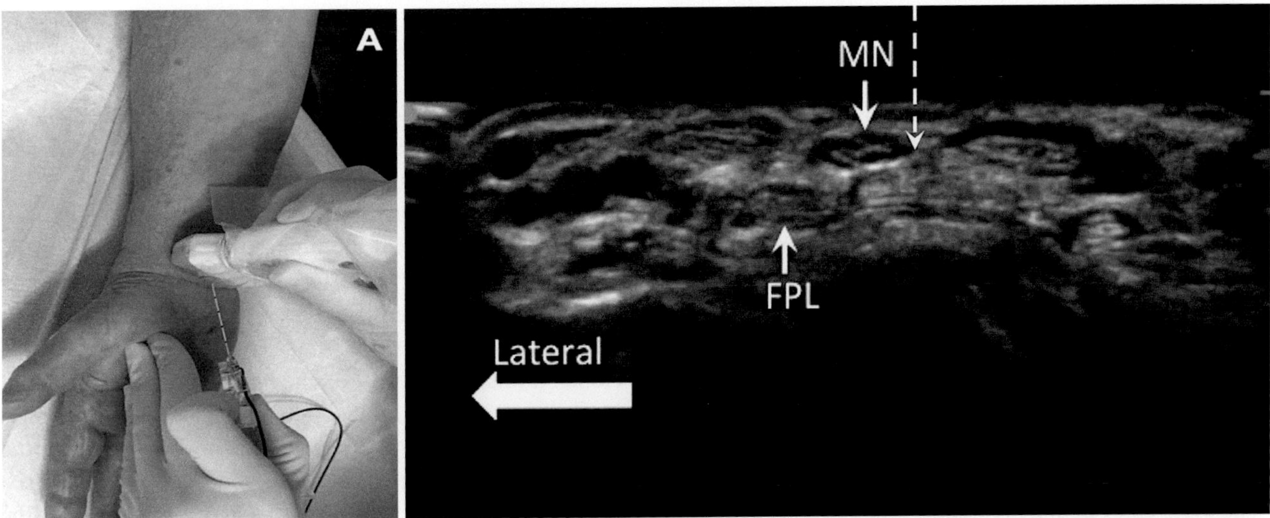

Fig. 27.13 Approach to the median nerve at the wrist level. *MN* median nerve, *FPL* flexor pollicis longus muscle. Dotted arrow, insertion point of the needle. Reproduced with permission from Philip Peng Educational Series

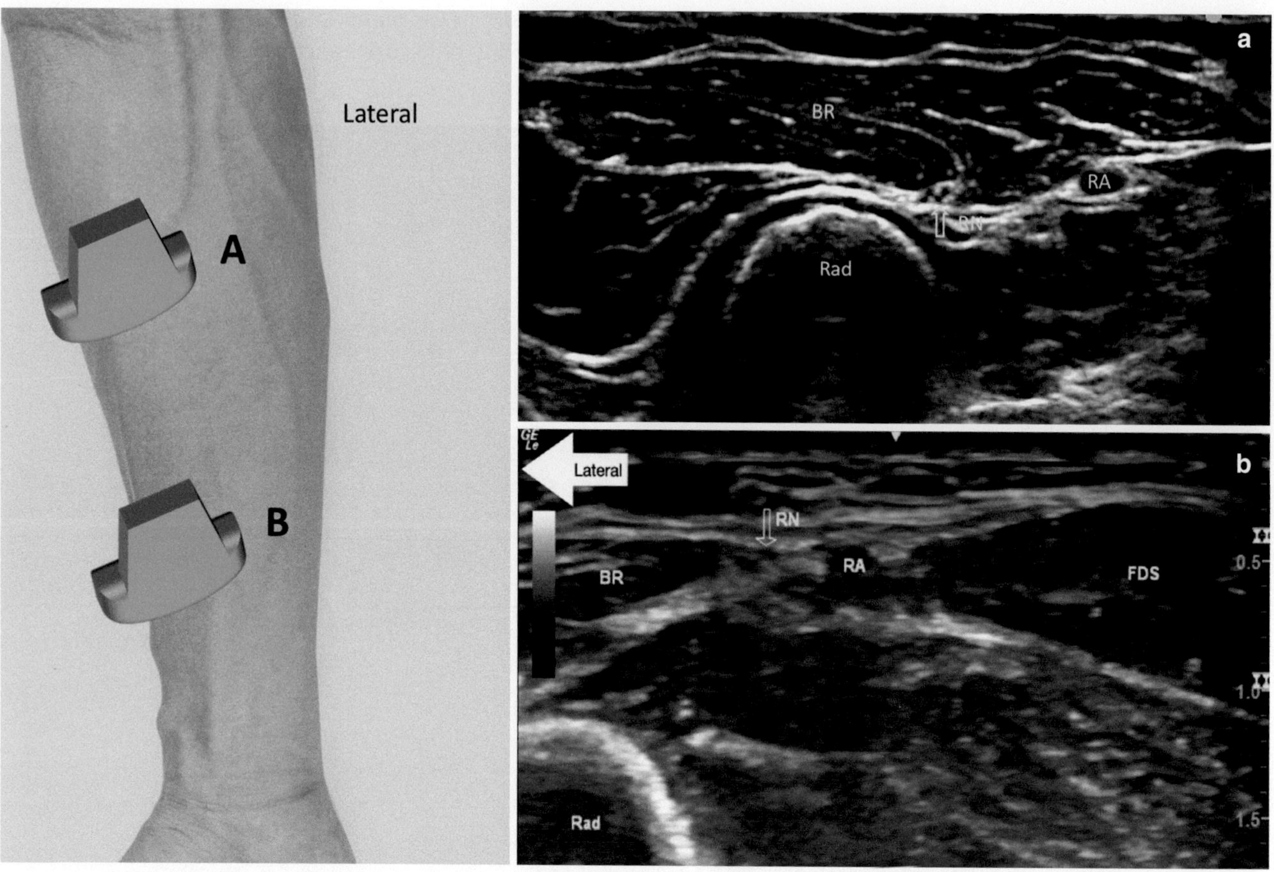

Fig. 27.14 Approach to the superficial radial nerve at the wrist level. Left panel: position of the ultrasound probe at the mid-forearm (A) and distal forearm (B). Right panel: sonogram corresponding to probe position A (upper figure) and position B (lower figure). *RN* superficial branch of radial nerve, *FDS* flexor digitorum superficialis muscle, *RA* radial artery, *BR* brachioradialis muscle, *Rad* radius. Reproduced with permission from Philip Peng Educational Series

Radial Nerve

At this level, the superficial branch of RN is superficial and lateral to the radial artery. If you scan at this distal level at the wrist, it might be very difficult to identify it, because it divides in very thin and superficial terminal branches. A skin wheal of local anesthetic around the styloid process of the radius bone might be sufficient.

If ultrasound is used, superficial branch of RN can be identified at two sites: one at approximately four finger-breadth proximal to the wrist crease and another at the mid-forearm (Fig. 27.14). In mid-pronation, the transducer is placed at the lateral aspect of the wrist. The RN is in close proximity of the radial artery deep to the brachioradialis (Fig. 27.14a). Scanning proximally might help to identify the RN as it can be readily seen deep to the brachioradialis (Fig. 27.14b). A volume of 3 mL is sufficient.

Ulnar Nerve

The upper limb is in supination and the transducer placed over the ventromedial aspect of the wrist at the proximal palmar crease. The UN is medial to the ulnar artery. The needle is carefully inserted using an out-of-plane approach to the medial aspect of the ulnar artery (Fig. 27.15). One should be aware that this artery is usually accompanied by two veins (easily seen if the pressure of the transducer is released). Injection of 3 mL of local anesthetic is sufficient. At this distal location, the palmar and dorsal cutaneous branches are not included in the block. These branches can be blocked with a subcutaneous infiltration along the ulnar aspect on both sides (volar and dorsal) of the wrist with 5 mL of local anesthetic. To avoid this mishap, the ulnar block can be performed at the elbow level (see above).

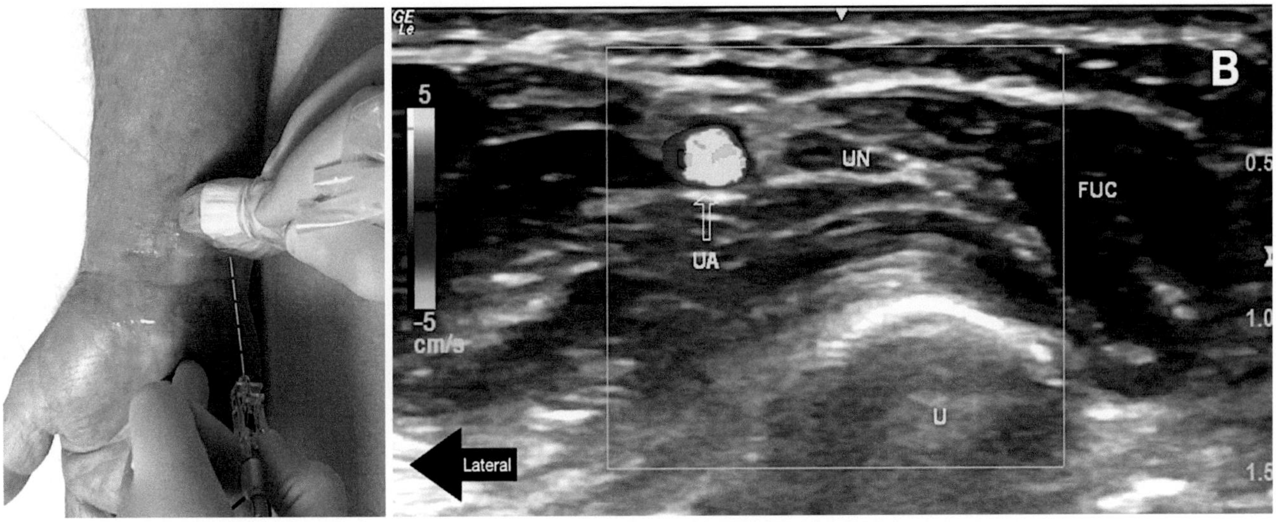

Fig. 27.15 Approach to the ulnar nerve at the wrist level. Left panel: diagram showing the position of the probe and needle insertion. Right panel: corresponding sonogram. *UN* ulnar nerve, *UA* ulnar artery, *U* ulna, *FUC* flexor carpi ulnaris muscle. Reproduced with permission from Philip Peng Educational Series

Complications

There are no major complications associated with these techniques. Intraneural injection can happen with the use of sharp needles, and the risk of intravascular injection can also occur as the nerves are usually close to arteries and veins.

Practical Tips

These are very superficial nerves and exhibit pronounced anisotropy, namely, the median nerve. Tilting will "light up" the nerve.

At the wrist level, the nerves might be identified as tendons and vice versa. In order to identify correctly, trace proximally. If it disappears into the muscle, it is a tendon. If the structure maintains, it is a nerve.

Subcutaneous injections can be painful.

Suggested Reading

Jankovic D, Peng P. Peripheral nerve blocks in the elbow region. In: Regional nerve blocks in anesthesia and pain therapy; 2015a. p. 423–30. https://doi.org/10.1007/978-3-319-05131-4.

Jankovic D, Peng P. Peripheral nerve blocks in the wrist region. In: Regional nerve blocks in anesthesia and pain therapy; 2015b. p. 431–6. https://doi.org/10.1007/978-3-319-05131-4.

Lin J-A, Bendtsen TF, Lopez AM, Jalil H. Ultrasound-guided blocks at the elbow. In: Hadzic A, editor. Hadzic's textbook of regional anesthesia and acute pain management. 2nd ed. New York: McGraw-Hill Education; 2017. p. 586–90.

Zhu W, Zhou R, Chen L, et al. The ultrasound-guided selective nerve block in the upper arm: an approach of retaining the motor function in elbow. BMC Anesthesiol. 2018;18(1):143. https://doi.org/10.1186/s12871-018-0584-7.

Pain Procedures Around the Elbow

28

Wesley Miller, Kyle Stoffers, and Marko Bodor

Contents

General Consideration

Chronic elbow pain may be secondary to overuse, a history of trauma, or osteoarthritis. The superficial anatomy of the elbow makes it amenable to diagnosing and treating problems using high-frequency ultrasonography. This chapter will serve to discuss some of the most common painful conditions and their treatments around the elbow.

W. Miller
Bodor Clinic, Napa, CA, USA

K. Stoffers
Department of Physical Medicine and Rehabilitation, University of California Davis, Davis, CA, USA

M. Bodor (✉)
Department of Neurological Surgery, University of California San Francisco, San Francisco, CA, USA

Indication/Patient Selection

Lateral epicondylosis or common extensor tendinosis, also known as "tennis elbow," is one of the most common causes of chronic elbow pain. Risk factors include frequent and forceful gripping activities. Ultrasonography may reveal a loss of the normal echotexture indicating degenerative tendinopathy or a tear. Other causes of chronic lateral elbow pain include radio-capitellar joint arthritis, rupture of the radial collateral ligament, and radial tunnel syndrome, involving compression of the radial nerve between the two heads of the supinator muscle.

Medial epicondylosis or common flexor tendinosis, also known as "golfer's elbow," is one of the most common causes of chronic medial elbow pain. Other causes include humero-ulnar joint arthritis, ulnar collateral ligament disruption, ulnar neuropathy at the elbow including symptomatic ulnar nerve subluxation over the medial epicondyle. Olecranon bursitis, triceps tendinosis, and humero-ulnar joint arthritis can cause posterior elbow pain, while distal biceps tendinosis may cause anterior elbow pain. Pain with joint swelling can occur secondary to osteoarthritis, rheumatoid arthritis, hemarthrosis, gout, and infection.

D. Jankovic, P. Peng (eds.), *Regional Nerve Blocks in Anesthesia and Pain Therapy*,
https://doi.org/10.1007/978-3-030-88727-8_28

Interventional treatment is indicated when a trial of ergonomic modifications and physiotherapy has not been successful at resolving chronic pain. The exception to this is acute effusions or hemarthroses which often benefit from early aspiration and injection. Pain with resisted wrist extension and flexion and tenderness to sonopalpation (palpation under live ultrasonography) can be used to diagnose lateral and medial epicondylosis, whereas anterior elbow pain with resisted supination indicates possible distal biceps tendinopathy and posterior pain with resisted elbow extension indicates possible triceps tendinopathy.

Anatomy

The elbow consists of the humeral trochlea and ulnar coronoid process (hinge joint) and the humeral capitellum and radial head (ball and socket joint). The elbow joint is stabilized laterally by the radial collateral and annular ligaments and medially by the ulnar collateral ligaments (Fig. 28.1). The lateral epicondyle is the origin of the common extensor tendon (CET) of the extensors carpi radialis brevis, digitorum communis, and carpi ulnaris muscles (Fig. 28.2), while the medial epicondyle serves as the origin of the common

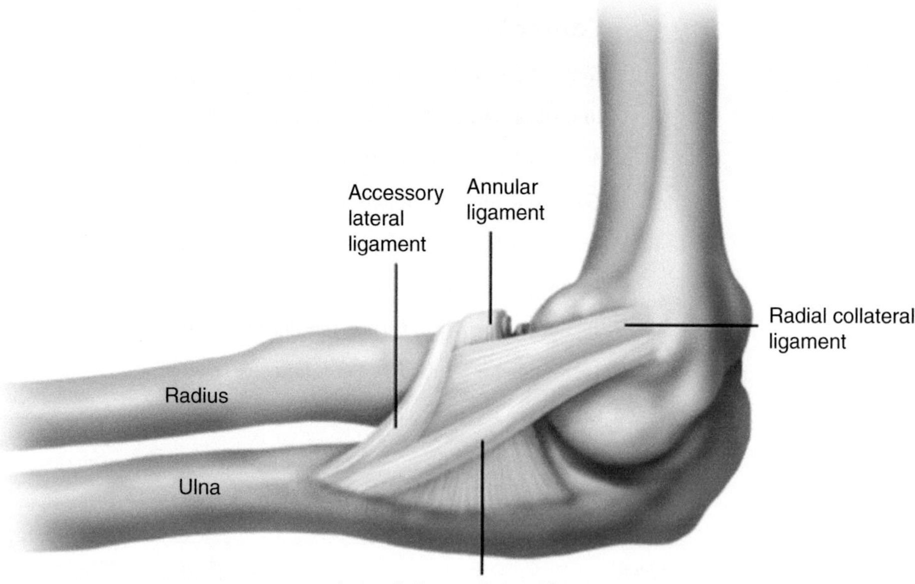

Fig. 28.1 The ligaments of the lateral elbow. Reprinted with permission from Philip Peng Educational Series

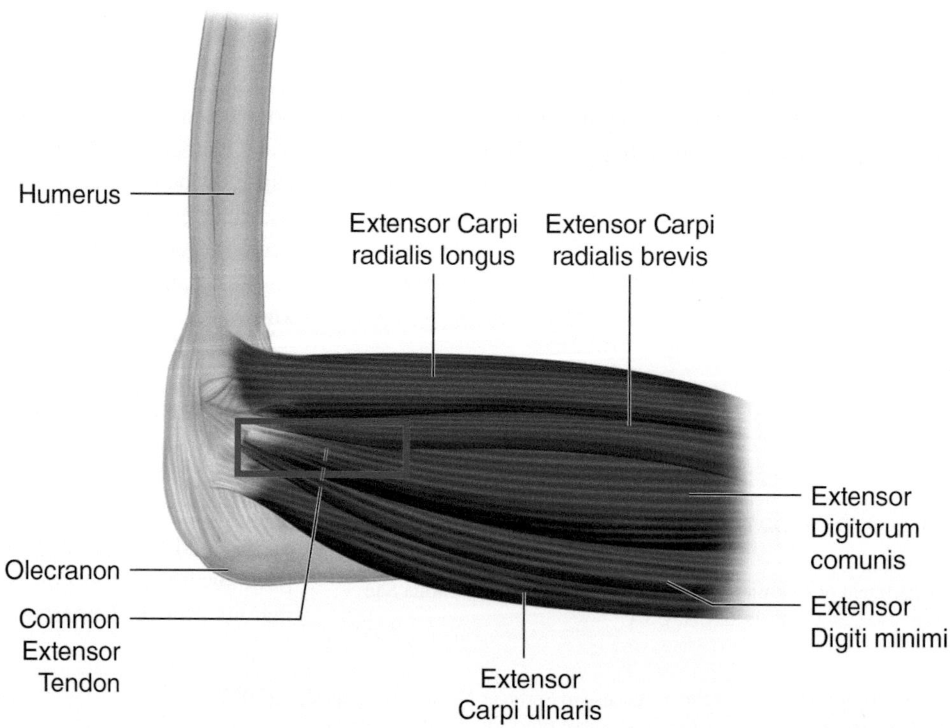

Fig. 28.2 Anatomy of the lateral elbow. The blue box is the region of the common extensor tendon and area of interest for ultrasound scanning

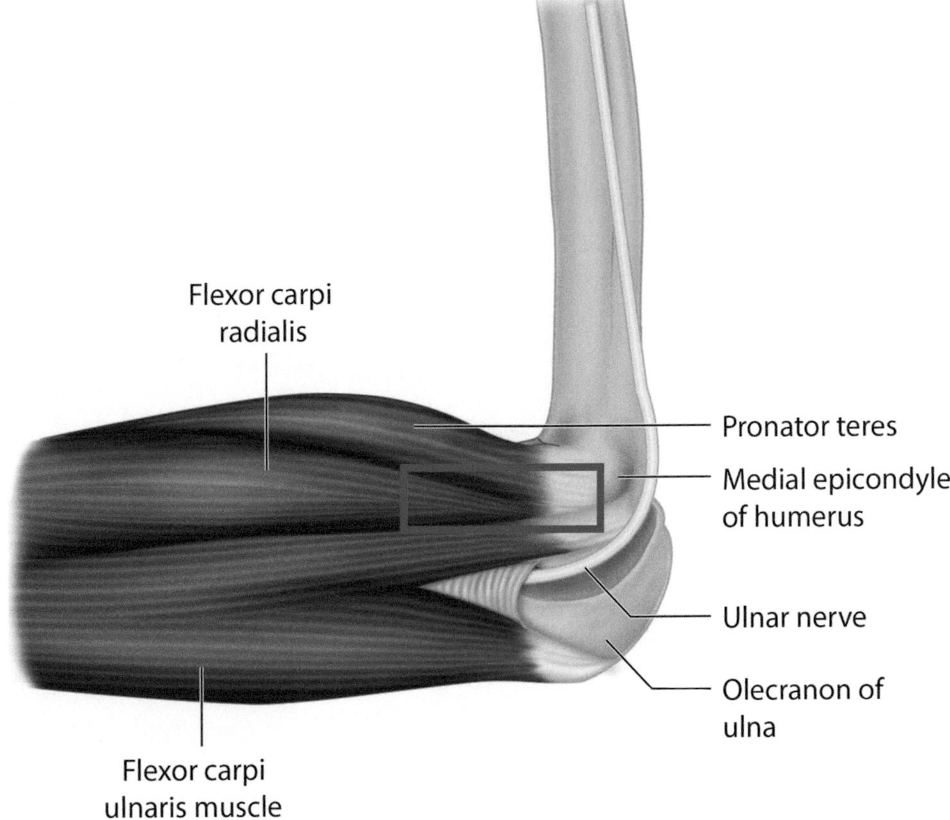

Fig. 28.3 Anatomy of the medial elbow. The blue box is the region of the common flexor tendon and area of interest for ultrasound scanning

flexor tendon (CFT) of the flexors carpi radialis, ulnaris, digitorum superficialis, palmaris longus, and pronator teres muscles (Fig. 28.3). The olecranon bursa lies superficial to the triceps tendon, which attaches to the olecranon process of the ulna. The distal biceps tendon inserts onto the radius, while the brachialis muscle inserts onto the ulna. The radial nerve courses through the radial tunnel, between the superficial and deep heads of the supinator muscle. The ulnar nerve passes behind the medial epicondyle, where it is vulnerable to stretch and external compression when leaning on the elbow, and then passes distally and enters the cubital tunnel under the aponeurosis of the two heads of the flexor carpi ulnaris muscle (ligament of Osborne), which can become thickened and compress the nerve internally. The median nerve is located at the anterior and medial elbow between the brachial artery and biceps tendon, from where it descends into the forearm between the superficial and deep heads of the pronator teres.

Technique for Lateral and Medial Epicondylosis/Tendinosis

For a lateral epicondyle/common extensor tendon procedure, the patient is seated with the elbow flexed and propped on a pillow (Fig. 28.4). For a medial epicondyle/common flexor tendon procedure, the patient is supine with the elbow flexed and supported, and it is imperative that the position of the ulnar nerve be checked to ensure that it is not subluxed over the medial epicondyle (Fig. 28.5). The ultrasound transducer is positioned along the long axis of the tendon with one end over the epicondyle. An in-plane distal to proximal approach is taken using a 25-G or 27-G needle targeting the tendon about 1 cm distal to the epicondyle. When doing regenerative procedures such as needle tenotomy (multiple passes of a needle through a tendon), lidocaine/dextrose or platelet-rich plasma (PRP) injections, the tendon attachment to the epicondyle is also targeted. Whenever injecting a tendon, the flow of injectate should be visualized in two planes by rotating the transducer 90 degrees. Injectate volume ranges from 0.25 to 0.5 ml to maximize specificity of diagnostic injections and 1.0–3.0 ml for therapeutic injections.

Technique for Radio-Capitellar Joint Injection

The patient is seated with the elbow flexed and propped up on a pillow (Fig. 28.6). One end of the transducer is positioned on the lateral epicondyle in line with the common extensor tendon. The radio-capitellar joint is visualized

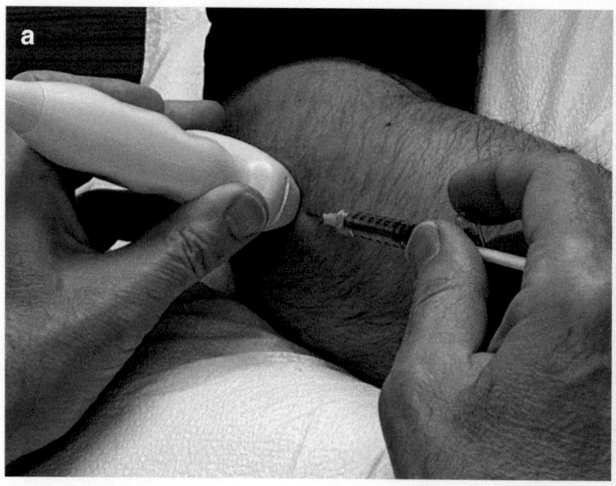

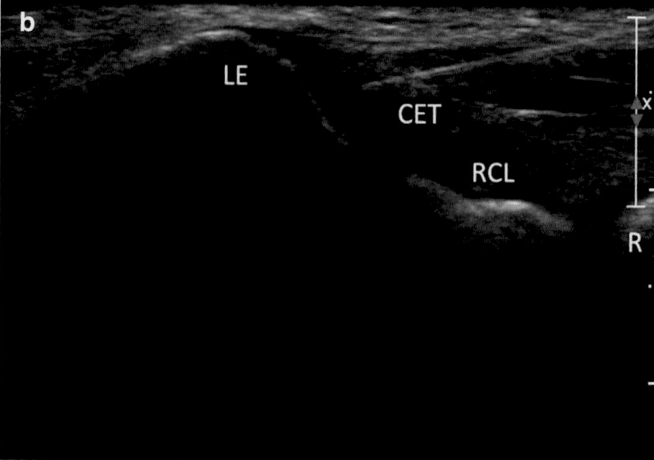

Fig. 28.4 Lateral epicondyle/common extensor tendon (CET) injection: (**a**) photo of patient, transducer and needle being inserted; the location of the transducer is the same indicated by the blue box in Fig. 28.2. (**b**) 17–5 MHz ultrasound image of the needle entering the tendon (CET) next to the lateral epicondyle (LE), radial collateral ligament (RCL), radius (R)

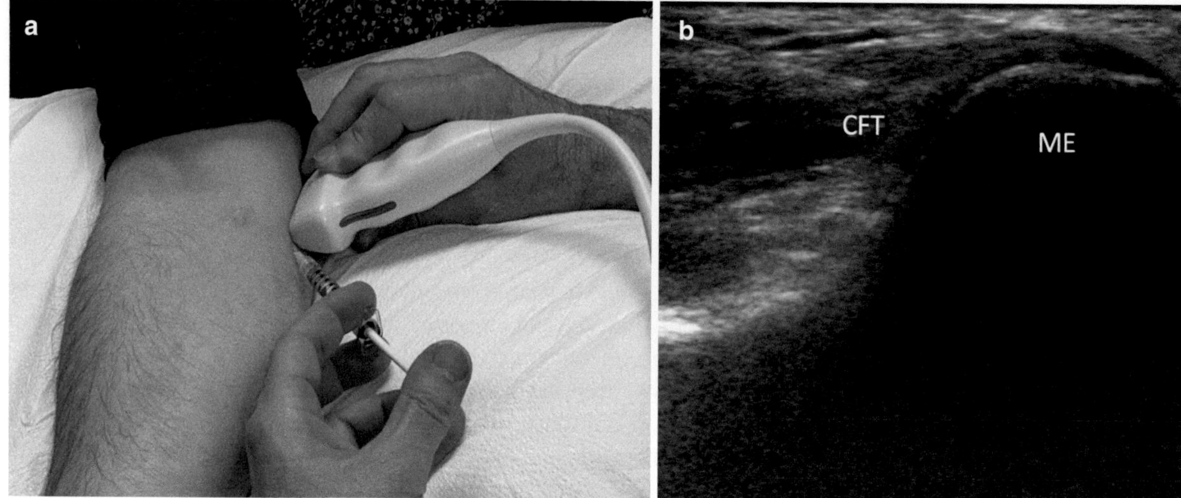

Fig. 28.5 Medial epicondyle/common flexor tendon (CFT) injection: (**a**) photo of patient, transducer and needle being inserted; the location of the transducer is indicated in Fig. 28.3, (**b**) 17–5 MHz ultrasound image of the needle entering CFT next to the medial epicondyle (ME)

below. A short-axis out-of-plane approach is used to pass the needle into the joint.

Technique for Humero-Ulnar Joint Injection/ Aspiration

The patient is seated or side-lying with the elbow completely flexed and the forearm propped up on a pillow (Figs. 28.7 and 28.8). One end of the transducer is positioned on the olecranon in line with the triceps tendon, and then the proximal end is rotated laterally until the humero-ulnar joint is seen. While keeping the joint in view, the transducer is translated distally to bring the joint closer to the proximal end of the transducer, reducing the distance the needle needs to be advanced to reach the joint.

Technique for Distal Biceps Tendon Injection

The patient is seated with the elbow flexed, elevated on a pillow, and maximally pronated (Fig. 28.9). The transducer is placed perpendicular to the long axis of the forearm over the proximal forearm, identifying the radius and ulna and the curved and tapered appearance of the distal biceps tendon insertion. Gentle pronation and supination can help to

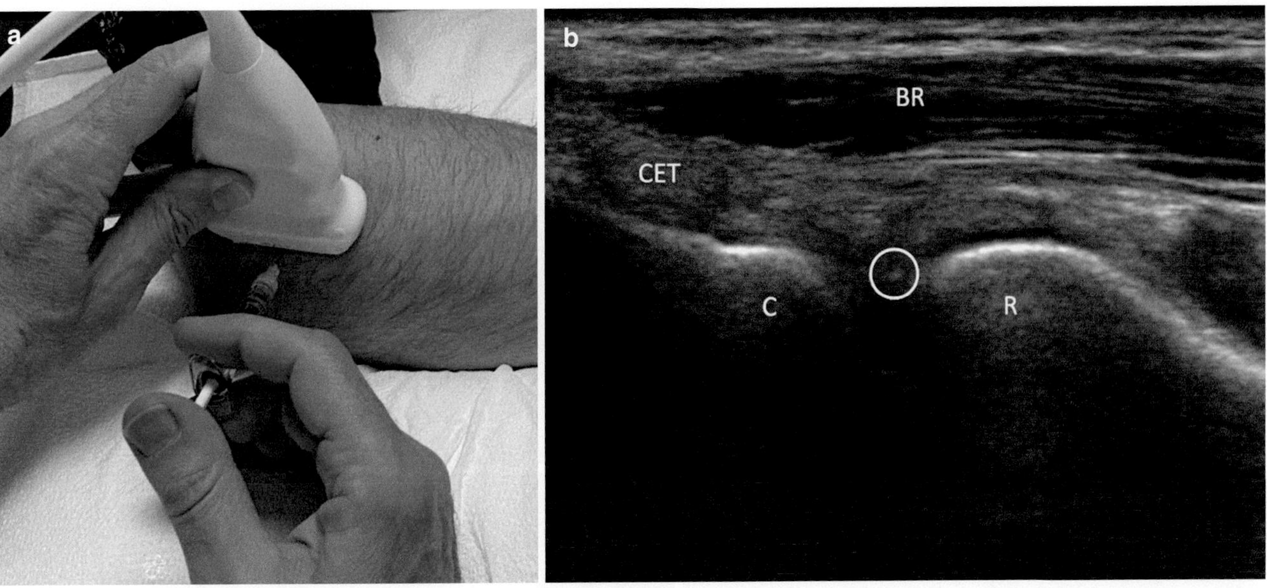

Fig. 28.6 (**a**) Radio-capitellar joint injection, and (**b**) 17–5 MHz ultrasound image of the needle tip (circle) within the joint; common extensor tendon (CET), capitellum (**c**), brachioradialis muscle (BR), radial head (R)

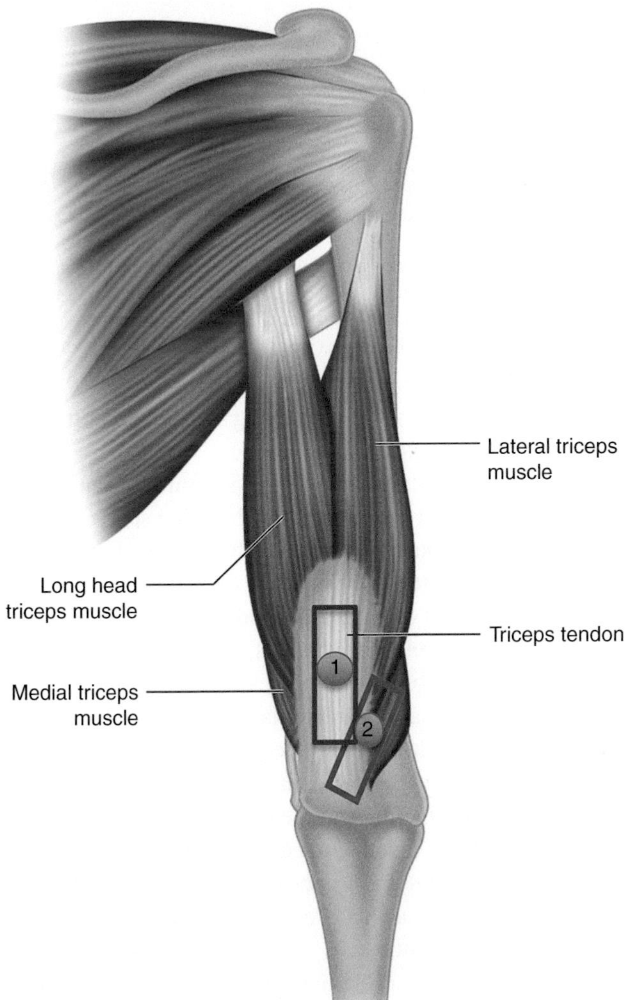

Fig. 28.7 Anatomy of the posterior elbow. The blue boxes are the areas of interest for ultrasound scanning

identify the tendon insertion. The radial nerve, coursing between the two heads of the supinator, should be avoided. The needle is advanced in plane to just outside the tendon for a peri-tendinous injection or into the tendon for an intra-tendon injection.

Technique for Ultrasonic Percutaneous Tenotomy

For chronic tendon pain and tendinopathy refractory to previous treatments for which surgery to remove pathologic tissue and stimulate healing would traditionally be the next step, ultrasound-guided percutaneous tenotomy can be performed. This procedure can be done using a device that oscillates and emulsifies (TX1, Tenex Health) or uses a high-pressure jet of water (TenJet, Hydrocision Inc.) to remove degenerated tissue. For lateral epicondylosis/common extensor tendinopathy, an in-plane approach is used. A stab incision is made through the skin and subcutaneous fascia to enable placement of the device (Fig. 28.10). Degenerated parts of the tendon, typically less echogenic and exhibiting loss of the normal tendon fibrillar pattern, are targeted. The vibrating tip of the device is advanced and retracted methodically in order to ensure that a single pass goes through all of the degenerated tissue or until microbubble artifact, a by-product of the procedure, is present throughout the targeted area. It is imperative that the treatment be limited to tendon and not go too deep and involve the underlying radial or ulnar collateral ligaments.

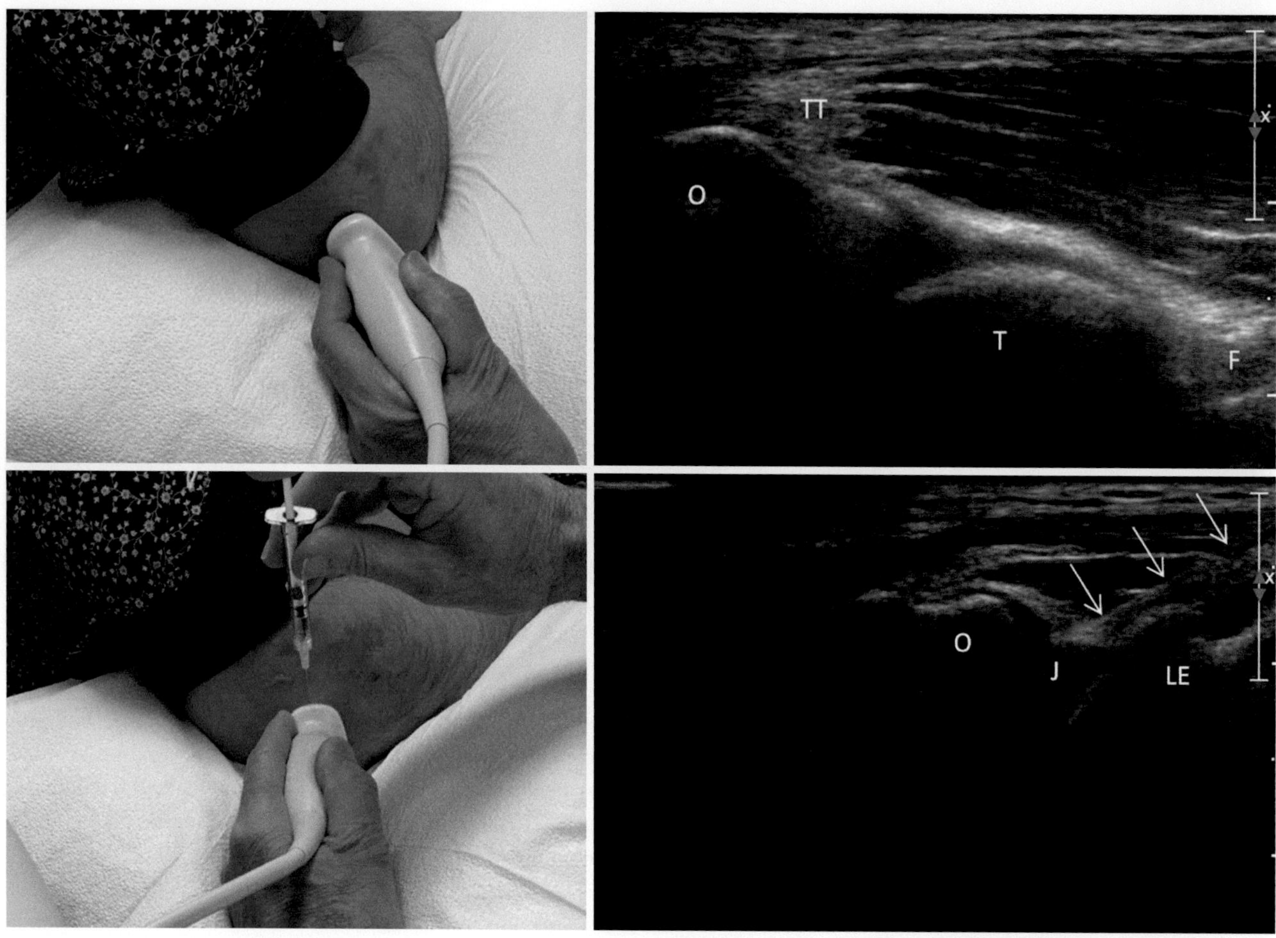

Fig. 28.8 Humero-ulnar joint injection: upper left panel, initial transducer position (box 1 in Fig. 28.7) over the olecranon of the ulna (O) and triceps tendon (TT); upper right panel, corresponding 17–5 MHz ultrasound image; lower left panel, transducer position after lateral rotation of its proximal end (box 2 in Fig. 28.7); and lower right panel, 17–5 MHz ultrasound image of the needle (arrows) advancing toward the joint space (J), trochlea (T), posterior fat pad (F), posterior aspect of lateral epicondyle of the humerus (LE)

Literature Review

For the initial treatment of lateral epicondylalgia, physiotherapy provides better long-term outcomes than corticosteroid injections. Corticosteroid injections typically provide relief up to 3 months, but patients receiving local anesthetic injections without corticosteroid are much more likely to have complete relief of symptoms at 1 year. When using corticosteroids, the lowest possible dose should be used (e.g., 5–10 mg triamcinolone acetonide or 1–2 mg dexamethasone). As an alternative to corticosteroids, dextrose 10% injections have been shown to have excellent long-term outcomes compared to normal saline in a Level I study with 24 patients whose symptoms ranged from 6 months to 10 years. Among 230 patients unresponsive to physical therapy, corticosteroid injections or NSAIDs for chronic lateral epicondylalgia, a Level I study showed that needle tenotomy plus leukocyte-rich platelet-rich plasma (PRP) injections resulted in >50% improvement in pain at 6 months in 82% of patients receiving PRP versus 60% receiving needle tenotomy and local anesthetic injection alone.

Medial epicondylalgia is much less common than lateral. Risk factors include participation in throwing sports and laxity of the ulnar collateral ligament. The treatment protocol is in general similar to that for lateral epicondylalgia, as it is also for triceps and distal biceps tendinopathy, consisting of physiotherapy, injection treatments, and surgery. However, the treatment outcomes are not expected to be the same because each one has different anatomical and biomechanical features. The outcomes of injection treatments for elbow joint arthritis are unknown at this time but, on the basis of studies on other joints such as the knee, might be expected to provide short-term benefit from corticosteroid and long term from dextrose or leukocyte-poor PRP injections. For chronic lateral epicondylalgia that would otherwise have required open surgery, percutaneous ultrasonic ultrasound-guided tenotomy in a series of 19 patients resulted in an average improvement of VAS scores from 6.4 to 0.7 at 1 year. This technique has also been used successfully for medial

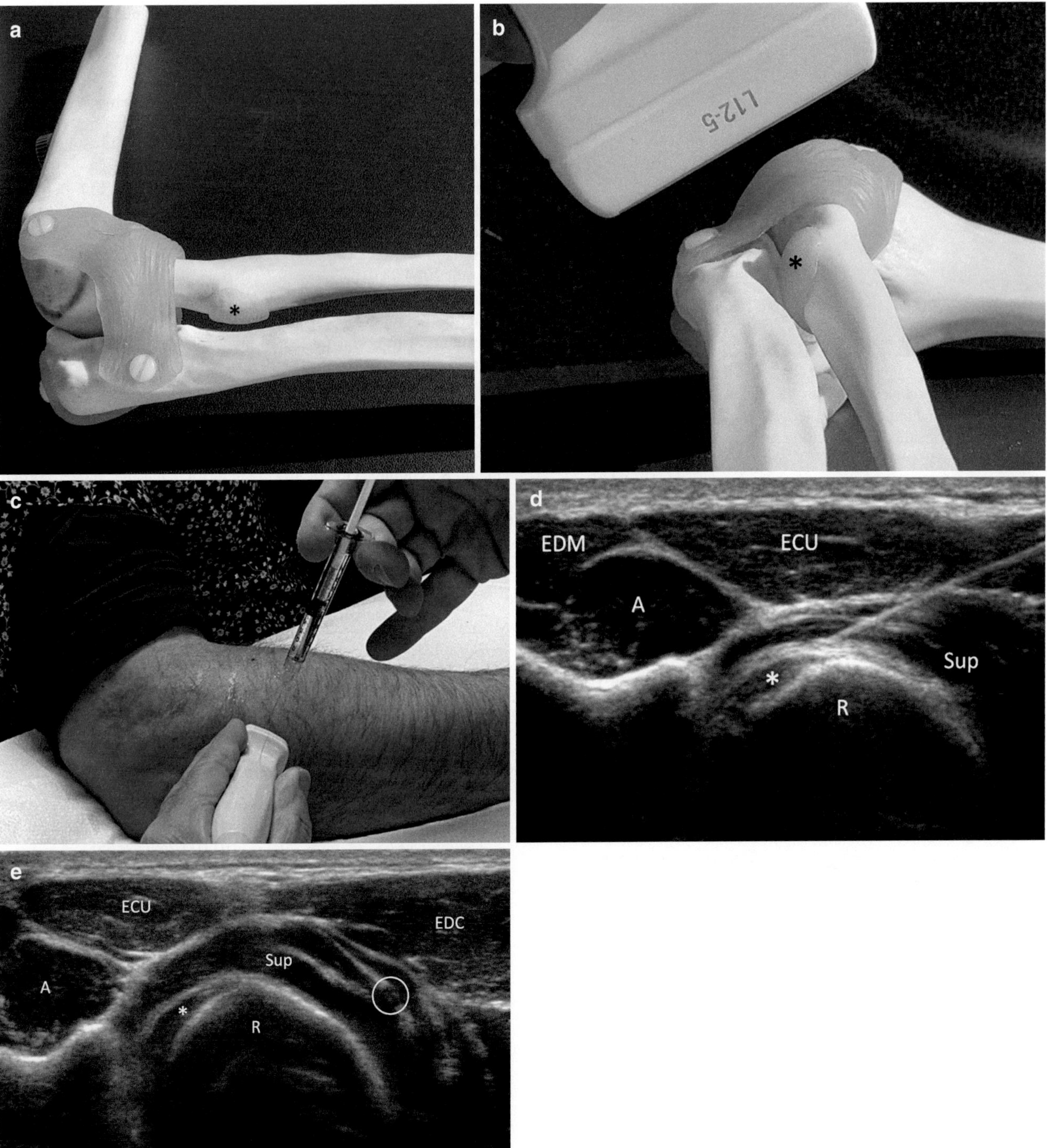

Fig. 28.9 Distal biceps brachii tendon injection: (**a**) lateral and (**b**) axial views of anatomical model of the elbow; (**c**) photo of patient, forearm fully pronated, transducer and needle being inserted; (**d**) 12–5 MHz ultrasound image of the needle approaching the distal biceps tendon insertion (asterisk), radial tuberosity (R), supinator muscle (Sup), anconeus (A), extensors carpi ulnaris (ECU) and digiti minimi (EDM); and (**e**) 12–5 MHz panoramic ultrasound image also showing deep radial nerve (circle) and extensor digitorum communis (EDC) muscles

epicondylalgia and triceps tendinopathy, but is not yet indicated for distal biceps tendinopathy.

Injection treatments for ulnar neuropathy at the elbow, radial tunnel, and pronator syndrome are currently not well researched. Ulnar neuropathy at the retrocondylar groove involves compression of the nerve by external forces (from outside the body), in which case a corticosteroid injection, which reduces swelling and adaptive enlargement of the nerve, could worsen symptoms. In the only randomized controlled trial, 5 ml perineural dextrose, 5% resulted in better

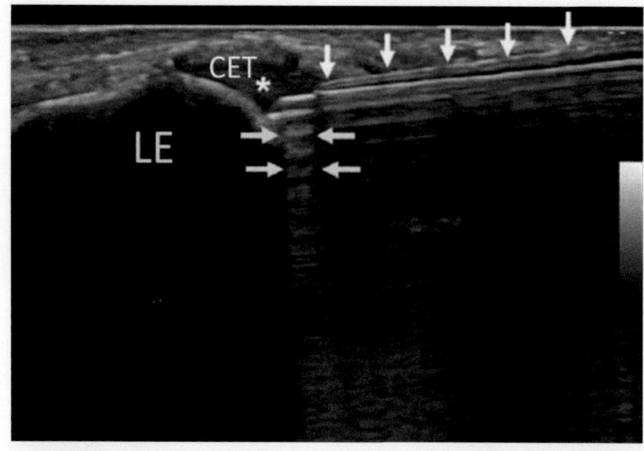

Fig. 28.10 Percutaneous ultrasonic tenotomy. Intraoperative ultrasound image. The outer sheath (vertical white arrows) is clearly visualized, with the metallic tip protruding from the sheath and located within the common extensor tendon (CET, asterisk). Horizontal yellow arrows demonstrate the reverberation artifact from the metal tip. (With permission from Barnes et al.)

outcomes than triamcinolone 10 mg injections for ulnar neuropathy at the elbow. By contrast, multiple studies have shown consistent and significant improvement of symptoms and median nerve function for carpal tunnel syndrome, likely on the basis of reduced tendon swelling and pressure on the nerve within the fibro-osseus tunnel.

Suggested Reading

Armstrong T, Devor W, Borschel L, Contreras R. Intracarpal steroid injection is safe and effective for short-term management of carpal tunnel syndrome. Muscle Nerve. 2004;29(1):82–8. https://doi.org/10.1002/mus.10512.

Barnes DE, Beckley JM, Smith J. Percutaneous ultrasonic tenotomy for chronic elbow tendinosis: a prospective study. J Shoulder Elb Surg. 2015;24(1):67–73. https://doi.org/10.1016/j.jse.2014.07.017.

Bianchi S, Martinoli C. Ultrasound of the musculoskeletal system. Berlin: Springer-Verlag; 2007.

Bisset L, Beller E, Jull G, Brooks P, Darnell R, Vicenzino B. Mobilisation with movement and exercise, corticosteroid injection, or wait and see for tennis elbow: randomised trial. BMJ. 2006;333(7575):939. https://doi.org/10.1136/bmj.38961.584653.AE.

Bodor M, Colio S, Khan J, Raj M. Ultrasound-guided injections for elbow pain. In: Peng P, Finlayson R, Lee S, Bhatia A, editors. Ultrasound for interventional pain management. Springer; 2020. p. 233–46.

Bodor M, Rojo-Manaute JM, Podnar S. Reply re: why do corticosteroid injections work for carpal tunnel syndrome but not ulnar neuropathy at the elbow. Muscle Nerve. 2016;54(2):344–5. https://doi.org/10.1002/mus.25170.

Chen LC, Ho TY, Shen YP, Su YC, Li TY, Tsai CK, et al. Perineural dextrose and corticosteroid injections for ulnar neuropathy at the elbow: a randomized double-blind trial. Arch Phys Med Rehabil. 2020 Aug;101(8):1296–303. https://doi.org/10.1016/j.apmr.2020.03.016.

Coombes BK, Bisset L, Brooks P, Khan A, Vicenzino B. Effect of corticosteroid injection, physiotherapy, or both on clinical outcomes in patients with unilateral lateral epicondylalgia: a randomized controlled trial. JAMA. 2013;309(5):461–9. https://doi.org/10.1001/jama.2013.129.

Fitzpatrick J, Bulsara M, Zheng MH. The effectiveness of platelet-rich plasma in the treatment of tendinopathy. Am J Sports Med. 2017;45:226–33. https://doi.org/10.1177/0363546516643716.

Huang K, Giddins G, Wu LD. Platelet-rich plasma versus corticosteroid injections in the management of elbow epicondylitis and plantar fasciitis: an updated systematic review and meta-analysis. Am J Sports Med. 2020 Aug;48(10):2572–85. https://doi.org/10.1177/0363546519888450.

Jacobson J. Fundamentals of musculoskeletal ultrasound. 3rd ed. Philadelphia: Elsevier; 2018.

Mishra AK, Skrepnik NV, Edwards SG, Jones GL, Sampson S, Vermillion DA, et al. Efficacy of platelet-rich plasma for chronic tennis elbow: a double-blind, prospective, multicenter, randomized controlled trial of 230 patients. Am J Sports Med. 2014 Feb;42(2):463–71. https://doi.org/10.1177/0363546513494359.

Ostergaard PJ, Meyer MA, Earp BE. Non-operative treatment of carpal tunnel syndrome. Curr Rev Musculoskelet Med. 2020;13(2):141–7. https://doi.org/10.1007/s12178-020-09616-0.

Podnar S, Omejec G, Bodor M. Nerve conduction velocity and cross-sectional area in ulnar neuropathy at the elbow. Muscle Nerve. 2017 Dec;56(6):E65–72. https://doi.org/10.1002/mus.25655.

Riboh JC, Saltzman BM, Yanke AB, Fortier L, Cole BJ. Effect of leukocyte concentration on the efficacy of platelet-rich plasma in the treatment of knee osteoarthritis. Am J Sports Med. 2016;44(3):792–800. https://doi.org/10.1177/0363546515580787.

Scarpone M, Rabago DP, Zgierska A, Arbogast G, Snell E. The efficacy of prolotherapy for lateral epicondylosis: a pilot study. Clin J Sport Med. 2008;18(3):248–54. https://doi.org/10.1097/JSM.0b013e318170fc87.

Stover D, Fick B, Chimenti RL, Hall MM. Ultrasound-guided tenotomy improves physical function and decreases pain for tendinopathies of the elbow: a retrospective review. J Shoulder Elb Surg. 2019 Dec;28(12):2386–93. https://doi.org/10.1016/j.jse.2019.06.011.

Pain Procedures Around the Hand and Wrist

29

David A. Spinner, Erica R. Eldon, and Rebecca A. Freedman

Contents

D. A. Spinner (✉)
Mount Sinai, Rehabilitation and Human Performance, New York, NY, USA
e-mail: David.spinner@mountsinai.org

E. R. Eldon · R. A. Freedman
Icahn School of Medicine at Mount Sinai, Rehabilitation and Human Performance, New York, NY, USA
e-mail: erica.eldon@mountsinai.org; rebecca.freedman@mountsinai.org

D. Jankovic, P. Peng (eds.), *Regional Nerve Blocks in Anesthesia and Pain Therapy*,
https://doi.org/10.1007/978-3-030-88727-8_29

Carpal Tunnel

General

The carpal tunnel is the most common compression neuropathy site. Carpal tunnel syndrome (CTS), also known as median nerve entrapment neuropathy, is classically described by a constellation of symptoms: pain, paresthesias, and thenar atrophy. Compression of the median nerve occurs when pressure increases through the carpal tunnel at the volar aspect of the wrist, either by edema or direct wrist trauma. Entrapment at the carpal tunnel will produce numbness or tingling in the median nerve distribution in the hand which includes the palmar aspect of the thumb, index finger, middle finger, and radial half of the ring finger (Fig. 29.1). Some may have sparing over the thenar palm and little finger. Pain is often worse at night and may be reported to improve with shaking of the hand or "flick sign." High body mass index (BMI) and repetitive wrist movement are associated with increased risk of developing CTS. Provocative maneuvers that reproduce symptoms include carpal compression test, Phalen's sign, and Tinel's sign because they compress the median nerve; however, they are neither sensitive nor specific. Diagnostic studies such as electromyography, nerve conduction studies, and cross-sectional area (CSA) of the median nerve on ultrasound assist in accurately diagnosing CTS. Thenar atrophy is strongly associated with ruling in CTS, but lack of thenar atrophy is not associated with ruling out CTS. Combined history, physical exam, and diagnostic studies support a clinical diagnosis of CTS.

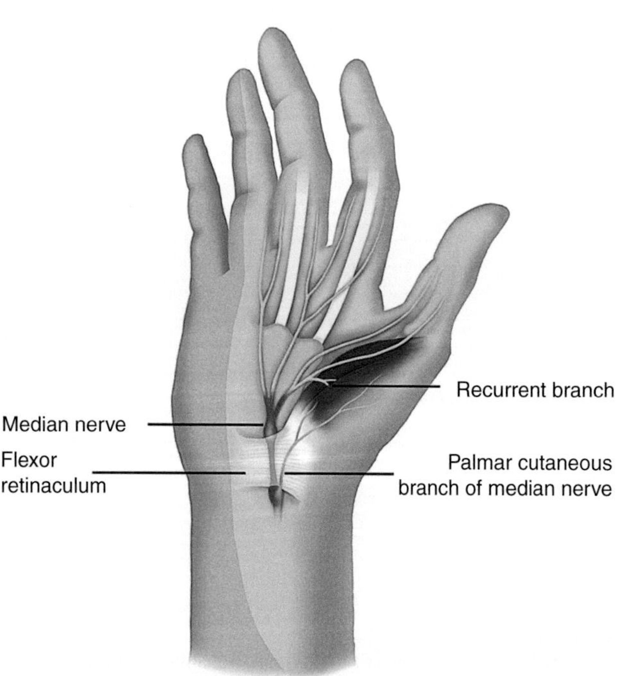

Fig. 29.1 Median nerve entrapment neuropathy. Reprinted with permission from Philip Peng Educational Series

Indications

Corticosteroid injection of the median nerve in the carpal tunnel should be considered in patients who have confirmed CTS based on history, physical exam, and diagnostic studies, who have failed conservative therapy. Conservative therapy includes immobilization with a splint, brace, or orthosis. Avoid injecting if a patient has infection near the injection site such as cellulitis of the overlying skin.

Functional Anatomy

The carpal tunnel is located just distal to the distal wrist crease when observing the volar aspect of the hand and wrist. The lateral border is formed by the scaphoid and trapezium, and the medial border is formed by the pisiform and hamate. The flexor retinaculum, also known as the transverse carpal ligament, extends from the hamate to the trapezium forming the superficial volar border. The median nerve runs within the volar radial area of the carpal tunnel, superficial to the flexor pollicis longus (FPL) tendon and radial to the flexor digitorum superficialis (FDS) tendons and flexor digitorum profundus (FDP) tendons (Fig. 29.2). Key anatomy outside of the carpal tunnel includes the palmaris longus (PL) tendon located at the midpoint of the median crease and the ulnar artery and nerve which lie volar to the flexor retinaculum near its attachment to the hamate. The radial artery is located radial to the trapezium at the distal wrist crease and is therefore not near the flexor retinaculum. The median nerve gives rise to the superficial palmar branch of the median nerve prior to entering the carpal tunnel leading to palmar sparing of sensation.

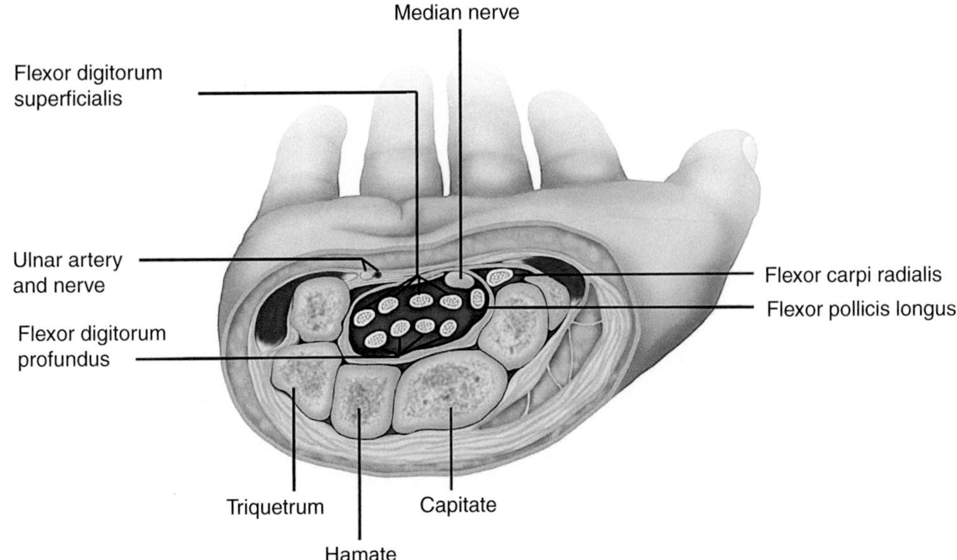

Fig. 29.2 Cross-section anatomy of the carpal tunnel. Reprinted with permission from Philip Peng Educational Series

Technique

Position Seated with arm supinated and resting comfortably on a flat surface. A towel roll can be placed under the wrist to assist in slight wrist extension.

Equipment Ultrasound probe: High-frequency linear array transducer or hockey stick linear probe.

- Needle: 25G or 27G 1.5in needle.
- Injectate: 1–3 mL local anesthetic, 0.5 mL steroid.

Scan Scan in short axis over the distal wrist crease. Identify key anatomy, including the carpal bones bordering the carpal tunnel, the hyperechoic tendons, and the median nerve which will appear as a hypoechoic honeycomb bundle (Fig. 29.3). Scan proximally and distally to clearly identify the course of the median nerve. Tilt the probe to correct for anisotropy. Flex and extend the fingers to observe movement of the tendons within the carpal tunnel. Use color flow to verify the location of the ulnar artery. The optimal position for injection will be where the median nerve is at the level of the pisiform and most superficial within the tunnel.

In-Plane Approach With the probe in short-axis position, in-plane approach is performed from the ulnar side with the needle entering the distal wrist crease parallel to the transducer and just radial or deep to the ulnar artery and nerve (Fig. 29.4). Using a shallow approach, advance the needle into the carpal tunnel toward the median nerve. The needle will appear as a hyperechoic line. When the tip is near the nerve, administer the injectate. Some practitioners prefer to hydrodissect the nerve off of the flexor retinaculum or tendons, while others inject anywhere in the carpal tunnel since it is a confined space and the injectate will spread and saturate the nerve.

Out-of-Plane Approach With the probe in short-axis position, out-of-plane approach is performed with the needle entering distal to the distal crease at a steep angle perpendicular to the transducer and just ulnar to the median nerve (Fig. 29.5). The needle will appear as a hyperechoic dot when the needle tip is directly under the transducer. Administer the injectate next to the median nerve. Hydrodissection is not performed in this approach because the entire needle path cannot be visualized and care should be taken to ensure the needle tip is maintained under the transducer.

Oblique Gel Standoff Technique Place a hockey stick probe in the oblique ulnar position over a thick layer of sterile gel. Stabilize the probe position with the holding hand to ensure the probe does not rest on the skin and maintains a gel buffering layer. Advance the needle in plane through the gel until the needle tip reaches the distal wrist crease. The needle is visualized in plane under the transducer before piercing the skin. Advance the needle into the skin, and continue to visualize the entire needle path as it approaches the median nerve, similar to the in-plane approach previously described. Administer injectate next to the nerve.

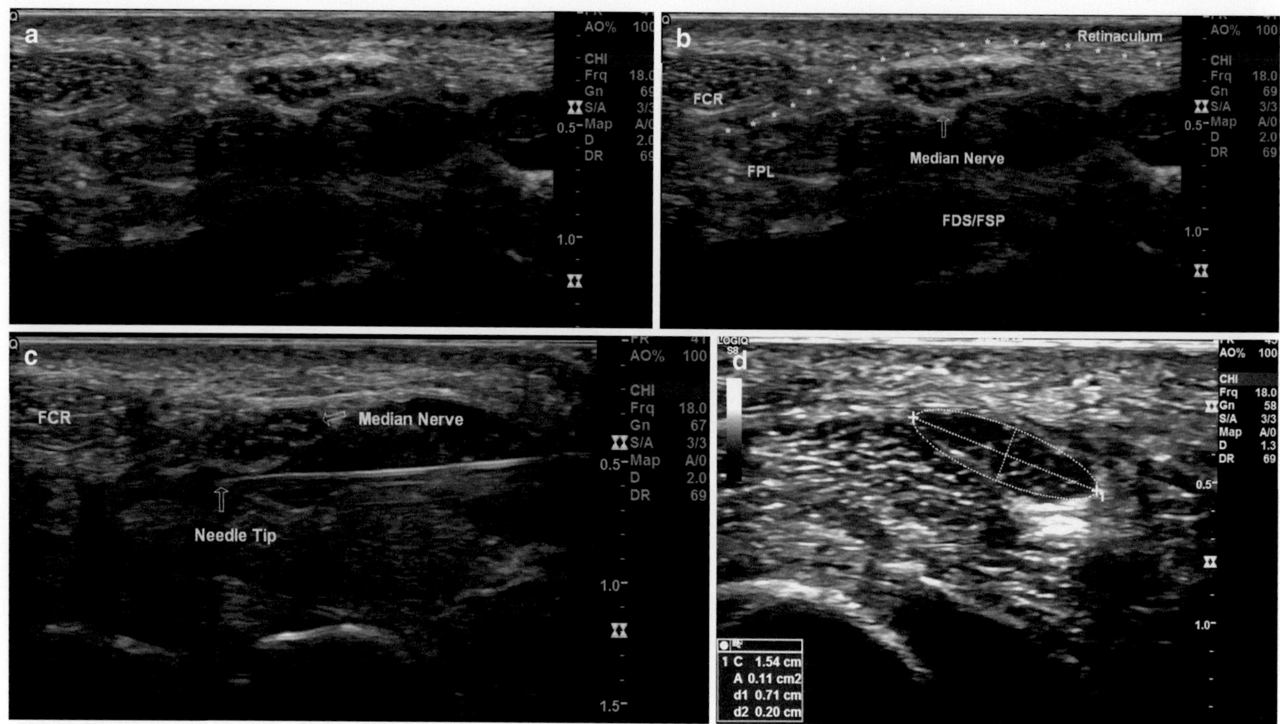

Fig. 29.3 (**a**) Axial view of the carpal tunnel. (**b**) Axial view of the carpal tunnel with structures labeled. Structures on the radial side is FCR and FPL. *FCR* flexor carpi radialis, *FPL* flexor pollicis longus, *FDS/FDP* flexor digitorum superficialis tendons and flexor digitorum profundus tendons, *stars* flexor retinaculum, *arrow* median nerve. (**c**) Axial view of the carpal tunnel with in-plane needle placement. *Arrow* identifies the needle tip. (**d**) Example of measuring cross-sectional area of the median nerve

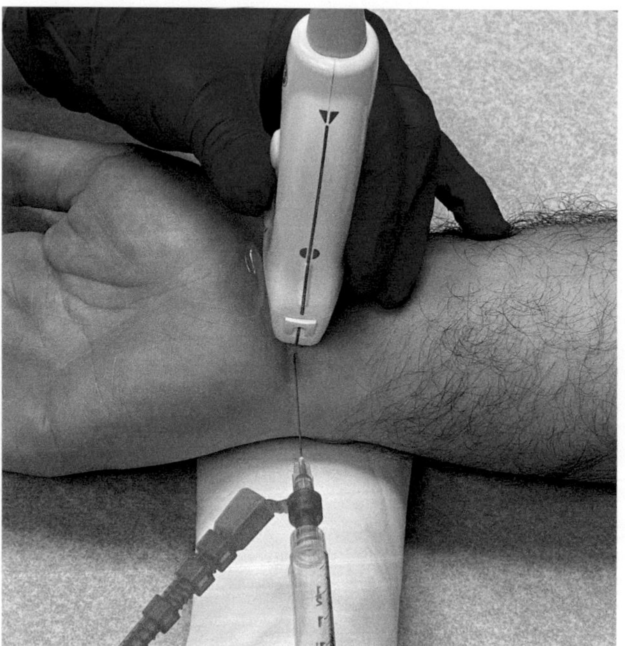

Fig. 29.4 Example of probe in short-axis position with in-plane approach

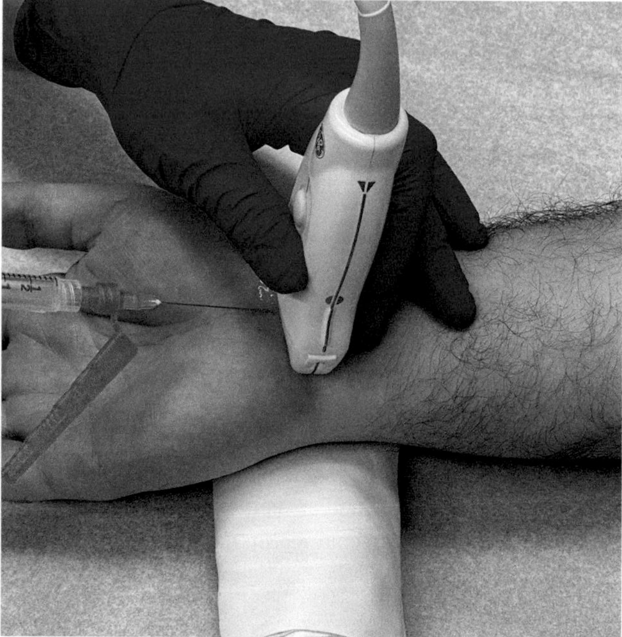

Fig. 29.5 Example of probe in short-axis position with out-of-plane approach

Complications

The palmar cutaneous branch of the ulnar nerve is superficial to the flexor retinaculum and is at risk of injury with the in-plane ulnar approach. Use color Doppler to identify vasculature in case of anatomical variants. The patient may experience hand numbness or weakness and should be advised not to drive.

Practical Tips

- Place a towel roll under the wrist to assist in slight wrist extension.
- Tilt the transducer to correct for anisotropy. The median nerve has less anisotropy than the tendons. Flex and extend the fingers to identify tendons and clearly visualize the nerve.
- Use color Doppler to identify vasculature.
- Oblique standoff technique is useful for small wrists.

Literature Review

The ulnar approach is preferred because a "safe zone" exists between the ulnar neurovascular bundle and the median nerve; however, a study investigating arteriole presence within the "safe zone" found that 38.9% of wrists had arterioles deep to the flexor retinaculum and the majority of deep arterioles were in close proximity to the median nerve, supporting the use of Doppler to identify vasculature. Median nerve CSA proximal and distal to the carpal tunnel, difference between cross-sectional areas, bowing of the retinaculum at the outlet, and outlet hypervascularity have been shown to have clinical utility in diagnosing CTS. A recent meta-analysis pooled median CSA values and determined that CSA correlated with severity in accordance with electrodiagnostic classification of CTS: mean CSA 11.64 mm for mild, 13.74 for moderate, and 16.80 for severe CTS.

Ganglion Cyst

General

Ganglion cysts are benign, soft tissue masses often found on the dorsal or volar surfaces of the wrist and hand. They are filled with mucoid material encapsulated in collagenous sheets without a synovial lining and communicate with a nearby joint via a stalk.

The exact mechanisms of ganglion cyst formation are unknown; however, it has been suggested that the cystic fluid may arise from within the joint itself due to joint motion and stress or from joint stress leading to mucinous degeneration of adjacent extra-articular soft tissues. The majority of ganglion cysts occur in the dorsal wrist, followed by the volar surface. Ganglia can also arise from tendons or tendon sheaths.

Diagnosis is largely based on clinical examination and symptoms. Ganglia of the wrist are typically 1–2 cm rubbery, transilluminating structures that are well attached to an underlying joint or tendon sheath. Many times, ganglia appear as a painless mass. However, if they are compressing on or irritating neighboring structures, they may become symptomatic. For example, patients may complain of aching in the wrist or hand, radiation of pain proximally through the arm, paresthesias from nerve compression, pain with activity or palpation of the mass, impaired grip strength, and decreased range of motion of the wrist and hand joint.

Indications

If a patient has failed conservative treatment options including observation and immobilization and symptoms are interfering with function, aspiration and/or injection of the ganglion cyst may be appropriate.

Functional Anatomy

On ultrasound, a ganglion cyst appears as a well-defined, anechoic or hypoechoic, fluid-filled mass, oftentimes connected to an adjacent joint or ligament via a communicating pedicle.

Sixty to seventy percent of ganglia are located on the dorsal wrist. Most commonly, ganglia are associated with the dorsal scapholunate ligament and joint. If present, it can impinge on the terminal branches of the posterior interosseous nerve in the fourth dorsal compartment.

About 20% of ganglion cysts occur on the volar aspect of the wrist. They usually are located in close proximity to the radial artery. On the palmar surface, ganglia frequently arise over the radiocarpal or scaphotrapezial joint. If found within the carpal tunnel or Guyon's canal, ganglia can cause a compression neuropathy of the median or ulnar nerves, respectively.

Technique

Position Patient seated with arm resting on the table. The forearm supinated for volar ganglion cyst, pronated for dorsal ganglion cyst. A towel roll can be placed under the wrist to assist in flexion or extension if needed.

Equipment High-frequency linear array transducer.

- 25G needle with 1–3 mL local anesthetic
- 16–18G 1.5-inch needle attached to a 3 cc syringe for aspiration
- 0.5 mL corticosteroid and local anesthetic solution in separate syringe.

Scan Visualize the ganglion cyst in both the long-axis view and short-axis view to assess position and depth. To assess the dorsal wrist, place the probe longitudinally over the distal radius and scan distally until the scaphoid is visualized, and then rotate the probe to axial position and visualize the scapholunate joint. To assess the volar wrist, place the probe longitudinally over the distal radius, and scan distally until the radiocarpal joint is visualized. Use color Doppler to visualize nearby vasculature, including the radial artery which is in close proximity to the radiocarpal joint.

In-Plane Longitudinal Approach Using the 25G needle, inject a wheel of local anesthetic at the skin entry location. Position transducer in the longitudinal axis with the hypoechoic cyst centered in the screen (Fig. 29.6). Using the in-plane approach, advance the 16–18G needle attached to a 1 cc or 3 cc syringe until the needle tip is within the cyst. Aspirate cyst contents. You will see the cyst collapse around the needle tip. With the needle stabilized and maintained in position within the cyst, change the syringe, and administer corticosteroid injectate under direct visualization.

Complications

Visualize vasculature using color Doppler. Vascular aneurysms can present as a painful lesion similar in appearance to a cyst on physical exam, and radiocarpal cysts can be located in close proximity to the radial neurovascular bundle. Volar radiocarpal cysts have a 59–66% recurrence rate at 9 months after aspiration.

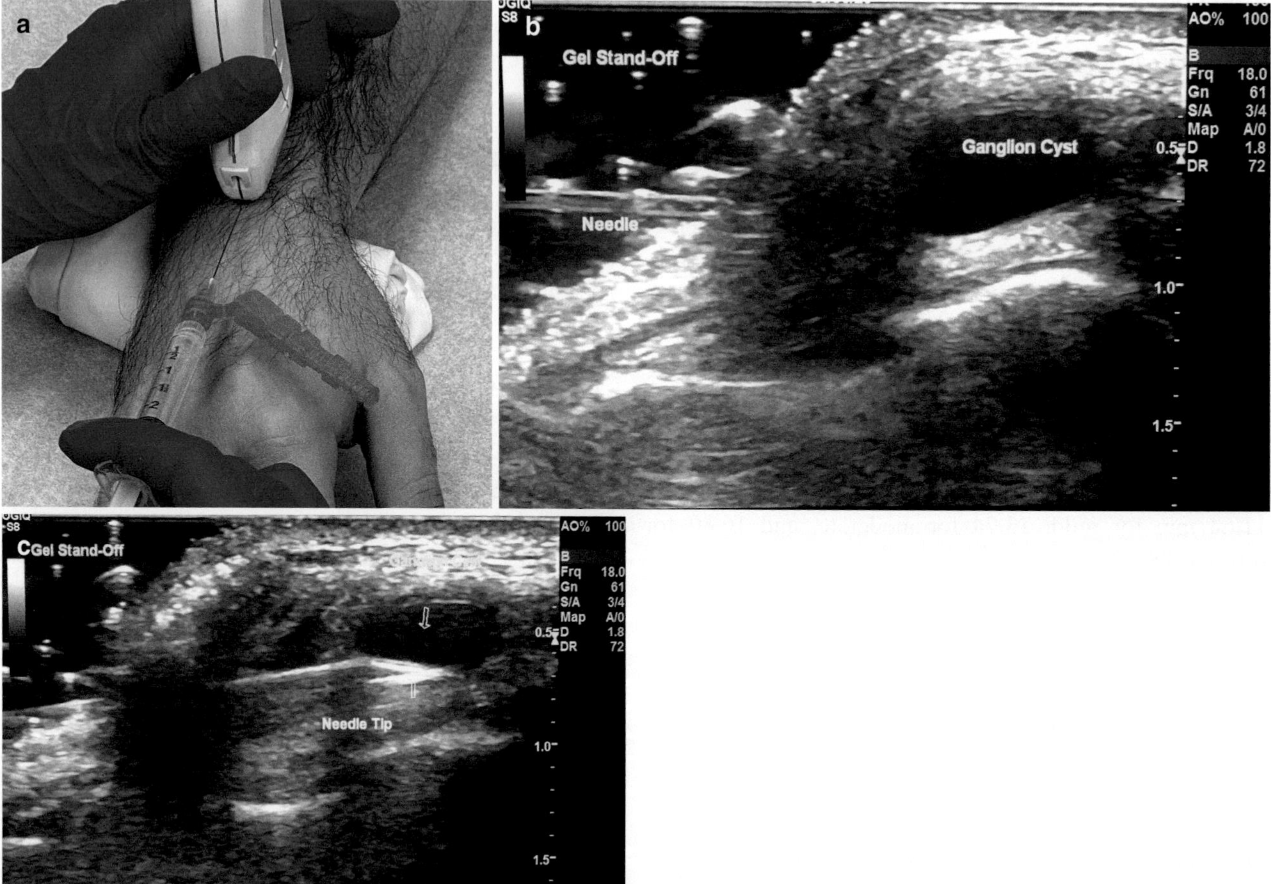

Fig. 29.6 (**a**) probe placement in longitudinal position with in-plane approach and gel standoff technique. (**b**) and (**c**) ultrasound images with the needle entering the skin and the needle inside the ganglion cyst. Arrows, needle tip and cyst

Practical Tips

- Place a towel roll under the wrist to assist in flexion/extension to open the carpal joints for better visualization.
- Use color Doppler to visualize nearby vasculature, including the radial artery.
- Use oblique gel standoff technique for small wrists or superficial cysts.

Literature Review

Variable success and recurrence rates have been observed for aspiration of ganglion cysts. Studies have investigated aspiration with injection of corticosteroid, using hyaluronidase in conjunction with a steroid, and aspiration with splinting. Surgical excision has demonstrated significantly lower recurrence rates in comparison to aspiration; however, it may be associated with an increased risk of complications, such as wound infections or damage to surrounding anatomical structures, and a prolonged recovery. Although limited studies exist investigating the benefit and techniques of ultrasound-guided aspiration of ganglion cysts, due to the ease of the procedure, aspiration with or without injectate still remains a widely used and acceptable treatment option.

Trigger Finger

General

Trigger finger (stenosing tenosynovitis) is caused by tenosynovitis of the flexor digitorum profundus (FDP) and flexor digitorum superficialis (FDS) tendons as they cross the metacarpal phalangeal (MCP) joint at the A1 pulley. Thickening of the A1 pulley due to chronic friction causes secondary flexor tendon inflammation, and the flexor tendons get mechanically stuck proximal to the annular tendon, locking the affected finger into flexion. Diagnosis is based on history and physical exam, which includes pain located over the volar MCP joint that can radiate down the affected digit or proximally into the palm, a palpable mass, a tightness of the flexor tendon, and the digit becoming locked in flexion or a sensation of catching when extending the digit from a flexed position. Diagnosis can be reinforced by visualization of hypoechoic thickening of the A1 pulley and a nodule on the flexor tendon. Have the patient flex, and extend the finger and observe for any dynamic abnormalities or catching as the flexor tendons slide under the A1 pulley. Trigger finger is more common in women and associated with diabetes and rheumatoid arthritis.

Indications

If a patient has failed conservative treatment options (observation, immobilization with a ring splint for 6–12 weeks, and NSAIDs) and symptoms are interfering with function, injection of the tendon sheath may be appropriate.

Functional Anatomy

The flexor pulley system is made of canals formed by retinacular sheaths on the volar surface of the fingers through which the FDP and FDS flexor tendons pass through. The system comprises five annular pulleys and three cruciform pulleys (Fig. 29.7). The FDP inserts on the base of the distal

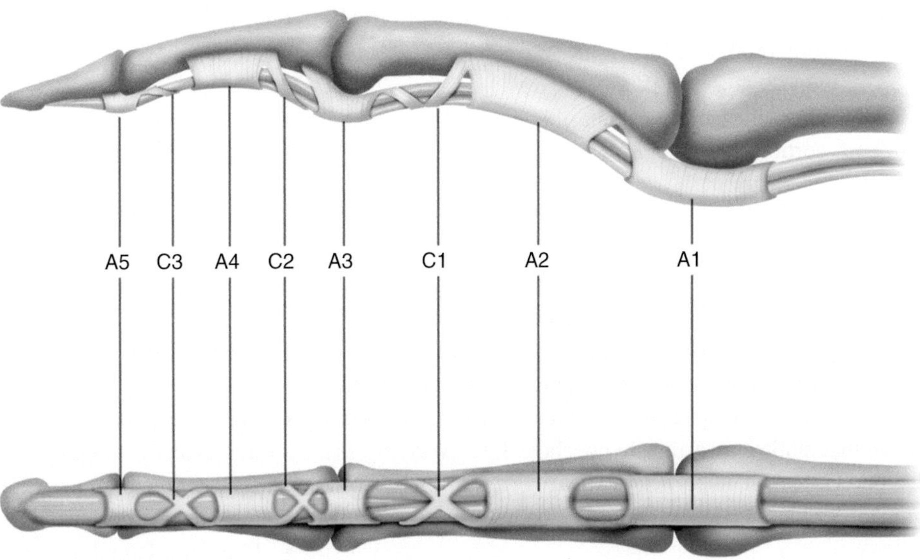

Fig. 29.7 Flexor tendon of the finger and the annular (A1–5) and cruciform (C1–3) pulleys Reprinted with permission from Philip Peng Educational Series

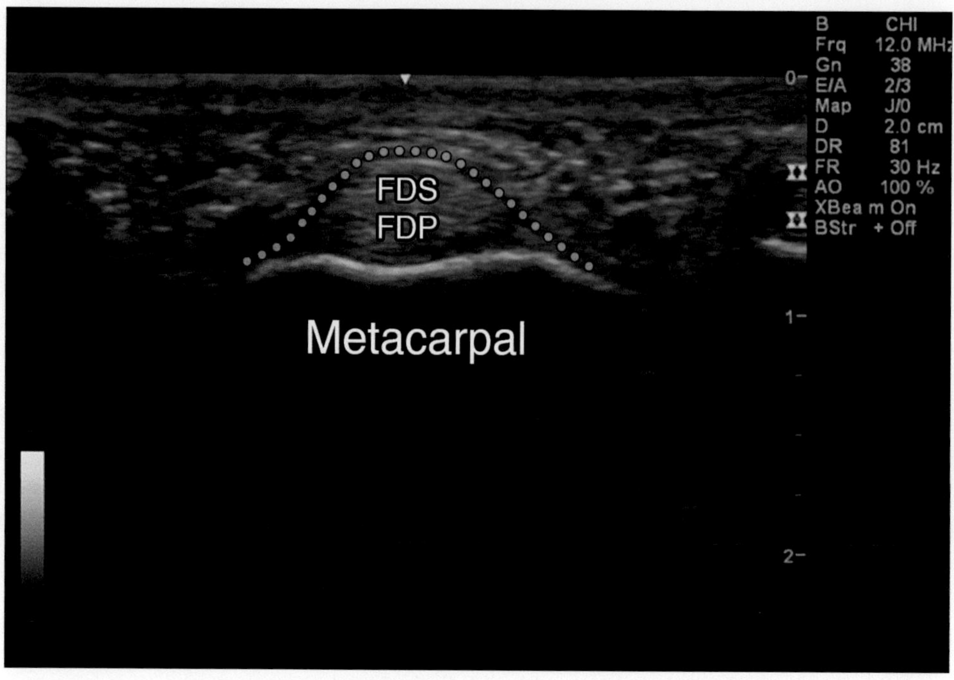

Fig. 29.8 Axial view of FDS and FDP overlying the metacarpal. *Green dotted* line represents the tendon sheath forming the A1 pulley

phalanx and flexes the distal interphalangeal joint (DIP). The FDS inserts on the body of the middle phalanx and flexes the proximal interphalangeal joint (PIP) and MCP. The A1 pulley overlies the volar surface of the MCP joint and is the most commonly affected pulley. Digital arteries and nerves run along the medial and lateral side of each phalanx.

Technique

Position Patient seated with arm resting on the table, the hand palm up.

Equipment High-frequency linear array transducer (10 Hz) or hockey stick probe.

- 25G needle with 1 mL local anesthetic
- 0.5 mL corticosteroid.

Scan Place the probe in a long-axis position over the affected MCP joint, and visualize the A1 pulley as it crosses superficial and proximal to the joint. The tendons of the flexor digitorum superficialis (FDS) and flexor digitorum profundus (FDP) can be seen overlying the phalanx. Rotate the probe into a short-axis position over the MCP joint. View the annular pulley as a thin hypoechoic line overlying the FDS and FDP, from superficial to deep (Fig. 29.8). Use color Doppler to identify digital arteries on either side of the phalanx.

Out-of-Plane Sagittal Approach: Center the probe over the MCP joint in short-axis view. Identify the A1 pulley overlying the FDS, FDP, and metacarpal, from superficial to deep. Using out-of-plane approach with a steep angle, insert the needle, and aim for the center of the probe (Fig. 29.9). When the needle tip, identified as a hyperechoic dot, is in the tendon sheath, administer the injectate. Do not inject directly into the tendon.

In-Plane Longitudinal Approach Center the probe over the MCP joint in a long-axis view. Using the in-plane approach, advance the needle parallel to the probe at a very shallow angle (Fig. 29.10). When the needle tip enters the superficial aspect of the tendon sheath, administer the injectate, and verify placement by observing distention of the sheath.

Complications

Fat necrosis, skin depigmentation, and tendon rupture can occur as a result of corticosteroid injection.

Practical Tips

- For small anatomy or if the high-frequency linear array transducer is too large, use the hockey stick probe and gel standoff technique for easier access and needle visualization.
- Use color Doppler to visualize nearby digital arteries.

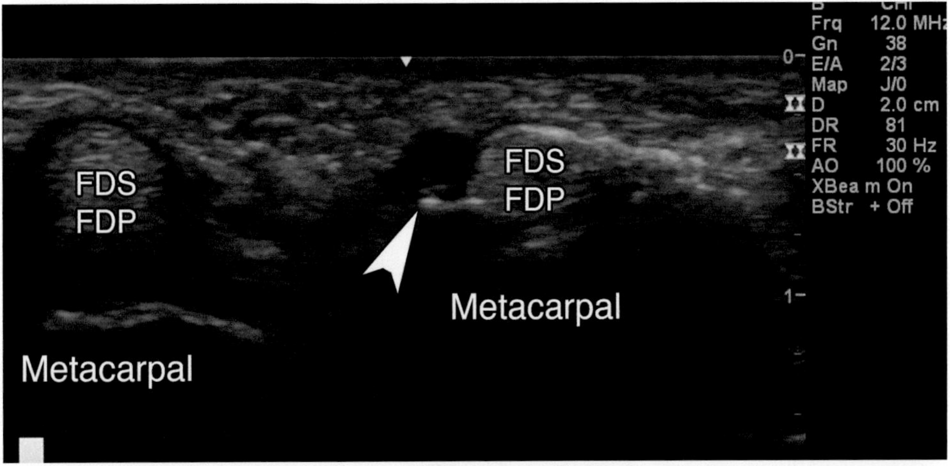

Fig. 29.9 Axial view of the A1 pulley with needle in out-of-plane approach. *Arrowhead* points to the needle

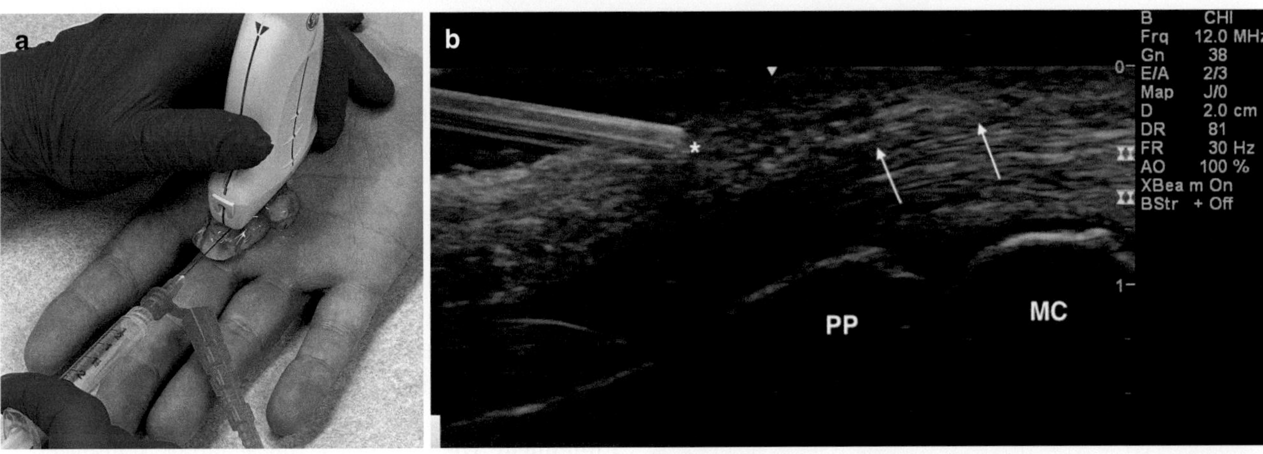

Fig. 29.10 (**a**) longitudinal probe placement over the MCP joint with in-plane gel standoff injection technique. (**b**) ultrasound image of a long-axis view of the flexor tendon over the MCP joint with in-plane needle approach. *Arrows* point to tendon sheath. *Star* identifies the needle tip. *MC* is the metacarpal and *PP* is the proximal phalanx

- Flex and extend the affected digit to visualize the tendon; look for hypoechoic thickening and/or a nodule.
- If resistance is felt, pull needle back to avoid injecting into the tendon.

Literature Review

Steroid injections treat trigger finger symptoms by decreasing inflammation of the FDS and FDP tendons, therefore reducing friction as they slide under the thickened A1 pulley. NSAIDs have been injected to reduce inflammation in patients who cannot tolerate steroids; however, studies have shown that steroids are more effective with 70% of patients reporting complete resolution of symptoms compared to 53% of patients treated with NSAID injection. Ultrasound guidance for intra-sheath steroid injection confirms correct placement of injectate and minimizes risk of tendon injury or rupture. Postinjection ultrasound has been used to compare preinjection and postinjection thickness of the A1 pulley and flexor tendons, with significant improvement in tendon thickness, VAS score, and Quinnell grading at 3 weeks postinjection, confirming the therapeutic effects of the steroid injection.

Dequervain's Tenosynovitis

General

De Quervain's tenosynovitis is a painful inflammation of the first dorsal extensor compartment of the wrist (Fig. 29.11), consisting of the abductor pollicis longus (APL) and extensor pollicis brevis (EPB). It is the most common tendinopathy of the wrist and hand. It most often occurs in middle-aged women and in occupations or athletes that require repetitive wrist bending or twisting. Patients present with a point of exquisite tenderness over the radial styloid process and the involved tendons. Typically, patients experience symptoms

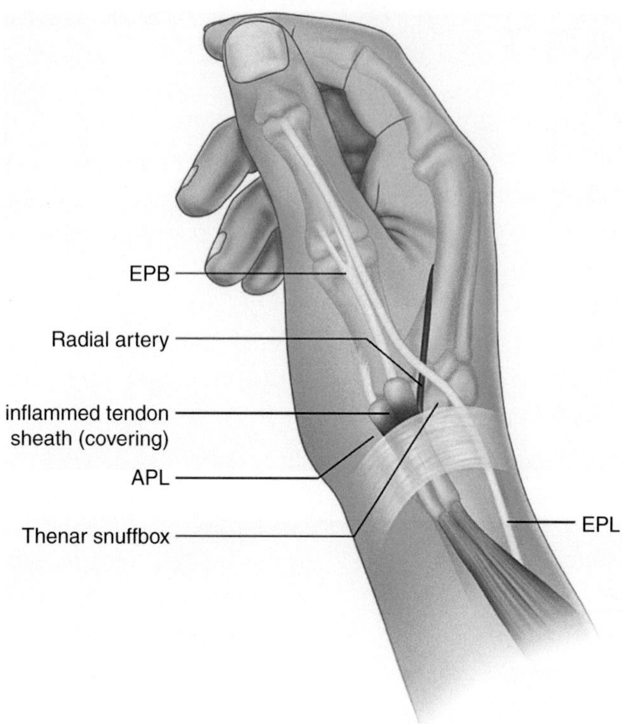

Fig. 29.11 Tenosynovitis of the first dorsal extensor compartment. EPB, extensor pollicis brevis, APL, abductor pollicis longus, EPL, extensor pollicis longus

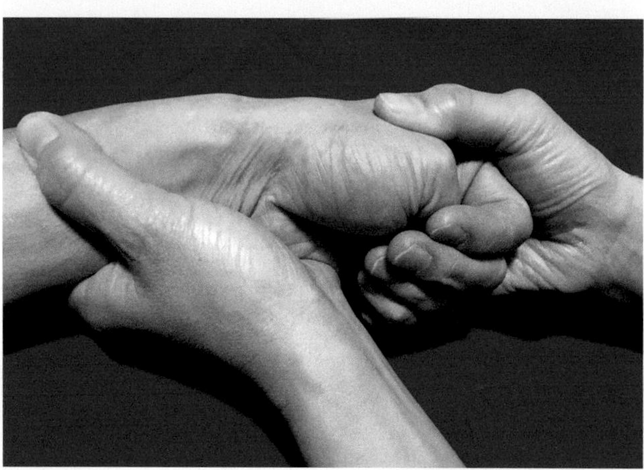

Fig. 29.12 Finkelstein's test

in their dominant wrist, usually from overuse rather than a direct trauma.

Finkelstein's test is a special maneuver to assist in diagnosing de Quervain's tenosynovitis (Fig. 29.12). Reproduction of symptoms occurs by flexing the thumb into the palm and applying an ulnar deviation to the wrist, stretching the two thumb tendons. X-rays are not routinely used as they are often unremarkable. Ultrasound can reveal swelling of the tendons or a thickened extensor retinaculum suggesting possible synovitis.

Indications

Patients with continued debilitating pain who have failed conservative treatment including splinting and NSAIDs may be candidates for ultrasound-guided injections. Stenosing tenosynovitis of the first dorsal compartment responds well to corticosteroid injections, with reported relief in up to 90% of patients.

Functional Anatomy

The first dorsal extensor compartment of the wrist consists of the APL and EPB and is located directly over the radial styloid process (Fig. 29.13). The APL originates on the posterior radius and ulna and inserts at the base of the first metacarpal. Its action includes abduction and extension of the thumb. The EPB originates on the posterior radius and inserts at the base of the proximal phalanx of the thumb. Its action is to extend the thumb, and it forms the radial border of the anatomical snuffbox. The APL lies more volar than the EPB. The compartment is surrounded by an extensor retinaculum.

Technique

Position Place the forearm resting comfortably on table surface in neutral position with radial styloid facing up.

Equipment High-frequency linear array transducer or hockey stick linear probe

- 25G 1.5 in needle with 1–3 mL local anesthetic
- 0.5 mL corticosteroid

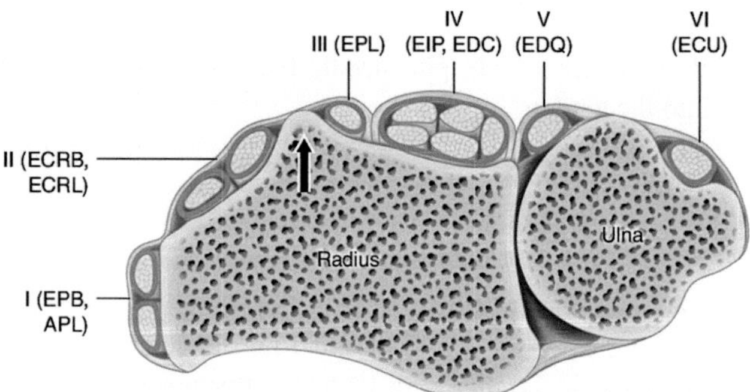

Fig. 29.13 Six compartments of the extensor tendons in the wrist. First compartment, abductor pollicis longus (APL) and extensor pollicis brevis (EPB); second compartment, extensor carpi radialis longus (ECRL) and extensor carpi radialis brevis (ECRB); third compartment, extensor pollicis longus (EPL); fourth compartment, extensor indicis proprius (EIP) and extensor digitorum (EDC); fifth compartment, extensor digiti quinti (EDQ); sixth compartment, extensor carpi ulnaris (ECU). Lister tubercle (arrow) separates the second from the third compartment

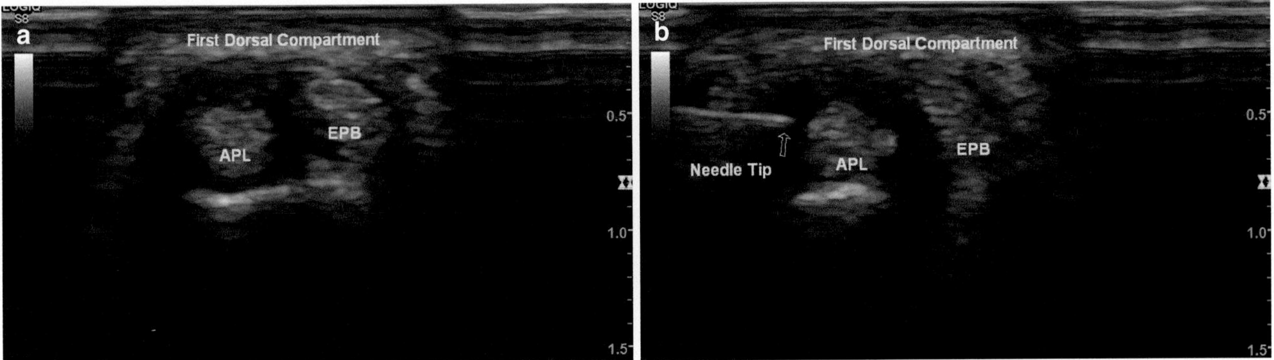

Fig. 29.14 (**a**) short-axis view of the first dorsal compartment with extensor retinaculum. *APL* abductor pollicis longus, *EPB* extensor pollicis brevis, and radius. (**b**) short-axis view of needle in plane and needle tip under the extensor retinaculum. *Arrow* identifies the needle tip

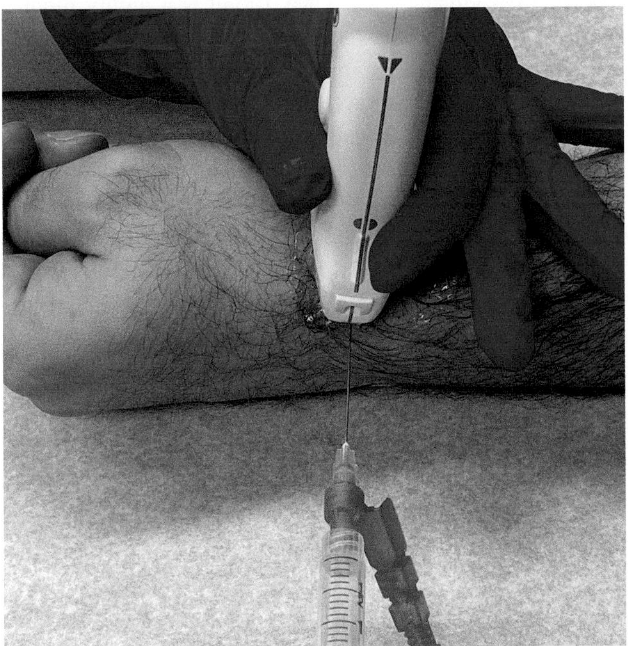

Fig. 29.15 Probe in short-axis position with in-plane approach

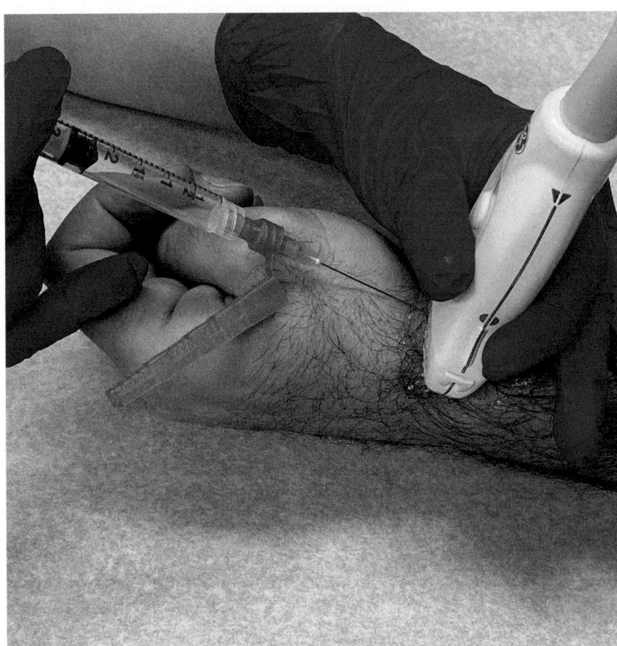

Fig. 29.16 Probe in short-axis position with out-of-plane approach (b)

Scan Place the probe in the short axis over the first extensor compartment at the level of the radial styloid (Fig. 29.14). Visualize the APL tendon volar to the EPB tendon with the superficial extensor retinaculum overlying the compartment. Deep to the APL and EPB is the radius. Identify and verify the location of the radial artery near the volar surface using color flow. Proximally the tendons will be side by side and will diverge distally. Tendon sheath thickening may be seen, and "donut sign" in short-axis view may indicate synovitis.

In-Plane Short-Axis Approach Place the probe in the short axis over the first extensor compartment at the level of the radial styloid. Advance the needle in plane to the transducer, from dorsal to volar, in a shallow trajectory until the needle tip is under the extensor retinaculum and above the APL and EPB tendons. Administer the injectate under direct visualization (Fig. 29.15).

Out-of-Plane Short-Axis Approach Place the probe in the short axis over the first extensor compartment at the level of the radial styloid as above. Advance the needle from distal to proximal out of plane with the needle entering the skin with a steep angle adjacent to and at the center of the transducer (Fig. 29.16). Observe the needle tip (hyperechoic dot) as it enters the extensor compartment and reaches the target under the extensor retinaculum and above the APL and EPB tendons. Administer the injectate under direct visualization.

Complications

When using corticosteroids, there is a risk of skin depigmentation. Injecting near tendons increases the risk of tendon rupture. The superficial branch of the radial nerve that lies over the extensor compartment is at risk of being blocked with resultant temporary hand numbness.

Practical Tips

- For small anatomy or if the high-frequency linear array transducer is too large, use the hockey stick probe and gel standoff technique for easier access and needle visualization
- Scan in the longitudinal view to visualize the APL and EPB in long axis. Thickening of the tendon sheath may suggest synovitis.
- Thoroughly scan the length of the tendons and their insertions. If a septum is noted, inject into both compartments to ensure adequate spread of injectate.
- Use color Doppler to visualize nearby vasculature, including the radial artery.

Literature Review

Ultrasound-guided injections have been shown to better and more precisely deliver corticosteroid in comparison to landmark-guided injections. US allows the practitioner to visualize the extensor retinaculum, the APL, and the EPB. It also allows for visualization of sub-compartmentalization of the first extensor compartment, an anatomical variant which requires a tailoring of injection technique. Ultimately, utilization of ultrasound permits for different injection techniques based on ultrasound findings of the first extensor compartment and has shown to be beneficial in the management of de Quervain's tenosynovitis.

CMC Joint

General

The first carpometacarpal (CMC) joint is a highly mobile, saddle joint. The joint space is formed between the trapezium and the first metacarpal bone (Fig. 29.17). The CMC joint allows for thumb movement in various planes and is a common site of arthritis and instability.

CMC joint pathology appears to be more frequent in females and is caused by repetitive stress. Patients with CMC joint pathology usually experience pain upon movement of the thumb as well as decreased range of motion and weakness. Grasping, pinching, or twisting motions typically elicit pain.

Two provocative tests which are useful when diagnosing CMC joint pathology are the grind test and the lever test (Fig. 29.18). For the grind test, axially load and rotate the CMC joint. For the lever test, hold the base of the metacarpal bone, and move the CMC joint in both radial and ulnar

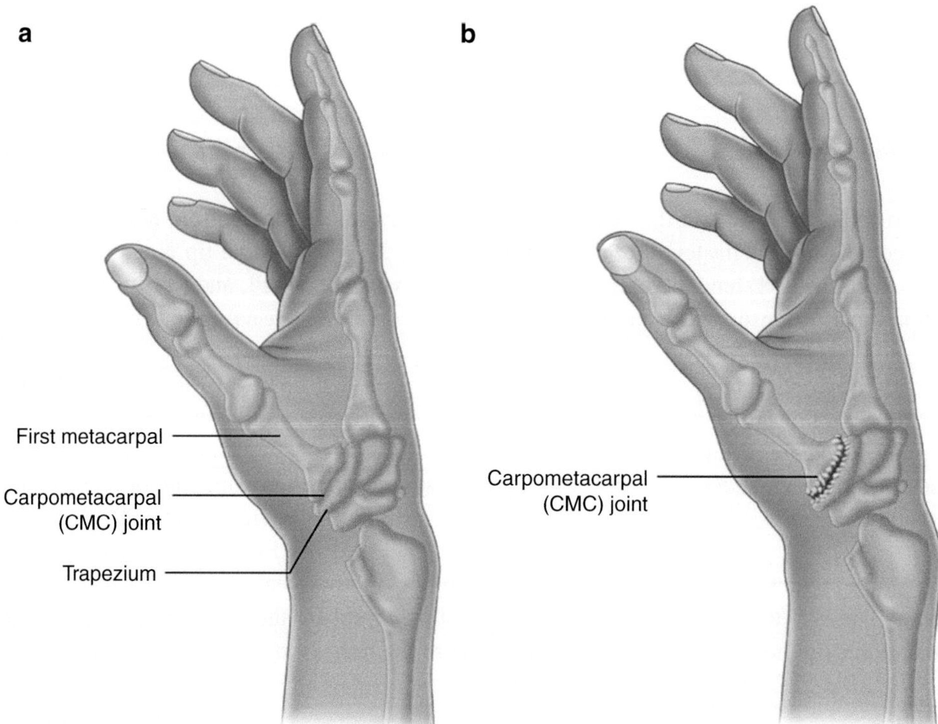

Fig. 29.17 Carpometacarpal joint, normal (**a**) and with arthritis (**b**)

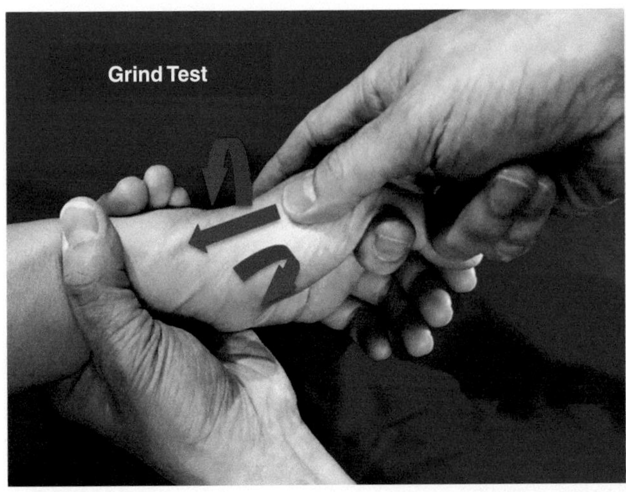

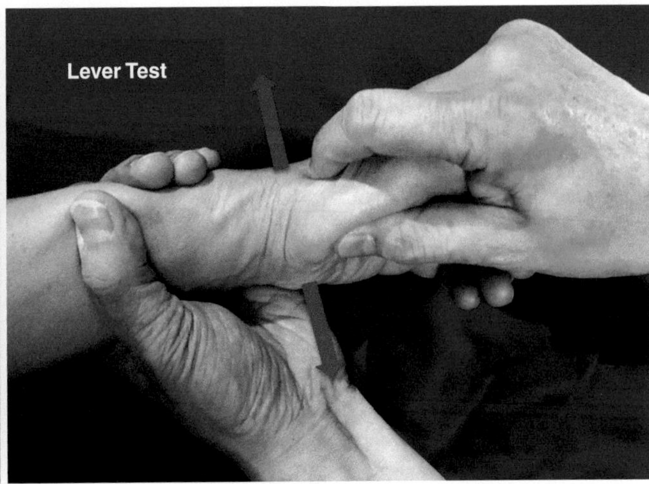

Fig. 29.18 Grind and level test

directions. These tests are positive if they reproduce pain or crepitus is appreciated.

Plain radiographs may demonstrate degenerative changes within the joint. Ultrasound evaluation can also show degenerative changes, such as joint space narrowing, synovitis, cortical irregularities, osteophytes, and effusions.

Indications

Patients who continue to experience pain that is refractory to conservative measures, such as a thumb spica, activity modification, nonsteroidal anti-inflammatory medications, and occupational therapy, may be appropriate for diagnostic or therapeutic injection to the CMC joint.

Functional Anatomy

The thumb is composed of the distal phalanges and the proximal phalanges, connecting to the first metacarpal bone. Attached to the first metacarpal bone is the trapezium, and this articulation forms the CMC joint. Movement through this joint allows for primary movements, including flexion, extension, adduction, and abduction, and more complex movements, including opposition, retropulsion, palmar abduction, radial abduction, and radial adduction.

Several important structures neighbor the CMC joint. The superficial radial nerve has terminal branches located on either side of the CMC joint. Also nearby are the superficial and deep palmar arteries, which branch off of the radial artery. They are found at the anatomic snuffbox, located just proximally to the CMC joint. Traversing the CMC joint are the abductor pollicis longus and extensor pollicis brevis tendons.

Technique

Position Place the forearm resting comfortably on a flat surface in neutral position with radial styloid facing up.

Equipment High-frequency linear array transducer or hockey stick linear probe.

- 25G 1.5 in needle with 1–3 mL local anesthetic
- 0.5 mL corticosteroid.

Scan Place the transducer in the longitudinal position over the CMC joint. Identify the first metacarpal distally, the base of the trapezium proximally, and the joint space (Fig. 29.19). The APL and EPB tendons are seen overlying the CMC joint.

Out-of-Plane Longitudinal Approach Place the transducer in the longitudinal position over the CMC joint. Note the first metacarpal and trapezium, and place the joint space in the center of view. With needle approaching from dorsal to volar and using a steep angle, enter the skin close to the center of the transducer, and advance toward the joint space (Fig. 29.20). When the needle tip is visualized as a hyperechoic dot in the joint space, administer the injectate under direct visualization, and confirm correct placement by observing capsular displacement.

In-Plane Longitudinal Gel Standoff Approach Place the transducer in the longitudinal position over the CMC joint as above. Identify the APL and EPB overlying the CMC joint, note the first metacarpal and trapezium, and place the joint space in the center of view. With the needle approaching from distal to proximal, visualize the needle within the gel, and enter the skin over the trapezium and advance into the

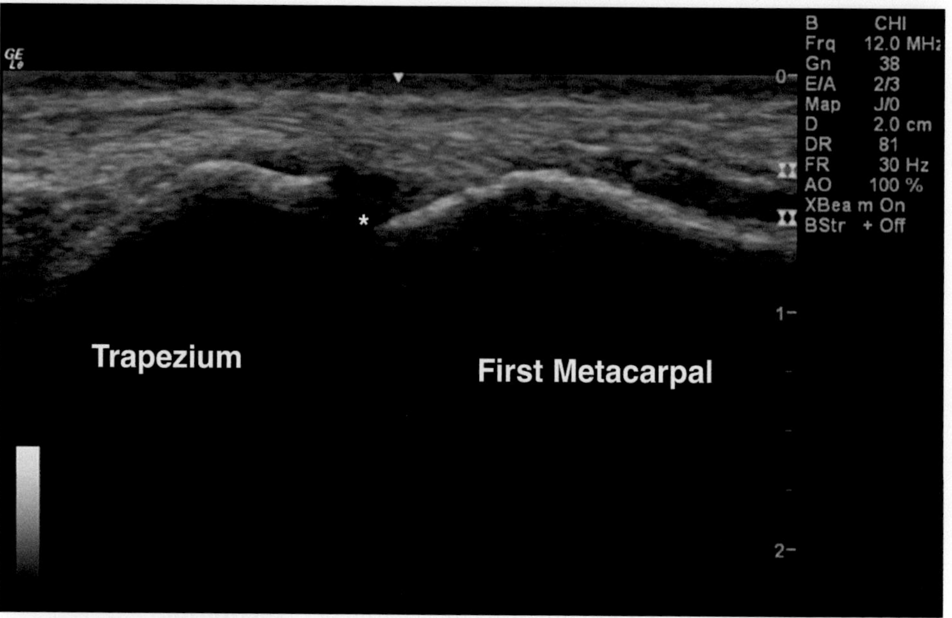

Fig. 29.19 Long-axis view of first CMC joint. *Asterisk* identifies the joint space. This is also the needle tip target for an out-of-plane approach

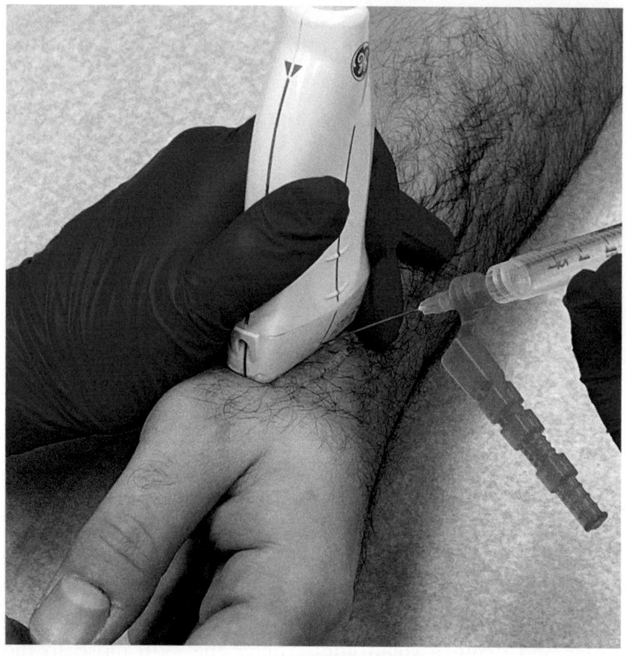

Fig. 29.20 Probe in longitudinal position over CMC joint with out-of-plane approach

joint (Fig. 29.21). Administer the injectate under direct visualization taking care not to pierce the overlying APL and EPB, and confirm correct placement by observing capsular displacement.

Complications

Avoid piercing the APL and EPB. Risks include bleeding, tendon rupture, infection, and skin depigmentation if corticosteroid is used.

Practical Tips

- Flex the thumb to open up the CMC joint.
- Avoid injecting into the tendons.
- Use the in-plane or oblique gel standoff technique for small anatomy.

Literature Review

Ultrasound guidance, when performed by an experienced user, has been found to improve the accuracy for thumb CMC injections, by assisting with correct needle placement in cases of severe joint space narrowing and osteoarthritis.

Intra-articular CMC joint injections are usually performed with corticosteroids and provide short-term relief. Alternative injectates, such as hyaluronate or nonsteroidal anti-inflammatories, can be considered alone or in combination for CMC joint osteoarthritis. PRP injections have also been postulated to offer longer relief of symptoms.

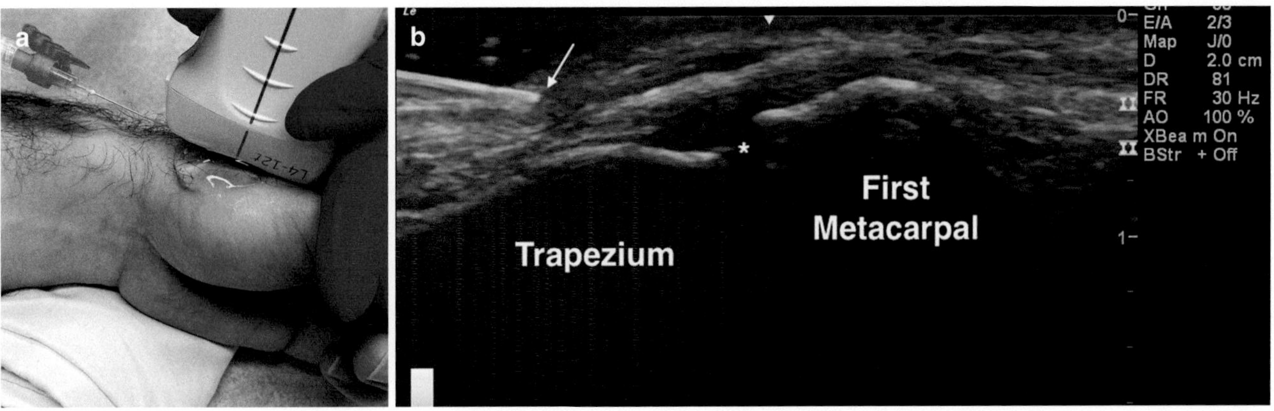

Fig. 29.21 (**a**) probe in longitudinal position over CMC joint with in-plane gel standoff approach. (**b**) ultrasound image of long-axis view of the first CMC joint with in-plane approach using gel standoff technique. *Asterisk* identifies the joint space. *Arrow* shows the needle tip

Suggested Reading

American Academy of Orthopaedic Surgeons. Management of carpal tunnel syndrome evidence-based clinical practice guideline. Published February 29, 2016. Available from: https://www.aaos.org/globalassets/quality-and-practice-resources/carpal-tunnel/cts_cpg_4-25-19.pdf

Bing J-H, Choi S-J, Jung S-M, Ryu D-S, Ahn J-H, Kang C-H, et al. Ultrasound-guided steroid injection for the treatment of de Quervain's disease: an anatomy-based approach. Skelet Radiol. 2018;47(11):1483–90.

Cartwright MS, Hobson-Webb LD, Boon AJ, Alter KE, Hunt CH, Flores VH, et al. Evidence-based guideline: neuromuscular ultrasound for the diagnosis of carpal tunnel syndrome. Muscle Nerve. 2012;46(2):287–93.

Colio SW, Smith J, Pourcho AM. Ultrasound-guided interventional procedures of the wrist and hand: anatomy, indications, and techniques. Phys Med Rehabil Clin N Am. 2016;27(3):589–605.

Danda RS, Kamath J, Jayasheelan N, Kumar P. Role of guided ultrasound in the treatment of De Quervain tenosynovitis by local steroid infiltration. J Hand Microsurg. 2016;08(01):034–7.

Egan M, Spinner D. Hand. In: Nelson B, Topol E, Bhagra A, Mulvagh S, Narula J, editors. . Cham: Atlas of Handheld Ultrasound. Springer; 2018. https://doi.org/10.1007/978-3-319-73855-0_7.

Gil JA, Hresko AM, Weiss A-PC. Current concepts in the Management of Trigger Finger in adults. J Am Acad Orthop Surg. 2020;28(15):e642–50.

Gitto S, Lee SC, Miller TT. Ultrasound-guided percutaneous treatment of volar radiocarpal ganglion cysts: safety and efficacy. J Clin Ultrasound. 2019;47(6):339–44.

Gonzalez-Suarez CB, Fidel BC, Cabrera JTC, Cruz FCD, Gesmundo MVT, Regala CFG, et al. Diagnostic accuracy of ultrasound parameters in carpal tunnel syndrome: additional criteria for diagnosis. J Ultrasound Med. 2019;38(11):3043–52.

Gude W, Morelli V. Ganglion cysts of the wrist: pathophysiology, clinical picture, and management. Curr Rev Musculoskelet Med. 2008;1(3):205–11.

Koh SH, Lee SC, Lee WY, Kim J, Park Y. Ultrasound-guided intra-articular injection of hyaluronic acid and ketorolac for osteoarthritis of the carpometacarpal joint of the thumb: a retrospective comparative study. Medicine. 2019;98(19):e15506.

Kuczmarski AS, Harris AP, Gil JA, Weiss A-PC. Management of Diabetic Trigger Finger. J Hand Surg Am. 2019;44(2):150–3.

Malahias M-A, Roumeliotis L, Nikolaou VS, Chronopoulos E, Sourlas I, Babis GC. Platelet-rich plasma versus corticosteroid intra-articular injections for the treatment of Trapeziometacarpal arthritis: a prospective randomized controlled clinical trial. CARTILAGE. 2021;12(1):51–61.

McDermott JD, Ilyas AM, Nazarian LN, Leinberry CF. Ultrasound-guided injections for de Quervain's tenosynovitis. Clin Orthop Relat Res. 2012;470(7):1925–31.

Mifune Y, Inui A, Sakata R, Harada Y, Takase F, Kurosaka M, et al. High-resolution ultrasound in the diagnosis of trigger finger and evaluation of response to steroid injection. Skelet Radiol. 2016;45(12):1661–7.

Ng AWH, Griffith JF, Lee RKL, Tse WL, Wong CWY, Ho PC. Ultrasound carpal tunnel syndrome: additional criteria for diagnosis. Clin Radiol. 2018;73(2):214.e11–8.

Roomizadeh P, Eftekharsadat B, Abedini A, Ranjbar-Kiyakalayeh S, Yousefi N, Ebadi S, et al. Ultrasonographic assessment of carpal tunnel syndrome severity: a systematic review and meta-analysis. Am J Phys Med Rehabil. 2019;98(5):373–81.

Sahler CS, Spinner DA, Kirschner JS. Ultrasound-guided first metatarsophalangeal joint injections: description of an in-plane, gel standoff technique in a cadaveric study. Foot Ankle Spec. 2013;6(4):303–6.

Sergeant A-C, Badr S, Saab M, Demondion X, Cotten A, Jacques T. Carpal tunnel ultrasound: is the "safe zone" on the ulnar side of the median nerve really avascular? Eur Radiol. 2020;30(2):887–94.

Spinner DA, Mazzola AJ. Intervention on wrist and hand. In: Peng P, Finlayson R, Lee S, Bhatia A, editors. Ultrasound for interventional pain management. Cham: Springer; 2020. https://doi.org/10.1007/978-3-030-18371-4_21.

Spinner DA, Rosado MI. Wrist and hand. In: Spinner D, Kirschner J, Herrera J, editors. Atlas of ultrasound guided musculoskeletal injections, Musculoskeletal medicine. New York: Springer; 2014. https://doi.org/10.1007/978-1-4614-8936-8_4.

Teh J, Vlychou M. Ultrasound-guided interventional procedures of the wrist and hand. Eur Radiol. 2009;19(4):1002–10.

Part V

Nerve Block for Regional Anesthesia and Pain Therapy in Chest, Abdomen and Pelvis

Ultrasound-Guided Thoracic Paravertebral Block

30

Ranjith Kumar Sivakumar and Manoj Kumar Karmakar

Contents

Abbreviations

IICM	Internal intercostal membrane
LA	Local anaesthetic
PICS	Posterior intercostal space
SCTL	Superior costotransverse ligament
TP	Transverse process
TPVB	Thoracic paravertebral block
TPVS	Thoracic paravertebral space
USG	Ultrasound-guided

General Consideration

Thoracic paravertebral block (TPVB) is the technique of injecting local anaesthetic (LA) alongside the thoracic vertebra and close to where the spinal nerves emerge from the intervertebral foramen. It produces ipsilateral, somatic and sympathetic nerve blockade in multiple contiguous thoracic dermatomes that culminate in high-quality afferent nociceptive blockade. The latter is evidenced as an abolition of somatosensory evoked potential, to intercostal nerve stimulation, from the blocked thoracic segments. The ipsilateral segmental thoracic anaesthesia is effective in managing pain of unilateral origin from the thorax and abdomen. TPVB has also been used, albeit in conjunction with intravenous sedation, to provide surgical anaesthesia for primary breast cancer and hernia surgery. Bilateral TPVB has also been described. TPVB is traditionally performed using surface anatomical landmarks, but recent years have seen an increase in interest in the use of ultrasound for TPVB, and several variations of the technique have been described. This chapter

R. K. Sivakumar · M. K. Karmakar (✉)
Department of Anaesthesia and Intensive Care, The Chinese University of Hong Kong, Prince of Wales Hospital, Shatin, NT, Hong Kong
e-mail: karmakar@cuhk.edu.hk

D. Jankovic, P. Peng (eds.), *Regional Nerve Blocks in Anesthesia and Pain Therapy*,
https://doi.org/10.1007/978-3-030-88727-8_30

briefly outlines the basic principles of TPVB, sonoanatomy of the TPVS and the technique of ultrasound-guided (USG) TPVB.

Indications

TPVB is indicated for anaesthesia and analgesia for surgical procedures where the afferent nociception is predominantly unilateral in origin from the thorax and abdomen. It has also been used for chronic pain management. Some of the commonly reported indications for a TPVB are listed in Table 30.1.

Functional Anatomy

The TPVS is a wedge-shaped space located on either side of the thoracic vertebral column and behind the parietal pleura (retropleural) (Fig. 30.1). The TPVS is wider on the left than on the right. The base of the TPVS is formed by the vertebral body, the intervertebral disc and the intervertebral foramen with its contents (Fig. 30.1). The parietal pleura forms the

Table 30.1 Indications of thoracic paravertebral block

A. Surgical anaesthesia
1. Breast surgery
2. Herniorrhaphy
3. Percutaneous radiofrequency ablation of liver tumours
B. Perioperative analgesia
1. Breast surgery
2. Thoracic surgery—Open thoracotomy, video-assisted thoracoscopic surgery
3. Minimally invasive cardiac surgery
4. Inguinal herniorrhaphy
5. Cholecystectomy
6. Appendicectomy
7. Renal and ureteric surgeries
8. Liver resection
C. Acute and chronic pain management
1. Acute postherpetic neuralgia
2. Fracture ribs
3. Pain due to stretching of liver capsule (trauma or liver mass)
4. Benign and malignant neuralgia
5. Complex regional pain syndrome
D. Miscellaneous
1. Therapeutic control of hyperhidrosis
2. Liver capsule pain after blunt abdominal trauma

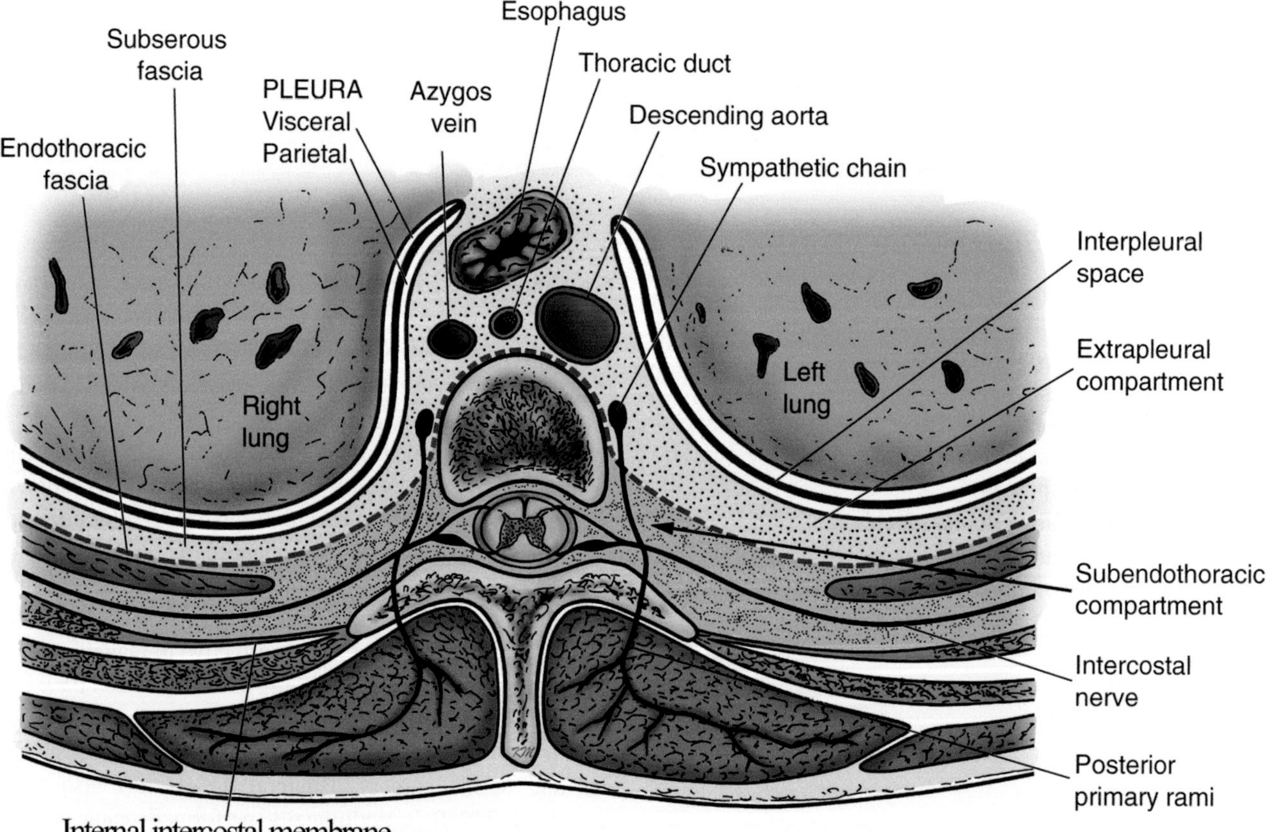

Fig. 30.1 Transverse anatomy of the thoracic paravertebral space. (The figure is reproduced with kind permission from www.aic.cuhk.edu.hk/usgraweb)

anterolateral boundary while the superior costotransverse ligament (SCTL), which extends from the lower border of the transverse process (TP) above to the upper border of the rib below, forms the posterior boundary of the TPVS (Figs. 30.2, 30.3, and 30.4). The inter-transverse ligament, which is much thinner than the SCTL, also extends between the adjacent transverse processes (Figs. 30.3 and 30.4). The SCTL is continuous laterally with the internal intercostal

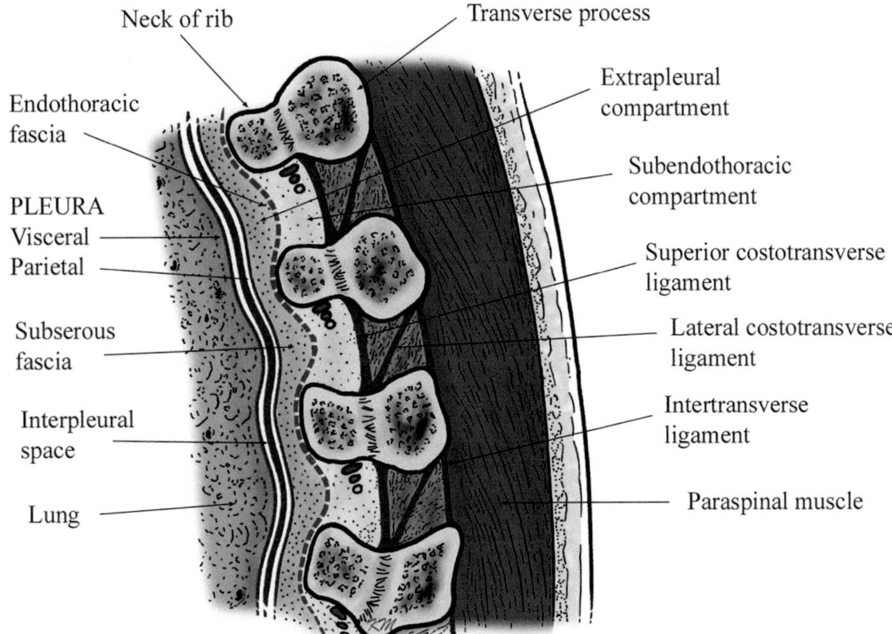

Fig. 30.2 Sagittal anatomy of the thoracic paravertebral space. (The figure is reproduced with kind permission from www.aic.cuhk.edu.hk/usgraweb)

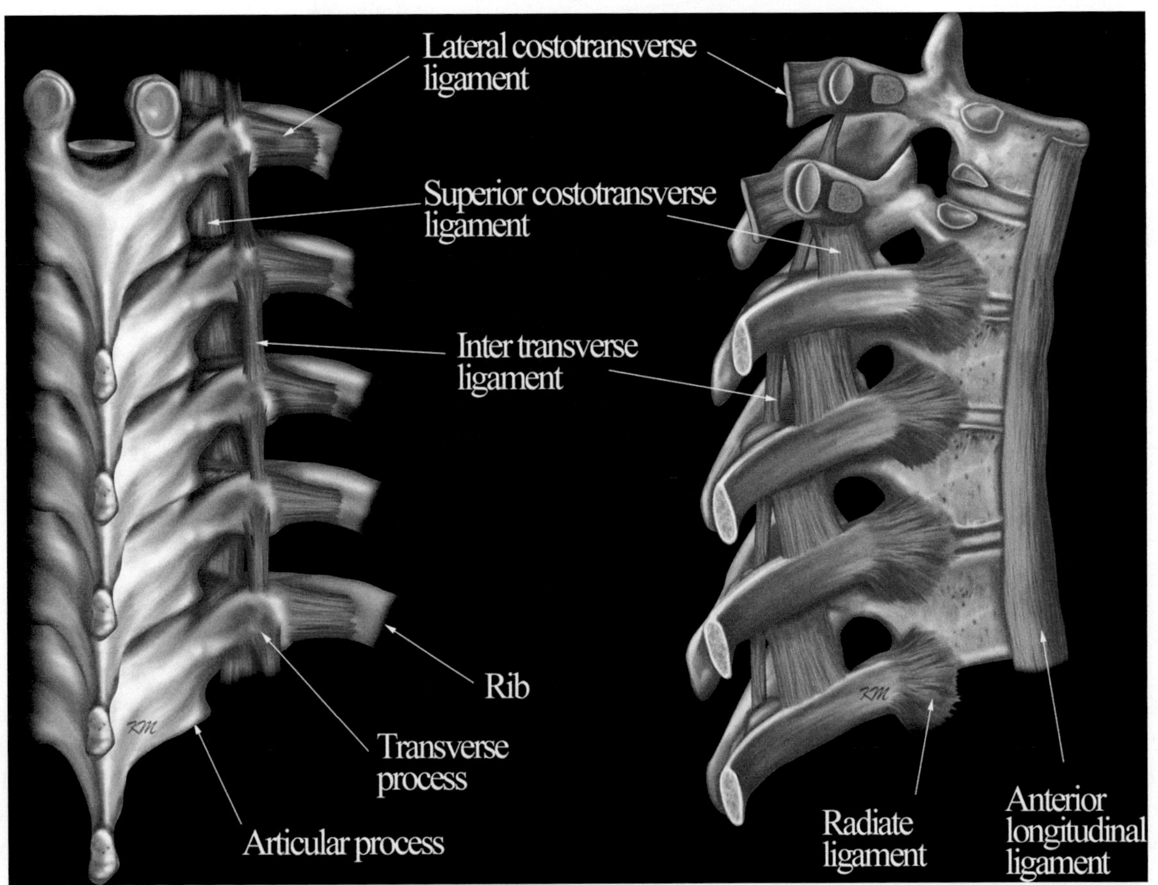

Fig. 30.3 Ligaments attached to the transverse process of the thoracic vertebra. (The figure is reproduced with kind permission from www.aic.cuhk.edu.hk/usgraweb)

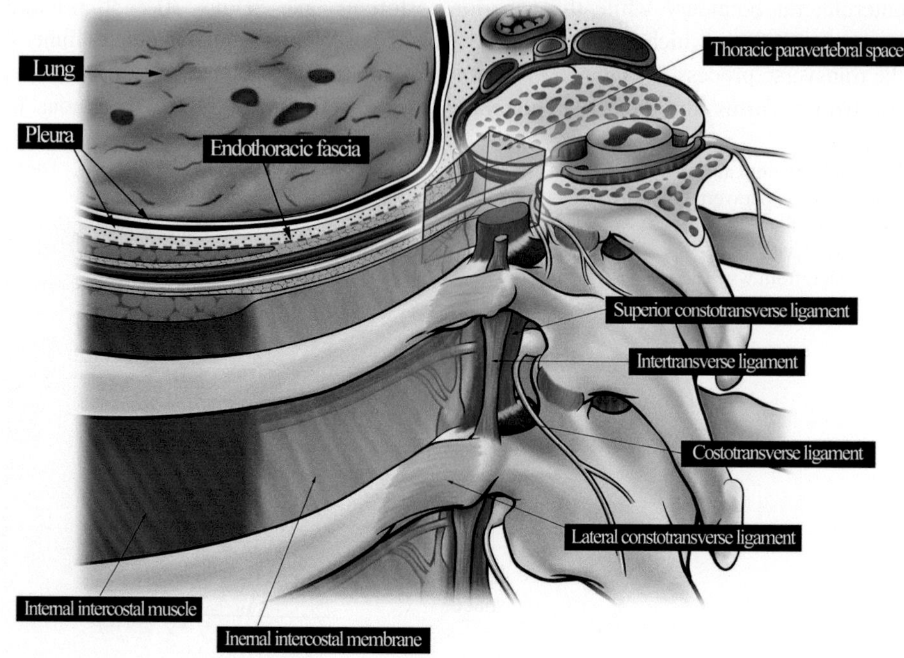

Fig. 30.4 Anatomy of the thoracic paravertebral region showing the various paravertebral ligaments and their anatomical relationship to the thoracic paravertebral space. (The figure is reproduced with kind permission from www.aic.cuhk.edu.hk/usgraweb)

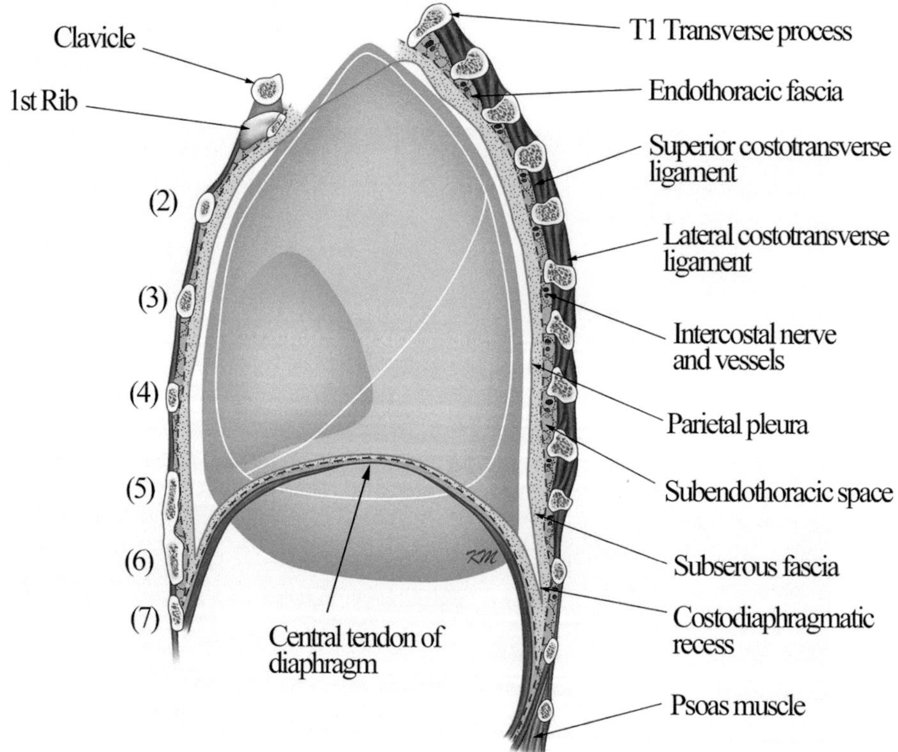

Fig. 30.5 Paravertebral sagittal section of the thorax showing how the endothoracic fascia, represented by the broken purple line, lines the internal aspect of the thoracic cage. Note the location of the neurovascular bundle in relation to the endothoracic fascia and its continuity with the psoas fascia inferiorly. (The figure is reproduced with kind pcrmission from www.aic.cuhk.edu.hk/usgraweb)

membrane (IICM) (Fig. 30.4), which is the medial extension of the internal intercostal muscle, and the apex of the TPVS is continuous with the posterior intercostal space (PICS) lateral to the tip of the TP (Fig. 30.4).

Interposed between the parietal pleura anteriorly and the SCTL posteriorly is a fibroelastic structure of the 'endothoracic fascia' (Figs. 30.1 and 30.2), which is the deep fascia of the thorax and lines the internal aspect of the thoracic cage (Figs. 30.5 and 30.6). At the TPVS, the endothoracic fascia is loosely attached to the ribs (Fig. 30.6) and the TP and fuses medially with the periosteum of the vertebral body close to its mid-point (Fig. 30.6). There is an intervening layer of loose areolar connective tissue, 'the subserous fascia', between the parietal pleura and the endothoracic fascia

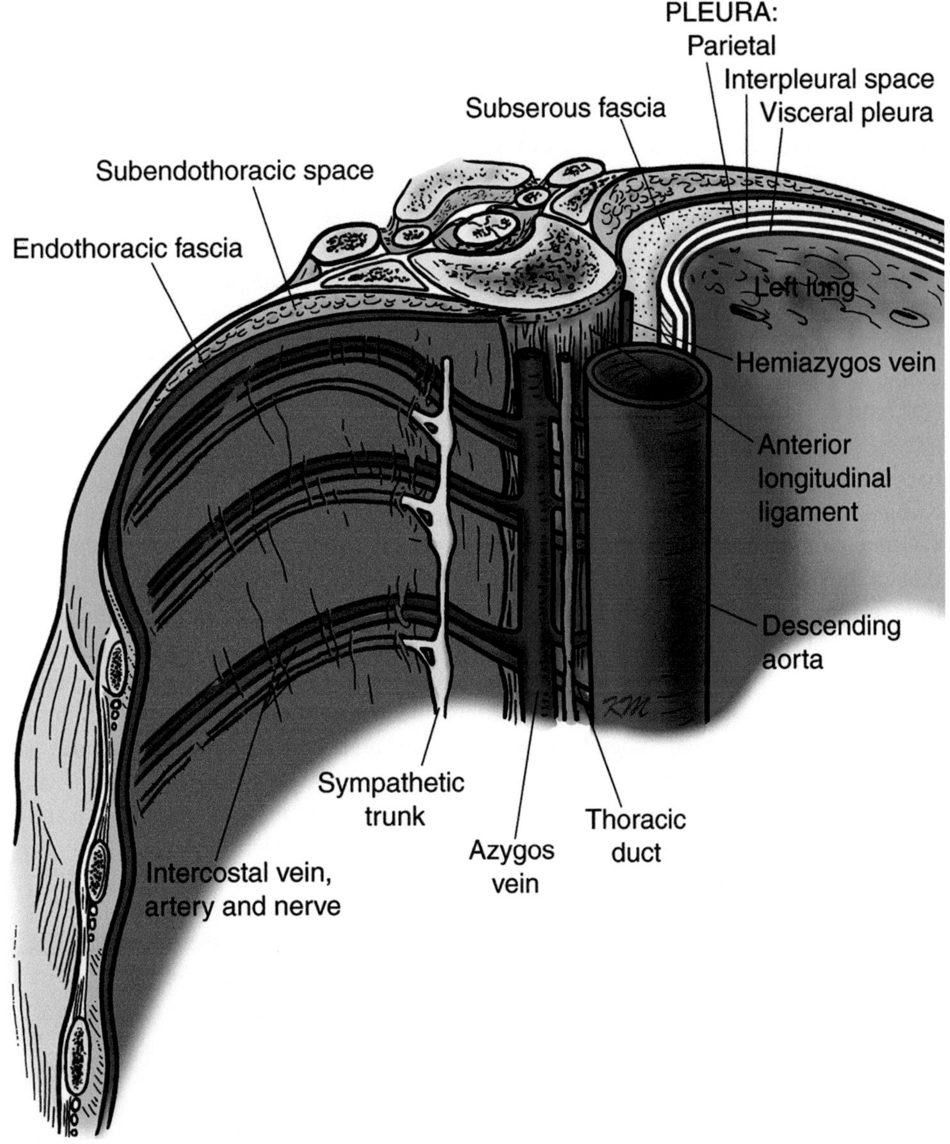

Fig. 30.6 The endothoracic fascia and its anatomical relationship to the thoracic paravertebral space. Note the fascial compartments and the location of the neurovascular structures in relation to the endothoracic fascia. (The figure is reproduced with kind permission from www.aic.cuhk.edu.hk/usgraweb)

(Figs. 30.1 and 30.2). The 'endothoracic fascia' thus divides the TPVS into two potential fascial compartments, the anterior 'extrapleural paravertebral compartment' and the posterior 'subendothoracic paravertebral compartment' (Figs. 30.1 and 30.2). The TPVS contains fatty tissue within which lie the intercostal (spinal) nerve, the dorsal ramus, intercostal vessels, rami communicantes and anteriorly the sympathetic chain (Fig. 30.1). The spinal nerves in the TPVS divide into multiple small bundles that lie freely among the fatty tissue. They are also devoid of a fascial sheath, which make them vulnerable to the effects of the injected LA during a TPVB. The intercostal nerve and vessels are located behind the endothoracic fascia, while the sympathetic trunk is located anterior to it in the TPVS (Figs. 30.4 and 30.6).

The TPVS is continuous with the epidural space medially via the intervertebral foramen, the intercostal space laterally; and the contralateral TPVS via the epidural and prevertebral space (Fig. 30.1). The cranial extension of the TPVS is still not defined, but we have observed direct paravertebral spread of radio-opaque contrast medium from the thoracic to the cervical region, indicating that there may be a direct anatomical continuity between the thoracic and cervical paravertebral regions. In clinical practice, ipsilateral Horner syndrome after thoracic paravertebral injections is also not uncommon. Nevertheless, the anatomical pathway for the spread of LA from the thoracic to the cervical paravertebral space is still not clear. The endothoracic fascia is continuous superiorly with the scalene or Sibson's fascia and attached to the medial border of the first rib anteriorly and the TP of the seventh cervical vertebra posteriorly. Therefore, an injection posterior to the endothoracic fascia in the subendothoracic paravertebral compartment of the upper thoracic region is unlikely to spread cranially via the paravertebral space because of the attachment of the endothoracic fascia to the TP. However, we believe that an injection anterior to the endothoracic fascia in the extrapleural paravertebral compartment may spread to the cervical paravertebral region via the subserous layer of connective tissue. The latter also provides the connective tissue support for the mediastinal structures and is continuous with the connective tissue investing the neurovascular structures at the root of the neck.

There is controversy about the caudal boundary of the TPVS. Caudal spread of a thoracic paravertebral injection is considered implausible as the TPVS is limited caudally by the origin of the psoas major muscle. However, ipsilateral lumbar spinal nerves are occasionally involved after a lower thoracic paravertebral injection. Saito and colleagues have also demonstrated ipsilateral thoracolumbar spread of coloured dye in cadavers. We have also observed radiological spread of contrast below the diaphragm and ipsilateral thoracolumbar anaesthesia after a TPVB. These observations challenge the concept of lumbar nerve root sparing following a TPVB. The exact mechanism for the ipsilateral thoracolumbar spread of LA or the contrast medium is still not clear, but it is suggested that it occurs either due to epidural spread or extended subendothoracic fascial spread (Fig. 30.7) to the retroperitoneal space, posterior to the facia transversalis, where the ilioinguinal and iliohypogastric nerves are located.

Sonoanatomy Relevant for Thoracic Paravertebral Block

Basic Considerations

An ultrasound scan for TPVB can be performed in the transverse (axial scan) or sagittal (longitudinal scan) axis and with the patient in the sitting, lateral decubitus or prone position. The prone position is preferred in patients undergoing USG TPVB for chronic pain procedure because it also allows the concurrent use of fluoroscopy. Currently, there are no data demonstrating an optimal axis for the ultrasound scan or the intervention. It is often a matter of individual choice or experience of the proceduralist. The transducer of choice for the ultrasound scan also depends on the body habitus of the patient. A review of the literature indicates that high-frequency ultrasound (12–5 MHz) is more frequently used for USG TPVB than low-frequency ultrasound. This may be because the relevant anatomical structures (TP, SCTL and pleura) are relatively shallow in location, and high-frequency ultrasound, despite its limited penetration, provides higher resolution of these structures than low-frequency ultrasound. However, in patients with large body habitus or when one has to scan at a depth, then a low-frequency ultrasound transducer (5–2 MHz) with a divergent beam and a wide field of view may be preferable. Published data using low-frequency ultrasound for

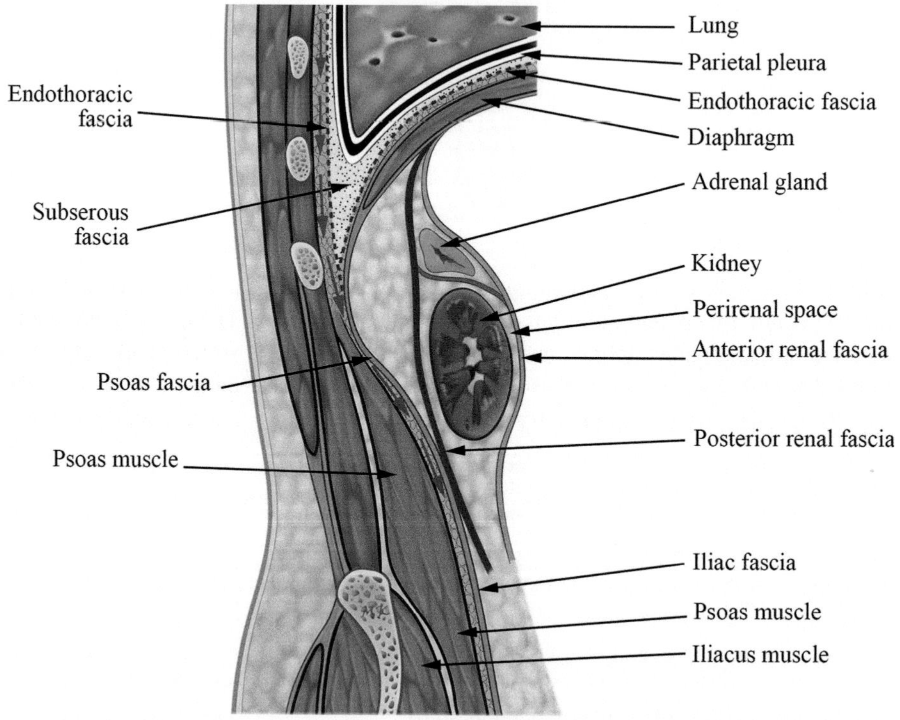

Fig. 30.7 Sagittal section of the thoracolumbar region showing the fascial relations of the lower thoracic paravertebral space and the retroperitoneal space. The pathway for the direct spread of local anaesthetic from the thoracic to the lumbar paravertebral region, along the subendothoracic paravertebral compartment, is shown using red arrows. (The figure is reproduced with kind permission from www.aic.cuhk.edu.hk/usgraweb)

TPVB in clinical practice is sparse, but contrary to common understanding (poor resolution), we have been using low-frequency ultrasound (2–5 MHz) to perform a transverse scan of the thoracic paravertebral region and guide the block needle in real-time with great success (details below).

Transverse Scan of the Thoracic Paravertebral Region

For a transverse scan of the thoracic paravertebral region, a high-frequency linear array transducer is positioned lateral to the thoracic spinous process, at the target vertebral level, with the orientation marker directed laterally (Fig. 30.8). On a transverse sonogram, the paraspinal muscles are clearly delineated and lie superficial to the TP. The TP is seen as a rounded hyperechoic structure, anterior to which there is a dark acoustic shadow which completely obscures the TPVS (Fig. 30.8). Lateral to the TP, the hyperechoic pleura that moves with respiration and exhibits the typical 'lung sliding sign' is seen. Comet tail artefacts, which are reverberation artefacts, may also be visualized deep to the pleura and within the lung tissue and are often synchronous with respiration. A hypoechoic space is also seen between the parietal pleura and the IICM laterally, which represents the medial limit of the PICS or the apex of the TPVS (Fig. 30.8), and the two communicate with each other (Fig. 30.4). Therefore, LA injected medially into the TPVS can often be seen to spread laterally to distend this space or vice versa. LA injected laterally into this space can spread medially to the paravertebral space. The latter is the anatomic basis for the intercostal approach for USG TPVB where the needle is inserted in the plane of the ultrasound beam from a lateral to medial direction (*see below*). The SCTL which forms the posterior border of the TPVS is also visible, and it blends laterally with the IICM, which forms the posterior border of the posterior intercostal space (Fig. 30.4). The communication between the TPVS and the PICS can also be visualized laterally (Fig. 30.9).

We have recently evaluated the use of a low-frequency (5–2 MHz) curved array transducer to perform a transverse scan of the thoracic paravertebral region and USG TPVB. To the best of our knowledge, there are limited published data describing the use of a low-frequency ultrasound for USG TPVB. Our preliminary experience is that excellent ultrasound images of the paravertebral region are obtained using a low frequency transducer (Fig. 30.10). Also the wide field of view, produced by the divergent ultrasound beam, is an added advantage when compared to the narrow rectangular field of view produced by a linear array transducer during the USG TPVB. Using a curved array transducer, the transverse scan is performed sequentially over three contiguous osseous anatomical sites at the target vertebral level (Fig. 30.11) for consistency and to better define the relevant sonoanatomy; (1) Position 1: at the level of the transverse process-rib complex (Fig. 30.11a, green box), (2) Position 2: at the level of the transverse process (Fig. 30.11a, yellow box) and (3) Position 3: at the level of the articular process (Fig. 30.11a, b, red box). Based on the underlying osseous and musculoskeletal

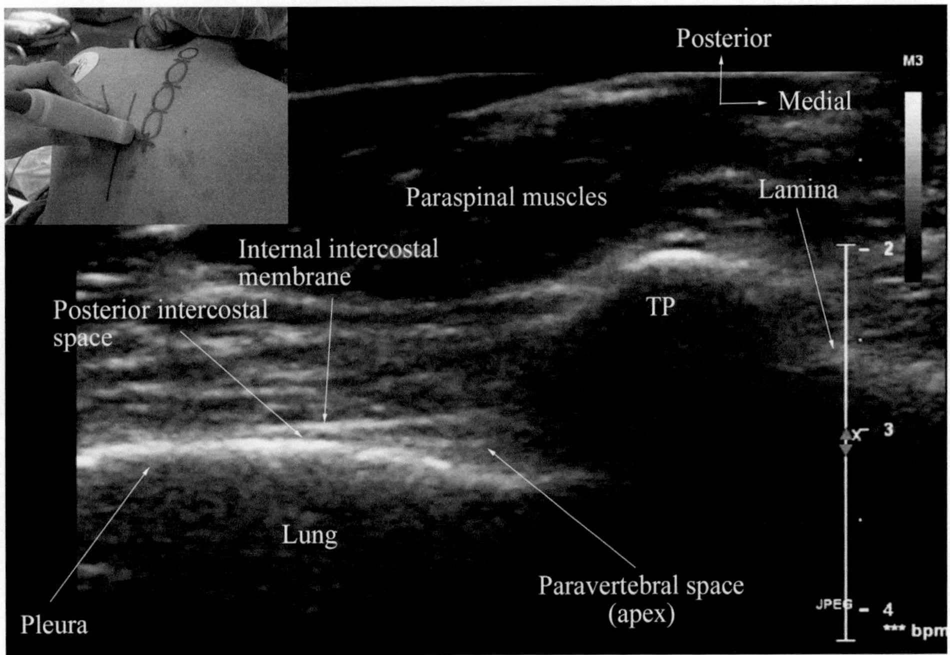

Fig. 30.8 Transverse sonogram of the right thoracic paravertebral region using a high-frequency linear transducer with the ultrasound beam being insonated over the transverse process (TP). Note how the acoustic shadow of the TP obscures the thoracic paravertebral space (TPVS). The hypoechoic space posterior to the parietal pleura and anterolateral to the TP is the apex of the TPVS or the medial limit of the posterior intercostal space. Inset image (top left) is showing the position and orientation of the ultrasound transducer with the patient in the sitting position. (The figure is reproduced with kind permission from www.aic.cuhk.edu.hk/usgraweb)

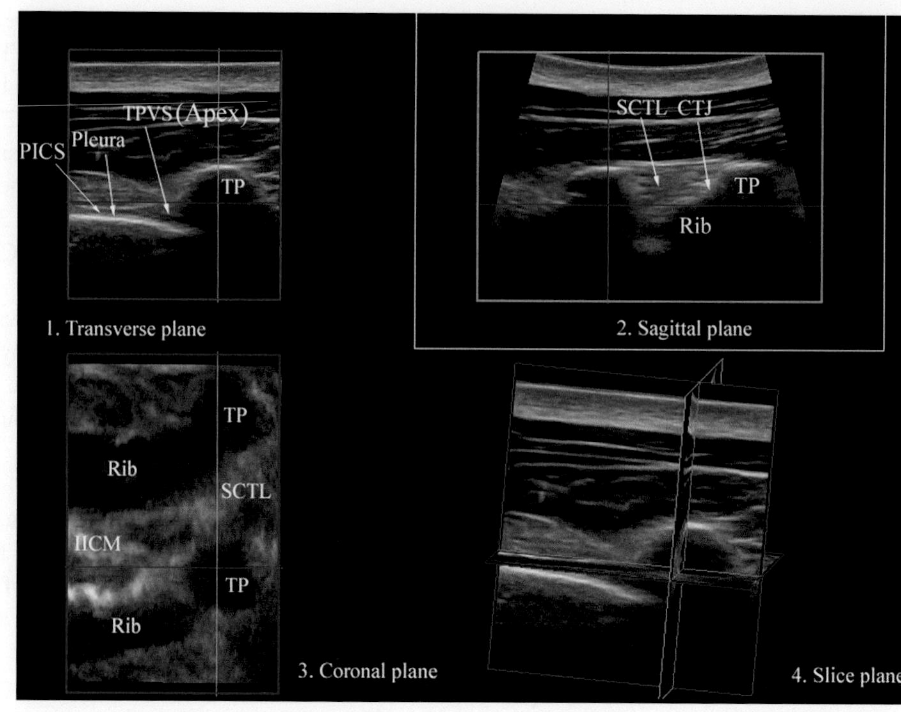

Fig. 30.9 A multiplanar 3D ultrasound view of the thoracic paravertebral region with the reference marker or 'marker dot' placed over the transverse process (TP). Note how the three slice planes (red—transverse, green—sagittal and blue—coronal) have been obtained and how the superior costotransverse ligament (SCTL) is continuous with the internal intercostal membrane (IICM) laterally in the coronal plane. *TPVS* thoracic paravertebral space, *PICS* posterior intercostal space, *CTJ* costotransverse junction. (The figure is reproduced with kind permission from www.aic.cuhk.edu.hk/usgraweb)

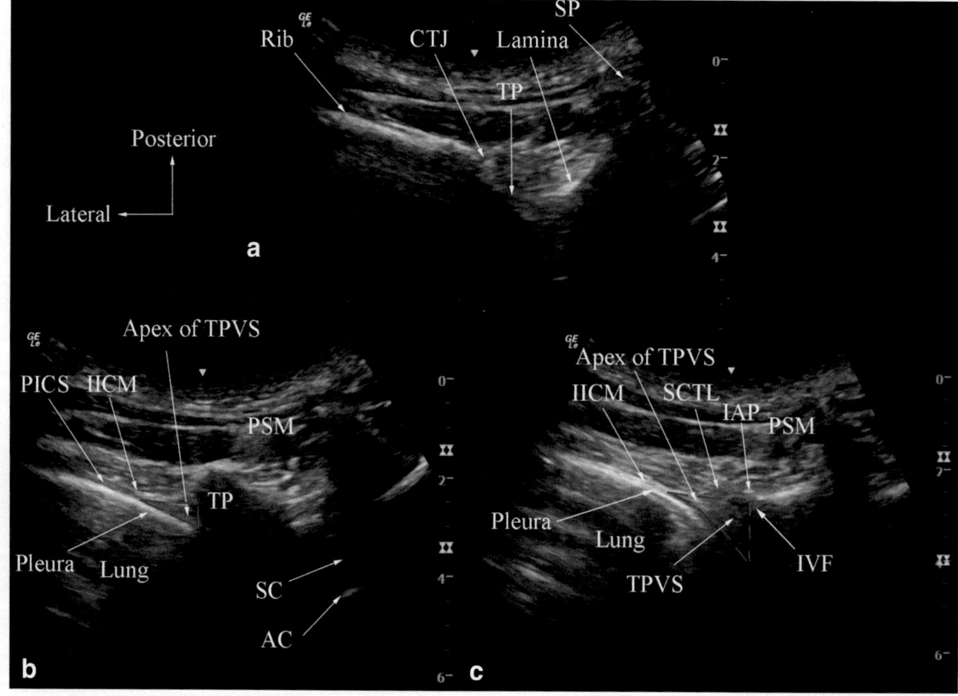

Fig. 30.10 Paramedian transverse sonograms of the thoracic paravertebral region with the ultrasound beam being insonated (**a**) at the level of the rib and transverse process (position 1 in Fig. 30.11), (**b**) at the level of the transverse process (position 2 in Fig. 30.11), and (**c**) at the level of the inferior articular process (position 3 in Fig. 30.11). *SP* spinous process, *TP* transverse process, *CTJ* costotransverse junction, *PSM* paraspinal muscles, *TPVS* thoracic paravertebral space, *IICM* internal intercostal membrane, *PICS* posterior intercostal space, *SC* spinal canal, *AC* anterior complex, *IAP* inferior articular process, *SCTL* superior costotransverse ligament, *IVF* intervertebral foramen. (The figure is reproduced with kind permission from www.aic.cuhk.edu.hk/usgraweb)

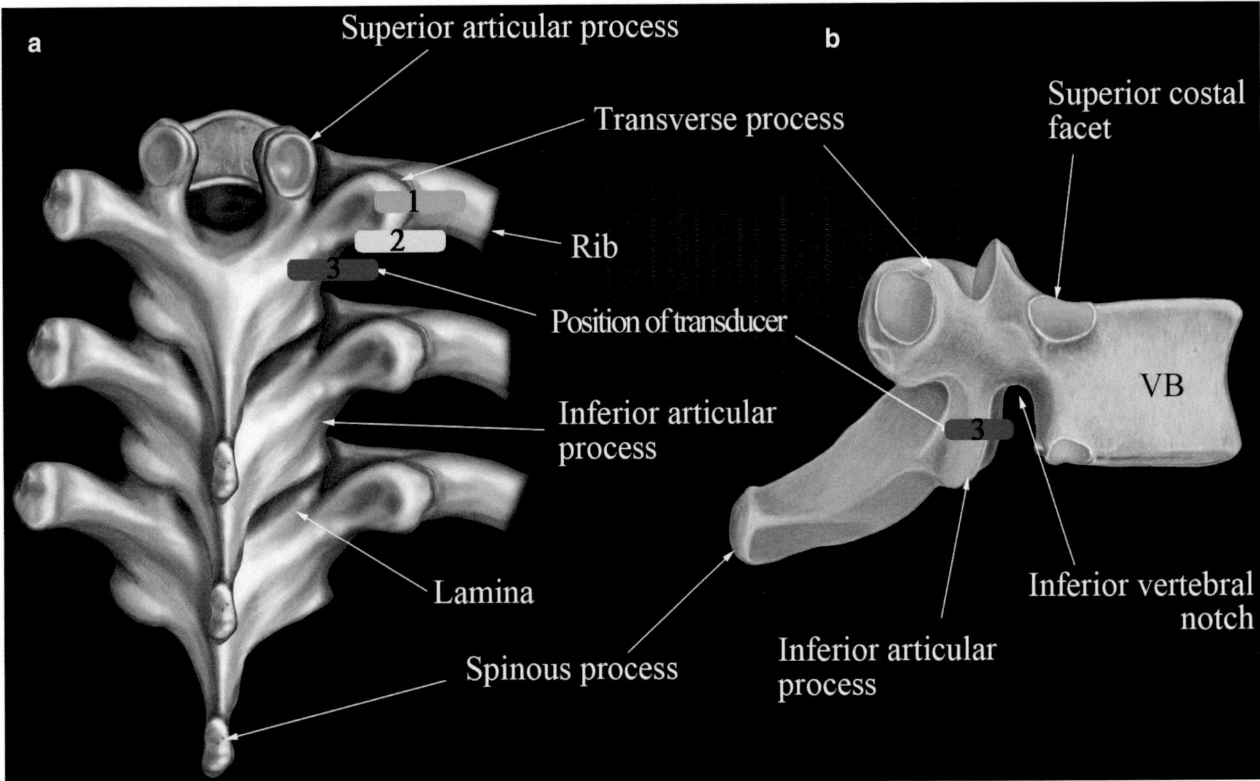

Fig. 30.11 (**a**) Posterior view: Figure illustrating the various positions of the ultrasound transducer, relative to the osseous structures of the thoracic spine, during the ultrasound scan sequence described. Position 1: at the level of the rib and transverse process; position 2: at the level of the transverse process; position 3: at the level of the inferior articular process. (**b**) Lateral view: Note the relationship of the inferior articular process to the inferior vertebral notch and the intervertebral foramen. (The figure is reproduced with kind permission from www.aic.cuhk.edu.hk/usgraweb)

anatomy, each of these three ultrasound scan windows produce three distinct sonograms (Fig. 30.10). Correlative cadaver anatomical-CT-MRI and ultrasound images for positions 2 and 3 of the transverse scan sequence described above are presented in Figs. 30.12 and 30.13.

Step 1: Transverse scan at the level of the transverse process-rib complex. The transducer is positioned 2–3 cm lateral to the midline, at the target vertebral level, in the transverse plane and over the rib and costotransverse articulation (position 1, green box). The hyperechogenic outlines of the spinous process, lamina, TP, costo-transverse junction and the rib with their corresponding acoustic shadows are clearly delineated from a medial to lateral direction (Fig. 30.10a). The posterior angulation of the TP of the thoracic vertebra (Fig. 30.14) is also easily recognized (Fig. 30.10a). This is in contrast to the TP of the lumbar vertebra which is more or less at right angles to the vertebral body (Fig. 30.14). This ultrasound window does not lend itself to visualizing the paravertebral anatomy because the acoustic shadow of the TP-rib complex completely obscures the TPVS (Fig. 30.10a). Therefore, it is used more as a starting point for the subsequent steps in the transverse scan sequence.

Step 2: Transverse scan at the level of the transverse process. From position 1, one can gently slide the transducer caudally until the acoustic shadow of the rib is no longer visualized (Fig. 30.11, position 2, yellow box), and the hyperechogenic outline of the lamina and TP with their acoustic shadow are visualized (Fig. 30.10b). Lateral to the TP, one can define the IICM posteriorly and the hyperechogenic pleura and lung anteriorly. Interposed between the two is the hypoechoic apical part of the TPVS (Fig. 30.10b). The PICS may also be visualized in continuity with the apex of the TPVS laterally (Fig. 30.10b).

Step 3: Transverse scan at the level of the articular process: Finally, if one now slides the transducer slightly caudally from position 2 (Fig. 30.11, position 3, red box), the acoustic shadow of the lamina and transverse process disappear, and the echogenic inferior articular process (Fig. 30.10c) with its acoustic shadow is now visualized medially. This acoustic window represents the transverse-intertransverse view of the TPVS. As in the scan at the level of the TP

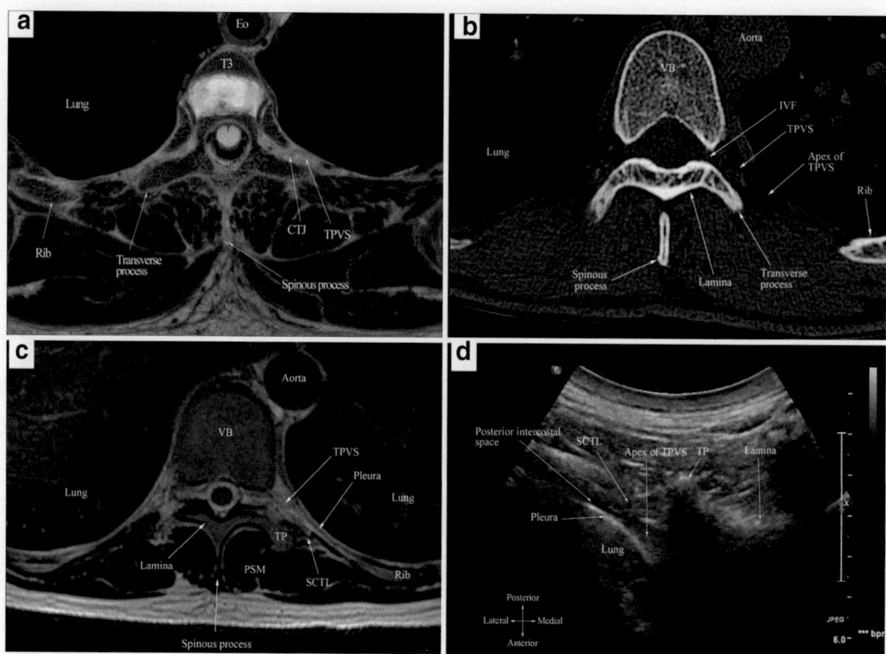

Fig. 30.12 Correlative transverse cadaver anatomic (**a**), CT (**b**), MRI (T1 weighted, **c**) and ultrasound (**d**) images of the thoracic paravertebral region from the level of the vertebral body and transverse process corresponding to the level at which the transverse scan is performed (position 2, Fig. 30.11). *Eo* oesophagus, *CTJ* costotransverse junction, *TPVS* thoracic paravertebral space, *VB* vertebral body, *PSM* paraspinal muscle, *IVF* intervertebral foramen, *TP* transverse process, *SCTL* superior costotransverse ligament. (The figure is reproduced with kind permission from www.aic.cuhk.edu.hk/usgraweb)

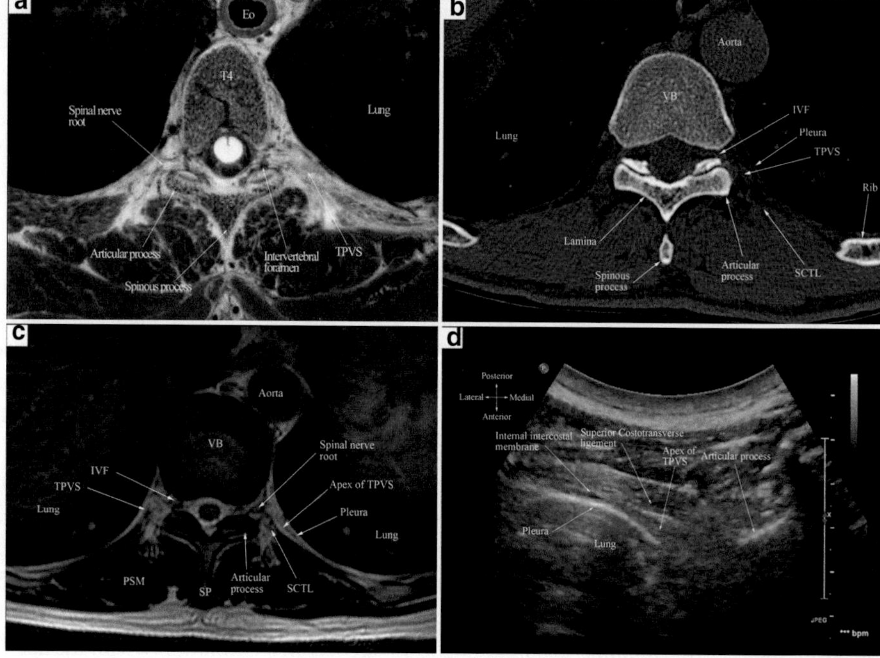

Fig. 30.13 Correlative transverse cadaver anatomic (**a**), CT (**b**), MRI (T1 weighted, **c**) and ultrasound (**d**) images of the thoracic paravertebral region from the level of the vertebral body and inferior articular process corresponding to the level at which the transverse scan is performed (position 3, Fig. 30.11). *TPVS* thoracic paravertebral space, *VB* vertebral body, *PSM* paraspinal muscle, *IVF* intervertebral foramen, *SCTL* superior costotransverse ligament, *SP* spinous process. (The figure is reproduced with kind permission from www.aic.cuhk.edu.hk/usgraweb)

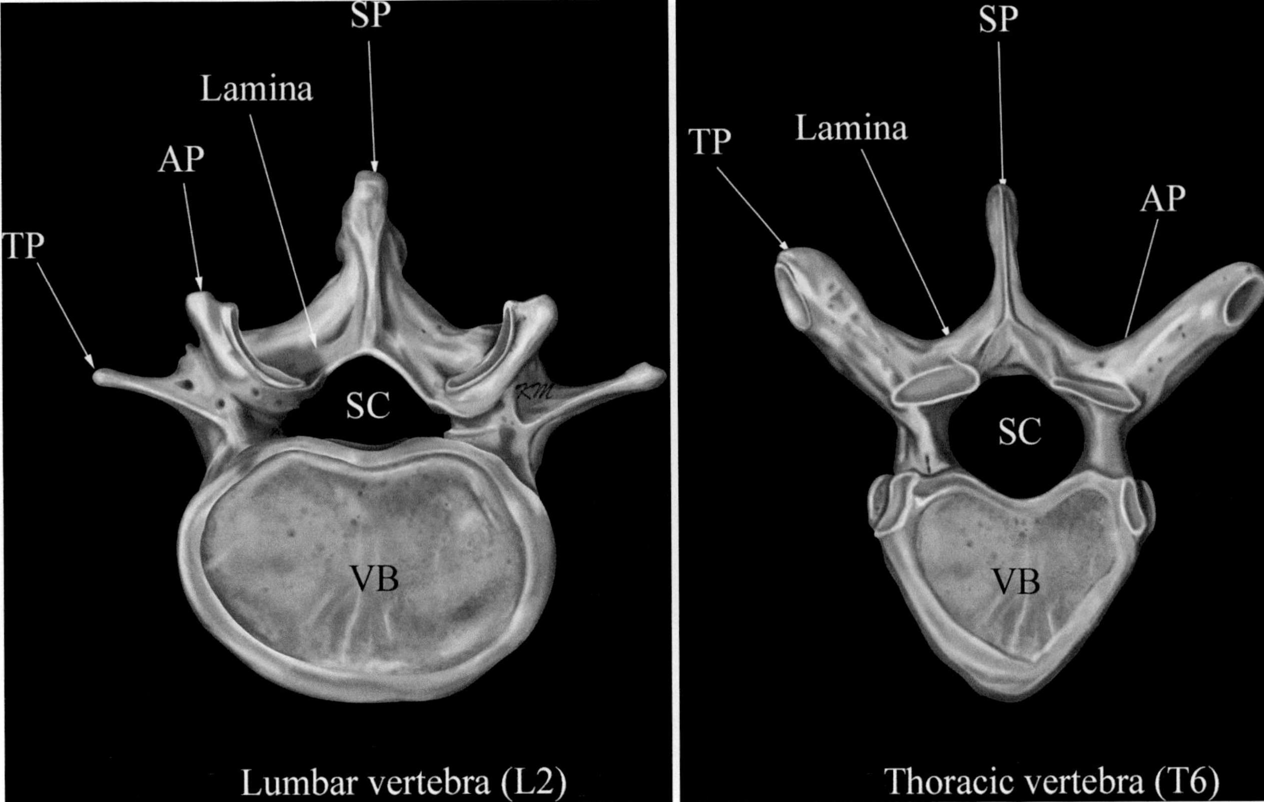

Fig. 30.14 Figure showing the difference in the size, shape and orientation of the transverse process (TP) of a thoracic and lumbar vertebra. Note how the TP of a thoracic vertebra is directed posteriorly. *SP* spinous process, *AP* articular process, *TP* transverse process, *SC* spinal canal, *VB* vertebral body. (The figure is reproduced with kind permission from www.aic.cuhk.edu.hk/usgraweb)

(Position 2, Fig. 30.10b), the SCTL, parietal pleura, lung and the apical part of the paravertebral space are clearly delineated. However, the area of the acoustic shadow at the level of the articular process is significantly less than that at the level of the TP. As a result, one can visualize majority of the TPVS with this view (Fig. 30.10c). Currently, there are limited published data describing the use of a transverse scan at the level of the articular process for USG TPVB.

Sagittal Scan of the Thoracic Paravertebral Region

For a sagittal scan of the thoracic paravertebral region, a high-frequency linear transducer (12–5 MHz) is positioned 2–3 cm lateral to the midline (paramedian), with its orientation marker directed cranially, at the target vertebral level (Fig. 30.15). This ultrasound window (paramedian sagittal) clearly delineates the transverse processes as rounded hyperechoic structures, with its acoustic shadow anteriorly, deep to the paraspinal muscles (Fig. 30.15). One can also appreciate the acoustic window between the contiguous transverse processes produced by reflections from the SCTL, intertransverse ligament, TPVS with its contents, hyperechoic parietal pleura and the underlying lung tissue, from a posterior to anterior direction. (Fig. 30.15). In the resultant sagittal sonogram, the TPVS is seen as a hypoechoic space between the SCTL and the parietal pleura (Fig. 30.15). Doppler ultrasound can be used to define the intercostal vessels lying caudal to the transverse process (Fig. 30.16), but we have not been able to delineate the intercostal nerve with current ultrasound technology.

We have observed that the underlying pleura and the TPVS are not clearly delineated in a true paramedian sagittal scan (Fig. 30.15). This may be due to 'anisotropy' because the ultrasound beam is not perpendicular to the anteromedial reflection of the parietal pleura near the vertebra in the paravertebral region. Loss of spatial resolution at the depth corresponding to the TPVS, from using high-frequency ultrasound, cannot also be excluded. Therefore, in order to

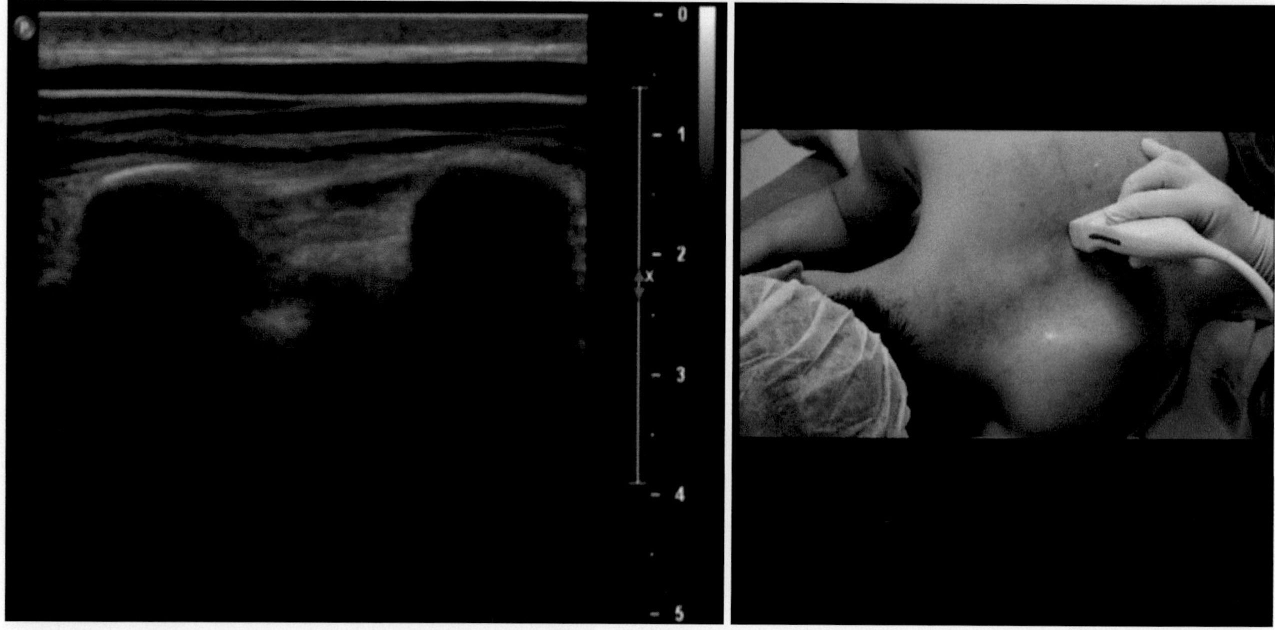

Fig. 30.15 Paramedian sagittal scan of the right mid-thoracic paravertebral region using a high-frequency linear transducer. Note the paravertebral structures including the parietal pleura and the paravertebral space are not clearly delineated in this image. *TP* transverse process, *SCTL* superior costotransverse ligament, *TPVS* thoracic paravertebral space. (The figure is reproduced with kind permission from www.aic.cuhk.edu.hk/usgraweb)

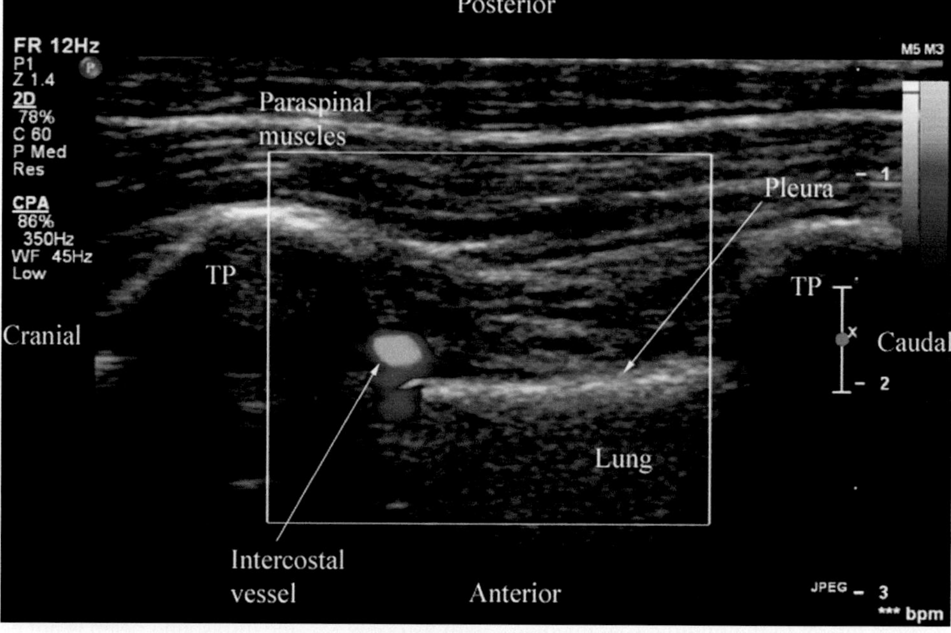

Fig. 30.16 Paramedian sagittal oblique sonogram of the thoracic paravertebral region showing the power Doppler signal from the intercostal artery at the apex of the paravertebral space. *TP* transverse process. (The figure is reproduced with kind permission from www.aic.cuhk.edu.hk/usgraweb)

minimize 'anisotropy' and to better visualize the underlying TP, SCTL, TPVS and the pleura, we recommend performing a 'paramedian sagittal oblique' scan. This is achieved by gently tilting the ultrasound transducer laterally (outward) until the underlying parietal pleura is clearly delineated (Fig. 30.17). We believe the lateral tilt directs the ultrasound beam perpendicular to the parietal pleura and thereby minimizes 'anisotropy'. A pitfall of the lateral tilt manoeuvre is that the proceduralist may unintentionally tilt or manipulate the transducer too far laterally so as to insonate the rib and posterior intercostal space rather than the TP and apical part of the TPVS (Fig. 30.18). The clinical implication is that the proceduralist may unknowingly perform a posterior intercostal injection instead of a paravertebral injection, and depending on the technique used, the potential for inadvertent pleural puncture may be greater with the intercostal

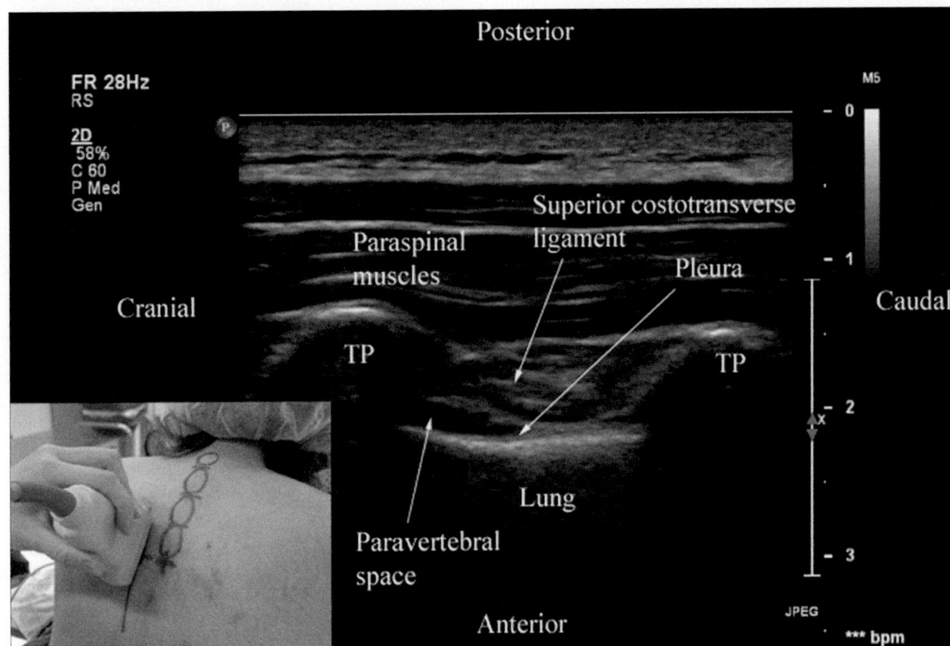

Fig. 30.17 Paramedian sagittal oblique sonogram of the thoracic paravertebral region. The picture in the inset shows how the ultrasound transducer is tilted slightly laterally (outwards) during the scan. Note the pleura, superior costotransverse ligament and the paravertebral space are clearly delineated in this sonogram. *TP* transverse process. (The figure is reproduced with kind permission from www.aic.cuhk.edu.hk/usgraweb)

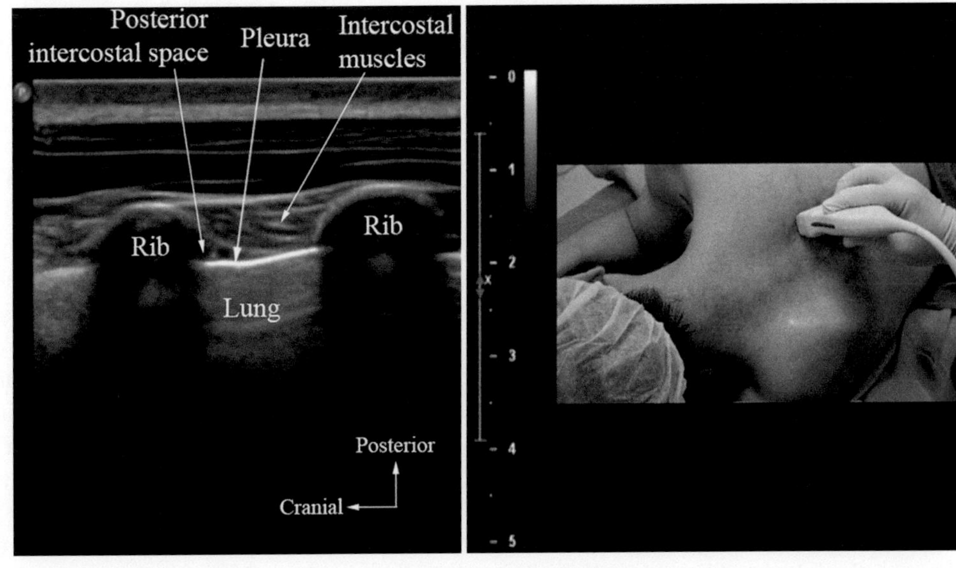

Fig. 30.18 Paramedian sagittal oblique scan of the right mid-thoracic paravertebral region, using a high-frequency linear transducer, whereby the ribs instead of the transverse processes are being insonated. Note the pleura is also very clearly delineated in this sonogram. (The figure is reproduced with kind permission from www.aic.cuhk.edu.hk/usgraweb)

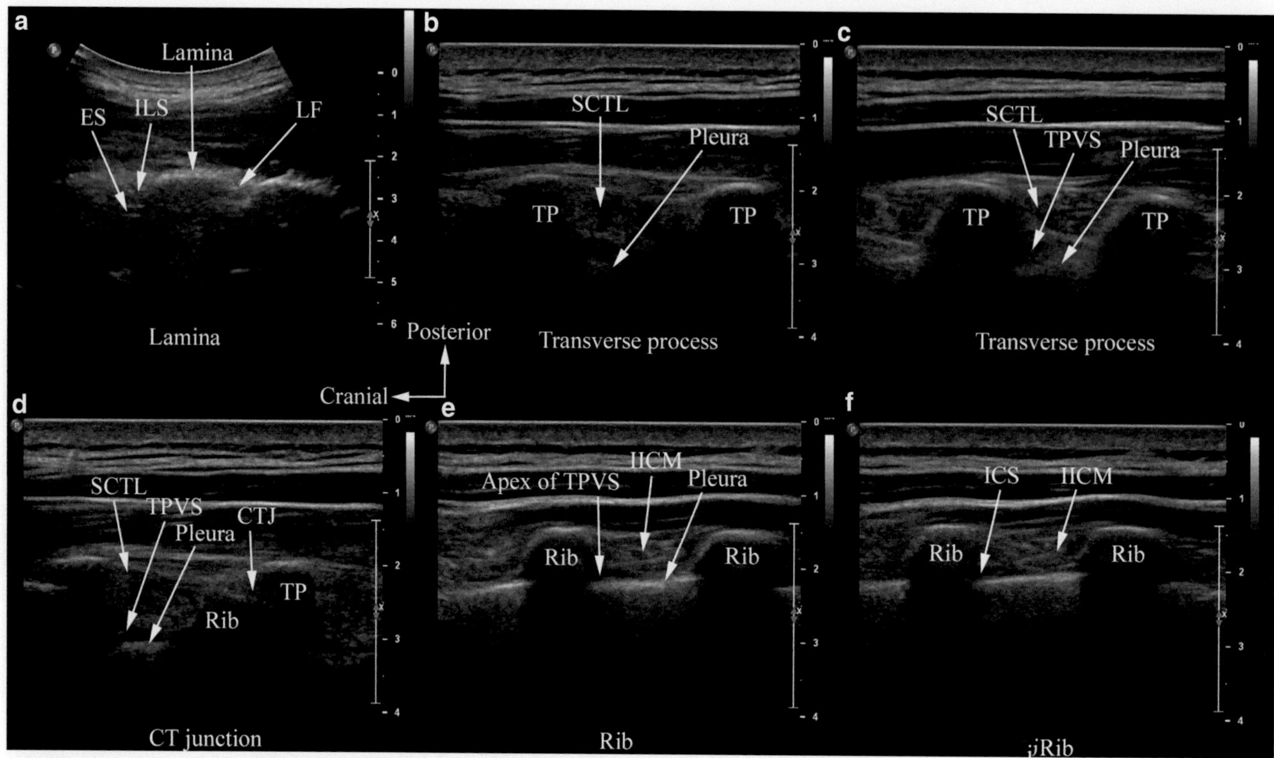

Fig. 30.19 A sequence of sagittal sonograms of the thoracic paravertebral region (from the same subject) showing the transition of the anatomy (medial to lateral) from the level of the lamina of the vertebra to the ribs. Note the difference in the sonographic appearance of the lamina (**a**), transverse process (TP) (**b**, **c**) and the ribs (**e**, **f**). Also note the relative depths at which each structure is located. The articulation of the rib with the transverse process at the CTJ (costotransverse junction) is also clearly delineated in (**d**). Also note that the pleura is not clearly visualized at the level of the TPs, but it is at the level of the ribs. *ES* epidural space, *ILS* interlaminar space, *LF* ligamentum flavum, *SCTL* superior costotransverse ligament, *TPVS* thoracic paravertebral space, *IICM* intercostal muscles, *ICS* intercostal space. (The figure is reproduced with kind permission from www.aic.cuhk.edu.hk/usgraweb)

injection. Also, the posterior intercostal injection may produce a totally different block dynamic, with limited segmental spread of the somatic and sympathetic nerve blockade, when compared to a TPVB. Therefore, when using a sagittal scan to perform USG TPVB, it is prudent to identify the subtle transition in sonoanatomy from the rib to the transverse process (Fig. 30.19).

Techniques Used for USG TPVB

Several different techniques have been described for USG TPVB. There are pros and cons of each technique, and they are highlighted in the following section. However, there is paucity of data comparing the safety and efficacy of the various approaches. Therefore, as described above, the choice of technique often depends on the preference and experience of the anaesthesiologist. Also although the literature indicates that USG TPVB is most frequently performed using a high-frequency linear transducer (12–5 MHz), the authors have been using a low-frequency curvilinear transducer (5–2 MHz) for USG TPVB for over a decade with excellent results and no major complications (details below). Overall USG TPVB can be performed using any one of the following five approaches.

Paramedian Sagittal Scan with Out-of-Plane Needle Insertion

This technique was originally described by Hara and colleagues. A paramedian sagittal scan is performed at the level of the TP at the target vertebral level as described above and the block needle is inserted out-of-plane. Since the block needle is inserted out-of-plane, and at a relatively steep angle, tracking the needle tip in real-time can be challenging. This may explain why Hara and colleagues used loss of resistance to saline injection, after contacting the TP, and sought sonographic evidence (turbulence within the TPVS and forward displacement of the parietal pleura) to confirm correct needle tip placement within the TPVS. Given that needle tip tracking is challenging, and there is the potential for inadvertent pleural puncture with this technique beginners should exercise caution when using this approach.

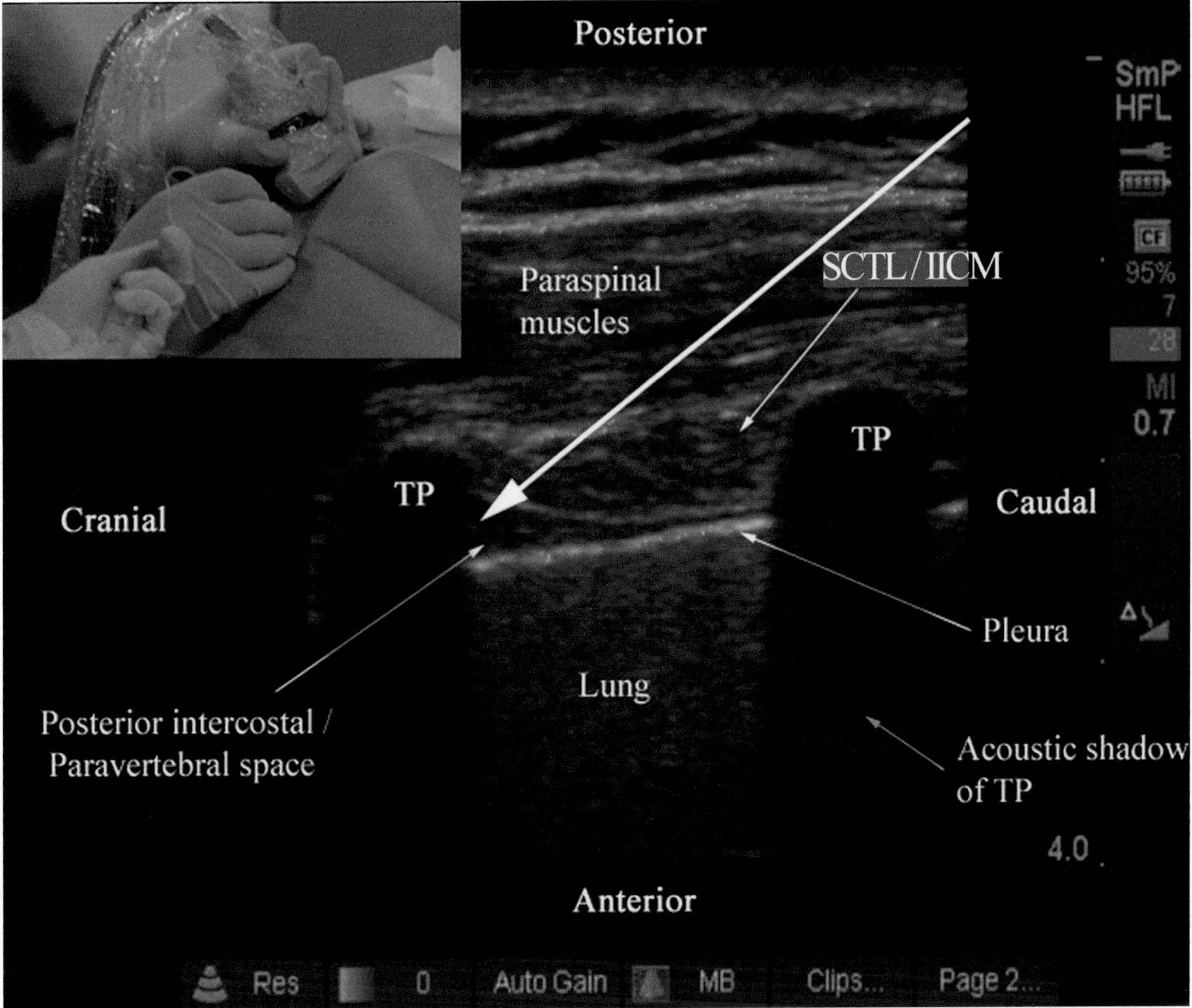

Fig. 30.20 Ultrasound-guided TPVB using a paramedian sagittal oblique scan. The long white arrow represents the direction in which the needle is inserted and the picture in the inset shows how the block needle is inserted in the long axis of the ultrasound plane. Visualizing the block needle with this approach can be very challenging. The picture in the inset also shows how the transducer is oriented and the direction in which the needle is inserted. *TP* transverse process, *SCTL/IICM* superior costotransverse ligament-internal intercostal membrane complex. (The figure is reproduced with kind permission from www.aic.cuhk.edu.hk/usgraweb)

Paramedian Sagittal Scan with In-Plane Needle Insertion

With this approach, a paramedian sagittal oblique scan is performed at the target vertebral level as described above, and the block needle is inserted in-plane and in a caudocranial direction (Fig. 30.20). Although the needle is inserted in-plane, visualizing and tracking the needle tip can be challenging with this technique. This may be because the block needle is inserted at an acute angle, and the ultrasound beam is also insonated with a slight outward (oblique) tilt for optimal ultrasound visibility of the pleura. Due to these limitations, we rarely use this approach although there are proponents of this technique. If one were to use this technique, then we recommend advancing the block needle under ultrasound guidance to deliberately contact the lower border of the TP after which the block needle is slightly withdrawn and re-advanced so as to pass under the lower border of the TP. A test bolus of normal saline (2–3 ml) is then injected, and sonographic evidence (pleural displacement) is sought to ensure that the tip of the block needle is in the TPVS (Fig. 30.21). A calculated dose of LA is then injected in small aliquots. Following the injection, it is common to see

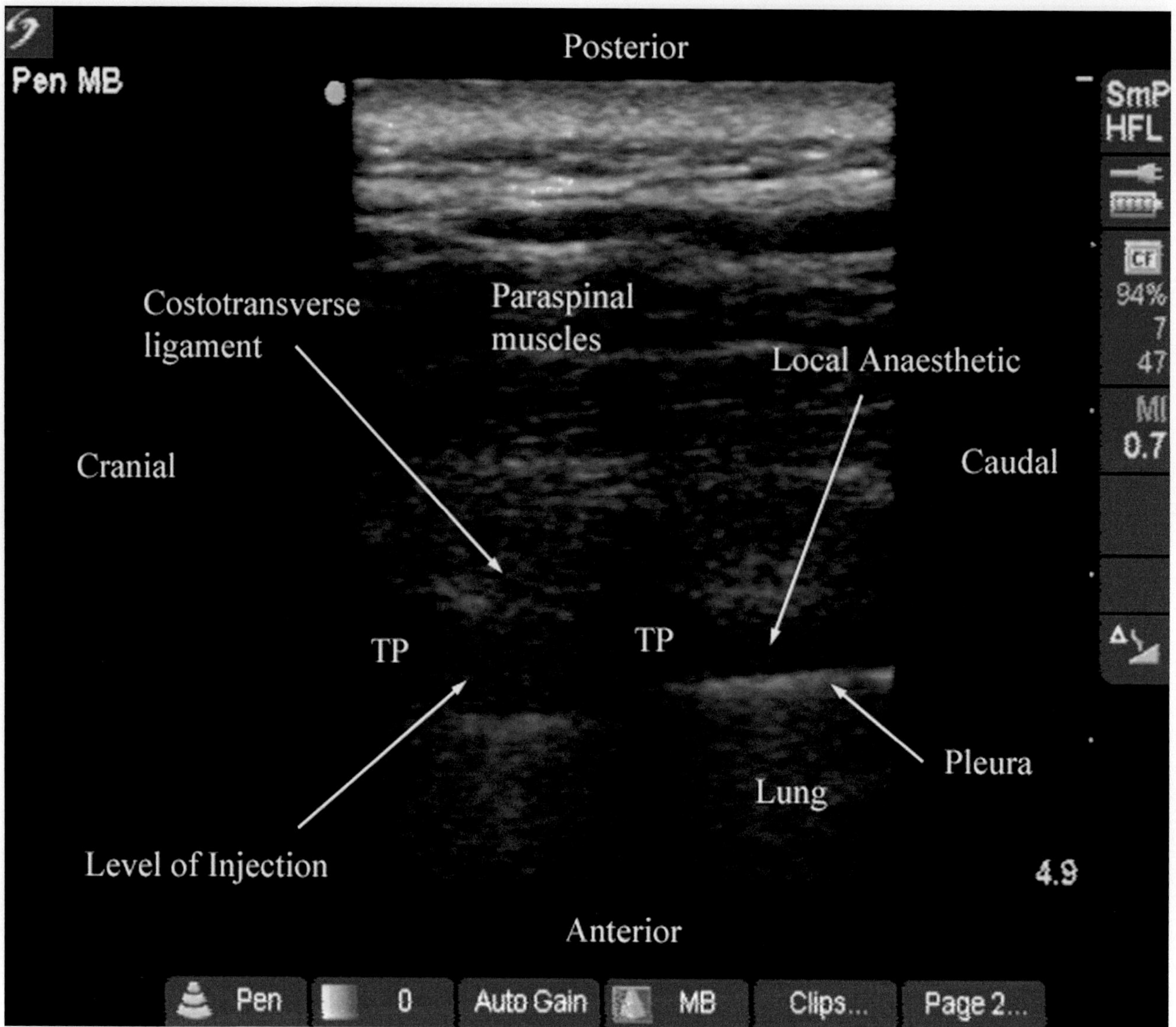

Fig. 30.21 Paramedian sagittal oblique sonogram of the TPVS after local anaesthetic injection. Note the widening of the paravertebral space and displacement of the parietal pleura. The local anaesthetic is also seen to have spread to the contiguous paravertebral space form the level of injection. *TP* transverse process. (The figure is reproduced with kind permission from www.aic.cuhk.edu.hk/usgraweb)

anterior displacement of the parietal pleura, widening of the paravertebral space and an increased echogenicity of the pleura (Fig. 30.21) that are objective signs of a correct injection into the TPVS. Spread of the injected LA to the contiguous paravertebral spaces may also be visualized in real-time (Fig. 30.21), confirming that the contiguous TPVS's communicate with each other.

Transverse Scan with Out-of-Plane Needle Insertion

With this technique, a transverse scan of the thoracic paravertebral region is performed at the desired vertebral level and at the level of the TP and the block needle inserted in the short axis of the ultrasound beam (Fig. 30.22). During the preview scan, the depth to the TP and pleura is determined. The direction of needle insertion with this approach mimics that with a surface anatomic landmark-based TPVB (Fig. 30.22). Since the needle is inserted in the short axis, it is visualized only as a bright spot, and needle tracking can be challenging. The aim of this approach is to guide the needle to the TP. Once the TP is contacted, the needle is withdrawn slightly and re-advanced by a predetermined distance of 1–1.5 cm so as to pass under the TP into the TPVS. Alternatively, the needle can be inserted laterally into

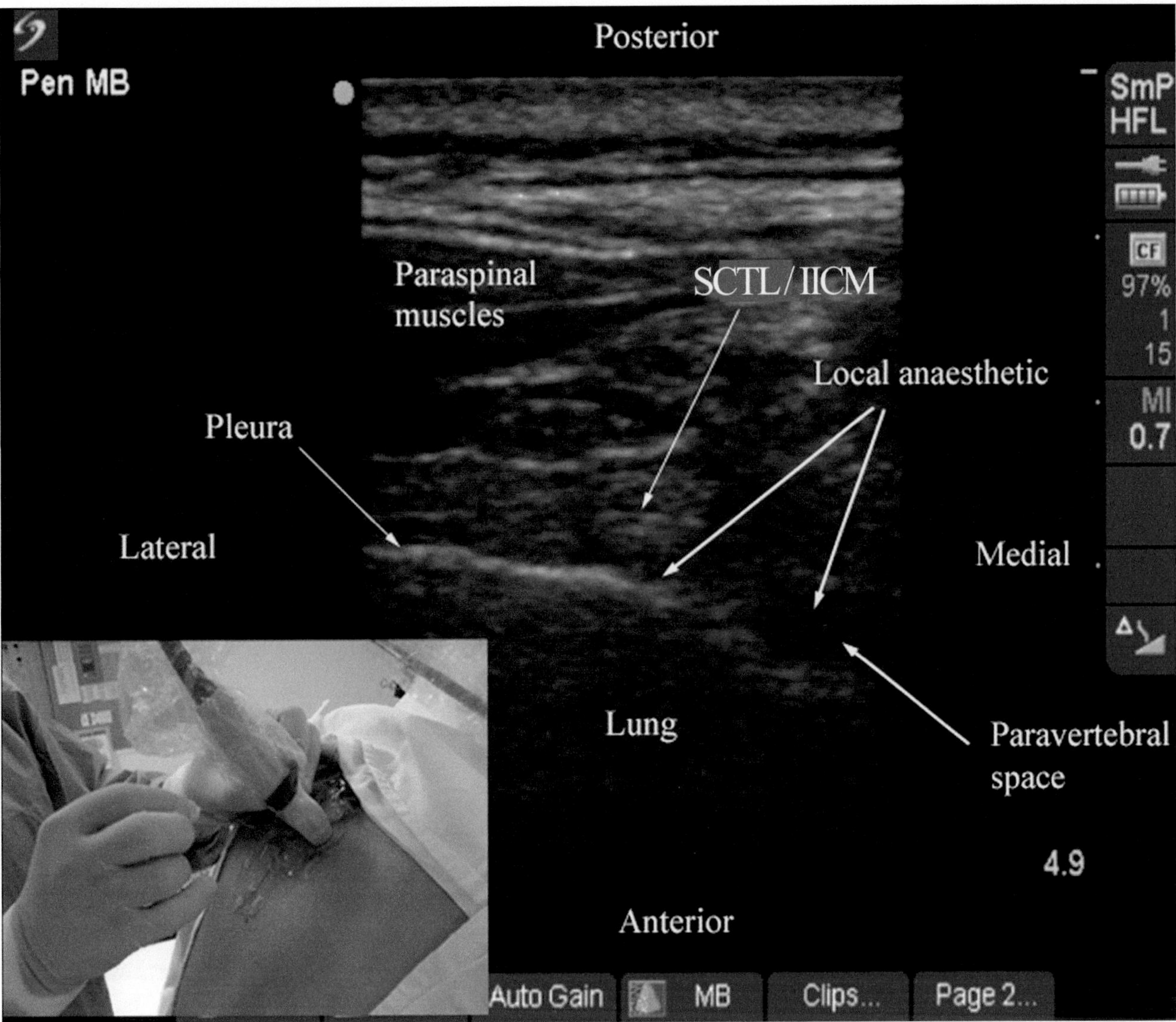

Fig. 30.22 Ultrasound-guided TPVB using a transverse scan in which the block needle is inserted in the short axis of the ultrasound plane. Note the widening of the paravertebral space and anterior displacement of the pleura by the local anaesthetic on the transverse sonogram. The local anaesthetic is also seen to spread to the posterior intercostal space laterally. The picture in the inset shows the orientation of the transducer and the direction in which the needle is inserted. *SCTL/IICM* superior costotransverse ligament. (The figure is reproduced with kind permission from www.aic.cuhk.edu.hk/usgraweb)

the apex of the TPVS. After negative aspiration for blood or CSF, the calculated dose of LA is injected in aliquots. Following the injection, it is common to see widening of the apex of the TPVS and anterior displacement of the pleura by the LA (Fig. 30.22). The LA may also spread to the posterior intercostal space laterally. Widening of the contiguous paravertebral spaces by the injected LA can also be visualized on a sagittal scan after the injection.

Intercostal Approach to the TPVS

With this approach, a transverse scan is performed at the target vertebral level as described above. Originally described by Shibata and Nishiwaki, the transverse scan is performed at the level of the TP, and the block needle is inserted in-plane from a lateral to medial direction (Fig. 30.23), aiming to place the needle tip at the apical part of the TPVS. A test bolus of normal saline (1–2 ml) is then injected, and sonographic evidence is sought to confirm correct needle tip placement in the TPVS. This is visualized as widening of the TPVS and anterior displacement of the parietal pleura (Fig. 30.23). A calculated dose of LA is then slowly injected in aliquots. Compared to the previously described techniques, the block needle is best visualized with this approach because the needle is inserted in the plane of the ultrasound beam. Shibata and Nishiwaki also suggest that since the block needle is advanced, tangential to the parietal pleura,

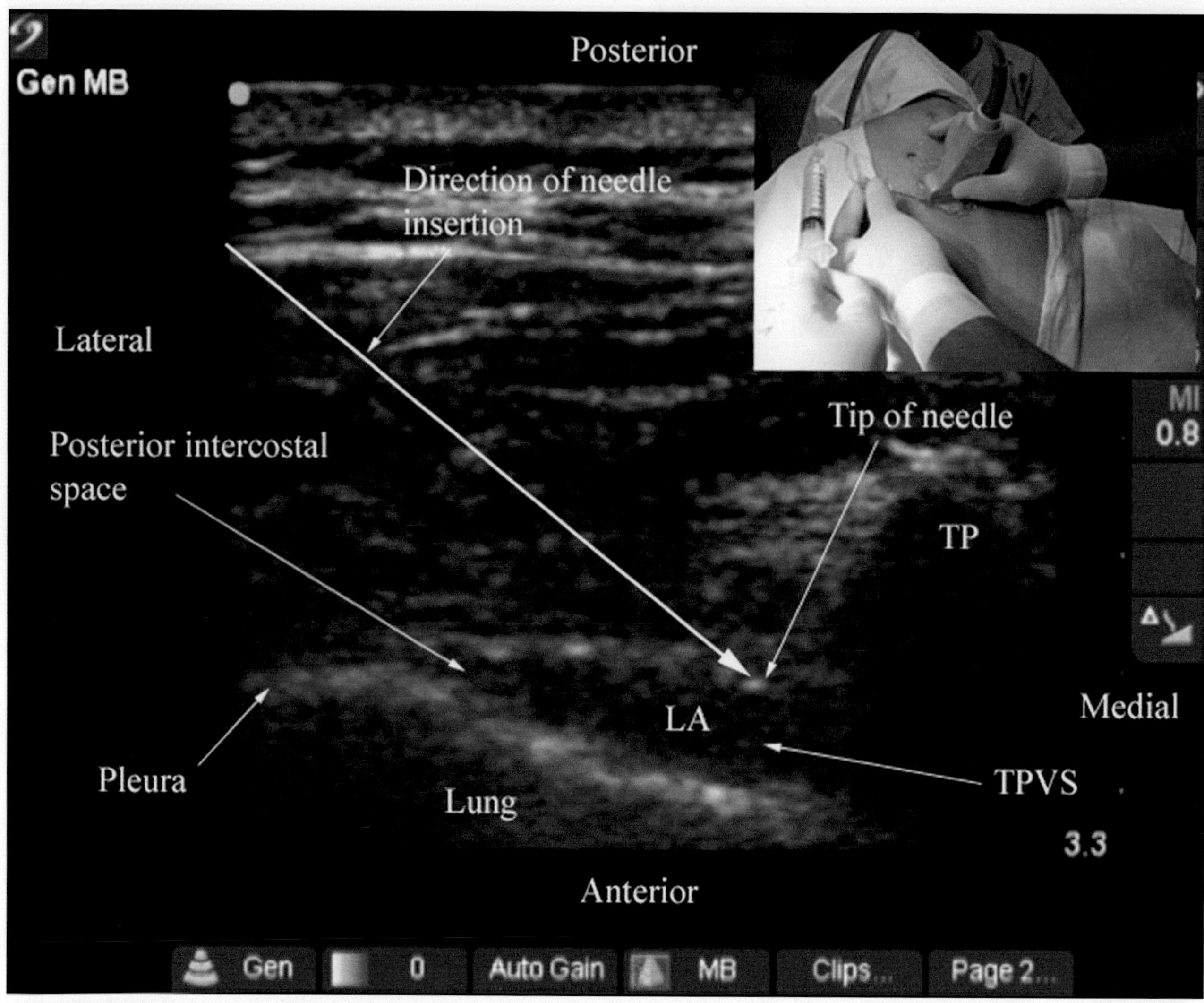

Fig. 30.23 Transverse sonogram of the TPVS (at the level of the TP) after the local anaesthetic injection. Note the widening of the paravertebral space, anterior displacement of the parietal pleura and spread of local anaesthetic (LA) to the posterior intercostal space laterally. The long white arrow represents the direction in which the block needle is inserted. The picture in the inset shows how the block needle is inserted in the plane of the ultrasound beam from a lateral to medial direction. *TP* transverse process, *LA* local anaesthetic, *TPVS* thoracic paravertebral space. (The figure is reproduced with kind permission from www.aic.cuhk.edu.hk/usgraweb)

this approach may have a lower potential for pleural puncture. However, since the block needle is inserted from a lateral to medial direction and towards the intervertebral foramen and the acoustic shadow of the transverse process obscures ultrasound visualization of the needle beyond the tip of the transverse process (Fig. 30.23), this approach may predispose to epidural injection or central neuraxial complications.

We have modified the intercostal approach, and instead of performing the ultrasound scan and injection at the level of the transverse process, as described above, the procedure is performed at the level of the articular process (Fig. 30.10). Without the transverse process in the path of the ultrasound beam, we believe this approach allows visualization of a greater part of the TPVS and also offers little bony obstruction to needle advancement (Fig. 30.24). Therefore, the tip of the nerve block needle can be seen passing through the SCTL/IICM complex to enter the apical part of the TPVS (Fig. 30.25). After the LA injection, there is widening of the TPVS, anterior displacement of the parietal pleura and increased echogenicity of the parietal pleura (Fig. 30.26). However, with the block needle being inserted from a lateral to medial direction and towards the intervertebral foramen, the technique may also predispose to epidural spread or central neuraxial complications. Since the intervertebral foramen is located immediately anterior to the inferior articular process (Figs. 30.11 and 30.13), one must avoid inserting the block needle too deep or perform the LA injection adjacent

Fig. 30.24 Paramedian transverse sonogram of the right thoracic paravertebral region (zoomed view) with the ultrasound beam being insonated through the inter-transverse space, i.e., between two adjoining thoracic transverse processes, and at the level of the articular process (position 3, Fig. 30.11). Note the hyperechogenic inferior articular process and its acoustic shadow medially, which obscures the underlying intervertebral foramen (IVF). As with the paramedian transverse scan at position 2 (refer to Fig. 30.10b), the apex of the thoracic paravertebral space (TPVS), parietal pleura and the superior costotransverse ligament (SCTL) are visualized laterally, but the area of the acoustic shadow is minimal in this ultrasound scan window when compared to that at the level of the transverse process (position 2, Fig. 30.10b). (The figure is reproduced with kind permission from www.aic.cuhk.edu.hk/usgraweb)

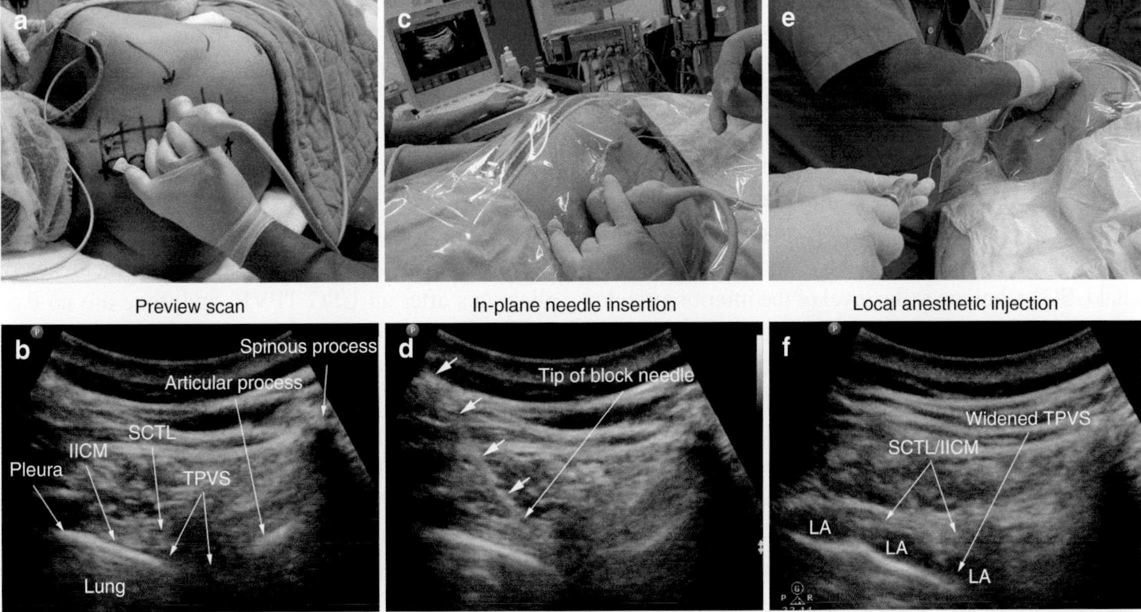

Fig. 30.25 A series of images illustrating ultrasound-guided thoracic paravertebral block (TPVB) using a transverse scan at the level of the inferior articular process (position 3, Fig. 30.11a). Figure showing (**a**) position of the patient, skin markings on the back, and position and orientation of the ultrasound transducer, (**b**) transverse sonogram at the level of the inferior articular process, (**c**) in-plane needle insertion from a lateral to medial direction, (**d**) transverse sonogram showing the path of the block needle, (**e**) local anaesthetic (LA) injection of LA by an assistant with the needle tip in the TPVS, (**f**) note widening of the paravertebral space and spread of the LA to the posterior intercostal space. *IICM* internal intercostal membrane, *SCTL* superior costotransverse ligament, *TPVS* thoracic paravertebral space, *SCTL/IICM* superior costotransverse ligament-internal intercostal membrane complex. (The figure is reproduced with kind permission from www.aic.cuhk.edu.hk/usgraweb)

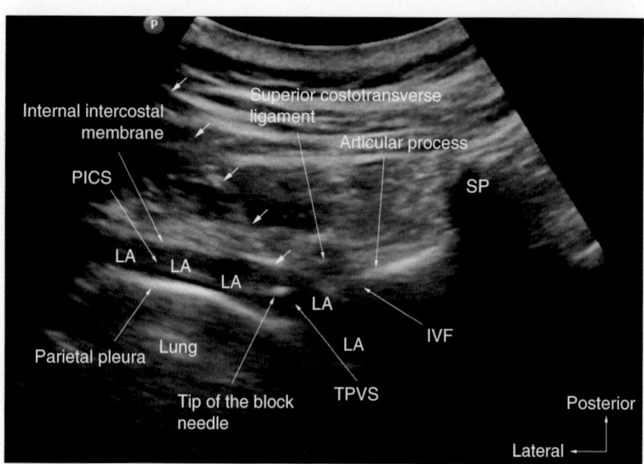

Fig. 30.26 Transverse sonogram of the thoracic paravertebral region after a single-injection ultrasound-guided thoracic paravertebral block (25 ml volume) at the level of the inferior articular process. Note the tip of the block needle is located near the apex of the thoracic paravertebral space (TPVS) and away from the intervertebral foramen (IVF). Also note there is widening of the TPVS and spread of the local anaesthetic (LA) to the medial aspect of the TPVS and laterally to the posterior intercostal space (PICS). *SP* spinous process. (The figure is reproduced with kind permission from www.aic.cuhk.edu.hk/usgraweb)

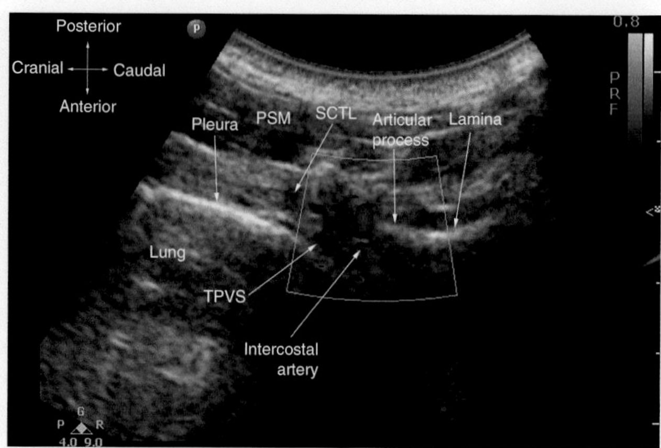

Fig. 30.27 Paramedian transverse sonogram of the thoracic paravertebral region at the level of the inferior articular process in colour (sepia tone) showing the power Doppler signal from the intercostal artery in the paravertebral space. *PSM* paraspinal muscle, *SCTL* superior costotransverse ligament, *TPVS* thoracic paravertebral space. (The figure is reproduced with kind permission from www.aic.cuhk.edu.hk/usgraweb)

to articular process. We consider this as the "no-go-zone" and perform the LA injection at the apical part of the TPVS. It is to be seen how our modification of the intercostal approach fares with regard to epidural spread and central neuraxial complications when compared to the traditional method of performing TPVB. Our preliminary clinical experience with the modified intercostal approach described above has been very encouraging, and we have experienced no major neuraxial complication despite more than a decade of use.

Paralaminar Approach to the TPVS

The paralaminar technique, recently described by Taketa and colleagues, is a medial variation of the intercostal approach (described above) and similar to the anatomic landmark-based "medial technique" described by Shaw and Hollis, and the medial USG technique at the level of the inferior articular process described by Gautier and Luyet. With the paralaminar approach, the transverse scan is performed at the target vertebral level using a micro-convex transducer (8–5 MHz), and the sonogram depicting the vertebral lamina, SCTL-IICM complex and the parietal pleura anteriorly is acquired. The block needle is then inserted in-plane, and nearly perpendicular to the skin, from the medial edge of the transducer and advanced until the needle tip enters the TPVS beyond the lateral edge of the lamina. Taketa and colleagues describe using 10 ml of normal saline to confirm correct needle tip position by observing anterior displacement of the parietal pleura. After negative aspiration for blood or CSF, a calculated dose of local anaesthetic is injected in aliquots via the needle or through a catheter placed 2 cm beyond the tip of the needle. Preliminary evidence suggests that the paralaminar approach may be preferable to the lateral intercostal approach for USG TPVB since it offers clinical advantages (discussed below). However, currently there is paucity of data on the safety of the paralaminar technique, and given that it places the needle tip close to the intervertebral foramen with vital neurovascular structures (Fig. 30.27), it may predispose to vascular and neuraxial complications. Therefore, until more safety data is available, it may be prudent to be cautious with the use of medial USG TPVB techniques.

Complications

Complications after a TPVB is relatively uncommon. Currently, there is paucity of data on the incidence of complications after an USG TPVB, and there are no data comparing complication after an anatomical landmark-based and USG TPVB. Preliminary evidence indicates that pleural puncture and postoperative pneumothorax after an USG TPVB are also rare. Neisen and colleagues report an overall incidence of 0.38% (3.6 per 1000 surgeries, 95% CI 0.5–13.6; 0.9 per 1000 levels blocked, 95% CI 0.1–3.3) for postoperative pneumothorax, which is consistent with the incidence (0.5%) previously reported for landmark-based TPVB. Other complications reported after an USG TPVB include hypotension, vascular puncture, ipsilateral brachial plexus and hemidiaphragmatic palsy, transient Horner's syndrome and local anaesthetic systemic toxicity.

Practical Tips

1. During a paramedian sagittal scan of the TPVS, a slight outward (lateral) tilt of the ultrasound transducer improves ultrasound visualization of the parietal pleura.
2. When using a paramedian sagittal oblique scan for the TPVB, it is important to have a clear understanding of the subtle transition in sonoanatomy from the level of the ribs to the lamina.
3. The transverse ultrasound scan at the level of the inferior articular process (inter-transverse view) provides minimal acoustic shadowing from the osseous structures and thus clear visualization of the TPVS.
4. The transverse scan should be performed in a sequential manner (as described above) to consistently and accurately identify the sonoanatomy of the TPVS at the level of the transverse process and inferior articular process of the vertebra.
5. If needle visualization proves difficult during an USG TPVB, then hydrodissection with 1–2 ml of normal saline may help improve visualization of the needle tip.
6. It is imperative to sonographically confirm correct needle tip position within the TPVS (saline test bolus) before the LA injection in small aliquots. The same may also reduce the potential for accidental intravascular injection.
7. Sonographic signs that confirm correct needle tip position within the TPVS after the saline test bolus injection include turbulence within the TPVS, anterior displacement of the parietal pleura, widening of the TPVS and increased echogenicity of the pleura.
8. When performing the intercostal approach for USG TPVB, it may be prudent to perform the LA injection at the apex of the TPVS and avoid unnecessary deep needle insertion.

Literature Review

Currently there are very few studies comparing outcomes after different techniques for USG TPVB. Uppal and colleagues compared dermatomal anaesthesia produced by a single (T3-T4) versus multiple (5 injection, T1–T5, 5 ml per segment) injection USG TPVB using a paramedian sagittal approach with in-plane needle insertion and a total of 25 ml of 0.5% ropivacaine. There was no difference in the median dermatomal spread of anaesthesia with the single-injection (5 [4–6] segments) when compared to the multiple-injection (5 [5, 6] dermatomes) technique. Duration of analgesia was also comparable, but the single-injection took less time to perform. Uppal and colleagues thus concluded that a single-injection may be preferable to a multiple-injection for USG TPVB. We believe this conclusion is valid when the single-injection USG TPVB is used for postoperative analgesia after primary breast cancer surgery, the outcome evaluated by Uppal and colleagues, but its efficacy as the sole anaesthetic technique for the same surgery will require future research validation.

Patnaik and colleagues compared anatomical landmark-based and USG multi-level TPVB (T1-T6, 5 ml of LA at each level) for surgical anaesthesia during a variety of breast surgery in 72 female patients. The paramedian sagittal oblique ultrasound window with in-plane needle insertion technique was used for the USG multi-level TPVB. They observed that significantly more dermatomes were blocked in the USG group when compared to the anatomical landmark group (median [range]; USG group 5[1–5] vs. landmark group 4 [2–5], $p = 0.0001$). More patients in the USG group also had successful block of the T2 ($p = 0.003$) and T3 ($p = 0.006$) dermatomes than the landmark group. Furthermore, more patient ($p = 0.024$) in the USG group (94%) had successful block for the breast surgery when compared to the anatomical group (72%). While these are encouraging results, the readers should note that a significant number of patients in both study groups still required supplementary analgesia (USG group 82% vs. anatomical landmark group 58%) at various stages of the breast surgery, indicating that a multi-level TPVB (T1–T6) in conjunction with light sedation is inadequate for surgical anaesthesia during major breast surgery (discussion beyond the scope of this chapter).

Fujii and colleagues aimed to determine the best approach for USG TPVB catheterisation and compared the transverse and parasagittal (paramedian sagittal) approach in 60 patients using a micro-convex transducer. Correct catheter placement was possible in 77% and 80% of patients using the transverse and paramedian sagittal approach, respectively. They conclude that both approaches achieved a high rate of successful catheter placement, and there is no clinically significant difference between the two approaches for paravertebral catheterization.

Seidal and colleagues compared the effect of different injection techniques and volume of injection on the patterns of dye spread after an USG TPVB in cadavers. They compared 10 vs. 20 ml, USG vs. landmark-based technique, and different approaches (transverse vs. sagittal, medial vs. lateral, and single vs. multiple injections). Seidal and colleagues conclude that a higher injection volume results in a larger number of intercostal nerves being stained. The sympathetic trunk was stained in 84.6% (100% with multiple-injection), and it was independent of the injection volume. Epidural spread was less likely if the injections were more lateral with the transverse approach or with a cranially directed needle with the sagittal approach.

Conclusion

USG TPVB is an attractive alternative to the traditional anatomical landmark-based technique for TPVB. With the currently available ultrasound technology, it is possible to accurately delineate the anatomy relevant for TPVB. During the preview scan, one is able to define the paravertebral anatomy prior to block placement and determine the depth to the TP or parietal pleura. Depending on the technique used, the latter defines the maximum safe depth for needle insertion or the structure to avoid, and thus may help reduce the incidence of pleural puncture. With real-time ultrasound guidance, one is able to accurately advance the block needle to the TPVS, avoid pleura puncture and visualize the distribution of the LA during the injection. This may translate into improved technical outcomes, higher success rates and reduced needle-related complications. Ultrasound is also an excellent teaching tool for demonstrating the anatomy relevant for TPVB and has the potential to improve the learning curve of this technique. Several different techniques have been described for USG TPVB to date, and the preliminary evidence suggests that a medial injection technique may be preferable to a lateral injection technique for efficacy. However, currently, there are limited outcome data after an USG TPVB and given that medial injection techniques for TPVB are performed close to the intervertebral foramen, with potential for central neuraxial complications, future research to establish an optimal technique for USG TPVB and to establish its role in clinical practice is warranted.

Acknowledgments The cadaver anatomical sections are courtesy of the Visible Human Server at École Polytechnique Fédérale de Lausanne, Visible Human Visualization Software (http://visiblehuman.epfl.ch) and Gold Standard Multimedia (www.gsm.org).

Suggested Reading

Abdallah FW, Brull R. Off side! A simple modification to the parasagittal in-plane approach for paravertebral block. Reg Anesth Pain Med. 2014;39:240–2.

Antonakakis JG, Sites BD, Shiffrin J. Ultrasound-guided posterior approach for the placement of a continuous interscalene catheter. Reg Anesth Pain Med. 2009;34:64–8.

Ben-Ari A, Moreno M, Chelly JE, Bigeleisen PE. Ultrasound-guided paravertebral block using an intercostal approach. Anesth Analg. 2009a;109:1691–4.

Ben-Ari A, Moreno M, Chelly JE, Bigeleisen PE. USG PVB using an intercostal approach. Anesth Analg. 2009b;109:1691–4.

Cheema SPS, Ilsley D, Richardson J, Sabanathan S. A thermographic study of paravertebral analgesia. Anaesthesia. 1995;50:118–21.

Conacher ID. Resin injection of thoracic paravertebral spaces. Br J Anaesth. 1988;61:657–61.

Conacher ID, Kokri M. Postoperative paravertebral blocks for thoracic surgery. A radiological appraisal. Br J Anaesth. 1987;59:155–61.

Coveney E, Weltz CR, Greengrass R, Iglehart JD, Leight GS, Steele SM, Lyerly HK. Use of paravertebral block anesthesia in the surgical management of breast cancer—experience in 156 cases. Ann Surg. 1998;227:496–501.

Dugan DJ, Samson PC. Surgical significance of the endothoracic fascia. The anatomic basis for empyemectomy and other extrapleural technics. Am J Surg. 1975;130:151–8.

Evans PJ, Lloyd JW, Wood GJ. Accidental intrathecal injection of bupivacaine and dextran. Anaesthesia. 1981;36:685–7.

Fagenholz PJ, Bowler GM, Carnochan FM, Walker WS. Systemic local anaesthetic toxicity from continuous thoracic paravertebral block. Br J Anaesth. 2012;109:260–2.

Fujii T, Shibata Y, Shinya S, Nishiwaki K. Transverse vs. parasagittal in-plane approaches in ultrasound-guided paravertebral block using a microconvex probe: a randomised controlled trial. Eur J Anaesthesiol. 2020;37:752–7.

Greengrass R, O'Brien F, Lyerly K, Hardman D, Gleason D, D'Ercole F, Steele S. Paravertebral block for breast cancer surgery. Can J Anaesth. 1996;43:858–61.

Hara K, Sakura S, Nomura T. [Use of ultrasound for thoracic paravertebral block]. Masui. 2007;56:925–31.

Hara K, Sakura S, Nomura T, Saito Y. Ultrasound guided thoracic paravertebral block in breast surgery. Anaesthesia. 2009;64:223–4.

Karmakar M. Thoracic paravertebral block. Anesthesiology. 2001;95:771–80.

Karmakar MK. Ultrasound-guided thoracic paravertebral block. Tech Reg Anesth Pain Manag. 2009;13:142–9.

Karmakar M, Chung D. Variability of a thoracic paravertebral block. Are we ignoring the endothoracic fascia? Reg Anesth Pain Med. 2000;25:325–7.

Karmakar MK, Kwok WH, Kew J. Thoracic paravertebral block: radiological evidence of contralateral spread anterior to the vertebral bodies. Br J Anaesth. 2000;84:263–5.

Karmakar M, Gin T, Ho A. Ipsilateral thoraco-lumbar anaesthesia and paravertebral spread after low thoracic paravertebral injection. Br J Anaesth. 2001;87:312–6.

Karmakar MK, Critchley LA, Ho AM, Gin T, Lee TW, Yim AP. Continuous thoracic paravertebral infusion of bupivacaine for pain management in patients with multiple fractured ribs. Chest. 2003;123:424–31.

Kittredge RD. Computed tomographic evaluation of the thoracic prevertebral and paravertebral spaces. J Comput Tomogr. 1983;7:239–50.

Klein SM, Greengrass RA, Weltz C, Warner DS. Paravertebral somatic nerve block for outpatient inguinal herniorrhaphy: an expanded case report of 22 patients. Reg Anesth Pain Med. 1998;23:306–10.

Krediet AC, Moayeri N, van Geffen GJ, Bruhn J, Renes S, Bigeleisen PE, Groen GJ. Different approaches to ultrasound-guided thoracic paravertebral block: an illustrated review. Anesthesiology. 2015;123:459–74.

Lichtenstein DA, Menu Y. A bedside ultrasound sign ruling out pneumothorax in the critically ill. Lung sliding. Chest. 1995;108:1345–8.

Lonnqvist PA, Hildingsson U. The caudal boundary of the thoracic paravertebral space—a study in human cadavers. Anaesthesia. 1992;47:1051–2.

Lonnqvist PA, Mackenzie J, Soni AK, Conacher ID. Paravertebral blockade—failure rate and complications. Anaesthesia. 1995;50:813–5.

Luyet C, Herrmann G, Ross S, Vogt A, Greif R, Moriggl B, Eichenberger U. Ultrasound-guided thoracic paravertebral puncture and placement of catheters in human cadavers: where do catheters go? Br J Anaesth. 2011;106:246–54.

Marhofer P, Kettner SC, Hajbok L, Dubsky P, Fleischmann E. Lateral ultrasound-guided paravertebral blockade: an anatomical-based description of a new technique. Br J Anaesth. 2010;105:526–32.

Marhofer D, Marhofer P, Kettner SC, Fleishmann E, Prayer D, Schernthaner M, Lackner E, Willschke H, Schwetz P, Zeitlinger M. Magnetic resonance imaging analysis of the spread of local anesthetic solution after ultrasound-guided lateral thoracic paravertebral blockade. Anesthesiology. 2013;118:1106–12.

Naja MZ, Ziade MF, Lonnqvist PA. General anaesthesia combined with bilateral paravertebral blockade (T5–6) vs. general anaesthesia for laparoscopic cholecystectomy: a prospective, randomized clinical trial. Eur J Anaesthesiol. 2004;21:489–95.

Niesen AD, Jacob AK, Law LA, Sviggum HP, Johnson RL. Complication rate of ultrasound-guided paravertebral block for breast surgery. Reg Anesth Pain Med. 2020;45:813–7.

Nunn JF, Slavin G. Posterior intercostal nerve block for pain relief after cholecystectomy. Anatomical basis and efficacy. Br J Anaesth. 1980;52:253–60.

O'Riain SC, Donnell BO, Cuffe T, Harmon DC, Fraher JP, Shorten G. Thoracic paravertebral block using real-time ultrasound guidance. Anesth Analg. 2010;110:248–51.

Pace MM, Sharma B, Anderson-Dam J, Fleischmann K, Warren L, Stefanovich P. Ultrasound-guided thoracic paravertebral blockade: a retrospective study of the incidence of complications. Anesth Analg. 2016;122:1186–91.

Pangthipampai P, Karmakar MK, Songthamwat B, Pakpirom J, Samy W. Ultrasound-guided multilevel thoracic paravertebral block and its efficacy for surgical anesthesia during primary breast cancer surgery. J Pain Res. 2020;13:1713–23.

Paraskeuopoulos T, Saranteas T, Kouladouros K, Krepi H, Nakou M, Kostopanagiotou G, Anagnostopoulou S. Thoracic paravertebral spread using two different ultrasound-guided intercostal injection techniques in human cadavers. Clin Anat. 2010;23:840–7.

Patnaik R, Chhabra A, Subramaniam R, Arora MK, Goswami D, Srivastava A, Seenu V, Dhar A. Comparison of paravertebral block by anatomic landmark technique to ultrasound-guided paravertebral block for breast surgery anesthesia: a randomized controlled trial. Reg Anesth Pain Med. 2018;43:385–90.

Pintaric TS, Veranic P, Hadzic A, Karmakar M, Cvetko E. Electron-microscopic imaging of endothoracic fascia in the thoracic paravertebral space in rats. Reg Anesth Pain Med. 2012;37:215–8.

Purcell-Jones G, Pither CE, Justins DM. Paravertebral somatic nerve block: a clinical, radiographic, and computed tomographic study in chronic pain patients. Anesth Analg. 1989;68:32–9.

Renes SH, Bruhn J, Gielen MJ, Scheffer GJ, Van Geffen GJ. In-plane ultrasound-guided thoracic paravertebral block: a preliminary report of 36 cases with radiologic confirmation of catheter position. Reg Anesth Pain Med. 2010;35:212–6.

Renes SH, van Geffen GJ, Snoeren MM, Gielen MJ, Groen GJ. Ipsilateral brachial plexus block and hemidiaphragmatic paresis as adverse effect of a high thoracic paravertebral block. Reg Anesth Pain Med. 2011;36(2):198–201.

Richardson J, Vowden P, Sabanathan S. Bilateral paravertebral analgesia for major abdominal vascular-surgery—a preliminary-report. Anaesthesia. 1995;50:995–8.

Richardson J, Jones J, Atkinson R. The effect of thoracic paravertebral blockade on intercostal somatosensory evoked potentials. Anesth Analg. 1998;87:373–6.

Saito T, Den S, Tanuma K, Tanuma Y, Carney E, Carlsson C. Anatomical bases for paravertebral anesthetic block: fluid communication between the thoracic and lumbar paravertebral regions. Surg Radiol Anat. 1999a;21:359–63.

Saito T, Den S, Tanuma K, Carlsson C. Extended unilateral anesthesia in humans. Reg Anesth Pain Med. 1999b;24:15.

Seidel R, Wree A, Schulze M. Thoracic-paravertebral blocks: comparative anatomical study with different injection techniques and volumes. Reg Anesth Pain Med. 2020;45:102–6.

Sharrock NE. Postural headache following thoracic somatic paravertebral nerve block. Anesthesiology. 1980;52:360–2.

Shaw WM, Hollis NY. Medial approach for paravertebral somatic nerve block. JAMA. 1952;148:742–4.

Shibata Y, Nishiwaki K. Ultrasound-guided intercostal approach to thoracic paravertebral block. Anesth Analg. 2009;109:996–7.

Taketa Y, Fujitani T. A novel paralaminar in-plane approach for ultrasound-guided continuous thoracic paravertebral block using microconvex array transducer. Reg Anesth Pain Med. 2015;40:390.

Taketa Y, Fujitani T, Irisawa Y, Sudo S, Takaishi K. Ultrasound-guided thoracic paravertebral block by the paralaminar in-plane approach using a microconvex array transducer: methodological utility based on anatomical structures. J Anesth. 2017;31:271–7.

Taketa Y, Irisawa Y, Fujitani T. Comparison of analgesic efficacy between two approaches of paravertebral block for thoracotomy: a randomised trial. Acta Anaesthesiol Scand. 2018;62:1274–9.

Uppal V, Sondekoppam RV, Sodhi P, Johnston D, Ganapathy S. Single-injection versus multiple-injection technique of ultrasound-guided paravertebral blocks: a randomized controlled study comparing dermatomal spread. Reg Anesth Pain Med. 2017;42:575–81.

Wu ZW, Ni HD, Hou XM, Lu YP, Zhou XY, Yao M. [Effects of lateral and medial points of thoracic paravertebral nerve block by ultrasound for rapid recovery after laparoscopic cholecystectomy]. Zhonghua Yi Xue Za Zhi. 2019;99:988–92.

Pectoral and Serratus Plane Blocks

31

Barbara Versyck

Contents

General Consideration

The ultrasound-guided interpectoral, pectoserratus, and serratus anterior plane blocks are nerve blocks for superficial surgery of the anterolateral chest wall and axillary region. These blocks focus on providing analgesia in the T2–T6 region (Fig. 31.1).

These blocks are the so-called fascial plane blocks, a newer class of regional anesthesia techniques in which a generous volume of local anesthetic at lower concentrations is injected into a fascial plane rather than directly around nerves. Analgesia is achieved by the passive spread of local anesthetic to nerves within these planes or in adjacent tissue compartments.

In 2011, Blanco described a technique to inject local anesthetic in between the pectoralis major and minor muscles, which he successfully performed in 50 patients

B. Versyck (✉)
AZ Turnhout, Department of Anesthesia and Intensive Care, Turnhout, Belgium

Department of Anesthesia, Intensive Care and Pain Medicine, Catharina Hospital, Eindhoven, The Netherlands

D. Jankovic, P. Peng (eds.), *Regional Nerve Blocks in Anesthesia and Pain Therapy*,
https://doi.org/10.1007/978-3-030-88727-8_31

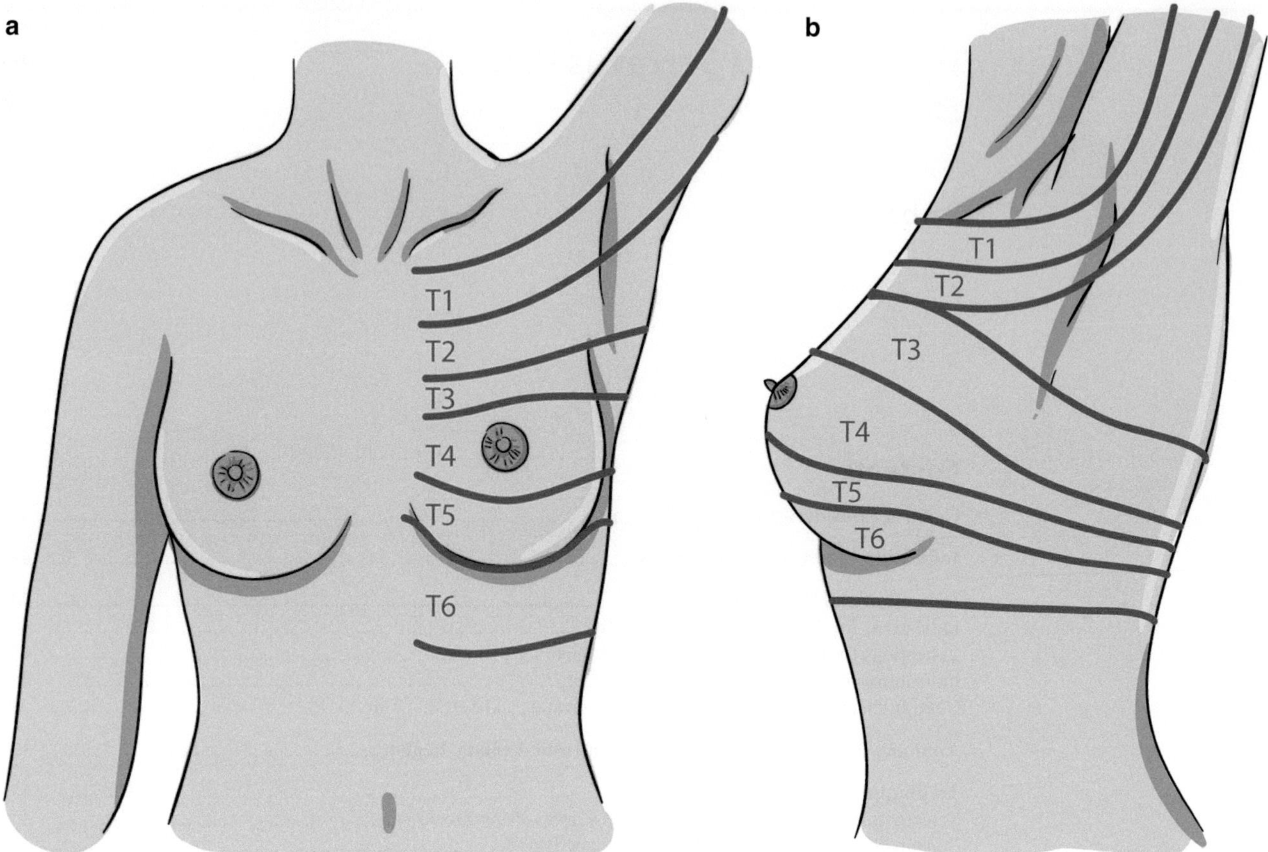

Fig. 31.1 Region of interest for interpectoral, pectoserratus, and serratus anterior plane blocks. (**a**) Anterior view; (**b**) lateral view. (Reproduced with permission of Dr. Barbara Versyck BV)

requiring analgesia after breast surgery. One year later, Blanco et al. described a modified version of this technique where they additionally injected local anesthetic between the pectoralis minor and serratus muscles (now the pectoserratus plane block). Upon introduction of the second block, Blanco et al. labeled the first block as the Pecs I (now the interpectoral plane block) and the later modified technique collectively as Pecs II (now the interpectoral-pectoserratus plane block). The interpectoral plane block is an injection between the major and minor pectoral muscles to block the medial and lateral pectoral nerves as well as the intercostobrachial nerve. The pectoserratus plane block is between the pectoralis minor and serratus muscle to target at least the II–VI intercostals and the long thoracic nerve. Lastly, in 2013, Blanco et al. described the serratus anterior plane block (SAPB). There are two variants of the serratus anterior plane block, a superficial and a deep variant, which involve an injection superficial or deep to the serratus anterior muscle, respectively, at the lateral chest wall. Both target the lateral cutaneous branches of the thoracic intercostal nerves. This superficial serratus anterior plane block is comparable to the pectoserratus plane block and additionally stains the thoracodorsal and long thoracic nerves (Table 31.1).

Due to their relative simplicity, safety, and efficacy, these three blocks have rapidly gained popularity. The blocks are generally used as an adjuvant to general anesthesia or occasionally with sedation.

Indications and Contraindications

See Tables 31.2 and 31.3.

Indication and Patient Selection

Indications for the Interpectoral Plane Block

Effect of the Blockade

The interpectoral plane block blocks the medial and lateral pectoral nerves as well as the intercostobrachial nerve. This blockade attenuates the stretch-induced pain of the pectoral muscles and provides sensory analgesia of the axilla through the intercostobrachial nerve. As it does not reach the intercostal nerves, there is no sensory blockade of the thoracic wall.

Table 31.1 Technique performance of the interpectoral, pectoserratus, and serratus anterior plane blocks

Technique	Technical performance
Interpectoral plane block	• Injection between pectoralis major and minor muscles • Level of the third rib underneath the lateral half of the clavicle
Interpectoral-pectoserratus plane block	• Interpectoral plane block and a second injection between the pectoralis major and serratus anterior muscles • Level of the third rib underneath the lateral half of the clavicle
Serratus anterior plane block (SAPB): superficial	• Injection superficial to serratus anterior muscle • Anywhere between the anterior and posterior axillary line and the third to sixth rib
Serratus anterior plane block (SAPB): deep	• Injection deep to serratus anterior muscle and superficial to ribs and intercostal muscles • Anywhere between the anterior and posterior axillary line and the third to sixth ribs

Table 31.2 Targeted nerves per block

	Cutaneous and subcutaneous innervation				Muscle innervation			
	Intercostal nerves			Cervical plexus	Brachial plexus			
Nerves	Lateral cutaneous branches	Anterior cutaneous branches	Intercostobrachial nerve	Supraclavicular nerves	Lateral pectoral nerve	Medial pectoral nerve	Thoracodorsal nerve	Long thoracic nerve
Innervation of	Lateral breast	Medial breast	Axilla and medial upper arm	Cranial breast	Pectoralis major muscle	Pectoralis major and minor muscles	Latissimus dorsi muscle	Serratus anterior muscle
Interpectoral plane block			√		√	√		
Interpectoral-pectoserratus plane block	√		√		√	√		√
Serratus anterior plane block (SAPB): superficial	√		√				√	√
Serratus anterior plane block (SAPB): deep	√		√					

Acute Therapeutic

- Minor breast surgery including subpectoral prostheses and insertion of breast expanders.
- Subpectoral device insertion including pacemakers and port-a-caths.

Indications for the Interpectoral-Pectoserratus Plane Block

Effect of the Blockade

The site and volume of injection influences the effect of the blockade, in particular the block of the intercostobrachial nerve. Assuming the procedure described below, the interpectoral-pectoserratus plane block provides analgesia to the lateral chest wall and axillary region (Fig. 31.2). There is no complete analgesia of the hemithorax as, for example, the anterior cutaneous branches of the intercostal nerves, which innervate the sternum, are not blocked.

Diagnostic

- Breast biopsy.

Acute Therapeutic

- Breast cancer surgery procedures such as lumpectomy, mastectomy, axillary clearance, and sentinel node dissection.
- Reconstructive breast surgery and breast augmentation.
- Subpectoral prostheses and devices including pacemakers and port-a-caths.
- Chest drains in T2–T6.
- Partial first rib resection.

Chronic Pain

- Persistent pain after breast cancer surgery.

Table 31.3 Nerves involved in frequently performed anterolateral and axillary region surgery

	Cutaneous and subcutaneous innervation				Muscle innervation			
	Intercostal nerves			Cervical plexus	Brachial plexus			
Nerves	Lateral cutaneous branches	Anterior cutaneous branches	Intercostobrachial nerve	Supraclavicular nerves	Lateral pectoral nerve	Medial pectoral nerve	Thoracodorsal nerve	Long thoracic nerve
Innervation of	Lateral breast	Medial breast	Axilla and medial upper arm	Cranial breast	Pectoralis major muscle	Pectoralis major and minor muscles	Latissimus dorsi muscle	Serratus anterior muscle
Tissue expander	√	√		√	√	√		
Lumpectomy	If lateral lumpectomy	If medial lumpectomy		If cranial lumpectomy				
Mastectomy	√	√		√				
Sentinel node or axillary dissection			√				√	√
Latissimus dorsi flap							√	
Device implementation e.g., port-a-cath, pacemaker				√	√	√		
Video-assisted thoracic surgery (VATS)	√						√	√
Trauma to lateral chest wall e.g., rib fracture	√							

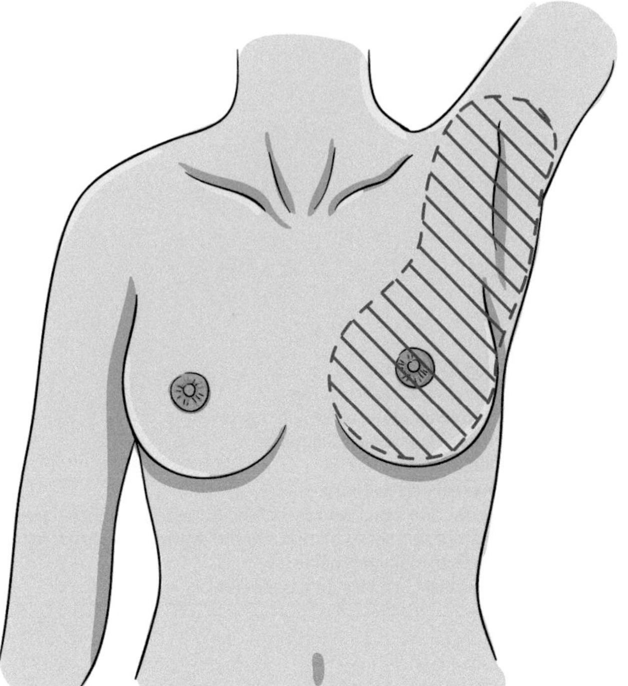

Fig. 31.2 Blockade achieved by the interpectoral-pectoserratus plane block. (Reproduced with permission of Dr. Barbara Versyck BV)

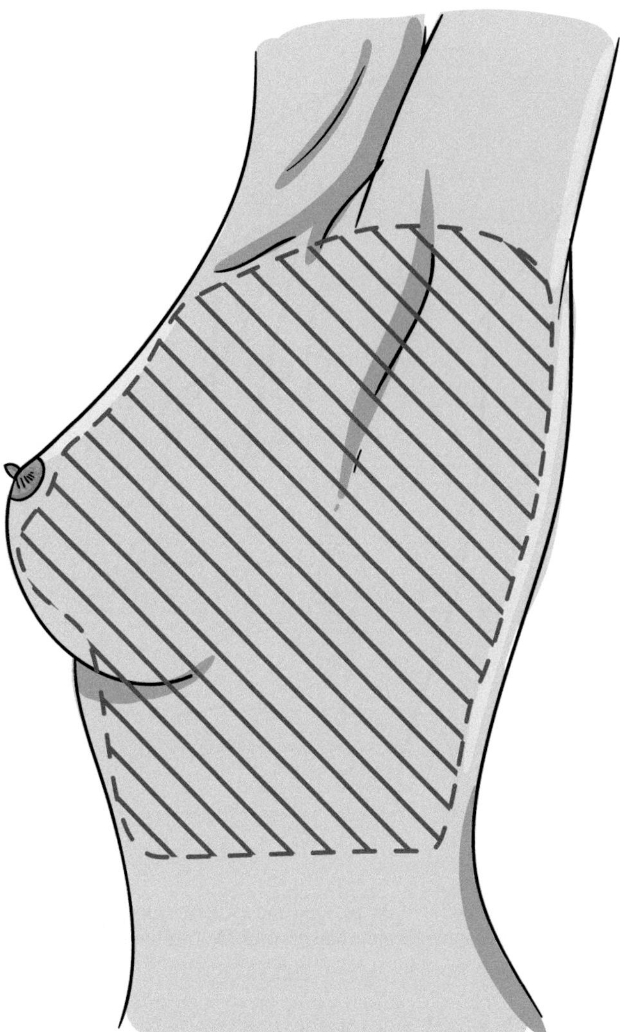

Fig. 31.3 Blockade achieved by the serratus anterior plane block upon performing the block at the level of r4 resulting in a maximal spread of T2–T6. (Reproduced with permission of Dr. Barbara Versyck BV)

Indications for Serratus Anterior Plane Block

Effect of the Blockade

The serratus anterior plane block can be performed anywhere between the anterior and posterior axillary lines and the third to sixth rib. The site and volume of injection influences the effect of this blockade, in particular in which intercostal nerve territories will be blocked. Assuming the procedure described below, the serratus anterior plane block typically achieves analgesia one to two levels cephalad and one to two levels caudad from the location of injection (Fig. 31.1). For instance, the T2–T6 blockade can be achieved by a block at the level of the fourth rib (Fig. 31.3).

Acute Therapeutic

- Mastectomy.
- Thoracotomy.
- Rib fractures.
- Chest drain insertions.

Chronic Pain

- Rib fractures.

Contraindications for Interpectoral, Pectoserratus, and Serratus Anterior Plane Blocks

These blocks are contraindicated in situation when a patient refuses or has a known history of allergy to the local anesthetics, a presence of abnormal anatomy or inflammation at the injection site, e.g., breast cancer.

Anatomy of the Anterolateral Chest Wall and Axillary Region

Five nerve groups are key for the sensory innervation of the anterolateral chest and axillary region: (1) the anterior cutaneous branches of the thoracic intercostal nerves, (2) the lateral cutaneous branches of the thoracic intercostal nerves, (3) the pectoral nerves, (4) the long thoracic nerve, and (5) the supraclavicular nerves (Fig. 31.4). These five groups originate from three different regions: the neuraxis, brachial plexus, and cervical plexus.

The anterior and lateral cutaneous branches of the thoracic intercostal nerves originate from the neuraxis. Generally, the anterior branches innervate the medial side of the breast T2–T6, while the lateral branches provide innerva-

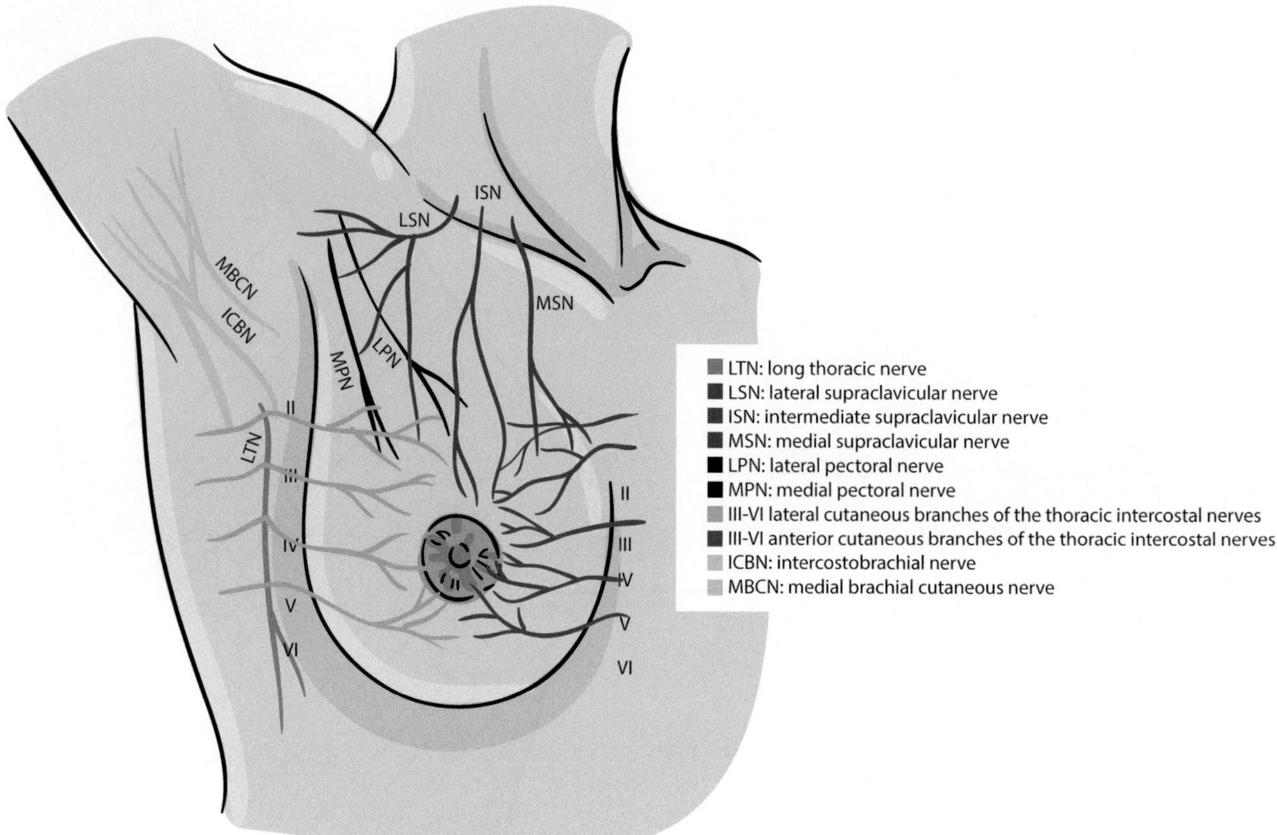

Fig. 31.4 Innervation of the pectoral and axillary region. *LPN* lateral pectoral nerve, *MPN* medial pectoral nerve, *MBCN* medial brachial cutaneous nerve, *ICBN* intercostobrachial nerve, *LTN* long thoracic nerve. (Reproduced with permission of Dr. Barbara Versyck BV)

tion of the lateral side of the breast T3–T6. The lateral cutaneous branch of T2 forms the intercostobrachial nerve and innervates the axilla and medial upper arm. In the axilla, the intercostobrachial nerve may merge with the medial brachial cutaneous nerve. The lateral cutaneous branches pierce the intercostal and serratus anterior muscles before dividing into an anterior and posterior branch.

The pectoral nerves and the long thoracic nerve originate from the brachial plexus. The medial and lateral pectoral nerves innervate the pectoral muscles. The long thoracic nerve is responsible for the innervation of the serratus muscle.

The supraclavicular nerves provide sensory innervation of the superior part of the breast region and originate from the cervical plexus.

Technique

While these techniques are not complex, they should only be carried out by anesthesiologists with experience in ultrasound-guided regional anesthesia or under their supervision. The pre-procedure preparation is summarized in Table 31.4.

Table 31.4 Pre-procedure preparation

General	Equipment
• Informed discussion and consent • Emergency equipment and drugs • Intravenous access • Standard monitoring • Sterile precaution	• Ultrasound machine at the head of patient with a linear high-frequency probe • 50-mm (ultrasound) needle • Sterile ultrasound cover and gel • Long-acting local anesthetic (bupivacaine or ropivacaine)

Sonoanatomy for the Interpectoral-Pectoserratus Plane Blocks

With the patient in supine position and arm either abducted or along the side of the body, a linear transducer is positioned in a similar position as for an infraclavicular block as it allows the visualization of the second rib caudal to the lateral part of the clavicle (Fig. 31.5a). The transducer is moved further caudally to the third rib and rotated about 45 degrees inferolateral to visualize both the third and the fourth rib (Fig. 31.5b). The corresponding ultrasound image should at least visualize pectoralis major, pectoralis minor, pectoral branch of the thoracoacromial artery, and the third and fourth rib (Fig. 31.5c).

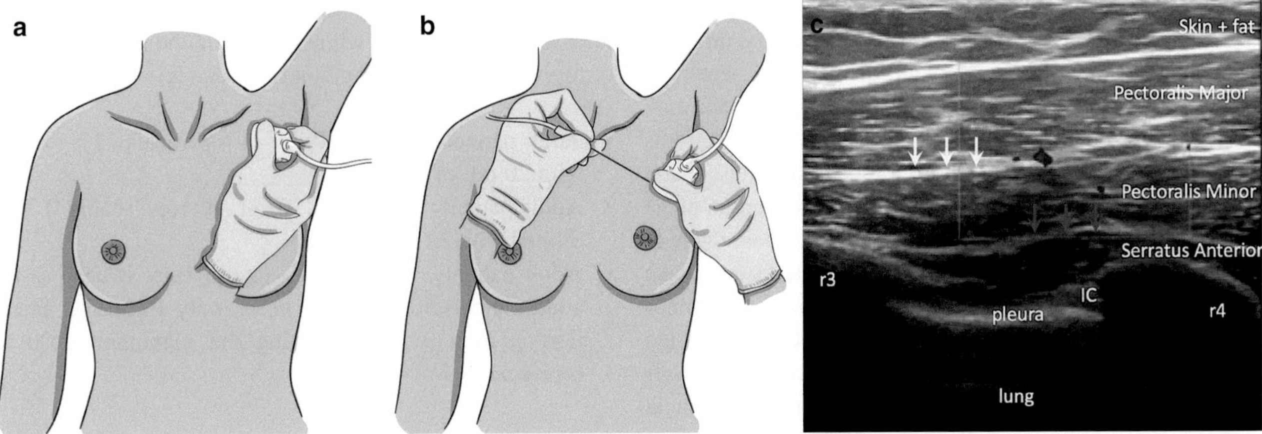

Fig. 31.5 (**a**) Initial position of the linear transducer for the interpectoral-pectoserratus plane block. (**b**) Ultrasound probe and needle positioning for the interpectoral-pectoserratus plane block. (**c**) Ultrasound image for the interpectoral-pectoserratus plane blocks. *Red* pectoral branch of the thoracoacromial artery, *r3* third rib, *r4* fourth rib, *IC* intercostal muscle, *White arrows* target for the interpectoral injectate, *red arrows* target for the pectoserratus injectate. (Reproduced with permission of Dr. Barbara Versyck BV)

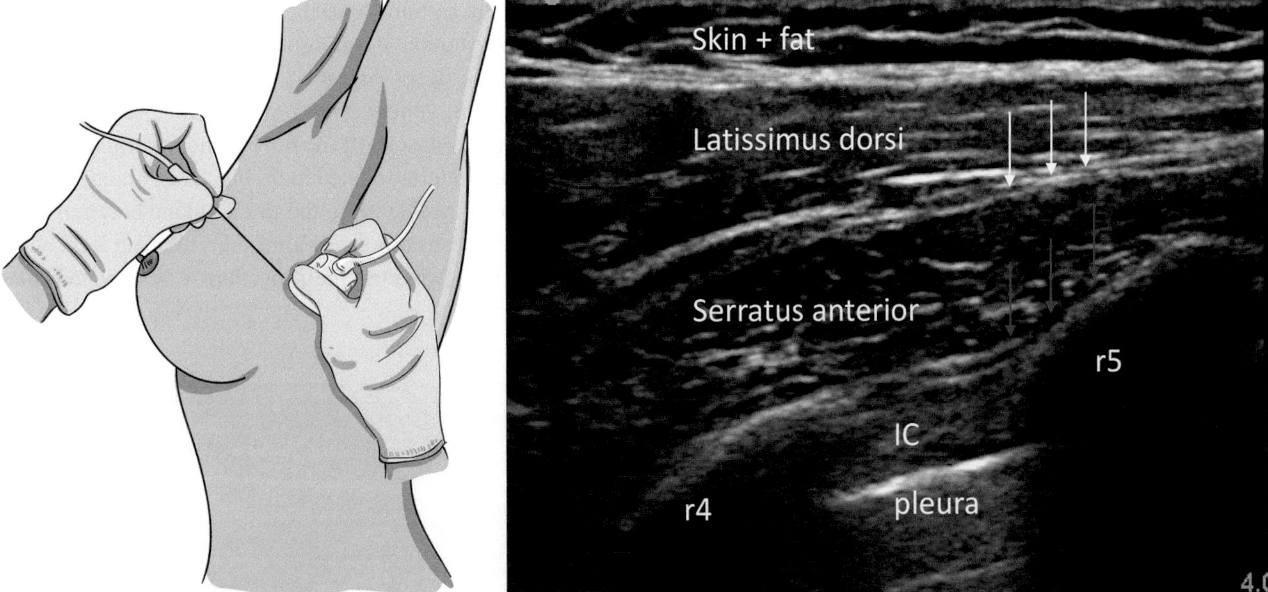

Fig. 31.6 Left: ultrasound probe and needle positioning for the serratus anterior plane block. Right: ultrasound image for the serratus anterior plane block at the level of r5. white arrows target for the superficial serratus anterior plane block, red arrows target for the deep serratus anterior plane block. r4 fourth rib, r5 fifth rib, IC intercostal muscle. (Reproduced with permission of Dr. Barbara Versyck B.V.)

Sonoanatomy for the Serratus Anterior Plane Block

The patient is typically placed in lateral decubitus position, with the arm flexed, adducted, and raised over the head. A linear transducer is placed initially caudal to the clavicle at the midclavicular line to visualize the second rib. The transducer is lowered inferolaterally toward the midaxillary line to the levels of the third, fourth, or fifth rib. The transducer is positioned to visualize both third and fourth ribs or fourth and fifth ribs (Fig. 31.6). The corresponding ultrasound image should at least visualize serratus anterior and intercostal muscles as well as the corresponding ribs and pleura. Depending on the probe position, the overlying muscle layer may be pectoralis minor or latissimus dorsi (Fig. 31.6).

Injection Technique

Interpectoral-Pectoserratus Plane Blocks

The needle is introduced in plane from medial to lateral aiming toward the underlying fourth rib. Such orientation is important to avoid puncturing the pleura. The needle is advanced medial from the thoracoacromial artery until the needle tip reaches the facial plane deep to the pectoralis minor muscle. Due to the anatomic variation, this plane may be between the pectoralis minor muscle and the serratus anterior muscle or between the pectoralis minor muscle and the intercostal muscle. At this level, the pectoserratus plane block is performed (Fig. 31.7, yellow arrow). Then, the needle is retracted until the needle tip reaches the fascial plane between the pectoralis major muscle and the pectoralis minor muscle where the interpectoral plane block is injected (Fig. 31.7, orange arrow). The procedure is completed after confirming the lateral spread of local anesthetic in both facial planes.

Optimal volumes and concentrations of local anesthetics for use for the interpectoral-pectoserratus plane block have yet to be determined. As with all facial plane blocks, the area of spread is related to the total volume of injectate used, rather than concentration. A balance must be found between achieving an optimal spread of sensory anesthesia and avoiding toxicity as well as minimizing the impact on the surgical field.

In adult patients over 50 kg, it is the author's practice to use a total volume of 40 mL instead of the initially proposed 30 mL by Blanco et al. for the interpectoral-pectoserratus plane block. Twenty mL of local anesthetic is injected in each fascial planc. The higher volume of the interpectoral injection ensures that the local anesthetic reaches the axilla and blocks the intercostobrachial nerve. The following mixtures are recommended while respecting the maximum dose of ropivacaine (2–3 mg/kg, not to exceed 225 mg per dose):

- Adult patients >70 kg: 20 mL of ropivacaine 1% diluted with 20 mL of saline.
- Adult patients 50–70 kg: 20 mL of ropivacaine 0.75% diluted with 20 mL of saline.
- Adult patients <50 kg: The same mixture is used as for adult patients 50–70 kg; however, only 15 mL per injection is used while respecting the maximum dose of ropivacaine.

Also for the interpectoral plane block, the author prefers 15–20 mL of the same mixture rather than the initially described 10 mL.

Serratus Anterior Plane Block

The needle is introduced in plane from medial to lateral aiming toward the serratus anterior muscle and the underlying rib. Such orientation is important to avoid puncturing the pleura. For the deep variant of the serratus anterior plane block (Fig. 31.8, yellow arrow), our target is separating the serratus anterior muscle off the rib. For the superficial variant of the serratus anterior plane block (Fig. 31.8, orange arrow), we position the needle tip in the fascial plane between latissimus dorsi and serratus anterior muscles to inject local anesthetic. For both variants, the procedure is completed after

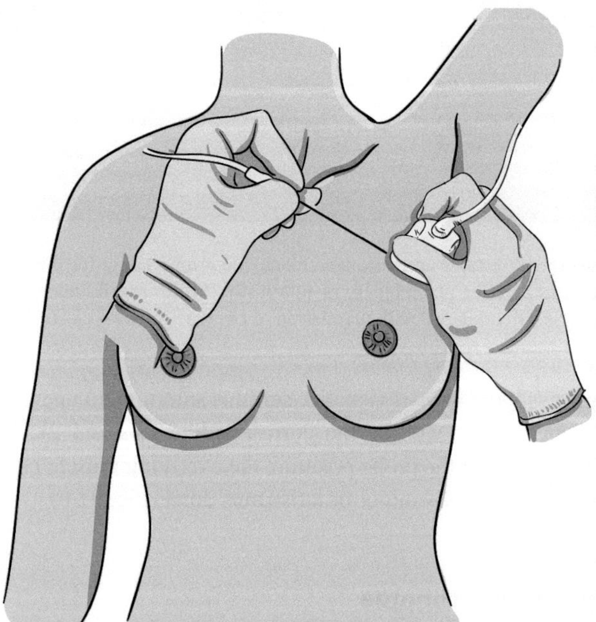

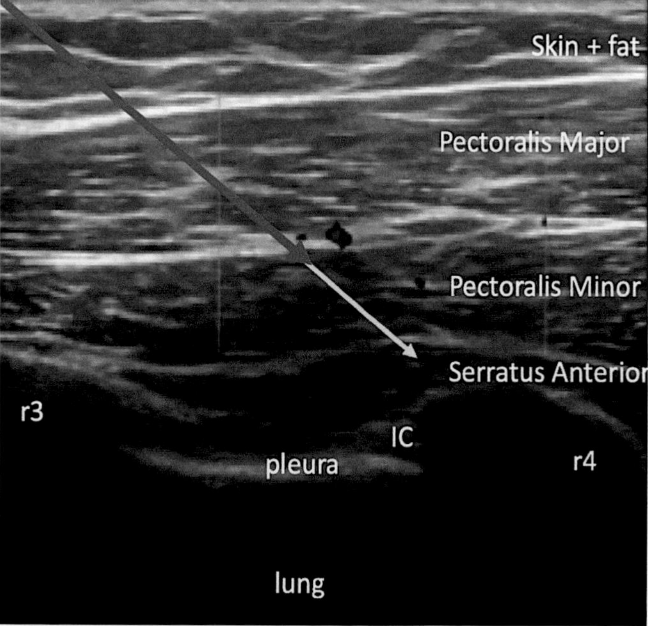

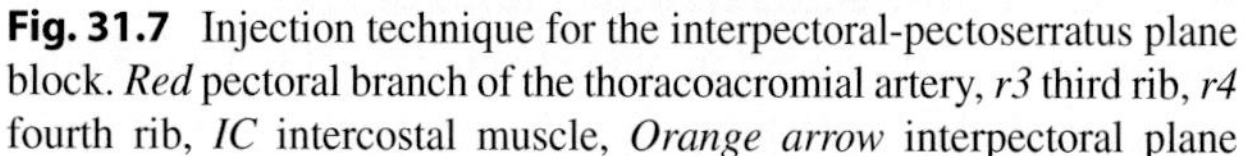

Fig. 31.7 Injection technique for the interpectoral-pectoserratus plane block. *Red* pectoral branch of the thoracoacromial artery, *r3* third rib, *r4* fourth rib, *IC* intercostal muscle, *Orange arrow* interpectoral plane block, *Yellow arrow* pectoserratus plane block. (Reproduced with permission of Dr. Barbara Versyck BV)

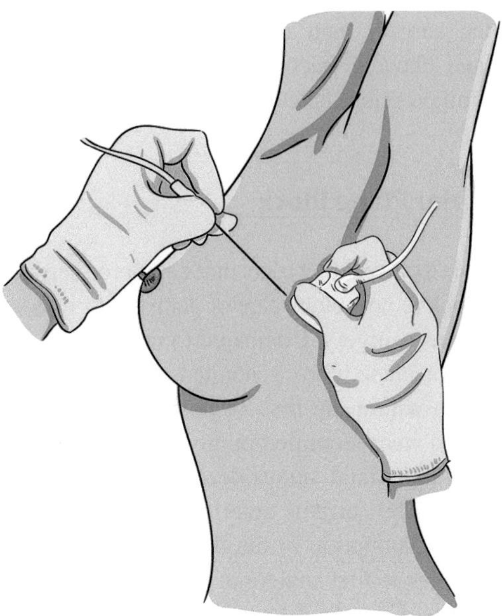

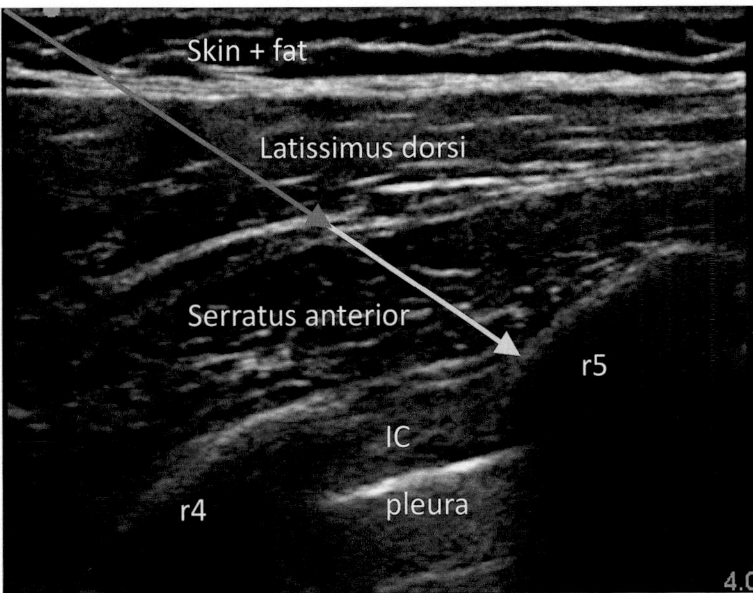

Fig. 31.8 Injection technique for the serratus anterior plane block at the level of r5. *r4* fourth rib, *r5* fifth rib, *IC* intercostal muscle, *Orange arrow* superficial variant, *Yellow arrow* deep variant of serratus anterior plane block. (Reproduced with permission of Dr. Barbara Versyck BV)

confirming the lateral spread of local anesthetic in the fascial plane.

Another variant is recommended by Biwas et al., which combines a deep and superficial serratus anterior plane block. Each injection contains half of a mixture of 20 mL of ropivacaine 1% and 20 mL of saline while respecting the maximum dose of ropivacaine.

Complications

Complications

- Intravascular injection (thoracoacromial artery) with toxic reactions when performing the Pecs blocks.
- Hematoma formation.
- Pleural puncture.

Side Effects

This technique may impact the surgical site by spreading local anesthetic in musculofascial planes.

Practical Tips

Application

The interpectoral, pectoserratus, and serratus anterior plane blocks are flexible in terms of the time of application. These blocks can be performed pre- and post-induction, before and after surgery, and as a rescue block. As clinical introduction of such regional anesthesia techniques may be challenging, it is recommended to choose the time of application that has the least impact on the existing way of working and fine-tune as soon as their benefits have been recognized by all stakeholders.

Tools

To perform the interpectoral, pectoserratus, and serratus anterior plane blocks, it is recommended to use short-length needle (50 mm). A shorter needle may reduce the risk of pleural puncture and produces greater agility to perform the block.

Local Anesthetic

In general, surgery of the anterolateral chest wall and axillary region may result in considerable acute postoperative pain over a longer period. Therefore, it is recommended to prefer a long-acting local anesthetic such as ropivacaine.

Procedure

To avoid pleural puncture, it is important to perform these techniques in plane while aiming the needle at an underlying rib.

Literature Review

Interpectoral Plane Block

Overall, little scientific research has been performed to study the interpectoral plane block. This might be due to its limited clinical applications as well as relatively short time between the introduction of the interpectoral plane and interpectoral-pectoserratus plane block. One meta-analysis on these blocks for modified radical mastectomy performed an interpectoral plane block subgroup analysis (interpectoral plane block, $n = 137$; GA, $n = 140$) and found that the block did not confer any benefit in terms of postoperative opioid consumption and pain scores.

Interpectoral-Pectoserratus Plane Block

The interpectoral-pectoserratus plane block is most commonly used as one component of a multimodal analgesia in oncological breast surgery. For this indication, multiple meta-analyses have concluded that the interpectoral-pectoserratus plane block significantly improves the quality of analgesia and reduces opioid consumption compared with systemic analgesia alone and may be used as an alternative to paravertebral block as regional analgesia technique.

A first group of meta-analyses studied the interpectoral-pectoserratus plane block either with systemic analgesia alone or with paravertebral block in patients undergoing breast cancer surgery in general (mastectomy or lumpectomy with axillary clearance or sentinel node dissection). These studies presented similar results: compared to systemic analgesia alone, interpectoral-pectoserratus plane block significantly reduced postoperative pain scores and opioid consumption within the first 24 postoperative hours and resulted in comparable postoperative pain scores and opioid consumption within the first 24 postoperative hours as the paravertebral block.

A second group of meta-analyses had a similar objective while focusing only on patients undergoing mastectomy. These findings were similar to the broader breast cancer surgery studies: interpectoral-pectoserratus plane block produced improved analgesic outcomes compared to systemic analgesia alone and comparable outcomes to the paravertebral block.

Based on this evidence, the 2020 PROSPECT guidelines for oncological breast surgery state, with Grade A, that the interpectoral-pectoserratus plane block may be used as an alternative to paravertebral block as regional analgesia technique.

Other indications for the interpectoral-pectoserratus plane block include implantation of cardiac devices, thoracotomy, sternotomy, transcatheter cardiac procedures, minimally invasive cardiac surgery, and traumatic thoracic injuries including rib and clavicle fractures. For such indications, there are only limited scientific evidence.

Serratus Anterior Plane Block

One meta-analysis examined 19 trials that compared serratus anterior plane block to non-block care or paravertebral block in breast and thoracic surgery. Compared to non-block care, the serratus anterior plane block generated a modest reduction in pain scores within the first 24 postoperative hours. Similar magnitudes were identified in the breast versus thoracic surgery and superficial versus deep serratus injection subgroup analyses. The serratus anterior plane block also decreased opioid consumption in the first 24 postoperative hours, prolonged time to first analgesia, and reduced rates of PONV and pruritus. Compared to the paravertebral block, there was no difference in pain scores at all time points except for the immediate postoperative period where serratus anterior plane block pain scores were slightly higher. All other outcomes were similar between groups.

One systematic review analyzed the effectiveness of the serratus anterior plane block in cardiothoracic surgery and trauma. The qualitative summary indicates that the block improves postoperative analgesia compared to systemic analgesia alone, particularly within the first 4–6 postoperative hours.

Suggested Reading

Biswas A, Castanov V, Li Z, Perlas A, Kruisselbrink R, Agur A, et al. Serratus plane block: a cadaveric study to evaluate optimal injectate spread. Reg Anesth Pain Med. 2018;43(8):854–8.

Chong M, Berbenetz N, Kumar K, Lin C. The serratus plane block for postoperative analgesia in breast and thoracic surgery: a systematic review and meta-analysis. Reg Anesth Pain Med. 2019;44(12):1066–74.

Grape S, El-Boghdadly K, Albrecht E. Analgesic efficacy of PECS vs paravertebral blocks after radical mastectomy: a systematic review, meta-analysis and trial sequential analysis. J Clin Anesth. 2020a;63:109745.

Grape S, Jaunin E, El-Boghdadly K, Chan V, Albrecht E. Analgesic efficacy of PECS and serratus plane blocks after breast surgery: a systematic review, meta-analysis and trial sequential analysis. J Clin Anesth. 2020b;63:109744.

Hussain N, Brull R, McCartney CJL, Wong P, Kumar N, Essandoh M, et al. Pectoralis-II myofascial block and analgesia in breast cancer surgery: a systematic review and meta-analysis. Anesthesiology. 2019;131(3):630–48.

Jack JM, McLellan E, Versyck B, Englesakis MF, Chin KJ. The role of serratus anterior plane and pectoral nerves blocks in cardiac surgery, thoracic surgery and trauma: a qualitative systematic review. Anaesthesia. 2020;75(10):1372–85.

Jacobs A, Lemoine A, Joshi GP, Van de Velde M, Bonnet F. PROSPECT working group collaborators#. PROSPECT guideline for oncological breast surgery: a systematic review and procedure-specific postoperative pain management recommendations. Anaesthesia. 2020;75(5):664–73.

Kunigo T, Murouchi T, Yamamoto S, Yamakage M. Spread of injectate in ultrasound-guided serratus plane block: a cadaveric study. JA Clin Rep. 2018;4(1):10.

Lovett-Carter D, Kendall MC, McCormick ZL, Suh EI, Cohen AD, Oliveira GSD. Pectoral nerve blocks and postoperative pain outcomes after mastectomy: a meta-analysis of randomized controlled trials. Reg Anesth Pain Med. 2019;44(10):923–8.

Versyck B, Groen G, Van Geffen G-J, Houwe PV, Bleys RL. The pecs anesthetic blockade: a correlation between magnetic resonance imaging, ultrasound imaging, reconstructed cross-sectional anatomy and cross-sectional histology. Clin Anat. 2019a;32(3):421–9.

Versyck B, van Geffen G-J, Chin K-J. Analgesic efficacy of the pecs II block: a systematic review and meta-analysis. Anaesthesia. 2019b;74(5):663–73.

Zhao J, Han F, Yang Y, Li H, Li Z. Pectoral nerve block in anesthesia for modified radical mastectomy: a meta-analysis based on randomized controlled trials. Medicine. 2019;98(18):e15423.

Transversus Abdominis Plane Blocks

32

Niall Cribben and John McDonnell

Contents

Definitions

The transversus abdominis plane (TAP) is a potential space, existing immediately superficial to the innermost muscle of the abdominal wall, the transversus abdominis. It is a neurovascular region which allows access to most of the nerves supplying the abdominal wall, hence its utility in regional nerve blocks. The deposition of local anaesthetic in this plane was first described and studied by Rafi and McDonnell in the early 2000s and has accelerated the investigation and development of other truncal and myofascial plane blocks.

It is worth noting the term 'TAP block' now encompasses several techniques, and although all refer to the administration of local anaesthetic into the neurovascular plane superficial to the TA muscle, they also involve different approaches and end results. Henceforth, we will use the following nomenclature:

Landmark TAP Block Although the lumbar triangle has been adopted as the traditional landmark for this approach, the key surface landmark for this technique is the insertion of the latissimus dorsi on the iliac crest. Immediately anterior to this is the 'latissomo-iliac point'. The needle is inserted immediately anterior to this point and superior to the iliac crest. The latissimo-iliac point may be a more reliable landmark than the lumbar triangle, which displays significant inter-individual variability.

Subcostal TAP Block Accessing the TAP inferior to the costal margin, inferior to the rectus abdominis muscle, at the point at which the TA muscle tapers off to become part of the rectus sheath.

N. Cribben · J. McDonnell (✉)
Department of Anaesthesia, Critical Care and Pain Management, University Hospital Galway, Galway, Ireland

D. Jankovic, P. Peng (eds.), *Regional Nerve Blocks in Anesthesia and Pain Therapy*, https://doi.org/10.1007/978-3-030-88727-8_32

Oblique Subcostal TAP Block Deposition of LA in the subcostal TAP region, along the entire costal margin. This is a dynamic technique requiring considerable skill.

Lateral TAP Block Block performed in the classic position, superior to the iliac crest, inferior to the costal margin, in the region of the midaxillary line.

Posterior TAP Block The authors recommend performing the TAP block as posterior as is practicably possible. The injection site for posterior TAP blocks is posterior to the midaxillary line. As discussed in Carney's radiological study, posterior deposition may offer access to the paravertebral space, thus providing additional sympathetic blockade which may in turn prolong analgesia.

Bilateral Dual TAP Block Combining subcostal and lateral TAP blocks on each side.

Background

The original approach to the TAP block was a landmark-based technique, using the lumbar triangle of Petit to identify the insertion point (Fig. 32.1). In this method, a needle is inserted posterior to the midaxillary line within the triangle, until two 'pops' are appreciated. The first positions the needle in the fascial plane between the external and internal oblique muscles, the second in the desired position between the internal oblique and transversus abdominis muscles.

Subsequent studies revealed significant inter-individual variability in the location of the lumbar triangle, which led to ultrasonography being incorporated to improve the block's success rate. The TAP block has been studied extensively since its introduction, leading to widely validated use as part of multimodal analgesia across a variety of surgical disciplines.

Functional Anatomy

A good understanding of the origins of the TA muscle, and the way it interacts with the nerves of the abdominal wall, is key to understanding the functional anatomy of this block.

The TA muscle is a bilateral paired muscle sheet, the innermost of the abdominal wall muscles. Laterally, the internal and external oblique muscles lie superficially, whilst medially, the rectus abdominis and pyramidalis muscles form the corresponding outer layers. In its lateral course, the TA muscle tapers off along with the internal oblique, back into its origin from the thoracolumbar fascia.

Medially, it blends with the aponeuroses of the internal and external oblique muscles to form the rectus sheath. The

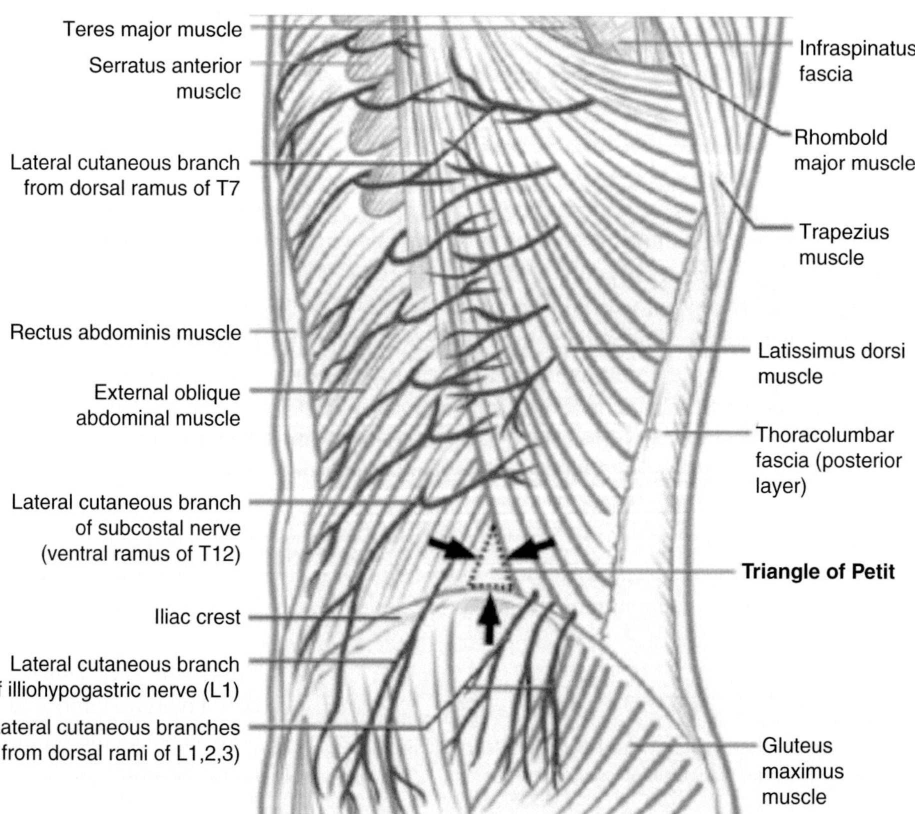

Fig. 32.1 Original representation of the lumbar triangle, McDonnell 2007. (Illustration produced by Theresa Sakno, with permission)

TA muscle also inserts into the anterior two-thirds of the iliac crest (Fig. 32.2).

Superiorly, the TA muscle attaches to the 7th–12th costal cartilages, as well as the xiphoid process. Inferiorly, the aponeurosis of the TA inserts into the pubic crest and pectineal line via the conjoint tendon.

The TA plane offers access to all of the nerves supplying the anterior and lateral abdominal wall. The innervation is derived from the anterior primary rami of the lower seven thoracic spinal nerves (the thoracoabdominal nerves, T6–T12), as well as the ilioinguinal and iliohypogastric nerves (L1).

Each of the thoracoabdominal nerves gives off a lateral cutaneous branch in the midaxillary line, supplying the lateral abdominal wall. The anterior divisions progress medially, emerging in the costal margin between the TA and the IO muscle to travel in the TA plane. The four uppermost of these, T6–T9, only enter the TAP medial to the anterior axillary line.

The anterior branch of T6 enters just proximal to the linea alba, with the anterior branch of each subsequent lower nerve entering the TAP incrementally more lateral. This has important implications for the pattern of nerve blockade seen at different injection sites whilst performing TAP blocks.

The lower segmental nerves (T9–L1) give off multiple communicating branches, forming a longitudinal TAP plexus from which the terminal anterior divisions arise.

Incorporating this knowledge into a given clinical scenario allows appropriate TAP block selection. For upper abdominal procedures in the T6–T9 region, such as open cholecystectomy or supraumbilical hernia repair, a subcostal TAP block is appropriate. Procedures around T9–T12, such as open appendicectomy, would benefit from coverage with a classic lateral or posterior TAP block, whilst a large midline incision can be covered with bilateral dual TAP blocks.

Indications

Approach	Nerves blocked	Area supplied
Lateral	T10–T12	Infraumbilical anterior abdominal wall
Posterior	T9–T12, with potential paravertebral spread	Infraumbilical anterior abdominal wall
Subcostal	T6–T9	Supraumbilical anterior abdominal wall
Oblique subcostal	T6–L1	Supraumbilical and infraumbilical anterior abdominal wall
Bilateral dual TAP block	T6–T12	Supraumbilical and infraumbilical anterior abdominal wall

TAP blocks are currently employed for a wide range of surgical procedures, primarily as part of a multimodal analgesia regimen (Fig. 32.3). Several case reports exist of the successful use of TAP blocks as anaesthesia for abdominal wall procedures, but it must be remembered that this block

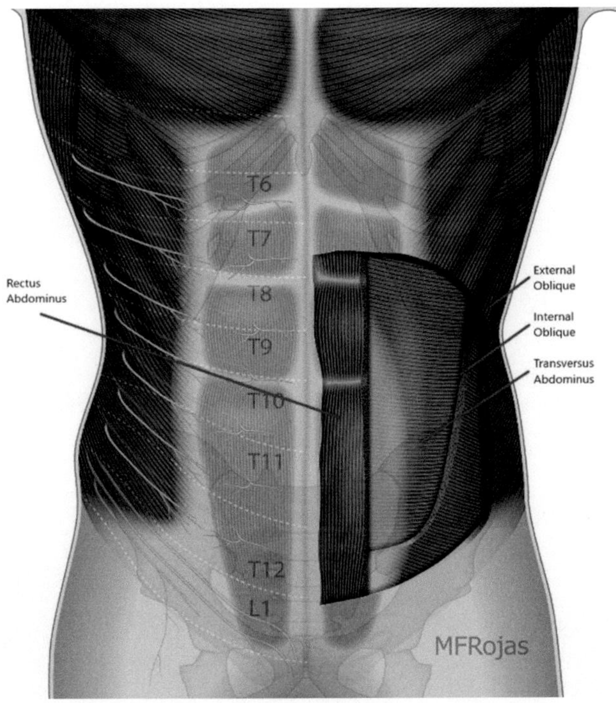

Fig. 32.2 Muscular layers of the abdominal wall. (With permission from Dr. Maria Fernanda Rojas)

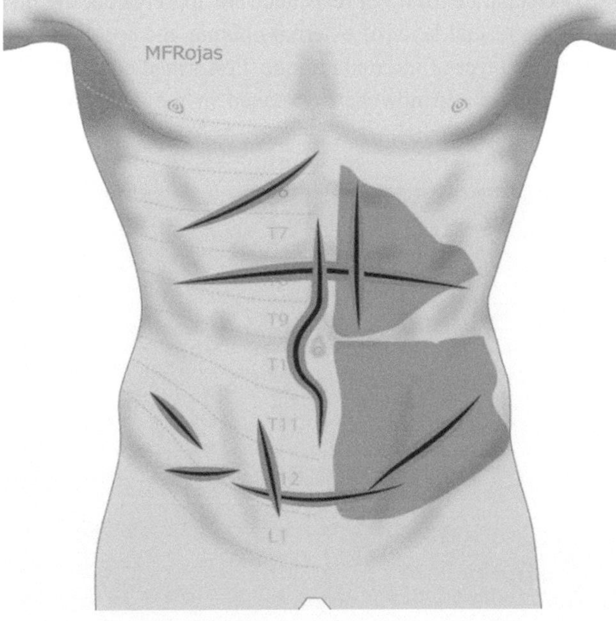

Fig. 32.3 Red areas indicate expected block coverage based on Borglum et al. (2012) results for bilateral dual TAP block. A number of common and uncommon surgical incisions are also shown. (With permission from Dr. Maria Fernanda Rojas)

will not provide abdominal visceral coverage, no matter the technique employed.

General Surgery—laparoscopic surgery, cholecystectomy, umbilical/incisional hernia repair, open appendicectomy, midline laparotomy procedures.
Urology—prostatectomy, nephrectomy.
Obstetrics/Gynaecology—total abdominal hysterectomy, caesarean section.
Chronic Pain—diagnosis of somatosensory chronic abdominal pain.

Technique

Landmark Approach

Although this block is now most commonly performed under US guidance, the authors recognise that this adjunct is not always available. There remains a large body of evidence demonstrating the safety and efficacy of the landmark approach, provided due care is taken to identify the requisite landmarks.

As mentioned previously, identification of the LIP is maybe more useful than the less specific target of the lumbar triangle. The iliac crest, posterior border of external oblique and anterior border of latissimus dorsi are identified (palpating the iliac crest in an anteroposterior direction until the border of LD is met is a useful technique here). Needle insertion is at the point where the anterior border of LD meets the iliac crest (Fig. 32.4).

Two separate losses of resistance are appreciated, the first being the fascial layer of external oblique, the second being the fascial layer of internal oblique. Performed correctly, the needle tip should now be positioned in the TAP. A blunt regional anaesthesia needle or Tuohy needle can be used to access the plane.

Additionally, the landmark approach may confer the additional benefit of a more posterior deposition of local anaesthetic, potentially augmenting and prolonging the analgesic efficacy of this block.

Subcostal TAP Block

This approach offers more reliable coverage of the upper thoracoabdominal nerves T6–T9 and is suitable for use in procedures where supraumbilical analgesia is desired.

The original technique employed a 100–150-mm needle, inserted in an inferolateral direction, with a single injection opening the TAP in the area immediately inferior and parallel to the costal margin, between the RA and TA muscles.

Injectate spread and resultant block may vary with insertion site. If the injection is made lateral to the linea semilunaris (at the lateral border of the RA muscle), the block will centre around the T10 and T11 dermatomes. However, if the desired area of blockade is T9 and above, the chosen site should be medial to the linea semilunaris, as close as possible to the xiphoid process (Fig. 32.5).

For this approach, the US probe can also be used to manipulate the injectate under the RA, moving it in a cephalad-caudad fashion along the linea alba, thus providing an additional rectus sheath block (Fig. 32.6).

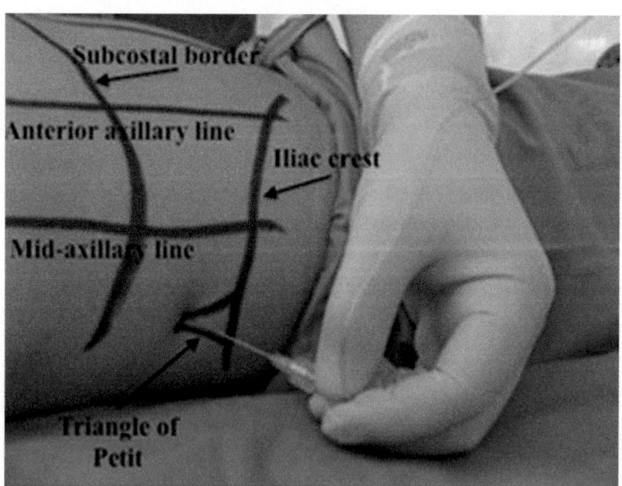

Fig. 32.4 Surface landmarks for the original approach. (With permission form Dr. John McDonnell)

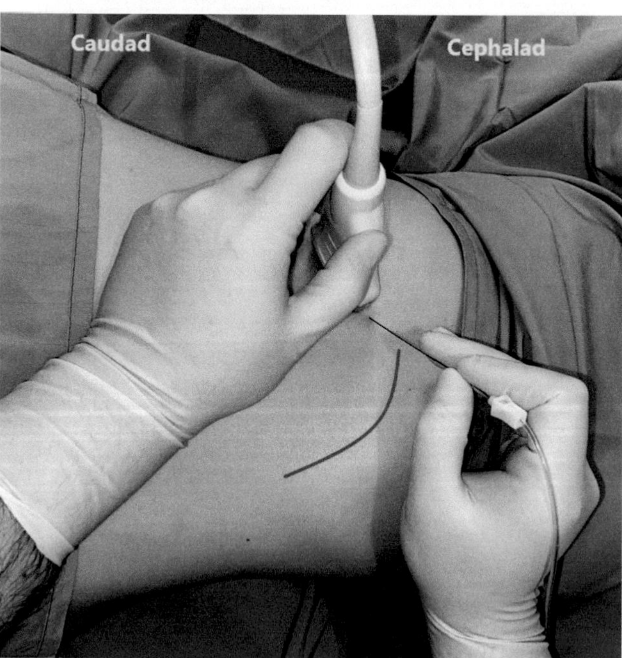

Fig. 32.5 Probe positioned immediately inferior to the costal margin on the block side. Contralateral costal margin outlined in red

Oblique Subcostal TAP Block

The oblique subcostal line runs from the xiphoid process to the anterior margin of the iliac crest. Deposition of local anaesthetic along this region has the potential to cover dermatomes from T6 to L1 within the TAP. This variant of TAP block is a development on the subcostal approach and requires considerable technical skill and sonographic knowledge to successfully execute (Fig. 32.7).

This approach requires a longer needle (150 mm) and larger volumes of local anaesthetic, to achieve to goal of hydro-dissection of the TAP along the entirety of oblique subcostal line. This can be achieved from a single insertion site (technically challenging), with the potential to site a catheter in the opened TA plane. Alternatively, this technique can be performed with dual or multiple insertions (Fig. 32.8).

These authors do not recommend the use of the original technique as described. Rather, this approach can be simplified by first depositing local in the TAP area desired, followed by the application of pressure from the US probe to move the fluid laterally.

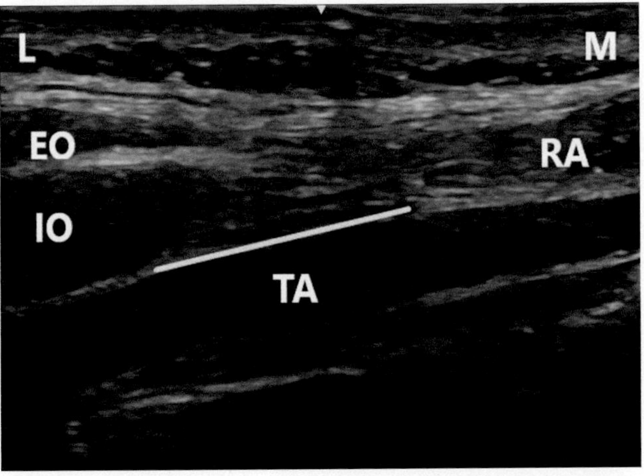

Fig. 32.6 Target area in yellow, lateral to the border of the rectus abdominis muscle

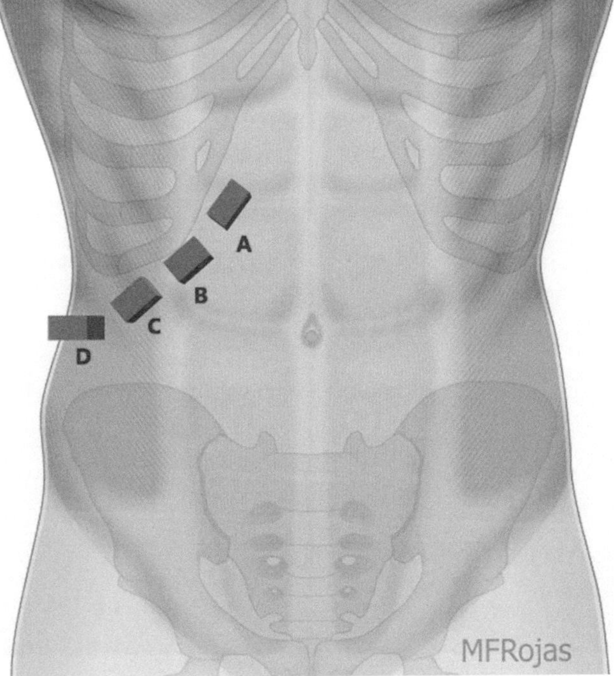

Fig. 32.7 Dynamic US probe positions, with likely subsequent views shown below. Note this is subject to significant variability in different individuals. (With permission from Dr. Maria Fernanda Rojas)

Lateral TAP Block

First described by McDonnell in 2007, for this approach, the probe is placed on the midaxillary line, parallel to the iliac crest and costal margin, at the midpoint between the two (Fig. 32.9). This region allows easy identification of the three muscle layers of the anterolateral abdominal walls (Fig. 32.10). A 100-mm needle is suitable in most patients.

This approach will reliably block the thoracoabdominal nerves T10, T11 and T12. Radiological studies have indicated injectate spread is limited to an area from the injection point in the midaxillary line, as far as the costal margin, with posterior spread minimal compared to the original landmark technique. T9 and above will not typically be blocked, as they enter the TAP medial to the anterior axillary line.

Posterior TAP Block

To overcome the limited spread of the lateral approach, the authors recommend moving the probe posteriorly until quadratus lumborum is seen and choosing an injection site as posterior as possible (Fig. 32.11). Views of QL offer a degree of assurance over the location of your injectate and the potential for paravertebral access.

Bilateral Dual TAP Block

Where analgesia for the entire abdominal wall is required (e.g. a large laparotomy incision), a bilateral dual TAP block is an appropriate choice. This will involve four separate injections, encompassing the lateral/posterior and subcostal approaches on each side.

The theoretical benefits of this approach add the blockade of the upper thoracoabdominal dermatomes produced by a medial subcostal TAP, to the consistent blockade of the T10–T12 dermatomes produced by the lateral TAP, to achieve a total coverage of T6–T12.

However, available studies show this approach will reliably block up to the T8 dermatomes, but not T6/T7 in most cases. Injectate spread is also limited to an area between the anterior and the midaxillary line, so lateral cutaneous branches will also be spared. Again, the focus should be on posterior placement of the lateral TAP blocks, in order to achieve potential paravertebral spread.

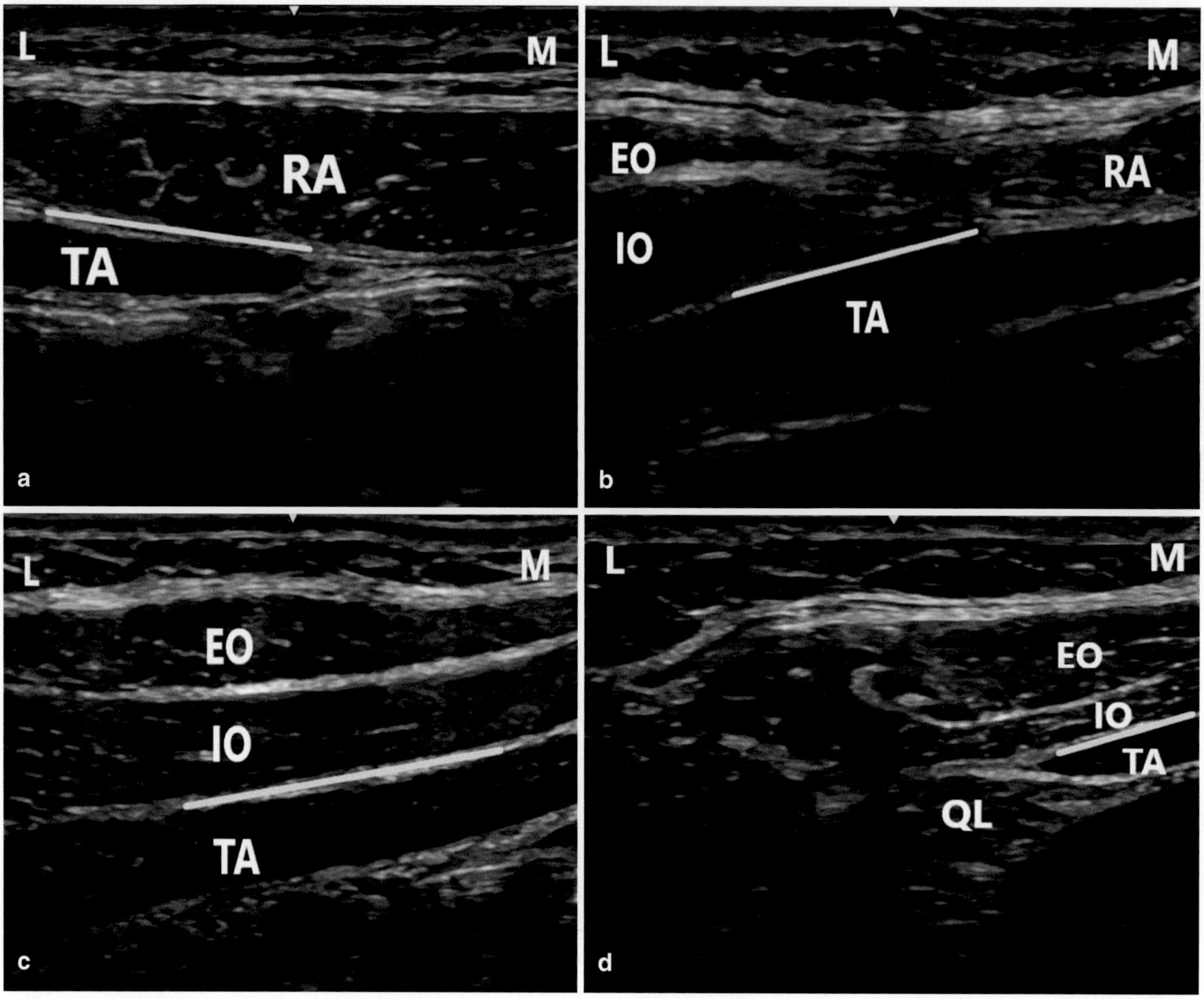

Fig. 32.8 Expected US images, with target areas for deposition of local anaesthetic highlighted in yellow. (*L* lateral, *M* medial)

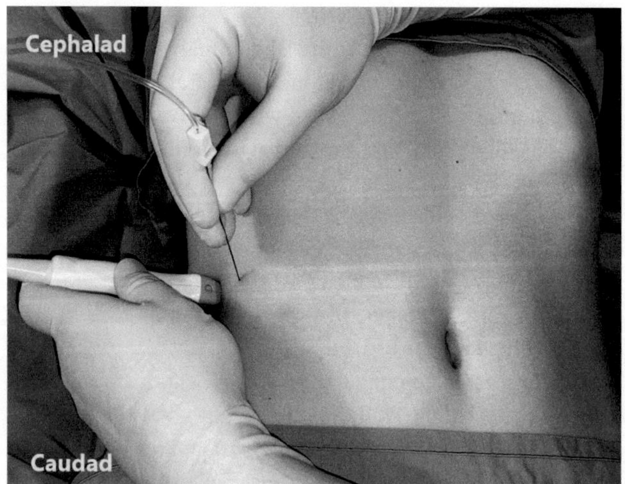

Fig. 32.9 Probe positioned in the midaxillary line for the lateral approach. Move the probe posteriorly until QL is viewed for a posterior TAP block

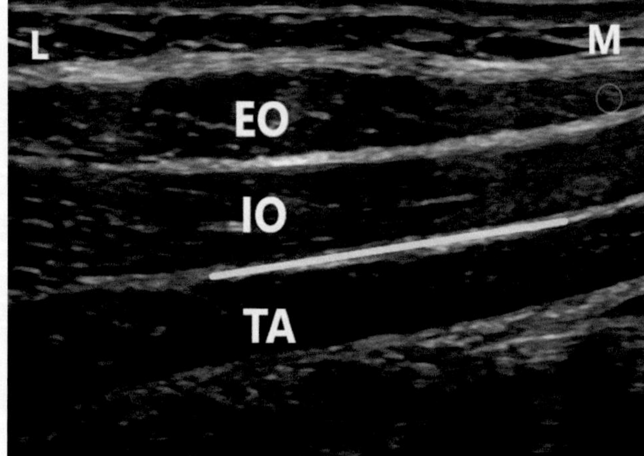

Fig. 32.10 Injectate site for classic lateral TAP block. (Figures 5, 6, 8, 9, 10 with permission from Dr. Niall Cribben)

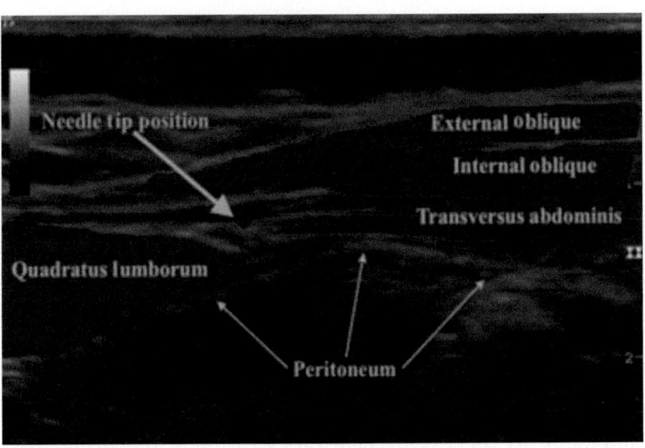

Fig. 32.11 Image from Carney, McDonnell et al. 2011 study on injectate spread within the TAP for a posterior TAP block. View of QL with posterior probe placement. (With permission from Dr. John McDonnell)

Continuous Techniques

A major limitation of TAP blocks to date has been the duration of analgesia provided by the block. Current evidence indicates reductions in pain scores and opioid consumption for up to 24–48 h. However, when investigated by first request for analgesia or offset of sensory block, TAP blocks are effective on average for 6–10 h.

Catheter techniques have been employed to overcome this but come with several practical difficulties. When sited preoperatively, there is the potential for disruption of the surgical field. Sited post-operatively, the procedure may become more technically challenging owing to the placement of dressings and the disruption of the muscle layers by the surgeons. Furthermore, larger midline incisions will require the insertion and management of four separate catheters. Evidence for using continuous infusions vs. intermittent boluses is also lacking.

Drugs and Dosing

The long-acting local anaesthetics ropivacaine (2.5–3.5 mg/kg) and bupivacaine/levobupivacaine (12 mg/kg) are the most commonly employed for TAP blocks. Available evidence suggests volume rather than dose is the main determinant of efficacy, as injectate spread is crucial. Even so, there appears to be little benefit of using volumes of local anaesthesia exceeding 15–20 mL per block.

Volumes should take into account maximum dose recommendations, and these in turn should be adjusted to lean body weight. In summary, in adult populations, the authors recommend 15–20 mL of 0.25–0.375% ropivacaine or 15–20 mL of 0.25% bupivacaine/levobupivacaine per side, with epinephrine added to reduce peak plasma concentrations. Paediatric data is limited.

Liposomal bupivacaine offers a novel potential solution to the time-limited nature of single-shot TAP blocks, but further studies are required.

Evidence for the use of adjuncts is mixed. A study by Singh and colleagues in 2016 suggested the addition of clonidine improves duration of analgesia in patients undergoing caesarean section, but other trials have failed to demonstrate similar results. Other studies showed lower pain scores in patients receiving dexmedetomidine as an additive. A recent systematic review of the addition of dexamethasone to TAP blocks in abdominal surgery also demonstrated efficacy.

The authors currently make no recommendation on the routine use of adjuncts and advise consideration on a case-by-case basis.

Procedure and Equipment

All procedures should be conducted with usual standards of monitoring, emergency drugs available and assistance where required. Sterile gloves, drapes, aseptic technique and probe cover as standard.

The authors recommend supine positioning, which can be augmented by placing a wedge (or a 1-L bag of IV fluid) under the patient's hip on the side to be blocked. This allows more posterior access.

For most patients, a 21-G, 50–100-mm short-bevelled needle will suffice. If performing a subcostal oblique approach, a longer needle (150 mm or more) may be required.

Complications

Reports exist in the literature of abdominal visceral damage from TAP block insertion, including liver and spleen puncture (especially in the setting of hepatosplenomegaly), bowel and flank haematomas and renal injury.

Accidental intravascular injection and plasma concentrations suggesting LAST have been reported. Cases of accidental co-administration of LA by anaesthetists (to the TAP) and surgeons (to the wound) have also occurred as a result of suboptimal communication. Overall, complication rates from TAP blocks are very low, and it is generally considered a safe and effective technique.

Tips to Improve Block Success

- Access to the area posterior to the midaxillary line allows avoidance of a common pitfall in TAP block performance, depositing LA too anteriorly. Placing a fluid bag (1–3 L depending on the size of the patient) under the hip on the block side offers easier access to the posterior structures.
- Hydro-dissection is a useful technique prior to the deposition of the full LA dose. Saline (or 1% lidocaine with epinephrine) may be used to open the TAP initially, improving success when the full volume is sited.

- As has been emphasised throughout this chapter, posterior is better. Anterior TAP injections are easier to visualise and perform and are a tempting endeavour (especially when first learning this block). However, for better results, it is best to aim posterior and for the potential benefits of paravertebral spread.

Literature Review

The TAP block has been well studied since its introduction, and a large body of evidence now exists to support its use in a variety of settings.

Upper Abdominal Surgery

TAP blocks have been compared with thoracic epidurals for post-operative analgesia in several studies (including catheter techniques). Results indicate the TAP block is a useful alternative where thoracic epidural insertion proves difficult or contraindications exist. TAP blocks are associated with fewer complications in this setting, most notably hypotension. Upper abdominal surgery is associated with significant visceral pain, in which TAP blocks will not cover. The nature of the incisions for upper GI procedures can make TAP block insertion challenging, and thoracic epidural is more likely to provide superior analgesia.

In the setting of laparoscopic cholecystectomy, evidence for the routine use of TAP blocks is limited. Pain control regimens for this procedure, incorporating multimodal analgesia and port-site infiltration with local anaesthetic, have rendered the benefit of additive TAP blocks questionable.

TAP blocks have recently been studied in the setting of bariatric surgery. One systematic review indicates TAP blocks are an effective additive to multimodal analgesia, contributing to lower pain scores and lower opioid consumption. Another recent review in this cohort revealed less post-operative nausea and vomiting, earlier ambulation, but similar pain scores in the TAP group. Overall, there is low to moderate evidence for the use of TAP blocks in bariatric surgery.

A recent systematic review and meta-analysis (limited to two RCTs) concluded that TAP blocks have a role in reducing opioid requirements in the 24-h period following liver transplant.

Lower Abdominal Surgery

The efficacy of TAP blocks in open and laparoscopic colorectal surgery has been well demonstrated. A high-quality early trial involving open procedures showed a significant reduction in pain scores and opioid use, with benefits seen at up to 48 h. For laparoscopic approaches, TAP blocks have consistently shown to be beneficial in reducing pain scores and opioid consumption, in many cases also allowing earlier mobilisation and return of bowel function. A recent systematic review comparing thoracic epidural to TAP blocks in laparoscopic colorectal surgery showed equivalent analgesia between the groups but shorter time to ambulation and passing flatus in the TAP group. As such, TAP blocks can be considered a safe and effective additive to enhanced recovery programmes after colorectal surgery.

Open appendicectomy is amongst the procedures most amenable to successful TAP block. Typical incisions cross the T11/T12 dermatomes, which are reliably covered by the lateral approach. The evidence for employing TAP blocks in laparoscopic appendicectomy is equivocal at best, possibly owing to a larger contribution to the pain score from visceral elements. In similar fashion to use in laparoscopic cholecystectomy, when combined with multimodal analgesia and port-site infiltration with local anaesthetic, there appears to be little additive benefit to a TAP block.

For inguinal hernia repair, the evidence is surprisingly conflicting. Despite an operative site seemingly suited to the TAP block, the literature suggests benefit for the early post-operative period but not beyond. Compared with ilioinguinal and iliohypogastric blocks, the TAP approach is likely not inferior, but again the benefits are limited to the first 24 h at best. A recent systematic review concluded these approaches lead to similar opioid consumption, with a similar complication rate.

Gynaecological Surgery

Two recent systematic reviews concluded that TAP blocks provide early benefit in terms of pain scores and opioid consumption in patients undergoing total abdominal hysterectomy. However, there was marked heterogeneity in the studies included. Many individual RCTs examining TAP blocks in the TAH have marked limitations. The evidence for use in laparoscopic approaches is lacking. As with laparoscopic approaches for other surgical disciplines, there appears to be a marginal benefit when combined with multimodal analgesia and local infiltration.

Obstetric Surgery

For the obstetric population, there appears to be several distinct circumstances under which TAP blocks are beneficial. With most caesarean sections performed under subarachnoid block, intrathecal morphine has become the gold standard for analgesia in the immediate 24 h after delivery. In this setting, the addition of a TAP block does not appear to confer any benefit.

For patients not receiving intrathecal morphine, early benefits in pain scores and opioid consumption have been demonstrated, as well as a consequential decrease in the incidence of PONV. Benefits appear to be limited to the early post-operative period, and a recent systematic review concluded wound infiltration is close to equivalent. There may also be a role for TAP blocks in rescue analgesia for uncontrolled pain and in settings where opioids or NSAIDs are contraindicated.

Urological Procedures

TAP blocks have been studied in the setting of renal transplantation, with little apparent benefit to routine use. Pain control in the study groups was sufficient without the addition of TAP blocks even in the setting of NSAID avoidance.

The same can be applied to open radical prostatectomy patients. Whilst there is evidence for an initial reduction in opioid use, when compared to optimal multimodal analgesia with wound infiltration, TAP blocks do not offer additional benefits.

Conclusions

There is now a large body of evidence studying TAP blocks, over two decades and in a variety of contexts. The authors recommend considering TAP blocks for open procedures such as appendicectomy and inguinal hernia repair, in relevant settings where the standard intervention is contraindicated (i.e. as an alternative to thoracic epidural or intrathecal morphine), or as a rescue technique for escalating pain scores. It is important to bear in mind benefits appear to be limited in laparoscopic surgery and will likely not extend beyond the initial 24-h period post-operatively in most cases. This may be improved by a more posterior deposition of local anaesthetic, potentially tracking retrograde into the paravertebral spaces.

Suggested Reading

Abdallah FW, Chan VW, Brull R. Transversus abdominis plane block: a systematic review. Reg Anesth Pain Med. 2012;37(2):193–209. PMID: 22286518. https://doi.org/10.1097/AAP.0b013e3182429531.

Aveline C, Le Hetet H, Le Roux A, et al. Comparison between ultrasound-guided transversus abdominis plane and conventional ilioinguinal/iliohypogastric nerve blocks for day-case open inguinal hernia repair. Br J Anaesth. 2011;106:380–6.

Bacal V, Rana U, McIsaac DI, Chen I. Transversus abdominis plane block for post hysterectomy pain: a systematic review and meta-analysis. J Minim Invasive Gynecol. 2019;26(1):40–52. Epub 2018 Apr 30. PMID: 29723644. https://doi.org/10.1016/j.jmig.2018.04.020.

Baeriswyl M, Kirkham KR, Kern C, Albrecht E. The analgesic efficacy of ultrasound-guided transversus abdominis plane block in adult patients: a meta-analysis. Anesth Analg. 2015;121:1640–54.

Baeriswyl M, Zeiter F, Piubellini D, Kirkham KR, Albrecht E. The analgesic efficacy of transverse abdominis plane block versus epidural analgesia: a systematic review with meta-analysis. Medicine (Baltimore). 2018;97(26):e11261. PMID: 29952997; PMCID: PMC6039642. https://doi.org/10.1097/MD.0000000000011261.

Børglum J, Maschmann C, Belhage B, Jensen K. Ultrasound-guided bilateral dual transversus abdominis plane block: a new four-point approach. Acta Anaesthesiol Scand. 2011;55:658–63.

Børglum J, Jensen K, Christensen AF, et al. Distribution patterns, dermatomal anesthesia, and ropivacaine serum concentrations after bilateral dual transversus abdominis plane block. Reg Anesth Pain Med. 2012;37:294–301.

Brogi E, Kazan R, Cyr S, Giunta F, Hemmerling TM. Transversus abdominal plane block for postoperative analgesia: a systematic review and meta-analysis of randomized-controlled trials. Can J Anaesth. 2016;63(10):1184–96. Epub 2016 Jun 15. PMID: 27307177. https://doi.org/10.1007/s12630-016-0679-x.

Carney J, McDonnell JG, Ochana A, Bhinder R, Laffey JG. The transversus abdominis plane block provides effective postoperative analgesia in patients undergoing total abdominal hysterectomy. Anesth Analg. 2008;107(6):2056–60.

Carney J, Finnerty O, Rauf J, Bergin D, Laffey JG, Mc Donnell JG. Studies on the spread of local anaesthetic solution in transversus abdominis plane blocks. Anaesthesia. 2011;66(11):1023–30. Epub 2011 Aug 18. https://doi.org/10.1111/j.1365-2044.2011.06855.x.

Charlton S, Cyna AM, Middleton P, Griffiths JD. Perioperative transversus abdominis plane (TAP) blocks for analgesia after abdominal surgery. Cochrane Database Syst Rev. 2010;(12):CD007705. Update in: Cochrane Database Syst Rev. 2020 Apr 9;4:CD007705. PMID: 21154380. https://doi.org/10.1002/14651858.CD007705.pub2.

Chin KJ, McDonnell JG, Carvalho B, et al. Essentials of our current understanding: abdominal wall blocks. Reg Anaesth Pain Med. 2017;42:133–83.

Favuzza J, Delaney CP. Outcomes of discharge after elective laparoscopic colorectal surgery with transversus abdominis plane blocks and enhanced recovery pathway. J Am Coll Surg. 2013;217:503–6.

Ganapathy S, Sondekoppam RV, Terlecki M, et al. Comparison of efficacy and safety of lateral-to-medial continuous transversus abdominis plane block with thoracic epidural analgesia in patients undergoing abdominal surgery: a randomised, open-label feasibility study. Eur J Anaesthesiol. 2015;32:797–804.

Grape S, Kirkham KR, Albrecht E. The analgesic efficacy of transversus abdominis plane block after bariatric surgery: a systematic review and meta-analysis with trial sequential analysis. Obes Surg. 2020;30(10):4061–70. PMID: 32572686. https://doi.org/10.1007/s11695-020-04768-x.

Griffiths JD, Middle JV, Barron FA, Grant SJ, Popham PA, Royse CF. Transversus abdominis plane block does not provide additional benefit to multimodal analgesia in gynecological cancer surgery. Anesth Analg. 2010;111:797–801.

Gulyam KSM, Mukhtar K, Singh SK. A randomised controlled trial of ultrasound-guided transversus abdominis plane block for renal transplantation. Anaesthesia. 2014;69:1222–6.

Hamid HKS, Marc-Hernández A, Saber AA. Transversus abdominis plane block versus thoracic epidural analgesia in colorectal surgery: a systematic review and meta-analysis. Langenbecks Arch

Surg. 2021;406(2):273–82. Epub ahead of print. PMID: 32974803. https://doi.org/10.1007/s00423-020-01995-9.

Hebbard P. Subcostal transversus abdominis plane block under ultrasound guidance. Anesth Analg. 2008;106:674–5.

Hebbard P. TAP block nomenclature. Anaesthesia. 2015;70:112–3.

Hebbard PD, Barrington MJ, Vasey C. Ultrasound-guided continuous oblique subcostal transversus abdominis plane blockade: description of anatomy and clinical technique. Reg Anesth Pain Med. 2010;35:436–41.

Jankovic ZB, du Feu FM, McConnell P. An anatomical study of the transversus abdominis plane block: location of the lumbar triangle of petit and adjacent nerves. Anesth Analg. 2009a;109:981–5.

Jankovic ZB, Pollard SG, Nachiappan MM. Continuous transversus abdominis plane block for renal transplant recipients. Anesth Analg. 2009b;109(5):1710–1.

Johns N, O'Neill S, Ventham NT, Barron F, Brady RR, Daniel T. Clinical effectiveness of transversus abdominis plane (TAP) block in abdominal surgery: a systematic review and meta-analysis. Colorectal Dis. 2012;14(10):e635–42. PMID: 22632762. https://doi.org/10.1111/j.1463-1318.2012.03104.x.

Kane SM, Garcia-Tomas V, Alejandro-Rodriguez M, Astley B, Pollard RR. Randomized trial of transversus abdominis plane block at total laparoscopic hysterectomy: effect of regional analgesia on quality of recovery. Am J Obstet Gynecol. 2012;207(419):e1–5.

Keller DS, Ermlich BO, Delaney CP. Demonstrating the benefits of transversus abdominis plane blocks on patient outcomes in laparoscopic colorectal surgery: review of 200 consecutive cases. J Am Coll Surg. 2014;219:1143–8.

Lee THW, Barrington MJ, Tran TM, Wong D, Hebbard PD. Comparison of extent of sensory block following posterior and subcostal approaches to ultrasound-guided transversus abdominis plane block. Anaesth Intensive Care. 2010;38:452–60.

Ma N, Duncan JK, Scarfe AJ, Schuhmann S, Cameron AL. Clinical safety and effectiveness of transversus abdominis plane (TAP) block in post-operative analgesia: a systematic review and meta-analysis. J Anesth. 2017;31(3):432–52. Epub 2017 Mar 7. PMID: 28271227. https://doi.org/10.1007/s00540-017-2323-5.

McDermott G, Korba E, Mata U, et al. Should we stop doing blind transversus abdominis plane blocks? Br J Anaesth. 2012;108:499–502.

McDonnell JG, O'Donnell B, Curley G, Heffernan A, Power C, Laffey JG. The analgesic efficacy of transversus abdominis plane block after abdominal surgery: a prospective randomized controlled trial. Anesth Analg. 2007a;104(1):193–7. Erratum in: Anesth Analg 2007 May;104(5):1108. https://doi.org/10.1213/01.ane.0000250223.49963.0f.

McDonnell JG, O'Donnell BD, Farrell T, et al. Transversus abdominis plane block: a cadaveric and radiological evaluation. Reg Anesth Pain Med. 2007b;32:399–404.

McDonnell JG, Curley G, Carney J, Benton A, Costello J, Maharaj CH, Laffey JG. The analgesic efficacy of transversus abdominis plane block after cesarean delivery: a randomized controlled trial. Anesth Analg. 2008;106(1):186–91, table of contents. https://doi.org/10.1213/01.ane.0000290294.64090.f3.

Mishriky BM, George RB, Habib AS. Transversus abdominis plane block for analgesia after cesarean delivery: a systematic review and meta-analysis. Can J Anaesth. 2012;59(8):766–78. Epub 2012 May 24. PMID: 22622954. https://doi.org/10.1007/s12630-012-9729-1.

Niraj G, Searle A, Mathews M, et al. Analgesic efficacy of ultrasound-guided transversus abdominis plane block in patients undergoing open appendicectomy. Br J Anaesth. 2009;103:601–5.

Niraj G, Kelkar A, Jeyapalan I, et al. Comparison of analgesic efficacy of subcostal transversus abdominis plane blocks with epidural analgesia following upper abdominal surgery. Anaesthesia. 2011;66:465–71.

Peltrini R, Cantoni V, Green R, Greco PA, Calabria M, Bucci L, Corcione F. Efficacy of transversus abdominis plane (TAP) block in colorectal surgery: a systematic review and meta-analysis. Tech Coloproctol. 2020;24(8):787–802. Epub 2020 Apr 6. PMID: 32253612. https://doi.org/10.1007/s10151-020-02206-9.

Petersen PL, Stjernholm P, Kristiansen VB, et al. The beneficial effect of transversus abdominis plane block after laparoscopic cholecystectomy in day-case surgery: a randomized clinical trial. Anesth Analg. 2012;115:527–33.

Rafi AN. Abdominal field block: a new approach via the lumbar triangle. Anaesthesia. 2001;56:1024–6.

Rafi AN. Abdominal field block via the lumbar triangle revisited. Anaesthesia. 2012;67:1399–401.

Røjskjaer JO, Gade E, Kiel LB, et al. Analgesic effect of ultrasound-guided transversus abdominis plane block after total abdominal hysterectomy: a randomized, double-blind, placebo-controlled trial. Acta Obstet Gynecol Scand. 2015;94:274–8.

Rozen WM, Tran TM, Ashton MW, Barrington MJ, Ivanusic JJ, Taylor GI. Refining the course of the thoracolumbar nerves: a new understanding of the innervation of the anterior abdominal wall. Clin Anat. 2008;21:325–33.

Shin HJ, Oh AY, Baik JS, Kim JH, Han SH, Hwang JW. Ultrasound-guided oblique subcostal transversus abdominis plane block for analgesia after laparoscopic cholecystectomy: a randomized, controlled, observer-blinded study. Minerva Anestesiol. 2014;80:185–93.

Skjelsager A, Ruhnau B, Kistorp TK, et al. Transversus abdominis plane block or subcutaneous wound infiltration after open radical prostatectomy: a randomized study. Acta Anaesthesiol Scand. 2013;57:502–8.

Sondekoppam RV, Brookes J, Morris L, Johnson M, Ganapathy S. Injectate spread following ultrasound-guided lateral to medial approach for dual transversus abdominis plane blocks. Acta Anaesthesiol Scand. 2015;59:369–76.

Tanggaard K, Jensen K, Lenz K, et al. A randomised controlled trial of bilateral dual transversus abdominis plane blockade for laparoscopic appendicectomy. Anaesthesia. 2015;70:1395–400.

Tolchard S, Davies R, Martindale S. Efficacy of the subcostal transversus abdominis plane block in laparoscopic cholecystectomy: comparison with conventional port-site infiltration. J Anaesthesiol Clin Pharmacol. 2012;28:339–43.

Wu Y, Liu F, Tang H, et al. The analgesic efficacy of subcostal transversus abdominis plane block compared with thoracic epidural analgesia and intravenous opioid analgesia after radical gastrectomy. Anesth Analg. 2013;117:507–13.

Zhao X, Tong Y, Ren H, Ding XB, Wang X, Zong JY, Jin SQ, Li Q. Transversus abdominis plane block for postoperative analgesia after laparoscopic surgery: a systematic review and meta-analysis. Int J Clin Exp Med. 2014;7(9):2966–75. PMID: 25356170; PMCID: PMC4211820.

Quadratus Lumborum Block

33

Jens Børglum, Christian Kruse Hansen, and Katrine Bayer Tanggaard

Contents

Background

With the first description of a (possible) quadratus lumborum (QL) block, Dr. Blanco did not even mention the QL muscle in the abstract submitted. Instead, the block was called a "TAP (transversus abdominis plane) block under ultrasound guidance: the description of a 'no pops' technique." With the passing of time, this description has evolved in block execution, clarity, and nomenclature. In a later magnetic resonance imaging (MRI) study using volunteers, Carney et al. again mention the ultrasound-guided (USG) *posterior* approach to the TAP block, in which local anesthetic (LA) was deposited close to the antero-lateral border of the QL muscle. With this technique, the authors reported predominantly posterior spread of contrast around the QL muscle to the paravertebral space from T5 to L1 vertebral levels. This finding was in contrast to a preceding study by the same research group, where the "blind and landmarked based" *posterior* approach to the TAP block with the "double pop" technique—presumably with the same point of injection—resulted in reliable deposition into the TAP. The sensory block extended from T7 to L1, and this finding was supported by MRI studies that showed a gradual reduction in contrast in the TAP over time, i.e., indicating an anterior spread of injectate.

The USG posterior TAP block described by Carney et al. was later investigated by Parras et al. in a randomized controlled trial (RCT) for postoperative analgesia in femoral neck fracture patients, i.e., the block technique was by now called a QL I block. This QL I block was defined as LA

J. Børglum (✉)
Department of Anesthesiology and Intensive Care, Zealand University Hospital, Roskilde, Denmark

Department of Clinical Medicine, Faculty of Health and Medical Sciences, University of Copenhagen, Copenhagen, Denmark

C. K. Hansen · K. B. Tanggaard
Department of Anesthesiology and Intensive Care, Zealand University Hospital, Roskilde, Denmark
e-mail: ckh@regionsjaelland.dk; kabt@regionsjaelland.dk

D. Jankovic, P. Peng (eds.), *Regional Nerve Blocks in Anesthesia and Pain Therapy*,
https://doi.org/10.1007/978-3-030-88727-8_33

injected very close to the antero-lateral part of the QL muscle. The mode of injection and execution did bear much resemblance to the fascia transversalis plane block technique described by Dr. Hebbard previously in 2009. As it were, the first QL block (QL I) was abandoned by Blanco et al. in favor of a new QL block called QL II.

The USG transmuscular QL (TQL) block was first described in 2013. The idea of the TQL block never had the intention that the injected LA would spread into the TAP. Rather, the TQL block had, from the beginning, the premise that if the injectate was deposited in the facial interspace *between* the QL and psoas major (PM) muscles (at the level of L3–L4), *and posterior to the transversalis fascia*, then the injectate would spread cephalad in the plane between the two muscles to reach the diaphragmatic openings and spread beyond further cranially into the thoracic paravertebral space to anesthetize the ventral rami of the segmental nerves and the sympathetic thoracic trunk. This theory was first documented in a cadaveric study by Dam et al.

Block Indications

Unilateral: Unilateral herniotomy, percutaneous nephrolithotomy, open appendicectomy, and as a rescue block in the Post Anesthesia Care Unit (PACU).

Bilateral: Laparoscopic procedures (nephrectomy, heminephrectomy, hemicolectomy, hysterectomy, cholecystectomy), cesarean section, mini-laparotomy, and as rescue blocks in the PACU.

Anatomy

The quadratus lumborum muscle is a paired muscle of the left and right posterior abdominal wall. Each of the two muscles is irregular and quadrilateral in shape. The QL muscles derive from the wings of the ilium, where they originate from the iliolumbar ligaments and the internal lips of the iliac crests. The QL muscle *insertions* are on the transverse processes of the upper four lumbar vertebrae and additionally at the lower posterior borders of the twelfth rib. The innervation of the QL muscles is with branches of the ventral rami of T12 to L4. The psoas major (PM) muscle lies adjacent and antero-medial to the QL muscle. The PM is innervated by direct branches of the anterior rami of the lumbar plexus at the levels of L1–L3. The superficial part of the PM muscle *originates* from the lateral surfaces of the last (T12) thoracic vertebra, the lumbar vertebrae (L1–L4), and from the neighboring intervertebral discs. Thus, the QL and PM muscles either insert or originate *within* the thoracic cage.

The muscles of the torso are embryologically divided into the hypaxial and epaxial muscle compartments. The epaxial (or paraspinal) muscles are the components of the erector spinae muscles. In the lumbar region that is the iliocostalis lumborum, the longissimus lumborum, and the spinalis dorsi muscles. The hypaxial muscles in the lumbar region include the QL and PM muscles, and these are in fact the posterior aspect of the abdominal wall. The distinction is relevant due to the difference in nomenclature, but also because the related fasciae have different properties. The transversalis fascia covers the deep side of all of the abdominal wall (hypaxial) muscles, i.e., rectus abdominis, transversus abdominis, as well as the QL and PM muscles.

Various anatomists disagree on the issue of layers from the thoracolumbar fascia (TLF). When describing the TLF as a 2-layer structure, the anterior part is what elsewhere (3-layer structure) is known as the middle part. Since the transversalis fascia is a marked structure of its own, and the embryologic origin of the two muscle compartments is apart, many anatomists advocate a 2-layer model of the TLF. The posterior layer encapsulates the paraspinal muscles, i.e., the erector spinae muscles. The anterior part of the TLF is attached to the transverse processes of the lumbar vertebrae, where it forms the intramuscular septum and a clear division between the two muscle compartments. Thus, the anterior part of the TLF separates the paraspinal/epaxial muscles from the hypaxial muscles in the posterior aspect of the abdominal wall, which consists of the QL and PM muscles.

The discovery of a pathway from the lumbar into the thoracic paravertebral region is not new. Injectate flow through the pathway has previously been described from a thoracic starting point, and understanding the pathway is crucial for accepting the pattern of injectate spread associated with the TQL block. The transversalis fascia covers the QL and PM muscles (anteriorly) below the diaphragm. At the level of the diaphragmatic openings, the transversalis fascia splits into an anterior layer covering the abdominal (deep) side of the diaphragm, and a posterior layer that covers the most cephalad parts of the QL and PM muscles, as they insert (QL) or originate (PM) within the thoracic cage. At this level, the transversalis fascia becomes continuous with the endothoracic fascia. Thus, any injected volume of LA deposited below the diaphragm, *posterior* to the transversalis fascia, *and* in the fascial interspace between the QL and PM muscles, could potentially spread cephalad and enter into the thoracic paravertebral space, i.e., with the injectate now *posterior* to the *endothoracic fascia*.

Why not inject directly into the (lower) thoracic paravertebral space? The benefits of a direct thoracic paravertebral block are evidently (potentially) many. There are several techniques described. However, since a direct USG thoracic paravertebral block is by many physicians considered to be a rather advanced block and to be associated with the potential—maybe perceived—risk of pneumothorax due to its close proximity to the pleura, an indirect way of reaching the thoracic paravertebral space is widely searched and research in this area has increased rapidly the last years.

Block Nomenclature

During the last decade, there has been a fluctuating nomenclature relative to the various QL block techniques. A suggestion for a common nomenclature was put forward by Elsharkawy et al. in 2019. These suggestions have now been broadly accepted with international consensus, and this has resulted in a novel manuscript which has been accepted for publication in Regional Anesthesia and Pain Medicine with the initial title "Standardizing nomenclature in regional anesthesia: An ASRA-ESRA Delphi consensus study of abdominal wall, paraspinal and chest wall blocks." This means that the QL I and QL II blocks are now called the lateral and posterior QL blocks, respectively (Figs. 33.1 and 33.2). The transmuscular QL block is now called the anterior QL block (Figs. 33.1 and 33.2). It is important to realize that the anatomy is changing relative to which level you are able to get the optimal sonographic image of all relevant anatomical structures.

Block Techniques

The QL I Block/The Lateral QL Block Approach

With the patient in a *supine* position a high frequency linear transducer is placed in a transverse position in the mid-axillary line at the lateral border of the anterior abdominal wall. The transducer is then moved posteriorly until the transversus abdominis and internal oblique aponeurosis are visualized. With a needle trajectory guided by ultrasound in an anterior to posterior direction, the point of injectate is at the antero-lateral border of the quadratus lumborum muscle, *superficial* to the transversalis fascia and deep to the transversus abdominis and internal oblique aponeurosis (Figs. 33.1 and 33.2).

The QL2 Block/The Posterior QL Block Approach

Same position for the patient and the same transducer as described for the QL I block, but the point of injection is postero-lateral to the QL muscle, deep to the latissimus dorsi muscle and superficial to the QL muscle (Figs. 33.1 and 33.2).

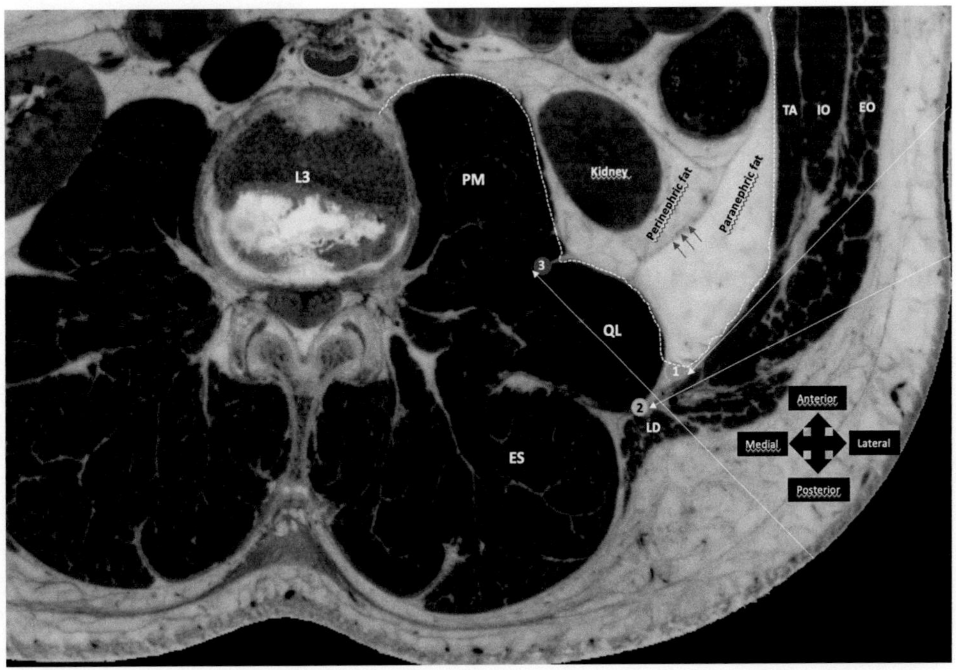

Fig. 33.1 Quadratus lumborum blocks at the level of L3. *EO* external oblique muscle, *IO* internal oblique muscle, *TA* transversus abdominis muscle, *LD* latissimus dorsi muscle, *QL* quadratus lumborum muscle, *PM* psoas major muscle, *ES* erector spinae muscles, *L3* vertebral body of L3. White dotted line depicts relevant parts of the transversalis fascia. Red arrows indicate the posterior renal fascia (Gerota's fascia). White arrows; needle trajectory with injections for the lateral QL block (number 1, blue circle), the posterior QL block (number 2, green circle), and the anterior QL block (number 3, red circle)

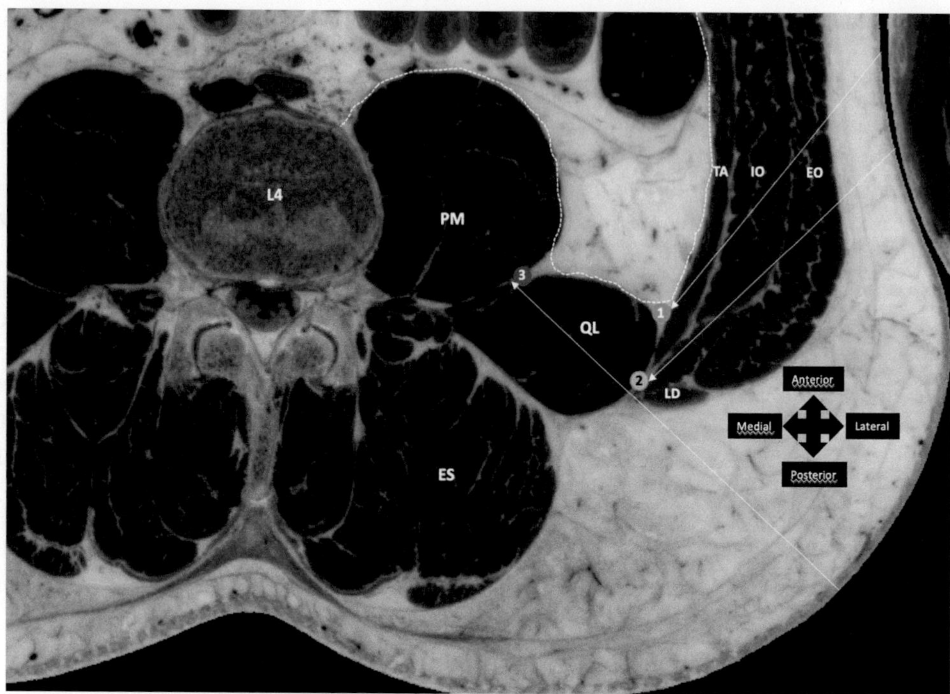

Fig. 33.2 Quadratus lumborum blocks at the level of L4. *EO* external oblique muscle, *IO* internal oblique muscle, *TA* transversus abdominis muscle, *LD* latissimus dorsi muscle, *QL* quadratus lumborum muscle, *PM* psoas major muscle, *ES* erector spinae muscles, *L3* vertebral body of L3. White dotted line depicts relevant parts of the transversalis fascia. Red arrows indicate the posterior renal fascia (Gerota's fascia). White arrows; needle trajectory with injections for the lateral QL block (number 1, blue circle), the posterior QL block (number 2, green circle), and the anterior QL block (number 3, red circle)

The Transmuscular QL Block/The Anterior QL Block Approach

The patient is placed in the lateral decubitus position. A low frequency curved array transducer is placed in the transverse position between the iliac crest and costal rim in the posterior axillary line. The transducer is then adjusted to visualize the Shamrock sign (the transverse process of L4, QL muscle, PM muscle, and erector spinae muscles). The needle is advanced in a posterior to anterior direction passing through the QL muscle. The point of injection is in the fascial interspace between the QL and PM muscles, *posterior* to the transversalis fascia (Figs. 33.1, 33.2, and 33.3).

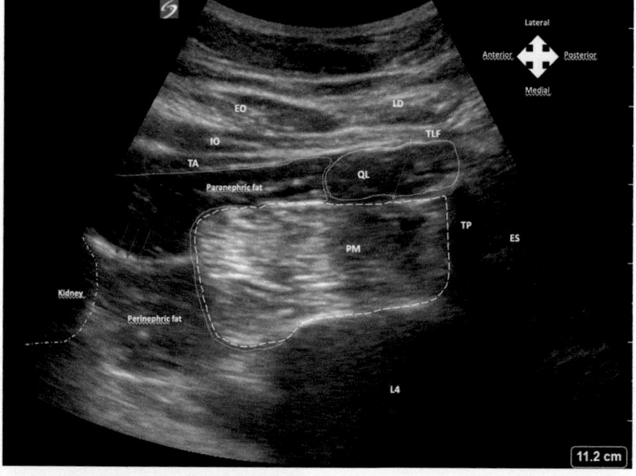

Fig. 33.3 Stepwise approach to the transmuscular quadratus lumborum block. Model photo. *EO* external oblique muscle, *IO* internal oblique muscle, *TA* transversus abdominis muscle, *LD* latissimus dorsi muscle, *TLF* thoracolumbar fascia, *QL* quadratus lumborum muscle, *PM* psoas major muscle, *ES* erector spinae muscles, *TP* transverse process of L4, *L4* vertebral body of L4. Yellow dotted line depicts relevant parts of the transversalis fascia. Red arrows indicate the posterior renal fascia (Gerota's fascia). Green arrow; needle trajectory with injection in the fascial interspace between the QL and PM muscles, posterior to the transversalis fascia

Block Complications (All QL Block Approaches)

Local systemic toxicity, vascular injection, injection of LA into the peritoneal cavity, lower limb weakness (if accidental piercing of the psoas muscle), Horner's syndrome (case rapport), and block failure.

Practical Tips

The transmuscular QL block is by many considered to be an advanced block. To improve the block success rate we recommend this stepwise approach (Fig. 33.3):

1. Identification of the antero-lateral abdominal wall muscles, i.e., transversus abdominis, internal and external oblique muscles. Notice the aponeurosis of the transversus abdominis and internal oblique muscles, which merges with the posterior part of the TLF at the postero-lateral aspect of the QL muscle (Fig. 33.3).

2. With real time ultrasound scanning, notice the respiratory movements of the para- and peri-renal fat compartments.
3. Locate the posterior part of the renal fascia (Gerota's fascia), separating the para- and peri-renal fat compartments, attaching to the hyperechoic antero-lateral part of the intrinsic fascia of the PM muscle. Often, the para-renal fat compartment can be difficult to distinguish from the likewise hypoechoic QL muscle, i.e., thus it is important to observe the respiratory movements of the para-renal fat, whereas the QL muscle will not move.
4. Observe the bony landmarks of the vertebral bodies (L3/4) and the hypoechoic shape of the transverse process, also known as the Shamrock sign. The OL muscle attaches to the apex of the transverse process.
5. The needle is advanced from the posterior side of the curved array transducer. Endpoint for injection is in the fascial interspace (or plane) between the QL and PM muscles, *posterior* to the transversalis fascia (Fig. 33.3). Advancing the needle in a postero-lateral to antero-medial direction through the QL muscle is key in order to avoid piercing the transversalis fascia and to ensure a muscular "backstop" for the needle when piercing the medial intrinsic fascia of the QL muscle.
6. After (or during) injection of LA, a subsequent longitudinal orientation (Fig. 33.4) of the transducer (turning the transducer 90° into the sagittal plane) enables visualization of intended cranial spread of LA between the QL and PM muscles.

Long lasting immobilization with muscle atrophy, osteoporosis, extensive abdominal circumference, anatomical variations, and air trapped intraabdominally may hinder an adequate ultrasound image prior to block execution. The transmuscular QL block should not be performed without a satisfactory visualization of some of the necessary internal landmarks.

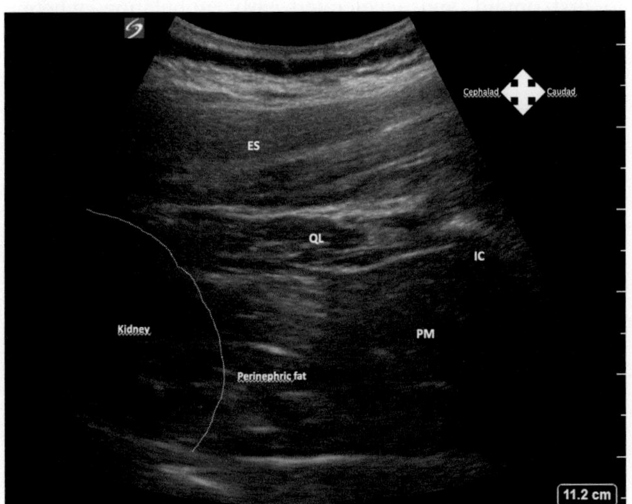

Fig. 33.4 Sagittal orientation of the transducer depicts relevant anatomical structures. Model photo. *ES* erector spinae muscles, *QL* quadratus lumborum muscle, *PM* psoas major muscle, *IC* iliac crest

Literature Review

In recent years, the number of randomized studies investigating the different QL blocks have increased. However, the common denominator of all studies is, they are single-center studies with inclusion of a rather small number of participants. No systematic review, where the three QL blocks are not pooled in the statistical analysis, has been published yet.

The QL1 Block/The Lateral QL Block Approach

Letters and articles by Blanco et al. have stipulated that the correct point of injection was between the transversus abdominis and internal oblique muscle aponeurosis and superficial to the transversalis fascia (Figs. 33.1 and 33.2). Mode of action has not entirely reached consensus. In a small MRI study by Carney et al., utilizing healthy young volunteers (when the block was still called an USG posterior approach TAP block), no spread of contrast into the TAP was found. Rather, contrast was observed to be pooled between the QL and PM muscles, and a resultant spread to the thoracic paravertebral space was observed. A later cadaveric study found spread of dye to the TAP but no spread to the thoracic paravertebral space. Using the QL I block, clinical studies have found a reduction in pain scores and opioid consumption in patients with femoral neck fracture (vs. femoral block), in patients undergoing cesarean section (vs. control), and also for lower abdominal surgery (vs. TAP block).

The QL2 Block/The Posterior QL Block Approach

Dr. Blanco et al. later abandoned the QL I block approach in favor of a more posterior approach (QL II block) (Figs. 33.1 and 33.2). The point of injectate with this technique is explained to be between the latissimus dorsi and QL muscle. It is stipulated that MRI (unpublished data and 3-D MRI reconstructions) show a spread of injectate into the paravertebral space, although a close examination of these 3-D image reconstructions seems to show rather scarce contrast spread limited to the lumbar paravertebral area reaching cephalad to the twelfth rib. Two cadaveric studies also refuted these findings and showed a variety of spread with dye reaching the subcostal, iliohypogastric, and ilioinguinal nerves and spread into the TAP (some cadavers) in one study, and in

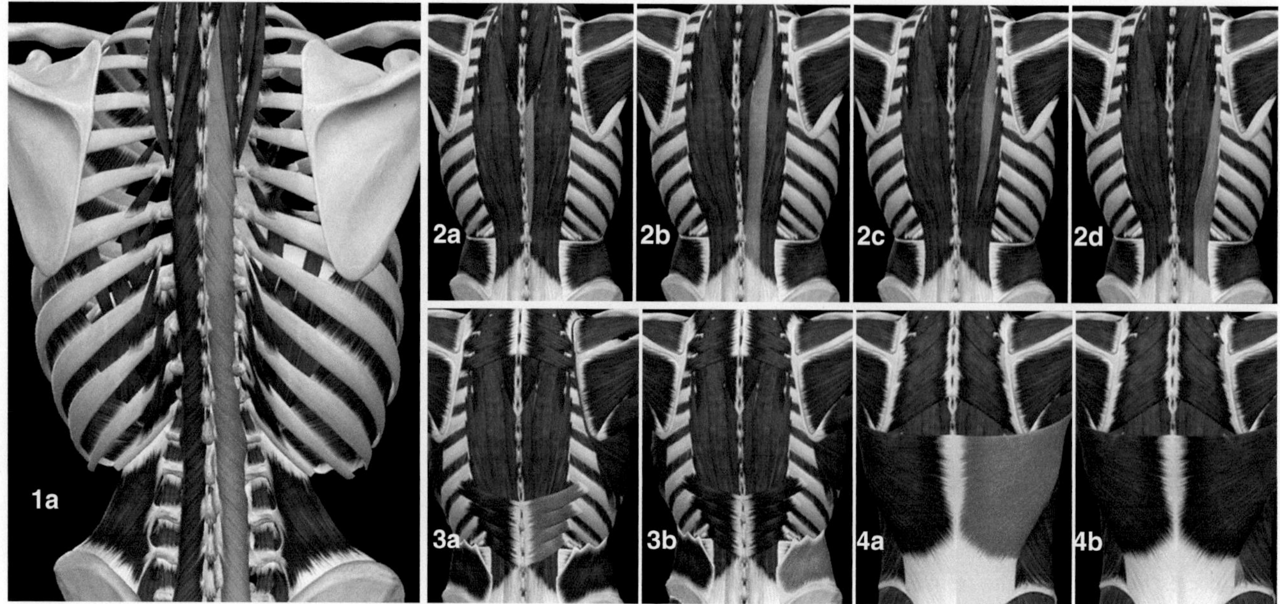

Fig. 33.5 Posterior paravertebral muscle compartments and adjacent muscular structures. First (deepest) muscular layer (orange color); multifidus muscle (1a). Second muscular layers (orange color) (2a–2d)—from medial to lateral; spinalis thoracis (2a), longissimus thoracis (2b), iliocostalis thoracis (2c), iliocostalis lumborum (2d) muscles. Third muscular layers (orange color) (3a–3b)—from medial to lateral; serratus posterior inferior (3a), internal (abdominal) oblique (3b). Fourth muscular layer (orange color) (4a left); latissimus dorsi muscle. Notice the appearance of the internal (abdominal) oblique (orange color) (4a right), deep to the overlying external (abdominal) oblique muscle (not marked). (The figure is a modified excerpt from Complete Anatomy, with permission from 3D4Medical (www.3d4medical.com))

the other study spread of dye reaching into the TAP, subcutaneous tissue or muscular spread.

From an *anatomical* point of view, it is quite challenging to fully elucidate, how spread of LA deep to the latissimus dorsi muscle would be able to advance cephalad and then to penetrate anterior into the thoracic paravertebral space from this posterior position, i.e., given the *massive* muscular "barrier" deep to the latissimus dorsi muscle. This is clearly illustrated in Fig. 33.5, which depicts the posterior paravertebral muscle compartments and adjacent muscular structures.

Nevertheless, it is also apparent that clinical studies investigating the QL II block have found a reduction in opioid consumption and NRS score following cesarean section, laparoscopic gynecological surgery, laparoscopic colorectal surgery, laparoscopic cholecystectomy, and abdominoplasty to name a few.

The Transmuscular QL Block/The Anterior QL Block Approach

A third approach to perform a QL block was proposed in 2013. The TQL block stipulates the endpoint of the injected LA as being in the fascial interspace between the QL and PM muscles, *posterior* to the transversalis fascia (Fig. 33.1). Cadaveric studies—both of them with a transmuscular approach—first by Dam et al. and subsequently later by Elsharkaway et al. (subcostal approach)—confirmed the spread of dye reaching into the thoracic paravertebral space. Further, spread of dye also reached the subcostal, iliohypogastric, and ilioinguinal nerves. Another two cadaveric studies could not reproduce these findings, but they were flawed in the block administration technique. Clinical RCTs have found a reduction in opioid consumption and NRS score following percutaneous nephrolithotomy (PNL), elective cesarean section, and laparoscopic nephrectomy. In one RCT, TQL block also reduced length of stay in hospital, prolonged time to first opioid, and accelerated early ambulation, whereas other trials also showed prolonged time to first opioid.

Suggested Reading

Adhikary SD, El-Boghdadly K, Nasralah Z, Sarwani N, Nixon AM, Chin KJ. A radiologic and anatomic assessment of injectate spread following transmuscular quadratus lumborum block in cadavers. Anaesthesia. 2017;72:73–9.

Bjelland TW, Yates TGR, Fagerland MW, Frøyen JK, Lysebråten KR, Spreng UJ. Quadratus lumborum block for postoperative analgesia after full abdominoplasty: a randomized controlled trial. Scand J Pain. 2019;19:671–8.

Blanco R. Tap block under ultrasound guidance: the description of a 'no pops' technique. Reg Anesth Pain Med. 2007;32:130.

Blanco R, McDonnell JG. Optimal point of injection: the quadratus lumborum type I and II blocks. 2014. http://www.respond2articles.com/ANA/forums/post1550.aspx. Accessed 28 Nov 2015.

Blanco R, Ansari T, Girgis E. Quadratus lumborum block for postoperative pain after caesarean section: a randomized controlled trial. Eur J Anaesthesiol. 2015;32:812–8.

Blanco R, Ansari T, Riad W, Shetty N. Quadratus Lumborum block versus transversus abdominis plane block for postoperative pain after cesarean delivery: a randomized controlled trial. Reg Anesth Pain Med. 2016;41:757–62.

Børglum J, Moriggl B, Jensen K, Lönnqvist PA, Christensen AF, Sauter A, et al. Ultrasound-guided transmuscular quadratus lumborum blockade. Br J Anaesth. 2013. http://bja.oxfordjournals.org/forum/topic/brjana_el%3b9919. Accessed 15 Jun 2015.

Carline L, McLeod GA, Lamb C. A cadaver study comparing spread of dye and nerve involvement after three different quadratus lumborum blocks. Br J Anaesth. 2016;117:387–94.

Carney J, Finnerty O, Rauf J, Bergin D, Laffey JG, Mc Donnell JG. Studies on the spread of local anaesthetic solution in transversus abdominis plane blocks. Anaesthesia. 2011;66:1023–30.

Chin KJ. Thoracic wall blocks: from paravertebral to retrolaminar to serratus to erector spinae and back again—a review of evidence. Best Pract Res Clin Anaesthesiol. 2019;33:67–77.

Chin KJ, McDonnell JG, Carvalho B, Sharkey A, Pawa A, Gadsden J. Essentials of our current understanding: abdominal wall blocks. Reg Anesth Pain Med. 2017;42:133–83.

Dam M, Moriggl B, Hansen CK, Hoermann R, Bendtsen TF, Børglum J. The pathway of injectate spread with the transmuscular quadratus lumborum block: a cadaver study. Anesth Analg. 2017;125:303–12.

Dam M, Hansen CK, Poulsen TD, Azawi NH, Wolmarans M, Chan V, et al. Transmuscular quadratus lumborum block for percutaneous nephrolithotomy reduces opioid consumption and speeds ambulation and discharge from hospital: a single centre randomised controlled trial. Br J Anaesth. 2019;123:e350–8.

Dam M, Hansen C, Poulsen TD, Azawi NH, Laier GH, Wolmarans M, et al. Transmuscular quadratus lumborum block reduces opioid consumption and prolongs time to first opioid demand after laparoscopic nephrectomy. Reg Anesth Pain Med. 2021;46:18–24.

Elsharkawy H, El-Boghdadly K, Kolli S, Esa WAS, DeGrande S, Soliman LM, et al. Injectate spread following anterior sub-costal and posterior approaches to the quadratus lumborum block: a comparative cadaveric study. Eur J Anaesthesiol. 2017;34:587–95.

Elsharkawy H, El-Boghdadly K, Barrington M. Quadratus Lumborum block: anatomical concepts, mechanisms, and techniques. Anesthesiology. 2019;130:322–35.

Gallaudet BB. A description of the planes of fascia of the human body: with special reference of the fascia of the abdomen, pelvis and perineum. New York: Columbia University Press; 1931. p. 1–32.

Hansen CK, Dam M, Steingrimsdottir GE, Laier GH, Lebech M, Poulsen TD, et al. Ultrasound-guided transmuscular quadratus lumborum block for elective cesarean section significantly reduces postoperative opioid consumption and prolongs time to first opioid request: a double-blind randomized trial. Reg Anesth Pain Med. 2019;44:896–900.

Hansen C, Dam M, Nielsen MV, Tanggaard KB, Poulsen TD, Bendtsen TF, et al. Transmuscular quadratus lumborum block for total laparoscopic hysterectomy: a double-blind, randomized, placebo-controlled trial. Reg Anesth Pain Med. 2021;46:25–30.

Hebbard PD. Transversalis fascia plane block, a novel ultrasound-guided abdominal wall nerve block. Can J Anaesth. 2009;56:618–20.

Ishio J, Komasawa N, Kido H, Minami T. Evaluation of ultrasound-guided posterior quadratus lumborum block for postoperative analgesia after laparoscopic gynecologic surgery. J Clin Anesth. 2017;41:1–4.

Karmakar MK, Gin T, Ho AM. Ipsilateral thoraco-lumbar anaesthesia and paravertebral spread after low thoracic paravertebral injection. Br J Anaesth. 2001;87:312–6.

Krediet AC, Moayeri N, van Geffen GJ, Bruhn J, Renes S, Bigeleisen PE, et al. Different approaches to ultrasound-guided thoracic paravertebral block: an illustrated review. Anesthesiology. 2015;123:459–74.

Krohg A, Ullensvang K, Rosseland LA, Langesæter E, Sauter AR. The analgesic effect of ultrasound-guided Quadratus Lumborum block after cesarean delivery: a randomized clinical trial. Anesth Analg. 2018;126:559–65.

Kumar GD, Gnanasekar N, Kurhekar P, Prasad TK. A comparative study of transversus abdominis plane block versus Quadratus Lumborum block for postoperative analgesia following lower abdominal surgeries: a prospective double-blinded study. Anesth Essays Res. 2018;12:919–23.

McDonnell JG, O'Donnell BD, Farrell T, Gough N, Tuite D, Power C, et al. Transversus abdominis plane block: a cadaveric and radiological evaluation. Reg Anesth Pain Med. 2007;32:399–404.

Mieszkowski MM, Mayzner-Zawadzka E, Tuyakov B, Mieszkowska M, Zukowski M, Waśniewski T, et al. Evaluation of the effectiveness of the Quadratus Lumborum block type I using ropivacaine in postoperative analgesia after a cesarean section—a controlled clinical study. Ginekol Pol. 2018;89:89–96.

Nielsen MV, Bendtsen TF, Børglum J. Superiority of ultrasound-guided shamrock lumbar plexus block. Minerva Anestesiol. 2018;84:115–21.

Ökmen K, Metin Ökmen B, Topal S. Ultrasound-guided posterior quadratus lumborum block for postoperative pain after laparoscopic cholecystectomy: a randomized controlled double blind study. J Clin Anesth. 2018;49:112–7.

Parras T, Blanco R. Randomised trial comparing the transversus abdominis plane block posterior approach or quadratus lumborum block type I with femoral block for postoperative analgesia in femoral neck fracture, both ultrasound-guided. Rev Esp Anestesiol Reanim. 2016;63:141–8.

Saito T, Den S, Tanuma K, Tanuma Y, Carney E, Carlsson C. Anatomical bases for paravertebral anesthetic block: fluid communication between the thoracic and lumbar paravertebral regions. Surg Radiol Anat. 1999;21:359–63.

Willard FH, Vleeming A, Schuenke MD, Danneel L, Schleip R. The thoracolumbar fascia: anatomy, function and clinical considerations. J Anat. 2012;221:507–36.

Zhu M, Qi Y, He H, Lou J, Pei Q, Mei Y. Analgesic effect of the ultrasound-guided subcostal approach to transmuscular quadratus lumborum block in patients undergoing laparoscopic nephrectomy: a randomized controlled trial. BMC Anesthesiol. 2019;19:154.

34 The Erector Spinae Plane (ESP) Block

Juan Felipe Vargas Silva, Vicente Roques, and Mauricio Forero

Contents

Introduction

In the last 10 years, there is an increase in the number of interfacial plane blocks developed, with the philosophy of targeting a bundle of nerves with a single injection. In 2016, the erector spinae plane (ESP) was described by Forero et al. for the management of chronic thoracic neuropathic pain. Since then, there was an outpouring interest in this block in acute and chronic pain. As of September 2020, there are more than 400 publications and 65 randomized controlled trials (RCT) published; and most importantly, there are 34 comparative trials evaluating the ESP block against other blocks. The multiple indications of the ESP block are linked to the widespread distribution of the erector spinae muscle from the neck to the lumbar region.

Indications and Choice of Level

The use of ESP blocks for upper and lower thoracic surgeries has decreased the use of epidural and paravertebral blocks. The rationale is augmented in less severe complications associated with the interfacial blocks, giving the potential to achieve greater patient access to regional analgesia. For major abdominal surgery, epidural analgesia continues to be highly used, but with enhanced recovery protocols, the practices are moving away from epidurals, so the use of interfacial plane blocks may represent an alternative.

J. F. Vargas Silva (✉)
Department of Surgery, Interventional Radiology and Pain Relief, Hospital Pablo Tobon Uribe, Medellin, Antioquia, Colombia

V. Roques
Department of Anesthesia and Chronic Pain Treatment, Hospital Universitario Virgen de la Arrixaca, Murcia, Spain

M. Forero
Department of Anesthesia, McMaster University, Hamilton, ON, Canada

D. Jankovic, P. Peng (eds.), *Regional Nerve Blocks in Anesthesia and Pain Therapy*, https://doi.org/10.1007/978-3-030-88727-8_34

Table 34.1 Level selection for erector spinae plane block, according to painful condition

Spinal level	Pain condition		Volume
	Acute	Chronic	
High thoracic T2 or T3	Postsurgical shoulder pain	Chronic shoulder pain syndrome	20–30 mL
		CRPS upper extremity	
Mid-thoracic T4 to T6	Rib fracture (midpoint of the level of rib fracture)	Chronic postherpetic neuralgia (level of segment involved)	20–30 mL
	Open thoracotomy and VATS lobectomy(T5)	Chronic post-thoracotomy pain (level of segments involved)	
	Rescue after TE failure for thoracic surgery(T5)	Metastatic rib cancer (level of segments involved)	
	Cardiac surgery sternotomy (T5)		
	Breast surgery with axillary lymph node dissections (T3)		
Low thoracic T7 to T12	Nephrectomies (T8) Hysterectomies (T10) Laparoscopic ventral hernia repair with mesh (T7) Laparotomies (T7)	Chronic postherpetic neuralgia (level of segment involved)	20–30 mL
		Chronic abdominal pain syndrome (T7 to T10)	
		Chronic pelvic pain syndrome (T10)	
Lumbar (L4)	Vertebral surgery (midpoint of levels involved)	Postsurgical hip replacement pain management (L4)	20–30 mL

The ESP block can be used to deliver regional analgesia (with a multimodal analgesic approach) for a wide variety of surgical procedures in the anterior, posterior, and lateral thoracic and abdominal areas, as well as for management of acute and chronic pain syndromes (Table 34.1). Also, the ESP block placed at the most upper thoracic segments (T1–T2) could provide coverage up to cervical nerve roots giving analgesia for shoulder pain.

Usually, the level chosen for thoracic indications is between T2 and T5 and for abdominal or pelvic indications is between T7 and T10. Despite its extensive spread, it is recommended to perform an ESP block at a vertebral level congruent to the thoracic or abdominal surgical incision, rather than relying on adequate spread of the local anesthesia.

Contraindications

Infection at the site of injection in the paraspinal region or near the puncture site.

Anticoagulation may be a relative contraindication to ESP block, although there are no specific guidelines.

Anatomy and Physiology

The Fascia

The fascia is composed of soft, collagen-containing, loose, and dense fibrous connective tissues and is ubiquitous in the whole body. Fascia over a muscle is composed of three layers in the human body: superficial, more dense deep fascia, and muscle-related layers (epimysium, perimysium, and endomysium) (Fig. 34.1). The deep fascia is composed of multiple layers and is the target for the interfacial plane blocks. This fascia is a membrane that extends throughout the whole body under basal tension where numerous muscular expansions attach and transmit the tension generated by muscle contraction to the neighboring areas. It forms sheaths for the nerves and vessels. The deep fascia is independent of the underlying muscle, separated from it by the epimysium and a layer of loose connective tissue.

Deep fascial planes are potential spaces transmitting forces around the whole body. These fascial planes are a continuum, with multiple potential points of injection in the same tissue plane at different craniocaudal anatomical levels. Local anesthetic injected within these potential spaces will spread widely along the path of least resistance. Other factors also influence the spread. The movement of the muscle encourage the spread via a pumping mechanism to the injectate. The negative intrathoracic pressure during respiration may also influence the spread (Fig. 34.2). This fascial sheath has multiple perforations in his anterior wall and is intermittently tethered to bony structures such as the spinous processes and transverse processes of the vertebrae, allowing passage of local anesthesia (Fig. 34.3).

The Erector Spinae Muscles

The architecture of the erector spinae muscle is complex, with three muscle bellies distributing in the lumbar, thoracic, and cervical area and surrounded by fascia.

The thoracolumbar fascia covers the deep muscles of the back and the trunk. Medially, it is attached to the spines of the thoracic vertebrae and laterally to the angles of the ribs. In the lumbar region, the thoracolumbar fascia is divided into three layers (posterior, middle, and anterior) attached at different levels. The posterior layer is attached to the spines of the lumbar and sacral vertebrae and to the supraspinous ligaments. The middle layer is attached to the tips of the lumbar transverse processes and the intertransverse ligaments. The anterior layer covers quadratus lumborum and is attached to the anterior surfaces of the lumbar transverse processes behind the psoas major. At its caudad portion, it is attached to the

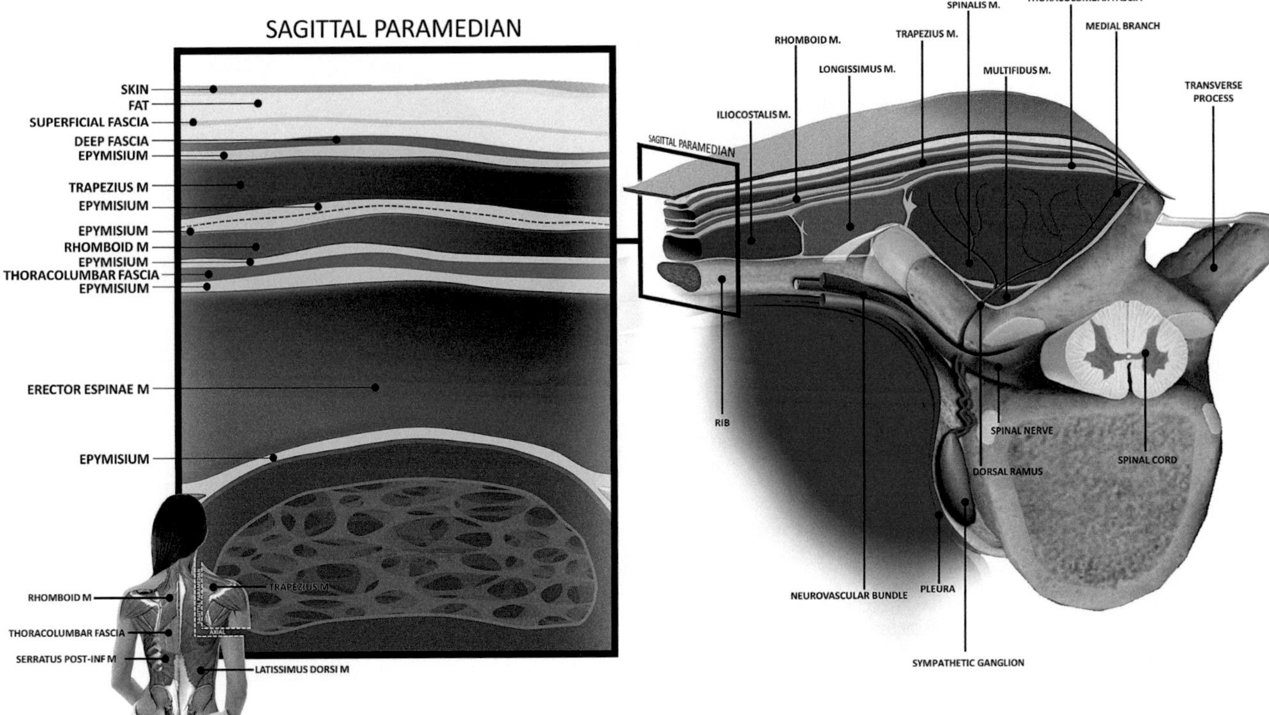

Fig. 34.1 Facial connective layers at the erector spinal plane. (Reprinted with permission from Dr. Vicente Roques from IMEDAR.com)

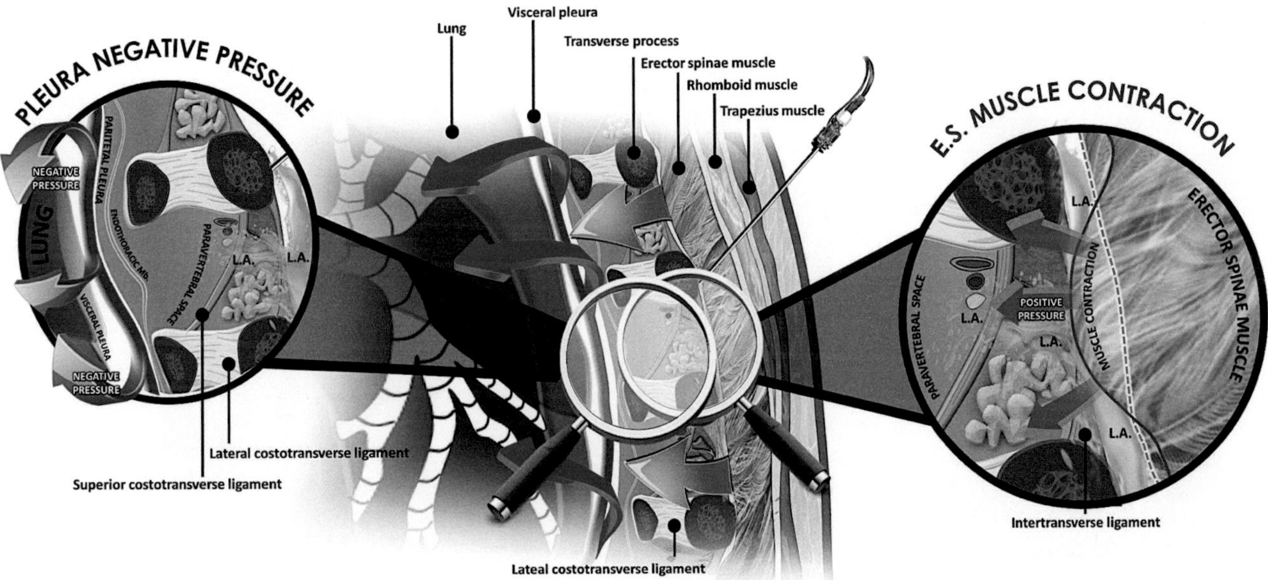

Fig. 34.2 Possible mechanism of in vivo erector spinae plane block, facilitating the spread of the injectate with muscle contraction and negative intrathoracic pressure during inspiration. (Reprinted with permission from Dr. Vicente Roques from IMEDAR.com)

iliolumbar ligament and the iliac crest. The posterior and middle layers unite to form a tough raphe at the lateral margin of erector spinae (the lateral border of quadratus lumborum) and join the anterior layer to form the aponeurotic origin of transversus abdominis.

Three muscles are in the plane of the ESP block at upper thoracic levels. Trapezius is the most superficial (posterior), rhomboid major in the middle, and erector spinae anterior (deeper). They are identified superficial to the tip of the hyperechoic transverse processes (Fig. 34.4).

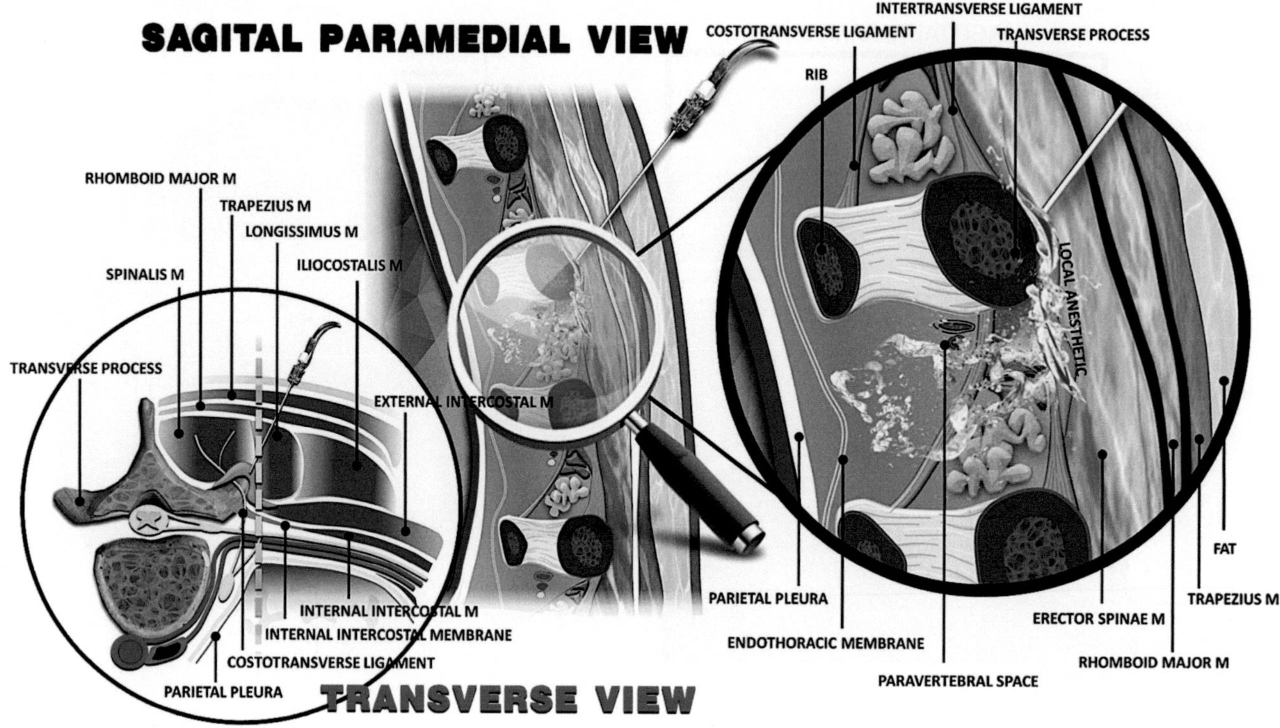

Fig. 34.3 Passage of local anesthesia through intermittent perforations in the anterior wall. (Reprinted with permission from Dr. Vicente Roques from IMEDAR.com)

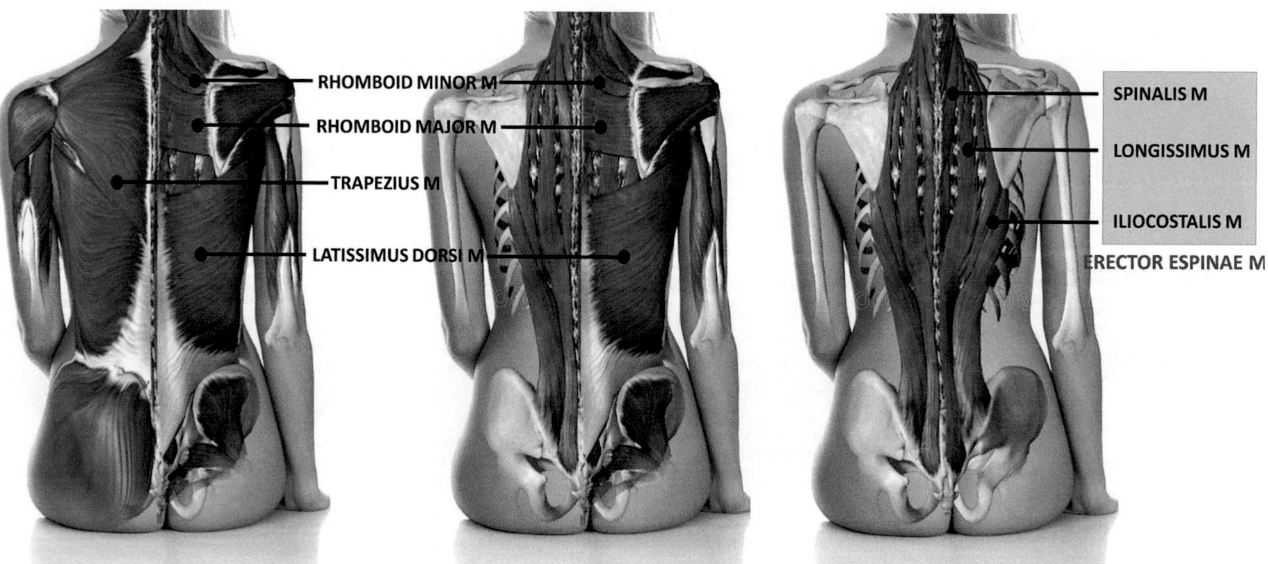

Fig. 34.4 Muscular anatomy of the back. Note the different muscle planes encountered at different spinal levels when the most superficial muscles are removed. (Reprinted with permission from Dr. Vicente Roques from IMEDAR.com)

The erector spinae muscles are a complex structure that forms the paraspinal column, composed of three muscles, iliocostalis, longissimus, and spinalis, and surrounded by muscular groups at different levels in the plane of the erector muscles (Fig. 34.5). They arise from and insert into various bony components of the vertebral column (from spinous process to spinous process, rib to rib, and transverse process to transverse process).

It originates from the sacrum and the lumbar spinous processes and extends upward as a gradually tapering column of muscle in the paravertebral groove on either side of the spinous processes, with insertions on the thoracic and cervical vertebrae as high as C2. This muscular column is encased in a retinaculum (blended aponeuroses and fasciae) that extends from the sacrum to the skull base. In the lower back, this retinaculum is referred to as the thoracolumbar

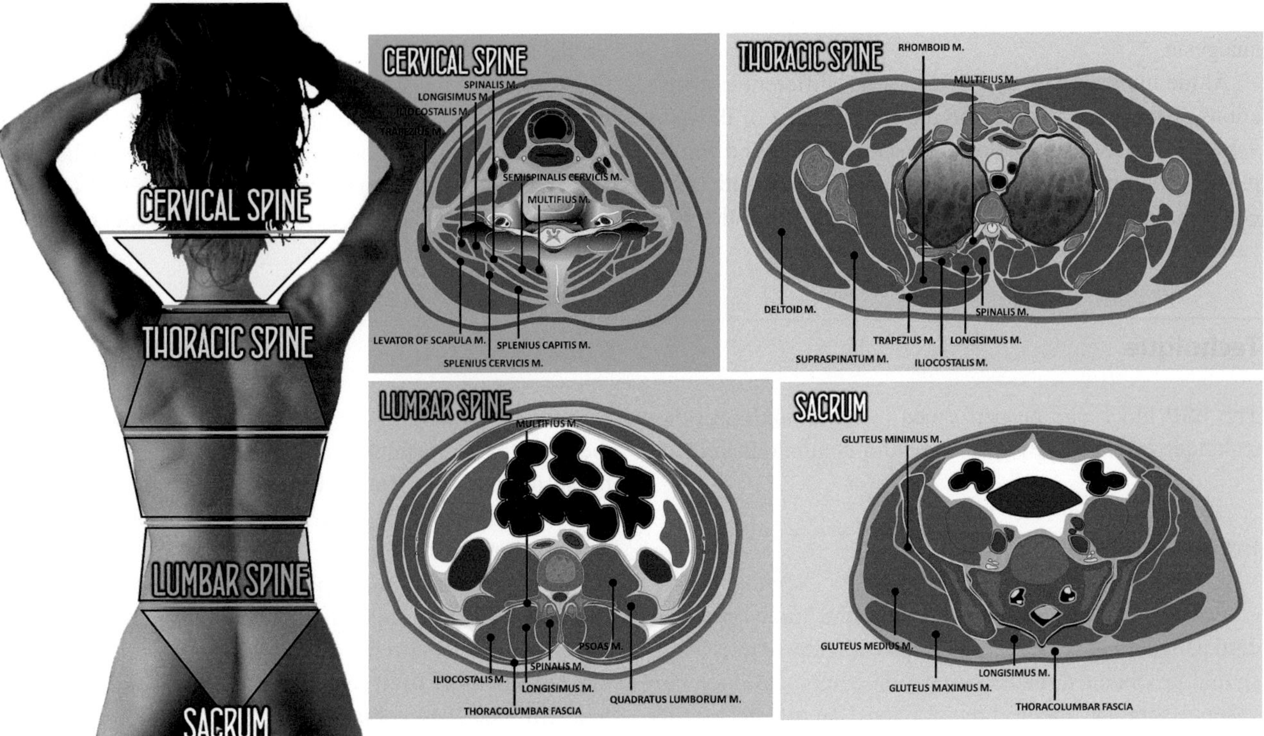

Fig. 34.5 Cross-sectional anatomy of paraspinal muscles. (Reprinted with permission from Dr. Vicente Roques from IMEDAR.com)

fascia. This thoracolumbar fascia, extending from the posterior thorax and abdomen in continuity with the nuchal fascia, facilitates the spread of the injectate or multiple thoracic and lumbosacral levels during ESP blocks at lower thoracic levels.

The target of the ESP block is to place the local anesthetic between the deepest layer (most anterior) of the erector spinae muscle and the tip of the transverse process. This place allows cranial-caudal spread in multiple spinal segments (Fig. 34.3). The injectate is placed in close relation to the intertransverse connective soft tissue, which allows the spread of the local anesthetic to the paravertebral or epidural space. This multilevel spread blocks the dorsal and ventral rami of the thoracic and abdominal spinal nerves allowing a multi-dermatomal sensory block. This multi-dermatomal sensory block is thought to be due to the cranial and caudal spread of the injected local anesthetic through the thoracolumbar fascia, aided by muscle tone and contraction. The cranial to caudal spread in the posterior wall is quite consistent in the spread study, but the extent in the anterior wall is quite variable as shown in multiple cadaver models and limited human studies.

Mechanism of Action

The mechanism of action has been examined through clinical and cadaveric studies. There is substantial evidence that the ESP block consistently anesthetizes the dorsal ramus (posterior hemi-body analgesia). Regarding the ESP block anterior spread (anterior hemi-body analgesia), the cadaveric data is less homogeneous. In fact, about 50% of cadaveric studies did not demonstrate paravertebral/intercostal/ or epidural spread, but 50% did. In contrast, imaging studies in live subjects (MRI-CT dye spread studies) found consistent anterior spread (anterior hemi-body analgesia) reaching the thoracic paravertebral space, the intercostal space, and in some cases also the epidural space. However, the extent of the cranial to caudal spread is inconsistent.

It is theorized that the volume (mass) of local anesthetic that reaches the nerves is small to be seen, but enough to produce analgesia, blocking preferentially unmyelinated C fibers over the larger A-δ and A-γ fibers, giving it the characteristic differential blockade (analgesia without motor block). If there is a passage of local anesthetic through the paravertebral space with ipsilateral and contralateral (bilateral) epidural spread, it provides abdominal visceral analgesia in the lower thoracic levels.

The craniocaudal spread has been found variable in both cadaveric and live subject imaging studies. However, most ESP block case studies described that 20 mL of local anesthetic produces clinical sensory blockade from 4 to 8 dermatomes in both anterior and posterior hemi-bodies. The authors advise performing the block at the level of the surgical incision to cover two dermatomes up and two dermatomes down consistently from the injection site when using

20 mL and inserting a perineural catheter to prolong analgesia.

At the lumbar level, an ESP block has different considerations. The spread is partial to the anterior area of the paravertebral space, surrounding the psoas muscle and lumbar plexus, leading to blockage of the nerves L2–L5, with different patterns of spread depending on volume, and therefore varying anesthetic effects.

Technique

The ESP block can be performed using a single-injection technique or via catheter placement for continuous infusion.

Preparation

After informed consent and peri-procedural "time-out," standard patient monitoring should be placed. Intravenous access should be obtained, and resuscitation equipment, including vasopressors and medications for local anesthetic toxicity, should be available. The procedure is performed with standard prep, the use of sterile gloves, surgical cap, mask, and sterile ultrasound probe cover for imaging. Linear probe (7–12 MHz) is usually sufficient. For high BMI, a curvilinear (2–6 MHz) is recommended. The typical needle is 22-gauge 50–100-mm needle (depending on body habitus). When catheter insertion is considered, perineural (catheter through needle or needle over catheter) or regular epidural catheter can be considered.

Procedure

Position the patient in sitting or prone position, depending on the operator and patient's comfort. A lateral decubitus could be an alternative when performing the block after general anesthetic induction or when the patient is unable to tolerate sitting or prone position.

The ultrasound probe is placed at the selected level of the spine using a longitudinal parasagittal approach, approximately 3 cm lateral to the spinous process. The level is identified by counting from cephalad to caudad, starting from the first rib and descending caudally to the desired level (Fig. 34.6). This level is followed medially to identify the

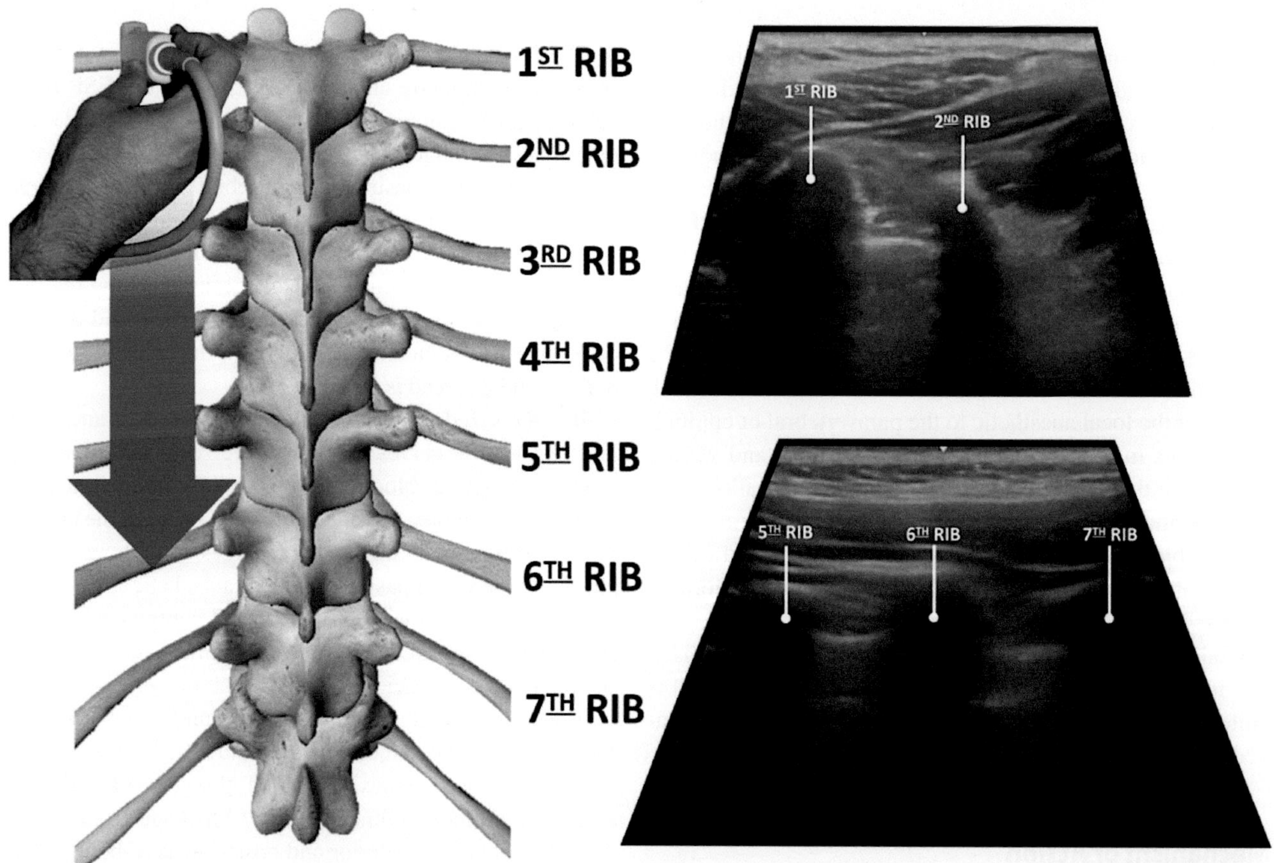

Fig. 34.6 Process for the recognition of the level before the realization of the erector spinae plane block. (Reprinted with permission from Dr. Vicente Roques from IMEDAR.com)

corresponding transverse process. The location could be established using the transverse process counting cephalad from the 12th rib.

The transverse process requires differentiation from the rib at that level. The transverse process will be more superficial, wider, and square-shaped, while the rib will be thinner and semicircular-shaped (Fig. 34.7a, b). Alternatively, the transverse process can be visualized by a transverse approach over the spinous process in the midline, and the lamina, transverse process, and rib are seen laterally (Fig. 34.8). After all the structures are seen, the probe is rotated in a parasagittal orientation with the tip of the transverse process as the target.

The trapezius, rhomboid major, and erector spinae muscles are identified superficial to the tip of the transverse process in the upper/mid-thoracic area (Fig. 34.7b). Following skin infiltration with lidocaine, insert the needle using an in-plane superior-to-inferior approach to place the tip into the fascial plane on the deep (anterior) aspect of erector spinae muscle. The location of the needle tip is confirmed by visible fluid lifting the erector spinae muscle off the bony shadow of the transverse process (Fig. 34.9). Any injection deeper to the anterior sheath wall does not permit craniocaudal spread of local anesthesia beyond that single intertransverse space, because of tight junctions between the sheath to the transverse processes, so the optimal plane for injection must be within the hyperechoic investing sheath, rather than deep to it. The injection superficial to this fascial layer, inside the muscle fibers, produces an erroneous image similar to that seen with an interfacial injection, known as lamination (Fig. 34.10).

A total of 20 to 30 mL of local anesthesia is injected in 5-mL aliquots through the needle with frequent aspiration to prevent intravascular injection. If a continuous technique is desired, insert the catheter trough the needle under direct vision 3 to maximum 5 cm beyond the needle tip keeping always in mind to leave the tip of the catheter at the surgical indicated level (Fig. 34.11). After the catheter is secured in place, a patient-controlled local anesthetic infusion regimen is started with a background infusion of at least 8 mL/h of 0.2% ropivacaine and 5 mL bolus with a lockout interval of 30 to 60 minutes.

Complications

Complications like pneumothorax, spinal cord injury, or spinal hematoma are unlikely as the injection target is away from the pleura, major blood vessels, and spinal cord. Local anesthetic toxicity has been reported when performing

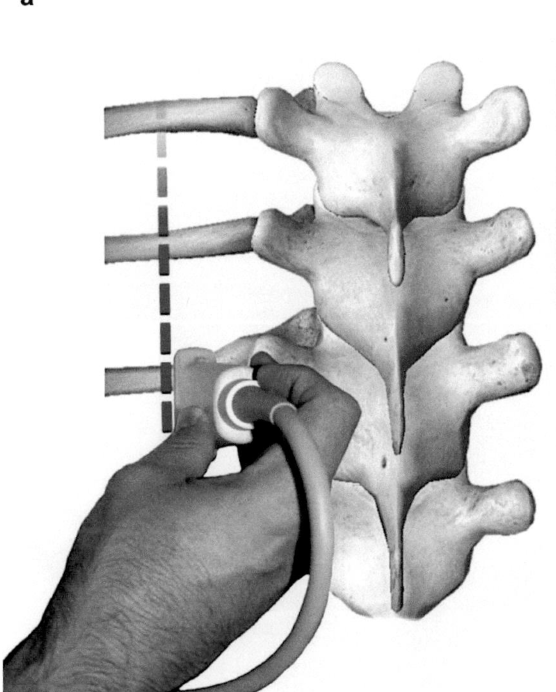

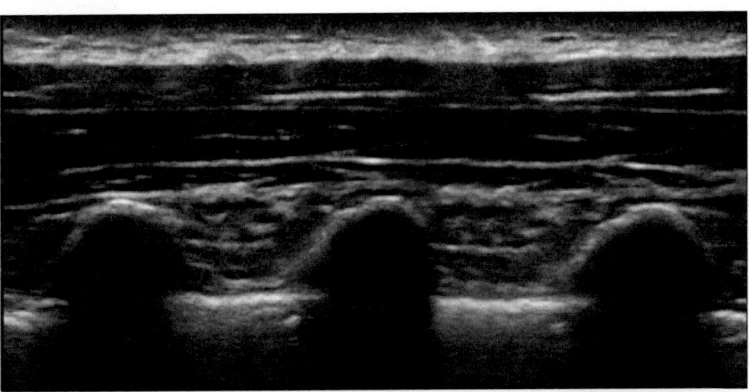

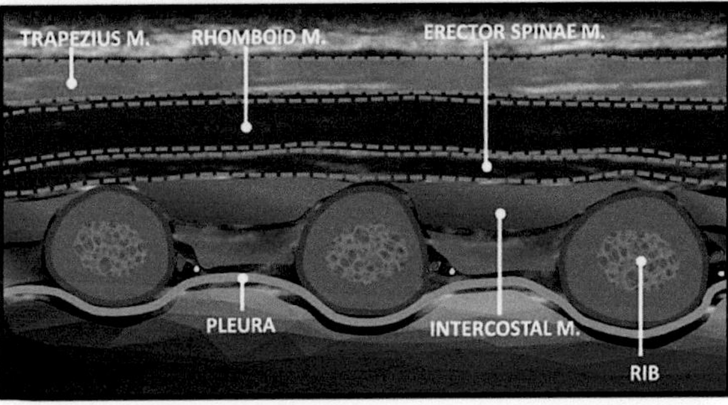

Fig. 34.7 (**a**) Sonographic appearance of the rib. The rib is smaller, thinner, and semicircular in shape and deepens toward the posteromedial planes. (**b**) The transverse process is more superficial, wider, and square-shaped. The structures in the sonogram are indicated in the schematic diagram. (Reprinted with permission from Dr. Vicente Roques from IMEDAR.com)

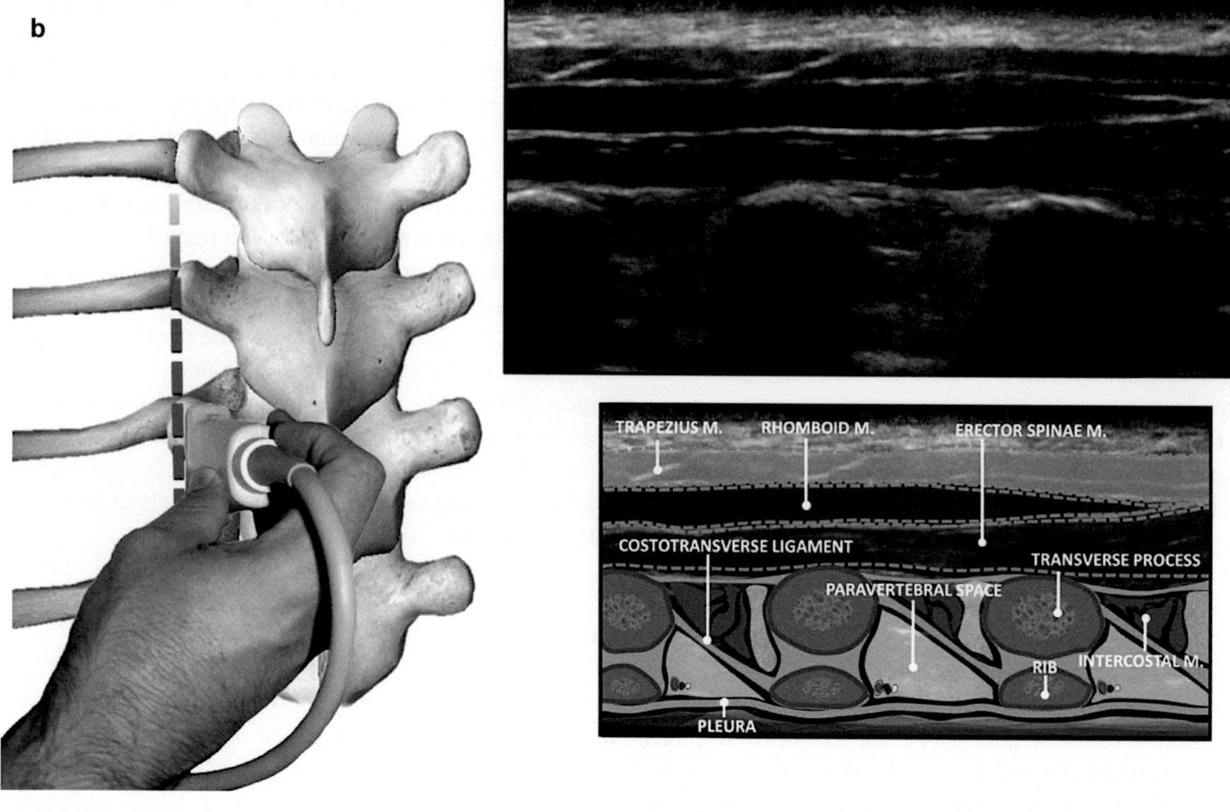

Fig. 34.7 (continued)

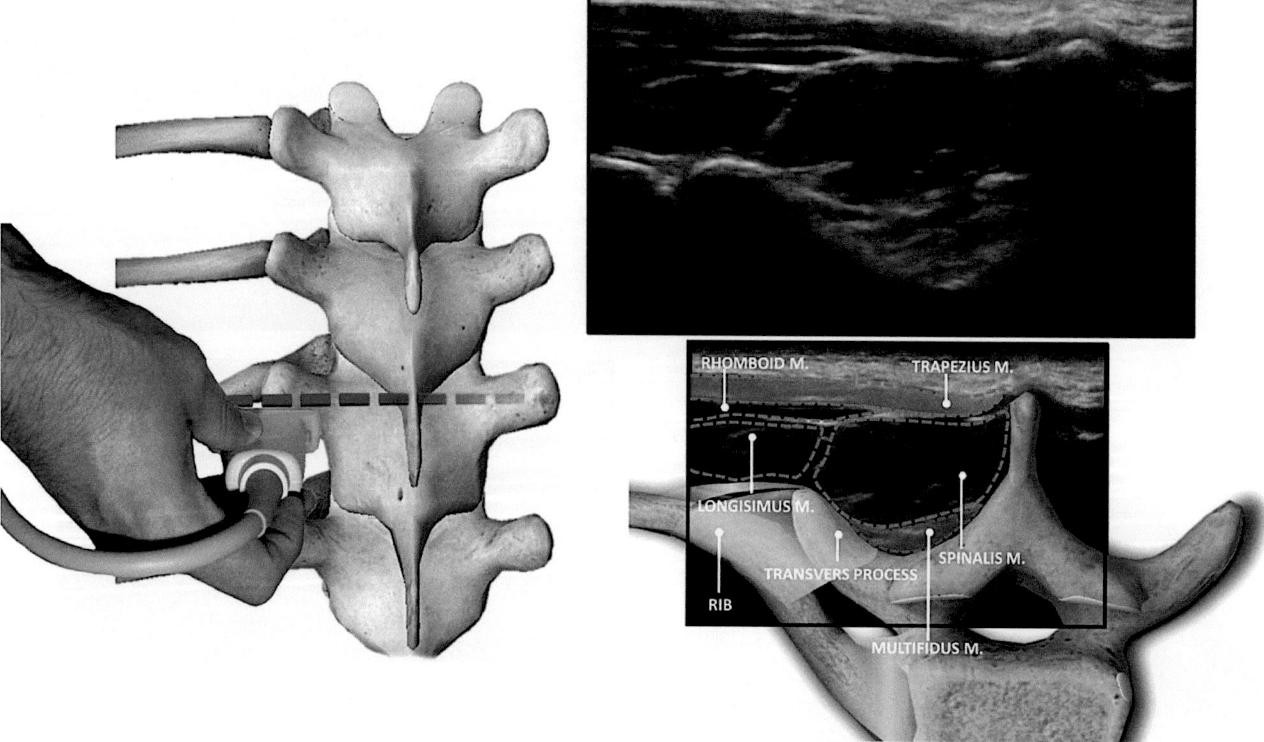

Fig. 34.8 Transverse view of the spine. This approach can help to better characterize the structures and differentiate the transverse process from adjacent structures, such as the lamina and rib. Once the transverse process is identified, the transducer can be rotated 90° in a sagittal orientation to perform the block. (Reprinted with permission from Dr. Vicente Roques from IMEDAR.com)

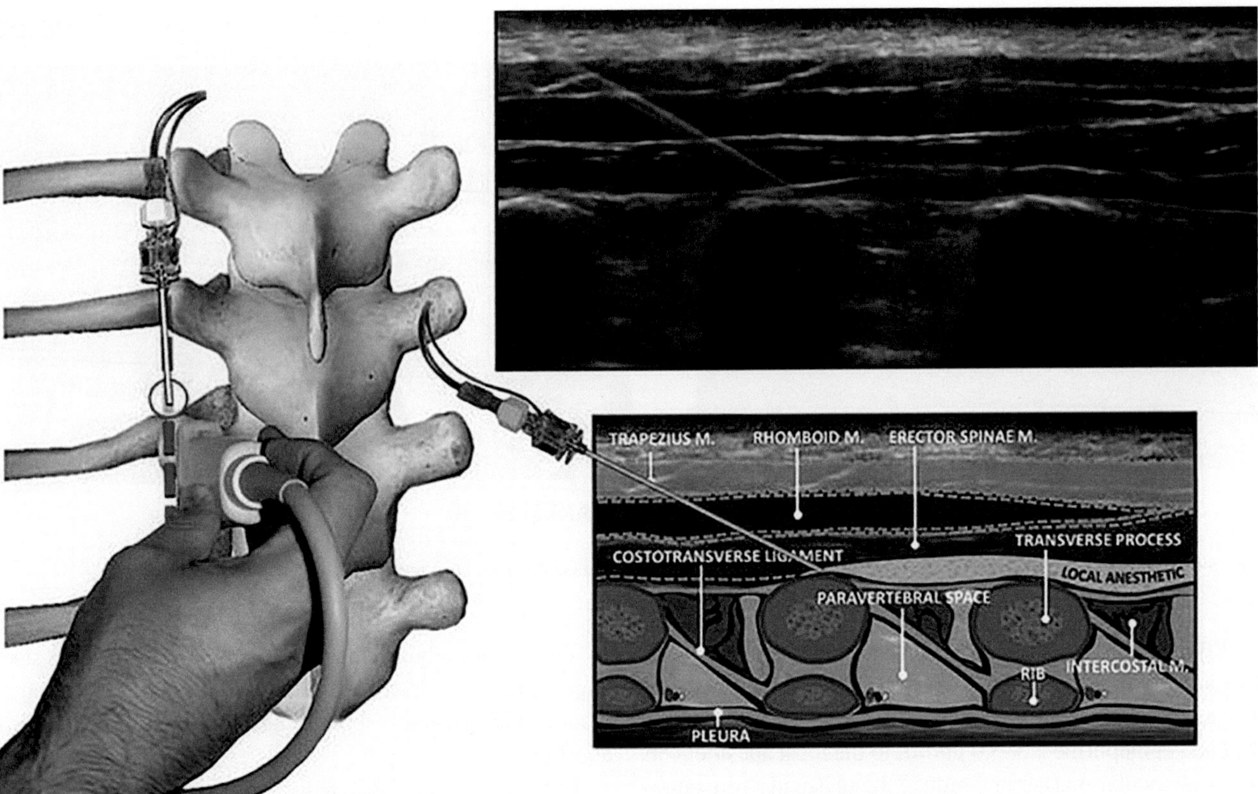

Fig. 34.9 Correct location of the injection during the erector plane block. Note the injection between the anterior fascia of the erector muscle and the intertransverse ligament. (Reprinted with permission from Dr. Vicente Roques from IMEDAR.com)

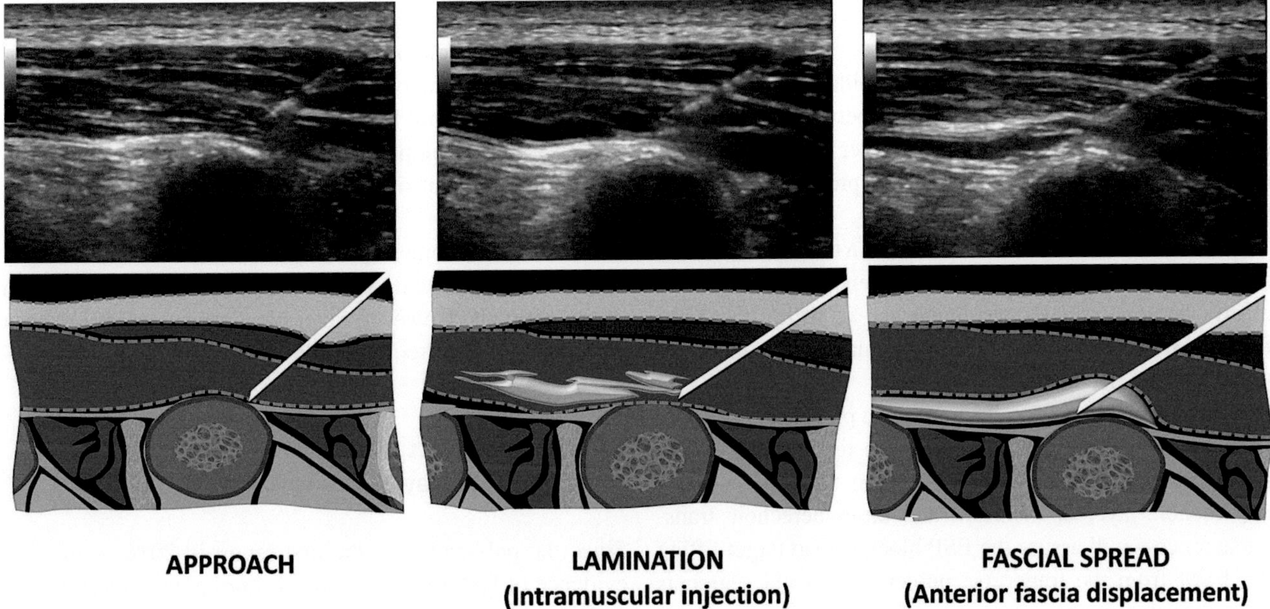

Fig. 34.10 In a parasagittal approach, lamination mimics an interfacial spread, but the injectate is inside the muscle and needs needle repositioning. With a transverse approach, the needle placed intramuscularly results in circumferential spread, which is less likely to be confused with interfacial spread, but need needle repositioning. (Reprinted with permission from Dr. Vicente Roques from IMEDAR.com)

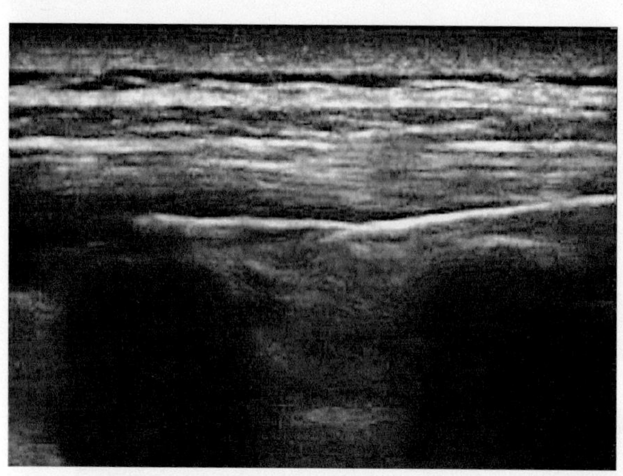

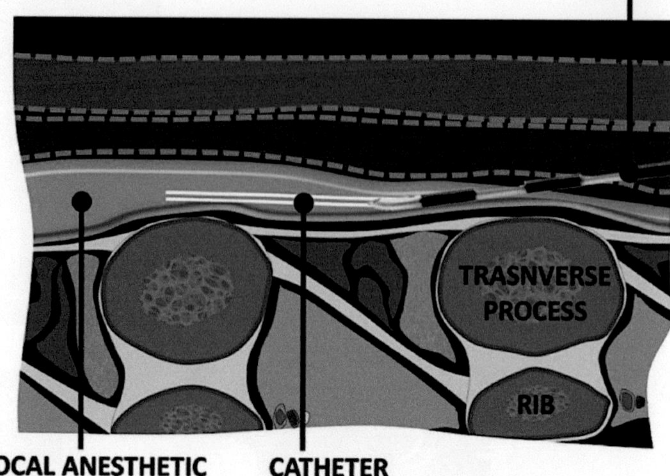

Fig. 34.11 Catheter in place of the erector spine plane. (Reprinted with permission from Dr. Vicente Roques from IMEDAR.com)

ESPB, and precaution must be taken as any other interfacial block using large volumes to avoid local anesthetic toxicity. It is advised to use lower doses than maximum recommended and add epinephrine 2.5–5.0 μg/mL to the local anesthetic as an intravascular marker and reduce the plasmatic concentration of the local anesthetic.

So far 65 RCTs have been published reporting no complications linked to the ESP block although more investigations are needed to reinforce the safety and complications rates of the ESP block.

Clinical Pearls

Intramuscular injection should be avoided. The injectate spread must be in the interfacial plane between two distinct hyperechoic layers, the most anterior layer of the erector spinae muscles (ESM) and the transverse process, rather than purely in the erector spine muscle.

The transverse process can be used as a target for ease and safety of the procedure. However, the endpoint that should always be sought is a clear linear spread lifting the ESM from the transverse process in both cranial and caudal directions from the needle tip.

The ESP block target is the transverse process. The needle must avoid piercing the intertransverse ligament or deeper structures. Keeping the needle between the most anterior hyperechoic layer of the ESM and the hyperechoic transverse process will assure the ESP block spread target lifting the ESM from the transverse process in several segments after a single injection. Sometimes, despite being in contact with the transverse process, there is intramuscular injection into the erector muscle (lamination) and requires repositioning of the needle.

The authors advise repositioning the needle to a less steep angle and hydrodissection using a non-active solution to assure the correct spread before injection of local anesthetic.

ESP block in pediatric patients is feasible, with volumes from 0.2 cc to 0.4 cc per kg. The clinician should avoid exceeding the maximum recommended dose of local anesthesia.

There is no evidence that the needle orientation impacts the clinical outcome. It can be performed either from cranial to caudal or vice versa.

Although there is extensive craniocaudal spread with multiple dermatomes involved, it is recommended to target the tip of the needle or catheter to the most painful or surgical incisional dermatome.

Consider bilateral blocks for incisions crossing the midline. Use with extreme caution in high thoracic ESP blocks due to the potential risk of hypotension or bilateral phrenic nerve palsy.

ESP block becomes an attractive alternative in anticoagulated patients, due to its extra-axial position without invasion of the neuraxis. However, other bleeding complications can ensue. Studies are required to evaluate safety in anticoagulated patients.

Literature Reviews

Since the publication of the first report in 2016, a growing evidence of ESP block developed, starting with case reports and anecdotal experience, followed by several RCTs that led to the possibility of systematic reviews. To date, there are 65 RCTs and 8 systematic reviews in different clinical scenarios, showing the versatility of the ESP block.

The efficacy of ESP block in breast surgery had been examined in four systematic reviews. The most recent two systematic reviews by Leong et al. and Hussain et al. covered 13 and 12 RCTs, respectively, and conveyed a number of important messages.

First, compared with no block, the literature consistently supported the superior analgesic efficacy of ESP block with decrease in pain scores and opioid consumption in the first postoperative 24 h.

Second, the clinical implication of the difference had been under scrutiny. For instance, the review by Hussain et al. showed that the mean differences in pain score (0–10) were −1.17, −1.17, −0.85, and −0.72 in recovery room and at 6-h, 12-h, and 24-h time points, respectively. The reduction in oral morphine equivalent consumption is 17.6 mg. The reduction in pain intensity represented 34–42% over the first 24-h postoperative period. Another review by Leong et al. represented with similar result. Hussian's group suggested a minimal reduction of 2 points in pain score as clinically meaningful. However, the mean pain scores of the control group were less than 3 in all time points in the first 24-h period.

Third, paravertebral used to be the standard regional anesthesia for breast surgery. The popularity faded with the advent of the newer interfascial plane block: pectoral nerve block and ESP block. Review of paravertebral block in breast surgery by Schnabel et al. in 2020 showed an impressive reduction in pain intensity: approximately 2.0–2.5 reduction in pain score when the control group pain score ranged between 4.0 and 7.0; but all studies were conducted at least 14 years ago. Hussain's review showed that all the mean pain scores in the control group (the group with no regional anesthesia block) were less than 3. Comparative studies between ESP block and paravertebral block did not find any difference in opioid consumption but the presence of four cases of pneumothorax in paravertebral group (none in ESP block group). The choice of regional anesthesia is a balance between the risk and benefit.

For analgesia in laparoscopic cholecystectomy, Daghmouri performed a systematic review and meta-analysis with five RCTs analyzed. Bilateral ESP block showed a lower postoperative pain score, a significant reduction of postoperative intravenous opioid consumption reported up to 24 h after surgery, and a longer time to first rescue analgesic. However, the opioid-sparing effect did not translate to reduction in postoperative nausea and vomiting.

In lumbar spinal surgery, Qui summarized the use of ESPB in a systematic review including all types of articles (case report, case series, retrospective cohort study, and randomized controlled trials). They included 171 participants from 11 publications (2 RCTs). The two RCTs found that ESP block significantly reduced lumbar postoperative pain scores and analgesic drug consumption, without operation-related adverse events. With the small number of RCT, the authors concluded that the effectiveness and safety of ESP block for lumbar spine surgery are still controversial because the evidence is insufficient. However, there are three more RCTs published since this review, all demonstrating the analgesic efficacy of ESPB for lumbar spine surgery vs. no blocks.

In conclusion, there is moderate quality evidence that erector spinae plane block is an effective strategy to improve postsurgical analgesia in adults in different surgical models. This conclusion needs to be interpreted with caution due to insufficient evidence. It will need large-scale RCTs to confirm this statement.

Suggested Reading

Aponte A, Sala-Blanch X, Prats-Galino A, Masdeu J, Moreno LA, Sermeus LA. Anatomical evaluation of the extent of spread in the erector spinae plane block: a cadaveric study. Can J Anesth. 2019;66(8):886–93.

Barrios A, Camelo J, Gomez J, Forero M, Peng PWH, Visbal K, Cadavid A. Evaluation of sensory mapping of erector spinae plane block. Pain Physician. 2020;23:E289–95.

Cai Q, Liu GQ, Huang LS, Yang ZX, Gao ML, Jing R, Liu Z, Pan LH. Effects of erector spinae plane block on postoperative pain and side-effects in adult patients underwent surgery: a systematic review and meta-analysis of randomized controlled trials. Int J Surg. 2020;80:107–16.

Chin KJ, Adhikary S, Forero M. Is the erector spinae plane (ESP) block a sheath block? A reply. Anaesthesia. 2017;72(7):916–7.

Chin KJ, Adhikary SD, Forero M. Understanding ESP and fascial plane blocks: a challenge to omniscience. Reg Anesth Pain Med. 2018;43(7):807–8.

Cornish PB. Erector spinae plane block: the "happily accidental" paravertebral block. Reg Anesth Pain Med. 2018;43(6):644–5.

Daghmouri MA, Akremi S, Chaouch MA, Mesbahi M, Amouri N, Jaoua H, Ben Fadhel K. Bilateral erector spinae plane block for postoperative analgesia in laparoscopic cholecystectomy: a systematic review and meta-analysis of randomized controlled trials. Pain Pract. 2020;21(3):357–65.

De Cassai A, Andreatta G, Bonvicini D, Boscolo A, Munari M, Navalesi P. Injectate spread in ESP block: a review of anatomical investigations. J Clin Anesth. 2020;61:109669.

ElHawary H, Abdelhamid K, Meng F, Janis JE. Erector spinae plane block decreases pain and opioid consumption in breast surgery: systematic review. Plast Reconstr Surg Glob Open. 2019;7(11):e2525.

Elsharkawy H, Pawa A, Mariano ER. Interfascial plane blocks: back to basics. Reg Anesth Pain Med. 2018;43(4):341–6.

Elsharkawy H, Bajracharya GR, El-Boghdadly K, Drake RL, Mariano ER. Comparing two posterior quadratus lumborum block approaches with low thoracic erector spinae plane block: an anatomic study. Reg Anesth Pain Med. 2019;44(5):549–55.

Forero M, Adhikary SD, Lopez H, Tsui C, Chin KJ. The erector spinae plane block: a novel analgesic technique in thoracic neuropathic pain. Reg Anesth Pain Med. 2016;41(5):621–7.

Forero M, Rajarathinam M, Adhikary SD, Chin KJ. Erector spinae plane block for the management of chronic shoulder pain: a case report. Can J Anesth. 2018;65(3):288–93.

Hamilton DL. Pneumothorax following erector spinae plane block. J Clin Anesth. 2019;52:17.

Hamilton DL, Manickam BP. Is the erector spinae plane (ESP) block a sheath block? Anaesthesia. 2017;72(7):915–6.

Huang J, Liu JC. Ultrasound-guided erector spinae plane block for postoperative analgesia: a meta-analysis of randomized controlled trials. BMC Anesthesiol. 2020;20:1–8.

Huang W, Wang W, Xie W, Chen Z, Liu Y. Erector spinae plane block for postoperative analgesia in breast and thoracic surgery: a systematic review and meta-analysis. J Clin Anesth. 2020;66:109900.

Ivanusic J, Konishi Y, Barrington MJ. A cadaveric study investigating the mechanism of action of erector spinae blockade. Reg Anesth Pain Med. 2018;43(6):567–71.

Jacobs A, et al. PROSPECT guideline for oncological breast surgery: a systematic review and procedure-specific postoperative pain management recommendations. Anaesthesia. 2020;75(5):664–73.

Klingler W, Velders M, Hoppe K, Pedro M, Schleip R. Clinical relevance of fascial tissue and dysfunctions. Curr Pain Headache Rep. 2014;18(8):439.

Kose HC, Kose SG, Thomas DT. Lumbar versus thoracic erector spinae plane block: similar nomenclature, different mechanism of action. J Clin Anesth. 2018;48:1.

Leong RW, Tan ESJ, Wong SN, Tan KH, Liu CW. Efficacy of erector spinae plane block for analgesia in breast surgery: a systematic review and meta-analysis. Anaesthesia. 2020;76(3):404–13.

López MB, Cadórniga ÁG, González JML, Suárez ED, Carballo CL, Sobrino FP. Erector spinae block. A narrative review. Cent Eur J Clin Res. 2018;1(1):28–39.

Macintosh JE, Bogduk N. 1987 Volvo award in basic science: the morphology of the lumbar erector spinae. Spine. 1987;12(7):658–68.

Nair AS, Seelam S. The risks associated with erector spinae plane block in patients with abnormalities of coagulation. Korean J Anesthesiol. 2019;72(3):275.

Narayanan M, Venkataraju A. Transverse approach to the erector spinae block: is there more? Reg Anesth Pain Med. 2019;44:529–30.

Papa P, Antunez-Maciel M, Asenjo JF. Cancer shoulder pain treated with a neurolytic erector spinae plane block. Can J Anesth. 2020;67:1262–3.

Pourkashanian A, Narayanan M, Venkataraju A. The erector spinae plane block: a review of current evidence. Education for anaesthesia providers worldwide; 2019. p. 27.

Qiu Y, Zhang TJ, Hua Z. Erector spinae plane block for lumbar spinal surgery: a systematic review. J Pain Res. 2020;13:1611.

Schnabel A, Reichl SU, Kranke P, Pogatzki-Zahn EM, Zahn PK. Efficacy and safety of paravertebral blocks in breast surgery: a meta-analysis of randomized controlled trials. Br J Anaesth. 2010;105:842–52.

Schnabel A, Weibel S, Meißner M, Reichl SU, Kranke P, Meyer-Frießem CH, Zahn PK, Pogatzki-Zahn E. Erector spinae plane block for postoperative pain. Cochrane Database Syst Rev. 2020;(10):CD013763.

Schwartzmann A, Peng P, Maciel MA, Forero M. Mechanism of the erector spinae plane block: insights from a magnetic resonance imaging study. Can J Anesth. 2018;65(10):1165–6.

Schwartzmann A, Peng P, Maciel MA, Alcarraz P, Gonzalez X, Forero M. A magnetic resonance imaging study of local anesthetic spread in patients receiving an erector spinae plane block. Can J Anaesth. 2020;67(8):942–8. https://doi.org/10.1007/s12630-020-01613-8.

Susan S. Gray's anatomy: the anatomical basis of clinical practice. 41th ed. Amsterdam: Elsevier Health Sciences; 2015.

Tulgar S, Selvi O, Ozer Z. Clinical experience of ultrasound-guided single and bi-level erector spinae plane block for postoperative analgesia in patients undergoing thoracotomy. J Clin Anesth. 2018;50:22–3.

Tulgar S, Ahiskalioglu A, De Cassai A, Gurkan Y. Efficacy of bilateral erector spinae plane block in the management of pain: current insights. J Pain Res. 2019;12:2597.

Tulgar S, Aydin ME, Ahiskalioglu A, De Cassai A, Gurkan Y. Anesthetic techniques: focus on lumbar erector spinae plane block. Local Reg Anesth. 2020;13:121.

Ueshima H. Pneumothorax after the erector spinae plane block. J Clin Anesth. 2018;48:12.

Vidal E, Giménez H, Forero M, Fajardo M. Erector spinae plane block: a cadaver study to determine its mechanism of action. Revista Española de Anestesiología y Reanimación. 2018;65(9):514–9.

Yang HM, Choi YJ, Kwon HJ, O J, Cho TH, Kim SH. Comparison of injectate spread and nerve involvement between retrolaminar and erector spinae plane blocks in the thoracic region: a cadaveric study. Anaesthesia. 2018;73(10):1244–50.

Intercostal Nerve Block

35

Rajendra Sahoo and Philip Peng

Contents

General Consideration

First described by Heinrich Braun in 1907 for pain control of the thorax and abdominal wall, intercostal nerve block has been in clinical use for a very long time. Before the emergence of interfascial plane blocks for the thorax, this block was the popular procedure for the management of acute rib fracture pain, perioperative thoracotomy pain, and chronic neuropathic pain of the chest wall.

R. Sahoo
Department of Anesthesia and Pain Management, Kalinga Institute of Medical Sciences, KIIT Deemed University, Bhubaneswar, Odisha, India

P. Peng (✉)
Department of Anesthesiology and Pain Medicine, Toronto Western Hospital, University of Toronto, Toronto, ON, Canada
e-mail: philip.peng@uhn.ca

Indications

This nerve block is considered in a wide array of conditions resulting in pain in the chest wall. One of the most common indications is the alleviation of pain from rib fractures. In perioperative setting, it is a useful blockade providing postoperative analgesia for thoracotomy and upper abdominal surgery. It can be used for other acute pain conditions such as pain from acute herpes zoster and insertion of chest drain. In patient with chronic pain in the chest wall, such as chest wall tumor, chronic thoracic neuropathic pain, or nerve entrapment, intercostal nerve block allows the interruption of the pain signal from the affected areas. In some situation, the blockade is prolonged with the use of radiofrequency (RF) ablation, cryoablation, or chemical ablation.

Contraindications

The procedure is absolutely contraindicated in patients refusing the procedure, with active infection at the injection site, known history of allergy to local anesthetic, or severe

D. Jankovic, P. Peng (eds.), *Regional Nerve Blocks in Anesthesia and Pain Therapy*,
https://doi.org/10.1007/978-3-030-88727-8_35

coagulopathy. Because of the risk of pneumothorax, it is relatively contraindicated in patients with poor lung reserve, single lung, or unknown anatomic changes on the side of injection. Clinician should exercise discretion of the intercostal block in patients with bleeding diathesis (from disease or drugs), previous nerve injury, and systemic infection, and they are relatively contraindicated.

Functional Anatomy

There are 12 pairs of thoracic spinal nerves. With the exception of the first two, these spinal nerves are smaller in size compared with the lower half of the cervical spinal nerves. These spinal nerves emerge from the spinal cord with two roots—the sensory dorsal root (posterior) and the motor ventral root (anterior) (Fig. 35.1). After leaving the dural sac, the two roots are surrounded by a dural sheath. The sensory root expands to accommodate the sensory neurons and forms the dorsal root ganglion. Beyond the ganglion, the roots form a common mixed spinal nerve trunk, which divides into four branches after exiting through the intervertebral foramen: the dorsal primary rami, the ventral primary rami, the meningeal branches which supply the spinal canal and the meninges, and the white and gray communicating branches, which anastomose with each neighboring ganglion of the sympathetic trunk and thus extend to the viscera and vessels, mediating and involving the sympathetic nervous system. They also carry sympathetic fibers to the spine.

The dorsal rami of the thoracic nerves pass between the two transverse processes to their area of distribution and divide into two typical branches, the medial and lateral branches; they give off muscular branches (back muscles) and cutaneous branches (spinous processes, posterior wall of the thorax, and lumbar region). The ventral rami of the thoracic nerves are also termed intercostal nerves, and they are distributed segmentally (Fig. 35.2).

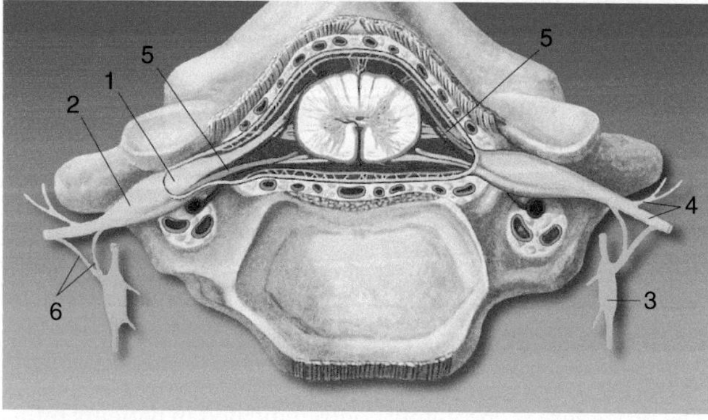

Fig. 35.1 Anatomy of the thoracic spinal nerves. (1) spinal ganglion, (2) spinal nerve, (3) ganglion of the sympathetic trunk, (4) dorsal and ventral branch, (5) dorsal and ventral root, (6) white and gray communicating branches. (Reprinted with permission from Danilo Jankovic)

The 11 upper nerves are (relative to the thoracic ribs) genuinely intercostal because the nerves at least partially run in the intercostal space. The 12th, however, lies caudal to the 12th rib and is known as the subcostal nerve. The six upper intercostal nerves run entirely in the intercostal spaces, as far as the edge of the sternum; the six lower ones reach the area of the linea alba. All the intercostal nerves, with the exception of the 12th, run in the relevant intercostal space in front of the superior costotransverse ligament and on the inner surface of the internal intercostal muscles. The internal intercostal muscles are absent from the spine as far as the costal angle and replaced by internal intercostal membrane (Fig. 35.3). Over this area, the intercostal nerves lie over the endothoracic fascia and costal or parietal pleura. Approaching the angle of the rib, the nerves lie between the internal and innermost intercostal muscles, and they are accompanied by the intercostal vessels (the intercostal artery and vein). They lie caudal to the vessels (Fig. 35.4). Special care needs to be taken during procedures, as due to the proximity of blood vessels to the nerves, toxic concentrations of local anesthetic can easily be reached.

The intercostal nerves give out various branches: muscular branches for various chest wall muscles such as serratus posterior and rectus abdominis muscles; lateral cutaneous branches supplying the skin of lateral sides of the thorax and abdomen, as well as skin of the axilla (first intercostal nerve); anterior cutaneous branches supplying the anterior side of the thorax; and pleural and peritoneal branches supplying the pleura and thoracic wall and the peritoneum of the lateral and anterior abdominal wall, as well as the pleural and peritoneal covering at the origin of the diaphragm (Fig. 35.5).

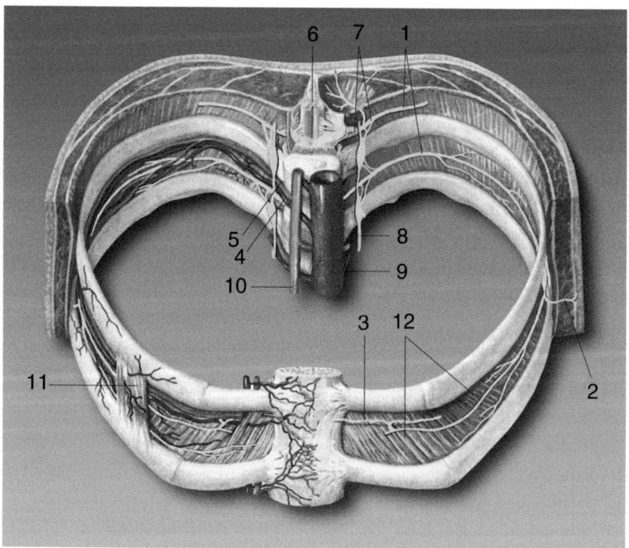

Fig. 35.2 Intercostal nerves (1). Ventral branches (intercostal nerves), (2) lateral cutaneous branch, (3) anterior cutaneous branch, (4) posterior intercostal artery, (5) posterior intercostal vein, (6) spinal cord, (7) spinal nerve, (8) sympathetic trunk, (9) thoracic aorta, (10) azygos vein, (11) external intercostal muscles, (12) internal intercostal muscles. (Reprinted with permission from Danilo Jankovic)

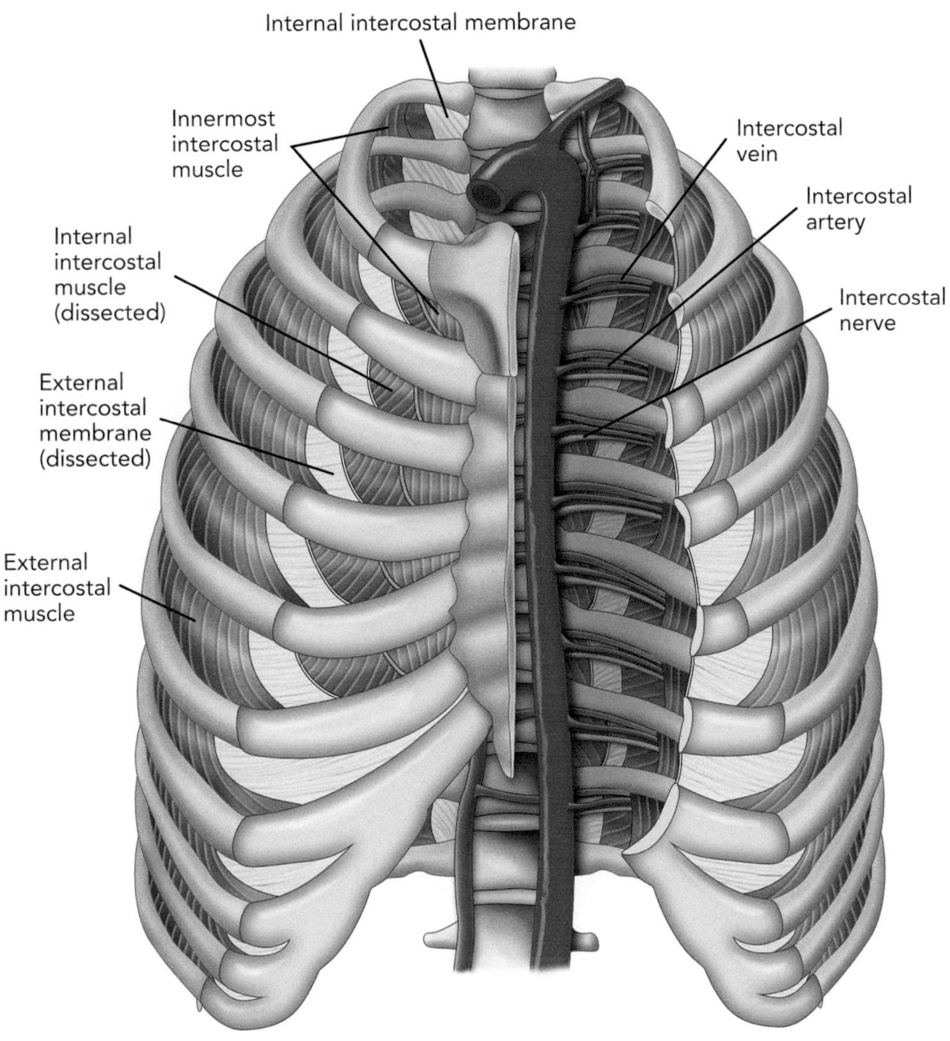

Fig. 35.3 Intercostal muscles in the chest wall. (Reprinted with permission from Philip Peng Educational Series)

Technique

Landmark Technique

The patient is placed in prone (preferred position for bilateral block) or lateral recumbent position (Fig. 35.6). When the procedure is performed in prone position, a pillow is placed under the mid-abdomen, between the arch of the ribs and the iliac crest line, with the patient's arms hanging (Fig. 35.6). The first four intercostal nerves are blocked paravertebrally, 3.5–4 cm or two fingerbreadths lateral to the spinous processes. For the other level, the target is the caudal boundary of the rib at costal angle (7–8 cm or four fingerbreadths lateral to the midline and lateral to the musculature of the erector muscle of the spine). The rib level is counted from 12th rib onward cranially.

The index and middle fingers of the left hand palpate the rib being blocked and press the skin around the contours of the ribs. The index finger locates the lower edge of the rib. A 3.5-cm 25-G-long needle is advanced at an angle of 80° to the skin surface until bone contact (costal periosteum) is made. Upon contact with bone, the needle is withdrawn slightly, and the skin and needle are then simultaneously pushed caudally until the needle slides under the lower edge of the rib (Fig. 35.7). After loss of bone contact, the needle must not be introduced beyond 2–3 mm deeper. The hub of the needle is fixed between the thumb and the index finger as this is done; the middle finger fixes the shaft and directs the needle. The side of the left hand (left hypothenar eminence) rests on the patient's back; initially, it serves as a brake, and then during the injection, it serves as fixation. After aspiration at various levels, the local anesthetic is injected on an incremental basis.

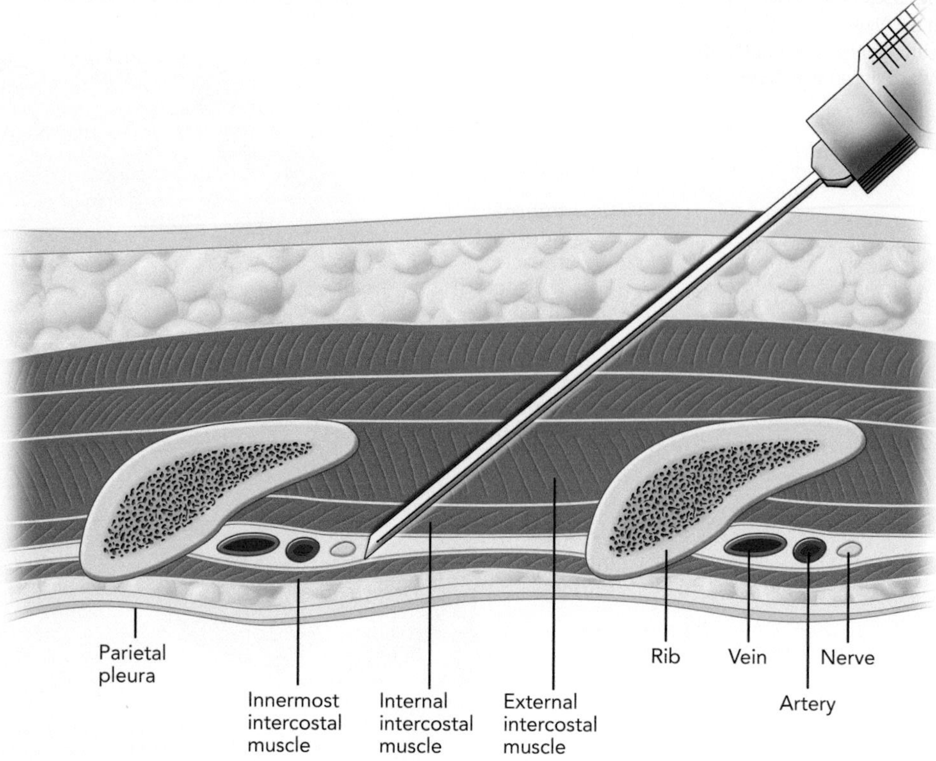

Fig. 35.4 Cross section of the chest wall showing intercostal muscles and neurovascular bundles. (Reprinted with permission from Philip Peng Educational Series)

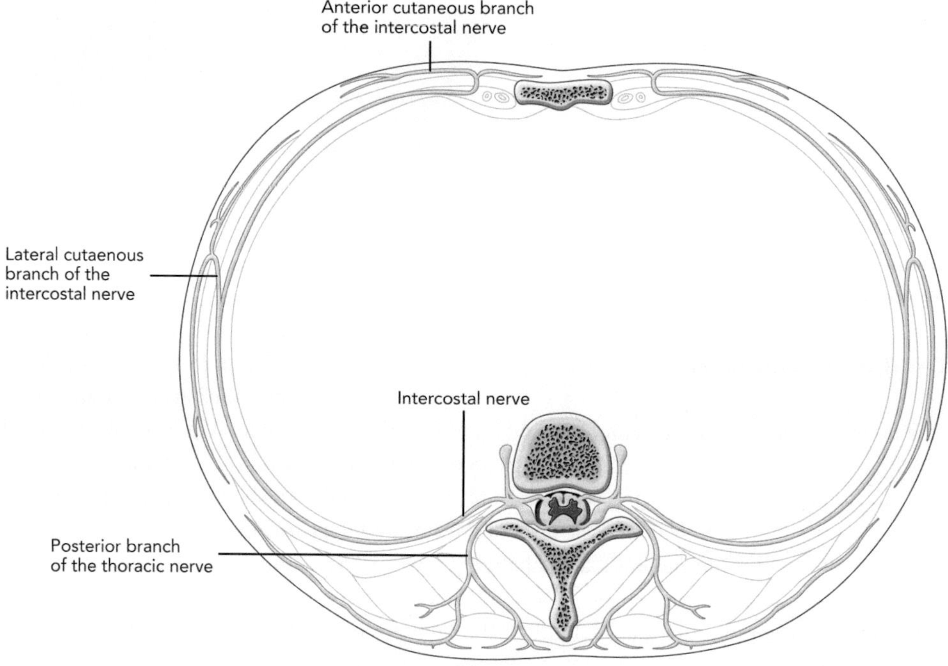

Fig. 35.5 Branches of the typical intercostal nerves. (Reprinted with permission from Philip Peng Educational Series)

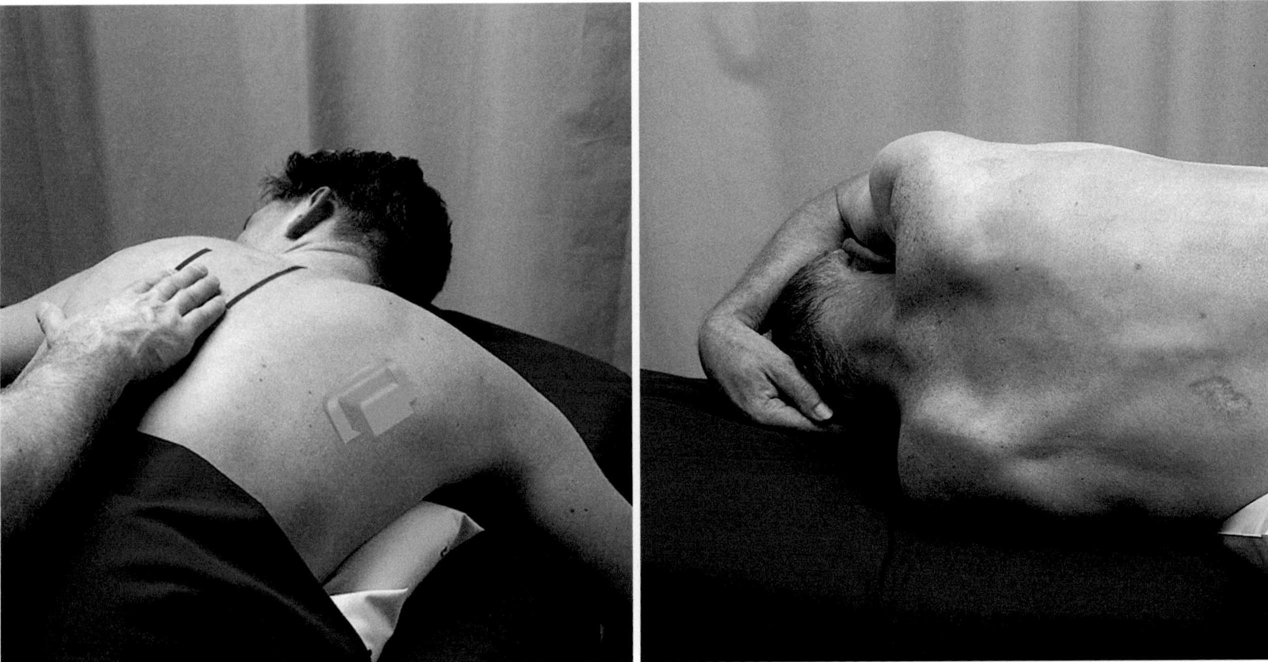

Fig. 35.6 Left: prone position. The red line indicates the midline and blue indicates line joining the angle of ribs. The ultrasound probe position is indicated on the right side. Right: lateral position. (Reprinted with permission from Danilo Jankovic)

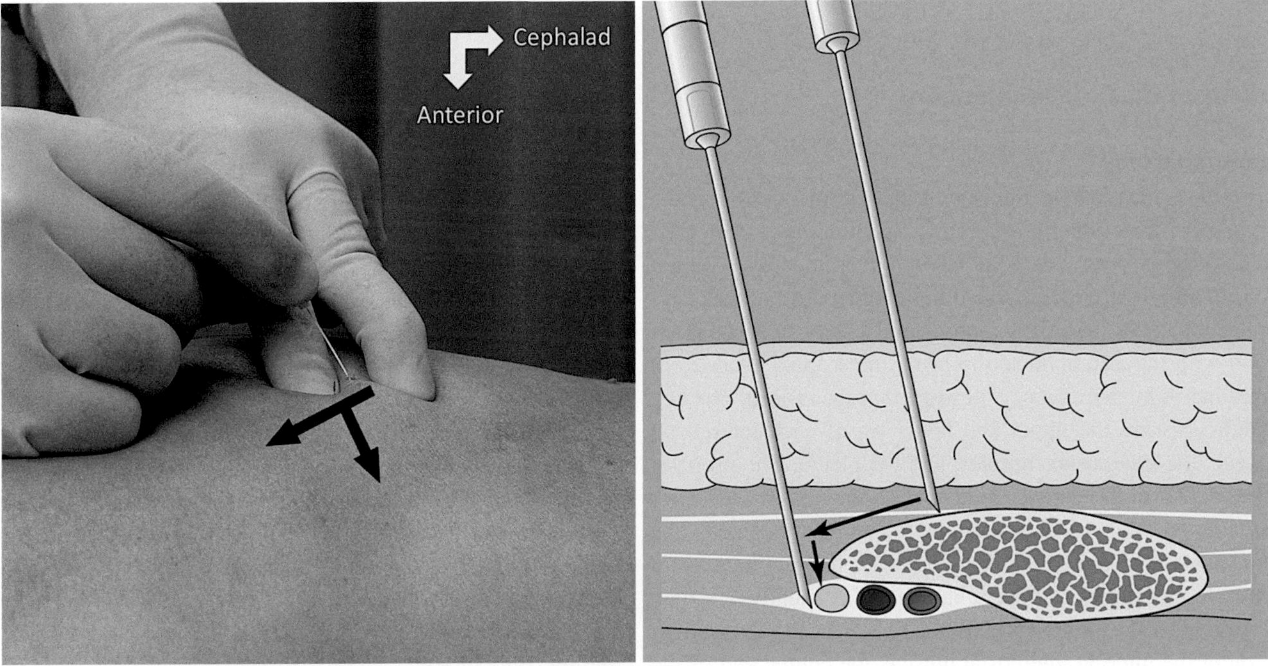

Fig. 35.7 Left: the needle position with landmark technique. Right: schematic diagram to show how the needle is moved. The skin and the needle are simultaneously pushed caudally, and the needle is then introduced a further 2–3 mm. (Reprinted with permission from Danilo Jankovic)

During the injection, the following points must be observed:

1. The person carrying out the injection must stand on the side being blocked.
2. The intercostal nerve runs dorsocaudal to the vessels in the inferior costal groove.
3. Start with the lowest rib.
4. The injection must only be carried out after definite identification of the rib being blocked.
5. Targeted paresthesias are not elicited.
6. If the patient coughs, it indicates pleural irritation. The procedure should be stopped.
7. Injection should be carried out on an incremental basis, with frequent aspiration.

Due to overlap, at least three nerves have to be blocked in order to achieve a complete segmental block. A volume of 3–5-mL local anesthetic is injected per segment, e.g., 0.5–0.75% ropivacaine and 0.25–0.5% bupivacaine (0.25–0.5% levobupivacaine). As intercostal block is the procedure in which the highest blood levels of local anesthetic per milligram injected are achieved (due to very fast absorption), there is a risk of overdose. The individual maximum dose must be carefully calculated and must never be exceeded.

Ultrasound-Guided Injection

Sonoanatomy

The ideal location for ultrasound-guided injection is at the level of angle of the rib because the internal intercostal muscle is formed from this point onward and the lateral cutaneous branch is still incorporated in the intercostal nerve.

The patient lies on the contralateral side or in prone position with the arm abducted to bring the scapula away from midline. A high-frequency ultrasound probe is used. The key landmarks are the upper and lower rib of each intercostal space, the intercostal muscles, and the pleura. The probe is placed 90° to the course of the ribs so that upper and lower ribs, intercostal muscles, and pleura can be visualized. The target is the intercostal nerve deep to the internal intercostal muscle just caudal to the cranial rib and is usually less than 5 mm from the pleura (Fig. 35.8). To enhance the visualization of the internal intercostal muscle, the cranial end of the ultrasound probe is tilted laterally to align with the muscle.

The preferred position for ultrasound-guided technique is prone position for two reasons: it is easier to count the level of ribs in this position, and it is the preferred position to diagnose the presence of pneumothorax as air tends to stay in the nondependent position. These two are also the advantages of the use of ultrasound over the landmark-guided technique. In addition, ultrasound guidance allows the target and the needle to be visualized, as well as the confirmation of the spread of injectate, avoiding inadvertent vascular injection.

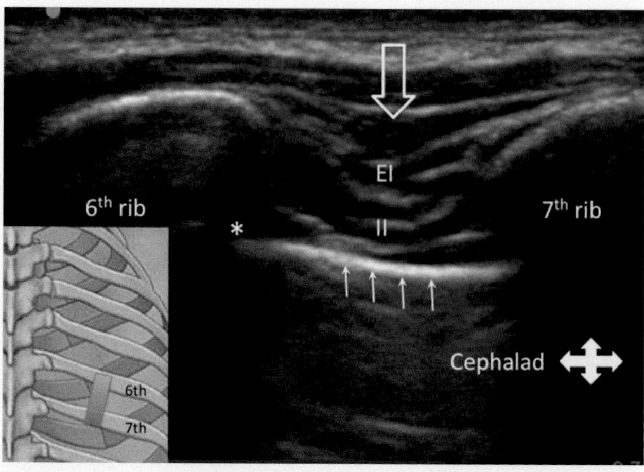

Fig. 35.8 Ultrasonographic image showing the intercostal muscles and pleura at the angle of the rib. EI, external intercostal muscle; II, internal intercostal muscle; *, intercostal neurovascular bundle; arrows, pleura, appears as a hyperechoic line. (Reproduced with permission from Philip Peng Educational Series)

Needle Insertion

With out-of-plane technique, the ultrasound probe is placed in short axis to the two ribs of the intercostal space. The target is the intercostal nerve deep to the internal intercostal muscle just caudal to the cranial rib and is usually less than 5 mm from the pleura. The ultrasound probe should be positioned so that this target is in the center of view in the ultrasound screen. A 25-G 1.5-in. needle is inserted out of plane in an angle almost parallel to the midpoint of the ultrasound probe. The hand holding the ultrasound probe should adjust the tilting of the probe constantly to follow the needle tip. When the needle is in the external intercostal muscle (Fig. 35.9), the position of the needle tip should be confirmed with hydrolocation technique by injecting a small amount of local anesthetic (0.1–0.2 mL). The needle is then carefully advanced to the target. If the tip is in the right location, the pleura is seen pushed down by the spread of injectate (Fig. 35.9). A volume of 1–2 mL is sufficient, contrast to the landmark-guided technique. Alternatively, an in-plane technique can be performed with the block needle inserted from caudad to cephalad targeting the caudal part of the costal margin (Fig. 35.10).

Following the injection of various levels, it is advisable to perform a scan of the pleura to document the absence of pneumothorax. It is important to scan the lung at the site when the needle is inserted. The feature to look for is the pleura which is a thin but densely hyperechoic structure gliding freely with B lines, which are bright, hyperechoic reverberation artifacts originating from the pleura and travelling all the way to the edge of the screen (Fig. 35.11). Absence of

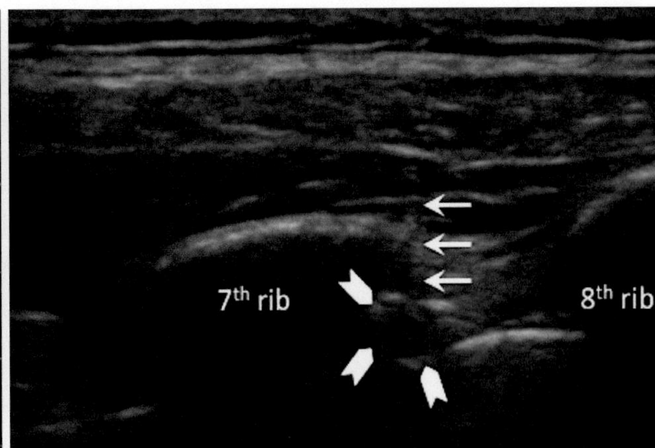

Fig. 35.9 Left: the arrows indicate the needle position inserted with out-of-plane technique. It indicates the needle tip is in external intercostal muscle. Right: further insertion of the needle results in the tip just deep to the internal intercostal muscle. Injection of local anesthetic will result in the appearance of pooling of local anesthetic (bold arrows), which pushes the pleura deeper. (Reproduced with permission from Philip Peng Educational Series)

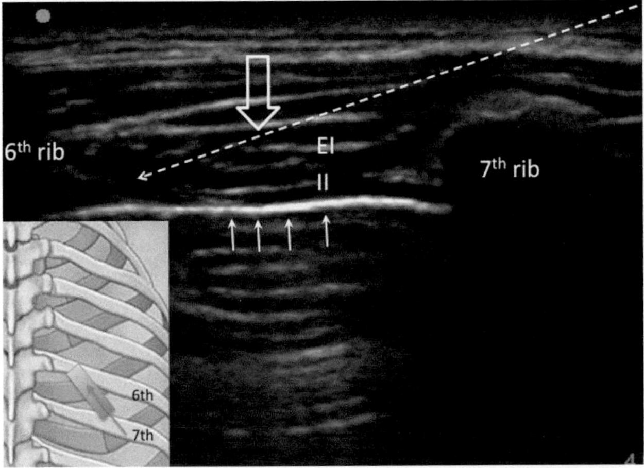

Fig. 35.10 Alternative probe position in a more oblique alignment to allow in-plane insertion of the needle (arrow). *EI* external intercostal muscle, *II* internal intercostal muscle, *arrows* pleura, appears as a hyperechoic line. (Reproduced with permission from Philip Peng Educational Series)

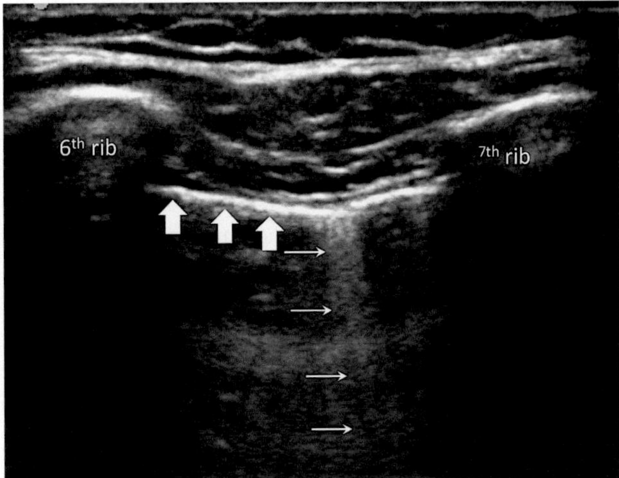

Fig. 35.11 Ultrasound image showing the B line (line arrows). The pleura is indicated by the bold arrows. (Reproduced with permission from Philip Peng Educational Series)

lung gliding, B lines, and conversion of "seashore sign" to "barcode sign" in M mode are diagnostic for the presence of pneumothorax (Fig. 35.12). The concept of lung point is important and is 100% diagnostic of pneumothorax. It represents a transition point where there is absence of the normal lung signs to the point when lung gliding reappears.

Complications

1. Pneumothorax.
2. Local anesthetic systemic toxicity due to high systemic absorption and overdosage.
3. Intravascular injection.
4. Infection.
5. Hematoma.

Practical Tips

1. Patient positioning is important. Intercostal nerve blocks can be performed with patient in prone, lateral decubitus, or sitting position, but it is best performed in prone position.
2. The target is the intercostal nerve deep to the internal intercostal muscle. Regardless of the body build, the tip of the needle is <5 mm to the pleura, and a successful injection will result in pushing the pleura. Therefore,

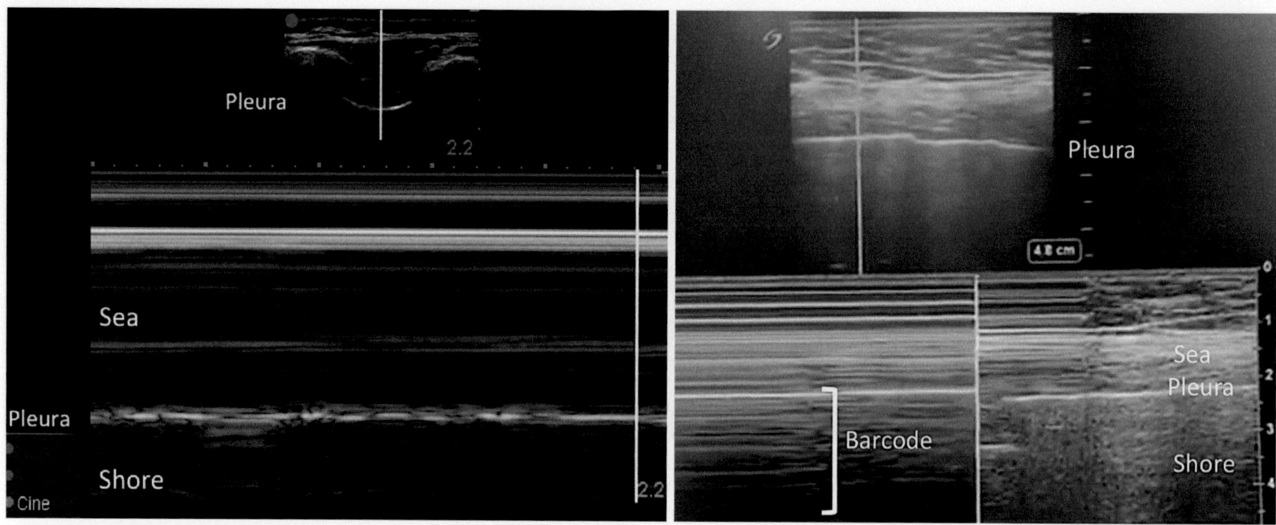

Fig. 35.12 Left: M mode showing the sea (soft tissue superficial to the pleura) shore sign. Right: with pneumothorax, the region deep the pleura will appear as the same as superficial to the pleura and gives the appearance of barcode sign. (Reproduced with permission from Philip Peng Educational Series)

when a clinician is using out-of-plane technique, a couple of caveats, have the needle 0.5 to 1 cm away from the probe, but insert at a steep angle (this allows early visualization of the needle and avoids the tip to advance to the other side of the probe); pay attention to the fascia joining the superficial surface of both adjoining ribs as movement of it signifying the needle is about to enter into the intercostal muscle. Then use hydrodissection to confirm the tip location from that point onward.

3. Intercostal blocks are best performed near the angle of the ribs. In the upper chest, the ipsilateral arm can be put on the contralateral shoulder to move the scapula away.
4. Postprocedure evaluation for pneumothorax is warranted. The scanning of the lung should be in the same position as injection.

Literature Review

In perioperative setting, intercostal nerve block provided superior pain control at rest and with movement (cough) after major surgery such as esophagectomy through thoracotomy when compared with opioids alone in early postoperative period. When added as part of multimodal analgesia technique, intercostal nerve block reduced opioid consumption and hospital stay in breast implant surgery. However, the effect size and analgesic duration are limited. In a randomized study, investigators evaluated the added benefit of intercostal nerve block to thoracic epidural analgesia performed by the surgeon at the end of the surgery (at the level of the thoracotomy and two levels up and down). The authors concluded that addition of intercostal block to epidural analgesia does not confer any benefit in terms of postoperative pain, opioid requirement, or inspiratory effect as measured by spirometry.

In addition, the fear of pneumothorax decreased the popularity of this block, and paravertebral block can provide the same type of analgesic benefit. A recent systematic review and meta-analysis compared the safety and efficacy of paravertebral block with intercostal nerve block in the setting of thoracotomy, thoracoscopic surgery, and breast surgery. The primary outcome was visual analog scale (VAS) at rest recorded at 1, 2, 12, and 24 h after surgery. The secondary outcomes included the rate of postoperative nausea and vomiting (PONV), rate of additional analgesia, and postoperative consumption of morphine. They included a total of 9 trials including 440 patients (paravertebral block, 222 patients; intercostal nerve block, 218 patients) and found that paravertebral block provided better analgesia and resulted in lower consumption of morphine after thoracic surgery and breast surgery.

The use of intercostal nerve block and subsequent thermal radiofrequency ablation (RFA) has been successfully described in chronic pain settings. Applying RFA to intercostal nerves showed promising result in palliative setting in either metastatic disease of the rib (nociceptive pain) or chest wall neuralgia (neuropathic pain). In one study, RFA of the intercostal nerve was used to treat 25 patients with uncontrollable breakthrough pain (BTP) arising out of the rib metastasis. Following the RFA treatment, there was more than 50% decrease in both intensity and frequency of BTP in more than 50% of patients for 3 months, and there was more than 50% decrease in BTP opioid dose in more than 50% of patients throughout the study period. There was also significant improvement in the background pain, functional status, and quality of life after the RFA. This group of investigators noted that the pain relief, opioid reduction, and functional status improvement were found mostly in patients with intercostal nerve involvement, i.e., neuropathic pain or mixed neuropathic and nociceptive pain. Similarly, thermal RFA has been reported providing long-lasting pain relief in patient with cancer-related refractory chest wall neuralgia.

Persistent chest wall neuralgic pain is not uncommon in the contact sports athletes and can limit their activity and participation in the sports. In a case series involving 18 patients with sports-related persistent intercostal neuralgic pain who underwent pulsed radiofrequency (PRF) neuromodulation, 16 of 18 (88%) patients had effective pain relief (NRS <3) following the PRF therapy from the baseline numeric pain score 8.5 ± 1.9 up to the 4-week follow-up. The PRF provides adequate and quick pain relief, enabling them to resume their sports activities. In addition, cryoanalgesia has been successfully used in the treatment of post-thoracotomy pain syndrome. Traditionally, it used to be done with landmark-guided technique but in recent times under ultrasound guidance which significantly reduces the possibility of pneumothorax and provides effective long-term pain relief.

In patient with refractory chest wall pain from tumor spread, another option is chemical neurolysis of the intercostal nerves. In a retrospective analysis of 146 patients who underwent intercostal nerve block, intercostal nerve chemical ablation provided pain relief in 62% of patient after a successful diagnostic blockade. Authors chose alcohol over phenol as the neurolytic agent due to a perceived decreased risk in deafferentation pain, whereas phenol may lead to nerve arborization and neuroma formation. Both local anesthetic and neurolytic agents have been described to enter the intrathecal space and cause anesthesia and paralysis, respectively. Hence, it is prudent that small amount of neurolytic solution (<1 mL) is used for neurolysis and ultrasound guidance allows the precise location of the target.

References

Abd-Elsayed A, Lee S, Jackson M. Radiofrequency ablation for treating resistant intercostal neuralgia. Ochsner J. 2018;18(1):91–3.

Ahmed A, Bhatnagar S, Khurana D, Joshi S, Thulkar S. Ultrasound-guided radiofrequency treatment of intercostal nerves for the prevention of incidental pain arising due to rib metastasis: a prospective study. Am J Hosp Palliat Med. 2017;34(2):115–24.

Bhatia A, Gofeld M, Ganapathy S, Hanlon J, Johnson M. Comparison of anatomic landmarks and ultrasound guidance for intercostal nerve injections in cadavers. Reg Anesth Pain Med. 2013;38:503–7.

Brown DL. Intercostal block. In: Brown DL, editor. Atlas of regional anesthesia. Philadelphia: WB Saunders; 1992. p. 211–7.

Byas-Smith MG, Gulati A. Ultrasound-guided intercostal nerve cryoablation. Anesth Analg. 2006;103(4):1033–5.

Curatolo M. Intercostal nerve block. In: Peng PW, editor. Ultrasound for pain medicine intervention: a practical guide. Peripheral structures. Philip Peng educational series. iBook, vol. 1. 1st ed. Cupertino, CA: Apple; 2013. p. 65–8.

Curatolo M, Bogduk N. Diagnostic and therapeutic nerve blocks. In: Fishman SM, Ballantyne JC, Rathmell JP, editors. Bonica's management of pain. Philadelphia: Lippincott William & Wilkins; 2010a. p. 1401–23.

Curatolo M, Bogduk N. Diagnostic blocks for chronic pain. Scand J Pain. 2010b;1:186–92.

Gulati A, Shah R, Puttanniah V, Hung JC, Malhotra V. A retrospective review and treatment paradigm of interventional therapies for patients suffering from intractable thoracic Chest Wall pain in the oncologic population. Pain Med. 2015;16:802–10.

Hashemi M, Mohseni G, Ataei MH, Zafari A, Keyhani S, Jazayeri SM. Intercostal nerves pulsed radiofrequency for intractable neuralgia treatment in athletes with sport trauma of the chest: a case-series study. Arch Trauma Res. 2017;6:37–40.

Haskins SC, Tsui BC, Nejim JA, et al. Lung ultrasound for the regional anesthesiologist and acute pain specialist. Reg Anesth Pain Med. 2017;42:289–98.

Huan S, Deng Y, Wang J, Ji Y, Yin G. Efficacy and safety of paravertebral block versus intercostal nerve block in thoracic surgery and breast surgery: a systematic review and meta-analysis. PLoS One. 2020;15(10):e0237363. https://doi.org/10.1371/journal.pone.0237363.

Jankovic D. Thoracic spinal nerve blocks. In: Jankovic D, editor. Regional nerve. Blocks & infiltration therapy. 3rd ed. Oxford: Blackwell; 2004. p. 171–85.

Jemal B, Woldeyohanes M, Shitemaw T, Ayalew N, Awoke Z, Abiy S. Effectiveness of thoracic paravertebral and intercostal nerve blocks as a part of postoperative analgesia in patients undergoing open cholecystectomy under general anesthesia in Addis Ababa, Ethiopia: a prospective cohort study. Int J Surg Open. 2019;18:1–8.

Moorjani N, Zhao F, Tian Y, Liang C, Kaluba J, Maiwand MO. Effects of cryoanalgesia on post-thoracotomy pain and on the structure of intercostal nerves: a human prospective randomized trial and a histological study. Eur J Cardiothorac Surg. 2001;20(3):502–7.

Peng P, Narouze S. Ultrasound-guided interventional procedures in pain medicine: a review of anatomy, sonoanatomy and procedures. Part I: non-axial structures. Reg Anesth Pain Med. 2009;34:458–74.

Ranganathan P, Tadvi A, Jiwnani S, Karimundackal G, Pramesh CS. A randomised evaluation of intercostal block as an adjunct to epidural analgesia for post-thoracotomy pain. Indian J Anaesth. 2020;64:280–5.

Shah A, Rowlands M, Krishnan N, Patel A, Ott-Young A. Thoracic intercostal nerve blocks reduce opioid consumption and length of stay in patients undergoing implant-based breast reconstruction. Plast Reconstr Surg. 2015;136:584e–91e.

Shankar H, Eastwood D. Retrospective comparison of ultrasound and fluoroscopic image guidance for intercostal steroid injections. Pain Pract. 2010;10:312–7.

Vlassakov KV, Narang S, Kissin I. Local anesthetic blockade of peripheral nerves for treatment of neuralgias: systematic analysis. Anesth Analg. 2011;112:1487–93.

Zhu M, Gu Y, Sun X, et al. Ultrasound-guided intercostal nerve block following esophagectomy for acute postoperative pain relief in the postanesthesia care unit. Pain Pract. 2018;18:879–83.

Ilioinguinal, Iliohypogastric, and Genitofemoral Nerve Blocks

36

Athmaja Thottungal and Philip Peng

Contents

General Consideration

Ilioinguinal nerve (IIN) and iliohypogastric nerve (IHN) along with genitofemoral nerve (GFN) and subcostal nerve (T12 intercostal nerve) provide sensory and motor supply to the lower abdominal walls (Figs. 36.1 and 36.2). Blocking these nerves can be used for anesthesia and analgesia as a part of acute and chronic pain management. Collectively, the IIN, IHN, and GFN are called the "border nerves," and the chronic pain originating from these nerves is called "border nerve syndrome." These nerves show very high rate of anatomical variability from the spinal nerve root origin, divisions, communication between the nerves, fascial plane penetration, and sensory contributions. Performing these nerve blocks using blind landmark techniques or nerve stimulating techniques has been used for many years with a high rate of failure and complications which is highly understandable due to the anatomical variability and location. Recently various ultrasound-guided techniques are described which showed to have a high success rate with reduced adverse incidents. The aims of this chapter is to give an overview of these nerve blocks with specific attention to the latest ultrasound-guided techniques which are useful for patients with acute, chronic, and palliative pain. For discussion, IIN/IHN and GFN block techniques are discussed under two separate headings.

A. Thottungal (✉)
Department of Anaesthesia and Pain Management, Kent and Canterbury Hospital, East Kent Hospitals University NHS Foundation Trust, Canterbury, UK

P. Peng
Department of Anesthesiology and Pain Medicine, Toronto Western Hospital, University of Toronto, Toronto, ON, Canada
e-mail: philip.peng@uhn.ca

D. Jankovic, P. Peng (eds.), *Regional Nerve Blocks in Anesthesia and Pain Therapy*,
https://doi.org/10.1007/978-3-030-88727-8_36

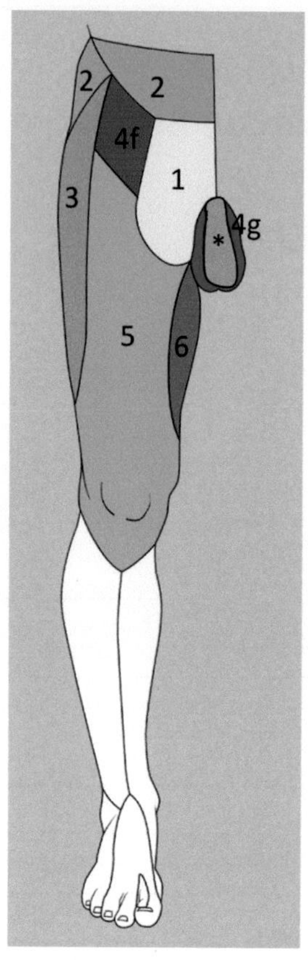

Fig. 36.1 Sensory innervation from the lumbar plexus. (Reprinted with permission from Philip Peng Educational Series)

Indications

Acute Pain

Local anesthetic block of these nerves provides analgesia for operations or trauma involving the lower part of the abdomen and anterior pelvic region.

Surgeries: Inguinal hernia repair, pelvic open and laparoscopic surgeries, trocar trauma from laparoscopic or robotic surgery, appendicectomy, hysterectomy, abdominoplasty, Pfannenstiel incision, orchiectomy, surgery of female or male external genitalia.

Trauma: Blunt abdominal trauma, femoral catheter placement, tearing of the lower external oblique aponeurosis in hockey or other sports players, stretch injury as in pregnancy or during lower segment Cesarean section, entrapment near the rectus border (anterior cutaneous nerve entrapment syndrome) and near the ilium or around psoas/quadratus lumborum muscles.

Chronic Pain

The nerve blockade of these nerves can be used to provide analgesia for persistent postsurgical pain following any of the above surgeries, neuropathic pain, or psoas spasm.

Cancer Pain

In patient with cancer pain originating from inguinal region or external genitalia region, blockade of GFN with or without IIN/IHN can be considered.

Functional Anatomy

The II and IH nerves originate from the anterior rami of L1 nerve roots with contributions from T12 or L2, emerging near the lateral border of the psoas major muscle. These two nerves extend diagonally toward the crest of the ilium. The GFN tends to originate predominantly from L1 and L2, and after the intrapelvic course, it enters the abdominal wall at the level of the deep inguinal ring.

The IHN pierces the transversus abdominis muscle above the iliac crest, midway between the iliac crest and the 12th rib. The IIN runs caudally and parallel to the IHN. Here, both nerves can be found consistently (90%) between the transversus abdominis and internal oblique muscles. Terminal branches of the IH nerve perforate the external oblique muscle aponeurosis approximately 4 cm lateral to the midline to supply the skin over the lower portion of the rectus abdominis. The IH nerve also provides sensory innervation to the skin above the tensor fasciae latae through a lateral cutaneous

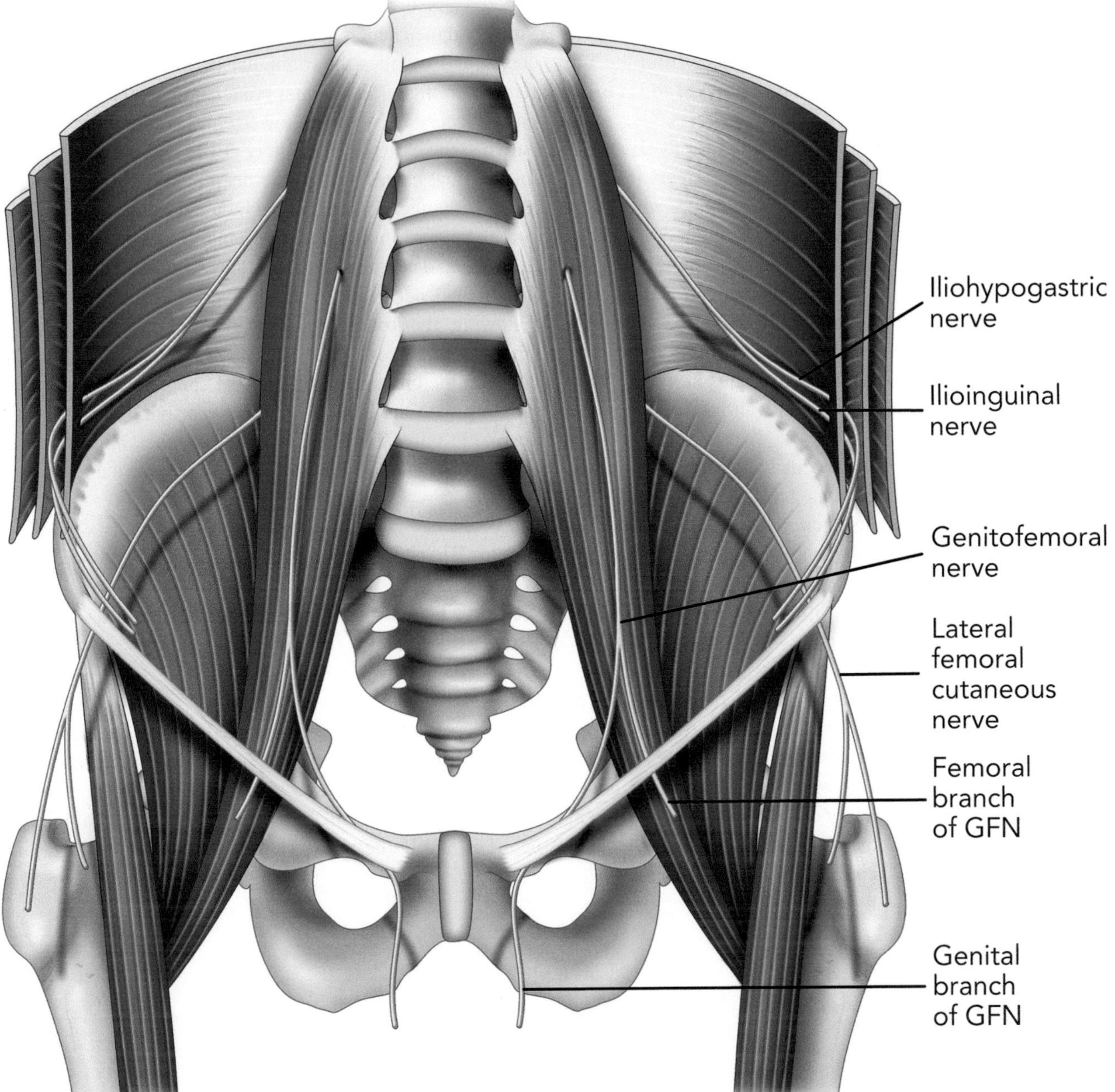

Fig. 36.2 The anterior abdominal wall muscles showing the relationship of "border nerves" and GFN. (Reprinted with permission from Philip Peng Educational Series)

branch. Terminal branches of the II nerve enter the inguinal canal through the deep inguinal ring; it may lie upon the cremaster muscle and fascial layer of the spermatic cord in men or the round ligament in women. Here, the II nerve is often accompanied by the genital branch of the GF nerve, and wide variations in the course of these nerves within the inguinal canal have been documented. The terminal sensory branches may innervate the skin of the mons pubis, inner thigh, inguinal crease, and anterior surface of the scrotum or anterior one-third of the labia (Fig. 36.1).

However, the main concept to remind when dealing with the "border nerves" is the high rate of variability they are associated with. Anatomic studies highlight this variability, which have been reported with respect to their origin and spinal contribution, communication between nerves, penetration of fascial layers, branching patterns, and dominance patterns; in some cases, one of the nerves may be entirely absent. Although the general anatomy of the IH and II nerves has been well documented in standard anatomy textbooks, recent studies related to nerve injury during surgery or based on cadaver dissections were able to identify multiple and different spinal nerves contributing to the formation of these nerves. The II and IH nerves mainly originate from the T12 and L1 nerve roots, but a contribution from T11 to L3 exists in a minority of patients.

The most consistent anatomical location for the II and IH nerves to perforate the abdominal muscular layers is lateral and superior to the anterior superior iliac spine, where they run between the transversus abdominis and internal oblique muscular layers, even though the distance from the ASIS to the point the nerves enter the fascial layer can widely vary. Also, communication between the GF, IH, or II nerves (as well as the lateral femoral cutaneous nerve) is common and results in sensory overlap. Finally, the sites at which the II and IH nerves pierce the abdominal wall muscle layers are significantly variable.

Special considerations are needed for pediatric patients. Anatomically, pediatric patients have varying II and IH nerves compared with adults; anatomical results from adults cannot be downscaled to infants and children, in whom the iliohypogastric and ilioinguinal nerves lie closer to the ASIS than originally thought, and differences have been noted according to different age groups.

The GFN originates from the L1 and L2 nerve roots (Figs. 36.1 and 36.2). It emerges on the anterior surface of the psoas muscle either as a single trunk or separate genital and femoral branches and crosses the ureter on its descent. The division could happen anywhere during its course above the inguinal ligament. It mainly carries sensory fibers except motor fibers to cremaster muscle. The femoral branch which is a sensory branch passes laterally over the external iliac artery and then penetrates the fascia latae to enter the femoral sheath and supplies the triangular dermatomal part over the femoral triangle. The genital branch crosses the inferior epigastric artery (IEA) at its lower end lateral to the junction between the external iliac artery (EIA) and the IEA to enter the inguinal canal through the deep inguinal ring. It travels along with other contents of the inguinal canal along with the spermatic cord in men and the round ligament of the uterus in women. The canal also contains inguinal branch of the ilioinguinal nerve and testicular vessels in men or vessels following the round ligament of the uterus in females (Fig. 36.3). Anatomical studies describe this branch running between the cremaster and internal spermatic fascia, incorporating with the cremasteric fascia, or lying outside of the spermatic cord. Terminal sensory branches may innervate the scrotum and possibly the upper, inner, medial thigh.

Nerve Block Techniques

Existing Landmark Techniques for Nerve Blockade

IIN/IHN

As discussed above, there is a high degree of anatomic variability in not only the course of the nerves but also their branching patterns, areas of penetration of the fascial layers, and dominance patterns. By far, the most consistent location of the II and IH nerves is lateral and superior to the ASIS,

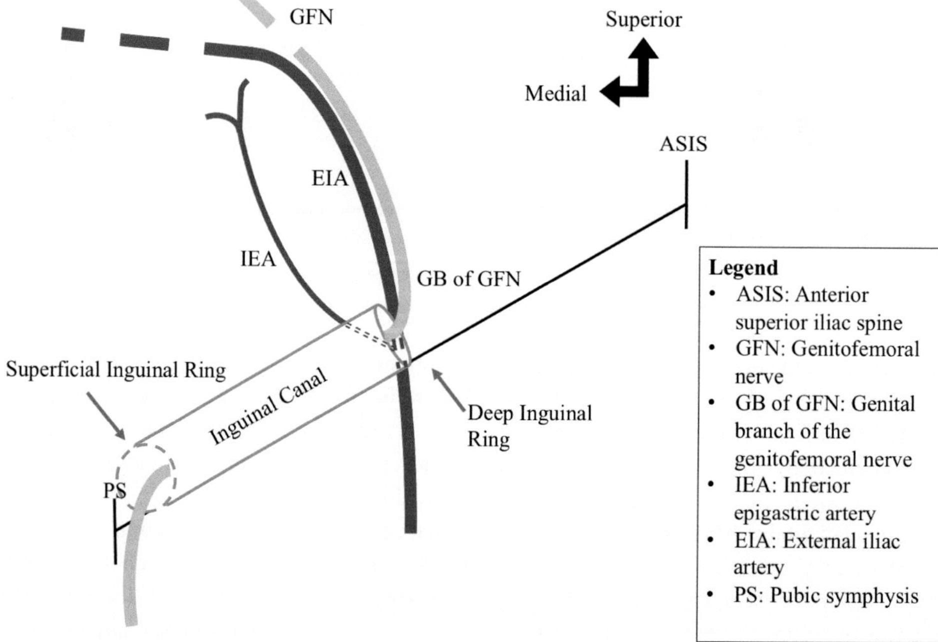

Fig. 36.3 The schematic diagram showing the relationship of the genital branch (GB) of the GFN to the external iliac artery (EIA) and inferior epigastric artery (IEA). (Reprinted with permission from Philip Peng Educational Series)

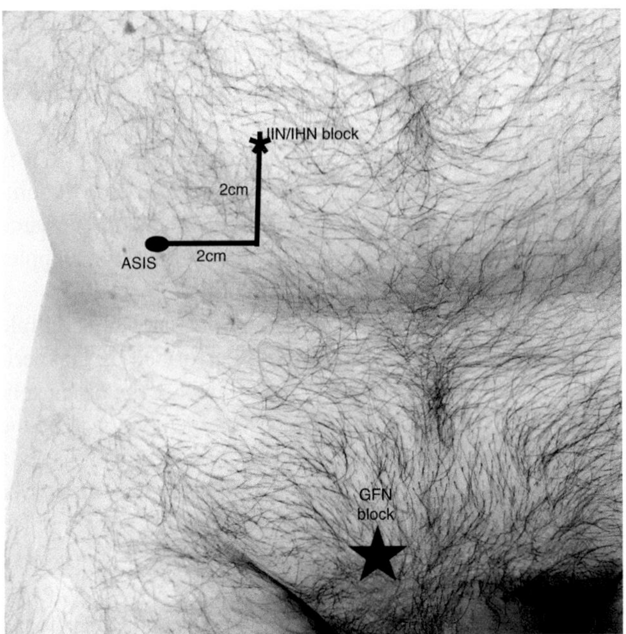

Fig. 36.4 Landmark points for ilioinguinal and iliohypogastric nerves (IIN/IHN) block (asterisk mark) and genitofemoral nerve (GFN) block (star mark). *ASIS* anterior superior iliac spine. (Reprinted with permission from Dr. Athmaja Thottungal)

where the nerves are found between the transverses abdominis and internal oblique muscular layers in nearly 90% of cases. While most of the anatomical variations occur medial to the ASIS, virtually all landmark-guided injection techniques described in the literature are performed in the anterior abdominal wall (Fig. 36.4). Because the existing landmark-based techniques rely on blind infiltration of local anesthetic through different layers, the risk of complications are well understandable: these include inadvertent femoral nerve block, colonic puncture, and vascular injury. Nevertheless, block failure is still an important matter of concern, and failure rate of the blind technique lies in the range of 10% to 40%. This is attributed to the potential for injecting local anesthetics into the wrong abdominal plane, and in some situation, it leads to injection inside the peritoneum. This is more common in pediatric population.

GFN

The conventional description of the blockade of genital branch of GF nerve is mainly a "blind" technique and relies on the pubic tubercle, inguinal ligament, inguinal crease, and femoral artery as landmarks. One involves infiltration of local anesthetic immediately lateral to the pubic tubercle caudal to the inguinal ligament. In another method, a needle is inserted into the inguinal canal to block the genital branch. The blind techniques described are essentially infiltration techniques and rely on high volumes of local anesthetic for consistent results. Although the basis of this landmark is not clear, the needle is likely directed toward the spermatic cord, and important structures of the spermatic cord (testicular artery and vas deferens) or the peritoneum are at risk. It is also worth remembering that the common site of nerve injury is proximal to the site of injection in these techniques which leads to high failure rate with these techniques (Fig. 36.4).

Ultrasound-Guided Block Techniques

Advantages of ultrasound guidance include the identification of muscular and fascial layers (including structures lying deeper to the peritoneum), the visualization of needle's trajectory and spread of injectate, and the detection of vascular structures. Ultrasound helps physicians to overcome the wide anatomical variability associated with the structures in this area, helping to identify the nerves themselves or the plane they lie within. Ultrasound guidance has demonstrated to improve accuracy in the injection of local anesthetics, with less risk of inadvertent injections in the wrong fascial plane, reduced amount of local anesthetics used for anesthesia, and lower consumption of systemic pain medications compared to landmark techniques. The identification of individual nerves is important for the success of blocks in chronic pain treatment modalities like pulsed radiofrequency denervation, cryotherapy, neuromodulation, or neurolysis.

IIN/IHN Block Technique

The IHN and IIN are very superficial nerves and best viewed with a linear probe of high frequency (6–13 MHz). In very obese patient, a curved medium-frequency probe may be useful.

The patient is usually placed in supine; in situations of high BMI or pendulous abdomen, the patient can be placed in lateral position with the affected side up to improve the visibility.

Most of clinical studies or reports used ASIS as landmark, and the position of the probe was above ASIS and moved along the line joining the ASIS and umbilicus. This approach carries some limitation: when the probe is placed too near to ASIS, the external oblique muscle layer may be missed; when the probe is too far away from the ASIS (the "bone shadow of the iliac crest" not in the scan), the nerve seen in between the transversus abdominis and internal oblique muscular layers is likely to be the 12th intercostal nerve or subcostal nerve instead.

The recommended area for ultrasound scanning of II and IH nerves is lateral and superior to the anterior superior iliac spine (Fig. 36.5), because the two nerves are detectable in this area in 90% of cases. When the probe is placed cranial and three fingerbreadths lateral to the ASIS with the transducer perpendicular to the inguinal ligament and its lateral end in contact with the iliac crest, three layers of the abdominal wall muscle can be seen. Below the transversus abdominis, peristaltic movements of the bowel may be detected. The IIN and IHN will be found in the split fascial plane between the internal oblique and transversus abdominis muscle layers. Both nerves should be within 1.5 cm of the iliac crest at this site, located on the "upsloping" split fascia close to the iliac crest, with the IIN closer to the iliac crest. In some cases, the nerves may run approximately 1 cm apart, and in many cases, they are so close together so that it is visualized as single neurovascular bundle. The deep circumflex iliac artery which is close to the two nerves in the same fascial layer can be revealed with the use of color Doppler (Fig. 36.6).

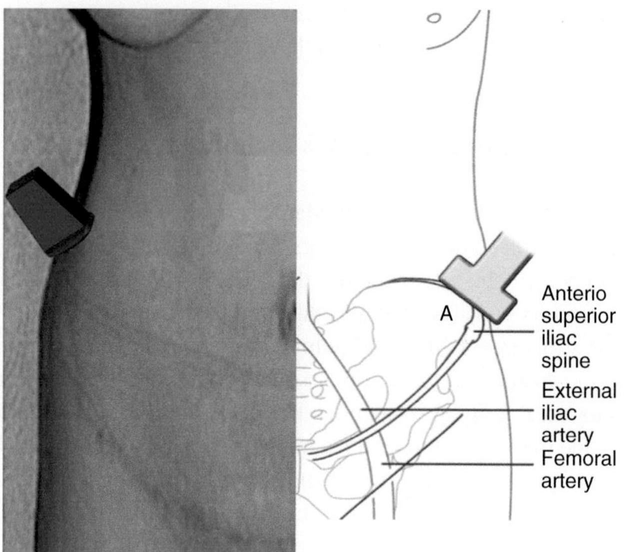

Fig. 36.5 The probe position for the ilioinguinal and iliohypogastric nerves. (Reprinted with permission from Philip Peng Educational Series)

In some patients (those with previous surgery, multiple childbirth) or when the procedure is performed by inexperienced practitioners, either the IIN and IHN or the fascia split is difficult to visualize; in these cases, the target will be the fascial plane between the internal oblique and transverse abdominal muscles. Neurostimulation to locate the nerves under the ultrasound can be used to locate the nerves which are essential for the chronic pain procedures.

Injection can be performed with either out-of-plane or in-plane (Fig. 36.7) techniques with a 50-mm echogenic needle. As the two nerves run very closely within the fascial plane (sometimes as a common trunk) and frequently overlap in sensory innervation, a selective block of one of the two nerves has recently been demonstrated to be impractical. In chronic pain settings, the out-of-plane technique helps to

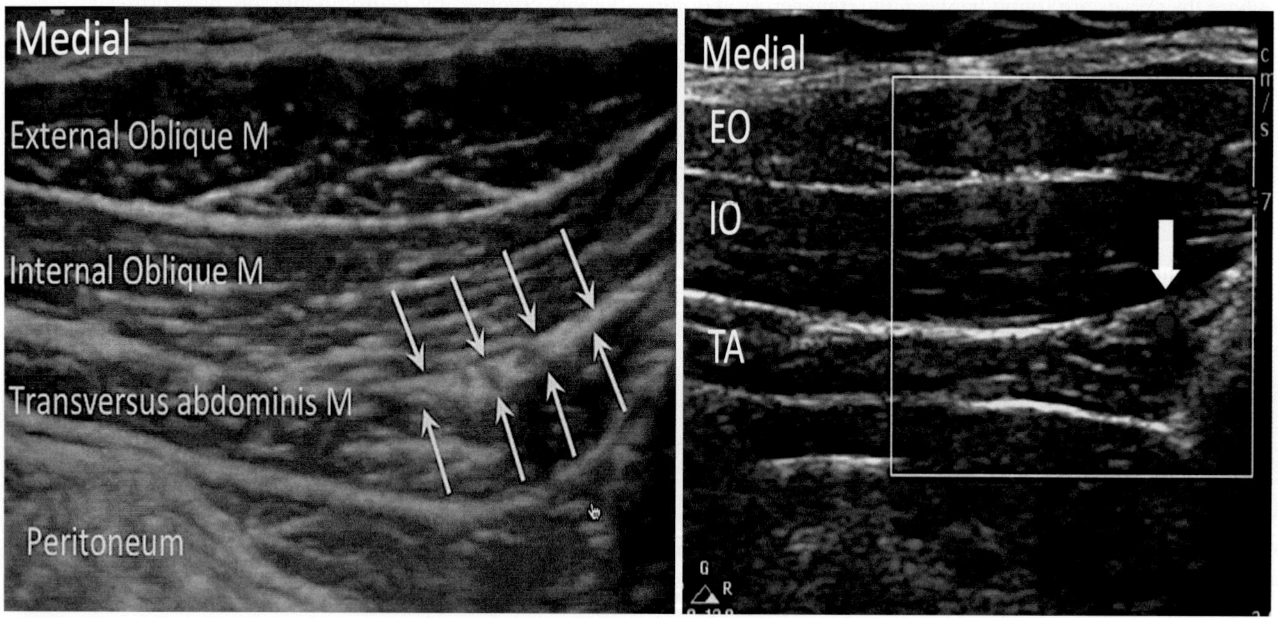

Fig. 36.6 Left figure. Sonoanatomy of the ilioinguinal and iliohypogastric nerves in the fascia plane (indicated by arrows) between internal oblique (IO) and transverse abdominis (TA) muscles. RIght figure. Sonogram showing the deep circumflex iliac artery (bold arrow) in the fascia layer where the ilioinguinal and iliohypogastric nerves are located. *EO* external oblique. (Reprinted with permission from Philip Peng Educational Series)

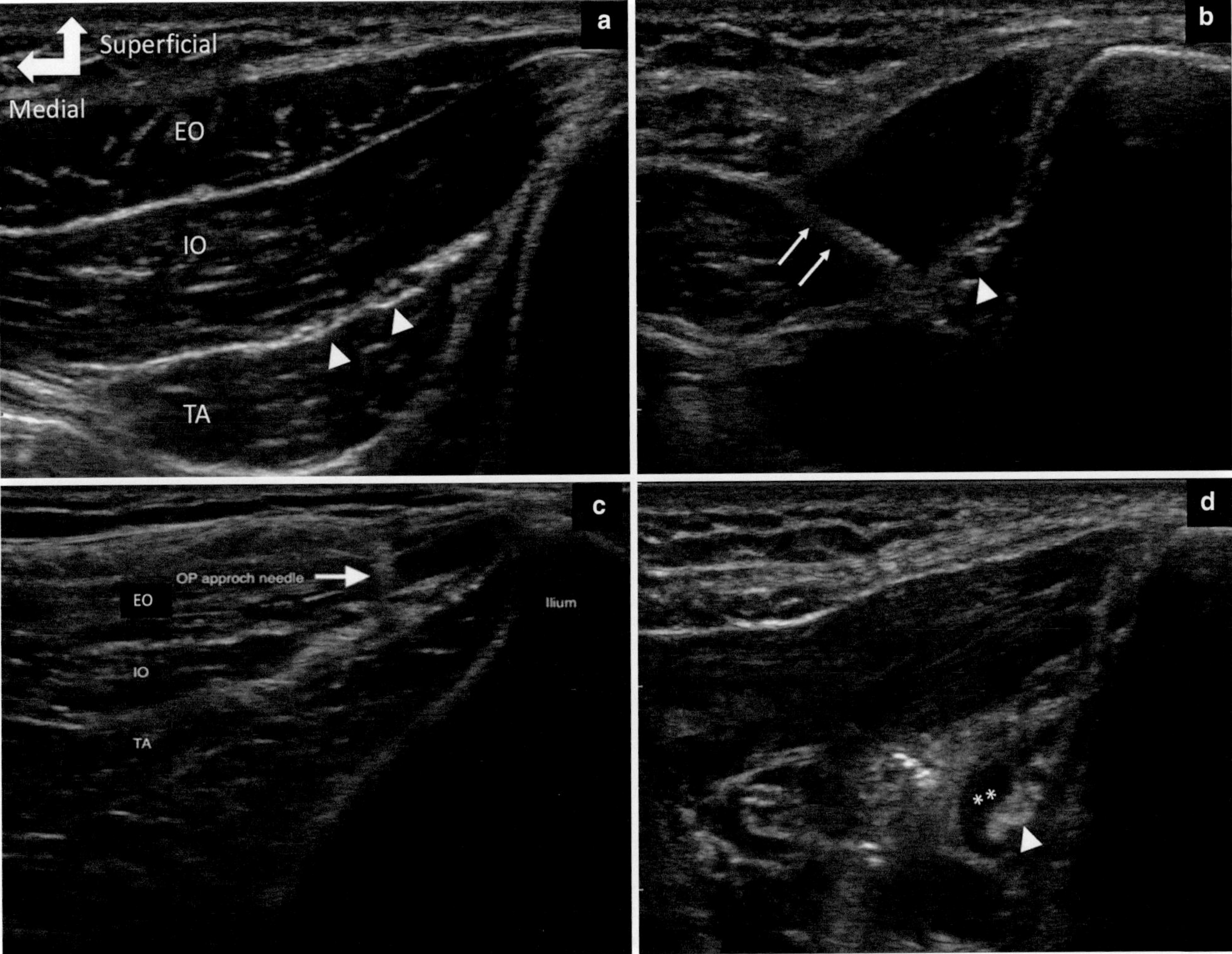

Fig. 36.7 (**a**) Ilioinguinal and iliohypogastric nerves (arrowheads) between the IO and TA (internal oblique and transversus abdominis muscles), *EO* external oblique; (**b**) in-plane needle insertion to Ilioinguinal and iliohypogastric nerves (arrowhead). Arrow shows the needle next to the nerve. (**c**) Out-of-plane (OP) approach. The needle is inserted perpendicular to the nerve (arrow); (**d**) local anesthetic (**) within the fascia expansion. (Reprinted with permission from Dr. Athmaja Thottungal)

keep the tip of radiofrequency cannula and neurostimulator catheters parallel to the nerves from cranial to caudal direction. The injectate that the author usually used is 2–4 mL of 0.25–0.5% levo or plain bupivacaine. In chronic pain, this can be mixed with 1-mL (3.8 mg) dexamethasone or 40-mg depomedrone. In addition to the injection, straight or curved radiofrequency needle with 5-mm active tip, cryoprobe, or stimulating catheter can be used appropriately.

GFN Block Technique

There are three different methods to scan and identify the genitofemoral nerve (GFN). No validated standardized technique has been described yet. Two methods are already described in the literature, and the third one is from author's clinical experience especially from scanning female patients. In all situations, the patient is put in supine position, and a high-frequency probe is used.

Method 1: GFN Blockade Proximal to Deep Inguinal Ring

This is from the author's clinical experience. The initial scanning starts at the rectus abdominis muscle at the lower abdomen in transverse plane to identify inferior epigastric artery (IEA) (Fig. 36.8). The probe is further moved caudally till the junction of the IEA with the external iliac artery (EIA) is identified. The lateral part of the probe is tilted cranially to align the probe position parallel to the inguinal ligament (Fig. 36.9). The deep inguinal ring area is visible lateral to the IEA and the GFN and spermatic cord or round ligament of the uterus entering into the inguinal canal. Once the GFN is located, a 20-G or 22-G 50-mm echogenic needle is inserted in plane in lateral to medial direction (Fig. 36.10). The injectate is 2–4 mL of 0.25–0.5% levo or plain bupivacaine. In chronic pain, this can be mixed with 1-mL (3.8 mg) dexamethasone or 40-mg depomedrone.

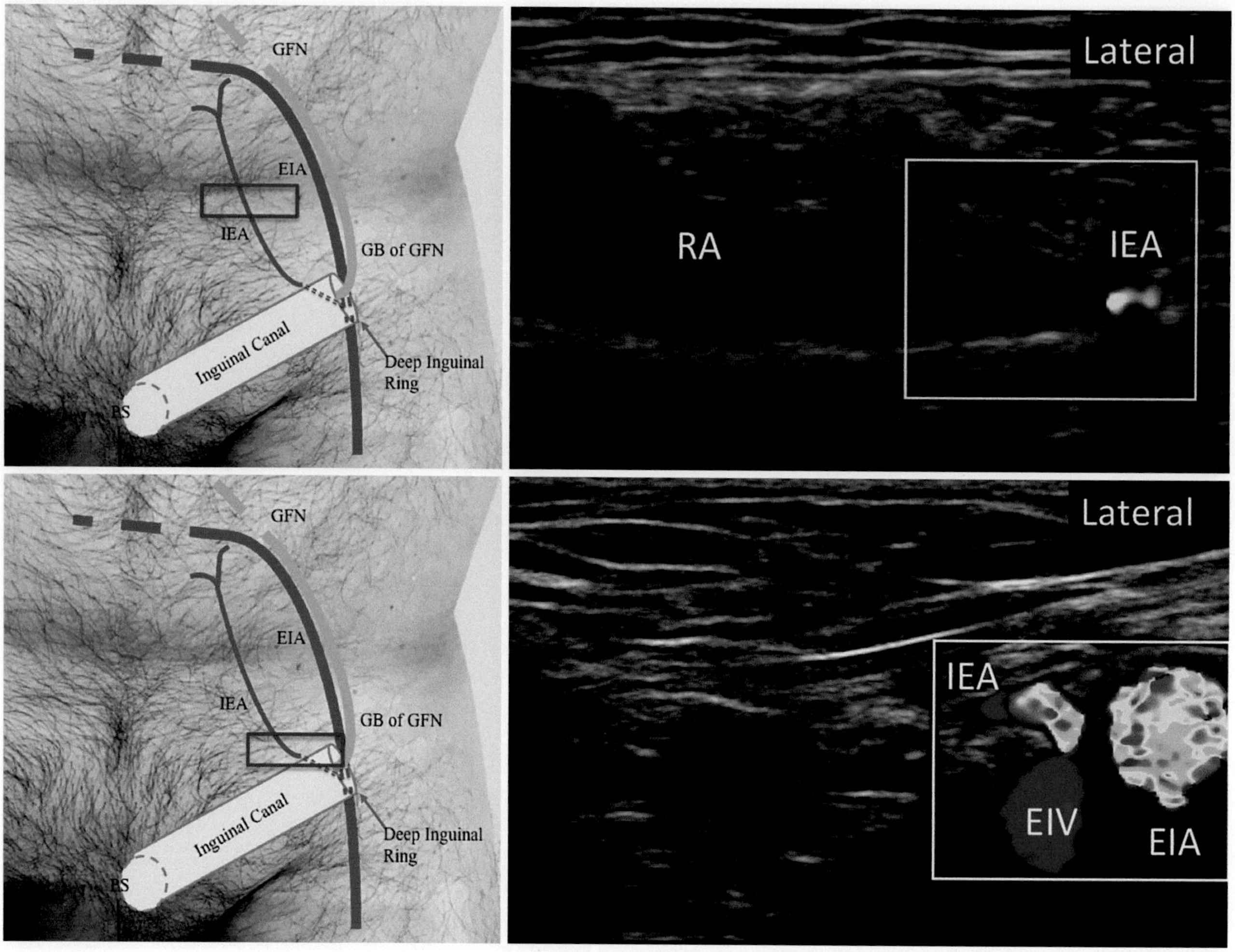

Fig. 36.8 Position of ultrasound probe (blue rectangle) with corresponding sonography. Upper panel: inferior epigastric artery (IEA) is seen deep to the rectus abdominis (RA) muscle. Lower panel: sonography when the ultrasound probe is moved lower to the junction of the IEA with the external iliac artery (EIA). *GFN* genitofemoral nerve, *GB* genital branch, *EIV* external iliac vein. (Reprinted with permission from Philip Peng Educational Series)

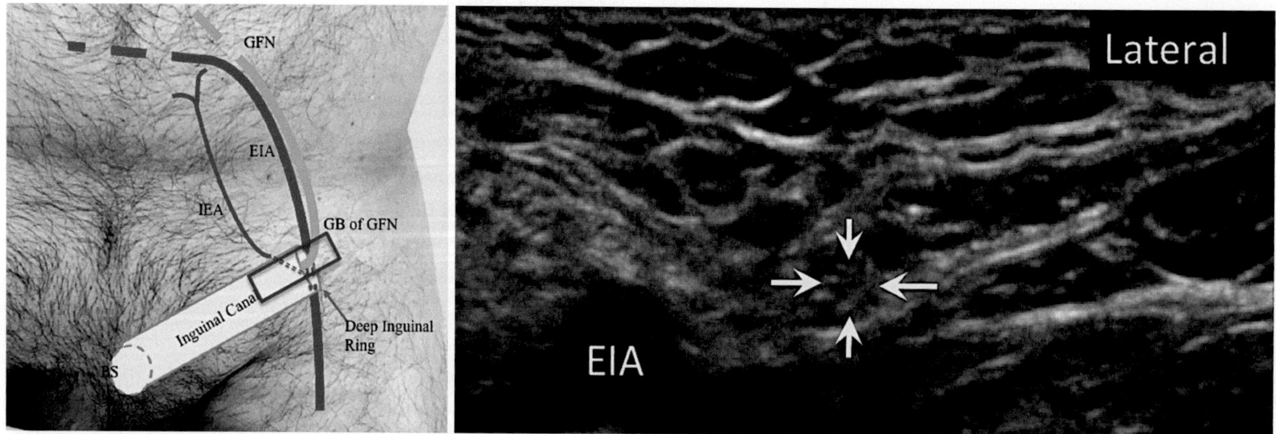

Fig. 36.9 Sonography when the ultrasound probe is aligned to the inguinal canal. The genital branch of the genitofemoral nerve (GFN) is indicated by arrows. (Reprinted with permission from Philip Peng Educational Series)

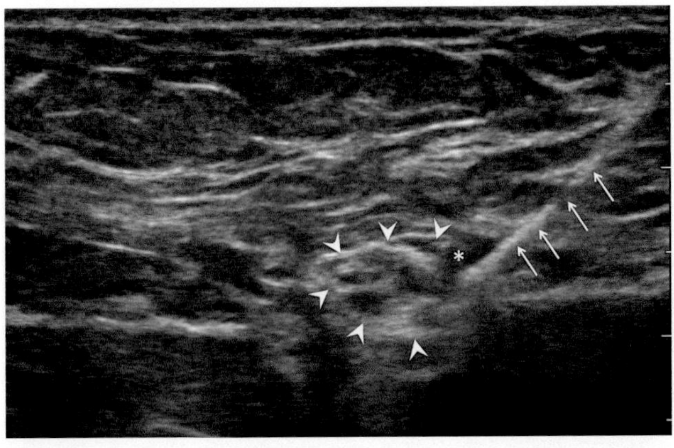

Fig. 36.10 Needle insertion in-plane approach from lateral to medial direction. The genital branch of genitofemoral nerve is indicated by the arrowheads and the local anesthetic by the *. (Reprinted with permission from Dr. Athmaja Thottungal)

Method 2: Using Femoral Artery to Identify the Inguinal Canal

The initial scan of this method is similar to that of the femoral nerve block. The probe is placed in transverse plane just below the inguinal ligament to identify femoral artery (FA), which is then kept in the middle of the screen (Fig. 36.11). The probe is then rotated to sagittal plane to visualize FA longitudinally, and the FA is traced cranially until it becomes EIA diving deep into the abdomen (Fig. 36.12). At this point, the inguinal canal is seen as an oval structure superficial to the FA with the spermatic cord or round ligament of the uterus inside (Fig. 36.13). The inguinal canal can be traced in medial direction for maximal visibility. Because of the superficial nature of the inguinal canal, the needle can be easily advanced with out-of-plane approach. The medication used is the same as above, but 2–4 mL of injectate is admin-

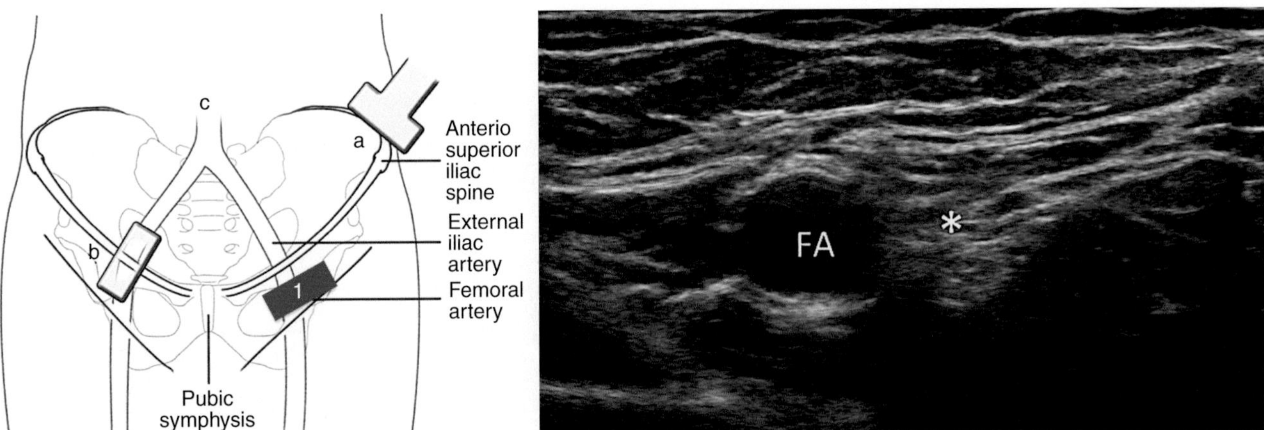

Fig. 36.11 Sonography of the femoral artery (FA) in short axis when the ultrasound probe is placed below the inguinal ligament (position 1). * femoral nerve. (Reprinted with permission from Philip Peng Educational Series)

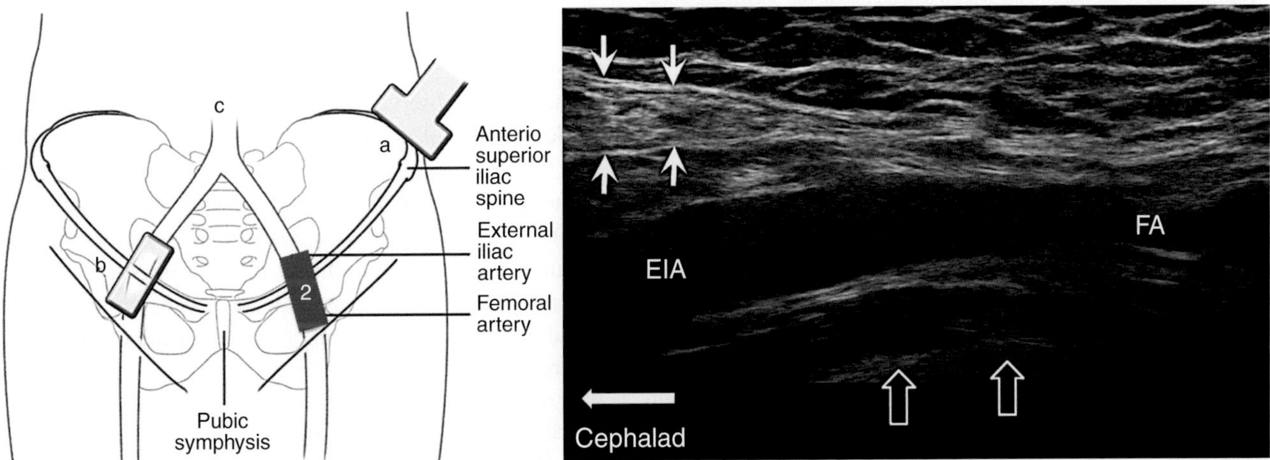

Fig. 36.12 Sonography of the femoral artery (FA) in long axis when the ultrasound probe is placed below the inguinal ligament (position 2). *EIA* external iliac artery, *arrows* inguinal canal, *bold arrows* pubic ramus. (Reprinted with permission from Philip Peng Educational Series)

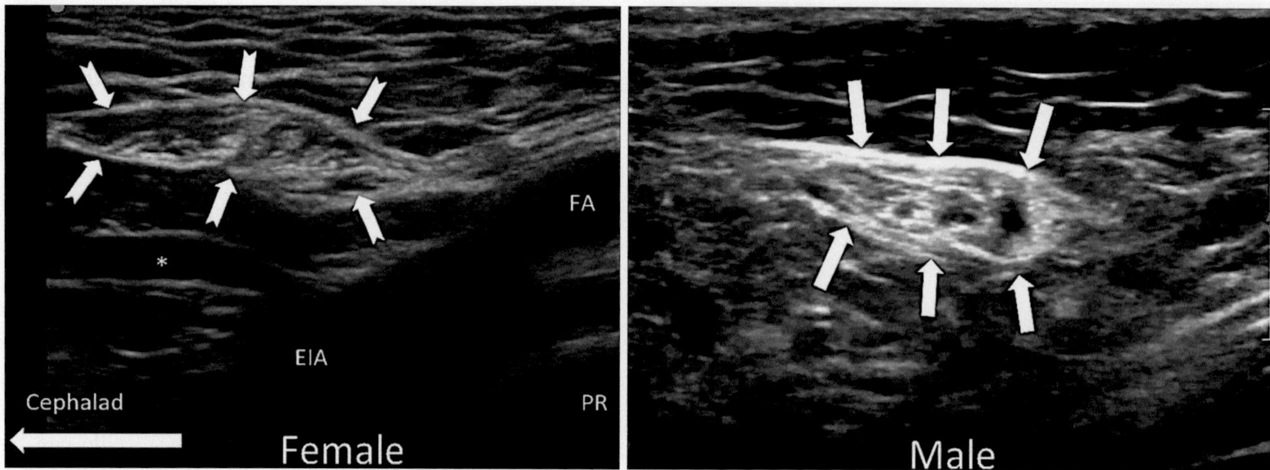

Fig. 36.13 Left: inguinal canal (bold arrows) in a female patient with a round ligament of the uterus. Right: inguinal canal (bold arrows) in a male patient with spermatic cord inside. (Reprinted with permission from Dr. Athmaja Thottungal)

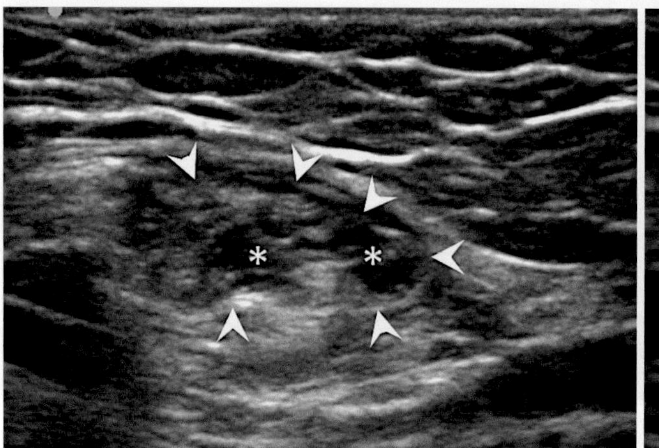

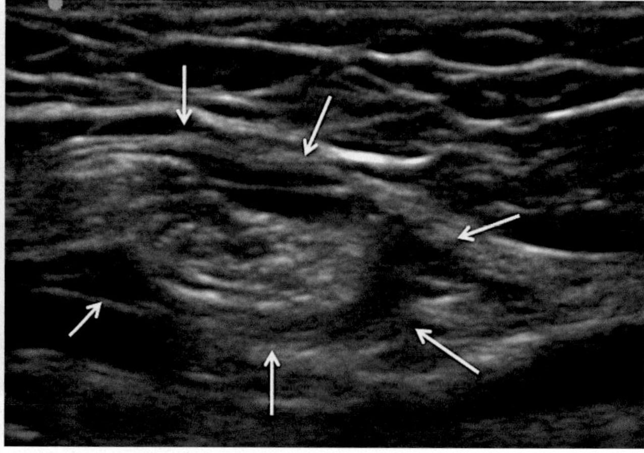

Fig. 36.14 Inguinal canal with the effect of injectate. Left: local anesthetic (**) is sent spread inside the spermatic cord (outlined by arrowheads). Right: local anesthetic is seen spread inside the spermatic cord (arrows) but outside the spermatic cord. (Reprinted with permission from Philip Peng Educational Series)

istered inside the inguinal canal and another 2–4 mL inside the spermatic cord. This is because the GFN may travel outside or within the spermatic cord (Fig. 36.14).

Method 3: Placing the Ultrasound Probe Right over the Spermatic Cord

This method applies to male patient since the spermatic cord can be seen next to superficial inguinal ring in surface anatomy. The initial probe is placed lateral and superior to the pubic tubercle and moved laterally till EIA is identified (Fig. 36.15). This is also known as "spermatic cord block" or "inguinal canal block."

Both in-plane and out-of-plane techniques may be used. Hydrodissection with saline should be utilized to confirm adequate spread within the inguinal canal or within the cord. Absence of any observed spread is indicative of intravascular injection or loss of needle tip visualization. Given the anatomic variability of the genital branch of the GF nerve, local anesthetic is injected within and outside of the spermatic cord in men; in women, local anesthetic is injected around the round ligament only. In males, the local anesthetic should not contain epinephrine so as to avoid vasoconstriction of the testicular arteries. Steroid can be added for the management of chronic pain syndromes.

Complications of IIN, IHN, and GFN Blocks

Vascular injury, nerve injury, perforation of the gut, spermatic cord injury, and infection.

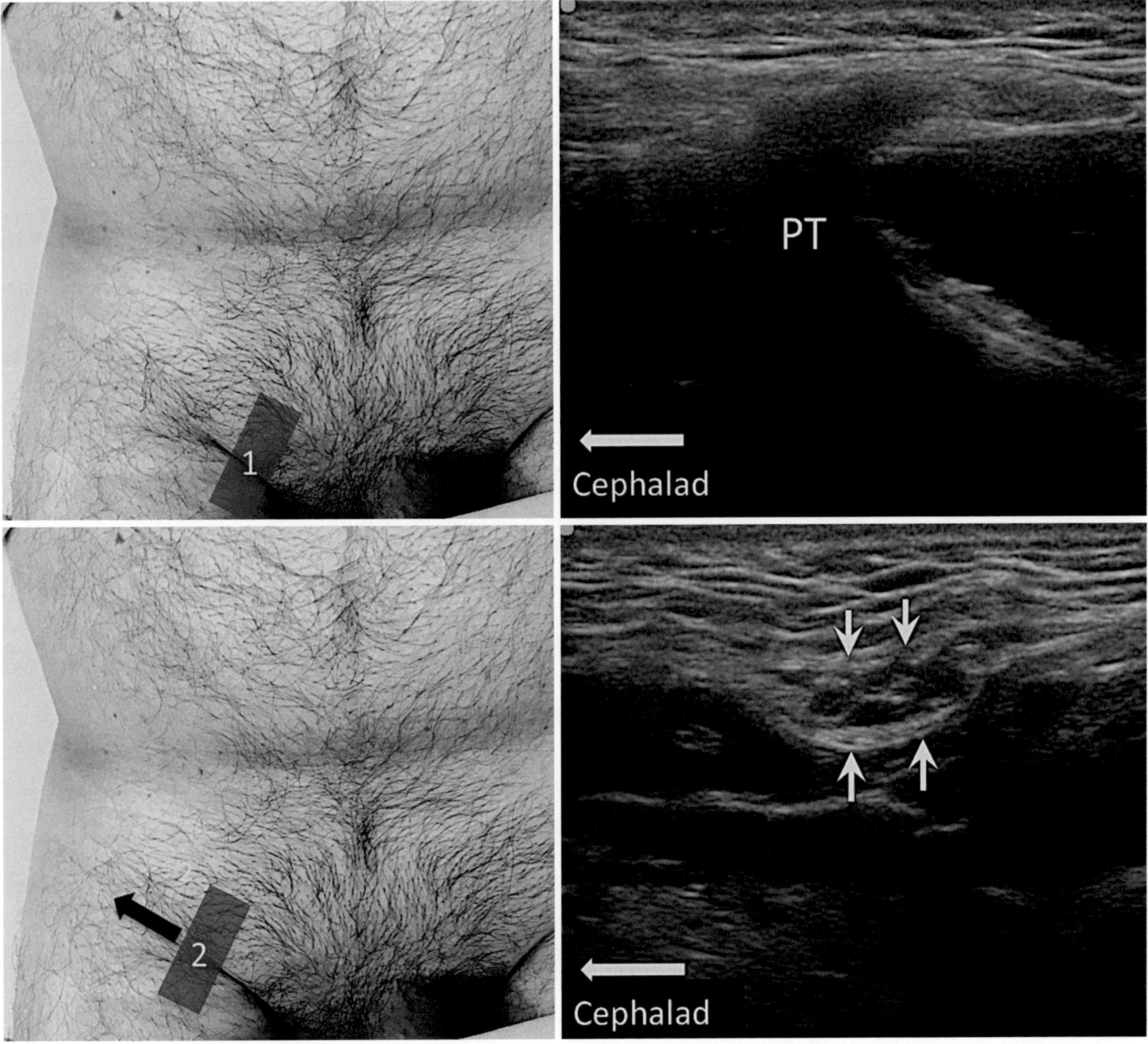

Fig. 36.15 Upper panel: probe position at pubic tubercle (PT) and corresponding sonography. Lower panel: lateral movement of the ultrasound probe revealed the spermatic cord outlined by arrows. (Reprinted with permission from Philip Peng Educational Series)

Practical Tips

II/IH Nerve Blocks

1. Make sure the probe is above ASIS enough so that all three layers of the abdomen, ilium, and iliacus muscle are visible all the time.
2. Apply pressure to the medial end of the probe which is pointing toward the umbilicus to "cave in" so that the ultrasound beam is falling on and reflecting from the iliacus muscle inside of the ilium which will make visibility of nerves much easier.
3. Put patients to lateral position with the affected side up for patients with high BMI and pendulous abdomen which will help to move tissue away from the ilium and visibility of the nerve and needling much easier.
4. Out-of-plane technique is much easier if patients have a high BMI and also for certain chronic pain procedures.
5. Using color Doppler to identify deep circumflex iliac artery is helpful if the facial planes are fibrosed after surgery to locate the plane.

GF Nerve Blocks

1. Method 1 is useful for both male and female patients, any age group, and size. If methods 2 and 3 are used in elderly women or women with high BMI, identifying the round ligament of the uterus can be technically difficult. In men, it is easier as the spermatic cord is easy to identify.
2. Method 1 is also a preferred position for neuromodulatory techniques like pulsed radiofrequency denervation and peripheral nerve stimulation.
3. In-plane needling is preferred as EIA and FA are closed by and can avoid bleeding.
4. Always use color Doppler prior to injection to identify testicular vessels and IEA pulsations.
5. GFN is a nerve of huge anatomical variation. It could also be originating from T12 or L3. L2 contribution tends to be more consistent.
6. The division of genital and femoral branch is very variable and can happen anywhere during the course of the nerve.
7. There is overlap between dermatomal supplies of the ilioinguinal nerve (IIN) and GFN. So, checking the IIN is also important when GFN pathology is suspected.
8. Do not use local anesthetic with epinephrine for this block if injected around the spermatic cord.

Literature Review

The IIN/IHN and GFN blocks are used for both anesthesia and analgesia purposes. In chronic pain situations, these are used for diagnostic and therapeutic purposes. There is a huge variability in the anatomical origin, course, location of penetration of various abdominal wall muscles, and dermatomal distribution. This leads to high failure rate and complications when blind techniques are used where ASIS is the only reliable landmark that can be used. When using ultrasound-guided technique for IIN/IHN, these nerves are found superior and lateral to ASIS between internal oblique and transverse abdominis muscles and are validated by a cadaver study with 95% accuracy. The genitofemoral nerve branches to genital and femoral branches. If distal branch blocking techniques are used, it blocks only the genital branch, not the entire GFN. The femoral branch of the GFN is spared. The inguinal canal contains both genital branch of the GFN and inguinal branch of the IIN. This makes it difficult to isolate the nerve for persistent postsurgical pain following hernia repair.

Suggested Reading

Alfieri S, Amid PK, Campanelli G, et al. International guidelines for prevention and management of post-operative chronic pain following inguinal hernia surgery. Hernia. 2011;15(3):239–49.

Bellingham G, Peng P. Ultrasound-guided interventional procedures for chronic pelvic pain. Tech Reg Anesth Pain Manag. 2009a;13(3):171–8.

Bellingham GA, Peng PWH. Ultrasound guided interventional procedures for chronic pelvic pain. Tech Reg Anesth Pain Manang. 2009b;13:171–8.

Campos NA, Chiles JH, Plunkett AR. Ultrasound-guided cryoablation for genitofemoral nerve for chronic inguinal pain. Pain Physician. 2009;12(6):997–1000.

Chan CW, Peng PWH. Ultrasound guided blocks for pelvic pain. In: Nauroze S, editor. Atlas of ultrasound guided procedures in interventional pain management. 1st ed. Berlin: Springer. p. 207–26.

Deer T. Interventional and neuromodulatory techniques for pain management. Philadelphia: Elsevier/Saunders; 2012.

Ducic I, Dellon A. Testicular pain after inguinal hernia repair: an approach to resection of the genital branch of genitofemoral nerve. J Am Coll Surg. 2004;198(2):181–4.

Huang Z, Xia W, Peng X, Ke J, Wang W. Evaluation of ultrasound-guided genitofemoral nerve block combined with Ilioinguinal/iliohypogastric nerve block during inguinal hernia repair in the elderly. Curr Med Sci. 2019;39(5):794–9.

Liu W, Chen T, Shyu J, Chen C, Shih C, Wang J, et al. Applied anatomy of the genital branch of the genitofemoral nerve in open inguinal herniorrhaphy. Eur J Surg. 2002a;168(3):145–9.

Liu WC, Chen TH, Shyu JF, et al. Applied anatomy of the genital branch of genitofemoral nerve in open inguinal herniorraphy. Eur J Surg. 2002b;168(3):145–9.

Narouze S. Atlas of ultrasound-guided procedures in interventional pain management. Berlin: Springer.

Oelrich T, Moosman D. The aberrant course of the cutaneous component of the ilioinguinal nerve. Anat Rec. 1977;189(2):233–6.

Pandav D. Ultrasound guided ilioinguinal & iliohypogastric nerve blocks combined with genital branch of genitofemoral nerve block for open inguinal hernia repair. J Med Sci Clin Res. 2020;8(7).

Peng PWH, Tumber PS. Ultrasound-guided interventional procedures for patients with chronic pelvic pain—a description of techniques and review of the literature. Pain Physician. 2008;11:215–24.

Rab M, Ebmer J, Dellon AL. Anatomic variability of the ilioinguinal and genitofemoral nerve: implications for the treatment of groin pain. Last Reconstr Surg. 2001;108(6):1618–23.

Rosendal F, Moir L, de Pennington N, Green A, Aziz T. Successful treatment of testicular pain with peripheral nerve stimulation of the cutaneous branch of the Ilioinguinal and genital branch of the genitofemoral nerves. Neuromodulation. 2012;16(2):121–4.

Seib R, Peng P. Ultrasound-guided peripheral nerve block in chronic pain management. Tech Reg Anesth Pain Manag. 2009;13(3):110–6.

Soneji N, Peng P. Ultrasound-guided pain interventions—a review of techniques for peripheral nerves. Kor J Pain. 2013;26(2):111.

Terkawi AS, Romdhane K. Ultrasound-guided pulsed radiofrequency ablation of the genital branch of the genitofemoral nerve for treatment of intractable orchalgia. Saudi J Anaesth. 2014;8(2):294–8. https://doi.org/10.4103/1658-354X.130755.

Thottungal AR, Peng P. Genitofemoral nerve. In: Peng P, editor. Ultrasound for interventional pain management—an illustrated procedural guide. Springer: Cham; 2019. p. 83–92.

Waldman SD. Atlas of pain management injection techniques. 3rd ed. Philadelphia: Elsevier Saunders; 2013. p. 340–1.

Piriformis and Obturator Internus Injection

37

Philip Peng and Danilo Jankovic

Contents

General Consideration

Because of the central location in greater sciatic notch in proximity to various neurovascular bundles including sciatic nerve, piriformis muscle is incriminated to the differential diagnosis of patient with back and leg pain. Yeoman was the first to attribute piriformis to sciatica, and a decade later, Beaton and Anson described the "spasm of piriformis" as the etiology factor for sciatic nerve compression through their observation of cadaver dissections. Since then, piriformis syndrome was used to refer to pain caused by impingement of the sciatic nerve by the piriformis muscle, resulting in buttock pain, sciatica, or both, and the prevalence is estimated between 5 and 8%.

However, the term piriformis syndrome has been scrutinized recently for a few reasons. First, piriformis is not the only muscle in the gluteal region that can contribute to posterior hip pain. Second, secondary causes had been well documented for the posterior hip pain and sciatica symptoms such as hematoma, abscess, or endometriotic deposits. Third, sciatic nerve irritation or compression can be caused by other pathologies in the vicinity: gemelli-obturator internus, ischiofemoral impingement, and proximal hamstring syndromes. Fourth, the incidence of piriformis syndrome between patients with typical anatomical arrangement of muscle and sciatic nerve is not different to that of anatomical variations. Finally, the sciatic symptoms can be related to fibrous or fibrovascular bands limiting the excursion movement of the sciatic nerve. Therefore, deep gluteal syndrome is the preferred term to broadly define the presence of pain in the buttock caused by non-discogenic and extrapelvic entrapment of the sciatic nerve. The boundary of the deep gluteal space is shown in Fig. 37.1. Piriformis or obturator internus syndromes are only the subset of the deep gluteal syndrome.

P. Peng (✉)
Department of Anesthesia and Pain Medicine, Toronto Western Hospital, University of Toronto, Toronto, ON, Canada
e-mail: philip.peng@uhn.ca

D. Jankovic
Pain Management Centre DGS – Cologne – Huerth, Cologne-Hürth, Germany
e-mail: danilo@jankovic1.de

D. Jankovic, P. Peng (eds.), *Regional Nerve Blocks in Anesthesia and Pain Therapy*,
https://doi.org/10.1007/978-3-030-88727-8_37

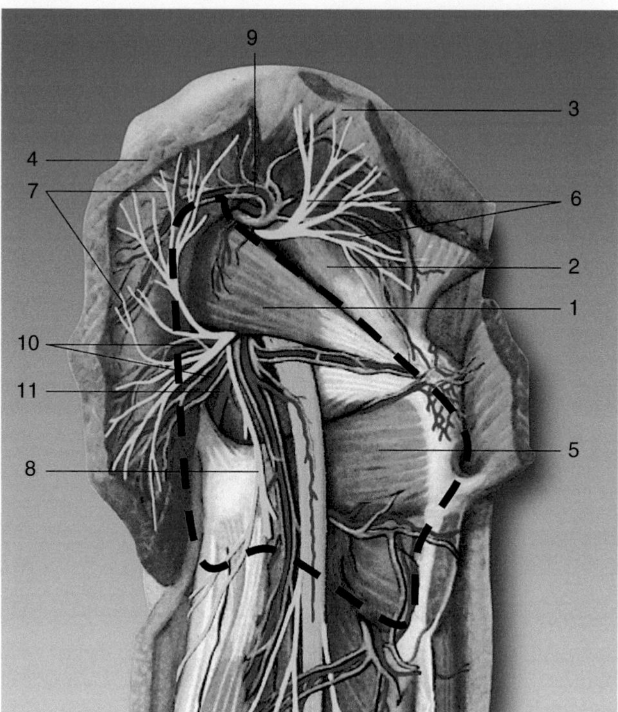

Fig. 37.1 The piriformis muscle (1) and neighboring muscles, nerves, and vessels: (2) gluteus minimus, (3) gluteus medius, (4) gluteus maximus, (5) quadratus femoris, (6) superior gluteal nerve, (7) inferior gluteal nerve, (8) posterior cutaneous femoral nerve, (9) superior gluteal artery, (10) inferior gluteal artery and vein, (11) internal pudendal artery. The black dotted line outlined the deep gluteal space. (Reproduced with permission from Danilo Jankovic)

Indication and Patient Selection

According to a recent review of the symptomatology of piriformis syndrome, the most common clinical features are buttock pain, pain aggravated on sitting, tenderness near the greater sciatic notch, pain on any maneuver that increases piriformis muscle tension, and limitation of straight leg raising. Different specific physical maneuvers have been developed, and the philosophy of those examinations is either to stretch the piriformis muscle or to enhance active contraction of the muscle (Fig. 37.2). Obturator internus muscle dysfunction may present with similar clinical pictures.

Functional Anatomy

The piriformis muscle (Latin: *pirum,* pear, *forma,* shape) was named by Flemish anatomist Adriaan van den Spieghel (Spigelius) (1578–1625). Originating from the anterior surface of the sacrum between first and fourth sacral foramina, the piriformis passes through the greater sciatic foramen and inserts on the upper edge of the greater trochanter. The piriformis is the only muscle that courses transversely through the greater sciatic notch, and it is the key landmark to all the important nerves and vessels that pass from the pelvis to the gluteal region, such as sciatic nerve, the pudendal nerve and artery, and the superior and inferior gluteal arteries and nerves (Figs. 37.1 and 37.3). It receives innervation from S1 and S2.

The function of the piriformis in the non-weight-bearing limb is external rotation of the thigh with the hip extended and abduction when the hip is fixed at 90°. In weight-bearing activities, the piriformis restrains vigorous or excessive medial rotation of the thigh. The other short lateral rotators of the thigh at the hip (the superior gemellus, obturator internus, inferior gemellus, and quadratus femoris muscle lying distal to the piriformis) may cause symptoms in piriformis syndrome, especially the obturator internus muscle, which is partly an intrapelvic muscle and partly a hip muscle. The sciatic nerve arises from the ventral branches of the spinal nerves, from L4 to S3. Exiting from pelvic cavity at the lower edge of the piriformis, the sciatic nerve runs between the ischial tuberosity and the greater trochanter; turns downward over the gemelli, the obturator internus tendon, and the quadratus femoris muscle, which separate it from the hip joint; and leaves the buttock to enter the thigh beneath the lower border of the gluteus maximus. This is the region where the course of sciatic nerve is intimately related to the piriformis and short rotators of the hip. There are six routes by which portions of the sciatic nerve may exit the pelvis, and these are illustrated in a schematic diagram (Fig. 37.4).

Technique

Various modalities have been described to help localize the piriformis or obturator internus muscle. These include imaging techniques such as ultrasound, CT, and fluoroscopy to guide the needle to the vicinity of the muscle and electrophysiologic techniques such as electromyography and nerve stimulation to confirm activation of the piriformis muscle or sciatic nerve. Contrast injection is commonly used in fluoroscopic-guided technique to confirm needle placement within the piriformis muscle, which has been shown to be unreliable. Ultrasound is an attractive imaging technique as it provides visualization of the soft tissue and neurovascular structures and allows real-time imaging of needle insertion toward the target. The accuracy of needle placement with ultrasound was estimated 95%. With the increasing popular-

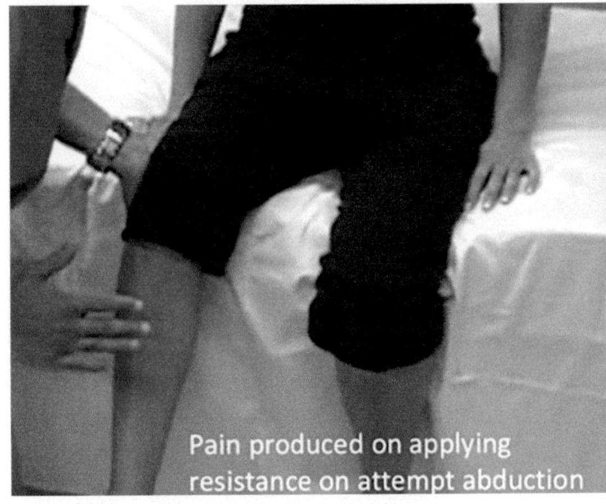

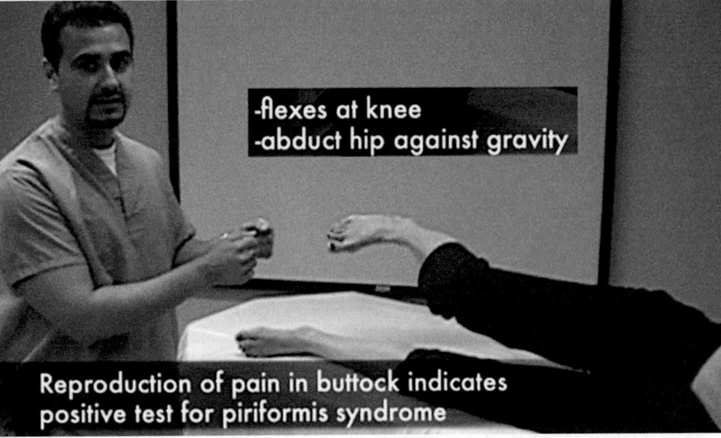

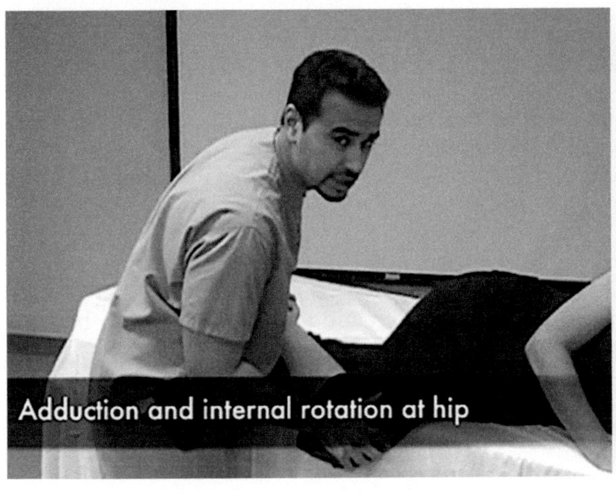

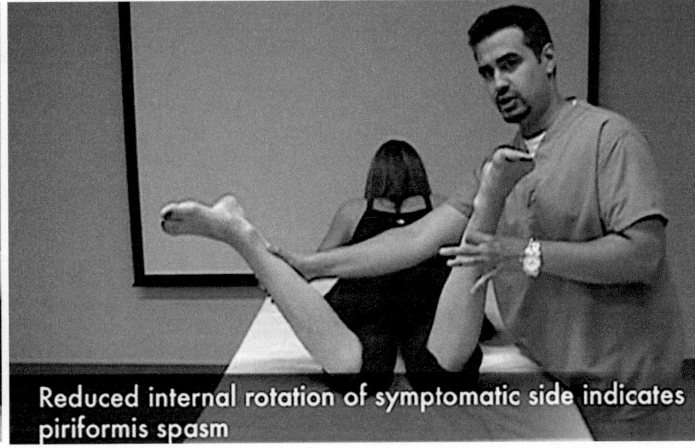

Fig. 37.2 Four different physical examinations for the piriformis syndrome. (Reproduced with permission from Philip Peng Educational Series)

ity of ultrasound for intervention, the ultrasound-guided technique will be described in details.

Specific Technique for Piriformis Muscle

With the patient in prone position, a low-frequency curvilinear probe (2–5 MHz) is initially placed caudal and lateral to the posterior inferior iliac spine (PSIS) to visualize the gluteal muscles and ilium (Fig. 37.5). With the angle of the probe orientated along the long axis of the piriformis muscle, the probe is moved in caudal direction until the medial half of the hyperechoic line (ilium) recedes. At this level, two separate muscular layers are identified: the gluteus maximus and the piriformis muscles (Fig. 37.5). By internal and external rotation of the patient's hip with the knee flexed, the piriformis muscle can be seen gliding underneath the gluteus maximus muscle. The sequence of scanning the PSIS first and then moving the probe caudally is important because the ultrasound image of the lesser sciatic notch may be confused with that of the greater sciatic notch.

Once the piriformis muscle is identified, a long 22-gauge 3.5-in. needle is directed toward the thickest part of the piriformis muscle in the sciatic notch and the tip position should be confirmed with hydrolocation (Fig. 37.6). The needle insertion can be made medially or laterally to the ultrasound probe. Some clinician prefers to inject in the tendinous part of the muscle.

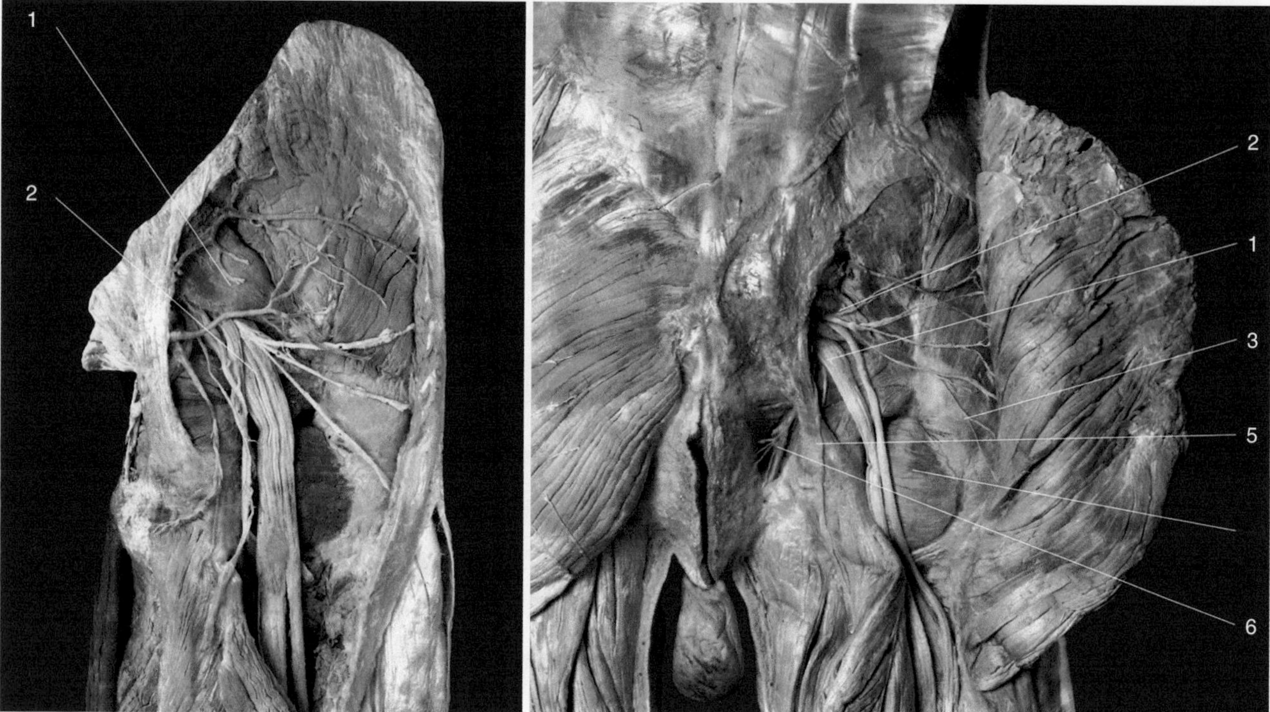

Fig. 37.3 (**Left panel**) Posterior view of the piriformis muscle (1) and sciatic nerve (2). (**Right panel**) High separation of the sciatic nerve (1): the common peroneal nerve courses through the piriformis and the tibial nerve through the infrapiriform foramen, (2) the piriformis muscle with the gluteal inferior nerve, (3) the greater trochanter, (4) quadratus femoris, (5) sacrotuberous ligament, (6) the pudendal nerve in the ischiorectal fossa. (Reproduced with permission from Danilo Jankovic)

For intramuscular injection, the literature describes a volume of 5 mL. However, in the author's opinion, only 1–2 mL of volume is enough to cover the main muscle bulk with ultrasound guidance. Too aggressive a volume will cause localized pain, and it defeats the purpose of the injection, which is to facilitate the rehabilitation and stretching of the piriformis. The injectate can be local anesthetic or a solution of botulinum toxin (50 units).

Specific Technique for Obturator Internus Muscle and Tendon

The position of patient and initially scanning are similar to what is described above. The probe is moved in caudal direction further until it is at the level of ischial spine (Fig. 37.7). At this level, the bony structure appears straight. From there, further caudal movement of the probe will reveal the lateral part of the lesser sciatic notch, and the bony configuration is very different from ischial spine. Medial to the bone, the hypoechoic shadow is the obturator internus muscle (Fig. 37.8). A 22-gauge 3.5-in. needle is inserted in plane from medial to lateral direction until contact with bone. A small volume (1 mL) of either local anesthetic or botulinum toxin (25–50 units) is administered once the tip of the needle is confirmed with hydrolocation.

Complication

Other than the general complication from any injection such as injection or hematoma and the complication related to the injectate such as allergic reaction or steroid-related side effects, two particular complications need to be included in the counseling of the procedures. One is the localized tenderness in an already spastic muscle. The potential factors that may minimize these side effects are avoidance of multiple needle entry and minimizing the volume of injectate. If local anesthetic is used, the duration is limited, and it will be counterproductive to have localized pain to prevent the patient from performing stretching or rehabilitation. Another is related to the sciatic nerve involvement, either because of the needle injury or spread of local anesthetic to the nerve with neurological complication.

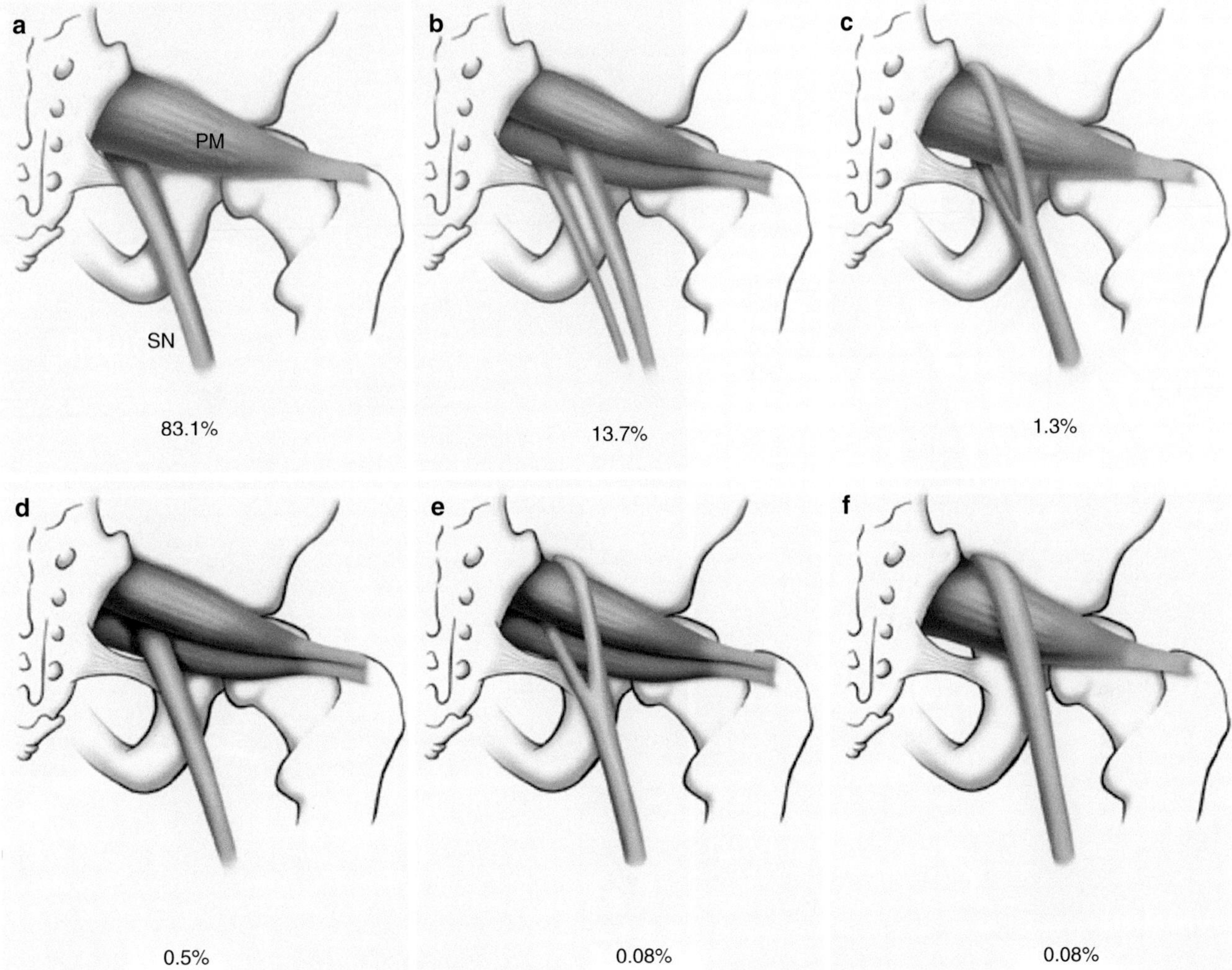

Fig. 37.4 The six routes (**a**–**f**) by which portions of the sciatic nerve may exit the pelvis. PM piriformis muscle. (Reproduced with permission from Philip Peng Educational Series)

Practical Tips

Start the scan from the ilium (caudal to PSIS) as it assures the "two-muscle" arrangement caudal to it as the greater sciatic notch. The view in lesser sciatic notch can mimic the picture as in greater sciatic notch.

In case one is not sure, the fascia plane between the gluteus maximus and piriformis (quite common in repeated Botox injection of the piriformis when the piriformis is atrophic), internal and external rotation of the piriformis muscle is a very useful manoeuver to differentiate the gluteus maximus and piriformis muscle.

The greater sciatic notch orientated posterolaterally. Therefore, the idea probe position is to tilt medially to optimize the view of the notch.

When injecting the obturator internus, turn on the Doppler to visualize the pudendal artery and avoid it.

Literature Review

Piriformis syndrome is a non-discogenic extrapelvic cause of sciatic nerve compression or irritation and is estimated to account for 6% to 8% of all cases of sciatica. There are no clear definite diagnostic criteria, and the diagnosis relies on exclusion of spinal and intrapelvic cause of sciatic and a constellation of clinical features. Systematic review of the clinical features revealed for consistent findings in piriformis syndrome in literature: buttock pain, pain aggravated on sitting, tenderness near the greater sciatic notch, pain on any

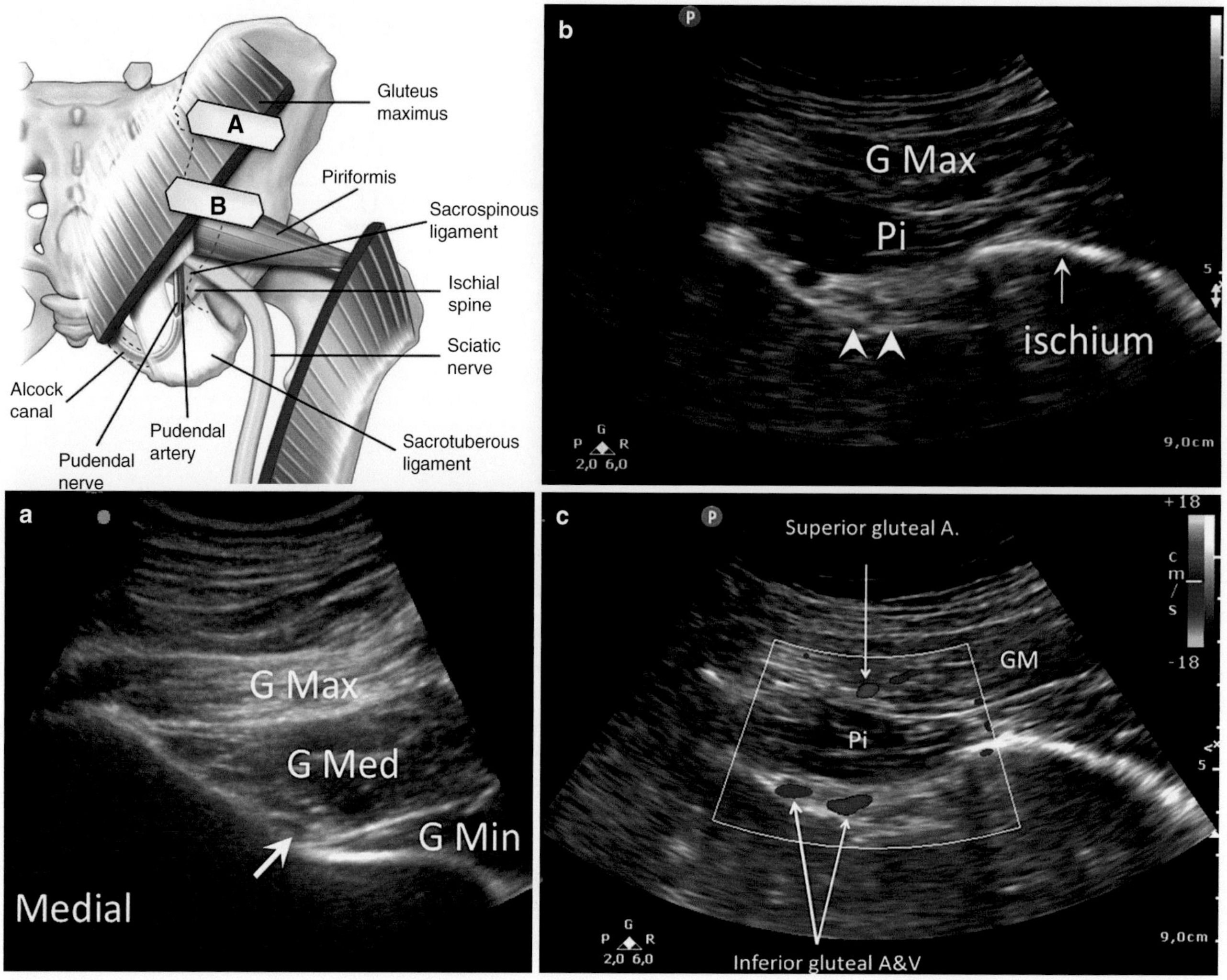

Fig. 37.5 The left upper figure shows the position of the scan. (**a**) The ultrasound image when the probe is in position A. The sonogram shows the iliac crest and the gluteus maximus (G Max), medius (G Med), and minimus (G Min) muscles. The arrow indicates the superior gluteal artery and nerve. (**b**) Ultrasound image corresponds to the scan **b** in the left upper figure. The scan can be optimized by aligning the probe with the long axis of piriformis and tilting the probe in medial orientation. *Pi* piriformis. (**c**) The Doppler scan as **b**. (Reproduced with permission from Philip Peng Educational Series)

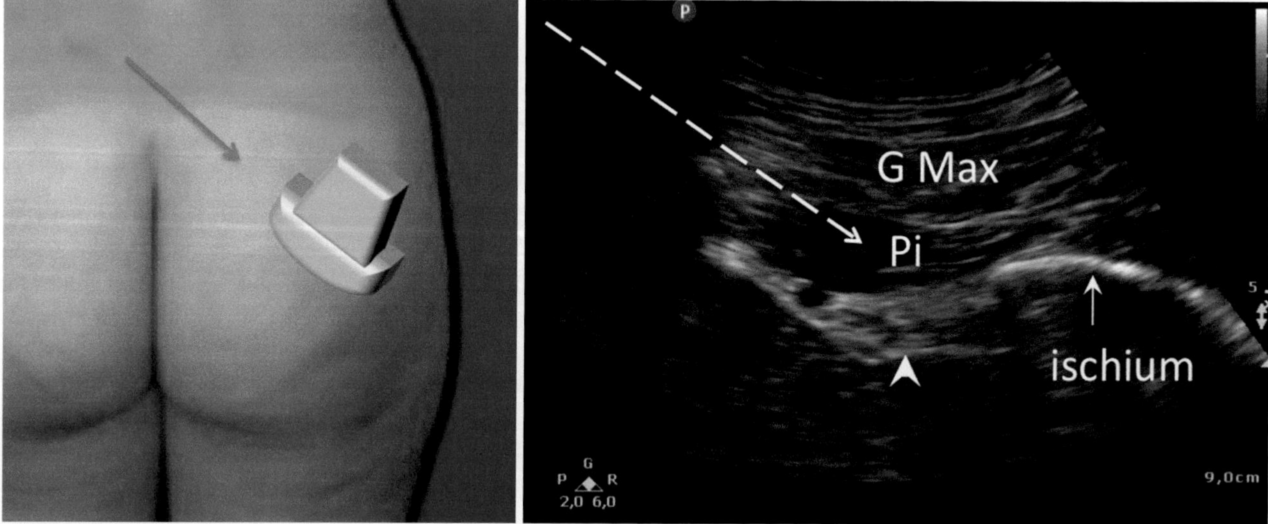

Fig. 37.6 Ultrasonography shows the position of the needle insertion. The needle is inserted in plan from medial to lateral position. *Pi* piriformis, *G Max* gluteus maximus. Arrowhead: sciatic nerve. (Reproduced with permission from Philip Peng Educational Series)

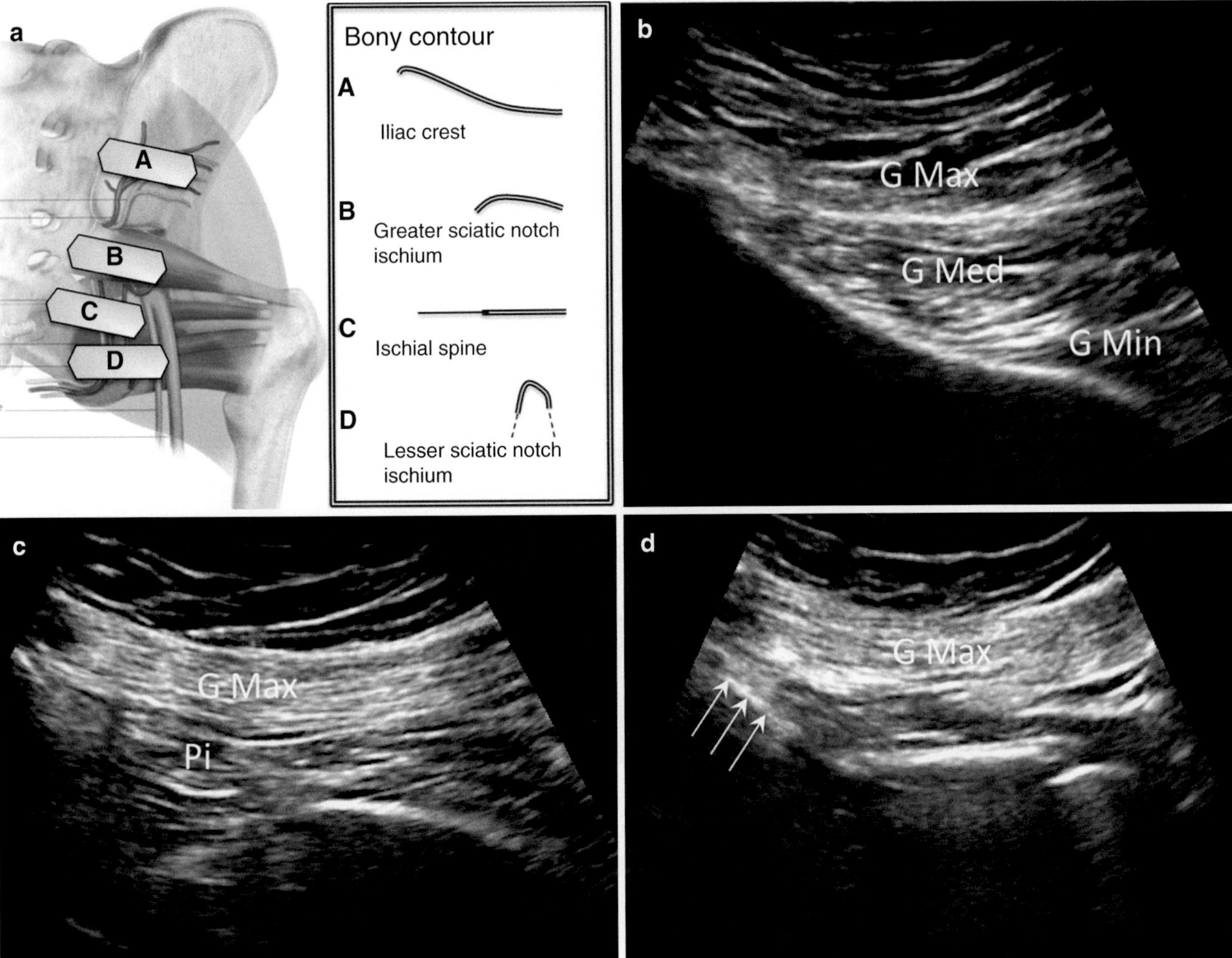

Fig. 37.7 (**a**) This figure shows the position of the probe in different position and the bone signatures in each scan. The scan sequence is similar to the scanning of piriformis, starting from the iliac crest, the greater sciatic notch, and then the ischial spine (**b–d**). (**b**) At the iliac crest, three gluteus muscles can be visualized. (**c**) At the greater sciatic fossa, the piriformis muscle (Pi) is seen. (**d**) At the ischial spine level, the bony contour is straight, and a hyperechoic line on the medial side of the ischial spine is the sacrospinous ligament (arrows in the right lower figure). G Max and Med Min stand for gluteus maximus and medius and minimus, respectively. The sonogram at position D is shown in Fig. 37.8. (Reprinted with reproduction from Philip Peng Educational Series)

maneuver that increases piriformis muscle tension, and limitation of straight leg raising. In physical examination, almost all of them had tenderness to deep palpation over the greater sciatic notch. The provocative test is helpful. The sensitivity and specificity of those tests are summarized in a recent review article by Probst et al.

Obturator internus syndrome may present with clinical features similar to that of piriformis syndrome. Both piriformis and obturator internus fuse together prior to the insertion in greater trochanter in 43% of patients, allowing simultaneous stretching of both tendons during hip rotations. In some individuals, it was shown that the obturator internus, not the piriformis, impinged on the sciatic nerve in early flexion. There is also report that patient with apparent piriformis syndrome received partial benefit from piriformis injection but the long-lasting pain relief increased to 100% when obturator internus was injected.

Other than clinical features, other investigations are mainly to exclude other causes of sciatica. Electrodiagnostic testing is usually normal in patient with piriformis syndrome but is usually to reveal lumbosacral radiculopathy or other source of pain in lower extremity. Likewise, CT scan and MRI are not specific in the diagnosis of piriformis syndrome but serve to exclude other pathologies.

By suppressing the signal of the tissue around the nerve, MR neurography improves visualization of peripheral nerves. In a large case series with patients who had pain in the sciatic nerve distribution with unclear diagnosis or failed response to lumbar spine surgery, MR neurography revealed edema or hyperintensity in the ipsilateral sciatic nerve rela-

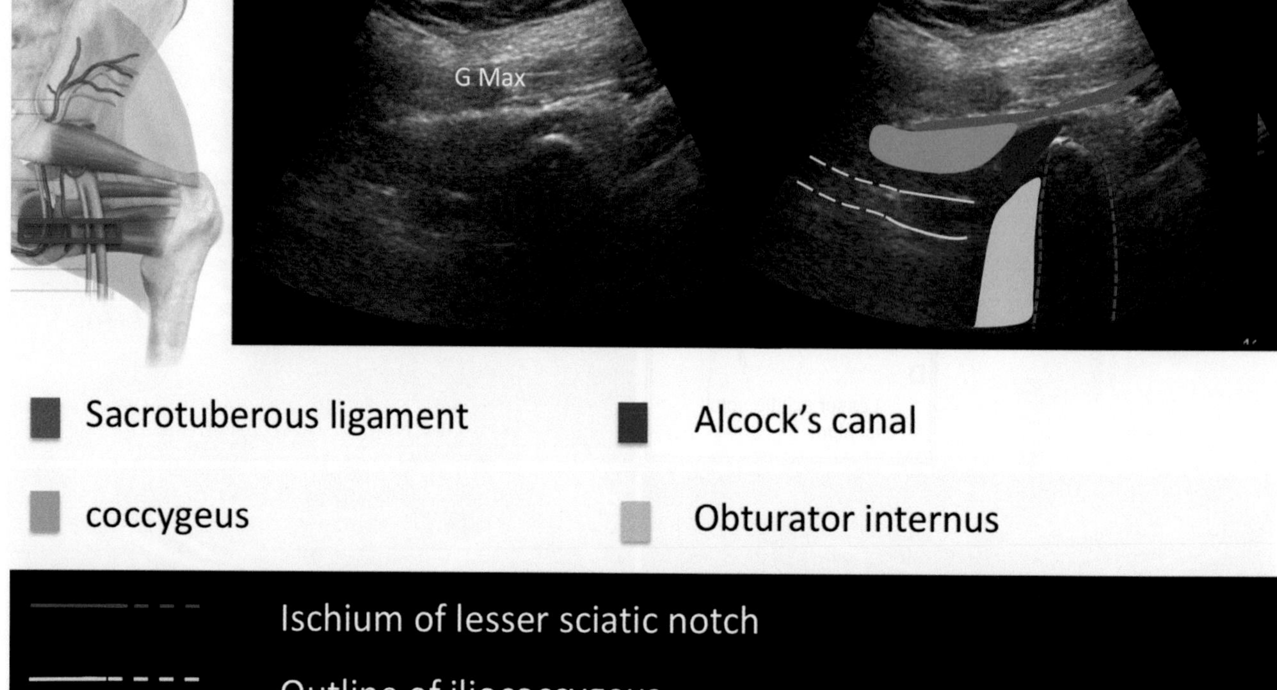

Fig. 37.8 From the ischial spine level (as in Fig. 37.7d), further caudal movement of the probe will reach the lesser sciatic notch. Please note the bony contour. Because of the orientation of the bone and obturator internus (OI) muscle is close to 90° to the ultrasound probe, the OI appears as a hypoechoic structure. If the clinician carefully observes the structures transitioned from the ischial spine to the less sciatic notch, the sacrotuberous ligament continues to be observed, and the pudendal neurovascular bundle will move close to the OI in the Alcock's canal. Deep to the sacrotuberous ligament, two pelvic floor muscles can be seen: coccygeus (labeled blue deep to the sacrotuberous ligament) and iliococcygeus muscle (outlined by yellow line). (Reprinted with permission from Philip Peng Education Series)

tive to the contralateral side in 94% of patients. Of these patients, 88% reproduced their symptoms with the flexion, adduction, and internal rotation (FAIR). Combining the finding of unilateral sciatic nerve hyperintensity at the sciatic notch and asymmetry of the piriformis had a specificity of 0.93 and sensitivity of 0.64 for predicting good-to-excellent outcome from piriformis muscle release surgery.

Piriformis syndrome causing sciatica usually responds to conservative treatments, including physical therapy; lifestyle modification; symptomatic relief of muscle and nerve pain with nonsteroidal anti-inflammatory agents, tricyclic antidepressants, muscle relaxants, neuropathic pain agents such as gabapentin, pregabalin, and carbamazepine; and psychotherapy. When patients fail to respond to simple conservative therapy, interventional modalities are considered. In rare circumstances, surgical release of the piriformis has been described for difficult cases of piriformis syndrome, but this is occasionally accompanied by morbidity.

Physical therapy should be considered as the initial treatment for piriformis syndrome. The primary consideration in treating piriformis with osteopathic manipulation is to relieve the contracture of the affected musculature and reduce connective tissue adhesions in the area. The techniques include relaxation exercises for the pelvic floor muscles, stretching exercises for the gluteal muscles, massage of the piriformis, and exercises to mobilize the sacroiliac articulation, and lumbar spine should be performed. Other recommended techniques include intermittent cold with stretching, internal transrectal or transvaginal massage of the muscle, ischemic compression with a tennis ball, ultrasound application, shortwave diathermy in conjunction with a full course of physical therapy, self-stretching of the muscle, corrective actions (e.g., for lower limb length differences), postural and activity stress reduction, and avoidance of prolonged immobilization of the affected lower limb when driving vehicles for long distances. Focused shock waves have been successfully used for couple decades now for common orthopedic indications. The treatment of trigger points in the piriformis muscle with focused shock waves is a new and promising noninvasive method as a part of multimodal therapy.

Mixing the local anesthetic solution with 20–40 mg of a long-acting corticosteroid (e.g., long-acting methylprednisolone) is also recommended. Experience shows that long-acting local anesthetics do not provide any substantial advantages over short-acting agents. In addition to the anti-inflammatory properties, steroids also have membrane-stabilizing properties. The response to these injectate can be immediate but may be of short duration. Benzon et al. reported that 16 of 19 patients responded to piriformis muscle injections over a short-term follow-up period of 3 months. However, the majority of these patients had associated diagnoses, including herniated disks, spinal stenosis, failed back surgery syndrome, and complex regional pain syndrome. Filler et al. reported on 46 patients who received local anesthetic injections. Sixteen percent had sustained pain relief for periods ranging from 8 months to 6 years; 8% had 2–4 months of relief but required a second injection; 37% had 2–4 months of relief but experienced recurrence after a second injection; 24% of the patients benefited for only 2 weeks; and 16% experienced no benefit.

Botulinum toxin type A inhibits the release of acetylcholine from peripheral cholinergic nerve endings, functionally denervates muscle fibers, and causes flaccid paralysis. The literature supports the analgesic efficacy of the use of botulinum toxin A. Compared with a mixture of lidocaine and steroid as well as normal saline (placebo), botulinum toxin provided superior pain relief in patients with piriformis syndrome in a double-blind, randomized, placebo-controlled trial. When combining the botulinum toxin injection with physical therapy, significant pain relief (>50% reduction in pain score) was achieved in 24 of 27 patients with piriformis syndrome. Furthermore, botulinum toxin injection resulted in "good to very good" pain relief in 77% of a large cohort of patients with piriformis syndrome who failed to respond to conservative management with medications and physical therapy. The main disadvantage of the botulinum toxin is related to its cost.

In summary, anesthesiologists are commonly involved in the management of piriformis syndrome due to their expertise in pain management and in carrying out nerve blocks. Injections of local anesthetics, steroids, and botulinum toxin into the piriformis muscle can serve both diagnostic and therapeutic purposes. The practitioner should be familiar with variations in the anatomy and the limitations of landmark-based techniques. An ultrasound-guided injection technique has recently been described, which offers improved accuracy in the nerve blockade. This technique has been shown to have both diagnostic and therapeutic values in the treatment of piriformis syndrome. The results of surgical treatment for piriformis are disappointing. Optimizing the therapeutic approach requires an interdisciplinary evaluation of treatment.

Suggested Reading

Abram SE. Treatment of lumbosacral radiculopathy with epidural steroids. Anesthesiology. 1999;91:1937–41.

Bartret AL, Beaulieu CF, Lutz AM. Is it painful to be different? Sciatic nerve anatomical variants on MRI and their relationship to piriformis syndrome. Eur Radiol. 2018;28:4681–6.

Beaton LE, Anson BJ. The sciatic nerve and the piriformis muscle. Their interrelation and possible cause of coccygodynia. J Bone Joint Surg Am. 1938;20-A:686–8.

Benzon HT, Katz JA, Benzon HA, Iqbal MS. Piriformis syndrome: anatomic considerations, a new injection technique, and a review of the literature. Anesthesiology. 2003;98:1442–8.

Carro LP, Hernando MF, Cerezal L, et al. Deep gluteal space problems: piriformis syndrome, ischiofemoral impingement and sciatic nerve release. Muscles Ligaments Tendons J. 2016;6:384–96.

Cassidy L, Walters A, Bubb K, Shoja M, Tubbs SR, Loukas M. Piriformis syndrome: implications of anatomical variations, diagnostic techniques, and treatment. Surg Radiol Anat. 2012;34:479–86.

Dalmau-Carola J. Myofascial pain syndrome affecting the piriformis and the obturator internus muscle. Pain Pract. 2005;5(4):361–3.

Durrani Z, Winnie AP. Piriformis muscle syndrome: an underdiagnosed cause of sciatica. J Pain Symptom Manage. 1991;6:374–9.

Filler AG, Haynes J, Jordan SE, et al. Sciatica of nondisc origin and piriformis syndrome: diagnosis by magnetic resonance neurography and interventional magnetic resonance imaging with outcome study of resulting treatment. J Neurosurg Spine. 2005a;2(2):99–115.

Filler AG, Haynes BA, Jordan SE, et al. Sciatica of nondisc origin and piriformis syndrome: diagnosis by magnetic resonance neurography and interventional magnetic resonance imaging with outcome study of resulting treatment. J Neurosurg Spine. 2005b;2:99–115.

Fishman LM, Anderson C, Rosner B. BOTOX and physical therapy in the treatment of piriformis syndrome. Am J Phys Med Rehabil. 2002;81:936–42.

Fishman LM, Konnoth C, Rozner B. Botulinum neurotoxin type B and physical therapy in the treatment of piriformis syndrome: a dose-finding study. Am J Phys Med Rehabil. 2004;83:42–50. quiz 51-43.

Hallin RP. Sciatic pain and the piriformis muscle. Postgrad Med. 1983;74(2):69–72.

Hernando MF, Cerezal L, Pérez-Carro L, Abascal F, Canga A. Deep gluteal syndrome: anatomy, imaging, and management of sciatic nerve entrapments in the subgluteal space. Skeletal Radiol. 2015;44:919–34.

Hopayian K, Danielyan A. Four symptoms define the piriformis syndrome: an updated systematic review of its clinical features. Eur J Orthop Surg Traumatol. 2018;28(2):155–64.

Jankovic D. Mit der Stosswellen gegen das Piriformis Syndrom. Schmerz. 2011;1:11–3.

Jankovic D, Peng P, van Zundert A. Piriformis syndrome: etiology, diagnosis and management. Can J Anesth. 2013;60:1003–12.

Johansson A, Hao J, Sjölund B. Local corticosteroid application blocks transmission in normal nociceptive C-fibres. Acta Anaesthesiol Scand. 1990;34:335–8.

Martin HD, Reddy M, Gómez-Hoyos J. Deep gluteal syndrome. J Hip Preserv Surg. 2015;2:99–107.

Meknas K, Christensen A, Johansen O. The internal obturator muscle may cause sciatic pain. Pain. 2003a;104:375–80.

Meknas K, Christensen A, Johansen O. The internal obturator muscle may cause sciatic pain. Pain. 2003b;104:375–80.

Michel F, Decavel P, Toussirot E, et al. Piriformis muscle syndrome: diagnostic criteria and treatment of a monocentric series of 250 patients. Ann Phys Rehabil Med. 2013;56:371–83.

Papadopoulos EC, Khan SN. Piriformis syndrome and low back pain: a new classification and review of the literature. Orthop Clin North Am. 2004;35:65–71.

Park JW, Lee YK, Lee YJ, Shin S, Kang Y, Koo KH. Deep gluteal syndrome as a cause of posterior hip pain and sciatica-like pain. Bone Joint J. 2020;102-B:556–67.

Peng PWH. Piriformis syndrome. In: Peng PWH, editor. Ultrasound for pain medicine intervention: a practical guide. Pelvic pain. Philip Peng educational series. iBook, vol. 2. 1st ed. Cupertino, CA: Apple; 2013.

Probst D, Stout A, Hunt D. Piriformis syndrome: a narrative review of the anatomy, diagnosis, and treatment. PM R. 2019;11(Suppl 1):S54–63.

Retzlaff EW, Berry AH, Haight AS, et al. The piriformis muscle syndrome. J Am Osteopath Assoc. 1974;73:799–807.

Smoll NR. Variations of the piriformis and sciatic nerve with clinical consequence: a review. Clin Anat. 2010;23:8–17.

Windisch G, Braun EM, Anderhuber F. Piriformis muscle: clinical anatomy and consideration of the piriformis syndrome. Surg Radiol Anat. 2007;29:37–45.

Yeoman W. The relation of arthritis of the sacroiliac joint to sciatica, with an analysis of 100 cases. Lancet. 1928;2(5492):1119–22.

Yoon SJ, Ho J, Kang HY, et al. Low-dose botulinum toxin type a for the treatment of refractory piriformis syndrome. Pharmacotherapy. 2007;27:657–65.

Pudendal Nerve

38

G. Bellingham and Philip Peng

Contents

General Considerations

The anatomical course of the pudendal nerve has been the subject of numerous investigations, and studies continue to report novel anatomic variations. These studies challenge the originally held belief of the pudendal nerve as a singular nerve with a consistent pathway through the pelvis. In contrast, nerve anatomy can be complex with several well-described variations. Knowledge of these variances can aid in the appropriate management of patients requiring intervention through nerve blockade or surgery.

G. Bellingham (✉)
Department of Anesthesia and Perioperative Medicine, St. Joseph's Health Care London, Schulich School of Medicine and Dentistry, London, Canada
e-mail: geoff.bellingham@sjhc.london.on.ca

P. Peng
Department of Anesthesia and Pain Medicine, Toronto Western Hospital, University of Toronto, Toronto, ON, Canada
e-mail: philip.peng@uhn.ca

Indication (Patient Selection)

Surgical and Obstetric Anesthesia and Analgesia

Pudendal nerve blockade can be used to confer analgesia and surgical anesthesia for pelvic surgical procedures involving structures innervated by the pudendal nerve. Surgical and obstetric procedures that have evaluated the use of pudendal nerve blockade are summarized in Table 38.1.

Pudendal Neuralgia

Pudendal neuralgia is an uncommon cause of perineal pain that may result from compression of the nerve or its trunks along its course through the pelvis. The use of pudendal

D. Jankovic, P. Peng (eds.), *Regional Nerve Blocks in Anesthesia and Pain Therapy*,
https://doi.org/10.1007/978-3-030-88727-8_38

nerve blockade may assist in facilitating a diagnosis of pudendal neuralgia or to confer periods of analgesia as a treatment option.

To assist in the identification of the subset of pudendal neuralgia-pudendal entrapment neuropathy (PNE), the Nantes criteria have been proposed which list clinical inclusion and exclusion criteria. Essential criteria include (1) pain in the anatomical territory of the pudendal nerve, (2) symptoms worsened by sitting, (3) patient not woken at night by pain, (4) no objective sensory loss on clinical examination, and (5) positive anesthetic pudendal nerve block.

Pudendal nerve blockade may satisfy the last essential Nantes criterion if the pain is relieved for the duration of the local anesthetic. However, as described in the original article, a positive diagnostic block may not be specific for pudendal neuralgia, as alternative causes of the perineal pain will be anesthetized if they are situated within the nerve's territory.

Table 38.1 Indications for pudendal nerve block

Surgical procedures	Obstetric anesthesia or analgesia
Hemorrhoidectomy Penile prosthesis surgery Hypospadias repair Circumcision Prostate biopsy Placement of prostate HDR brachytherapy Suburethral tape placement Colpoperineorrhaphy Transvaginal pelvic reconstructive surgery	Augment analgesia when sacral sparing occurs during epidural catheter use Instrumented deliveries Episiotomies Repair of perineal tears McDonald cerclage

Functional Anatomy

The ventral rami of S2, S3, and S4 commonly form the pudendal nerve, yet contributions from S1 and S5 nerve roots have been documented. Contributing nerve roots may either combine to form a single pudendal nerve or form between 2 and 3 "trunks," which may or may not combine to form the pudendal nerve and its terminal branches (inferior rectal, perineal, and dorsal branches).

Once formed, the pudendal nerve and its trunks briefly exit the pelvis to enter the gluteal region, beneath the piriformis muscle via the infrapiriform notch (Figs. 38.1 and 38.2).

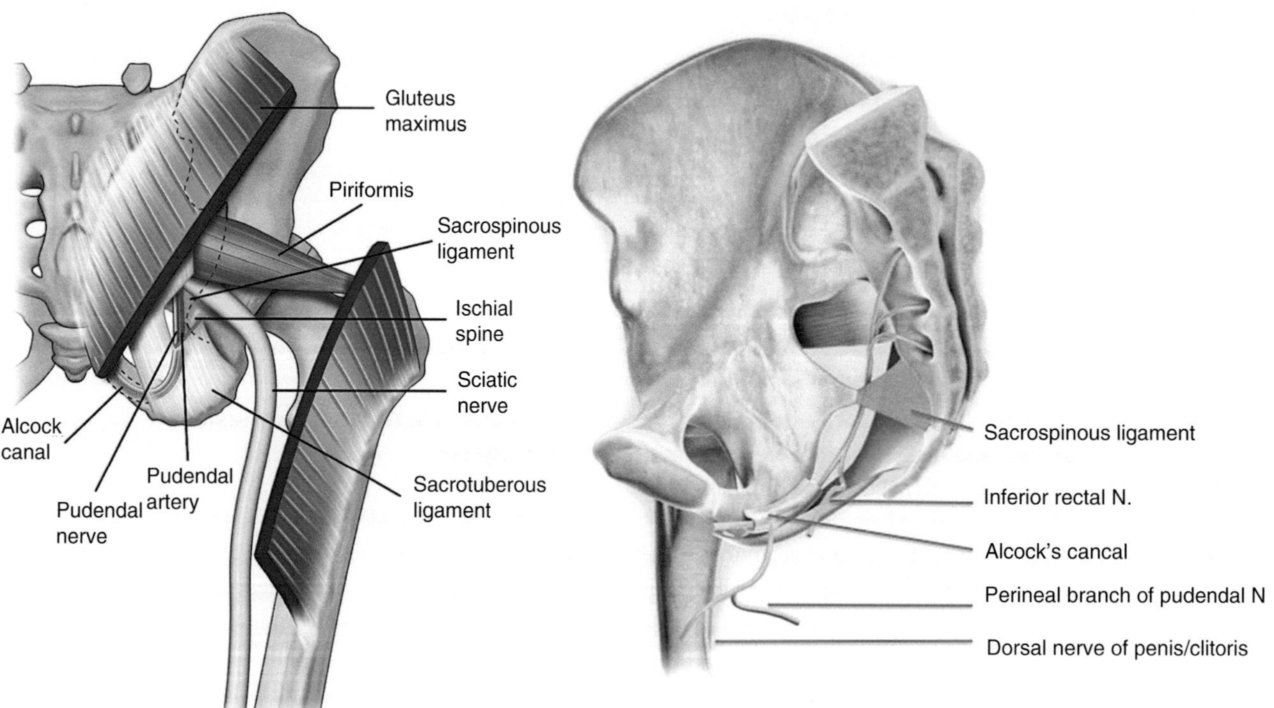

Fig. 38.1 Left: posterior view of the pelvis showing the piriformis muscle and the neurovascular bundle deep to it. The pudendal nerve and artery run between the sacrospinous and sacrotuberous ligaments. Right: anterior view of the pelvis showing the pudendal nerve arising from S2 to S4 and exiting the pelvis to enter the gluteal region through the greater sciatic foramen. The nerve gives rise to the inferior rectal nerve, the perineal nerve, and the dorsal nerve of the penis or clitoris. The inferior rectal nerve branches from the pudendal nerve prior to Alcock's canal. *N* nerve. (Reproduced with permission from Philip Peng Educational Series)

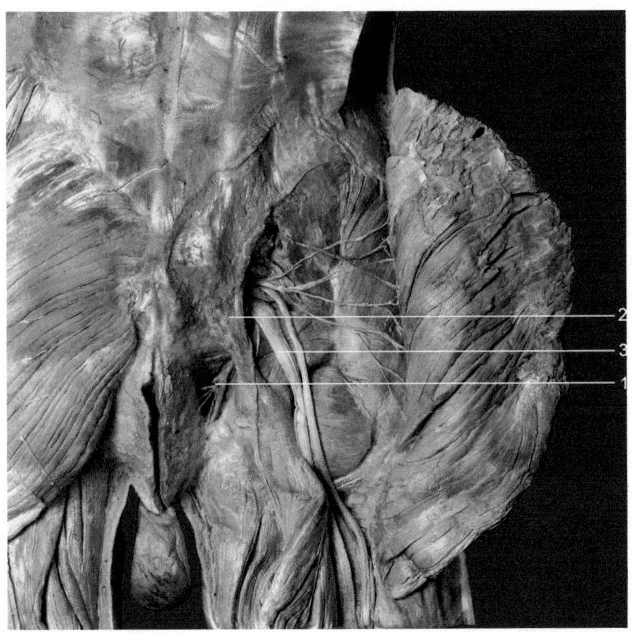

Fig. 38.2 Anatomic specimen. (1) Pudendal nerve and pudendal vessels in the ischiorectal fossa, (2) sacrotuberous ligament, (3) sciatic nerve. (Reproduced with permission from Dr. Danilo Jankovic)

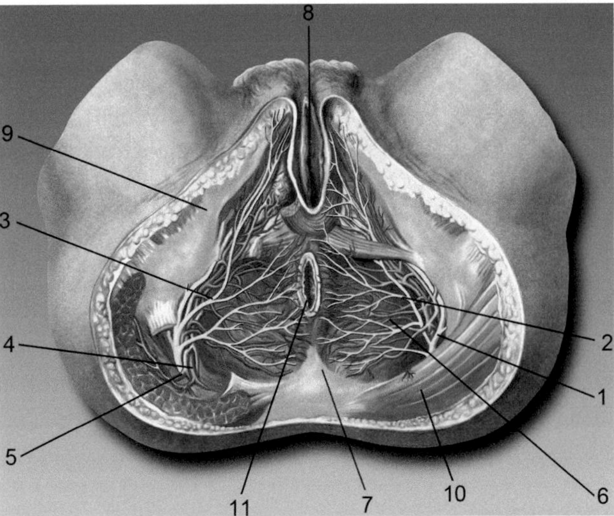

Fig. 38.3 Anatomy of the perineum (1). Pudendal nerve, (2) inferior rectal nerves, (3) perineal nerves, (4) internal pudendal artery, (5) internal pudendal veins, (6) inferior rectal artery, (7) ischiorectal fossa, (8) vaginal orifice, (9) ischial tuberosity, (10) gluteus maximus muscle, (11) anus. (Reproduced with permission from Dr. Danilo Jankovic)

The nerve then courses between the sacrospinous and sacrotuberous ligaments, adjacent to the ischial spine. At this point, the nerve may cross over the posterior aspect of either the sacrospinous ligament or the ischial spine. Anatomical study has revealed that the nerve crosses the sacrospinous ligament in 80% of cases, while in 15% of cases, it crosses the ischial spine. Remaining variations contained multi-trunked nerves crossing both the ischial spine and sacrospinous ligament.

The relationship of the pudendal artery to the nerve has also been examined from anatomical study. In 80% of cases, the pudendal nerve lies medial to the artery, while in 10% of cases, the nerve lies lateral to the artery. Remaining anatomical relationships observed include having the artery lie between two trunks, and in 7.5% of cases, the artery crossed the nerve.

After passing at the level of the ischial spine, the nerve reenters the pelvis through the lesser sciatic foramen to continue its course anteriorly through a fascial tunnel formed along the medial border of the obturator internus muscle known as Alcock's canal (Fig. 38.1). Alcock's canal lies medial to the obturator internus muscle and is formed by a splitting of the muscle's fascia into a medial and lateral layer. The medial layer covers the pudendal neurovascular bundle and fuses below with obturator fascia. The lateral layer is continuous with the obturator fascia. The length of the canal has been measured from 1.4 to 1.8 cm in adults, ending at a distance of 2 to 3 cm from the inferior border of the symphysis pubis.

The pudendal nerve divides into three branches: the inferior rectal branch, the perineal branch, and the dorsal nerve of the penis/clitoris (Figs. 38.1 and 38.3).

The inferior rectal branch descends to occupy the lower half of the ischiorectal fossa. It subdivides into cutaneous branches that supply sensory innervation to the anal canal and the skin around the anus. Sensory innervation may include the skin of the scrotum. The inferior rectal branch provides the main motor innervation to the external anal sphincter, and investigations have also documented occasional motor innervation to the levator ani muscle as well, through an "accessory rectal nerve." The inferior rectal branch can pierce through the sacrospinous ligament as it proceeds to the ischiorectal fossa, which can be a possible site of entrapment.

The perineal branch of the pudendal nerve divides into superficial and deep branches. The superficial branch provides sensory innervation through the posterior scrotal/posterior labial nerve, which contributes to the innervation of the posterior aspect of the scrotum or labia majora. This branch may join the sensory branches of the inferior rectal branch. The deep branch supplies motor innervation to the muscles of the pelvic floor and the deep perineal pouch. The external urethral sphincter receives voluntary innervation from this branch. Other muscles that receive motor innervation include the transverse perinei, bulbospongiosus, and ischiocavernosus muscles. Motor innervation has also been reported to include the anterior part of the external anal sphincter and the levator ani muscle.

The dorsal nerve of the penis or clitoris is the final branch of the pudendal nerve. This branch pierces through the superior fascia of the urogenital diaphragm once it reaches the inferior pubic ramus. Beyond this point, the nerve travels in a pouch that is defined by the crus of the penis/clitoris anteriorly and inferiorly. The branch may then pierce either the inferior fascia of the urogenital diaphragm or pierce above the inferior transverse pubic ligament. Once exited the pelvis at this point, the nerve travels anterior to the pubic bone in a groove known as the "sulcus nervi dorsalis penis/clitoris." It then deflects ventrally to innervate the penis or clitoris.

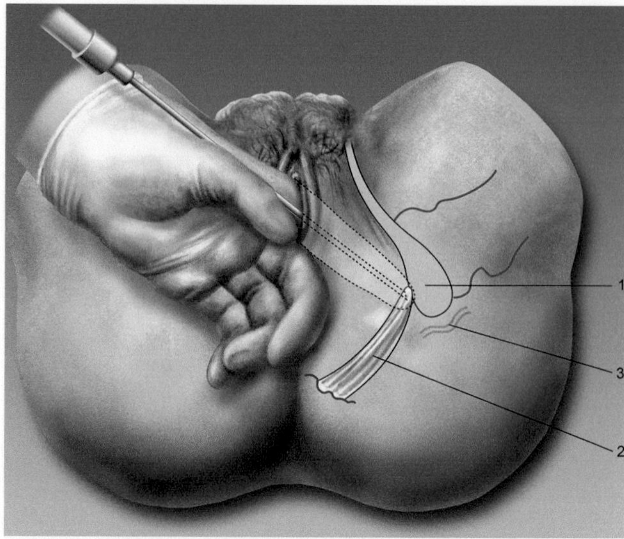

Fig. 38.4 Transvaginal access. (1) Ischial spine, (2) sacrospinous ligament, (3) pudendal nerve. (Reproduced with permission from Dr. Danilo Jankovic)

Technique

Transvaginal Technique

The pudendal nerve can be blocked transvaginally through a "blind" technique using the ischial spine as an anatomic landmark (Fig. 38.4). The distal end of an introducer kit is used to guide the needle toward the pudendal nerve, which allows for infiltrating needles to be advanced 1.0 to 1.5 cm beyond their distal openings. Introducers described in the literature include the Iowa trumpet or Kobak needle and needle guide.

The introducer is first placed against the vaginal mucosa, inferior to the ischial spine. In obstetrical anesthesia literature, the guide is to be held parallel to the delivery table. The needle is advanced into the vaginal mucosa, and 1 mL of local anesthetic is infiltrated. The needle is then advanced further until contact is made with the sacrospinous ligament, where another 3 mL of local anesthetic is injected. Care should be taken at this point to first aspirate for blood to help exclude intravascular injection prior as the pudendal vessels will be in close proximity. The needle is then passed through the ligament into the loose areolar tissue posterior to it, where another 3 mL of local anesthetic is deposited prior to aspiration. These steps are then repeated, but with the introducer placed superior to the ischial spine so as to ensure adequate spread around the pudendal nerve.

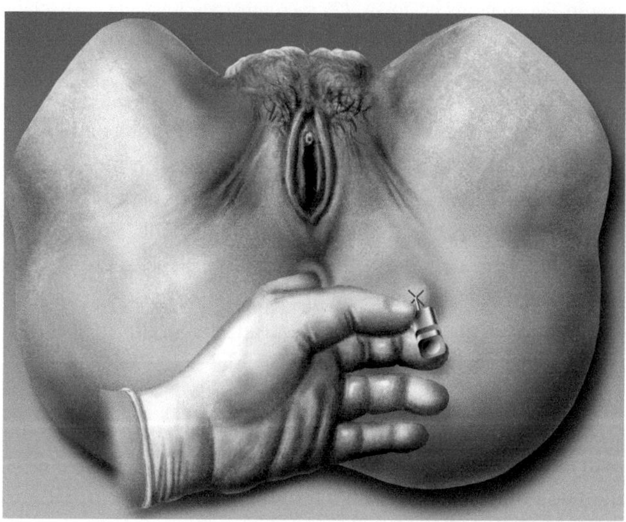

Fig. 38.5 Transperineal access. Rectal palpation of the ischial spine with the index finger. The needle is introduced into the ischiorectal fossa. (Reproduced with permission from Dr. Danilo Jankovic)

Transperineal Technique

This approach has been described in the literature together with the use of nerve stimulation and has mainly focused on providing analgesia either for perineal surgical procedures or for management of pudendal neuralgia.

The techniques described commonly include stimulation of the pudendal nerve adjacent to the ischial spine to elicit a contraction of the external anal sphincter and perineal muscles. The ischial spine can be localized by palpation of the ischial spine by inserting a finger through the vagina or rectum. Once this anatomic landmark is identified, a needle is guided to this point through the skin overlying the ischiorectal fossa (Fig. 38.5). The skin entry point can vary between descriptions. However, maintaining anal sphincter and perineal muscle contraction while diminishing the stimulating current to 0.5–0.6 mA is typically used to optimize the final needle tip position.

It should be noted that anal sphincter contraction alone might not be sufficient for a satisfactory pudendal nerve block, as this may indicate that only the inferior rectal nerve branch is being stimulated. Contraction of the pelvic floor muscles is more desirable as it indicates that the perineal branch is also being stimulated, signifying that the pudendal nerve itself, rather than individual branches, is being contacted.

Transgluteal Approach

Fluoroscopy-Guided

Blockade of the nerve is accomplished by targeting the nerve within the gluteal region as it courses adjacent to the ischial spine (Fig. 38.6).

Patients are placed in a prone position. A fluoroscope is then positioned over the targeted side of blockade to obtain an oblique view 5–20° to the side to be blocked. This view exposes the ischial spine more clearly, avoiding the overlapping with the pelvic brim. Once the ischial spine is identified, a skin entry point on the buttock is marked at the tip of the ischial spine. After skin infiltration with local anesthetic is achieved, a spinal needle can be advanced, coaxial to the fluoroscopic beam, until it contacts the bony surface of the spine. Once satisfied, 1 mL of contrast medium can be injected to confirm appropriate soft tissue spread. Once complete, injection of the chosen solution can take place.

Contrast spread patterns described include spread in an irregular or round pattern at the tip of the ischial spine. Additionally, spread can occur along the ipsilateral obturator internus muscle, sacrotuberous ligament, or sacrospinous ligament. Investigators have not described any particular correlation between pattern of spread and success of sensory blockade.

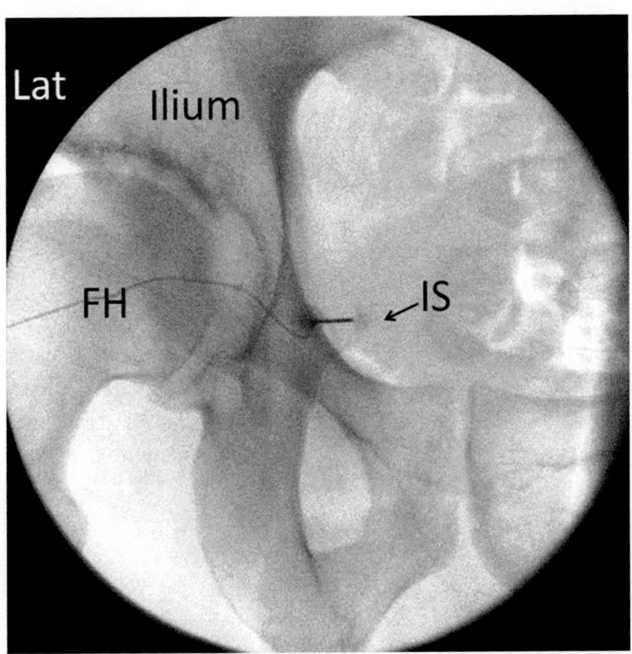

Fig. 38.6 Fluoroscopy-guided pudendal nerve block. *FH* femoral head, *Lat* lateral, *IS* tip of the ischial spine. (Reproduced with permission from Philip Peng Educational Series)

Ultrasound-Guided

The use of an ultrasound-guided approach to block the pudendal nerve has been described in the literature. The use of ultrasound allows for the visualization of soft tissues, needle advancement, and live spread of injectate around the target structures. The use of ultrasound guidance has been described for blockade of the pudendal nerve at the level of the ischial spine as well as at Alcock's canal.

Level of the Ischial Spine

Patients are placed in a prone position, and a curvilinear transducer with a low frequency (2–5 MHz) is required because of greater tissue depths. The transducer is first positioned over the ilium at the level of the posterior superior iliac spine (PSIS). The ilium appears as a straight, hyperechoic line descending laterally (Fig. 38.7). As scanning continues caudally to the level of greater sciatic notch, the hyperechoic line of the ilium starts to regress from the medial aspect of the screen. The lateral aspect of the ultrasound screen transitions to a curved hyperechoic line revealing the posterior aspect of the acetabulum. At this point, two muscular layers can be identified: the gluteus maximus and the piriformis muscles.

Moving the probe in the caudal direction to the ischial spine reveals four changes in the sonographic image: the transition of curved posterior portion of the acetabulum to the straight ischial spine, disappearance of the piriformis muscle, appearance of a dense hyperechoic line extending medially from the ischial spine, and appearance of the pudendal artery. The most likely location of the pudendal nerve is medial to this artery, and careful scanning may reveal its fascicular structure.

Once the anatomy is identified as best possible, a needle is advanced medial to the probe at a steep angle, using an in-plane approach. Owing to the steep angle of needle advancement, the needle insertion point should be 2 cm away from the probe. Movement of the tissues or spread of injectate may be used to act as surrogate markers for locating the needle tip position.

The needle will pierce through the sacrotuberous ligament, which may provide sturdy resistance to advancement. One may feel a "pop" sensation as the needle passes through. At this juncture, injection can begin under direct ultrasound visualization. Ideally, the spread of the injectate is medial to the pudendal artery and is contained between the sacrotuberous and sacrospinous ligaments. If the injectate does not follow this pattern, the needle can be repositioned. There is no

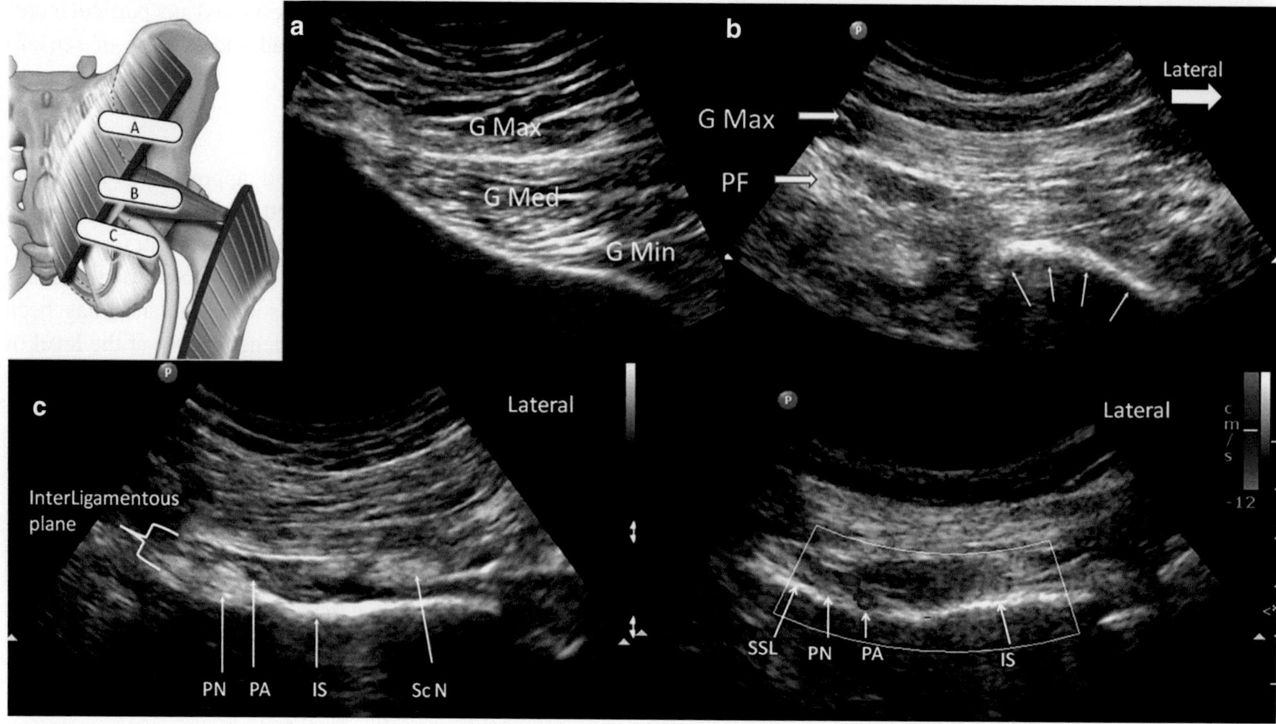

Fig. 38.7 Upper panel. Left: three positions of the ultrasound probe (**a**–**c**). Middle: sonography corresponding to position A, which shows the ilium at the level of the posterior superior iliac spine. Right: sonography corresponding to position B, which is at the level of the greater sciatic notch (arrows). Lower panel. Left: sonography corresponding to position C, which is at the level of the ischial spine. Right: same sonography with Doppler scan. *G Max* gluteus maximus, *G Med* gluteus medius, *G Min* gluteus minimus, *PF* piriformis, *ScN* sciatic nerve, *IS* ischial spine, *PN* pudendal nerve, *PA* pudendal artery, *SSL* sacrospinous ligament. (Reproduced with permission from Philip Peng Educational Series)

investigation on the optimal injectate. The authors preferred plain bupivacaine (to avoid jeopardizing circulation to the entrapped nerve) and steroid, e.g., 4-mL 0.25% bupivacaine and 40-mg Depomedrol®.

Alcock's Canal

Recent publications have reported the use of ultrasound to inject the pudendal nerve at the entrance of Alcock's canal. This technique has been described in anatomical studies and a limited case series of three patients diagnosed with pudendal neuralgia.

This method is an extension of the ultrasound technique used to identify the pudendal nerve at the level of the ischial spine. When the ultrasound probe is shifted caudally from this level, the scanning continues to the lesser sciatic notch. At this level, the straight, hyperechoic line of the ischial spine transitions in morphology to a smooth and rounded morphology indicative of the ischium at the level of the lesser sciatic notch. The soft tissue of the obturator internus tendon can be seen emerging from within the pelvis, wrapping around this bony landmark to extend laterally toward the greater trochanter of the femur.

Moving the probe further inferiorly, the pudendal nerve, artery, and vein can be visualized inside the proximal aspect Alcock's canal, lying superficial and medial to the obturator internus muscle. This neurovascular bundle can be identified by finding the pulsatile pudendal artery with the hyperechoic pudendal nerve laterally situated (Fig. 38.8). The artery can be further highlighted using color Doppler.

The injection technique has been described as advancing a needle to the pudendal nerve using an in-plane approach. A medial-to-lateral approach is recommended to avoid needle contact with the ischial tuberosity and to reduce the risk of rectal perforation.

Using this ultrasound-guided technique, Bendtsen et al. reported that in two study cadavers, all four pudendal nerves were successfully targeted three patients obtained pain relief with bilateral injections. Soucy et al. reported 81% accuracy targeting pudendal nerves at Alcock's canal in cadaveric specimens.

Equipment and Solutions

Reports describing the use of pudendal nerve blockade have tremendous variability in the types and volumes of injectates used. Needle types are also inconsistent but typically depend on the type of guidance employed to perform the block (e.g., transvaginal with introducer, ultrasound, or MRN).

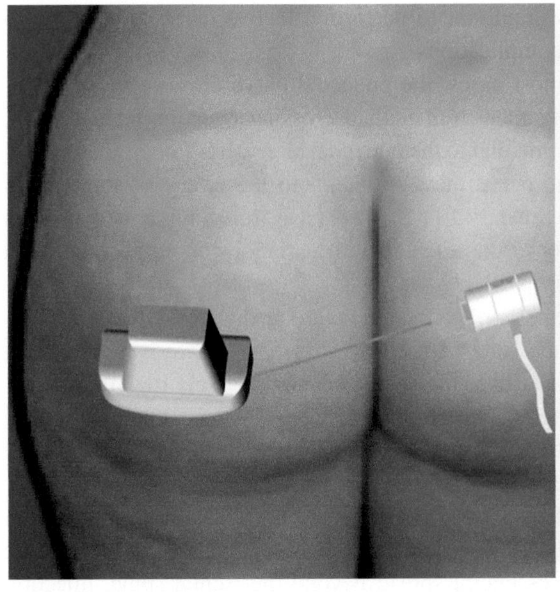

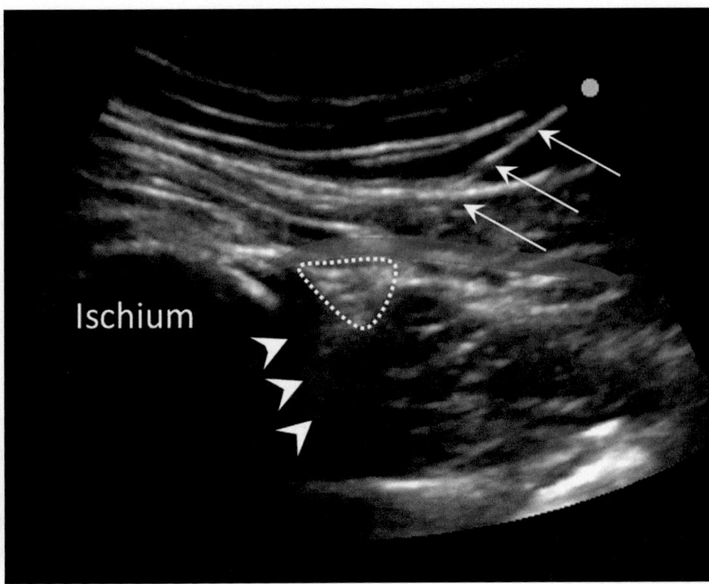

Fig. 38.8 Left: position of the probe and needle injection. Right: corresponding sonography. The obturator internus is seen as an hypoechoic structure medial to the ischium as indicated by arrowheads, and the pudendal neurovascular bundle at the entrance of the Alcock's canal is outlined in dotted line. The sacrotuberous ligament is shaded in green color, and the needle is indicated by arrows. (Reproduced with permission from Philip Peng Educational Series)

Table 38.2 Needle types and injectate for different approaches

Approach	Indication	Needle gauge and type	Injectate
Transvaginal	Obstetrical analgesia Obstetrical analgesia Obstetrical analgesia Obstetrical analgesia	22-gauge, 150-mm needle via tubular introducer Not specified Not specified Not specified	9-mL 1% lidocaine 20-mL 1% lidocaine 20-mL 1% mepivacaine 5-mL 2% prilocaine
Transperineal	Colpoperineorrhaphy Episiotomy analgesia Chronic pelvic pain and anorectal surgery Transrectal ultrasound-guided prostate biopsy	100-mm stimulating needle 100-mm stimulating needle 22-gauge, 100-mm stimulating needle 22-gauge spinal needle	10-mL 0.25% bupivacaine 15-mL 0.75% ropivacaine 5-mL 0.25% bupivacaine 10-mL 1% prilocaine
Transgluteal fluoroscopy	Chronic perineal pain	25-gauge, 3.5″ spinal needle	3-mL 0.38% ropivacaine and 20-mg triamcinolone
Transgluteal ultrasound	Pudendal neuralgia	22-gauge, 120-mm insulated stimulating needle	5-mL, 0.25% bupivacaine in 1:200,000 epinephrine and 40 mg methylprednisolone

Table 38.2 provides a survey of needle types and injectates used to perform pudendal nerve blocks according to the approach used.

Complications

When performing pudendal nerve blockade for obstetrical anesthesia, the most frequently reported complication has been block failure. When used during the second stage of labor, failure rates of the block have ranged from 10 to 50% in the literature. This may be due to failure of the local anesthetic to reach the nerve or improper timing of the block placement. If the block is placed as the fetal head is crowning, nerve blockade may not be effective in time for an episiotomy, and may only be fully established in time for the repair.

Other more common complications can include unintended blockade of adjacent nerves. If pudendal nerve blockade is performed at the ischial spine, local anesthetic spread to the sciatic nerve may lead to sensory and motor blockade of the lower limb. Depending on the patient setting, this could lead to delays in ambulation, risk of falls, or delayed discharge from hospital or clinic. A randomized controlled study comparing fluoroscopic- and ultrasound-guided pudendal nerve blockade through a transgluteal approach revealed an incidence of sciatic nerve sensory loss in 7/23 fluoroscopy-guided procedures and 3/23 ultrasound-guided procedures. Motor weakness in the form of foot drop was noted in two patients for each group.

The posterior femoral cutaneous nerve is another nerve near the pudendal nerve at the level of the ischial spine that also provides sensory innervation to the perineum. If a pudendal nerve blockade is being used to assist in the diagnosis of a pelvic pain syndrome, local anesthetic spread to the posterior femoral cutaneous nerve may lead to false-positive results.

The pudendal nerve provides motor innervation to the urethral sphincter and external anal sphincter, and loss of muscle tone may lead to temporary incontinence of bladder or bowel function. In the study comparing fluoroscopic- to ultrasound-guided techniques of pudendal nerve blockade, only 1 patient of 23 experienced bladder incontinence with bilateral pudendal nerve blockade. Although this may be an infrequent occurrence, patients should be made aware of this possibility.

Practitioners and patients should also be made aware of the uncommon, yet serious complications that are possible through pudendal nerve blockade. When used for labor analgesia, cases of fetal distress and neonatal local anesthetic toxicity have been documented. Presentations of the neonates with local anesthetic toxicity have included hypotonia, apnea, bradycardia, cyanosis, prolonged QT interval, and seizure activity. Factors that may increase the risk of this event include fetal ion trapping in the presence of acidosis and increased local anesthetic vascular uptake from the perineum during labor.

Introduction of infection after transvaginal blocks for labor analgesia has been reported due to seeding of bacteria into soft tissues from vaginal mucosa. This can lead to serious morbidity and mortality, with two deaths having been reported in the literature. Abscess formation has been reported posterior to the hip joint, into the gluteal musculature, or the retropsoal space. Of note, authors of these reports have highlighted the risk of delays in diagnosis as the clinical presentation can be initially confused with normal postpartum pain from sacroiliac joint strain or trochanteric bursitis.

The formation of significant hematoma after pudendal artery puncture has also been described in the literature in conjunction with infection. After blind infiltration for labor analgesia, an infected retroperitoneal hematoma along the iliac and psoas muscles has been reported, which extended from the midpelvis to the infrarenal fossa. Infection rather than blood loss was the principal concern in this case, however.

Practical Tips

An important anatomical landmark for performing a pudendal nerve block is the ischial spine. This is a common location for nerve infiltration for obstetrical, perioperative, and chronic pain purposes. Knowledge of anatomy at this location is important to perform effective nerve blocks and to avoid complications.

In most cases, the pudendal nerve crosses the sacrospinous ligament, rather than crossing over the ischial spine, and lies medial to the pudendal artery. It is important to recall that the nerve may lie lateral to the artery in some cases (approximately 1 in 10) or exist as trunks lying medially and laterally to the artery. These variations could account for a failed or partial block.

The authors suggest injecting medial to the pudendal vessel at the level of the ischial spine. If there is a prominent vessel lateral to the ischial spine, it is likely the inferior gluteal artery instead of the pudendal artery. Care should be taken to perform a color Doppler scan in this area to avoid mistaking these vessels.

If the injection is performed under ultrasound, attention should be paid to spread of the injectate laterally. When one witnesses lateral spread beyond the ischial spine, injection should be stopped to prevent the spread to the sciatic nerve given its proximity.

The authors recommend a systematic approach to ultrasound scanning for anatomical landmarks to facilitate pudendal nerve blocks through a transgluteal approach. This is best accomplished by first scanning for the iliac crest since it is easily recognized as a single hyperechoic line. Scanning then continues caudally toward the greater sciatic notch and then to the ischial spine.

Since the plane of greater sciatic notch is laterally oriented, the probe should ideally be tilted medially, so that the ultrasound beam is directed toward the notch. This allows for better visualization of the greater sciatic notch and its contents and the changes in sonoanatomy as scanning continues caudally.

Due to the stiffness of the sacrotuberous and sacrospinous ligaments, care should be taken not to overshoot the placement of the needle tip. This may occur if initial resistance to needle advancement is met with a "give way" of the needle once it passes through the ligament. If this occurs, the needle should be pulled back or carefully imaged to ensure proper placement between the ligaments.

Literature Review

Perioperative Pain Control

There have been a number of investigations evaluating the utility of this block for hemorrhoidectomy, as the postoperative pain of this procedure can be very severe. Pudendal nerve blockade has been found to confer substantial benefits for pain control over other types of analgesia, such as neuraxial blocks, general anesthesia, or nonspecific local anesthetic infiltration to the soft tissues of the perineum. In additional, the use of this block is associated with reduced length of patient stay in hospital, reduced oral analgesic consumption, and improved patient satisfaction over other methods of analgesia.

Urinary retention after hemorrhoidectomy is a common and undesirable side effect of anal surgery, as well as with neuraxial anesthetic techniques. The use of pudendal nerve blockade has been shown to significantly reduce this particular postoperative complication.

The evaluation of benefits of pudendal nerve blockade has also been investigated for urological procedures such as penile prosthesis surgery, hypospadias repair and circumcision in pediatric population, prostate biopsy, and placement of prostate HDR brachytherapy. The use of pudendal nerve blockade has been described for gynecologic surgical procedures such as placement of suburethral tape and colpoperineorrhaphy. Pudendal nerve blockade, however, has not proven useful to reduce pain after transvaginal pelvic reconstructive surgery.

Obstetrical Practice

The use of pudendal nerve blockade during labor has typically been reserved for the second stage of labor. During this stage, pain is experienced in the perineum and becomes somatic, innervated by the S2 to S4 nerve roots and the pudendal nerves.

Pudendal nerve block was likely used prior to the introduction of epidural anesthesia techniques. However, it can still be employed when neuraxial techniques are contraindicated or if sacral sparring occurs during epidural catheter use. This nerve block has been described for facilitating instrumented deliveries, episiotomies, repair of perineal tears, and McDonald cerclages for incompetent cervices.

The literature examining the effectiveness of local anesthetic infiltration during the second stage of labor has primarily focused on the use of paracervical blocks. However, pudendal nerve infiltration has been evaluated in several studies. There have been two studies that have directly compared the effectiveness of a single-shot spinal anesthetic to pudendal nerve blockade during the second stage of delivery. The investigation by Pace et al. sought to compare the effectiveness of these interventions for women requesting analgesia during advanced labor, defined as cervical dilation greater than 7 cm. The investigation by Hutchins compared these two techniques for instrumental delivery. In both studies, the neuraxial technique demonstrated superiority to pudendal nerve blockade for degree of analgesia and patient satisfaction.

Although neuraxial techniques for labor analgesia may offer superior pain relief compared to the use of pudendal blockade alone, concern for prolonging the second stage of labor has been raised when epidural analgesia is used. Increased dosing of epidural analgesia with local anesthetic during the second stage of labor can lead to increased weakness of abdominal muscles, thereby diminishing forces required to facilitate a delivery.

Xu et al. sought to determine if the use of pudendal nerve blockade during the second stage of labor reduced supplemental epidural dosing, thereby helping to prevent a prolonged second stage of labor in nulliparous women. Pudendal nerve blockade was performed using ultrasound guidance, and the study was conducted as a prospective, double-blind, randomized controlled trial. The group receiving the pudendal nerve block required significantly less hourly bupivacaine boluses through their epidural catheter and reduced the length of the second stage of labor by 33.8 min.

Pudendal Neuralgia

Pudendal nerve blocks have been employed for patients suffering from pudendal neuralgia and have failed conservative techniques. Targets for nerve infiltration are possible sites of entrapment such as at the level of the ischial spine between the sacrospinous and sacrotuberous ligaments or Alcock's canal.

Studies have investigated the effectiveness of pudendal nerve infiltration for relief of this chronic pain syndrome but have been heterogeneous in methodology. For example, variations exist in the chosen technique to perform the block (e.g., CT guidance or landmark-guided infiltration), single or repeated injections, choice of outcome measures, or duration of follow-up.

Investigations have also had considerable variability in the way in which patients are diagnosed and included to study this condition. For example, some investigations adhere to the Nantes criteria to establish the diagnosis of pudendal neuralgia, while others only presume a diagnosis of the condition without taking any confirmatory steps for patient study inclusion. These are considerable limitations when attempting to make conclusions about effectiveness of this block from the literature.

Despite these challenges, a recent systematic review of the literature has attempted to extract some generalizations for the effectiveness of interventions for drug-resistant pudendal neuralgia. For nerve infiltration, an immediate improvement in pain intensity is achieved in 77% to 82% of patients. Data analysis further revealed that improvement in pain intensity is experienced in 62% of patients at 3 months and 6.8% to 12.2% of patients at 1-year, post-procedure. Functional outcome measures were not reported in this review.

Notably, there has been one randomized controlled trial evaluating the role of the addition of steroid to pudendal nerve blockade via CT guidance for pudendal neuralgia. Injections were performed at the sacrospinous ligament and Alcock's canal as two possible sites of entrapment. Study participants had to meet the first four of the Nantes criteria to be included in the study (the fifth criteria being a positive response to pudendal nerve block which was being evaluated). Patients were randomized to three groups: (a) 1% lidocaine only, (b) 1% lidocaine followed by injection of corticosteroids using 20 mg of methylprednisolone per injection site, and (c) same procedure as group B with the addition of large volume of normal saline to evaluate benefits of hydrodissection. A total of 201 patients were included in the study. The primary endpoint of the study was pain intensity score at 3 months. Patients were defined as responders with at least a 30-point improvement on a100-point visual analogue scale of mean maximum pain over a 2-week period. At 3 months, 11.8% of patients in Arm A were responders, while 14.3% were responders in Arms B and C. The study concluded that there is no benefit to the addition of corticosteroids to the block for pudendal neuralgia, and no significant effect is produced using hydrodissection.

Suggested Reading

Abramov Y, Sand PK, Gandhi S, Botros SM, Miller JJ, Koh EK, et al. The effect of preemptive pudendal nerve blockade on pain after transvaginal pelvic reconstructive surgery. Obstet Gynecol. 2005;106(4):782–8.

Adsan O, Inal G, Ozdogan L, Kaygisiz O, Ugurlu O, Cetinkaya M. Unilateral pudendal nerve blockade for relief of all pain during transrectal ultrasound-guided biopsy of the prostate: a randomized, double-blind, placebo-controlled study. Urology. 2004;64(3):528–31.

Aissaoui Y, Bruyere R, Mustapha H, Bry D, Kamili ND, Miller C. A randomized controlled trial of pudendal nerve block for pain relief after episiotomy. Anesth Analg. 2008;107(2):625–9.

Arslan M, Yazici G, Dilek U. Pudendal nerve block for pain relief in episiotomy repair. Int J Gynaecol Obstet. 2004;87(2):151–2.

Bellingham GA, Bhatia A, Chan CW, Peng PW. Randomized controlled trial comparing pudendal nerve block under ultrasound and fluoroscopic guidance. Reg Anesth Pain Med. 2012;37(3):262–6.

Bendtsen TF, Parras T, Moriggl B, Chan V, Lundby L, Buntzen S, et al. Ultrasound-guided pudendal nerve block at the entrance of the pudendal (Alcock) canal: description of anatomy and clinical technique. Reg Anesth Pain Med. 2016;41(2):140–5.

Bharucha AE. Pelvic floor: anatomy and function. Neurogastroenterol Motil. 2006;18(7):507–19.

Bolandard F, Bazin JE. Nerve stimulator guided pudendal nerve blocks. Can J Anaesth. 2005;52(7):773; author reply -4.

Bozynski ME, Rubarth LB, Patel JA. Lidocaine toxicity after maternal pudendal anesthesia in a term infant with fetal distress. Am J Perinatol. 1987;4(2):164–6.

Castellvi J, Sueiras A, Espinosa J, Vallet J, Gil V, Pi F. Ligasure versus diathermy hemorrhoidectomy under spinal anesthesia or pudendal block with ropivacaine: a randomized prospective clinical study with 1-year follow-up. Int J Colorectal Dis. 2009;24(9):1011–8.

Chan CL, Ponsford S, Scott SM, Swash M, Lunniss PJ. Contribution of the pudendal nerve to sensation of the distal rectum. Br J Surg. 2005;92(7):859–65.

Choi SS, Lee PB, Kim YC, Kim HJ, Lee SC. C-arm-guided pudendal nerve block: a new technique. Int J Clin Pract. 2006;60(5):553–6.

Cunningham FG, Williams JW. Williams obstetrics. 23rd ed. New York: McGraw-Hill Medical; 2010. p. 444–63.

Dos Reis JM, Glina S, Da Silva MF, Furlan V. Penile prosthesis surgery with the patient under local regional anesthesia. J Urol. 1993;150(4):1179–81.

Fadel MG, Peltola L, Pellino G, Frunza G, Kontovounisios C. The role of pudendal nerve block in colorectal surgery: a systematic review. J Invest Surg. 2020;34:1238–45.

Furtmuller GJ, McKenna CA, Ebmer J, Dellon AL. Pudendal nerve 3-dimensional illustration gives insight into surgical approaches. Ann Plast Surg. 2014;73(6):670–8.

Gabrielli F, Cioffi U, Chiarelli M, Guttadauro A, De Simone M. Hemorrhoidectomy with posterior perineal block: experience with 400 cases. Dis Colon Rectum. 2000;43(6):809–12.

Grigorescu BA, Lazarou G, Olson TR, Downie SA, Powers K, Greston WM, et al. Innervation of the levator ani muscles: description of the nerve branches to the pubococcygeus, iliococcygeus, and puborectalis muscles. Int Urogynecol J Pelvic Floor Dysfunct. 2008;19(1):107–16.

Gruber H, Kovacs P, Piegger J, Brenner E. New, simple, ultrasound-guided infiltration of the pudendal nerve: topographic basics. Dis Colon Rectum. 2001;44(9):1376–80.

Hruby S, Ebmer J, Dellon AL, Aszmann OC. Anatomy of pudendal nerve at urogenital diaphragm—new critical site for nerve entrapment. Urology. 2005;66(5):949–52.

Hutchins CJ. Spinal analgesia for instrumental delivery. A comparison with pudendal nerve block. Anaesthesia. 1980;35(4):376–7.

Imbelloni LE, Beato. L, Beato C, Cordeiro JA, de Souza DD. Bilateral pudendal nerves block for postoperative analgesia with 0.25% S75:R25 bupivacaine. Pilot study on outpatient hemorrhoidectomy. Rev Bras Anestesiol. 2005;55(6):614–21.

Inal G, Adsan O, Ugurlu O, Kaygisiz O, Kosan M, Cetinkaya M. Comparison of four different anesthesia methods for relief of all pain during transrectal ultrasound-guided prostate biopsy. Int Urol Nephrol. 2008;40(2):335–9.

Iremashvili VV, Chepurov AK, Kobaladze KM, Gamidov SI. Periprostatic local anesthesia with pudendal block for transperineal ultrasound-guided prostate biopsy: a randomized trial. Urology. 2010;75(5):1023–7.

Ismail MT, Elshmaa NS. Pre-emptive analgesia by nerve stimulator guided pudendal nerve block for posterior colpoperineorrhaphy. Eur J Obstet Gynecol Reprod Biol. 2012;163(2):200–3.

Kaufman JJ. Penile prosthetic surgery under local anesthesia. J Urol. 1982;128(6):1190–1.

Kim J, Lee DS, Jang SM, Shim MC, Jee DL. The effect of pudendal block on voiding after hemorrhoidectomy. Dis Colon Rectum. 2005;48(3):518–23.

Kim SH, Song SG, Paek OJ, Lee HJ, Park DH, Lee JK. Nerve-stimulator-guided pudendal nerve block by pararectal approach. Colorectal Dis. 2012;14(5):611–5.

King JC, Sherline DM. Paracervical and pudendal block. Clin Obstet Gynecol. 1981;24(2):587–95.

Kovacs P, Gruber H, Piegger J, Bodner G. New, simple, ultrasound-guided infiltration of the pudendal nerve: ultrasonographic technique. Dis Colon Rectum. 2001;44(9):1381–5.

Kurzel RB, Au AH, Rooholamini SA. Retroperitoneal hematoma as a complication of pudendal block. Diagnosis made by computed tomography. West J Med. 1996;164(6):523–5.

Labat JJ, Riant T, Robert R, Amarenco G, Lefaucheur JP, Rigaud J. Diagnostic criteria for pudendal neuralgia by pudendal nerve entrapment (Nantes criteria). NeurourolUrodyn. 2008;27(4):306–10.

Labat JJ, Riant T, Lassaux A, Rioult B, Rabischong B, Khalfallah M, et al. Adding corticosteroids to the pudendal nerve block for pudendal neuralgia: a randomised, double-blind, controlled trial. BJOG. 2017;124(2):251–60.

Mahakkanukrauh P, Surin P, Vaidhayakarn P. Anatomical study of the pudendal nerve adjacent to the sacrospinous ligament. Clin Anat. 2005;18(3):200–5.

Mamlouk MD, van Sonnenberg E, Dehkharghani S. CT-guided nerve block for pudendal neuralgia: diagnostic and therapeutic implications. AJR Am J Roentgenol. 2014;203(1):196–200.

Naja Z, Ziade MF, Lonnqvist PA. Nerve stimulator guided pudendal nerve block decreases posthemorrhoidectomy pain. Can J Anaesth. 2005;52(1):62–8.

Naja Z, El-Rajab M, Al-Tannir M, Ziade F, Zbibo R, Oweidat M, et al. Nerve stimulator guided pudendal nerve block versus general anesthesia for hemorrhoidectomy. Can J Anaesth. 2006;53(6):579–85.

Naja Z, Al-Tannir MA, Faysal W, Daoud N, Ziade F, El-Rajab M. A comparison of pudendal block vs dorsal penile nerve block for circumcision in children: a randomised controlled trial. Anaesthesia. 2011;66(9):802–7.

Naja ZM, Ziade FM, Kamel R, El-Kayali S, Daoud N, El-Rajab MA. The effectiveness of pudendal nerve block versus caudal block anesthesia for hypospadias in children. Anesth Analg. 2013;117(6):1401–7.

Novikova N, Cluver C. Local anaesthetic nerve block for pain management in labour. Cochrane Database Syst Rev. 2012;4:CD009200.

Pace MC, Aurilio C, Bulletti C, Iannotti M, Passavanti MB, Palagiano A. Subarachnoid analgesia in advanced labor: a comparison of subarachnoid analgesia and pudendal block in advanced labor: analgesic quality and obstetric outcome. Ann N Y Acad Sci. 2004;1034:356–63.

Pages H, de la Gastine B, Quedru-Aboane J, Guillemin MG, Lelong-Boulouard V, Guillois B. Lidocaine intoxication in newborn following maternal pudendal anesthesia: report of three cases. J Gynecol Obstet Biol Reprod (Paris). 2008;37(4):415–8.

Peng PW, Tumber PS. Ultrasound-guided interventional procedures for patients with chronic pelvic pain—a description of techniques and review of literature. Pain Physician. 2008;11(2):215–24.

Petros JG, Bradley TM. Factors influencing postoperative urinary retention in patients undergoing surgery for benign anorectal disease. Am J Surg. 1990;159(4):374–6.

Pirro N, Sielezneff I, Le Corroller T, Ouaissi M, Sastre B, Champsaur P. Surgical anatomy of the extrapelvic part of the pudendal nerve and its applications for clinical practice. Surg Radiol Anat. 2009;31(10):769–73.

Prat-Pradal D, Metge L, Gagnard-Landra C, Mares P, Dauzat M, Godlewski G. Anatomical basis of transgluteal pudendal nerve block. Surg Radiol Anat. 2009;31(4):289–93.

Pybus DA, D'Bras BE, Goulding G, Liberman H, Torda TA. Postoperative analgesia for haemorrhoid surgery. Anaesth Intensive Care. 1983;11(1):27–30.

Rofaeel A, Peng P, Louis I, Chan V. Feasibility of real-time ultrasound for pudendal nerve block in patients with chronic perineal pain. Reg Anesth Pain Med. 2008;33(2):139–45.

Schelhorn J, Habenicht U, Malessa R, Dannenberg C. Magnetic resonance imaging-guided perineural therapy as a treatment option in young adults with pudendal nerve entrapment syndrome. Clin Neuroradiol. 2013;23(2):161–3.

Schenck M, Schenck C, Rubben H, Stuschke M, Schneider T, Eisenhardt A, et al. Pudendal nerve block in HDR-brachytherapy patients: do we really need general or regional anesthesia? World J Urol. 2013;31(2):417–21.

Schierup L, Schmidt JF, Torp Jensen A, Rye BA. Pudendal block in vaginal deliveries. Mepivacaine with and without epinephrine. Acta Obstet Gynecol Scand. 1988;67(3):195–7.

Schraffordt SE, Tjandra JJ, Eizenberg N, Dwyer PL. Anatomy of the pudendal nerve and its terminal branches: a cadaver study. ANZ J Surg. 2004;74(1–2):23–6.

Shafik A. Neuronal innervation of urethral and anal sphincters: surgical anatomy and clinical implications. Curr Opin Obstet Gynecol. 2000;12(5):387–98.

Shafik A, Doss SH. Pudendal canal: surgical anatomy and clinical implications. Am Surg. 1999;65(2):176–80.

Shafik A, El-Sherif M, Youssef A, Olfat ES. Surgical anatomy of the pudendal nerve and its clinical implications. Clin Anat. 1995;8(2):110–5.

Shah AP, Mevcha A, Wilby D, Alatsatianos A, Hardman JC, Jacques S, et al. Continence and micturition: an anatomical basis. Clin Anat. 2014;27(8):1275–83.

Shmueli A, Salman L, Orbach-Zinger S, Aviram A, Hiersch L, Chen R, et al. The impact of epidural analgesia on the duration of the second stage of labor. Birth. 2018;45(4):377–84.

Soucy B, Luong DH, Michaud J, Boudier-Reveret M, Sobczak S. Accuracy of ultrasound-guided pudendal nerve block in the ischial spine and Alcock's canal levels: a cadaveric study. Pain Med. 2020;21(11):2692–8.

Svancarek W, Chirino O, Schaefer G Jr, Blythe JG. Retropsoas and subgluteal abscesses following paracervical and pudendal anesthesia. JAMA. 1977;237(9):892–4.

Tepetes K, Symeonidis D, Christodoulidis G, Spyridakis M, Hatzitheofilou K. Pudendal nerve block versus local anesthesia for harmonic scalpel hemorrhoidectomy: a prospective randomized study. Tech Coloproctol. 2010;14(Suppl 1):S1–3.

Tricard T, Munier P, Story F, Lang H, Saussine C. The drug-resistant pudendal neuralgia management: a systematic review. NeurourolUrodyn. 2019;38(1):13–21.

Volmanen P, Palomaki O, Ahonen J. Alternatives to neuraxial analgesia for labor. Curr Opin Anaesthesiol. 2011;24(3):235–41.

Wenger DR, Gitchell RG. Severe infections following pudendal block anesthesia: need for orthopaedic awareness. J Bone Joint Surg Am. 1973;55(1):202–7.

Xu J, Zhou R, Su W, Wang S, Xia Y, Papadimos T, et al. Ultrasound-guided bilateral pudendal nerve blocks of nulliparous women with epidural labour analgesia in the second stage of labour: a randomised, double-blind, controlled trial. BMJ Open. 2020;10(8):e035887.

Paracervical (Uterosacral Block)

39

Danilo Jankovic

Contents

General Consideration

Before the established popularity of epidural anesthesia for labor and delivery, paracervical block was one of the most frequently used regional techniques administered for analgesia during the first stage of labor (see Chap. 42).

This block is rarely performed in contemporary obstetric practice because of its associated high rate of fetal bradycardia. Perhaps the most common use of this block is for cervical dilation and uterine curettage (d&c). In combination with light sedation, a paracervical block provides good analgesia for d&c in patients who are not optimal candidates for spinal and general anesthesia.

Functional Anatomy

Pain from the uterus passes in sequence through uterine plexus, the pelvic ganglia and plexus, the hypogastric nerve, the superior hypogastric plexus, the lumbar and lower thoracic sympathetic chain, and the white rami communicans, associated with the eleventh and twelfth nerves. Then, the pain stimuli pass through the posterior roots of these spinal nerves (T11 and T12) to enter the spinal cord (Figs. 39.1 and 39.2). Frankenhauser's ganglion, which contents all the visceral sensory nerve fibers from the uterus, cervix, and upper vagina, is located in the lateral fornix of the upper vaginal canal. It is that ganglion or plexus of nerves that is blocked by a paracervical block.

D. Jankovic (✉)
Pain Management Centre DGS – Cologne – Huerth, Cologne-Hürth, Germany
e-mail: danilo@jankovic1.de

D. Jankovic, P. Peng (eds.), *Regional Nerve Blocks in Anesthesia and Pain Therapy*,
https://doi.org/10.1007/978-3-030-88727-8_39

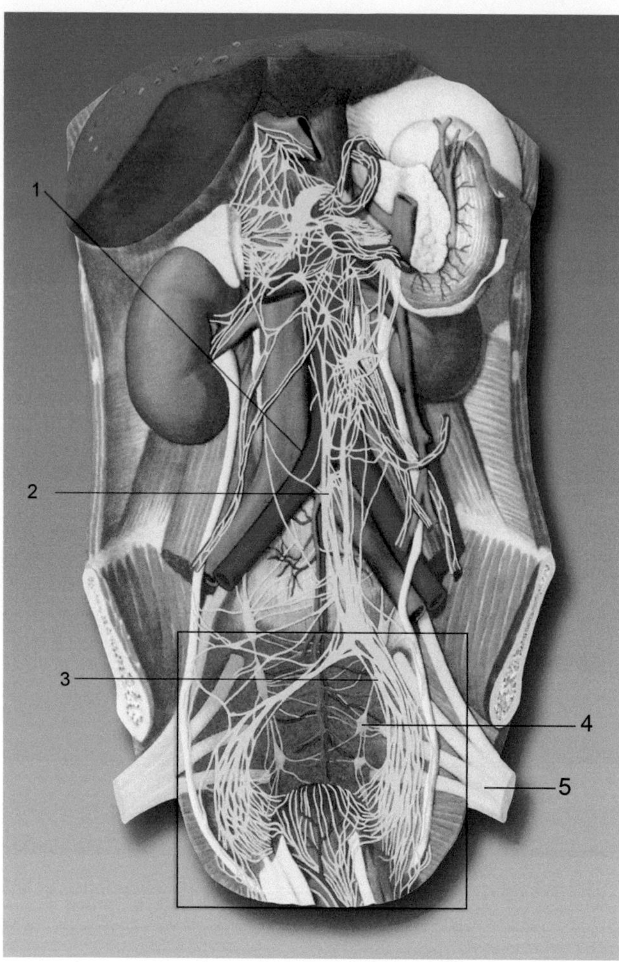

Fig. 39.1 Anatomy. *(1)* Aorta and inferior vena cava, *(2)* superior hypogastric plexus, *(3)* pelvic (inferior hypogastric plexus), *(4)* lumbosacral sympathetic ganglia, *(5)* lumbosacral plexus. (Reproduced with permission from Danilo Jankovic)

Indications

Paracervical block has a limited role in modern obstetric practice, except in cases where central neural blockade is not feasible or is unavailable.

Surgical

- Bilateral block may be used for dilatation of the cervix and uterine curettage.
- Occasionally, it may be combined with pudendal nerve block and local infiltration to perform a vaginal hysterectomy.

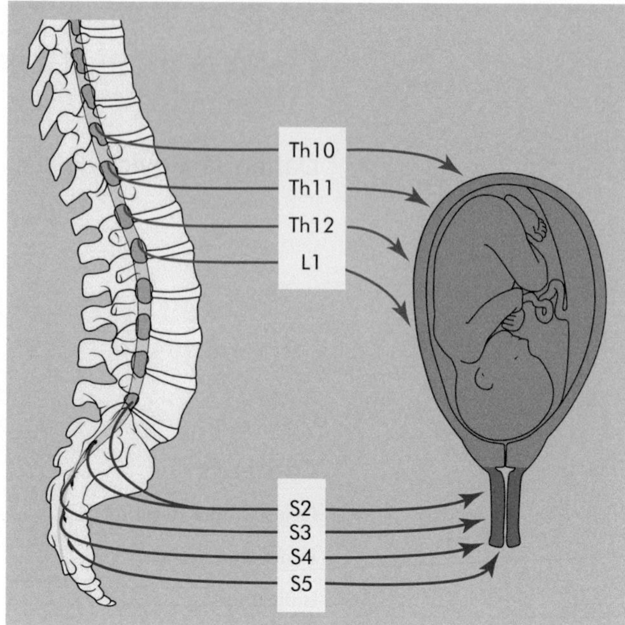

Fig. 39.2 Peripheral pain pathways during labor. (Reproduced with permission from Danilo Jankovic)

Vaginal Delivery

Bilateral paracervical block alleviates the pain of the first stage of labor, and this is the most frequent use of this block.

- Avoid: In prematurity, fetal distress, and uteroplacental insufficiency.

Therapeutic

- Relief of severe dysmenorrhea.
- Endometritis and parametritis.

Diagnostic

Differentiation of severe dysmenorrhea from other similar complaints which may be associated with menstruation.

Materials

The IOWA trumpet, Kobak instrument is used as a guide for the placement of the needle (20-gauge, 12–14 cm needle) (see Chap. 38).

Technique

Paracervical and uterosacral blocks are identical procedures and the local anesthetic solution bathes the same plexus and ganglia. If the solution is deposited at the 3 and 9 o'clock positions, the block is termed paracervical, and if solution is deposited at the 4 and 8 o'clock positions, the block is termed uterosacral (Fig. 39.4). The pelvic (inferior hypogastric) ganglia and plexus are anesthetized when this block is performed.

Position and Landmarks

The patient is placed in the supine position with her legs apart and partially in the lithotomy.

position. The injection is made in the lateral fornices of the vagina.

- Vaginal examination should be performed immediately before the block to determine the precise position of the presenting part.
- Maternal and fetal vital signs should be determined immediately before the block.

Procedure

1. The needle is introduced through the submucosa into the lateral vaginal fornix (Fig. 39.3).

   The guide, with needle tip protected, is directed into the lateral fornices between 3 and 4 o'clock and between 8 and 9 o'clock, by the index and middle fingers, so that the tip of the guide does not depress the vaginal mucosa excessively and to determine the precise location of the needle and to protect the vaginal tissues and the fetal presenting part from inadvertent puncture by the advancing needle (Fig. 39.4).
2. The needle is then introduced into the uterosacral ligament.

   The needle should be inserted with a guard (e.g., an Iowa Trumpet) so that the needlepoint cannot protrude beyond the guard for more than 5–7 mm. This maneuver prevents inadvertent intravascular injection and also prevents damage to the fetal presenting part.
3. After careful aspiration at various levels (blood), the local anesthetic is injected on an incremental basis. Approximately 5–10 mL of the chosen local anesthetic should be used in each fornix for satisfactory paracervical block.
4. The needle is removed, the guide redirected to the other side of the cervix, and the injection repeated.

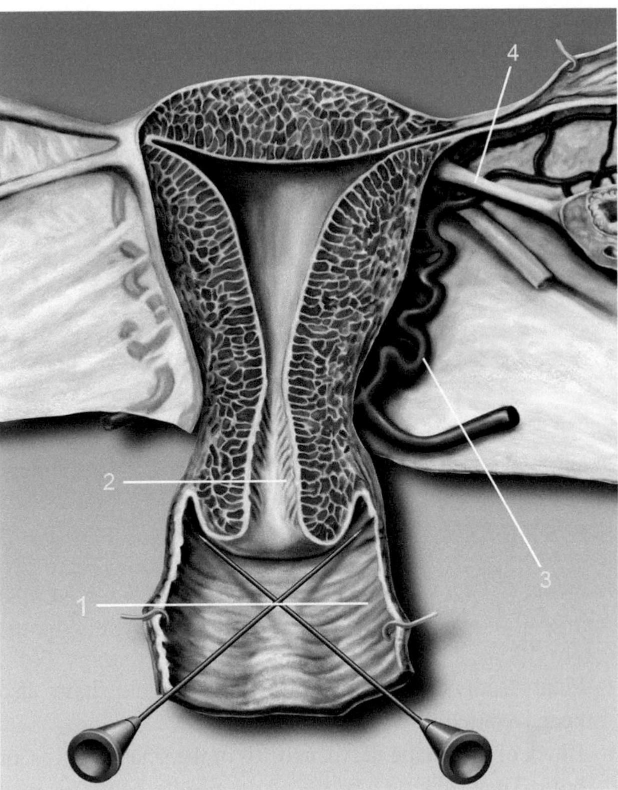

Fig. 39.3 The needle is introduced through the submucosa into the lateral vaginal fornix. (*1*) Lateral vaginal fornix, (*2*) ostium uteri, (*3*) uterine artery, (*4*) round ligament of uterus. (Reproduced with permission from Danilo Jankovic)

Dosage

The duration of the analgesia will vary with the local anesthetic, its concentration, and the total dose used:

- 0.25% Bupivacaine provides 90–150 min of analgesia.
- 1% mepivacaine provides 90–150 min of analgesia.
- 1% procaine or 2% chloroprocaine provides 40 to 50 min of analgesia.
- When performing a paracervical block, fetal heart rate and maternal uterine contractions should be monitored immediately preceding and for some time following the block.

Complications

- Systemic toxic reactions (see Chap. 5).
- Fetal distress, bradycardia, fetal acidosis, neonatal depression, and low Apgar scores. Paracervical injection may lead to high levels of local anesthetics in the fetus, up to 70% of fetuses will have arrhythmias (principally bradycardia) within 10 min of injection.

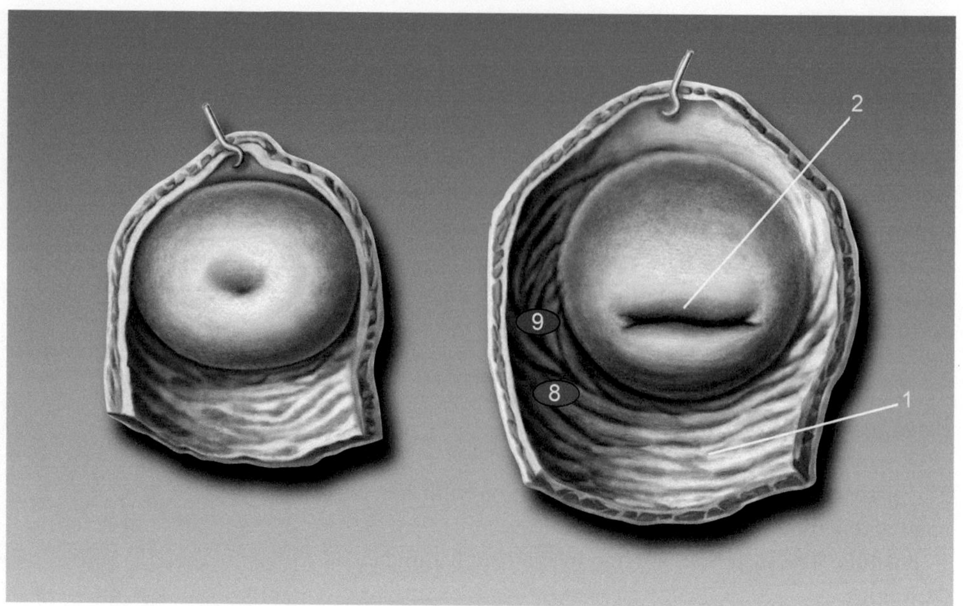

Fig. 39.4 The guide, with the needle tip protected, is directed into the lateral fornices between 3 and 4 o'clock and between 8 and 9 o'clock. *(1)* Vaginal fornix, *(2)* ostium uteri. (Reproduced with permission from Danilo Jankovic)

- Fetal deaths from bupivacaine cardiotoxicity have also been reported.
- Block of the sciatic nerve, neuritis of the sciatic nerves, or both. They may be a result of the needle being inserted further than 1.5 cm beyond the vaginal mucosa, the use of great volume of local anesthetic solution, or a combination of these.
- Hematoma of the parametrium. This occurs from trauma to a blood vessel during execution of the block. Finally, uterine artery hematoma, cervical abscess, and uternal trauma have been reported.
- Injections have occasionally been made directly into the fetal scalp.
- A transient decrease in intensity and/or frequency of uterine contractions could be associated with the local anesthetic, especially when epinephrine is used to perform the block.

Literature Review

Cervical dilation and uterine interventions (such as hysteroscopy, endometrial biopsies, fractional curettage, and suction terminations) can be performed without any analgesia or anesthesia, with regional anesthetic injections as with paracervical block, using oral or intravenous analgesics and sedatives, or under general anesthesia. Many gynecologists use paracervical local anesthesia but its effectiveness is unclear. The paracervical block with lidocaine is a commonly used part of analgesia in many outpatient gynecologic procedures, including suction d&c. The majority of abortions are performed using a paracervical block (without general anesthesia). It is important to recognize that the block itself causes considerable discomfort. Adding sodium bicarbonate to lidocaine results in decreased pain during injection (1 mL of 8.4% sodium bicarbonate per 10 mL of local anesthetic). The addition of fentanyl to lidocaine may improve pain control. In addition, anecdotally, the smaller the needle size (e.g., 25G vs. 22G), the less pain experienced with injection. Until recently, however, despite its frequent use, the data were conflicting on paracervical block efficacy for cervical dilation pain. The number of injection sites did not seem to make a difference in the pain experienced with cervical dilation. A 20 mL block is superior to a 10 mL volume block. The multiple injections at the 2, 4, 8, and 10 o'clock positions are not necessary. The 4 and 8 o'clock positions allow one to reach the nerve plexuses traveling along the uterosacral ligaments. The available evidence does not show if paracervical block is inferior, equivalent, or superior to the alternative analgesic techniques, either in terms of efficacy or safety. Some women are likely to experience anesthesia is hazardous, for example, when patients are frail, unwell, or when no anesthesiologist is available. Paracervical local anesthesia offers an alternative for cervical dilation and uterine intervention as it does not require general anesthetic equipment or personnel trained to give general anesthesia. Twenty-six studies involving 2790 women compared paracervical block and other anesthetic and analgesia methods for women undergoing uterine interventions.

There was evidence that paracervical block reduced the risk of severe pain but not any pain. There was little evidence to support the belief that paracervical block made any consistent difference to any outcome.

Suggested Reading

Aldridge CW, Nanzig RP, Beaton JH. Uterosacral block and the obstetrical anesthesia problem. Am J Obstet Gynecol. 1961;81:941–7.

Allen R, Kumar D, Fitzmaurice G, et al. Pain management of first-trimester surgical abortion: effects of selection of local anesthesia with and without lorazepam or intravenous sedation. Contraception. 2006;74(5):407–13. https://doi.org/10.1016/i:contraception.2006.06.002.

Asling JH, Shnider SM, Margolis AJ, et al. Paracervical block anesthesia in obstetrics. II. Etiology of fetal bradycardia following paracervical block anesthesia. Am J Obstet Gynecol. 1971;107:626.

Baken MP, Freeman DW, Barno A. Transvaginal regional block anesthesia in labor. Surg Gynecol Obstet. 1962;114:375–8.

Bloom SL, Horswill CW, Curet LB. Effects of paracervical blocks on the fetus during labour. A prospective study with the use of direct fetal monitoring. Am J Obstet Gynecol. 1972;114:218.

Brownridge P, Cohen SE, Ward E. Neural blockade for obstetrics and gynecologic surgery. In: Cousins M, Bridenbaugh PO, editors. Neural blockade. 3rd ed. Philadelphia, PA: Lippincott-Raven; 1998. p. 574–5.

Cibils LA, Santonja-Lucas JJ. Clinical significance of fetal heart rate patterns during labour. III: effect of paracervical block anesthesia. Am J Obstet Gynecol. 1978;130:73.

Glanz JC, Shomento S. Comparison of paracervical block techniques during first trimester pregnancy termination. Int J Gynaecol Obstet. 2001;72:171.

Goins JR. Experience with mepivacaine paracervical block in an obstetric private practice. Am J Obstet Gynecol. 1992;167:342.

Grimes DA, Gates J. Deaths from paracervical anesthesia used first trimester abortion. N Engl J Med. 1976;295:1397.

Ireland LD, Allen RH. Pain management for gynecologic procedures in the office. Obstet Gynecol Surv. 2016;71:89–98.

Kobak AJ, Sadove MS, Mazeros WT. Anatomic studies of transvaginal regional anesthesia. Roentgenographic visualization of neural pathways. Obstet Gynecol. 1962;19:302–10.

Lopez LM, Bernholc A, Zeng Y, Allen R, et al. Interventions for pain with intrauterine device insertion. Cochrane Database Syst Rev. 2015;(7):CD007373. https://doi.org/10.1002/14651858.CD007373.pub3.

Mody SK, Farala JP, Jimenez B. Paracervical block for intrauterine device placement among nulliparous women: a randomized controlled trial. Obstet Gynecol. 2018;132:575.

Moore DC. Paracervical (uterosacral block). In: Moore DC, editor. Regional block. Springfield, IL: Charles Thomas; 1976. p. 21–187.

Murphy PJ, Wright JD, Fitzgerald TB. Assessment of paracervical nerve block anesthesia. during labour. Br Med J. 1970;1:526.

Page EP, Kamm ML, Chappell CC. Usefulness of paracervical block in obstetric. Am J Obstet Gynecol. 1961;81:1094–8.

Parris WCV. Paracervical nerve. In: Hahn M, McQuillan PM, Sheplock GJ, editors. Regional anesthesia. St. Louis, MO: Mosby; 1996. p. 273–7.

Renner RM, Ensen JT, Nichols MD, et al. Pain control in first trimester surgical abortion. Cochrane Database Syst Rev. 2009;(2):CD006712.

Renner RM, Jensen JT, Nichols MD, et al. Pain control in first trimester surgical abortion: a systematic review of randomized controlled trials. Contraception. 2010;81:372–88.

Renner RM, Nichols MD, Jensen JT. Paracervical block for pain control in first trimester surgical abortion: a randomized controlled trial. Obstet Gynecol. 2012;119:1030–7.

Rosefsky JB, Petersiel ME. Perinatal deaths associated with mepivacaine paracervical block anesthesia in labor. N Engl J Med. 1968;278:530.

Seeds AE, Stein-Messinger P, Dorsey JH. Paracervical blocks: results of a double-blind evaluation. Obstet Gynecol. 1962;20:462–7.

Shnider SM, Asling JH, Hall JW, et al. Paracervical block anesthesia in obstetrics: I. Fetal. complications and neonatal morbidity. Am J Obstet Gynecol. 1970;107:619.

Tangsiriwatthana T, Sangkomkamhang U, Lumbiganon P, et al. Paracervical local anesthesia for cervical dilatation and uterine intervention. Cochrane Database Syst Rev. 2013;(9):CD005056. https://doi.org/10.1002/14651858.CD005056.pub3.

Van Praagh IG, Povey WG. Paracervical block anesthesia in labour. Can Med Assoc J. 1966;94(6):262–7.

Viscomi CM. Obstetric anesthesia. Paracervical block. In: Rathmell JP, Neal J, Viscomi CM, editors. Regional anesthesia. Philadelphia: Elsevier–Mosby; 2004. p. 173–85.

White CA, Pitkin RM. Paracervical block anesthesia in obstetric. Postgrad Med. 1963;33:585–9.

Part VI

Nerve Block for Regional Anesthesia and Pain Therapy in Neuraxial Region

Neuraxial Anatomy and Sonoanatomy

40

Danilo Jankovic and Ki Jinn Chin

Contents

Intimate knowledge of the anatomy of the vertebral column and its contents is the keystone to successful, safe neuraxial anesthesia, not only in terms of the performance of lumbar puncture but also in terms of the spread of local anesthetics in CSF and the level of anesthesia achieved.

D. Jankovic (✉)
Pain Management Centre DGS – Cologne – Huerth, Cologne-Hürth, Germany
e-mail: danilo@jankovic1.de

K. J. Chin
Department of Anesthesiology and Pain Medicine, Toronto Western Hospital, University of Toronto, Toronto, ON, Canada
e-mail: kijinn.chin@uhn.ca

D. Jankovic, P. Peng (eds.), *Regional Nerve Blocks in Anesthesia and Pain Therapy*,
https://doi.org/10.1007/978-3-030-88727-8_40

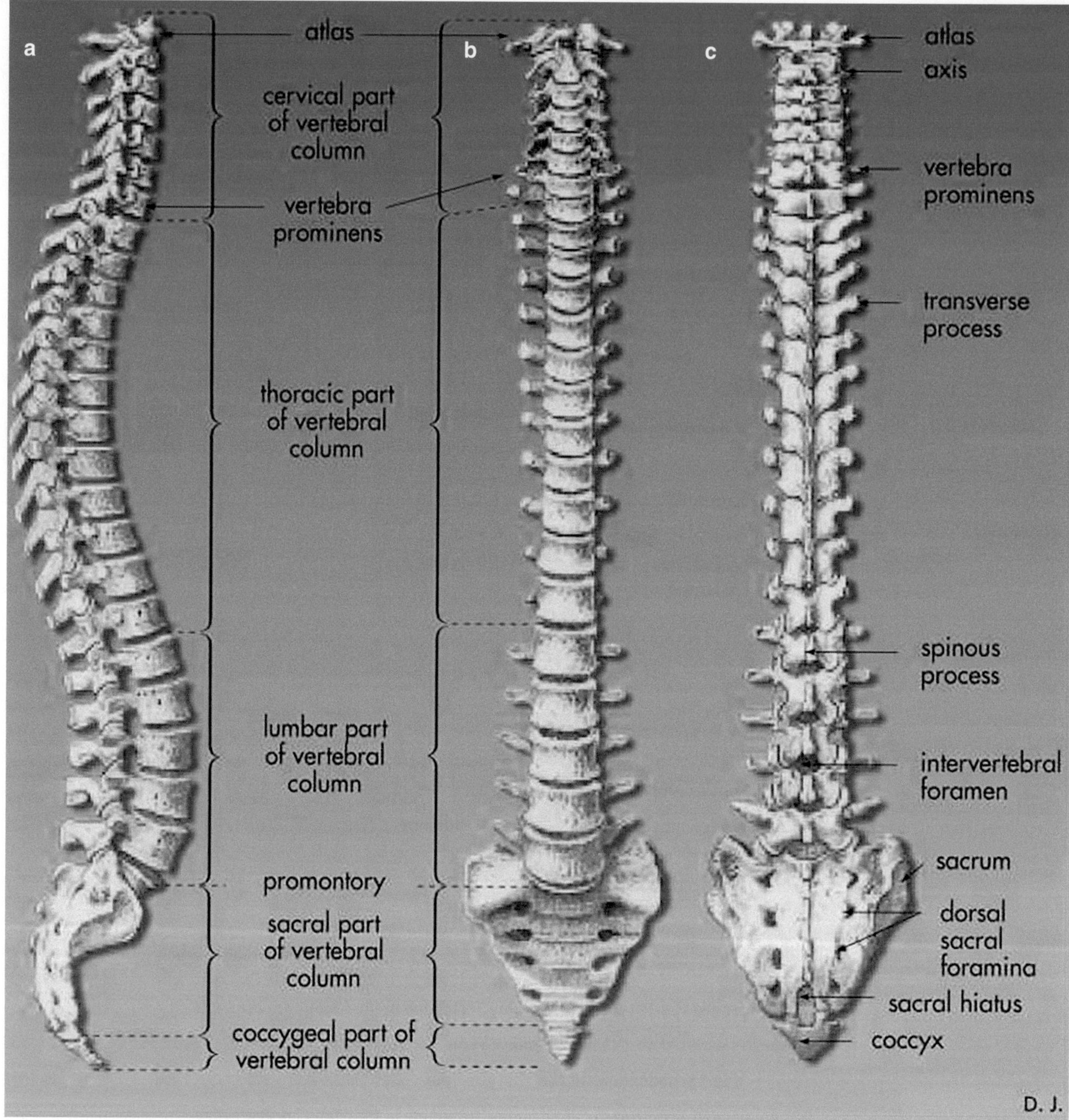

Fig. 40.1 (**a–c**) Spine. (**a**) Lateral, (**b**) Ventral, (**c**) Dorsal. (Reproduced with permission from Danilo Jankovic)

Spine and Sacrum Spine

The spinal column consists of 33 vertebrae—seven cervical vertebrae; 12 thoracic vertebrae; five lumbar vertebrae; the sacrum, consisting of five fused sacral vertebrae; and the coccyx, consisting of four fused coccygeal segments (Fig. 40.1a–c).

According to research findings, the mean length of the spinal column, from the foramen magnum to the tip of the coccyx, is 73.6 cm (range 67.4–78.8 cm), while in women it is 7–10 cm shorter.

All of the vertebrae have the same basic shape, which is subject to certain variations in the individual sections of the spine. The basic shape consists of an anterior body (the body of the vertebra) and a dorsal arch (the vertebral arch), which consists of pedicles and laminae (Fig. 40.2).

The laminae of the vertebral arch join dorsally to form the spinous process. A transverse process branches off on each side of the vertebral arch, as well as a superior and an inferior articular process.

The vertebrae in the cervical region are smaller, but their size increases from cranial to caudal. The angle of inclination of the spinous processes—important topographic signposts for neuraxial injections—varies at different levels of the spine.

The cervical spinous processes, the first two thoracic spinous processes and the lumbar spinous processes lie at the same level as their vertebrae. From T3 to L1, the spinous processes are angled caudally (particularly in the T4–T9 area) (Fig. 40.3a–c).

The vertebral canal (which provides excellent protection for the spinal cord) and the spinal cord, with its meningeal covering, extend throughout the whole length of the spine terminating in the cauda equina.

The spinal vessels and nerves emerge laterally through openings at the upper and lower margins of the roots of the arches of the adjoining vertebrae (the intervertebral foramina).

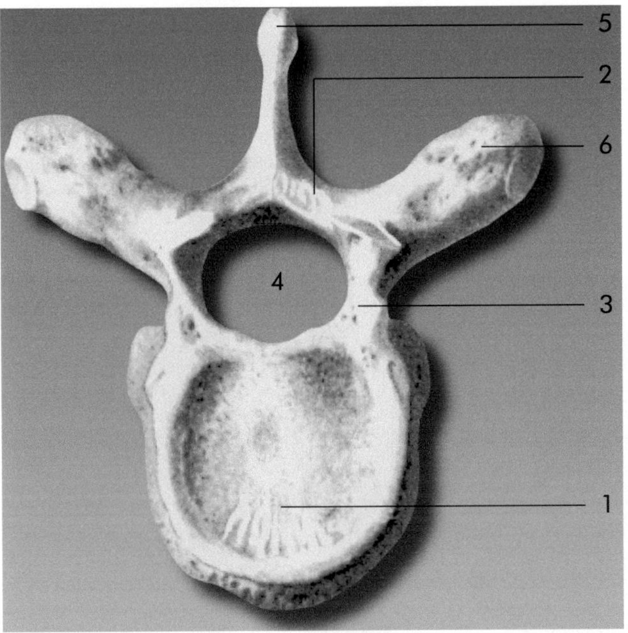

Fig. 40.2 Basic shape of a vertebra. (1) Vertebral body, (2) vertebral arch, (3) pedicle of the vertebral arch, (4) vertebral foramen, (5) spinous process, and (6) transverse process. (Reproduced with permission from Danilo Jankovic)

Sacrum

The sacrum is wedge-shaped and consists of five vertebrae fused together. It lies distal to the fifth lumbar vertebra and is connected distally, at its apex, to the coccyx. Dorsally, the sacrum has a convex surface, in the middle of which the median sacral crest stands out (Fig. 40.4a).

The crest is produced by the fusion of the rudimentary spinous processes of the upper third or fourth sacral vertebrae. Normally, the arch of the fifth and occasionally also of the fourth sacral vertebra is absent, so that there is a sacral hiatus at this point. The hiatus is bounded by the sacral horn as a remnant of the caudal articular process, and it is used as a passage by the five small sacral nerves and by the coccygeal nerves. Between the median sacral crest and the lateral sacral crest lie the four sacral openings (the posterior sacral foramina), through which the dorsal branches of the sacral spinal nerves emerge. The anterior view shows a concave aspect. Alongside the transverse lines (fused vertebrae), there are large anterior openings (the anterior pelvic sacral foramina), through which the primary anterior parts of the sacral nerves emerge (Fig. 40.4b).

Spinal Ligaments

The vertebrae are supported from the axis to the cranial sacrum by intervertebral disks and by various ligaments (Fig. 40.5a, b). The intervertebral disks lie between neighboring vertebrae and function as fixed connecting elements and pressure-absorbing buffers. The disks are at their thinnest in the area of T3–T7 and thickest in the lumbar area.

The anterior longitudinal ligament (Figs. 40.6 and 40.7) is attached at the anterior edge of the vertebral bodies and intervertebral disks and is at its thickest in the thoracic area. The posterior longitudinal ligament (Figs. 40.6 and 40.7) is wider cranially than it is caudally and it lies behind the vertebral bodies in the medullary canal. The supraspinous

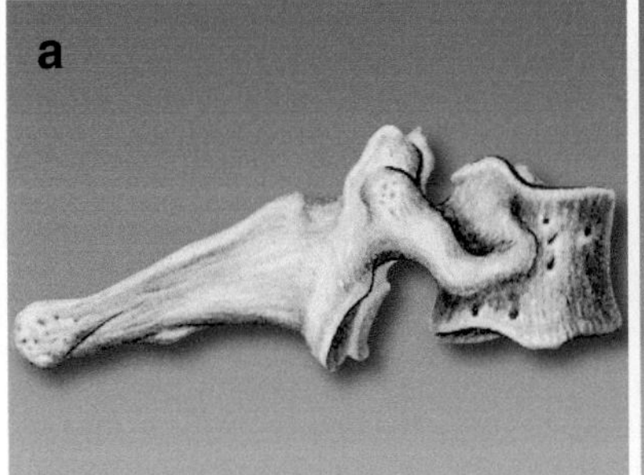

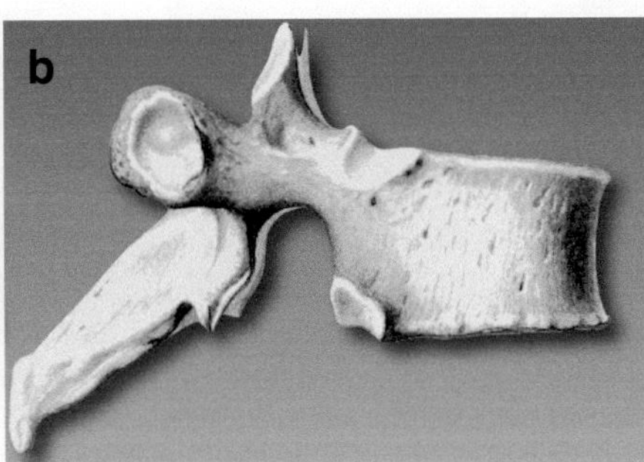

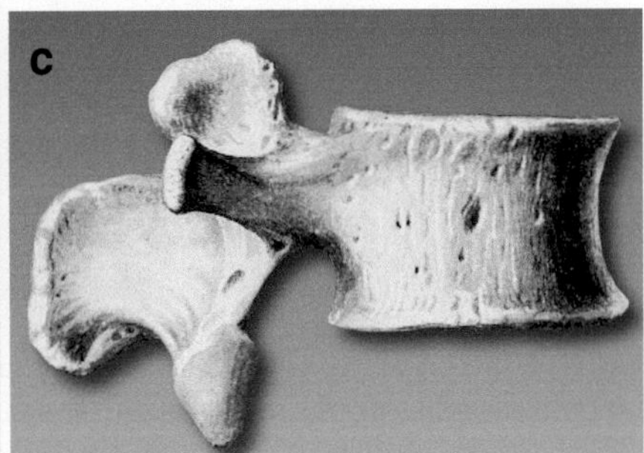

Fig. 40.3 (**a**–**c**) Cervical, thoracic, and lumbar spinous processes. (**a**) C7 cervical vertebra (vertebra prominens, nuchal tubercle). (**b**) T8 thoracic vertebra. (**c**) L3 lumbar vertebra. (Reproduced with permission from Danilo Jankovic)

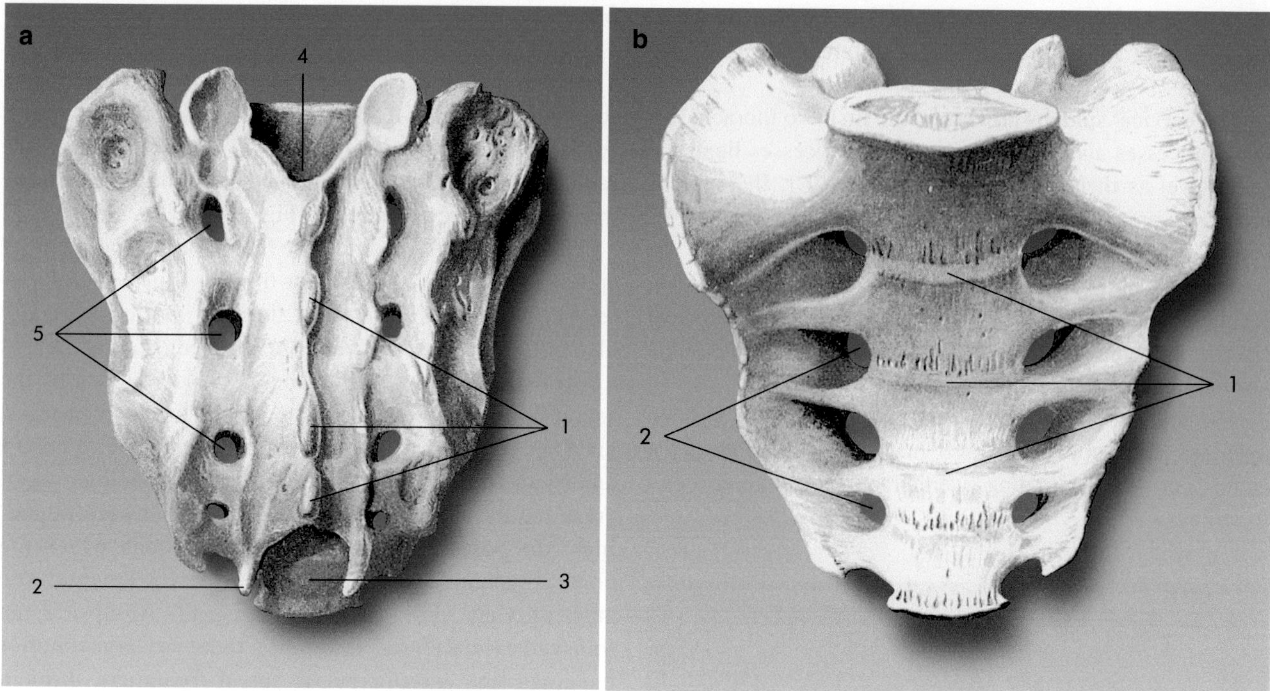

Fig. 40.4 (**a**) Sacrum (dorsal view). (1) Median sacral crest, (2) sacral horn, (3) sacral hiatus, (4) sacral canal, (5) posterior sacral foramina (Reproduced with permission from Danilo Jankovic). (**b**) Sacrum (ventral view). (1) Transverse lines, (2) anterior pelvic sacral foramina. (Reproduced with permission from Danilo Jankovic)

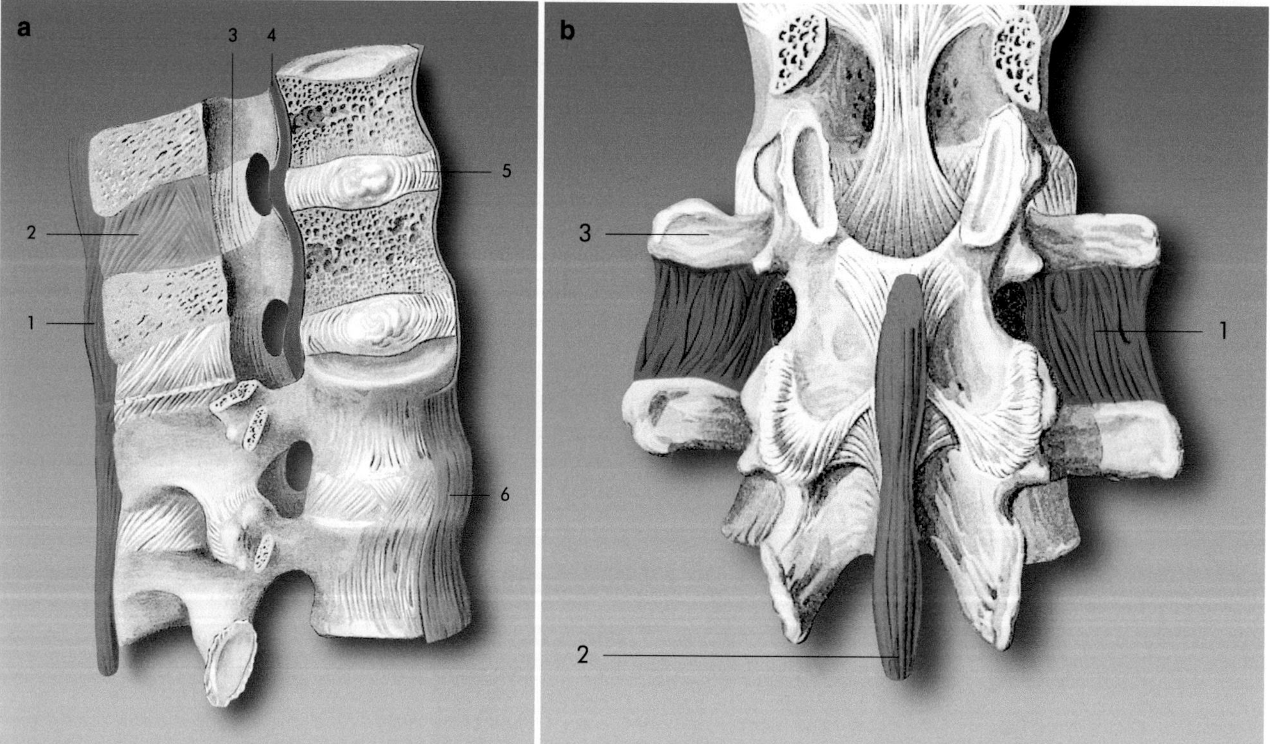

Fig. 40.5 (**a**) Ligaments of the spinal cord. (1) Supraspinous ligament, (2) interspinous ligament, (3) ligamentum flavum, (4) posterior longitudinal ligament, (5) intervertebral disk, (6) anterior longitudinal ligament (Reproduced with permission from Danilo Jankovic). (**b**) Ligaments of the spinal cord. (1) Intertransverse ligament, (2) supraspinous ligament, (3) transverse process. (Reproduced with permission from Danilo Jankovic)

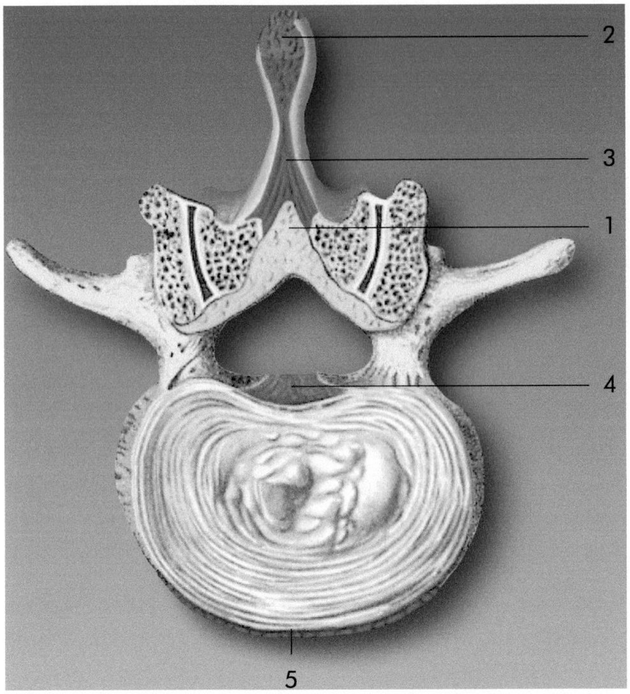

Fig. 40.6 Ligaments of the spinal cord. (1) Ligamentum flavum, (2) supraspinous ligament, (3) interspinous ligament, (4) posterior longitudinal ligament, (5) anterior longitudinal ligament. (Reproduced with permission from Danilo Jankovic)

ligaments extend as far as the sacrum along the tips of the spinous processes, with which they are connected, and continue cranially in the nuchal ligament and caudally in the interspinous ligament. They become thicker from cranial to caudal. The interspinous ligaments connect the roots and tips of the spinous processes.

The intertransverse ligaments serve to connect the transverse processes (Fig. 40.5b).

The ligamentum flavum largely consists of yellow, elastic fibers and it connects the neighboring laminae (Figs. 40.6 and 40.7). It is at its thinnest in the midline (small fissure spaces exist for the veins running from the internal vertebral venous plexus to the external vertebral venous plexus), and its thickness increases laterally. The size and shape of the ligamentum flavum vary at the various levels of the spine. Caudally, for example, it is thicker than in the cranial direction.

There are usually only 22 genuine ligamenta flava, as they do not develop between the atlas and occiput or between the atlas and the axis. The mean length of the ligamentum flavum is 0.84 cm in the cervical spine, 1.03 cm in the thoracic spine, and 1.61 cm in the lumbar spine. The mean width is 2.30 cm in the cervical region, 2.0 cm in the thoracic region, and 3.22 cm in the lumbar region. The ligamenta flava have a mean thickness of 1.37 mm in the cervical spine, 1.75 mm in the thoracic spine, and 2.55 mm in the lumbar spine. According to Yong-Hing et al. (1976), the human ligamentum flavum consists of 50%–80% elastin and 20%–50% collagen.

Iliolumbosacral Ligaments (Sacroiliac Joints)

The stability of the iliolumbosacral region is ensured by lumbosacral and sacroiliac connections that transfer the entire weight of the trunk via the hip bones to the lower extremities. These ligamentous connections serve to connect the vertebrae with one another and to stabilize the sacrum.

Clinically important ligaments: interspinous, supraspinous, iliolumbar, interosseous sacroiliac, sacrospinous and sacrotuberous ligaments (Figs. 40.8a, b).

Spinal Cord

The mean length of the spinal cord from the foramen magnum downward is 45.9 cm in men and 41.5 cm in women. The conus medullaris continues in the threadlike median filum terminale as far as the posterior side of the coccyx (Figs. 40.7, 40.9a–c, and 40.13).

Rootlets: Cauda Equina

The cauda equina is generally regarded as consisting of the thick, horsetail-shaped fascicle of nerve fibers in the lower part of the dural sac, containing the paired rootlets of the lowest thoracic and entire lumbar and coccygeal medulla. All of the motor and sensory fibers of the lumbosacral plexus, pudendal nerve, and coccygeal nerve course inside the lumbosacral subarachnoid space. A constant increase in the thickness of the root fascicle is seen between the L1 and L3 segments. The terminal filum of the spinal cord is approximately 153 mm long (range 123–178 mm) (Figs. 40.9b, 40.11, 40.13 and 40.14).

The dura mater and arachnoid, and consequently the subarachnoid space as well, extend downward as far as the level of the second sacral vertebra.

Meninges

The spinal cord is surrounded and protected by the meninges (the dura mater, arachnoid mater, and pia mater) and by cerebrospinal fluid, epidural fatty tissue and veins (Figs. 40.10 and 40.11).

The meninges form a connected, unified organ with important protective functions for the brain and spinal cord; they provide mechanical, immunological, and thermal protection and are also important for metabolism in the

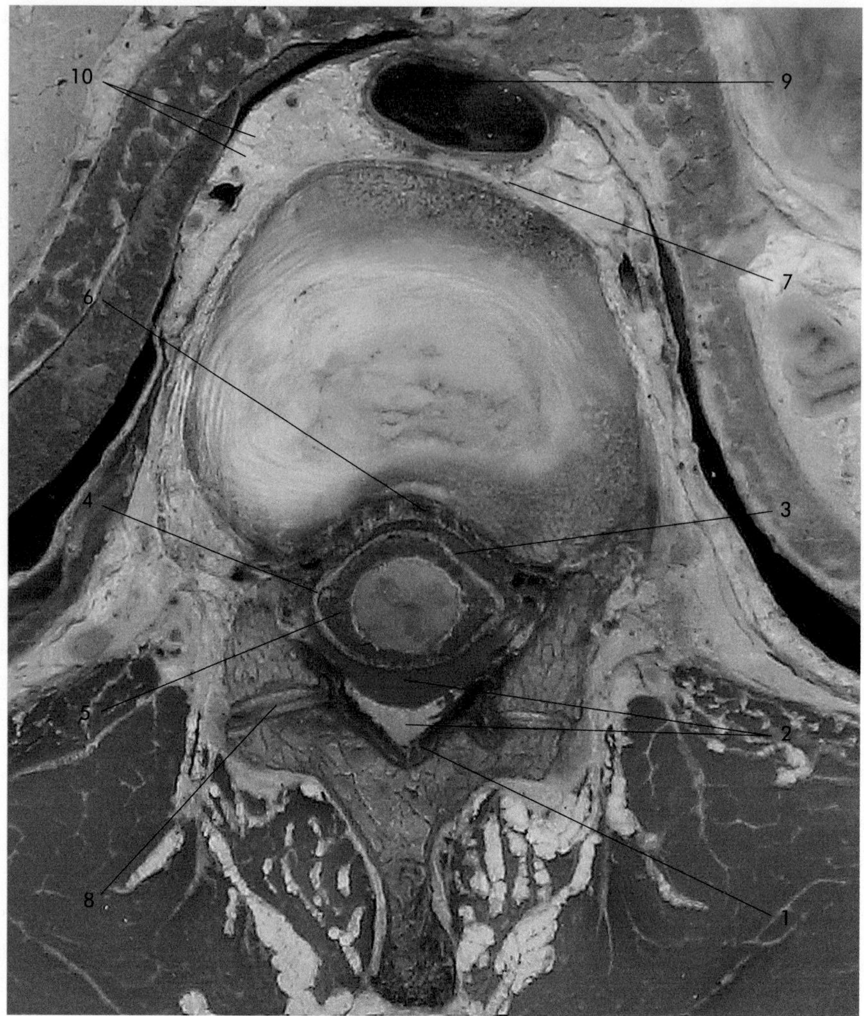

Fig. 40.7 Transverse section through the thorax at the level of T9. (1) Ligamentum flavum, (2) posterior epidural space, (3) anterior epidural space, (4) spinal dura mater, (5) subarachnoid space and spinal cord, (6) posterior longitudinal ligament, (7) anterior longitudinal ligament, (8) zygapophysial joint, (9) aorta, (10) sympathetic trunk ganglion. (Reproduced with permission from Danilo Jankovic)

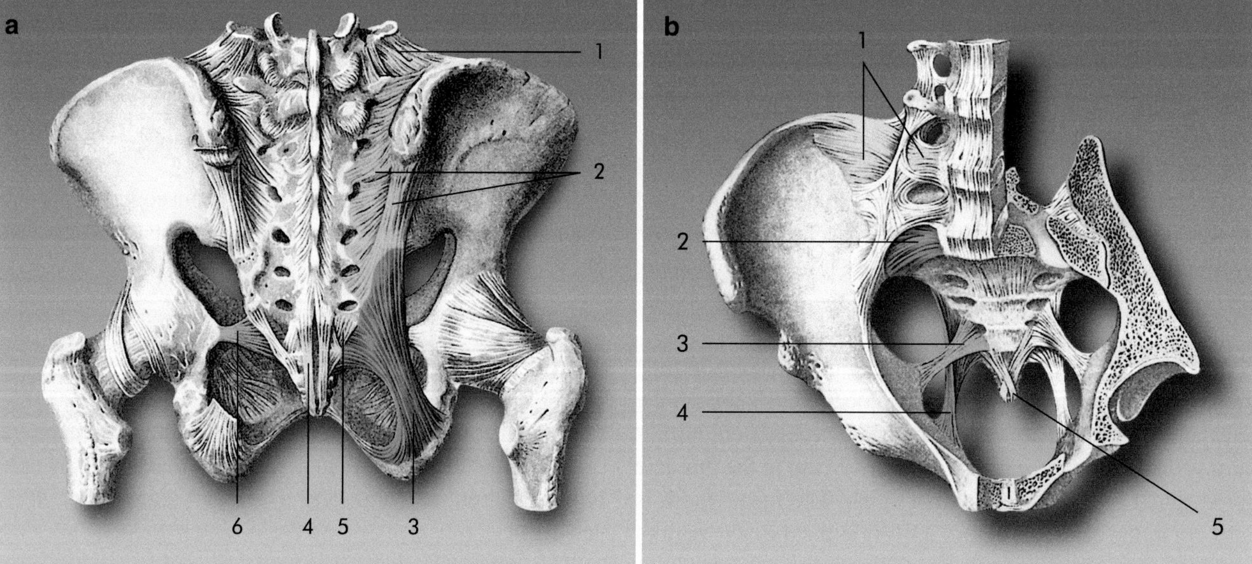

Fig. 40.8 (**a**) Iliolumbosacral ligaments (dorsal view). (1) Iliolumbar ligament, (2) dorsal sacroiliac ligament, (3) sacrotuberous ligament, (4) superficial dorsal and deep dorsal sacrococcygeal ligaments, (5) lateral sacrococcygeal ligament, (6) sacrospinous ligament(Reproduced with permission from Danilo Jankovic). (**b**) Iliolumbosacral ligaments (ventral view). (1) Iliolumbar ligament, (2) ventral sacroiliac ligament, (3) sacrospinous ligament, (4) sacrotuberous ligament, (5) ventral sacrococcygeal ligament. (Reproduced with permission from Danilo Jankovic)

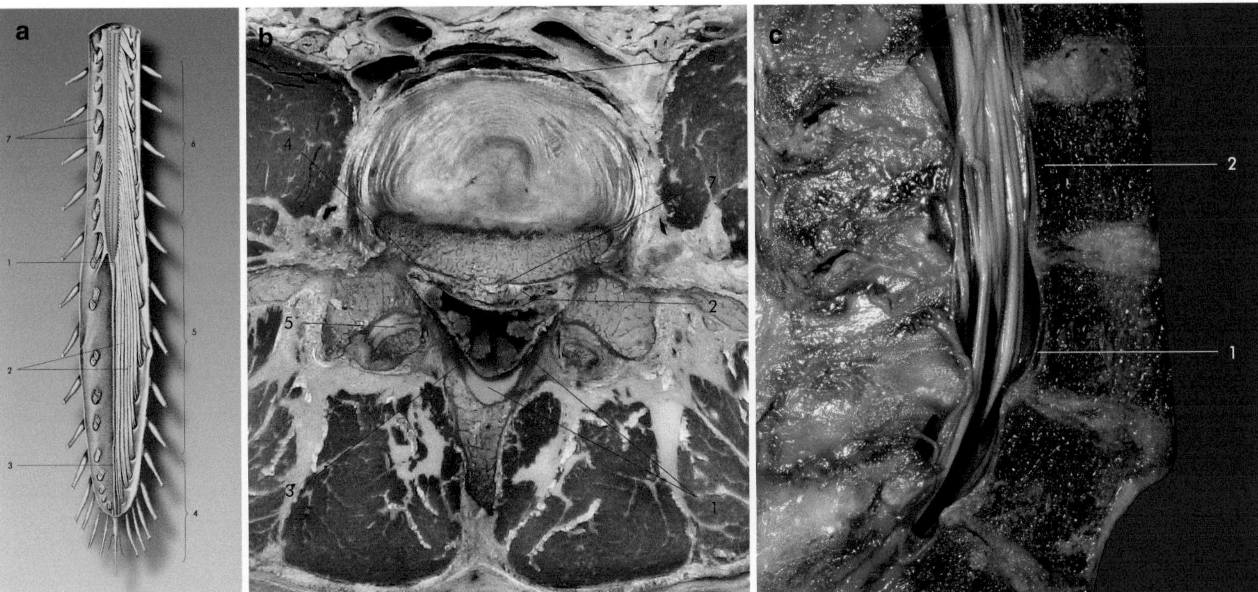

Fig. 40.9 (**a**) Spinal cord (lower half). (1) Conus medullaris, (2) cauda equina, (3) filum of spinal dura mater (filum terminale), (4) sacral nerves, (5) lumbar nerves, (6) thoracic nerves, (7) dura mater. (Reproduced with permission from Danilo Jankovic). (**b**) Transverse section at the level of L4/5. (1) posterior epidural space with fat, (2) anterior epidural space with veins, (3) spinal dura mater, (4) subarachnoid space and cauda equina, (5) zygapophysial joint, (6) anterior longitudinal ligament, (7) posterior longitudinal ligament. (Reproduced with permission from Danilo Jankovic). (**c**) The cauda equina at the level of L2–5. Lateral view. (1) Spinal dura mater, (2), epidural space. (Reproduced with permission from Danilo Jankovic)

CNS. The mechanical function of the meninges consists of providing fixation for the brain in the cranium and for the spinal cord in the vertebral canal, as well as in forming a highly adaptable fluid mantle that functions like a water-bed. The fixation is provided by the dura mater.

Dura Mater of the Spinal Cord (Figs. 40.7, 40.10, 40.11, 40.12, 40.13 and 40.14)

The dura mater of the spinal cord, a fibroelastic membrane, extends as far as the second sacral vertebra, where it ends in a blind sac. It encloses the anterior and posterior spinal nerve roots.

It surrounds the anterior and posterior spinal nerve roots. It consists of collagenous fibers and a few elastic fibers; it is 0.1–0.5 mm thick and is usually thinner anteriorly than it is posteriorly. The dural sac is often enlarged in the area between L4 and S1, and also between T12 and L1 (Spischarny's terminal cystoma). The thickness of the spinal dura mater declines from medial to lateral. The dura mater is often thinner ventrally than dorsally, and it sends off leaves and fibers into the epidural space. It shows notable foliation near the intervertebral foramina, where it passes on the one hand into the epineurium of the peripheral nerves and into the capsule of the spinal ganglia, and on the other radiates into the cavernous body of the vascular plexus characterizing this area. One of the major characteristics of the dura mater is its extremely marked vascularization. Particularly in the boundary zone with the arachnoid, numerous capillaries and venules are fenestrated, promoting the exchange of various metabolites and cells between the blood and dura. The vascularization increases strongly in the lateral areas, particularly in the area of the dural infundibulum. The dural vessels are connected with the epidural vascular plexus and thus with the internal and external vertebral vein plexus as well. There are numerous nerve fibers in close proximity to the dural vessels. In terms of size, C fibers predominate. In terms of function, the dural nerves consist of sympathetic, parasympathetic, and sensory fibers. A whole range of neurotransmitters and neuropeptides have been identified in the dural nerves, such as acetylcholine, serotonin, substance P, calcitonin gene-related peptide (CGRP), neuropeptide Y, vasoactive intestinal polypeptide (VIP), etc. In addition to vasoactive nerves, local factors also play a role in the regulation of dural perfusion, such as adenosine, which has been found abundantly in the dura. Via a multilayered cell cluster known as the subdural nerve papilla (neurothele), the arachnoid membrane is directly connected with the innermost lamellae of the dura. A "subdural fissure"—often presents postmortem and only arising during life in specific circumstances—must be regarded as an artefact.

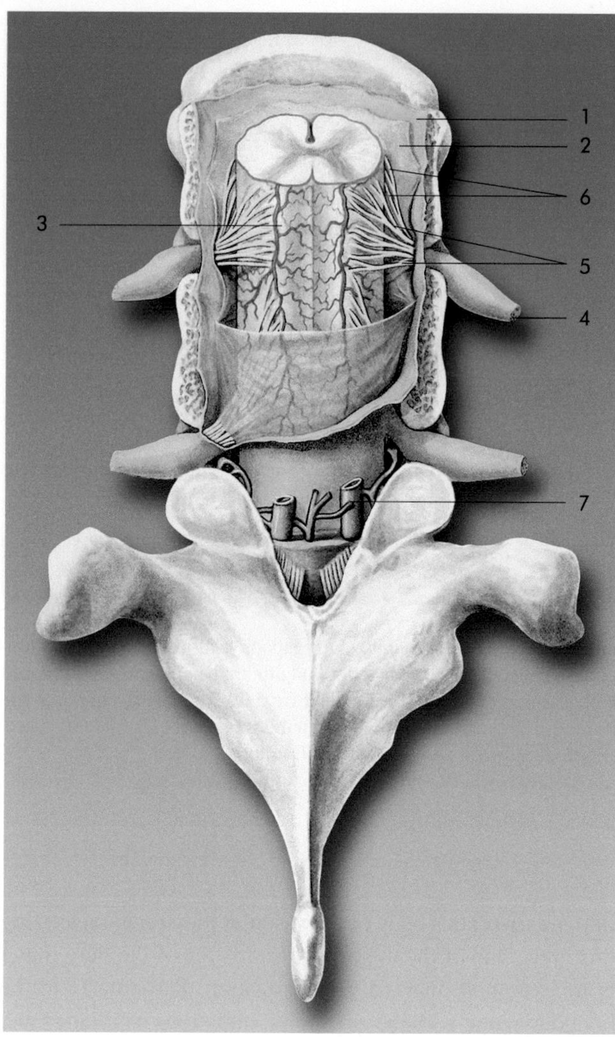

Fig. 40.10 Meninges. (1) Dura mater, (2) arachnoid mater, (3) pia mater, (4) spinal nerve, (5) dorsal (posterior) root, (6) ventral (anterior) root, (7) internal vertebral venous plexus. (Reproduced with permission from Danilo Jankovic)

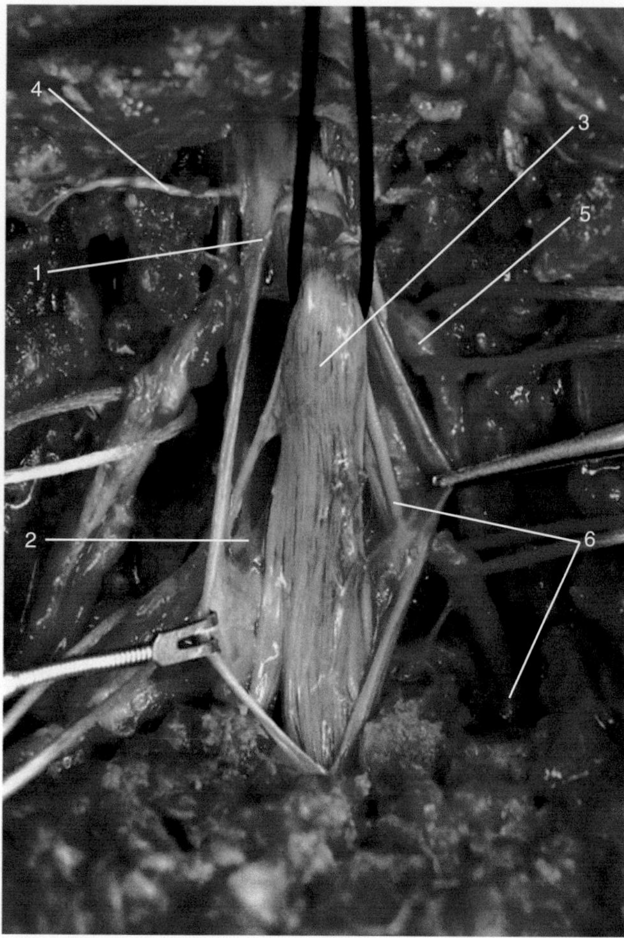

Fig. 40.11 A lumbar vertebral canal opened from posterior in the area of L3 and L4. The cauda equina has been exposed by partial resection of the spinal dura mater and arachnoid mater. (1) Spinal dura mater, (2) arachnoid mater, (3) with posterior and anterior roots, (4) dorsal root, (5) spinal ganglion, (6) posterior and anterior spinal branches. (Reproduced with permission from Danilo Jankovic)

Between the dura mater and the arachnoid, there is a space, the subdural space, in which a small amount of lymph-like fluid is located.

The arachnoid mater (Figs. 40.10 and 40.11), a non-vascularized membrane, also ends at the level of the second sacral vertebra. Between the arachnoid mater and the pia mater lies the subarachnoid space, which is filled with cerebrospinal fluid (see section "Cerebrospinal Fluid"). The expansion forces present here reduce the weight of the brain "floating" in the cerebrospinal fluid to just under 50 g.

This protects the brain from harmful acceleration forces.

The same applies to the spinal cord. There is a substantial amount of exchange between the cranial and spinal cerebrospinal fluid. Magnetic resonance studies have confirmed Du Boulay's older view that there are fluid waves synchronous with cardiac systole that move the cerebrospinal fluid from the basal cisterns into the cervical subarachnoid space, respiration-synchronous fluid movements are superimposed. The spinal subarachnoid space, with the extremely elastic spinal dura and adaptable arachnoid, makes it possible to absorb these rhythmic fluid waves (compliance). Artificial losses of cerebrospinal fluid undoubtedly have severe effects on the system's natural mechanism and reduce the water-bed function of the exterior subarachnoid space. The subarachnoid space is important for thermoregulation of the CNS, as it acts as a temperature buffer both against excessive external temperatures and also against functional or pathological increases in temperature in the CNS. The normal basic temperature of the cerebrospinal fluid is approximately 37 °C. It is important to note that the cerebrospinal fluid does not represent "standing water" but is instead constantly in movement and continually being freshly produced, mainly in the choroid plexus. It is reabsorbed over a wide surface, not only via the arachnoid

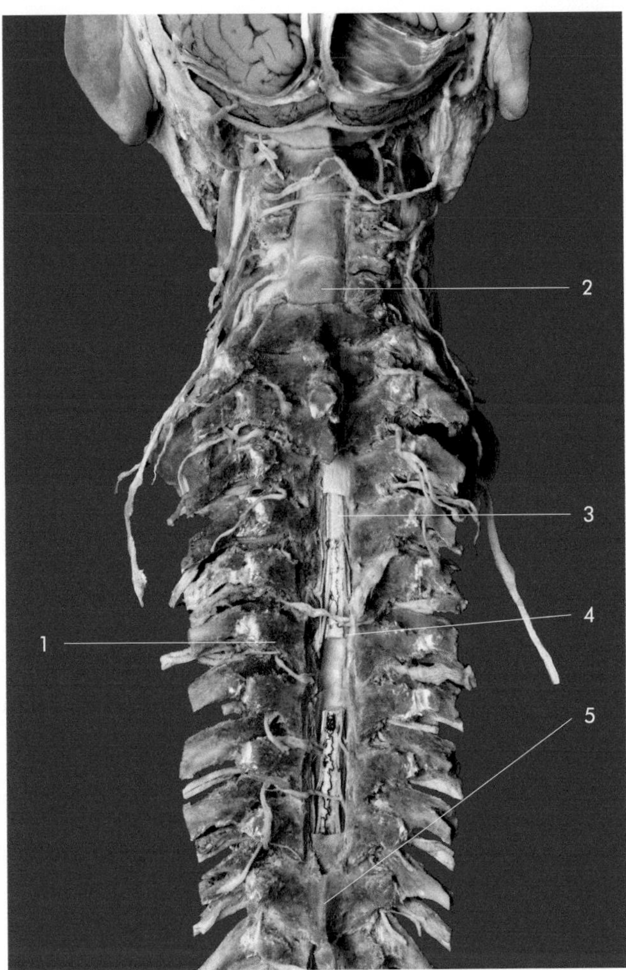

Fig. 40.12 Thoracic region of the spine. (1) Transverse process, (2) spinal dura mater (note the covering of the spinal ganglion), (3) spinal cord with vessels lying above it; the denticulate ligament is located to the left and right, (4) the spinal dura mater has been removed; posterior longitudinal ligament, (5) thoracic spinous process; note the epidural space above. (With permission from Danilo Jankovic)

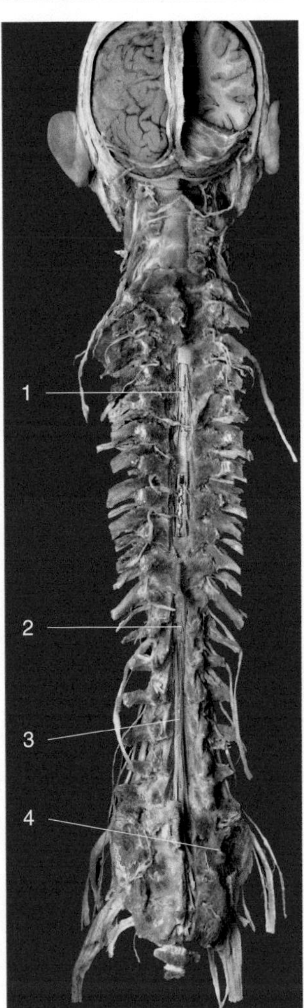

Fig. 40.13 The spinal cord. (1) Spinal cord with vessels on it; the denticulate ligament is located to the right and left, (2) conus medullaris, (3) terminal filum with cauda equina, (4) sacrum. (Reproduced with permission from Danilo Jankovic)

granulations or villi in the area of the nerve exit sites, but also diffusely through the arachnoid into the dural vascular system and via the pia into the vessels of the pial vascular network. The choroid plexus is not only a production organ, but also a site for reabsorption of cerebrospinal fluid.

The spinal pia mater (Figs. 40.10 and 40.13) is a thin, very well vascularized membrane that tightly encloses the spinal cord.

Caudal to the medullary cone, it develops into the thin filum terminale, which descends medial to the cauda equina, penetrates the final part of the dural sac and arachnoid, and fuses with the connective tissue posterior to the first coccygeal segment.

The pia mater sends off 22 denticulate ligaments on each side, which attach to the dura mater and thus stabilize the spinal cord (Figs. 40.10, 40.12 and 40.13).

Spinal Nerves

There are 31 pairs of spinal nerves in the human: eight cervical pairs, 12 thoracic pairs, five lumbar pairs, five sacral pairs, and one coccygeal pair. These are connected to the spinal cord by a series of ventral and dorsal radicular filaments, which combine to form the nerve roots (Figs. 40.7, 40.10, 40.11, 40.12, 40.15, and 40.16).

The thicker dorsal (posterior) root is responsible for conducting afferent impulses (pain, temperature, touch, position). Each of the dorsal spinal nerve roots has a sensory spinal ganglion incorporated in it.

The ventral (anterior) root is responsible for conducting efferent impulses (muscles, glands). The nerve roots in the lower segments of the spinal cord descend in the horsetail-like cauda equina to their exit openings.

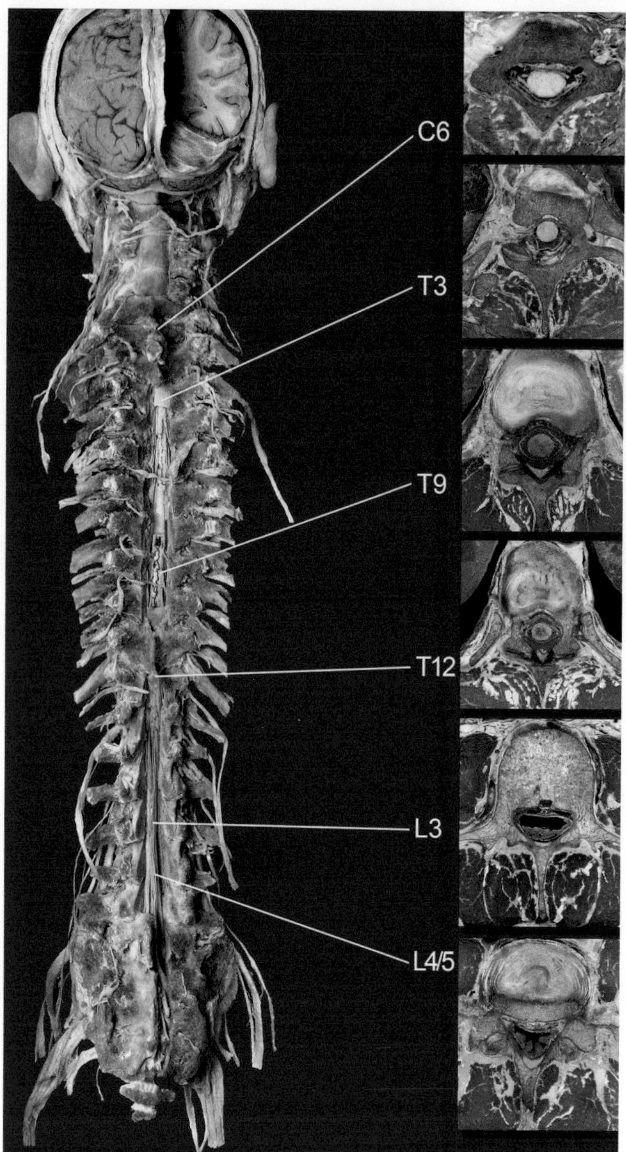

Fig. 40.14 The spinal cord. Cervical, thoracic, and lumbar. Serial transverse sections at the levels of C6, T3, T9, T12, L3, and L4/5. Note the conus medullaris (T12) and cauda equina (L3, L4/5). (Reproduced with permission from Danilo Jankovic)

After exiting from the subarachnoid space, the ventral and dorsal roots cross the epidural space.

In spinal anesthesia, the nerve roots are the principal targets for local anesthesia (Figs. 40.7, 40.14 and 40.15).

Spinal Dermatomes

Via its branching spinal nerves, each segment of the spinal cord provides the sensory supply for a specific area of skin, known as the dermatome. These areas of skin, which often overlap, are very important for checking and verifying the spread of anesthesia (Fig. 40.16a, b).

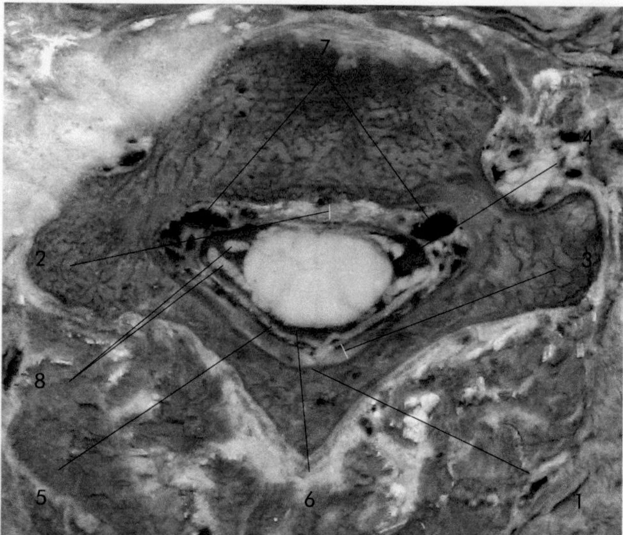

Fig. 40.15 Transverse section at the level of the C6 segment. (1) Ligamentum flavum, (2) anterior epidural space, (3) posterior epidural space, (4) subarachnoid space with the spinal cord, (5) spinal dura mater, (6) spinal pia mater, (7) epidural veins, (8) anterior and posterior spinal nerve roots. (Reproduced with permission from Danilo Jankovic)

Arteries of the Spinal Cord

The spinal cord is supplied by numerous radicular arteries, which form the anterior spinal artery and twin posterior spinal arteries.

The radicular arteries branch off from the cervical vertebral artery, the thoracic intercostal arteries and the abdominal lumbar arteries (Figs. 40.17 and 40.18).

The anterior spinal artery, which arises from the fourth segment of the vertebral arteries, accompanies the spinal cord in the midline (anterior median fissure) along its entire course.

Via the central branches and small branches of the arterial pial network, the anterior spinal artery supplies the anterior two-thirds of the spinal cord.

The cervical and first two thoracic spinal cord segments receive blood from the radicular branches of subclavian artery branches.

In the mediothoracic spinal cord region (T3–T7), there is a radicular branch at the level of T4 or T5.

The thoracolumbar segment of the spinal cord (T8 to the medullary cone) draws its arterial supply mainly from the large-caliber arteria radicularis magnus. The artery of Adamkiewicz (the major anterior radicular artery) has a large anterior and a smaller posterior radicular branch.

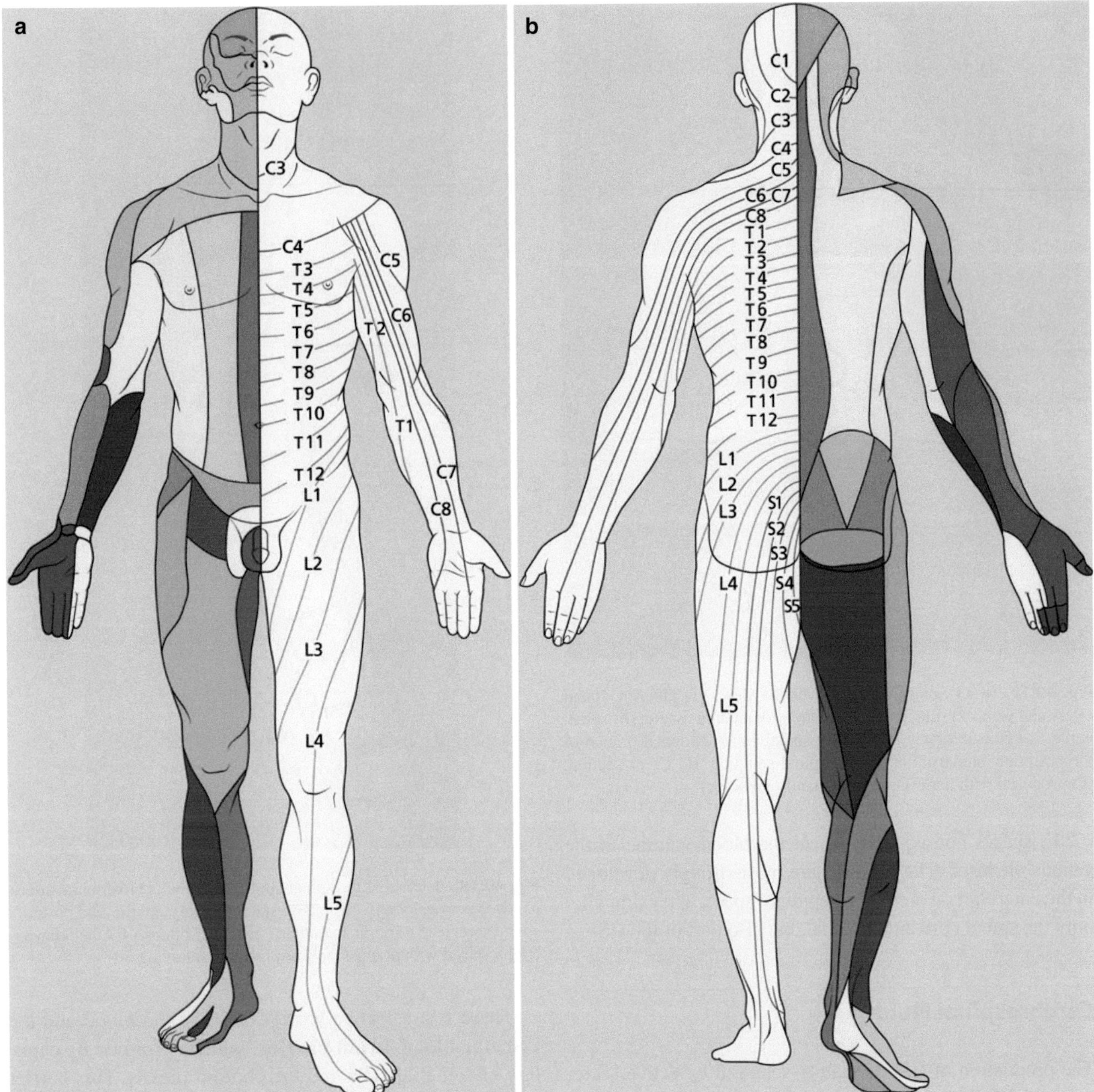

Fig. 40.16 (**a**) Spinal dermatomes and the corresponding spinal cord segments. (Reproduced with permission from Danilo Jankovic). (**b**) Cutaneous innervation areas (detailed descriptions are given in the relevant chapters). (Reproduced with permission from Danilo Jankovic)

The cauda equina is supplied by branches of the lumbar, iliolumbar, and lateral or median sacral arteries.

These also supply the medullary cone.

The paired posterior spinal arteries arise from the fourth segment of the vertebral artery, receiving flow from 10 to 23 posterior radicular branches, and supply the dorsal third of the spinal cord.

Thin pial branches run from the spinal arteries, forming a network on the surface of the spinal cord known as the arterial pial network.

Veins of the Spinal Cord and Vertebrae

The entire spinal canal is traversed by two venous plexuses, the internal and external vertebral venous plexuses (Fig. 40.19a, b).

Together, these form a ring around each vertebra, freely anastomosing with one another and receiving flow from the vertebrae, ligaments, and spinal cord. They are largely avalvular. Pressure changes in the thoracic or cerebrospinal fluid

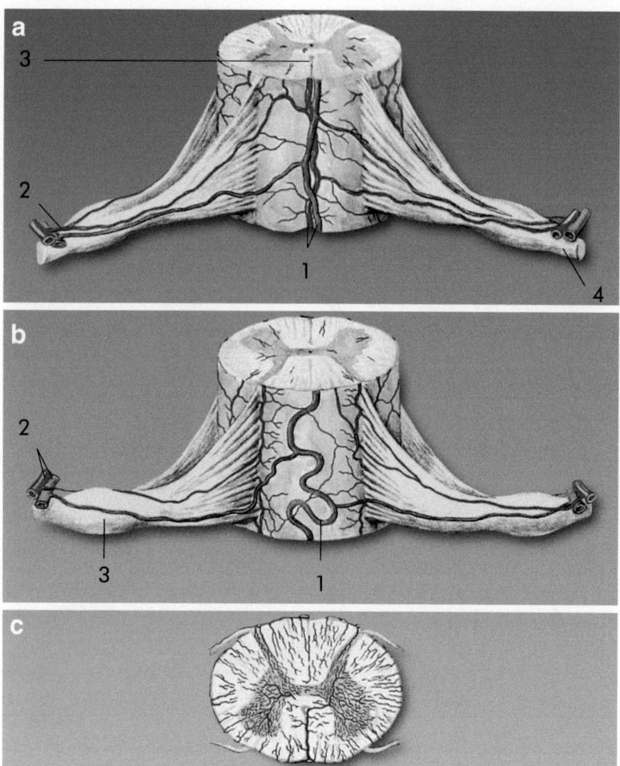

Fig. 40.17 (a–c) Spinal cord. (a) Ventral view: (1) anterior spinal artery and vein, (2) spinal branch, (3) anterior median fissure, (4) spinal nerve. (b) Dorsal view: (1) posterior spinal vein, (2) dorsal branch of the posterior intercostal artery, (3) spinal ganglion. (c) Cross-section. (Reproduced with permission from Danilo Jankovic)

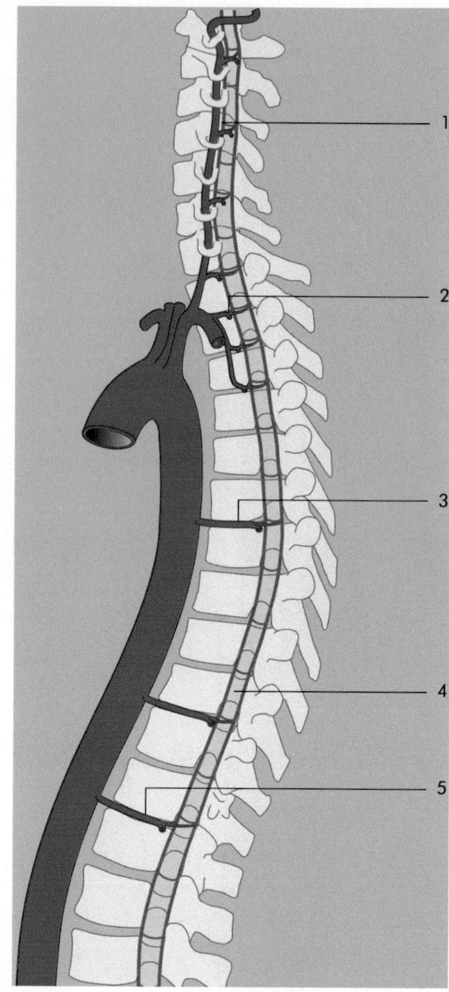

Fig. 40.18 Arteries of the spinal cord (side view). (1) Vertebral artery, (2) deep cervical artery, (3) intercostal artery, (4) anterior and posterior spinal artery, (5) arteria radicularis magnus: artery of Adamkiewicz. (Reproduced with permission from Danilo Jankovic)

(CSF) spaces consequently affect the blood volume in the venous plexuses. The plexuses are most strongly developed in the anterolateral area of the epidural space. They drain not only the spinal cord and its canal, but also part of the CSF.

Cerebrospinal Fluid

The production of CSF is mainly achieved by active secretion and diffusion through the epithelial cells of the **choroid plexus**, but also to a small extent in the **subarachnoid space** and **perivascularly**.

The main tasks of the cerebrospinal fluid are as follows:

- To function as a hemodynamic buffer and physical protection against forces affecting the spinal cord and brain.
- To substitute for the function of the lymphatic vessels, which are absent in the central nervous system.
- To allow metabolic exchange between blood and neural tissue.

There is a selective barrier between the blood and the CSF, the **blood–brain barrier**, which is formed by capillary endothelial cells and the choroid plexus. This barrier is clinically significant, as it is impermeable to many drugs.

The total quantity of the CSF in the adult is about 120–150 mL (with about 20–35 mL below the foramen ovale and about 15 mL below T5).

Approximately 400–450 mL of CSF is produced every day, and complete exchange of the fluid takes place every 10–12 h.

Lumbar **CSF pressure** in a supine position is about 6–10 cmH_2O, while in a seated position it is about 20–25 cmH_2O.

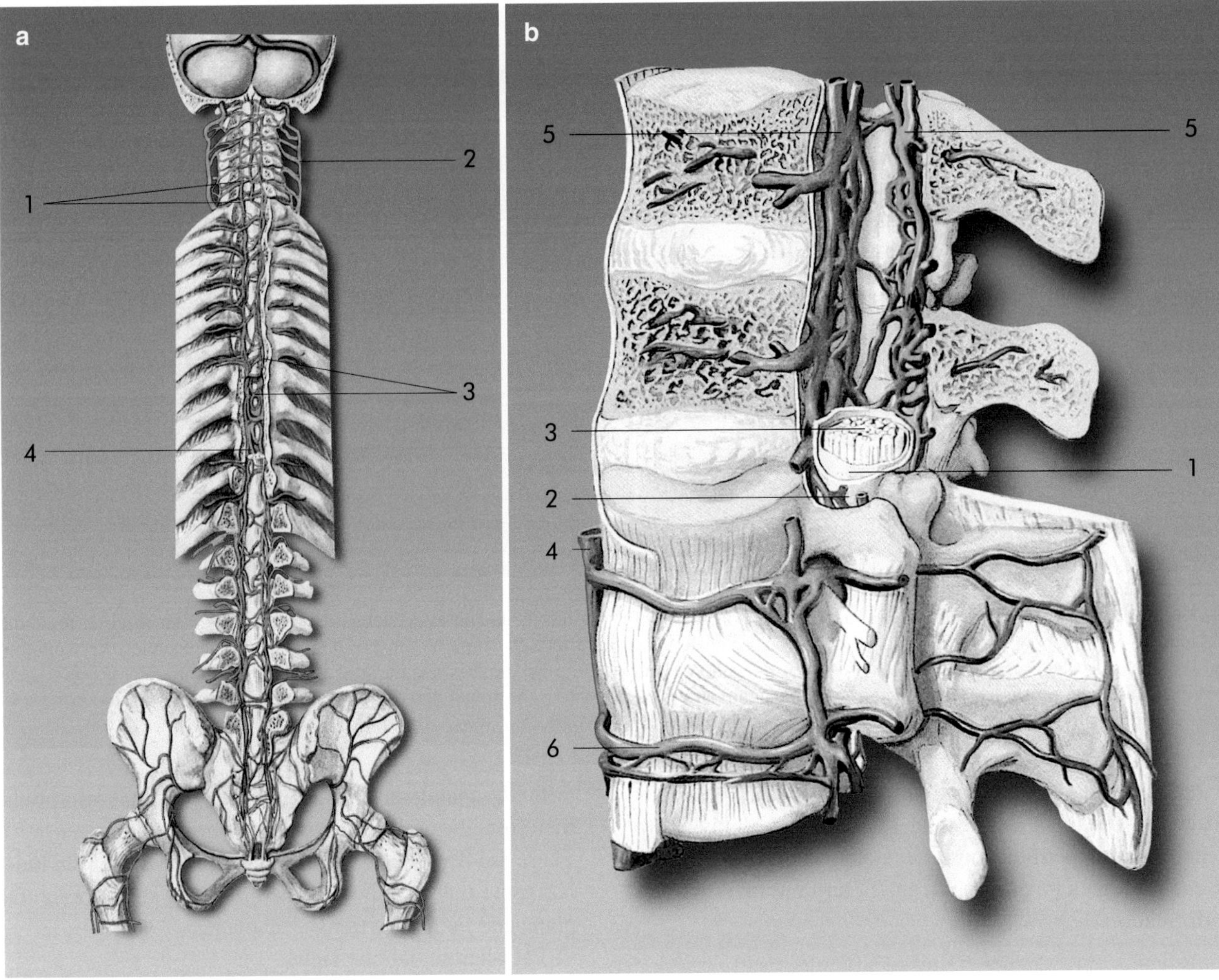

Fig. 40.19 (**a**) Veins of the spinal cord. (1) Vertebral veins, (2) deep cervical vein, (3) internal vertebral venous plexus, (4) spinal veins (Reproduced with permission from Danilo Jankovic). (**b**) Veins of the spinal cord (lumbar region). (1) Arachnoid, (2) dura mater, (3) cauda equina, (4) inferior vena cava, (5) internal vertebral venous plexus, (6) lumbar vein. (With permission from Danilo Jankovic)

The **specific gravity** of the CSF is 1.007 (1.003–1.009), and this must be taken into account in relation to the local anesthetic being used.

The **osmolarity** of CSF is comparable with that of the blood plasma (300 osmol/L), and the pH value is approximately the same as the physiological value. Injected drugs mainly spread by diffusion, since CSF in the spinal canal circulates very little, if at all. **Resorption** of CSF into the blood takes place via the **arachnoid granulations** and through the walls of the capillary vessels in the central nervous system and pia mater.

The liquid in the CSF sheaths of the cranial nerves and in the root pockets of the spinal nerves is an exception to the above rule. This liquid can enter the extradural lymphatic vessels directly.

Ultrasound Imaging for Central Neuraxial Blockade

Introduction

The main technical challenge in central neuraxial blockade is to identify a soft-tissue window into the vertebral canal. This is usually inferred from palpation of the spinous processes and tactile feedback from the needle tip as it is inserted. However, this can be difficult if surface landmarks are obscured, altered, or absent, or if the interspinous and interlaminar spaces are narrowed by age-related changes. Technical difficulty and multiple needle insertion attempts are associated with patient discomfort, and more importantly, with serious complications including spinal hematoma and neurologic injury.

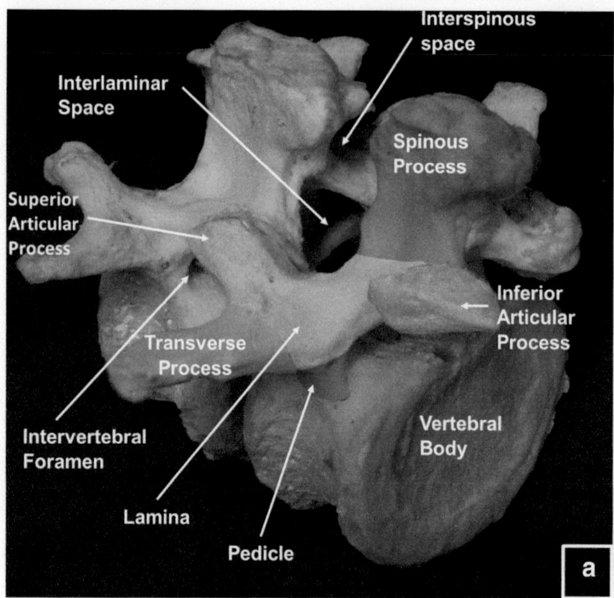

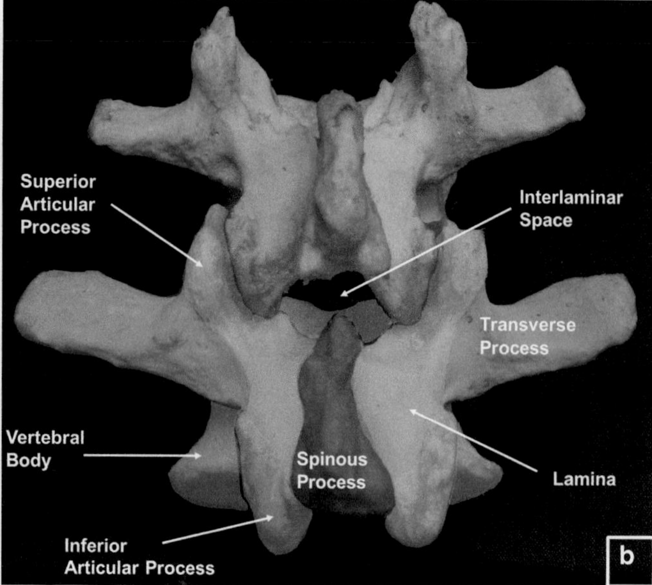

Fig. 40.20 Three-quarter oblique view (**a**) and posterior view (**b**) of adjacent lumbar vertebrae. The interlaminar space is located posteriorly and is bounded by the bases of the spinous processes, the laminae, and the inferior articular processes. It is roofed over by the ligamentum flavum. The interspinous space lies in the midline and is filled by the supraspinous and interspinous ligaments. The intervertebral foramina are located laterally and are bounded by the pedicles, the vertebral body, the laminae, and the superior and inferior articular processes and contain the spinal nerve roots and their accompanying blood vessels. (Courtesy of www.usra.ca)

Pre-procedural ultrasound imaging of the spine is extremely useful in delineating the spinal anatomy more clearly, which permits more accurate planning of needle insertion, trajectory, and depth, and in turn improves ease of performance.

Anatomy and Sonoanatomy of the Lumbar Spine

- Knowledge of the gross bony anatomy of the spine is essential for interpretation of neuraxial ultrasound. It is particularly important to appreciate the contours of the posterior bony surfaces of the spine (Fig. 40.20) as these are responsible for the characteristic shapes of the acoustic dropout shadows seen on ultrasound.
- A curvilinear low-frequency ultrasound probe with its wider field of view and better beam penetration is recommended for use in all adult patients.
- Two planes and ultrasound probe orientations are commonly used to image the spine (Fig. 40.21):
  - Transverse (or axial).
  - Parasagittal (or longitudinal).
- The transverse plane is most useful in determining an appropriate needle insertion point for a midline approach. The parasagittal plane on the other hand provides valuable additional information on the location and identity of interlaminar spaces, particularly in the patient with more difficult anatomy. The ultrasound examination should therefore always utilize both probe orientations.
- There are five typical ultrasonographic views of the lumbar spine that may be obtained: three in the parasagittal plane and two in the transverse plane.
  - Parasagittal oblique view.
  - Parasagittal transverse process view.
  - Parasagittal articular process view.
  - Transverse midline interlaminar view.
  - Transverse midline spinous process view.
- The parasagittal oblique (PSO) and transverse midline (TM) interlaminar views are the two most important views to obtain.

Parasagittal Oblique (PSO) View

- The probe is placed in a longitudinal parasagittal orientation and angled towards the midline to direct the beam through the paramedian interlaminar spaces.
- The beam transects the sloping laminae of the lumbar vertebrae, producing a characteristic "sawtooth" pattern of acoustic shadows (Fig. 40.22).
- Two hyperechoic linear structures are seen in the interlaminar gap between the "sawteeth." The more superficial one that adjoins the bases of adjacent "sawteeth" is the **posterior complex** and represents the ligamentum flavum, epidural space, and posterior dura. The deeper hyperechoic

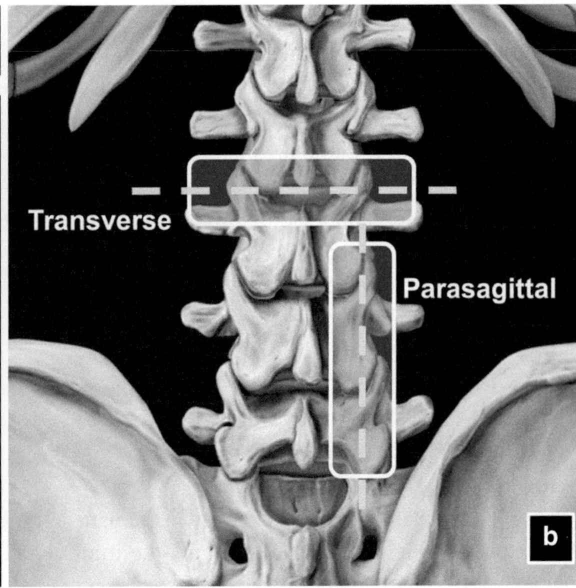

Fig. 40.21 Figure **a** is a lateral view, and Figure **b** is a posterior view, of the surface placement of the ultrasound probe over the lumbar spine The ultrasound probe may be placed in two basic orientations: transverse or parasagittal, which determines the "cut" of the spine that will be visualized. (Courtesy of www.usra.ca)

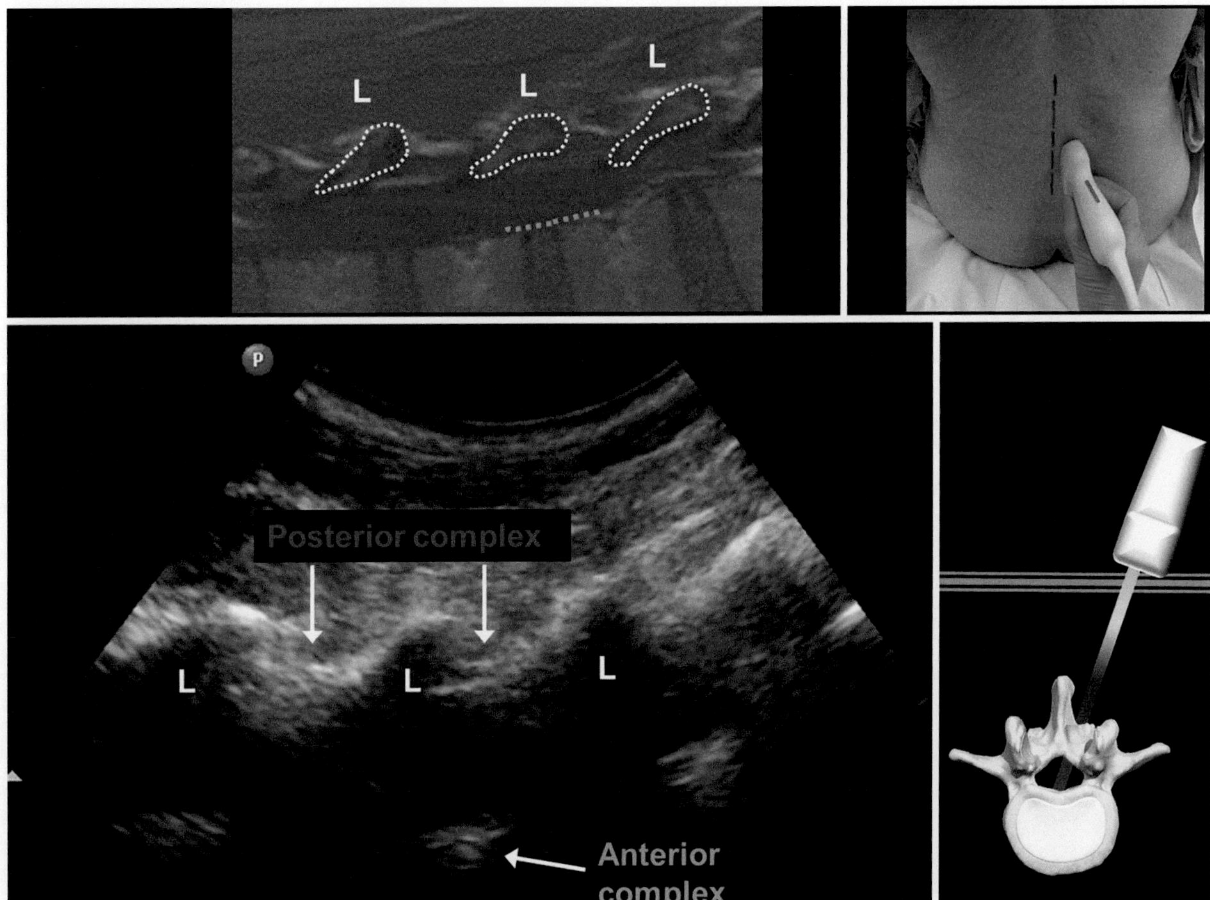

Fig. 40.22 Parasagittal oblique (PSO) view of the lumbar spine with corresponding magnetic resonance image above. The laminae (L) are visible in cross-section as sloping hyperechoic lines with acoustic shadowing beneath and form a "sawtooth" pattern. The hyperechoic posterior complex, consisting of ligamentum flavum, posterior epidural space, and posterior dura, is visible between laminae; these structures cannot always be distinguished from one another. The deeper hyperechoic linear structure is the anterior complex, consisting of anterior dura, anterior epidural space, posterior longitudinal ligament, and the posterior aspect of the vertebral body and intervertebral disc. (Courtesy of www.usra.ca)

structure is the **anterior complex** and represents the anterior dura, posterior longitudinal ligament, and posterior aspect of the vertebral body and intervertebral disc, which together constitute the anterior wall of the vertebral canal.
- The intervening hypoechoic area is the intrathecal space. The conus medullaris has the same echogenicity as cerebrospinal fluid and cannot be distinguished in the adult patient. Pulsatile hyperechoic streaks may occasionally be seen within the intrathecal space and most likely represent elements of the cauda equina.

Parasagittal Views of the Articular Processes and Transverse Processes

- If the probe is positioned more laterally in the parasagittal plane or is insufficiently angled towards the midline, an image of the articular processes or transverse processes may be obtained instead. Recognition of these two views will indicate the appropriate manipulation of the probe required to obtain the PSO view.
- The overlapping superior and inferior articular processes can be recognized as a continuous, wavy hyperechoic line with a dense acoustic shadow beneath (Fig. 40.23).
- The transverse processes, on the other hand, cast characteristic "finger-like" acoustic shadows with the psoas major muscle visible in between (Fig. 40.24).

Transverse Midline (TM) Interlaminar View

- The most important characteristic of the TM interlaminar view is visualization of the hyperechoic **anterior complex**, which signifies that the ultrasound beam has penetrated the vertebral canal through the interspinous and interlaminar spaces (Fig. 40.25).
- The **posterior complex** is usually visible as well but is generally less distinct compared to the PSO view.

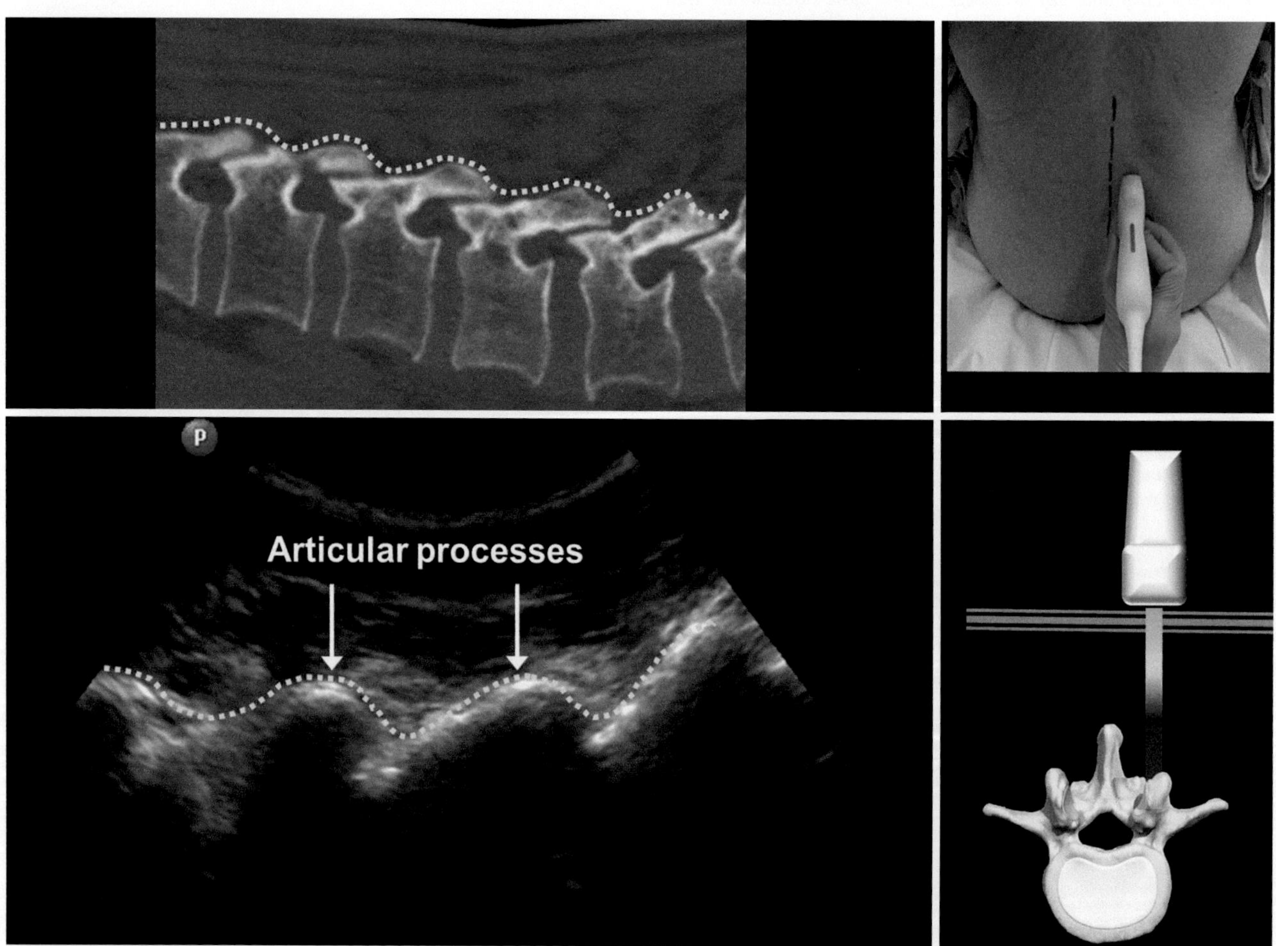

Fig. 40.23 Parasagittal articular process view of the lumbar spine and corresponding computed tomography image (above). The overlapping bony superior and inferior articular processes are seen as a continuous hyperechoic line of "humps" with acoustic shadowing beneath. (Courtesy of www.usra.ca)

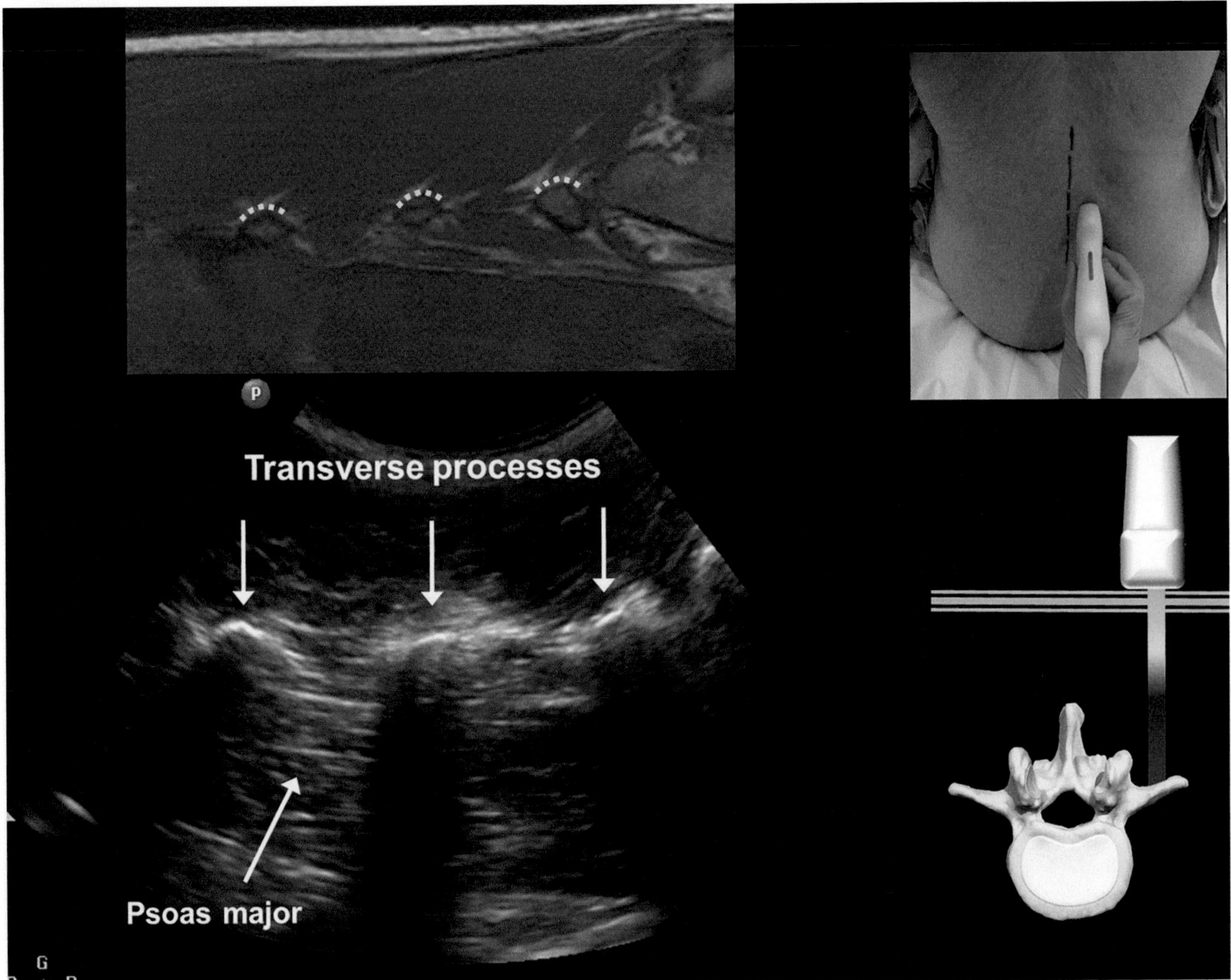

Fig. 40.24 Parasagittal transverse process view of the lumbar spine and corresponding magnetic resonance image (above). The probe is placed over the tips of the transverse processes (TP), which appear as hyperechoic curvilinear structures with "finger-like" acoustic shadowing beneath. The erector spinae muscle and the psoas muscle lie superficial and deep to the transverse processes, respectively. (Courtesy of www.usra.ca)

- The articular processes and transverse processes lie in the same transverse plane and their bony contours are usually visible lateral to the posterior and anterior complexes. In the obese patient, these are important surrogate markers of the interlaminar space as the posterior and anterior complexes may be poorly visible due to soft-tissue attenuation of the ultrasound beam.

TM Spinous Process View

- The TM spinous process view is easily recognized by the hyperechoic appearance of the tip of the spinous process and adjacent lamina, and the dense acoustic dropout shadow that they cast (Fig. 40.26).
- This view is a cue to manipulate the ultrasound probe cephalad or caudad to obtain the TM interlaminar view.
- It may also be used to definitively establish and mark the position of the spinous process and midline, which in itself can be helpful in performing neuraxial block if an adequate TM interlaminar view cannot be obtained.

Recommended Pre-Procedural Scanning Technique in the Lumbar Spine

Patient, machine, and operator positioning

- The operator stands or sits behind the patient, who may be placed in the sitting or lateral decubitus position.
- The ultrasound machine is ideally placed on the opposite side of the bed from the operator.

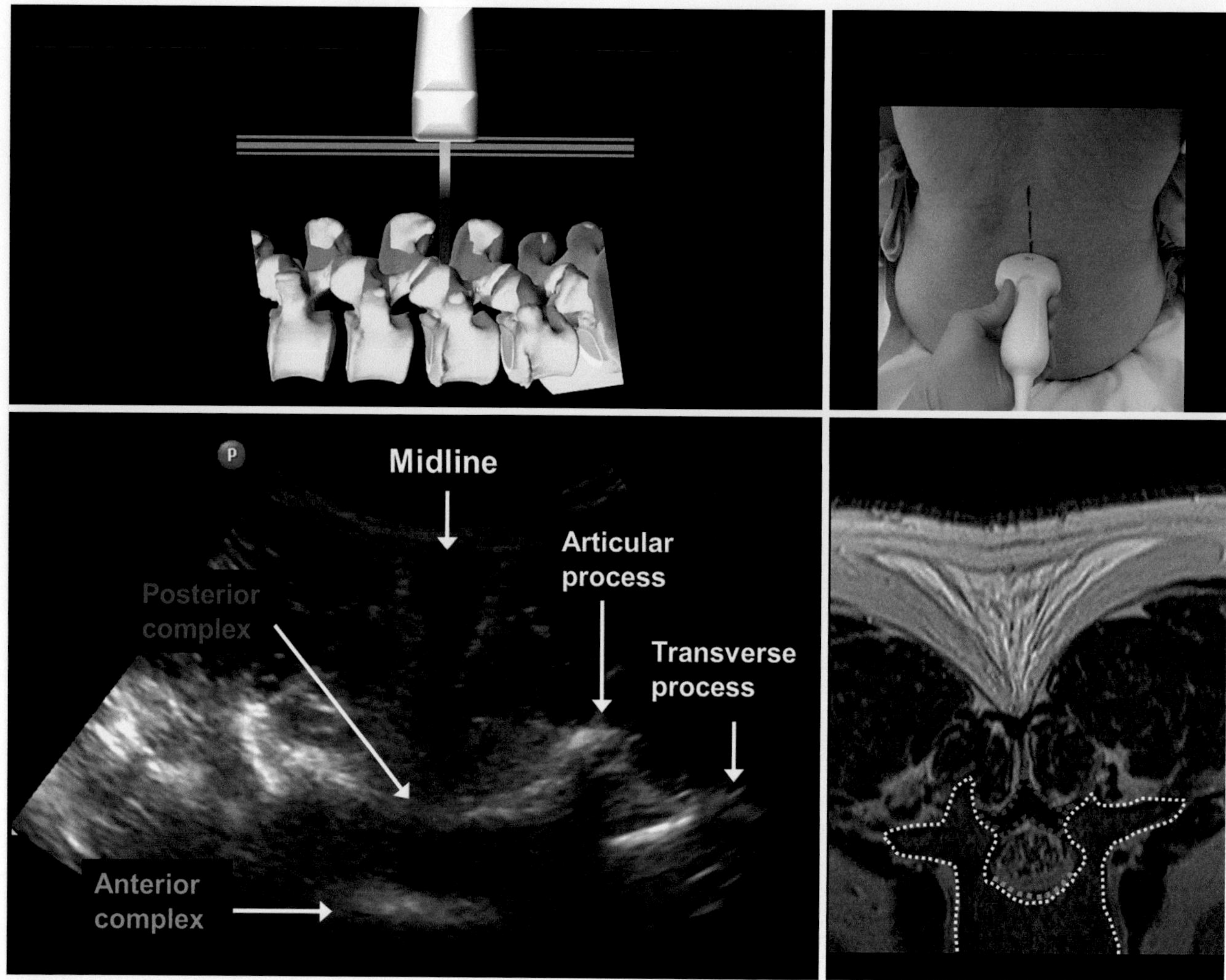

Fig. 40.25 Transverse midline interlaminar view of the lumbar spine and corresponding magnetic resonance imaging scan (right). The intrathecal space is a dark hypoechoic band sandwiched between the hyperechoic posterior and anterior complex. The transverse processes and articular processes lie in the same transverse plane and are usually visible. The ligamentum flavum, posterior epidural space, and dura usually cannot be distinguished from one another in the transverse view. The midline is indicated by the dark vertical stripe of the interspinous ligament. (Courtesy of www.usra.ca)

Parasagittal and parasagittal oblique scan

- The probe is first placed in a parasagittal orientation over the sacrum of the patient. The sacrum is easily recognizable as a continuous hyperechoic line with acoustic shadowing beneath (Fig. 40.27).
- The probe is slid in a cephalad direction and angled toward the midline to obtain a PSO view of the L5–S1 interlaminar space. Successive interlaminar spaces are identified by continuing to slide the probe in a cephalad direction.
- Each interlaminar space should be centered on the ultrasound screen and a corresponding mark made on the patient's skin in the middle of the long edge of the probe (Fig. 40.28). These marks serve to confirm the identity of the intervertebral level being imaged when scanning in the transverse plane. In the event an adequate TM interlaminar view cannot be obtained, these marks also indicate the approximate location of the interlaminar space and can thus guide needle insertion.

Transverse scan

- The probe is then rotated into the transverse plane and manipulated to obtain the TM interlaminar views at the relevant interspaces. Slight cephalad tilting of the probe may be required to optimize image quality in patients with limited spine flexion.
- When the appropriate view is obtained, skin marks made at the mid-points of the long and short edges of the probe will indicate the locations of the neuraxial midline and interlaminar space respectively (Fig. 40.29). The intersection of these two marks is an appropriate needle insertion point for a midline approach to the vertebral canal.

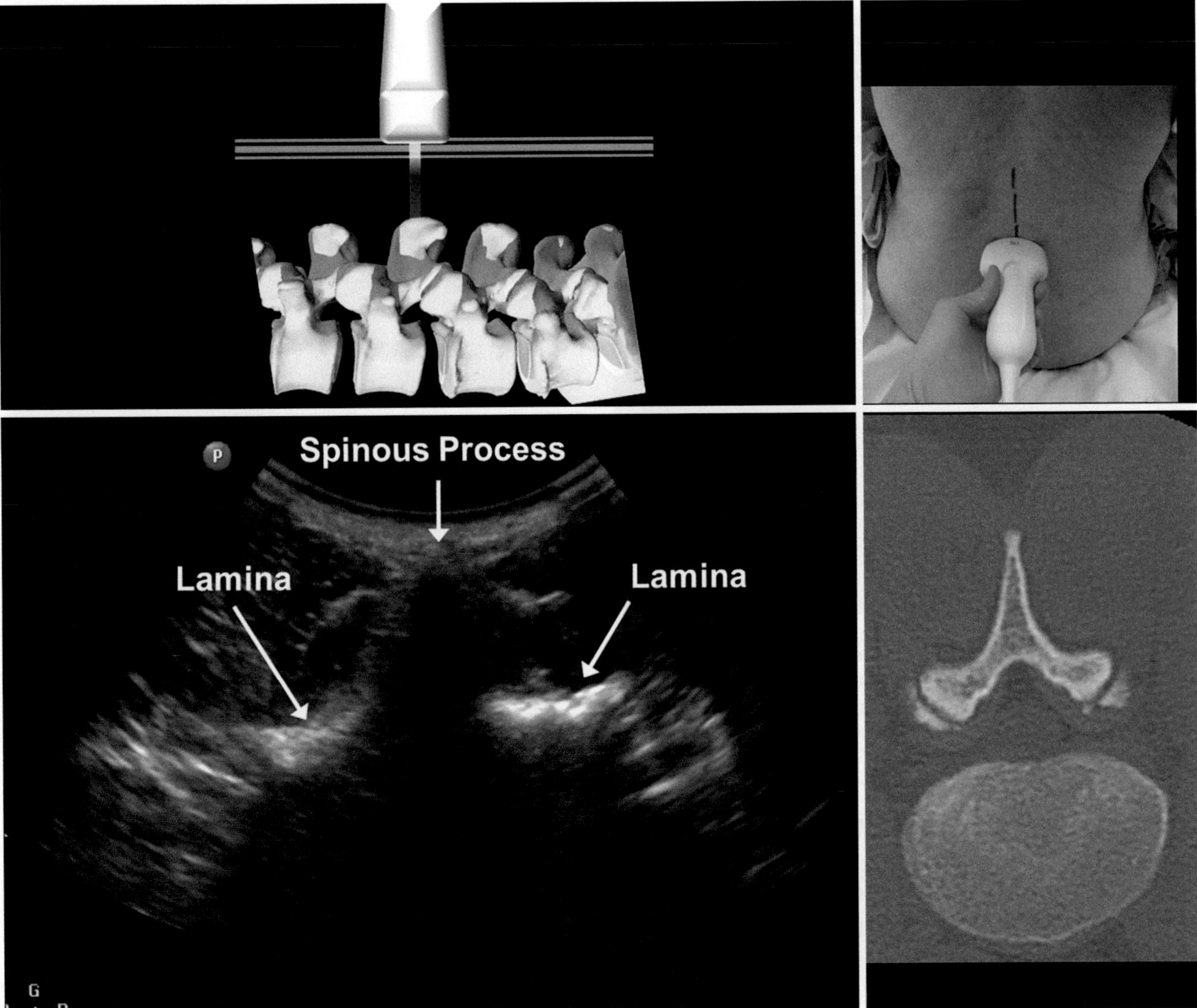

Fig. 40.26 Transverse midline spinous process view of the lumbar spine and corresponding computed tomography image (right). The tip of the spinous process and the lamina are brightly hyperechoic on ultrasound with pronounced acoustic shadowing that obscures all deeper structures. (Courtesy of www.usra.ca)

- The depth to the deep aspect of the posterior complex may be measured in either the PSO or TM interlaminar view, and correlates well with actual needle depth to the epidural and intrathecal space.

Strategies in Subjects with Poor-Quality Views

The obese patient

- Obese patients are primarily a challenge because attenuation of the ultrasound by the increased depth reduces the echogenicity of the relevant anatomical structures.
- In the obese patient, image quality may be improved by adjustments in gain and focus, and reducing frequency to enhance penetration.
- Firm probe pressure helps by enhancing skin-probe contact and reducing the effective depth to the structures of interest.
- Experience in scanning and image interpretation will also facilitate recognition of more subtle appearances of the characteristic patterns described above (Fig. 40.30).

The elderly patient

- Elderly patients may present a challenge due to narrowing of the interspinous and interlaminar spaces associated with age-related degenerative changes. The probe must be manipulated in a careful and controlled manner to try and direct the beam through these narrowed spaces.
- Prominent spinous processes in a thinner elderly patient may hinder adequate skin-probe contact and contribute to poor visualization of neuraxial structures. In such patients,

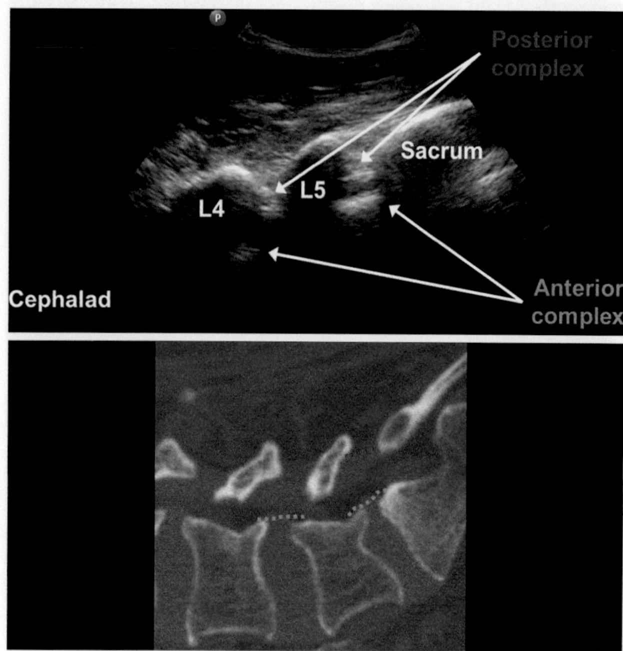

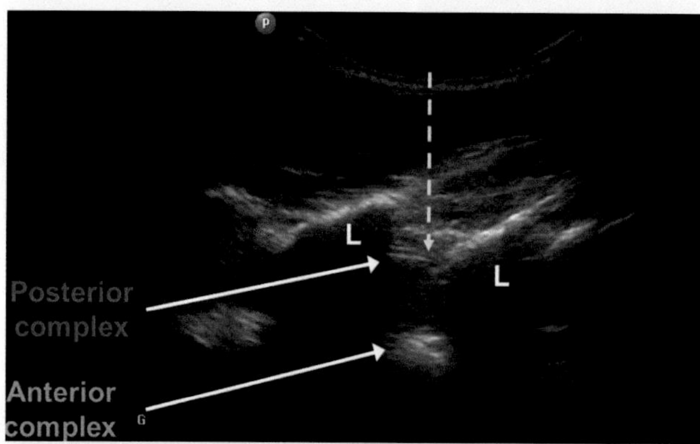

Fig. 40.27 Parasagittal oblique view of the L5–S1 junction and corresponding computed tomography image (below). The sacrum is recognizable as a horizontal hyperechoic linear structure, and the L5 lamina has the typical "sawtooth" appearance. The posterior and anterior complexes are visible through the intervening gap. (Courtesy of www.usra.ca)

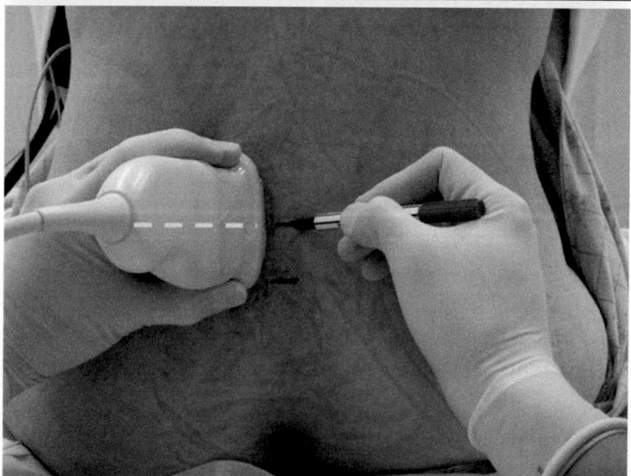

Fig. 40.28 In the parasagittal oblique view, each interlaminar space is centered in turn on the ultrasound screen. A corresponding skin mark is made at the midpoint of the probe's long edge to mark its position. (Courtesy of www.usra.ca)

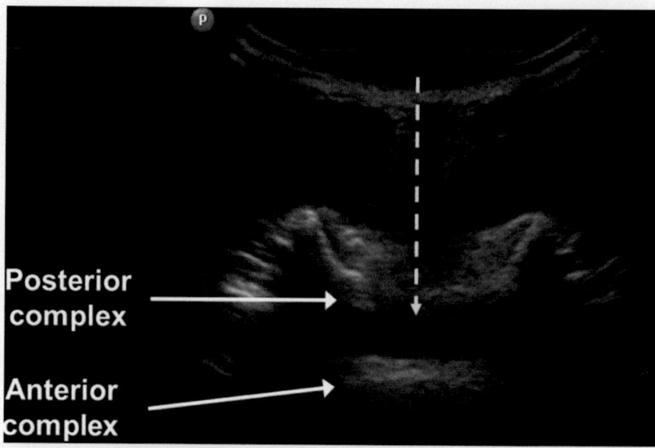

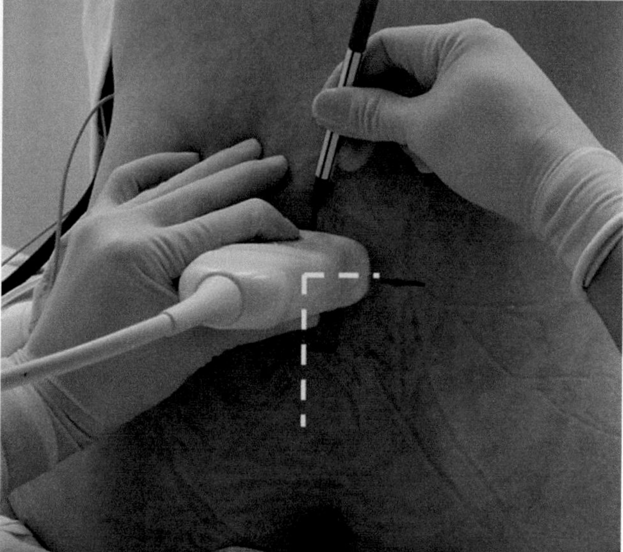

Fig. 40.29 In the transverse midline interlaminar view, the midline is centered on the ultrasound screen, and skin marks are made at the midpoint of the probe's long and short edges. The intersection of these two marks provides an appropriate needle insertion point for a midline approach to the epidural or intrathecal space at that level. (Courtesy of www.usra.ca)

a TM interlaminar view may be physically difficult or impossible to obtain; and the PSO view may be a better alternative. Contact may also be improved by using a probe with a smaller footprint.

Anatomy and Sonoanatomy of the Thoracic Spine

- There are significant differences in the morphology of the thoracic spine relative to the lumbar spine (Fig. 40.31).
- In the mid-thoracic spine (T5–8), the spinous processes angle steeply in a caudad direction such that the inferior border of the spinous process overlies the midpoint of the lamina below. The thoracic laminae also lie closer together and the interlaminar spaces are therefore much narrower.
- The lower 4 thoracic vertebrae (T9–12) are similar to lumbar vertebrae in that their spinous processes that are broad, flat, and only slightly angled.

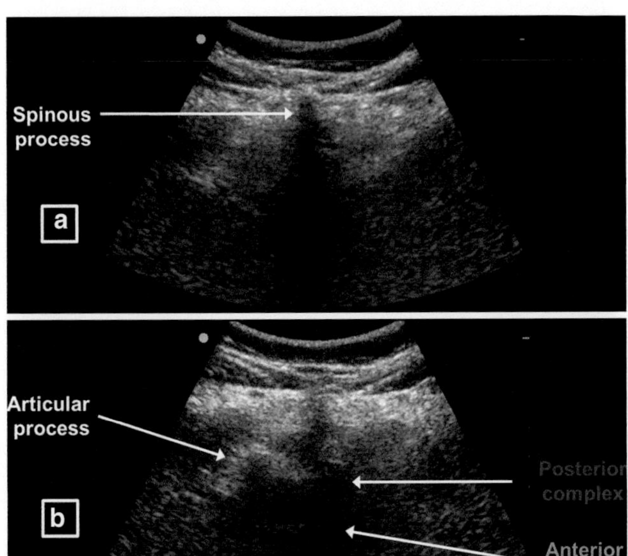

Fig. 40.30 An example of poor-quality transverse midline spinous process (**a**) and interlaminar (**b**) views in one individual. In the interlaminar view (**b**), the posterior and anterior complexes are only faintly hyperechoic, but nevertheless are visible, especially when contrasted with the dense acoustic shadow cast by the spinous process and lamina in (**a**). The other visual cue that (**b**) is an interlaminar view as opposed to a spinous process view is the contour of the tip of the articular process which lies in the same transverse plane as the interlaminar space. (Courtesy of www.usra.ca)

- A curvilinear low-frequency probe is generally recommended; however, in slimmer individuals, a linear high-frequency probe may also produce adequate images.
- As in the lumbar spine, the two most important views are the PSO and TM interlaminar views.
- In the lower thoracic spine, these views are similar to those of the lumbar spine except that the interlaminar spaces tend to be narrower. The mid-thoracic views are quite different however and are described below.

Recommended Pre-Procedural Scanning Technique in the Mid-Thoracic Spine

Patient, machine, and operator positioning

- The operator stands or sits behind the patient, who may be placed in the sitting or lateral decubitus position.
- The ultrasound machine is ideally placed on the opposite side of the bed from the operator.

Parasagittal oblique scan

- The mid-thoracic laminae appear as almost horizontal hyperechoic linear structures, separated by narrow gaps which represent the paramedian interlaminar spaces (Fig. 40.32).
- Due to the narrow interlaminar spaces, the posterior complex and anterior complex are rarely visible, and are usually smaller and fainter than in the lumbar spine.
- The interlaminar spaces are identified and marked using the PSO view in a process similar to that described for the lumbar spine.
- The depth to the lamina or posterior complex is measured to estimate needle depth to the epidural space.
- Identification of intervertebral level can be achieved by counting upwards from the L5-S1 junction. Alternatively the spaces can also be counted down from T1 or up from T12, having first identified the articulation of the first rib with T1 or the 12th rib with T12, respectively.

Transverse midline scan

- The overlapping spinous processes in the mid-thoracic spine make it impossible to obtain a TM interlaminar view of posterior and anterior complexes.
- The visible structures are the hyperechoic bony contours of the spinous process, lamina and transverse processes; and more laterally, the ribs and pleura (Fig. 40.33).
- The TM view is therefore used mainly to map and mark out the location of the neuraxial midline particularly if it cannot be palpated or if it is distorted, e.g. by scoliosis. With this additional information, the needle approach to the thoracic epidural space can be triangulated more accurately.

Learning Strategies in Neuraxial Ultrasound

Familiarization with the gross anatomy and sonoanatomy of the spine is essential prior to performing the ultrasound-guided neuraxial blockade in clinical practice.

- This can be done by the following:
  - reviewing didactic material,
  - attending educational workshops,
  - repetitive practice on a water-based spine phantom or human volunteers.
- An additional educational resource is an interactive 3-dimensional digital spine model available online at http://www.usra.ca/vspine.php.
- Competency in the technique of pre-procedural scanning and marking should be acquired in normal patients before attempting it in patients with more challenging anatomy.

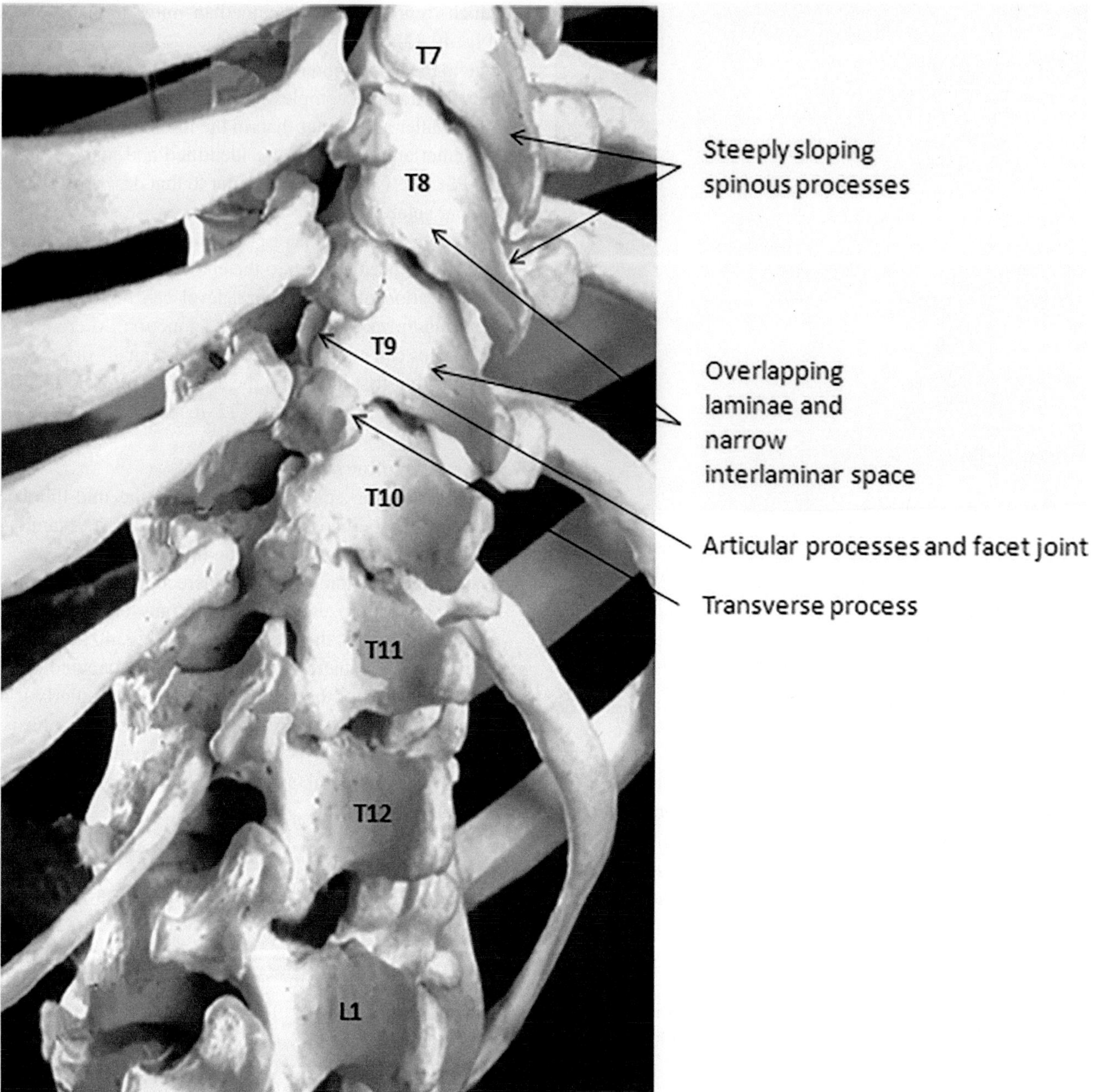

Fig. 40.31 The lower thoracic vertebrae (T10–T12) are similar in morphology and ultrasonographic appearance to lumbar vertebrae. The middle thoracic vertebrae have steeply sloping spinous processes that make it impossible to obtain a transverse interlaminar view. The interlaminar spaces are also small, and the paramedian sagittal oblique view into the vertebral canal is limited as a result. (Courtesy of www.usra.ca)

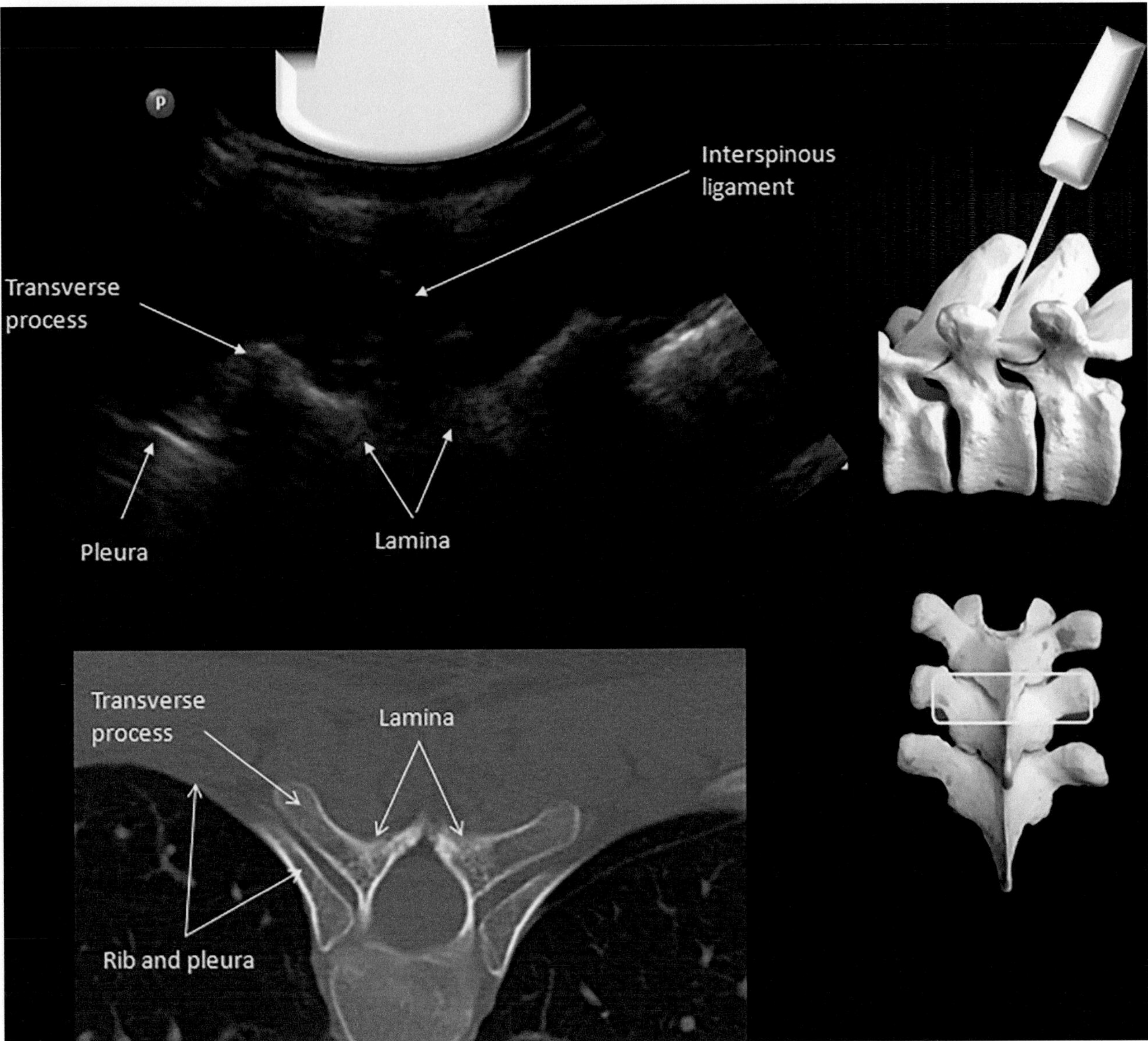

Fig. 40.32 Transverse view of the midthoracic spine and corresponding computed tomography image. An *interlaminar* view into the vertebral canal cannot be obtained because of the steeply sloping spinous processes and overlapping laminae. (Courtesy of www.usra.ca)

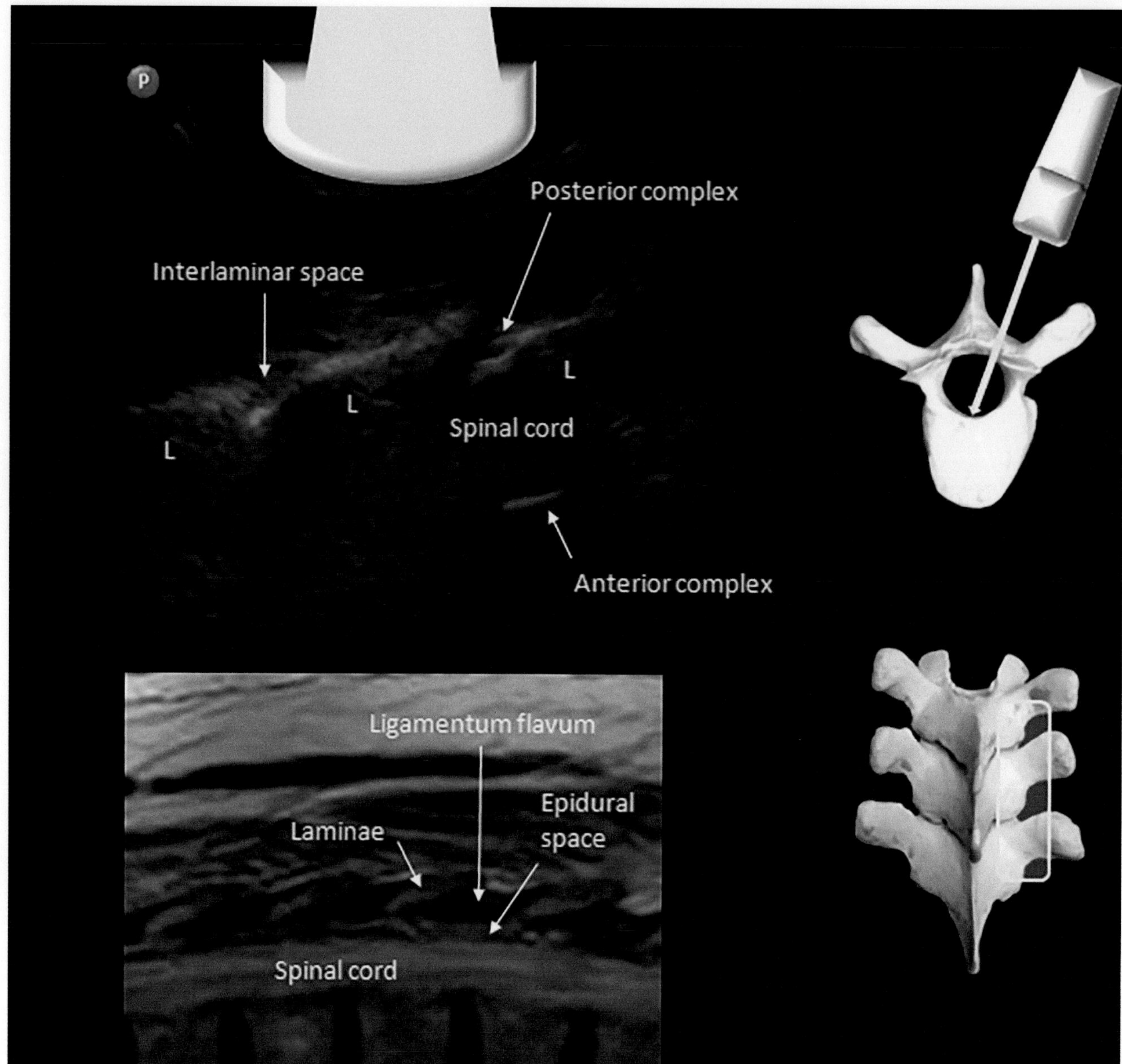

Fig. 40.33 Paramedian sagittal oblique view of the midthoracic spine and corresponding magnetic resonance image. Despite the narrow interlaminar space, it is possible to visualize the posterior and anterior complex at one or more levels. At a minimum, the location of the interlaminar space can be determined by the dip or gap between successive laminae (L). Note that the spinal cord is hypoechoic and cannot be distinguished from the surrounding cerebrospinal fluid. (Courtesy of www.usra.ca)

Suggested Reading

Andres KH. Über die Feinstruktur der Arachnoidea und Dura mater von Mammalia. Z Zellf Mikr Anat. 1967;79:272–95.

Balki M. Locating the epidural space in obstetric patients-ultrasound a useful tool: continuing professional development. Can J Anaesth. 2011;57:1111–26.

Chin KJ, Karmakar MK, Peng P. Ultrasonography of the adult thoracic and lumbar spine for central neuraxial blockade. Anesthesiology. 2011;114:1459–85.

de Sèze M, Sztark F, Janvier G, Joseph P. Severe and long-lasting complications of the nerve root and spinal cord after central neuraxial blockade. Anesth Analg. 2007;104:975–9.

Drug Safety Communications. Updated recommendations to decrease risk of spinal column bleeding and paralysis in patients on low molecular weight heparins (Safety Announcement). 2013. http://www.fda.gov/downloads/Drugs/DrugSafety/UCM373735.pdf.

Du Boulay GH. Pulsatile movements in the CNS pathways. Br J Radiol. 1966;39:255–62.

Düring MV, Bauersachs M, Böhmer B, et al. Neuropeptide Y- and substance P-like immunoreactive nerve fibers in the rat dura mater encephali. Anat Embryol. 1990;182:363–73.

Faraci FM, Kadel KA, Haistad DD. Vascular responses of dura mater. Am J Physiol. 1989;257:H157–61.

Frederickson RG. The subdural space interpreted as a cellular layer of meninges. Anat Rec. 1991;230:38–51.

Groen GJ, Baljet J, Drukker J. The innervation of the spinal dura mater: anatomy and clinical applications. Acta Neurochir. 1988;92:39–46.

Karmakar MK, Li X, Kwok WH, Ho AM, Ngan Kee WD. Sonoanatomy relevant for ultrasound-guided central neuraxial blocks via the paramedian approach in the lumbar region. Br J Radiol. 2012;85:e262–9.

Keller JT, Marfurt CF. Peptidergic and serotoninergic innervation of the rat dura mater. J Comp Neurol. 1991;309:515–34.

Lang J. Funktionelle Anatomie der Halswirbelsäule und des benachbarten Nervensystems. In: Hohman D, Kügelgen B, Liebig K, Schirmer M, editors. Neuroorthopädie 1. Berlin, Heidelberg: Springer; 1983.

Lang J. Klinische Anatomie der Halswirbelsäule. Stuttgart, New York: Thieme Verlag; 1991.

Schroth G, Klose U. Cerebrospinal fluid flow. I. Physiology of cardiac-related pulsations. Neuroradiology. 1992a;35:1–9.

Schroth G, Klose V. Cerebrospinal fluid flow. II. Physiology of respiration-related pulsations. Neuroradiology. 1992b;35:10–5.

Vandermeulen EP, Van Aken H, Vermylen J. Anticoagulants and spinal-epidural anesthesia. Anesth Analg. 1994;79:1165–77.

Zenker W. Einige neue Aspekte zu Feinbau und Funktion der Dura mater und des Subarachnoidalraumes. Symposium über Spinalanästhesietechnik. Bad Säckingen; 1994.

Zenker W. Anatomisches Institut der Universität zu Zürich. Personal communication. 2005.

Neuraxial Blocks: Spinal and Epidural Anesthesia

41

Hywel-Gethin Tudur Evans, Donogh Burns, and Ki Jinn Chin

Contents

H.-G. T. Evans · D. Burns · K. J. Chin (✉)
Department of Anesthesiology and Pain Medicine, Toronto Western Hospital, University of Toronto, Toronto, ON, Canada
e-mail: kijinn.chin@uhn.ca

D. Jankovic, P. Peng (eds.), *Regional Nerve Blocks in Anesthesia and Pain Therapy*,
https://doi.org/10.1007/978-3-030-88727-8_41

Introduction

Central neuraxial techniques are among the most reliable regional anesthesia techniques at the disposal of the anesthesiologist. Although relatively simple to perform, a thorough knowledge of neuraxial anatomy and the factors determining the spread and duration of anesthesia is important to their success. Similarly, an understanding of the physiological effects and potential complications of these neuraxial techniques is paramount for patient safety.

Spinal anesthesia is the administration of local anesthetic (and optional adjuncts) into the cerebrospinal fluid within the subarachnoid space. This results in the rapid onset of a dense sensory and motor block of the lower torso and legs that is suitable for surgical anesthesia.

Epidural anesthesia involves the instillation of local anesthetic into the fat-filled epidural space, usually through an indwelling catheter. This results in a slower-onset block and one which is generally less dense. This is most often used to provide analgesia rather than surgical anesthesia.

Spinal anesthesia is usually only performed at the lower lumbar intervertebral levels in order to avoid spinal cord injury. Epidural anesthesia may, however, be performed at the lumbar, thoracic, or even cervical levels depending on the desired area of sensory blockade.

Combined spinal-epidural anesthesia is a technique that takes advantage of the rapid onset of spinal anesthesia as well as the ability to extend the duration of the block with further local anesthetic administration through an epidural catheter.

Applied Functional Anatomy

A three-dimensional understanding of spinal anatomy serves to improve success of neuraxial blockade, particularly when difficulty is encountered. This most commonly occurs in patients with pathology of the spine (e.g. scoliosis, vertebral collapse, calcified spinal ligaments) or in those with a high body mass index, which can make patient positioning and palpation of bony landmarks more challenging. The previous chapter presents a detailed discussion of spinal anatomy. Here, we will briefly review only the most important aspects relevant to neuraxial blockade.

Surface Anatomy

Surface landmarks can be used to locate a particular vertebral level. Figure 41.1 illustrates these landmarks and the vertebral levels to which they correspond. It should be noted that these landmarks only provide an approximate estimation of vertebral level. Many factors, including normal anatomical variation, subcutaneous fat and patient positioning can render the identification of vertebral levels by surface landmarks somewhat inaccurate. It is recommended that radiological

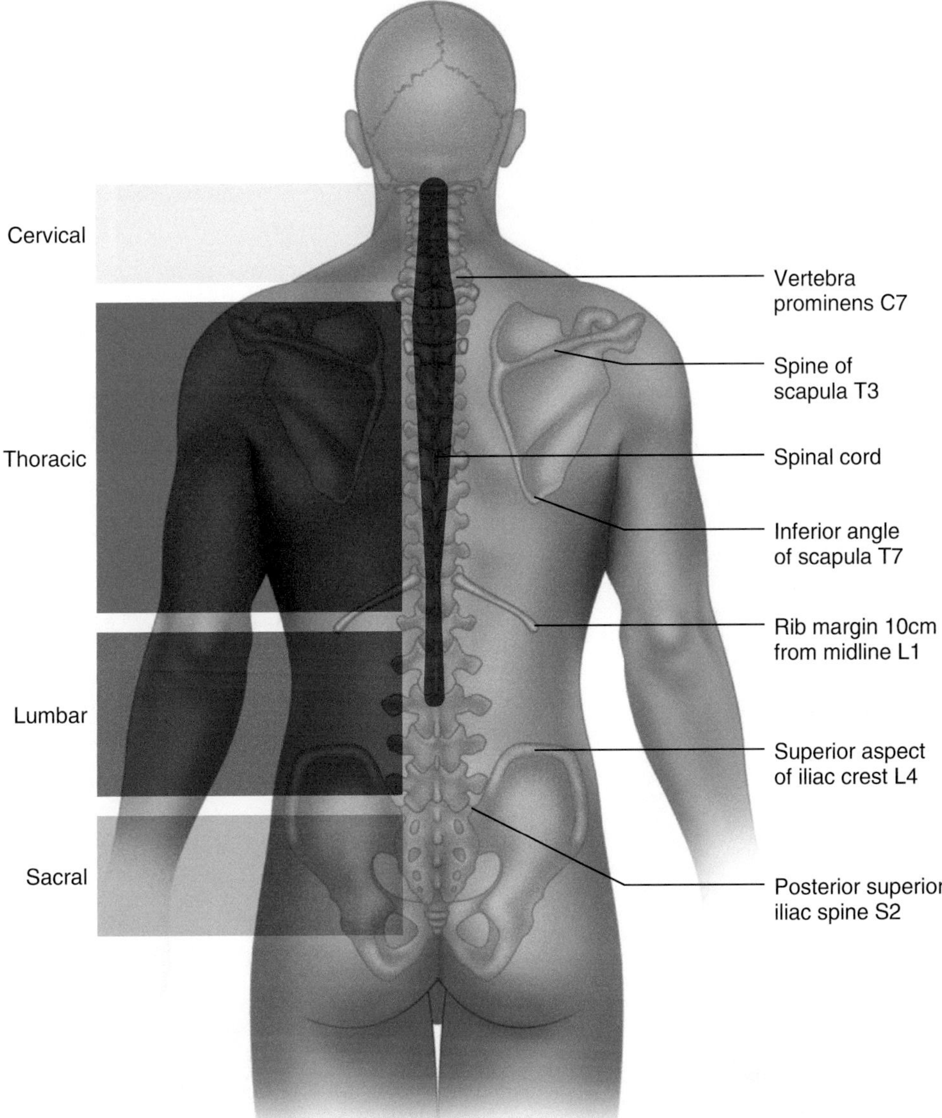

Fig. 41.1 Illustration showing the surface landmarks used to locate a particular vertebral level

imaging, e.g. using ultrasound or fluoroscopy, be used to confirm the surface location of specific intervertebral spaces in scenarios where precision and accuracy are essential.

Spinous Processes

The lumbar vertebrae have spinous processes that are nearly horizontal, whereas thoracic vertebrae have spinous processes that are angled caudally (Fig. 41.2b, c). As a result, needle insertion should always start perpendicular to the skin when performing spinal anesthesia or a lumbar epidural via a midline approach through the interspinous space; little to no cranial angulation is usually needed to enter the interlaminar space. In contrast, greater cranial angulation of the needle will be required when performing an epidural in the thoracic region (Fig. 41.3a).

Spinal Curves

The kyphotic thoracic curve and the lordotic lumbar curve can influence the spread of local anesthetic injected into the subarachnoid space. Hyperbaric local anesthetic injected at the midpoint of the lumbar lordosis will spread both caudad and cranial when the patient is supine (Fig. 41.3b). The cranial extent of this spread is limited by the upward slope of the mid-thoracic concavity. (A useful illustration of this concept can be found at https://www.youtube.com/watch?v=XQ7zh5rdu6o).

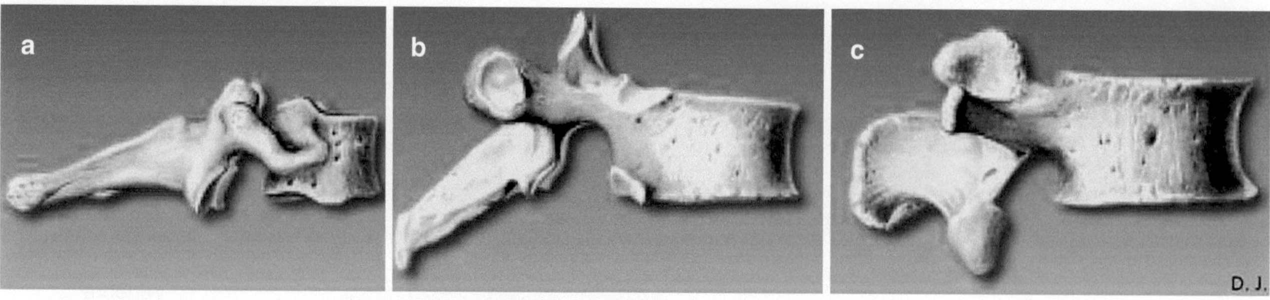

Fig. 41.2 (**a**) Cervical (**b**) Thoracic and (**c**) Lumbar spinous processes. (Reproduced with permission from Dr. Danilo Jankovic)

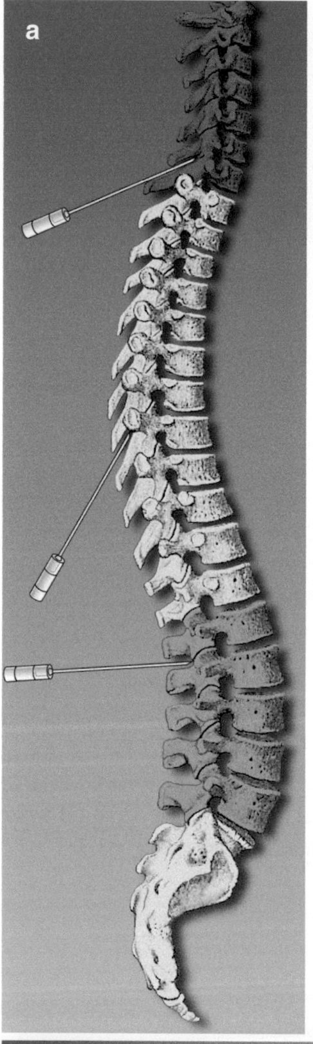

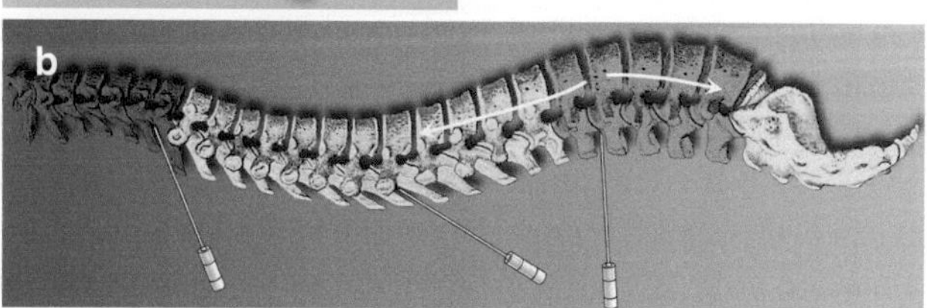

Fig. 41.3 (**a**) Degree of needle angulation required at the lumbar, thoracic, and cervical intervertebral spaces. (**b**) White arrows show spread of hyperbaric local anesthetic within intrathecal space following lumbar intrathecal injection when the patient is supine. (Reproduced with permission from Dr. Danilo Jankovic)

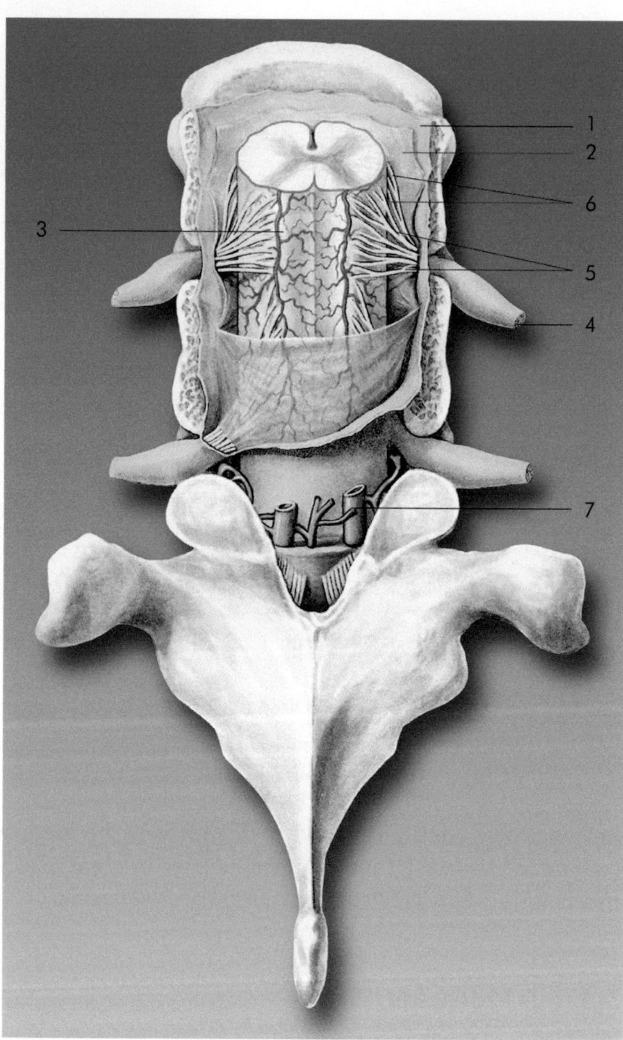

Fig. 41.4 (1) Dura mater, (2) arachnoid mater, (3) pia mater, (4) spinal nerve, (5) dorsal (posterior) nerve root, (6) ventral (anterior) nerve root, and (7) internal vertebral venous plexus. (Reproduced with permission from Dr. Danilo Jankovic)

Meninges

The three meningeal layers—the dura, arachnoid, and pia mater—envelop and protect the spinal cord (Fig. 41.4). The dura mater is the tough, outermost meningeal layer. The epidural space is superficial to this layer and is the target for epidural anesthesia. The subdural space lies between the dura and the arachnoid mater. Unintentional deposition of local anesthetic into the subdural space produces an unpredictable and patchy block. The arachnoid mater encloses the subarachnoid space which contains the cerebrospinal fluid (CSF). Both the spinal cord and the spinal nerve roots are exposed to cerebrospinal fluid. These are the sites of action of local anesthetic deposited within the subarachnoid space during a spinal anesthetic.

Spinal Ligaments

A needle inserted in the midline will traverse the following structures to access the subarachnoid space (Fig. 41.5a, b):

- Skin.
- Subcutaneous tissue.
- Supraspinous ligament.
- Interspinous ligament.
- Ligamentum flavum.
- Epidural space.
- Dura mater.
- Subdural space.
- Arachnoid mater.

There is a characteristic "feel" to the different tissue structures as the needle tip is advanced through skin, subcutaneous tissue (a loose sensation), supraspinous and interspinous ligament (a gritty, tearing sensation with firmer resistance to advancement), and ligamentum flavum (a firm, rubbery resistance). A paramedian needle insertion (discussed later in the chapter) bypasses the supraspinous and interspinous ligaments, passing instead through the paraspinal muscles to enter the ligamentum flavum. This approach can be useful in older patients who may have calcified ligaments, or patients in whom the interspinous space is narrowed because of suboptimal positioning (e.g. in hip fracture) or degenerative disease.

The Location of the Conus Medullaris

This varies with age. In the fetus, the spinal cord extends to the end of the vertebral column. The vertebrae grow more quickly than the spinal cord such that by birth, the terminal end of the cord, the conus medullaris, extends only to L3. In the majority of adults, the conus ends at L1. To avoid the risk of spinal cord injury, spinal anesthetics should be performed at the L2–3 intervertebral space or lower.

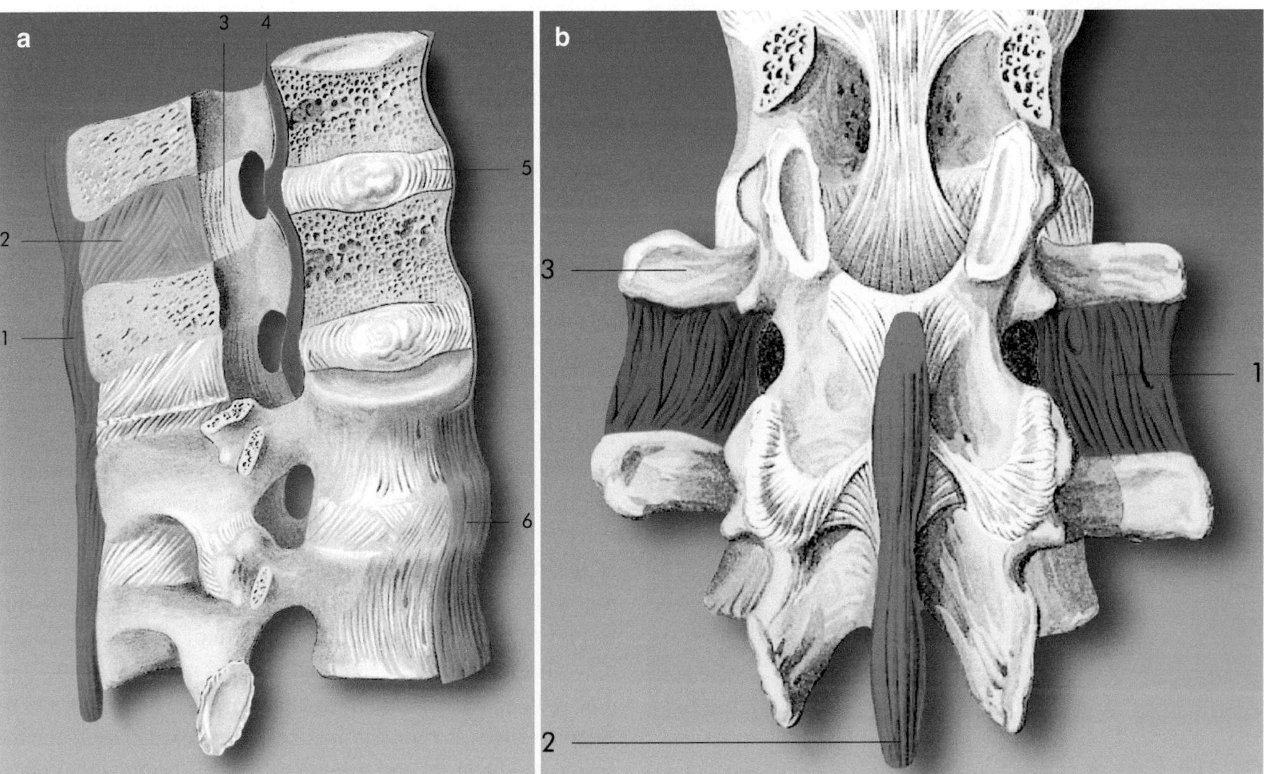

Fig. 41.5 (**a**) Sagittal section of the vertebral column illustrating the ligaments of the spinal cord. (1) Supraspinous ligament, (2) interspinous ligament, (3) ligamentum flavum, (4) posterior longitudinal ligament, (5) intervertebral disk, and (6) anterior longitudinal ligament. (**b**) Ligaments of the spinal cord. (1) Intertransverse ligament, (2) supraspinous ligament, (3) transverse process. (Reprinted with permission from Danilo Jankovic)

Epidural Space

The depth of the epidural space from the skin varies with body habitus, being deeper in obese and pregnant individuals. Ultrasound is a useful tool for measuring this and predicting actual needle insertion depth.

The epidural space is not a continuous space but is segmented along its length. Cryomicrotome sectioning and imaging has shown that the various compartments of the epidural space are segmented by areas where the dura is directly fused with the bone. The lateral epidural compartment is divided by intervening pedicles which are in contact with dura. The posterior epidural compartment is divided by dural contact with bone beneath the cranial half of each lamina. The anterior epidural compartment is divided by the attachment of the posterior longitudinal ligament to the intervertebral disc at each level. These posterior, lateral, and anterior compartments of the epidural space may impede the movement of injectate and may explain the unpredictable spread (or lack thereof) of epidural blockade that is occasionally seen.

Epidural fat in the epidural space (Fig. 41.6) may play an important role in the pharmacokinetics of lipophilic drugs administered here by acting as a reservoir. This may result in a delayed onset and a longer duration of action. A reduction in the epidural fat with age may partly explain the age-related changes in epidural dose requirements.

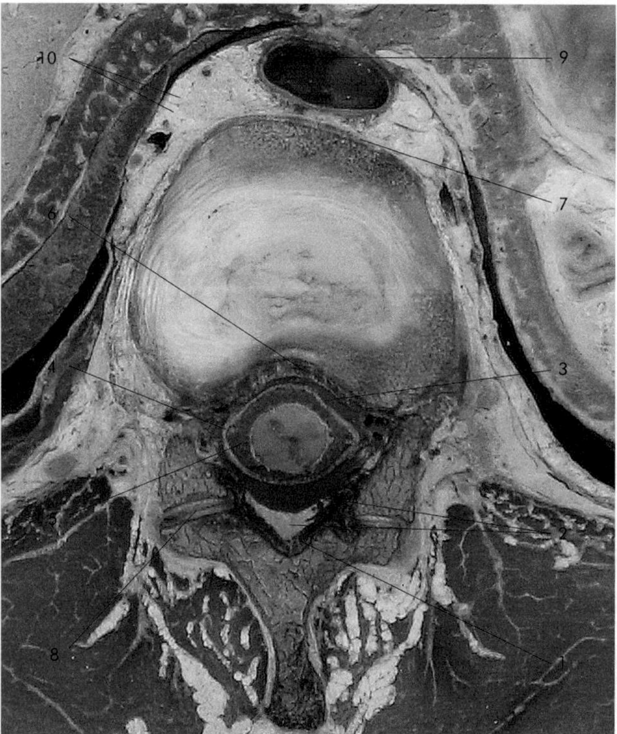

Fig. 41.6 Transverse dissection at the level of the T9 vertebra. (1) Ligamentum flavum, (2) posterior epidural space with fat, (3) anterior epidural space with veins, (4) spinal dura mater, (5) subarachnoid space with spinal cord, (6) posterior longitudinal ligament, (7) anterior longitudinal ligament, (8) zygapophysial joint, (9) aorta, and (10) sympathetic ganglion. (Reprinted with permission from Danilo Jankovic)

Physiology of Neuraxial Blockade

The physiological effects of both subarachnoid and an epidural block are similar. However, the effects of an epidural block have a slower onset and are usually confined to a segmental range of spinal nerves with an upper and lower limit, whereas spinal anesthesia blocks all of the nerve roots below a particular level. These effects are summarizes below.

Neurological Blockade

The injection of local anesthetic within the intrathecal or epidural space produces nerve blockade. Generally, the speed of onset of nerve blockade is inversely related to the nerve's diameter and degree of myelination. Thus, **sympathetic** blockade manifests before **sensory** block, which in turn precedes the **motor** block. Among the sensory modalities, the sequence of blockade is initially temperature, followed by pain, light touch, pressure and finally proprioception. Sensory block usually extends for two to four segments higher than the motor block, while sympathetic block extends two to four segments higher still. Block offset occurs in the reverse manner with autonomic sympathetic fibers being the last to recover.

Cardiovascular Effects

Blockade of the thoracolumbar sympathetic nerves manifests as the cardiovascular effects that follow a neuraxial block, including **hypotension** and **bradycardia**. These effects are in proportion to the extent of the block produced. They may be exaggerated in patients who are hypovolemic or those that are taking medications that affect the cardiovascular system such as antihypertensives and beta-blockers. Hypotension is the result of arteriolar vasodilatation and venous pooling which diminishes cardiac preload. Bradycardia is due in part to blockade of cardiac accelerator fibers (T1–T5). It may also result from decreased preload which activates cardiac reflexes involving intra-cardiac stretch receptors. The **Bezold–Jarisch reflex** is invoked as an explanation for the severe bradycardia and even asystole following spinal anesthesia that is occasionally observed in young healthy adults.

In general, the sympathetic block following a spinal anesthetic is more rapid in onset and greater in extent compared to an epidural. Thus, a gradually dosed epidural anesthetic may be useful in providing hemodynamic stability in patients with risk factors for cardiovascular compromise following neuraxial blockade.

Respiratory Effects

In a patient with normal lung function, neuraxial blocks usually have a negligible impact on respiratory function. However, with a high thoracic blockade or in a patient with pre-existing respiratory compromise, this effect may be significant. The paralysis of abdominal and intercostal muscles can negatively impact **expiratory** function causing a reduction in peak expiratory flows, expiratory reserve volume, and maximal minute ventilation. This may manifest as dyspnea. Nevertheless, these effects are usually outweighed by the pain relief obtained following thoracic or abdominal surgery, and thus thoracic epidural analgesia is associated with an overall improvement in postoperative outcome and a reduction in postoperative pulmonary complications.

Spread of local anesthetic to cervical segments can affect **inspiratory** effort due to blockade of the phrenic nerve and subsequent loss of diaphragmatic function.

A **total spinal** is a rare complication of spinal anesthesia in which there is excessive cranial spread of local anesthetic within the intrathecal space. Apart from respiratory distress from thoracic wall and diaphragmatic paralysis, it can lead to respiratory arrest due to medullary hypoperfusion rather than an effect of local anesthetics per se.

Gastrointestinal Function

The splanchnic blockade (T6–L2) produced following a neuraxial block leads to unopposed parasympathetic activity. This results in increased gastrointestinal secretions, increased intestinal motility and relaxation of sphincters. This prevents bowel distension and allows better access during abdominal surgery. Vasodilation increases visceral perfusion, which may improve healing, and contribute to an earlier return of bowel function following surgery.

Nausea and vomiting, if observed, are usually secondary to unopposed vagal tone and hypotension, and resolve with vasopressor treatment and restoration of normal blood pressure.

Genitourinary Effects

Neuraxial anesthesia does not directly affect renal blood flow since it is autoregulated. Sacral blockade produces an atonic bladder and an increased bladder sphincter tone. This not infrequently results in urinary retention until the resolution of the block.

Thermoregulation

Redistribution of heat following sympathetic block and vasodilation of the lower body results in mild hypothermia. This induces thermoregulatory vasoconstriction and shivering above the level of the neuraxial block.

Neuroendocrine Effects

Neuraxial block effectively inhibits the afferent innervation from the surgical site and it is responsible for the inhibition of the surgical stress response that involves release of a variety of mediators (including catecholamines, vasopressin, growth hormone, renin, angiotensin, glucose, antidiuretic hormone, and thyroid stimulating hormone). The magnitude of the stress response correlates with postoperative morbidity and thus its attenuation may be of benefit in enhancing post-surgical recovery.

Spinal Versus Epidural Anesthetic

Both spinal and epidural anesthesia provide a temporary blockade of nerve conduction in the autonomic (sympathetic), sensory, and motor fibers. There are, however, some important differences between the two. These are summarizes in Table 41.1.

Table 41.1 Important differences between a spinal and an epidural anesthetic

Variable	Spinal anesthetic	Epidural anesthetic
Space accessed	Subarachnoid space	Epidural space
Time needed to perform	Takes less time (since it is usually a single-injection) technique)	Takes more time (since it is usually a catheter technique)
Onset of conduction block	Faster	Slower
Nature of conduction blockade	Denser, therefore, mainly employed as an anesthetic technique	Less dense, therefore, mainly employed as an analgesic technique. Sufficient volume and concentration of local anesthetic will produce an anesthetic block
Duration of conduction blockade	Fixed duration unless a catheter is inserted; the length of this is dependent on dose administered and the local anesthetic drug used	Duration is flexible as a catheter is usually inserted and local anesthetic can be infused as required
Cardiovascular effect	Rapid drop in blood pressure	A more gradual and limited drop in blood pressure

Comparison to General Anesthesia

Compared to an opioid-based general anesthetic, the central neuraxial anesthesia techniques offer the following advantages:

- Avoidance of airway manipulation.
- Avoidance of side effects of a general anesthetic (sore throat, nausea and vomiting, dental damage, aspiration of gastric contents, malignant hyperthermia, etc.).
- Predictable physiological changes.
- Minimal metabolic disturbances (in hepatic or renal disease).
- Preservation of consciousness.
- Extension into postoperative analgesia (with insertion of an epidural catheter).
- Enhanced gastrointestinal perfusion and motility.
- Reduced postoperative nausea and vomiting.
- Reduced adverse cardiovascular events, perioperative pulmonary complications, thromboembolic events, development of chronic pain, surgical stress response, immune dysfunction, and morbidity and mortality.

However, general anesthesia is advantageous over neuraxial block when better control over hemodynamics is desired (such as in severe or critical aortic stenosis). It also offers definitive control of the airway and it allows for immediate assessment of the adequacy of postoperative analgesia.

Indications

The indications for spinal and epidural anesthetic are considered in Table 41.2. Figure 41.7a, b illustrate the required sensory levels for different procedures, and how to test for them.

Table 41.2 Indications for spinal and epidural anesthesia

Spinal anesthetic	Epidural anesthetic
Surgical indications Most surgical procedures below the level of the umbilicus are amenable to spinal anesthesia • Surgical procedures in the area of the lower extremities, hip joint, and inguinal region • Urological procedures (prostate, bladder) • Gynecological and obstetric procedures • Surgery in the perineal and perianal region • Lumbar spinal surgery	*Surgical indications* • Surgical procedures in the area of the lower extremities, hip joint, and inguinal region • Upper abdominal and thoracic procedures, in combination with general anesthesia • Urological procedures (prostate, bladder) • Gynecological and obstetric procedures • Procedures in the perineal and perianal region *Postoperative and post-traumatic pain therapy* Usually in combination with local anesthetics and opioids

Combined Spinal Epidural (CSE)

These have the advantage of providing a rapid anesthetic block which can subsequently be prolonged either as an anesthetic or analgesic block. This is particularly advantageous when the duration of a surgical procedure is likely to be longer than the expected duration of spinal anesthesia. For example, CSEs may be used for bilateral total hip or knee arthroplasty or complex revisions where the operative time is expected to be prolonged.

Continuous Spinal Anesthesia (CSA)

This is another technique that can be used to provide extended neuraxial anesthesia. It is, however, less-commonly used than CSE as it requires a specialized needle and catheter kit, and it carries a higher risk of post-dural puncture headache compared to a single-injection spinal anesthetic with a small-gauge needle. It may occasionally be employed in obstetric practice when there is an inadvertent dural puncture during attempted labor epidural analgesia; the catheter can be inserted into the subarachnoid space and with appropriate dosing, used to provide analgesia for labor and delivery.

Contraindications

The absolute and relative contraindications to spinal and epidural anesthesia are summarizes in Table 41.3.

Coagulopathy

Whether secondary to anticoagulants or a disease process, impaired coagulation is an important contraindication to neuraxial blockade. The primary concern is that patients may develop a spinal hematoma which can lead to compressive ischemia of the spinal cord and, consequently, permanent neurological disability. In Table 41.3, it has been classified as a relative contraindication, only because there is a spectrum of severity. There are certain thresholds for coagulation parameters and anticoagulation therapy, beyond which the majority of practitioners would consider it to be an absolute contraindication. Decision-making in individual patients should be based upon balancing the small but very real risk of a spinal hematoma against the potential benefits of neuraxial blockade. The American Society of Regional Anesthesia and Pain Medicine has published expert consensus guidelines to help guide treatment decisions; the key messages are summarizes below (see Chap. 1).

- Neuraxial blockade may be undertaken 4–6 h after the last dose of **IV unfractionated heparin** provided that a normal coagulation result is obtained.
- 12 h should pass from the last dose of **prophylactic SC low molecular weight heparin** (LMWH) and 24 h if a **treatment dose** is used.
- Isolated **non-steroidal anti-inflammatory drug** (NSAID) therapy, including low dose aspirin (81 mg), is not a contraindication to neuraxial blockade. However, needle insertion should be limited to one or two attempts, as the risk of a spinal hematoma increases with the degree of trauma.
- Neuraxial blockade should be avoided for 7 days after **clopidogrel** and 14 days after **ticlopidine**.
- Neuraxial blockade is considered safe with an **internationalized ratio (INR) < 1.5**.
- Administration of anticoagulants should be timed not only to provide a suitable window for inserting an epidural catheter but also to ensure the safe timing of epidural catheter removal.
- If an epidural vein is punctured, subcutaneous heparin administration should be held for at least 2 h, and LMWH held for at least 24 h.
- **GIIa/IIIb inhibitors** should be withheld for at least 4 weeks prior to epidural placement.

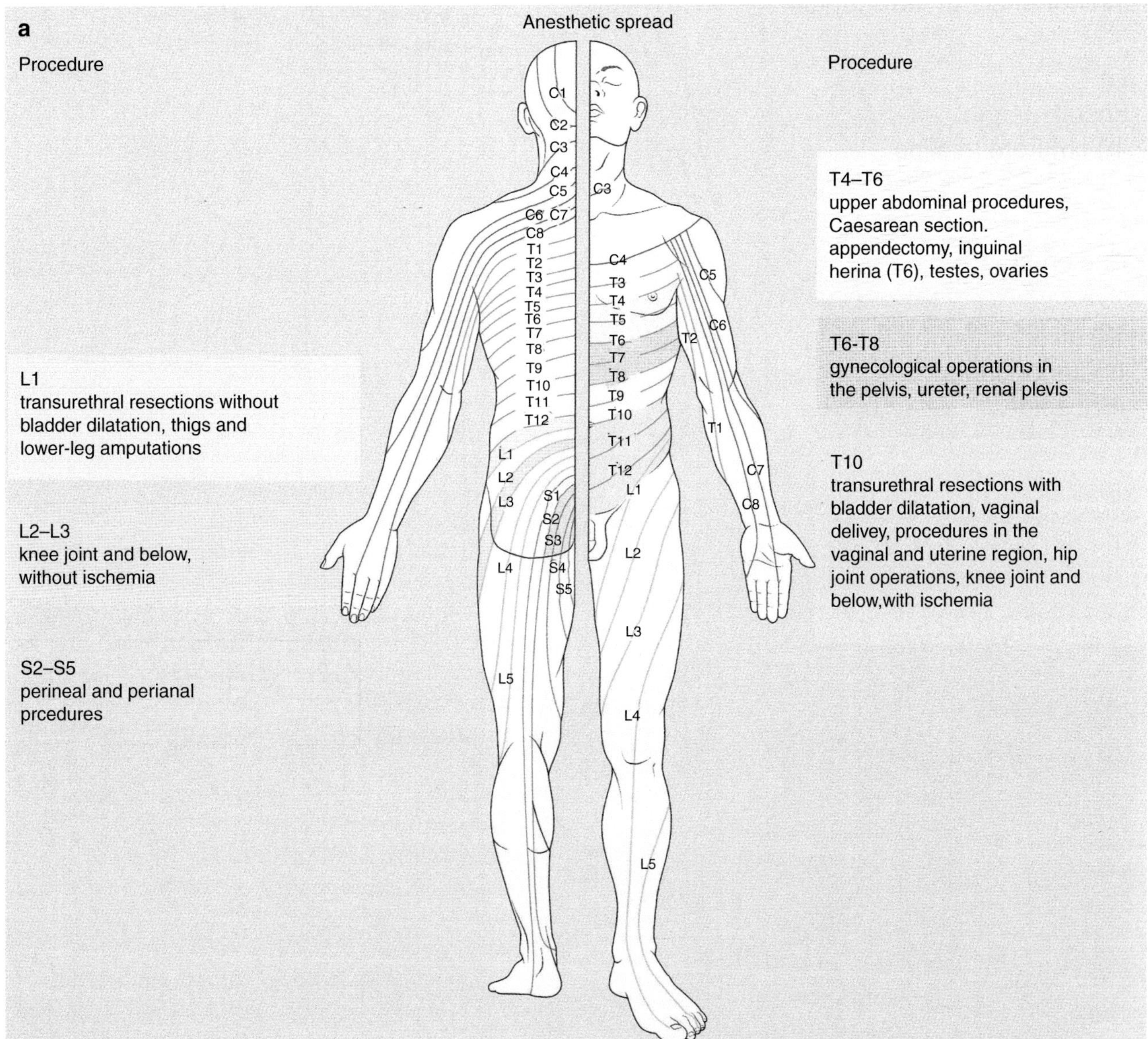

Fig. 41.7 (**a**) Location of the procedure and required sensory spread of local anesthetic. (Reprinted with permission from Danilo Jankovic). (**b**) Landmarks for testing the spread of local anesthetic after neuraxial anesthesia. (Reprinted with permission from Danilo Jankovic)

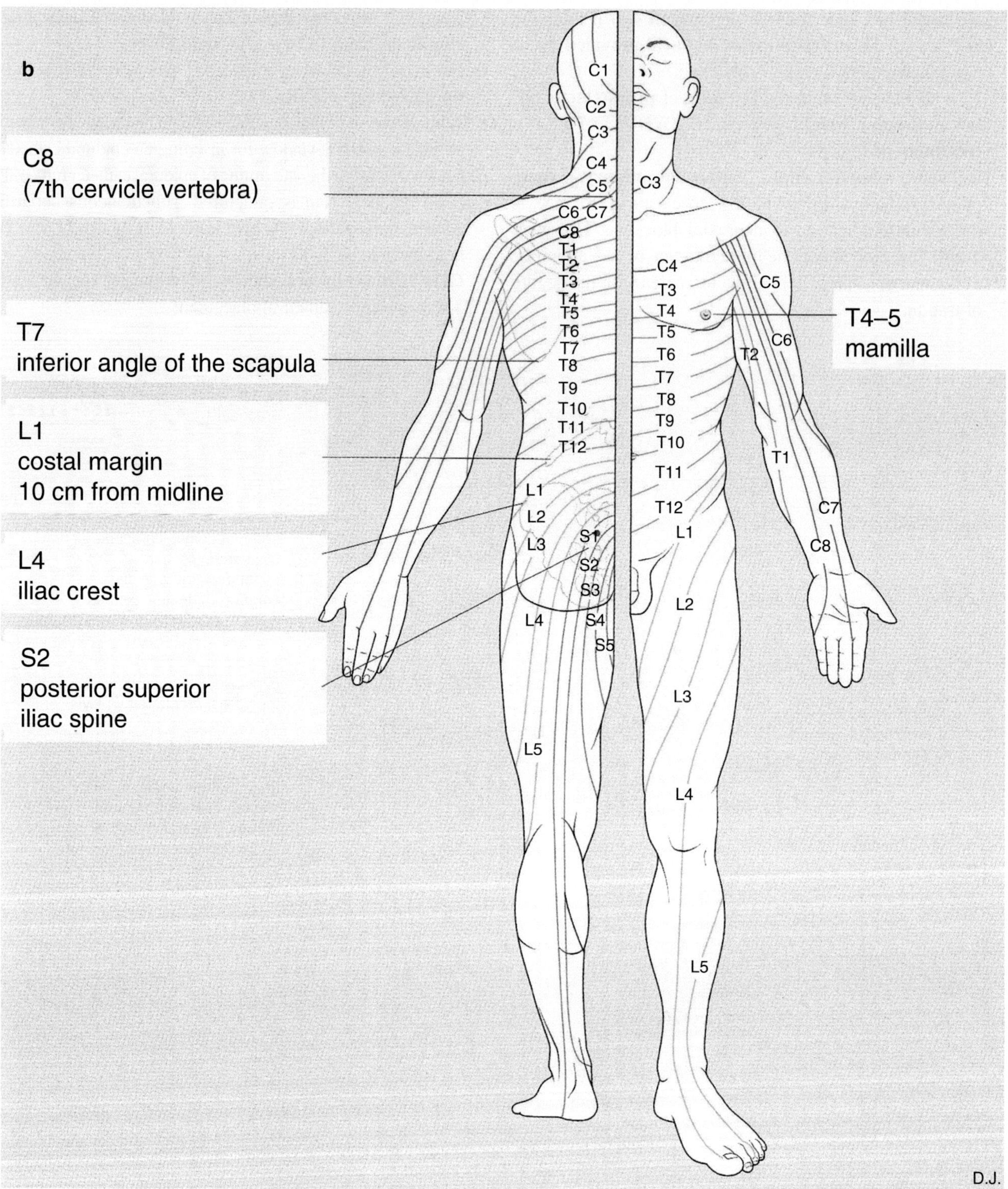

Fig. 41.7 (continued)

Table 41.3 Contraindications to neuraxial blockade

Absolute	Relative
• Patient refusal • Sepsis or local infection at the injection site • Severe decompensated hypovolemia • Acute cerebral or spinal cord diseases • Increased intracranial pressure • Uncooperative patient	• Coagulopathy: Coagulation disorders or anticoagulant therapy • Spinal pathology including severe spinal deformities, arthritis, osteoporosis, intervertebral disk prolapse, spinal canal stenosis, post spinal surgery, and spinal metastases • Unknown duration of surgery • Severe cardiovascular diseases of myocardial, ischemic, or valvular origin • Pre-existing neurological deficits (radiculopathies, peripheral neuropathies, multiple sclerosis)

Cardiovascular Disease

Patients with aortic stenosis deserve special mention. The concern in these patients is that they have a fixed cardiac output which cannot be increased in response to a reduction in intravascular resistance. They are therefore at risk of hypotension, myocardial ischemia, and cardiovascular collapse following the disruption to sympathetic outflow seen following neuraxial blockade. However, decades of clinical experience indicate that this is only of concern in patients with severe or critical aortic stenosis; hence it is a relative contraindication. Neuraxial techniques can be used safely, especially in mild-moderate degrees of aortic stenosis, with appropriate monitoring and preparation to promptly treat or pre-empt any hypotension. Intra-arterial blood pressure monitoring should be instituted before the neuraxial block is performed. Ensuring availability of vasopressor drugs (as boluses or continuous infusion), maintaining normovolemia, and appropriate dosing of local anesthetic, are also essential.

Consent for Neuraxial Blockade

In addition to a description of the procedure itself, the following risks and complications should be discussed with patients as part of the consent process.

Benefits

- Avoidance of airway manipulation and invasive ventilation.
- Reduced post-operative nausea and vomiting.
- Reduced risk of DVT and PE.
- Reduced postoperative drowsiness, especially if judicious sedation is used.
- Improved post-operative analgesia (particularly if opiate adjuncts are used).

Risks and Complications

- Pain and bruising at site of injection.
- Hypotension.
- Nausea and vomiting.
- Urinary retention.
- Inadvertent dural puncture (epidural anesthesia only).
- Post-dural puncture headache.
- Failure or insufficient efficacy with need to repeat the procedure or revert to a general anesthetic.
- High or complete spinal.
- Temporary nerve injury.
- Permanent nerve injury (1 in 24,000 to 1 in 51,000).

Performing Neuraxial Blockade

Preparation and Equipment

- Check that the emergency equipment is complete and in working order (intubation kit, emergency drugs, anesthetic machine).
- Obtain intravenous access and start an IV infusion. Consider volume loading (250–500 mL of a balanced electrolyte solution).
- Vasopressors such as ephedrine, phenylephrine, or metaraminol should be readily available.
- ECG, non-invasive blood pressure and pulse oximetry monitoring are essential.
- Skin preparation using an alcohol, iodine or chlorhexidine. If chlorhexidine is used, extreme care must be taken to prevent its inadvertent introduction into the neuraxis, as it has been implicated in chemical arachnoiditis. Chlorhexidine concentration should not exceed 0.5%. Sterile precautions including drape with fenestration and full sterile gown, gloves, facemask.
- Local anesthetic for skin infiltration.
- Appropriate medication for injecting into the intrathecal or epidural space—usually a combination of local anesthetic and opiate. These must be preservative free.
- Local anesthetic systemic toxicity management kit including 20% lipid emulsion and instructions for use.

Spinal Needles

These are usually of the following two types (Fig. 41.8a–c):

25–27 G spinal needles with a conical tip (pencil-point)—e.g. Sprotte, Pencan, and Whitacre. When the dura is penetrated with these needles, the dural fibers are separated (rather than cut) and then close together again. This reduces the risk of postdural puncture headache.

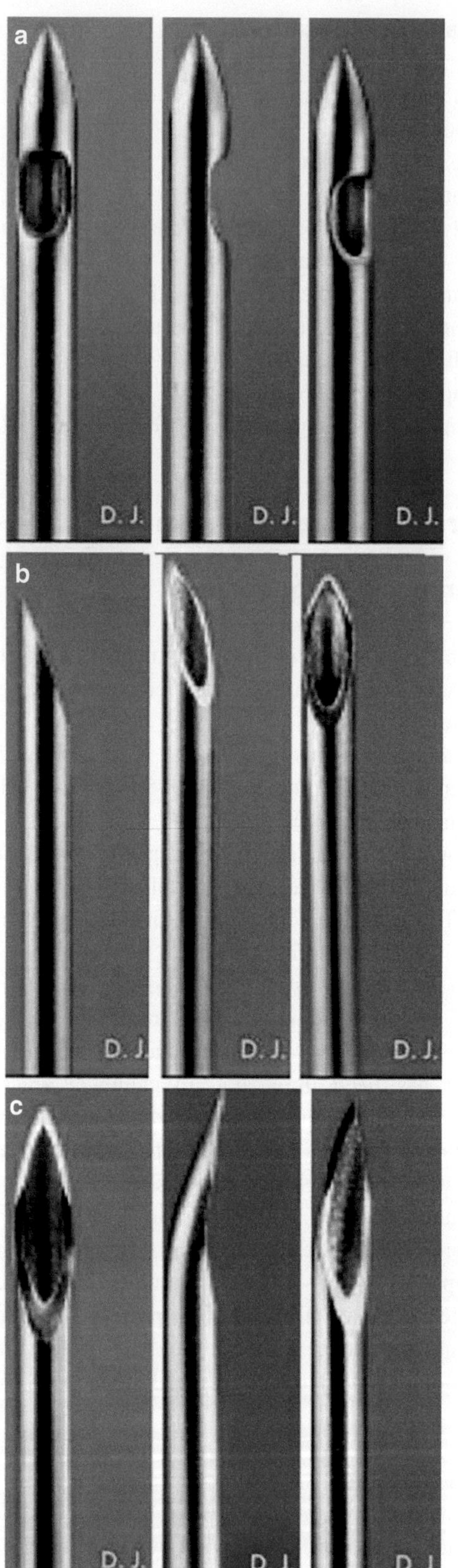

Fig. 41.8 (**a–c**) Spinal needles. (**a**) Pencil-point, 25G; (**b**) Quincke tip, 27G; (**c**)Atraucan Special Cut, 26G. (Reprinted with permission from Danilo Jankovic)

25–27 G spinal needles with Quincke tip. The advantage of the Quincke tip is that it will pierce skin, and dense or calcified tissues with less effort, and with less risk of the needle bending and deviating from the intended trajectory.

A thicker 22-G Quincke tip needle is advantageous for similar reasons—the increased stiffness of the shaft makes it easier to handle and to redirect in small increments and may be used in patients with more challenging anatomy—e.g. narrowed interlaminar spaces, or suboptimal positioning, as well as obese patients with a large amount of overlying soft tissue.

The types of epidural needles are discussed later in the chapter.

Patient Positioning

Optimal patient positioning both prior to and immediately after performing neuraxial anesthesia is essential for ensuring block success. The most common positions used are the sitting or the lateral decubitus position. The prone or jack knife position is another alternative but one that is rarely utilized in modern anesthetic practice.

Lateral Decubitus Position

The assistant stands in front of the patient to help with stabilization and to prevent any falls. The patient's legs are flexed at the hips and knees as far as possible without causing discomfort, and the chin is flexed down onto the chest (Fig. 41.9). This reverses the lumbar lordosis and widens the lumbar interspinous and intervertebral spaces.

It may be easier for novices to maintain an appropriate needle trajectory if the patient is kept in a strict lateral position. However, with larger patients, allowing them to tilt anteriorly towards the assistant may improve the stability of their position. In this case, the operator must compensate by angling the needle towards the surface of the bed when advancing in a midline approach, to maintain the needle in the sagittal plane of the patient (Fig. 41.10a, b). This slightly tilted position is also advantageous when employing a paramedian approach from the dependent side of the spine as it creates more room between the needle hub and the surface of the bed.

A key point to note is that gravity will cause the soft tissues to sag downwards and thus the surface midline groove of the back will be slightly lateral to the bony midline and spinous processes. This must be taken into account when palpating the spinous processes and choosing a skin insertion site. The position of the overlying skin and subcutaneous tissues must be controlled with the fingers of the non-dominant hand during needle insertion (Fig. 41.11).

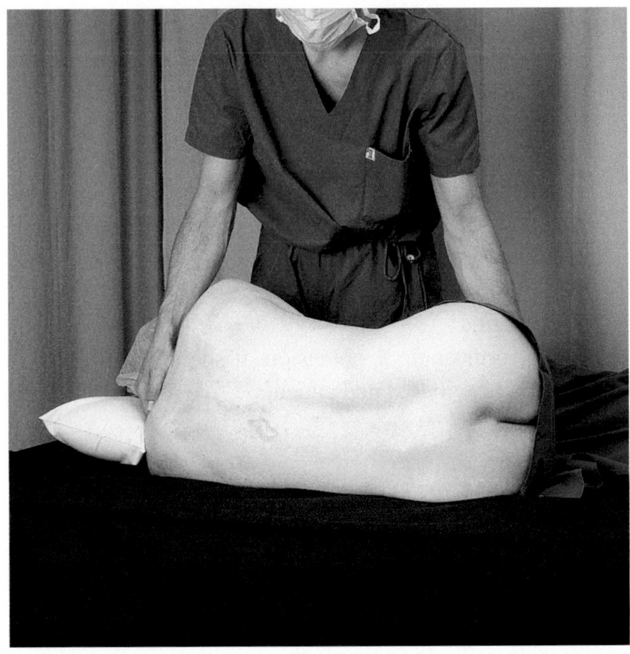

Fig. 41.9 Lateral decubitus position. (Reprinted with permission from Danilo Jankovic)

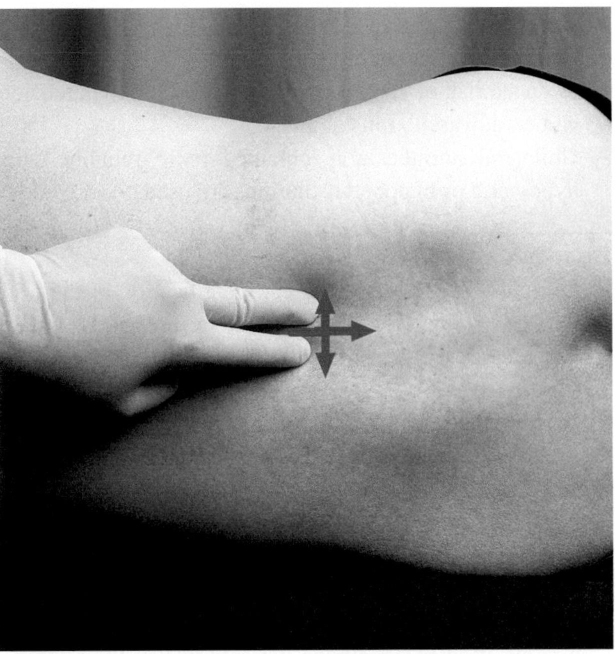

Fig. 41.11 Palpation of the intervertebral space. (Reprinted with permission from Danilo Jankovic)

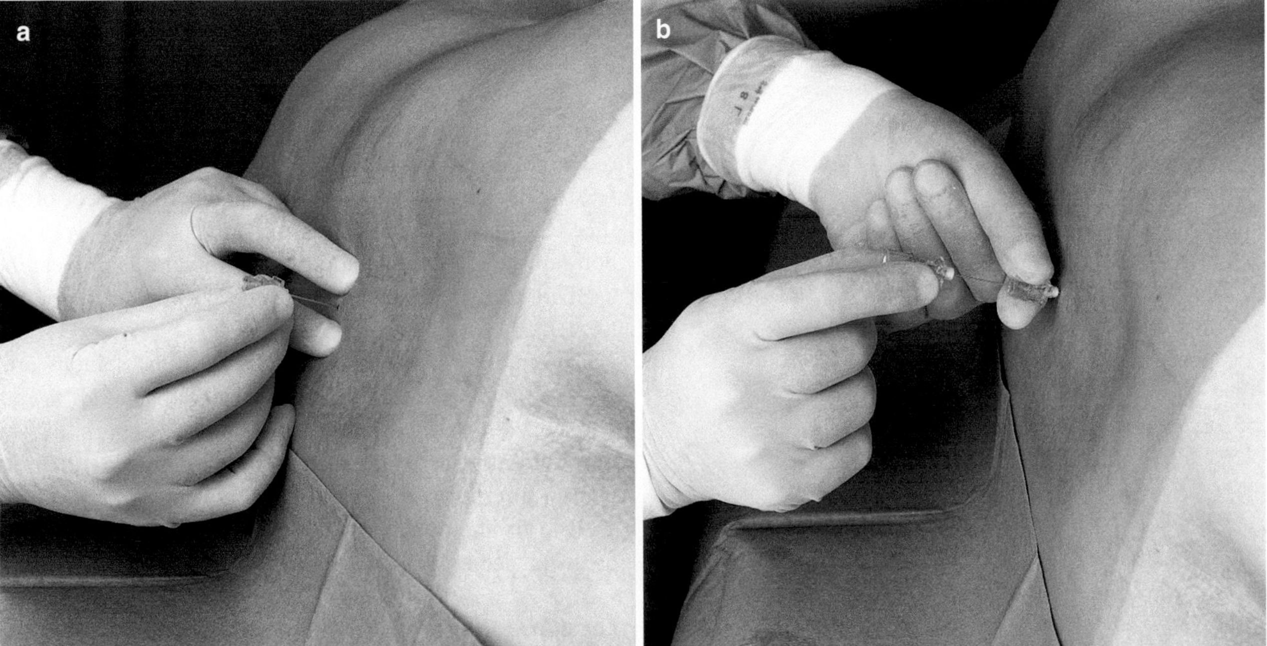

Fig. 41.10 (**a** and **b**) Tilting the patient away from the operator can provide a more stable position, but the trajectory must be adjusted downwards relative to the bed surface as needed to keep the needle advancing in the midline. (Reprinted with permission from Danilo Jankovic)

Advantages

- Increased patient comfort.
- Reduced risk of venous pooling, orthostatic hypotension, and cardiovascular instability.
- Unilateral anesthesia is obtained more reliably when hyperbaric or hypobaric solutions are used.

Disadvantages

- Difficulty may arise in correct identification of the midline, especially if the pelvis is tilted too anteriorly or there is extensive subcutaneous tissue.

Sitting Position

The patient is seated on the edge of the operating table, supported by an assistant standing in front of them (Fig. 41.12). The patient's feet rest flat on a stool placed on the floor in front of them. It may also be helpful to provide a padded Mayo stand, adjustable table or similar device for the patient to lean on for additional support. Various audio cues are commonly used to encourage patients to flex their lumbar spine and correct the lordosis, such as "arch your back like an angry cat/prawn/shrimp" or "slouch like a sulky teenager." A visual demonstration sometimes improves patient positioning.

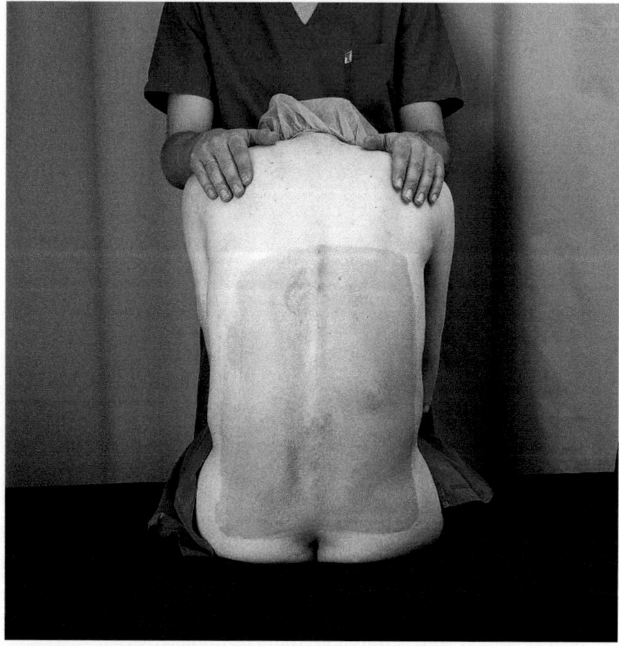

Fig. 41.12 Sitting position. (Reprinted with permission from Danilo Jankovic)

Advantages

- Easier to locate the midline, particularly in obese patients, as the tissue falls away to the sides rather than over the midline as in the lateral position.
- Optimal position for performing a saddle block whereby only the S2 to S5 dermatomes are anesthetized. This facilitates surgery in the perineal region while preserving power and sensation in the legs.

Disadvantages

- Risk of orthostatic hypotension. It should be avoided in frail and heavily sedated patients.

Spinal Anesthesia

Injection Technique

The subarachnoid space may be accessed using a midline, paramedian or Taylor's approach.

Midline Approach

Landmarks

The injection is carried out in the midline below the level of the conus medullaris, usually between the spinous processes of the L2–3, L3–4, or L4–5 vertebrae. L5-S1 may also be an option, especially in the older patient with degenerative narrowing of intervertebral spaces. Tuffier's line (or intercristal line) is determined by palpating the superior aspect of the iliac crests on each side. This line bisects the L4 vertebral body in roughly half of adults. Ultrasound imaging can be used to more precisely identify the desired intervertebral level.

The midline is identified by palpating the spinous processes above and below the intervertebral space. It is recommended that **the index and middle fingers of the non-dominant hand be used to palpate and identify the chosen interspace**, as they can subsequently be parted and used to **fix** the overlying skin (Fig. 41.11). This improves precision and accuracy in needle insertion.

Local Anesthesia Infiltration to Skin and Soft Tissues

The skin and the supraspinous and interspinous ligaments are anesthetized with 1–2 mL of a local anesthetic (e.g. 1% lidocaine). The injection is carried out between the spread index and middle fingers of the left hand (Fig. 41.13). The local anesthetic needle may be used to explore the under-

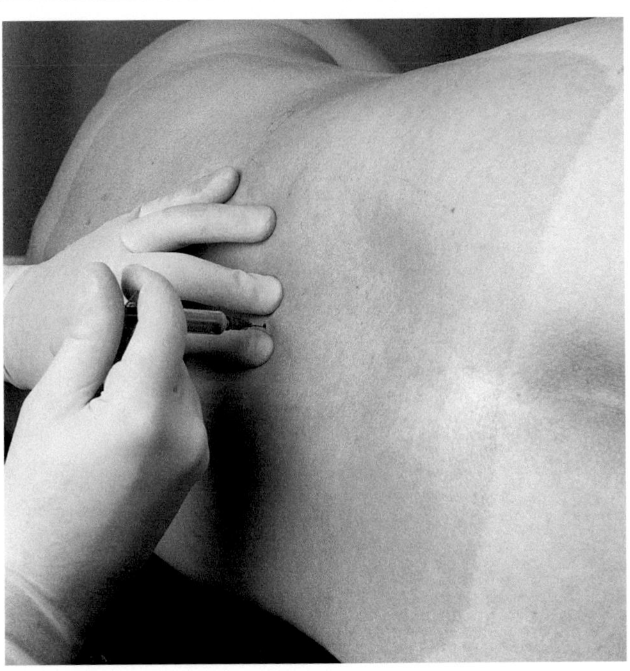

Fig. 41.13 Infiltration of the subcutaneous tissue with local anesthesia. (Reprinted with permission from Danilo Jankovic)

lying anatomy. Bony contact at a relatively shallow depth indicates contact with the tip of the spinous process and the location of the midline. Firm resistance to further injection of local anesthetic indicates that the needle tip lies in the midline within the interspinous ligament, and not in the paraspinous muscles on either side.

Advancing the Introducer Needle

An introducer needle is used with 25–27G pencil-point needles to facilitate skin puncture and avoid bending or deviation during insertion. Without moving the spread index and middle finger of the left hand away from the intervertebral space (which prevents inadvertent movement of the skin overlying the chosen interspace), the introducer is grasped between the thumb and index finger of the right hand and advanced in the sagittal plane until it is felt to be sitting firmly in the interspinous ligament (Fig. 41.14). In very obese patients, however, the length of the introducer needle may be insufficient to reach the ligament. Insertion of a 22G needle does not require an introducer, but the same principle of skin fixation with the index and middle fingers of the non-dominant hand should be adhered to, to ensure the needle is travelling in the sagittal plane towards the bony midline rather than off to one side.

It is recommended keep cranial angulation to a minimum to start with, since the lumbar spinous processes are largely horizontal, especially if there is good flexion of the lumbar spine. Incremental cranial angulation is undertaken as needed if there is bony contact with the spinous process

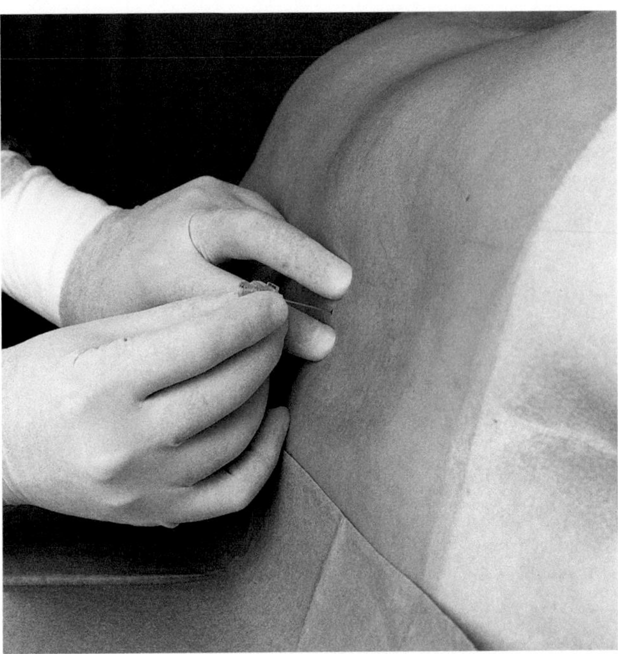

Fig. 41.14 Advancing the introducer needle in a midline approach. Note that the patient is tilted slightly anteriorly such that the surface of the back is not perpendicular to the surface of the bed. Keeping the needle in the sagittal plane during advancement therefore requires that the needle is angled slightly downwards towards the bed surface (see also Fig. 41.15). (Reprinted with permission from Danilo Jankovic)

(Fig. 41.14). Once in place, the introducer is controlled with the thumb and index finger of the left hand, with the dorsum of the hand lying firmly on the patient's back.

Introducing the Spinal Needle and Dural Puncture

The spinal needle, held between the thumb and index finger (or middle finger) of the right hand, is inserted via the introducer needle (if used), through the interspinous ligament, ligamentum flavum, epidural space, dura, and arachnoid mater and into the subarachnoid space (Figs. 41.15 and 41.16). Each of these tissues has a characteristic "feel" as described above. Penetration of the interlaminar space and ligamentum flavum is usually evident by the "rubbery" resistance to needle advancement. A characteristic "dural click" may be felt when the subarachnoid space is reached; however, this does not always occur. It is therefore recommended that the stylet be intermittently withdrawn between incremental advancements to check for CSF backflow (see below) once the ligamentum flavum has been engaged by the needle tip.

Experience shows that failure to locate and enter the interlaminar space is usually due to deviation of the needle from the midline or excessive cranial angulation of the needle.

Removing the Stylet

The following may occur here:

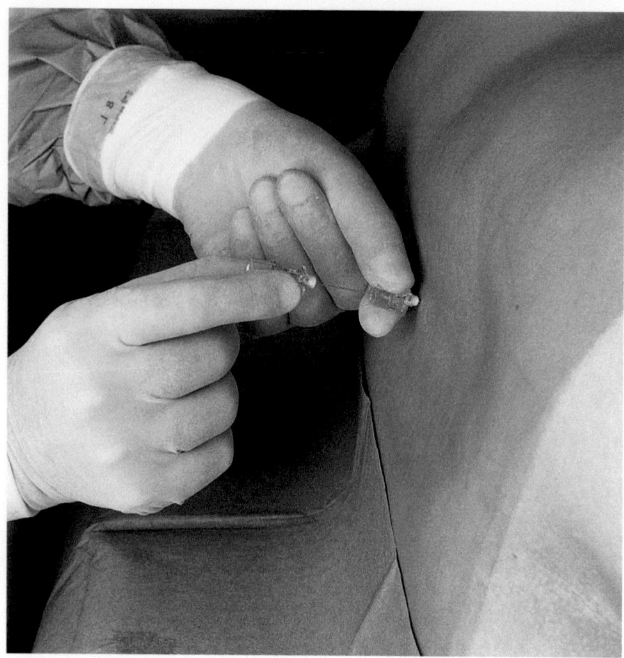

Fig. 41.15 Introducing the spinal needle and puncturing the subarachnoid space in a midline approach. Note the slight downward angle of the needle which is required due to the slight anterior tilt of the patient (see Fig. 41.14). (Reprinted with permission from Danilo Jankovic)

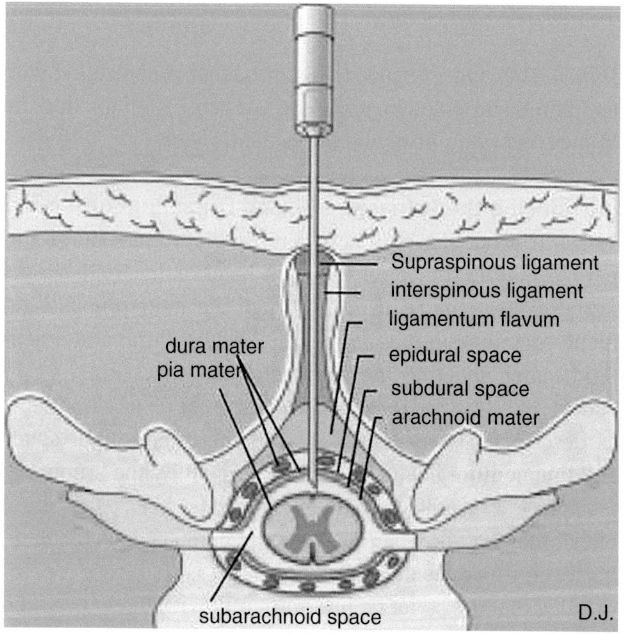

Fig. 41.16 Subarachnoid position of the needle. (Reprinted with permission from Danilo Jankovic)

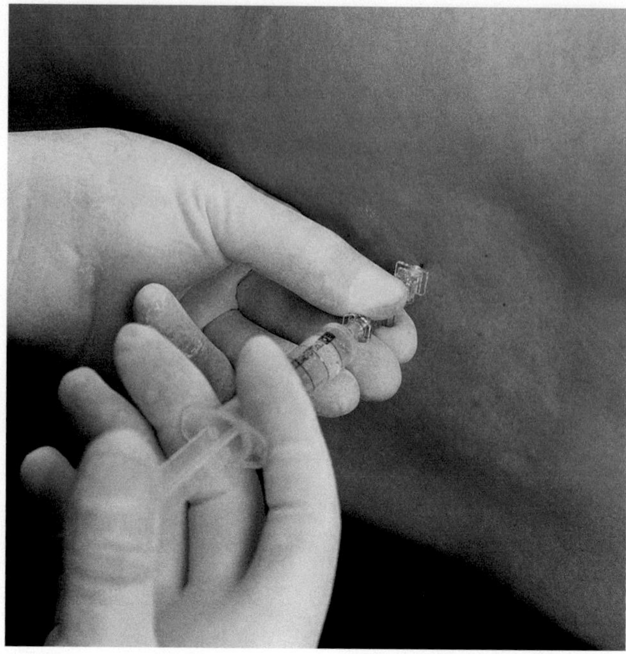

Fig. 41.17 Subarachnoid injection. (Reprinted with permission from Danilo Jankovic)

CSF Flows Freely

The injection needle is fixed between the thumb and index finger of the left hand, which is braced on the patient's back. The syringe containing the local anesthetic mixture is carefully and firmly attached to the needle (Fig. 41.17). Aspiration of CSF (0.1 mL) should be attempted immediately before and after injection of local anesthetic to confirm that the needle orifice is within the subarachnoid space. The rate of injection is not thought to play a significant part in determining the height of the block.

Blood in the CSF

Slightly bloodstained CSF which clears quickly (spontaneously, or after aspiration) usually occurs after penetration of an epidural vein on the way into the subarachnoid space. The local anesthetic can be injected if this is the case. However, backflow of frank blood indicates that the injection needle is likely positioned within a vein. A new attempt at puncture must be made, possibly in a different intervertebral space.

CSF Present in the Needle Hub But Does Not Flow Freely

This is more likely in elderly or dehydrated patients who may have low CSF pressure. It may also be caused by part of the cauda equina occluding the orifice of the needle, especially when negative pressure is applied to the syringe. Rotation of the needle to all four quadrants and careful gentle aspiration may improve flow. If aspiration continues to be impossible, it is recommended that the syringe be disconnected from the hub, and the fluid meniscus in the hub of the needle observed to see if the meniscus extrudes, signifying slow but positive CSF backflow. If this occurs, the syringe may be carefully reattached and injection performed without further reattempts at aspiration (which will only increase the risk of dislodgement of the orifice out of the subarachnoid space).

If no CSF flows in spite of all these measures, the needle should be removed and the procedure repeated with a different needle direction or at a different interspace.

Unexpectedly deep bony contact, or bony contact after the ligamentum flavum has been penetrated, suggests that the anterior wall of the vertebral canal or an intervertebral disk has been reached. The stylet should be removed, and the needle slowly and carefully withdrawn in small increments, pausing in between to observe for CSF backflow as the orifice re-enters the subarachnoid space. If CSF is not observed during this process, the bony contact may have been the base of the spinous process rather than the anterior wall of the vertebral canal, in which case further cranial redirection is required to enter the interlaminar space.

Pain or Paresthesia During Puncture

Pain or paresthesia prior to entry into the epidural or intrathecal space, especially if localized to one side, is most often due to needle contact with the facet joint, which forms the lateral border of the interlaminar space. The location of the midline should be reassessed, and the needle should be directed slightly more medially, away from the side on which the pain or paresthesia occurred.

It is not uncommon for a transient paresthesia radiating down one leg to occur upon needle entry into the intrathecal space; this signals contact with the cauda equina. The stylet should always be withdrawn at this point to check for CSF backflow. If the paresthesia or pain is persistent, the needle must be withdrawn slightly or repositioned, before any injection is performed. The local anesthetic must never be injected without evidence of CSF. The location and distribution of any paresthesia arising during the puncture procedure should be recorded.

Paramedian Approach (Lateral, Paraspinal)

In this technique (Figs. 41.18 and 41.19), the supraspinous and interspinous ligaments are avoided. The ligamentum flavum becomes the primary target on the way into the subarachnoid space.

Procedure

This technique can be used in all the patient positions mentioned above. Flexion of the spine to widen the interspinous spaces is not essential as the needle will bypass these—this is a major advantage of the technique. It may therefore be helpful in patients with degenerative changes of the spine, older patients with calcification of the supraspinous and interspinous ligaments and in patients who find it difficult to flex the lumbar spine.

The cranial edge of the lower spinous process of the desired interspace is marked (Fig. 41.20). The injection site is located in-line with this edge and not more than 1 cm lateral to the spinous process, which avoids the need for a large lateral-to-medial angle; this should be kept within 5–10°. The needle is inserted with a slight cranio-caudal angle of about 10–15°. It is not unusual to contact the lamina on the

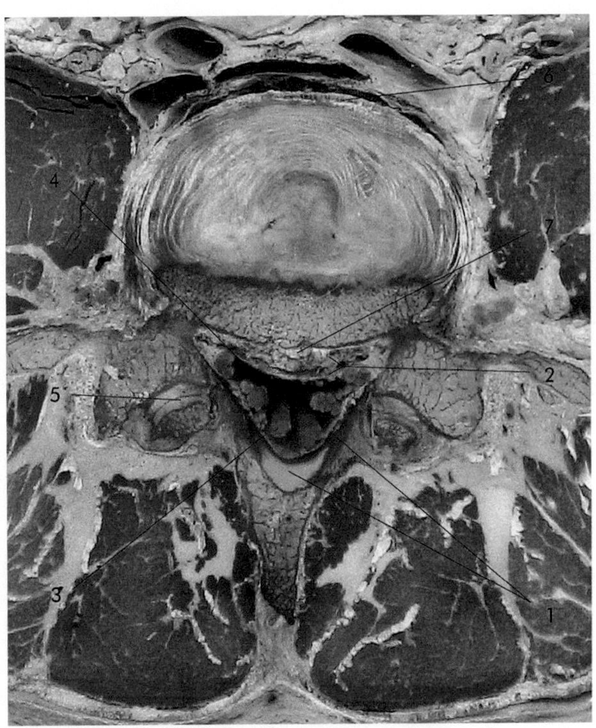

Fig. 41.18 Transverse dissection at the level of the L4/5. (1) Posterior epidural space with fat, (2) anterior epidural space with veins, (3) spinal dura mater, (4) subarachnoid space and cauda equine, (5) zygapophysial joint, (6) anterior longitudinal ligament, and (7) posterior longitudinal ligament. (Reprinted with permission from Danilo Jankovic)

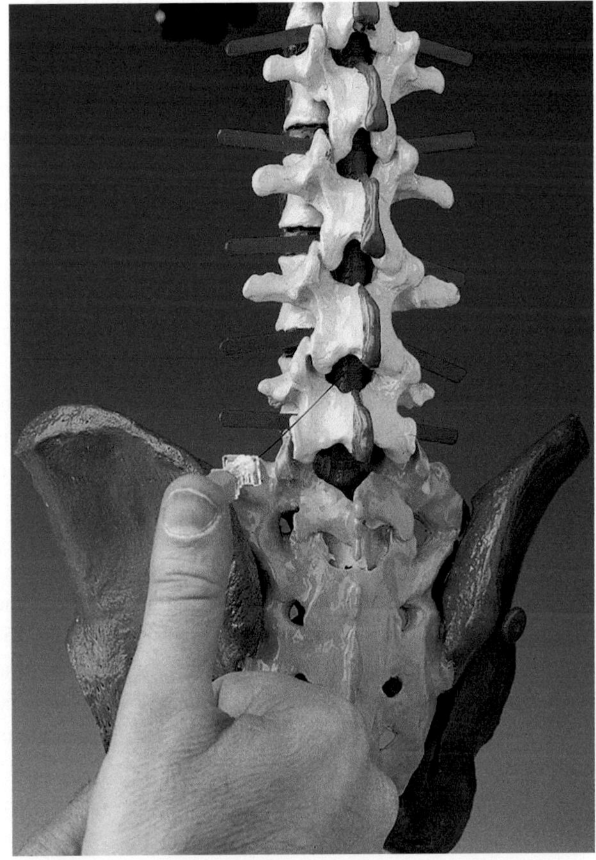

Fig. 41.19 Paramedian approach. (Reprinted with permission from Danilo Jankovic)

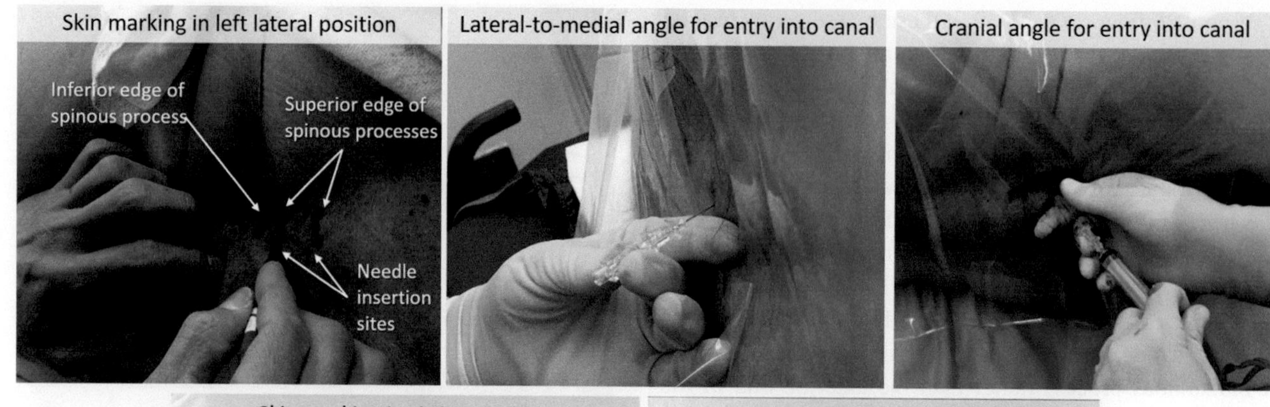

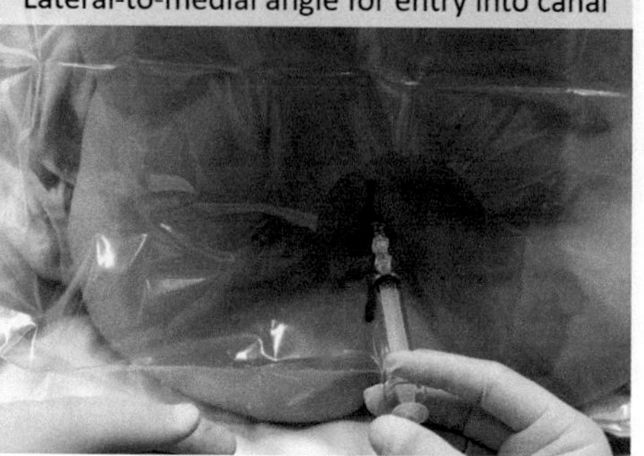

Fig. 41.20 Top row of images illustrates the paramedian (paraspinous) approach to spinal anesthesia in the lateral position; the bottom row illustrates the same approach in the sitting position. A suitable needle insertion site is approximately 1–1.5 cm lateral to the midline or just lateral to and superior to the superior edge of the spinous process. The lateral-to-medial angle should not exceed 10–15°, and maintained constant while the cranial angle of the needle trajectory is incrementally adjusted as needed, starting perpendicular to the skin, to walk off the lamina and into the vertebral canal. The exact angles required for success will vary depending on patient anatomy and the precision of the needle skin insertion site. (Reprinted with permission from Dr. Ki Jinn Chin)

first needle pass. The needle tip is then walked cranially in small increments until it slips off the lamina and deeper into the interlaminar space and ligamentum flavum; this will be signaled by the characteristic feel. Failure arises most commonly when the needle is angled too cranially or when the needle entry point is too lateral.

Taylor's Approach

This lumbosacral (L5–S1) approach (Figs. 41.21 and 41.22) is a paramedian injection via the intervertebral space of L5 and S1, the largest interlaminar space in the spinal region. As with the paramedian approach described above, this approach is somewhat more forgiving when patient positioning is suboptimal.

Procedure

The injection site is located 1 cm medial and inferiorly to the posterior superior iliac spine. The needle is directed 45°–55° cranially and medially. Initial resistance will be felt when the needle contacts the ligamentum flavum and subsequently the dura. If bony resistance is felt, this most likely reflects contact

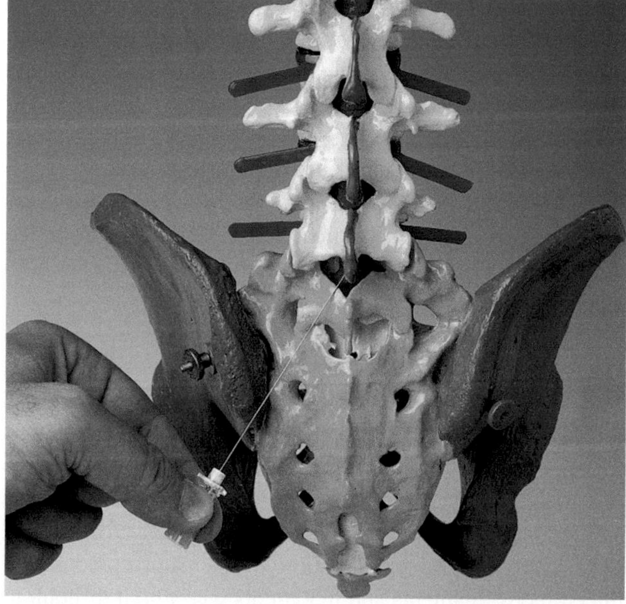

Fig. 41.21 Taylor's approach. (Reprinted with permission from Danilo Jankovic)

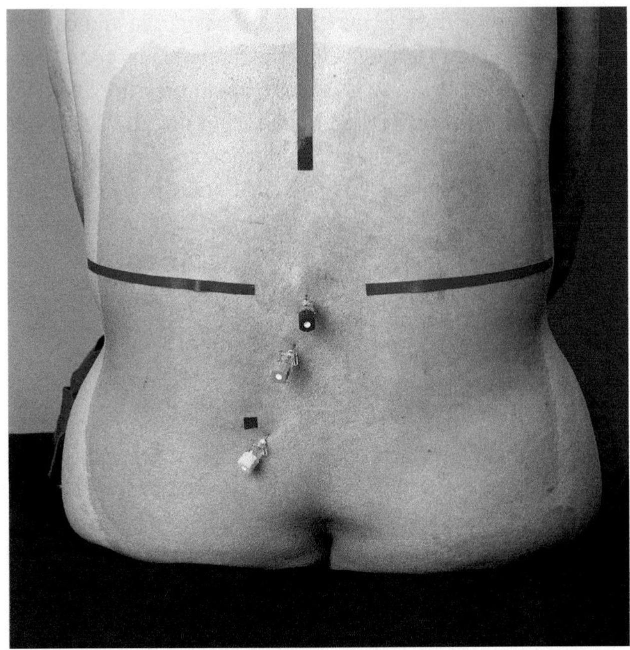

Fig. 41.22 Puncture of the subarachnoid space: (1) median, (2) paramedian, (3) Taylor. (Reprinted with permission from Danilo Jankovic)

with the sacrum. Withdraw the needle and redirect it medially and cranially. Spread of local anesthetic to higher spinal segments can be achieved more easily if hyper- or hypobaric solution is used and the patient is appropriately positioned.

Unilateral Spinal Anesthesia

Unilateral spinal anesthesia is intended to block only the anterior and posterior spinal nerve roots on the side being operated on, while the contralateral side—and particularly its sympathetic fibers—remains unblocked. This leads to a reduced incidence of hypotension.

Indications

Surgical procedures on the lower limbs.

Procedure

Patient positioning: lateral decubitus position, lying on the side that is to be operated on if a hyperbaric local anesthetic solution is used and on the opposite side if a hypobaric solution is used. Hyperbaric solutions usually have 8% glucose added to them and are commercially available, while hypobaric solutions can be concocted by 2:1 or 3:1 dilution with sterile water.

Injection technique: this is the same as for conventional spinal anesthesia. After piercing the dura, the opening of the pencil-point needle may be rotated to the operating side and the desired amount of local anesthetic is injected slowly. The patient remains in the same position for 15–20 min.

Advantages

- Reduced sympathetic block (by about 70%) as smaller volumes of local anesthetic can be used and fewer spinal segments are blocked.
- Improved hemodynamic stability.
- Faster recovery from anesthesia.
- Suitable for outpatient procedures.
- Greater acceptance by patients.

Disadvantages

True unilateral anesthesia is only achieved if adequate time (10–15 min) is allowed for the local anesthetic to settle on the operative side. However, a differential block of some degree can almost always be achieved.

Continuous Spinal Anesthesia

The insertion of a catheter into the subarachnoid space allows a continuous or repeated intermittent dosing of local anesthetic.

Indications

- Lower abdominal and lower limb surgery in elderly patients and high-risk patients.
- Postoperative pain relief.
- Chronic pain relief (in cancer patients).

Procedure

The procedure is similar to a standard spinal anesthetic. Usually, a 20–22 G spinal needle is used to gain access to the subarachnoid space, and a 25–27 G catheter is threaded (usually 2–3 cm) into the subarachnoid space (Fig. 41.23).

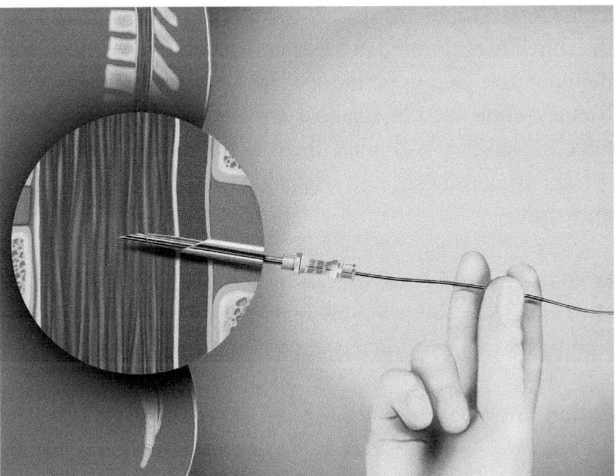

Fig. 41.23 Introducing the catheter in the subarachnoid space. (Reprinted with permission from Danilo Jankovic)

Advantages

- A smaller initial dose of local anesthetic can be injected without concern about inadequate block height or duration. This helps prevent hypotension due to excessive sympathetic block caused by large doses or greater spread of local anesthetic.
- Ability to prolong spinal anesthetic as needed.

Disadvantages

- Higher risk of post dural puncture headache as a higher gauge spinal needle is used.
- Use of small micro catheters (less than 24 G) may predispose to sacral pooling of local anesthetic leading to cauda equina syndrome.

Management of the Patient After Intrathecal Injection

Patient Positioning

The spread of local anesthetic to different vertebral levels is influenced by positioning the patient. It is checked with cold tests at intervals of 2–5 min.

Hyperbaric Spinal Anesthesia

Lateral decubitus position: the patient remains on the side of surgery for 10–15 min if unilateral anesthesia is desired. The patient is laid supine if bilateral anesthesia is required.

Sitting position: the patient is immediately laid supine to allow the anesthetic to spread cranial. The patient remains sitting if only sacral spread is desired (saddle block).

Hypobaric Spinal Anesthesia

The hypobaric technique has gained popularity in major hip surgery, which is often performed in the lateral position. Thus, repositioning of the patient will not be required when the spinal is performed in the lateral decubitus position, with the operative side uppermost. If the sitting position is used, it is recommended to sit them on the side of the operating table or bed that will allow them to lie down directly, once the spinal anesthesia is completed, with the operative side uppermost.

Isobaric Spinal Anesthesia

Horizontal positioning is adequate; other positions have no significant influence on the spread of the anesthesia.

Patient Monitoring

Sympathetic block following a spinal anesthetic usually results in a drop in blood pressure. This may be profound in patients who are elderly or fluid deplete. Bradycardia may occur after the peak of sympathetic block is achieved (30–60 min after spinal injection) due to the blockade of cardiac accelerator fibers. Unexpected bradycardia and cardiac arrest may occur in young healthy patients. Thus, continuous monitoring of the vitals (heart rate, blood pressure and oxygen saturation) is advocated both during the procedure and for the duration of the block. Supplemental oxygen administration is recommended after a spinal anesthetic, especially if sedation is used for patient comfort. Capnometry is also recommended if sedation is used.

Postoperatively, the patient should be monitored until the effects of spinal anesthetic have receded.

Block Assessment

The spread of anesthesia should be checked at short intervals. The first sign of an effect on the spinal nerve roots is a subjective sensation of warmth in the gluteal region and feet. The further development of the block encompasses touch, deep pressure, motor function, vibration sensitivity, and positional sense.

Motor function is completely blocked at the site of the greatest concentration of the local anesthetic. Sensory block extends two to four segments higher than motor block, and the sympathetic block extends for a further two to four segments higher than the sensory block.

Resolution of the block is marked by a return of motor function, followed by the sensory modalities. The autonomic function is the last to recover. This sometimes explains why patients continue to have a degree of hypotension in the post anesthetic care unit even after the sensory and motor block have resolved.

Pharmacology of Drugs Used for Spinal Anesthesia

There is a fairly limited range of local anesthetic agents and adjuvant medications commonly used for spinal anesthesia. The specific medication and dosage used will help to determine the spread, duration, and intensity of the block.

Pharmacokinetics of Intrathecal Local Anesthetics

Determinants of Intrathecal Distribution

Local anesthetic deposited within the subarachnoid space spreads to the nerves via bulk flow. Many factors have been proposed to influence the spread of local anesthetics within the subarachnoid space. These may be classified as follows:

Characteristics of the Injected Drug

Baricity: this is defined as the ratio of the density of the local anesthetic solution relative to the patient's CSF at 37 ° C. *Isobaric, hyperbaric,* and *hypobaric* solutions have the same, greater, and lesser density than the CSF, respectively.

While hyperbaric solutions will sink to the most dependent areas within the subarachnoid space, the hypobaric solutions rise upwards towards the nondependent areas. In general, hyperbaric solutions will produce a greater spread than isobaric or hypobaric solutions.

Mass: mass, volume, and concentration have been investigated for their effects on the spread of the local anesthetics in the intrathecal compartment. For plain solutions, the effect of drug mass injected is more important than the volume or the concentration. For hyperbaric solutions, this may not always be true, with some studies finding no effect.

Effect of additives: while the addition of vasoconstrictors prolong the block duration, the addition of opioids may increase spread and delay block recession. All additives must be labeled as preservatives carry a risk of causing adverse neurological outcomes.

Technical Considerations

Patient positioning immediately after a spinal anesthetic influences the extent of spread of local anesthetic. This is governed by gravity and is further influenced by the curvatures of the spine.

Level of injection: for an isobaric solution, a higher level of injection results in a greater cranial spread of the block. This is not consistently observed with hyperbaric solutions where the effect of gravity may be more profound.

Needle direction: turning the needle aperture cranial may result in a higher spread of the drug, with a shorter duration of action and faster resolution of the block. Cranial angulation of insertion has shown similar results.

Speed of injection: Has clinically minimal effects.

Barbotage: may shorten the time of onset with hyperbaric solutions.

Patient Factors

Individual patient factors such as age, height, body mass index, and sex do not help to predict the spread of intrathecal local anesthetics. However, excessive lordosis in pregnancy may promote cranial spread and lowering doses is recommended.

Uptake of Local Anesthetics

The local anesthetic deposited in the subarachnoid space spreads within the CSF. It is then taken up by the nerve roots in the cauda equina, resulting in neuronal block. This uptake is affected by the following factors:

- Concentration of the local anesthetic in the CSF.
- The surface area of the nerve root exposed to the CSF.
- The lipid content of the nerve root (since local anesthetics are lipid soluble).
- The blood flow within the nerve.

Elimination of Local Anesthetics

The elimination of local anesthetics from the subarachnoid space is determined by the following factors:

- Vascular absorption of the local anesthetic (this is the most important route).
- Escape of the drug to the epidural space, with subsequent vascular absorption.
- Lipophilicity of the local anesthetic (highly lipophilic drugs such as bupivacaine have a slower elimination due to greater binding with the neuronal tissue).

Determinants of Duration

Elimination of local anesthetics from the intrathecal space determines the duration of their neural block. The factors influencing this are as follows:

Physicochemical properties of the local anesthetic chosen: prilocaine is a short acting agent whereas lignocaine and mepivacaine are short to intermediate acting local anesthetics. Bupivacaine, levo-bupivacaine, and ropivacaine are longer acting agents.

Dose injected: in general, the duration of the block is increased with an increase in the dose (or mass) of the local anesthetic injected.

Block spread: for a given dose of the local anesthetic, a block with a greater spread (i.e. higher peak sensory block) will regress faster, thereby shortening the duration of action.

Addition of adjuvants: as mentioned above, the addition of vasoconstrictors and opioids may delay the regression of the block.

Intrathecal Local Anesthetics

The physicochemical properties of local anesthetics such as lipid solubility and protein binding impact the duration of block. They may be classified as follows:

Short Acting Agents

Procaine: It is an amino ester with a rapid onset (3–5 min) but short duration (50–60 min) of block. This is due to its poor lipid solubility and protein binding. Compared to lignocaine, it has a higher rate of block failure but a lower rate of transient neurologic syndrome (TNS).

2-Chloroprocaine: It is an amino ester with a rapid onset and short duration (60 min) of spinal block comparable to lignocaine. It has a lower incidence of TNS.

Prilocaine: It is a short acting amino amide with a short duration of action (60–120 min). It has been recently used for ambulatory surgery, with shorter recovery times when compared to lignocaine. It is not currently available in North America.

Short to Intermediate Acting Agents

Lignocaine: It is an amino amide with a rapid onset and short to intermediate duration of action (60 min, depending upon dose). Its use has dramatically declined due to higher frequency of TNS observed with its use (15–33%).

Mepivacaine: It is an amino amide with similar profile to lignocaine, but lower incidence of TNS (3–6%). It is seeing a resurgence in its use, particularly in the context of ambulatory surgery.

Long Acting Agents

Tetracaine: It is a long acting (3 h) amino ester with a high lipid solubility. It has been almost entirely replaced by bupivacaine due to poor reliability.

Bupivacaine: It is a prototypical amino amide with a long duration of action due to high lipid solubility. It is the most widely used intrathecal local anesthetic. It has an onset time of 10 min and a block duration of 3–4 h. Reducing the doses for unilateral spinal, or ambulatory surgery shortens the duration of action, but may also increase incidence of block failures.

Levo-bupivacaine: this less cardiotoxic stereoisomer of bupivacaine is almost identical to bupivacaine in its spinal anesthetic profile.

Ropivacaine: It is a long acting amino-amide which has gained popularity by virtue of its less cardiotoxic potential. When compared to bupivacaine, it is less potent and produces a block of shorter duration.

Doses

Dosages and duration of commonly used local anesthetics are summarizes in Tables 41.4 and 41.5.

Intrathecal Adjuvants

Additives are often used along with intrathecal local anesthetics to prolong or intensify their block. Although many drugs have been used and evaluated for this, the commonly used intrathecal additives include opioids, vasoconstrictors, and the α2-adrenergic agonists.

Opioids

These act synergistically with the local anesthetics by blocking the opioid receptors at the spinal level.

Morphine It is the most commonly used hydrophilic opioid. Because of its slow distribution within the CSF and a slow plasma clearance, it has a long duration of action when given intrathecally. Used in the doses of 100–400 μg, it provides good postoperative analgesia up to 24 h. However, the intrathecal use of morphine has been implicated in delayed respiratory depression due to rostral migration within the CSF. Higher doses of intrathecal morphine are associated with higher incidence of side effects such as nausea, vomiting, pruritus, urinary retention, and respiratory depression.

Fentanyl It is the most commonly used lipophilic opioid having a rapid onset (5–10 min) and an intermediate duration (1–2 h) of action. In the dose range of 10–25 μg, it increases the intensity of the block without prolonging it. This makes it a suitable option for ambulatory surgery. It should be noted, however, that there is a risk of nausea and vomiting, and pruritus, especially at higher doses.

Sufentanil It is a lipophilic opioid used in the dose range of 2.5–7.5 μg. It has been used in orthopedic surgery and labor analgesia.

Table 41.5 Dosages of isobaric local anesthetic

Local anesthetic	Dose	Duration of effect
Prilocaine 2%	3–4 mL (60–80 mg)	60–120 min
Mepivacaine 2%	3–5 mL (60–100 mg)	30–90 min
Lidocaine 2%	3–5 mL (60–100 mg)	30–90 min
Bupivacaine 0.5%	3–4 mL (15–20 mg)	160 min
Ropivacaine 0.5%	3–5 mL (15–25 mg)	60–120 min

Table 41.4 Dosages of hyperbaric local anesthetics

	0.5% Bupivacaine (5–8% glucose)		5% Lignocaine (7.5% glucose)		4% Mepivacaine (9.5% glucose)		1% Tetracaine (5% glucose)	
Local anesthetic	mL	mg	mL	mg	mL	mg	mL	mg
T6-high	2.5–4.0	12.0–20.0	1.5–2.0	75–100	1.5–2.0	60–80	1.5–2.0	7.5–10.0
T10-medium	2.0–2.5	10.0–12.5	1.0–1.5	50–75	1.0–1.5	40–60	1.0–1.5	5.0–7.5
L1-deep	1.5	7.5	1.0–1.2	50–60	1.0–1.2	40–48	1.0–1.2	5.0–6.0
S1–S5 saddle block	1.0	5.0	0.6–1.0	30–50	0.6–1.0	24–40	0.5–1.0	2.5–5.0
Onset of effect (min)	10–20		5–10		5–10		10–20	
Duration of effect (min)	Up to 160		Up to 60		Up to 60		Up to 150	
Prolongation with vasopressors	No clinically significant prolongation						Up to 180–240 min	

Vasoconstrictors

These drugs reduce the vascular uptake of intrathecal local anesthetics, thereby prolonging their duration. They include phenylephrine and epinephrine. The effect is seen primarily with tetracaine and is rarely utilized.

α2-Adrenergic Agonists

Clonidine and **dexmedetomidine** act on α2-adrenergic receptors in the **substantia gelatinosa** in the spinal cord, intensifying and prolonging both sensory and motor block produced by intrathecal local anesthetics. Clonidine also prolongs spinal block when given orally or intravenously. This, however, is accompanied by a higher incidence of undesirable side effects such as bradycardia, hypotension, and sedation, when compared with the intrathecal route. The recommended dose of clonidine is 15–150 μg (lower doses are advocated), while that of dexmedetomidine is 3 μg.

Ambulatory Surgery

Many surgical procedures are increasingly being performed as day cases. These include hip and knee arthroplasties, as well as minor general and urological procedures. Short acting spinal anesthesia is a useful tool to facilitate this, in conjunction with the principles of enhanced recovery; the prophylactic use of antiemetics, judicious use of opiate medications, etc.

Mepivacaine 2% and prilocaine 2% (the latter is not available in North America) at a dose of up to 3mls are particularly useful in this setting. The addition of sterile water (1-part water to 2-parts local anesthetic) enables a more unilateral block to be performed, thus reducing the total dose of local anesthetic and facilitating a faster recovery. A saddle block with as little as 0.4 mL of heavy bupivacaine 0.75% will reliably enable anal fistula and perineal surgery.

Epidural Anesthesia and Analgesia

Preparation and patient positioning for performing an epidural are the same as for spinal anesthesia.

Epidural Needles

The epidural needles required to perform an epidural block are generally large gauge (16–18G) needles with distinct tip design to facilitate entry into the epidural space and introduction of the catheter. Some of these are depicted below in Fig. 41.24. Of these, Tuohy tip epidural needles are most commonly used.

Needle Insertion: Midline Versus Paramedian (Paraspinous) Approach

The spinous processes of lumbar and lower thoracic vertebrae are directed horizontally. However, those of the upper to mid-thoracic vertebrae are angulated steeply downwards. Thus, while a midline approach is appropriate and commonly used at the lumbar and lower thoracic levels, a paramedian (or paraspinous) approach becomes increasingly useful at the upper to mid-thoracic levels. The midline approach has the advantage of a clear anatomical landmark, provided the relevant spinous processes are easily palpable. A paramedian approach may be preferable at the lumbar level in patients with significant narrowing of the space between adjacent spinous processes. The interlaminar space lateral to the spinous processes typically provides a larger window for needle entry compared to the interspinous space.

Occasionally, there is a failure of the left- and the right-sided ligamentum flavum to fuse in the midline. This anatomical anomaly has been implicated in inadvertent dural puncture and difficulty in localizing the epidural space with the "loss-of-resistance" technique when using a midline approach. The ligamentum flavum remains intact lateral to the midline even in cases where a midline gap is present. Thus, a paramedian approach which enters the epidural space lateral to the midline may offer higher sensitivity in determining loss of resistance compared to a midline approach.

Midline Approach Lumbar Epidural

As for spinal anesthesia, a lumbar epidural needle is inserted below the L2 vertebra, distal to the termination of the spinal cord.

Local Anesthesia

Infiltration of the skin and ligaments with lidocaine serves both to increase patient comfort and to allow exploration of the underlying anatomy as described earlier. Securing the skin with the index and middle finger of the non-dominant hand improves precision and accuracy in needle insertion (Fig. 41.25).

Epidural Needle Insertion

The following sequence of photos indicate midline lumbar epidural placement, with the patient in a left sided lateral decubitus position.

Without moving the index and middle fingers of the left hand from the intervertebral space, the local infiltration needle is removed and an epidural needle is held between

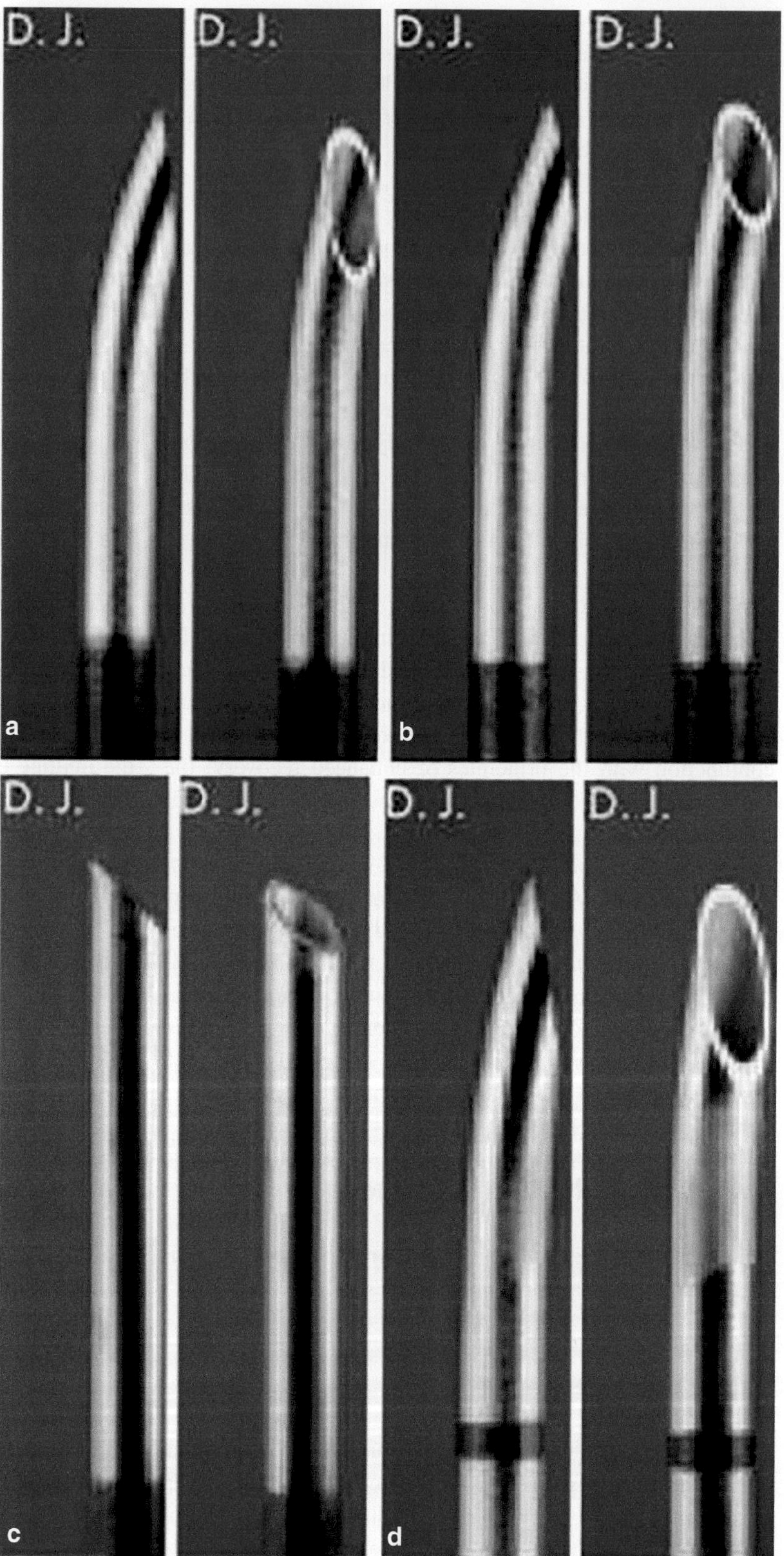

Fig. 41.24 Epidural needles. (**a**) Tuohy, (**b**) Hustead, (**c**) Crawford, (**d**) Weiss. Reprinted with permission from Danilo Jankovic)

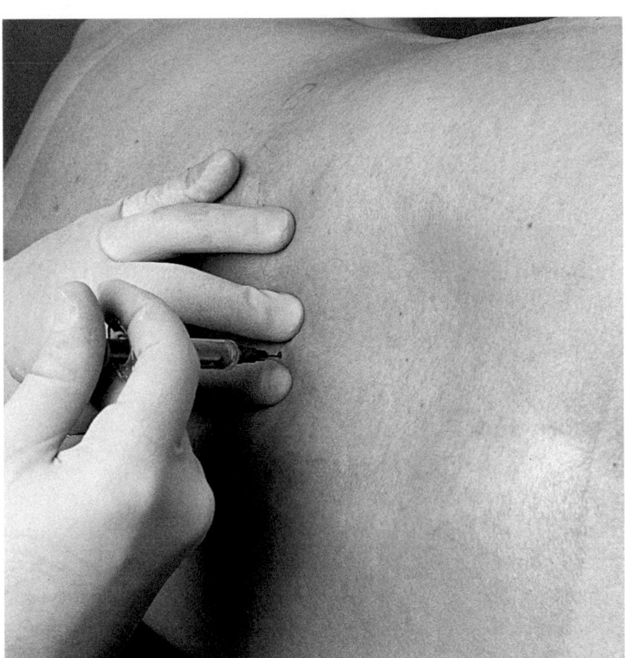

Fig. 41.25 Local anesthesia infiltration of soft tissues. (Reprinted with permission from Danilo Jankovic)

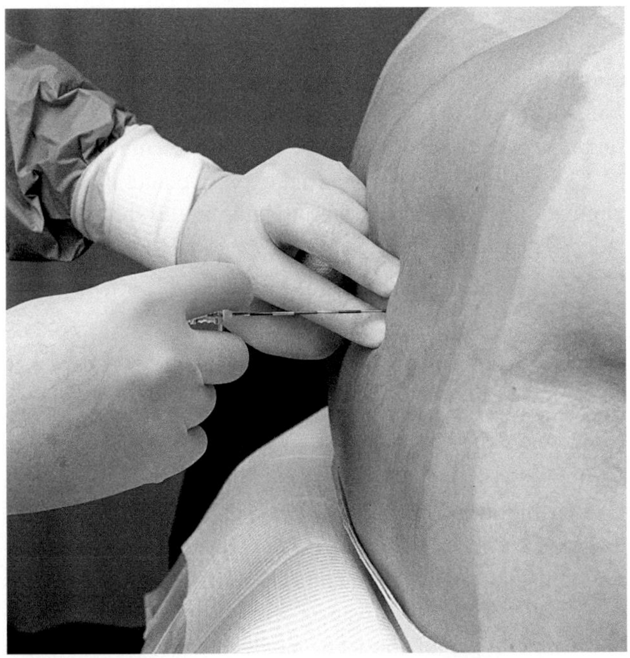

Fig. 41.26 Introducing the epidural needle while continuing to fix the skin with the left hand. (Reprinted with permission from Danilo Jankovic)

the thumb of the right hand (hub) and the index and middle finger (shaft) is advanced through the skin at the same site and trajectory with the bevel facing cephalad (Fig. 41.26). After traversing the supraspinous ligament, which is about 1 cm thick, the needle, the needle is slowly advanced a further 2–3 cm (depending on the anatomy), until it rests firmly in the interspinous ligament. Advancing through the interspinous ligament often produces a in a "gritty" sensation from the tip of the needle, especially in older patients. At this point the stylet is removed from the needle and a low friction (loss of resistance) syringe is attached (Fig. 41.27).

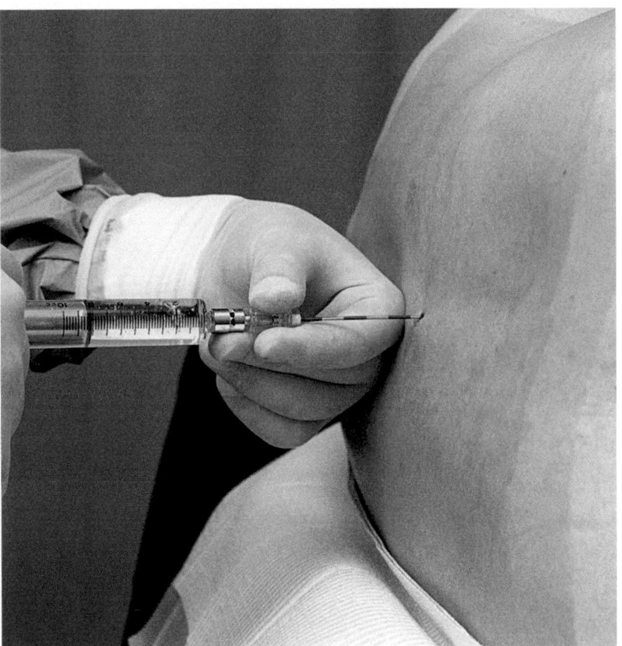

Fig. 41.27 Removing the stylet and attaching a low-friction syringe. (Reprinted with permission from Danilo Jankovic)

Locating the Epidural Space

With the dorsum of the left hand resting firmly on the patient's back, the left thumb and index finger (1) secure the needle, (2) advance it millimeter by millimeter, and (3) serve as a "brake" to prevent inadvertent forward movement. The thumb of the right hand applies pressure on the syringe plunger (Fig. 41.28). *Loss of resistance* indicates that the epidural space has been reached. The contents of the syringe are easily injected.

Care should be taken to ensure that the needle is kept in the midline. Inadvertent deviation from the midline leads to the needle passing the supraspinous ligament, with an angled entry into the interspinous ligament with only brief resistance and a subsequent false loss of resistance. This type of puncture ends in the paravertebral musculature and is accompanied by localized back pain.

Variations in the Loss of Resistance Technique

Saline only technique: The low-friction syringe is filled with a saline solution. Pressure is applied to the plunger as the needle is advanced and upon entry to the epidural space, a loss of resistance is detected with an ability to inject saline easily. Some operators advocate deliberately injecting

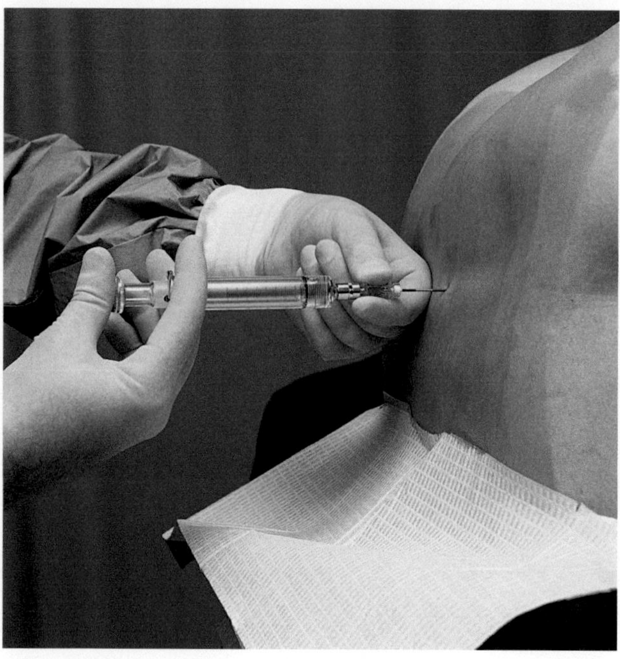

Fig. 41.28 Identifying the epidural space (loss of resistance). (Reprinted with permission from Danilo Jankovic)

approximately. 3 mL of saline to "open" the space and facilitate introduction of the catheter. However, excessive fluid injection may dilute subsequent injected agents (test dose and loading dose).

Loss of Resistance with Air

In this technique, the syringe is filled with air. Proponents of this technique argue that it allows clearer identification of an accidental dural puncture, as any fluid that emerges from the hub of the needle must be CSF. However, using air to locate epidural space has been associated with patchy blocks, venous air embolism, and pneumocephalus.

Saline with an Air Bubble

The low-friction syringe is filled with a saline solution, but a small air bubble is retained within the syringe as an additional visual indicator of the resistance to attempted injection. Visual compression of the bubble corresponds to tactile resistance to pressure on the syringe plunger (Fig. 41.29a). When the epidural space is reached, the bubble re-expands to its normal shape, the plunger is depressed with little resistance and the saline is injected (Fig. 41.29b).

Hanging Drop Technique

This technique is only advocated for use in thoracic epidural placement due to more consistent negative pressures in the epidural space in this region. After the interspinous ligament has been reached *(in midline approach)* or interlaminar space reached *(in paramedian approach)*, a drop of saline is placed within the hub of the needle (Fig. 41.30a). After the ligamentum flavum has been passed and the epidural space has been reached, the drop is "sucked in" due to the negative pressure in the epidural space caused by tenting of the epidural space by the needle (Fig. 41.30b). As both hands can grip the needle, needle advancement may be more controlled. By only advancing the needle during inspiration, negative pressure in the epidural space is maximized, to improve the sensitivity of this technique.

Paramedian Approach Epidural

This is performed using the same landmarks as for spinal anesthesia (Fig. 41.20), just with an epidural needle rather than a spinal needle. In the lumbar region where the spinous processes are close to horizontal in orientation, the skin puncture site is 0.5–1 cm lateral to the superior border of the lower spinous process of the intervertebral space being entered. The needle is advanced in a cranio-medial direction at a lateral to medial angulation of about 5–10° to the sagittal plane with a slight cranial angulation of 0–10° to the skin surface. If the lamina is encountered, the needle should be redirected with a slight increase in cranial angle, without altering the lateral to medial angulation to enter the interlaminar space. The only ligament that needs to be penetrated on the way to the epidural space is the ligamentum flavum.

Care should be taken to avoid excessive lateral to medial angulation to prevent crossing the midline to the ipsilateral side. The needle should essentially pass alongside the spinous process.

Catheter Placement into Epidural Space

Having reached the epidural space, the loss of resistance syringe is removed. The catheter is introduced, provided no CSF or blood is seen to drain from the needle. The thumb and index finger of the left hand secure the epidural needle, with the back of the hand lying firmly on the patient's back. The catheter is advanced cranially, using the thumb and index finger of the right hand, to a depth of 4–5 cm beyond the tip of the needle (Fig. 41.31). Advancing it further than this can lead to lateral deviation of the catheter and consequently a unilateral block. It is also associated with greater risk of intravascular placement. After placement of the catheter in the desired position, the needle is slowly withdrawn (Fig. 41.32), while the thumb and index finger of the left hand secures the catheter at the injection site (Fig. 41.33).

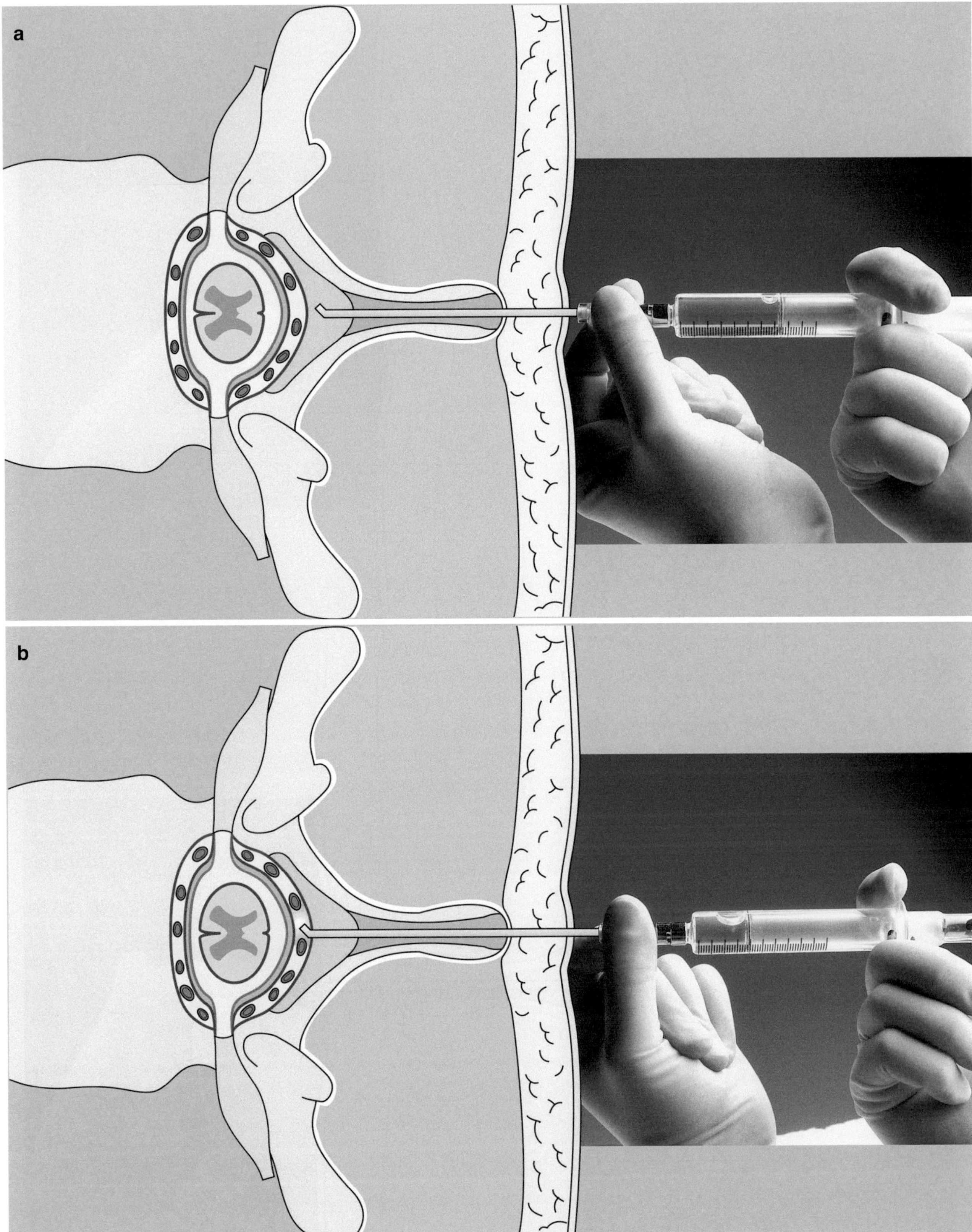

Fig. 41.29 (**a**) Loss-of-resistance technique with saline. The air bubble is compressed by pressure on the syringe plunger. (Reprinted with permission from Danilo Jankovic). (**b**) Loss-of-resistance technique with saline. The epidural space has been reached. The air bubble has returned to its normal shape and saline has been injected. (Reprinted with permission from Danilo Jankovic)

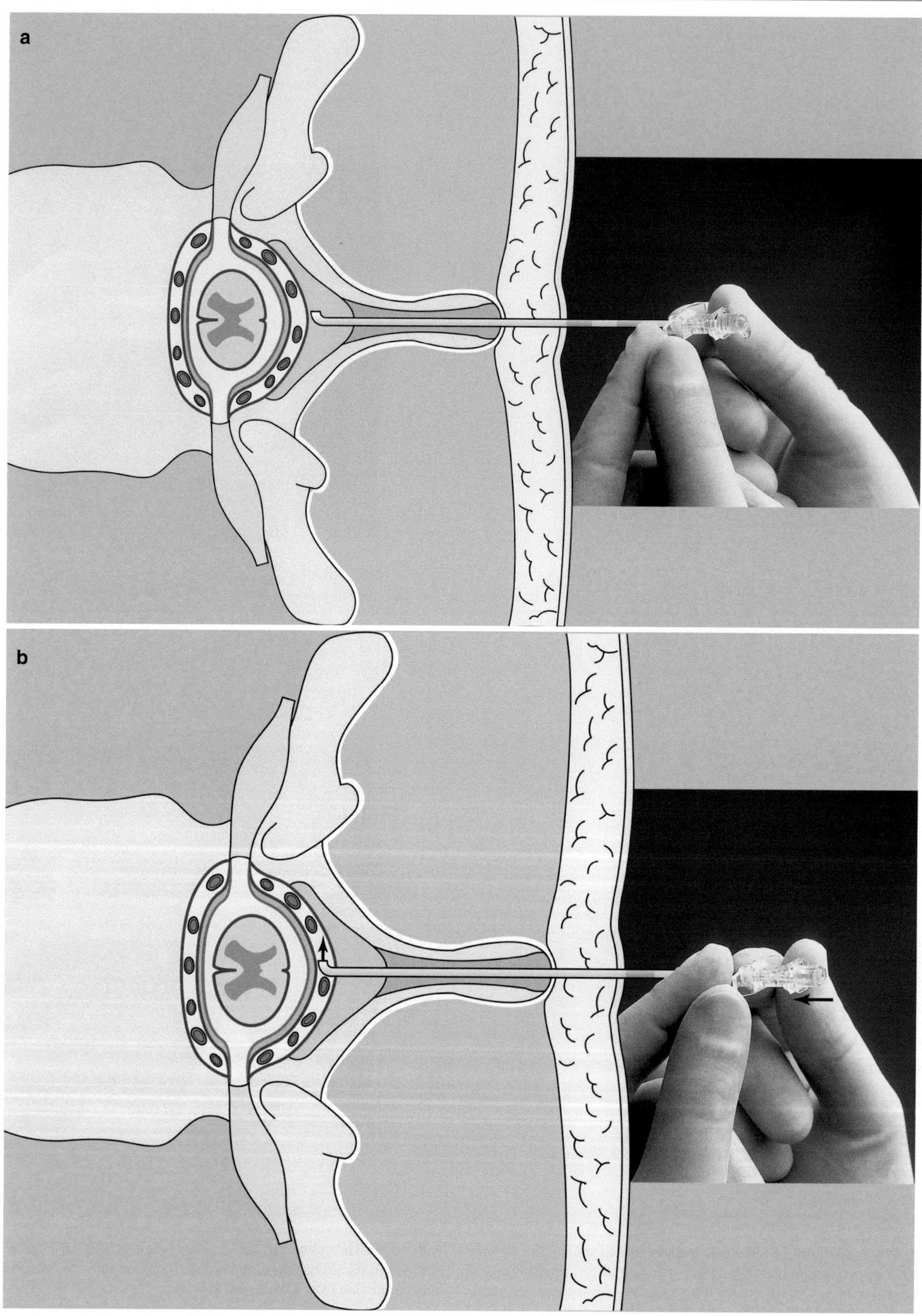

Fig. 41.30 (**a**) "Hanging drop" technique. The epidural needle is positioned in the ligamentum flavum. (Reprinted with permission from Danilo Jankovic). (**b**) "Hanging drop" technique. The epidural space has been reached. The drop is sucked back in. (Reprinted with permission from Danilo Jankovic)

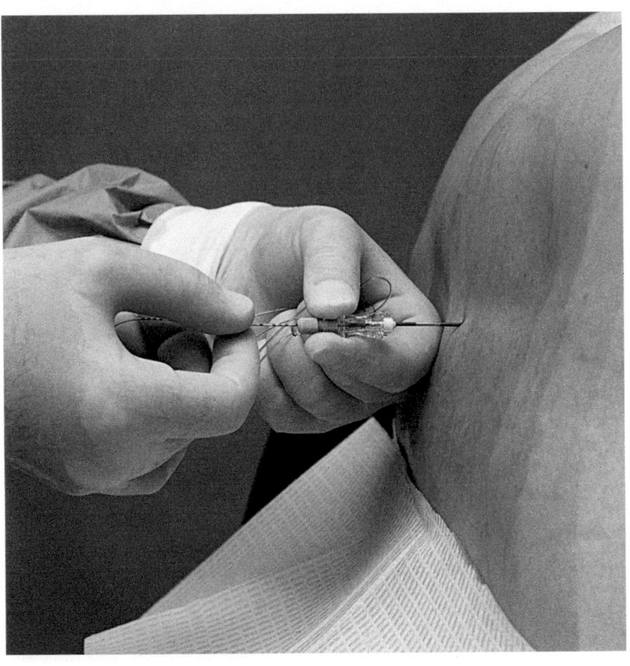

Fig. 41.31 Introducing the catheter. (Reprinted with permission from Danilo Jankovic)

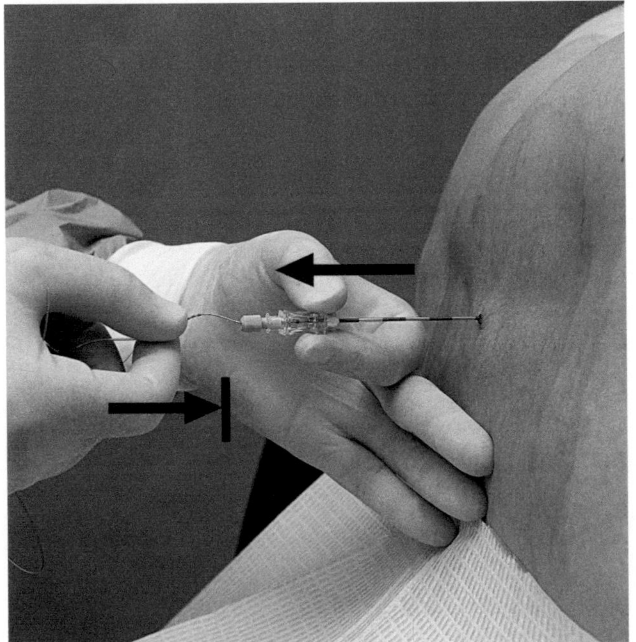

Fig. 41.32 Withdrawing the injection needle. (Reprinted with permission from Danilo Jankovic)

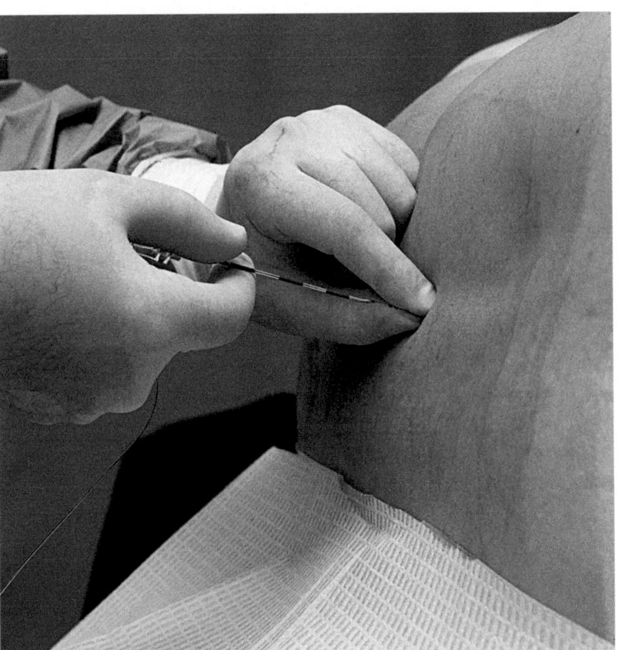

Fig. 41.33 The catheter is secured at the injection site with the thumb and index finger. (Reprinted with permission from Danilo Jankovic)

Length of Catheter Placement

The optimal length for catheter advancement is subject to conflicting views, with recommended distances for catheter insertion in the literature ranging from 2 to 6 cm. There is evidence that resistance is encountered at a mean distance of catheter insertion of only 2.5 cm. In theory, any further advancement has an increased risk of coiling, transforaminal exit or vascular puncture and some sources advocate a minimal insertion approach. However, studies have supported 5 cm insertion as non-inferior to 3 cm in terms of performance and complication rates.

The proximal orifice in multi-orifice catheters typically lies approximately 1.5 cm from the tip and this should also be taken into account as all orifices should remain in the epidural space. As catheter migration of up to 1–2 cm is common in the post-operative period, it is prudent to thread a small excess length of catheter to avoid migration out of the epidural space. This also provides a margin of safety for inadvertent dislodgement during epidural placement as the Tuohy needle is being removed and the catheter is being fixed to the skin. Based on this rationale, a 4–5 cm catheter insertion is advocated.

An adapter is attached to the proximal end of the catheter. Patency of the catheter is tested by injecting 1–2 mL of saline (Fig. 41.34). After aspiration, the syringe and adaptor are disconnected and the open end of the catheter is placed on a sterile drape below the puncture site. Attention must be given to any escaping fluid (CSF or blood) (Fig. 41.36). The catheter is then held vertically above the needle insertion point (Fig. 41.35). A rapid fall of the meniscus or fluid level within the catheter is a sensitive (though not specific) indicator of correct placement of the catheter within the epidural space.

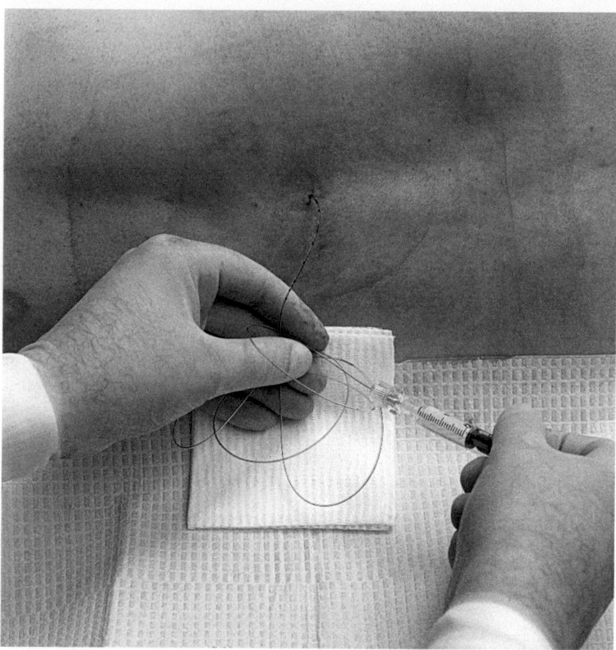

Fig. 41.34 Injection of 1 mL saline. (Reprinted with permission from Danilo Jankovic)

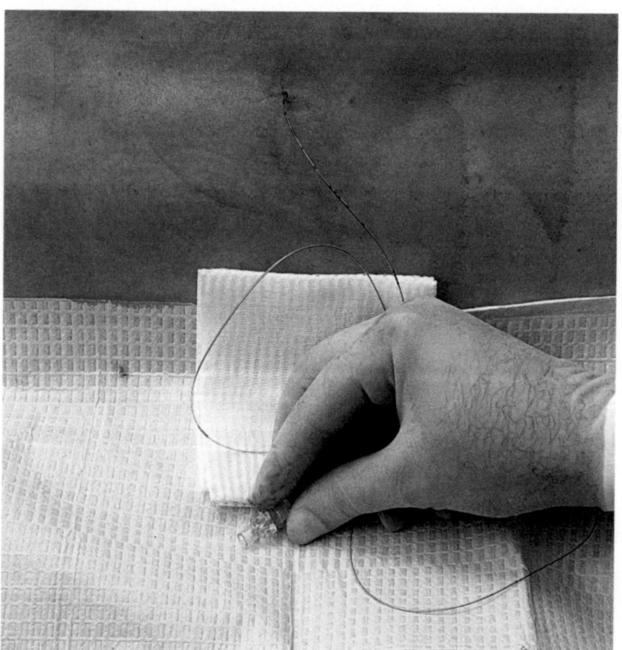

Fig. 41.35 The end of the catheter is placed below the injection site. (Reprinted with permission from Danilo Jankovic)

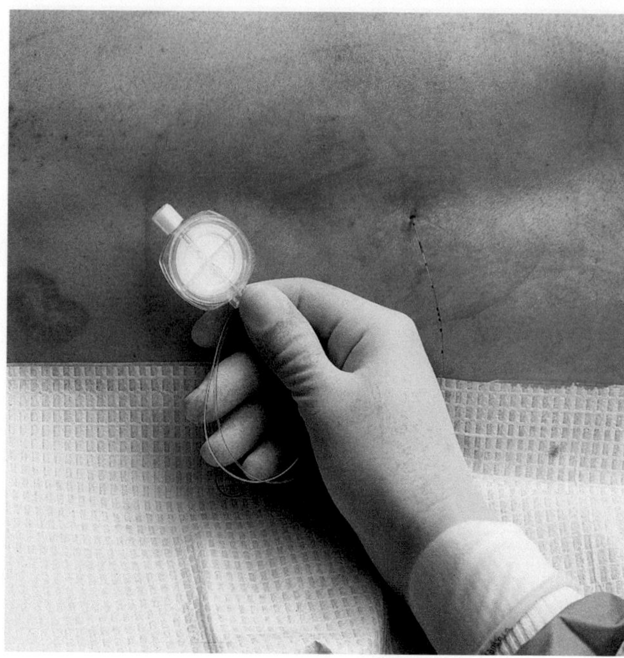

Fig. 41.36 Placing a bacterial filter

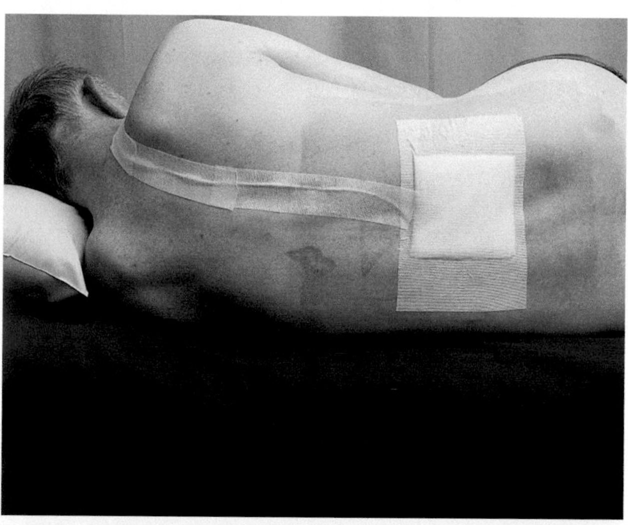

Fig. 41.37 Securing the catheter and dressing. (Reprinted with permission from Danilo Jankovic)

Test Dose and Fixation of Catheter

A bacterial filter is attached (Fig. 41.36) and a test dose (for example 45 mg lidocaine and an optional 15 µg epinephrine) is administered. The catheter is secured and dressed to prevent dislodgement and ensure sterility (Fig. 41.37). The patient is then placed in the desired position. Fixation of the catheter can be accomplished in a variety of ways (see section "Catheter Fixation").

The test dose allows detection of intrathecal injection (rapid development of spinal block) or intravascular injection (tachycardia, hypertension or T-wave changes on ECG). The addition of epinephrine can lead to unreliable results in patients taking beta-blockers, patients under general anesthesia, and pregnant patients. Due caution must be exercised while adding epinephrine in pregnant patients (as may cause transient fetal bradycardia due to reduced uterine blood flow), older patients with coronary artery disease and hypertensive patients. The use of epinephrine is best avoided in patients with closed angle glaucoma, and tachyarrhythmias.

Following test dose administration, it is important to maintain verbal contact with the patient, to conduct careful cardiovascular monitoring and to check the spread of the anesthesia in order to exclude the ever-present risk of inadvertent intrathecal injection. After 5 min, if no evidence of intrathecal or intravascular spread has occurred, the loading dose, adjusted for the individual patient, can be administered on an incremental basis until the desired level of anesthesia is reached. It may take 15—20 min for the test dose to produce a clinical block confirming correct epidural placement. In practice, this time may not be readily available, particularly if the epidural is being used in combination with general anesthesia and induction occurs soon after epidural placement.

Catheter Fixation

Epidural catheter migration and/or dislocation is a common phenomenon. Significant catheter migration (>20 mm inwards or outwards) is associated with diminished analgesia, early termination of epidural anesthesia and may contribute to more serious complications such as spinal hematoma or predispose to bacterial contamination (Ref: Sellman). Although evidence supports tunneling and suturing the catheter to minimize movement, this adds time and it has its own potential complications and it is not a widely practiced technique.

Methods for epidural fixation range from simple adhesive dressings to proprietary epidural fixation systems. There is insufficient evidence to support the use of a specific dressing. All may be compromised by perspiration or leakage of fluid or blood from the puncture site. Clean, dry skin is paramount for effective fixation regardless of the dressing used, as is attention to detail and examination of the site in the peri-operative period. Daily checks should be carried out post-operatively, and if any doubt on the integrity of the dressing, re-fixation in a sterile manner should take place.

Considerations regarding choice of fixation method include expense and ease of use in addition to efficacy of fixation. As an example, in a recent study, tissue glue (2-Ethyl cyanoacrylate adhesive) was associated with an absence of thoracic epidural catheter movement and also with decreased fluid leakage at the skin requiring refixation of dressings. These advantages have to be weighed against the cost of tissue glue.

Troubleshooting Needle/Catheter Entry

Fluid backflow from the needle hub: after the epidural space has been identified or after administration of the test dose, a few drops of fluid may still drip from the positioned needle. This may be saline from the syringe or CSF if intrathecal space has been punctured. A higher viscosity, higher temperature (Fig. 41.38), near neutral pH, higher glucose content and turbidity with thiopentone help identify the fluid as CSF. If the fluid is not CSF, one can proceed with the procedure.

Blood backflow from the needle hub or catheter: in this case (Figs. 41.39 and 41.40) it is best to withdraw the needle or the catheter. One may attempt another insertion at a segment higher or lower; or abandon the procedure and choose to administer general anesthesia and/or alternative regional anesthetic technique.

CSF backflow from the needle hub: The options in the event of accidental dural puncture include conversion to a spinal anesthetic by injecting an appropriately reduced dose of local anesthetic, or inserting a continuous spinal catheter (which must clearly be labeled as such, to avoid inadvertent overdosing with subsequent top-ups). Another attempt at insertion can also be made keeping in mind the possibility of another dural tap, and that an epidural dose of local anesthetic may unpredictably spread intrathecally through the first dural puncture site and lead to a total spinal anesthesia. Finally, one may choose to abandon the procedure and administer general anesthesia. In any case, the patients must be informed about the possibility of a postdural puncture headache. Insertion of a spinal catheter or further attempts at

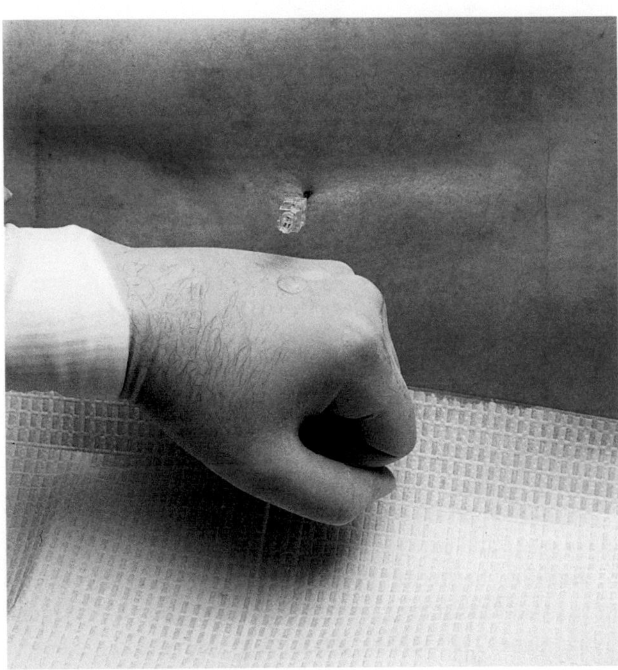

Fig. 41.38 Escaping fluid: is it cold or warm? (Reprinted with permission from Danilo Jankovic)

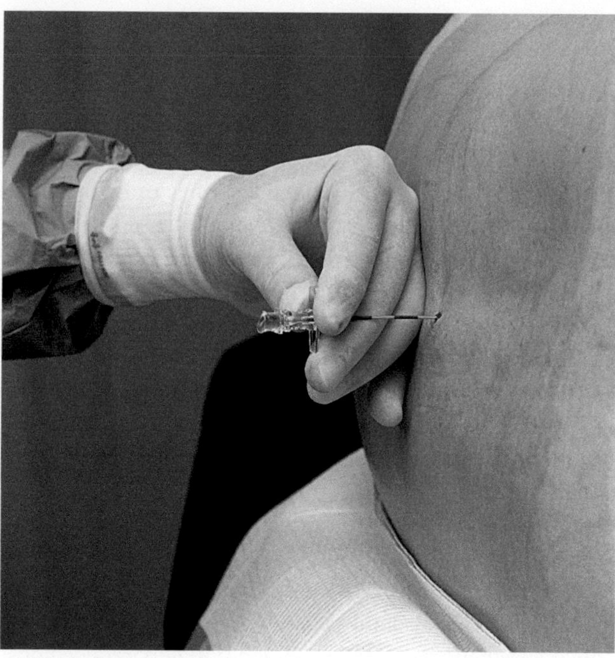

Fig. 41.39 Blood-tinged fluid. (Reprinted with permission from Danilo Jankovic)

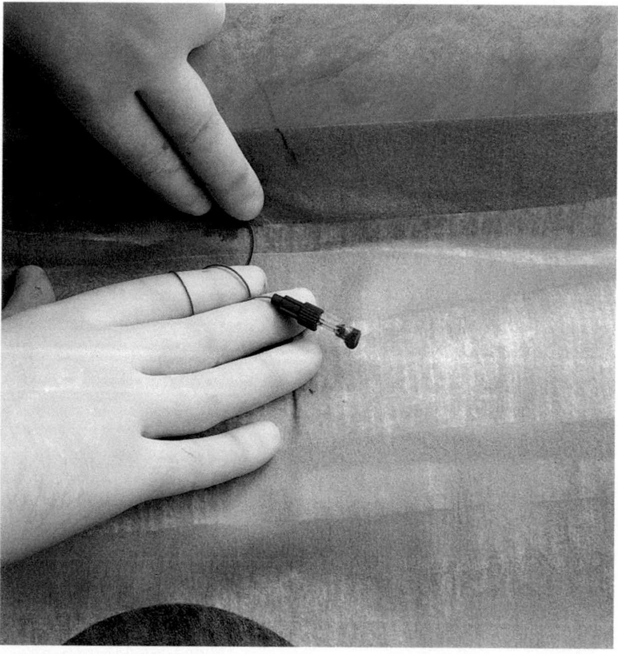

Fig. 41.40 Blood from the catheter hub. (Reprinted with permission from Danilo Jankovic)

insertion are not recommended in the thoracic region in the event of a dural puncture.

Inability to thread the catheter: this may happen when a false loss of resistance has been encountered in a superficial tissue plane. The catheter should be removed and the procedure reattempted, aiming to obtain a convincing loss of resistance. If the catheter is withdrawn through the needle, there is a potential risk of shearing of the catheter tip against the bevel of the needle. Gentle withdrawal of the needle through the catheter may be attempted; though if any resistance is encountered, we recommend that the needle and catheter are withdrawn en-bloc.

Thoracic Epidural Placement

While the general approach for thoracic epidural analgesia is as described in the preceding section in terms of preparation, equipment, catheter insertion, and fixation, there are notable differences between lumbar and thoracic epidural placement. Placement of thoracic epidurals is a fundamental anesthetic skill but is nonetheless considered a technically challenging procedure. This is reflected in the high primary failure rate of up to 22% (incorrect placement of the thoracic epidural catheter), as well as the potential for secondary failure (catheter migration or suboptimum dosing).

Thoracic epidurals are most often used to provide analgesia for thoracic or major abdominal surgery. The analgesic efficacy of thoracic epidural analgesia is well established as being superior to parenteral opioid administration. Additional benefits include improved perioperative outcomes relating to cardiac, respiratory, and gastrointestinal function. Adverse side effects of epidural analgesia include hypotension, urinary retention, pruritis, and motor block.

The level at which an epidural catheter is optimally sited is dependent on the desired area of sensory blockade. The catheter tip is typically located at a vertebral level corresponding to the midpoint of the surgical incision on a dermatomal map.

A needle inserted in the midline will traverse the skin, subcutaneous tissue, supraspinous ligament, interspinous ligament, and ligamentum flavum to access the epidural space (Fig. 41.41). A paramedian insertion of the needle, on the other hand, bypasses the supraspinous and interspinous ligaments. Bony resistance is expected when the lamina is encountered and may be “walked off” in a cephalad direction to access the interlaminar space, ligamentum flavum, and epidural space.

Paramedian Approach for Upper to Mid-Thoracic Levels

Skin Puncture Site

At this level, the puncture site is located about 0.5–1 cm lateral from the caudal edge of the superior spinous process of space being entered (Fig. 41.42) and 1–2 cm caudal to the interlaminar space which is being targeted. This target may be identified by ultrasound (see previous chapter). These guidelines apply to the region of mid to upper thoracic spine

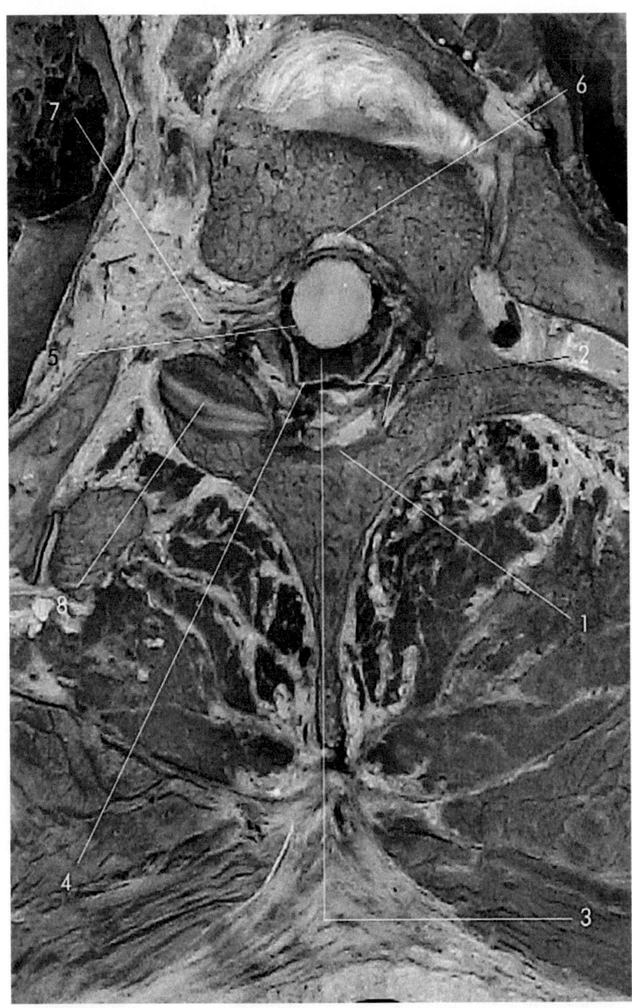

Fig. 41.41 Transverse dissection at the level of the T3. (1) Ligamentum flavum, (2) epidural space, (3) subarachnoid space with spinal cord, (4) spinal dura mater, (5) spinal pia mater, (6) posterior longitudinal ligament, (7) neural foramen with spinal nerves, and (8) zygapophysial joint. (Reprinted with permission from Danilo Jankovic)

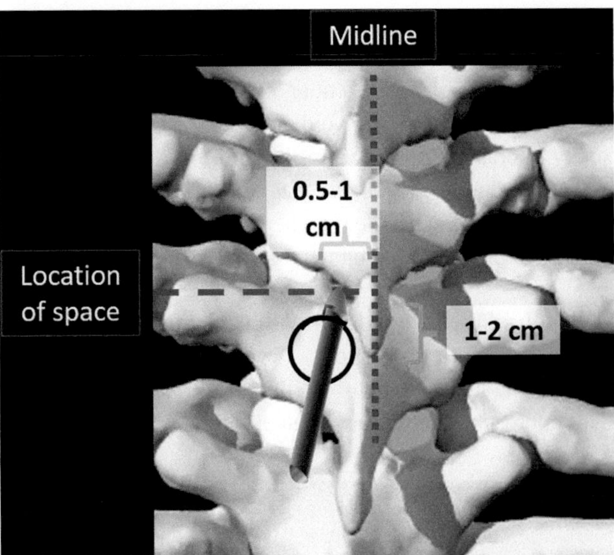

Fig. 41.42 The recommended insertion site for a paramedian approach to the thoracic epidural space in a typical adult patient is approximately 1–2 cm inferior to the tip of the spinous process, and not more than 1 cm lateral to the midline (just enough to avoid and pass alongside the spinous process). The needle should be angled not more than 5–10° towards the midline. It can be advanced initially at 90-degrees to the patient's back to contact the lamina, and then the tip walked cranially to enter into the space, maintaining the slight degree of lateral-medial angulation. (Reproduced with permission from Dr. Ki Jinn Chin)

where spinous processes are steeply angled and interlaminar spaces overlap.

A fan-shaped local anesthesia infiltration is used to anesthetize the skin. The local infiltration needle may also be used to explore the contours of the spinous processes/depth to lamina and to confirm the optimal trajectory. The epidural needle is introduced in a *cranio-medial direction* at a lateral to medial angulation of about 5–10° to the sagittal level and a cranial angulation of about 35–45° to the skin surface (Fig. 41.43) is required.

The only ligament that needs to be penetrated on the way to the epidural space is the ligamentum flavum. The initial needle advancement may be carried out with minimal cranial angulation with the intention of contacting the lamina. Upon bone contact, the needle is withdrawn by 0.5 cm, walked off the bone in a medial/cephalad direction to access the interlaminar space, while maintaining the same lateral-medial

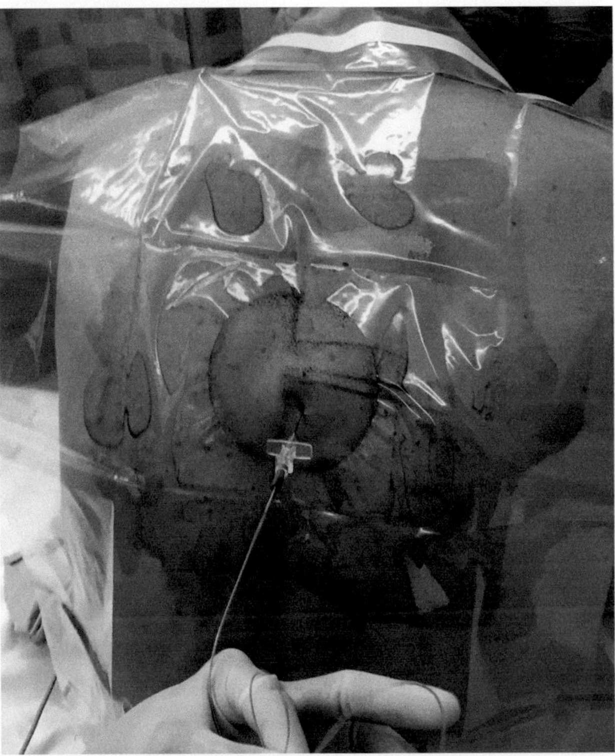

Fig. 41.43 Paramedian approach at T7/8 level. (Reprinted with permission from permission from Dr. Ki Jinn Chin)

angulation throughout. The stylet is then removed from the puncture needle and identification of the epidural space is carried out using a low friction/"loss of resistance" syringe.

It is recommended to avoid entering the skin at an excessively lateral point relative to the midline. The shallow lateral to medial approach advocated is useful for estimating the position of the needle tip when advancing the needle and it helps to prevent crossing the midline to the ipsilateral side.

Ultrasound Technique for the Identification of the Interlaminar Space

Preprocedural ultrasound of the thoracic spine with a paramedian approach has been associated with a decreased number of skin punctures and improved pain scores versus a palpation based paramedian approach. This technique allows the practitioner to determine an optimal skin entry point and to estimate the distance to the ligamentum flavum. The procedure for ultrasound scanning of the thoracic spine is described in Chap. 40.

The midline may be identified in the transverse view, and the interlaminar spaces are identified and marked using the parasagittal oblique view as indicated in Fig. 41.44. The depth from the skin to the interlaminar space or posterior complex is measured. This is the safe needle insertion depth. The actual depth to enter the epidural space will be greater due to needle angulation and the additional distance from lamina to the epidural space.

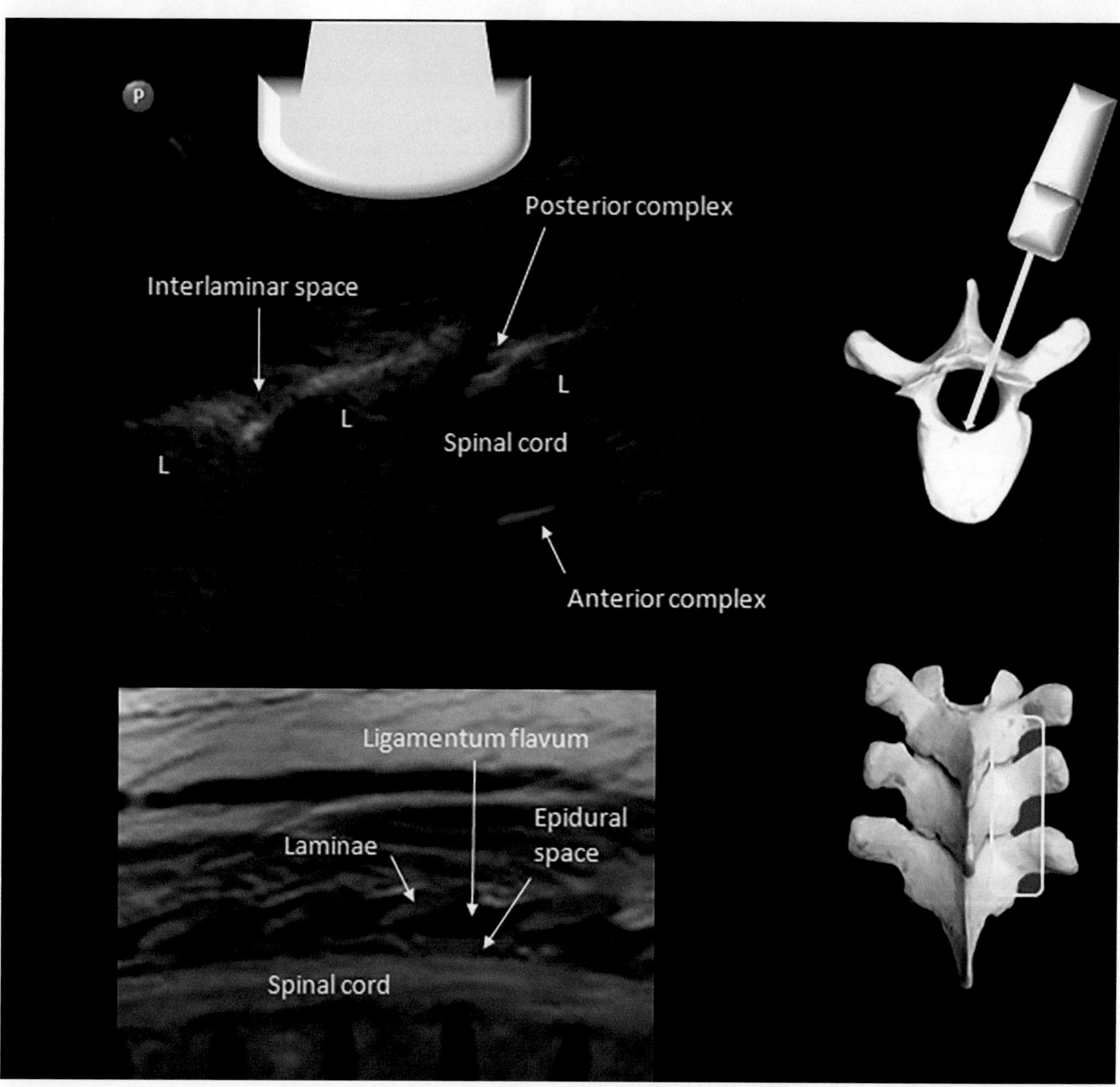

Fig. 41.44 Paramedian sagittal oblique view of the mid-thoracic spine and corresponding magnetic resonance image. Despite the narrow interlaminar space, it is possible to visualize the posterior and anterior complex at one or more levels. At a minimum, the location of the interlaminar space can be determined by the dip or gap between successive laminae (L). Note that the spinal cord is hypoechoic and cannot be distinguished from the surrounding cerebrospinal fluid

With this additional information, the needle approach to the thoracic epidural space can be triangulated more accurately. Marking a needle entry site approximately 0.5 cm lateral to the midline and 2 cm caudal to the identified interlaminar space will facilitate the required 55° cranial and 5–10° lateral to medial needle angulation. The shallow lateral to medial angle means that the needle is almost parallel to the spinous process and decreases the risk of the needle tip inadvertently crossing the midline to the contralateral paravertebral muscles or pleural space (Fig. 41.45).

Once the entry site has been identified, the preparation of the skin and the entry of the needle with the LOR technique is identical to that of the landmark technique. Real-time ultrasound-assisted thoracic epidural placement has also been described. However, this is not commonly practiced.

Test Dose for Thoracic Epidural

A test dose of 30 mg Lidocaine (3 mL 1.0% Lidocaine) and 15mcg epinephrine is advocated for thoracic epidurals. While the evidence base for an ideal test dose is lacking, the risk of high spinal with conventional lumbar test dose (45 mg lidocaine) warrants use of a lower test dose.

Drug Administration

Loading Dose

In adults, approximately 1–2 mL of local anesthetic is typically required per vertebral segment to be blocked. A maximum of 3–4 mL of loading dose should be injected at a time at thoracic levels. Use of a larger volume may lead to profound hypotension due to a widespread sympathetic block. It has been shown that with the same dose a greater number of segments are blocked in elderly patients compared to younger adults. As the autonomic effects of epidural analgesia are both more marked and often more poorly tolerated in older patients, they should be loaded more judiciously.

Clinical Testing of Loading Dose

A loading dose is typically given prior to induction of general anesthesia in epidurals placed for postoperative analgesia. The loading dose may be omitted at this timepoint in certain patients due to concerns that sympathectomy related hypotension would complicate induction. Clinical assessment of the efficacy of the epidural anesthesia via sensory testing requires approximately 15 min to demonstrate blockade in most patients (including 5 min for test dose assessment prior to loading dose). In the case of inadequate block following sufficient passage of time, the epidural should be reattempted, if time and circumstances allow. If this is not possible, alternative regional anesthetic options or increased parenteral opioid dosing should be considered.

Pharmacology of Drugs Used for Epidural Anesthesia and Analgesia

The local anesthetic injected spreads both cephalad and caudad in the epidural space. Since the band of anesthesia produced cannot be predicted accurately in a given patient, clinicians must be aware of major factors determining this spread. These are discussed below.

Drug mass, concentration, and volume: both total drug dose and volume are independent determinants of the spread of epidural block. However, they are not linearly related. A higher concentration produces a profound block of both motor and sensory nerves. Lower concentrations provide a more selective sensory block. In adults, approximately 1–2 mL of local anesthetic is usually required per vertebral segment to be blocked.

A higher dose (concentration and volume) also increases the degree of sympathetic block resulting in both reduced systematic vascular resistance and direct cardiac depressant effects (if sufficiently cephalad distribution). This results in hypotension.

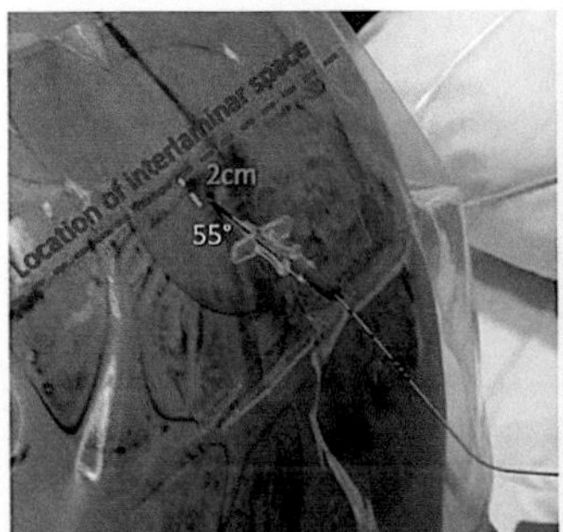

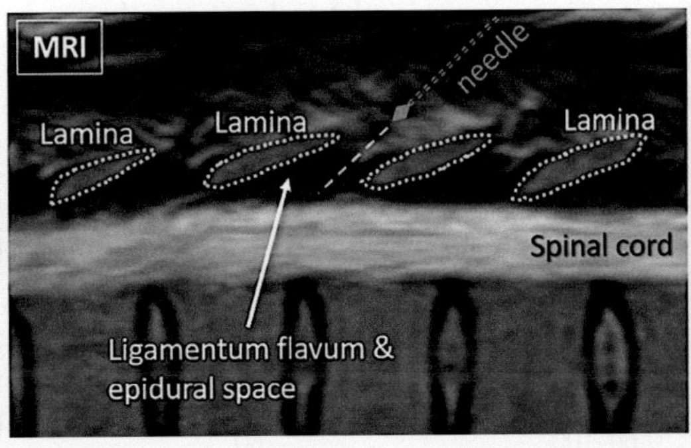

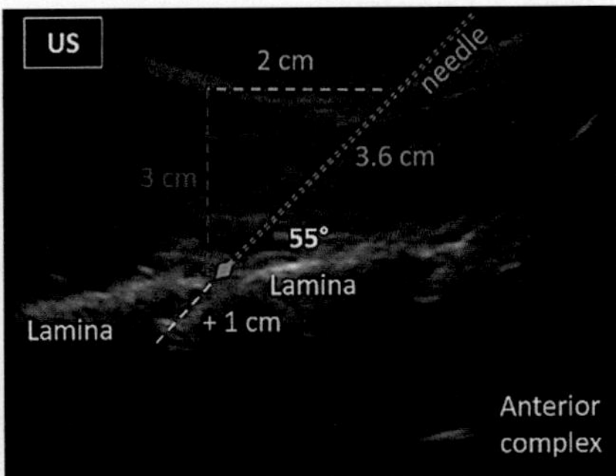

Fig. 41.45 Parasagittal ultrasound and MRI images of the thoracic spine illustrating the geometry of the thoracic epidural approach. Examples of measurements are provided. Ultrasound allows the laminae, the interlaminar space, and the vertical depth from skin to be identified. Needle insertion should be at a site approximately 2 cm inferior to the interlaminar space. A 55-degree angle to the patient's surface is recommended to pass through the interlaminar gap. The epidural space is usually reached within another 1 cm of needle insertion depth. This means that needle insertion depth to the epidural space usually exceeds the measured depth to the laminae by approximately 1.5–2 cm. (Reprinted with permission from Dr. Ki Jinn Chin)

Site of injection: this is a major determinant of the epidural spread. For example, the same volume of drug in the caudal space covers less dermatomes when compared to the thoracic level.

Other technical factors: patient position, needle angulation, direction of needle opening, and the speed of injection are not clinically significant.

Length of catheter in space: threading an epidural catheter more than 5 cm may lead to lateral placement of the catheter tip, resulting in missed segments or unilateral block.

Patient factors: increasing age, shorter height, and increased body mass index are associated with increased spread, but this is highly variable and it cannot be accurately predicted. The epidural spread is not affected by the sex of the patient.

Local Anesthetics Used for Epidurals

Local anesthetics used for epidural blocks are commonly classified by their duration of action. "*Time for two segment regression*" is the time taken for the block to recede by two dermatomes from its maximal extent, while the "*time for complete resolution*" is the time taken for the recovery from sensory block. While the former helps to time the repeating of an epidural dose intraoperatively, the latter is used to estimate the time for discharge of outpatients. Commonly used agents with doses are mentioned in Table 41.6.

In general, more dilute concentrations suffice for analgesia, while higher concentrations are used for a surgical block. The total dose and volume needed depend upon the surgery, patient factors, and the use of adjuvants medications.

Adjunct Medications Used in Epidural Anesthesia and Analgesia

Similarly to spinal anesthesia, adjuvant medications are used to improve the quality of an epidural block. These are summarizes below.

Alpha-1 Agonists

Epinephrine: in a concentration of 2.5–5 μg/mL (1:400,000–1:200,000), epinephrine prolongs both the sensory and motor block when added to short to intermediate acting local anesthetics. It reduces the vascular uptake of local anesthetics into the systemic circulation. It may also exert an analgesic effect through α2-adrenergic receptors, reducing pain transmission within spinal cord. The addition of epinephrine in an epidural block produces a vasodilatation secondary to β2-adrenergic effects in the periphery. This decreases the mean arterial pressure, but also increases the cardiac output.

Alpha-2 Agonists

Clonidine: It prolongs the sensory block only, when added to epidural local anesthetics. It is used in doses of 150–300 μg (2 μg/kg). Hypotension and sedation are common secondary to systemic uptake.

Dexmedetomidine: It possesses sedative and analgesic properties by activating α_2 receptors in the spinal cord. It produces a prolonged analgesic effect, with mostly sensory effects, although increased motor block has been noted at concentrations of 1 μg/mL. Hypotension, bradycardia, and sedation are associated side effects. Infusion dose: 0.5 μg/mL (range 0.25–1.0 μg/mL).

Opioids

While it has been established that epidural administration of opioid alone is of limited advantage over parenteral opioids, in combination with local anesthetics a synergistic effect exists. The use of opioids increases the speed of onset of block and the number of segments blocked. Opioid related side effects include nausea, pruritus, sedation, and respiratory depression.

Commonly used epidural opioids include fentanyl (0.5–0.15 μg/kg), sufentanil (0.3–0.7 μg/kg), hydromorphone (0.8–1.5 mg), and morphine (4–6 mg).

Alkalizing Agents

Bicarbonate: the addition of sodium bicarbonate (0.1 mEq/mL) to local anesthetics has been proposed as a means to hasten the onset of the blocks. While some studies have shown a faster onset, others have found no difference.

Table 41.6 Commonly used local anesthetic agents for a surgical epidural block

Drug and concentration	Dose (mL)	Onset time (min)	Time for two segment resolution (min)	Recommended "top-up" time (min)	Time for complete resolution (min)
Short acting agents					
Chloroprocaine 2–3%	15–25	6–12	45–60	45	100–160 min
Intermediate acting agents					
Lignocaine 1–2%	10–20	10–20	60–100	60	160–200
Mepivacaine 1.5–2.0%	15–30	10–30	60–100	60	160–200
Long acting agents					
Ropivacaine 0.2–1.0%	10–20		90–180	120	180–360
Bupivacaine 0.25–0.5%	10–20	5–20	120–240	120	300–480
Levobupivacaine 0.25–0.5%	10–20	5–20	120–240	120	300–480

Drug Regimens for Continuous Epidural Analgesia

Conclusions about the optimum anesthetic agents and combinations are difficult to make due to the wide ranges of drugs and concentrations used in various studies, however several typical and recommended regimens are listed below. The side effects of epidural local anesthetics and opioids differ from one another and are mostly dose dependent. By administering a combination of these agents in low concentrations, analgesia may be optimized while minimizing adverse effects. Opioids may be omitted if a history of allergy or sensitivity to opioids exists or if there is particular concern regarding respiratory depression.

Suggested Dosing Regimens for Continuous Thoracic Epidural Analgesia

Local Anesthetic

- Ropivacaine 0.15–0.2%.
- Bupivacaine 0.05–0.125%.

Opiates

- Fentanyl 2–5 μg/mL.
- Hydromorphone 5–10 μg/mL.

Rate

- 3–10 mL/h.

The evidence supporting either patient controlled epidural analgesia (PCEA) or continuous epidural infusions as being superior is conflicting for specific procedures. A meta-analysis indicates that continuous infusion produces superior analgesia but is associated with a higher incidence of nausea, vomiting, and motor block. Concurrent background infusion alongside PCEA is a further option.

Regardless of the regimen used, careful and methodical monitoring of the patient with assessment of analgesic efficacy and adverse effects must occur while the catheter remains in situ. Particular vigilance should be exercised following bolus dose administration or a change in the infusion rate.

Management of the Patient After an Epidural Block

Patient Positioning

Gravity does not play a clinically significant role in determining the spread of local anesthetic in the epidural space. Thus, the patient is generally placed supine after the block.

Patient Monitoring

- The patient should be monitored during and after the placement of an epidural block, just like a spinal block. However, the cardiovascular changes seen with an epidural block are generally slower and less profound when compared to a spinal anesthetic. Fluids and vasopressors are used to treat hypotension.
- Supplemental oxygen administration is recommended, especially if sedation is used for patient comfort.
- End-tidal carbon dioxide monitoring may be used to monitor the respiratory rate.
- Postoperatively, the patient should be monitored until the effects of epidural anesthetic have receded and the epidural catheter is removed.

Assessment of the Block

Epidural block leads to sensory, autonomic, and motor blockade which are assessed as follows:

Sensory Block

This can be assessed by testing for loss of touch, temperature, or pin-prick sensation. A differential block is noted between the complete loss of cold sensation which is one to two dermatomes more cephalad than the loss of both pinprick and light touch sensation.

Autonomic Block

This can be subjectively assessed by sensing the skin temperature in the area of the block and the extent of the drop in blood pressure (sympathetic block). Digital plethysmogram and skin conductance are used in research settings to test this objectively.

Motor Block

Lumbar Epidural

This can be assessed by using the **Bromage scale**, as summarizes in Table 41.7.

Thoracic Epidural

This can be assessed using the Rectus Abdominus Muscle (RAM) scale, as summarizes in Table 41.8.

Alternative Techniques for Confirmation of Needle Entry to Epidural Space

The most frequently used method to identify the needle entry into the epidural is the loss of resistance technique which is described earlier. A major shortcoming of this method is the non-specificity of the loss of resistance endpoint. A false positive loss of resistance may occur due to age related cysts in the interspinous ligaments, the needle tip entering paraspinous muscles or other intermuscular planes if needle misdirection occurs. Several methods have been developed to confirm correct catheter placement to overcome this problem.

Table 41.7 Bromage scale for assessment of motor block

Grade	Criteria	Degree of block
I	Free movement of legs and feet	Nil (0%)
II	Just able to flex knees with free movement of feet	Partial (33%)
III	Unable to flex knees, but with free movement of feet	Almost complete (66%)
IV	Unable to move legs or feet	Complete (100%)

Table 41.8 RAM test of abdominal muscles

Power	Criteria
100%	Able to rise from supine to sitting position with hands behind the head
80%	Can sit only with arms extended
60%	Can lift only head and scapulae off the bed
0%	Can lift only shoulders off the bed
20%	An increase in abdominal muscle tension can be felt during effort; no other response seen

Epidural Pressure Waveform Analysis

Epidural Pressure Waveform analysis is based upon the distinctive pulsatile pressure waveform obtained when a needle or catheter located in the epidural space is transduced. The epidural space has a low or negative pressure which pulsates in synchrony with the arterial pressure. Application of this characteristic may be used to determine needle entry into the epidural space in place of loss of resistance or else as a confirmatory adjunct for a needle or catheter already sited in the presumed epidural space.

The equipment required is often readily available and this technique is relatively simple to use. A pressure transducer, saline filled rigid tubing form part of the standard arterial blood pressure monitoring kit and the same patient monitor can be used.

There is randomized control trial evidence for a reduction in the failure rate as well as improved patient satisfaction in patients with pressure waveform guided epidural catheter placement (PWEP) compared to the conventional loss of resistance method.

Further studies have demonstrated the utility of epidural waveform analysis as a confirmatory adjunct by transducing either the epidural needle or catheter sited in the presumed epidural space following the LOR technique. After injecting saline (5 mL) through the needle and connecting it to a pressure transducer, the presence of waveforms synchronized with arterial pulsations serves as a confirmatory end point. If waveforms are still not present following a further 2.5 mL saline, it is deemed that the needle is not located in the epidural space and removal and reattempt is indicated. However, some waveforms are difficult to assess and false negatives are likely to occur to some extent with the potential for unnecessarily repeated procedures.

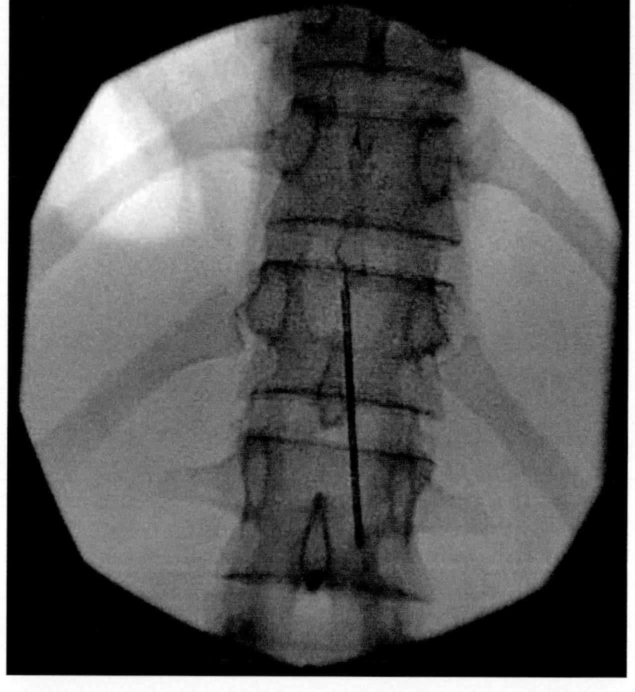

Fig. 41.46 Epidural Needle fluoroscopic guidance. (Reprinted with permission from Philip Peng Educational Series)

Fluoroscopy

Fluoroscopic techniques have been well established to successfully guide needle entry into interlaminar or interspinous spaces followed by standard loss of resistance to enter the epidural space. This is most often used in the context of chronic pain interventions and not for peri-operative epidural placement (Fig. 41.46 and 41.47). Advantages of fluoroscopy include clear identification of the appropriate vertebral level and avoidance of excessive needle to bone contact. Fluoroscopy has also been studied as a confirmatory adjunct for correct catheter placement in the epidural space via contrast injection, though it is not routinely used for this indication.

The main disadvantage of fluoroscopy is the additional equipment and personnel required for its use. Radiation exposure is also a consideration. Training in fluoroscopic

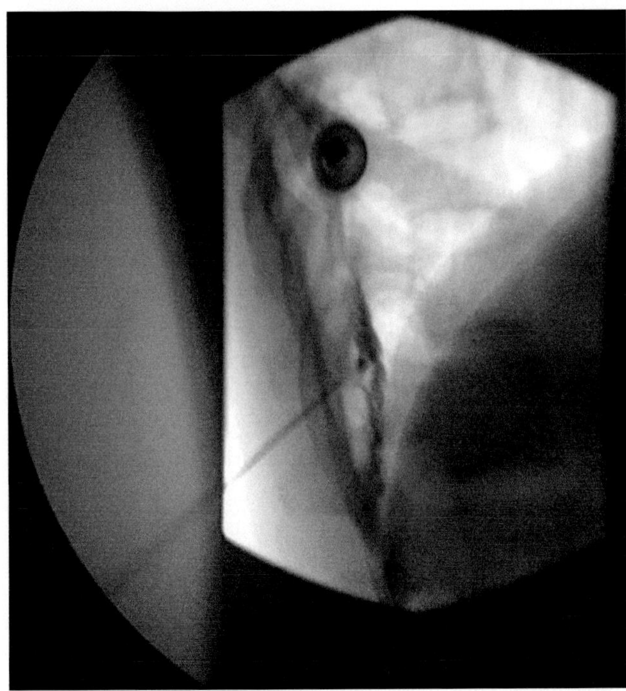

Fig. 41.47 Lateral View: Injection of radiopaque dye. (Reprinted with permission from Philip Peng Educational Series)

guidance of epidural needles is routine in the specialty of chronic pain, but not more widely amongst anesthesiologists. Therefore, the use of fluoroscopy is limited for general surgical settings unless trained staff and equipment are readily available.

Electrical Stimulation

The epidural electrical stimulation test (EEST) or Tsui test involves the application of low-amplitude electrical current to the epidural catheter following its insertion. A motor response in the truncal muscles is sought for thoracic epidural catheters. Response at a current range of 1–15 mA is a positive for correct epidural tip placement, whereas a motor response to a current of <1 mA indicates catheter tip placement in an intrathecal, subdural or foraminal position. A high level of sensitivity is associated with EEST which exceeds that of the local anesthetic test dose method. A further advantage compared to the clinical test dose is speed of testing, with confirmation of catheter position available immediately following placement.

Additional equipment required to conduct the EEST includes a nerve stimulator with a current range of 0.1–15 mA, a pulse width of 0.1–0.2 ms, a pulse frequency of 1–2 Hz, a digital current readout, and appropriate connectors (anode to an ECG electrode and a cathode to a Johans ECG adaptor). A stainless-steel wire reinforced catheter primed with saline or a stimulating catheter is required for conduction.

An additional benefit of electrical stimulation is the ability to determine the vertebral level of the epidural needle tip by correlating it to the motor response. Although this method is reliable and safe, it has not been widely adopted. Certain technical difficulties such as the need for frequent saline flushing and pain/paresthesia during stimulation have been reported. Nonetheless, it provides an objective measure of successful catheter placement which may be particularly useful in a teaching environment.

Practical Tips

Trajectory: While the midline may easily be found by palpation or ultrasound, operator error in terms of needle trajectory is relatively common, particularly in the lateral position. It may be helpful to get the perspective of a colleague or to stand back to identify the correct plane of approach and the needle trajectory.

Inadequate sensory block: this may require repeat dosing if the block fails to reach adequate sensory height after 30 min of the initial dose. Addition of opioids (such as fentanyl) to local anesthetic solution may speed the onset and extend the number of segments blocked.

Missed segments: this may be due to an inadequate volume of initial dose used. A repeat dose often improves this. If the missed segment is unilateral, turning the patient on the spared side before dosing can help. A 2% lignocaine solution with epinephrine is most effective in dealing with missed segments or an inadequate block.

Considerations in Patients with Challenging Anatomy

Performing a neuraxial block can be technically challenging in certain patient groups. This includes patients with a high body mass index, patients with spinal pathology and those who have undergone spinal surgery. Altered anatomy makes performing the block technically challenging, while spinal stenosis or postoperative epidural fibrosis (associated with spinal surgery) can impair the spread of spinal anesthetics in subarachnoid or epidural space, resulting in failed blocks.

Patients with a High Body Mass Index The anthropometric changes associated with obesity can make performing a neuraxial block more challenging. This is due to difficulty in patient positioning, obscured anatomical landmarks, increased depth of ligamentum flavum and the occasional inadequacy of usual equipment, e.g. the needle is too short. Ultrasound may help in the correct identification of the midline and the intervertebral spaces. Ultrasound also estimates the depth of the epidural space. It has been successfully used to improve the success rate of epidural placement in obese parturients.

Patients with Scoliosis Lateral deviation of the spine is accompanied by the rotation of the vertebral bodies towards the convex side of the curvature, while the spinous processes are rotated towards the concave side. This makes performing a neuraxial block more difficult. Ultrasound assists in identifying the lateral curvature and the degree of rotation. The usual approach to this situation is to perform the block using a paramedian injection on the convex side, which provides a more direct access to the neuraxis. Alternatively, if a midline insertion is used, the needle should be directed in a transverse plane, towards the convex side.

Patients with Previous Spinal Surgery Epidural fibrosis following spinal surgery, altered spinal anatomy, and the possibility of worsening neurological symptoms make this patient subset a challenge. Despite this, there have been several reports and reviews of successful neuraxial blocks in patients with previous spine surgery. While the absence of spinous processes makes it hard to locate intervertebral spaces, laminectomy may actually increase the chances of obtaining a successful dural puncture by increasing the size of the interlaminar gap. However, performing an epidural at the level of previous spinal surgery poses additional challenges due to spinal stenosis immediately above the fusion or decompression and tethering of the dura to the ligamentum flavum by scar formation. The epidural space may also be scarred which reduces the reliability of the loss-of-resistance technique. Thus, performing the epidural injection one or two spaces above or below the level of the surgery is advocated to reduce the chances of accidental dural puncture and ineffective block. Note that scarring of the epidural space may also lead to a patchy block.

Ultrasound can help immensely to locate the intervertebral space, identify the interlaminar window, visualize and estimate the depth of the ligamentum flavum.

Complications of Neuraxial Blocks

Complications arising from a spinal or an epidural anesthetic are mostly cardiovascular and neurological. However, practically they can be classified as early or late.

Early Complications

These include complications seen immediately following a neuraxial block and in the early perioperative period.

Cardiovascular

These are the most prominent complications of a central neuraxial anesthetic, and occur as a consequence of profound sympathetic block.

Hypotension Arteriolar dilatation and venous pooling lead to hypotension, which occurs commonly (16–33%). Risk factors for hypotension after neuraxial blockade include a block above T5, emergency surgery, age greater than 40, and chronic hypertension. Epidural anesthesia is associated with a more gradual fall in blood pressure compared to spinal anesthesia, making it a better choice in certain circumstances. Prophylactic fluid administration (20 mL/kg) and the use of vasopressors such as ephedrine (in 5–10 mg increments) or phenylephrine (50–100 μg increments) can be used to effectively counteract hypotension.

Bradycardia It usually results from a high block, as a consequence of blockade of the cardiac accelerator fibers (T1–T4), or more commonly from a vagal reflex associated with intracardiac stretch receptors in the presence of decreased cardiac filling (Bezold–Jarisch reflex). Apart from a high block, a younger age, ASA class 1 status, preoperative use of beta blockers, and male gender are risk factors for bradycardia. Anticholinergics such as atropine and adrenergics such as ephedrine are commonly used to treat this.

Cardiovascular Collapse Asystole and cardiac arrest following a spinal is a known complication. It is usually preceded by bradycardia resulting from the mechanisms described above.

Nausea and Vomiting This is associated with hypotension (hypoperfusion of the chemoreceptor trigger zone) and the use of opioid adjuncts (direct stimulation of chemoreceptor trigger zone). A sympathetic-parasympathetic imbalance may also have a role to play in the causation of nausea. It can be effectively treated with dexamethasone and ondansetron.

Tissue Trauma and Back Pain Multiple attempts at a neuraxial block lead to trauma to soft tissue and ligaments. This can contribute to persistent back ache. However, other factors may have a role to play as well.

Total Spinal This may result due to inappropriate dosing during a spinal anesthetic, positioning error or unintended passage of local anesthetic from epidural space to subarachnoid space (secondary to an unrecognized dural tap or catheter migration). It manifests as a rapidly ascending motor-sensory block, hypotension, bradycardia, and respiratory compromise. Medullary paralysis may result in a respiratory arrest and loss of consciousness. It is a life-threatening emergency. Management involves prompt recognition, securing the airway, ventilation, and supporting the hemodynamics until spontaneous recovery of the patient. To mitigate the risk of aspiration of gastric contents, the airway should be promptly secured with endotracheal intubation. This will require a rapid sequence induction dose of a muscle relaxant (succinylcholine or rocuronium) as the muscles of mastication may still be contracting, hindering effective laryngoscopy. Some advocate the use of a small amount of an induction agent to mitigate the risk of awareness. Ventilation will be required. Profound hypotension may rapidly ensue. Elevation of the legs is sometimes the most immediate intervention available. This should be accompanied by a generous dose of a vasopressor such as phenylephrine and the rapid administration of a fluid bolus. Cardiac arrest may ensure necessitating cardiopulmonary resuscitation.

Subdural Anesthetic This presents as widespread but ineffective and patchy anesthesia (Fig. 41.48). The subdural space does not end at the great foramen as does the epidural space but continues cranially. Warning signs include an unusually high sensory block which develops very slowly (even after 20 min) and a much less marked motor block. The clinical picture resembles that of total spinal anesthesia and is characterized by moderate hypotonia, breathing difficulties with retained consciousness, and often involvement of the cranial and cervical nerves. It may warrant similar intervention to that as total spinal anesthesia (see above).

Trigeminal Nerve Palsy Paresthesia in the area supplied by the nerve and transient weakness of the muscles of mastication is occasionally observed after high epidural anesthesia or subdural spread.

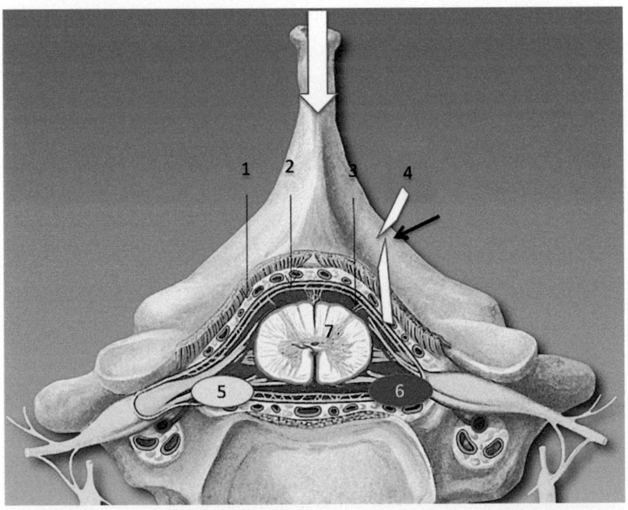

Fig. 41.48 Complications. (1) Intravascular injection, (2) subdural injection, (3) subarachnoid injection, (4) catheter shearing, (5) epidural abscess, and (6) epidural hematoma, and (7) injury to the spinal cord and nerve roots. (Reprinted with permission from Danilo Jankovic)

Horner's Syndrome This is produced after neuraxial anesthesia with a high spread of the injected local anesthetic and block of the sympathetic nerve fibers in the areas of segments T4-C8. Most often, Horner's syndrome is seen after a high spinal or epidural anesthesia in obstetrics and when there is subdural spread of the local anesthetic. Symptoms usually resolve fairly rapidly.

Inadvertent Dural Puncture During Epidural Catheter Insertion This usually presents as a gush of CSF through the epidural needle or upon aspiration through the catheter (Fig. 41.48). Management options include passing a catheter through the puncture made or reattempting the epidural in another space. In over 75% of the cases, use of an epidural needle is associated with the development of post dural puncture headache—this is likely to require a blood patch. There may be a reduction in the incidence of post-dural puncture headache if the catheter remains in the intrathecal space for at least 24 h.

Local Anesthetic Toxicity Inadvertent deposition of drug into a vein or systemic absorption of local anesthetic following epidural infusions may lead to local anesthetic toxicity.

Delayed Complications

These present usually after a few days or weeks of having performed a neuraxial block.

Nerve Injury

The following mechanisms are involved:

Direct Needle Trauma this commonly occurs at the time of performance of the block and is associated with severe paresthesia in the dermatomal distribution of the nerve root injured.

Neurotoxicity All local anesthetics are potentially neurotoxic. Despite this, local anesthetic induced neural damage is rarely seen clinically.

Transient Neurological Syndrome This presents as low back pain that radiates to the lower extremities after a spinal anesthetic. The symptoms last for a week and are treated supportively using simple analgesics. Risk factors such as outpatient procedures, the lithotomy position, obesity, and the use of lidocaine have been implicated in their development.

Cauda Equina Syndrome This presents as motor weakness and loss of bladder and bowel function, following the use of continuous spinal anesthesia. The pooling of local anesthetic around sacral nerves is thought to be the causative mechanism in its development.

Infections Infections such as localized skin infections, a spinal abscess, an epidural abscess or meningitis can rarely occur following a neuraxial anesthetic (Fig. 41.45). A spinal or epidural abscess presents as localized back pain, tenderness upon palpation, with sensory or motor deficits and fever. A magnetic resonance imaging of the vertebral canal is considered best for establishing a diagnosis. Intravenous antibiotics and surgical drainage or decompression may be needed. Diagnosis and definitive treatment should be urgently sought to limit long-term neurological impairment.

Post Dural Puncture Headache (PDPH)

This is a relatively common complication of spinal or an epidural anesthetic. The incidence of PDPH with the use of smaller gauge spinal needle (25–26G) is 0.5–1%, while puncture with an epidural needle (17–18G) results in PDPH in over 75% of cases.

Mechanism The proposed mechanism of the headache is the loss of CSF causing decrease in CSF pressure. This causes sagging of intracranial structures, with consequent traction on pain sensitive structures (such as meninges, cranial nerves, and veins). A second hypothesis suggests that decreased CSF pressure leads to intrathecal hypotension and painful vasodilatation of the intracranial blood vessels. Mainly when the patient is in a standing position, painful areas dilate (meninges, tentorium, vessels) and there is further pain transmission via the cerebral nerves and upper cervical nerves.

Clinical Presentation PDPH presents as a positional headache, worse on sitting up, 12–48 h after a dural puncture. PDPH is bilateral, predominantly frontal-temporal, and dull or throbbing in nature. Its severity varies, and it may be accompanied by associated symptoms such as nausea, vomiting, photophobia, diplopia, and hearing impairment. While younger females and parturients are at a higher risk of PDPH, older males are at a lower risk.

CSF Hypotension Syndrome and Involvement of the Cranial and Cervical Nerves All of the cranial nerves, with the exception of the olfactory nerve, glossopharyngeal nerve and vagus nerve, can be affected by low CSF pressure. The abducens nerve and vestibulocochlear nerve are most frequently affected. The long intracranial course of the abducens nerve leads to traction and consequent irritation of the nerve when there are changes in intracranial pressure. The patient complains of double vision, with parallel horizontal images and difficulties in focusing on objects. When precise audiometric examinations are carried out, unilateral or bilateral hyperacusis (vestibulocochlear nerve involvement) can be observed in 0.4–40% of patients with CSF hypotension syndrome. The prognosis is good.

Differential Diagnosis This includes migraine, tension headache, cervical myofascial pain (particularly in the sternocleidomastoid muscle, with what is known as "pseudospinal headache"), CNS infections (bacterial meningitis), sinus thrombosis (in the second half of pregnancy or in the puerperium, frequently in preeclampsia), and pneumocephalus (if the dura is breached when using the loss of resistance to air epidural insertion technique).

Initial Management This is conservative and includes simple analgesics and oral hydration. The majority of patients experience marked improvement in the symptoms or complete recovery after 5–7 days with this form of treatment. Other drugs such as caffeine, sumatriptan and ACTH have been found useful. Caffeine produces cerebral vasoconstriction and consequent decrease in cerebral blood flow providing a transient relief from headache. ACTH may stimulate the adrenal gland to increase cerebrospinal fluid production. Sumatriptan, a serotonin type 1d receptor agonist, may relieve headache by producing cerebral vasoconstriction.

Invasive Management The gold standard for the treatment of PDPH remains an autologous blood patch (Figs. 41.49 and 41.50). Its mechanism appears to be the tamponade of a dural leak, with subsequent improvement of CSF pressures. It produces a rapid relief of symptoms in between 70 and 98% of patients if performed after 24 h after the dural puncture. Repeating the procedure has a similar success rate.

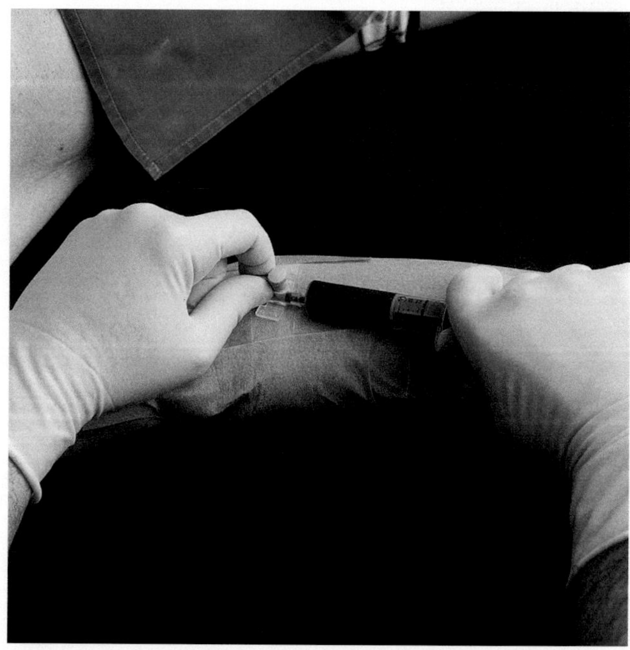

Fig. 41.49 Sterile withdrawal of blood. (Reprinted with permission from Danilo Jankovic)

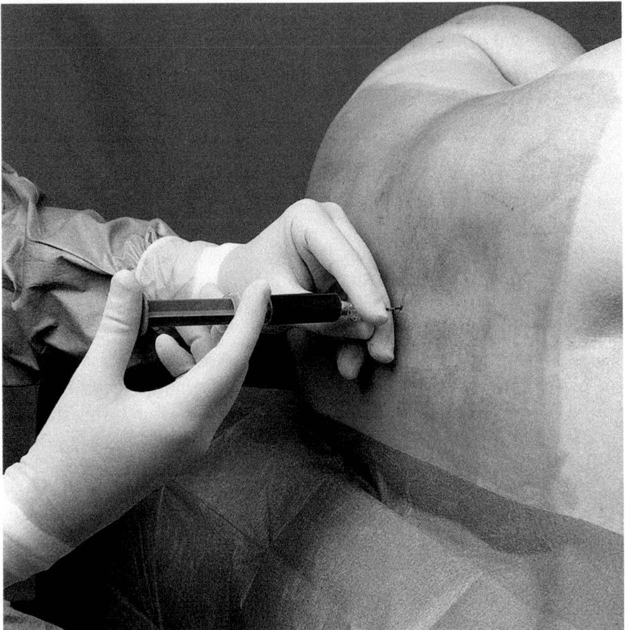

Fig. 41.50 Epidural Injection of homologous blood. (Reprinted with permission from Danilo Jankovic)

Spinal or Epidural Hematoma

Although rare, this is the most feared complication of a central neuraxial block (Fig. 41.45). Because the vertebral canal is a confined space, any bleeding may result in compression of the spinal cord resulting in a sensory-motor loss below the level of the compression. Patients with altered hemostasis and ongoing antiplatelet or anticoagulant therapy are at increased risk of developing a spinal or epidural hematoma. This usually presents as a sensory-motor impairment of unusually prolonged duration. Confusing this with an ongoing effect of local anesthetic often delays the correct diagnosis and management. Back pain and bladder or bowel dysfunction may also point towards the possibility of neural damage. Prompt imaging and neurosurgical consult should be arranged, as the prognosis is poor if the delay between the onset of paralysis and surgical decompression is more than 6–8 h. Guidelines concerning neuraxial anesthesia in anticoagulated patents should be followed to minimize the risks of this devastating complication.

Suggested Reading

Arendt K, Segal S. Why epidurals do not always work. Rev Obstet Gynecol. 2008;1(2):49–55.

Balki M, Lee Y, Halpern S, Carvalho JCA. Ultrasound imaging of the lumbar spine in the transverse plane: the correlation between estimated and actual depth to the epidural space in obese parturients. Anesth Analg. 2009;108(6):1876–81.

Berkowitz S, Gold MI. Spinal anesthesia for surgery in patients with previous lumbar laminectomy. Anesth Analg. 1980;59(11):881–2.

Bernards CM, Shen DD, Sterling ES, Adkins JE, Risler L, Phillips B, et al. Epidural, cerebrospinal fluid, and plasma pharmacokinetics of epidural opioids (part 1): differences among opioids. Anesthesiology. 2003;99(2):455–65.

Boon JM, Prinsloo E, Raath RP. A paramedian approach for epidural block: an anatomic and radiologic description. Reg Anesth Pain Med. 2003;28(3):221–7.

Breivik H, Bang U, Jalonen J, Vigfússon G, Alahuhta S, Lagerkranser M. Nordic guidelines for neuraxial blocks in disturbed haemostasis from the Scandinavian society of Anaesthesiology and intensive care medicine. Acta Anaesthesiol Scand. 2010;54(1):16–41.

Camorcia M, Capogna G. Sensory assessment of epidural block for caesarean section: a systematic comparison of pinprick, cold and touch sensation. Eur J Anaesthesiol. 2006;23(7):611–7.

Campagna JA, Carter C. Clinical relevance of the Bezold-Jarisch reflex. Anesthesiology. 2003;98(5):1250–60.

Casati A, Fanelli G. Unilateral spinal anesthesia: state of the art. Minerva Anestesiol. 2001;67(12):855–62.

Chakraverty R, Pynsent P, Isaacs K. Which spinal levels are identified by palpation of the iliac crests and the posterior superior iliac spines? J Anat. 2007;210(2):232–6.

Chan YK, Gopinathan R, Rajendram R. Loss of consciousness following spinal anaesthesia for caesarean section. Br J Anaesth. 2000;85(3):474–6.

Cook TM, Counsell D, Wildsmith JAW. Major complications of central neuraxial block: report on the third National Audit Project of the Royal College of Anaesthetists. Br J Anaesth. 2009;102(2):179–90.

Dahlgren N, Törnebrandt K. Neurological complications after anaesthesia. A follow-up of 18,000 spinal and epidural anaesthetics performed over three years. Acta Anaesthesiol Scand. 1995;39(7):872–80.

Denny NM, Selander DE. Continuous spinal anaesthesia. Br J Anaesth. 1998;81(4):590–7.

Faust A, Fournier R, Van Gessel E, Weber A, Hoffmeyer P, Gamulin Z. Isobaric versus hypobaric spinal bupivacaine for total hip arthroplasty in the lateral position. Anesth Analg. 2003;97(2):589–94, table of contents.

Gehling M, Tryba M. Risks and side-effects of intrathecal morphine combined with spinal anaesthesia: a meta-analysis. Anaesthesia. 2009;64(6):643–51.

Gosch UW, Hueppe M, Hallschmid M, Born J, Schmucker P, Meier T. Post-dural puncture headache in young adults: comparison of two small-gauge spinal catheters with different needle design. Br J Anaesth. 2005;94(5):657–61.

Graham AC, McClure JH. Quantitative assessment of motor block in labouring women receiving epidural analgesia. Anaesthesia. 2001;56(5):470–6.

Guay J. The epidural test dose: a review. Anesth Analg. 2006;102(3):921–9.

Hermanides J, Hollmann MW, Stevens MF, Lirk P. Failed epidural: causes and management. Br J Anaesth. 2012;109(2):144–54.

Hocking G, Wildsmith JAW. Intrathecal drug spread. Br J Anaesth. 2004;93(4):568–78.

Hogan QH. Lumbar epidural anatomy. A new look by cryomicrotome section. Anesthesiology. 1991;75(5):767–75.

Hogan Q. Distribution of solution in the epidural space: examination by cryomicrotome section. Reg Anesth Pain Med. 2002;27(2):150–6.

Horlocker TT, McGregor DG, Matsushige DK, Chantigian RC, Schroeder DR, Besse JA. Neurologic complications of 603 consecutive continuous spinal anesthetics using macrocatheter and microcatheter techniques. Perioperative Outcomes Group. Anesth Analg. 1997;84(5):1063–70.

Horlocker TT, Wedel DJ, Rowlingson JC, Enneking FK. Executive summary: regional anesthesia in the patient receiving antithrombotic or thrombolytic therapy: American Society of Regional Anesthesia and Pain Medicine evidence-based guidelines (third edition). Reg Anesth Pain Med. 2010;35(1):102–5.

Huang J. Paramedian approach for neuroaxial anesthesia in parturients with scoliosis. Anesth Analg. 2010;111(3):821–2; author reply 822.

Janik R, Dick W, Stanton-Hicks MD. Influence of barbotage on block characteristics during spinal anesthesia with hyperbaric tetracaine and bupivacaine. Reg Anesth. 1989;14(1):26–30.

Kettner SC, Willschke H, Marhofer P. Does regional anaesthesia really improve outcome? Br J Anaesth. 2011;107(Suppl):i90–5.

Kim J-T, Bahk J-H, Sung J. Influence of age and sex on the position of the conus medullaris and Tuffier's line in adults. Anesthesiology. 2003;99(6):1359–63.

Kim JE, Kim NY, Lee HS, Kil HK. Effects of intrathecal dexmedetomidine on low-dose bupivacaine spinal anesthesia in elderly patients undergoing transurethral prostatectomy. Biol Pharm Bull. 2013;36(6):959–65.

Lirk P, Kolbitsch C, Putz G, Colvin J, Colvin HP, Lorenz I, et al. Cervical and high thoracic ligamentum flavum frequently fails to fuse in the midline. Anesthesiology. 2003;99(6):1387–90.

Liu S, Kopacz DJ, Carpenter RL. Quantitative assessment of differential sensory nerve block after lidocaine spinal anesthesia. Anesthesiology. 1995;82(1):60–3.

Margarido CB, Mikhael R, Arzola C, Balki M, Carvalho JCA. The intercristal line determined by palpation is not a reliable anatomical landmark for neuraxial anesthesia. Can J Anaesth. 2011;58(3):262–6.

Motiani P, Chaudhary S, Bahl N, Sethi AK. Intrathecal sufentanil versus fentanyl for lower limb surgeries—a randomized controlled trial. J Anaesthesiol Clin Pharmacol. 2011;27(1):67–73.

Nair GS, Abrishami A, Lermitte J, Chung F. Systematic review of spinal anaesthesia using bupivacaine for ambulatory knee arthroscopy. Br J Anaesth. 2009;102(3):307–15.

Neal JM. Hypotension and bradycardia during spinal anesthesia: significance, prevention, and treatment. Tech Reg Anesth Pain Manag. 2000;4(4):148–54.

Nelson KE, Rauch T, Terebuh V, D'Angelo R. A comparison of intrathecal fentanyl and sufentanil for labor analgesia. Anesthesiology. 2002;96(5):1070–3.

Ousley R, Egan C, Dowling K, Cyna AM. Assessment of block height for satisfactory spinal anaesthesia for caesarean section. Anaesthesia. 2012;67(12):1356–63.

Panjabi MM, Takata K, Goel V, Federico D, Oxland T, Duranceau J, et al. Thoracic human vertebrae. Quantitative three-dimensional anatomy. Spine (Phila Pa 1976). 1991;16(8):888–901.

Panjabi MM, Goel V, Oxland T, Takata K, Duranceau J, Krag M, et al. Human lumbar vertebrae. Quantitative three-dimensional anatomy. Spine (Phila Pa 1976). 1992;17(3):299–306.

Pollard JB. Cardiac arrest during spinal anesthesia: common mechanisms and strategies for prevention. Anesth Analg. 2001;92(1):252–6.

Pollock JE. Neurotoxicity of intrathecal local anaesthetics and transient neurological symptoms. Best Pract Res Clin Anaesthesiol. 2003;17(3):471–84.

Pysyk CL, Persaud D, Bryson GL, Lui A. Ultrasound assessment of the vertebral level of the palpated intercristal (Tuffier's) line. Can J Anaesth. 2010;57(1):46–9.

Rabinowitz A, Bourdet B, Minville V, Chassery C, Pianezza A, Colombani A, et al. The paramedian technique: a superior initial approach to continuous spinal anesthesia in the elderly. Anesth Analg. 2007;105(6):1855–7.

Raffaeli W, Marconi G, Fanelli G, Taddei S, Borghi GB, Casati A. Opioid-related side-effects after intrathecal morphine: a prospective, randomized, double-blind dose-response study. Eur J Anaesthesiol. 2006;23(7):605–10.

Reina MA, Franco CD, López A, Dé Andrés JA, van Zundert A. Clinical implications of epidural fat in the spinal canal. A scanning electron microscopic study. Acta Anaesthesiol Belg. 2009;60(1):7–17.

Reynolds F. Damage to the conus medullaris following spinal anaesthesia. Anaesthesia. 2001;56(3):238–47.

Saberski LR, Kondamuri S, Osinubi OY. Identification of the epidural space: is loss of resistance to air a safe technique? A review of the complications related to the use of air. Reg Anesth. 1997;22(1):3–15.

Salinas FV, Sueda LA, Liu SS. Physiology of spinal anaesthesia and practical suggestions for successful spinal anaesthesia. Best Pract Res Clin Anaesthesiol. 2003;17(3):289–303.

Sharrock NE, Urquhart B, Mineo R. Extradural anaesthesia in patients with previous lumbar spine surgery. Br J Anaesth. 1990;65(2):237–9.

Singh H, Yang J, Thornton K, Giesecke AH. Intrathecal fentanyl prolongs sensory bupivacaine spinal block. Can J Anaesth. 1995;42(11):987–91.

Sultan P, Gutierrez MC, Carvalho B. Neuraxial morphine and respiratory depression: finding the right balance. Drugs. 2011;71(14):1807–19.

Turnbull DK, Shepherd DB. Post-dural puncture headache: pathogenesis, prevention and treatment. Br J Anaesth. 2003;91(5):718–29.

Walker DS, Brock-Utne JG. A comparison of simple tests to distinguish cerebrospinal fluid from saline. Can J Anaesth. 1997;44(5 Pt 1):494–7.

Zaric D, Pace NL. Transient neurologic symptoms (TNS) following spinal anaesthesia with lidocaine versus other local anaesthetics. Cochrane Database Syst Rev. 2009;(2):CD003006.

Neuraxial Anesthesia and Analgesia for Obstetric Practice

42

Frederik Marynen and Marc Van de Velde

Contents

General Considerations

Women in labor should be offered effective labor analgesia whenever they request analgesia. Neuraxial analgesia is one of the options. Modern clinical guidelines suggest that neuraxial analgesia should not be denied to women in labor when a request is made.

In 2007, the National Institute for Health and Care Excellence (NICE) published a guideline about "intrapartum care" and gave the following advice: "Women in labor who desire regional analgesia should not be denied it, including women in severe pain in the latent first stage of labor."

F. Marynen · M. Van de Velde (✉)
Section Anesthesiology, Department of Cardiovascular Sciences, KULeuven and University Hospitals Leuven, Leuven, Belgium
e-mail: frederik.marynen@uzleuven.be; marc.vandevelde@uzleuven.be

The American College of Obstetricians and Gynecologists (ACOG) in 2006 and the American Society of Anesthesiologists in 2007 stated that if no contra-indications are present, neuraxial analgesia should not be denied if a woman in labor asks for it.

For many years, the effects of neuraxial analgesia on the labor and birth process were discussed. It is now clear that with modern forms of analgesia, these effects are minimal.

Indication

Women in labor should not be denied neuraxial labor analgesia in the absence of contraindications. Absolute contraindications include severe coagulopathy, infection at the site of epidural insertion, acutely raised intracranial pressure, uncorrected severe hypovolemia, and of course patient refusal. Relative contraindications include mild coagulopathy,

D. Jankovic, P. Peng (eds.), *Regional Nerve Blocks in Anesthesia and Pain Therapy*,
https://doi.org/10.1007/978-3-030-88727-8_42

chronically increased intracranial pressure, systemic infection, stenotic valvular disease, pulmonary hypertension from the Eisenmenger type, and preexisting neurological problems. An individual assessment and evaluation should be performed by the anesthesiologist in every patient.

Neuraxial anesthesia for cesarean section is also recommended for most operative deliveries. The degree of urgency of the C-section or uncontrolled preeclampsia might be additional contraindications to perform neuraxial anesthesia.

Functional Anatomy

Pregnancy influences the functional anatomy making modification to our neuraxial technique necessary. Firstly, since the uterus is growing, lumbar lordosis increases. As a result, the distance between the skin and the dura mater posterior also increases. Hence, the L2–L3 and L3–L4 interspaces seem the most ideal interspaces to perform obstetric neuraxial anesthetic techniques. Preference goes to the L3–L4 interspace because of the conus medullaris that might end as low as L2, making neurologic injury more likely when the neuraxial technique is performed at the L2–L3 level.

Secondly, the epidural venous plexus enlarges during pregnancy, which reduces the volume of the epidural space and reduces the amount of liquor in a spinal segment. Because of these changes, the spread of a neuraxial blockade will be greater for a given dose of local anesthetic. This is the anatomical reason why the dose of local anesthetic during pregnancy has to be reduced. Additionally, the engorged venous epidural plexus makes bloody epidural punctures and inadvertent intravascular placement of epidural catheters more likely.

Also, the pregnancy-associated increase in adipose tissue and fluid retention might complicate the neuraxial procedure. Fixation of the epidural catheter is more problematic because of increased mobility during labor of the pregnant patient.

Finally, because of the enlarged uterus and the accompanying aorto-caval syndrome, side effects such as spinal-induced hypotension are more likely to occur in pregnancy.

Technique

Neuraxial Analgesia for Labor

When neuraxial analgesia for labor is performed, the anesthesiologist needs to consider different aspects: How will we initiate analgesia? How will we maintain analgesia? And which drugs are we going to administer? In the majority of cases, analgesia will be initiated through an epidural catheter or through a combined spinal-epidural (CSE) technique. Single-shot spinal anesthesia, caudal anesthesia, or continuous spinal anesthesia can be used but are exceedingly rare. Worldwide epidural analgesia is the preferred option, but the CSE technique is gaining popularity.

Neuraxial Techniques

Conventional Epidural Versus Combined Spinal-Epidural Technique

For 30 years, the preferred technique to initiate labor analgesia has been discussed in obstetric anesthesia literature. A Cochrane review could not identify major differences between both techniques, apart from a faster onset of analgesia and more pruritus with CSE. However, a detailed comparison might be useful, since subtle differences exist between both techniques that might be important in specific patient populations.

Analgesia Induction Time

Onset of analgesia is more rapid with the CSE technique. With CSE, analgesia is achieved consistently within 5–10 min with low patient variability, regardless of the intensity and the stage of labor. With epidural analgesia, there is good analgesia only after a median 20 to 30 min, with great variability between patients. In more advanced labor, it might even take 45 min or longer to reach a satisfying level of analgesia.

Quality of Analgesia and the Reliability of the Epidural Catheter

Visual analogue scores (VAS) for pain are lower with CSE and then with epidural analgesia. The most important advantage of the CSE technique is that the epidural catheter functions more reliably than an epidural catheter placed as part of a conventional epidural technique. There is less breakthrough pain and there is less need of replacement of the catheter. Also, thanks to the identification of the cerebrospinal fluid, a midline insertion of the epidural catheter is more likely to occur.

Consumption of Local Anesthetic

The consumption of local anesthetic is 20–30% less with the CSE technique compared to the conventional epidural technique. The most important reason is that the initial epidural dose is avoided. Secondly, the perforated dura will allow for subclinical spinal analgesia, and hence less breakthrough pain and less additional top-ups are required. A recent investigation from Patel et al. indicated that when the initial spinal dose has worn off, the epidural bolus that has to be given subsequently might possibly be marginally higher in the CSE technique. However, the methodology of this study does not reflect routine clinical practice, in which an epidural maintenance dose is immediately given before reoccurrence of pain. Patel et al. withheld the first epidural dose until pain was reoccurring.

Duration of the Spinal Analgesia Component

Usually the original spinal dose will provide analgesia for approximately 120 min, which is comparable with the first epidural dose in conventional epidural analgesia. With the addition of adjuvants, the duration of action can be prolonged up to 4 h.

Failure of the Spinal Component

The inability to administer the spinal dose might occur because the dura and subsequently the intrathecal space cannot be identified. Of course, the epidural catheter might offer a solution in this case. However, when the dura has not been identified, chances are higher that the epidural catheter will fail as well since the epidural catheter might be introduced off midline. Also, epidural catheters placed as part of the conventional epidural technique might end up off midline. However, the anesthesiologist lacks knowledge of a previous failed spinal puncture.

Dural Puncture Epidural Technique

The dural puncture epidural (DPE) technique is the most recent neuraxial technique developed in the setting of labor analgesia. DPE is a modification of CSE, where a dural perforation is made through a spinal needle but intrathecal administration of medication is withheld. An epidural catheter is then inserted through which analgesia is initiated. The idea of this technique is improving the quality of analgesia by allowing leakage of drugs from the epidural space to the intrathecal space through the perforation made. Some studies suggest an improved quality of analgesia with DPE compared to a standard epidural technique (improved caudal spread and bilateral pain relief). Also, studies suggest fewer maternal and fetal side effects with DPE compared to CSE. However, a recent systematic review performed by Heesen et al. concludes that currently a lack of evidence exists regarding the benefits and risks of DPE, necessitating further investigation concerning this technique.

Maintenance of Analgesia

Following initiation, analgesia has to be maintained throughout the entire duration of labor and delivery. Ideally, this is achieved with a modality in which the woman herself can adjust the level of analgesia according to her needs. Furthermore, the method of maintenance has to anticipate to the constantly changing circumstances with increasing intensity of pain throughout labor. Maintenance can be achieved using different modalities such as (1) intermittent top-ups (by midwife or doctor), (2) continuous epidural infusions, or (3) patient-controlled analgesia. Many studies have demonstrated that intermittent top-ups and certainly PCEA are superior compared to continuous epidural infusions. There is less breakthrough pain (and so less interventions needed by the anesthesiologist), less consumption of local anesthetics, and less requirement for instrumental delivery. Thereafter, the satisfaction of the women is higher with the PCEA mode.

In recent years, another modality of maintenance has become available: programmed intermittent automatic epidural bolus (PIEB), which can be combined with PCEA. A programmed bolus of a sufficient volume injected at a high infusion speed achieves a better spread in the epidural space compared to a continuous epidural infusion or a PCEA bolus with a lower volume and lower injection speed. Also, the automatic timing of the bolus prevents the recurrence of breakthrough pain, and the patient is less required to activate the PCEA system herself. This PIEB mode has been compared in several studies with continuous epidural infusions. A meta-analysis concerning these studies indicates a lower consumption of local anesthetics, a higher rate of satisfaction of the woman, and a lower chance of instrumental delivery with PIEB. In addition, Capogna et al. clearly demonstrated a significant and clinically relevant lower incidence of motor block with PIEB, compared to a continuous epidural infusion.

Recently, Roofthooft et al. were the first to compare PIEB with PCEA without background infusion. They noted higher local anesthetic consumption with PIEB but significantly less breakthrough pain and a significantly lower need for anesthesiologists to intervene.

Subsequently, other modes for maintenance of analgesia are currently being developed in which the continuous infusion rate, the PIEB-bolus lockout time, or the volume of the PIEB bolus are automatically adapted based on the number of PCEA boluses the woman has asked in the previous hour of labor. This technique is called computer-integrated PCEA. Since labor and delivery are dynamic processes with a varying intensity of pain, the analgesia should also be adaptable. The limited research that is currently available is positive and demonstrates a higher patient satisfaction and an even lower consumption of local anesthetics (Table 42.1).

Neuraxial Medication

Choice of Local Anesthetic

Several local anesthetics are available for analgesia during labor. Lidocaine does not seem very useful given the relatively short duration of action. Long-acting amide local anesthetics (bupivacaine, levobupivacaine, and ropivacaine) are the preferred local anesthetics. The risk of toxicity is lower with ropivacaine, but given the low concentrated solutions, this is not an important argument. It is important to consider the sensory-motor separation between these three long-acting amides. The literature demonstrates that ropivacaine in low concentrations is clearly superior concerning motor

Table 42.1 Modalities to maintain neuraxial analgesia

Modality	Advantages	Disadvantages
PCEA	Individualized analgesia	No prevention of breakthrough pain
CEI	Prevention of breakthrough pain	– No individualized analgesia – Poor spread
PIEB	– Prevention of breakthrough pain – Good spread – Reduced motor block – Less instrumental delivery	No individualized analgesia
PIEB + PCEA	– Low workload for practitioners – Good maternal satisfaction – Combines advantages of both techniques	
PIEB + CEI	Combines advantages of both techniques	– Less maternal satisfaction – Higher workload – Higher anesthetic consumption compared to PIEB + PCEA

block compared to bupivacaine in low concentrations. A recent meta-analysis of Guo et al. confirms this finding.

Dose and Volume of the Local Anesthetic Mixture

Spinal Component

The dose of local anesthetic administered in the spinal component of CSE to initiate analgesia has been determined empirically. The dose of bupivacaine suggested is 2–3 mg. Similar doses have been described for levobupivacaine. For ropivacaine, the originally used dose was determined empirically and expected to be 3.5 mg. A full dose-response study comparing levobupivacaine, ropivacaine, and bupivacaine (combined with sufentanil) was conducted by Van de Velde et al. This study demonstrates that levobupivacaine and ropivacaine are less potent than bupivacaine and that the previous empirically used doses for these three local anesthetics were lower than the ED95. The ED95 was 3.5 mg for bupivacaine and 4.5 mg for ropivacaine and levobupivacaine.

Epidural Component

When starting epidural analgesia, the first dose of local anesthetic has to be sufficiently large to saturate the whole epidural space from T10 to S3 with local anesthetic. Hence, the volume is more important than concentration, and a low concentrated solution (<0.15%) is preferred to a higher concentrated mixture. This results in nicely spread local anesthetic, with less consumption of local anesthetics and less motor block. The volume that will be injected at first has to be a minimum of 10 to 15 mL. In addition, with breakthrough pain, it is very important to administer a high-volume bolus of a low concentrated solution. A small volume bolus with a high concentration is completely pointless. This will induce motor block and analgesia with poor epidural spread. This will never provide analgesia to the lowest sacral roots (which are the main cause of breakthrough pain).

Adjuvants

Several adjuvants are available to potentially improve the action of local anesthetics during neuraxial analgesia for labor and delivery. However, most of these adjuvants are not part of the routine neuraxial analgesia because of their side effects.

The adjuvants can be divided into two groups: opioids and non-opioids.

Opioids

Opioids potentiate the action of local anesthetics allowing a significant reduction in the dose of local anesthetics that is administered spinally or epidurally. This results in less side effects (less motor block, less hypotension) and better analgesia quality. The disadvantage of the addition of opioids consists of pruritus and the possibility of changes in fetal heart rate when administered intrathecally.

Conventionally, 1 to 3 μg/mL fentanyl or 0.5–1 μg/mL sufentanil is used epidurally. Intrathecally the dose of fentanyl is 10–25 μg and sufentanil 2–5 μg. Higher intrathecal doses are not advised because of previously described changes in fetal heart rate.

Non-opioid Adjuvants

Clonidine and Dexmedetomidine

Both these alpha-agonists can potentially optimize the analgesic effect of local anesthetics. Intrathecal clonidine is not recommended. Analgesia was strengthened and prolonged, but significant hypotension occurred. Hence, most obstetric anesthesiologists do not recommend the intrathecal administration of clonidine.

Epidurally doses of 30–150 μg have been tested. A good analgesic effect was described. However, with higher-dose (>75 μg) sedation, changes in fetal heart rate, hypotension, and bradycardia did occur. Lower doses (30–75 μg) have little side effects. Currently, epidural clonidine is not recommended for routine epidural use. We use epidural clonidine in a dose of 75 μg to treat breakthrough pain (in the clinical situation in which the epidural catheter is confirmed to be in the epidural space).

Recently, Zhang et al. performed a study in which dexmedetomidine was compared with sufentanil as an adjuvant to local anesthetic for epidural labor analgesia. Dexmedetomidine seemed to be superior to sufentanil in analgesic effect when combined with 0.1% ropivacaine. No significant differences in side effects were noted, except for a higher value on the Ramsay Sedation Scale for dexmedetomidine.

Neostigmine

Also, the neuraxial application of neostigmine has been studied. It provides good analgesia when administered both intrathecally and epidurally. However, the intrathecal administration causes severe nausea and vomiting. When administered through epidural route, nausea and vomiting has not been demonstrated, and in doses of 500–750 μg, it produces good analgesia. Therefore, it can be used in the management of breakthrough pain. However, it is not recommended for routine use.

Neuraxial Anesthesia in Caesarean Section

Neuraxial Techniques

Single-shot spinal anesthesia (SSSA) is the most used neuraxial technique to provide anesthesia for a cesarean section (when an epidural catheter is not yet in place). This technique is easy to perform and cheap and achieves a profound block rapidly. However, there are important disadvantages to this technique. Firstly, the duration of the spinal block is limited. Since a certain amount of time of anesthesia has to be guaranteed, the spinal anesthetic has to be overdosed, resulting in significant maternal hypotension.

Secondly, in 6% of the cases where the SSSA technique is used, there seems to be insufficient anesthesia. This results in the need to administer additional anesthesia/analgesia (e.g., intravenous opioids) or convert to general anesthesia.

Compared to the SSSA technique, CSE can produce prolonged anesthetic conditions, and the spinal dose can be reduced producing less hemodynamic perturbations. By combining spinal anesthesia with insertion of an epidural catheter, the advantages of the spinal component (deep block with fast onset) are combined with the flexibility of an epidural catheter (possibility for epidural top-ups during the operation and an access for postoperative analgesia). Besides, this extra tool to provide analgesia results in the possibility to reduce the dose of the initial spinal component, which decreases the incidence of spinal-induced hypotension.

For women in labor who already received an epidural catheter for analgesia and who are unexpectedly planned for a cesarean section, an epidural top-up is the technique of choice. In this technique, a local anesthetic (possibly combined with an opioid) is carefully titrated and administered through the epidural catheter. This top-up can be initiated in the delivery room, in the presence of an anesthesiologist. This practice might save important time, especially in cases of emergent deliveries. Ideally before administering the top-up dose, the epidural catheter is tested by administering a test dose.

In every neuraxial technique, it is crucial to test the level of the sensory block correctly before starting surgery. For cesarean section, a complete blockade of the nerve fibers of T4 and lower is mandatory, including all sacral nerve fibers. Practically, this means the complete absence of any cold feeling from level T4 and lower. A common pitfall exists in the blurred zone where cold feeling is blunted but not absent. This degree of blockade is not enough for any level lower than T3.

Neuraxial Medication

Concerning the spinal component in SSSA and CSE, hyperbaric bupivacaine is the most used local anesthetic. The dose administered into the spinal space is typically 10–15 mg. In modern practice, a lipofilic opioid is added to the spinal mixture to increase the quality of anesthesia intra-operatively. Fentanyl (15–30 μg) or sufentanil (2–5 μg) are routinely used for this purpose.

In the scenario of an epidural top-up (for an unplanned caesarean section with an epidural catheter already in place), several pharmacological options are listed in Table 42.2. Hillyard et al. performed a meta-analysis concerning the local anesthetic mixtures used in this setting. They concluded that based on the quality of analgesia, the pharmacological properties and the toxicity profiles of ropivacaine 0.75% and lidocaine 2% are the most ideal local anesthetic mixtures for the epidural top-up (2-chloroprocaine 3% was not routinely used at that time).

Table 42.2 Epidural local anesthetics for epidural top-up in setting of unplanned caesarean section

Local anesthetic mixture	Dose (mg)	Onset (min)	Duration of action (min)
Lidocaine 2% + bicarbonate	300–500	5–7	75–100
Lidocaine 2% + adrenaline	300–500	7–11	75–100
Bupivacaine 0.5% or levobupivacaine 0.5%	75–125	10–15	120–180
Ropivacaine 0.75%	75–150	10–15	120–180
2-chloroprocaine 3%	450–750	2–10	45

Complications

Spinal-Induced Hypotension

Hypotension can occur following every neuraxial anesthetic technique. Hence, monitoring of the maternal vital parameters is mandatory in order to be able to provide a fast and thorough treatment of this hypotension.

Spinal hypotension is a common side effect, particularly following neuraxial anesthesia in the setting of caesarean section. Several strategies exist to prevent this spinal hypotension in caesarean section:

- Positioning the patient in a left lateral tilt (supine), since this allows the uterus to shift away from the great vessels in the abdomen.
- The use of a hyperbaric solution of local anesthetic to perform the spinal anesthesia results in a smaller spread with a lower blockade, resulting in less hypotension.
- Lowering the spinal dose. However, this is only possible with CSE, since this results in a shorter duration of anesthesia.
- Administering intravenous fluid: Loading of crystalloids or colloids at the time of neuraxial placement is useful to reduce hypotension. Also, preloading colloids is a good strategy. However, preloading a crystalloid solution is considered to be less effective.
- Administering vasopressors: The prophylactic use of phenylephrine is recommended. Also, phenylephrine is the gold standard to treat spinal hypotension in C-section, since this leads to less fetal acidosis compared to ephedrine. Recently, also noradrenaline was tested and found to be effective and safe in the initial clinical trials. However, more work is required.

Spinal-Epidural Hematoma

A hemorrhage into the neuraxis is a serious complication but luckily very rare. It is more likely to occur in patients with bleeding disorders and in patients who are treated with anticoagulants. According to a large nationwide data analysis in the United States, the incidence of spinal hematoma was 0.6 per 100,000 epidural catheterizations in obstetric patients. Because of the severity of the potential consequences of this complication, a high index of suspicion must be maintained. Spinal-epidural hematoma produces severe bilateral back pain and neurological sensory and motor deficit. Rapid decompression of the hematoma is required if complete recovery needs to be achieved.

Postdural Puncture Headache (PDPH)

The incidence of PDPH following epidural analgesia is 0.5–2%. Although it is a theoretical concern that the spinal component in the CSE technique increases this risk, findings in clinical practice nor in several studies could establish this concern. CSE does not seem to increase the risk for PDPH. The full range of prophylactic and therapeutic measures that can be taken is not within the scope of this chapter.

Neurological Complications

Since important neurological structures are located nearby the target of neuraxial anesthesia, neurological complications are possible. Fortunately, these complications are very rare.

Other Complications

- Pruritus, nausea.
- Maternal motor block.
- Changes in fetal heart rhythm.
- Respiratory depression.
- Total spinal anesthesia.
- Local anesthetic systemic toxicity.

Practical Tips

Neuraxial Ultrasound

To improve the success rate and to minimize the risk of complications, the clinician might perform an ultrasound of the neuraxial structures before performing the procedure. This technique allows the clinician to identify some important anatomical landmarks and to gather relevant information about the procedure: the midline of the spine, the vertebral level, the distance from the puncture site toward the epidural space, the insertion point of the needle, and the optimal angle of the needle trajectory.

A recent meta-analysis of Young et al. demonstrated that the use of preprocedural ultrasound increased the first-pass success rate (a single skin puncture with no needle redirections) significantly. Besides, they did not find evidence of a prolongation in total time of the procedure performing preprocedural ultrasound compared to that with conventional landmark palpation. More specifically, this meta-analysis highlights the increased benefit of preprocedural ultrasound for those cases in which the neuraxial procedure was predicted to be difficult. Complications, including postpartum back pain and headache, were decreased with the performance of preprocedural ultrasound.

Given its potential to increase efficacy and reduce complications, the use of preprocedural ultrasound is recommended.

Malpositioning of the Epidural Catheter: Aspiration Test

The epidural catheter can unintentionally be located in the intrathecal or intravascular space. A crucial step to exclude an intrathecal or intravascular location of the catheter is the aspiration test performed on the epidural catheter following placement. This is performed with a 2-cc syringe to evaluate if blood or cerebrospinal fluid can be aspirated through the catheter. This test identifies most of the wrongly located catheters. Besides this, the possibility of an epidural test dose exists.

Although general opinion is growing that administering an epidural test dose through an epidural catheter that showed a negative aspiration test is not necessary, however, the epidural catheter should be tested by administering a test dose when used for a cesarean section.

Suggested Reading

Buyse I, Stockman W, Columb M, et al. Effect of sufentanil on minimum local analgesic concentrations of epidural bupivacaine, ropivacaine and levobupivacaine in nullipara in early labour. Int J Obstet Anesth. 2007;16(1):22–8.

Capogna G, Camorcia M, Stirparo S, et al. Programmed intermittent epidural bolus versus continuous epidural infusion for labor analgesia: the effects on maternal motor function and labor outcome. A randomized double-blind study in nulliparous women. Anesth Analg. 2011;113(4):826–31.

Cappiello E, O'Rourke N, Segal S, et al. A randomized trial of dural puncture epidural technique compared with the standard epidural technique for labor analgesia. Anesth Analg. 2008;107(5):1646–51.

Chau A, Tsen LC. Update on modalities and techniques for labor epidural analgesia and anesthesia. Adv Anesth. 2018;36(1):139–62.

Chau A, Bibbo C, Huang CC, et al. Dural puncture epidural technique improves labor analgesia quality with fewer side effects compared with epidural and combined spinal epidural techniques: a randomized clinical trial. Anesth Analg. 2017;124(2):560–9.

Gambling D, Berkowitz J, Farrell TR, et al. A randomized controlled comparison of epidural analgesia and combined spinal-epidural analgesia in a private practice setting: pain scores during first and second stages of labor and at delivery. Anesth Analg. 2013a;116(3):636–43.

Gambling D, Berkowitz J, Farrell TR, et al. A randomized controlled comparison of epidural analgesia and combined spinal-epidural analgesia in a private practice setting: pain scores during first and second stages of labor and at delivery. Anesth Analg. 2013b;116(3):636–43.

George RB, Allen TK, Habib AS. Intermittent epidural bolus compared with continuous epidural infusions for labor analgesia: a systematic review and meta-analysis. Anesth Analg. 2013;116(1):133–44.

Guo S, Li B, Gao C, et al. Epidural analgesia with bupivacaine and fentanyl versus ropivacaine and fentanyl for pain relief in labor: a meta-analysis. Medicine (Baltimore). 2015;94(23):e880.

Hallworth SP, Fernando R, Columb MO, et al. The effect of posture and baricity on the spread of intrathecal bupivacaine for elective cesarean delivery. Anesth Analg. 2005;100(4):1159–65.

Heesen M, Rijs K, Rossaint R, et al. Dural puncture epidural versus conventional epidural block for labor analgesia: a systematic review of randomized controlled trials. Int J Obstet Anesth. 2019;40:24–31.

Hillyard SG, Bate TE, Corcoran TB, et al. Extending epidural analgesia for emergency caesarean section: a meta-analysis. Br J Anaesth. 2011;107(5):668–78.

Kinsella SM. A prospective audit of regional anaesthesia failure in 5080 caesarean sections. Anaesthesia. 2008;63(8):822–32.

Kinsella SM. Anaesthesia. 2019. Recommendations vasopressors.

Kinsella SM, Carvalho B, Dyer RA, et al. International consensus statement on the management of hypotension with vasopressors during caesarean section under spinal anaesthesia. Anaesthesia. 2018;73(1):71–92.

Langesaeter E, Rosseland LA, Stubhaug A. Continuous invasive blood pressure and cardiac output monitoring during cesarean delivery: a randomized, double-blind comparison of low-dose versus high-dose spinal anesthesia with intravenous phenylephrine or placebo infusion. Anesthesiology. 2008;109(5):856–63.

Lee AJ, Ranasinghe JS, Chehade JM, et al. Ultrasound assessment of the vertebral level of the intercristal line in pregnancy. Anesth Analg. 2011;113(3):559–64.

Leo S, Ocampo CE, Lim Y, et al. A randomized comparison of automated intermittent mandatory boluses with a basal infusion in combination with patient-controlled epidural analgesia for labor and delivery. Int J Obstet Anesth. 2010;19(4):357–64.

Loubert C. Fluid and vasopressor management for cesarean delivery under spinal anesthesia: continuing professional development. Can J Anaesth. 2012;59(6):604–19.

Lyons GR, Kocarev MG, Wilson RC, et al. A comparison of minimum local anesthetic volumes and doses of epidural bupivacaine (0.125% w/v and 0.25% w/v) for analgesia in labor. Anesth Analg. 2007;104(2):412–5.

Missant C, Teunkens A, Vandermeersch E, et al. Intrathecal clonidine prolongs labour analgesia but worsens fetal outcome: a pilot study. Can J Anaesth. 2004;51(7):696–701.

Orbach-Zinger S, Jadon A, Lucas D, et al. Intrathecal catheter use after accidental dural puncture in obstetric patients: literature review and clinical management recommendations. Anaesthesia. 2021;76(8):1111–21. https://doi.org/10.1111/anae.15390.

Patel NP, Armstrong SL, Fernando R, et al. Combined spinal epidural vs epidural labour analgesia: does initial intrathecal analgesia reduce the subsequent minimum local analgesic concentration of epidural bupivacaine. Anaesthesia. 2012;67(6):584–93.

Roofthooft E. Neuraxiale anesthesie voor keizersnede. In: Schryns-van den Berg X, Van de Velde M, editors. Anesthesie en de normale zwangerschap. Leuven: Acco; 2017. p. 139–55.

Roofthooft E, Barbé A, Schildermans J, et al. Programmed intermittent epidural bolus vs. patient-controlled epidural analgesia for maintenance of labour analgesia: a two-centre, double-blind, randomised study. Anaesthesia. 2020;75(12):1635–42.

Roofthooft E, Joshi GP, Rawal N, et al. PROSPECT guideline for elective caesarean section: updated systematic review and procedure-specific postoperative pain management recommendations. Anaesthesia. 2021;76(5):665–80.

Rosero EB, Joshi GP. Nationwide incidence of serious complications of epidural analgesia in the United States. Acta Anaesthesiol Scand. 2016;60(6):810–20.

Russell IF. At caesarean section under regional anaesthesia, it is essential to test sensory block with light touch before allowing surgery to start. Int J Obstet Anesth. 2006;15(4):294–7.

Simmons SW, Taghizadeh N, Dennis AT, et al. Combined spinal-epidural versus epidural analgesia in labour. Cochrane Database Syst Rev. 2012;10:CD003401.

Van de Velde M. Neuraxiale analgesie voor arbeid en bevalling. In: Schryns-van den Berg X, Van de Velde M, editors. Anesthesie en de normale zwangerschap. Leuven: Acco; 2017. p. 99–121.

Van de Velde M, Teunkens A, Hanssens M, et al. Post dural puncture headache following combined spinal epidural or epidural anaesthesia in obstetric patients. Anaesth Intensive Care. 2001;29(6):595–9.

Van de Velde M, Dreelinck R, Dubois J, et al. Determination of the full dose-response relation of intrathecal bupivacaine, levobupivacaine, and ropivacaine, combined with sufentanil, for labor analgesia. Anesthesiology. 2007a;106(1):149–56.

Van de Velde M, Dreelinck R, Dubois J, et al. Determination of the full dose-response relation of intrathecal bupivacaine, levobupivacaine, and ropivacaine, combined with sufentanil, for labor analgesia. Anesthesiology. 2007b;106(1):149–56.

Van De Velde M, Vercauteren M, Stockman W, et al. Recommendations and guidelines for obstetric anesthesia in Belgium. Acta Anaesthesiol Belg. 2013;64(3):97–104.

Van der Marel C. Fysiologische veranderingen door zwangerschap en Hun implicaties voor de anesthesie. In: Schryns-van den Berg X, Van de Velde M, editors. Anesthesie en de normale zwangerschap. Leuven: Acco; 2017. p. 43–57.

van der Vyver M, Halpern S, Joseph G. Patient-controlled epidural analgesia versus continuous infusion for labour analgesia: a meta-analysis. Br J Anaesth. 2002;89(3):459–65.

Young B, Onwochei D, Desai N. Conventional landmark palpation vs. preprocedural ultrasound for neuraxial analgesia and anaesthesia in obstetrics—a systematic review and meta-analysis with trial sequential analyses. Anaesthesia. 2021;76(6):818–31. https://doi.org/10.1111/anae.15255.

Zhang T, Yu Y, Zhang W, Zhu J. Comparison of dexmedetomidine and sufentanil as adjuvants to local anesthetic for epidural labor analgesia: a randomized controlled trial. Drug Des Dev Ther. 2019;13:1171–5.

Thoracic Facet Pain

43

Andre Marques Mansano

Contents

General Consideration

The lifetime prevalence of thoracic musculoskeletal pain is close to 20%. Almost one-fourth of these patients refer to significant disability. The differential diagnosis of thoracic pain is usually challenging, including visceral conditions (e.g. coronary, aortic, or esophageal diseases), or various musculoskeletal problems (e.g. disc degeneration, enthesitis, zygapophyseal, costovertebral or costochondral joints inflammation or degeneration). The thoracic zygapophyseal joints are the leading cause of pain in 43% of cases and can provoke different patterns of pain (Fig. 43.1).

The treatment includes conservative measures as physical therapy and a pharmacological approach. Options of great value for the diagnose and treatment of recalcitrant thoracic facet pain are intra-articular and medial branch block or percutaneous medial branch ablation.

A. M. Mansano (✉)
Department of Interventional Pain Management, Hospital Israelita Albert Einstein, São Paulo, Brazil

Indication (Patient Selection)

- Refractory thoracic facet pain (intra-articular/ medial branch block).
- Refractory thoracic facet pain with a previous positive diagnostic block (medial branch ablation).

Functional Anatomy

The thoracic facet joints, also called thoracic zygapophyseal joints, are real diarthrodial synovial joints with a richly innervated capsule. They are quite different from lumbar or cervical facet joints as their orientation is more coronal. The superior and inferior facets come from the superior and inferior parts do the pedicle of the thoracic vertebra, respectively.

Understanding the thoracic facet joint innervation is crucial to carry out interventional pain management as medial branch blocks or ablation. Chua and Bogduk showed that the thoracic medial branch from T1 to T3 and T9–T10 are seated on the superolateral corner of the thoracic transverse pro-

D. Jankovic, P. Peng (eds.), *Regional Nerve Blocks in Anesthesia and Pain Therapy*,
https://doi.org/10.1007/978-3-030-88727-8_43

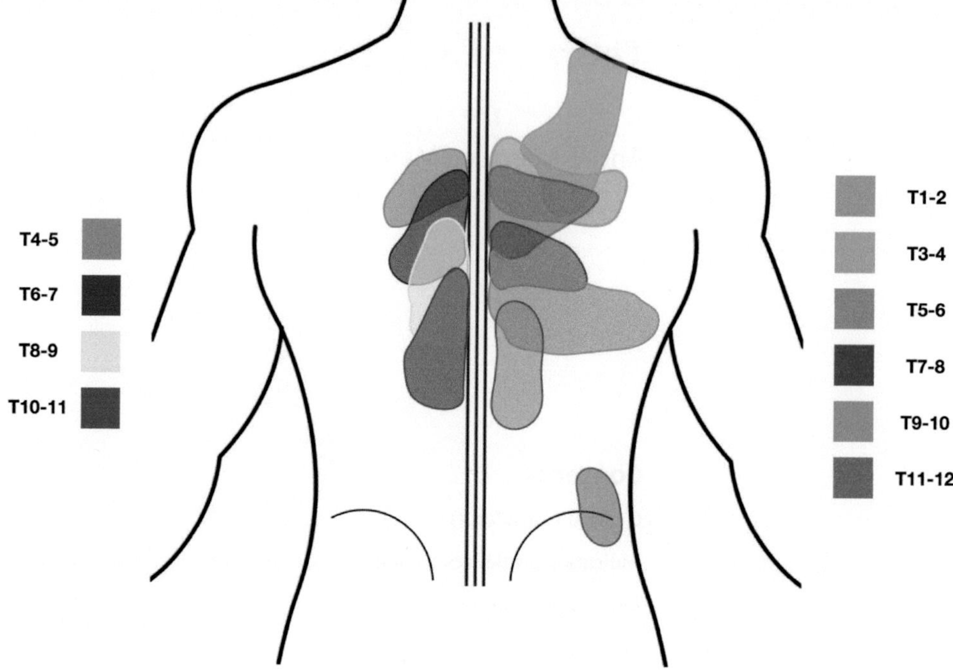

Fig. 43.1 Area of pain and corresponding thoracic level. (Reproduced with permission from Dr. Andre Marques Mansano)

cess. This relationship between the nerve and a bony structure would allow a reliable landmark for fluoroscopic or ultrasound-guided blocks/ablation. The other medial branches, from T4 to T8, are commonly founded in the tissue between the thoracic transverse processes, limiting the use of consistent fluoroscopic techniques. Ishizuca et al. found that no articular branches are originating from the medial branches. Instead of it, they found articular branches from the first branch of the thoracic dorsal rami, also called the descending branch.

In the most recent study, Joshi showed that the articular branches from T4 to T8 arise close to the intervertebral foramen and require partial, lateral laminectomy for full exposure in all specimens. In 88% of the samples, the articular branches arise from the dorsal ramus and 11% from the medial branch. They also confirmed what Ishizuca et al. found that the articular branches to T4–8 facet joint are found in the tissue plane of intertransverse space.

Table 43.1 Most common anticoagulants and antiplatelets drugs and their need of withdrawal before thoracic facet joints/medial branches procedures

Drug	When to stop	When to restart
Aspirin Primary prophylaxis	No need to stop	–
Aspirin Secondary prophylaxis	No need to stop	–
Clopidogrel	Share assessment and risk stratification	Share assessment and risk stratification
Warfarin	Share assessment and risk stratification	Share assessment and risk stratification
Dabigatran Pradaxa®	Share assessment and risk stratification	Share assessment and risk stratification
Rivaroxaban Xarelto®	Share assessment and risk stratification	Share assessment and risk stratification
Apixaban Eliquis®	Share assessment and risk stratification	Share assessment and risk stratification
IV heparin	6 h	2 h
Subcutaneous heparin	6 h	2 h
Enoxaparin (prophylatic)	12 h	4 h
Enoxaparin (therapeutic)	24 h	4 h

Technique

Medial Branch Block: Technique from T1 to T3 and T9–T12

Based on Chua and Bogduk anatomical study, the rationale of medial branch block from T1 to T3 and from T9 to T12 is touching the superior and lateral aspect of the thoracic transverse process. This can be accomplished under fluoroscopic or ultrasound guidance.

Before treatment, informed consent is required, and all advantages and disadvantages of the procedure should be discussed with the patient and his/her relative(s). Use of anticoagulants and antiplatelets should be accessed according to the last guidelines that consider percutaneous trigeminal procedures as low-risk serious bleeding (Table 43.1).

An IV line and ASA standard monitors are mandatory. Little or no sedation is desired once sedatives can cause false-positive results and decrease the procedure safety.

Fluoroscopic Guided Technique

The patient should be placed in a prone position on a radiolucent table. The thoracic transverse process must be identified in an anteroposterior—AP view. The target is the superolateral aspect of the transverse process (Fig. 43.2).

The lateral view must show the needle touching bone posterior to the transverse process (Fig. 43.3).

Either 25G or 22G spinal needles can be used for diagnostic blocks with a volume not higher than 0.5 cc to decrease false-positive results. There are some options for thoracic facet joint denervation as conventional or bipolar radiofrequency (22 to 18G, 10 mm active tip needle), tripod needles, and even cooled radiofrequency. For bipolar lesions, needles should be inserted 10 mm apart (Fig. 43.4) to allow a more significant denervation area.

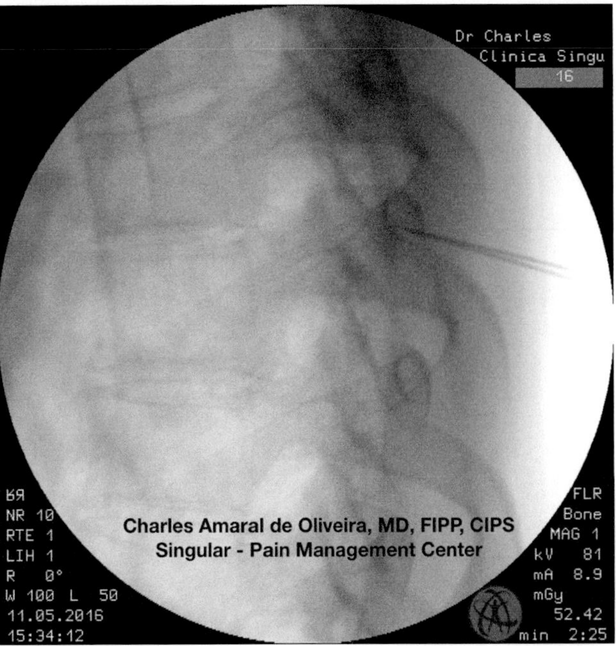

Fig. 43.3 Lateral X-ray of thoracic spine. Needle at the posterior aspect of the transverse process. (Reproduced with courtesy of Dr. Charles Amaral de Oliveira)

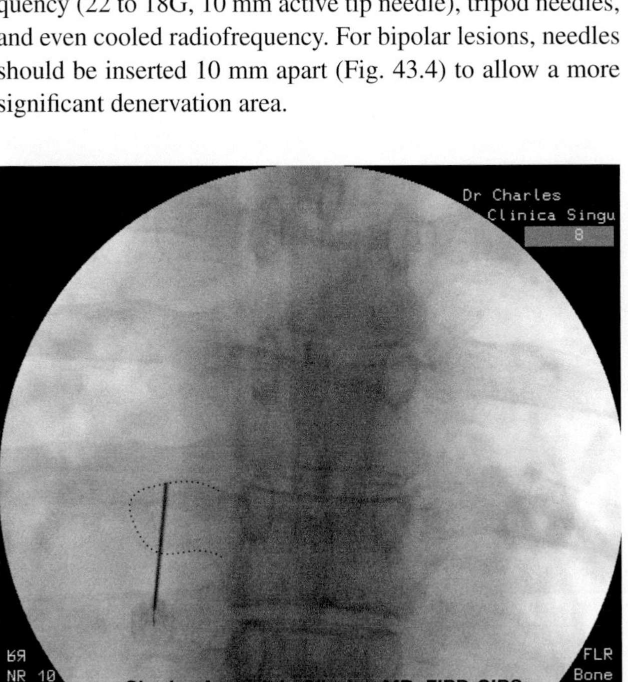

Fig. 43.2 Fluoroscopic image of thoracic spine. Dotted line—Thoracic transverse process. (Reproduced with courtesy of Dr. Charles Amaral de Oliveira)

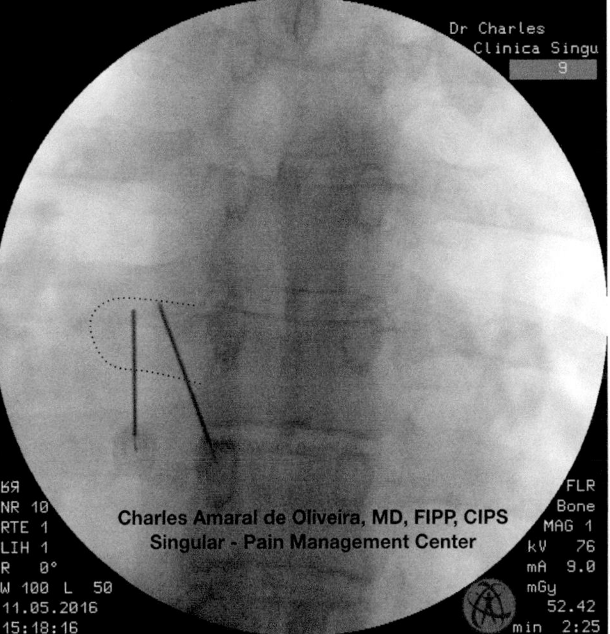

Fig. 43.4 Two RF needles, 1 cm apart, to promote bipolar lesion. (Reproduced with courtesy of Dr. Charles Amaral de Oliveira)

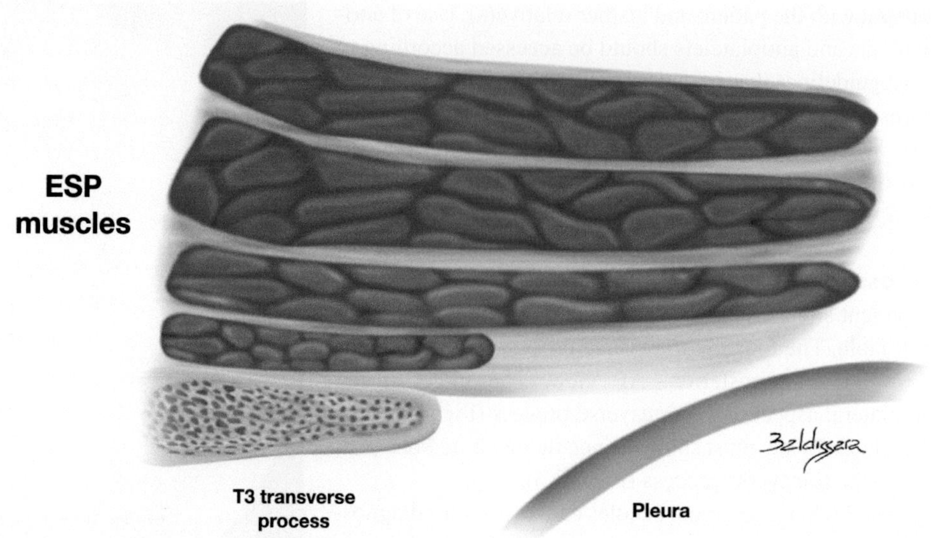

Fig. 43.5 Schematic diagram showing the thoracic paravertebral muscles, transverse process and pleura. (Reproduced with permission from Dr. Andre Marques Mansano)

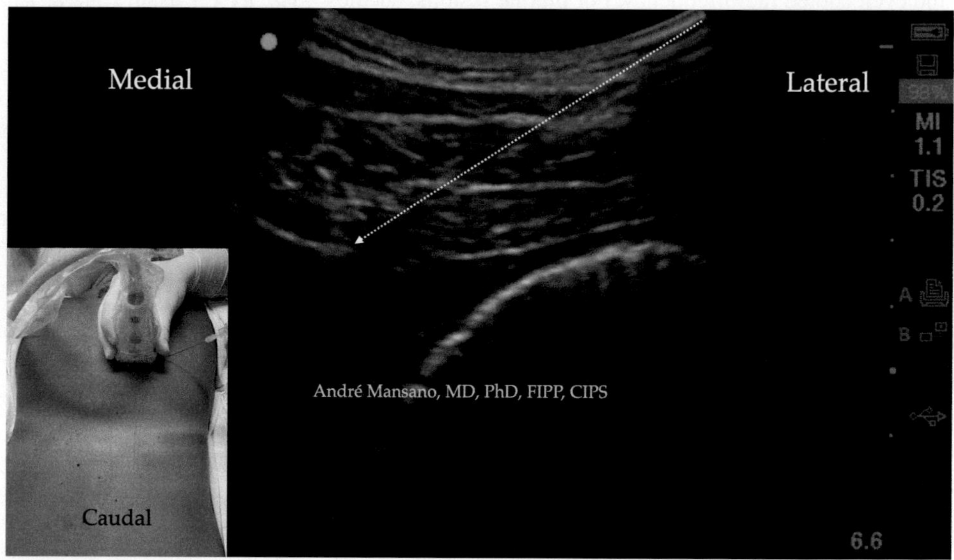

Fig. 43.6 Ultrasound-guided thoracic medial branch block. The dotted line is showing the needle path. (Reproduced with permission from Dr. Andre Marques Mansano)

Ultrasound-Guided Technique: Long Axis—In-Plane Approach

The patient should be placed in the prone position. The thoracic transverse process and parietal pleura must be identified in a long axis view (Fig. 43.5).

The target is the superolateral aspect of the transverse process—in-plane approach (Fig. 43.6).

Ultrasound-Guided Technique: Short Axis—In-Plane Approach

The patient should be placed in a prone position. We usually start scanning the ribs on the short axis (Fig. 43.7a, b). On moving the probe in medial direction, the transverse process can be easily differentiated from the rib by the rectangular appearance (Fig. 43.8a, b). The needle is inserted in-plane from cephalad or caudal direction (Figs. 43.9 and 43.10).

Medial Branch Block: Technique from T4 to T8

Based on the same anatomical studies, the rationale of the thoracic medial branch block should be aiming at the tissue between the thoracic transverse process (Figs. 43.10 and 43.11), which is more suitable under ultrasound guidance.

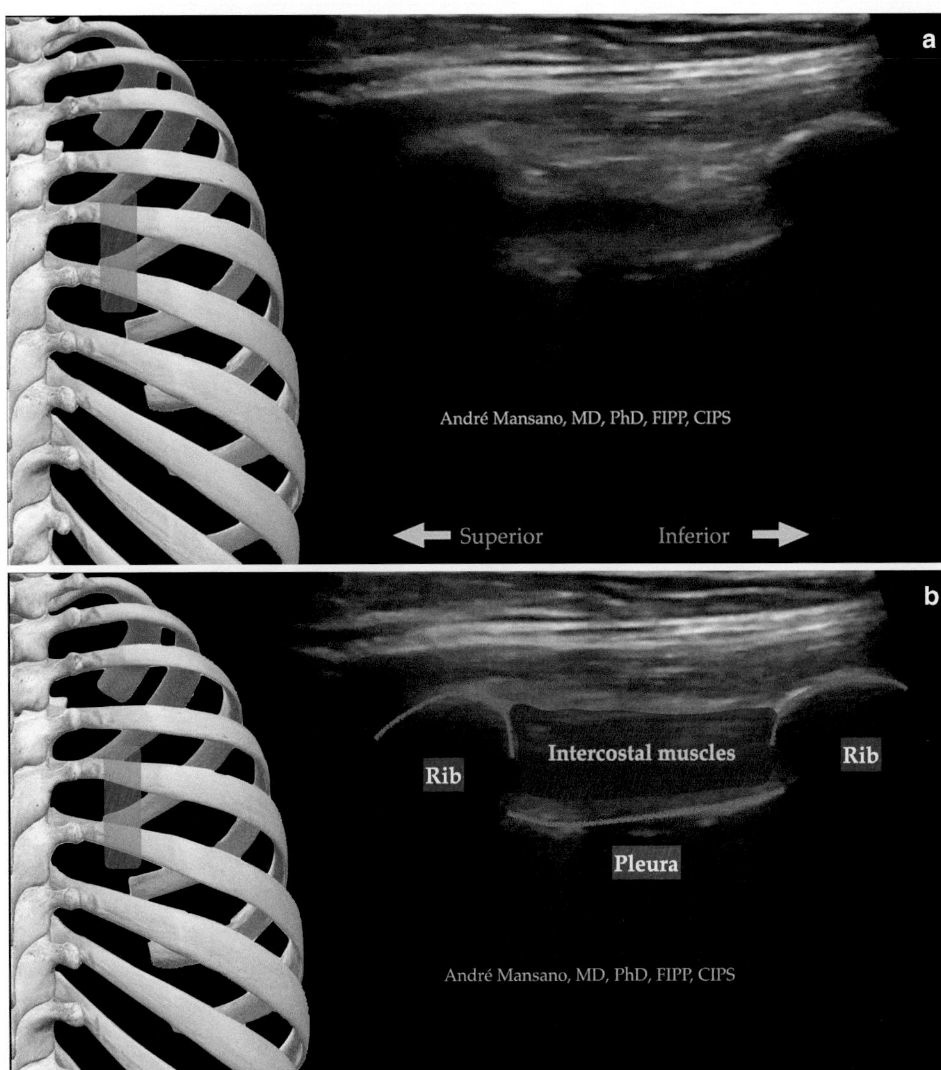

Fig. 43.7 (**a**) Short axis ultrasonographic view of the ribs. (Reproduced with permission from Dr. Andre Marques Mansano). (**b**) Short axis ultrasonographic view of the ribs with label. (Reproduced with permission from Dr. Andre Marques Mansano)

The ultrasonographic scanning is the same as the technique from T1 to T3 or T9 to T12.

Intra-Articular Thoracic Facet Joint Block

The cephalad caudal orientation of the thoracic facet joint and the bone overlap between the superior and inferior articular process make fluoroscopic guided intra-articular injection extremely challenging. The ultrasound-guided technique is more suitable for this procedure.

The patient should be placed in the prone position. We usually start scanning from the ribs on the short axis. The next step is to examine medially reaching the transverse process. And then, the thoracic facet joint is founded gently scanning medially (Fig. 43.12). The injection is done in an "in-plane" approach, from inferior to superior.

Complications

The main thoracic facet joint/medial branch complications are infections, hematoma, and pneumothorax. Keeping the needle away from the lung is crucial, and ultrasound is beneficial to do it. Rare and more severe complications include spinal cord damage, and this is more probable during an ultrasound or fluoroscopic guided intra-articular injections, especially if the needle slips off medially.

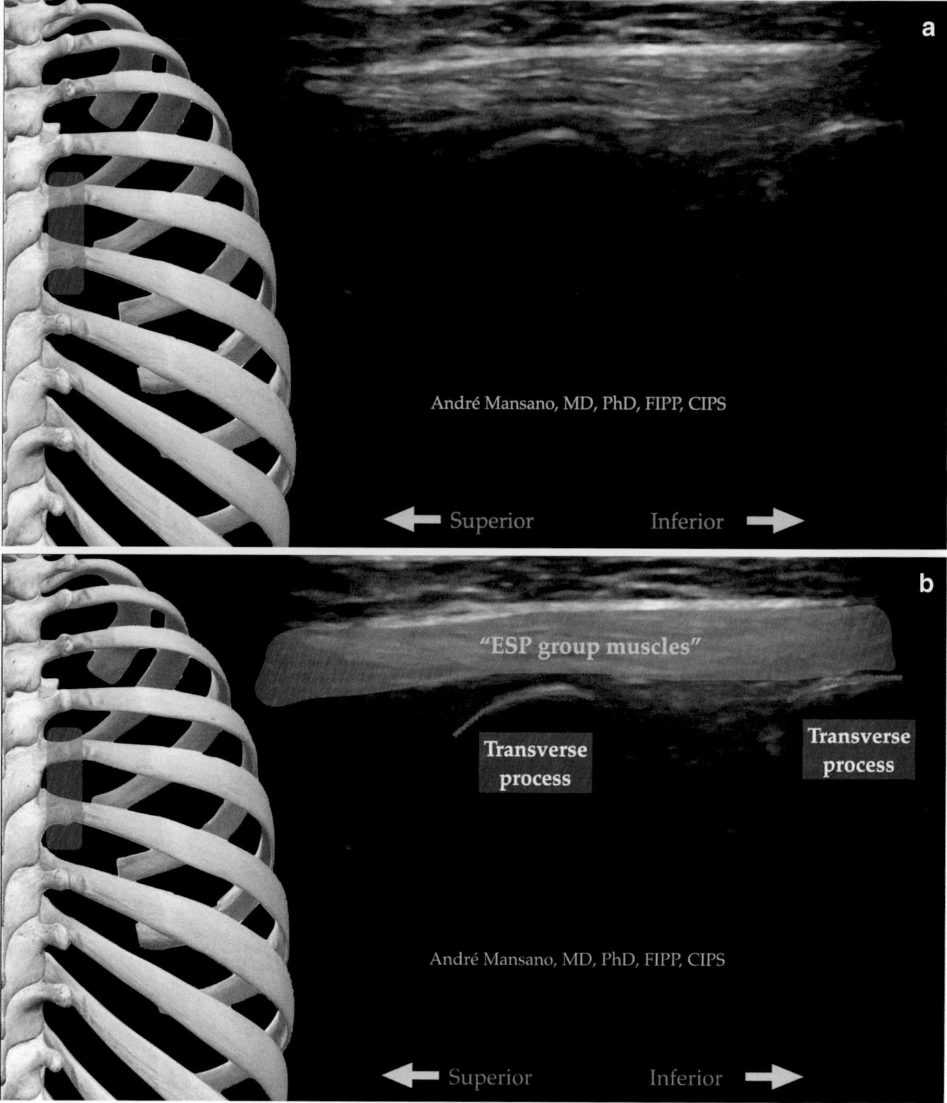

Fig. 43.8 (**a**) Short axis ultrasonographic view of the thoracic transverse process. (Reproduced with permission from Dr. Andre Marques Mansano). (**b**) Short axis ultrasonographic view of the thoracic transverse process with label. (Reproduced with permission from Dr. Andre Marques Mansano)

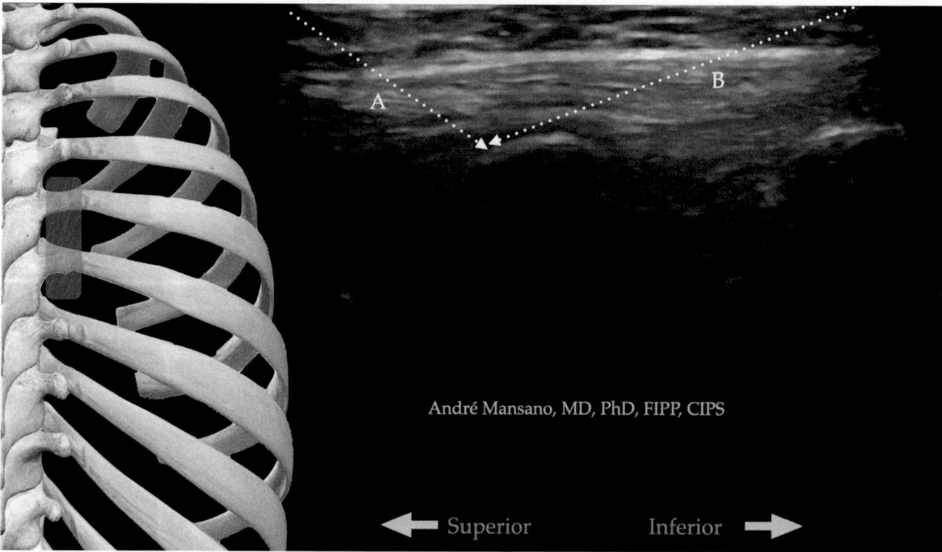

Fig. 43.9 Dotted line showing the in-plane path of the needle from superior (A) and from inferior (B). (Reproduced with permission from Dr. Andre Marques Mansano)

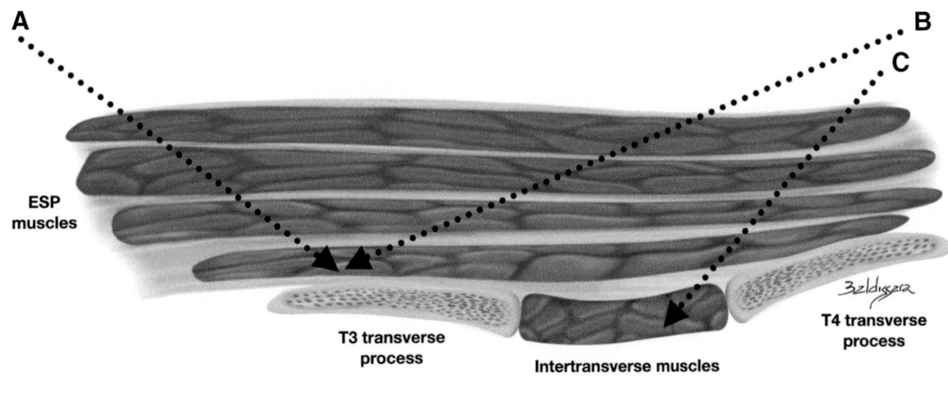

Fig. 43.10 Schematic diagram showing the erector spinae (ESP) muscles. And the intertransverse soft tissue. A and B: needle path-T1-T3 and T9 to T12 medial branch block. C-needle path-T4 to T8 articular branches block (see Fig. 43.11). (Reproduced with permission from Dr. Andre Marques Mansano)

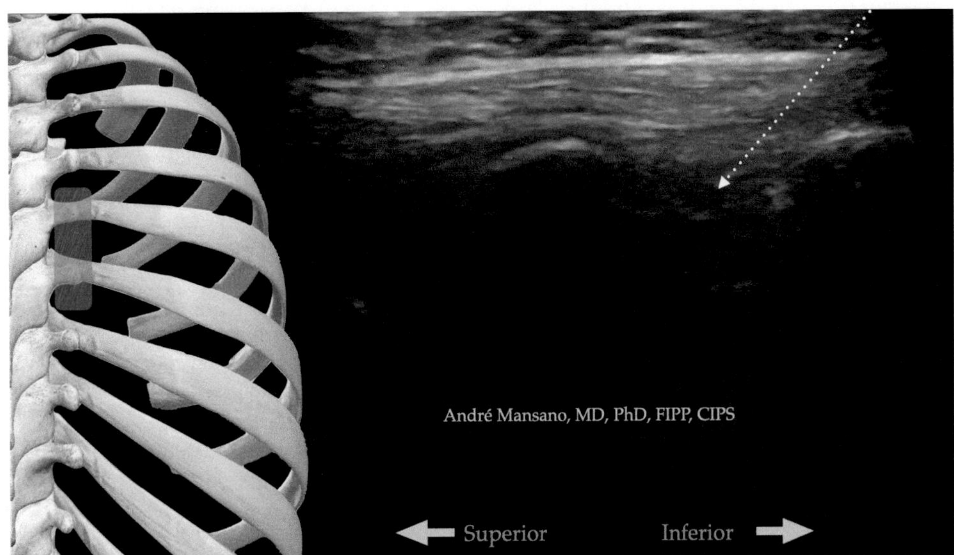

Fig. 43.11 Dotted line showing the in-plane path of the needle, reaching the intertransverse space. (Reproduced with permission from Dr. Andre Marques Mansano)

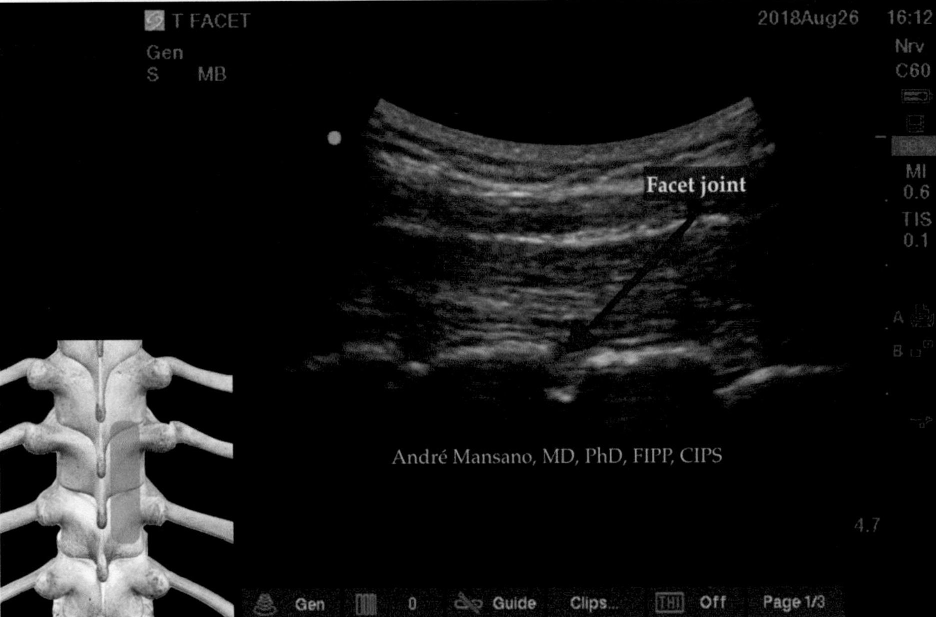

Fig. 43.12 Thoracic facet joint—ultrasound view. (Reproduced with permission from Dr. Andre Marques Mansano)

Table 43.2 Summary of thoracic facet joint studies

Study/methods	Participants	Intervention(s)	Outcome(s)	Result(s)	Conclusion(s)
Stolker et al. (1993) Observational study	40 patients with thoracic facet pain	Radiofrequency denervation of thoracic medial branch	Pain relief	After 2 months 47.5% of patients were pain free and 35% had more than 50% pain relief	Percutaneous thoracic medial branch denervation can be a safe and beneficial therapy
Manchikanti et al. (2006) Prospective observational study	55 patients with thoracic facet pain	Medial branch block	Numeric pain scores at 3, 6, 12, 24, and 36 months	Significant pain relief (50% decrease) in 71% of the patients at 3 and 6 months, 76% at 12 months, 71% at 24 months, and 69% at 36 months	Therapeutic medial branch blocks were an effective modality to treat thoracic facet pain
Manchikanti et al. (2010) Randomized trial	100 patients with thoracic facet pain	Medial branch blocks with bupivacaine or bupivacaine plus betamethasone	Numeric rating score and Oswestry disability scale after 1 year	In both groups exhibits 90% of the patients exhibits significant pain relief	Therapeutic thoracic medial branch blocks, with or without steroid, may provide significant pain relief
Kim (2014) Case series	9 patients with thoracic facet disease confirmed by MRI	Bipolar radiofrequency ablation in the inferior aspect of the facet joint	Visual analog scale after 1 month	47.6% VAS reduction	Technically easy and valid method of treating mid back pain of thoracic facet origin
Hambraeus et al. (2017) Observational study	82 patients with thoracic facet pain	Radiofrequency denervation of thoracic medial branch	Health-related quality of life	Improvement in quality of life in 51% after 12 months	Thoracic medial branch denervation can lead to long term improvement of quality of life
Lee et al. (2018) Randomizes trial	40 patients with thoracic facet pain	Intra-articular (IA) or medial branch block (MBB) with bupivacaine and dexamethasone	Numeric rating score at 6 months	65% of the patients in the IA group reported successful pain relief (pain relief ≥50%), and 40% of the patients in the MBB group showed successful pain relief	Both IA TFJ steroid injection and therapeutic MBB significantly relieved TFJ pain
Chang (2018) Observational study	72 patients with thoracic facet pain	Thoracic medial branch pulsed radiofrequency	Numeric rating score at 1, 2, and 3 months	The NRS scores changed significantly over time (pretreatment, 6.0 ± 1.0; 1 month, 3.3 ± 2.2; 2 months, 3.9 ± 2.1; and 3 months, 4.0 ± 2.2	PRF on the thoracic medial branch is an effective and safe interventional technique for the control of chronic TFJ pain
Gungor (2020) Retrospective study	23 patients with thoracic facet pain	Cooled radiofrequency denervation (CRFA) of thoracic medial branch	Average % improvement from baseline	Improvement of average pain level was 20.72% in the first follow-up (FU) (4–8 weeks), 53% in the second FU (2–6 months), and 37.58% in the third FU (6–12 months)	CRFA procedure is an effective treatment modality for thoracic facet-related pain

Literature

Unfortunately, the level of evidence and recommendation for thoracic facet joint procedures is still weak to moderate once we don't have any randomized study comparing any procedure with a sham group. The main studies related to thoracic facet joint procedures are summarized in Table 43.2.

Suggested Reading

Atluri S, Datta S, Falco FJ, Lee M. Systematic review of diagnostic utility and therapeutic effectiveness of thoracic facet joint interventions. Pain Physician. 2008;11(5):611–29.

Atluri S, Singh V, Datta S, Geffert S, Sehgal N, Falco FJ. Diagnostic accuracy of thoracic facet joint nerve blocks: an update of the assessment of evidence. Pain Physician. 2012;15(4):E483–96.

Briggs AM, Smith AJ, Straker LM, Bragge P. Thoracic spine pain in the general population: prevalence, incidence and associated factors in children, adolescents and adults. A systematic review. BMC Musculoskelet Disord. 2009;10(1):77.

Chang MC. Effect of pulsed radiofrequency treatment on the thoracic medial branch for managing chronic thoracic facet joint pain refractory to medial branch block with local anesthetics. World Neurosurg. 2018;111:e644–8.

Dreyfuss P, Tibiletti C, Dreyer SJ. Thoracic zygapophyseal joint pain patterns: a study in normal volunteers. Spine (Phila Pa 1976). 1994;19(7):807–11.

Ebraheim NA, Xu R, Ahmad M, Yeasting RA. The quantitative anatomy of the thoracic facet and the posterior projection of its inferior facet. Spine (Phila Pa 1976). 1997;22(16):1811–8.

Fukui S, Ohseto K, Shiotani M. Patterns of pain induced by distending the thoracic zygapophyseal joints. Reg Anesth. 1997;22(4):332–6.

Gungor S, Candan B. The efficacy and safety of cooled-radiofrequency neurotomy in the treatment of chronic thoracic facet (zygapophyseal) joint pain. Medicine (Baltimore). 2020;99(14):e19711.

Hambraeus J, Hambraeus KS, Persson J. Radiofrequency denervation improves health-related quality of life in patients with thoracic zygapophyseal joint pain. Pain Med. 2018;19(5):914–9.

Joshi A, Amrhein TJ, Holmes MA, Talsma J, Shonyo M, Taylor AB. The source and the course of the articular branches to the T4-T8 zygapophysial joints. Pain Med. 2019;20(12):2371–6.

Kim D. Bipolar intra-articular radiofrequency thermocoagulation of the thoracic facet joints: a case series of a new technique. Korean J Pain. 2014;27(1):43–8.

Lee DG, Ahn SH, Cho YW, Do KH, Kwak SG, Chang MC. Comparison of intra-articular thoracic facet joint steroid injection and thoracic medial branch block for the management of thoracic facet joint pain. Spine (Phila Pa 1976). 2018;43(2):76–80.

Manchikanti L, Manchikanti KN, Manchukonda R, Pampati V, Cash KA. Evaluation of therapeutic thoracic medial branch block effectiveness in chronic thoracic pain: a prospective outcome study with minimum 1-year follow up. Pain Physician. 2006;9(2):97–105.

Manchikanti L, Singh V, Falco FJE, Cash KA, Pampati V. Comparative effectiveness of a one-year follow-up of thoracic medial branch blocks in management of chronic thoracic pain: a randomized, double-blind active controlled trial. Pain Physician. 2010;13(6):535–48. https://pubmed.ncbi.nlm.nih.gov/21102966/.

Manchukonda R, Manchikanti KN, Cash KA, Pampati V, Manchikanti L. Facet joint pain in chronic spinal pain: an evaluation of prevalence and false-positive rate of diagnostic blocks. J Spinal Disord Tech. 2007;20(7):539–45.

Narouze S, Benzon HT, Provenzano D, Buvanendran A, De Andres J, Deer T, et al. Interventional Spine and Pain Procedures in Patients on Antiplatelet and Anticoagulant Medications (Second Edition): Guidelines from the American Society of Regional Anesthesia and Pain Medicine, the European Society of Regional Anaesthesia and Pain Therapy, the American Academy of Pain Medicine, the International Neuromodulation Society, the North American Neuromodulation Society, and the World Institute of Pain. In: Regional anesthesia and pain medicine, vol. 43. Philadelphia, PA: Lippincott Williams and Wilkins; 2018. p. 225–62.

Niemeläinen R, Videman T, Battié MC. Prevalence and characteristics of upper or mid-back pain in Finnish men. Spine (Phila Pa 1976). 2006;31(16):1846–9.

Rohof O, Chen CK. The response to radiofrequency neurotomy of medial branches including a bipolar system for thoracic facet joints. Scand J Pain. 2018;18(4):747–53.

Stolker RJ, Vervest AC, Groen GJ. Percutaneous facet denervation in chronic thoracic spinal pain. Acta Neurochir. 1993;122(1–2):82–90.

van Eijs F, Stanton-Hicks M, Van Zundert J, Faber CG, Lubenow TR, Mekhail N, et al. Evidence-based interventional pain medicine according to clinical diagnoses. 16. Complex regional pain syndrome. Pain Pract. 2011;11(1):70–87.

Celiac Plexus Block

44

Arash Yousefi, Neal Rakesh, Amitabh Gulati, and Sushma Bhatnagar

Contents

Background

In 1914, Kappis and his colleagues published their study on intraoperative splanchnic and celiac plexus blockade, using a percutaneous technique which remained the gold standard to date. Ever since, the technique has had various modifications. Several imaging modalities including fluoroscopy, ultrasound, computed tomography (CT), and magnetic resonance imaging (MRI) have been used to improve procedural guidance, but there is still no consensus regarding the best technique.

Celiac plexus block (CPB) is a safe and effective technique which targets the afferent nociceptive fibers of the celiac plexus. It is helpful in diagnosing and treating chronic abdominal pain (CAP). Benign disorders such as visceral upper abdominal pain, chronic pancreatitis, cirrhosis, and inflammatory bowel disease and malignant disorders such as colorectal, hepatic, gastric, intestinal, biliary, ovarian, esophageal, pulmonary, or appendiceal cancers and malignancies with retroperitoneal nodal metastases may benefit from CPB. This technique has also been used for the treatment of refractory hypertension and postoperative pain. Finally, patients suffering from malignant abdominopelvic cancers and metastasis, who suffer from substantial pain which is frequently irresponsive to medical pain management, would benefit greatly from a CPB.

The need for better pain control advocates for minimally invasive interventional techniques. Celiac plexus block (CPB) is the temporary disruption of the pain signals through the celiac plexus by injecting corticosteroids and anesthetics. Celiac plexus neurolysis (CPN) is a more permanent treatment that involves injecting phenol, ethanol, or

The original version of this chapter was revised: authorship has been updated to include the first author. The correction to this chapter can be found at https://doi.org/10.1007/978-3-030-88727-8_77

A. Yousefi
Neurology, Mount Sinai Downtown, New York, NY, USA

N. Rakesh · A. Gulati (✉)
Department of Anesthesiology and Critical Care, MSKCC, New York, NY, USA
e-mail: gulatia@mskcc.org

S. Bhatnagar
Department of Onco-Anesthesia and Palliative Medicine, AIMS, New Delhi, Delhi, India

D. Jankovic, P. Peng (eds.), *Regional Nerve Blocks in Anesthesia and Pain Therapy*,
https://doi.org/10.1007/978-3-030-88727-8_44

other neurolytic substances, with rare instances of thermal or cryoablation, into the plexus to induce fibrosis and disrupt signal transmission. Interventional approaches including CPN and CPB can control pain and improve quality of life without significant medication-induced adverse effects.

Anatomy

The celiac plexus is the largest autonomic plexus in the human body. It supplies the sympathetic, parasympathetic, and visceral sensory fibers of the upper abdominal organs including the liver, biliary tract, gallbladder, pancreas, spleen, adrenals, kidneys, distal esophagus, and bowel to the level of the distal transverse colon. It is comprised of a network of ganglia (a pair of celiac, superior mesenteric, and aortorenal ganglia) forming a substantial network of interconnecting fibers that regulate the upper abdominal viscera

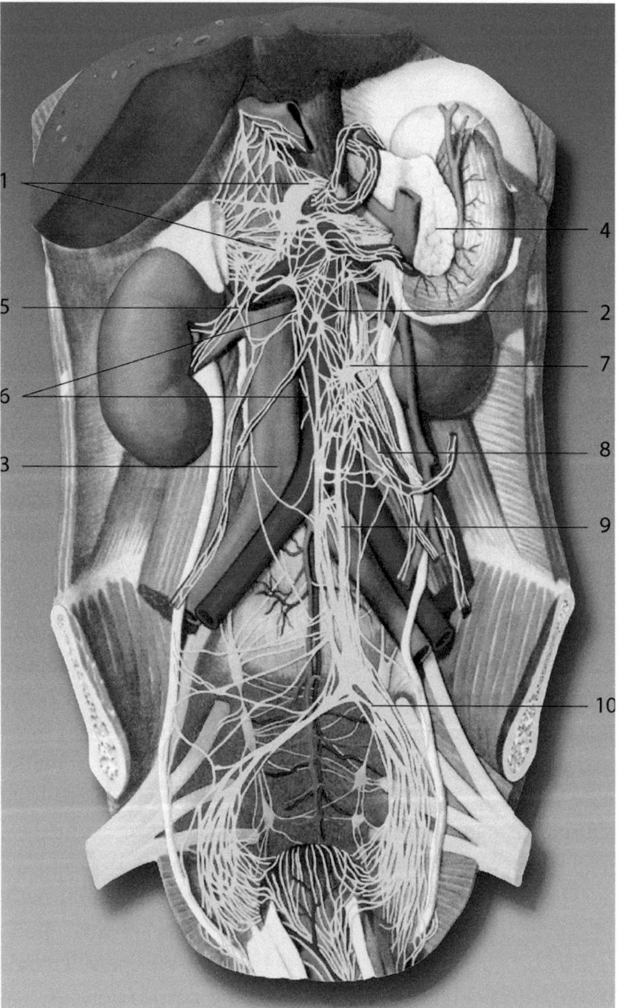

Fig. 44.1 Anatomy. (1) Celiac plexus, (2) aorta, (3) inferior vena cava, (4) pancreas, (5) renal plexus, (6) abdominal aortic plexus, (7) inferior mesenteric ganglion, (8) inferior mesenteric plexus, (9) superior hypogastric plexus, (10) inferior hypogastric plexus. (Reproduced with permission from Danilo Jankovic)

(Fig. 44.1). It is referred to as the solar plexus because of its vast web of nerve fibers.

It is located deep in the retroperitoneal fat, anterior to the aorta, inferior to the celiac trunk and superior mesenteric artery (SMA), and posterior to the stomach and pancreas (Figs. 44.2 and 44.3). It extends in front of and around the aorta for several centimeters. The location is variable between the level of T12 and L2, but the most common location is at the level of T12. The celiac artery has the most consistent anatomy in the area, and it is a more reliable landmark for localizing the celiac plexus compared to the vertebral column. The left and right ganglions lie 0.9 and 0.6 cm caudal to the celiac artery, respectively.

The celiac plexus contains sympathetic, parasympathetic, and visceral sensory (nociceptive) fibers. The sympathetic innervation of the plexus is formed by preganglionic sympathetic efferent fibers of the greater, lesser, and least splanchnic nerves, originating from the anterolateral horn of the spinal cord at the level of T5 to T12. The parasympathetic input to the plexus originates mainly from the preganglionic fibers of the posterior branch of the vagus nerve providing autonomic supply to the abdominal organs. Traversing visceral sensory fibers pass through the plexus and are the primary target for the plexus blockade. As the plexus carries the nociceptive signals, it is a key target point of pain transmission of the upper abdominal organs. Therefore, CPB and CPN are effective interventional techniques in controlling pain from these organs.

Indication and Contraindications

Common disease states which may benefit from a CPB or CPN	Common causes
Malignant abdominopelvic pain	Cancer of the foregut, midgut, and pelvic organs (e.g., pancreas, liver, kidney, adrenal, stomach, small bowel, gallbladder, and pelvic organs)
Benign syndromes	Chronic pancreatitis, pancreatic pseudocyst, liver cirrhosis, gastric syndromes (emptying syndromes, etc.)
Cardiovascular	Renal hypertension, refractory hypertension
Contraindications	
Bleeding disorder	Thrombocytopenia and coagulopathy increase the risk of bleeding; thus, low platelet (plt) count (plt <50,000), uncorrected coagulopathy (INR > 1.5), and anticoagulation use are relative contraindications for these procedures
Infectious disease	Cancer patients undergoing chemotherapy or radiotherapy may be neutropenic, immunocompromised, and susceptible to infection after the procedures. In addition, the procedure increases the risk of spreading the preexisting local or intra-abdominal infections and are contraindication for the procedure
Bowel obstruction	Celiac plexus block and neurolysis result in inhibition of the sympathetic activity of the bowel and consequently increase the parasympathetic activities and peristalsis and therefore are contraindicated in bowel obstruction

Contraindications	
Disulfiram use	Disulfiram can accumulate ethanol in the form of acetaldehyde, resulting in tachycardia, nausea, vomiting, and headaches. Therefore, patients on disulfiram are not good candidates for ethanol blocks
Aortic disease	A transaortic approach should be avoided in patients with abdominal aortic aneurysm or extensive atherosclerotic calcification of the abdominal aorta
Abnormal anatomy	Abnormal anatomy along the trajectory of the needle from prior surgeries or congenital abnormalities may increase complication risks and reduce success rates and need to be considered before the procedure

Pancreatic Cancer Pain

Pancreatic cancer pain is complex and multifactorial, and the pain management strategy for it also needs to be multifactorial. Pain commonly starts in the occult stage of the cancer and gradually increases, and it is observed in 90% of the patients.

The pathophysiology of the pain is characterized by a mixture of somatic, visceral, central, and neuropathic pain. Somatic pain occurs after direct invasion or metastasis of cancer cells to the peritoneum, retroperitoneum, or bones. Retroperitoneal spread of cancer cells can involve the celiac plexus and cause severe visceral pain and dysfunction. The cancer cells can block the pancreatic ducts increasing the pressure in the parenchyma and on the nerves. Tissue edema, neovascularization, and alteration in expression of signaling molecules can contribute to the pain. In addition, pancreatic cancer has the tendency for direct perineural invasion which is estimated to occur in 70–90% of patients and result in neuropathic pain.

The pain is typically located in the epigastrium with radiation to the back. It is usually diffused, deep-seated, and poorly localized. It is often crampy or colicky in nature, increased by lying down, and relived by bending forward. Interventional approaches are not the primary approach for the pain management but are a vital element of a multimodal pain management strategy.

CPN is a very effective invasive treatment for pancreatic cancer pain management. It inhibits pain signal transmission to the CNS and results in treating pain with different mechanisms. The neuropathic and bony metastasis pain is especially resistant to conventional medical management. Interventional approaches, especially CPB and CNP, can minimize these types of pain without significant side effects and reduce the need for conventional analgesics. The procedure is more effective in early stages of the cancer before it has developed substantial somatic components. It can have approximately 80% efficacy for weeks to months.

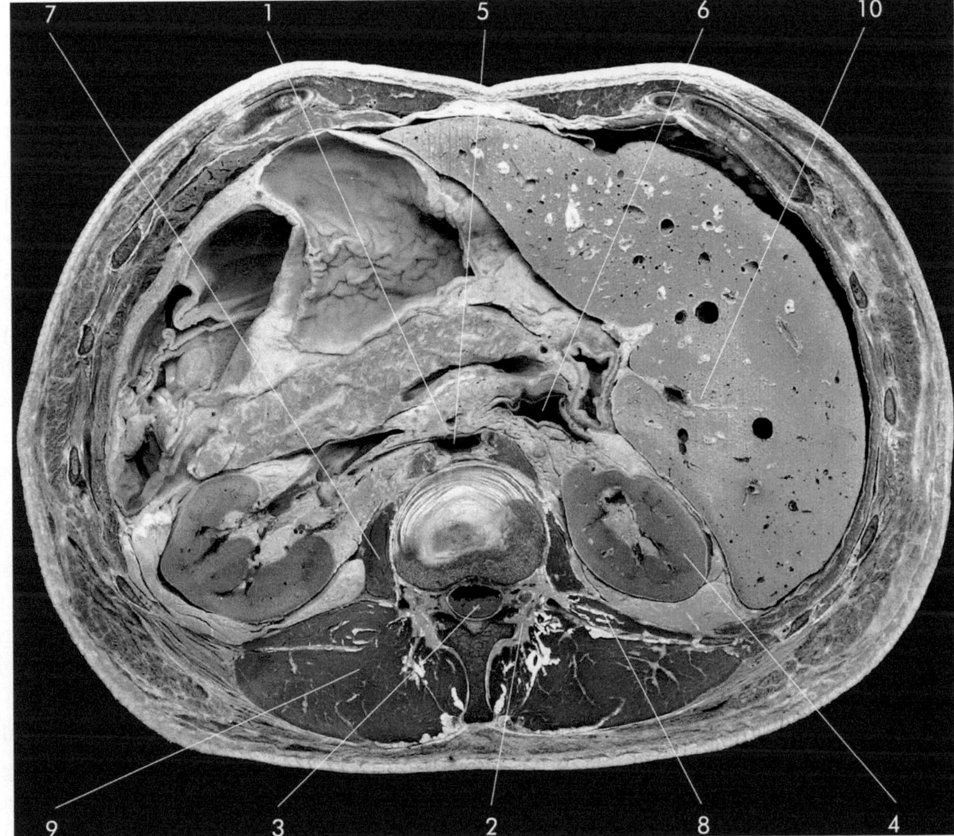

Fig. 44.2 Transversal section through the abdomen at the level of the first lumbar vertebra. (1) Celiac plexus with ganglion celiacum, (2) spinal ganglion , (3) cauda equina, (4) medulla renalis, (5) aorta, (6) inferior vena cava, (7) psoas muscle, (8) quadratus lumborum muscle, (9) erector spinae muscle, (10) liver. (Reproduced with permission from Danilo Jankovic)

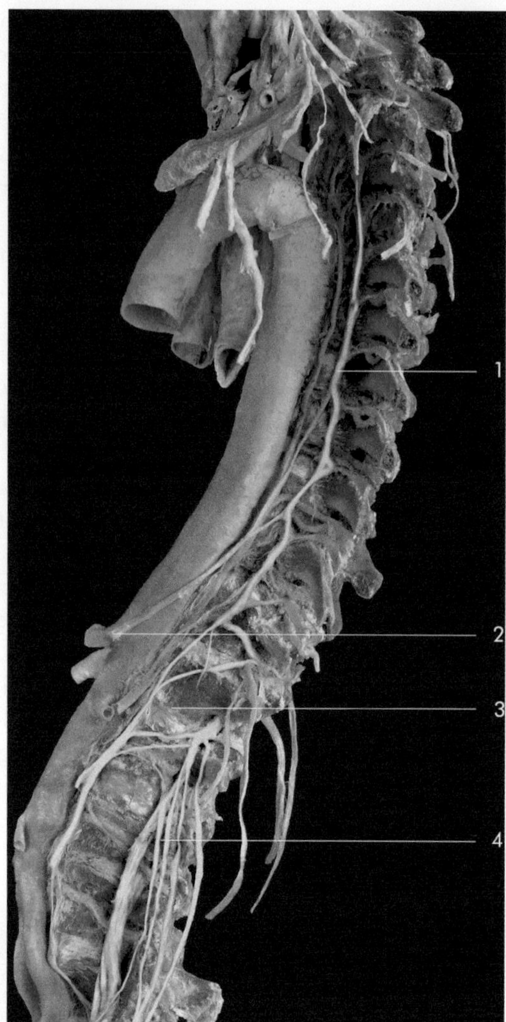

Fig. 44.3 (1) Sympathetic trunk (underneath: greater and minor splanchnic nerves), (2) celiac plexus (underneath: superior mesenteric artery and renal artery), (3) vertebral body of the first lumbar vertebra with right communicantes albi, (4) lumbar plexus. (Reproduced with permission from Danilo Jankovic)

Technique

Preprocedural Workup and Evaluations

Patients need to be selected appropriately, and the procedure should be explained in detail. Consent forms must be signed, and patients should be aware of risks, benefits, and alternative therapies. Reasonable understanding and realistic expectations are necessary for better outcomes. Patients should be questioned regarding their allergies and recent anticoagulation use. Anticoagulation medications should be discontinued in accordance with standard procedural guidelines. Short-acting pain medications can confound pain evaluation during the procedure and should be discontinued, but long-acting pain medications can be continued. Basic lab works, bleeding time, platelet count, and coagulation panels should be reviewed and, if necessary, optimized. Available images should be reviewed to determine patient positioning for the procedure, needle trajectory, and injection site. To safely sedate patients for CPN, they will need to fast for 6–8 h prior to the procedure. Sedation is minimized for CPB to assess intraprocedural pain relief and treatment efficacy, so fasting is usually not necessary for CPB. After the celiac block or neurolysis, patients are prone to hypotension due to loss of sympathetic tone in the vessels. Vital signs should be closely monitored before, during, and after the procedure. If post-procedural hypotension is anticipated, it is recommended to provide preprocedural fluid bolus and 12-h bed rest post-procedure.

The Injectate

Injectate mixture and the amount injected are variable in different approaches and at different institutes. In general, patients with benign pathologies are injected with local anesthetics and corticosteroids. Benign processes causing pain (such as chronic pancreatitis) commonly induce inflammation which can improve with steroid injection. Ethanol and phenol are neurolytics which may damage axons and myelin and are usually reserved for management of malignant pain. Typically, ethanol and steroids are injected mixed with local anesthetics to decrease injection pain. The injectate can be mixed with iodinated contrast for better visualization, but phenol's viscosity makes it more difficult to mix well with the contrast material used for needle guidance.

Relative to phenol, ethanol can be mixed more easily with the anesthetics and iodinated contrasts and is easier to inject due to its lower viscosity. Phenol has an immediate anesthetic effect so it is less painful when injected without using anesthetics. Ethanol can cause temporary pain when injected alone and should be injected with a long-acting anesthetic such as bupivacaine for better tolerance. Usually, ethanol is the preferred first-line agent for the block.

In malignant diseases, ethanol is used at 50–100% concentration and phenol at 3–20% concentration. Concentrations above 50% for ethanol and above 3% for phenol have been shown to cause irreversible nerve damage. At concentrations above the minimum, neurolysis depends on distribution rather than concentration. In benign diseases and temporary blocks, a commonly used mixture contains 20 mL of bupivacaine 0.025% and 6 mL of triamcinolone 80 mg/mL. The most common injectate used in malignant diseases is a mixture of 95–100% ethanol with bupivacaine and iodinated contrast in 6:3:1 ratio.

Injected volume is variable depending on the needle tip position and whether the single or double technique is used. Antecrural space can embed larger volumes of injectate compared to the retrocrural space. Studies have recommended 30–60 mL of injectate for the antecrural and 15–30 mL for retrocrural space. The injections are performed through one needle or split between two needles.

Various Approaches

Regardless of the approach, CPB and CPN are shown to have analgesic benefits and result in opioid use reduction. The procedures can be performed by laparotomy, by thoracotomy, or by percutaneous techniques. The procedures can be guided by fluoroscopy, CT, MRI, or endoscopic ultrasound (EUS).

While there is no clear advantage among various image-guided procedures, the technique should be selected considering patients' comfort, anatomy, and comorbidities as well as interventionist expertise, preference, and available resources.

EUS is a more recent method and has unique benefits over the percutaneous approaches. The plexus and adjacent structures can be visualized with EUS with decreased risk of unwanted damage. Injection under a CT guide has rapidly become one of the favorite procedures. CT guidance allows optimum tissue distinction, trajectory planning, localization of the needle tip during the procedure, and visualizing the diffusion of the medication. MR guidance is also feasible and effective, though more expensive and less accessible.

Several approaches have been described for performing the procedure. Based on the patient's position and the site of needle insertion, the approaches are divided into anterior and posterior.

In general, posterior approaches are more common with multiple variations which include antecrural, retrocrural, transintervertebral disc (intradiscal), transaortic, and para-aortic techniques with single or bilateral needle placements. Posterior approaches have lower risk of damage to visceral organs.

Neurological complications due to direct needle injury or by neurolytic spread of the injectate in the retrocrural space are less likely in the anterior approaches.

Posterior Para-aortic (Retrocrural) Approach

The posterior para-aortic approach is the traditional approach for accessing the celiac plexus. This procedure is performed with the patient in a prone or lateral decubitus position, draped and disinfected, while thoracic kyphosis is increased by adding extra support under the abdomen. Evaluating Pre-Procedural images will assist in selecting the needle, the insertion site, and a safe path to the plexus. A 20–24-gauge bevel-tipped needle is introduced at the inferior border of the 12th rib, 5–8 cm from the midline under fluoroscopic guidance (Fig. 44.4). If CT guidance, the entry vertebral level may be modified for optimum placement of the neurolytic in the retrocrural space (Fig. 44.5). The needle entry point is slightly more lateral on the right side compared to the left. With a 45-degree angle medially and 15-degree cephalad, the needle is advanced cautiously to the ventral surface of the T12–L1

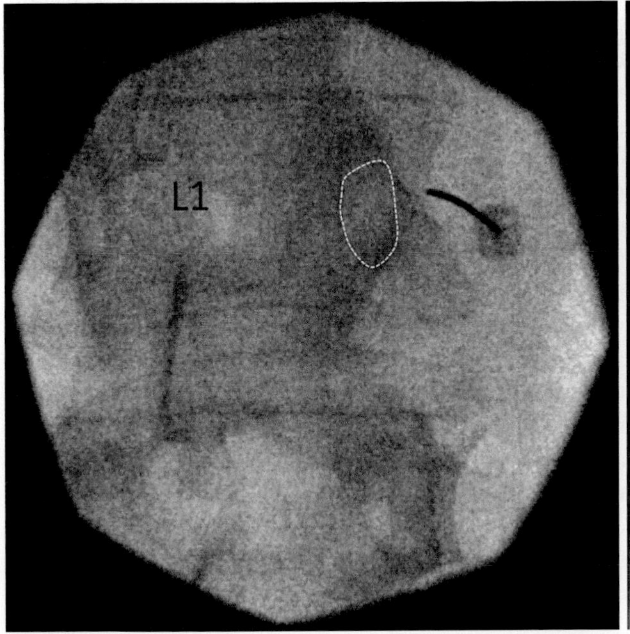

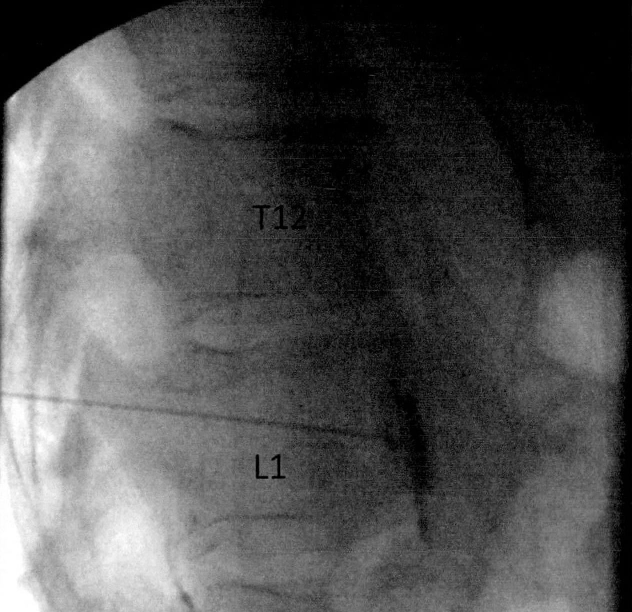

Fig. 44.4 Fluoroscopic image of the retrocrural approach. Left panel: oblique radiograph with needle inserted above the transverse process to the lateral border of the vertebrae. Right panel: lateral radiograph to show the spread of contrast in the retrocrural region. Pedicle is highlighted in dotted line

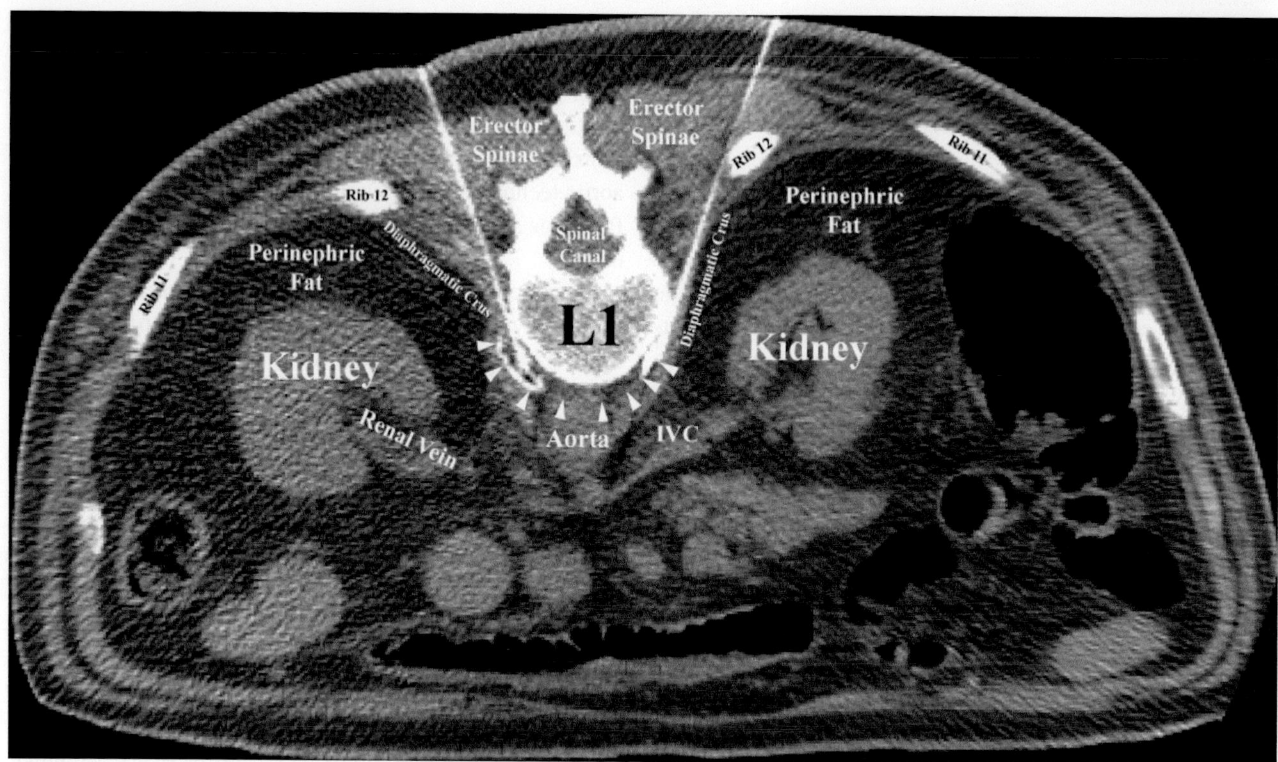

Fig. 44.5 Arrowheads represent retrocrural region where contrast and neurolytic agent is injected for a celiac block. *IVC* inferior vena cava. (Reproduced with permission from Dr. Amitabh Gulati and Neal Rakesh)

intervertebral space avoiding the transverse processes, the vasculatures, and the kidneys. After contact, the needle is slightly withdrawn, laterally redirected, and advanced along the vertebral body to reach the retrocrural space (the needle will pierce the diaphragmatic crura to become retrocrural and behind the aorta and/or IVC). The needle tip should ultimately be positioned 1–2 cm anterior and lateral to the aorta, between the celiac trunk and the superior mesenteric artery, and posterior to the diaphragmatic crura. The right side approach may require approximately 2 cm further advancement compared to the left side. Continuous aspiration is required as the needle might puncture the aorta or adjacent vasculatures. The location is confirmed under imaging, by visualizing free contrast spread, without any resistance, on the anterior surface of the aorta bilaterally. After confirming the correct location, either celiac plexus block or celiac necrolysis can be performed. After injecting the prepared injectate, normal saline or local anesthetics can be injected as the needle is withdrawn, to prevent neurolytic tracking along the needle trajectory. A unilateral approach is usually performed on the left side, and if it is unsuccessful, the procedure can be performed bilaterally.

Note: The retrocrural approach targets the splanchnic nerves which supply the celiac plexus. For better results, block needs to be attempted on both sides.

Posterior Antecrural Approach

A posterior antecrural approach is the most used technique with the goal of direct celiac plexus block. The plexus is blocked by injecting into the antecrural space via a posterior paravertebral route and passing through the diaphragmatic crura. This technique is similar to the retrocrural approach in terms of needle positioning and trajectory, except that in this technique the needle is advanced 1–2 cm further to pass the crura and enter the antecrural space. Ultimately, the needle tip should be placed anterolateral to the aorta in between the celiac trunk and SMA, anterior to the crura, and posterior to the pancreas. Crura may cause resistance, but after piercing them, the injection should be free of resistance. Contrast spread may help distinguish crural spread. Location is confirmed by diffusion of contrast along the anterolateral wall of the aorta. The antecrural space is larger compared to the retrocrural and can accommodate more injectate volume. An antecrural approach targets the celiac plexus with good contrast spread confirmation; the technique can be attempted only on one side (usually the left side). Splanchnic and celiac blocks are performed concurrently in some cases for enhanced analgesic effects.

Posterior Transintervertebral Disc Approach

This alternative approach is usually performed when the paravertebral approach is not anatomically feasible. This approach decreases the risk of visceral damage in the paravertebral approaches but may cause disc, cord, and aortic injuries, discitis, or retroperitoneal hematomas. Given the serious risks with this approach, it is usually not considered a first option. The technique is performed with the patient in a prone or lateral decubitus. The needle is introduced at the level of T12–L1 or L1–L2 and passes through the intervertebral disc with a unilateral or bilateral needle placement. The needle is advanced until the tip is placed anterior to the aorta adjacent to the celiac plexus. Given the proximity of the needle tip to the plexus, smaller volume (20–30 mL) of injectate is required compared to the paravertebral approaches. As the needle passes through the intervertebral disk, the risk of visceral organ injury is decreased. Nonetheless, there is a higher risk for spinal cord injury and disc herniation. The approach is not ideal for patients with degenerative disease or patients with tumor invasion to the spine.

Posterior Transaortic Approach

In this posterior approach, the needle transverses the abdominal aorta to reach the celiac plexus. This approach can theoretically minimize the neurolytic spread causing injury to the spinal cord and spinal plexus. Pre-procedural imaging is required to explore aortic aneurysms, mural calcifications, or thromboses, any of which can preclude the patient from this approach. The needle is introduced at the level of the first vertebrae, inferior to the 12th rib, 4–7 cm lateral to the midline on the left side. The needle is advanced similarly to the paravertebral approach until aortic pulsation is felt in the needle. After traversing both aortic walls, the needle tip will be in the preaortic space. Location is confirmed first with aspiration and then with contrast injection observing its diffusion in the space. Due to needle proximity to the plexus, low injectate volume (~15–30 mL) would be sufficient for this block. It is reported that about 0.5% of patients develop retroperitoneal hemorrhages, with higher risk in patients with hypertension and coagulopathy.

Anterior Approach

This approach was introduced in 1918 and has remained a second-line procedure due to higher risk of visceral organ injuries compared to the posterior approaches. Visceral organ damage can result in hemorrhage, infection, perforation, or fistula formation. However, the procedure is relatively easy and fast. It may be the preferred approach in patients with altered anatomy or when the posterior approach is restricted by tumor invasion. Patients with abdominal pain, recent abdominal surgery, or colostomy or ileostomy are generally more comfortable with this approach. In addition, as the retrocrural space is intact, chances of epidural or subarachnoid spread, and consequently neurological adverse effects, are lower in this approach.

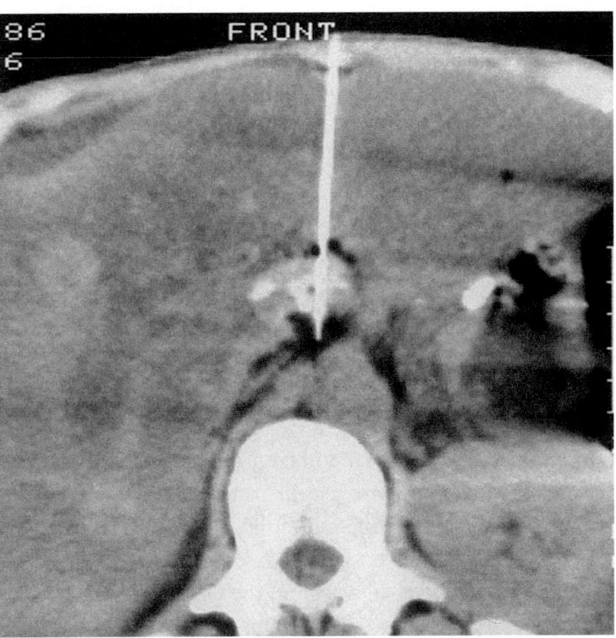

Fig. 44.6 Ventral transhepatic CT-guided injection. Several access routes are possible in celiac plexus injection. In this case, the injection was carried out using a ventral transhepatic approach. The tip of the needle lies directly alongside the celiac trunk. The alcohol spreads precisely within the celiac plexus. (Reproduced with permission from Danilo Jankovic)

The procedure can be performed using a single- or double-needle approach. The patient is positioned in a supine position and the needle is introduced vertically, approximately at the level of the T12 vertebral body to target the space between the SMA and celiac artery (Fig. 44.6). Imaging is necessary to visualize patients' anatomy and map needle trajectory. After the tip position in the antecrural space, 1–2 cm anterolateral to the aorta, is confirmed by imaging and contrast injection, 30–50 mL injectate is injected. The needle is then withdrawn while injecting normal saline or anesthetics to prevent irritation of the organs by the injectate.

In this approach, the visceral organs, most commonly the stomach, bowel, and liver, are traversed. Major vessels, biliary ducts, pancreas, and colons should be avoided given the risk of bleeding, pancreatitis, and infection. Needle repositioning increases the risk of complications and should be avoided.

Guidance to Intervention

Endoscopic Approach

Wisere, Faigel, et al. performed the first case of endoscopic ultrasound (EUS) celiac plexus block/necrolysis in 1996. This technique benefits from proximity to the posterior gastric wall, celiac plexus, and large vascular landmarks, particularly the aorta and celiac artery. The procedure is relatively easy and fast, requiring only a few minutes after staging or sampling of a pancreatic tumor. The needle is positioned precisely, close to the celiac trunk, and the needle's trajectory is significantly shorter than in other approaches.

This approach is likely to have lower complication rates, arguably due to the anterior approach of the procedure, a shorter needle trajectory, and consequently avoiding visceral and neural structures. In addition, real-time vascular Doppler prevents major vascular damage in this approach.

A meta-analysis published in 2008 showed that about 80% of patients with pancreatic cancer experience pain relief with this approach. A randomized clinical trial comparing EUS-CPB and morphine use in pancreatic cancer patients showed higher pain reduction in the EUS-CPB group in the first and third months post-procedure.

The EUS scope is advanced in the GI tract to the level of the celiac artery. The scope is then rotated clockwise until the celiac artery is out of view. At this point, the celiac plexus should be localized under the ultrasound guide as a constellation of hypoechoic clusters. Then, the needle punctures the posterior gastric wall and the needle tip is positioned anterolateral to the aorta. The needle is flushed with normal saline to remove any tissue in the needle. Once aspiration confirms that the needle is out of vessels, bupivacaine followed by absolute alcohol is injected. The needle is again flushed with normal saline before withdrawing to prevent alcohol trach, which can cause post-procedural pain and discomfort.

EUS can be performed with a unilateral or bilateral approach. A bilateral approach requires a higher skill level. It is more sophisticated, takes longer to perform, and consequently has higher risks. In a study comparing unilateral and bilateral approaches, there was no significant difference in short-term pain relief among the two groups. However, only patients who had undergone a bilateral procedure had statistically significant reduction in postoperative analgesic use.

Santosh et al. in 2009 assessed the efficacy of fluoroscopy-guided CPB with EUS-guided CPB in chronic pancreatitis. They disclosed that pain relief in the EUS-guided group was about 70% compared to 30% in the fluoroscopy-guided group; thus, outcomes were significantly superior in the EUS-guided group.

CT-Guided Approach

Celiac block is traditionally performed with a posterior approach by a pain medicine physician under fluoroscopy guidance. However, fluoroscopy provides limited soft tissue visualization. It mainly displays bony structures and visceral organs and needle trajectory is hardly visualized.

The needle is introduced in the exact desired spot with CT imaging assistance. The needle is then directed to the celiac plexus while internal organs are visualized and avoided as much as possible. After reaching the target, contrast spread is closely visualized under CT imaging guidance (Fig. 44.5). The technique is similar to fluoroscopic approaches but with the refinement of imaging to decide appropriate anatomic location for the neurolytic placement.

MRI-Guided Approach

MRIs have been shown to precisely guide various interventional procedures such as percutaneous biopsies. MRI-guided celiac block and neurolysis are shown to be practical for pain management of pancreatic cancer. An MRI can demonstrate retroperitoneal structures without the need for contrast. It does not involve risks of ionized radiation, provides near real-time imaging, and has multiplanar capability. It can visualize critical organs in the needle trajectory and assist in needle maneuvering. Open MRIs are more convenient for procedural approaches and have enough space for adjusting the needle during the procedure. Some of the new optical tracking systems such as Ipath200 can display the needle route and enable precise needle trajectory tracking with an MRI.

Ultrasound-Guided Approach

Ultrasound-guided CPN is performed at bedside using anterior approach with real-time needle visualization. It is cost-effective, fast, and suitable for claustrophobic patients who cannot tolerate CT or MRI. Unlike fluoroscopy- and CT-guided procedures, ultrasound does not involve any radiation. The ultrasound device is portable and is suitable for bedside procedures. Since the procedure is performed in supine position, patients with painful abdominal malignancy, mass, or distention tolerate it better. Similar to other anterior approaches, this approach has lower risk of neurological complications.

Ultrasound-guided approach is limited in obese patients, abdominal abscess, and those with unprepared bowels. Prior abdominal surgery or large intra-abdominal masses can distort the land marks and limit needle access to the plexus. The interventionist has limited view of the retroperitoneal structures in this approach, and in 20% of the cases, the celiac plexus may not be visible. In addition, procedure success is largely dependent on operator skills and requires expertise in needle manipulation under ultrasound guide.

Prior to the procedure, patients typically fast for at least 8 h to ensure GI preparedness. While in supine position, insertion site and needle approach are determined by ultrasound visualization (Fig. 44.7). A 22-G Chiba needle is then inserted, and the needle tip is tracked in real time until the celiac plexus (Fig. 44.8). After aspiration, the injectate which is a mixture of ethanol, bupivacaine, and non-iodinated contrast is injected. The procedure can be confirmed after injec-

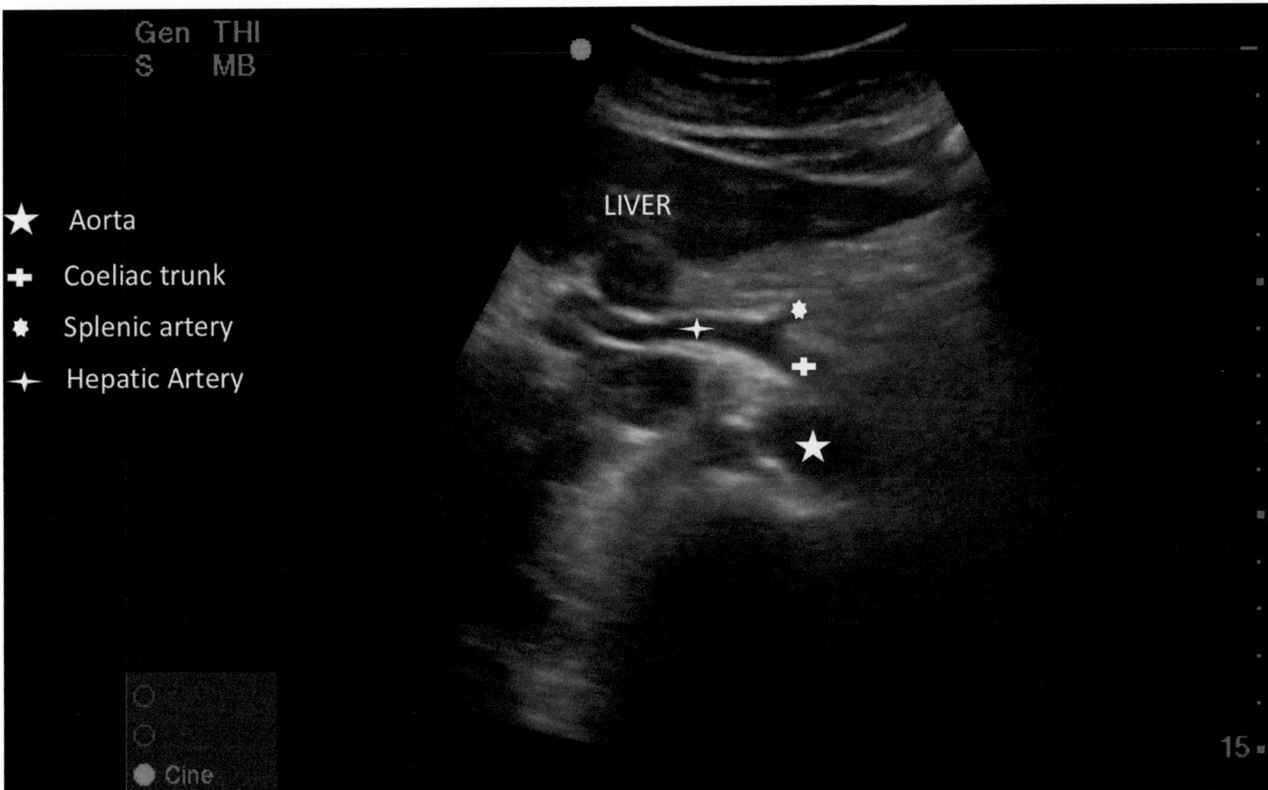

Fig. 44.7 Sonoanatomy of the target at the optimal scan. The coeliac trunk is visualized which branches out to the hepatic artery on the right and the splenic artery on the left. (Reproduced with permission from Dr. Sushma Bhatnagar)

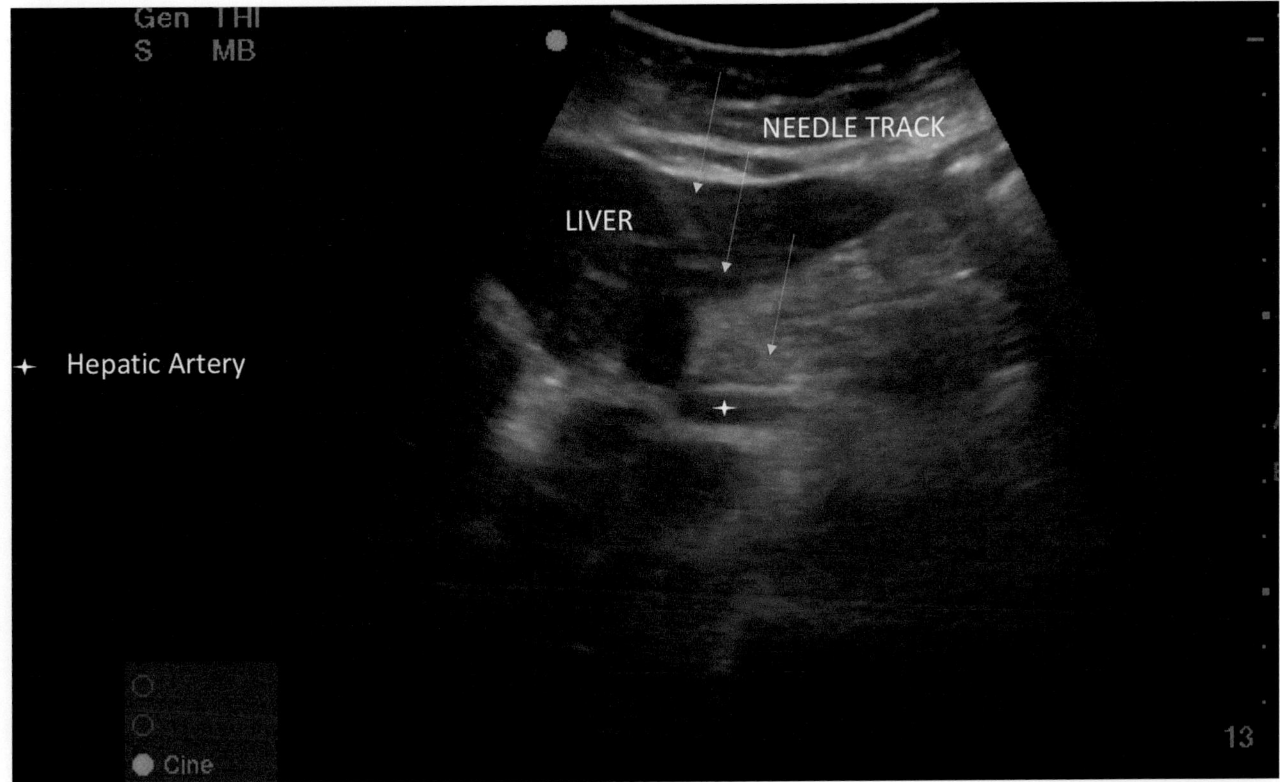

Fig. 44.8 Injection of the coeliac plexus. The needle (arrows) is inserted in plane from right to left in front of the hepatic artery. (Reproduced with permission from Dr. Sushma Bhatnagar)

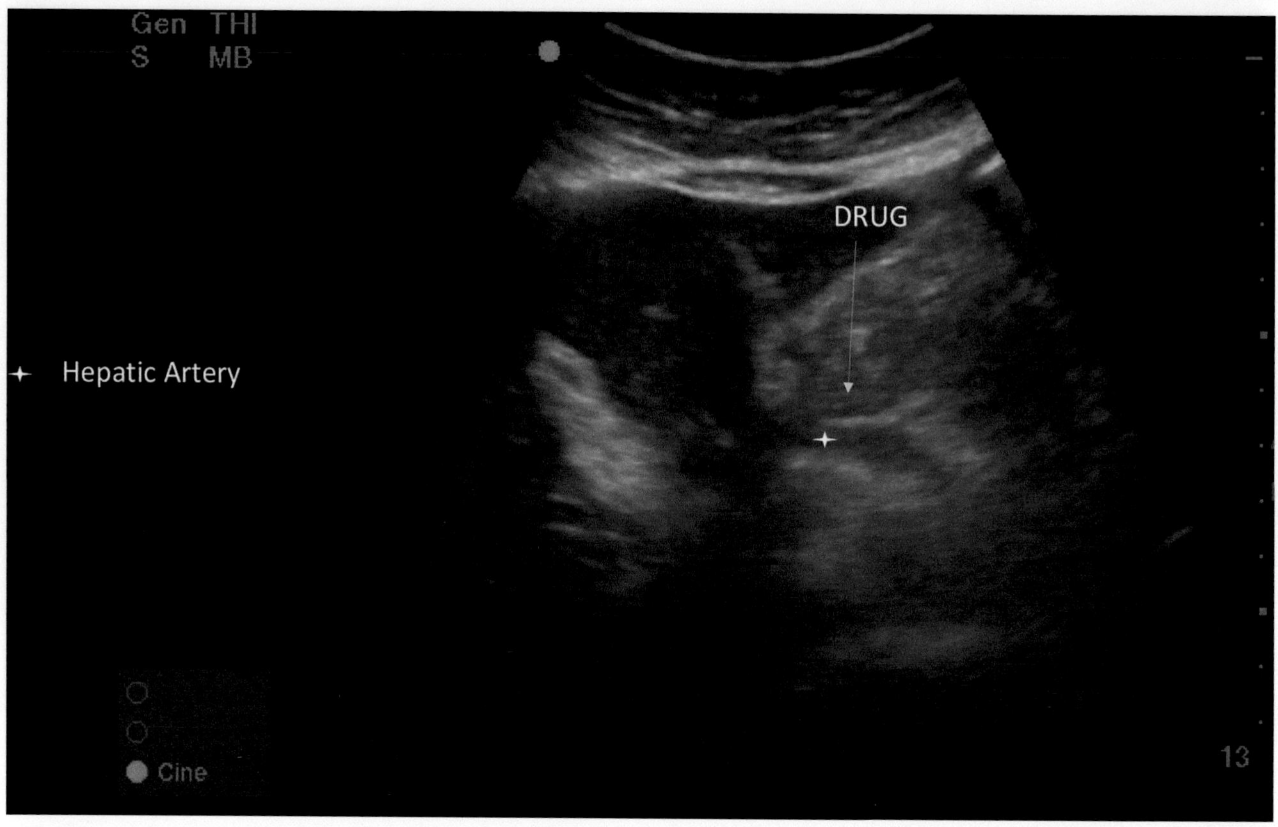

Fig. 44.9 Same scan as in Fig. 44.7. The drug is seen localized ventral to the hepatic artery. (Reproduced with permission from Dr. Sushma Bhatnagar)

tion by visualization of an echogenic cloud under ultrasound in the majority of the cases (Fig. 44.9). Prior to needle removal and after the injection, a CT scan can further confirm the needle position and solution spread following the injection.

Complications

Overall significant clinical and practical complications in CPB and CPN are rare. Studies have suggested the frequency of major complications to be approximately 1–2%. Various procedural approaches have different complication rates. Image-guided approaches are usually safer and more precise compared to blind procedures.

Transient local back pain has been frequently reported as the most common complication. Back pain may radiate to the shoulder and improves in fewer than 72 h. Ethanol injection during the procedure can also cause pain and irritation which can be prevented by flushing the needle before removal or by adding a long-acting anesthetic to the injectate.

Diarrhea and orthostatic hypotension can commonly occur following the blockade or destruction of the celiac plexus. Their incidences in different studies have rated from 10 to 60%. Blockade of the celiac plexus leads to sympathetic denervation and subsequently increases the bowel peristalsis due to unopposed parasympathetic signals. Diarrhea is self-limiting and usually resolves within 24–48 h.

Orthostatic hypotension is typically transient and occurs as a result of splanchnic vasculature dilation. It usually resolves in 6–12 h and can be managed by lying flat or with IV fluid.

Poor needle positioning and trajectory can lead to injury to nerve roots, internal organs, and vasculatures. Good detail visualization of anatomical structures and use of tracking navigation can decrease these procedure-related complications.

Spinal cord ischemia is rare but can cause the most severe complications of this procedure including paralysis or paresis. It is frequently caused by embolic occlusion of the Adamkiewicz artery or vasospasm of the radicular arteries. Direct puncture of the spinal cord or anterior spinal artery or direct neurolytic injection can lead to this complication. Image-guided approaches, especially EUS-guided procedures and anterior approaches, can decrease the chance of spinal cord injury.

Renal injury can cause hematuria and pleural puncture can cause pneumothorax. Retroperitoneal hematoma can happen after puncturing the vessels. Infection and abscess formation are possible and can be minimized with proper aseptic techniques.

There are reported cases of hepatic, splenic, and bowel infarction after vasospasm or thrombosis of the internal organ vessels after the procedures. Other reported complications include anesthetic toxicity, chylothorax, pericarditis, aortic dissection, pseudoaneurysm, intervertebral disc injury, retroperitoneal fibrosis, and pulmonary embolism.

Efficacy

The efficacy of CNB and CPB for pain control is usually dependent on the underlying disease. Most studies of CBP in chronic pancreatitis are small and show slight pain benefit. However, multiple studies have confirmed that celiac plexus neurolysis in pancreatic cancer is effective and reliable in terms of pain reduction and decreasing opioid use and their side effects. Studies have also suggested that decreasing opioid-related side effects in cancer patients undergoing the procedures will result in improving their functionality and quality of life. A meta-analysis of EUS-guided CPB and CPN has shown higher pain reduction in pancreatic cancer compared to chronic pancreatitis but minimal reduction in pain medication use.

The procedure is usually more effective in tumors of the pancreatic head compared to the ones in the body or tail. Lower preprocedural opioid use, CT guidance compared to fluoroscopy, performing the procedure without sedation, and local anesthetic administration for the block are shown to be correlated with a better response rate. In pancreatic cancer as the disease progresses, it affects anatomical structures of the abdominal wall and result in somatic type of pain. This type of pain is usually not transmitted through the celiac plexus and is, consequently, less responsive to plexus neurolysis. Therefore, patients with worse survival rate are shown to have lower chance of remaining pain free after neurolysis.

CPB is shown to have temporary effect on pain reduction. Most studies report that CPB is effective for a duration of about 3 months. However, repeated CPB procedure is shown to be safe and effective. An EUS-guided celiac plexus block study showed that positive response to the first CBP predicts response to future CBP procedures. Current data does not suggest a significant difference in pain duration or pain medication use reduction in unilateral versus bilateral techniques.

CPB and CBN only affect sympathetic pain mechanisms. Usually, patients undergoing the procedure, especially cancer patients, have mixture of somatic, sympathetic, and neuropathic pain due to the widespread invasion of the cancer cells to the peritoneum, lymph nodes, internal organs, and nervous system. Literatures suggest that pain management in these patients becomes exceedingly difficult as the cancer progresses. In addition, as tumors grow, they displace nearby structures and affect the spread of injectate to the plexus. It is suggested to use higher doses of injectate and attempt a bilateral approach in these patients for better response. However, the interventionist should be aware of the side effects of using high doses of injectate in this vulnerable population.

Future Recommendations

Because of the lack of robust evidence, we still could not find the final recommendation in terms of the best available approach. There is a need for a well-designed RCT to give final recommendations in this regard. Nonetheless, the CPB and CPN have a breath of evidence supporting its use as an early pain treatment option for malignant abdominopelvic visceral pain and refractory benign abdominal visceral pain.

Lumbar Sympathetic Block

45

Juan Felipe Vargas Silva and Philip Peng

Contents

General Consideration

Development of lumbar sympathetic block was first credited to Brunn and Mandl in 1924 as a component of their paravertebral approach. Later, the technique gained importance for the treatment of causalgia and post-traumatic reflex dystrophies. Roberts in 1986 initially used the term "sympathetic mediated pain" as the pain characterized by continuous burning pain with mechanical hyperalgesia/allodynia following a history of physical trauma to the painful area and relief of pain by sympathetic blockade. Also, lumbar sympathectomy was part of the treatment of arterial occlusive disease before the development of recently surgical and endovascular procedures, and now it has gained new interest when the occlusion is not revascularizable.

Lumbar sympathetic block is commonly performed to manage pain pathologies of the lower extremity, with diagnostic, prognostic, and therapeutic indications. As diagnostic blocks, lumbar sympathetic block stratifies the nature of the pain as a sympathetically mediated pain or sympathetically independent pain. As a prognostic block, they help to identify those patient candidates for

J. F. Vargas Silva (✉)
Department of Surgery, Interventional Radiology & Pain Relief, Hospital Pablo Tobon Uribe, Medellin, Antioquia, Colombia

P. Peng
Department of Anesthesia and Pain Medicine, Toronto Western Hospital, University of Toronto, Toronto, ON, Canada
e-mail: philip.peng@uhn.ca

D. Jankovic, P. Peng (eds.), *Regional Nerve Blocks in Anesthesia and Pain Therapy*, https://doi.org/10.1007/978-3-030-88727-8_45

neurolytic or surgical sympathectomy. They also aid in treatment a myriad of painful conditions as a therapeutic procedure.

Sympathetic Mediated Pain (SMP)

The term sympathetic mediated pain was described by Roberts in 1986 as pain maintained by sympathetic efferent innervation or by circulating catecholamines. Under normal conditions, the sympathetic nervous system (SNS) does not activate nociceptors in the sensory nervous system. The existence of SMP implies an interaction between sympathetic nerves and nociceptive sensory nerves in some diseased states.

It is hypothesized that a painful stimulus gives rise to a regional sympathetic reflex that may facilitate nociceptive transmission from the painful region, allowing an interaction between nociceptive and autonomic neural structures. Such abnormal interactions between sympathetic nerves and nociceptive nerves could be mediated either non-synaptically with electrical current passing between nerves (ephaptic coupling) or chemically by catecholamines (primarily noradrenaline) released by sympathetic nerve endings. There is no convincing solid evidence for ephaptic sympathetic–sensory interactions. Instead, they revealed an altered sensitivity to catecholamines rather than an altered sympathetic nerve traffic.

The patient response to sympathetic blockade may be used to differentiate sympathetic mediated pain from other pain types, although the validity of this method is controversial with lack of well-designed randomized controlled trials. However, the weight of evidence favors the existence of sympathetic mediated pain in a subgroup of patients with CRPS. In these patients, sympathetic blocks relieve pain and hyperalgesia.

A number of different peripheral neuropathic pain syndromes may be aggravated or maintained by actions of the sympathetic nervous system, including postherpetic neuralgia or neuroma pain and then could be potentially relieved by a sympathetic block.

Patient Selection

Lumbar sympathetic chain blocks serve as a diagnostic and prognostic procedure, to determine if the pain is sympathetically maintained or whether it is independent of sympathetic function. Sometimes, these procedures are used to predict the effects of definitive (neurolytic or surgical) sympathectomy (Table 45.1).

Table 45.1 Indication of lumbar sympathetic block

Pain related indications	
Sympathetic mediated pain	Interstitial cystitis
Severe ischemic lower limb pain[a]	Renal colic
Complex regional pain syndrome I or II	Postherpetic neuralgia
Raynaud's disease	Phlegmasia alba dolens
Polyneuropathy	Erythromelalgia
Burning-feet syndrome	Acrocyanosis
Postherpetic neuralgia	Trench foot
Phantom pain/postamputation pain	
Non-pain related indications	
Plantar hyperhidrosis	Frostbite

[a] In patient with rest pain and concurrent non-reconstructable peripheral arterial disease

Contraindications

- Infections
- Wet gangrene
- Bleeding diathesis
- Local infection

Anatomy of the Sympathetic Chain

The sympathetic nervous system consists of preganglionic and postganglionic efferent fibers that innervate deep somatic structures, skin, and viscera. The preganglionic fibers pass by way of their corresponding nerves as white rami communicans, which joins with postganglionic efferent to the pelvic viscera, although some postganglionic fibers communicate directly to the aortic plexus and the superior and inferior hypogastric plexuses. The cell bodies responsible for vasoconstriction in the lower limbs are in the lower three thoracic and first three lumbar segments. Also, intermediate ganglia found in the psoas and iliacus muscles communicate with postganglionic fibers that pass through the lumbar and sacral nerves and are responsible for vasomotor, pilomotor, and sudomotor functions.

The lumbar sympathetic trunk usually contains four interconnected ganglia (rarely five), extraperitoneal and anterolateral to the lumbar vertebrae along the medial margin of psoas major (Fig. 45.1). They are typically at L1–L4, with the L1 and L2 ganglia commonly fused. The size, number, and precise location of the sympathetic ganglia are known to be variable. It is continuous with the thoracic sympathetic trunk superiorly, and inferiorly, it is continuous with the sacral sympathetic trunk. The L2 ganglion is situated at the junction of the lower third and upper two-thirds of the L2 vertebral body. The L3 ganglion is situated at the junction of the lower two-thirds and upper third of the vertebral body. The L4 ganglion is variable in position.

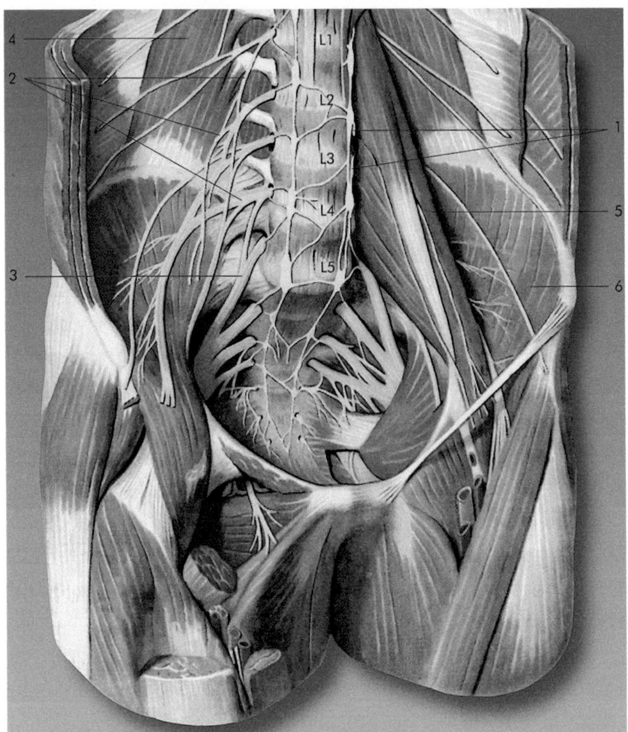

Fig. 45.1 Anatomy (anterior view): (1) sympathetic trunk with communicating branches, (2) lumbar plexus, (3) lumbosacral trunk, (4) quadratus lumborum muscle, (5) psoas major muscle, (6) iliac muscle. (Reprinted with permission from Dr. Danilo Jankovic)

The inferior vena cava maintains a close association along the anterior margin of the right lumbar sympathetic chain, and the aorta is similarly positioned slightly anterior and medial to the left lumbar sympathetic chain (Fig. 45.2). The psoas muscle is situated posteriorly deep to the fibrous arcades. The white and gray rami communicans passing to their respective ganglia at each level.

Technique

Preparation for the Procedure

The needle for insertion is a 15 cm 20–22-gauge Chiba needle or 3.5-in./5-in. Quincke needle. If the latter is used, the end of the needle is bent (Fig. 45.3). Imaging equipment is required and this procedure is commonly performed under fluoroscopy but ultrasound-guided technique has been described. Other equipment include water-soluble contrast, extension tube, and 25-gauge needle for skin infiltration.

For diagnostic or therapeutic block purpose, 12 mL of local anesthetic (0.5% ropivacaine, 0.5% bupivacaine, or 2% lidocaine) is used. For neurolytic block, the agents are either 6–10% aqueous phenol (5–8 mL) or 50–100% alcohol (5–8 mL).

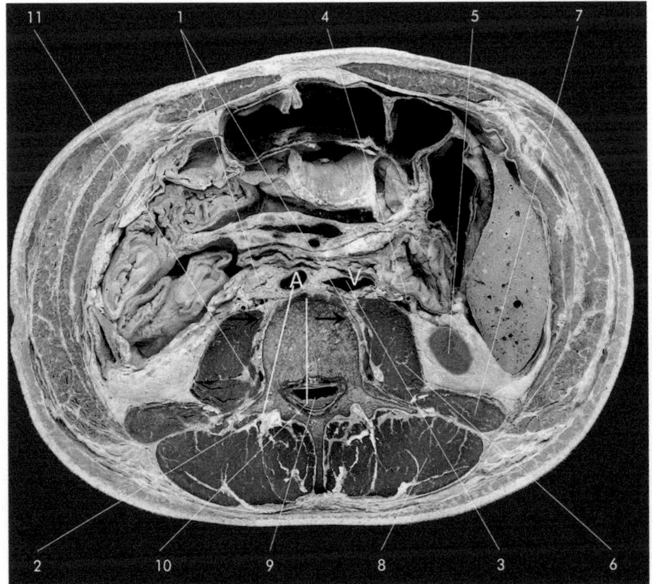

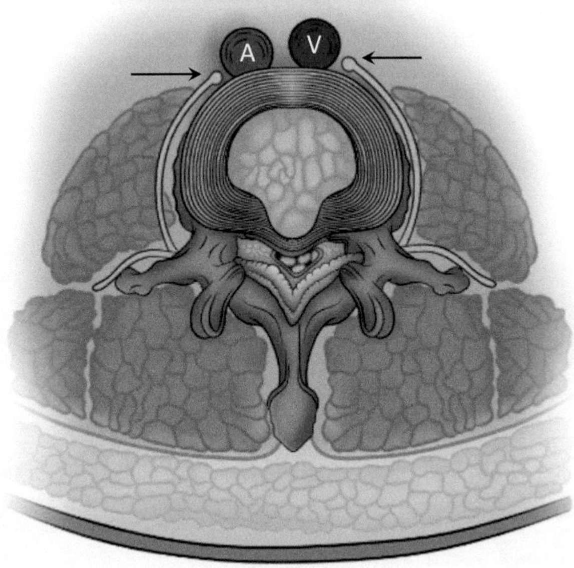

Fig. 45.2 Cross section anatomy at the level of L3. Left. Dissection. (1) Sympathetic trunk, (2) aorta, (3) inferior vena cava, (4) ureter, (5) kidney, (6) psoas major muscle, (7) quadratus lumborum muscle, (8) erector spinae muscle, (9) cauda equina, (10) anterior longitudinal ligament, (11) lumbar plexus (reprinted with permission from Danilo Jankovic). Right. Schematic diagram of the same cross section at L3 (reprinted with permission from Philip Peng Educational Series). A—aortic; V—inferior vena cava; sympathetic ganglion indicated by the arrow

Procedure (Fluoroscopy)

All procedures must be performed after an informed consent and routine surgical time-out to verify patient, procedure, and the site, and to rule out any allergy to the medications employed.

The patient is positioned prone with sterile skin preparation of the lumbar spine region. A pillow under the lower abdomen and pelvis reduces the lumbar lordosis (Fig. 45.4a). Prophylactic antibiotics are not generally administered. The targets are the anterolateral aspects of the ipsilateral L2–L4 vertebrae and are revealed using an oblique fluoroscopy projection (Fig. 45.4b). Usually, L3 is chosen, with the intent of having a spread of contrast over the L2–L4 sympathetic ganglions.

After aligning the vertebral endplates and obtaining an oblique view of 20–30° approximately until the tip of the transverse process overlies the anterolateral margin of the vertebral body, a 15 cm 20 or 22 gauge needle is advanced just inferior to the transverse process targeting the lateral aspect of the vertebral body (Fig. 45.5). Typically, the skin entry point is approximately 7 cm lateral from midline, depending on body habitus. The needle is advanced under intermittent biplane (oblique and lateral) fluoroscopy until making a gentle contact with the vertebral body. An additional 1–2 mL of local anesthesia is placed on the vertebral body to keep walking off the needle.

With a lateral fluoroscopy view, the final needle adjustments can be made to ensure the final needle position. Because the vertebral body cortex is contacted, the needle needs to be walked-off to reach the anterolateral aspect of the vertebral body, into the prevertebral space, medial to the perimysium of the psoas muscle, and lateral to the great vessels (Fig. 45.5). A curved needle-tip could facilitate the process to navigate and walk in or walk off the vertebral body. The needle is navigated until the tip of the needle is over the anterior 1/3 of the vertebral body on a lateral projection.

After needle aspiration to exclude inadvertent intravascular position, a small volume of water-soluble contrast is injected to identify the correct tissue plane. The dye should spread craniocaudal anterior to the vertebral bodies over L2–L4 levels (Fig. 45.6a–c). Minimal resistance upon injection should be noted.

If a myogram of the psoas is noted (the needle is in the interior of the psoas muscle), it should alert an intramuscular injection and the needle must be advanced further (Fig. 45.7a, b). An extension line helps to avoid moving the needle during the procedure. Intermittent aspiration during the final injection excludes the possibility of inadvertent intravascular injection.

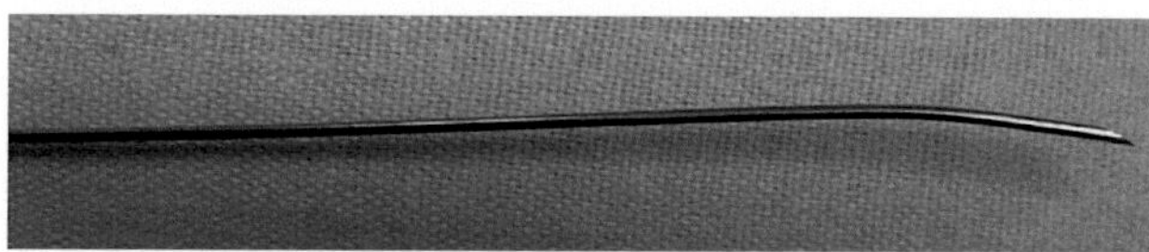

Fig. 45.3 Quincke needle bended at the end

Procedure (Ultrasound)

Currently, fluoroscopy-guided lumbar sympathetic block is the preferred interventional approach. Kirvelä in 1992

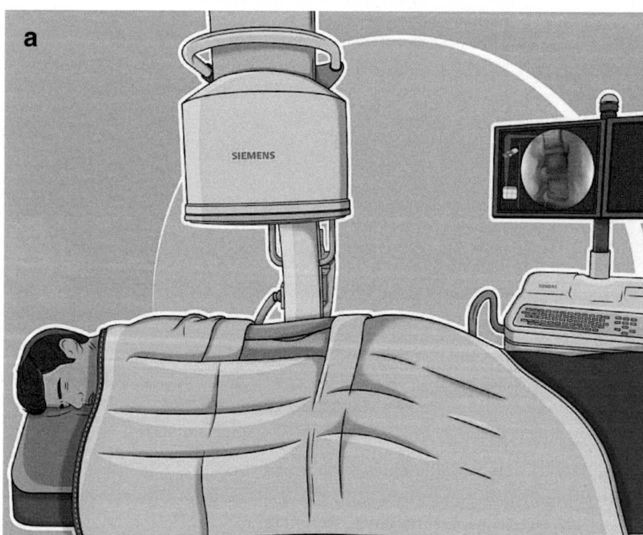

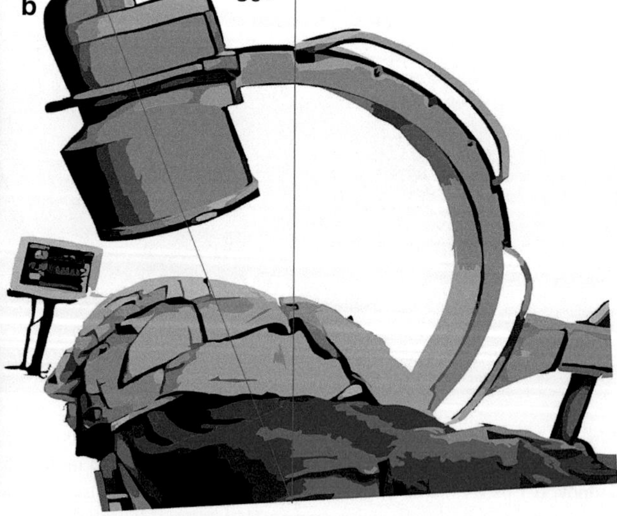

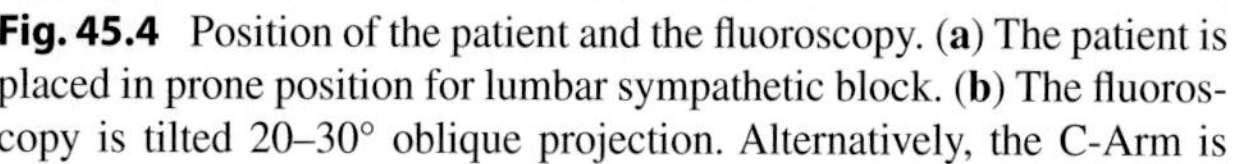

Fig. 45.4 Position of the patient and the fluoroscopy. (**a**) The patient is placed in prone position for lumbar sympathetic block. (**b**) The fluoroscopy is tilted 20–30° oblique projection. Alternatively, the C-Arm is rotated until the tip of the transverse process overlies the anterolateral margin of the vertebral body. (Reprinted with permission from Philip Peng Educational Series)

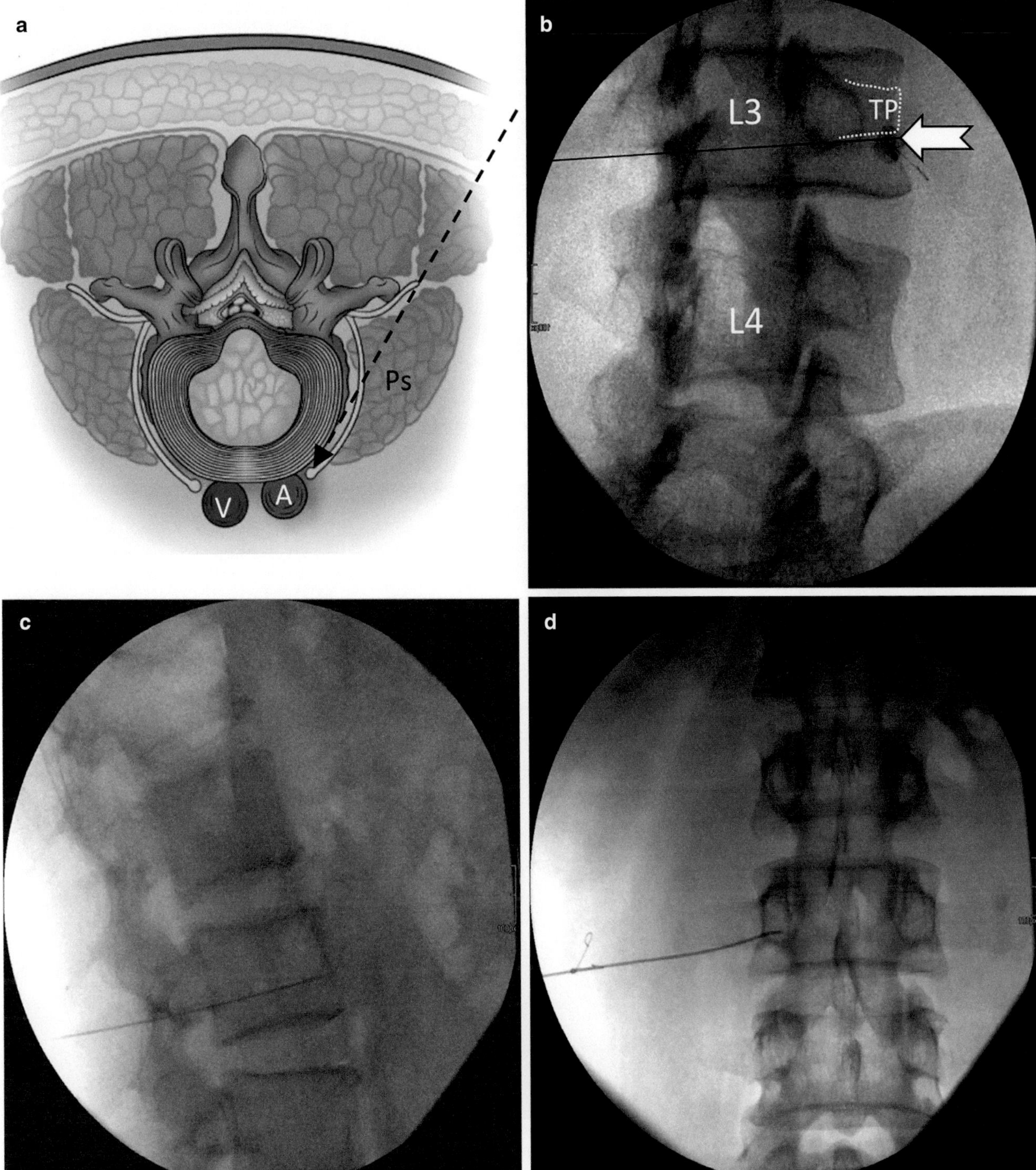

Fig. 45.5 (**a**) Dotted line is the trajectory of the needle. (**b**) Oblique view of lumbar spine with the target indicated by the bold arrow. TP-transverse process which is outlined by the dotted line. (**c**) Lateral view. The tip of the needle is at the anterior border of the vertebra. (**d**) Anteroposterior view. Usually, the tip of the needle is in front of the pedicle. (Reprinted with permission from Philip Peng Educational Series)

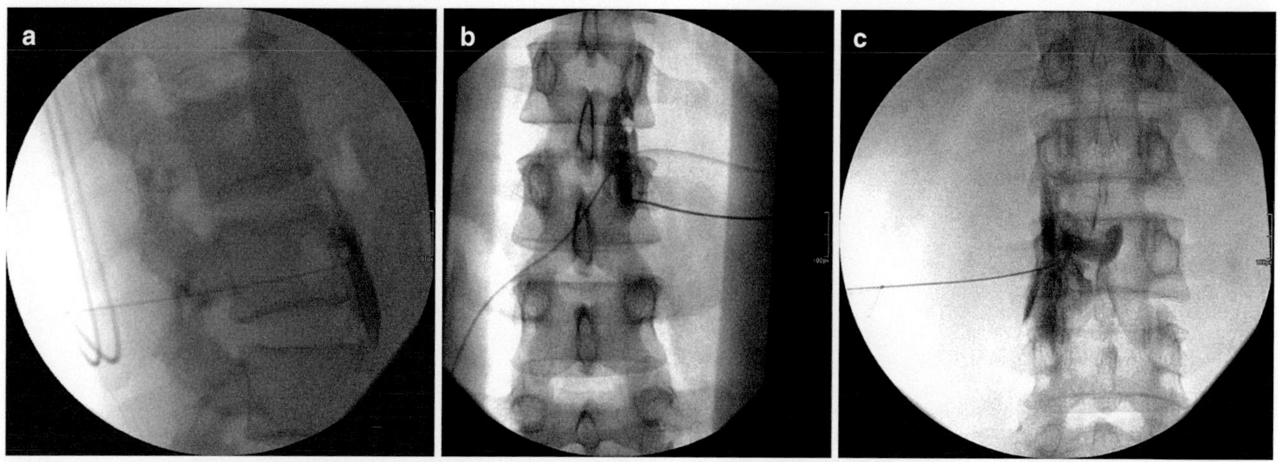

Fig. 45.6 (**a**) Lateral fluoroscopy image of contrast spread anterior to the vertebral body. (**b**, **c**) Anteroposterior view shows the contrast pattern spread in the anterolateral region of the vertebrae on the left and right sides. (Reprinted with permission from Philip Peng Educational Series)

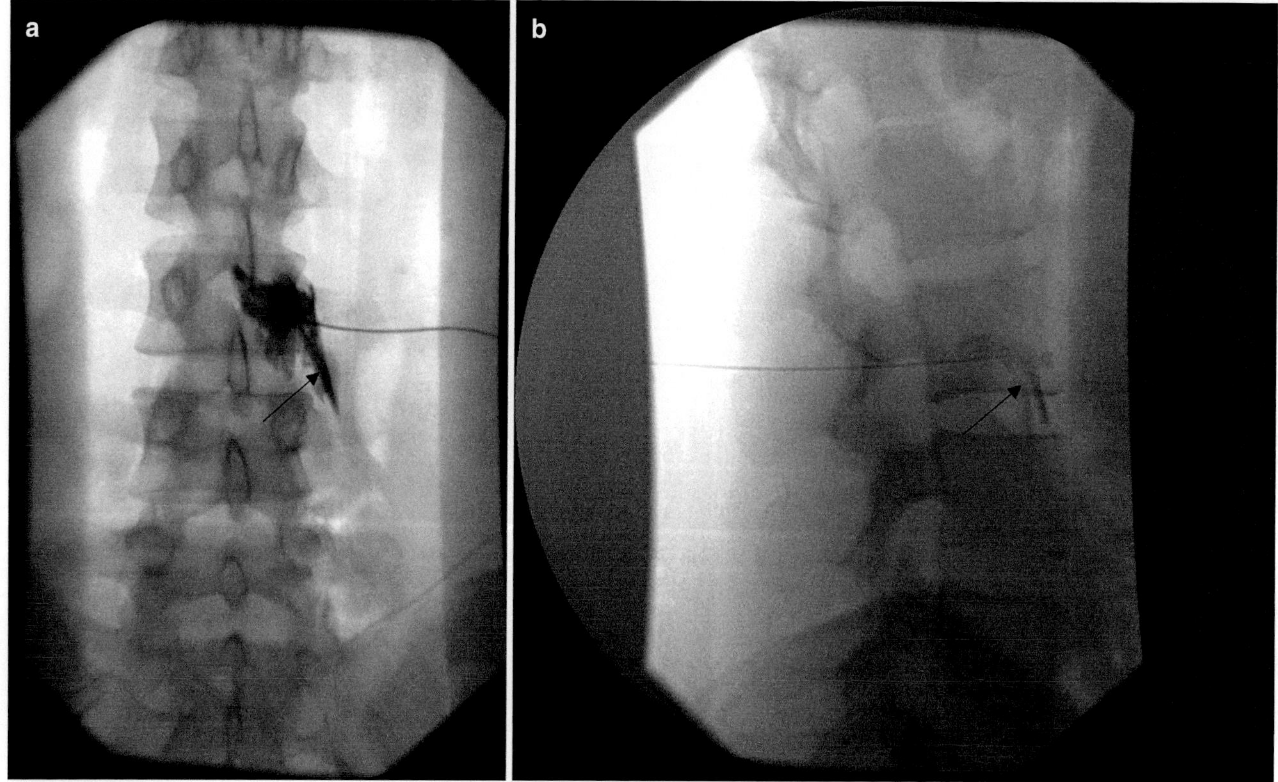

Fig. 45.7 (**a**) A linear spread, band-like with visibly present muscular striations moving away from cephalic to lateral and caudad, indicates a psoas muscle injection (arrow). (**b**) In the lateral view, a claw-like pattern is evident, confirming injection into the psoas muscle and the needle needs to be advanced further. (Reprinted with permission from Philip Peng Educational Series)

reports a case series with ultrasound guidance, but it was never reproduced again until recent years.

The scanning is started with the patient placed in lateral decubitus position with the affected limb in the nondependent side and the ultrasound placed in front of the patient for an ergonomic reason (Fig. 45.8). The spine level can be counted with the parasagittal view of the spine using a low frequency (2–6 MHz) curved probe. Once the level is counted, the curved probe can be placed in short-axis view over the mid-axillary line just above the iliac crest (similar to the Shamrock approach of quadratus lumborum block) and the level selected. Usually, the most caudal level vertebra level when the kidney shadow is seen will be L3. In the far field of the screen, the acoustic shadow of the transverse process (TP) is identified with the lateral border of the vertebral body anterior to it (Fig. 45.9a). In between the vertebral body and the transverse process, the psoas muscle is well seen in short axis. Other important structures amenable to be seen in this approach are the abdominal musculature, the major vessels (aorta and inferior vena cava), the kidney in front of the psoas (sometimes only seen with a deep breath), the erector spinae muscles and quadratus lumborum. The color Doppler helps to determine the presence of vascular structures and to plan a needle trajectory (Fig. 45.9b).

The target (the lumbar sympathetic chain) in the sonography is found as a hyperechoic virtual space on the anteromedial edge of the vertebra lateral to the aorta (left side) or the inferior vena cava (right side). Once the structures are identified, the probe is tilted slightly cephalic or caudal to get rid of the TP view. That will help to facilitate the approach with a flatten angulation of the needle and a better view once it is in its trajectory towards the sympathetic chain. With full aseptic technique, a 12 or 15 cm long needle is inserted in-plane from posterior to anterior towards the target aiming the anteromedial edge of the psoas muscle in contact with the vertebral body. Once the needle gets in contact with the bone, the needle is rolled until the psoas epimysium is through, to reach the target in front of the vertebral body and lateral to the major vessels (Fig. 45.10).

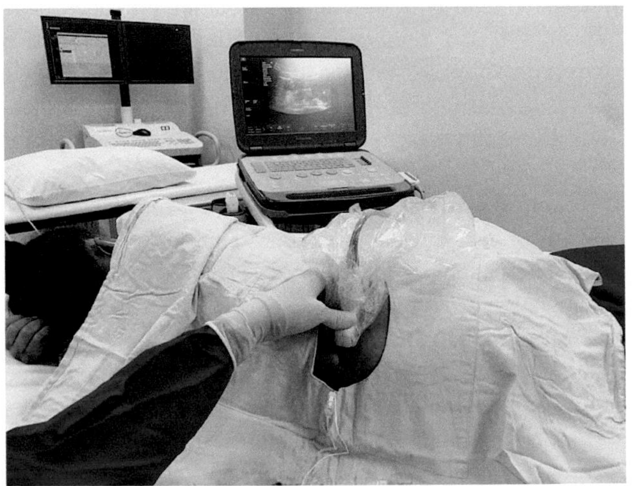

Fig. 45.8 A lateral position to facilitate an ergonomic procedure. (Reprinted with permission from Philip Peng Educational Series)

Several factors could affect the ultrasound-guided procedure. One factor in particular is the body mass index (BMI), and the procedure is generally limited to patient of a low BMI. The angle of needle trajectory is also important because a very steep angle of the needle could impair the visualization during the procedure. Consider using echogenic needles and a flat needle position.

Evaluation of the Sympathetic Block

It is important to evaluate the presence of the sympathetic blockade because technical failure might lead to absence of therapeutic response and false negative result. Skin temperature monitoring is an easy way to test sympathetic blockade and is inexpensive, painless, and sensitive method for measuring cutaneous blood flow. With vasodilatation after a sympathetic blockade, the skin temperature will approximate to core body temperature.

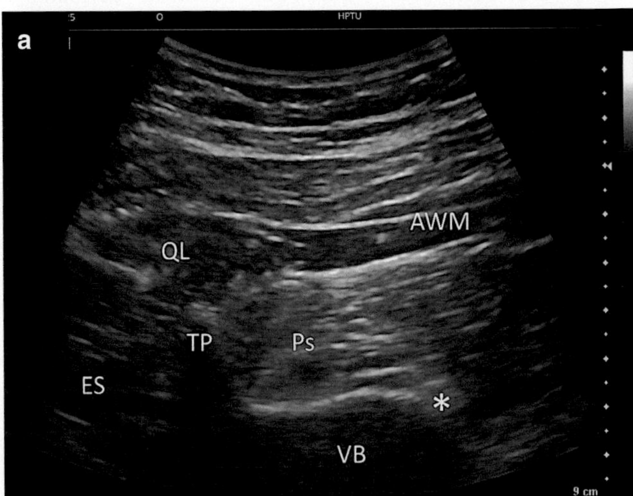

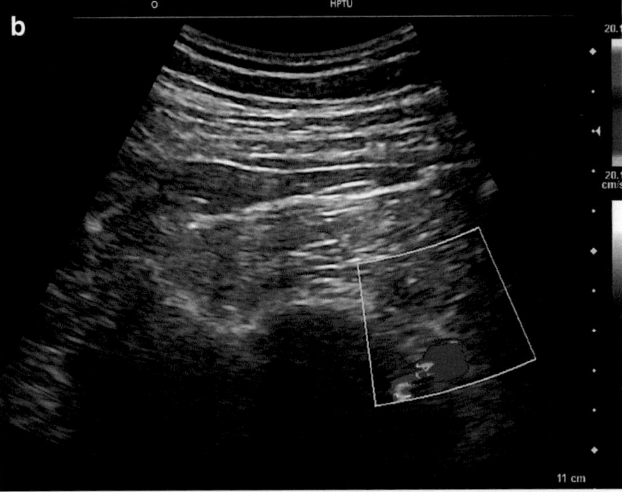

Fig. 45.9 (**a**) Sonograph at L3 with transverse process in view (Shamrock appearance). With a slight tilt, the transverse process is absent to facilitate the entrance of the needle. *TP* transverse process, *VB* vertebral body, *Ps* psoas muscle, *QL* quadratus lumborum muscle, *ES* erector spinae muscles, *AWM* anterior abdominal wall muscles. * sympathetic chain. (**b**) Color Doppler showing the major vessels—inferior vena cava/aorta. (Reprinted with permission from Philip Peng Educational Series)

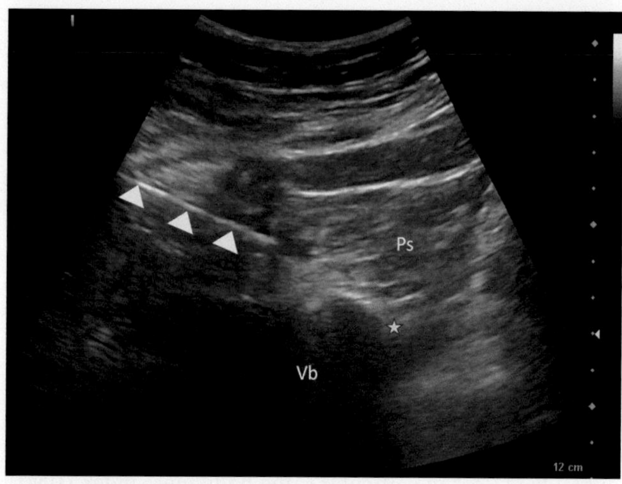

Fig. 45.10 Needle (arrow tips) approaching the target at the sympathetic chain (star) beyond the anterior part of the psoas muscle (Ps). (Vb): Vertebral body. (Reprinted with permission from Philip Peng Educational Series)

Lower extremity temperature at the acral regions of the body, including the toes and the foot, is particularly useful for indicating sympathetic tone because of the unique control of blood flow in these regions, which have a predominance of arteriovenous anastomoses. It is recommended to measure skin temperatures before and after the block of both affected and unaffected sides. If an infrared thermometer is used, the change in skin temperature must be at least of 2 °C after sympathetic block. Sometimes this may not occur despite appropriate blockade. Some CRPS already have a warm extremity that does not become warmer after a sympathetic blockade.

The evidence of sympatholysis (i.e. vasodilation, increased temperature) is important, but the effect of the block on the preexisting symptoms, such as pain, allodynia, or hyperalgesia also requires assessment after sympatholysis. Pain relief can be reported immediately after block or can be delayed for several hours in some patients. Placebo responses and systemic effect (after absorption) of local anesthetics could affect the pain response.

Chemical Neurolytic Block

Neurolysis of the lumbar sympathetic chain is considered only after a positive response to the local anesthetic block of the lumbar sympathetic chain. A longitudinal (cephalad and caudad) spread of drugs along the sympathetic chain in the anterolateral border of the vertebral body in a tight, linear fashion is required for adequate neurolysis. If contrast diffuses laterally it is usually deposited either in the psoas muscle or on the fascia (Fig. 45.7).

Phenol or alcohol can be used. Phenol produces a lower incidence of neuralgia than do equivalent volumes of alcohol. Instead of using a single needle technique as in the diagnostic block, two separate needles at L2 and L3 are inserted and a volume as small as 2 mL is injected through each needles. Larger volumes (6 mL total) through a single needle have been equally efficacious. Avoid using higher volumes to prevent spread to genitofemoral nerve.

Radiofrequency Lesioning

Compared with chemical sympathectomy, potential advantages of radiofrequency include the reduced risk of genitofemoral nerve and third lumbar nerve neuritis from the spread of neurolytic solution. The latter produces pain, dysesthesia, and numbness around the knee area, and if neurolytic solution spreads to the dural cuff, paraplegia can result. Also, with RF lesioning, the risk of complications due to intravascular injection of a neurolytic agent is absent.

Technical consideration includes a good knowledge of the anatomy of the sympathetic chain and the surrounding structures. The pattern of the contrast spreads is crucial to the identification of accurate needle placement in the anterolateral aspect of the vertebral body medial to the psoas sheath. Radiofrequency thermal ablation outside this position could result in damage to the lumbar plexus nerves.

Electrical stimulation is aimed to test proximity to sensory and motor nerves. Low-frequency motor stimulation should not cause muscle contraction. Because the sympathetic nerves carry afferent pain fibers, patients might complain of tingling in the anterior compartment of the thigh and knee. However, this would not be in a dermatomal distribution.

Complications

Comparing with landmark guidance, the complication rates are reduced with image guidance technique (fluoroscopy or computed tomographic/CT scan). The possible complications can be reduced if meticulous attention is paid to the technique.

Intraspinal Injection

Injection in the spinal canal is rare, but theoretically possible. This complication could occur after puncture of either an extended dural cuff or the intraspinal dura.

Intravascular Injection

Intravascular injection is rarely reported but possible in a clinical scenario, due to the anterior position of both the aorta and inferior vena cava and its close proximity to the sympathetic chain. Puncture to the vertebral venous plexus is also a risk, as it is close to the trajectory of the needle. This risk of intravascular injection is minimized by appropriate use of fluoroscopy and contrast medium before the injection of local anesthetics or neurolytic agents. Negative aspiration should not be relied upon prior to injection, as it provides false safety, with a sensitivity of only 40.7%, due to collapse of the venous system with aspiration.

Needle Trauma

One of the risks of "blind" technique is needle trauma to the kidney, ureter, and bowel. These events can be minimized with the utilization of fluoroscopic-guidance.

Drug Effects

These complications are associated to the use of either local anesthetics or neurolytic agents. Cardiovascular effects are frequent with postural hypotension as a result of significant sympathetic blockade. Another possible undesirable effect is sexual dysfunction in male patients, although it must be remembered that vascular insufficiency can cause sexual dysfunction by itself and vascular insufficiency is one of the main indications of a sympathetic blockade. If there is a critical fixed stenosis of the arterial supply to one region, vasodilatation after the sympathetic block could give rise to a "steal" syndrome with deterioration of the perfusion to the ischemic area.

One of the most common complication following a chemical sympathectomy is genitofemoral neuralgia. At the levels of L1 and L2, the genitofemoral nerve arises from the lumbar plexus and lies on the ventral surface of the psoas muscle and is in close proximity to the sympathetic chain. It emerges from the anterior aspect to supply the groin and upper thigh. Thus, it is susceptible to the spread of neurolytic agent if high volume is used. The incidence is variable, between 5% and 40% and most cases are transient, lasting less than 6 weeks. To minimize neuralgia or genitofemoral blockage, a careful technique is required, avoiding intramuscular injection into the psoas muscle and, more importantly, limiting the volume of the neurolytic agent. A transdiscal approach to lumbar sympathetic block has been advocated to avoid genitofemoral neuralgia because the needle does not pass through the psoas muscle.

Table 45.2 Possible complications associated to lumbar sympathetic block and neurolysis

Types	Remarks
Intraspinal injection	Dural cuff, direct spinal needle positioning
Intravascular injection	Aorta, vena cava, vertebral venous plexus
Needle trauma	Kidney, ureter, bowel
Intraspinal injection	
Drug effects	Hypotension
	Sexual dysfunction
	Steal syndrome
	Genitofemoral neuralgia
	Ureteric or kidney injury
Post procedure discomfort	Approximately 5 days
Bleeding	2:2000
Infection	
Nerve root injury	
Retrograde ejaculation	Rare. Do not perform bilateral sympathectomy

The ureters and somatic nerves are also located in close proximity to the sympathetic chain and kidney is close to the trajectory of the needle especially if the needle entry point is too lateral. Although ureteric injury is uncommon, it can occur following chemical sympathectomy. Whether injury is related to needle trauma or ureterolysis from the neurolytic agents is unclear. The delayed presentation of urological symptoms suggests that injury is more likely related to the neurolytic agent, highlighting the importance of limiting the amount of neurolytic agent applied (Table 45.2).

Literature Review

Despite the long history of its use, lumbar sympathetic block lacks a strong evidence, and their efficacy for providing analgesia has been sparsely reported. Many case reports and series have been published, but few placebo-controlled, blinded studies exist.

Haynsworth in 1991 published a case series of 17 patients to evaluate duration of sympathetic block with phenol compared to radiofrequency. At 8 weeks, 89% of patients in the phenol group showed signs of sympathetic blockade compared to 12% at the radiofrequency group and the incidence of post-sympathectomy neuralgia was 22% with phenol and 0% with radiofrequency denervation.

Alexander reported a large retrospective review of neurolytic lumbar sympathetic blocks for peripheral vascular disease over a 13-year period. The observational review included 544 fluoroscopy-assisted procedures in 489 patients (bilateral blocks were performed at different times). He found improvement in rest pain, skin blood flow, and ischemic ulcers in 72% of patients. In this cohort, 148 patients were followed up during a mean period of 8 months and 35% in this subgroup had good long-term improvement in the treated limb with healing of ischemic ulcers and relief of rest pain.

Manjunath performed a randomized controlled trial in 20 patients with CRPS type 1 lasting more than 6 months and unresponsive to medical pharmacologic management. They compared the radiofrequency thermal lumbar sympathectomy with lumbar sympathetic neurolysis with phenol. There were no statistically significant differences in pain scores between the two treatment groups and there was no evidence of nerve injury during follow-up. However, the sample size was small.

Several systematic reviews have evaluated the effectiveness of sympathetic blocks and neurolysis over the years. Nath in 1996 reviewed on surgical sympathectomy for reflex sympathetic dystrophy/CRPS patients and concluded that sympathectomy was somewhat effective and sympathectomy should be reserved for patients with severe CRPS refractory to other treatment modalities. Kingery in 1997 reviewed the literature of controlled clinical trials for peripheral neuropathic pain and CRPS and found no placebo-controlled trials to evaluate either local anesthetic blocks of sympathetic ganglia or surgical sympathectomy. In 2002, Mailis-Gagnon and Furlan showed in a Cochrane Systematic Review that sympathectomy is based on poor quality, uncontrolled studies, and personal experience. Jackson and Gaeta in 2008 reviewed the literature and found poor evidence for neuroablation and concluding that no agent was demonstrably better than any other and limit this treatment for last resort after careful consideration. Day in a systematic review published in 2008 found low-quality evidence to support the use of sympathetic block but the procedure was strongly recommended for situations where analgesics were ineffective for controlling pain. These procedures could be offered to patients whose pain has been refractory to conservative therapy albeit 1A studies may be few or lacking. These blocks can help reduce the requirement for oral analgesics while decreasing tolerance and side effects.

Straube in a Cochrane Systematic review in 2013 found only 1 RCT with no significant differences between groups in mean pain scores. They concluded that the practice of sympathectomy (surgical and chemical) for neuropathic pain and CRPS is based on very little high-quality evidence and it should be used cautiously as a last resource after failure of other treatment options.

Clinical Pearls

Avoid injection of local anesthetic (and even more of neurolytic substances) in the muscle mass of the psoas to avoid a psoas compartment/lumbar plexus block or neurolysis.

With ultrasound, it is useful to follow the needle trajectory anteriorly as the needle approaching the target, making small adjustments with the probe tilting towards the belly button to improve the visualization of the needle, the position of the sympathetic chain and the great vessels. Consider using the electronic zoom of the machine to get a bigger field of view once the needle is approaching the sympathetic chain, and precisely reach the target in deep areas.

Understanding variations in anatomy of the lumbar sympathetic chain is important to achieve the best results for lumbar sympathetic blocks.

The incidence of genitofemoral neuralgia is decreased when the block is performed at L2 as compared to L4 and limiting the volume of the neurolytic agent.

Suggested Reading

Alexander JP. Chemical lumbar sympathectomy in patients with severe lower limb ischaemia. Ulst Med J. 1994;63(2):137.

Bandyk DF, Johnson BL, Kirkpatrick AF, Novotney ML, Back MR, Schmacht DC. Surgical sympathectomy for reflex sympathetic dystrophy syndromes. J Vasc Surg. 2002;35(2):269–77.

Bonica JJ. The management of pain. Philadelphia, PA: Lea & Febiger; 1953.

Bonica JJ. The management of pain. Philadelphia, PA: Lea & Febiger; 1990. p. 407–46, 915–66, 1047–72.

Bruehl S, Harden RN, Galer BS, Saltz S, Bertram M, Backonja M, et al. External validation of IASP diagnostic criteria for complex regional pain syndrome and proposed research diagnostic criteria. Pain. 1999;81(1):147–54.

Brunn F, Mandl F. Die paravertebrale Injektion zur Bekampfung visceraler Schmerzen. Wien Klin Wochenschr. 1924;37:511.

Crockett A, Panickar A. Role of the sympathetic nervous system in pain. Anaesth Intens Care Med. 2011;12(2):50–4.

Cross FW, Cotton LT. Chemical lumbar sympathectomy for ischemic rest pain: a randomized, prospective controlled clinical trial. Am J Surg. 1985;150(3):341–5.

Day M. Sympathetic blocks: the evidence. Pain Pract. 2008;8(2):98–109.

Dellon L, Andonian E, Rosson GD. Lower extremity complex regional pain syndrome: long-term outcome after surgical treatment of peripheral pain generators. J Foot Ankle Surg. 2010;49(1):33–6.

Dotson RM. Causalgia—reflex sympathetic dystrophy—sympathetically maintained pain: myth and reality. Muscle Nerve. 1993;16(10):1049–55.

van Eijs F, Stanton-Hicks M, Van Zundert J, Faber CG, Lubenow TR, Mekhail N, et al. 16. Complex regional pain syndrome. Pain Pract. 2011;11(1):70–87.

Elam M. What lies above and beyond the concept of "sympathetically maintained pain"? Clin Auton Res. 2001;11(6):331–3.

Feigl GC, Kastner M, Ulz H, Breschan C, Dreu M, Likar R. Topography of the lumbar sympathetic trunk in normal lumbar spines and spines with spondylophytes. Br J Anaesth. 2011;106(2):260–5.

Flamer D, Seib R, Peng P. Chapter 16. Complications of regional anesthesia in chronic pain therapy. In: Finucane BT, Tsui BCH, editors. Complications of regional anesthesia: principles of safe practice in local and regional anesthesia. Cham: Springer International Publishing; 2017.

Gibbs GF, Drummond PD, Finch PM, Phillips JK. Unravelling the pathophysiology of complex regional pain syndrome: focus on sympathetically maintained pain. Clin Exp Pharmacol Physiol. 2008;35(7):717–24.

Harden RN, Bruehl S, Galer BS, Saltz S, Bertram M, Backonja M, et al. Complex regional pain syndrome: are the IASP diagnostic criteria valid and sufficiently comprehensive? Pain. 1999;83(2):211–9.

Haynsworth RF, Noe CE. Percutaneous lumbar sympathectomy. A comparison of radiofrequency denervation versus phenol neurolysis. Anesthesiology. 1991;74(3):455–63.

Jackson TP, Gaeta R. Neurolytic blocks revisited. Curr Sci. 2008;12:7–13.

Kingery WS. A critical review of controlled clinical trials for peripheral neuropathic pain and complex regional pain syndromes. Pain. 1997;93:123–39.

Kirvelä O, Svedström E, Lundbom N. Ultrasonic guidance of lumbar sympathetic and celiac plexus block: a new technique. Reg Anesth. 1992;17(1):43.

Leriche R. De la causalgie envisagée comme une névrite du sympathique et de son traitement par la dénudation et l'excision des plexus nerveux péri-artériels. Presse Méd. 1916;24(178–180):19.

Mailis-Gagnon A, Furlan AD. Sympathectomy for neuropathic pain. Cochrane Database Syst Rev. 2002;(1):CD002918.

Mandl F. Die Paravertebrale Injektion. Vienna: J Springer; 1926.

Manjunath PS, Jayalakshmi TS, Dureja GP, Prevost AT. Management of lower limb complex regional pain syndrome type 1: an evaluation of percutaneous radiofrequency thermal lumbar sympathectomy versus phenol lumbar sympathetic neurolysis—a pilot study. Anesth Analg. 2008;106(2):647–9.

Murata Y, Takahashi K, Yamagata M, et al. Variations in the number and position of human lumbar sympathetic ganglia and rami communicantes. Clin Anat. 2003;16:108–13.

Nath RK, Mackinnon SE, Stelnicki E. Reflex sympathetic dystrophy. The controversy continues. Clin Plast Surg. 1996;23(3):435–46.

O'Connell NE, Wand BM, McAuley J, Marston L, Moseley GL. Interventions for treating pain and disability in adults with complex regional pain syndrome. Cochrane Database Syst Rev. 2013;(4):CD009416.

Raj PP, Lou L, Erdine S, Staats PS, Waldman SD, Racz G, Hammer M, et al. Interventional pain management. London: Elsevier Health Sciences; 2008.

Rathmell JP, Nelson GJ. Atlas of image-guided intervention in regional anesthesia and pain medicine. Philadelphia, PA: Lippincott Williams & Wilkins; 2012.

Reid W, Watt JK, Gray RG. Phenol injection of the sympathetic chain. Br J Surg. 1970;57:45.

Roberts WJ. A hypothesis on the physiological basis for causalgia and related pains. Pain. 1986;24:297–311.

Ryu JH, Lee CS, Kim YC, Lee SC, Shankar H, Moon JY. Ultrasound-assisted versus fluoroscopic-guided lumbar sympathetic ganglion block: a prospective and randomized study. Anesth Analg. 2018;126(4):1362–8.

Standring S, Gray H. Gray's anatomy: the anatomical basis of clinical practice. Amsterdam: Elsevier; 2015.

Stanton-Hicks M. Reflex sympathetic dystrophy: a sympathetically mediated pain syndrome or not? Curr Rev Pain. 2000;4(4):268–75.

Stanton-Hicks M, Jänig W, Hassenbusch S, Haddox J, Boas R, Wilson P. Reflex sympathetic dystrophy: changing concepts and taxonomy. Pain. 1995;63(1):127–33.

Straube S, Derry S, Moore RA, Cole P. Cervico-thoracic or lumbar sympathectomy for neuropathic pain and complex regional pain syndrome. Cochrane Database Syst Rev. 2013;9:CD002918.

Zechlinski JJ, Hieb RA. Lumbar sympathetic Neurolysis: how to and when to use? Tech Vasc Interv Radiol. 2016;19(2):163–8.

Lumbar Facet Joint and Nerve Blocks

46

Zhongxi Zheng and Anuj Bhatia

Contents

General Consideration

Low back pain (LBP) is ranked as the single leading cause of disability worldwide. There are numerous potential sources of LBP, with the contribution of lumbar facet (zygapophyseal) joints to low back pain ranging from as low as 4.8% to over 50% with incidence rising with age. The wide range of reported prevalence is a reflection of the lack of accuracy of diagnostic testing in the absence of any noninterventional diagnostic reference standard. There is also a poor correlation between facet joint pathology detected on imaging and clinical symptoms reported by patients. It is not surprising that lumbar facet joint interventions comprise the second most common procedure performed for patients with LBP. In this chapter, we review fluoroscopy and ultrasound-guided approaches to intra-articular facet joint injections and diagnostic blocks that target the sensory innervation to these joints.

Pain arising from lumbar facet joints generally presents as LBP that can be associated with non-dermatomal referred pain in the lower limbs above the knees. Facet loading maneuvers (hyperextension and lumbar rotation) are often painful as is local paraspinal pressure over the facet joints. Motor function and reflexes in the lower limbs are usually preserved, and nerve irritation tests (e.g., straight leg raise) are usually negative. There are, however, no specific clinical symptoms or physical examination signs that can reliably diagnose lumbar facet joints as the cause of mechanical

Z. Zheng
Department of Anaesthesia and Surgical Intensive Care, Changi General Hospital, Singapore Health Services, Singapore, Singapore

Anesthesia and Pain Medicine, Toronto Western Hospital, University of Toronto, Toronto, ON, Canada
e-mail: zheng.zhongxi@singhealth.com.sg

A. Bhatia (✉)
Anesthesia and Pain Medicine, Toronto Western Hospital, University of Toronto, Toronto, ON, Canada
e-mail: anuj.bhatia@uhn.ca

D. Jankovic, P. Peng (eds.), *Regional Nerve Blocks in Anesthesia and Pain Therapy*,
https://doi.org/10.1007/978-3-030-88727-8_46

chronic LBP. Paraspinal pain and tenderness with pressure on the skin overlying the lumbar facet joints appear to be weakly associated with positive response to facet joint interventions. Likewise, the presence of radicular symptoms and signs (e.g., pain worse on coughing and straining, pain radiating below the knee, positive straight leg test) may suggest an etiology for LBP other than the facet joints.

Pain from the upper lumbar facet joints can be referred into the flank, hip, and upper lateral thighs, while pain from the lower lumbar facet joints can be referred to the groin. In less than 5% of patients, pain from the lower lumbar facet joints may also extend into the lower lateral leg and even to the foot. In surgically naïve patients, the L5/S1 facet joint is the most likely affected joint. Mechanical loads are redistributed to adjacent segments after lumbar stabilization operations, and these adjacent facet joints can often be the pain generators in patients who have undergone lumbar spine fusion surgery.

Regarding the contribution of imaging to diagnosing facet joint disease, fluoroscopy, scintigraphy, magnetic resonance imaging (MRI), and computerized tomography (CT) can be useful but are not mandatory prior to facet joint interventions. While there are studies that show weak positive correlations between the presence of facet degeneration or hypertrophy on MRI and the positive response to facet joint interventions, the evidence remains weak. Single photon emission CT (SPECT) has shown promise with identifying painful lumbar facet joints that are associated with a positive response to diagnostic lumbar medial branch blocks (MBB) and pain relief with intra-articular (IA) facet joint injections (FJI) although cost and radiation exposure are an issue with SPECT.

Diagnosis of facetogenic pain is thought to be reliably established only after evidence of reduction in pain and improvement in mobility after lumbar MBB with local anesthetics (LA). The decision regarding selection of target levels for FJI should be based on the synthesis of clinical presentation (local tenderness on palpation, pain referral patterns) and radiological findings when available.

Indications (Patient Selection)

Lumbar Facet Joint Innervation Blocks

Diagnostic blocks to the innervation of lumbar FJ, also known as lumbar medial branch blocks (MBB), are the most reliable means for diagnosing facet joints as pain generators. A positive response refers to 50% or greater reduction in pain following the MBB that is concordant with the expected duration of action of the LA (e.g., up to 2 h with 2% lidocaine and 3–6 h with 0.5% bupivacaine). Dual LA comparative blocks (with a short-acting LA on one occasion and a long-acting LA on another) are associated with a significant false-negative rate and have not been shown to be cost-effective. Current guidelines and evidence suggest that a single block is adequate for diagnosing facet joint pain.

Lumbar Facet Joint Intra-Articular (IA) Injections

Although facet joint IA injections meet criteria for diagnostic interventions for facet-mediated pain, they are less predictive than MBB for response to medial branch RFA and are characterized by a high technical failure rate. Current multisociety guidelines recommend MBB should be the prognostic screening test of choice before lumbar facet RFA. There is however a role for therapeutic IA injections in patients who have suspected inflammatory facetogenic pain and in whom denervation may be relatively contraindicated (pacemaker or implanted defibrillator-dependent) or those who have previously failed radiofrequency denervation despite analgesic benefit from IA injections.

Functional Anatomy

The lumbar facet joint is a true synovial joint containing a hyaline cartilaginous surface, a synovial membrane, and a fibrous capsule. The joint space is small, with a volume of about 1–1.5 mL. In contrast to the upper lumbar facet joints, the lower facet joints (in particular, the L5/S1 joint) have an orientation that is significantly more oblique to the anteroposterior sagittal plane. Entry into the joint space may thus require a greater oblique tilt when utilizing fluoroscopy for IA injection. Each facet joint is innervated by the medial branches of the dorsal rami from the same vertebral level and from the vertebral level above. For example, the L3–L4 facet joint receives dual innervations from L2 and L3 medial branches, which are typically blocked on the transverse processes of L3 and L4, respectively (Fig. 46.1). The medial branches of the L1–L4 dorsal rami run in a similar fashion across the groove formed by the junction of the transverse process and SAP of the vertebral level below (e.g., L3 crosses the transverse process of L4) beneath the mamillo-accessory ligament before innervating the multifidus muscle, interspinous ligament, and the periosteum of the neural arch. The L5 dorsal ramus differs from the other lumbar dorsal rami in that it (and not its medial branch) runs along the junction of the sacral ala and superior articular process of the sacrum and gives off the medial branch only as it reaches the caudal aspect of the L5–S1 facet joint.

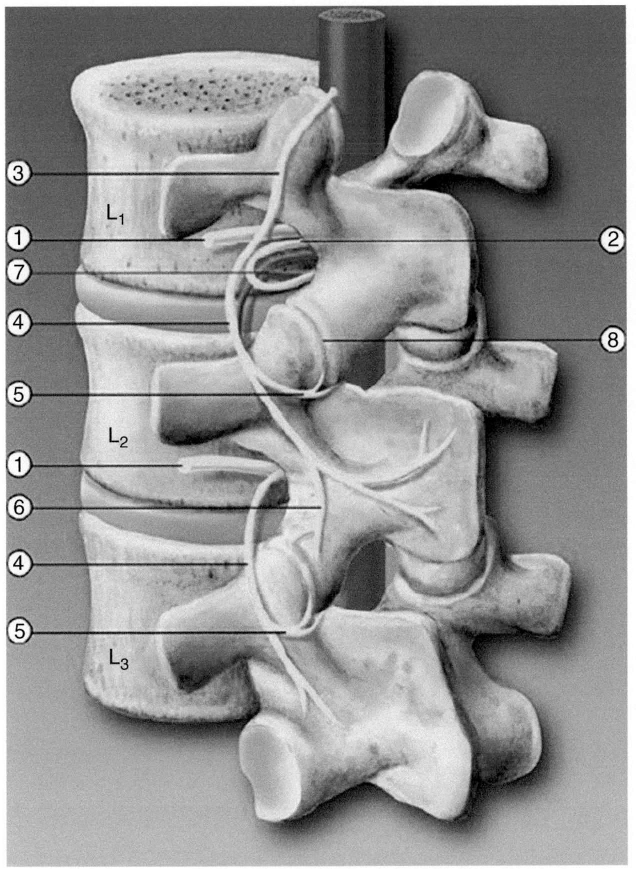

Fig. 46.1 Anatomical diagram of the facet joint: dual neural supply of the facet joint. Oblique parasagittal view of overlapping segmental innervation of the facet joint. (*1*) Ventral branch of spinal nerve, (*2*) dorsal branch of spinal nerve, (*3*) ascendant branch of dorsal ramus, (*4*) medial branch of dorsal ramus, (*5*) distal branch of medial ramus to facet joint, (*6*) proximal branch of medial ramus to facet joint, (*7*) posterior ramus (sinuvertebral nerve of Luschka), (*8*) facet joint. (Reproduced with permission from Danilo Jankovic)

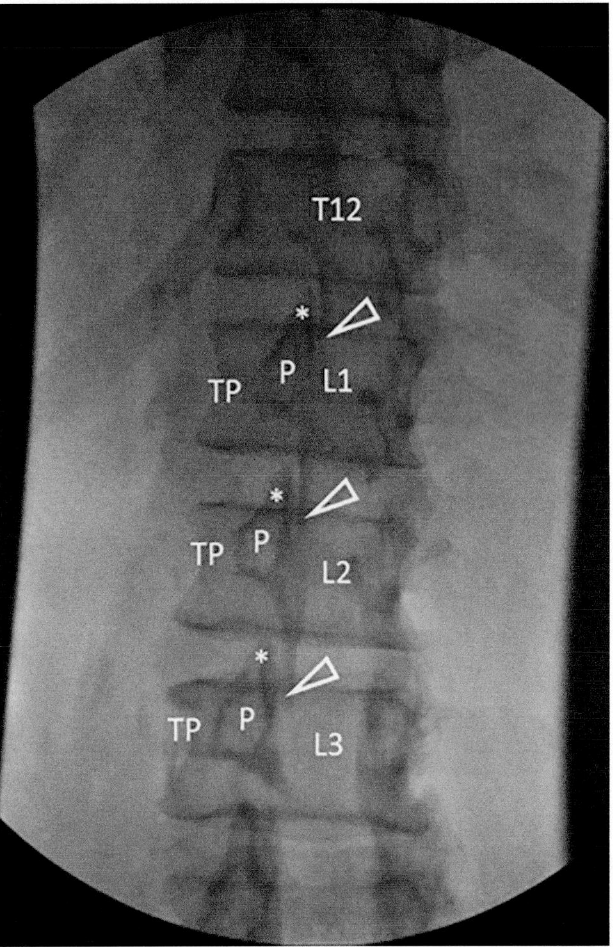

Fig. 46.2 A "scotty dog" view of the lumbar spine achieved with a left oblique tilt of the fluoroscopy arm. Note the superior endplates of the first and the second vertebral body are squared. Empty arrow—facet joint. Asterisk—superior articulating process. *TP* transverse process, *P* pedicle

Technique

Lumbar Facet Joint Innervation Blocks

Fluoroscopy-Guided Technique

The patient is placed in a prone position on a fluoroscopy (C-arm) table with a pillow under the pelvis for comfort and to obliterate the lumbar lordosis. The technique for the blockade of L1–L4 medial branches is the same. The first step is to count the appropriate level. This is usually done from the T12 level, or alternatively from the lumbosacral junction, taking into account anatomical differences with either sacralization of L5 or lumbarization of the S1. Once the appropriate vertebral level is identified, the superior end plate of the target vertebral body is squared, i.e., the anterior and posterior silhouettes of the superior end plate should be at the same level. This is usually achieved by a caudal tilt of the C-arm for the upper lumbar levels and a cephalad tilt for the lower lumbar levels. The C-arm is then rotated ipsilaterally to the side of injection to obtain an oblique view. In this view, the outline of the "scotty dog" is clearly evident (Fig. 46.2). The target is the junction of the superior border of transverse process with the superior articular process (Fig. 46.3).

Alternatively, another target point has been described (Fig. 46.2), which is the midpoint between the mamillo-accessory notch and the target point described above. This target point has been shown to minimize the inadvertent spread of injectate into the intervertebral foramen or the epidural space. For blocking the L5 dorsal ramus, the target point is the ala of the sacrum at the base of the superior articular process of the sacrum in an anteroposterior view (Fig. 46.4). The ipsilateral oblique tilt of the C-arm is sometimes limited (especially in males) by the large iliac crest that can superimpose on the target in oblique views.

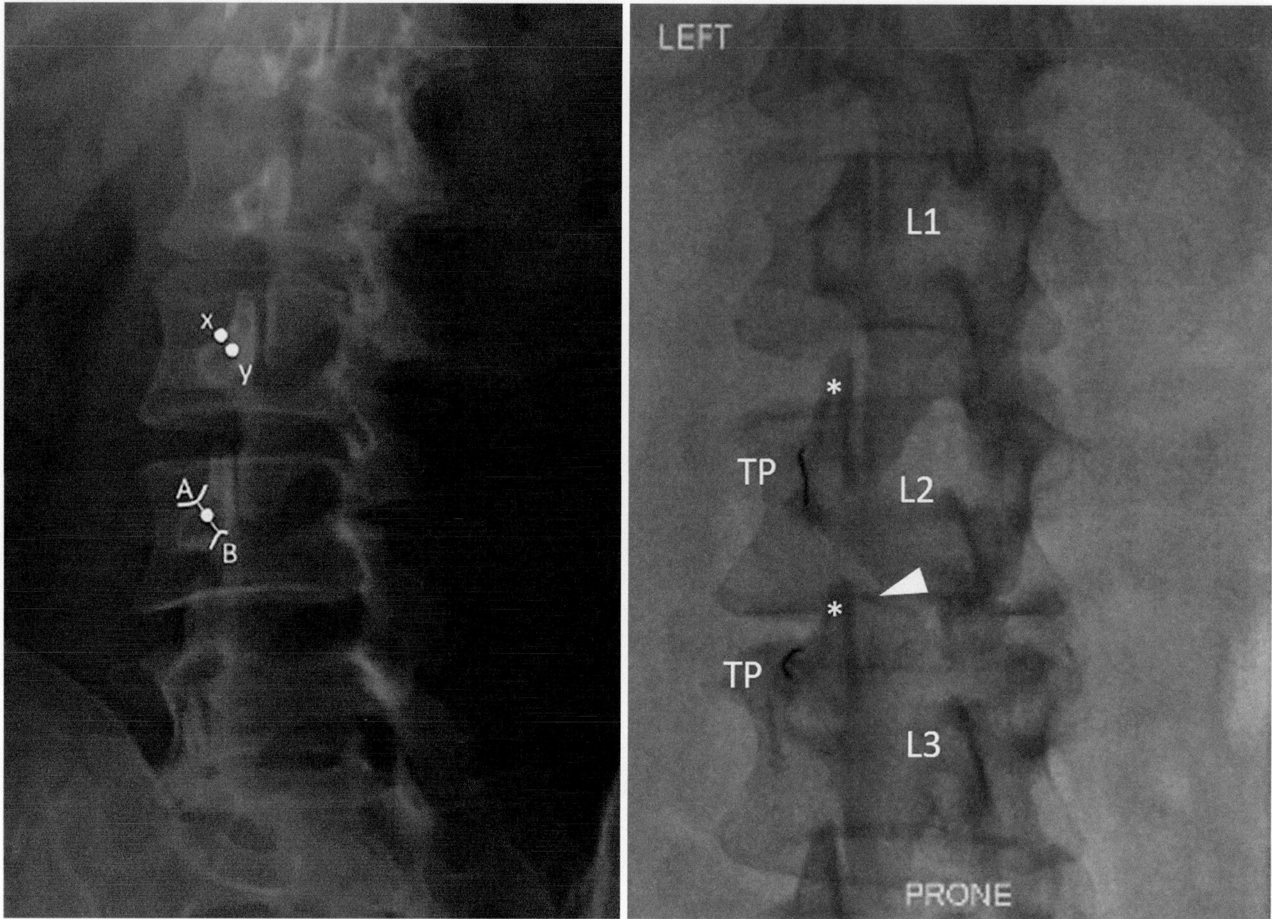

Fig. 46.3 Left. Two targets for the medial branches (*x* and *y*). *X*-junction of superior articular process and transverse process. *Y*-midpoint of *A* and *B*, where *A* is junction of superior articular process and transverse process and *B* is mamillo-accessory notch. Right. Appropriate sites for needle placement at the junction of the left second and third lumbar superior articular processes and transverse processes for performing medial branch blocks of the innervation to the left L2–3 facet joint. (Reproduced with permission from Philip Peng Educational Series)

A 22-gauge spinal needle (length 8 or 12 cm, depending on the patient's body habitus) is inserted following minimal LA infiltration of the skin. Once the bone is contacted at the target point, an anteroposterior fluoroscopic view should be obtained to check appropriate position of the needle tip. A lateral view can also be obtained to ensure the needle tip is not positioned anterior to the base of the SAP. This is followed by injection of a small amount of contrast (0.2 mL) to detect possible venous uptake (injection under live or digital subtraction fluoroscopic imaging has more sensitivity for detecting intravascular placement of the needle tip but it results in a greater exposure to radiation). A small volume of 0.5 mL of LA is then injected if the contrast appears in an appropriate location (Fig. 46.5) and if there is no evidence of venous uptake.

Ultrasound-Guided Technique

The patient is positioned the same as for the fluoroscopy-guided technique. The target point for the medial branch (or dorsal ramus) is the junction between the superior articular process and transverse process. A curvilinear ultrasound probe (2–5 MHz) is used to first obtain a parasagittal oblique view. In this scan, both the sacrum and lamina can be seen and the vertebral level of interest is identified by counting (Fig. 46.6). The probe is then moved laterally to visualize the transverse process (Fig. 46.7). Once the appropriate level is identified, the probe is rotated to a transverse orientation to obtain a short-axis view of the spine to identify the transverse process and the corresponding SAP (the two-step sign). The probe is moved in cephalad direction until the cephalad aspect of the transverse process disappears. The

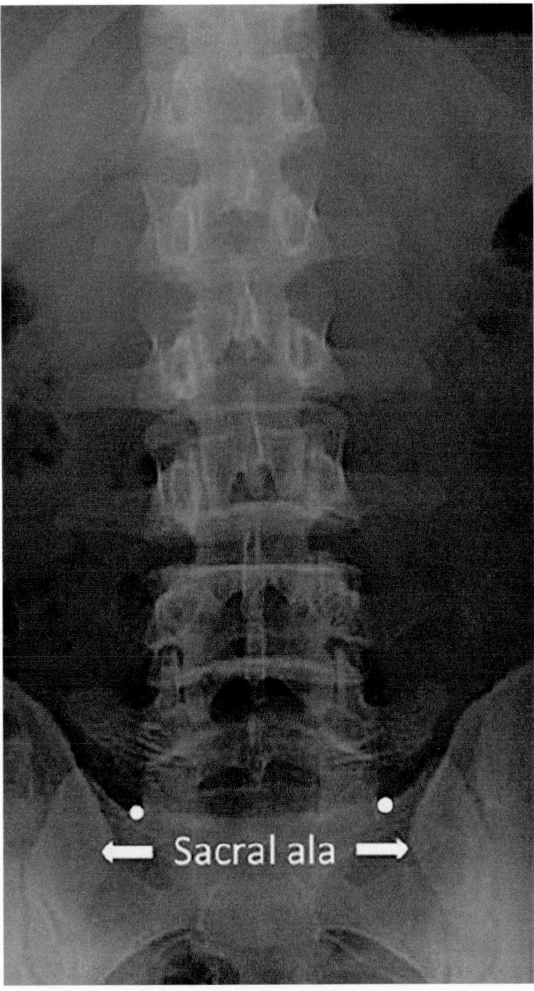

Fig. 46.4 The target points for L5 dorsal rami was indicated by the white dots, which are at the junction of the ala of the sacrum with the base of the superior articular process of the sacrum. (Reproduced with permission from Philip Peng Educational Series)

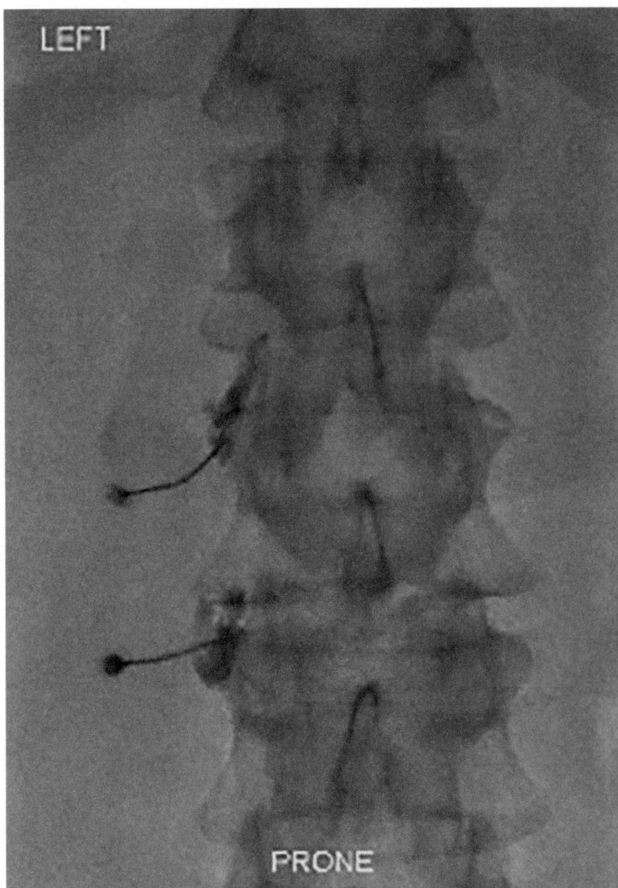

Fig. 46.5 A fluoroscopy image of injected contrast following placement of a needle for a medial branch block

target point for the injection (junction of the superior edge of the transverse process with the SAP) is confirmed when this part of the transverse process reappears on sliding the probe caudally (Fig. 46.8).

A 22-gauge spinal needle is inserted in-plane using a lateral-to-medial approach to access the target. The entire shaft of the inserted needle should be visible in this view as it is advanced toward the target. Once this is achieved, the probe is turned back to a parasagittal orientation to ensure the needle is at the cephalad part of the transverse process (Fig. 46.9). It is important to appreciate this is an out-of-plane view and the needle will be visualized as a hyperechoic dot when the ultrasound beam encounters the needle. Jiggling the needle with a small but rapid to-and-fro motion can help to identify the location of its tip.

The L5 dorsal ramus is usually difficult to assess with ultrasound guidance because of the ilium. To access this structure, obtain a paramedian sagittal view to determine the cephalad part of the sacrum (Fig. 46.10a). Then rotate the transducer to a transverse orientation but with the medial part slightly cephalad to the lateral part (Fig. 46.10b). This results in a view with all the necessary bony landmarks in a continuous hyperechoic line. They are (from medial to lateral) spinous process (SP) of L5, facet joint (FJ), sacral ala (SA), and iliac crest (IC). The junction between the SA and the sacral SAP is the target for the injection. To ensure the transducer is at the right location, simply move the transducer in cephalad position (Fig. 46.10c). A discontinuation of the hyperechoic shadow will be appreciated (line arrows). The needle is inserted with an oblique out-of-plane (arrow) approach with the tip (asterisk) at the upper edge of the sacral ala (SA) medial to the iliac crest (IC) in the groove just lateral to the SAP of the L5/S1 facet joint (FJ) (Fig. 46.11).

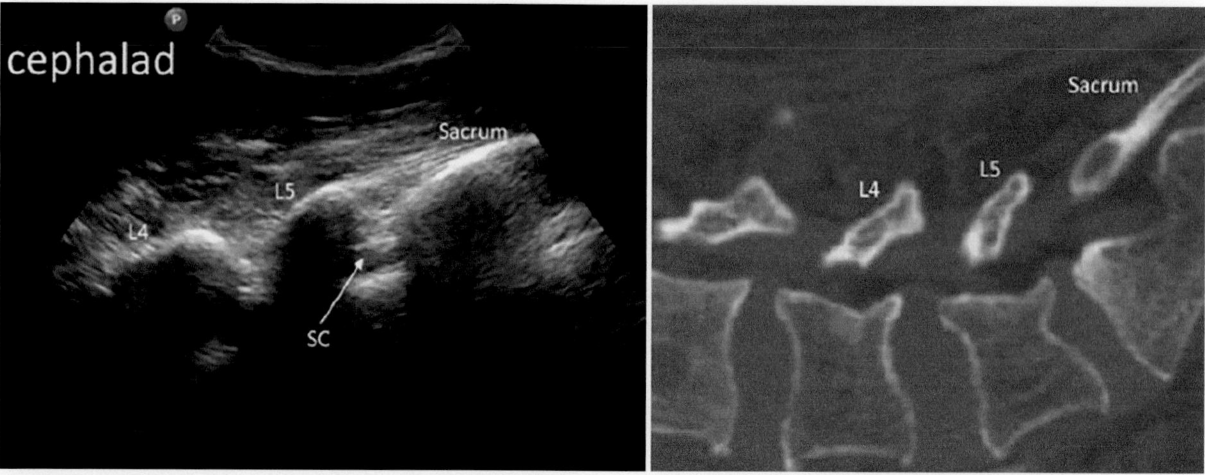

Fig. 46.6 Parasagittal oblique ultrasound view of the spine at the lumbosacral junction on the left and the corresponding magnetic resonance image on the right. *SC* spinal canal. L4 and L5 are the lamina of the fourth and the fifth lumbar vertebra, respectively. (Reproduced with permission from Philip Peng Educational Series)

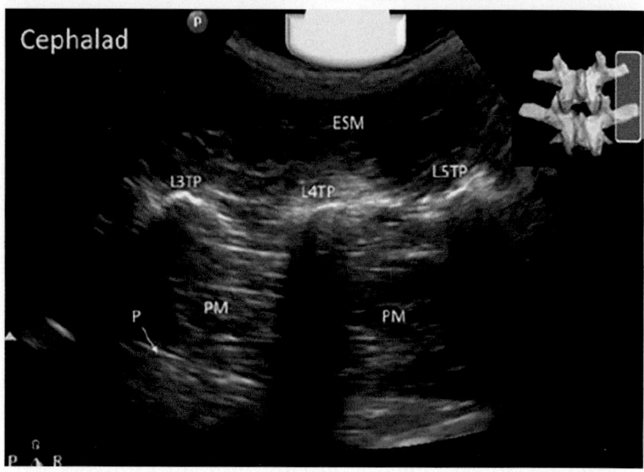

Fig. 46.7 Parasagittal ultrasound scan of the transverse process. The insert shows the position of the ultrasound probe. *ESM* erector spinae muscle, *PM* psoas muscle, *L3TP* transverse process of L3. (Reproduced with permission from Philip Peng Educational Series)

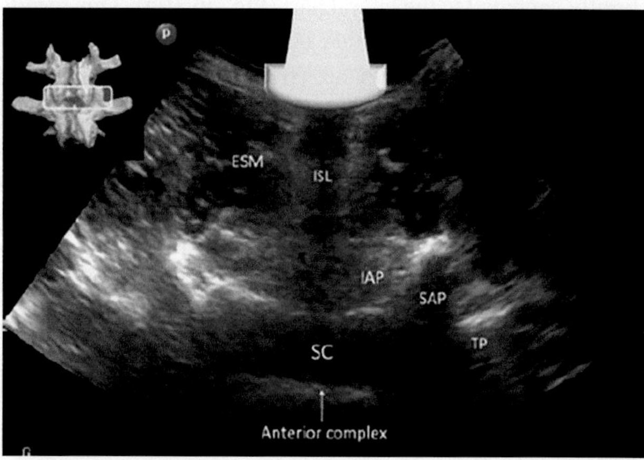

Fig. 46.8 Transverse scan of the spine at the interlaminar space. The insert showed position of the ultrasound probe. *ISL* interspinous ligament, *ESM* erector spinae muscle, *SAP* superior articular process, *IAP* inferior articular process, *TP* transverse process, *SC* spinal canal. (Reproduced with permission from Philip Peng Educational Series)

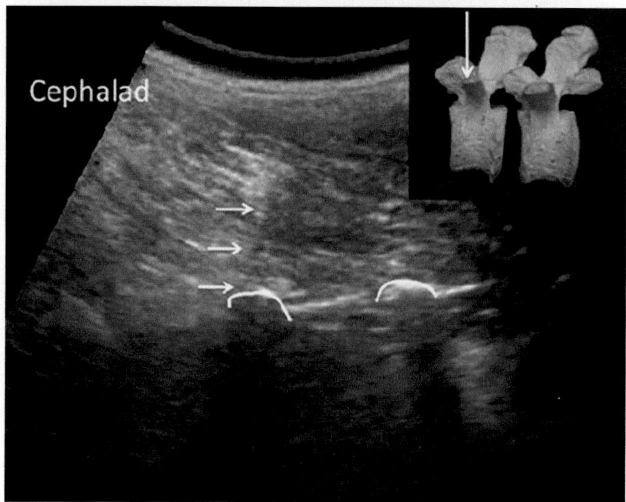

Fig. 46.9 Parasagittal view of the transverse process showing the needle (indicated by the arrows; out-of-plane in this scan) on the cephalad aspect of the transverse process. The transverse process is indicated by the curved lines, and the insert shows the position of the needle. (Reproduced with permission from Philip Peng Educational Series)

Lumbar Facet Joint Intra-Articular Injection

Fluoroscopy-Guided Technique

The patient is positioned as described for the facet medial branch block. An ipsilateral oblique view is obtained until the joint space formed between the articular processes is clearly seen (Fig. 46.12). It may be difficult to visualize the joint cavity if the joint is hypertrophied or if it has an osteophyte across its surface. A 22-gauge spinal needle is then inserted into the apical part of the joint using a coaxial technique. A small amount of contrast (0.2 mL) is injected to confirm intra-articular placement of the needle tip. A volume of 0.5–1 mL injectate containing 20 mg of methylprednisolone or triamcinolone is adequate. In patient with advanced disease, the joint space may be further obliterated, and a periarticular injection may then be performed.

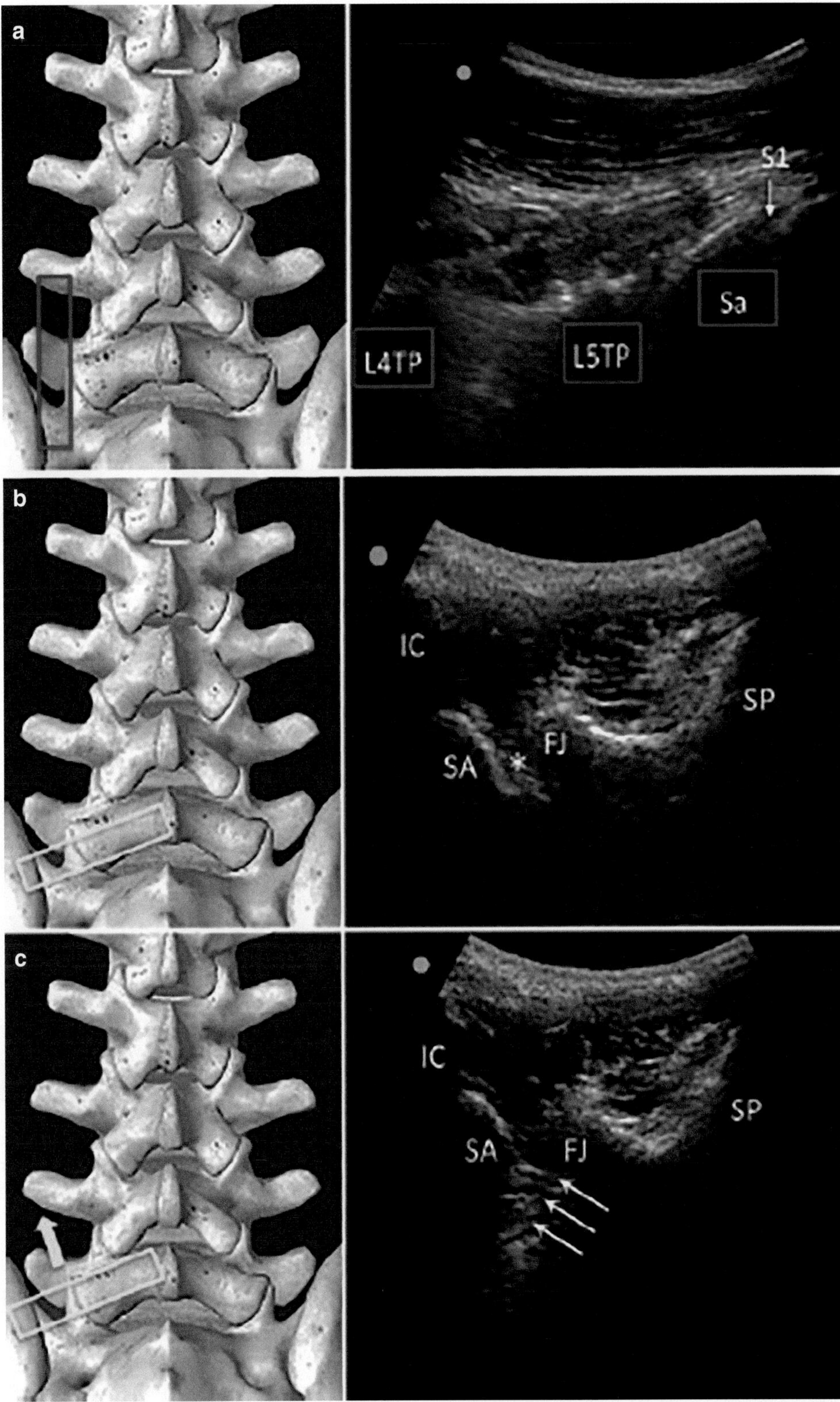

Fig. 46.10 (**a**) Paramedian sagittal transverse process view of the lumbosacaral junction. (**b**) Oblique view of lumbosacral junction. The target is marked by the asterisk, as the junction between sacral ala (SA) and the superior articular process. (**c**) same view as in b but with the. needle inserted in oblique out-of-plane (OOOP) and the entry of the needle is indicated by the needle. TP-transverse process, Sa-sacrum, FJ-facet joint, SP-spinous process, IC-iliac crest. (Reprinted with permission from Philip Peng Educational Series)

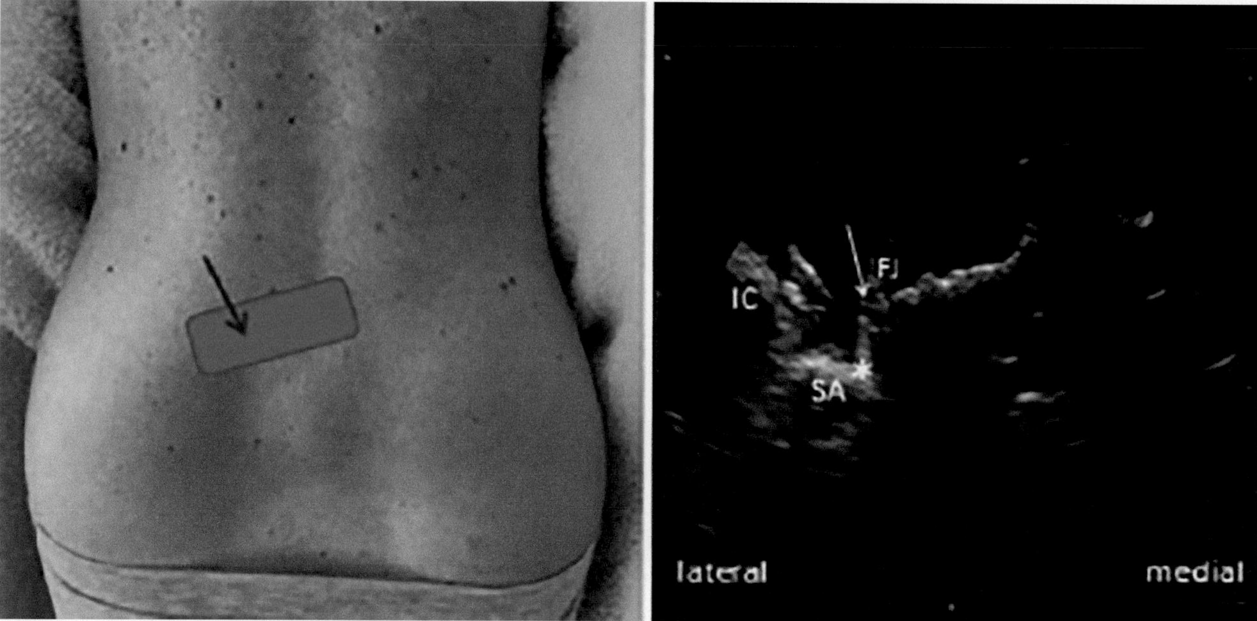

Fig. 46.11 Needle insertion for the L5 dorsal ramus block. (Reprinted with permission from Philip Peng Educational Series)

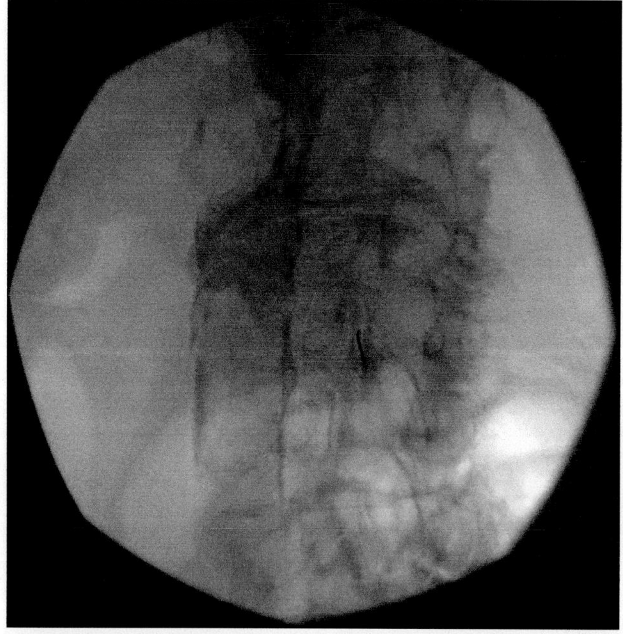

Fig. 46.12 A needle tip placed in a lumbar facet joint cavity for an intra-articular injection

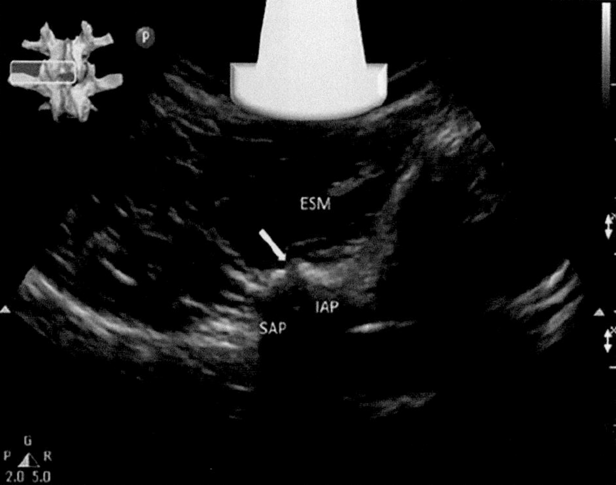

Fig. 46.13 Sonograph shows the facet joint indicated by the bold arrow (left side of the scan is lateral). *ESM* erector spinae muscle, *SAP* superior articular process, *IAP* inferior articular process. The insert showed the position of the probe. (Reproduced with permission from Philip Peng Educational Series)

Ultrasound-Guided Technique

The initial scanning technique is similar to that for blocking the lumbar medial branch. Once the transverse axis scan of the spine shows the transverse process and the superior articular process, the final position of the probe is tilted in cephalad and caudal direction until a joint space opening is clearly seen between the superior and inferior articular process (Fig. 46.13). This is the lateral edge of the first step. A 22-gauge spinal needle is inserted in-plane from a lateral-to-medial direction to access the target. In patients with limited joint space, advancing the needle into the joint space can be difficult, and a periarticular injection is acceptable.

Complications

Vascular Penetration and Injury

The incidence of intravascular positioning of the needle tip during lumbar MBB varies from 3.7% to upward of 20%. Arterial and venous punctures may occur during the procedures, with the latter more difficult to detect by aspiration alone due to the small caliber in comparison to aspirating pressures. Without identification, they may affect the result of the block by producing a false-negative result. Injection of particulate steroids into feeder radicular arteries can result in spinal cord ischemia. Use of a small volume of contrast <0.5 mL is suggested to identify venous injectate. Although real-time fluoroscopy is more sensitive than compared to spot radiographs, digital subtraction angiography is considered the reference standard for vascular uptake. For ultrasound-guided procedures, the presence of vessels should be checked with Power Doppler along the intended needle trajectory and observed in real-time volume spread at the needle tip during injection.

Post-block Numbness or Weakness in the Lower Limb

Transient numbness or weakness may occur following a medial branch block due to spillage of the LA toward the nerve roots that are immediately cephalad and caudad to the target or into the epidural space. This is more likely with largely volumes of injectate. Current recommendations suggest limiting injectate to a maximum of 0.5 mL at each level when performing medial branch blocks.

Joint Rupture

The lumbar facet joint is a tight and limited space, more so in diseased states, with generally a volume of less than 2 mL. Injections greater than 1.5 mL risk rupture of the facet joint capsule and can result in worsening of the pain. In situations where intra-articular pressures are high or limited injectate is administered, pericapsular or periarticular injection has also been found to be just as effective.

Practical Tips

- Reviewing relevant imaging before performing procedures on lumbar facet joints is essential for identifying aberrant anatomy. This is more relevant for ultrasound-guided injections, because of the limited view available during the procedure. Lumbarization or sacralization of the vertebra and the presence of spondylolisthesis can affect the fidelity of localizing the target.
- The combined use of ultrasonography and fluoroscopy may be useful in patients with challenging spine anatomy (e.g., severe facet arthritis, scoliosis, previous instrumentation) to ensure the appropriate site is targeted.
- Optimal positioning of the patient is vital for achieving good fluoroscopy and ultrasound images. Ensure the target area is centered on the screen and lumbar lordosis is minimized (commonly with a pillow) underneath the abdomen. This will reduce any further angulations and tilt that may be required to square the vertebral level of interest.
- Specifically for ultrasound-guided lumbar medial branch blocks, ensure that the most cephalad part of the transverse process is visualized by moving the transducer further cephalad over the intertransverse space to identify the psoas muscle and intertransverse ligament. Mistaking the intertransverse ligament as transverse process may lead to needle entry into the neuroforamen and trauma to the ventral nerve root.

Literature Review

Use of ultrasound for neuraxial procedures: Ultrasound may be useful in patients in whom radiation exposure may be associated with potential harm (e.g., pregnancy) or in patients with a normal body mass index when radiographic or radiological imaging is unavailable.

However, apart from a steep learning curve, the chief limitation to use of ultrasound for procedures on the lumbar spine is the limited visualization of the lumbar neuraxis, particularly in patients with a high body mass index and existing instrumentation. Other drawbacks of using ultrasound include the possibility of targeting an incorrect segment without fluoroscopic confirmation, as well as inadvertent vascular uptake.

Patients on anticoagulant therapy: Both medial branch and intra-articular facet joint blocks are procedure classifieds as low risk as per ASRA and SIS guidelines. It is currently recommended that non-heparin anticoagulants be continued in the peri-procedure period for patients undergoing either lumbar medial branch or facet joint blocks, especially in patients at high risk of thromboembolic complications.

Suggested Reading

Carette S, Marcoux S, Truchon R, et al. A controlled trial of corticosteroid injections into facet joints for chronic low back pain. N Engl J Med. 1991;325:1002–7.

Cohen SP, Moon JY, Brummett CM, et al. Medial branch blocks or intra-articular injections as a prognostic tool before lumbar facet radiofrequency denervation: a multicenter, case-control study. Reg Anesth Pain Med. 2015;40:376–83.

Cohen SP, Doshi TL, Constantinescu OC, et al. Effectiveness of lumbar facet joint blocks and their predictive value before radiofrequency denervation: the facet treatment study (FACTS). Anesthesiology. 2018;129:517–35.

Cohen SP, Bhaskar A, Bhatia A, et al. Consensus practice guidelines on interventions for lumbar facet joint pain from a multispecialty, international working group. Reg Anesth Pain Med. 2020;45:424–67.

Fairbank JCT, Park WM, McCall IW, et al. Apophyseal injection of local anesthetic as a diagnostic aid in primary low-back pain syndromes. Spine. 1981;6:598–605.

Falco FJE, Manchikanti L, Datta S, et al. An update of the systematic assessment of the diagnostic accuracy of lumbar facet joint nerve blocks. Pain Physician. 2012;15:E869–907.

Greher M, Moriggl B, Peng PWH, et al. Ultrasound-guided approach for L5 dorsal ramus block and fluoroscopic evaluation in unpreselected cadavers. Reg Anesth Pain Med. 2015;40:713–7.

International Spine Intervention Society. Lumbar medial branch blocks. In: Bogduk N, editor. Practice guidelines for spinal diagnostic and treatment procedures. 2nd ed. San Francisco, CA: International Spine Intervention Society; 2013. p. 457–88.

Kennedy DJ, Mattie R, Scott Hamilton A, et al. Detection of intravascular injection during lumbar medial branch blocks: a comparison of aspiration, live fluoroscopy, and digital subtraction technology. Pain Med. 2016;17:pnv073–6.

Manchikanti L, Malla Y, Wargo BW, et al. Complications of fluoroscopically directed facet joint nerve blocks: a prospective evaluation of 7,500 episodes with 43,000 nerve blocks. Pain Physician. 2012;15:E143–50.

Narouze S, Benzon HT, Provenzano D, et al. Interventional spine and pain procedures in patients on antiplatelet and anticoagulant medications (second edition): guidelines from the American Society of regional anesthesia and pain medicine, the European Society of regional anaesthesia and pain therapy, the American Academy of pain medicine, the International neuromodulation Society, the North American neuromodulation Society, and the world Institute of pain. Reg Anesth Pain Med. 2018;43:225–62.

Purcell-Jones G, Pither CE, Justins DM. Paravertebral somatic nerve block: a clinical, radiographic, and computed tomographic study in chronic pain patients. Anesth Analg. 1989;68:32–9.

Rauch S, Kasuya Y, Turan A, et al. Ultrasound-guided lumbar medial branch block in obese patients: a fluoroscopically confirmed clinical feasibility study. Reg Anesth Pain Med. 2009;34:340–2.

Schwarzer AC, Wang S-C, O'Driscoll D, et al. The ability of computed tomography to identify a painful zygapophysial joint in patients with chronic low back pain. Spine. 1995;20:907–12.

Stojanovic MP, Sethee J, Mohiuddin M, et al. MRI analysis of the lumbar spine: can it predict response to diagnostic and therapeutic facet procedures? Clin J Pain. 2010;26:110–5.

Lumbar Percutaneous Facet Denervation

47

Robert Jan Stolker, Hans van Suijlekom, André van Zundert, and Gerbrand Groen

Contents

General Consideration

The technique of lumbar facet denervation was first described by Shealy in 1974. Later several authors modified this technique. Anatomical studies revealed more exactly the place where the block had to be performed. In this chapter the most common technique will be described using fluoroscopy and bony landmarks. The procedure can be performed in an outpatient setting with the patient awake. Most patients are sufficiently cooperative. Administration of a sedative is rarely required. As the innervation of the joint and other structures in the dorsal compartment is regarded as two-leveled, the procedure should be performed at two levels. Consequently, considering that one vertebra has two facet joints, one with the superior and one with the inferior articular process, when both facet joints are involved, three subsequent medial branches should be targeted. The procedure can be performed uni- or bilaterally.

R. J. Stolker (✉)
Department of Anesthesiology, Erasmus University Medical Center, Rotterdam, The Netherlands
e-mail: r.stolker@erasmusmc.nl

H. van Suijlekom
Department of Anesthesiology, ICU & Pain Therapy, Catharina-ziekenhuis, Eindhoven, The Netherlands

A. van Zundert
Department of Anaesthesia & Perioperative Medicine, Royal Brisbane & Women's Hospital, Brisbane, QLD, Australia

G. Groen
Pain Center, University Medical Center Groningen, University of Groningen, Haren, The Netherlands

Indications

In the literature there is doubt about the existence of a specific facet syndrome but in Table 47.1 some signs and symptoms are listed, suggesting pain originating from facet joints.

Uni- or bilateral pain lasting longer than 3–6 months not reacting on physical therapy and other conservative management could be an indication for percutaneous facet denervation (PFD). In the absence of a specific facet syndrome, most authors advocate to perform a diagnostic block prior to a PFD. The diagnostic block can be in the form of a medial branch block or an intra-articular block with local anesthetic. The volume of local anesthetic should be limited to 0.5 mL

D. Jankovic, P. Peng (eds.), *Regional Nerve Blocks in Anesthesia and Pain Therapy*,
https://doi.org/10.1007/978-3-030-88727-8_47

Table 47.1 Possible signs and symptoms of facet pain in the lumbar region

• Back pain with or without irradiation to the groin, buttock, leg, and sometimes abdomen
• Pain aggravated by rest in any posture (standing, sitting, lying in bed)
• Pain relieved by movement
• Radiculopathy is absent (no neurological deficit)
• Pain should not radiate below the knee
• Morning stiffness
• Awakening by turning in bed
• Pain on anteflexion and/or rotation of the spine
• Paravertebral tenderness

Table 47.2 Contraindications

• Sensory loss
• Lack of cooperativeness
• Bleeding disorders or use of anticoagulants
• Signs of local infection
• Signs of local malignancy
• Presence of osteosynthesis material
• Allergy to local anesthetics

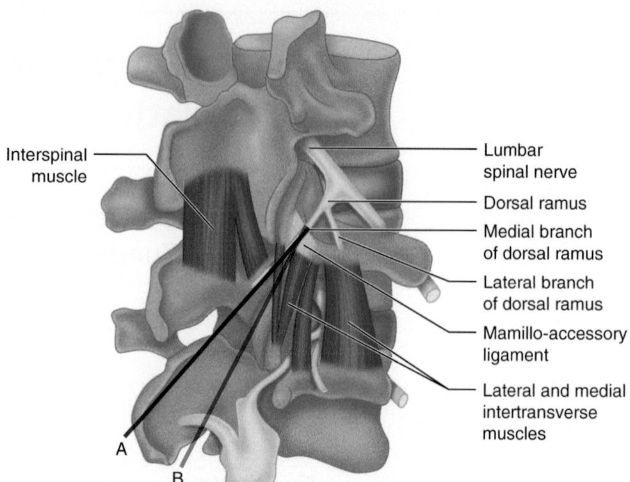

Fig. 47.1 Schematic drawing of dorsal lumbar branches and adjacent spinal muscles. (1) lumbar spinal nerve; (2) dorsal ramus; (3^1) medial branch of dorsal ramus; (3^2) lateral branch of dorsal ramus; (4) mamillo-accessory ligament; (5, 6) lateral and medial intertransverse muscles; (7) interspinal muscle. The blue lines depict a parallel (A) and near-parallel (B) insertion of the electrodes. (Cohen et al. 2020. *Redrawn after Paturet* (Paturet G. Traité d'Anatomie Humaine, Tome IV, Système Nerveux. Masson et Cie, Paris 1964)

per level in order to achieve a block as selective as possible. The risk of low volume blocks is a lower sensitivity. In the literature a medial branch block is considered to have more predictive value than an intra-articular joint block. Some authors advocate the use of double blocks with local anesthetic with a different duration of action or control blocks with saline in order to rule out placebo response. This is applied in some trials but not common in daily practice. Some patients benefit for a long time after injection of local anesthetic.

Some authors adjust steroids in order to achieve a longer lasting effect of the test procedure, since adding steroids would reduce any coexisting inflammation. Furthermore, the steroids prolong the action of local anesthetic by several hours. Radiological findings per se, such as facet arthritis, are no indication for a PFD. Contraindications are shown in (Table 47.2).

Anatomy

The goal of a lumbar percutaneous facet denervation procedure is to block the medial branch of the dorsal ramus of the spinal nerve (Fig. 47.1). When the dorsal and ventral roots come together, the spinal nerve is formed, which splits up into a ventral and a dorsal ramus. This dorsal ramus divides into a medial and a lateral ramus (=branch). The dorsal or posterior ramus supplies the so-called dorsal compartment of the back, which consists of structures of the back situated behind the intervertebral foramen. This dorsal compartment contains muscles, ligaments, blood vessels, and the facet joints. The facet or zygapophyseal joints are joints between the inferior articular process of a vertebra and the superior articular process of the vertebra below. Lumbar facet joints are small joints located in pairs on the back of the spine, providing stability and guiding motion in the lower back. These joints at the dorsal side of the spine form together with the intervertebral disk at the ventral side, the three moving parts of a motion segment.

The facet joints are innervated by medial branches of the dorsal ramus from the corresponding level and the super adjacent level. As such, the facet joint L5–S1 is innervated by the dorsal rami L4 and L5. Furthermore, the medial branches innervate the skin, ligaments, and lumbar muscles as well, whereas at level L5 the medial branch mostly consists of sensory fibers. The lateral branches innervate muscles. The advocated manner to block the medial branches is in the groove between the superior articular process and the transverse process (Fig. 47.1). The anatomy of the back and the innervation of the posterior compartment are described elsewhere more extensively (see reference 1 in the reference section).

If the joints become painful, they may cause pain in the low back, abdomen, buttocks, groins, or legs. The lumbar zygapophyseal joints are a potential source of low back pain and referred leg pain. However, there are doubts about the existence of a specific facet syndrome. This pain also may originate from other structures (muscles and ligaments) situated in the dorsal compartment.

Table 47.3 Equipment for the procedure

• 2–4 10 cm 22 G radiofrequency (RF) needles with 5 mm blank tip
• Local infiltration (e.g., lidocaine 1–2%)
• Thermocouple 10 cm
• Radiofrequency lesion generator
• Ground plate
• Connecting wires

Technique

This procedure should be performed by an experienced anesthesiologist specialized in invasive pain medicine or under his/her supervision. The equipment is summarized in Table 47.3. The patient is positioned in the prone position on a special table allowing the use of fluoroscopy.

The fluoroscope is directed in anteroposterior view. Sometimes a 5–10° oblique view is needed to obtain more reliable pictures. There is some debate about the angle between the needle and the medial branch. There is debate about the angle of insertion. In the ideal situation the target position of the needle is assumed to be parallel to the medial branch. However, the target position is not always visible in anteroposterior view. As a more lateral approach leads to a less parallel position, the angle of insertion should be as minimal as possible. The insertion place is marked at the skin by using a plastic calliper with a radiopaque ring, which should be placed at the site of the projection of the junction of the transverse and superior articular process. After disinfection of the skin, the needle is inserted following the local infiltration of the skin with 1 mL lidocaine 1–2%, and its position is controlled by fluoroscopic viewing. The direction of the needle is, if necessary, corrected and the needle is advanced until bone contact is made. After correcting the needle position slightly, the tip of the needle is advanced just a little more, keeping bone contact. The depth of the needle is controlled by a fluoroscopic lateral view. The projection of the needle may not be ventral to the dorsal rim of the intervertebral foramen (Figs. 47.2, 47.3, and 47.4).

After obtaining the correct anatomical position, the stylet of the needle is removed, and a thermocouple electrode inserted. The electrode has to be connected to the lesion generator. The ground plate is connected. Stimulation with a 50 Hz current is performed, and the patient is asked to warn if a tingling feeling laterocaudal to the insertion site of the needle and/or at the buttock will be felt. Stimulation threshold must be less than 1 V. The lower the threshold the better the outcome, as the value of the threshold reflects the distance to the nerve. A tingling feeling in the leg refers to a too anterior position of the needle (too close to the spinal nerve), which has to be withdrawn. The same stimulation procedure can be done with a 2 Hz current. As the medial branch is a mixed nerve (possible exception L5), a response at the same threshold (or 0.1 V higher) is expected. Local contractions will occur. Contractions of the leg are a sign of a too anterior position, close to the spinal nerve. A threshold for motor response of the leg at 2 V or less, must never be accepted.

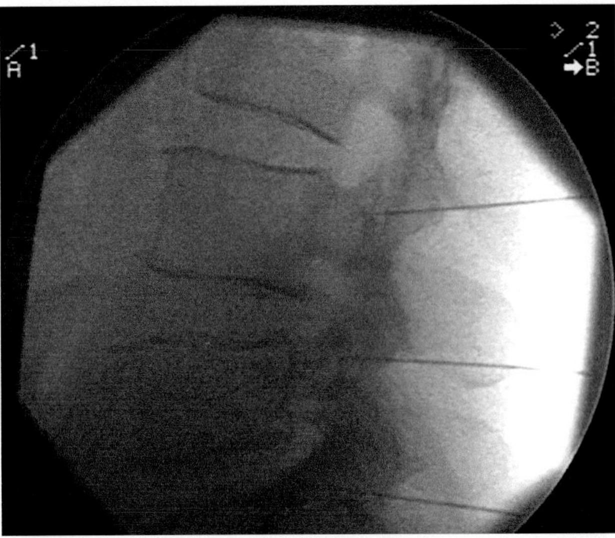

Fig. 47.2 Lumbar facet denervation (X-ray lateral view)

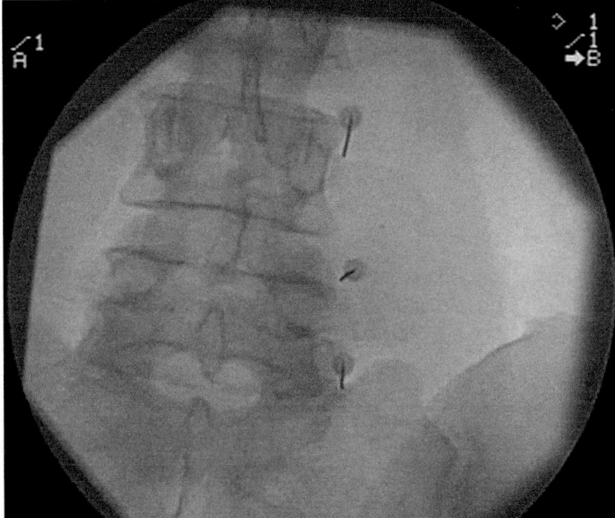

Fig. 47.3 Lumbar facet denervation (X-ray anteroposterior view)

If these thresholds are met, 0.5 mL lidocaine 1% (some recommend ≤0.5 mL) must be injected after careful aspiration in each needle in order to anesthetize the site of the thermolesion.

After a waiting period of 1–2 min, the radiofrequency lesion at 80 °C for 60 s can be made. In the thoracic spine a similar technique can be used. The position of the needle is somewhat more lateral compared to the lumbar procedure.

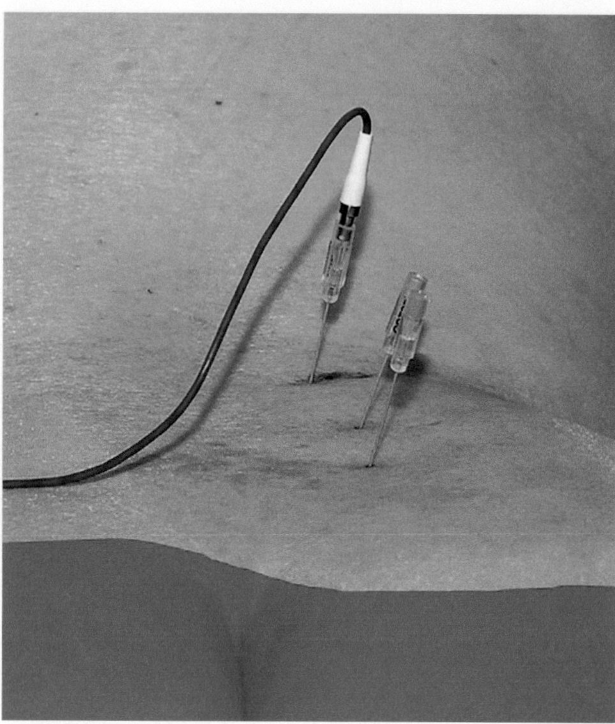

Fig. 47.4 Lumbar facet denervation: positioning needles L4–L5–S1

Instructions to Patients

Patients have to give their (written) informed consent. If patients are using acetylsalicylic acid or other thrombocyte aggregation inhibitors, they are informed to stop 5 days before the procedure. In case of the use of coumarin derivates, the intake of these drugs should be interrupted and the INR controlled before the procedure. An INR of 1.8 or less is appropriate.

Patients are advised to take a light meal before the procedure. Diabetic patients should not change their habits. Intake of food is free after the procedure. Because of possible temporary leg numbness and/or weakness, it is recommended the patients stay in the hospital at least 1 h following the procedure. Sometimes discharge must be postponed if the patient is unable to walk properly. In all cases the patient has to be driven home accompanied by a competent adult and they are not allowed to participate in the traffic (e.g., drive a car) or take important decisions during the day of operation for legal and liability reasons.

Complications and Side Effects

The main complication is postoperative pain. Not only pain of the needle lasting for a few days but also serious burning pain may occur in 20% of the patients. Patients should be informed that they can experience pain 7–9 days after the procedure, which can last for a couple of weeks. This pain will subside within 4–6 weeks. Bruising and hematomas at the back occur in a low percentage and are rarely serious. Neurological damage is very rare if the positioning and stimulation have been performed carefully but local numbness may infrequently occur despite a correct technique. The procedure has three preventive moments avoiding neurological deficits: (1) the lateral view (although not completely reliable), (2) electrostimulation, and (3) the injection of 0.5 mL or less lidocaine 1% is too small to anesthetize a spinal nerve when the electrode is accidentally placed too close. Sometimes a leg is numb and/or weak after the procedure due to overflow of the local anesthetic. This will subside spontaneously within a few hours.

Literature Review

Outcome

A recent meta-analysis (including eight studies with 303 patients) shows positive results on short term but limited results on longer term. According to the authors, most studies were of low quality, mainly due to heterogeneity. Inclusion criteria and the use of medial branch or intra-articular blocks with local anesthetics as selection for the procedure are still subject of discussion. Some authors use single test blocks; others double blocks whereas others perform no blocks at all as selection for the PFD. Their patient selection is fully based on clinical signs and symptoms.

Furthermore, technical differences, such as the exact positioning, angle of insertion of the needles, size of the electrodes (larger needles may cause a higher success rate and longer duration but also increase the risk of side effects) making one or more lesions, applied temperature and exposure time, use of electrical stimulation (sensory), are still subject of debate and may be the cause of variable and differing outcomes. Finally, in the studies up to now, also criteria for success (VAS-score, use of medication, inability scales, global perceived effect, or combinations of these) are not equivalent, which hampers a reliable comparison of results.

Technical Issues

At present the main parameters that are considered to increase the efficacy rate of radiofrequency lumbar facet denervation are patient selection and procedural factors. Which patients are to benefit from the procedure? In this regard, it is important to emphasize that pain derived from the locomotor apparatus is relayed on a manner similar to visceral pain, i.e., as pain referred to areas corresponding to the spinal cord segments where the nociceptive input is

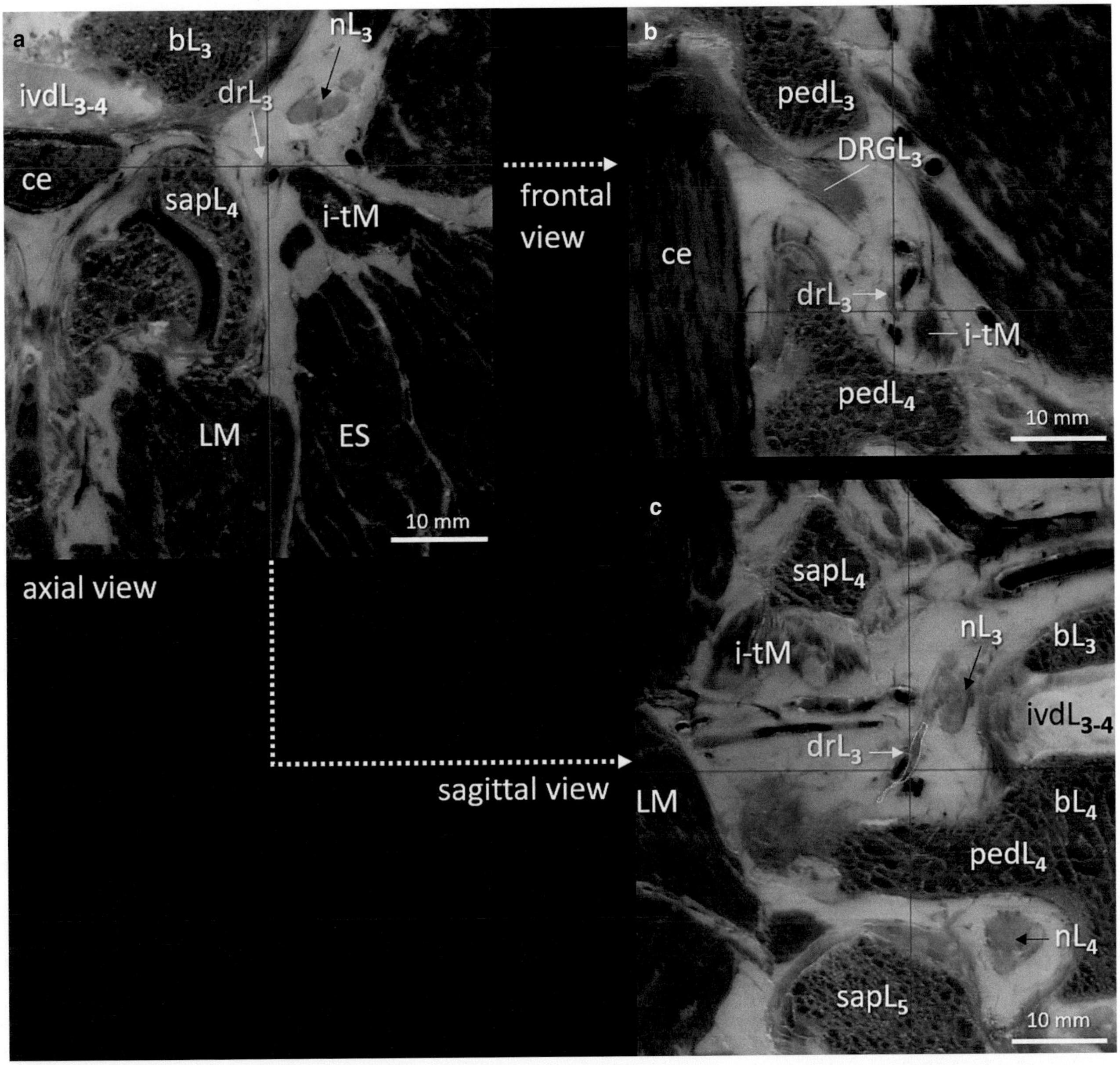

Fig. 47.5 Detailed views of digitized anatomical cross-sections of the spine in the three orthogonal planes *within the same* specimen, i.e., (**a**) axial, original; (**b**) frontal, reconstructed; and (**c**) sagittal, reconstructed. The small red lines depict the level of each cross-section, and the dorsal ramus of L3 (drL3) is highlighted in yellow. Section A is at the lowest part of the intervertebral foramen L3–L4 and shows the third lumbar spinal nerve (nL3) distal to the dorsal root ganglion (DRGL3). *bL3, bL4* body L3, L4, *ce* cauda equina, *ES* erector spinae, *i-tM* intertransverse muscles, *ivd* intervertebral disc, *LM* lumbar multifidus muscle, *ped* pedicle, *sap* superior articular process. Bar represents 10 mm

received. Because of the multisegmental nerve supply of structures of the spine, the overlap in referral pain areas hinders a precision diagnosis of the pain source. Thus, facetogenic pain may not be easily discriminated from pain of other adjacent locomotor sources.

With regard to the technical procedures, low volume diagnostic blocks with local anesthetics are advocated, single vs. double. However, in a recent paper it is put forward that the credibility of randomized, placebo-controlled blocks is higher than that of randomized, comparative local anesthetic blocks (95% vs. 75%). Furthermore, it is generally assumed that the medial branch of the dorsal ramus of the spinal nerve has a more or less constant trajectory, in which the L1–L4 branches bypass the subjacent transverse process, under the mamillo-accessory ligament (MAL) at the junction of the superior articular process and the root of the transverse process, in a medio-dorsal course. This is also shown in Figs. 47.5 and 47.6 from a digitized series of an anatomically obtained spine of a 43-year-old male, which demonstrate not only the extremely small sizes of the dorsal ramus and its medial branch but also their distance to the adjacent bony structures, which may amount up to 5 mm.

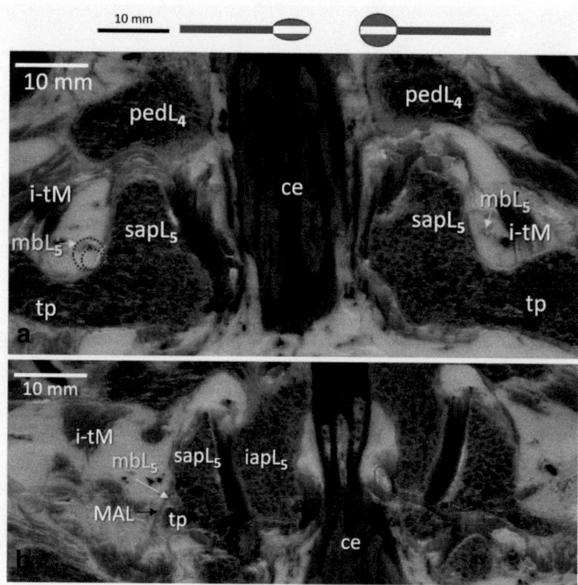

Fig. 47.6 Consecutive frontal views of a digitized spine at the level of L4–L5 showing the more distal trajectory of the medial branch of the dorsal ramus (mbL5) in the groove between superior articular process L5 (sapL5) and the transverse process. It runs between the intertransverse muscles (i-tM) and the bony structures and is accompanied by blood vessels (**a**); more distal it crosses beneath the mamillo-accessory ligament (MAL) (**b**). The figure above depicts the relative size of a RF lesion with a 22 G RF needle with 5 mm tip at 80 °C during 60 s. in egg white (2.9 mm max) and meat (4.5 mm max) according to Buijs et al. 2004; Bogduk et al. 1987; Lau et al. 2004. In (**a**) both lesions are depicted near the medial branch (red dashed lines). *Ce* cauda equina, *iap* inferior articular process. Bar represents 10 mm

In addition, it can be seen that the branches run adjacent to accompanying small blood vessels and lie close to small intrinsic spinal (intertransverse) muscles.

These factors partly may explain the variance in technical denervation of the medial branch when using small diameter RF needle (22 G) and the increase in chance of success with larger lesions as has been reported (some advocate even needle sizes of at least 18 G, enough to hit the target nerve).

Regarding the size of lesion, a RF lesion with a 10 cm RF needle, 5 mm tip, 22 G, and 80 °C for 60 s, the maximum effective radius in vitro (transverse diameter outside needle tip) has been measured as 1.1 ± 0.25 mm in egg white and 1.9 ± 0.30 mm in meat. In case of a 0.7 mm diameter needle, this would mean a cross-sectional diameter of the in vitro lesion 2.9 mm and 4.5 mm max, respectively, as shown above in Fig. 47.6, and at the left in Fig. 47.6a at its highest transverse cross-section near the medial branch.

The same accounts for duration of the lesioning. It was observed that after 60 s, about 87% of the maximal lesion is reached and that a longer duration and a higher temperature will increase the lesion size as well, sometimes even significantly.

Moreover, from the figures it can be deducted that a larger lesion, although advocated for a longer lasting clinical effect, also would include adjacent nonneural tissues, thus potentially increasing adverse effects and leading to unwanted local tissue destruction with unknown long-term side effects.

Conclusion

A selected group of patients with disabling low back pain, not relieved by conservative measures, attributed to the facet joints, can be successfully treated by lumbar facet joint denervation. Adequate patient selection and the use of an accurate lesioning technique under fluoroscopy are essential elements to get good long-term results following radiofrequency denervation. This minimally invasive technique, however, is appealing given the rather easy accessibility of the medial branch of the dorsal ramus and the reassurance of virtually nonexistent complications.

Suggested Reading

Bogduk N, Macintosh J, Marsland A. Technical limitations to the efficacy of radiofrequency neurotomy for spinal pain. Neurosurgery. 1987;20:529–35.

Buijs EJ, van Wijk RMAW, Geurts JWM, Weeseman RR, Stolker RJ, Groen GJ. Radiofrequency lumbar facet denervation: a comparative study to the reproducibility of lesion size following two current radiofrequency techniques. Reg Anesth Pain Med. 2004;29:400–7.

Chappell ME, Lakshman R, Trotter P, Abrahams M, Lee M. Radiofrequency denervation for chronic back pain: a systematic review and meta-analysis. BMJ Open. 2020;10:e035540. https://doi.org/10.1136/bmjopen-2019-035540.

Cohen SP, Huang JHY, Brummett C. Facet joint pain—advances in patient selection and treatment. Nat Rev Rheumatol. 2013;9:101–16.

Cohen SP, Bhaskar A, Bhatia A, et al. Consensus practice guidelines on interventions for lumbar facet joint pain from a multispecialty, international working group. Reg Anesth Pain Med. 2020;45:424–67.

Cosman ER, Dolensky JR, Hoffman RA. Factors that affect radiofrequency heat lesion size. Pain Med. 2014;15:2020–36.

Engel AJ, Bogduk N. Mathematical validation and credibility of diagnostic blocks for spinal pain. Pain Med. 2016;17:1821–8.

Juch JNS, Maas ET, Ostelo RWJG, et al. Effect of radiofrequency denervation in pain intensity among patients with chronic low back pain. The Mint randomized trials. JAMA. 2017;318:68–81.

Lau P, Mercer S, Bogduk N. The surgical anatomy of lumbar medial branch neurotomy (facet denervation). Pain Med. 2005;5:289–98.

Provenzano DA, Watson TW, Somers DL. The interaction between the composition of preinjected fluids and duration of radiofrequency on lesion size. Reg Anesth Pain Med. 2015;40:112–24.

Stolker RJ, Vervest ACM, Groen GJ. Percutaneous facet denervation in chronic thoracic spinal pain. Acta Neurochir. 1993;122:82–90.

Superior Hypogastric Plexus and Ganglion Impar Block

48

Amitabh Gulati, Sushma Bhatnagar, Neal Rakesh, Arash Yousefi, and Carolina Hernandez-Porras

Contents

Superior Hypogastric Plexus Block

Introduction

The visceral afferent branches of the pelvis, the sympathetic efferent fibers of the aortic plexus, and the splanchnic nerves form the superior hypogastric plexus.

A. Gulati (✉)
Memorial Sloan Kettering Cancer Center, Department of Anesthesiology and critical care, New York, NY, USA
e-mail: gulatia@mskcc.org

S. Bhatnagar
Onco-Anesthesia and Palliative Medicine, AIMS, New Delhi, India

N. Rakesh
Anesthesiology and Critical Care, MSKCC, New York, NY, USA

A. Yousefi
Neurology, Mount Sinai Downtown, New York, NY, USA

C. Hernandez-Porras
Palliative Care, Instituto Nacional De Cancerologia, Mexico City, Mexico

Indications

This blockade can be used for either malignant or benign pelvic pains, but studies have shown higher success rate in malignant conditions. Specifically, patients with cervical or bladder cancers have shown pain reduction with this procedure. There is evidence showing greater effectiveness in individuals over the age of 59 compared to younger patients. The procedure has shown a decrease on the visual analogue pain score in approximately 70% of the cancer patients. The group of patients successfully treated with this procedure have shown a 22% reduction in mean opioid use compared to the failure group.

Contraindications and Complications

Superior hypogastric plexus block can be performed safely with rare, but serious, complications. The blood supply to the anterior spinal cord is less likely to be compromised at this level, consequently, several neurological complications are less likely to occur compared to more cephalad blocks, such as the

D. Jankovic, P. Peng (eds.), *Regional Nerve Blocks in Anesthesia and Pain Therapy*,
https://doi.org/10.1007/978-3-030-88727-8_48

celiac plexus block. Nonetheless, given the ganglion is anterior to the psoas, psoas hematoma is a known complication. Furthermore, proximity to the L4, L5, and S1 nerve roots lend to the possibility of neural injury, especially with neurolytics.

Bilateral neurolysis, which may lead to complete sympathectomy of pelvic organs, may result in sexual dysfunction in men and should be avoided. Other possible complications include subarachnoid or epidural injections, nerve injury, or damage to structures such as the kidneys or urethra or muscular injury.

Critical Anatomy

The superior hypogastric plexus is a retroperitoneal plexus, located at the level of the lower third of the L5 and upper third of the S1 vertebrae. The superior hypogastric plexus contains both sympathetic and parasympathetic fibers. Sympathetic fibers innervate all pelvis organs except the ovaries and fallopian tubes. The inferior mesenteric ganglion and lumbar splanchnic nerves also contribute to the plexus with the fibers that travel with aorta. Visceral afferent fibers of the pelvic organs travel through the plexus and enter the spinal cord with the lumbar or sacral nerve roots.

Equipment and Patient Preparation

The procedure does not require any special monitoring. Supplemental oxygen, an AMBU bag, suction, ACLS drugs, and other resuscitation equipment must be available for emergencies. Peripheral IV access is not necessarily needed for this procedure. The patient should receive 1 g cefalexin/cefazolin or 1 g vancomycin for prophylaxis, and antiseptic techniques must be used before and during the procedure. The procedure will be performed under fluoroscopic guidance. The patient will be placed in a prone position. A 22 or 25-gauge, 7-in. needle will be used for the injections. Two to 3 mL of 1–2% lidocaine will be used for skin analgesia. Ten milliliter of 0.25–0.5% ropivacaine or bupivacaine, with 40–80 mg of particulate steroid (i.e. 40 mg/mL Triamcinolone), will be used for temporary blockade. Six to 8 mL of 10% phenol, or 8–10 mL of 50–100% ethanol, unilaterally will be injected for neurolysis.

Step-by-Step Technique

Fluoroscopy Technique

Classic or Posterolateral Approach

1. Patient is placed in a prone position, with the head turned to one side. When using a C-arm, Lumbar lordosis can be reduced using a pillow under the lower abdomen.
2. When the lower L5 and upper S1 endplates are squared in the AP view the transverse process is located ~10–15 mm lateral to the spinous process.
3. The needles will be inserted lateral to the right and left transverse process.
4. Needles are inserted 30-degree caudad (off the medial sagittal plane) and 45-degree obliqued.
5. After contacting the lower border of the outer third of the transverse process, the needle is removed 30 mm and redirected caudally.
6. A lateral view is necessary to verify the needle depth relative to the vertebral body.
7. The medial path is continued cautiously, avoiding the intervertebral disc.
8. Lateral position is proceeded until 1–2 mm before the end of the intervertebral disc, then the needle is connected to a 3- or 5-mL syringe for loss of resistance.
9. Needle path is verified in an AP view (Fig. 48.1).
10. Needle placement is verified by applying 2–3 mL of nonionic contrast under dynamic fluoroscopy in lateral plane (Fig. 48.2).
11. In patients with L5 mega-apophysis, or Bertolotti Syndrome, the procedure can be performed in the L4–L5 intervertebral space.
12. An AP X-ray is taken to visualize retroperitoneal contrast spread on the right and left sides.

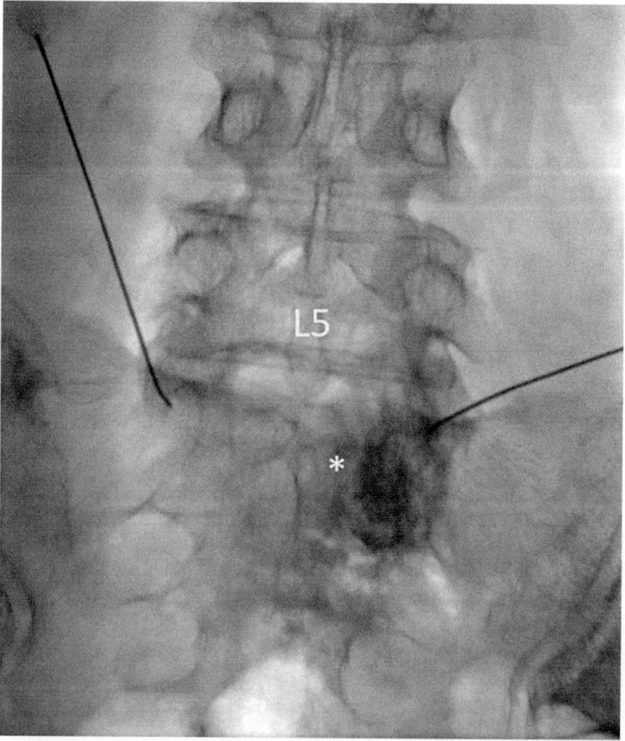

Fig. 48.1 AP view of bilateral needle placement for superior hypogastric plexus block under fluoroscopic guidance. (*) shows adequate left side spread which does remain lateral to the midline in an amorphous shape not following the contours of the psoas or organs (such as bowel)

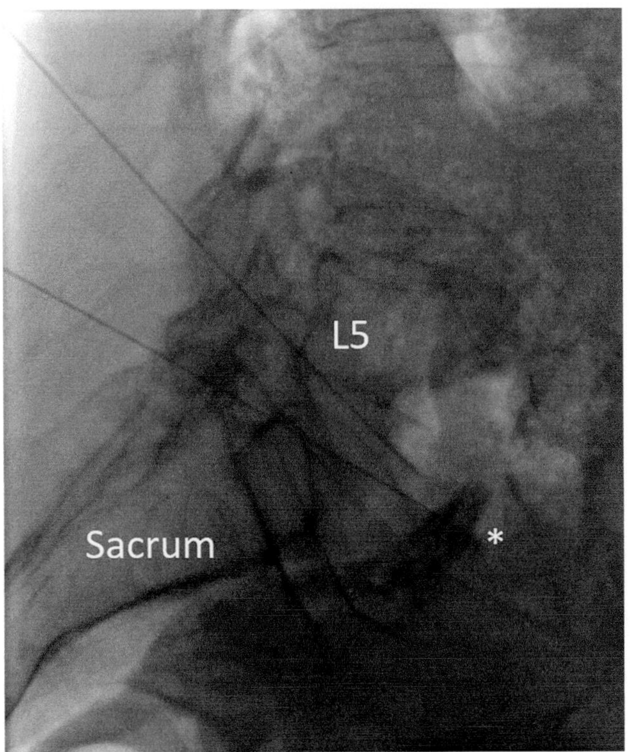

Fig. 48.2 Lateral view of bilateral needle placement for the superior hypogastric block under fluoroscopic guidance with good anterior spread along the sacral promontory (*)

13. Neurolysis is performed by injection of 8–10 mL of 10% phenol on each side. Diagnostic block is performed by using 0.25% bupivacaine with a similar volume.

Transdiscal Approach

1. Patient is placed in a prone position, with the head turned to one side. When using a C-arm, Lumbar lordosis can be reduced using a pillow under the lower abdomen.
2. The spinous process must be placed in the middle of the image by squaring off the lower L5 and upper S1 end-plates in an AP view.
3. By using an oblique view, the superior articular process of S1 should be visualized.
4. A 22 gauge spinal needle will be introduced through the oblique view in the caudal part of the intervertebral disc.
5. After advancing 3–5 cm (depending on the patient's morphological characteristics), a clear lateral view must be taken, which is crucial while advancing the needle through the disc. In a perfect lateral view the intervertebral foramen would be seen as a unique round image, while the L5 and sacrum are squared off.
6. If the needle touches the L5 root the patient may complain of pain as the needle advances. The needle can be retracted 5 mm, and a lateral view can be obtained to confirm the needle position at the entry of the foramina. If the needle is touching the root, the needle tip should turn up or down to avoid the root. If the needle enters the intervertebral disc, the patient will experience discogenic pain, which can be mitigated by injecting 0.5 mm lidocaine and advancing the needle.
7. The needle is advanced to the lateral third or the middle of the disc and then is connected to a 3- or 5-mL syringe for loss of resistance. Loss of resistance indicates that the needle has reached retroperitoneum. In order to prevent the needle from potentially puncturing the bowls, if resistance is not felt after advancing 3 cm, a lateral view should be obtained.
8. 1–2 mL nonionic contrast must be applied while visualizing the anterior spread of the contrast in a linear fashion over the anterior surface of the L5–S1 intervertebral discs.
9. In addition, 5–10 mL of air can be injected and visualized in the lateral view along the anterior sacrum body.
10. Retroperitoneal contrast spread can be visualized with an AP radiograph. If bilateral spread is not visualized, an additional 5 mL of air and 2 mL of contrast can be applied.
11. Transdiscal needles can achieve a more medial injectate distribution which is especially important in cancer patients with extensive retroperitoneal tumoral activity.
12. In a diagnostic block, 15 mL of bupivacaine 0.35% can be applied. Neurolysis can be done with 10–15 mL of 10% phenol. In a bilateral transdiscal approach, 8–10 mL of 10% phenol or alcohol can be applied with each needle.

CT Guided

1. Patient is placed in a prone position, and in order to reduce lumbar lordosis a pillow can be placed under the lower abdomen.
2. A topogram of the lumbosacral region should be obtained before the procedure, unless the CT software helps with needle path.
3. The needle trajectory must be planned prior to starting the procedure. The distance and angulation from the skin to the inferior border of the transverse process should be measured with a CT ruler in sagittal plane (distance *b*). The external laser beam can provide the skin entrance needle point but cannot provide the distance from the spinous process or the needle angulation. In order to measure angulation, the paravertebral distance from the anterolateral margin of the L5 vertebrae and the psoas major should be measured in axial plane. The distance should be calculated by measuring the distance between the L5 spinous process and distance *b*.
4. Needles are introduced in the planned direction. In order to confirm direction and depth, multiple low X-ray dose CT can be obtained if needed.
5. After the needle tip reaches the anterior vertebral body of the sacrum or the L5 (depending on the needle angulation)

air and contrast will be applied, followed by a new CT to confirm the location.

6. Air and contrast should not be visible in any of the foraminal levels. In the case that they are visible, the needle tip should be slightly advanced, followed by the application of more contrast until the spread is visible at the retroperitoneum. Phenol should not be applied without this confirmation.
7. After confirming air and contrast spread in retroperitoneum, 8–10 mL of 10% phenol will be applied through each needle. Alternatively, 8–10 mL of alcohol can be applied for this procedure. In the final reconstruction, contrast-air-lytic agent distribution should be visualized.

Tips

- Given the cost and difficulty of phenol injection due to its high viscosity, 8–10 mL of 50–100% ethanol can be used as an alternative to phenol for neurolysis.
- Increasing the caudal tilt can improve visibility if the iliac wing obstructs the view.
- Given the amount of caudal and lateral tilt required for this procedure, longer needles may be needed, especially for obese patients.

Radio-Frequency Lesioning

In a case report, pulsed radio-frequency (PRF) of the superior hypogastric plexus was performed for a patient with interstitial cystitis. She received two sessions of PRF at 6-month intervals, with a frequency of 2 Hz and a width of 20 ms for 120 s. The authors reported that following the treatment her pain improved for more than 2 years.

Other reported radio-frequency ablations studies are performed with classic techniques, using 20-gauge, 10 cm cannulas, and 10 mm active tip RF needles.

High quality literature supporting radio-frequency use for PRF in the sympathetic nervous system, particularly for superior hypogastric plexus, is limited.

Retroperitoneal location of the SHPB and its proximity to the aortic bifurcation makes this procedure challenging and supports further cadaveric studies to confirm the feasibility of RF in this case.

Ganglion of Impar Nerve Block

Introduction

The ganglion of impar is the most caudal ganglion of the sympathetic chain which innervates the lower pelvic structures. A pair of paravertebral sympathetic chains are fused close to the sacrococcygeal junction and form this ganglion in the retroperitoneum. The ganglion supplies the sympathetic and visceral innervation of the lower third of the rectum, including the vagina, vulva, urethra, and coccyx. The ganglion of impar mediates the pain from these structures through its sympathetic nervous system, making it a suitable target for pain relief. Perineal pain produced by pelvic tumors can be worsened by defecation. Opiate-induced constipation can increase perineal pressure and discomfort and can place these patients in a vicious cycle. The ganglion of impar receives the visceral pain of the pelvic structures through the sympathetic fibers. The pain is then transmitted to the sympathetic trunk, sacral nerve roots, and spinal cord and finally terminates in the brain.

Indications

The ganglion of impar lock has been shown to be effective in many benign and malignant conditions. Perineal and coccygeal pain, originating from tumors or post-radiation and post-surgical changes of the perineal structures, have been safely improved with this block. It has shown benefits in treating radiation-induced prostatitis or proctitis. Coccydynia, resulting from degenerative changes, trauma, or infection, can also be treated with this block. Nonmalignant conditions, such as post-herpetic neuralgia, rectal tenesmus, vulvodynia, cystitis, and idiopathic perineal and coccygeal pain, can also be treated with this block.

Critical Anatomy

The ganglion of impar is a solitary retroperitoneal ganglion that is about 5 mm long. It is a midline structure located anterior to the coccyx and posterior to the rectum. Its position may vary from the level of the sacrococcygeal junction to the second coccygeal vertebrae.

Equipment and Patient Preparation

The procedure does not require any special monitoring. Supplemental oxygen, an AMBU bag, suction, ACLS drugs, and other resuscitation equipment must be available for emergencies.

The procedure will be performed under fluoroscopic guidance. The patient will be placed in a prone position. A 25-gauge, 2- to 3.5-in. needle will be used for the injections. Four milliliter of 1–2% lidocaine or 0.25–0.5% ropivacaine or bupivacaine will be used for local anesthesia. 0.5–1 mL of particulate corticosteroid (i.e., 40 mg/mL triamcinolone) will be used as an adjuvant for this block.

Step-by-Step Technique

Fluoroscopic-Guided Approach

1. Patient is placed in a prone position, with the head turned to one side. When using a C-arm, lumbar lordosis can be reduced using a pillow under the lower abdomen.
2. The sacrococcygeal region is prepped and draped sterilely.
3. The junction between the S5 and first coccygeal vertebrae is located in both the anterior-posterior (AP) and lateral positions, using fluoroscopy.
4. The skin and subcutaneous tissue overlaying the sacrococcygeal junction is anesthetized with local anesthetics using a midline entry point which has already been identified via fluoroscopy.
5. Under fluoroscopic guidance in the lateral view, the needle is inserted and advanced to the sacrococcygeal disc.
6. Needle advancement is continued through the sacrococcygeal disc until the needle tip is located anterior to the sacrococcygeal ligament.
7. 1–2 mL of contrast is injected to confirm the needle tip position in the retroperitoneal space (Fig. 48.3).
8. If the needle is in the correct position, contrast spread will produce a "reverse comma" shape in the lateral view. The AP view must not show any vascular or epidural spread (Fig. 48.3).
9. Aspiration should be done prior to injection for any blood or CSF.

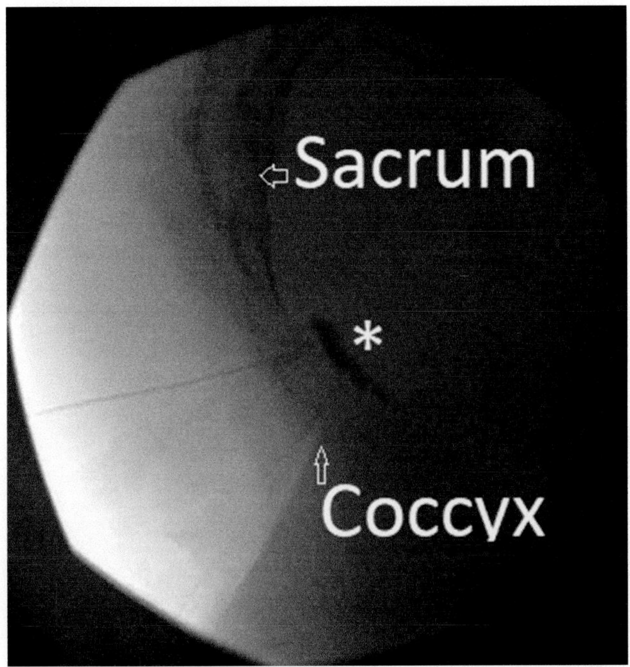

Fig. 48.3 Lateral fluoroscopic view of ganglion of impar block. (*) showing good anterior sacral spread of contrast agent, comma sign

CT-Guided Approach

The procedure can be performed with CT guidance. In an axial CT section of the sacrococcygeal disc, the needle trajectory from sacrum to the sacrococcygeal junction is planned off midline on both the sides. In order to prevent accidental rectal puncture and to have a better view of the sacrococcygeal junction, if rectal gas or stool obscures the view, a para-sagittal, CT-guided approach can be used.

Tips

- After traversing the sacrococcygeal ligament, a loss of resistance may be felt.
- Long-term relief may be achieved with chemical ablation, pulsed radiofrequency, or cryoablation.
- Prolonged pain relief has been shown to be achieved with 25–100 U of botulinum toxin.
- A calcified or fused sacrococcygeal disc may occasionally prevent the access to the ganglion. In these circumstances, a different approach such as the ano-coccygeal or intra-coccygeal approach may be selected. In this approach, a needle is inserted through the ano-coccygeal ligament and advanced against the sacrum and coccyx to contact the ventral coccyx. This approach has higher risk of rectal perforation and infection.

Safety Considerations

- The needle must not advance too far from the anterior surface of the coccyx, as rectal preformation is possible due to the proximity of the rectum and coccyx.
- It is possible that the needle breaks while traversing the disc since the disc is rigid and a small-bore needle is used for the procedures.
- If the sacral nerve roots are in proximity of the ganglion of impar, they may be damaged in the case of ganglion ablation. This proximity can be identified prior to the procedure with motor testing identifying gluteus spasms.

Post-procedure Management

The patient must be informed about the expected results and potential complications of the procedure. Some of the potential complications include rectal perforation, bleeding, nerve injury, parasympathetic denervation, infection, discitis, and epidural spread of the injectate.

Suggested Reading

Choi JW, Kim WH, Lee CJ, Sim WS, Park S, Chae HB. The optimal approach for a superior hypogastric plexus block. Pain Pract. 2018;18:314–21. https://doi.org/10.1111/papr.12603.

Datir A, Connell D. CT-guided injection for ganglion impar blockade: a radiological approach to the management of coccydynia. Clin Radiol. 2010;65:21–5. 20103417.

Khosla A, Adeyefa O, Nasir S. Successful treatment of radiation-induced proctitis pain by blockade of the ganglion impar in an elderly patient with prostate cancer: a case report. Pain Med. 2013;14(5):662–6. https://doi.org/10.1111/pme.12065.

Kim JH, Kim E, Kim BI. Pulsed radiofrequency treatment of the superior hypogastric plexus in an interstitial cystitis patient with chronic pain and symptoms refractory to oral and intravesical medications and bladder hydrodistension: a case report. Medicine (Baltimore). 2016;95(49):e5549.

Kraima AC, van Schaik J, Susan S, van de Velde CJ, Hamming JF, Lakke EA, DeRuiter MC. New insights in the neuroanatomy of the human adult superior hypogastric plexus and hypogastric nerves. Auton Neurosci. 2015;189:60–7. https://doi.org/10.1016/j.autneu.2015.02.001. PMID: 25704391.

Kroll CE, Schartz B, Gonzalez-Fernandez M, Gordon AH, Babade M, Erdek MA, Mekhail N, Cohen SP. Factors associated with outcome after superior hypogastric plexus neurolysis in cancer patients. Clin J Pain. 2014;30(1):55–62. https://doi.org/10.1097/AJP.0b013e3182869d68.

Le Clerc QC, Riant T, Levesque A, Labat JJ, Ploteau S, Robert R, Perrouin-Verbe MA, Rigaud J. Repeated ganglion impar block in a cohort of 83 patients with chronic pelvic and perineal pain. Pain Physic. 2017;20(6):E823–8.

de Leon-Casasola OA. Critical evaluation of chemical neurolysis of the sympathetic axis for cancer pain. Cancer Control. 2000;7(2):142–8. https://doi.org/10.1177/107327480000700204. PMID: 10783818.

Lim SJ, Park HJ, Lee SH, Moon DE. Ganglion impar block with botulinum toxin type A for chronic perineal pain - a case report. Korean J Pain. 2010;23:65–9. https://doi.org/10.3344/kjp.2010.23.1.65.

Malec-Milewska M, Horosz B, Kolęda I, et al. Neurolytic block of ganglion of Walther for the management of chronic pelvic pain. Wideochir Inne Tech Maloinwazyjne. 2014;9(3):458–62. https://doi.org/10.5114/wiitm.2014.43079.

Noor NA, Urits I, Viswanath O, Alexandre L, Kaye AD. Radiofrequency ablation of the splanchnic nerve and superior hypogastric plexus for chronic abdominal pain status post-abdominal surgery. Cureus. 2020;12(12):e12189.

Oh CS, Chung IH, Ji HJ, Yoon DM. Clinical implications of topographic anatomy on the ganglion impar. Anesthesiology. 2004;101:249–50.

Plancarte R, Amescua C, Patt RB. Presacral blockade of the ganglion of Walther (ganglion impar). Anesthesiology. 1990;73:A751.

Plancarte R, Amescia C, Patt R, Aldrete JA. Superior hypogastric plexus block for pelvic cancer pain. Anesthesiology. 1990;73(2):236–9.

Stogicza AR. Superior hypogastric plexus block – transdiscal approach. In: Stogicza AR, Mansano AM, Trescot AM, Staats PS, editors. Interventional pain. Cham: Springer; 2020.

Warfield CA, Bajwa ZH. Principles and practice of pain medicine. 2nd ed. New York, NY: McGraw-Hill; 2004.

Zacharias NA, Karri J, Garcia C, et al. Interventional radiofrequency treatment for the sympathetic nervous system: a review article. Pain Ther. 2021;10:115.

Sacroiliac Joint Pain

49

Charles Amaral de Oliveira, Karen Santos Braghiroli, Thais Kouri Vanetti, and Philip Peng

Contents

General Consideration

Sacroiliac joint (SIJ) pain is one of the differential diagnoses of low back pain. Approximately 90% of the population will present to a health service with low back pain during their lifetime, and 10–25% of these patients will have SIJ pain. It is more common after the fifth decade of life, especially in obese and sedentary patients. Risk factors for SIJ pain include but not limited to sacroiliac dysfunction, pregnancy, older age, pelvic alignment pathologies, degeneration, joint mobility pathologies, core muscle weakness, inflammation, and trauma.

There are various primary causes of SIJ pain, the most common of which is degenerative arthritis that is characterized by joint space narrowing, osteophyte formation, and joint sclerosis. It is also caused by abnormal motion (hypermobile) or malalignment of the joint. In patients manifesting other symptoms, a diagnosis of inflammatory arthropathy (sacroiliitis) should be considered. This includes the spondyloarthropathies—notably ankylosing spondylitis, reactive arthritis, and psoriatic arthritis. Other major causes are trauma (that results in ligament strain and fractures) and infections. Secondary conditions that may generate SIJ pain are spinal fusion procedures, scoliosis, or leg length discrepancy. Lumbar spine arthrodesis can also be responsible for SIJ pain since it increases impact load on the SIJ, causing mechanical overload and subsequently sacroiliitis.

C. A. de Oliveira (✉)
Singular Pain Management Center, Campinas, SP, Brazil
e-mail: charles@singular.med.br

K. S. Braghiroli
Clinica Unio and Hospital Alemão Oswaldo Cruz, São Paulo, SP, Brazil

T. K. Vanetti
Singular Pain Management Center, Campinas, SP, Brazil

Centro Médico de Campinas, Campinas, SP, Brazil

P. Peng
Department of Anesthesiology and Pain Medicine, Toronto Western Hospital, University of Toronto, Toronto, ON, Canada
e-mail: philip.peng@uhn.ca

D. Jankovic, P. Peng (eds.), *Regional Nerve Blocks in Anesthesia and Pain Therapy*, https://doi.org/10.1007/978-3-030-88727-8_49

Indication (Patient Selection)

Many attempts have been made to improve accuracy in diagnosing SIJ pain, mainly through physical examination, imaging techniques, and local anesthetic blocks. An incorrect diagnosis may lead to treatment failure and waste of healthcare resources.

Patients will complain of pain upon prolonged sitting or standing, on climbing stairs, or while lying down on the painful side. Pain is usually localized to the buttock region, but multiple pain referral patterns may occur, including from the posterior thigh and knee, radiating into the foot and mimicking radicular pain. The literature shows that the prevalence of pain among cases was 94% in the ipsilateral buttock region and 74% in the lower lumbar area, of which up to 50% have radiation to the lower extremity—6% to the upper lumbar area, 4% to the groin, and 2% to the lower abdomen. The pain is described as sharp, stabbing, or shooting. The patient often points to the area between the gluteal folds and posterior iliac crests.

There are several specific physical tests to improve accuracy in diagnosing SIJ pain; however, none are considered the gold standard. Patrick's test (or FABER) is done with the patient lying supine. The hip and knee are flexed to 90°, and the thigh is abducted and then externally rotated. If pain is elicited over contralateral SIJ, the test is considered positive. Though not specific for SIJ pain, provocation tests (Gaenslen's, distraction, thigh thrust, and others) may prove useful. Three or more positive provocation tests have a sensitivity of 91% and a specificity of 78% for SIJ pathology. The physical examination can reveal pelvic asymmetry, confirmed by the measurement of the limbs, and the spinal examination can identify abnormal curvatures or movement abnormalities. Despite citing referred pain, the patient generally has normal spinal range of motion, normal neurological exam, and negative straight leg raising test.

Diagnosing SIJ pain is quite challenging since low back pain and pain around the hips and the gluteal region may be attributed to other causes. Imaging studies are recommended to exclude alternative sources of pain such as malignancy, infection, and fracture. The main diagnostic tool is the SIJ injection, which is also therapeutic because of its target specificity. These injections can be done using fluoroscopy, ultrasound, or CT guidance.

In the literature, landmark-guided injections are not recommended because the incidence of real intra-articular injection is only 22%, while those of epidural or sacral foraminal injection are 24% and 44%, respectively. The low rate of intra-articular injection using landmark-guided techniques warrants the use of image guidance. Ultrasound guidance is more readily available and feasible in clinical practice. Reportedly, its success rate was 60% in the first 30 injections, gradually improving to attain 93% in the last 30 injections.

Although there are no reference standards to confirm diagnosis, greater than 50–75% post-injection pain relief has been recommended.

Diagnostic blocks must be target-specific in order to improve diagnostic accuracy because SIJ innervation is complex and variable. Hence, it is sometimes challenging to perform the blocks. Additionally, if the injection is periarticular, it can miss the innervation, prompting inaccurate interpretation of injection, leading to unreliable predictive values concerning response to further treatment.

Functional Anatomy

The sacroiliac joint is a true diarthrodial joint that lies between the ilium and the sacrum within the S1-S3 topography in an oblique coronal orientation (Fig. 49.1). The surface of the SIJ measures 1.5 cm^2 at birth, 7.0 cm^2 at puberty, and it attains 17.5 cm^2 in adulthood. It is a synovial joint lined by hyaline cartilages and covered with dense fibrous connections. Only the anterior portion is considered a true synovial joint because the posterior connection is a syndesmosis consisting of the interosseous ligament (Fig. 49.2). The SIJ is broader cephalad and narrower in its inferior one-third. Stabilized by muscles (gluteus and paraspinal muscles) and ligaments, its main function is to transfer weight from the upper body to the lower limbs. This joint has a limited range of motion, allowing for only minimal rotation and gliding. The upper two-thirds of the joint becomes fibrotic in adulthood.

The posterior innervation stems from the S1-S3 dorsal rami via lateral branches and from the L4-L5 rami, respec-

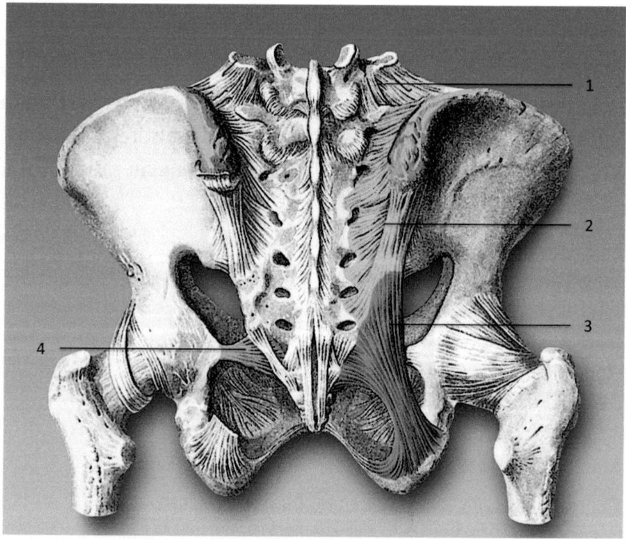

Fig. 49.1 Anatomy. (1) Iliolumbar ligament, (2) dorsal sacroiliac ligament, (3) sacrotuberous ligament, (4) sacrospinous ligament. (Reproduced with permission from Dr. Danilo Jankovicp)

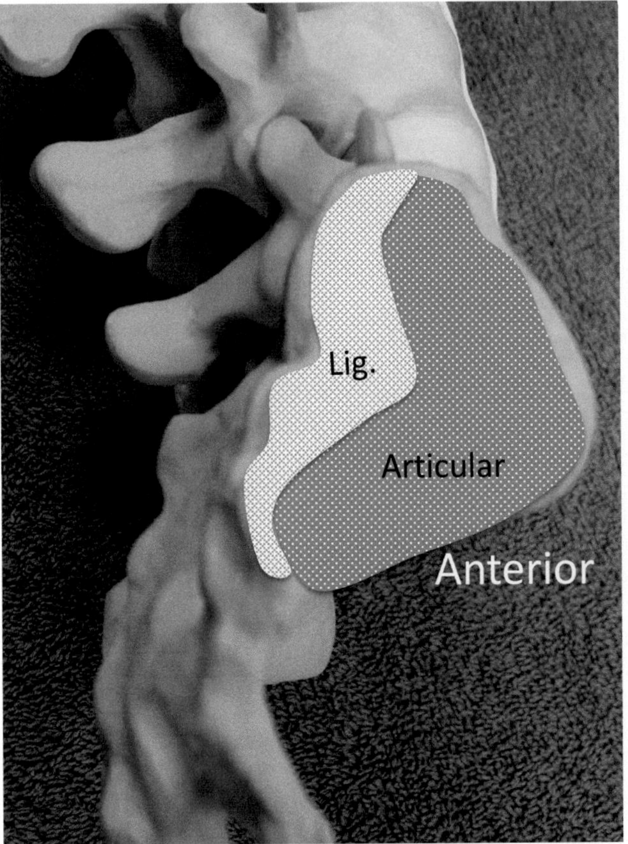

Fig. 49.2 Lateral view of the sacroiliac joint with the synovial surface (blue) and the ligamentous (lig) area. In the ligamentous area, the joint surfaces are connected with an intricate set of ligamentous connection. (Reproduced with permission of Philip Peng Educational Series)

tively, via medial and dorsal branches. The anterior innervation is provided by the lumbosacral plexus through the lateral branches of the anterior primary rami traveling from L2-S2. Contributions from the superior gluteal nerve as well as the obturator nerve have also been reported in the literature.

The anterior sacroiliac ligament is a thickening of the anterior joint capsule which connects the anterior surfaces of the sacrum and the ilium. The joint capsule is absent posteriorly, and the interosseous ligament forms the posterior border of the joint space. Accessory ligaments are comprised of the iliolumbar, sacrotuberous, and sacrospinous ligaments (Fig. 49.1). This ligament complex immobilizes the sacrum, thereby preventing x-axis rotation of the latter when it is subjected to gravitational forces.

Techniques

Fluoroscopy-Guided Technique

There are different techniques to access the SIJ using fluoroscopy. One of these involves placing the patient in prone position with the C-arm positioned posteroanteriorly, oriented toward the lumbosacral region. In this view, the SIJ is seen in addition to its posterior and anterior joint lines. The posterior joint line is usually the medial one (Fig. 49.3a, b). The C-arm should be adjusted to contralateral oblique view (approximately 5°–20°) in order to superimpose anterior and posterior joint lines (Fig. 49.3c, d). Under image intensifier control, a 25- or 22-gauge spinal needle is directed into the inferior one-third of the joint using a posterior approach (Fig. 49.4). Once the needle has entered the joint, intra-articular placement is confirmed by contrast medium injection (Figs. 49.5 and 49.6). In the posteroanterior view, the contrast medium travels rostrally along the joint line, whereas in the lateral view, it outlines the joint, confirming needle position.

Another technique is to perform a tunnel view injection with the C-arm in true posteroanterior view. The target is the medial line of the inferior one-third of the joint.

Total injected volume should be limited to 1.5–3 mL of solution.

Ultrasound-Guided Technique

The patient is placed in prone position, and the posterior superior iliac spine (PSIS) is palpated. The low-frequency curved transducer is placed over the PSIS in the axial plane and then slowly advanced, scanning caudad. The SIJ can be observed when the step-off between the sacrum and ilium is less pronounced. The upper SIJ appears as an iliac prominence, and then the dorsal sacroiliac ligament comes into view (Fig. 49.7). Moving the probe caudad, the S1 and S2 neural foramina can be identified medially to the SIJ cleft. The lower third of the SIJ becomes evident from the flat contour of the iliac crest and the presence of the S2 foramen that is located 2–3 cm above the caudal pole of SIJ (Fig. 49.8). Color Doppler scan is used to distinguish vascular structures. The target is the cleft between the lateral border of the sacrum and the medial border of the ilium, representative of the posterior aspect of the SIJ. If an in-plane technique is chosen, medial to lateral needle insertion is recommended after the probe is tilted medially to allow an optimal trajectory of the needle (Figs. 49.9 and 49.10).

Complications

Blockade of the sacral plexus may occur due to aggressive advancement of needle or ventral capsular defect, dorsal leakage from the joint capsule (potentially anesthetizing posterior structures), communication between the joint and the S1 foramen, and difficult access to joint in as many as 10% of patients.

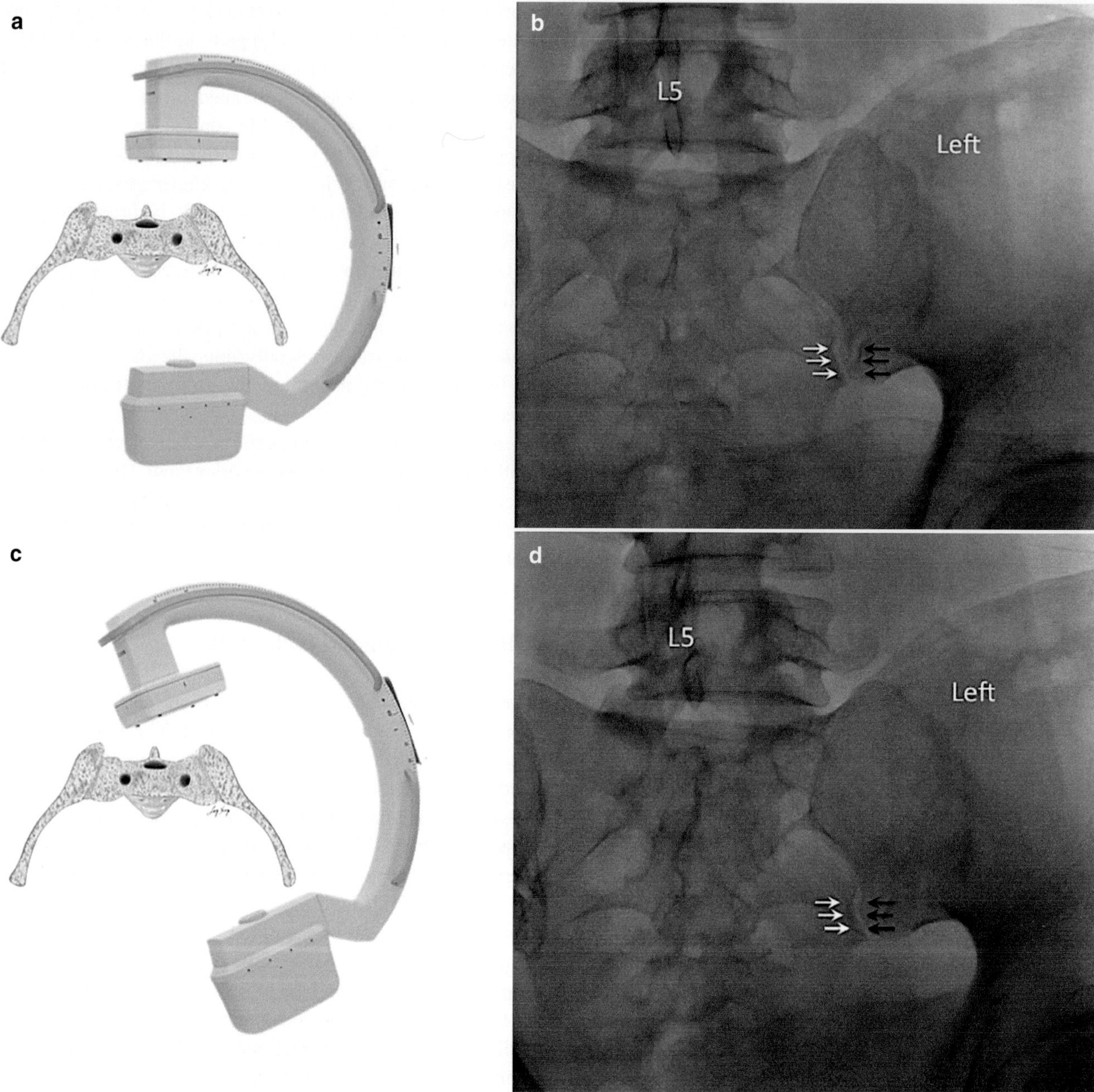

Fig. 49.3 Straight posteroanterior X-ray of the sacroiliac joint. (**a**) Position of C-arm with respect to the sacrum. (**b**) Corresponding fluoroscopic image. In this view, both anterior (black arrows) and posterior joint (white arrows) lines are seen. The posterior joint line (white arrows) is usually the more medial one. Contralateral oblique X-ray of the sacroiliac joint. (**c**) Position of C-arm with respect to the sacrum. (**d**) Corresponding fluoroscopic image. The anterior and posterior joint lines aligned to form a crisp silhouette of the joint. (Reproduced with permission of Philip Peng Educational Series)

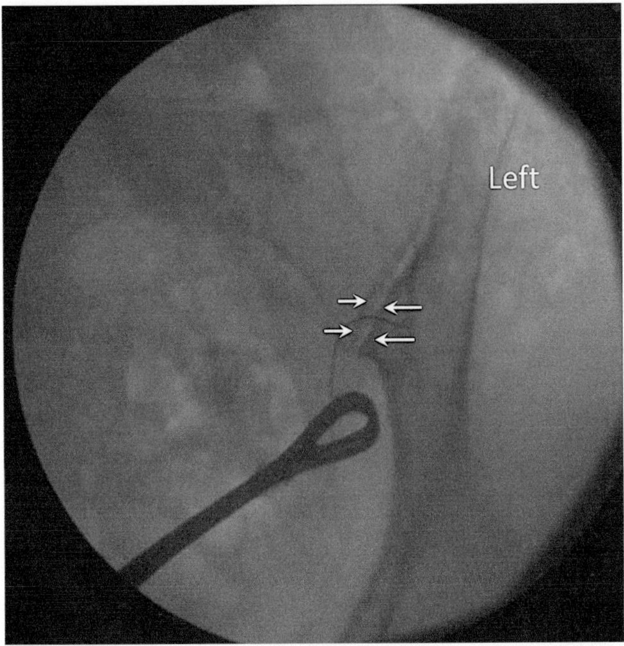

Fig. 49.4 Insertion of needle into the sacroiliac joint (SIJ). The needle is slightly bended by a swap forceps, the site of angulation was at the entrance of SIJ, and the needle inside the SIJ was only a few millimeters in length. (Reproduced with permission of Philip Peng Educational Series)

Practical Tips

1. The diagnostic blocks should always be performed under image guidance. This minimizes the probability of an extra-articular injection.
2. The total injected volume should not exceed 1.5–3 mL. This prevents extra-articular injection and false-positive results.
3. Contrast medium should be injected under fluoroscopic guidance when performing arthrograms to confirm intra-articular needle position.
4. Sacral lateral branch injection is more accurate when patients likely to respond better to radiofrequency are selected, since this technique selects only the posterior innervation. This is described in detail in the next chapter.

Literature Review

Intra-articular (IA) steroid injections have beneficial effects in 79–93% of the patients with average duration of effects lasting 9.9 months, according to various observational studies in the literature. However, owing to a lack of controlled randomized trials, the evidence is limited.

Murakami et al. observed in a prospective comparative study that improvement in pain was significantly higher in patients who had received periarticular (PA) injections after failed response to IA injections than in patients who had received IA injections alone. However, Nacey et al. concluded that there is no significant difference between IA and PA injections in the pain relief provided. There are studies in the literature comparing the effects of IA and PA injections, of which two double-blind studies showed the effectiveness of PA infiltrations in short-term pain relief. PA infiltration can be used if IA injection proves to be difficult. There is limited (or poor) evidence for PA injections of local anesthetic and steroid.

The level of evidence for conventional radiofrequency (RF) is limited, mostly due to limitations in needle positioning owing to the heterogeneous innervation of SIJ. RF ablation has shown limited efficacy due to its inability to denervate anterior neural structures and to provide long-lasting pain relief on denervation of posterior structures because these nerves regenerate within a few months.

In the setting of a negative IA anesthetic injection via sacral lateral branch block, the posterior ligaments may be considered potential pain generators. Recently, a randomized controlled trial compared ultrasound- and fluoroscopy-guided sacral lateral branch blocks in 40 patients and concluded that pain relief was similar in both the groups 30 days after the procedure. However, the study did reveal that the ultrasound technique had some advantages such as shorter times and fewer needle punctures, lower radiation exposure, and a lower risk of vascular breach. Another study compared the same two methods and also found no significant difference in pain scores after 1 and 3 months as well as similar functional outcomes.

A 2015 systematic review with a meta-analysis of the effectiveness of RF ablation for the treatment of SIJ pain concluded that RF is an effective treatment at 3 and 6 months, but its conclusions are limited by little available literature and a lack of randomized controlled trials. Diagnostic accuracy is Level 2 for dual diagnostic blocks with at least 70% pain relief as the criterion standard and Level 3 for single diagnostic blocks with at least 75% pain relief as the criterion standard. The evidence for cooled radiofrequency is Level 2–3; however, it is limited for conventional RF, IA steroid injections, and PA injections with steroids or botulinum toxin, which are rated as Level 3–4.

A prior systematic review of the therapeutic effectiveness of all SIJ interventions (IA injections, PA injections, conven-

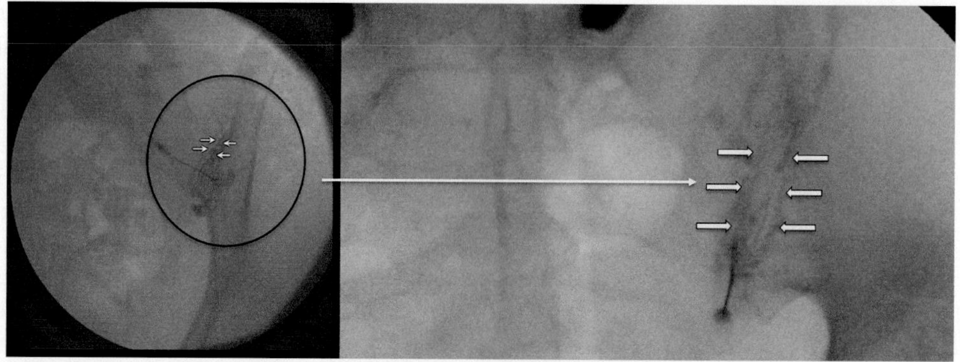

Fig. 49.5 Fluoroscopic image showed the contrast traveling in the rostral direction (white arrow heads). Right image is the zoomed image of the left. (Reproduced with permission of Philip Peng Educational Series)

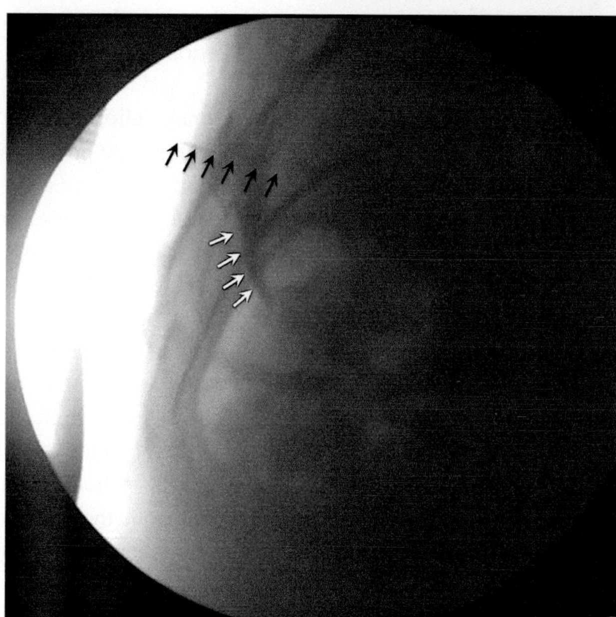

Fig. 49.6 Lateral view of the sacroiliac joint. The needle was marked by black arrows. The lower perimeter of the joint space was marked by the white arrows. (Reproduced with permission of Philip Peng Educational Series)

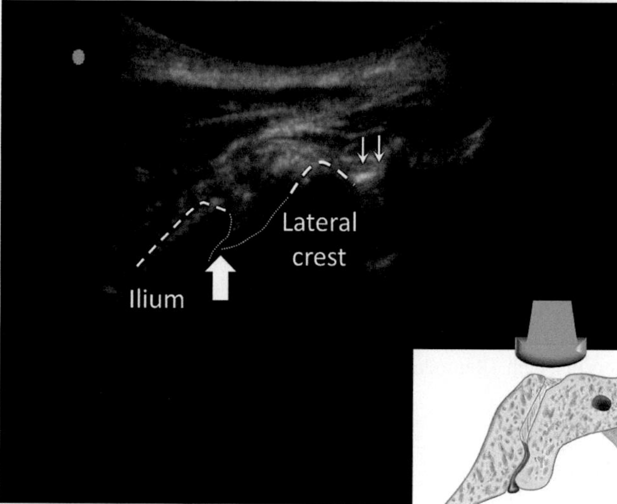

Fig. 49.8 Sonography of the lower sacroiliac joint (SIJ). The probe position was indicated in the insert in the lower right corner. The SIJ was indicated by the bold arrow, which is typically lateral to the lateral crest. Note the flat appearance of the ilium. The S2 foramen was indicated by the line arrows. The bold dotted line outlines the hyperechoic shadow of the bone while the fainted dotted line outlines the bone contour that is not seen. (Reproduced with permission of Philip Peng Educational Series)

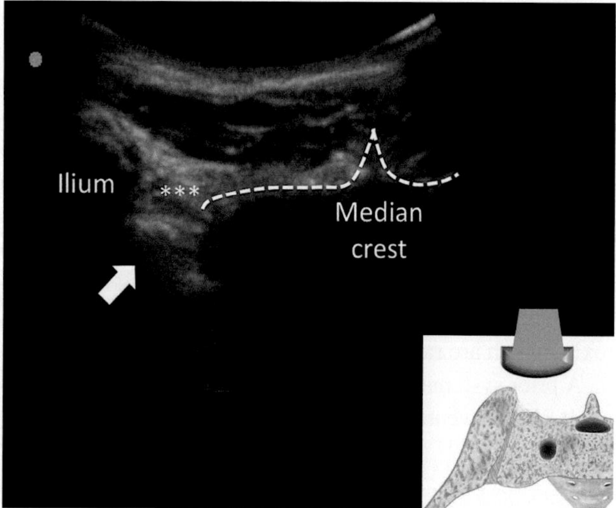

Fig. 49.7 Sonography of the upper sacroiliac joint (SIJ). The probe position was indicated in the insert in the lower right corner. The SIJ was indicated by the bold arrow. Note the prominence of the ilium. The median crest is outlined by the dotted line. **—dorsal sacroiliac ligament. (Reproduced with permission of Philip Peng Educational Series)

tional RF, cooled RF) had found the greatest amount of supporting evidence for cooled RF lateral branch blocks based on two randomized controlled trials and two observational studies. Other interventions have weaker proof of their effects.

In light of the complexity of the SIJ joint, multifactorial causes may lead to SIJ dysfunction, making it a challenge to diagnose. Accordingly, diagnostic workup should include physical examination, laboratory and radiological tests, and diagnostic blocks. The latter are considered the gold standard though some controversy still surrounds their application (use of single or dual injections) and selection (choice of intra-articular or peri-articular injections, or intra-articular or lateral sacral branch injections). Treatment involves various interventions and rehabilitation therapies; but the evidence is limited for most of them, mainly because higher-quality studies are still needed.

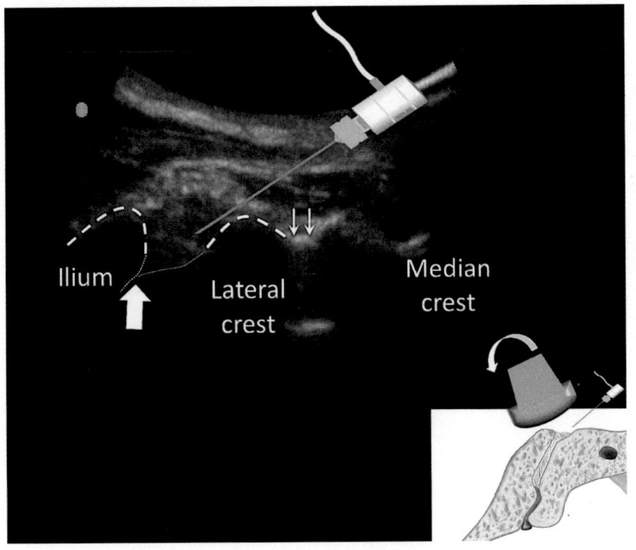

Fig. 49.9 Sonography of the lower sacroiliac joint (SIJ) similar to Fig. 49.8, but the ultrasound probe was tilted toward the midline to allow a steeper angle of the needle. The probe position was indicated in the insert in the lower right corner. The SIJ was indicated by the bold arrow and the needle trajectory is shown with a simulated needle. (Reproduced with permission of Philip Peng Educational Series)

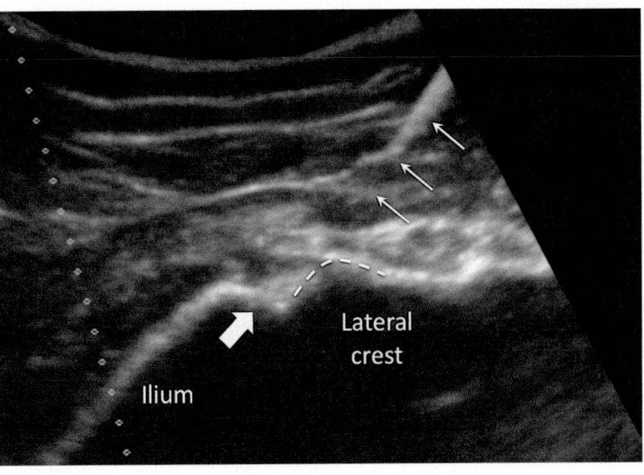

Fig. 49.10 Sonography of the lower sacroiliac joint (SIJ) with the needle (line arrows) inserting in-plane in a medial to lateral direction. The SIJ was indicated by the bold arrow. (Reproduced with permission of Philip Peng Educational Series)

Suggested Reading

Aydin SM, Gharibo CG, Mehnert M, et al. The role of radiofrequency ablation for sacroiliac joint pain: a meta-analysis. PM R. 2010;2(9):842–51.

Bernard TN Jr, Cassidy JD. The sacroiliac joint syndrome, pathophysiology, diagnosis and treatment. In: Frymoyer JW, editor. the adult spine: principles and practice. New York, NY: Raven Press; 1991. p. 2107–30.

Bollow M, Braun J, Taupitz M, Häberle J, Reibhauer BH, Paris S, et al. CT-guided intraarticular corticosteroid injection into the sacroiliac joints in patients with spondyloarthropathy: indication and follow-up with contrast-enhanced MRI. J Comput Assist Tomogr. 1996;20:512–21.

Cheng J, Pope JE, Dalton JE, Cheng O, Bensitel A. Comparative outcomes of cooled versus traditional radiofrequency ablation of the lateral branches for sacroiliac joint pain. Clin J Pain. 2013;29:132–7.

Cohen SP, Strassels SA, Kurihara C, Crooks MT, Erdek MA, Forsythe A, et al. Outcome predictors for sacroiliac joint (lateral branch) radiofrequency denervation. Reg Anesth Pain Med. 2009;34:206–14.

Cohen SP, Chen Y, Neufeld NJ. Sacroiliac joint pain: a comprehensive review of epidemiology, diagnosis and treatment. Expert Rev Neurother. 2013;13(1):99–116.

Cox RC, Fortin JD. The anatomy of the lateral branches of the sacral dorsal rami: implications for radiofrequency ablation. Pain Physic. 2014;17(5):459–64.

DePhillipo NN, Corenman DS, Strauch EL, Zalepa King LA. Sacroiliac pain: structural causes of pain referring to the SI joint region. Clin Spine Surg. 2019;32(6):E282–8.

Dreyfuss P, Dreyer SJ, Cole A, Mayo K. Sacroiliac joint pain. J Am Acad Orthop Surg. 2004;12:255–65.

Ferrante FM, King LF, Roche EA, Kim PS, Aranda M, Delaney LR, et al. Radiofrequency sacroiliac joint denervation for sacroiliac syndrome. Reg Anesth Pain Med. 2001;26:137–42.

Finlayson RJ, Etheridge JP, Elgueta MF, et al. A randomized comparison between ultrasound- and fluoroscopy-guided sacral lateral branch blocks. Reg Anesth Pain Med. 2017;42(3):400–6.

Fortin JD, Washington WJ, Falco FJ. Three pathways between the sacroiliac joint and neural structures. AJNR Am J Neuroradiol. 1999;20(8):1429–34.

Grob KR, Neuhuber WL, Kissling RO. Innervation of the sacroiliac joint of the human. Z Rheumatol. 1995;54:117–22.

Hansen HC. Is fluoroscopy necessary for sacroiliac joint injections? Pain Physic. 2003;6:155–8.

Hansen H, Manchikanti L, Simopoulos TT, Christo PJ, Gupta S, Smith HS, et al. A systematic evaluation of the therapeutic effectiveness of sacroiliac joint interventions. Pain Physic. 2012;15:E247–78.

Kennedy DJ, Engel A, Kreiner DS, et al. Fluoroscopically guided diagnostic and therapeutic intra-articular sacroiliac joint injections: a systematic review. Pain Med. 2015;16(8):1500–18.

Luukkainen RK, Wennerstrand PV, Kautiainen HH, Sanila MT, Asikainen EL. Efficacy of periarticular corticosteroid treatment of the sacroiliac joint in non-spondylarthropathic patients with chronic low back pain in the region of the sacroiliac joint. Clin Exp Rheumatol. 2002;20(1):52–4.

Magee DJ. "Pelvis." Orthopedic physical assessment. 6th ed. St Louis, MO: Elsevier Saunders; 2014. p. 649–88.

Maigne JY, Aivaliklis A, Pfefer F. Results of sacroiliac joint double block and value of sacroiliac pain provocation tests in 54 patients with low back pain. Spine. 1996;21(16):1889–92.

Manchikanti L, Singh V, Pampati V, Damron KS, Barnhill RC, Beyer C, et al. Evaluation of the relative contributions of various structures in chronic low back pain. Pain Physic. 2001;4:308–16.

Murakami E, Tanaka Y, Aizawa T, Ishizuka M, Kokubun S. Effect of periarticular and intraarticular lidocaine injections for sacroiliac joint pain: prospective comparative study. J Orthop Sci. 2007;12:274–80.

Nacey NC, Patrie JT, Fox MG. Fluoroscopically guided sacroiliac joint injections: comparison of the effects of intraarticular and periarticular injections on immediate and short-term pain relief. AJR Am J Roentgenol. 2016;207:1055–61.

Polly D, Cher D, Whang PG, et al. INSITE Study Group. Does level of response to SI joint block predict response to SI joint fusion? Int J Spine Surg. 2016;10:4.

Rashbaum RF, Ohnmeiss DD, Lindley EM, Kitchel SH, Patel VV. Sacroiliac joint pain and its treatment. Clin Spine Surg. 2016;29(2):42–8.

Rosenberg JM, Quint TJ, de Rosayro AM. Computerized tomographic localization of clinically guided sacroiliac joint injections. Clin J Pain. 2000;16(1):18–21.

Rupert MP, Lee M, Manchikanti L, Datta S, Cohen SP. Evaluation of sacroiliac joint interventions: a systematic appraisal of the literature. Pain Physic. 2009;12(2):399–418.

Schmidt GL, Bhandutia AK, Altman DT. Management of sacroiliac joint pain. J Am Acad Orthop Surg. 2018;26(17):610–6.

Schwarzer AC, Aprill CN, Bogduk N. The sacroiliac joint in chronic low back pain. Spine. 1995;20(1):31–7.

Simopoulos TT, Manchikanti L, Gupta S. Systematic review of the diagnostic accuracy and therapeutic effectiveness of sacroiliac joint interventions. Pain Physic. 2015;18:E713–56.

Soneji N, Bhatia A, Seib R, et al. Comparison of fluoroscopy and ultrasound guidance for sacroiliac joint injection in patients with chronic low back pain. Pain Pract. 2015;16(5):537–44.

Stelzer W, Aiglesberger M, Stelzer D, Stelzer V. Use of cooled radiofrequency lateral branch neurotomy for the treatment of sacroiliac joint-mediated low back pain: a large case series. Pain Med. 2013;14:29–35.

Thawrani DP, Agabegi SS, Asghar F. Diagnosing sacroiliac joint pain. J Am Acad Orthop Surg. 2019;27(3):85–93.

Tilvawala K, Kothari K, Patel R. Sacroiliac joint: a review. Indian J Pain. 2018;32:4.

Vallejo R, Benyamin RM, Kramer J, Stanton G, Joseph NJ. Pulsed radiofrequency denervation for the treatment of sacroiliac joint syndrome. Pain Med. 2006;7:429–34.

Van der Wurff P, Buijs EJ, Groen GJ. Intensity mapping of pain referral areas in sacroiliac joint pain patients. J Manip Physiol Ther. 2006;29:190–5.

Young S, Aprill C, Laslett M. Correlation of clinical examination characteristics with three sources of chronic low back pain. Spine J. 2003;3(6):460–5.

Sacroiliac Joint Lateral Branch Block and Radiofrequency Ablation

50

Eldon Loh, Taylor Burnham, Anne M. Agur, and Robert S. Burnham

Contents

General Considerations

10 to 27% of low back pain originates from the sacroiliac joint (SIJ), and the prevalence increases with age and in the context of lumbar fusion. SIJ radiofrequency ablation (RFA) is a common intervention that interrupts nociceptive pain signals originating from the SIJ through neural tissue thermocoagulation. Different needle placement locations and lesioning techniques have been described for SIJ RFA. Needle placement locations can be broadly catego-

E. Loh (✉)
Department of Physical Medicine and Rehabilitation, Schulich School of Medicine and Dentistry, Western University, London, ON, Canada

Parkwood Institute Research, Lawson Health Research Institute, London, ON, Canada

Parkwood Institute, St. Joseph's Health Care London, London, ON, Canada
e-mail: eldon.loh@sjhc.london.on.ca

T. Burnham
Division of Physical Medicine and Rehabilitation, University of Utah, Salt Lake City, UT, USA
e-mail: taylor.burnham@hsc.utah.edu

A. M. Agur
Division of Anatomy, Department of Surgery, University of Toronto, Toronto, ON, Canada
e-mail: anne.agur@utoronto.ca

R. S. Burnham
Division of Physical Medicine and Rehabilitation, Faculty of Medicine, University of Alberta, Edmonton, AB, Canada

Central Alberta Pain and Rehabilitation Institute, Lacombe, AB, Canada

Vivo Cura Health, Calgary, AB, Canada
e-mail: rburnham@capriclinic.ca

D. Jankovic, P. Peng (eds.), *Regional Nerve Blocks in Anesthesia and Pain Therapy*,
https://doi.org/10.1007/978-3-030-88727-8_50

rized as linear strip lesioning and periforaminal techniques. RFA lesioning techniques also vary and include conventional thermal, cooled, monopolar/multipolar approaches and specialized probe designs (e.g., multitined electrodes, multilesion probes). Extensive ablation of the SIJ posterior innervation is a fundamental goal of all techniques. Clinical studies do not demonstrate that a particular technique is superior to others, but the lack of large controlled trials with standardized selection criteria and procedural protocols limit comparison between techniques. Additionally, most clinical studies evaluating the effectiveness of SIJ RFA preceded the more recent cadaveric studies that more completely describe posterior SIJ innervation. Anatomical modeling suggests that linear strip lesion techniques utilizing multipolar lesioning optimize posterior innervation capture in general. Linear strip lesion techniques will therefore be the focus of this chapter.

Indication (Patient Selection)

Selection criteria for SIJ RFA are not standardized in practice. SIJ intra-articular injections are not sufficient to select patients for SIJ RFA. Capsular defects in the SIJ may lead to extra-articular spread and anesthetization of surrounding structures not impacted by SIJ RFA. Pain mediated by ventral innervation may improve after intra-articular SIJ injections but may not improve significantly after SIJ RFA, as only the posterior innervation is targeted. Additionally, pain-generating structures associated with the SIJ (e.g., the dorsal sacroiliac and interosseous sacroiliac ligaments) may not be anesthetized by intra-articular SIJ injection.

Two validated techniques for diagnostic block of the posterior SIJ innervation include an ultrasound (US)-guided technique, along the lateral sacral crest (LSC) at a single depth, and a fluoroscopic (FL)-guided multisite multi-depth technique. Anesthetization of the SIJ and surrounding structures have been demonstrated to be similar between both methods. Based on this and anatomical studies, single-depth injections along the LSC at the level of the periosteum should be sufficient to anesthetize the posterior SIJ innervation for diagnostic blocks.

The ability of any diagnostic block to predict RFA response is partly dependent on the magnitude of relief that is used as a criterion. Clinically, a cutoff of at least 50% relief of index pain for the anesthetic duration is often used to select patients for RFA. Using higher cutoff criteria (e.g., 75–90% relief post-block) increases the specificity of diagnostic blocks, but decreases sensitivity. The optimal number of blocks (i.e., single or double) required to select patients for SIJ RFA is yet to be determined.

Functional Anatomy

The posterior sacral network (PSN) is the plexus of nerves that innervates the SIJ posteriorly. The PSN originates most often from the S1 through S3 lateral branches, with occasional contribution from the L5 and S4 lateral branches (Fig. 50.1). The lateral branches and PSN lie at the level of the periosteum.

S1–S3 Lateral Branches

The S1–S3 lateral branches that comprise the PSN arise from the S1 to S3 posterior sacral foramen (PSF). The S1 lateral branches primarily exit at the inferolateral quadrant of the PSF, although a superior branch may exit in the superolateral quadrant. The S2 lateral branches exit from the superolateral

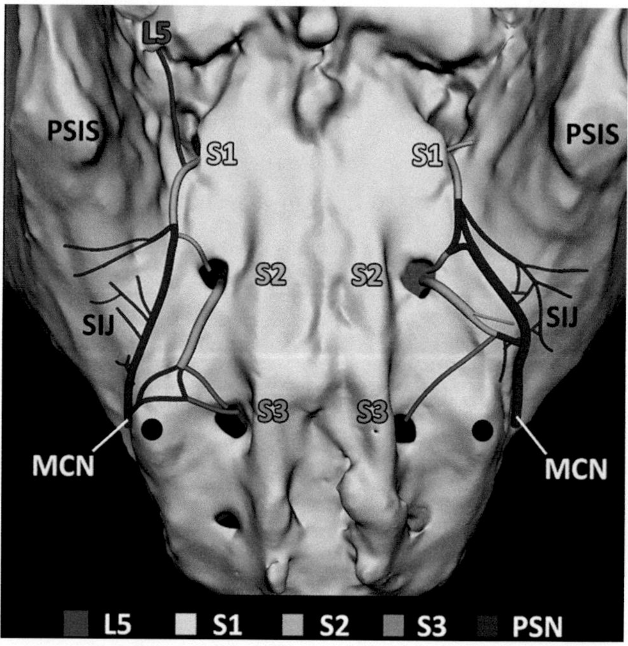

Fig. 50.1 Posterior innervation of the sacroiliac joint from the PSN. S1, S2, and S3 indicate the S1, S2, and S3 PSF. Lateral branches from S1 to S3 (S1, yellow; S2, green; and S3, blue) form the posterior sacral network laterally (purple). Occasionally, a branch from the L5 dorsal ramus (red) and/or the S4 lateral branches (not pictured) also contribute to the network. (Adapted by permission from BMJ Publishing Group Limited, Regional Anesthesia & Pain Medicine, Roberts SL et al. 39(6), 456–464, 2014)

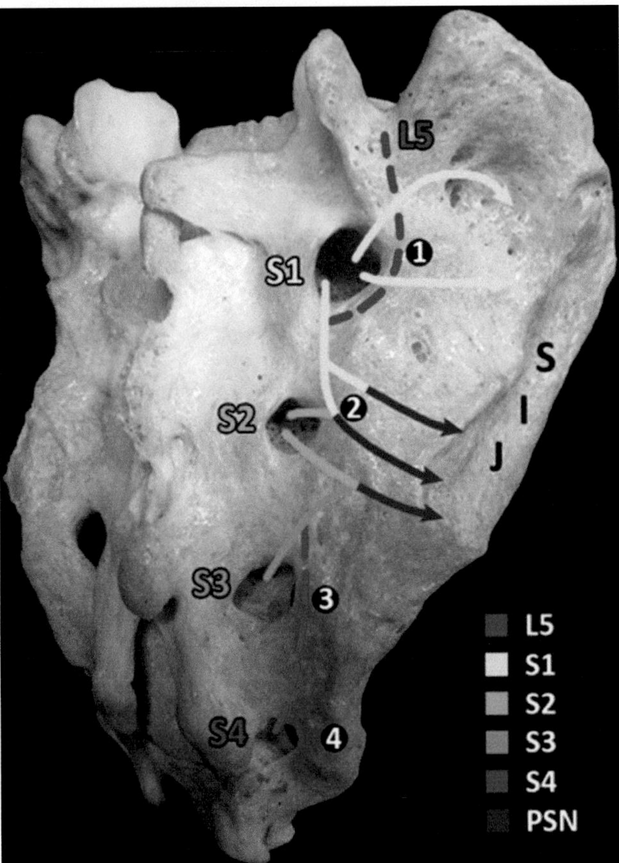

Fig. 50.2 A model illustrating the course of the posterior innervation (lateral branches of S1—yellow, lateral branches of S2—green, lateral branches of S3—blue, branches from L5 dorsal ramus and lateral branches of S4—dotted red, posterior sacral network—purple) to the SIJ relative to the TST (circled numbers). The common locations from which the lateral branches exit the PSF at each level are also illustrated. (Adapted by permission from BMJ Publishing Group Limited, Regional Anesthesia & Pain Medicine, Roberts SL et al. 39(6), 456–464, 2014)

and/or inferolateral quadrants of the PSF. The S3 lateral branches usually exit from the superolateral quadrant (Fig. 50.2).

PSN Landmarks

The transverse sacral tubercles (TST) delineate the borders of the PSN at the level of the LSC. The TST are approximately 6–9 mm lateral to the lateral margin of the PSF. Most of the time, the PSN is located between the second and third TST. The proximal border could extend to between the first and second TST. On occasion, some of the S1 lateral branches may innervate the SIJ directly without anastomosing with the PSN. These branches are most often located inferior to the first TST but could be located just above it as well.

L5 Dorsal Ramus

SIJ RFA often includes ablation of the L5 dorsal ramus. When the lateral branch of L5 contributes to the PSN, it anastomoses with the PSN and travels between the PSN landmarks described above.

Medial Cluneal Nerve

The medial cluneal nerve arises from the PSN (Fig. 50.1), so RFA of the PSN will impact this nerve. This may result in numbness to the medial buttock region.

Relevance to SIJ RFA

Based on the anatomy above, SIJ RFA using a strip lesion from the first TST to the third TST should capture the relevant posterior SIJ innervation in most cases. If it is difficult to access the first TST due to the location of the iliac crest/PSIS, a lesion extending from TST2 to TST3 may be sufficient as the PSN is most often located in this region.

Technique

Diagnostic Blocks

Goal

To anesthetize the SIJ posterior innervation by injecting local anesthetic along the LSC (under US) or lateral to the PSF (under FL).

US Technique

Probe: C5–C2 MHz curved transducer (most cases); 15–6 MHz linear transducer (in a very slender patient).

Position: Prone

Landmarking

Start with a transverse scan of the sacrum in a caudad to cephalad direction to identify transverse sacral tubercles (TST) 1–4. Identify the sacral cornua, and then move the probe laterally to identify PSF4 and TST4. Moving proximally, identify the third transverse sacral tubercle (TST3) and the third posterior sacral foramen (PSF), TST2 and PSF2, and finally TST1 and PSF1 (Figs. 50.3 and 50.4). Perform a sagittal scan to confirm PSF1 to PSF3 are correctly identified.

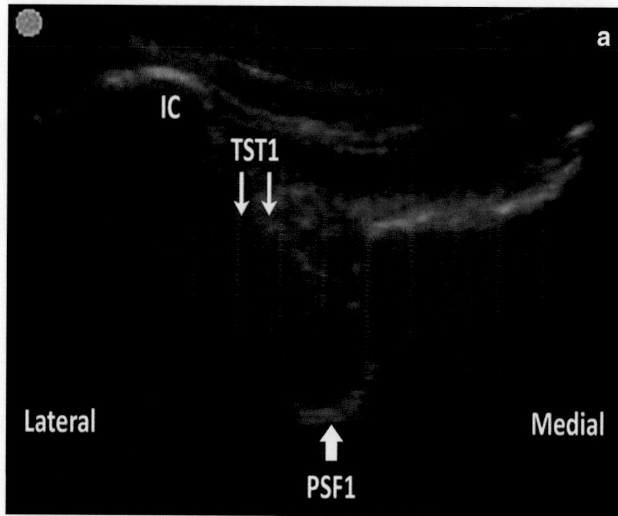

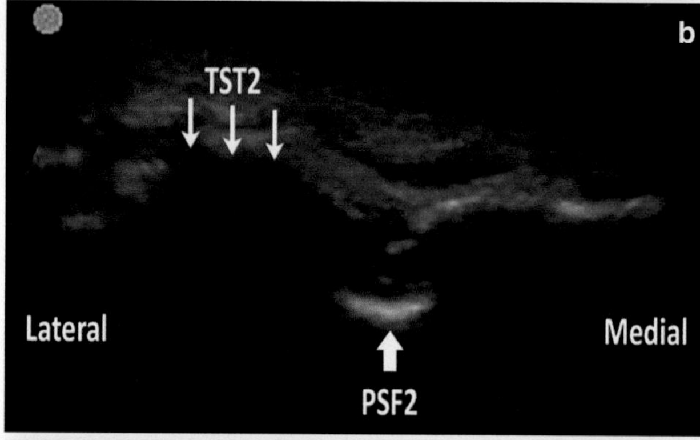

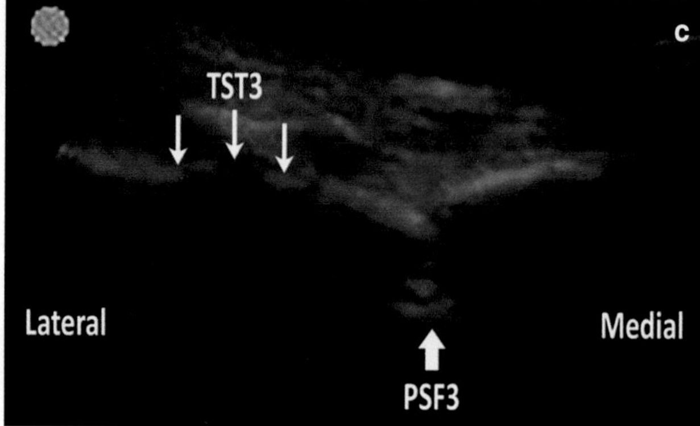

Fig. 50.3 Transverse US images of the first through third TST (**a**–**c**, respectively). (Adapted by permission from BMJ Publishing Group Limited, Regional Anesthesia & Pain Medicine, Roberts SL et al. 42(1):69–74, 2017)

Targets

Needles are placed using an in-plane approach from medial to lateral. Use the landmarks above to identify the targets outlined below; volumes of local anesthetic to inject are provided in parentheses.

1. On the LSC, at the midpoint between TST2 and TST3 (1.5 mL)
2. On the LSC, just proximal to TST2 (0.5 mL)
3. At TST1 (0.5 mL)

FL Technique

Position: Prone

Landmarking

On an anteroposterior (AP) view, square off the S1 superior end plate. Identify PSF1 and PSF3, and mark a point a few millimeters lateral to the lateral margin of PSF1 to PSF3. Mark 1 cm divisions between the marks lateral to PSF1 and PSF3 (Fig. 50.5).

Targets

Using the AP view, needles are inserted in sequence using a down-the-barrel approach at each skin mark identified on landmarking. Local anesthetic of 0.2–0.5 mL should be injected at each site. A lateral view should be obtained to ensure that the needle is not within the foramen and will also confirm that the correct levels are targeted.

Based on cadaveric studies, this FL-guided approach should encompass the areas targeted using the US-guided approach described in the previous section and areas targeted with SIJ RFA strip lesioning techniques.

Radiofrequency Ablation

Goal

To create a strip lesion lateral to PSF1 to PSF3 at the level of the periosteum (Fig. 50.6). Using US guidance, this will be along the LSC; with FL, this will be a few millimeters lateral to the lateral border of the PSF.

Fig. 50.4 US scanning protocol for landmark identification of targets for lateral branch blocks and SIJ RFA. (**a**) Transverse plane scan over the distal sacrum to identify the sacral cornua (SC), and the fourth transverse sacral tubercle (TST4); (**b**) the probe is moved proximally along the LSC until the third transverse sacral tubercle (TST3) is identified; (**c**) continuing proximally, the second transverse sacral tubercle (TST2) is identified; (**d**) the most proximal needle insertion site for diagnostic blocks/RFA (TST1) is identified. (Adapted by permission from Springer Nature: Springer, Sacroiliac Joint Radiofrequency Ablation by Loh E., Burnham R.S. in Ultrasound for Interventional Pain Management, Peng P., Finlayson R., Lee S., Bhatia A. (eds) (2020))

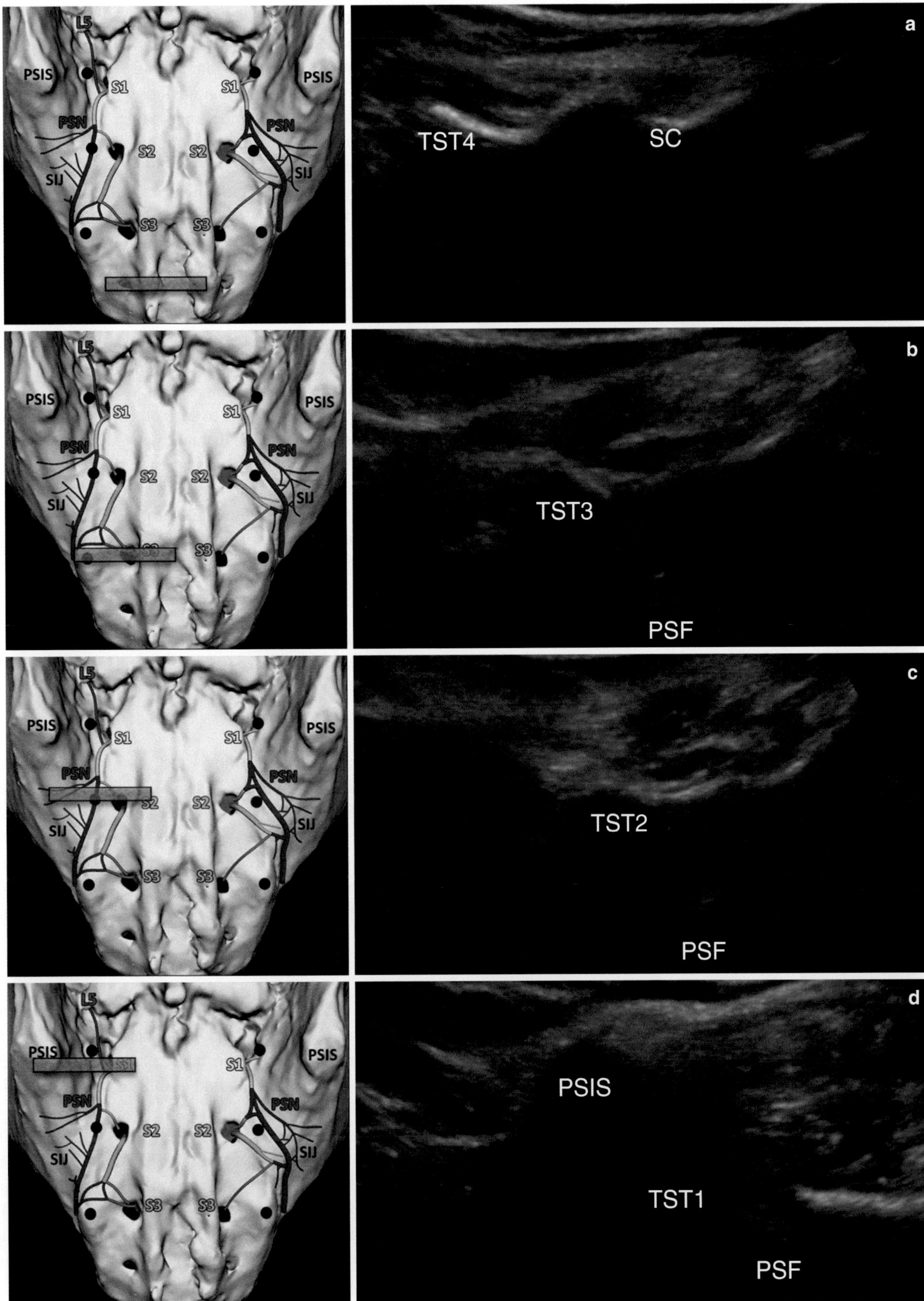

a
L5
PSIS
PSIS
S1
S1
PSN
PSN
S2
S2
SIJ
SIJ
S3
S3
TST4
SC
b
TST3
PSF
c
TST2
PSF
d
PSIS
TST1
PSF

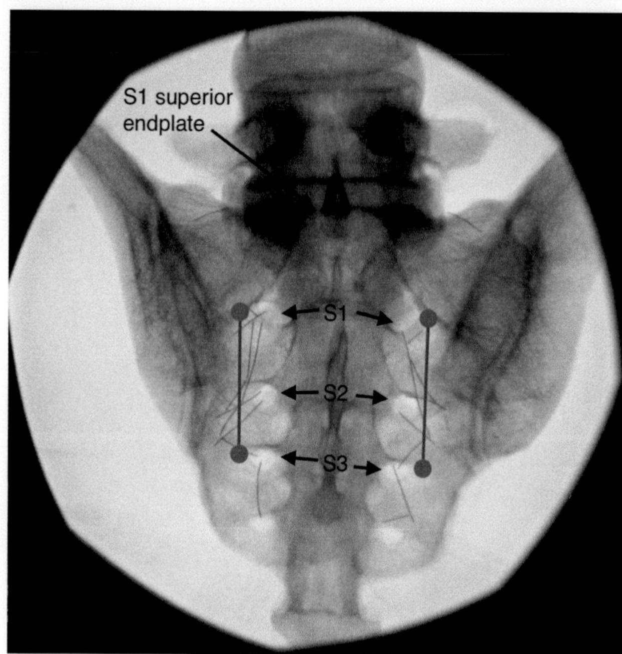

Fig. 50.5 A fluoroscopic AP view of a dissected cadaveric specimen of a sacrum. Radiopaque wires have been sutured onto the L5–S4 lateral branches and the medial portion of the PSN. The S1 superior end plate is squared off. The arrows from S1 through S3 indicate the PSF at each respective level. The green dots indicate locations for the most proximal and distal needle placements for RFA or diagnostic blocks. Additional needle placements are made along the red line 1.0 cm apart for diagnostic blocks; needle placement spacing varies along the red line for RFA depending on lesion parameters and techniques

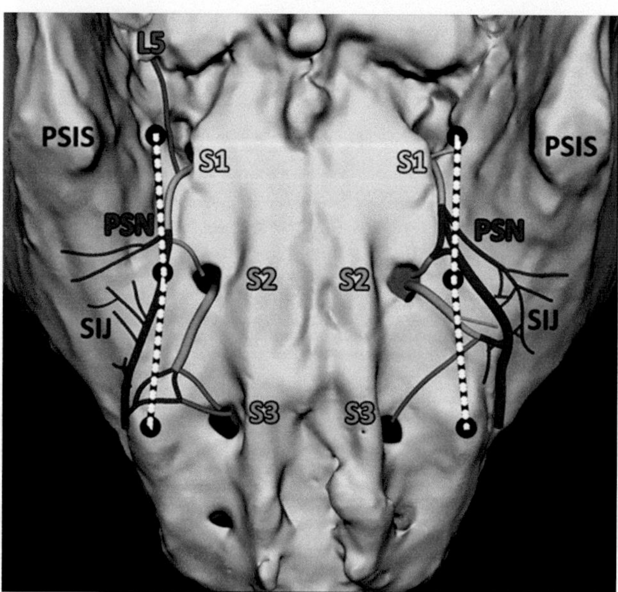

Fig. 50.6 Illustration of a lesion (dotted line) extending from the first to third TST along the LSC, which is the goal of strip lesion SIJ RFA. A lesion in this location should capture the posterior innervation of the sacroiliac joint. (Adapted by permission from BMJ Publishing Group Limited, Regional Anesthesia & Pain Medicine, Roberts SL et al. 39(6), 456–464, 2014)

Lesioning techniques

Multipolar lesioning techniques are more likely to capture a greater proportion of the SIJ innervation. The type of RFA cannula used and lesioning parameters will determine the distance needed between probes (e.g., larger gauge or multi-tined cannulae, higher thermal lesion temperatures, and longer lesion duration allow for larger intercannulae distances). Conventional thermal monopolar lesioning is not recommended.

The techniques described in this section focus on perpendicular placements to the sacral surface, using conventional thermal lesioning in a multipolar configuration. Using conventional 16- or 18-gauge cannulae, a lesion time of 3 min at a maximum temperature of 80–90° and an intercannulae distance of 10 mm should generate a contiguous lesion along the periosteum between cannulae. It is essential to ensure cannulae are placed as parallel to each other as possible, with minimal offset, to ensure the distance between needle tips at the periosteum is the same as measured at the skin; this will optimize the strip lesion that is generated.

Alternate methods of achieving a strip lesion besides multipolar lesioning, such as placing an RFA cannula along the surface of the sacrum, are possible.

US Technique

Probe: C5–C2 MHz curved transducer (most cases); 15–6 MHz linear transducer (in a very slender patient).

Position: Prone

Landmarking

Anatomical landmarking follows the same process as the US-guided block technique (Figs. 50.3 and 50.4). After identifying TST1 and TST3, mark the skin at these points. A line overlying the LSC between these points can be drawn on the skin as a guide. Measure 1.0 cm intervals along the LSC between TST1 and TST3 (distance between marks may differ depending on the lesioning technique and parameters used).

Targets

For a right-handed interventionalist, a distal to proximal approach while situated to the left side of the patient is most practical. Starting at the mark that indicates TST3, use an out-of-plane approach and a transverse sonographic view to insert an RFA cannula at this level. If using two needles, insert the second cannula at the next proximal skin mark, 1.0 cm away. Perform a bipolar RFA, and then move the most distal needle to the next available proximal skin mark in a "leapfrogging" manner, keeping the most proximal cannula in place. Repeat RFA and leapfrogging cannula placements until reaching the most proximal skin mark indicating TST1.

A prominent iliac crest can hinder cannula placement at the level of TST1 and may require a more medial to lateral insertion angle instead of a perpendicular approach. This may lead to a suboptimal strip lesion between TST1 and TST2 when using a multipolar technique.

FL Technique
Position: Prone

Landmarking
Landmarks are identified and marked in the same way as for FL diagnostic blocks (Fig. 50.5). Again, mark 1 cm divisions between the marks lateral to PSF1 and PSF3 (this assumes that the lesion parameters and cannulae outlined in ***Lesioning Techniques*** are used. Changing these parameters may require altering the distance between skin marks).

Targets
Using the AP view, needles are inserted in sequence using a down-the-barrel approach at each skin mark identified on landmarking. A proximal to distal approach, or vice versa, can be used. If using a proximal to distal approach and two needles, insert a needle at the most proximal mark lateral to PSF1. Insert the second needle at the next mark 1 cm distal to this; a lateral view should be checked to ensure that the probe is at the right location (i.e., not within the foramen or on the iliac crest) and to confirm that the appropriate levels are targeted (e.g., the first needle should be near the S1–S2 vestigial disc space for the S1 level) (Fig. 50.5).

Once the placement is confirmed, the initial bipolar RFA is completed. Using a leapfrogging approach, move the proximal needle to the next available distal skin mark while keeping the already placed distal needle in place, and repeat bipolar RFA. This sequence of moving the proximal needle in a leapfrogging manner and bipolar RFA is repeated until the most distal mark lateral to PSF3 is reached.

Complications

- Adequate capture of the PSN may lead to numbness post-block or post-RFA into the medial buttock region as the medial clunial nerve originates from the PSN.
- Despite the proximity of the PSF to the RFA lesion on the LSC/lateral to the PSF, incursion on the dorsal root is very rare. It is heralded by severe ipsilateral leg radicular pain as the lesion temperature increases.
- If needles are placed too far medially, there is a chance that they will enter the sacral foramen—the risk may be greater under FL, where the PSF can be difficult to identify at times.
- Checking a lateral view on FL is particularly important on placements around PSF1 to ensure the needle does not lie too far laterally on the iliac crest or too medially within the foramen.
  - The available space for needle placement between the iliac crest and PSF can be limited, particularly in males.
- Under FL, a lateral view is helpful to confirm that the probe is not within the foramen
  - Depending on the shape of the sacral surface, however, the needle may appear to lie beyond the surface of the periosteum on a lateral view under FL, even when it is not within the foramen. The interventionalist will need to determine whether the needle is truly within the foramen based on its position relative to other landmarks on AP and lateral views and the positions of any neighboring needles.
- If intraforaminal cannula placement is suspected (i.e., the depth of one cannula is significantly deeper than the adjacent cannula by observation or on lateral fluoroscopy), pre-lesion motor and sensory stimulation can be useful.
- At the level of TST1 under US, a prominent iliac crest may require placement at the LSC that utilizes an approach that is between a transverse and sagittal plane (i.e., between an out-of-plane and in-plane approach).
  - This approach may decrease the chances that a proper bipolar lesion is generated at this level as it is more challenging to have RFA probes parallel to each other.
- Even ideally placed needles in a multipolar configuration may not generate an adequate strip lesion at the level of the periosteum.
  - Because of the undulating surface of the sacrum, RFA probes may lie at different depths along the periosteum, resulting in a higher chance that two separate monopolar lesions form instead of a single, contiguous bipolar lesion.

Practical Tips (How to Improve Success and Avoid Complications)

1. When using a multipolar approach, place the needles as parallel to each other to ensure that the distance between needles measured at the skin is maintained at the periosteum level.
2. As cadaveric studies have shown that the nerves of the posterior sacral network are most commonly found between TST2 and TST3, particular attention should be paid to this area when performing denervation procedures.
   (a) If needle placement is difficult at and around the TST1/PSF1 region given the proximity of the iliac crest, an adequate RFA could still be performed with a strip lesion from the S2 to S3 levels (TST2/lateral to PSF2 to TST3/lateral to PSF3).

3. If L5 contributes to the SIJ posterior innervation, it will traverse with the PSN (whose proximal border usually extends only as proximal as TST1 at the LSC), so a separate L5 dorsal ramus RFA is often not necessary for targeted SIJ RFA.
   (a) If targeted L5 dorsal ramus block improves index pain, the inclusion of L5 dorsal ramus RFA may be appropriate but does not necessarily localize pain to the SIJ complex itself.
4. On FL, segment-specific imaging (through the vestigial sacral disc spaces) does not improve capture of the posterior SIJ innervation using cooled monopolar RF, and may increase the proportion of lateral branches missed.
   (a) Squaring of the S1 superior end plate is sufficient to orient the AP image under FL for SIJ RFA.

Literature Review

A systematic review noted that after SIJ RFA, 32–89% of patients achieved at least 50% pain relief for 6 months, while 11–44% achieved 100% pain relief for the same period. Meta-analyses have demonstrated that different SIJ RFA techniques, utilizing different lesioning types (e.g., conventional thermal, cooled, and pulsed RFA) and needle placements (e.g., periforaminal and strip lesion techniques), improve pain intensity and disability for up to 12 months post-procedure. Conclusions regarding the success of SIJ RFA from these meta-analyses should be interpreted with caution given the limited quantity and quality of included studies. Anatomic modelling studies have helped clarify the posterior innervation of the SIJ, which has led to the refinement of SIJ diagnostic block and RFA techniques. Anatomical models have also provided estimates of the proportion of S1–S3 lateral branches captured by current SIJ RFA techniques; bipolar techniques were estimated to capture 93.4–99.7% of lateral branches, compared to 49.6–99.1% for monopolar techniques. Bipolar linear strip lesion techniques targeting the LSC (using US-guidance) and the palisade technique (using FL-guidance) were found to have the highest capture rates.

Although multipolar strip lesion techniques are estimated to capture a greater proportion of the posterior SIJ innervation, superiority in clinical trials has not been demonstrated. Higher-quality randomized controlled trials may better demonstrate differences in clinical success between SIJ RFA techniques.

Suggested Reading

Finlayson RJ, Etheridge J-PBPB, Elgueta MF, Thonnagith A, De Villiers F, Nelems B, et al. A randomized comparison between ultrasound- and fluoroscopy-guided sacral lateral branch blocks. Reg Anesth Pain Med. 2017;42(3):400–6.

King W, Ahmed SU, Baisden J, Patel N, Kennedy DJ, MacVicar J, Duszynski B. Diagnosis and treatment of posterior sacroiliac complex pain: a systematic review with comprehensive analysis of the published data. Pain Med. 2015;16(2):257–65. https://doi.org/10.1111/pme.12630.

Roberts SL, Burnham RS, Ravichandiran K, Agur AM, Loh EY. Cadaveric study of sacroiliac joint innervation: implications for diagnostic blocks and radiofrequency ablation. Reg Anesth Pain Med. 2014;39(6):456–64. https://doi.org/10.1097/AAP.0000000000000156.

Roberts SL, Burnham RS, Agur AM, Loh EY. A cadaveric study evaluating the feasibility of an ultrasound-guided diagnostic block and radiofrequency ablation technique for sacroiliac joint pain. Reg Anesth Pain Med. 2017;42(1):69–74. https://doi.org/10.1097/AAP.0000000000000515.

Roberts SL, Stout A, Loh EY, Swain N, Dreyfuss P, Agur AM. Anatomical comparison of radiofrequency ablation techniques for sacroiliac joint pain. Pain Med. 2018;19:1924. https://doi.org/10.1093/pm/pnx329.

Robinson TJG, Roberts SL, Burnham RS, Loh E, Agur AM. Sacroiliac joint sensory block and radiofrequency ablation: assessment of bony landmarks relevant for image-guided procedures. Biomed Res Int. 2016;2016:1432074. https://doi.org/10.1155/2016/1432074.

Selective Sacral Nerve Root Block

51

Alexandra Bite, David Flamer, and Danyela Lee

Contents

General Considerations

S1 radiculopathy from nerve root compression or irritation from a herniated disc is widely known to be a cause of lower back and lower extremity pain. S2–S4 radiculopathy can also cause pain in the pelvic, rectal, perineal, or urogenital area, in a constellation of symptoms that make up intrapelvic nerve root entrapment syndrome endometriosis. In this syndrome, intrapelvic portions of the sacral nerve roots become compressed by various etiologies, such as endometriosis, vascular entrapments, or fibrosis. A selective sacral nerve root block via the sacral transforaminal approach may be used for both diagnostic and therapeutic purposes for S1 or S2–S4 radicular symptoms.

A. Bite · D. Flamer
University of Toronto, Toronto, ON, Canada
e-mail: david.flamer@sinaihealth.ca

D. Lee (✉)
Anesthesiology, University of Toronto, Toronto, ON, Canada
e-mail: danyela.lee@sinaihealth.ca

Indications

The sacral plexus is heterogenous and may contribute to many types of radicular pain, including back and leg pain from S1 radiculopathy, as well as S2–S4 symptoms including bladder sphincter spasm; bladder dysfunction; or pelvic, perineal, suprapubic, or genital pain. Pelvic pain can arise from the musculoskeletal, nervous, genitourinary, gastrointestinal, or gynecologic systems which complicates the diagnosis and treatment of these conditions. The pelvis is innervated by both somatic and visceral sources, making it difficult to delineate the exact etiology of poorly localized chronic pelvic pain. Involvement of multidisciplinary practitioners, a thorough pain history, neuropelviologic exam, and imaging are all key to selecting patients who may benefit from a selective sacral nerve root block for treatment of pelvic pain.

D. Jankovic, P. Peng (eds.), *Regional Nerve Blocks in Anesthesia and Pain Therapy*,
https://doi.org/10.1007/978-3-030-88727-8_51

S1 Selective Nerve Root Block

Diagnostic: S1 nerve root block is frequently performed for patients with radicular pain of unknown origin from lumbosacral nerve roots.

Therapeutic: Sciatic radicular pain with S1 transforaminal injection for mechanical or chemical irritation of the nerve root by a herniated intervertebral disc.

S2–S4 Selective Nerve Root Blocks

Diagnostic: S2–S4 nerve root blocks can be used to differentiate between pain states in the pelvis when the etiology is suspected intrapelvic nerve root entrapment syndrome.

Therapeutic: S2–S4 nerve root blocks can be used to treat symptoms of intrapelvic nerve root entrapment syndrome. As the sacral nerve roots give rise to both somatic and parasympathetic fibers (see below), the entrapment of these nerve roots can cause both dermatomal and visceral pain symptoms, such as sciatica associated with urinary symptoms (urgency, frequency, and dysuria); gluteal pain; perineal, vaginal, or penile pain; dysuria and/or painful ejaculation or orgasm; refractory urinary symptoms; or refractory pelvic and perineal pain.

Contraindications to sacral nerve root blocks include patient refusal, the presence of a bleeding diathesis (either coagulopathy or drug-related), or active infection over the site of injection.

Functional Anatomy

Thorough knowledge of pelvic neuroanatomy is mandatory for performing selective sacral nerve root blocks. The sacrum is a triangle-shaped bone composed of five fused vertebrae, with a concave, flat surface anteriorly. Dorsally, there are three sacral crests: median, intermediate, and lateral. There are four pairs of posterior sacral foramina located on each side of the median crest through which the dorsal branches of the sacral nerves emerge (Fig. 51.1). There are also four pairs of anterior sacral foramina through which the ventral rami of the sacral nerves emerge (Fig. 51.2).

The sacral plexus is formed on the anterior surface of the piriformis muscle, from the convergence of the lumbosacral trunk (L4 and L5) and S1–S3 ventral branches. Motor branches arising from the sacral plexus supply muscles of the pelvic region, including piriformis, gemelli, obturator internus, and quadratus femoris. In some individuals, the sacral nerve roots (mostly S2 or S3) course through the piriformis muscle, and this can be a potential site of sacral nerve root entrapment.

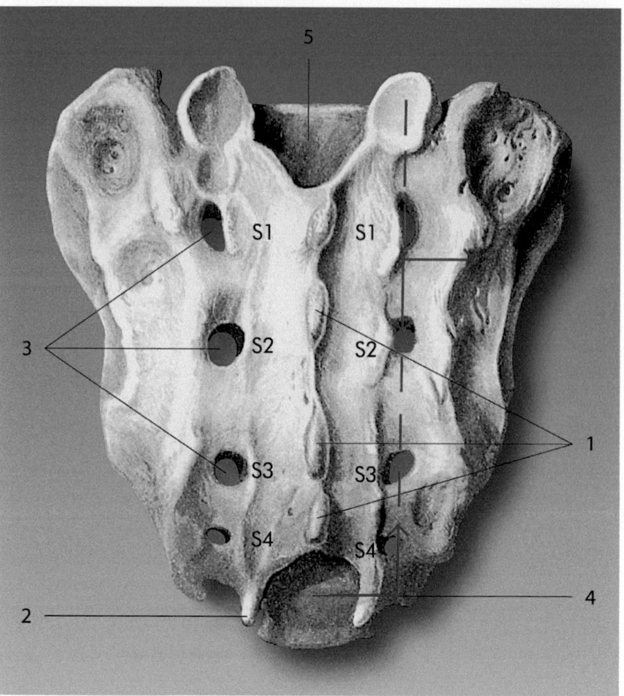

Fig. 51.1 The sacrum and paired foramina. (1) Median sacral crest; (2) sacral cornu; (3) posterior sacral foramina; (4) sacral hiatus; (5) sacral canal. The fourth sacral foramina are located approximately 1 cm lateral and cephalad to the sacral cornu. (Reprinted with permission from Philip Peng Educational Series)

The sacral canal contains 5 paired sacral nerves, which course caudally and exit through the sacral foramina. The sciatic nerve arises from ventral branches of spinal nerves L4–S3, and after its formation, it exits the pelvis and enters the gluteal region via the greater sciatic foramen, where it innervates the muscles of the posterior thigh and the hamstring portion of the adductor magnus. The superior gluteal nerve arises from L4 to S1, and supplies the gluteus medius and minimus muscles, while the inferior gluteal nerve arises from L5 to S2 and supplies the gluteus maximus. The posterior cutaneous nerve of the thigh (S1–S3) is purely sensory and gives off branches to the lower edge of buttocks (inferior cluneal nerves) and perineal region (perineal branches).

Finally, the pudendal nerve (S2–S5) leaves the pelvis through the infrapiriformis foramen, courses dorsally around the ischial spine, and passes through the lesser sciatic foramen into the ischiorectal fossa. In the fossa, it courses along the lateral wall to below the symphysis, where its terminal branch supplies the dorsal side of the penis or clitoris. The inferior rectal nerves (may also arise directly from S2 to S4) provide motor supply to the external anal sphincter and sensory supply to the perianal skin and lower two-thirds of the anal canal. The perineal nerves innervate the external anal sphincter and bulbospongiosus, ischiocavernosus, and superficial transverse perineal muscles, and the muscular branches

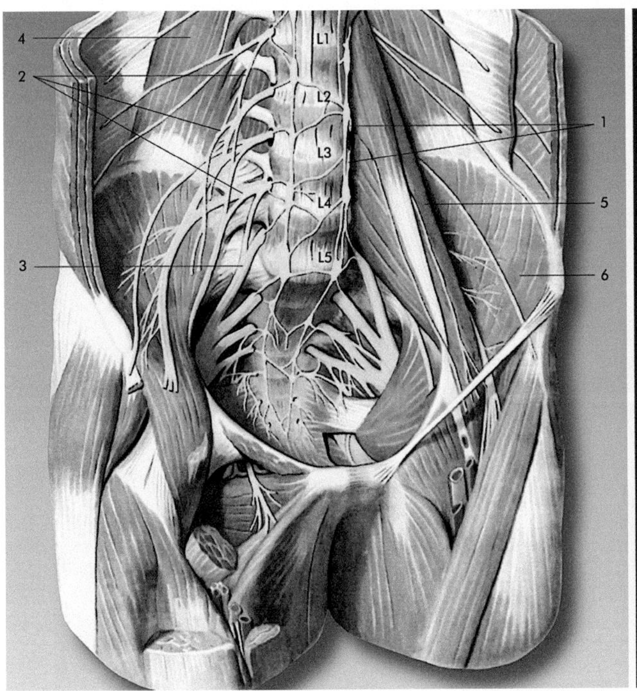

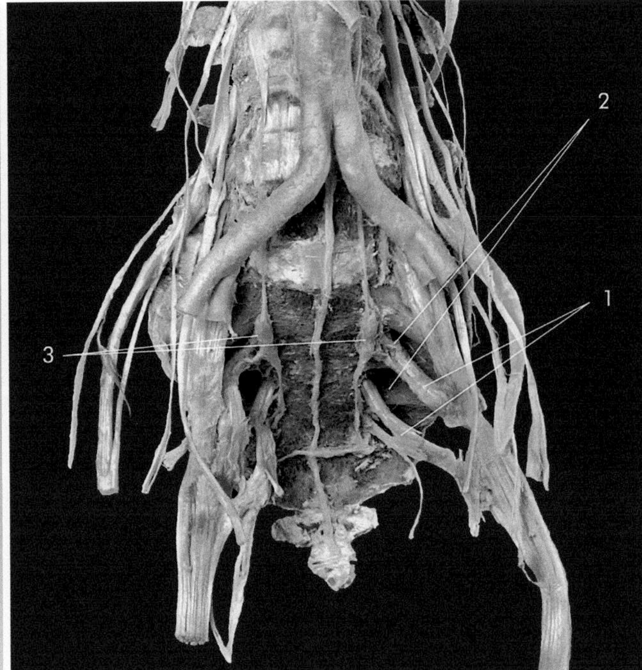

Fig. 51.2 Anterior view of sacrum: Left. Schematic drawing. (1) Sympathetic trunk with communicating branches, (2) lumbar plexus, (3) lumbosacral trunk, (4) quadratus lumborum muscle, (5) psoas major muscle, (6) iliac muscle. Right. Dissection. (1) Sacral plexus, (2) anterior sacral foramina, (3) sympathetic trunk. (Reprinted with permission from Dr. Danilo Jankovic)

(S3, S4) supply the levator ani and coccygeal muscles. The urinary bladder, urethra, and external genitalia are mainly innervated by the nerves from S2 to S4. Notably, the external genitalia, bladder, and rectum contain both the autonomic smooth muscle and voluntary striated muscle and therefore contain both autonomic and somatomotor fibers.

Technique

Transforaminal S1 Nerve Root Block

Before beginning the procedure, ensure that resuscitation equipment and drugs are available. The patient is placed in the prone position with a cushion under the anterior pelvis to reduce lordosis of the lower spine, and the area for injection is fully prepared in sterile manner. The target point for this injection is the lateral aspect of the posterior S1 neural foramen on the caudal border of the S1 pedicle. Under fluoroscopy, the S1 foramen should be located close to Charlie's line. The anterior and posterior S1 foramen should be superimposed by rotating the image intensifier in a cephalad direction. Occasionally, ipsilateral oblique tilt may also be required (Fig. 51.3).

Once the S1 foramen have been superimposed, the needle punctures the skin directly over the target with the needle curve facing the lateral and superior border of the foramen. The needle therefore follows the trajectory of the curved needle tip until contact is made with the bone of the superolateral border of the S1 foramen. This maneuver ensures the practitioner can appreciate the depth of the foramen and avoid accidentally penetrating the exiting nerve.

Upon bony contact, the needle is rotated medially to "walk off" the bone. Once the needle passes through the dorsal aspect of the foramen, the needle is then rotated with the curve toward the superolateral aspect of the foramen and advanced no more than a few millimeters. A lateral view is obtained to ensure the needle tip is within the S1 foramen but not ventral to the floor of the sacral canal. Confirmation of needle placement is made by injection 0.25–0.5 mL of contrast during AP and lateral fluoroscopic visualization. Contrast should be seen delineating the S1 nerve, spreading in a cephalocaudal direction (Fig. 51.4). Presence of vascular uptake is detected by either real-time fluoroscopy or digital subtraction angiography. Once the needle position is satisfactory, a mixture of 2 mL of local anesthetic (lidocaine 1%) plus 1 mL of steroid (preservative-free dexamethasone 10 mg) is administered.

S2–S4 Nerve Root Block

The procedure is usually carried out with the patient in the prone position, with a cushion under the pelvis and legs

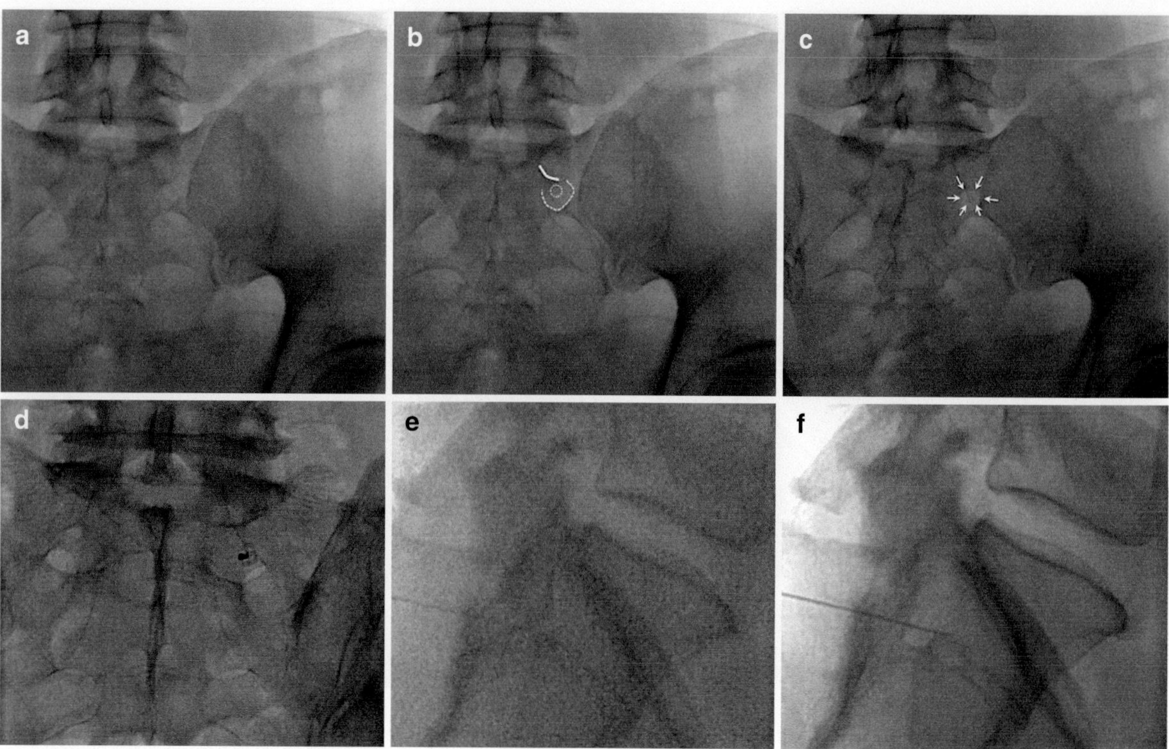

Fig. 51.3 (**a**) Radiograph of the lumbosacral spine. (**b**) The pedicle of S1 is indicated with the solid line. Caudal to this, the dorsal silhouette of the S1 foramen is indicated by the smaller circle, and ventral silhouette by the surrounding larger circle. (**c**) In the ipsilateral oblique view, the dorsal silhouette of the S1 foramen is better appreciated. (**d**) A 22-G spinal needle was inserted to the lateral and cephalad aspect of the S1 foramen. (**e**) Lateral view of the sacrum showing the spinal needle just entering the sacral canal. (**f**) advancing the needle toward the anterior foramen. (Reprinted with permission from Philip Peng Educational Series)

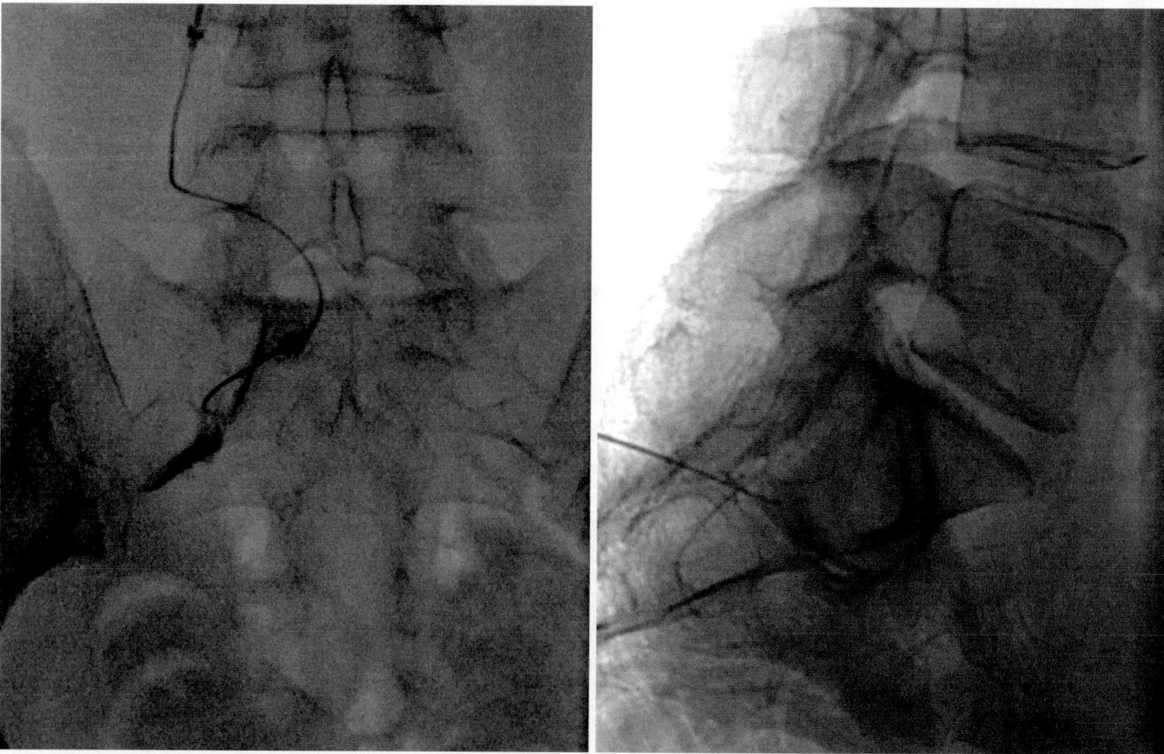

Fig. 51.4 Anteroposterior and lateral view of the sacrum showing the spread of contrast outlining the S1 nerve root. (Reprinted with permission from Philip Peng Educational Series)

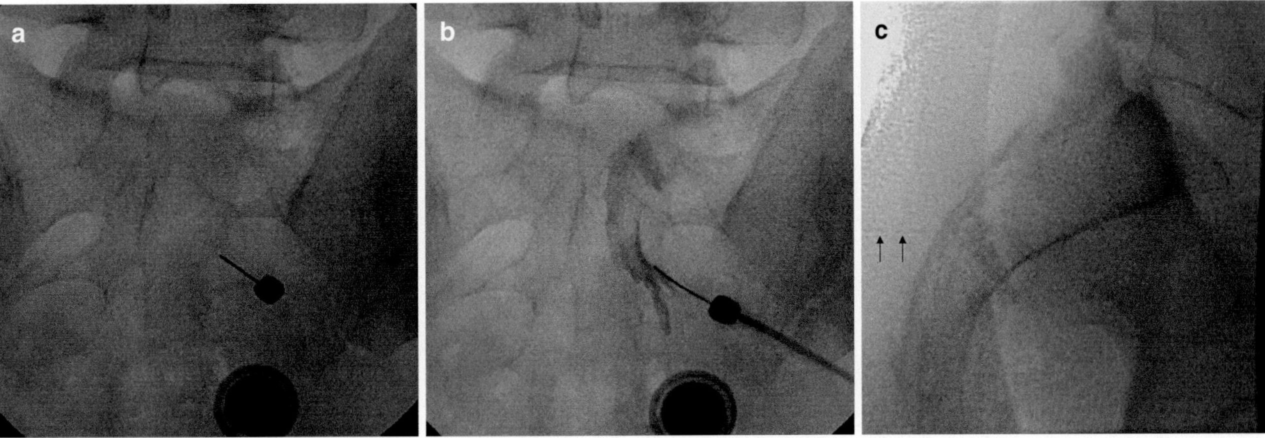

Fig. 51.5 (**a**) AP view of correct needle placement in the S2 foramen. (**b**) Contrast is injected in the AP view, and the dye is visualized tracking along the nerve root. (**c**) Lateral view of contrast tracking along the S2 nerve root. The needle is indicated by the arrows. (Reprinted with permission from Philip Peng Educational Series)

abducted with heels rotated outward and toes pointing inward. Gauze or a towel should be placed in the gluteal sulcus to protect the perianal area from disinfectants.

The procedure begins with localization of each of the sacral foramina via an AP fluoroscopic view. The anterior and posterior foramina of S2 will both be visible, with the posterior foramina appearing more medial. A small 25 G freezing needle is placed over the posterior foramina, and the fluoroscopy is rotated to obtain a lateral image. Following local anesthesia at the injection site, the 22 G spinal needle with a curved tip is introduced vertically to the skin surface until there is contact with the periosteum. The needle is then withdrawn slightly, and the needle trajectory is corrected (superior and medially), until the corresponding foramen is located ("hunt and peck" technique). The needle is then advanced through the posterior foramen under fluoroscopic visualization in the coaxial view, until the tip is just beyond the posterior sacrum in the lateral view. Following negative aspiration, confirmation of needle placement is made by injection 0.25–0.5 mL of contrast during lateral and AP fluoroscopic visualization (Fig. 51.5). Contrast should be seen delineating the exiting nerve root, spreading in a cephalocaudal direction. Presence of vascular uptake is detected by either real-time fluoroscopy or digital subtraction angiography. Once needle position has been confirmed, a mixture of 1 mL of local anesthetic and 1 mL steroid is injected fractionally.

The above steps can be repeated for S3 and S4, starting with identifying the targeted foramen in an AP view. The S3 foramen will be located just caudal to the line joining the lowest points of the sacroiliac joints, and the S4 foramen will appear at the level of the sacral cornu. The initial step is to take an anteroposterior X-ray and project a line joining all foramina. Then, another line is drawn joining the lowest point of sacroiliac joints (Fig. 51.6). The intersection is the suggested entry point to the S3 foramen. The best way to appreciate all sacral foramina is via a lateral X-ray (Fig. 51.7). The fourth sacral foramen is adjacent to the sacral cornu. Quite often, the contrast of the fluoroscopy needs to be adjusted to visualize the upper foramina (Fig. 51.8).

Complications

Motor blockade is a known complication of S1–S4 nerve root blocks and a long-lasting block can occur, up to 10–18 h, even after administration of low-dose local anesthetics. The patient must therefore use walking aids during this period, and simultaneous performance of bilateral S1–S4 nerve blocks should be avoided. Spillage to other nerve roots is common if the volume of local anesthetic is large, and thus using less than 3 mL per injection site is recommended. Another common complication is vascular puncture of surrounding vessels. Less common complications include subarachnoid or epidural injection, hematoma, infection, bowel and urinary incontinence, bowel perforation (for S2–S4), or breakage of puncture needles.

Practical Tips

- During the procedure, the operator should stand ipsilateral to the side being blocked.
- The line connecting both second sacral foramina marks the level of the dural sac in most patients, so the operator should be aware of the possibility of subarachnoid puncture above this level.

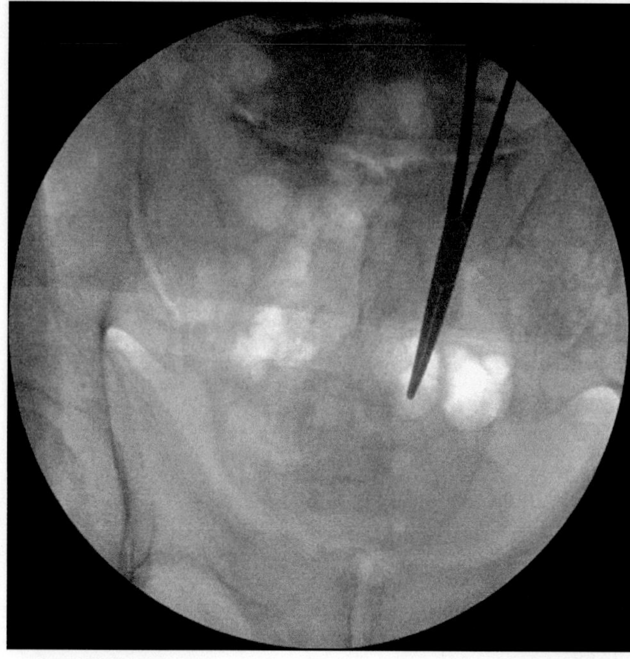

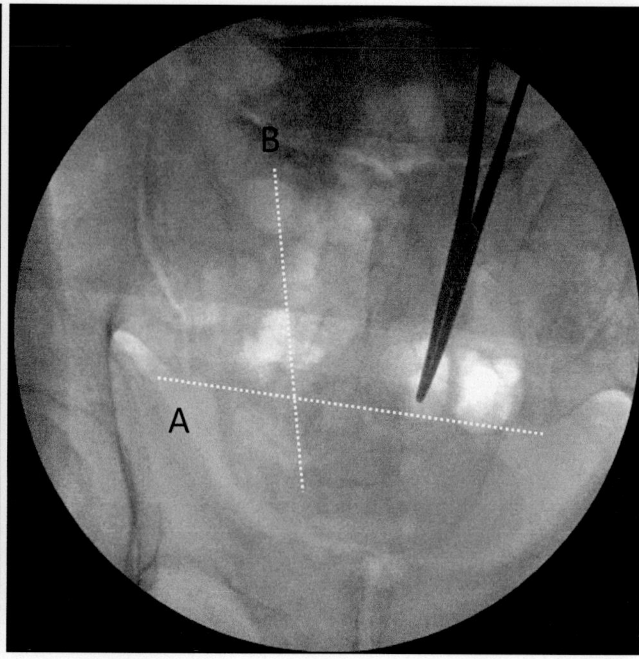

Fig. 51.6 Anteroposterior view of the lumbosacral spine. The bowel gas shadow makes it hard to comprehend the location of foramina (left). The location of S1 and S2 can be estimated, and a line (A) is drawn joining all the possible locations of foramina. Another line (B) joins the lowest point of the sacroiliac joints (right). The intersection of these two lines estimates the location of S3. (Reprinted with permission from Philip Peng Educational Series)

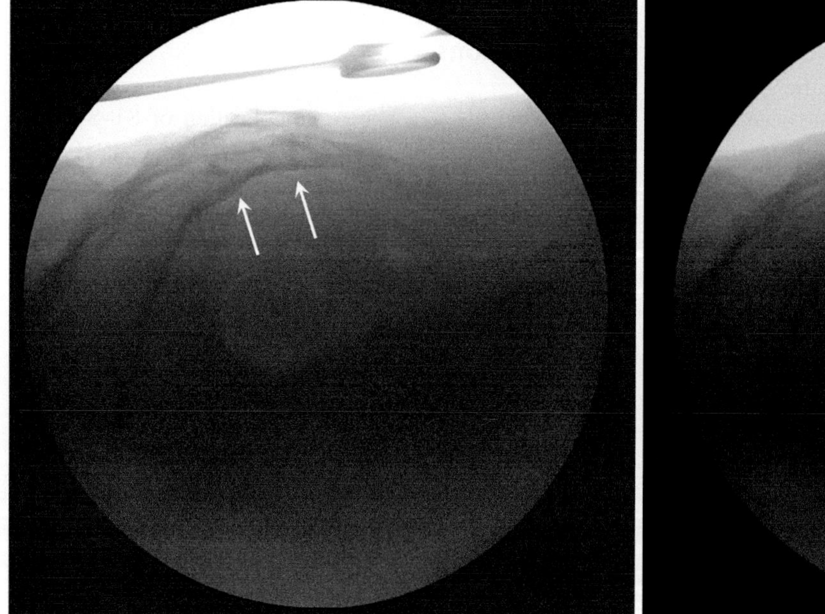

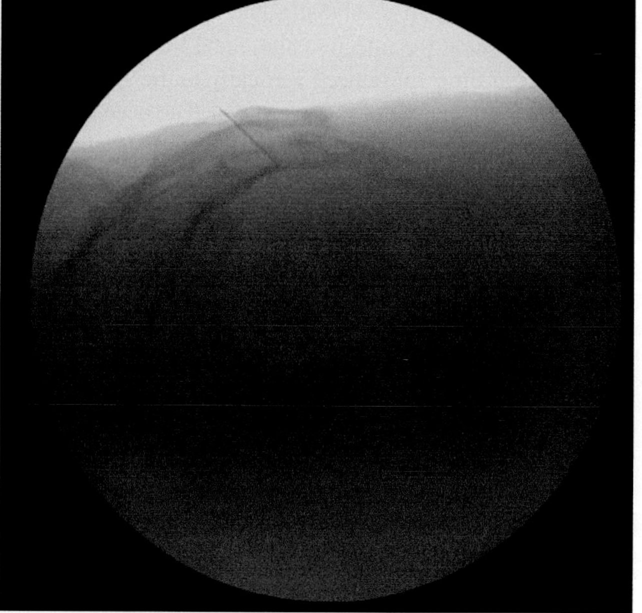

Fig. 51.7 Left. Lateral X-ray shows the S3 and S4 foramina (arrows). Right. Insertion of needle into the S4 foramen. (Reprinted with permission from Philip Peng Educational Series)

Literature Review

Lumbosacral nerve root pain has been widely recognized as a cause of chronic low back and leg pain, with the incidence of lumbosacral radicular pain varying between 9.9% and 25% in different studies. Sacral radicular pain is defined as pain caused by an irritation of the exiting sacral nerve roots, leading to a dysfunction of the sensory and, less commonly, motor fibers. Sensory abnormalities predominate and include paresthesia, dysesthesia, and pain in the corresponding der-

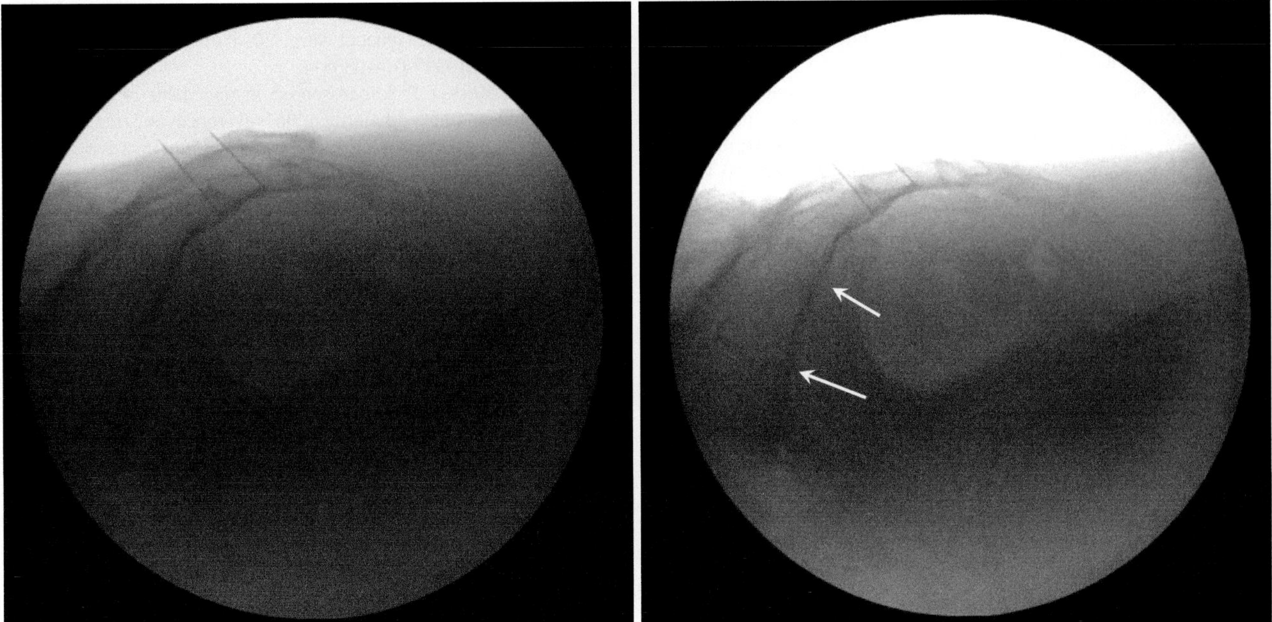

Fig. 51.8 Left. Lateral X-ray showing the needles into the S3 and S4 foramina. Right. Adjustment of contrast of the image shows the S1 and S2 foramina (arrows). (Reprinted with permission from Philip Peng Educational Series)

matomal distribution. While S1 radicular pain and associated interventions have been extensively described, sacral nerve root irritation as a possible cause of chronic pelvic pain (CPP) has gained traction in recent years. Recent epidemiologic studies have indicated a high population prevalence of CPP, with 14.7% in the United States and 24% in the United Kingdom.

To date, there have been no studies that describe the incidence of lumbosacral nerve root irritation as an etiology of CPP. However, several case reports have implicated lumbosacral radicular pathology in a wide variety of pelvic pain syndromes, including sacral nerve root schwannomas causing intractable vulvococcygodynia, several cases of lumbar disc herniation or spondylolisthesis causing scrotal or testicular pain, and a case of a sacral Tarlov cyst causing extreme penile pain. Lemos et al. have described intrapelvic nerve root entrapment syndrome as a heterogenous collection of pelvic symptoms caused by entrapment of the intrapelvic portions of sacral nerve roots. A series of case reports have described various etiologies for the underlying entrapment, including endometriosis, surgery for pelvic organ prolapse, fibrosis, vascular entrapment, and neoplasms. Management of intrapelvic nerve root entrapment syndrome has included selective sacral nerve root blocks for diagnostic and therapeutic indications, as well as laparoscopic surgery to decompress the nerve roots involved. Selective sacral nerve root blocks, electrical stimulation, and rhizotomy have also been used successfully in patients in with medically refractory neurogenic bladder dysfunction after spinal cord injury.

The efficacy and safety of selective sacral nerve root blocks have not been rigorously established. A review of selective nerve root blocks (cervical, lumbar, and sacral) in the treatment of radicular pain found that overall, 70% of patients experienced some pain relief by Day 7 postinjection with steroids, with no significant difference in the outcome between the types of procedure. Overall, the complication rate for lumbar nerve root blocks is low, with a study by Stalcup et al. describing a 5.5% complication rate, with most complications being minor. Most common complications described include dizziness, leg weakness, and increased pain. Incidence of complications for sacral nerve root blocks is unknown. Future research is needed to determine efficacy and complications of sacral nerve root blocks in treating a variety of radicular pain syndromes.

Suggested Reading

Alloussi SH, Lang C, Eichel R, et al. Videourodynamic changes of botulinum toxin A in patients with neurogenic bladder dysfunction (NBD) and idiopathic detrusor overactivity (IDO) refractory to drug treatment. World J Urol. 2012;30(3):367–73. https://doi.org/10.1007/s00345-011-0736-6.

Baranowski A, Mordecai L. Nerve blocks. In: Moldwin RM, editor. Urological and gynaecological chronic pelvic pain. Cham: Springer International Publishing; 2017. p. 271–81. https://doi.org/10.1007/978-3-319-48464-8_18.

Burnett CJ, Anderson J. Sacral injections. In: Sackheim KA, editor. Pain management and palliative care. New York, NY: Springer; 2015. p. 315–23. https://doi.org/10.1007/978-1-4939-2462-2_42.

Elkins N, Hunt J, Scott KM. Neurogenic pelvic pain. Phys Med Rehabil Clin N Am. 2017;28(3):551–69. https://doi.org/10.1016/j.pmr.2017.03.007.

Goldstein I, Komisaruk BR, Rubin RS, et al. A novel collaborative protocol for successful management of penile pain mediated by radiculitis of sacral spinal nerve roots from tarlov cysts. Sex Med. 2017;5(3):e203–11. https://doi.org/10.1016/j.esxm.2017.04.001.

Lemos N, Possover M. Laparoscopic approach to intrapelvic nerve entrapments. J Hip Preserv Surg. 2015;2(2):92–8. https://doi.org/10.1093/jhps/hnv030.

Mallinson PI, Tapping CR, Bartlett R, Maliakal P. Factors that affect the efficacy of fluoroscopically guided selective spinal nerve root block in the treatment of radicular pain: a prospective cohort study. Can Assoc Radiol J. 2013;64(4):370–5. https://doi.org/10.1016/j.carj.2013.03.001.

Nouri KH, Abdi S. Lumbosacral radicular pain. In: Cheng J, Rosenquist RW, editors. Fundamentals of pain medicine. Cham: Springer International Publishing; 2018. p. 203–8. https://doi.org/10.1007/978-3-319-64922-1_22.

Peng B, Li D, Pang X. Degenerative lumbar spondylolisthesis with testicular pain. Pain Med. 2014;15(1):169–70. https://doi.org/10.1111/pme.12246.

Possover M. The sacral LION procedure for recovery of bladder/rectum/sexual functions in paraplegic patients after explantation of a previous Finetech-Brindley controller. J Minim Invasive Gynecol. 2009;16(1):98–101. https://doi.org/10.1016/j.jmig.2008.09.623.

Possover M, Forman A. Neuropelveological assessment of neuropathic pelvic pain. Gynecol Surg. 2014;11(2):139–44. https://doi.org/10.1007/s10397-014-0838-4.

Possover M, Kostov P. Laparoscopic management of sacral nerve root schwannoma with intractable vulvococcygodynia: report of three cases and review of literature. J Minim Invasive Gynecol. 2013;20(3):394–7. https://doi.org/10.1016/j.jmig.2012.12.011.

Possover M, Lemos N. Risks, symptoms, and management of pelvic nerve damage secondary to surgery for pelvic organ prolapse: a report of 95 cases. Int Urogynecol J. 2011;22(12):1485–90. https://doi.org/10.1007/s00192-011-1539-4.

Stalcup ST, Crall TS, Gilula L, Riew KD. Influence of needle-tip position on the incidence of immediate complications in 2,217 selective lumbar nerve root blocks. Spine J. 2006;6(2):170–6. https://doi.org/10.1016/j.spinee.2005.08.009.

Terada Y. Sacral nerve root block (X-ray fluoroscopy-guided method, ultrasound-guided method). In: Ohseto K, Uchino H, Iida H, editors. Nerve blockade and interventional therapy. Tokyo: Springer; 2019. p. 341–4. https://doi.org/10.1007/978-4-431-54660-3_84.

Trautman N, Sabia M. Lumbar and sacral radiculitis. In: Sabia M, Sehdev J, Bentley W, editors. Urogenital pain. Cham: Springer International Publishing; 2017. p. 91–103. https://doi.org/10.1007/978-3-319-45794-9_6.

Wouda EJ, Leenstra S, Vanneste JAL. Scrotal pain as the presenting symptom of lumbar disc herniation: a report of 2 cases. Spine. 2005;30(2):E47–9. https://doi.org/10.1097/01.brs.0000150633.36777.c8.

52 Caudal Canal Injections

Juan Felipe Vargas Silva and Philip Peng

Contents

Introduction

Caudal canal injections refer to the application of medications (usually local anesthetics and steroids) into the epidural space via the sacral hiatus. It is useful when there are radicular symptoms originated from the lumbosacral spine, especially when the lumbar spine has difficult anatomy, such as previous lumbar surgery or degenerative changes, limiting transforaminal or interlaminar access to the epidural space. It could be helpful in cases of coccygodynia to assist local infiltration of coccygeal nerves and surrounding structures (sacrococcygeal ligament).

Success of caudal epidural injections depends on the appropriate placement of a needle into the epidural space, through the sacrococcygeal ligament, as the hiatus directly communicates with the epidural space. Without image assistance, the success rate could be as low as 75% even in experienced hands. Bony landmarks (e.g., sacral cornu and hiatus) can be difficult to identify, especially in obese patients. Fluoroscopy with an epidurogram could be an alternative to guide its placement; however, the radiation exposure close to the gonadal area is a major drawback, particularly in patients of reproductive age.

With ultrasound guidance, there is a 100% accuracy in caudal epidural needle placement. However, the needle (or catheter) could not be visualized beyond the sacral hiatus,

J. F. Vargas Silva (✉)
Department of Surgery and Image Guided Therapy, Pain Clinic, Hospital Pablo Tobon Uribe, Medellin, Antioquia, Colombia

P. Peng
Department of Anesthesiology and Pain Medicine, Toronto Western Hospital, University of Toronto, Toronto, ON, Canada
e-mail: philip.peng@uhn.ca

D. Jankovic, P. Peng (eds.), *Regional Nerve Blocks in Anesthesia and Pain Therapy*,
https://doi.org/10.1007/978-3-030-88727-8_52

and it cannot provide information to the depth of the inserted needle so inadvertent dural puncture could occur.

Patient Selection

There is evidence supporting this procedure for short- and long-term pain control for the following indications:

- Chronic back pain and lower limb pain secondary to herniated disc and/or radicular pain.
- Discogenic pain without herniated disk or radiculitis.
- Management of back and leg pain due to postlaminectomy syndrome and spinal stenosis.

Caudal canal injection has been used in the management of coccydynia and pain related to sacral nerve root irritation, but the evidence is scant.

Functional Anatomy

Sacrum

The sacrum is formed by the fusion of five vertebrae and the coccyx by the fusion three or four small vertebrae. It has two sets of foramens—the four posterior sacral foramina and the four anterior sacral foramina. Unlike the posterior sacral foramina, which is covered by a tight band of musculature (multifidus muscle), the anterior foramina offer no containment of injectate administered in the sacral canal. The sacral canal contains the epidural venous plexus and epidural fat. The termination of the thecal sac varies depending on age and varies between the lower border of the S1 foramen in adults and the S3 foramen in children. In 1–5% of patients, the dural sac terminates at S3 or below. This is important to consider the optimum placement of the epidural needle tip in order to avoid dural puncture and postdural puncture headache. The distance between the tip of the sacral hiatus and the edge of the dural sac is about 4.5 cm.

The first coccygeal vertebra articulates with the sacrum via the sacro-coccygeal intervertebral joint, which is usually a symphysis but may be fused or rarely synovial. This joint is reinforced by anterior, posterior, and lateral sacro-coccygeal ligaments and ligaments which connect the sacral cornu with the ipsilateral transverse process of the first coccygeal vertebra.

Sacral Hiatus

The sacral hiatus is a natural defect in the fusion between S4 and S5 and is bordered by the sacral cornua laterally. The sacral cornua are vestigial remnants of the fifth sacral vertebra, equivalent to the superior and inferior articular processes seen in proximal vertebrae and presented as two bony prominences at the caudal end of sacrum.

The sacral hiatus is covered by the skin, subcutaneous fat, and sacrococcygeal ligament, followed by the epidural space. The floor of the sacral hiatus is the vertebral body of S5. The sacral hiatus contains lower sacral and coccygeal nerve roots (passing through the sacral hiatus), filum terminale externa, and fibro-fatty tissue.

The mean anterior-posterior diameter of sacral hiatus at its apex is 5 ± 1.6 mm and the intercornual distance has a mean of 16.9 ± 2.7 mm. The apex of sacral hiatus is usually found at the S4 vertebra (65%), but it can be located at the S3 (15%) or S5 level (15%). The sacral hiatus could be palpable as a dimple between its cornua, but it is impalpable in 14.3–54% of isolated adult sacral bone, explaining the high failure rate associated with the blind technique.

Sacrococcygeal Ligament

Posteriorly, the sacral hiatus is covered by the skin, subcutaneous fat, and posterior sacrococcygeal ligament which is attached to the margins of the hiatus and the deep posterior sacrococcygeal ligament (Fig. 52.1). The superficial part of the posterior sacrococcygeal ligament extends between the free margin of the sacral hiatus and the dorsal surface of the coccyx and forms the roof of the sacral canal.

Innervation

The innervation of the coccyx is derived from the lower sacral spinal nerves and the coccygeal nerves, which derive from the lower sacral nerve roots. Anteriorly, the innervation is derived from the coccygeal plexus which is formed as an anastomosis between S4, S5, and coccygeal nerve (Fig. 52.2).

The first coccygeal nerve emerges from the conus medullaris, descends within the cauda equina, and exits the sacral hiatus to unite anteriorly with S4 and S5. Its role innervating the surrounding structures is controversial and debated, possibly giving anococcygeal nerves to supply the skin of the anal triangle, and sometimes supplying motor innervation to ischiococcygeus, part of elevator ani, and the posterior extremity of the external anal sphincter and the sacrococcygeal joint.

Anatomical Variants

Variations in the anatomy of the sacrococcygeal area (up to 10%) could make identification of landmark difficult, such

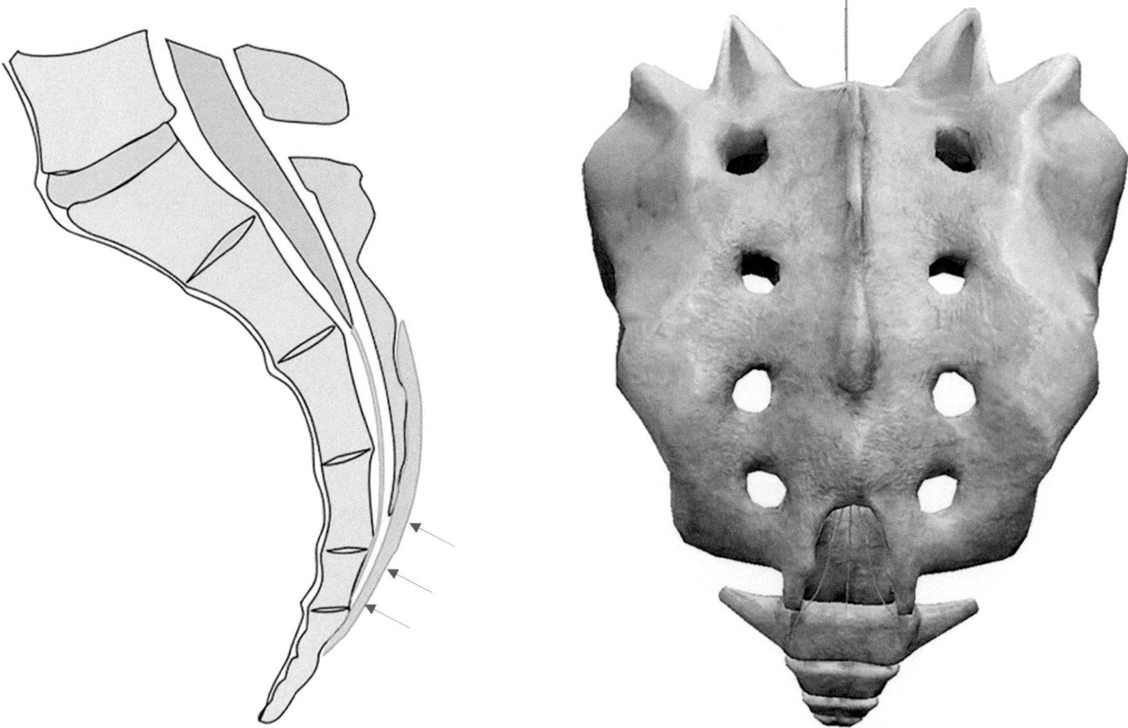

Fig. 52.1 Relevant anatomy of the sacrum. Arrows: Posterior sacrococcygeal ligament. (Reprinted and reproduced with permission from Philip Peng Educational Series)

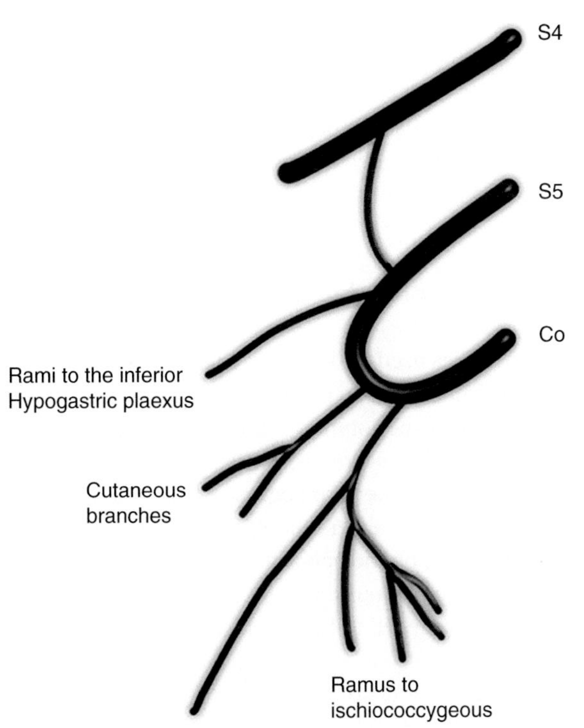

Fig. 52.2 Coccygeal plexus. (Reprinted and reproduced with permission from Philip Peng Educational Series)

as variations in the shape of the sacral hiatus (normally U or V inverted shape but could be M shape, bifida shape, dumb-bell shaped, or irregular) or even total absence of the posterior wall of the sacral canal (Fig. 52.3). The apex of sacral hiatus is located below the S3 level in 95% cases, but it can be located as a variant cephalad to this level. The incidences of the apex of sacral hiatus located at the level of S1 is 1% and 4% at S2 level. Complete agenesis of posterior wall of sacral canal (failure of fusion of sacral laminae) is described in 1% of cases. This situation of spina bifida should be suspected in situations in which a prominent sacrococcygeal ligament is evidenced in a long cephalic course, without the evidence of acoustic shadow of the posterior sacral bone (Fig. 52.4). This image should alert in advance the physician of the risk of inadvertent dural puncture, due to a cephalic entry point in the search of an acoustic shadow of the sacral bone. It should be noted that the more cephalad the entry point, it will be shorter the distance between it and the dural sac termination. The procedure sometimes could be difficult because of excess weight, aging, metastatic bone involvement of the sacrum, congenital and geometrical abnormalities. The sacral epidural space is highly vascular. Inadvertent intravenous injection is relatively common during caudal block, occurring in about 5–10% of these procedures.

There is little information about the ossification of the sacrococcygeal ligament or absence of the sacral hiatus.

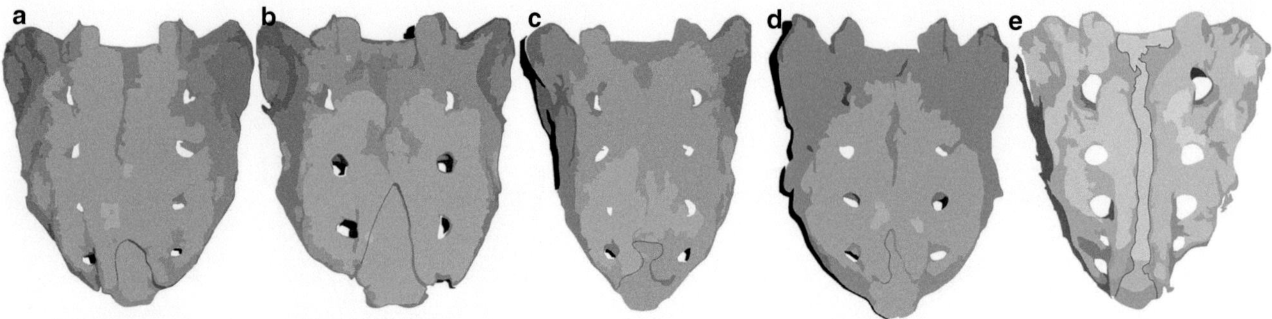

Fig. 52.3 Anatomical variations of sacral hiatus. (**a**) Inverted "U" shaped. (**b**) Inverted "V" shaped. (**c**) Dumbbell shaped. (**d**) Irregular shaped. (**e**) Complete agenesis of spinal bone or spina bifida (could be complete or incomplete). (Reprinted and reproduced with permission from Philip Peng Educational Series)

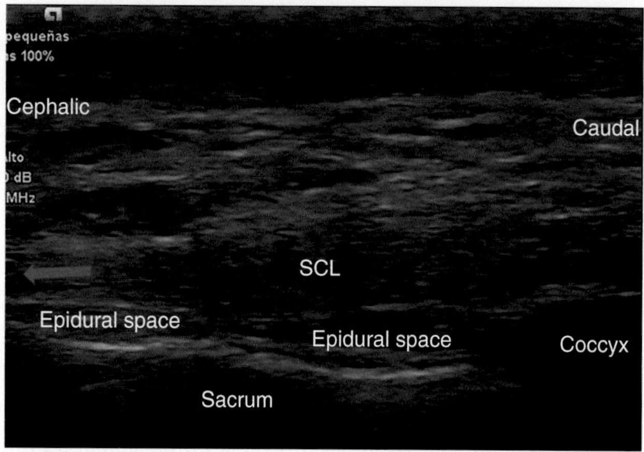

Fig. 52.4 Ultrasound image of a spina bifida. Note the absence of bone even beyond the solid arrow. *SCL* sacrococcygeal ligament. (Reprinted and reproduced with permission from Philip Peng Educational Series)

Sekiguchi in 2004 estimated an absence of sacral hiatus in 4% of specimens evaluated. However, both authors of this chapter with personal experience of more than 200 caudal injection, have not encountered a single patient with complete fusion of the intercornual space.

Although cyst in sacrum and sacral hiatus are not anatomic variants (they are pathological entities), they need to be mentioned due to their high incidence in asymptomatic patients, with possible complications of epidural injection through the sacral hiatus. The most frequent cyst in the sacral canal are perineural or Tarlov cysts, with an incidence of 4–9%, which are extradural meningeal cysts of the spinal nerve root. These cysts are mostly asymptomatic and are more frequently found at the S2 or S3 levels. Other possible cysts found in sacrum canal found are extradural meningeal cysts outside the spinal nerve root fibers and spinal intradural meningeal cysts.

Technique

In this chapter, we described the ultrasound technique for initial needle placement. In patient where the sacral landmark cannot be palpated or the presence of bowel gas shadow, the ultrasound technique is valuable. However, the needle cannot be visualized beyond the sacral hiatus with ultrasound, and the subsequent needle advancement and catheter positioning will be performed under fluoroscopic guidance.

Initial Preparation

Patient is placed in prone or Kraske position with the buttocks separated. The lateral decubitus position can also be used, if the patient cannot be placed in the prone position. Linear probe is generally used. A convex probe is rarely needed, except in cases of obese patients.

Ultrasound Needle Advancement

The examined area needs to be prepared and draped in a sterile field. The probe needs to be protected with a sterile cover and sterile gel or saline solution is used as interface between the skin and the transducer/cover. It is not recommended to use chlorhexidine as interface because of the risk of arachnoiditis if the solution enters the epidural space. Place the ultrasound machine on the opposite side as the interventionist and in line with the transducer.

The structures needed to be identified are (Fig. 52.5):

- The two sacral cornua (C)
- The apex of the sacral hiatus (A)
- The sacrococcygeal ligament (L)

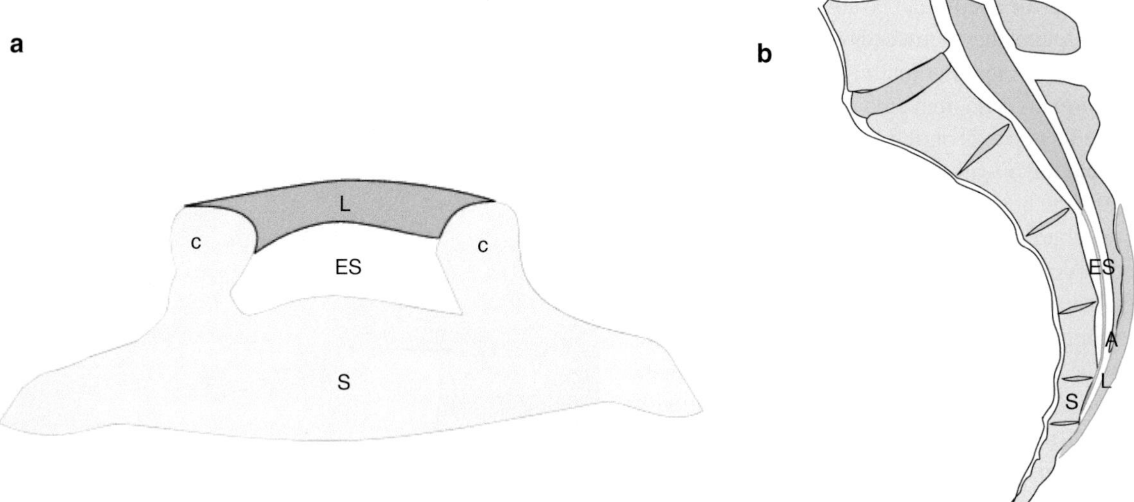

Fig. 52.5 Anatomical structures to be identified. (**a**) Transverse view of the spine. (**b**) Sagittal view of the spine. C: Cornua of the sacrum. L: Sacrococcygeal ligament. ES: Epidural space. S: Sacrum bone. A: apex of sacral hiatus. (Reprinted and reproduced with permission from Philip Peng Educational Series)

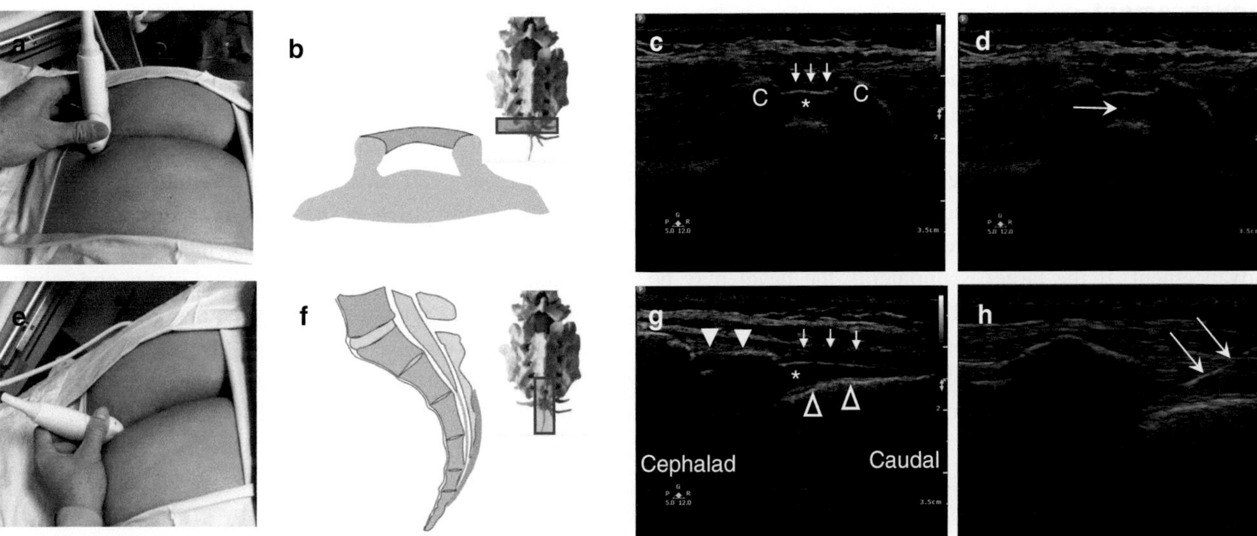

Fig. 52.6 Procedure description of the technique for caudal canal injections. (**a**–**d**) Out-of-plane landmark position of the probe and osseous anatomy. (**a**) Position of the probe. (**b**) Cross-sectional anatomy (transverse) of the sacrum at the sacral hiatus. (**c**, **d**) Short axis of the structures and out of plane needle visualization inside the epidural space. (**e**–**h**) In-plane landmark position of the probe, osseous, and sonoanatomy. (**e**) Position of the probe. (**f**) Cross-sectional anatomy of the sacrum (sagittal) at the sacral hiatus. (**g**, **h**) Long axis of the structures and in-plane needle visualization of the needle inside the epidural space. C, cornu; *, sacral canal; short arrows, sacrococcygeal ligament; long arrow, needle; solid arrowheads, posterior sacral wall; void arrowheads, anterior sacral wall. (Reprinted and reproduced with permission from Philip Peng Educational Series)

In the short axis of the spine, the two cornua (acoustic shadow) is found and the sacrococcygeal ligament (band-like structure) is found superiorly in between, and the dorsal bony surface of the sacrum anteriorly could be identified (Fig. 52.5a). The epidural space is the hypoechoic area in between the surface of the sacrum and the sacrococcygeal ligament.

The probe is initially placed in a short axis view of the sacrum at the level of S1 approximately to image the median crest (Fig. 52.6 upper panel). Afterwards, the probe is moved in a caudal direction until the sacral cornua are visible. A hyperechogenic line, which corresponds to the sacrococcygeal ligament, is observed between the cornua. Local tissue infiltration is performed at the puncture site. The needle is inserted out-of-plane until its tip is observed between the sacral cornua. Here, the needle can be advanced out-of-plane until piercing through the sacrococcygeal ligament or the probe can be rotated longitudinally to guide the needle advancement in-plane into the epidural space. The entry angle of the needle depends on the depth of the sacrococcygeal ligament and the longitudinal axis of the sacral canal.

Alternatively, the needle can be inserted in-plane. An initial transverse (short axis) image for the sacral hiatus and dorsal sacrococcygeal ligament between the bilateral sacral cornua is obtained first, then the transducer is rotated 90° to examine in a longitudinal view (long axis) the sacral hiatus and the sacrococcygeal ligament (Fig. 52.6, lower panel). Under real-time ultrasonography, local tissue infiltration is performed at the puncture site. The needle is inserted in plane at an approximate 45° angle piercing the dorsal sacrococcygeal ligament until the tip disappears deep to the dorsal sacrum shadow.

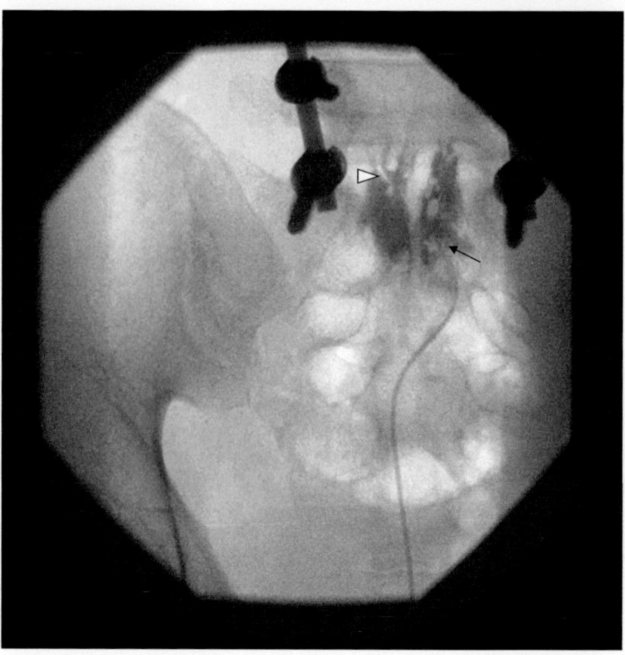

Fig. 52.7 Post injection epidurogram at the caudal canal. Arrow: Catheter tip position at S1 right side. Arrowhead: Epidurogram at L5-S1 junction. (Reprinted and reproduced with permission from Philip Peng Educational Series)

Fluoroscopy-Guided Needle and Catheter Advancement

Once the needle is inside the sacral canal, contrast is injected to confirm and the best view is lateral view. Upon confirmation, the needle is advanced the S2-3 level. Before the insertion of catheter, the authors suggested to make sure the bevel of the needle is facing posterior because the proximity of the bevel to the anterior sacral wall can hinder the catheter advancement. If the target is unilateral, the bevel may be directed to the target side. The catheter is advanced for 3–5 cm to the L5-S1 level (Fig. 52.7). Contrast is administered to confirm the proximity of the catheter tip to the target. Upon satisfactory positioning of the catheter, the medication is injected.

Drugs

The procedure is not selective; volumes as high as 10–20 mL could be used to reach more superior lumbar structures with a diluted local anesthetic and a steroid (e.g., methylprednisolone, dexamethasone).

Complications

Direct needle damage to spinal cord and spinal nerve, massive subdural spread, incidental dural tear, epidural hematoma, infection or epidural abscess, anterior spinal anterior syndrome, and ischemia could be caused with a caudal approach. Injury to sacral nerve(s) is rare during caudal epidural steroid injection. Inadvertent dural puncture during the caudal approach can occur if cystic structures are present at the lower sacrum, such as sacral meningocele or perineural cyst/Tarlov. It can also occur if the dural sac terminates abnormally low or the apex of the sacral hiatus ends abnormally high. Post injection pain at the sacral hiatus site of entry may be prolonged (up to 6 months when present).

Difficult entrance is encountered in patients with the AP diameter of sacral hiatus at apex of less than 1.6 mm.

Intravascular or intraosseous injection may lead to toxicity of local anesthetic. The incidence of accidental intravascular injections as confirmed by contrast enhanced fluoroscopy ranged between 11% and 42% in patients who had received caudal epidural injections, which is reduced administering the injectate right after penetrating the sacrococcygeal ligament and confirmed with fluoroscopy. Yoon in 2005 demonstrated the feasibility of ultrasound as a reliable imaging modality for caudal epidural steroid injection. Injections were successful if unidirectional flow (observed as one dominant color) of the solution was observed with color Doppler ultrasonography through the epidural space underneath the sacrococcygeal ligament, with no flows being observed in other directions (observed as multiple colors) (Fig. 52.8). If the injection flow was not seen heading mainly in the cephalad direction and color doppler spectrum was detected multicolored, it is considered that the medication is intravascular.

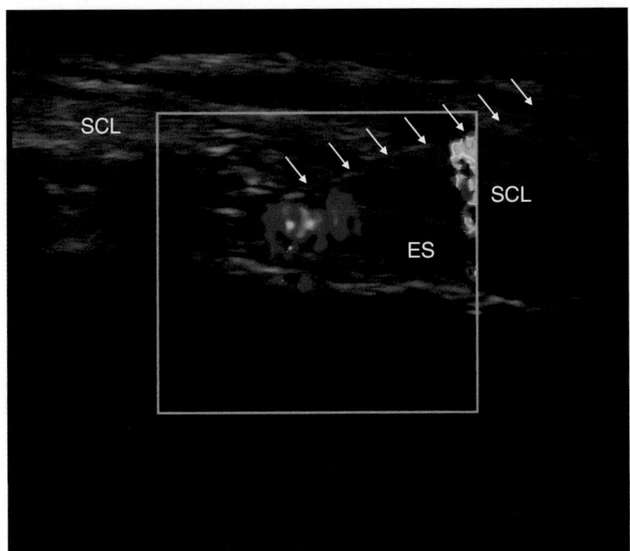

Fig. 52.8 Unidirectional flow shows predominantly one color spectrum. *ES* epidural space, *SCL* sacrococcygeal ligament. Arrow: needle trajectory. (Reprinted and reproduced with permission from Philip Peng Educational Series)

Literature Review

As part of a nonsurgical approach, lumbar epidural injections often are used in the management of radicular pain and lumbar disc herniation, mitigating inflammatory mediators that irritate the roots at the epidural space. The interlaminar or transforaminal approaches for epidural steroid injection are commonly used for this purpose. Transforaminal injection has been the preferred method to administer epidural steroids, aiming the ventral surface of the dorsal root ganglion and the nerve root. However, major complication has been associated with this technique such as paraplegia due to spinal cord infarct. Caudal epidural injection emerges as a safer alternative, especially in patients with anatomical alterations or distorted spine, mainly after surgery, in which the other approaches can be technically difficult.

Conn in 2009 performed a systematic review including 11 randomized trials and 20 observational non-RCT (prospective and retrospective evaluations). They found positive 1A/1B recommendation for caudal epidural steroid injections in managing disc herniation, radiculitis, and discogenic pain without disc herniation with moderate- to high-quality evidence, with benefits outweighing risks. They found 1B or 1C evidence for managing patients with post-lumbar laminectomy syndrome and spinal stenosis.

Iversen in 2010 published an RCT with three arms, comparing caudal epidural injections of triamcinolone vs. caudal epidural injections vs. subcutaneous saline injection in patients with lumbar radiculopathy. Oswestry Disability Index was the primary outcome measure. Pain score was a secondary outcome. They followed up 116 patients up to 52 weeks. The treatment groups did not differ significantly for the primary and secondary outcomes.

Meng, in a systematic review and metanalysis of 13 studies, compared epidural steroid injection with local anesthesia alone in patients with lumbar spinal stenosis up to 6 months. Five of the RCTs included used the caudal approach to inject the epidural steroids. They showed similar results in pain scores and functional improvement in both groups.

In patients with central spinal stenosis, Manchikanti found level II evidence for long-term results improving pain and functionality in patients receiving caudal epidural steroid injections based on seven randomized controlled trials.

In 2015, Manchikanti et al. performed a systematic review of RCT studying all types of epidural injections in managing chronic or chronic and subacute lumbar disc herniation. They elected 23 articles determining short- and long-term efficacy (pain relief and functional improvement) of the different approaches (caudal, lumbar interlaminar, and transforaminal) for epidural injections in the treatment of disc herniation, considering only placebo-controlled and active-controlled trials. Five of the 23 trials evaluated caudal epidural injections. Four of the five trials in total (three fluoroscopic, two non-fluoroscopic) showed efficacy of caudal epidural injections in the management of lumbar disc herniation, with strong evidence in the short term (<6 months) and moderate evidence in the long term (>6–12 months). Two of the articles were considered high-quality trials and the remaining tree as moderate-quality trial.

Park et al., in a case-controlled, retrospective study, compared 110 patients treated with ultrasound or fluoroscopy to guide caudal epidural steroid injection of dexamethasone. They did not find any significant statistical difference in Oswestry Disability Index, verbal numeric pain scale at 3, 6, and 12 months after the injections between both the groups.

Liu in a systematic review (2016) compared the effectiveness of transforaminal epidural steroids injections with caudal epidural injections, measuring pain and functional improvements in the treatment of radiculopathy. They initially found 1013 articles screened for review, and eight studies were ultimately included in the meta-analysis (six prospective, two retrospective). Follow-up periods were variable (from 2 weeks to 24 months). In the studies included, different types of corticosteroids were used, including triamcinolone, betamethasone, and methylprednisolone. Heterogeneity between studies was high, no differences were noted after 2 weeks, 3, 6, and 12 months of follow-up, although there was a trend toward higher pain indices in the caudal epidural group, not statistically significant.

Lee in 2018 performed a systematic review evaluating whether transforaminal epidural injections were more useful than caudal epidural steroid injections, including articles incorporating patients with low back and radicular leg pain, and diagnosis of lumbar disc herniation. They included six articles (four RCT and two non-RCT). The follow-up period was variable, ranging from 2 weeks to 1 year. Three of the RCT studies reported that transforaminal epidural steroids injections obtained better clinical outcomes than caudal epidural steroids injection at 6 months and one RCT showed superiority of caudal approach. One non-RCT study demonstrated better clinical efficacy of transforaminal approach than caudal, whereas the other study indicated no significant difference between the two techniques. They concluded that transforaminal approach was non-inferior or superior to caudal epidural steroid injection in the treatment of patients with lumbar disc herniation.

Ultrasound has proved to prevent vascular injection, reduce needle passes, and improve the accuracy up to 100% to place the needle into the epidural space with the advantage of an easier procedure with added safety and the avoidance of radiation exposure.

Clinical Pearls

- Remove the excess and let dry completely chlorhexidine to avoid its entrance into the epidural space in order to prevent arachnoiditis. Use sterile gel or saline solution as interface between the skin and the transducer/cover.
- Place the medication just piercing the sacrococcygeal ligament or use fluoroscopic guidance to advance the needle or threaten a catheter cephalic to the sacral hiatus and achieve specific epidural spread targeting a particular root or location with lower volumes.
- Avoid advancing the needle too deep into the sacral canal to prevent inadvertent dural puncture or vascular infections.
- Injection in the caudal epidural space is seen as distention of the space, displacement of the dura, findings on color Doppler, rising of the sacrococcygeal ligament as the caudal epidural space distends.
- Contemplate in advance, the possible variations in anatomy of the sacral hiatus. Remember to be especially careful with a high level of suspicion in spine bifida due to the risk of puncturing the dural sac, in the absence of posterior sacral bone.
- Consider to use the color doppler to confirm accurate position of the needle

Suggested Reading

Bagheri H, Govsa F. Anatomy of the sacral hiatus and its clinical relevance in caudal epidural block. Surg Radiol Anat. 2017;39(9):943–51.

Chen CP, Tang SF, Hsu T, Tsai W, Liu H, Chen MJ, et al. Ultrasound guidance in caudal epidural needle placement. Anesthesiology. 2004;101(1):181–4.

Chen Y, Huang-Lionnet JH, Cohen SP. Radiofrequency ablation in coccydynia: a case series and comprehensive, evidence-based review. Pain Med. 2017;18(6):1111–30.

Conn A, Buenaventura RM, Datta S, Abdi S, Diwan S. Systematic review of caudal epidural injections in the management of chronic low back pain. In: Database of Abstracts of Reviews of Effects (DARE): Quality-assessed review. York: Centre for Reviews and Dissemination; 2009.

Fukazawa K, Matsuki Y, Ueno H, Hosokawa T, Hirose M. Risk factors related to accidental intravascular injection during caudal anesthesia. J Anesth. 2014;28(6):940–3.

Iversen C. Effect of caudal epidural steroid or saline injection inchronic lumbar radiculopathy: multicentre, blinded, randomised controlled trial. BMJ. 2011;343:d5278. https://doi.org/10.1136/bmj.d5278.

Kao SC, Lin CS. Caudal epidural block: an updated review of anatomy and techniques. Biomed Res Int. 2017;2017:9217145.

Lee JH, Shin KH, Bahk SJ, Lee GJ, Kim DH, Lee CH, et al. Comparison of clinical efficacy of transforaminal and caudal epidural steroid injection in lumbar and lumbosacral disc herniation: a systematic review and meta-analysis. Spine J. 2018;18(12):2343–53.

Liu J, Zhou H, Lu L, Li X, Jia J, Shi Z, et al. The effectiveness of transforaminal versus caudal routes for epidural steroid injections in managing lumbosacral radicular pain: a systematic review and meta-analysis. Medicine (Baltimore). 2016;95(18):e3373.

Manchikanti L, Benyamin RM, Falco FJ, Kaye AD, Hirsch JA. Do epidural injections provide short-and long-term relief for lumbar disc herniation? A systematic review. Clin Orthop Relat Res. 2015a;473(6):1940–56.

Manchikanti L, Kaye AD, Manchikanti K, Boswell M, Pampati V, Hirsch J. Efficacy of epidural injections in the treatment of lumbar central spinal stenosis: a systematic review. Anesthesiol Pain Med. 2015b;5(1):e231392.

Meng H, Fei Q, Wang B, Yang Y, Li D, Li J, Su N. Epidural injections with or without steroids in managing chronic low back pain secondary to lumbar spinal stenosis: a meta-analysis of 13 randomized controlled trials. Drug Des Dev Ther. 2015;9:4657.

Ogoke BA. Caudal epidural steroid injections. Pain Physician. 2000;3(3):305–12.

Park GY, Kwon DR, Cho HK. Anatomic differences in the sacral hiatus during caudal epidural injection using ultrasound guidance. J Ultrasound Med. 2015a;34(12):2143–8.

Park KD, Kim TK, Lee WY, Ahn J, Koh SH, Park Y. Ultrasound-guided versus fluoroscopy-guided caudal epidural steroid injection for the treatment of unilateral lower lumbar radicular pain: case-controlled, retrospective, comparative study. Medicine. 2015b;94(50):e2261.

Porzionato A, Macchi V, Parenti A, De Caro R. Surgical anatomy of the sacral hiatus for caudal access to the spinal canal. In: Advances in minimally invasive surgery and therapy for spine and nerves. New York, NY: Springer; 2011. p. 1–3.

Rho ME, Tang C. The efficacy of lumbar epidural steroid injections: transforaminal, interlaminar, and caudal approaches. Phys Med Rehabil Clin N Am. 2011;22(1):139–48.

Saluja PG. The incidence of ossification of the sacrococcygeal joint. J Anat. 1988;156:11.

Sekiguchi M, Yabuki S, Satoh K, Kikuchi S. An anatomic study of the sacral hiatus: a basis for successful caudal epidural block. Clin J Pain. 2004;20(1):51–4.

Singh M, Mahajan A. An anatomical study of variations of sacral hiatus in sacra of north Indian origin and its clinical significance. Int J Morphol. 2013;31(1):110.

Woon JT, Stringer MD. Clinical anatomy of the coccyx: a systematic review. Clin Anat. 2012;25(2):158–67.

Woon JT, Stringer MD. Redefining the coccygeal plexus. Clin Anat. 2014a;27:254–60.

Woon JT, Stringer MD. The anatomy of the sacrococcygeal cornual region and its clinical relevance. Anat Sci Int. 2014b;89(4):207–14.

Wooten C. Anatomy of the Coccygeal plexus. In: Nerves and nerve injuries. London: Academic Press; 2015. p. 659–61.

Yoon JS, Sim KH, Kim SJ, Kim WS, Koh SB, Kim BJ. The feasibility of color Doppler ultrasonography for caudal epidural steroid injection. Pain. 2005;118(1-2):210–4.

Lumbosacral Epiduroscopy

53

Hemmo Bosscher

Contents

Introduction

Epiduroscopy is endoscopy of the epidural space. The spinal canal can be entered through different routes, but this chapter will only discuss flexible fiberoptic endoscopy using the trans-sacral approach to the epidural space, as initially described and developed by Heavner and further developed by Saberski and more recently by Bosscher et al.

Most complaints of back pain are nonspecific, and the cause of pain is often not known. Epiduroscopy of the spinal canal in patients with idiopathic low back pain is therefore appealing. Epiduroscopy allows for direct observation of epidural structures with minimal disruption of the anatomy. Suspect pathology can be touched with the tip of the epiduroscope, which may produce pain concordant with the pain for which the patient sought treatment. Specific tools can be passed or medications injected through the side port of the epiduroscope and thus be used to treat local pathology directly. Using the flexibility of the endoscope, different vertebral levels on both sides of the spinal canal can be examined in one session. Consequently, epiduroscopy is a versatile procedure that can be used for both diagnosis and treatment of a number of epidural pathologies.

While broadly useful, epiduroscopy has several drawbacks. First, the epidural space is small and the equipment not well-designed to work in such a narrow space. Moreover, epidural fat or fibrous strings may hinder views of anatomical structures. Frequently, fibrosis after back surgery or spinal stenosis may block advancement of the epiduroscope into areas of interest. While epidural fluid injections can dilate the epidural space and may bring epidural structures

H. Bosscher (✉)
Pain Management, Grace Health System/TTU HSC, Lubbock, TX, USA

D. Jankovic, P. Peng (eds.), *Regional Nerve Blocks in Anesthesia and Pain Therapy*, https://doi.org/10.1007/978-3-030-88727-8_53

into better focus, incorrect fluid management can cause serious complications. However, areas that are difficult to access with an open surgical approach can often be easily reached with epiduroscopy. Yet in doing so, important epidural tissues may be placed at risk. For example, damage to small but critical blood vessels may cause major neurological deficit.

In order to use epiduroscopy effectively and safely, detailed knowledge of the spinal anatomy and pathology is required to avoid causing damage while recognizing significant abnormalities and potential pitfalls. Unfortunately, significant gaps in our knowledge exist. In addition, a priori ideas of what preconceived spinal pathology is supposed to look like may bias the interpretation of images by the epiduroscopist.

The effectiveness of epiduroscopy has been reported by a number of investigators. Unfortunately, most of the publications have significant limitations. They often do not provide sufficient information in their Methods section for the reported procedures to be replicable, while the Result sections of the papers often give an interpretation rather than a description of their observations. For published reports on epiduroscopy to be useful, the reports should contain the following: (1) description or direct observation of pathological changes in the epidural space, (2) evidence that these changes are associated with the patient's complaint, and (3) evidence that targeted treatment of these pathological changes results in relief of back pain.

This chapter attempts to provide the reader with a reproducible method as to how to perform epiduroscopy systematically and effectively without relying on a preoperative and often incorrect diagnosis regarding the cause of low back pain. In the first section, pertinent anatomy and pathology for the epiduroscopist will be reviewed. In the second section, several applications of epiduroscopy for the treatment of low back pain are presented. Most importantly, the epiduroscopist must be ever mindful of the potential to cause severe complications that are specific to epiduroscopy and remain vigilant in the prevention and detection of these potential harms. This latter point is a rather extensive topic beyond the scope of this chapter.

Epiduroscopy: The Normal Epidural Space

Anatomy for Epiduroscopy

The spinal dura mater forms a longitudinal tube in the spinal canal that runs from the foramen magnum to the sacrum. The sacral dural sack terminates at the level of S2 but may extend as low as S4. The spinal cord terminates between the longitudinal level of T12 and L2 (please refer to Chap. 40 on Neuraxial Anatomy). The lumbosacral dural sac contains cerebrospinal fluid (CSF), nerve roots, blood vessels, and the internal filum terminalis (Fig. 53.1). In the lumbar spinal canal, the dura mater appears as a trigonal structure on an axial cut, with the base of the equilateral triangle in the anterior spinal canal. The posterior angle is formed by a dural fold in the midline that contains the internal filum. The posterior dural fold is most pronounced in the lumbar spinal canal. The lateral angles of the triangle are formed by folds that contain traversing lumbosacral nerve roots (Fig. 53.2). Following the dura in caudad direction, these lateral folds start to angulate laterally, to give rise to the exiting nerve root sleeves (Figs. 53.2 and 53.3). This angulation of the traversing nerve root starts just below the axilla of the adjacent exiting nerve root sleeve above. The exiting nerve root and dorsal root ganglion wrap around the medial and inferior aspect of the pedicle and can be followed into the superior compartment of the neural foramen. It continues as the spinal nerve just lateral and anterior to the inferior compartment of the neural foramen. The lateral recess is defined as the region between the lateral margin of the spinal dura and the lateral wall of the spinal canal but proper lateral recess can only be found over a very short distance between the axilla and the take-off of the next nerve root sleeve.

Fluoroscopy is required for the precise localization of the epiduroscope tip and to aid in the recognition of intraspinal anatomical structures. The axilla resides at the inferior margin of the pedicle on AP fluoroscopy. The lateral nerve root angulation starts near the superior end plate of the disc on AP fluoroscopy. In caudad direction, the nerve root fold closely follows the outline of the pedicle, leaving only a small space between the dura and the bony margin of the pedicle.

The wall of the canal consists of the posterior vertebral body, vertebral arch, the paired ligamentum flavum, and the intervertebral disc. The peridural membrane (PDM) is a continuous sheath within the spinal canal that contains the epidural venous plexus within its body and covers the walls of the spinal canal (Fig. 53.4). In the neural foramen, the peridural membrane forms a perineural evagination containing the spinal nerve and neural foraminal fat tissue that is continuous with epidural fat tissue in the posterior epidural space. Anteriorly, the peridural membrane covers the transverse fibers of the posterior longitudinal ligament that cover the intervertebral disc. Posteriorly, the peridural membrane covers the pars inferior and pars superior of the facet joint. More lateral, the peridural membrane forms a tubular sheath around the spinal nerve. A small inferior and superior space is formed between the pedicles and the perineural evagination of the peridural membrane in the neural foramen—the infra- and suprapedicular compartments. The intervertebral disc forms part of the anterior border of this compartment. The facet joint forms the posterior bor-

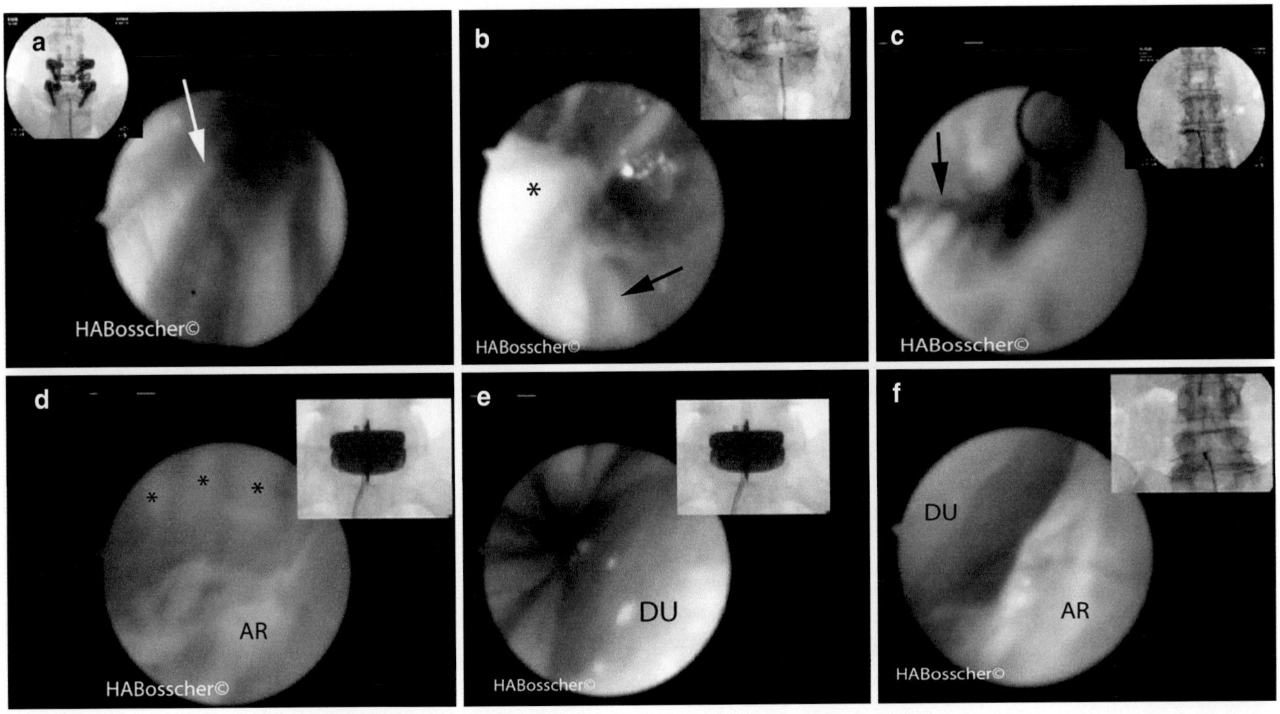

Fig. 53.1 Nerve roots in the epidural, subdural, and subarachnoid space. (**a**) Subdural placement of the epiduroscope. Notice "railroad track" configuration of subarachnoid nerve roots. (**b**) View of the cauda equina in the sacral epidural space. Star—posterior midline fold. Arrow aims at nerve roots contained in the lateral folds. (**c**) Caution. Unclear location of the epiduroscope. Possible subdural space. Arrow may aim at subarachnoid nerve roots. (**d**) Subdural placement of the epiduroscope. *AR* arachnoid membrane. Stars—subarachnoid nerve roots. (**e**) Subarachnoid placement of the epiduroscope. *DU* dura mater. (**f**) Subdural placement of the epiduroscope. *DU* inner aspect of the dural mater, *AR* arachnoid membrane

der. A suprapedicular segment of the peridural membrane in the spinal canal separates the suprapedicular compartment from the spinal canal.

In the spinal canal, multiple anterior, lateral, and posterior vertebro-meningeal ligaments connect the dura mater to the peridural membrane and the wall of the spinal canal. Thin fibrous connections between the dura mater and blood vessels are present at the midline in the posterior epidural space; however, there is no septum dividing both sides of the epidural space (Figs. 53.5 and 53.6). Multiple veins, an occasional small artery, and a network of lymphatics cross the epidural space and connect the dura with the peridural membrane. The peridural membrane, in turn, has numerous fibrous and vascular connections to the wall of the spinal canal. The posterior longitudinal ligament may be considered part of the peridural membrane and covers the ventral central spinal canal and the intervertebral discs. The anterior epidural venous plexus (Batson plexus) is also part of the peridural membrane and covers the extra-ligamentous sections of the anterior wall of the spinal canal and the transverse fibers of the posterior longitudinal ligament that cover the intervertebral disc in the neural foramen (Figs. 53.3 and 53.4).

Epiduroscopy in the Normal Spinal Canal

Attachment of the external part of the filum terminalis to the sacrococcygeal ligaments forces the scope introducer into the posterior epidural space. Although there is no dividing ventral or dorsal septum in the midline of the spinal canal, fibrous connections and the presence of the posterior epidural fold make examination of the contralateral posterior epidural space difficult. On introduction of the epiduroscope into the sacral spinal canal, the scope should therefore be directed to the side of interest. In approximately one out of ten men and one out of 20 women, the bony spinal canal is too narrow and epiduroscopy cannot be performed without sacral laminotomy. A preoperative lateral radiograph of the sacrum is often useful in the evaluation of the patency of the sacral spinal canal.

Once in the sacral spinal canal, the epiduroscope should not encounter any resistance. An occasional smooth-walled Tarlov's cyst can usually be bypassed. Sacral neural foramina are large, but abundant epidural fat makes examination of the sacral nerve roots difficult. Fortunately, the sacral spinal canal and sacral foramina are rarely the site of interest.

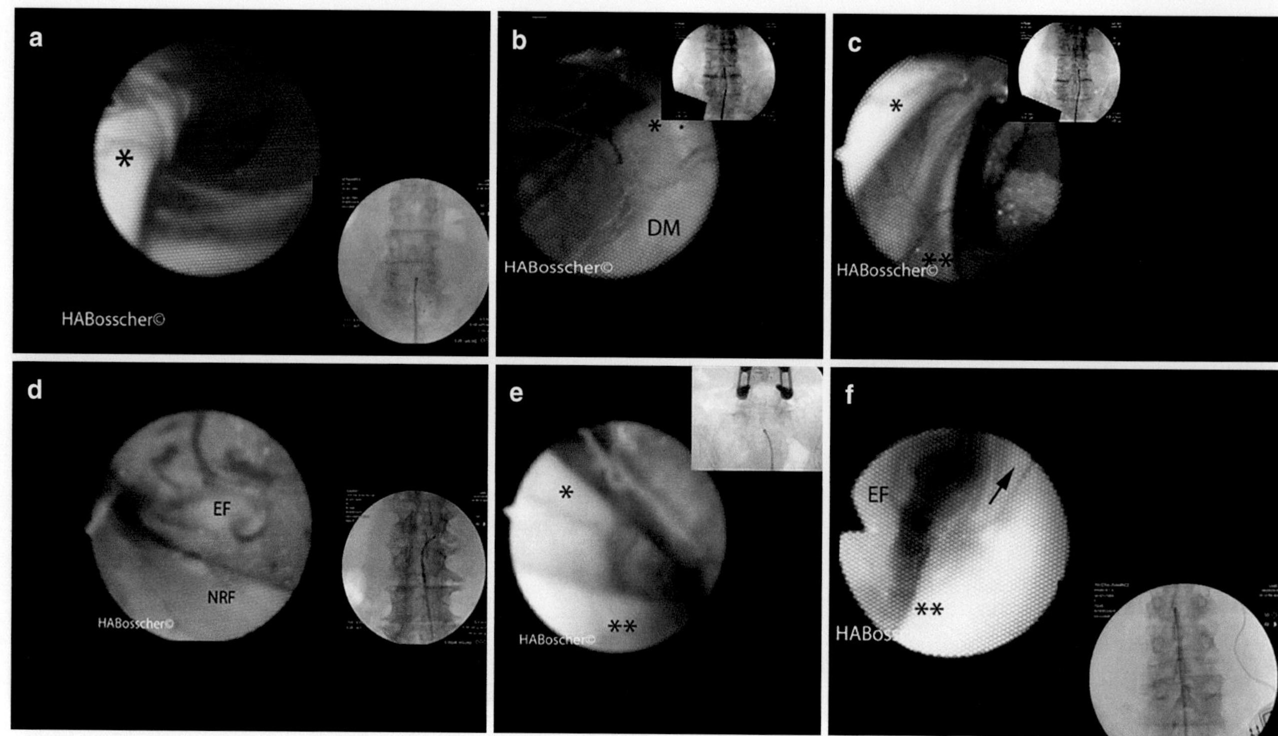

Fig. 53.2 Dural folds. (**a**) Posterior midline fold containing the terminal filum. (**b**) Midline fold with left posterior surface of the dura mater. (**c**) Posterior midline and lateral dural folds. (**d**) Lateral dural fold containing the sensory nerve root of L3 on the right. (**e**) Posterior midline and lateral dural folds in the sacral spinal canal. (**f**) Upper lumbar spinal canal. Posterolateral surface of the dura mater and lateral dural fold containing the nerve root of L3. *DM* dura mater, *EF* epidural fat tissue, *NRF* nerve root fold. Single star—posterior midline dural fold. Double star—lateral dural fold

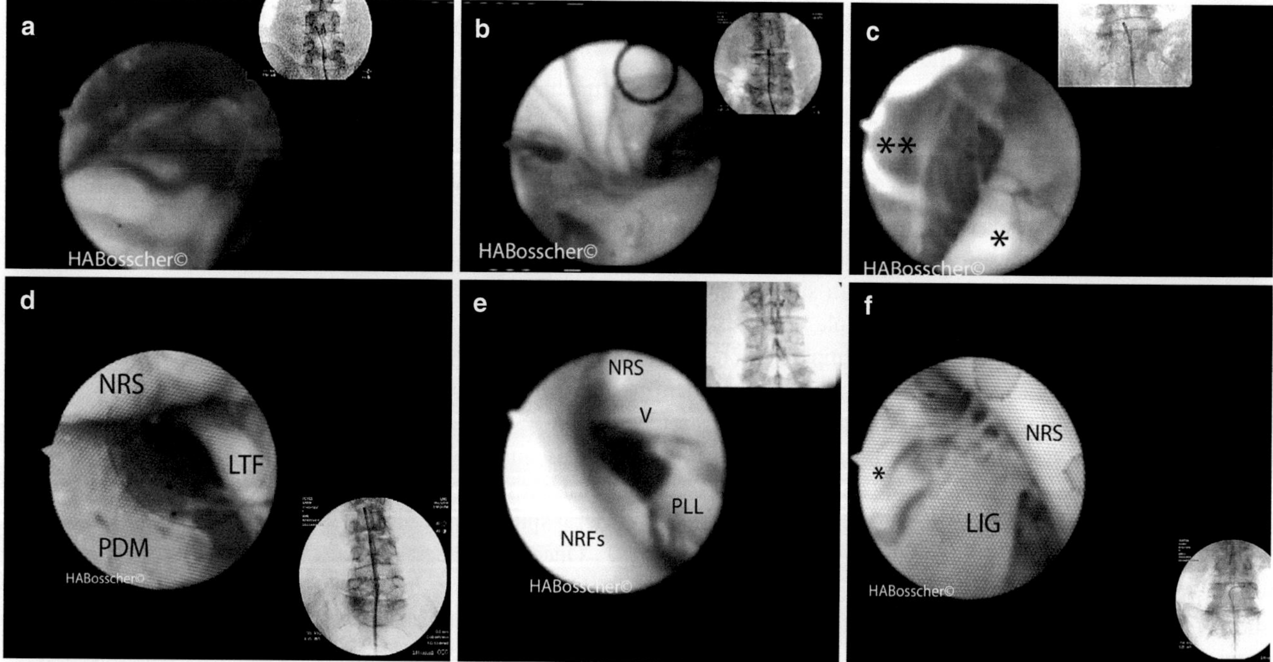

Fig. 53.3 Nerve root and dorsal root ganglion. (**a**) Dorsal root ganglion of L4. (**b**) Numerous "clumped" dural folds containing nerve roots. (**c**) Lateral dural fold containing the nerve root of L5 (single star) and pedicular peridural membrane (double star). (**d**) Axilla of the exiting nerve of L3 on the left, LTF—lateral dural fold, NRS—nerve root sleeve, PDM—anterior peridural membrane. (**e**) Axilla of the exiting nerve of L3 on the right. NRFs—nerve root folds of L4, NRS—nerve root sleeve L3, PLL—posterior longitudinal ligament, V—vein. (**f**) Nerve root fold of L5 on the left. LIG—anterior meningo-vertebral ligament, NRS—nerve root sleeve. Star—anterior peridural membrane

Fig. 53.4 Peridural membrane. (**a**) Detached posterior peridural membrane at L4–L5. EF—epidural fat tissue, PDM—posterior peridural membrane. (**b**) DU—dura mater, PDM—posterolateral peridural membrane. (**c**) Anterior peridural membrane at L4 on the right. Notice the irregular surface of the membrane. (**d**) Dura mater (DU) at L4 on the right. Star—vascular posterolateral peridural membrane. (**e**) Peridural membranous cover of a foraminal herniated disc at L3–L4. (**f**) Suprapedicular compartment of L5 on the left. Notice the pale-appearing aspect of the compartment and the presence of compressed suprapedicular transforaminal veins. Absence of epidural fat tissue is also a characteristic of the compartment

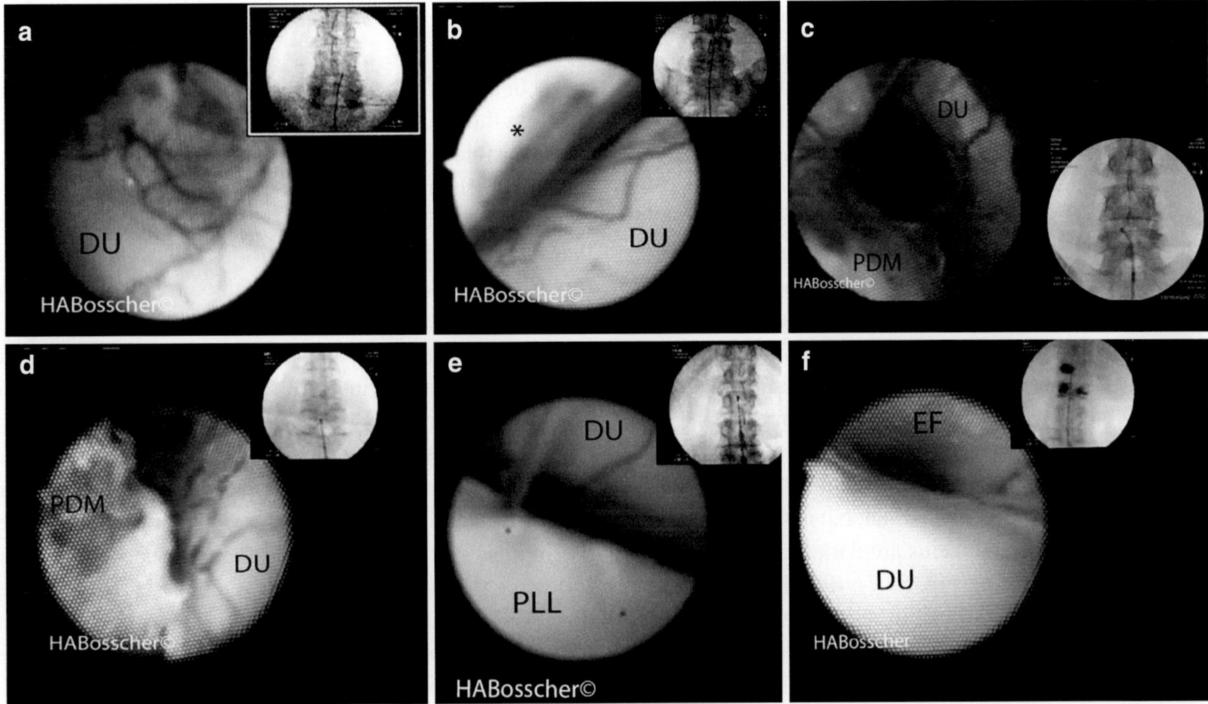

Fig. 53.5 Dura mater. (**a–f**) *DU* dura mater, *EF* epidural fat tissue, *PDM* peridural membrane, *PLL* posterior longitudinal ligament. Star—peridural membrane covering ligamentum flavum. Single star—posterior midline dural fold

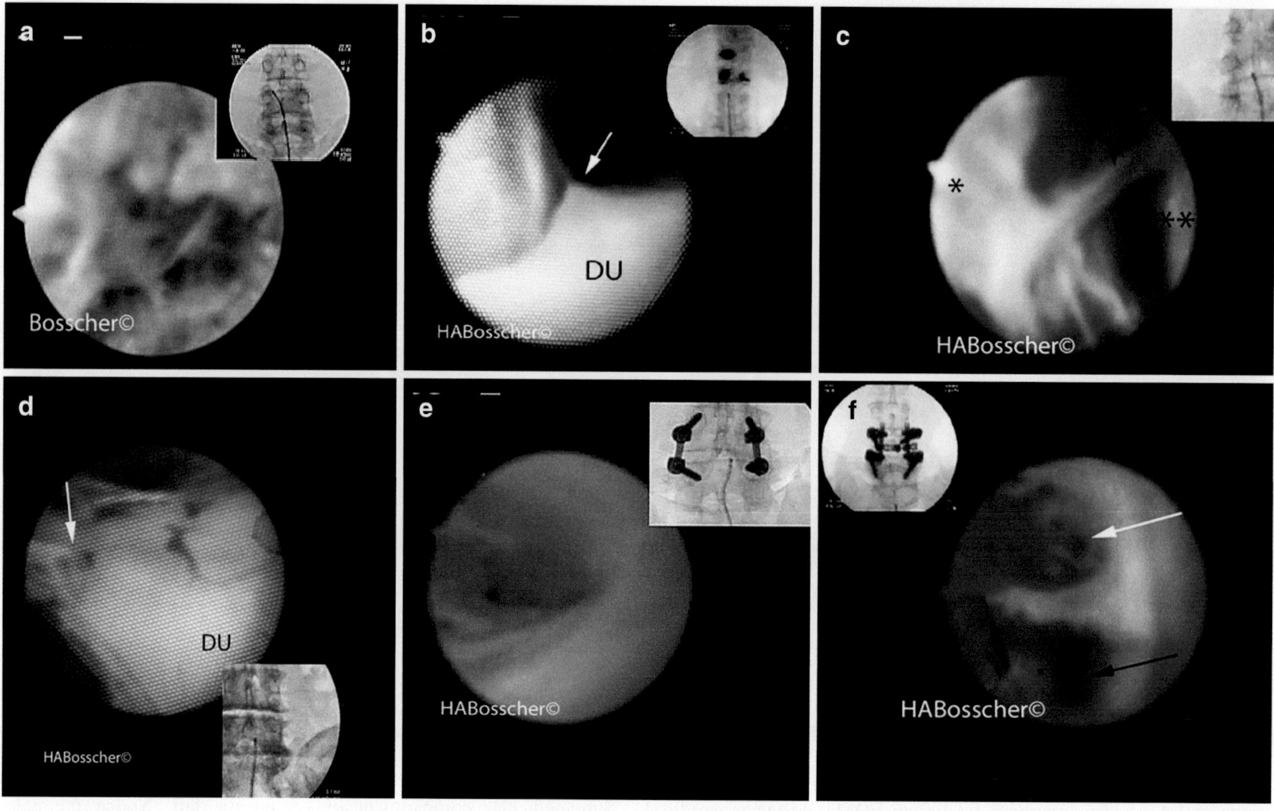

Fig. 53.6 Epidural fibrosis. (**a**) Hyperemia and fibrosis of suprapedicular peridural membrane at L4 on the left. (**b**) Tenting of the dura mater caused by a very small fibrous string between the pedicle of L3 and the dura mater. (**c**) Larger fibrous band connects hyperemic posterolateral peridural membrane (single star) with the dura mater (double star). Relative motion of the dura in the spinal canal (e.g., during straight leg raise testing) may cause back pain through traction on inflamed and painful peridural membrane. (**d**) Large adhesion deforming the posterior dura. (**e**) Severe epidural fibrosis after back surgery with complete obliteration of the epidural space. (**f**) Severe epidural fibrosis after back surgery. The white arrow aims at intact epidural adhesion. The black arrow aims at the site where the epiduroscope perforated the dura mater

Therefore, the epiduroscope is best immediately advanced into the lumbar epidural wherein most patients with back pain the nidus of pain generation can be found. Since lumbar vertebral segments are similar with respect to epiduroscopy, evaluation is described for a general lumbar segment.

The first observation that can be readily recognized in the posterior epidural space is the yellow-white granular-appearing epidural fat tissue with white strings or sheets of fibrous tissue. The tip of the epiduroscope should then be directed and advanced anteriorly without much resistance until the white/gray aspect of the dura mater can be seen (Fig. 53.4). Fluoroscopy should be used to identify the precise location of the endoscope tip within the spinal canal. The dura mater is relatively avascular, but isolated blood vessels may cross its surface. Veins are dark red, while arteries are bright red and pulsate (Fig. 53.7). Rotating the scope in the opposite or posterior direction, the posterior wall of the spinal canal can be studied in detail, although epidural fat may prevent clear views in some patients. In the sacral spinal canal, the posterior wall covering seems as a smooth white layer. In the lumbar spine canal, the lamina (white) and ligamentum flavum (yellow) are covered by the peridural membrane, visible as a thin, transparent vascular layer (Fig. 53.4). Blood vessels in the posterior peridural membrane are often sparse but can be abundant, showing multiple large dilated veins under pathological conditions. Between lamina, the ligamentum flavum forms a smooth convex indentation into the spinal canal. Ligamentum flavum hypertrophy may exacerbate this indentation and prevent the epiduroscope from further advancement into the spinal canal or from entering the neural foramen (Fig. 53.8).

To investigate the nerve roots and the dorsal root ganglion, the scope needs first be placed at the posterior dural fold in the midline and at the level of the inferior end plate of the lumbar vertebral body on AP fluoroscopy. By visually following the dura mater with the epiduroscopy tip in lateral direction, the lateral fold of the dura mater that contains the traversing sensory nerve root and more anteriorly the traversing motor nerve root can be identified (Figs. 53.2 and 53.3). When the scope is advanced in the cephalad direction, the

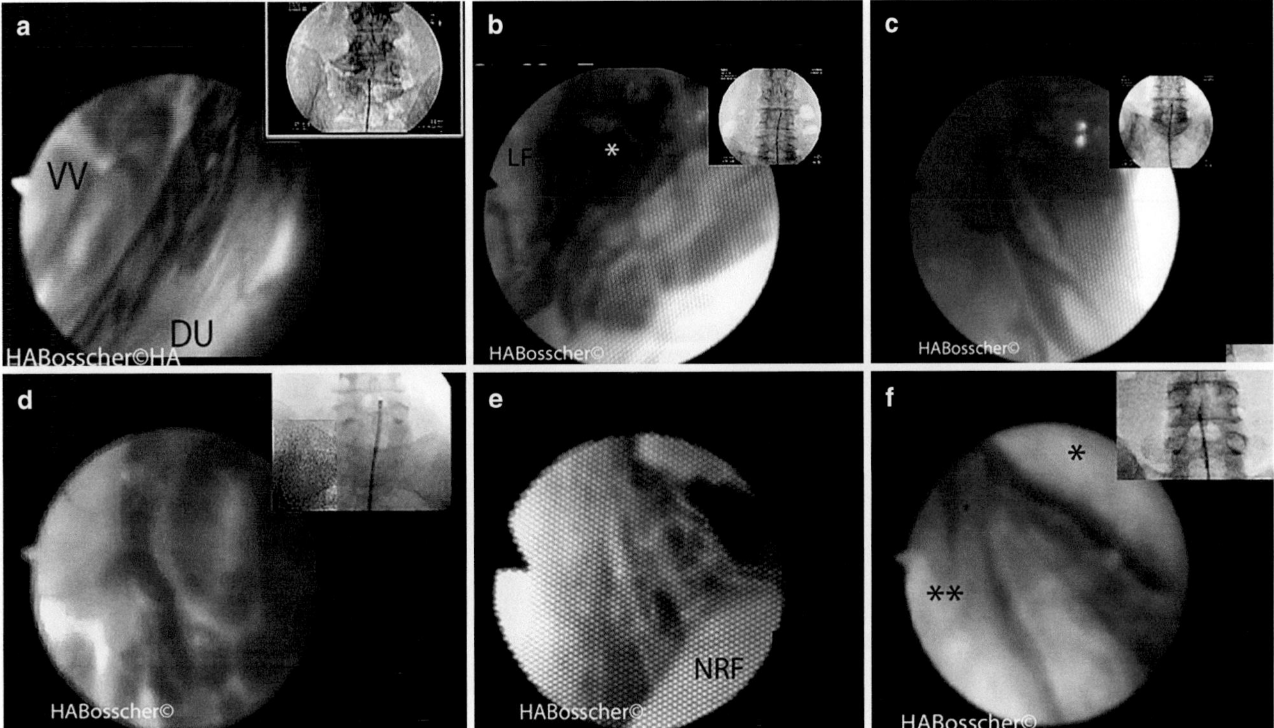

Fig. 53.7 Vascularity. (**a**) Marked increased vascularity (VV) within the left posterolateral peridural membrane at L5–S1. Notice an increase of vascularity on the surface of the dura mater (DU) as well. (**b**) Marked dilatation of veins on the surface of the dura mater in a region of severe spinal stenosis. LF—hypertrophic ligamentum flavum. Star—residual epidural space in the dorsal central spinal canal. (**c**) Isolated vein and small artery in the epidural space at L4–L5 on the right. (**d**) Varicose dilatation of an epidural vein at L4–L5 on the right. (**e**) Possible artery connecting the nerve root fold (NRF) to the wall of the spinal canal. Notice the presence of fibrous tissue. (**f**) Marked increased vascularity (double star) of the anterior peridural membrane at L4–L5 on the right. Single star—anterior dura mater

axilla of the exiting nerve root can be investigated. It is often difficult to view the take-off of the exiting nerve root, but the characteristic increase in vasculature in the axilla may be of aid. Moving the scope in caudad direction, the lateral fold containing the nerve roots, can be followed as it follows the contour of the pedicle and disappears in neural foraminal fat tissue, where it transitions into the dorsal root ganglion (DRG). The complete nerve root sleeve or DRG can rarely be seen in its entirety but can be studied in sections. Moving in the caudad direction, the start of the dural fold of the traversing root of the next vertebral segment can be identified (Fig. 53.3).

In the neural foramen, the epiduroscope can be placed anteriorly in the ventral spinal canal, but epidural fat in the perineural evagination of the peridural membrane often makes identification of ligaments, the intervertebral disc, and dorsal root ganglion difficult. However, starting more medially inside the spinal canal, the posterior longitudinal ligament can be seen as a white, smooth structure and can be followed over the disc more laterally. Moving the scope slightly more cephalad or caudad, the edge of the posterior longitudinal ligament may impress as a fold. It can be differentiated from the dura by the absence of blood vessels and a slightly smoother, white or pinkish appearance (Figs. 53.4, 53.5, and 53.9).

The extra-ligamentous part of the anterior wall of the spinal canal is covered by thick peridural membrane (Figs. 53.4 and 53.7). Here the membrane is a continuous sheath, containing multiple smaller and larger blood vessels, giving it a characteristic mottled appearance. The lateral edge of the posterior longitudinal ligament follows the contour of the pedicle. The pedicle is covered with thin peridural membrane that extends cephalad to form the medial wall of the suprapedicular compartment. This part of the PDM is easily mistaken for pedicular periosteum but deserves special attention, since it plays an important role in the pathogenesis of back pain. The scope can be advanced through this part of the membrane into the suprapedicular compartment as described above (Figs. 53.4, 53.9, and 53.10). On AP fluoroscopy, the suprapedicular compartment is in the area between the inferior end plate of the intervertebral disc and the superior margin of the pedicle. The suprapedicular compartment is bounded by suprapedicular transforaminal blood vessels and fibrous tissue and does not contain fat tissue.

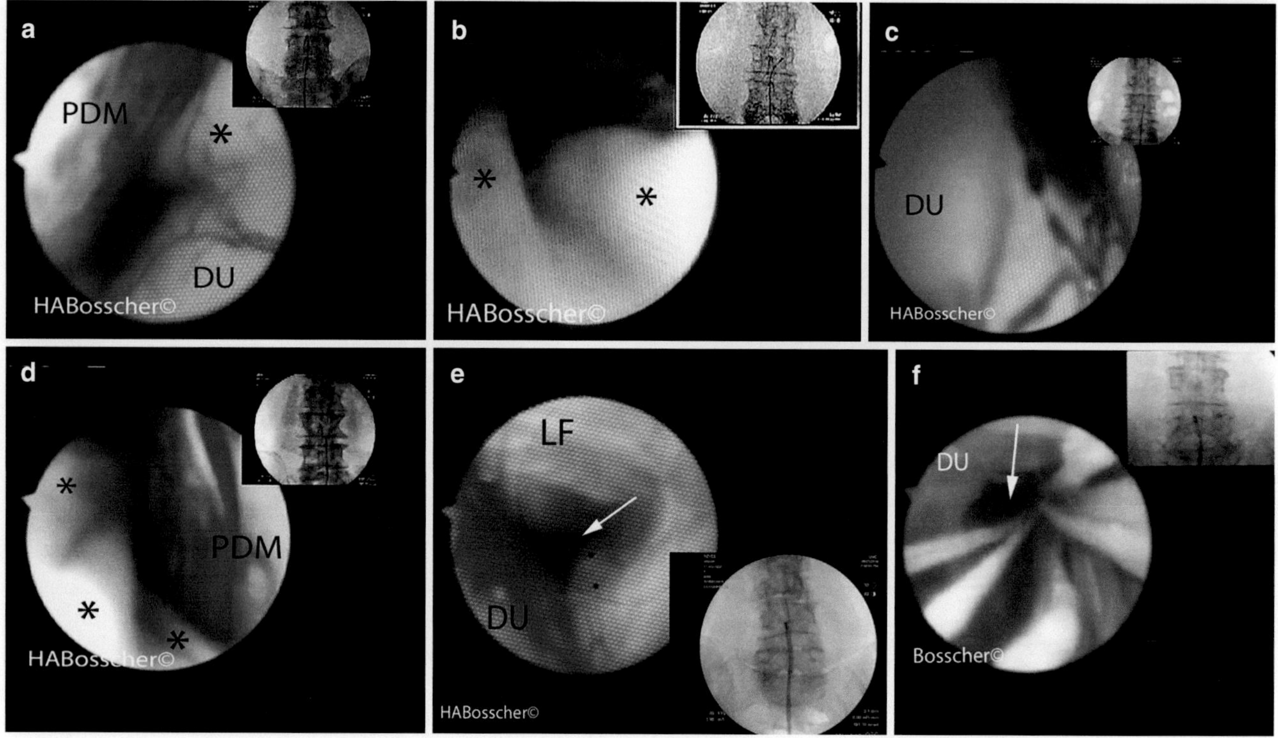

Fig. 53.8 Spinal stenosis. (**a**) Congenital narrow spinal canal. Notice the close proximity of the posterolateral wall of the spinal canal to the dura mater (DU) and the compromised position of the nerve root fold (star). *PDM* posterior peridural membrane. (**b**) Typical compressed configuration of nerve root folds in an area of spinal canal stenosis. (**c**) Vascular congestion of the right L3 nerve root fold cephalad to severe spinal canal stenosis at L4–L5. (**d**) Typical "corkscrew" configuration of nerve root folds in an area of severe spinal canal stenosis (L3–L4). Stars—nerve root folds. (**e**) Severe spinal stenosis. *DU* dura mater, *LF* ligamentum flavum. White arrow aims at the narrow residual epidural space. (**f**) Subarachnoid view of a region of spinal canal stenosis (L4–L5). Notice that only *critical* central spinal canal stenosis will cause compression of a subarachnoid nerve root

This gives the compartment a characteristic pale appearance on epiduroscopy. If the inferior compartment of the neural foramen is wide enough, the epiduroscope can traverse the entire compartment and enter the paraspinous tissues.

The ventral aspect of the spinal canal can be further investigated by advancing the scope tip underneath the anterior dural leaf of the axilla of the exiting nerve root. The anterior aspect of the exiting root sleeve and axilla may show transdural blood vessels (Figs. 53.1, 53.4, and 53.5). The central anterior epidural space does not contain fat tissue and can be inspected with ease. The posterior longitudinal ligament is located anteriorly and is white. The anterior dura mater has a white-yellowish appearance. Fibrous bands or strings and ligaments connect the two structures but offer usually very little resistance to scope advancement. Intervertebral discs, even when "bulging," are difficult to discern. Moving the scope laterally, the anterior epidural space may contain fat tissue and blood vessels. At the junction of the superior and medial margin of the pedicle on fluoroscopy, the suprapedicular compartment can be entered by moving the epiduroscope anterior to the motor root contained in the traversing nerve root fold into the neural foramen.

Diagnostic Epiduroscopy

Central Spinal Stenosis

Starting as described above in the midline of the posterior epidural space, with the tip of the epiduroscope approximately at the infra-pedicular level, the lamina and posterior fold of the dura mater can be identified. Following the posterior fold in cephalad direction, various degrees of ligament flavum hypertrophy may be seen, causing indentation of the lateral aspect of the posterior dura mater (Fig. 53.8). Even in severe central spinal stenosis, the scope can often still follow the posterior dural fold in cephalad direction through the narrow triangular opening between the two bulging ligamentum flavum and the dura mater. Fibrous tissue or inflamed PDM may be present in the narrowed spinal canal. In severe spinal stenosis, the nerve root folds can often be seen as posterior and lateral folds organized in a "corkscrew" fashion. This configuration appears to protect the nerve roots in areas of severe spinal stenosis from direct compression. Marked vascular congestion and hyperemia can often be observed in areas of spinal stenosis. Attempts to advance the scope into these tissues are often painful and suggest the presence of inflamed peridural membrane.

Lateral Recess Stenosis and Neural Foraminal Narrowing

Lateral recess stenosis and neural foraminal narrowing may be caused by a combination of facet joint and ligamentum flavum hypertrophy and intervertebral disc degeneration. The effect of these changes may be amplified by a congenital narrow lateral recess caused by short pedicles. Even minimal lateral recess stenosis may prevent scope for advancement into the lateral recess (Fig. 53.10). Surprisingly, MRI findings of lateral recess stenosis do not always correlate with epiduroscopic findings. The presence or absence of spinal stenosis on MRI does not necessarily predict the ability to pass the scope into the neural foramen. However, epiduroscopic lateral recess stenosis, i.e., inability to pass the epiduroscope through the neural foramen, independent of MRI findings, was a major predictor of the outcome of treatment of low back pain using epiduroscopy in one study and may also be an important predictor of the overall long-term outcome of treatment of chronic low back.

Hyperemia and Abnormal Vascularity

The normal epidural space is well vascularized. Hyperemia or increased perfusion of epidural tissues is visible as abnormally pronounced redness (Fig. 53.9). Hyperemia of tissues in the epidural space is a common finding and often not of clinical significance. Hyperemia may represent inflammation if hyperemic tissues are also painful to touch. In most patients with back pain, epiduroscopy does not show signs of inflammation of the dura, root sleeve, and dorsal root ganglion. However, hyperemia of the lining of the spinal canal and neural foramen is common. Hyperemia and pain to touch are most often encountered in the suprapedicular region of the neural foramen at L4–L5 and L3–L4 and probably represent inflamed and sensitized suprapedicular peridural membrane.

Increased vascularity is characterized by an increase in size and number of blood vessels and an abnormal pattern of

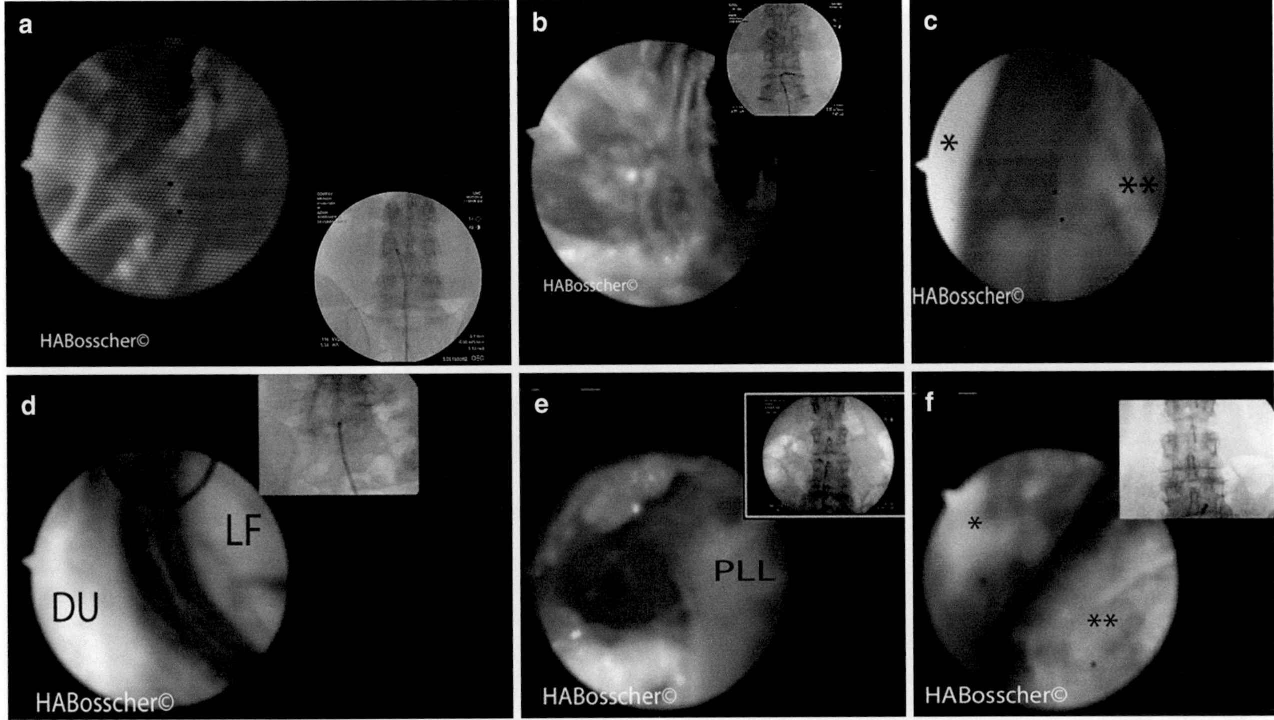

Fig. 53.9 Hyperemia. (**a**) Hyperemic peridural membrane at the left L4 vertebral pedicle. (**b**) Hyperemia of the suprapedicular membrane at L5 on the right. Notice the perforation of the peridural membrane caused by the epiduroscope. (**c**) Hyperemia of the right L5 suprapedicular membrane (double star). When the hyperemic suprapedicular peridural membrane is touched with the epiduroscope, back pain complaints can often be reproduced. Notice the absence of hyperemia of the nerve root fold of L5 (single star). Also notice hyperemia of the anterior peridural membrane (in the middle). (**d**) Hyperemia of posterolateral peridural membrane between hypertrophic ligamentum flavum (LF) at L5–S1 and the indentation of the dura mater (DU) on the right. (**e**) Hyperemia/increased vascularity of anterior peridural membrane (star). DU—anterior dura mater. (**f**) Hyperemia of the nerve root sleeve of L5 on the right (single star) is an unusual finding. Double star—anterior peridural membrane

blood vessels in the epidural space (Fig. 53.7 Vascularity). Increased vascularity, in an otherwise normal-appearing epidural space, suggests the presence of inflammation, causing a chemically induced dilatation of blood vessels, but can also be observed when venous outflow from the spinal canal is obstructed. Venous obstruction may occur in areas of stenosis or when extra-spinous venous pressure is elevated due medical conditions, such as abdominal tumors, constipation, or congestive heart failure. Varicose, tortuous dilatation of dark red epidural veins can sometimes be observed. Bright red arteriovenous malformations may be present and may appear as dilated pulsating blood vessels. One would expect significant congestion in postsurgical regions, where severe fibrosis obliterates the epidural space. Instead, postsurgical areas are characterized by a marked decrease or absence of blood vessels.

Pain to Touch

The dorsal root ganglion in the upper part of the neural foramen is painful to touch (Figs. 53.1 and 53.10). This pain is sharp and "electrical" and follows a dermatomal pattern but is rarely concordant with the patient's usual symptoms. Epiduroscopic exploration of the upper compartment of the neural foramen is better avoided, because dysesthesia caused by damage to the dorsal root ganglion may last weeks to months after surgery and damage to critical blood vessels in the superior compartment of the neural foramen may cause severe neurological complications. Pain in the distribution of a nerve root can also be caused by direct pressure on subarachnoid nerve roots when the scope passes through areas of central spinal or lateral recess stenosis or in areas of severe fibrosis, where nerve roots may be held in a fixed position. Epidural adhesions can be painful, particularly if the epiduroscopist attempts to enter a postsurgical region or when adhesions attached to inflamed peridural membrane are manipulated with the scope. Although inflammation of a nerve root or dorsal root ganglion has been reported, painful hyperemic tissues are predominantly present in the lateral recesses and the suprapedicular region of the neural foramen of L4–L5, occasionally L3–L4, and rarely elsewhere in the spinal canal. Inflamed-appearing, thin PDM that separates the suprapedicular compartment from the spinal canal will often reproduce concordant pain when gently touched with the epiduroscope. Painful, hyperemic peridural membrane,

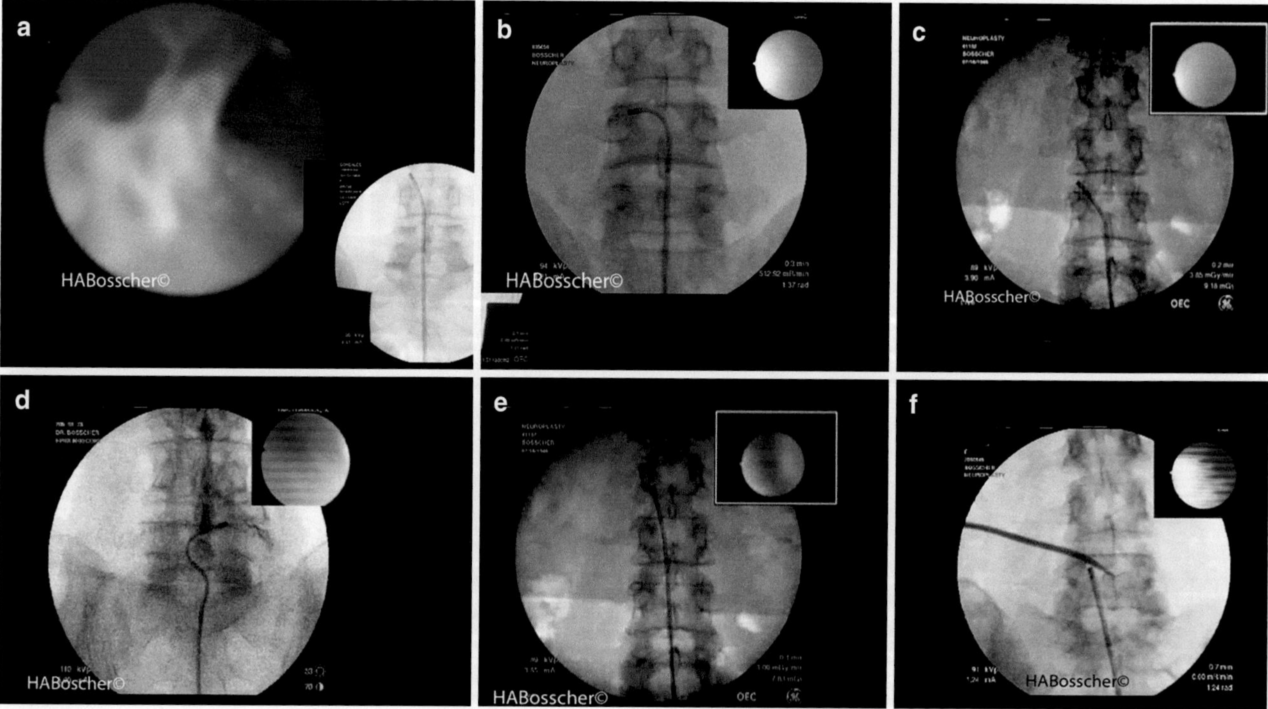

Fig. 53.10 Pain to touch and patency of the inferior neural foramen. (**a**) Hyperemic suprapedicular peridural membrane at L4 on the left. (**b**) Pain originating from inflamed suprapedicular membrane is the most common cause of back pain. Gentle touch with the epiduroscope will reproduce back pain in most patients undergoing epiduroscopy. (**c**) Passing the epiduroscope through inflamed suprapedicular peridural membrane, over the pedicle, often results in complete and sustained relief of back pain. (**d**) Inability to pass the epiduroscope through inflamed suprapedicular peridural membrane is a predictor of a poor long-term prognosis. (**e**) Touching the dorsal root ganglion produces dysesthesias in the corresponding nerve root distribution. This type of pain is rarely concordant with the patient's usual back pain. (**f**) A percutaneously placed dilator, passed through inflamed suprapedicular membrane in the inferior neural foramen, may be of aid when the tip of the epiduroscope is too large

"squeezed" into the narrow space between the hypertrophic ligamentum flavum and dura mater, is also a common site of concordant pain in patients with lateral recess stenosis (Fig. 53.8).

Epidural Fibrosis

Numerous fibrous tissue bands connecting the dura mater to the peridural membrane can be seen (Fig. 53.6). These tissue bands are considered abnormal when traction deforms the regular shape of the dura mater. Manipulation of isolated tissue bands or adhesions are usually not painful. Significant fibrosis around the dorsal root ganglion or nerve root sleeve, as observed with epiduroscopy, is uncommon. If present, manipulation of fibrous connections around the dorsal root ganglion causes dysesthesias but not concordant pain. In areas of spinal canal stenosis or neural foraminal narrowing, fibrosis is usually associated with increased vascularity and pain to touch (i.e., inflammation). Increases in fibrotic epidural bands in areas of increased vascularity suggest the presence of chronic inflammation. Severe epidural fibrosis is almost always associated with back surgery. Removal of the wall of the spinal canal also removes peridural membrane. The peridural membrane is essential for the maintenance and lubrication of the epidural space. Absence of peridural membrane will lead to fibrosis and complete obliteration of the epidural space, preventing access with the epiduroscope. Dense epidural bands and septa can often be seen in proximity to postsurgical regions and are often painful to touch but rarely show signs of inflammation (Fig. 53.6). Significant fibrosis, after multiple epidural corticosteroid injections, has been reported. In general, mild fibrosis is not a major determinant of epidural pathology and is usually not of much interest, while severe fibrosis has profound clinical implications but cannot be treated with epiduroscopy. Thus, for the epiduroscopist, epidural fibrosis plays a relatively minor role.

Herniation of the Intervertebral Disc and Juxta Facet Cyst

Small or moderately large disc herniation may be seen when the scope is placed in the anterior epidural space (Fig. 53.6e). However, even large disc herniations are surprisingly difficult to identify and usually require the assistance of fluoroscopy. Disc herniations compressing nerve roots in the dural sac or more lateral disc herniations compressing a nerve root sleeve or dorsal root ganglion have been reported but have not been observed by the author in some 2000 epiduroscopic investigations. In the neural foramen, large protruding discs or extruded disc material impress as a continuous fibrous tissue mass, similar to the severe fibrosis seen in postsurgical regions, is usually difficult to evaluate and treat. A large central disc herniation causes central spinal canal stenosis, which may be investigated if scope passage is possible. However, disc herniations, large enough to cause neurological deficit, make scope passage often impossible and of little use (Fig. 53.8). Large geometrical deformations of the spinal canal and neural foramen distort the normal anatomy and make interventions, such as forceful injections or ablations, potentially dangerous (Fig. 53.3c). Therefore, it is the author's opinion that epiduroscopy is not indicated in the presence of disc herniation with objective neurological deficit. In these cases, rigid endoscopy or open spine surgery is recommended.

Large disc herniation without neurological deficit can be investigated using epiduroscopy. With epiduroscopy, it can often be shown that a known disc herniation is not the cause of back pain or referred radiating pain but that the pain originates from inflamed peridural membrane elsewhere, usually at L4–L5. On occasion, a disc herniation or juxta facet cyst may cause positional radicular symptoms or cause pain through sensitization of peridural membrane adjacent to a spinal deformation. In such cases, the exact localization and evaluation of the nidus of low back pain, using epiduroscopy, may be helpful in the medical decision-making process.

Miscellaneous

In the absence of neurological deficit, epiduroscopy is a very useful tool for the evaluation and diagnosis of other specific spinal pathologies that may cause of back pain, such as lipomatosis, disc degeneration and disc herniation, spondylolisthesis, spinal stenosis, autoimmune disorders, neoplasm, chronic compression fractures, and many other pathologies that are usually diagnosed using conventional diagnostic methods. Moreover, pathologies that cannot be diagnosed with conventional methods are especially well suited for evaluation with epiduroscopy. Indeed, direct observation of intraspinal pathology and reaction to touch using epiduroscopy often do not support the original diagnosis. For example, elimination of nerve compression as a cause of concordant pain may prevent unnecessary back surgery or interventional procedures. Instead, localization and a precise diagnosis of causative pathology direct the interventionalist to where interventions may be performed effectively (Figs. 53.9 and 53.10).

Epiduroscopy can also be used for the diagnoses and evaluation of spinal pathologies that are not primarily related to back pain. Tissue abnormalities of the peridural membrane, epidural fat and dura mater may be caused by a plethora of medical diseases, such as neoplasms, metabolic and immune disorders, infections, or vascular abnormalities, can be observed directly and further analyzed using cytology brushes or biopsies forceps or other diagnostic instruments. Based on the correct diagnosis, an appropriate treatment with or without the use of endoscopy can then be instituted.

Therapeutic Epiduroscopy

Targeted Injections

Pharmacological agents can be injected through the side port of the epiduroscope and directly applied to the site of pathology. The first requirement for treatment using epiduroscopy is that the correct pathology is identified using the methods described above. Multiple areas of pathology may be identified, but maximal pain reproduction is usually confined to one area. Local epidurography, by injecting a small amount of contrast material at the specific site of interest, may further delineate relevant anatomy but is not necessary in all cases (Fig. 53.10). It is important to realize that pathology as diagnosed by conventional diagnostic methods, such as radiological imaging and electrophysiological studies, does not correlate well with epiduroscopy findings and should not bias the operator. A number of agents, such as hyaluronidase, hypertonic saline, or ozone, have been injected, but the most commonly used medications are crystalline corticosteroids and local anesthetics.

Although the use of epiduroscopy for targeted injections seems rational, there are no proper studies that meet the abovementioned criteria that prove the use of epiduroscopy offers an advantage over conventional injections. Considering the cost and potential for complications, the use of epiduroscopy for targeted injections should be reserved for patients in whom more conventional treatments are ineffective.

Adhesiolysis

A number of studies describe the use of epiduroscopy for breaking perineural adhesions. Putative objectives have included the restoration of normal physiology by decreasing traction on nerve tissue, the increase in blood flow and lymphatic or venous outflow, and the improved ability for pharmacological agents to reach the site of pathology. Although a number of studies claim effectiveness, none meet the abovementioned criteria for the use of epiduroscopy. In the nonsurgical epidural space, strings and sheets of fibrous tissue are a normal finding and are usually not painful to touch. On occasion, fibrous adhesions may appear hyperemic, possibly the result of chronic inflammation. Manipulation of these fibrous bands with the tip of the epiduroscope may cause pain, but the pain may not be concordant with the patient's usual back pain.

Proper identification of the nerve root with epiduroscopy is often difficult, separating the nerve from perineural adhesion is even harder, and breaking perineural adhesions without causing damage to the nerve root or dorsal root ganglion is almost impossible. Given that in most patients the nerve root is not the primary site of pathology, the contribution of epiduroscopy to the effectiveness of perineural adhesiolysis is difficult to prove. Severe epidural fibrosis occurs in areas where the wall of the spinal canal has been removed (e.g., laminectomy). This leads to complete obliteration of the local epidural space. Attempts to advance the scope in such areas is often impossible, even when the surgical excision was small. Rigorous attempts to advance the epiduroscope lead almost invariably to dural puncture or tear (Fig. 53.6e, f). Back pain commonly originates from the traction of fibrous connections to inflamed and sensitized peridural membrane. Adhesiolysis of these fibrous connections between the dura mater and the peridural membrane in the nonsurgical spinal canal, using the mechanical action of the scope tip, forceful injections, destructive chemicals, laser, or radiofrequency thermocoagulation, may therefore be useful. However, none of the currently reported studies using these approaches for adhesiolysis fulfill the previously defined requirements to support the use of epiduroscopy. Therefore, epiduroscopy for the treatment of epidural fibrosis in nonsurgical regions is, at this time, only recommended if adhesions can be shown to be clinically significant. In the author's opinion, epiduroscopy is ineffective for the treatment of severe epidural fibrosis in postsurgical regions and does not offer an advantage over less invasive interventions, such as the Racz procedure.

Discectomy

Compression of a nerve root is not a common cause of low back pain, yet classical theory dictates discectomy as the main treatment for radiating leg pain. Unfortunately, it is difficult to identify nerve compression using epiduroscopy. Pathology that leads to nerve root compression is often too severe and too extensive to be treated effectively and safely with epiduroscopy. Open spine surgery or transforaminal rigid endoscopy is a more suitable approach for reduction of disc herniations that cause neurological deficit or pain. Current technology makes the use of mechanical tools that can be advanced through the side port of the epiduroscopy difficult to impossible. Laser has been used to reduce disc size through evaporation of disc material. In these reports, the epiduroscope was mostly used as a probe and as a visual guide to monitor disc reduction and use was restricted to safe regions of the spinal canal, such as the central anterior epidural space, where nerve tissue is unlikely to cross the path of the laser beam. There is little evidence that the procedure treats back pain through the proposed mechanism of disc reduction, since most central disc protrusions are unlikely to cause intradural nerve root compression without significant neurological deficit and disc tissue itself is not well innervated and is thus itself not a likely source of pain (Fig. 53.8). However, laser may be an effective means of destruction and denervation of well-innervated inflamed and sensitized peridural membrane in areas adjacent to damaged tissue, such as a ruptured disc or arthritic facet joint. Unfortunately, low back pain most often originates from the peridural membrane in the inferior compartment of the neural foramen, where close proximity to the traversing and exiting nerve root makes the use of laser unsafe. Few studies on the use of laser meet the above criteria for the effective use of epiduroscopy. Therefore, epiduroscopic-guided laser treatment of epidural pathology is promising but needs refinement and should be used with caution.

PACIF (Percutaneous Ablation, Curettage, and Inferior Foraminotomy)

The most common cause of low back pain is painful sensitization of peridural membrane in the inferior neural foramen of L4–L5. Low back pain generally "diagnosed" as nonspecific or even "psychosomatic" can often be reproduced by touching hyperemic-appearing PDM just cephalad to the pedicle of L5 with the epiduroscope. Common low back pain may be explained by the accumulation of inflammatory mediators in the suprapedicular compartment. Tissue breakdown products, released from a damaged intervertebral disc or facet joint, may cause inflammation and sensitization of the well-innervated peridural membrane that forms the boundaries of the suprapedicular compartment. Removal of the peridural membrane by passing the epiduroscope directly over the pedicle has been shown to give profound and sustained pain relief in many patients with common low back pain (Fig. 53.10c). The exact mechanism of pain relief is unknown, but removal of inflammatory material from the suprapedicular compartment, denervation of painful PDM, and allowing inflammation to dissipate are additional proposed mechanisms of action. Unfortunately, the tip of the epiduroscope is delicate and not designed to be used as a dissection instrument and the ligamentum flavum hypertrophy or a bulging intervertebral disc often prevents complete passage of the epiduroscope through the neural foramen. Therefore, percutaneous ablation, curettage, and inferior foraminotomy (PACIF I) has been developed to overcome this obstruction. This procedure is a modification of the Seldinger technique. A dilator is placed over a percutaneously placed guide wire, itself passed over the pedicle into the anterior epidural space (Fig. 53.10f). PACIF has been shown to be highly effective in patients with nonspecific low back pain. Other tools such as laser may also be effective in removal of the peridural membrane, but close proximity to the traversing and exiting nerve root should caution the interventionalist. Removal of peridural membrane through rigid transforaminal endoscopy (PACIF II) is a highly effective alternative to PACIF I and may in the future become the treatment of choice for the treatment of severe and disabling chronic low back pain.

Miscellaneous Therapeutic Applications of Epiduroscopy

The science of epiduroscopy is just in its infancy. Technological limitations; incomplete knowledge of spinal anatomy, physiology, and pathology and inertia of the medical society to accept promising but unverified new methods have hindered the development of epiduroscopy into a full-fledged highly effective minimally invasive surgical spine procedure. This is regrettable, because:

1. Epiduroscopy allows for direct observation of pathological changes in the epidural space.
2. Epiduroscopy can be performed in a responsive patient and therefore can provide direct evidence that these pathological changes are associated with the patient's complaints.
3. Epiduroscopy allows for targeted and dynamic treatment of these pathological changes and has the potential to markedly reduce suffering in the large population of patients with pathology of the spine.

Unfortunately, many conventional and often expensive pain management methods lack these advantages and may lead to less favorable outcomes. Fortunately, epiduroscopy is also a powerful research tool, so that the many obstacles to the clinical application of epiduroscopy can each in turn be overcome with additional high-quality scientific investigation.

Few reports are available on the use of epiduroscopy for reasons other than back pain. Epiduroscopy has been used to assist in the placement of epidural catheters and electrodes but has the potential to be used for far more complicated medical problems, such as the evacuation of epidural hematomas and control of intraspinal hemorrhage, repair of dural tears, removal of cysts, retrieval of damaged hardware such as fractured DRG electrodes or sheared epidural catheters, as well as the repositioning or repair of nonfunctioning spinal cord stimulator leads, debridement and irrigation of intraspinal infections, biopsy and removal of intraspinal neoplasms, targeted chemotherapy, clipping of arteriovenous malformations, and so on.

Epiduroscopy can also be used to assist in common open surgical procedures of the spine, such as discectomies and reconstructive spine surgery, or to assist in minimally invasive spine surgery, such as the PACIF procedure, rigid transforaminal endoscopy, or vertebroplasty of complicated vertebral fractures. Similar to laparoscopy, additional large-bore needles can be placed into the epidural space to treat specific epidural pathologies and is a technique that deserves further exploration. Epiduroscopy has been used for the diagnosis and treatment of pathology in the thoracic and cervical spinal canal and endoscopy may be preferred over an open surgical approach. Presence of the spinal cord, with its vulnerable blood supply, requires a better understanding of the anatomy, physiology, and pathology of the cervical and thoracic spine. At this time, considering the potential of devastating neurological complications, epiduroscopy of the thoracic and cervical epidural space is not recommended and should be performed with great caution. Indeed, the number of potential applications of epiduroscopy seems endless, but close proximity to the central nervous system makes the occurrence of serious complications an ever-present possibility. However, this should not hamper further progress in the field of epiduroscopy but instead emphasizes the need for proper patient selection, careful preparation, and diligence when performing this promising but still mostly unexplored procedure.

Acknowledgment The author would like to thank Dr. Craig Hartrick for his contributions to the manuscript.

Suggested Reading

Akbas M, Babun H, Hamdy Salem H, Hussien Emara T, Elmosly S, Gunduz E, Karsli B, Asik F. One-year evaluation of epiduroscopy in chronic back pain with and without radiculopathy: a retrospective study. Egypt J Neurol Psychiat Neurosurg. 2020;56(4):1–5.

Ansari S, Heavner JE, McConnell DJ, Azari H, Bosscher HA. The peridural membrane of the spinal canal: a critical review. Pain Pract. 2012;12(4):315–25. https://doi.org/10.1111/j.1533-2500.2011.00510.x.

Avellanal M. [Epiduroscopy]. Rev Esp Anestesiol Reanim. 2011;58(7):426–33. doi:https://doi.org/10.1016/s0034-9356(11)70107-4

Avellanal M, Diaz-Reganon G. Interlaminar approach for epiduroscopy in patients with failed back surgery syndrome. Br J Anaesth. 2008;101(2):244–9. https://doi.org/10.1093/bja/aen165.

Avellanal M, Diaz-Reganon G, Orts A, Soto S. One-year results of an algorithmic approach to managing failed back surgery syndrome. Pain Res Manag. 2014;19(6):313–6. https://doi.org/10.1155/2014/474510.

Avellanal M, Diaz-Reganon G, Orts A, Gonzalez-Montero L, Riquelme I. Transforaminal epiduroscopy in patients with failed back surgery syndrome. Pain Physician. 2019;22(1):89–95. https://www.ncbi.nlm.nih.gov/pubmed/30700072.

Bogduk N. On the definitions and physiology of back pain, referred pain, and radicular pain. Pain. 2009;147(1–3):17–9. https://doi.org/10.1016/j.pain.2009.08.020.

Bosscher HA. Complications of epiduroscopy. In: Staats P, Erdine S, editors. Complications of pain management. New York, NY: Wiley; 2021.

Bosscher HA, Heavner JE. Incidence and severity of epidural fibrosis after back surgery: an endoscopic study. Pain Pract. 2010;10(1):18–24. https://doi.org/10.1111/j.1533-2500.2009.00311.x.

Bosscher HA, Heavner JE. Diagnosis of the vertebral level from which low back or leg pain originates. A comparison of clinical evaluation, MRI and epiduroscopy. Pain Pract. 2012;12(7):506–12. https://doi.org/10.1111/j.1533-2500.2012.00549.x.

Bosscher HA, Heavner JE. Lumbosacral epiduroscopy findings predict treatment outcome. Pain Pract. 2014;14(6):506–14. https://doi.org/10.1111/papr.12112.

Bosscher HA, Heavner JE. Treatment of common low back pain: a new approach to an old problem. Pain Pract. 2015;15(6):509–17. https://doi.org/10.1111/papr.12224.

Bosscher HA, Heavner JE, Grozdanov P, Warraich IA, Wachtel MS, Dertien J. The peridural membrane of the human spine is well innervated. Anat Rec (Hoboken). 2016;299(4):484–91. https://doi.org/10.1002/ar.23315.

Bosscher HA, Grozdanov PN, Warraich II, MacDonald CC, Day MR. The anatomy of the peridural membrane of the human spine. Anat Rec (Hoboken). 2020a;304:677. https://doi.org/10.1002/ar.24476.

Bosscher HA, Grozdanov PN, Warraich II, MacDonald CC, Day MR. The peridural membrane of the spine has characteristics of synovium. Anat Rec (Hoboken). 2020b;304:631. https://doi.org/10.1002/ar.24474.

Ceylan A, Asik I, Ozgencil EG, Erken B. Evaluation of the efficacy of epiduroscopic adhesiolysis in failed back surgery syndrome. Turk J Med Sci. 2018;49:249–57.

Chen M, Lin C. Is contrast media really a necessity in lumbar epiduroscopic procedures? Neuropsychiatry (London). 2018;8(5):1652–4.

Choi YK. Lumbar foraminal neuropathy: an update on non-surgical management. Korean J Pain. 2019;32(3):147–59. https://doi.org/10.3344/kjp.2019.32.3.147.

Depauw P, Groen RJM, Van Loon J, Peul WC, Malbrain M, De Waele JJ. The significance of intra-abdominal pressure in neurosurgery and neurological diseases: a narrative review and a conceptual proposal. Acta Neurochir. 2019;161(5):855–64. https://doi.org/10.1007/s00701-019-03868-7.

Epter RS, Helm S II, Hayek SM, Benyamin RM, Smith HS, Abdi S. Systematic review of percutaneous adhesiolysis and management of chronic low back pain in post lumbar surgery syndrome. Pain Physician. 2009;12(2):361–78. https://www.ncbi.nlm.nih.gov/pubmed/19305485.

Fai KR, Engleback M, Norman JB, Griffiths R. Interlaminar approach for epiduroscopy in patients with failed back surgery syndrome. Br J Anaesth. 2009;102(2):280; author reply 280–1. https://doi.org/10.1093/bja/aen371.

Geurts JW, Kallewaard JW, Richardson J, Groen GJ. Targeted methylprednisolone acetate/hyaluronidase/clonidine injection after diagnostic epiduroscopy for chronic sciatica: a prospective, 1-year follow-up study. Reg Anesth Pain Med. 2002;27(4):343–52. https://doi.org/10.1053/rapm.2002.27175.

Hazer DB, Acarbas A, Rosberg HE. The outcome of epiduroscopy treatment in patients with chronic low back pain and radicular pain, operated or non-operated for lumbar disc herniation: a retrospective study in 88 patients. Korean J Pain. 2018;31(2):109–15. https://doi.org/10.3344/kjp.2018.31.2.109.

Heavner JE, Bosscher H. Epiduroscopy and radiation exposure. Reg Anesth Pain Med. 2009;34(1):79; author reply 79. https://doi.org/10.1097/AAP.0b013e3181933fc0.

Heavner J, Chokhavatia S, Kizelshteyn G. Percutaneous evaluation of the epidural and subarachnoid space with a flexible fiberscope. Reg Anesth. 1991;15(1):85.

Heavner JE, Bosscher H, Dunn D, Lehman T. Xanthosis in the spinal epidural space--an epiduroscopy finding. Pain Pract. 2004;4(1):39–41. https://doi.org/10.1111/j.1530-7085.2004.04005.x.

Heavner JE, Wyatt DE, Bosscher HA. Lumbosacral epiduroscopy complicated by intravascular injection. Anesthesiology. 2007;107(2):347–50. https://doi.org/10.1097/01.anes.0000271867.77686.f5.

Heavner JE, Bosscher HA, Wachtel MS. Cell types obtained from the epidural space of patients with low back pain/radiculopathy. Pain Pract. 2009;9(3):167–72. https://doi.org/10.1111/j.1533-2500.2009.00272.x.

Helm S II, Racz GB, Gerdesmeyer L, Justiz R, Hayek SM, Kaplan ED, et al. Percutaneous and endoscopic adhesiolysis in managing low back and lower extremity pain: a systematic review and meta-analysis. Pain Physician. 2016;19(2):E245–82. https://www.ncbi.nlm.nih.gov/pubmed/26815254.

Igarashi T, Hirabayashi Y, Seo N, Saitoh K, Fukuda H, Suzuki H. Lysis of adhesions and epidural injection of steroid/local anaesthetic during epiduroscopy potentially alleviate low back and leg pain in elderly patients with lumbar spinal stenosis. Br J Anaesth. 2004;93(2):181–7. https://doi.org/10.1093/bja/aeh201.

Jin HS, Bae JY, In CB, Choi EJ, Lee PB, Nahm FS. Epiduroscopic removal of a lumbar facet joint cyst. Korean J Pain. 2015;28(4):275–9. https://doi.org/10.3344/kjp.2015.28.4.275.

Jo DH, Yang HJ, Kim JJ. Approach for epiduroscopic laser neural decompression in case of the sacral canal stenosis. Korean J Pain. 2013;26(4):392–5.

Ju JH, Ha HG, Jung CK, Kim HW, Lee CY, Kim JH. Patterns of epidural venous varicosity in lumbar stenosis. Korean J Spine. 2012;9(3):244–9. https://doi.org/10.14245/kjs.2012.9.3.244.

Jung CK. Sacral epiduroscopic laser decompression for complex regional pain syndrome after lumbar spinal surgery. Medicine. 2018;97(19):1–4.

Kallewaard JW, Vanelderen P, Richardson J, Van Zundert J, Heavner J, Groen GJ. Epiduroscopy for patients with lumbosacral radicular pain. Pain Pract. 2014;14(4):365–77. https://doi.org/10.1111/papr.12104.

Kim SK, Lee SC, Park SW. Trans-sacral epiduroscopic laser decompression versus the microscopic open interlaminar approach for L5-S1 disc herniation. J Spinal Cord Med. 2020;43(1):46–52. https://doi.org/10.1080/10790268.2018.1442285.

Magalhaes FN, Soares SC, Torres JM, Ungaretti A, Cacciacarro MF, Teixeira MJ, Fonoff ET. Effects of ozone applied by spinal endoscopy in patients with chronic pain related to failed back surgery syndrome: a pilot study. Neuropsychiatr Dis Treat. 2013;9:1759–66. https://doi.org/10.2147/NDT.S48663.

Moon BJ, Lee HY, Kim KN, Yi S, Ha Y, Yoon DH, Shin DA. Experimental evaluation of percutaneous lumbar laser disc decompression using a 1414 nm Nd:YAG laser. Pain Physician. 2015;18(6):E1091–9. https://www.ncbi.nlm.nih.gov/pubmed/26606022.

Oh J, Jo DH. Epiduroscopic laser neural decompression as a treatment for migrated lumbar disc herniation. Medicine. 2018;97:1–9.

Raffaeli W, Righetti D. Surgical radio-frequency epiduroscopy technique (R-ResAblator) and FBSS treatment: preliminary evaluations. Acta Neurochir Suppl. 2005;92:121–5. https://doi.org/10.1007/3-211-27458-8_26.

Ruetten S, Meyer O, Godolias G. Endoscopic surgery of the lumbar epidural space (epiduroscopy): results of therapeutic intervention in 93 patients. Minim Invasive Neurosurg. 2003;46(1):1–4. https://doi.org/10.1055/s-2003-37962.

Saberski LR. Advances in pain medicine: epiduroscopy. J Back Musculoskelet Rehabil. 1998;11(2):131–40. https://doi.org/10.3233/BMR-1998-11203.

Shimada N, Igarashi T, Murai K, Hara T, Kuramochi T, Takeuchi M. Adhesions in the epidural space caused by frequent epidural blocks. JA Clin Rep. 2017;3(1):57. https://doi.org/10.1186/s40981-017-0128-z.

Son S, Lee SG, Ahn Y, Kim WK. Clinical outcomes of trans-sacral epiduroscopic laser decompression (SELD) in patients with lumbar disc herniation. Pain Res Manag. 2020;2020:1537875. https://doi.org/10.1155/2020/1537875.

Tardieu GG, Fisahn C, Loukas M, Moisi M, Chapman M, Oskouian JM, Tubbs SR. The epidural ligaments (of Hofmann): a comprehensive review of the literature. Cureau. 2016;8(9):1–8.

54 Percutaneous Epidural Neuroplasty

James L. Morgan and Miles R. Day

Contents

General Consideration

Percutaneous epidural neuroplasty, also known as epidural neurolysis, epidural adhesiolysis or the Racz procedure, was originally described in 1989. It is a minimally invasive interventional pain procedure used to treat neuraxial pain, radiculopathies, or both. This procedure has been used in the cervical, thoracic, and lumbar spine safely and effectively. Certain forms of cervicogenic headaches have also been treated using this procedure as well.

This procedure has been implemented in pain practices worldwide and studied extensively throughout the years since the introduction by Dr. Gabor Racz in the late 1980s. This has led to the recognition of epidural neuroplasty as being a safe and effective treatment option for intractable neuraxial/radicular pain, when performed by properly by trained physicians with appropriate equipment. Cost-effectiveness has also been demonstrated and studied as well. Modifications have been implemented throughout the years regarding equipment and medication selection (volumes and dosing.) However, all modifications follow the general concept that leads to the introduction of percutaneous epidural neuroplasty. These modifications have led to a more in-depth understanding of potential complications and how to prevent them.

Pertaining to cost-effectiveness, percutaneous epidural neuroplasty was originally described as a three-infusion procedure (one infusion per day for 3 days) but has shown efficacy as a single infusion procedure all done in 1 day. This chapter will discuss both procedures.

The percutaneous epidural neurolysis procedure was developed and is widely accepted due to the following factors: (1) improved understanding of the anatomical structures involved in the etiology of pain regarding the epidural

J. L. Morgan · M. R. Day (✉)
Department of Anesthesiology and Pain Management, Texas Tech University Health Sciences Center, Lubbock, TX, USA
e-mail: james.morgan@ttuhsc.edu; miles.day@ttuhsc.edu

D. Jankovic, P. Peng (eds.), *Regional Nerve Blocks in Anesthesia and Pain Therapy*,
https://doi.org/10.1007/978-3-030-88727-8_54

space, (2) structural changes of epidural and intervertebral space in the development of neuraxial pain and radiculopathies, (3) location and patterns of pain due to stimulation of certain pathological structures of the epidural space, (4) reliable and reproducible techniques to access the epidural space, (5) interpretation of epidurography for diagnosis and treatment, (6) theoretical justifications and clear guidelines regarding the technical aspect of the procedure and doses, (7) evidence of the treatment regarding effectiveness, and (8) USCPT code provided for the procedure. The goals of percutaneous epidural neuroplasty are as follows:

- Diagnose pathological changes of the epidural space that could prevent medications from being delivered to identifiable pathological areas (e.g., epidural fibrosis.) Injection of radiographic contrast media is used to identify these filling defects and provide a target for neuroplasty.
- Eliminate the pathological obstructions and scar tissue using physiological saline mixed with hyaluronidase injected at the observed filling defect.
- Identify that the pathological obstructions leading to pain have been eliminated after the procedure by readministration of radiographic contrast media at the same-targeted area.
- Administer medication directly at the area of pathology for treatment of pain. Medications used include local anesthetics, steroids, and hypertonic saline.

Functional Anatomy

Neuraxial pain and radicular pain can be broken down into regional structures surrounding the spinal cord. This most commonly includes the intervertebral disk, composed of the nucleus pulposus and annulus fibrosus, and the structures surrounding the nerve roots. Studies have shown that radiculopathies can be caused by irritation of edematous, overextended, or compressed nerve roots. Back pain could be reproduced by stimulation of the outer layer of the annulus fibrosus and posterior longitudinal ligament. These structures have a vast innervation of meningeal branches called the sinuvertebral nerves. Surgical interventions such as a laminectomy result in fibrosis and scar tissue in the epidural space and perineural region. The fibrosis itself is not sensitive but is hypothesized to immobilize the nerve, which leads to irritability and increased pain with traction or pressure. Entrapment is not the only mechanism that can lead to pain going down the leg or neuraxial pain. Pressure, whether high or low, can lead to nerve irritation and pain. High pressure tends to lead to direct mechanical effects on the nerve tissue and can damage the anatomy of the nerve itself (distort nerve fibers, disrupt the nodes of Ranvier, or press in the paranodal myelin sheath).

Lower pressures lead to disruption of blood flow and ischemia to the nerve. Animal studies have shown that compression of the cauda equina, via a balloon attached to the spinal cord, equivalent to arterial pressure will interrupt the blood flow. Venous blood flow is reduced with a pressure of 5–10 mmHg, while 10 mmHg showed a reduced transport of nutrients to nerve roots by 20–30%. This compression can also lead to edema formation in the endoneurial capillaries in the nerve roots via changes or the permeability and transmural pressures. Animal studies showed this after 2 min of compression at 50 mmHg. Chronic nerve injury due to intraneural edema is associated with development of neural fibrosis, which may contribute to the slow rate of improvement in patients with nerve compression. Compound muscle action potentials have been demonstrated to be reduced by 65% with compression of spinal nerves at 10 mmHg for 2 h by two adjacent balloons that simulate compression of multiple nerve roots. However, compression using a single balloon at the same pressure for the same duration did not alter the compound muscle action potentials. Pressures of 10 mmHg only appeared to cause changes of nerve function if multiple segments are compressed.

Chemical substances, such as glycoproteins, lactic acid, cytokines, and histamines, have been studied to cause irritation of the surrounding structures after tears of the annulus fibrosis. These substances being released in the vertebral canal can cause inflammation of the nerve roots and meninges leading to pain. It is also theoretically possible that components of the nucleus pulposus itself can act as a foreign body and trigger an autoimmune response leading to pain. This pain generator is without any compression of the nerve roots via an intervertebral disk protrusion.

Structural changes of the spine, such as degenerative changes, disk protrusions, herniations, and facet arthropathies, can lead to construction of the intervertebral space and thus increased pressure on the spinal nerves causing pain. The posterior longitudinal ligament runs along the posterior aspect of the vertebral body and can be stretched or irritated by protruding intervertebral disks, leading to axial back pain. More severe protrusions or disk herniations can cause pressure on the local nerve roots causing radicular pain.

In theory, excessive fibrosis is believed to tether the dura and the nerve roots, chemically excite and/or compress the nerve roots, damage microvessels, and potentially lead to ischemia, edema, demyelination, and C-fiber activation. Chronic neuraxial and/or radiculopathy is involved with one or more pathologies, such as inflammation, edema, fibrosis, venous engorgement, mechanical pressure on the abovementioned structures, ischemia, and central sensitization. Inflammatory tissue along with mechanical stimuli can activate nociceptors and nociceptive axons that transmit information to the CNS. Inflamed neural structures seem to be more sensitive to pressure and entrapment by fibrous tissue.

Therefore, it is justifiable to treat neuraxial and radicular pain by local administration of medications (anti-inflammatory, edema reducing, local anesthetics, and tissue dissolving medications such as hyaluronidase.)

Indication (Patient Selection)

The selection criteria for patients who are candidates for percutaneous epidural neuroplasty include the following.

1. Patients who have exhausted all conservative treatments for persistent neuraxial pain, radicular pain, post-spinal surgery syndrome, and spinal stenosis
2. Presence of pathological changes in the facet joints, intervertebral disks, or sympathetic nerves
3. Positive selective nerve root block at the suspected level of pathology

Medications

Moore studied hyaluronidase in the 1950s for hernia repair procedures. Hyaluronidase breaks down the viscous mucopolysaccharides in the interstitial matrix and allows greater spread of substances injected. The previously reported incidence of allergies was 1:2000, but the formulation of hyaluronidase was animal derived. These preparations have been replaced with recombinant human PH20 hyaluronidase. No cases of allergic reactions have been reported. Recombinant human PH20 hyaluronidase has been extensively studied and shown not to elicit an immune response. It has also been extensively utilized intrathecally, in Bangalore, for treatment of arachnoiditis caused by tuberculosis and other noninfectious etiologies. Two high-quality studies have shown effectiveness with the use of hyaluronidase in neuroplasty procedures. It has been shown to improve pain outcomes, reduce procedures, and be cost-effective. Recombinant human hyaluronidase is also currently being studied as an alternative postoperative anti-edema agent compared to dexamethasone. Koc et al. studied traumatic edema formation in the hind paws of rats and compared paw volumes after injection of dexamethasone or recombinant human hyaluronidase. They concluded the hyaluronidase more effectively reduced the traumatic edema compared to dexamethasone. Fronza et al. evaluated the anti-inflammatory potential of bovine hyaluronidase (HYAL) by creating carrageenan-inflamed air pouches in the subcutaneous tissue of mice. Phosphate saline solution or HYAL was then injected into the air pouches. They showed HYAL inhibited cellular recruitment, edema formation, and pro-inflammatory mediator production, resulting in decreased adherence of leukocytes and tissue infiltration. Helm and Racz conducted a literature review regarding the use of hyaluronidase in neuroplasty. They concluded, based on enhanced efficacy, safety, and decreased number of procedures, hyaluronidase should be considered when deciding which medications to use during neuroplasty.

Birkenmaier and colleagues studied the effects of hyaluronidase, bupivacaine, and hypertonic saline in a human fibroblast cell culture model. Hyaluronidase was found not to have a relevant effect on fibroblast proliferation. Bupivacaine and hypertonic saline were found to have a time- and concentration-dependent effect on cell viability and proliferation, even at concentrations well below the ones used clinically.

Technique: Caudal Epidural Neuroplasty

Prior to any procedure, full informed written and verbal consent should be obtained. Risks, benefits, and technical aspects should be discussed with the patient. See complications at the end of the chapter.

Materials include the following: a 16-gauge or 15-gauge RX Coude' needle with fluoropolymer-coated epidural catheter made of stainless steel with a spiral tip TunL Kath or TunL-XL (stiffer) (Epimed International, Inc., Irving Texas, USA) (Figs. 54.1 and 54.2). Do not use a Tuohy needle for this procedure. Touhy needles are designed for unidirectional, forward advancement of the catheter into the epidural space. It is not designed for withdrawing the catheter through the needle as this can lead to shearing of the catheter and a retained catheter fragment.

Intravenous access is necessary to treat potential complications as well as administer analgesia and sedation for the procedure and antibiotics postoperatively. Sedation and analgesia are recommended prior to the procedure at the discretion of the performing physician or anesthesia personnel. Recommended medications for sedation include 1–2 mg midazolam and 25–50 μg fentanyl. On rare occa-

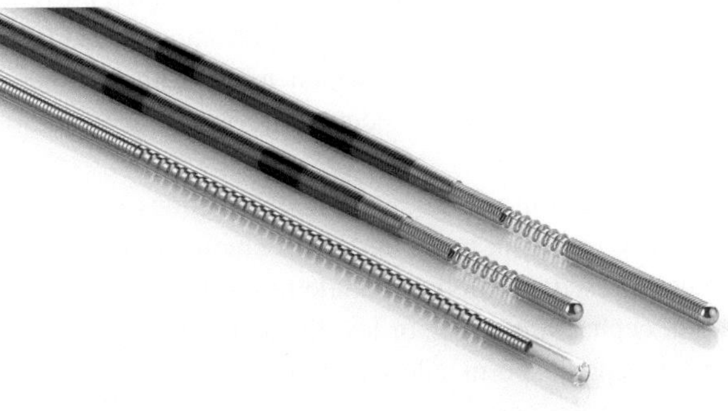

Fig. 54.1 Flexible catheters used in the epidural lysis of adhesions procedure. (Photograph courtesy of Epimed International and used with permission)

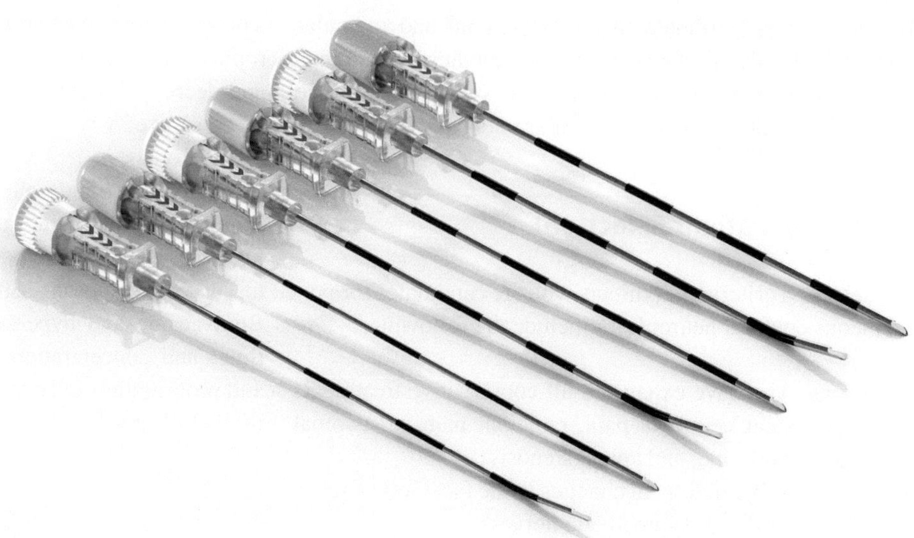

Fig. 54.2 Straight and Coude needles (18-, 16-, and 15-gauge) used in the lysis of adhesions procedure. (Photograph courtesy of Epimed International and used with permission)

sions, propofol may be necessary but must be used cautiously. Deep sedation is not recommended to ensure the patient is able to respond during the procedure to avoid any signs of spinal cord damage (weakness or paralysis). Pain from injection is likely due to stretching of nerve roots and corresponding cutaneous innervations regions. All procedures should be conducted under spot and continuous fluoroscopic guidance to optimize correct needle positioning, identification of contrast filling defect, and correct position of the catheter.

Radiographic contrast media should include a water-soluble, nonionic contrast medium, i.e., iohexol 240, to prevent subarachnoid injection. Non-water-soluble, ionic contrast can lead to spinal cord irritation, seizures, arachnoiditis, paralysis, or death. Epidural adhesions can increase the risk of subdural and/or subarachnoid injections due to anatomical variations.

Local anesthetic recommendation is 0.2% ropivacaine or 0.25% bupivacaine. Ropivacaine causes less of a motor block as compared to bupivacaine. The choice of corticosteroid used largely depends on availability. Long-acting steroid emulsions have a larger particle size (20 μm), which prevents injection through bacterial filters. Hypertonic saline (10%) has a local anesthetic effect, which helps with prolonged pain relief and reduces edema through its osmotic properties.

For the three-infusion procedure, intravenous antibiotics are given 30 min prior to the initial placement of the catheter. Commonly used antibiotics include the following: ceftriaxone 1 g, cephazolin 1–2 g, or levofloxacin 500 mg for penicillin or cephalosporin allergic patients. This is repeated every 24 h if the patient is admitted to the hospital. This is necessary, since the catheter is left in place overnight. For a single infusion procedure, antibiotics are not necessary, although some practitioners may choose to administer them.

The patient is placed in the prone position on the procedure table. The sacral region is then prepped in the usual sterile fashion. The sacral cornu and hiatus are then palpated, and the needle insertion target is located in the gluteal cleft opposite the affected side, approximately 1 cm lateral and 2.5 cm inferior to the sacral hiatus. This entry site allows easier maneuverability of the needle and catheter toward the affected side and reduces the risk of penetrating the dural sac or subdural space. An anteroposterior (AP) fluoroscopic image can be taken if there is difficulty locating the sacral hiatus through palpation. Lidocaine 1% is used to anesthetize the overlying skin of the target area. An 18-gauge A-bevel needle is used to puncture the skin initially, and then an epidural (16- or 15-gauge RX2-Coudé) needle is introduced and advanced through the sacral hiatus. In some patients, it is helpful to keep the tip of the index finger or thumb on the sacral hiatus to help guide the needle tip through the sacral hiatus. The needle should be advanced no further than the S3 foramen. This avoids dural puncture in patients who may have a low-lying dura. Confirmation of needle placement in the osseous canal is obtained using a lateral fluoroscopic view. Obtaining a lateral can also be helpful if there is difficulty advancing the needle through the sacral hiatus on the AP view. Returning to the AP view helps confirm the direction of the needle tip heading toward the affected side. Once needle placement is satisfactory, aspiration of CSF or blood is performed prior to injection of any medication. Once negative aspiration has been confirmed, 10 mL iohexol (Omnipaque 240 or Isovue-M 240) is injected under live fluoroscopy. A "Christmas tree"-shaped distribution pattern should be seen to confirm needle placement in the epidural space (Fig. 54.3). In the presence of epidural adhesions, filling defects will be seen and the entire "Christmas tree" pattern may not be visualized. If the needle is located in the subarachnoid space, the contrast will spread

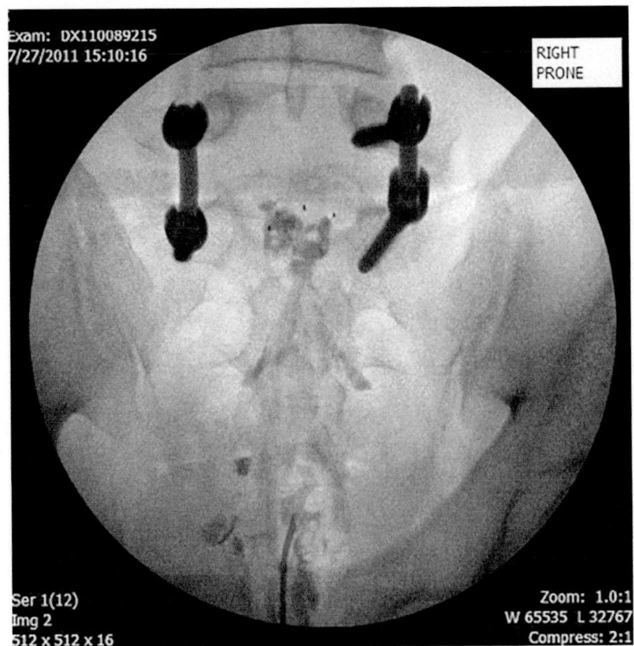

Fig. 54.3 Caudal epidurogram. The patient has a right S1 radiculopathy

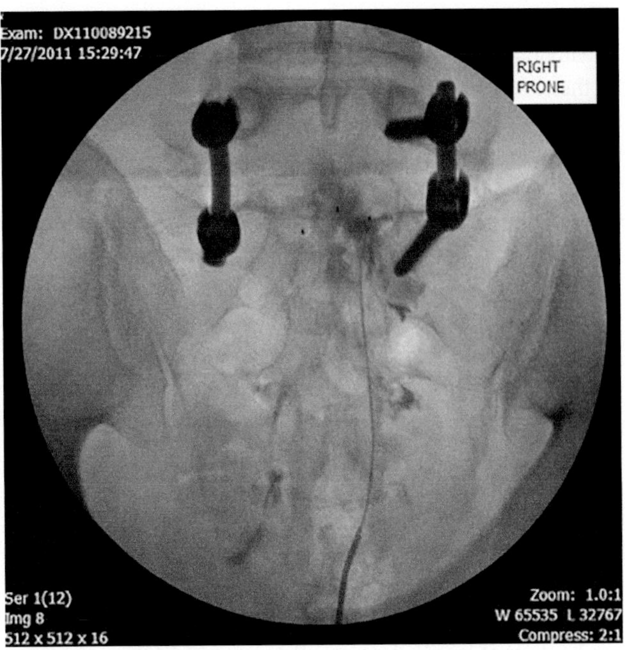

Fig. 54.4 Anteroposterior fluoroscopic image with a TunL-XL™ catheter in the bottom of the L5–S1 foramen for an S1 radiculopathy. The catheter could not be advanced further due to presumptive epidural scar tissue. Note the spread of contrast out of the inferior aspect of the right L5–S1 and S1 foramina after injection of hyaluronidase

in a central and cranial direction. Subdural placement would lead to a similar pattern but not as large of a spread as with subarachnoid placement. However, nerve roots can still be visualized due to lesser-resistant subdural space. Local anesthetic injected into the subarachnoid or subdural space will lead to a motor block much stronger and faster onset than injection into the epidural space. If aspiration is positive for blood, the needle should be repositioned until no more blood is aspirated. If CSF is aspirated, the procedure should be aborted and rescheduled. Allergic reactions to iodine containing contrast agents injected should be treated as needed with corticosteroids and antihistamines.

A fluoropolymer-coated epidural catheter made of stainless steel, with a spiral tip (TunL Kath) or less flexible (TunL-XL Kath), is then introduced into the adhesions through the needle. Multiple adjustments of the catheter are usually required due to the irregularity of adhesions. Therefore, it is recommended to use a 16- or 15-gauge RX-2 Coudé epidural needle to facilitate necessary corrections of the catheter tip and prevent shearing. Tuohy epidural needles should not be used given this fact.

Once the catheter tip has been confirmed to be in the correct position (ventral-lateral epidural space) and after negative aspiration, 1–2 mL of the contrast is injected a second time allowing visualization (filling) of the previous filling defects along the targeted spinal nerves or nerve roots (Fig. 54.4). Hyaluronidase is the slowly injected after negative aspiration. Recommended doses are 1500 units of animal-derived hyaluronidase or 150 units human recombinant hyaluronidase dissolved in 10 mL of preservative-free normal saline to further open up previous filling defects. An additional 2–3 mL of contrast can be injected to visualize the opening of previously scarred areas. Following this, a 3 mL test dose of a mixture of 9 mL 0.2% ropivacaine or 0.25% bupivacaine and 1 mL soluble or non-soluble corticosteroids is injected through the catheter. See Table 54.2 for injected solutions according to location. If after 5 min there is no evidence of subarachnoid injection, the remaining 7 mL of the aforementioned solutions is injected under live fluoroscopy. The location of the epidural adhesions should be documented. After waiting 30 min and placing the patient in the lateral decubitus position on the affected side, 10 mL of hypertonic saline solution (10%) is then injected after negative aspiration via an infusion pump over 30 min. The indwelling catheter is then flushed with 2 mL normal saline. This will result in decreased edema formation of previously scarred or inflamed nerve roots. This injection can be painful without the use of local anesthetic prior to injection. Hypertonic saline can also spread beyond the desired segments, in which local anesthesia was previously applied causing extreme pain that can be treated with IV sedatives or additional local anesthetic. Pain rarely lasts more than 5 min. Patients with known allergies to contrast or iodine can undergo the procedure without the administration of contrast. A test dose of local anesthetic is used to exclude subarachnoid or subdural positioning of the needle or catheter. Patients tend to experience pain in the skin area corresponding to the scarred epidural region. Resistance, due to adhesions, will be noted when advancing the catheter, and slow advancement is recommended to avoid entering the subarachnoid or subdural space. The catheter is then secured to the skin with a suture. The catheter insertion point is then covered with antibiotic ointment and covered with two split compresses (5 × 5 cm). Benzoin tincture is then spread on the surrounding tissue and secured with a Tegaderm transparent dressing (10 × 12 cm). Hypafix, a porous tape, is then used to cover the area and prevent the patient from sweating off the plaster. Additionally, an injection syringe adapter and bacterial filter are attached to the catheter which is then attached to the patient's side. Prophylactic antibiotics continue throughout the hospital stay as previously mentioned and 5 days after discharge. Two subsequent injections are done on the second day of admission, 6–8 h apart. This involves repeat injection of the previously mentioned test dose mixture, see table, followed by the full solution of local anesthetic and steroid mixture. After waiting 30 min, hypertonic saline (10%) is slowly infused as previously stated. Following the third injection, 10 min is allowed to elapse prior to removing the catheter and application of sterile dressing. Patients are discharged with a 5-day course of antibiotics, 500 mg oral cephalexin twice a day or oral levofloxacin 500 mg daily for penicillin allergic patients. Patients are also instructed to keep the catheter insertion site as dry as possible for 48 h to avoid infections.

Depending on size, large epidural adhesions cannot always be fully dissolved and require repeat procedures at 3-month intervals due to the use of steroids. Physical therapy, focusing on neural flossing exercises, is very important to improve muscle strength and tone. These exercises allow the nerve root to be mobilized by sliding in and out of the neural foramen that was previously limited by adhesions. These exercises should be performed 3–4 times per day for months following the procedure.

A transforaminal approach can also be used for catheter placement should there be a necessity to place two catheters above and below the level of interest. An oblique, infraneural approach is utilized using the same epidural needles and catheters used for the caudal approach (Figs. 54.5 and 54.6). The order and timing of medications injected is the same as in the caudal approach, but the volumes are reduced by 50%. These are in addition to what is injected caudally.

Table 54.1 describes a modified procedure for injecting hypertonic saline (10%) painlessly over a shortened period of time.

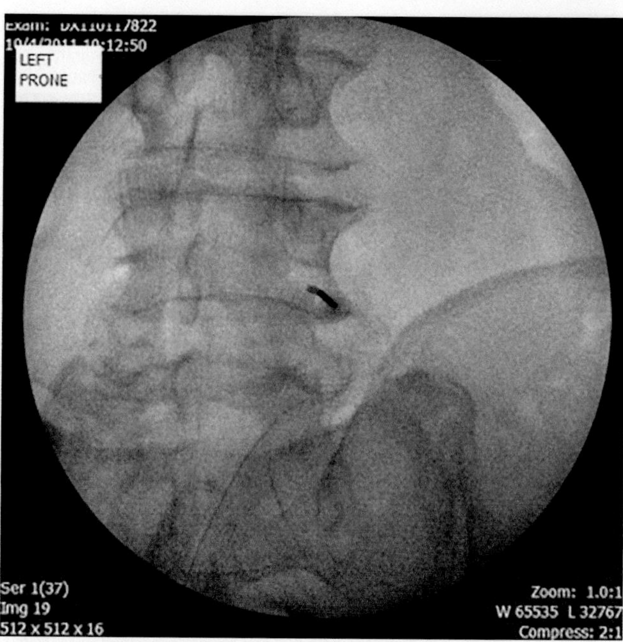

Fig. 54.5 Oblique fluoroscopic image of needle placement for a transforaminal catheter at L4–L5

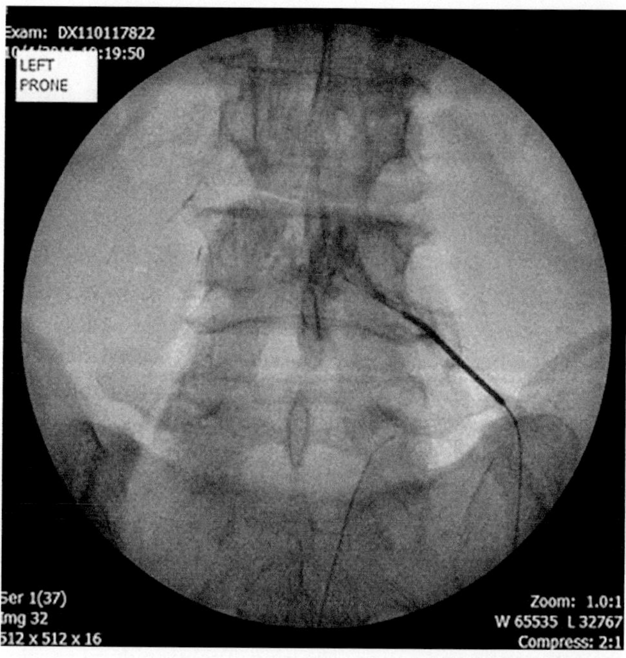

Fig. 54.6 Anteroposterior fluoroscopic image of a caudal catheter at right L5–S1 and a transforaminal catheter at right L4–L5

Technique: Cervical, Thoracic, or Lumbar Epidural Neuroplasty

Modifications have been made regarding injection technique and volumes to account for the spinal cord and avoidance of compression. The patient is placed prone or in the left lateral decubitus position on the procedure table. The "3D" technique (direction, depth, direction) to enter the epidural space is used. This will be highlighted in the following text. Preoperatively, the patient is examined, and needle puncture area is identified. Laboratory tests should be obtained pertaining to neuraxial blocks and reviewed. Intraoperatively, the area is prepped and draped in the usual sterile fashion. Needle insertion site is T1–T2, or T2–T3. A

Table 54.1 Pain-free hypertonic saline volumes and pharmacological adjustments

First series of injections: caudal catheter
1. 10 mL caudal epidural Omnipaque 240 contrast
2. 10 mL PF normal saline w/ 150 units hyaluronidase (Hylenex—human recombinant) or 1500 units hyaluronidase animal extract
3. 0.25% bupivacaine with 40 mg triamcinolone under fluoroscopic A/P and lateral observation. Lateral view [essential to rule out intravenous or subdural injection or spread through a partial surgical tear]. Observe patient for 20–30 min for delayed onset of motor block that would indicate subdural placement
**Abandon procedure if motor block develops.* Subdural motor block usually develops in 14–15 min later. *Shorter observations not recommended!*
Start flexion-rotation exercises
New—20–30 min later. Lidocaine 1% 1.5 mL injection, followed by 2–3 min later 10 mL of 10% sodium chloride in 0.6% lidocaine, injected in 1 mL increments fairly rapidly, over 3–5 min. The small volume, pre-hypertonic lidocaine, seems to cover the periphery of the injection site, therefore no pain from the hypertonic. Remember to flush at the end with 1 mL PF saline. Frequent check for motor function—postoperative observation requirements, maybe 2–4 h
Transforaminal catheter volumes are reduced to 5 mL (local and hypertonic)
Second series of injections: caudal catheter usually same day, 4–6 h later
1. 10 mL of bupivacaine 0.125%. No motor block → Wait 20–30 min if no motor block
2. 1.5 mL—1% lidocaine → Wait 2–3 min
3. Inject 10 mL (6 mL 1% lidocaine, 4 mL of 23.4% NaCl) = 10% sodium chloride in 0.6% lidocaine, fairly rapidly, over 3–5 min. Flush after observing patient for 30 min
Transforaminal catheter volumes are reduced to 5 mL [local and hypertonic]. Pre-hypertonic lidocaine: 1% 1 mL
If there is no motor block and patient is able to ambulate, patient can go home in 45–60 min. *Cost saving*
Third series of injections: caudal catheter usually same day, 4–6 h later
1. 10 mL of bupivacaine 0.125%. No motor block → Wait 20–30 min if no motor block
2. 1.5 mL—1% lidocaine → Wait 2–3 min
3. Inject 10 mL (6 mL 1% lidocaine, 4 mL of 23.4% NaCl) = 10% sodium chloride in 0.6% lidocaine, fairly rapidly, over 3–5 min. Flush after observing patient for 30 min
Transforaminal catheter volumes are reduced to 5 mL [local and hypertonic]. Pre-hypertonic lidocaine: 1% 1 mL
If there is no motor block and patient is able to ambulate, patient can go home in 45–60 min

paramedian approach is used by targeting the insertion site 1 cm or less lateral to midline and one intervertebral space below the epidural access point. The overlying skin of our insertion target is anesthetized with 1% lidocaine. The skin is then punctured using an 18-gauge needle prior to introducing a 16- or 15-gauge RX-2 Coudé needle. The **direction** of the needle (medial or lateral) is assessed using anteroposterior fluoroscopy. **Depth** is then obtained using a lateral view. The needle is advanced to the base of the spinous processes. The injection depth corresponds to the position of the lamina of the vertebral arch in the vicinity of the posterior epidural space. This technique has been improved with the use of the RX-2 Coudé needle, which has a second interlocking stylet that protrudes slightly beyond the tip of the needle. This allows the dura to be pushed away from the needle tip as it is turned 180° cephalad. Once needle placement is confirmed near the epidural space on a lateral view, the stylet is removed and a pulsator syringe (low friction) filled with 3 mL of normal saline and 2 mL of air is attached. The epidural space is then confirmed with loss of resistance technique. An AP view is obtained to check the final **direction** of the needle. A cervical epidurogram is performed with 1–2 mL of radiographic contrast. The catheter is then introduced the epidural needle in the direction of the filling defect and targeted nerve root of the lateral epidural space. Anterolateral positioning of the catheter is key giving the location of nociceptors concentrated in this space. After negative aspiration, 1500 units of animal-derived hyaluronidase or 150 units human recombinant hyaluronidase mixed with 4–6 mL normal saline is injected. Next, a mixed solution of 5 mL local anesthetic and 1 mL soluble or non-soluble corticosteroid is injected. A test dose of 2 mL should be administered first and then slow increments of 2–4 mL solution for a total of 4–6 mL. The needle is then carefully removed under live fluoroscopy, while the catheter remains in place. A bacterial filter is then attached to the end of the catheter, and the catheter is secured to the skin with a suture. Lastly, apply antibacterial and antimycotic ointment, followed by clean sterile dressing.

Postoperatively, the patient is carefully monitored for 30 min after the procedure to check the spread of anesthesia and exclude inadvertent subarachnoid or subdural injection. Six milliliter of hypertonic Saline (10%) is then administered through the catheter via an infusion pump. The catheter is then rinsed with 2 mL preservative-free normal saline (0.9%). The following day, patients can receive the second and third infusion that was discussed earlier. After negative aspiration, a test dose of 2 mL 0.2% ropivacaine is injected. Five minutes is allowed to elapse, excluding subarachnoid or subdural injection, prior to injection of an additional 4 mL of local anesthetic. Then, 20–30 min is allowed to elapse prior to infusion of 6 mL hypertonic saline (10%) over 30 min via an infusion pump. The catheter is then rinsed with 2 mL normal saline once the infusion is complete. The catheter is then removed 10–15 min after completion of the third infusion and dressings are applied. Patients should always be informed about the risks of infection. Meningitis can develop 2–4 weeks postoperatively due to the long-lasting effects of corticosteroids. The same post-procedure antibiotics are prescribed.

Percutaneous thoracic epidural neuroplasty is carried out using the same paramedian approach and sequence of steps described above. Volumes and dosages for all of the techniques are listed in Table 54.2.

Table 54.2 Injected solutions according to spinal cord section (volume in milliliter) in the injection sequence

Solution	Cervical	Thoracic	Lumbar	Caudal
Iohexol	2–3	4–6	10	10
Iohexol	1–2	2–3	3	3
Saline 0.9% + 1500 IU hyaluronidase or 150 units human recombinant hyaluronidase	4–6	6–8	10	10
Ropivacaine 0.2% + corticosteroid[a] (test dose)	2	2	3	3
Ropivacaine 0.2% + corticosteroid[a]	2–4	4–6	7	7
Hypertonic saline	4–6	6–8	10	10
Saline 0.9%	2	2	2	2
Then, on each of the following 2 days:				
Ropivacaine 0.2% + corticosteroid[a] (test dose)	2	2	3	3
Ropivacaine 0.2%	4	6	7	7
Hypertonic saline	4–6	6–8	10	10
Saline 0.9%	2	2	2	2

[a] 4 mg dexamethasone or 40 mg methylprednisolone or triamcinolone

Technique: Sacral 1 Neuroplasty

In 2011, Teske et al. identified a unique, triangular space in the sacrum. It measured 0.9–1.1 mL on each side. The boundaries are medial to the L5 nerve root, lateral to the S1 nerve root, and the base of the triangle is above the disk of L5–S1. This space is large enough to accept the average loose disk fragment. This space tends to collect leaky disk material, a common result of trauma and surgery. Due to the curvature of the sacrum and the formation of dense scarring, regular epidural catheters and scopes have not been able to enter this scarred epidural area. Matsumoto et al. realized that entering from the posterior aspect of the S1 neural foramen with an 18-gauge RX-2™ Coudé needle and then rotating it, the curved tip allows for ventral epidural projection of a 21-gauge VERSA-KATH®.

The scarring triangle is located in-between the L5 DRG and the S1 nerve root and above the L5–S1 disk. Dense scarring can present clinically as the following: ipsilateral back pain (due to the dura and posterior longitudinal ligament adhering together), L5 radiculopathy, numbness and dysesthesia in the lateral calf to the lateral ankle and foot, and weakness on dorsal flexion of the foot. In advanced cases, foot drop may be evident. The opening of the scarring triangle with the recommended volumes can reverse these clinical symptoms. An S2 component will present as radiculopathy along the posterior aspect of the thigh and calf. Stretch-induced ischemia of the involved nerve roots is likely the cause of foot drop and can be reversed following the scarring triangle neuroplasty.

Place the patient in the prone position. Fluoroscopically, with a true A-P view, the four sacral neural foramina will be seen as eight foramina because of the curvature of the sacrum. The posterior neural foramina will be seen more cephalad, while the anterior foramina will be seen more caudal. To align the neural foramina, rotate the c-arm in a cephalad direction until the S1 ventral and dorsal neural foramina line up. The 18-gauge needle has a curve near the tip, but one still needs a gentler angle to allow cephalad advancement of the catheter. The needle entry point is from the lateral side of the posterior S2 aiming toward the medial side of S1. Apply topical anesthesia and advance the needle through the skin. Curve the needle down to and contact bone between the S1 and S2 on the sacrum. After contact is made, continue to advance until a penetrative "pop" is felt, indicating foraminal entry. Remove the original stylet and interlock the atraumatic, blunt stylet. With the aid of lateral fluoroscopic visualization, rotate the needle tip dorsally and medially. Position the c-arm with a cephalad tilt to reduce radiation exposure to the operator's hand, leaving only the needle tip visible. Advance the styletted VERSA-KATH® into the sacral canal under fluoroscopic visualization after removing the second stylet (Figs. 54.7 and 54.8). The catheter needs to cross the L5–S1 disk space and advance into the fibrotic tissue (scar) near the top of the L5 neural foramen. The catheter should not advance medial or lateral inside the imaginary triangle between L5 and S1. For more accurate placement, the VERSA-KATH® can be rotated during advancement. Attach the connector and inject 5–10 cm^3 of iohexol 240 within the scarred area. Injection of contrast may require significant pressure for a complete spread due to its viscosity. It will open up the ventral epidural space, slowly crossing over, and spread from L4 down to S2 bilaterally. Inject a mixture of 10 cm^3 of preservative-free saline and 150 units of human recombinant hyaluronidase; this will disperse the contrast. Carefully observe for a potential spread into the subdural and subarachnoid spaces, especially in failed surgery cases where the possibility of a dural tear may exist. Slowly inject a mixture of 10 cm^3 of 0.2% ropivacaine and 40 mg triamcinolone. Ask the patient to move their feet and to report any pain at any time other than during injection. Subdural injectate accumulation in the scarred area may produce bilateral pain

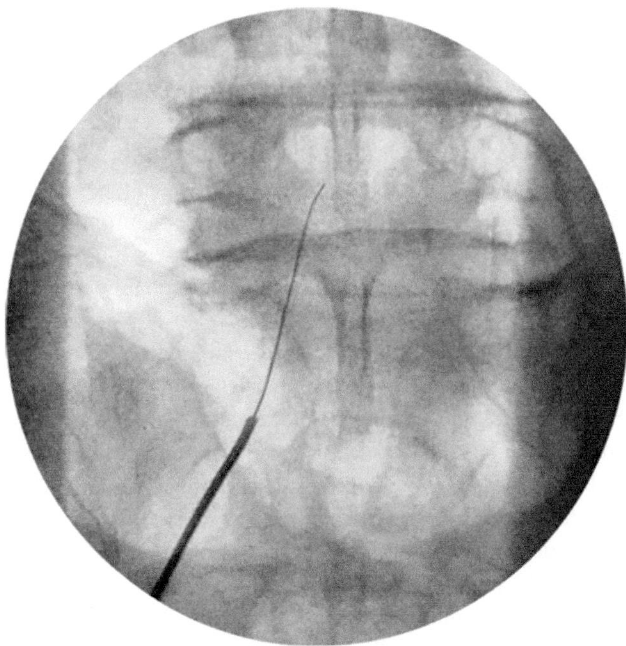

Fig. 54.7 Anteroposterior fluoroscopic image of a left trans S1 catheter. Image courtesy of Gabor Racz MD

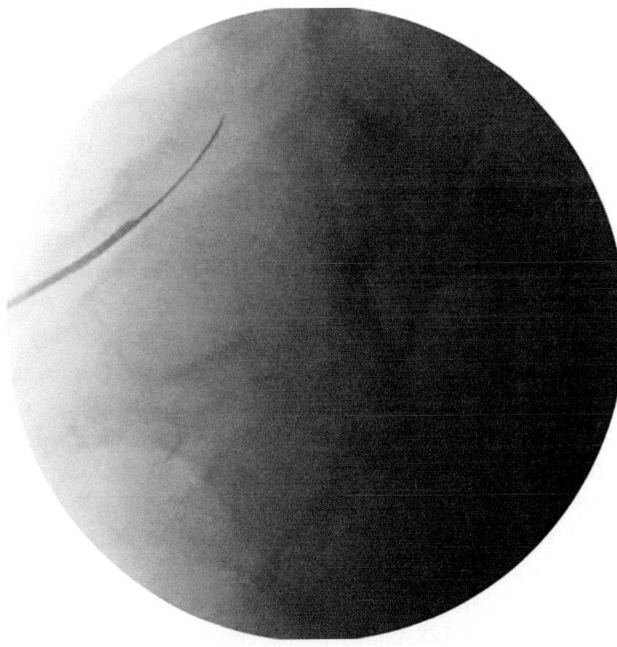

Fig. 54.8 Lateral fluoroscopic image of a left trans S1 catheter. Image courtesy of Gabor Racz MD

and has atypical appearance. If subdural loculation occurs, it can be aspirated with an interlaminar needle placement. After local anesthetic injection, observe the patient for 20–30 min and make sure they are able to perform a 90-degree straight leg raise without any evidence of motor block. Infuse 10% saline over a 15-min period. Then flush with local anesthetic or normal saline at completion. If the patient develops a motor block, he or she may need to be admitted into the hospital for observation.

A one-time injection into the scarring triangle is effective for a short period of time; however, three repeat injections, 6–8 h apart, have been reported as more effective for many months to over a year. Instruct the patient to perform neural flossing exercises to the patient for the sciatic area. There are also separate instructions for the upper lumbar area.

Complications

Potential complications and side effects of percutaneous epidural neuroplasty include inadvertent subarachnoid or subdural injection of local anesthetic or 10% hypertonic saline. This can lead to cardiac arrhythmia, paralysis, or sphincter dysfunction. Other complications are as follows: epidural abscess, epidural hematoma, paralysis, bowel or bladder dysfunction, infection, and catheter shearing. Loculation is another potential complication when injections are made into a confined space in the epidural space. Patients typically report pain during the injection and visualized with confined spread of contrast. Loculations are associated with increased epidural pressure, which can lead to injury of the central nervous system. For cervical neuroplasty, slow flexion and rotation of the neck can help prevent loculation while injecting the hyaluronidase and steroid solutions. Patients commonly have undiagnosed neurogenic bowel or bladder dysfunction from previous back surgeries or spinal cord compression. This should be properly evaluated and documented prior to the procedure to prevent any unwanted adverse effects from being attributed to the procedure itself. Constrictive arachnoiditis can frequently lead to bowel or bladder dysfunction. All injections should be slow. Fast injections into the epidural space can lead to increased CSF pressures. This will increase the risk of cerebral hemorrhage, visual disturbances, headaches, and disruption or blood flow in the spinal cord. Infections can occur 2–6 weeks after the procedure due to the procedure itself and the immunosuppressive nature of the corticosteroids. Red flag symptoms include—nausea, vomiting, neck stiffness, severe pain, weakness, numbness, or paralysis—and must be evaluated promptly, as these are linked to the procedure until proven otherwise. Patients should be advised to contact the physician who performed the procedure or their general practitioner immediately if they experience any red flag symptoms. Appropriate inpatient treatment may be immediately required, given the serious sequelae of an unrecognized epidural abscess.

Practical Tips

If the needle is located in the subarachnoid space, the contrast will spread in a central and cranial direction. Should his occur, cancel the procedure and schedule for another day.

When introducing the catheter, the beveled side of the needle should be directed toward the ventrolateral side of the caudal canal. The catheter should also be bent at a 15–30-degree angle, ~2.5 cm below the catheter tip. This allows for the tip of the catheter to reach the desired anterolateral position and reduce the risk of catheter shearing. Precise location of the needle is key for optimal efficacy. Medications injected in the posterior or posterolateral epidural space will not reach the pathological changes of the intervertebral foramina or anterior epidural space. Bending the catheter tip for easier guidance can better access the anterolateral epidural space. A transforaminal approach could also be used.

Literature Review

Multiple indications have been evaluated for epidural neuroplasty throughout the literature. Systematic review and meta-analysis from Helm and Racz have identified ten moderate to high-quality studies of lumbar neuroplasty as a treatment option for post-back surgery syndrome, spinal stenosis, neuraxial, and radicular pain. Gerdesmeyer et al. performed a landmark, randomized, double-blinded, placebo-controlled study to analyze the clinical efficacy of percutaneous epidural lysis of adhesions in chronic radicular pain. Ninety out of 381 screened patients were randomized to receive either percutaneous neurolysis or placebo after failing conservative therapy. The primary outcome measure was the difference in percent change of the Oswestry Disability Index (ODI) XE "Oswestry Disability Index (ODI)" scores 3 months after intervention. Secondary outcome measures were difference in percent change of ODI scores and visual analog scale (VAS) 6 and 12 months after intervention and success rates defined as at least 50% reduction in ODI scores and VAS (mean change from baseline) at 3, 6, and 12 months after treatment. The ODI and VAS scores as well as the success rates for ODI vs. VAS were significantly better 3, 6, and 12 months in the lysis group vs. the control group. Akbas et al. did a comparison study of 60 patients using three different approaches (caudal, S1 transforaminal, and L5–S1 transforaminal) of percutaneous epidural adhesiolysis. This case control, blinded study concluded that all three approaches lead to decreased pain scores and improved functionality and patient satisfaction. Kalagac et al. performed a study in 54 patients divided into two separate groups: pain from failed back surgery syndrome vs. chronic radicular pain without previous spinal surgery. Significant pain reduction was observed in both groups at 4- and 12-week follow-up. Manchikanti et al. completed systematic reviews and meta-analysis regarding epidural percutaneous neuroplasty in patients with post-lumbar surgery syndrome, central lumbar spinal stenosis, and chronic low back and lower extremity pain in post-surgery syndrome. They concluded there is level 2 evidence for the efficacy of percutaneous neuroplasty for post-laminectomy syndrome based on three high-quality randomized controlled trials and one low-quality randomized controlled trial. They also noticed over 70% of patients with spinal stenosis or post-lumbar surgery syndrome had clinically significant improvement of pain and function. Helm et al. reviewed the literature via a systematic review and meta-analysis and identified seven randomized controlled trials along with three observational studies. They concluded level 1 evidence or strong evidence for percutaneous neuroplasty in the treatment of chronic refractory low back and radicular pain. Aoi et al., using a retrospective study of mechanical adhesiolysis with a Cordis catheter, demonstrated statistically significant improvement of pain, functional status, and decreased medication use in 112 patients with degenerative chronic low back pain and radiculopathy treated by epidural neuroplasty. Brito-Garcia et al. conducted a systematic review to evaluate the efficacy, effectiveness, safety, and cost-effectiveness of epidural neuroplasty in 2019. They concluded that methodological flaws and bias were prevalent and led to insufficient evidence on efficacy and nonexistence of cost-effectiveness regarding percutaneous epidural neuroplasty. This was argued by Dr. Helm in his letter to the editor. Helm summarizes that Brito-Garcia et al. inappropriately excluded the most powerful literature by artificially narrowing the indications for percutaneous adhesiolysis.

Park et al. conducted a preliminary, prospective study on patient with cervical central stenosis treated with percutaneous cervical epidural adhesiolysis on 39 patients. They concluded percutaneous adhesiolysis is an effective management strategy in patients with chronic posterior neck and upper extremity pain due to cervical central spinal stenosis, although there was no correlation between therapeutic response and grade of stenosis. In addition, Park et al. conducted a retrospective study on clinical outcomes of epidural neuroplasty on 128 patients with cervical disk herniation. They showed good clinical outcomes in the treatment of cervical disk herniation and should be considered as a treatment option for cervical disk herniation refractory to conservative treatment. Hyun Oh et al. conducted a retrospective observational study in order to evaluate the efficacy of cervical percutaneous neuroplasty for single-level cervical disk disease. One hundred patients underwent cervical percutaneous neuroplasty and 58 required additional block therapy. They showed more than 80% and 40% of all patients with and without additional block therapy had good to excellent outcomes according to Odom's criteria at 12-month follow-up along with no severe complications. Han et al. conducted a retrospective study to examine the correlation between the contrast spread pattern and pain reduction in cervical epidural neuroplasty using a Racz catheter. They defined contrast runoff as the spread of contrast from the neural foramen to a nerve root. If the contrast did not spread in this manner, then there was no contrast runoff. They concluded cervical epidural neuroplasty with a contrast runoff pattern had a higher success rate at 1, 3, 6, and 12 months post-procedure. They recommend contrast runoff should be observed during neuroplasty, even in the presence of foraminal stenosis.

Conclusion

Percutaneous epidural neuroplasty, aka the Racz Procedure, is a useful procedure that should be added to every pain medicine physician's armamentarium for the treatment of persistent radicular pain and spinal stenosis. Although originally designed to treat continuing pain after surgery, it should be considered as the next step after epidural steroids have failed. Multiple studies have demonstrated its efficacy, but research must continue to make it a more effective and even safer procedure.

Suggested Reading

Akbas M, Elawamy AR, Salem HH, Fouad AZ, Abbas NA, Dagistan G. Comparison of 3 approaches to percutaneous epidural adhesiolysis and neuroplasty in post lumbar surgery syndrome. Pain Physician. 2018;21:E501–8.

Aoi I, Chen HC, Lui TN, Lin TJ. Outcomes of epidural neuroplasty utilizing adhesiolysis by means of hydraulic and mechanical force. J Biomed. 2018;3:26–31.

Brito-García N, García-Pérez L, Kovacs FM, Del Pino-Sedeño T, Pérez-Ramos J, Imaz-Iglesia I, Serrano-Aguilar P. Efficacy, effectiveness, safety, and cost-effectiveness of epidural adhesiolysis for treating failed back surgery syndrome. A systematic review. Pain Med. 2019;20:692–706.

Cho PG, Ji GY, Yoon YS, Shin DA. Clinical effectiveness of percutaneous epidural neuroplasty according to the type of single-level lumbar disc herniation: a 12-month follow-up study. J Korean Neurosurg Soc. 2019;62:681–90.

Fronza M, Muhr C, da Silveira DS, Sorgi CA, Rodrigues SF, Farsky SH, Paula-Silva FW, Merfort I, Faccioli LH. Hyaluronidase decreases neutrophils infiltration to the inflammatory site. Inflamm Res. 2016;65:533–42.

Gerdesmeyer L, Wagenpfeil S, Birkenmaier C, et al. Percutaneous epidural lysis of adhesions in chronic radicular pain: a randomized, double-blind, placebo-controlled trial. Pain Physician. 2013;16:185–96.

Gourie-Devi M, Satish P. Hyaluronidase as an adjuvant in the treatment of cranial arachnoiditis (hydrocephalus and optochiasmatic arachnoiditis) complicating tuberculous meningitis. Acta Neurol Scand. 1980;62:368–81.

Gourie-Devi M, Satish P. Intrathecal hyaluronidase treatment of chronic spinal arachnoiditis of noninfective etiology. Surg Neurol. 1984;22:231–4.

Gourie-Devi M, Satishchandra P. Hyaluronidase as an adjuvant in the management of tuberculous spinal arachnoiditis. J Neurol Sci. 1991;102:105–11.

Han YJ, Lee MN, Cho MJ, Park HJ, Moon DE, Kim YH. Contrast runoff correlates with the clinical outcome of cervical epidural neuroplasty using a racz catheter. Pain Physician. 2016;19:E1035–40.

Helm S. Percutaneous adhesiolysis is an effective, safe procedure. Pain Med. 2020;21:206–7.

Helm S, Knezevic NN. A review of the role of epidural percutaneous neuroplasty. Pain Manag. 2019;9:53–62.

Helm S, Racz G. Hyaluronidase in neuroplasty: a review. Pain Physician. 2019;22:555–60.

Kalagac FL, Šuput A, Gusić N, Mamontov P. Epidural adhesiolysis in the management of chronic low back pain in failed back surgery syndrome and in lumbar radicular pain: first year of experience in General Hospital Pula - Croatia, a randomized trial. J Anaesth Ther. 2018;1:102.

Koç O, Er N. Can hyaluronidase be an alternative postoperative antiedema agent to dexamethasone? Preliminary results of an animal study. J Oral Maxillofac Surg. 2018;76:1653–9.

Manchikanti L, Soin A, Boswell MV, Kaye AD, Sanapati M, Hirsch JA. Effectiveness of percutaneous adhesiolysis in post lumbar surgery syndrome: a systematic analysis of findings of systematic reviews. Pain Physician. 2019a;22:307–22.

Manchikanti L, et al. Effectiveness of percutaneous adhesiolysis in managing chronic central lumbar spinal stenosis: a systematic review and meta-analysis. Pain Physician. 2019b;22:E523–50.

Manchikanti L, Knezevic NN, Sanapati SP, Sanapati MR, Kaye AD, Hirsch JA. Is percutaneous adhesiolysis effective in managing chronic low back and lower extremity pain in post-surgery syndrome: a systematic review and meta-analysis. Curr Pain Headache Rep. 2020;24:30.

Matsumoto T, Kitagawa H. Treatment of lower back and leg pain using Racz Catheter-Matsumoto Way (via S1 intervertebral foramen). In: Poster presentation. 2014 WIP World Congress Maastricht, Netherlands; 2014.

Oh CH, Ji GY, Shin DA, Cho PG, Yoon SH. Clinical course of cervical percutaneous epidural neuroplasty in single-level cervical disc disease with 12-month follow-up. Pain Physician. 2017;20:E941–9.

Park CH, Lee SH, Lee SC. Preliminary results of the clinical effectiveness of percutaneous adhesiolysis using a Racz catheter in the management of chronic pain due to cervical central stenosis. Pain Physician. 2013a;16:353–8.

Park EJ, Park SY, Lee SJ, Kim NS, Koh DY. Clinical outcomes of epidural neuroplasty for cervical disc herniation. J Korean Med Sci. 2013b;28:461–5.

Racz G. Trans S1 infralaminar scarring triangle step by step: poster presentation ASIPP 21st Annual Meeting, Las Vegas, NV, 2019

Racz G, Heavener J. Introduction to lysis of adhesions. In: Racz GB, Noe CE, editors. Techniques of neurolysis. 2nd ed. Cham: Springer; 2016. p. 1–12. Chapter 1.

Racz G, Candido K, Helm S. Neuroplasty is a safe, effective procedure. Anesth Analg. 2018;126:363.

Teske W, Zirke S, Nottenkamper J, et al. Anatomical and surgical study of volume determination of eh anterolateral epidural space nerve root L5/S1 under the aspect of epidural perineural injection in minimal invasive treatment of lumbar nerve root compression. Eur Spine J. 2011;20:537–41.

Part VII

Nerve Block for Regional Anesthesia and Pain Therapy for Lower Limb

Lumbar Plexus Block Via Anterior Approach (Femoral Nerve, 3-in-1, Fascia Iliaca Block)

55

Angela Lucia Balocco, Imré Van Herreweghe, Ana M. Lopez, Catherine Vandepitte, and Admir Hadzic

Contents

The Femoral Nerve Block

General Considerations

The femoral nerve block is a well-established regional anesthesia technique. It is the single most powerful analgesic method to treat pain after major knee surgery, either as a single injection or continuous block. However, the recent use of protocols for enhanced recovery after surgery include early mobilization as an important goal, where a femoral nerve block may interfere with. A femoral nerve block invariably results in quadriceps muscle paresis, impeding early active mobilization and ambulation. Alternatively, more distal interventional analgesia techniques with less ambulation impairment may be better suited for some patients and surgeries. These options include blocks of the distal branches of the femoral nerve at different levels in the subsartorial space or soft tissue infiltration with a local anesthetic. Lower doses and concentrations of local anesthetics for femoral nerve blocks and periarticular infiltration of local anesthetics can also be used.

Indications (Patient Selection)

A femoral nerve block is indicated to provide anesthesia and analgesia after hip, femur, anterior thigh, knee, and patella

A. L. Balocco (✉) · A. M. Lopez · C. Vandepitte
Department of Anesthesiology, Ziekenhuis Oost-Limburg, Genk, Belgium
e-mail: lucia@nysora.com; catherine@nysora.com

I. Van Herreweghe
Department of Anesthesiology, Ziekenhuis AZ Turnhout, Turnhout, Belgium

A. Hadzic
Department of Anesthesiology, Ziekenhuis Oost-Limburg, Genk, Belgium

St.Luke's-Roosevelt Hospital Center, College of Physicians and Surgeons, Columbia University, New York, USA
e-mail: admir@nysora.com

D. Jankovic, P. Peng (eds.), *Regional Nerve Blocks in Anesthesia and Pain Therapy*, https://doi.org/10.1007/978-3-030-88727-8_55

procedures. It is still widely used in patients with hip or femur fractures, both as an analgesic modality in the emergency department and to facilitate patient positioning for spinal anesthesia.

Functional Anatomy

The femoral nerve originates from the dorsal divisions of the ventral rami of the L2–L4 lumbar nerves. Approximately at the level of the fifth lumbar vertebral body, the femoral nerve exits the psoas muscle in a medial-to-lateral direction deep to the fascia iliaca. It continues caudally and enters the anterior compartment of the thigh, passing deep to the inguinal ligament, anterior to the iliopsoas muscle and lateral to the femoral artery and vein (Fig. 55.1). At the femoral triangle, the nerve divides quickly into multiple terminal branches. Deep branches innervate the anterior aspect of the hip, femur, and knee; muscular branches innervate the iliacus, psoas major, pectineus, rectus femoris, vastus lateralis, vastus intermedius, vastus medialis, and sartorius muscles; cutaneous branches innervate the skin on the anterior aspect of the thigh and knee. The saphenous nerve also arises from the femoral nerve and continues to travel with the femoral artery on the medial side of the leg down to the midfoot, innervating the skin during this trajectory. It divides into the main saphenous branch, which continues down to the ankle, and the infrapatellar branch that crosses the knee below the patella. The latter further divides into three branches that combine with cutaneous nerves of the thigh and form the patellar plexus.

Sonoanatomy

At the level of the femoral crease, the femoral nerve lies superficial to the iliacus muscle enveloped by the fascia iliaca just lateral to the vascular compartment. The disposition of the nerve, lateral to the femoral artery and vein, is relatively consistent. On ultrasound, the nerve is seen as a flattened triangular or oval group of fascicles enveloped within two layers of the fascia iliaca, typically at a depth of 2–4 cm (Fig. 55.2). The superficial circumflex iliac artery takes off from the femoral artery in the femoral triangle and courses lateral and cephalad superficial to the fascia iliaca. The take-off of the profunda femoris (deep femoral artery) and the femoral nerve branching can be identified by scanning more distally.

Technique

Patient Position

The patient is positioned supine with the lower extremity fully extended and slightly rotated externally. In obese

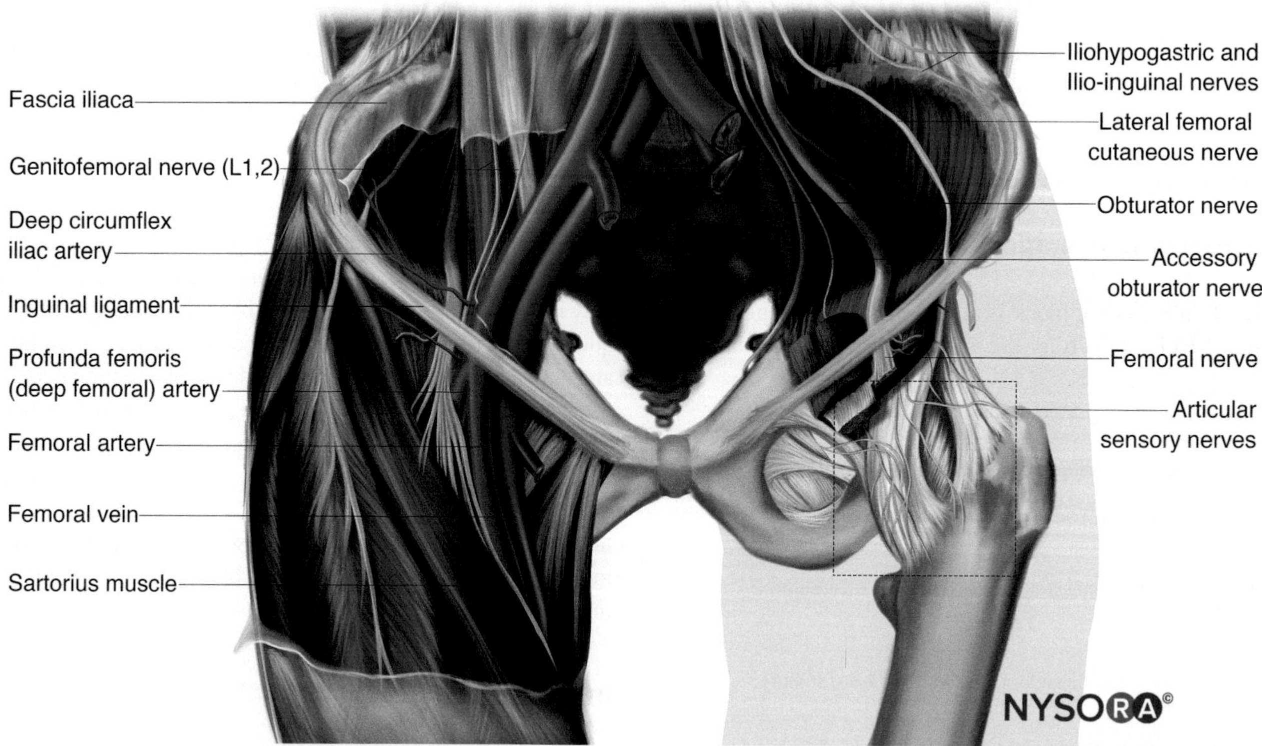

Fig. 55.1 Anatomy of the terminal branches of the lumbar plexus and their relationship with the fascia iliaca. (Reproduced with permission from NYSORA)

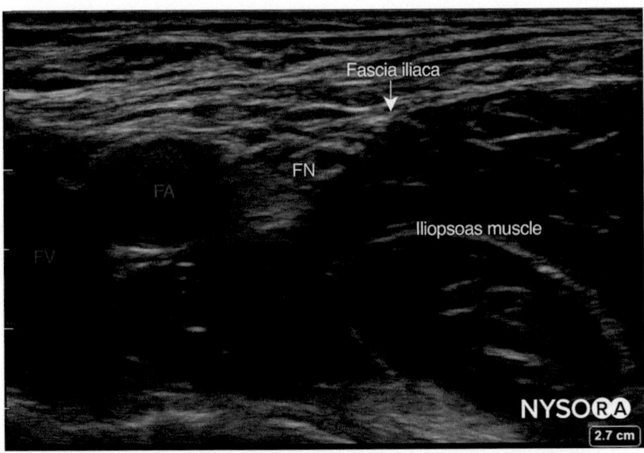

Fig. 55.2 Sonoanatomy of the femoral nerve (FN) at the femoral crease. FV, femoral vein; FA, femoral artery; GnFN, genitofemoral nerve. (Reproduced with permission from NYSORA)

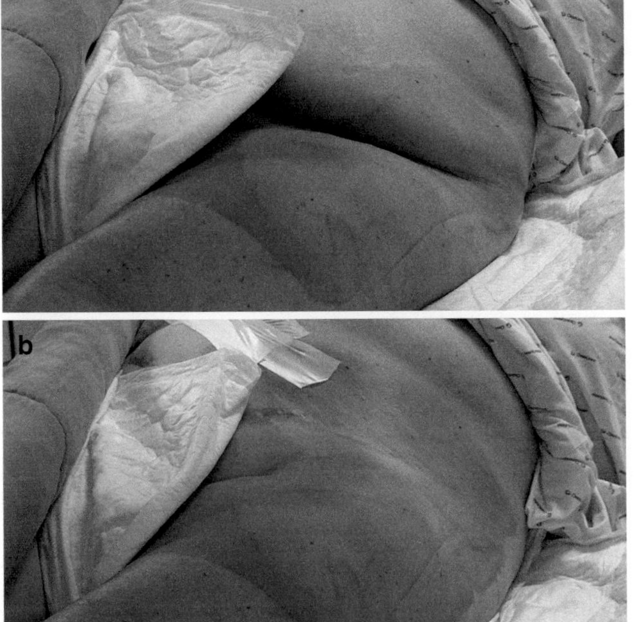

Fig. 55.3 (**a**, **b**) Tapping technique to facilitate exposure to the femoral crease in obese patients. (Reproduced with permission from NYSORA)

patients, access to the inguinal crease may be facilitated by tapping away the abdominal adipose tissue (Fig. 55.3).

Scanning Technique and Needle Insertion

The transducer is placed in a transverse orientation over the inguinal crease to identify the femoral artery. The artery is visualized as a round anechoic pulsating structure with the easily compressible femoral vein located medial to it (Fig. 55.4). When the bifurcation of the femoral artery and profunda femoris is seen, the transducer should be moved proximally until only one artery is identified. This maneuver increases the chance of achieving a complete block of the femoral nerve, since it begins to divide also at the level where the femoral artery bifurcates. Applying pressure to the transducer and adjusting the tilt will improve the ultrasound visualization of the femoral nerve and the fascia iliaca.

After a clear visualization of the femoral nerve, the needle is inserted in-plane from lateral to medial and toward the lateral edge of the nerve (Fig. 55.5). The goal is to pierce the superficial layer of the fascia iliaca enveloping the femoral nerve. At this point and after ruling out intravascular needle placement, 1–2 mL of local anesthetic is injected to evaluate the distribution of injectate, which will result in the displacement of the femoral nerve from the adjacent fascia and muscle (Fig. 55.6). When the correct position of the needle has been confirmed, complete the block with 8–15 mL of local anesthetic.

Complications

The femoral nerve block has been associated with a risk of postoperative falls in the ward due to the quadriceps muscle weakness. Protocols for specifying the risk and risk prevention are important whenever lower extremity nerve blocks are used, particularly for femoral and sciatic blocks. The incidence of femoral nerve injury reported in the literature is lower than that of upper extremity nerve blocks. However, the disability associated with a femoral nerve injury is significant. Therefore, we advise strict adherence to triple monitoring during block performance (ultrasound, nerve stimulation, opening injection pressure monitor).

Practical Tips

- Tilting the transducer cranially-caudally helps to optimize the image of the nerve.
- Try to pierce the fascia iliaca lateral to the edge of the femoral nerve to avoid landing on and injuring the nerve.
- Nerve stimulation should be used as a monitoring tool and set at 0.5 mA, 0.1 ms. The contact of the needle tip with the femoral nerve is associated with a motor response of the quadriceps muscle group. If a motor response is present, redirect the needle and make sure no motor response is present before injecting the local anesthetic.
- Beware of the motor weakness of the quadriceps—risk of falls.
- Circumferential local anesthetic spread around the nerve is not necessary to achieve a successful block.

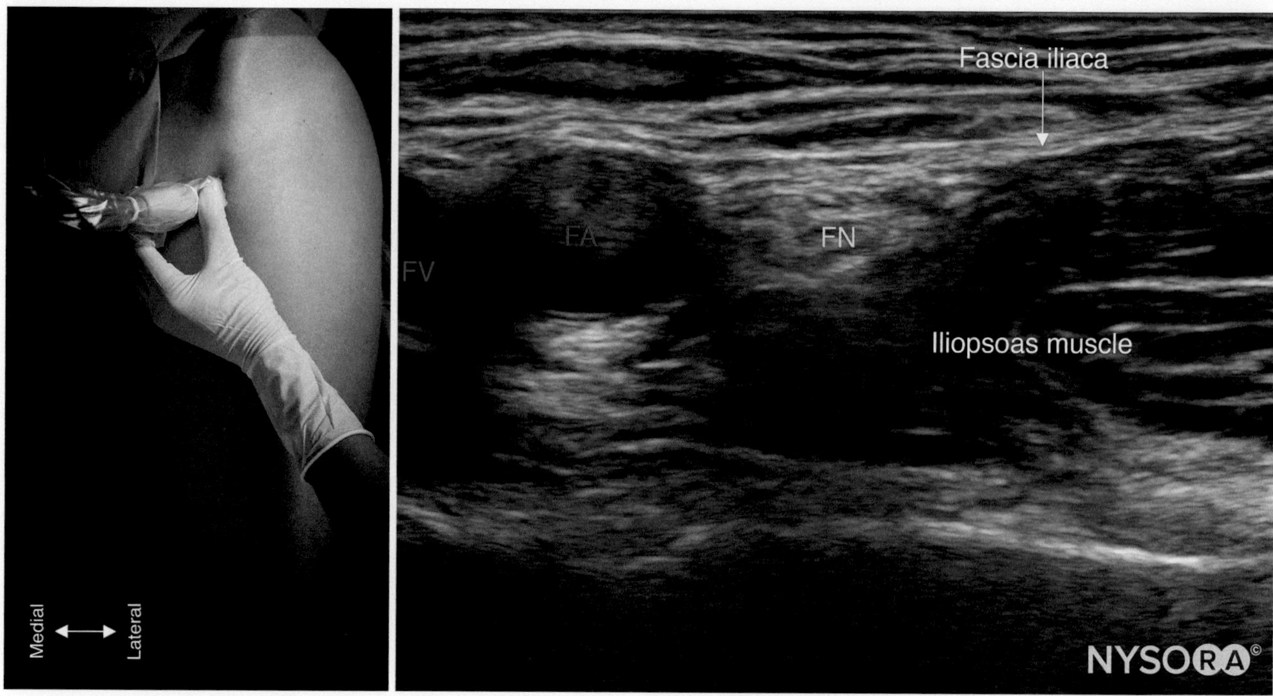

Fig. 55.4 Transducer position and sonoanatomy of the femoral nerve (FN) at the femoral crease. *FV* femoral vein, *FA* femoral artery, *GnFN* genitofemoral nerve. (Reproduced with permission from NYSORA)

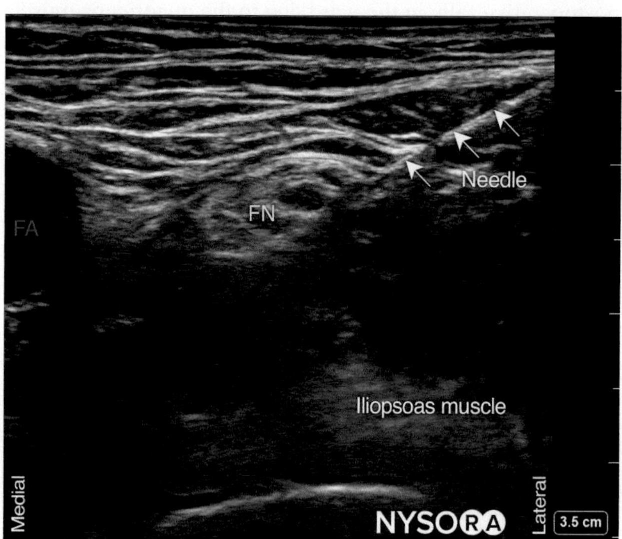

Fig. 55.5 Femoral nerve block showing needle insertion in-plane toward the lateral edge of the nerve. *FN* femoral nerve, *FV* femoral vein, *FA* femoral artery. (Reproduced with permission from NYSORA)

The 3-in-1 Block

General Considerations

The 3-in-1 block was described by Winnie et al. as a regional anesthesia technique in which three nerves of the lumbar plexus could be blocked with one paravascular injection. The technique is based on the rationale that placing a large local anesthetic volume in the femoral nerve sheath could spread proximally under the fascia iliaca reaching the femoral, lateral femoral cutaneous, and obturator nerves. Initially, the femoral nerve was localized using anatomical landmarks and eliciting paresthesias to determine the injection site. This was later replaced by nerve stimulation and eventually by ultrasound. The ability of the 3-in-1 block to effectively block the obturator and lateral femoral cutaneous nerves was challenged in anatomical and clinical studies, where it failed to provide adequate anesthesia in the areas supplied by these nerves. Over time and in search of an alternative technique that could consistently block all three nerves, the 3-in-1 block has transitioned toward the fascia iliaca compartment block.

The Fascia Iliaca Block

General Considerations

The fascia iliaca block, also called the fascia iliaca compartment block, is a regional analgesia technique that has evolved as a better alternative to posterior lumbar plexus, femoral nerve, or 3-in-1 blocks to provide analgesia for hip procedures. Its effectiveness in the preoperative pain management of hip fracture patients has been well-documented, prompting the National Institute for Health and Care Excellence and

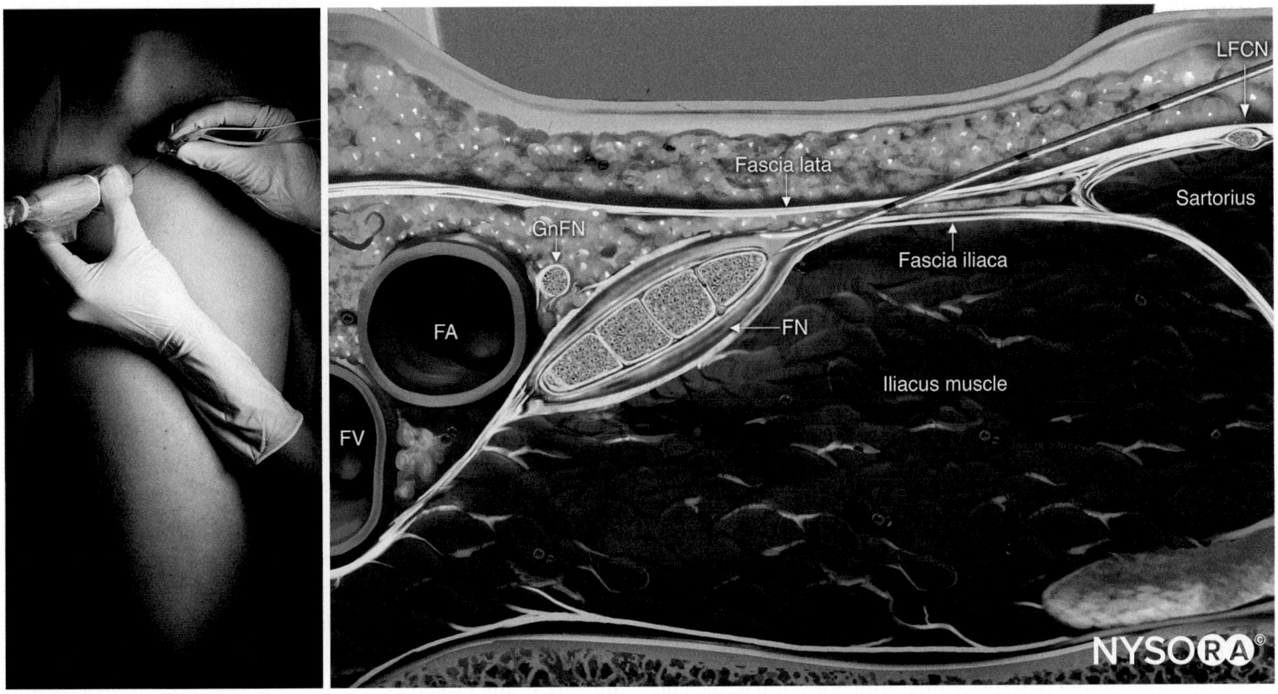

Fig. 55.6 Reverse ultrasound anatomy of a femoral nerve (FN) block showing needle insertion in-plane. *FV* femoral vein, *FA* femoral artery, *GnFN* genitofemoral nerve. (Reproduced with permission from NYSORA)

the Association of Anaesthetists of Great Britain and Ireland to recommend its use as part of the routine multimodal analgesic protocols for this indication.

The analgesic efficacy of this technique depends on the local anesthetic spread beneath the fascia iliaca in order to reach the femoral, lateral femoral cutaneous, and obturator nerves. However, the spread toward the obturator nerve is not consistent. This block has been performed for decades using landmarks and loss of resistance technique. With the introduction of ultrasound, it became apparent that many of such "blind" injections do not always occur in the proper plane. The fascia iliaca block has evolved from the infrainguinal "classic" approach to a suprainguinal technique with the aim to spread the local anesthetic injection cranially, more consistently reaching the lumbar plexus and resulting in a more superior analgesic efficacy compared to the infrainguinal or transverse approach.

Indications (Patient Selection)

The distribution of the sensory and motor block after a fascia iliaca block depends on the cranial extent of the local anesthetic and the nerves involved. Coverage of the femoral and lateral femoral cutaneous nerves is consistently achieved with this technique. Therefore, it is indicated as an analgesic method for hip and femur fractures and patient positioning before spinal anesthesia. Furthermore, it is also used for analgesia after hip and knee surgery and procedures performed on the anterior thigh.

Functional Anatomy

The fascia iliaca covers the iliacus muscle throughout its descent from the pelvic crest into the upper thigh and merges medially with the fascia overlying the psoas muscle. The femoral nerve (L2–L4) and lateral femoral cutaneous nerve (L2–L3) emerge from the lateral border of the psoas major muscle and travel under the fascia iliaca over the ventral surface of the iliacus muscle in their intrapelvic and inguinal course (Fig. 55.1). The femoral nerve gives off several sensory and motor nerves to the quadriceps and sartorius muscles as it descends distal to the inguinal ligament. However, the articular branches to the hip joint leave both proximal and distal to the inguinal ligament to innervate to the anterolateral surface of the hip capsule.

The obturator nerve (L2–L4) emerges from the medial border of the psoas muscle and travels posteriorly behind the common iliac arteries toward the obturator foramen. During its intrapelvic course, it is separated from the fascia iliaca compartment by the psoas muscle. Therefore, it is not consistently anesthetized by a fascia iliaca block. The articular branches arise before passing the obturator foramen to supply the inferomedial aspect of the hip capsule (Fig. 55.1).

When present (10–50% depending on the studies), the accessory obturator nerve leaves the obturator nerve laterally, proximally in the pelvic fossa, and crosses over the pubic ramus. In those cases, it contributes to the innervation of the anteromedial aspect of the hip capsule.

Sonoanatomy

The iliacus muscle appears at its most superficial location at the level of the inguinal ligament, making it the most convenient place to access the fascia iliaca compartment. Cranially and medially, the muscle lines the iliac bone and is covered by the abdominal wall muscles. Caudally and laterally, the iliopsoas muscle is covered by the sartorius muscle. The femoral nerve is located just deep to the fascia iliaca and separated from the femoral vessels by the iliopectineal arch. The deep and superficial iliac circumflex arteries course cranially and laterally superficial to the fascia iliaca at this level.

With the transducer placed perpendicular to the inguinal ligament, the fascia iliaca is seen as a hyperechoic line covering the rounded hypoechoic iliopsoas muscle. The sartorius can be seen as a superficial triangular shape on the lateral-caudal side, and the internal oblique muscle is visualized on the cranial-medial side (Fig. 55.7). The deep circumflex iliac artery appears between this muscle and the fascia iliaca. With the transducer placed distally and parallel to the inguinal ligament, the femoral nerve and femoral vessels are readily apparent on the medial side of the fascia iliaca.

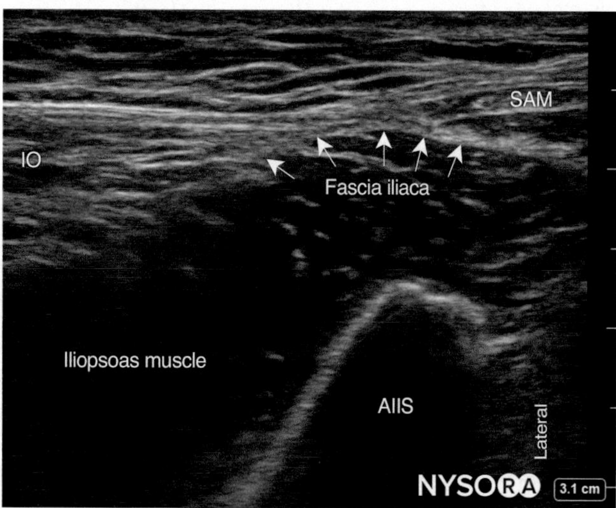

Fig. 55.7 Sonoanatomy of a suprainguinal fascia iliaca block. *AIIS* anterior inferior iliac spine, *SaM* sartorius muscle, *IO* internal oblique muscle. (Reproduced with permission from NYSORA)

Technique

Patient Position

The patient is positioned supine with the bed flattened to maximize access to the inguinal area. As for the femoral block, access to the inguinal crease in obese patients may be facilitated by taping away the abdominal adipose tissue.

Infrainguinal Fascia Iliaca Block

Scanning Technique and Needle Insertion

The transducer is placed in a transverse orientation over the femoral crease, parallel to the inguinal ligament. The goal is to identify the femoral artery and nerve, the iliopsoas muscle, and the fascia iliaca (Fig. 55.8). Tilting and applying pressure to the transducer help to optimize the image of the fascia iliaca which appears as a hyperechoic layer covering the hypoechoic iliopsoas muscle. The femoral nerve lies deep to the fascia and lateral to the femoral artery. When the above structures have been identified, the transducer is moved laterally until the triangular-shaped sartorius muscle appears in the image.

At this point, the needle is inserted in-plane from a lateral to medial direction, through the sartorius muscle, and toward the fascia iliaca, at a distance of approximately two-thirds away from the femoral nerve. As the needle encounters the fascia iliaca, indented by the needle, a loss of resistance follows when the needle tip pierces the fascial plane. After negative aspiration, 1–2 mL of local anesthetic is injected to confirm a proper local anesthetic distribution between the fascia iliaca and iliopsoas muscle (Fig. 55.9).

Local Anesthetic Distribution

The local anesthetic spread should occur in the medial-lateral and cranial-caudal direction from the injection point, separating the fascia from the muscle. The needle tip should be repositioned when the injection occurs above the fascia, between the fascia layers (intrafascial injection), or within the muscle.

Suprainguinal Fascia Iliaca Block

Scanning Technique and Needle Insertion

To perform a suprainguinal fascia iliaca block, two different transducer orientations can be used:

- Sagittal oblique orientation: For this approach, the anterior superior iliac spine (ASIS) is palpated and the transducer placed medial to it in a sagittal and oblique orientation, perpendicular to the inguinal ligament, and in a line between the ASIS and pubic tubercle. The trans-

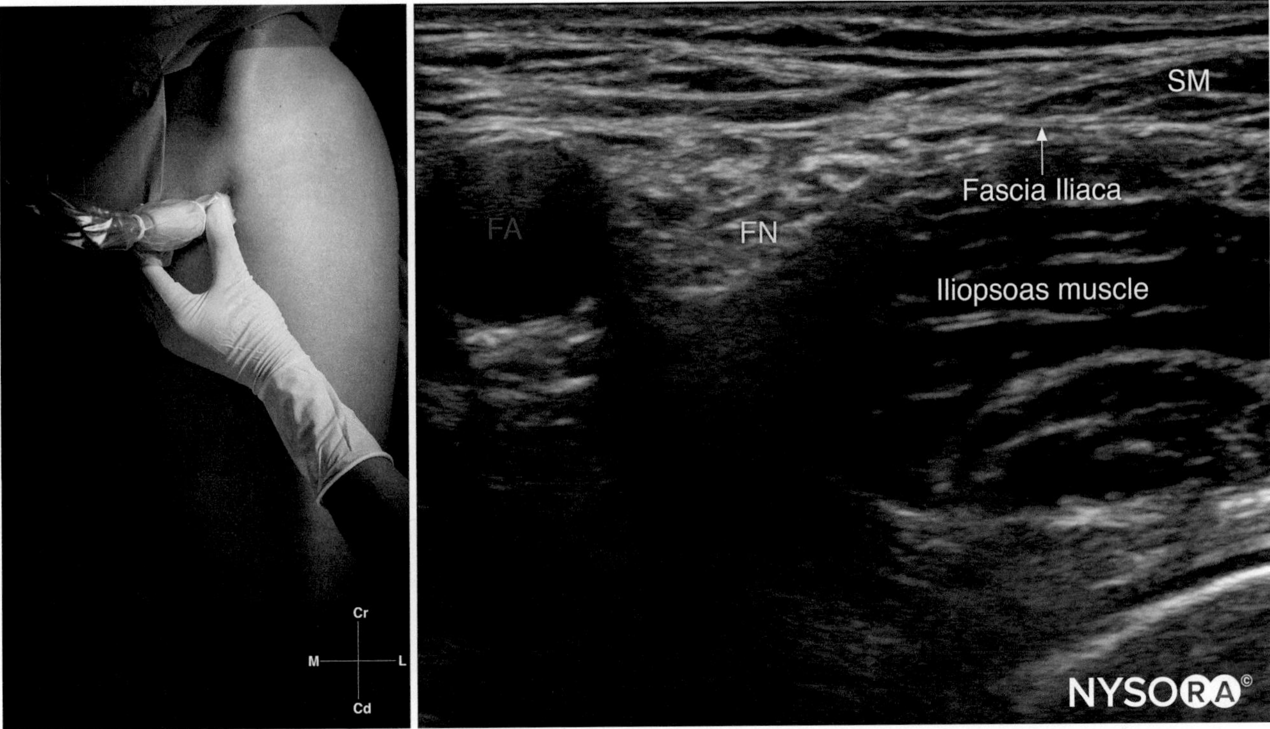

Fig. 55.8 Transducer position and sonoanatomy of an infrainguinal fascia iliaca block. *FV* femoral vein, *FA* femoral artery, *FN* femoral nerve. (Reproduced with permission from NYSORA)

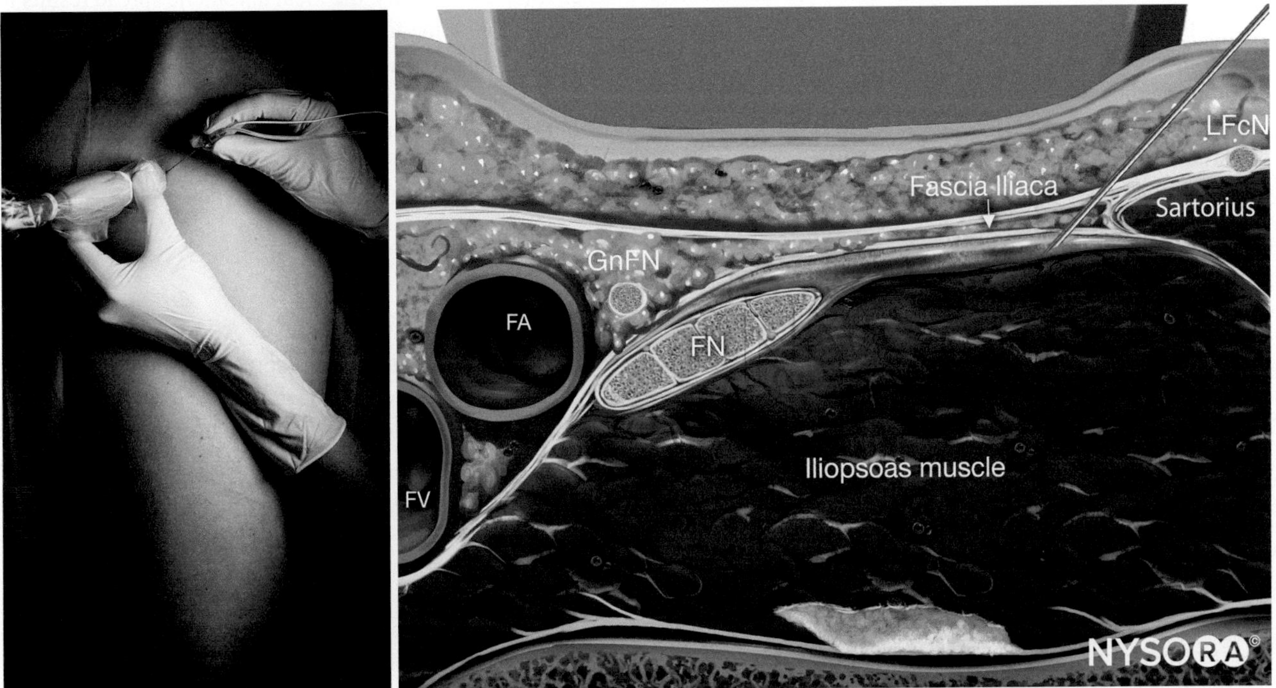

Fig. 55.9 Reverse ultrasound anatomy of an infrainguinal fascia iliaca block showing needle insertion in-plane. *FV* femoral vein, *FA* femoral artery, *FN*, femoral nerve. (Reproduced with permission from NYSORA)

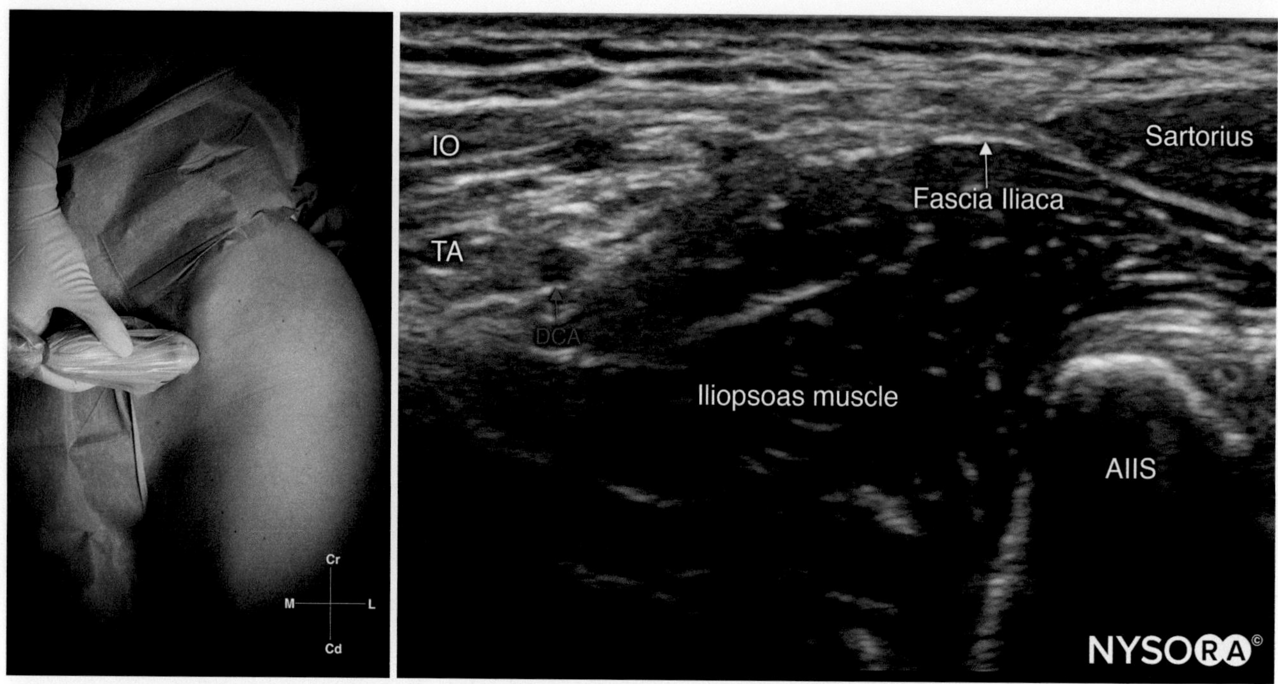

Fig. 55.10 Transducer position and sonoanatomy of a suprainguinal fascia iliaca block. *IO* internal oblique muscle, *TA* transversus abdominis muscle, *DCA* deep circumflex artery, *AIIS* anterior inferior iliac spine. (Reproduced with permission from NYSORA)

ducer is then slid caudally and medially along the inguinal ligament until the triangular shape of the anterior inferior iliac spine (AIIS) is visualized. At this location, the sartorius muscle is seen laterally and the internal oblique medially, forming the so-called "bowtie" or "hourglass" image (Fig. 55.10). Occasionally, the deep circumflex iliac artery can be identified between the abdominal muscles and fascia iliaca.

- Transverse orientation: For this approach, the transducer is placed in a transverse orientation over the femoral crease to identify the femoral artery, femoral nerve, iliopsoas muscle, and fascia iliaca. From here, and keeping the fascia iliaca image on ultrasound, the transducer is moved laterally until the sartorius muscle is identified. Then, it is moved cranially until the AIIS is visualized deep to the iliacus muscle. The ultrasound image is the same as described for the oblique approach and may be easier to obtain, in particular, in patients who are obese or cannot be well-positioned.

After identifying the correct injection site, the needle is inserted in-plane from lateral to medial and through the fascia iliaca at its most superficial point. After negative aspiration, 1–2 mL of local anesthetic is injected to confirm a proper local anesthetic distribution between the fascia iliaca and iliopsoas muscle (Fig. 55.11).

Local Anesthetic Distribution

When injected correctly, the local anesthetic spread results in the separation of the fascia iliaca and iliacus muscle, deep to the muscles of the abdominal wall (internal oblique and transversus abdominis) and the circumflex iliac artery, which is often seen displaced anteriorly with the injection. When the correct position of the needle has been confirmed, complete the block with 30–40 mL of local anesthetic.

Complications

Although the local anesthetic spread toward the femoral nerve can be confirmed by ultrasound, the extent of the local anesthetic proximal toward the lumbar plexus cannot be monitored or assured. Because the spread cannot be entirely controlled, this technique is primarily used for analgesia, not anesthesia.

Specific Risks

Overall complications involving the fascia iliaca compartment block are low. Being considered a fascial plane technique, intravascular injections or neurologic injury is uncommon as the injection site is remote from the major neurovascular structures. The most commonly reported complications include hematomas at the injection point and local

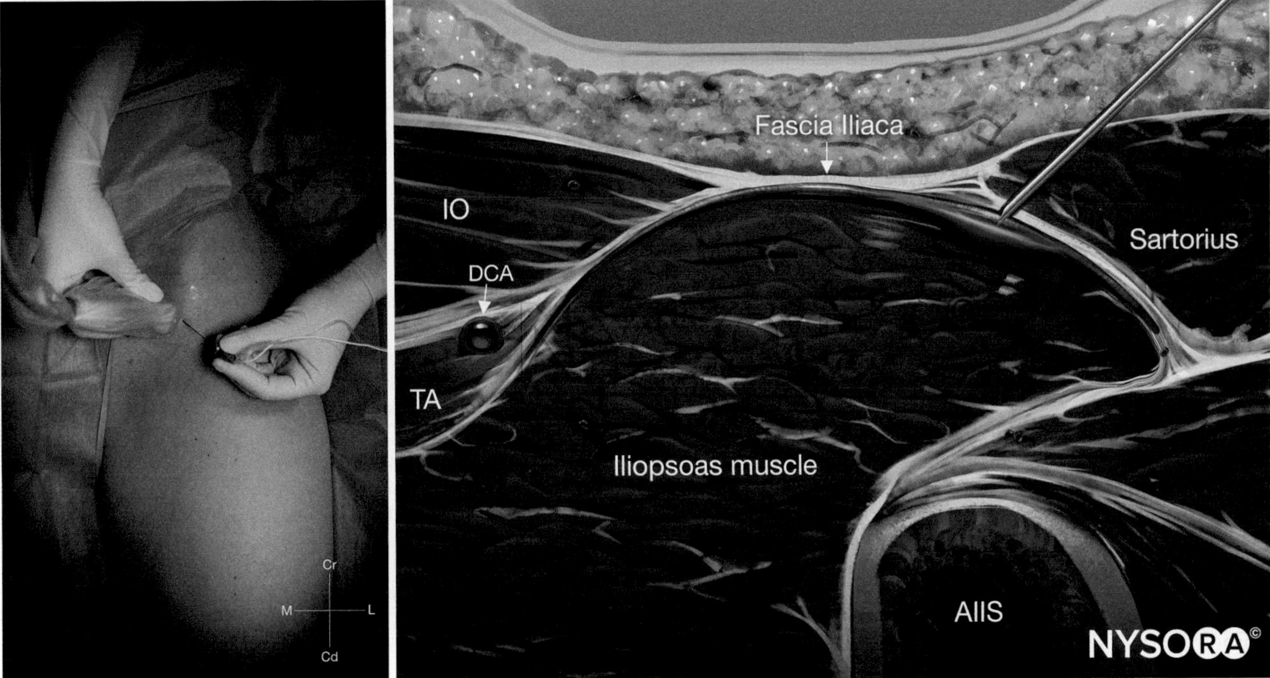

Fig. 55.11 Reverse ultrasound anatomy of a suprainguinal fascia iliaca block showing needle insertion in-plane. *IO* internal oblique muscle, *TA* transversus abdominis muscle, *DCA* deep circumflex artery, *AIIS* anterior inferior iliac spine. (Reproduced with permission from NYSORA)

anesthetic systemic toxicity. The plasma levels after an injection of 30 mL of 0.25% levobupivacaine are below the toxic threshold, even in elderly patients, who are the most common beneficiaries of the technique. However, pneumoperitoneum and bladder puncture have been reported.

Practical Tips

- In obese patients, it is useful to tape away the abdominal redundant tissue to facilitate access to the inguinal area.
- Correct local anesthetic distribution, deep to the fascia iliaca, can be monitored by sliding the transducer medially in search of the femoral artery and nerve and verifying that the local anesthetic reaches the nerve.
- If the spread occurs into the iliacus muscle, the needle is withdrawn and directed more superficially.

Suggested Reading

Behrends M, Yap EN, Zhang AL, Kolodzie K, Kinjo S, Harbell MW, Aleshi P. Preoperative fascia iliaca block does not improve analgesia after arthroscopic hip surgery, but causes quadriceps muscles weakness. Anesthesiology. 2018;129:536–43.

Blackford D, Westhoffen P. Accidental bladder puncture: a complication of a modified fascia iliaca block. Anaesth Intensive Care. 2009;37:140–1.

Cai L, Song Y, Wang Z, She W, Luo X, Song Y. The efficacy of fascia iliaca compartment block for pain control after hip arthroplasty: a meta-analysis. Int J Surg. 2019;66:89. https://doi.org/10.1016/j.ijsu.2018.12.012.

Capdevila X, Biboulet P, Bouregba M, Barthelet Y, Rubenovitch J, D'Athis F. Comparison of the three-in-one and fascia iliaca compartment blocks in adults. Anesth Analg. 1998;86:1039–44.

Chan EY, Fransen M, Parker DA, Assam PN, Chua N. Femoral nerve blocks for acute postoperative pain after knee replacement surgery. Cochrane Database Syst Rev. 2014;(5):CD00994.

Cooper AL, Nagree Y, Goudie A, Watson PR, Arendts G. Ultrasound-guided femoral nerve blocks are not superior to ultrasound-guided fascia iliaca blocks for fractured neck of femur. Emerg Med Aust. 2019;31(3):393–8.

Dalens B, Vanneuville G, Tanguy A. Comparison of the fascia iliaca compartment block with the 3-in-1 block in children. Anesth Analg. 1989;69:705–13.

Desmet M, Vermeylen K, Van Herreweghe I, Carlier L, Soetens F, Lambrecht S, Croes K, Pottel H, Van de Velde M. A longitudinal suprainguinal fascia iliaca compartment block reduces morphine consumption after total hip arthroplasty. Reg Anesth Pain Med. 2017;42:327–33.

Desmet M, Balocco AL, Van Belleghem V. Fascia iliaca compartment blocks: different techniques and review of the literature. Best Pract Res Clin Anaesthesiol. 2019;33:57–66.

Ee-Yuee C, Fransen M, David AP, Pryseley NA, Chua N. Femoral nerve blocks for acute postoperative pain after knee replacement surgery (Review). Cochrane Database Syst Rev. 2016;(13):CD009941.

Gabriel RA, Kaye AD, Nagrebetsky A, Jones MR, Dutton RP, Urman RD. Utilization of femoral nerve blocks for total knee arthroplasty. J Arthroplast. 2016;31:1680–5.

Gasanova I, Alexander JC, Estrera K, Wells J, Sunna M, Minhajuddin A, Joshi GP. Ultrasound-guided suprainguinal fascia iliaca compartment block versus periarticular infiltration for pain management after total hip arthroplasty: a randomized controlled trial. Reg Anesth Pain Med. 2019;44:206–11.

Grevstad U, Mathiesen O, Valentiner LS, Jaeger P, Hilsted KL, Dahl JB. Effect of adductor canal block versus femoral nerve block on quadriceps strength, mobilization, and pain after total knee arthroplasty: a randomized, blinded study. Reg Anesth Pain Med. 2015;40:3–10.

Gupta M, Kamath SS. Comparison of preoperative ultrasound guided fascia iliaca block versus femoral nerve block for proximal femur fractures before positioning for spinal anesthesia: an observational study. Korean J Pain. 2020;33:138–43.

Hadzic A, Houle TT, Capdevila X, Ilfeld BM. Femoral nerve block for analgesia in patients having knee arthroplasty. Anesthesiology. 2010;113:1014–5.

Horn J-L, Pitsch T, Salinas F, Benninger B. Anatomic basis to the ultrasound-guided approach for saphenous nerve blockade. Reg Anesth Pain Med. 2009;34:486–9.

Ilfeld BM, Duke KB, Donohue MC. The association between lower extremity continuous peripheral nerve blocks and patient falls after knee and hip arthroplasty. Anesth Analg. 2010;111:1552–4.

Jæger P, Nielsen ZJK, Henningsen MH, Hilsted KL, Mathiesen O, Dahl JB. Adductor canal block versus femoral nerve block and quadriceps strength: a randomized, double-blind, placebo-controlled, crossover study in healthy volunteers. Anesthesiology. 2013;118:409–15.

Kuang M-J, Ma J-X, Fu L, He W-W, Zhao J, Ma X-L. Is adductor canal block better than femoral nerve block in primary total knee arthroplasty? A GRADE analysis of the evidence through a systematic review and meta-analysis. J Arthroplast. 2017;32:3238–3248.e3.

Marhofer P, Schrögendorfer K, Koinig H, Kapral S, Weinstabl C, Mayer N. Ultrasonographic guidance improves sensory block and onset time of three-in-one blocks. Anesth Analg. 1997;85:854–7.

Ogami K, Murata H, Sakai A, Sato S, Saiki K, Okamoto K, Manabe Y, Hara T, Tsurumoto T. Deep and superficial circumflex iliac arteries and their relationship to the ultrasound-guided femoral nerve block procedure: a cadaver study. Clin Anat. 2017;30:413–20.

Riddell M, Ospina M, Holroyd-Leduc JM. Use of femoral nerve blocks to manage hip fracture pain among older adults in the emergency department: a systematic review. Can J Emerg Med. 2016;18:245–52.

Ritter JW. Femoral nerve “sheath” for inguinal paravascular lumbar plexus block is not found in human cadavers. Surv Anesthesiol. 1996;40:185.

Shariat AN, Hadzic A, Xu D, Shastri U, Kwofie K, Gandhi K, McCally CM, Gratenstein K, Vandepitte C, Gadsden J, Unis D. Fascia iliaca block for analgesia after hip arthroplasty: a randomized double-blind, placebo-controlled trial. Reg Anesth Pain Med. 2013;38:201–5.

Shelley B, Haldane G. Pneumoretroperitoneum as a consequence of fascia iliaca block. Reg Anesth Pain Med. 2006;31:582–92.

Sia S, Pelusio F, Barbagli R, Rivituso C. Analgesia before performing a spinal block in the sitting position in patients with femoral shaft fracture: a comparison between femoral nerve block and intravenous fentanyl. Anesth Analg. 2004;99:1221–4.

Steenberg J, Møller AM. Systematic review of the effects of fascia iliaca compartment block on hip fracture patients before operation. Br J Anaesth. 2018;120:1368–80.

Strid JMC, Sauter AR, Ullensvang K, Andersen MN, Daugaard M, Bendtsen MAF, Søballe K, Pedersen EM, Børglum J, Bendtsen TF. Ultrasound-guided lumbar plexus block in volunteers; A randomized controlled trial. Br J Anaesth. 2017;118:430–8.

Vermeylen K, Soetens F, Leunen I, Hadzic A, Van Boxtael S, Pomés J, Prats-Galino A, Van de Velde M, Neyrinck A, Sala-Blanch X. The effect of the volume of supra-inguinal injected solution on the spread of the injectate under the fascia iliaca: a preliminary study. J Anesth. 2018;32:908–13.

Vermeylen K, Desmet M, Leunen I, Soetens F, Neyrinck A, Carens D, Caerts B, Seynaeve P, Hadzic A, Van de Velde M. Supra-inguinal injection for fascia iliaca compartment block results in more consistent spread towards the lumbar plexus than an infra-inguinal injection: a volunteer study. Reg Anesth Pain Med. 2019;44:483–91.

Winnie A, Ramamurthy S, Durrani Z. The inguinal paravascular technique of lumbar plexus anesthesia: the “3-in-1 block”. Anesth Analg. 1973;52:989–96.

Zhang X, Ma J. The efficacy of fascia iliaca compartment block for pain control after total hip arthroplasty: a meta-analysis. J Orthop Surg Res. 2019;14:1–10.

Posterior Approach of Regional Nerve Block in the Lumbar Region

56

Matthias R. Braehler, Jens Kessler, and Andrew T. Gray

Contents

Abbreviations

ESPB	Erector spinae plane block
ESM	Erector spinae muscle
TP	Transverse process
LAST	Local anesthetic systemic toxicity

M. R. Braehler
Clinical Anesthesia, University of California,
San Francisco, CA, USA
e-mail: matthias.braehler@ucsf.edu

J. Kessler
Department of Anaesthesiology, University Hospital Division Center for Pain Therapy and Palliative Medicine,
Heidelberg, Germany
e-mail: jens.kessler@med.uni-heidelberg.de

A. T. Gray (✉)
Department of Anesthesia and Preoperative Care, University of California San Francisco, San Francisco General Hospital,
San Francisco, USA
e-mail: andrew.gray@ucsf.edu

Lumbar Erector Spinae Plane Block (Lumbar ESPB)

General Considerations

Erector spinae plane block (ESPB) was first described in patients with chronic thoracic neuropathic pain and following video-assisted thoracoscopic surgery. This block has rapidly gained popularity due to the simplicity of the approach and its perceived safety profile. In the thoracic region, the injections are relatively shallow and the muscle layers well-defined. These sonographic landmarks are easy to identify, even in patients with higher BMI. This general approach has now been applied throughout the spine, including the lumbar region.

Indications and Patient Selection

Lumbar approaches to ESPB can provide analgesia for a wide variety of surgeries, including those in the hip, femur, and knee regions. Bilateral lumbar ESPBs are part of a mul-

D. Jankovic, P. Peng (eds.), *Regional Nerve Blocks in Anesthesia and Pain Therapy*,
https://doi.org/10.1007/978-3-030-88727-8_56

timodal opioid-free pathway for lumbar spine surgery. Other reported applications include analgesia for inguinal hernia repair.

Functional Anatomy

The ultrasound approach to classic erector spinae plane block at T5 shows three muscle layers over the transverse process: the trapezius, rhomboid major, and erector spinae muscles. Below T6, only two muscle layers remain, the trapezius and erector spinae (below the inferior angle of the scapula). Since the trapezius inserts on the spinous process of T12, only the erector spinae muscle lies on the transverse process in the lumbar region. The erector spinae muscle has a deep fascia that must be punctured with the block needle in order to achieve spread of local anesthetic within the erector spinae plane (refer to Figs. 34.4 and 34.5 of Chap. 34). Compared to the thoracic region, the transverse processes are deeper and more lateral in the lumbar region. This means that lumbar ESPB is more difficult to perform, and a medium-frequency curvilinear probe may be necessary to identify the relevant structures and "trident sign".

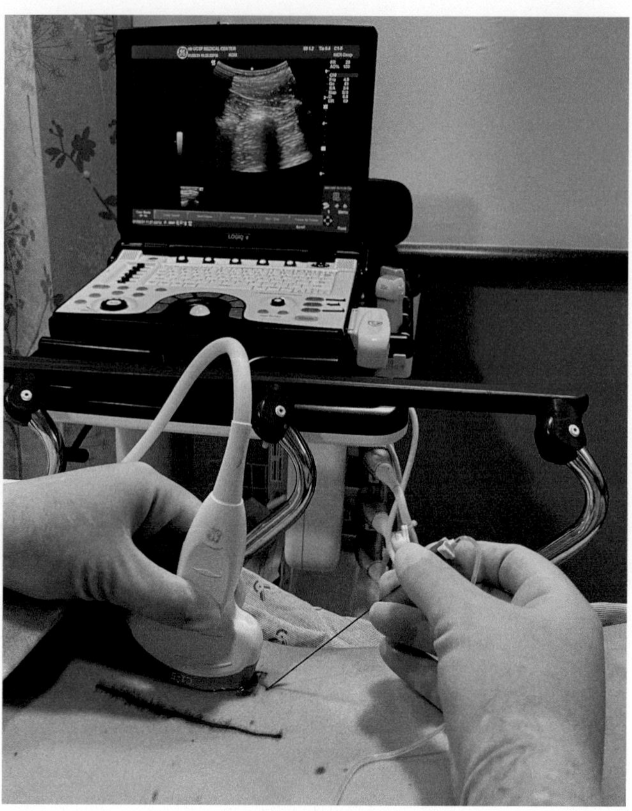

Fig. 56.1 Ultrasound-guided lumbar ESPB. With the patient in prone position, a parasagittal image showing the "trident sign" is obtained. In this example, the needle approaches in-plane from cephalad to caudad. The goal is for the injection to lift the erector spinae muscle off the transverse process of L3. The midline is marked on the skin

Technique

Lumbar ESPB can be performed in prone, lateral decubitus, or sitting positions. The most comfortable and stable position is prone, with a pillow or blanket placed underneath the lower abdomen to reduce the lumbar lordosis (Fig. 56.1). Lateral decubitus position (with the operative side up) is most often used when prone positioning is not possible. Routine monitors should be applied and a time-out utilizing a checklist performed prior to the block.

Most commonly, the block is performed with the lateral tip of the transverse process in parasagittal view. Initially, the spinous processes and sacrum are identified in longitudinal midline view. Then, the transducer is slowly slid laterally over the lamina, articular process, and transverse process (Fig. 56.2). In-plane approach from caudal to cephalad (or vice versa) can be used. Recent studies have shown that the spread of local anesthetic does not depend on the direction of approach. For catheter placement, we prefer to thread the catheter 3–4 cm beyond the tip of the needle at the transverse process above or below the desired level (depending on the direction of approach).

Several alternative approaches to the lumbar ESPB have been described. A transverse view with in-plane approach is possible (lateral to medial or medial to lateral). Another approach is to use a transverse view in lateral decubitus position to target the transverse process from posterior to anterior. The disadvantage of this approach is limited assessment of the longitudinal spread of local anesthetic within the erector spinae plane as well as difficulty threading an indwelling catheter.

Complications

Lumbar ESPB is a relatively new anesthetic technique, and only a few case reports concerning complications or adverse events have been published at this time. There are case reports of pneumothorax following thoracic ESPB, and this could potentially happen with high lumbar approach and caudal to cephalad needle trajectory. There also are isolated reports of unintended lower extremity motor blockade and adverse effects on spinal biomechanics following ESPB.

Lumbar ESPB, like all other nerve blocks, is an invasive procedure that has inherent risks (such as bleeding, infection, nerve injury, damage to adjacent anatomic structures). While no such complications have been reported, there is certainly some potential. However, we feel these events are highly unlikely to occur if the needle is only advanced when the tip is clearly identified on the ultrasound screen.

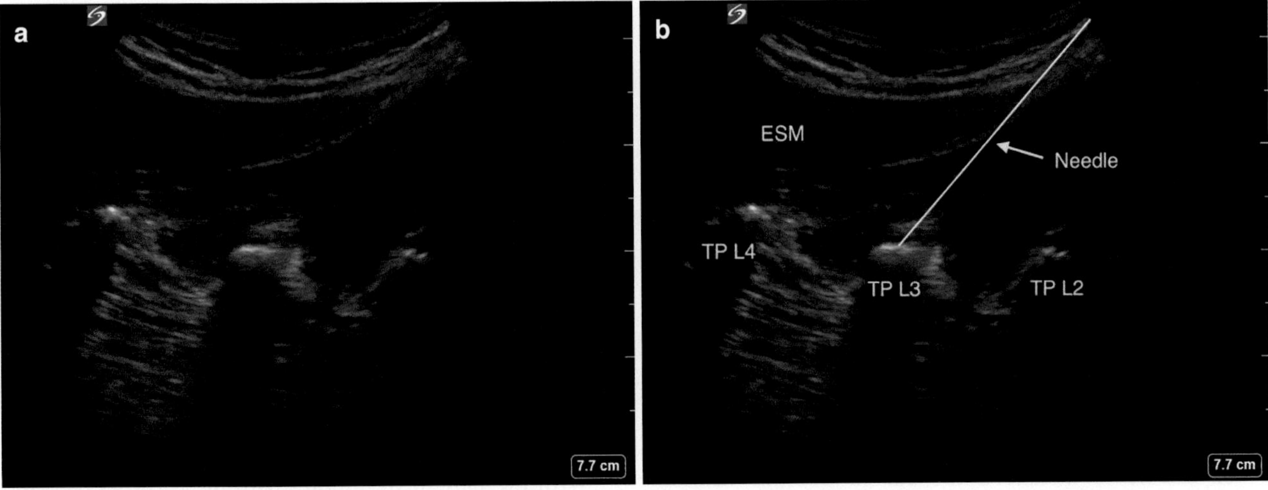

Fig. 56.2 (**a**, **b**) Corresponding sonograms shown without (panel **a**) and with labels and the approximate needle tip position (panel **b**). *ESM* erector spinae muscle, *TP* transverse process

The target of ESPB is the lateral tip of the transverse process, which is relatively far from neuraxial structures. This is why some authors have referred to these new interfascial plane blocks as "minimally invasive". There is some clinical evidence that ESPB is safe in anticoagulated patients. However, formal guidelines regarding ESPB and anticoagulation have not yet been given.

In smaller patients, and especially when bilateral blocks are performed, close attention should be paid to the total dose of local anesthetic relative to the maximum recommended dose. There are no specific studies yet available to evaluate the plasma concentrations of local anesthetic after ESPB. However, local anesthetic systemic toxicity (LAST) can occur, especially in susceptible patients (such as preexisting cardiac conditions, sarcopenia, etc.).

Unlike neuraxial anesthetic techniques, ESPB has not been associated with hypotension or urinary retention.

Practical Tips

In patients where the depth of the transverse process is more than 4–5 cm, a low- or medium-frequency curvilinear ultrasound probe may be advantageous. A high-frequency linear probe will not be able to penetrate the tissues and reach the pertinent structures to perform this block under these conditions. One limitation of the curvilinear probe is limited needle tip visibility.

Use a musculoskeletal preset on the ultrasound machine. The goal is not to identify individual nerves but rather bony contours and muscle borders in the lumbar region.

If the provider encounters difficulties to identify the transverse processes in the parasagittal view, a transverse approach can be utilized first to identify the spinous process, the lamina, and the transverse process. Once the transverse process has been identified, the depth from the skin can be measured and then a parasagittal view can be obtained, confirming that the depth of the TP is similar to the depth found in the transverse view. The transverse processes are the last bony structures when scanning from medial to lateral. They are best seen if the ultrasound beams hit the bone in a right angle, since the beams will be reflected straight back to the probe (a specular reflection with acoustic shadowing). Since the transverse processes do not necessarily travel parallel to the skin surface, slight tilting of the ultrasound probe may be necessary to obtain the best view of the TPs. Once this view has been achieved, the probe should no longer been moved, and the needle needs to be entered into this ultrasound plane.

Dissect the deep fascia of the erector spinae muscle off the transverse process, giving 20–30 mL of local anesthetic. Depending on the depth of the transverse processes, the spread of local anesthetic may not be visualized as clearly as in the thoracic region.

Initially, use normal saline to confirm the position of the needle tip underneath the deep fascia of the erector spinae muscle, which will lead to longitudinal distribution of fluid in both directions. If the spread is limited and no longitudinal spread is obtained, the injection is likely made into the erector spinae muscle itself, which will most likely lead to a failed block. Two maneuvers can be applied in this case: either the needle can be advanced against the TP with slight pressure and some rotational movement ("corkscrewing"), to eventually penetrate the deep fascia, or the needle can be walked off the TP in order to lift up this fascia. If the needle is walked off the TP, this can be done either toward or away from the needle entry site. The latter approach may facilitate placement of an indwelling catheter, should catheter placement be desired. Once longitudinal spread in both directions is confirmed, switch over to the local anesthetic syringe and inject the planned volume of 20–30 mL in the ES muscle plane.

Given that vital structures are relative far away from the target, there is a reasonable safety margin when performing ESPB in the lumbar region. However, all safety precautions that are adhered to with all other nerve blocks must be applied. A time-out prior to performing the block is important and sterile technique should be used. While there have been case reports of pneumothorax in thoracic ESPB, the pleura is usually not in the needle path, unless a high lumbar ESPB from caudad to cephalad is performed. However, the lumbar plexus, the peritoneum, the kidneys, and other structures could be potentially injured if the block needle is advanced too far in a blind fashion. Therefore, it is of paramount importance to ensure the needle is visualized at all times prior to advancing it. Echogenic needles are very useful for this block.

If bilateral blocks are performed, the provider can stay in the same position and perform both blocks from the same side of the patient by just sliding the probe right and left from midline. We recommend to always mark the midline and also pre-scan and mark the ultrasound probe footprint prior to the skin prep.

Lumbar Plexus Block

Indications

Posterior approach to lumbar plexus block can be useful for some lower extremity surgical procedures, including revision hip arthroplasty. Because this block can be challenging, it is most often used in small adults who can be positioned lateral. The block is especially beneficial in opioid-tolerant patients. This block can provide significant analgesia of the hip region.

Advantages

Lumbar plexus block has some advantages

over neuraxial techniques, including better ambulation, as well as less hypotension and urinary retention.

Disadvantages

The posterior approach is a deeper block that is not definitive for surgery. It therefore has limited utility in clinical practice.

Risks

The risks of posterior approach to lumbar plexus block include central distributions, systemic toxicity, and bleeding complications. Ultrasound imaging probably reduces these risks, although clinical evidence of this is lacking at this time.

Scanning Technique

A medium-frequency linear or curved transducer can be used for imaging. The initial scanning depth is 8 cm in small adults (about half the torso with).

With the patient in lateral position, a transverse view of the L3 transverse process is obtained (TP viewed en face). The transducer is then slid or tilted caudally to view the interspace between L3 and L4 (Fig. 56.3). The quadratus lumborum muscle is hypoechoic and attaches to the lateral edge of the TP. The psoas muscle is hyperechoic and lies between the vertebral body and transverse process in a chair configuration (Fig. 56.4). This muscle contracts with hip flexion. Pre-scanning Doppler is recommended to scout for adjacent blood vessels. The lumbar ventral rami that contribute to the lumbar plexus are 5–7 mm in diameter but difficult to image with ultrasound in adults.

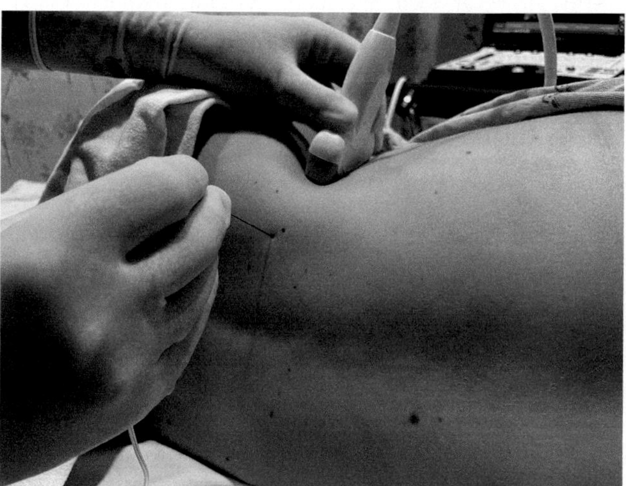

Fig. 56.3 Ultrasound-guided lumbar plexus block. With the patient in lateral decubitus position, the transducer is placed between the costal margin and iliac crest. The lateral tip of the transverse process is imaged en face. The transducer then tilts slightly caudal for an intertransverse view. A posterior in-plane approach is shown

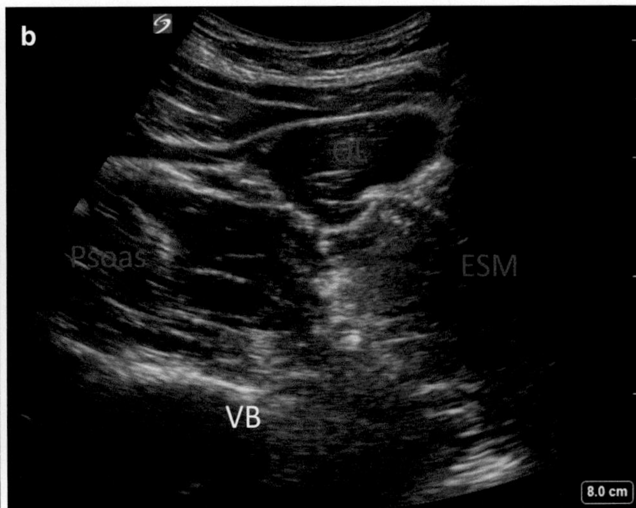

Fig. 56.4 (**a**, **b**) Corresponding sonograms showing the lateral tip of the transverse process (**a**, TP L3) and intertransverse view (**b**). Panel (**a**): The lateral tip of the transverse process points to the hypoechoic quadratus lumborum (QL) muscle (the "shamrock sign"). Panel (**b**): The lumbar plexus (not labeled) lies within the psoas muscle that lies over the vertebral body, VB. The lumbar plexus is difficult to distinguish from hyperechoic striations within the psoas muscle. The needle approaches in-plane nearly parallel to the active face of the transducer (through the erector spinae muscle, ESM). The goal is to approach the lumbar plexus within the psoas muscle and elicit a quadriceps twitch by combining nerve stimulation with ultrasound imaging as described in the text

Approach and Strategy

The goal is to place the needle tip within the psoas muscle and obtain a lower extremity evoked motor response (ultrasound combined with nerve stimulation, typically eliciting a femoral nerve motor response). The nerves of the lumbar plexus emerge between the vertebral bodies and transverse processes to enter the bottom center of the psoas muscle. Because the needle enters nearly parallel to the active face of the transducer, needle tip visibility is usually adequate. With this approach, bilateral epidural distributions are possible, particularly if high volume and high pressures are used.

Typical threshold stimulating currents are 0.5–1.0 mA. Relatively high volumes (20–30 mL ropivacaine 0.5%) are required for complete lumbar plexus block. Incremental injection technique with meticulous intermittent aspiration is required. The same approach is used for catheter placement.

Comments

The posterior approach is a deep block that has significant bleeding risks. Anticoagulation guidelines are the same as for neuraxial interventions. New technology is being developed to enhance needle tip visibility for this deeper block.

Acknowledgments The authors would like to thank Drs. Ed Labovitz and Ashley Sharp for their help with the images.

Suggested Reading

Adhikary SD, Prasad A, Soleimani B, Chin KJ. Continuous erector spinae plane block as an effective analgesic option in anticoagulated patients after left ventricular assist device implantation: a case series. J Cardiothorac Vasc Anesth. 2019;33(4):1063–7. PMID: 29753668.

Aksu C, Gürkan Y. Aksu approach for lumbar erector spinae plane block for pediatric surgeries. J Clin Anesth. 2019;54:74–5. PMID: 30408620.

Aksu C, Şen MC, Akay MA, Baydemir C, Gürkan Y. Erector spinae plane block vs quadratus lumborum block for pediatric lower abdominal surgery: a double blinded, prospective, and randomized trial. J Clin Anesth. 2019;57:24–8. PMID: 30851499.

Auroy Y, Benhamou D, Bargues L, Ecoffey C, Falissard B, Mercier FJ, Bouaziz H, Samii K. Major complications of regional anesthesia in France: the SOS Regional Anesthesia Hotline Service. Anesthesiology. 2002;97(5):1274–80. PMID: 12411815.

Boretsky K, Hernandez MA, Eastburn E, Sullivan C. Ultrasound-guided lumbar plexus block in children and adolescents using a transverse lumbar paravertebral sonogram: initial experience. Paediatr Anaesth. 2018;28(3):291–5. PMID: 29359366.

Callen PW, Filly RA, Marks WM. The quadratus lumborum muscle: a possible source of confusion in sonographic evaluation of the retroperitoneum. J Clin Ultrasound. 1979;7(5):349–52. PMID: 114538.

Chin KJ, Barrington MJ. Erector spinae block: a magic bullet for postoperative analgesia? Anesth Analg. 2019;129(1):8–9. PMID: 31206445.

Ebraheim NA, Xu R, Huntoon M, Yeasting RA. Location of the extraforaminal lumbar nerve roots. An anatomic study. Clin Orthop Relat Res. 1997;(340):230–5. PMID: 9224261.

Forero M, Adhikary SD, Lopez H, Tsui C, Chin KJ. The erector spinae plane block: a novel analgesic technique in thoracic neuropathic pain. Reg Anesth Pain Med. 2016;41(5):621–7. PMID: 27501016.

Gadsden JC, Lindenmuth DM, Hadzic A, Xu D, Somasundarum L, Flisinski KA. Lumbar plexus block using high-pressure injection leads to contralateral and epidural spread. Anesthesiology. 2008;109(4):683–8. PMID: 18813048.

Harbell MW, Seamans DP, Koyyalamudi V, Kraus MB, Craner RC, Langley NR. Evaluating the extent of lumbar erector spinae plane block: an anatomical study. Reg Anesth Pain Med. 2020;45(8):640–4. PMID: 32546551.

Horlocker TT, Vandermeuelen E, Kopp SL, Gogarten W, Leffert LR, Benzon HT. Regional anesthesia in the patient receiving antithrombotic or thrombolytic therapy: American Society of Regional Anesthesia and Pain Medicine evidence-based guidelines (Fourth Edition). Reg Anesth Pain Med. 2018;43(3):263–309. PMID: 29561531.

Hruschka J, Arndt CD. Transverse approach to the erector spinae block. Reg Anesth Pain Med. 2019;44(3):422–3. PMID: 30777908.

Kåsine T, Romundstad L, Rosseland LA, Ullensvang K, Fagerland MW, Kessler P, Bjørnå E, Sauter AR. The effect of needle tip tracking on procedural time of ultrasound-guided lumbar plexus block: a randomised controlled trial. Anaesthesia. 2020;75(1):72–9. PMID: 31506918.

King AD, Hine AL, McDonald C, Abrahams P. The ultrasound appearance of the normal psoas muscle. Clin Radiol. 1993;48(5):316–8. PMID: 8258221.

Kinjo S, Schultz A. Continuous lumbar erector spinae plane block for postoperative pain management in revision hip surgery: a case report. Rev Bras Anestesiol. 2019;69(4):420–2. PMID: 31362881.

Kline J, Chin KJ. Modified dual-injection lumbar erector spine plane (ESP) block for opioid-free anesthesia in multilevel lumbar laminectomy. Korean J Anesthesiol. 2019;72(2):188–90. PMID: 30392347.

Kose HC, Kose SG, Thomas DT. Lumbar versus thoracic erector spinae plane block: similar nomenclature, different mechanism of action. J Clin Anesth. 2018;48:1. PMID: 29649625.

Missair A, Flavin K, Paula F, Benedetti de Marrero E, Benitez Lopez J, Matadial C. Leaning Tower of Pisa? Avoiding a major neurologic complication with the erector spinae plane block. Reg Anesth Pain Med. 2019;44(7):713–4. PMID: 30918086.

Sauter AR, Ullensvang K, Niemi G, Lorentzen HT, Bendtsen TF, Børglum J, Pripp AH, Romundstad L. The Shamrock lumbar plexus block: a dose-finding study. Eur J Anaesthesiol. 2015;32(11):764–70. PMID: 26426575.

Selvi O, Tulgar S. Ultrasound guided erector spinae plane block as a cause of unintended motor block. Rev Esp Anestesiol Reanim. 2018;65(10):589–92. PMID: 30001858.

Sondekoppam RV, Tsui BCH. “Minimally invasive” regional anesthesia and the expanding use of interfascial plane blocks: the need for more systematic evaluation. Can J Anaesth. 2019;66(8):855–63. PMID: 31114940.

Tulgar S, Balaban O. Spread of local anesthetic in erector spine plane block at thoracic and lumbar levels. Reg Anesth Pain Med. 2019;44(1):134–5. PMID: 30640667.

Tulgar S, Senturk O. Ultrasound guided Erector Spinae Plane block at L-4 transverse process level provides effective postoperative analgesia for total hip arthroplasty. J Clin Anesth. 2018;44:68. PMID: 29149734.

Lateral Femoral Cutaneous Nerve Blockade

57

Guy Feigin and Philip Peng

Contents

General Consideration

Lateral femoral cutaneous nerve (LFCN) block is useful in the diagnosis and treatment of the entrapment neuropathy of the lateral femoral cutaneous nerve (LFCN), which is known as meralgia paresthetica (MP), a mononeuropathy of the LFCN that can lead to significant disability. The LFCNB can also be used for surgical anesthesia and/or postoperative pain control for procedures on the anterolateral thigh such as skin graft harvesting and to alleviate tourniquet pain from lower extremity orthopedic procedures. The prevalence of MP in the primary care setting is estimated at 4.3 per 10,000 person-years.

Indications (Patient Selection)

Indications for LFCN block include part of the multimodal analgesia for hip surgery, diagnosis and management of patient with meralgia paresthetica, and muscle biopsy of the proximal lateral thigh.

When the differential diagnosis of anterolateral or lateral thigh pain is not conclusive, a nerve entrapment of the lateral cutaneous nerve lateral, which may cause pain, paresthesias, and sensory loss within its distribution of the thigh, should be considered (Fig. 57.1).

The prevalence of MP peaks between 30- and 40-year-olds and the overall prevalence rate is 4.3 cases per 10,000 patients in the general population and 24.7 cases per 10,000 patients in individuals with diabetes mellitus. It is more common in males than females and can technically occur at all ages. Physical examination may reveal tenderness over the lateral aspect of the inguinal ligament with Tinel sign elicited at the site of entrapment. Hypoesthesia over the area innervated by the LFCN is commonly found with or without allodynia.

G. Feigin (✉)
Department of Anesthesia and Pain Management, University of Toronto, Toronto Western Hospital, Women's College Hospital, Wasser Pain Management Clinic, Mount Sinai Hospital, Toronto, ON, Canada

Department of Anesthesiology, Critical Care and Pain Management, Meir Medical Center, Kfar-Saba, Israel

P. Peng
Department of Anesthesia and Pain Management, University of Toronto, Toronto Western Hospital, Women's College Hospital, Wasser Pain Management Clinic, Mount Sinai Hospital, Toronto, ON, Canada
e-mail: philip.peng@uhn.ca

D. Jankovic, P. Peng (eds.), *Regional Nerve Blocks in Anesthesia and Pain Therapy*,
https://doi.org/10.1007/978-3-030-88727-8_57

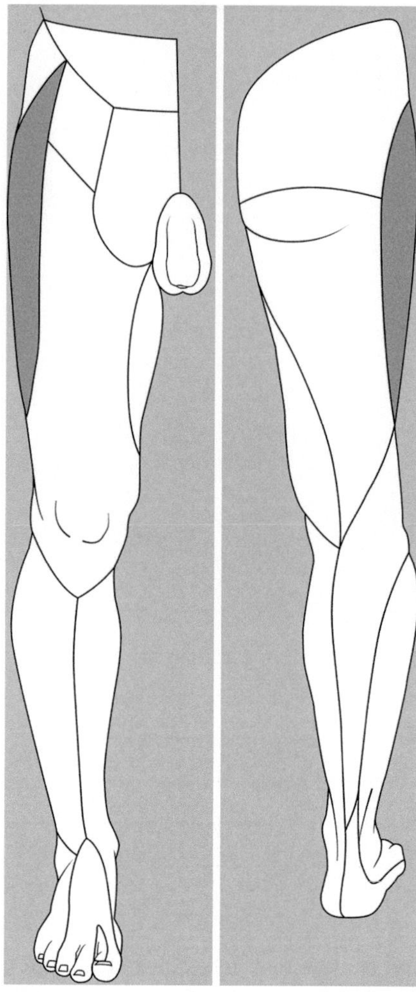

Fig. 57.1 The skin area supplied by LFCN. Reprinted with permission from Dr. Danilo Jankovic

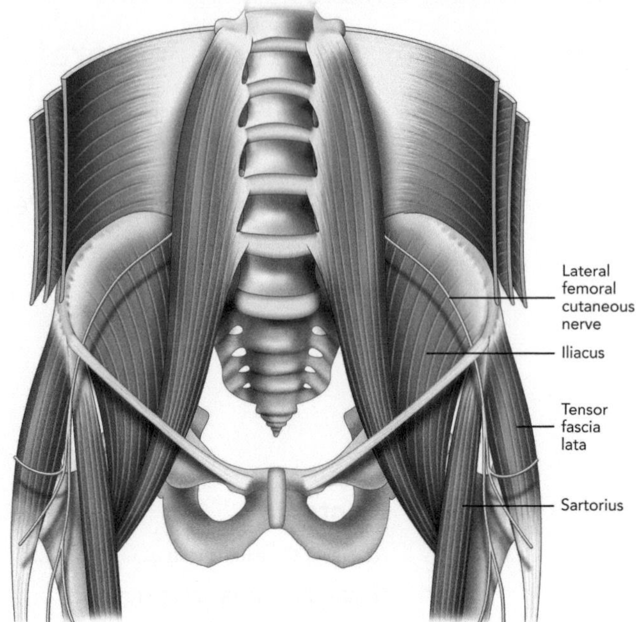

Fig. 57.2 Schematic diagram showing the pathway of a typical course of the lateral femoral cutaneous nerve. Reprinted with permission from Philip Peng Educational Series

Clues suggestive of the etiology may be revealed during the examination, such as the surgical scars, raised intra-abdominal pressure, or low-rise jean (hip-hugger). Because the LFCN is a peripheral sensory nerve, the presence of dermatomal sensory loss and motor and sphincter dysfunctions should alert the clinicians to the spinal etiology.

Anatomy

The LFCN is a pure sensory nerve, originating in most cases from L2 to L3 nerve roots and is a branch of the lumbar plexus. After exiting from the lumbar plexus, the LFCN emerges from the lateral border of the psoas major muscle and then moves alongside and cephalad to the iliac crest. It then crosses in an oblique fashion over the iliacus muscle toward the anterior superior iliac spine (ASIS) and exits the lesser pelvis by passing under the inguinal ligament (IL), superficial and medial to the sartorius muscle at a variable distance from ASIS (average 29 mm; range 0 mm to 73 mm) (Figs. 57.2 and 57.3). In 22% of cases, the nerve can travel through the sartorius.

From there, the LFCN runs to the lateral thigh consistently in a "fat-filled groove" between the tensor fascia lata muscle (TFL) and the sartorius muscle.

A few anatomical variations that one should bear in mind in scanning the LFCN: it may course over or through the IL rather than under it; it may branch before crossing the IL in up to 28% of cases; and it may pass over or posterior the ASIS in 4–29%. The average diameter of LFCN was found to be 3.2 ± 0.7 mm, although there is no established standard value for the cross-sectional area.

The LFCN divides into two branches: anterior and posterior. The anterior branch exits the fascia lata distally to the posterior branch and provides sensation to the anterolateral thigh until the knee. Together with the anterior division of the femoral nerve and the infrapatellar branch of the saphenous nerve, it forms part of the peripatellar plexus. The posterior division pierces the fascia lata more proximal than the anterior portion and provides sensation to the lateral thigh, covering the area from the greater trochanter (and sometimes the gluteal region) to mid-way down the thigh. The pain in patient with MP is presented more commonly in the distribution of the anterior division.

Technique

Comparing with the success rate of landmark approach, the ultrasound-guided approach is superior in accuracy (5% vs 84%, respectively), and therefore we will focus on the

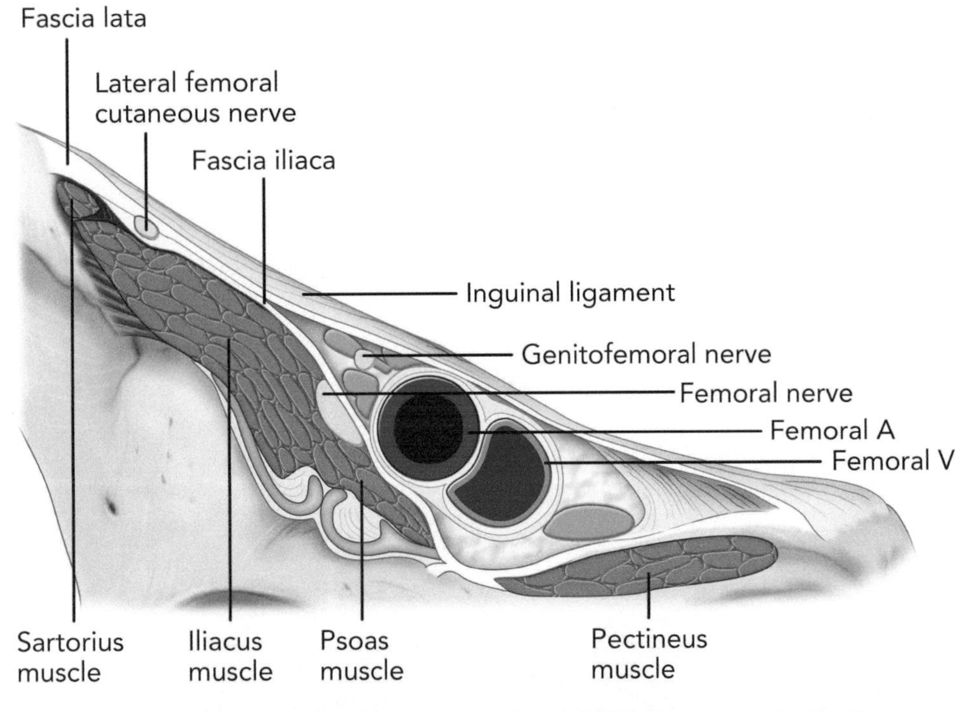

Fig. 57.3 Nerves at the inguinal area. Reprinted with permission from Philip Peng Educational Series

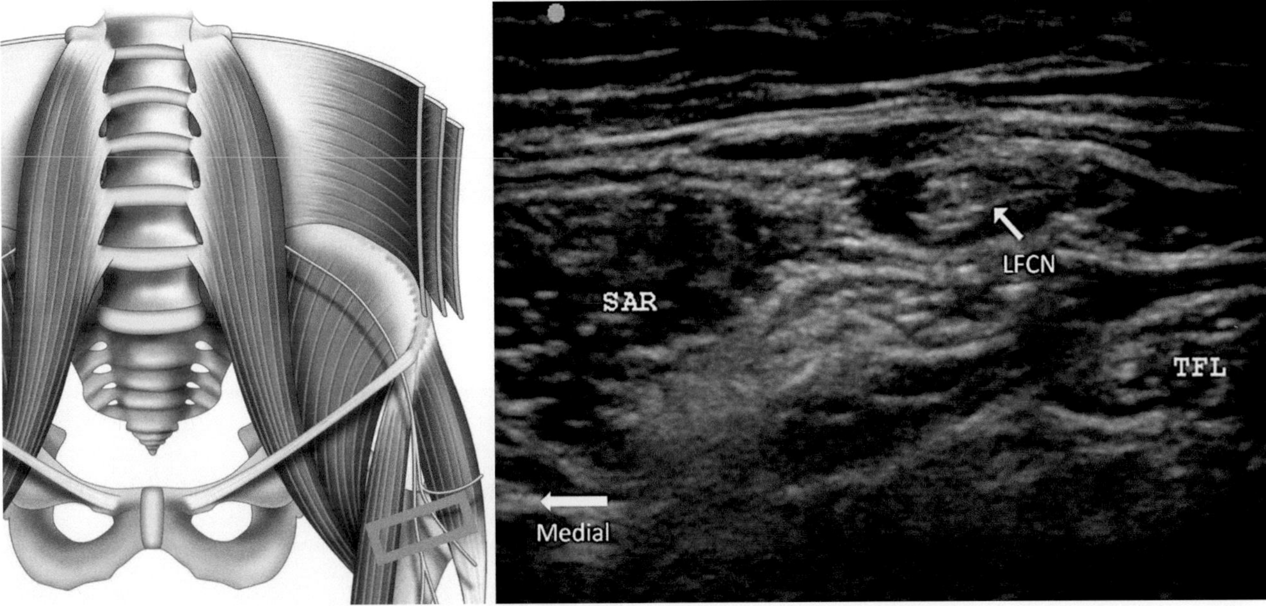

Fig. 57.4 Scanning at the fat-filled grove between sartorius and tensor fascia lata. Reprinted with permission from Philip Peng Educational Series

ultrasound-guided approach only. The LFCN is a small hyperechoic nerve that can be seen in the fat-filled groove between the TFL laterally and the sartorius medially. The authors suggest the starting point for scanning is four finger breadth inferior to ASIS in the fat-filled groove with the use of a high-frequency (6–15 MHz) linear probe (Fig. 57.4). In patient who has MP, the portion of the nerve distal to the entrapment usually appears swollen or enlarged. When performing a LFCN block, it is essential to perform dynamic scan. Once the LFCN is identified in the fat-filled groove, it should be traced proximally, and the nerve usually migrates medially toward the sartorius (Fig. 57.5).

For maximum therapeutic benefit, it is important to block the LFCN as close to the IL as the IL is commonly considered the source of irritation or compression of the nerve. A quick survey of the presence of vessel in the needle trajectory either by paying attention to the pulsatile structure with light compression or with the color Doppler imaging is

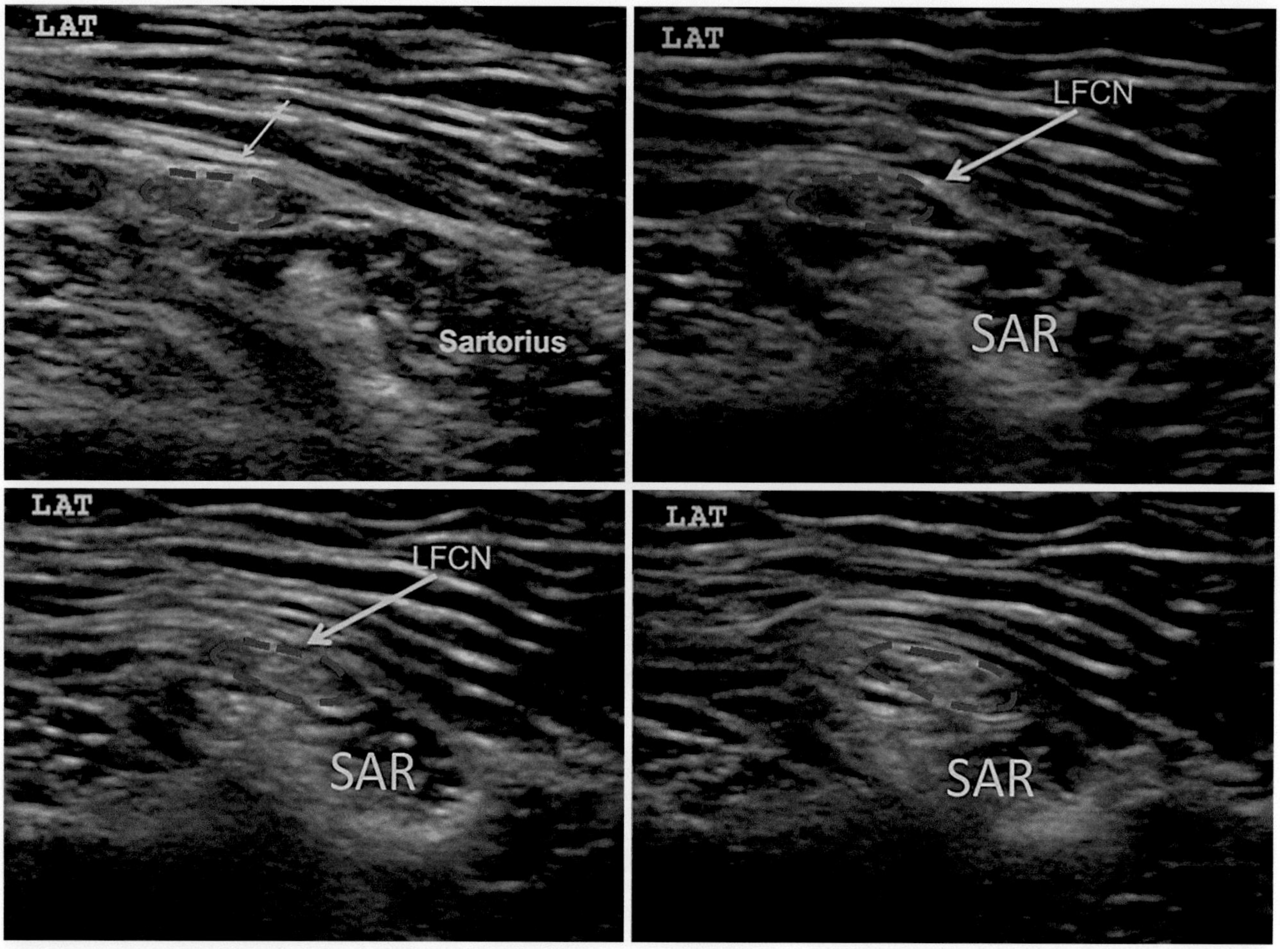

Fig. 57.5 Tracing the lateral femoral cutaneous nerve (LCFN) proximally. The LFCN can be seen moving medially toward the sartorius muscle. Reprinted with permission from Philip Peng Educational Series

usually a good clinical practice. Since the LFCN is a superficial structure, a 25G 1.5-in. needle is used and inserted in-plane or out-of-plane to the target after local infiltration of skin. Once the tip of needles is confirmed with hydrolocation, a volume of 2–3 mL of bupivacaine 0.25% with 20 mg depo-medrol is injected around the nerve (Fig. 57.6).

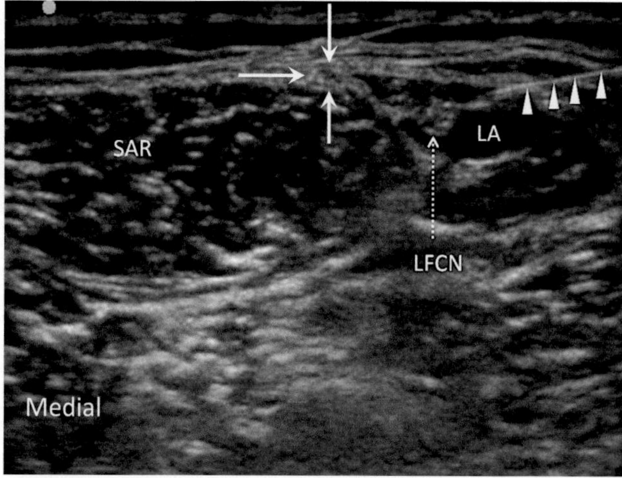

Fig. 57.6 Post-injection ultrasonographic picture of LFCN; the needle was inserted in-plane and was indicated by arrowheads. Following the injection of the LFCN, another small branch was seen (indicated by line arrows). LA local anesthetic, SAR sartorius muscle. Reproduced with permission from Philip Peng Educational Series

Complications

Because of the lack of major vascular structures and organs in the LFCN region, it is considered a safe block with minimal risk involved.

However, some of the possible complications may include:

- Concomitant femoral nerve blockade (most of the time is related to a high volume of injectate)
- No pain relief and the possibility of an increase in pain following the procedure

- Ecchymosis/hematoma at the injection site
- Infection
- Injury to the LFCN or femoral nerve and other anatomical structures resulting in permanent loss of muscle power (paralysis) and numbness
- Adverse reactions to local anesthetics
- Steroid exposure can be associated with:
  – Muscle weakness, transient increase in blood glucose and blood pressure, and rare risk of avascular necrosis. Furthermore, repeated steroid injection may be associated with bone loss, muscle atrophy, cataracts, psychosis, and weakness.

Practical Tips

The LFCN will course the fat-filled groove at a certain point distal to the ASIS. If the nerve is not seen on the initial scan at 4 finger breadth below the ASIS, one should continue to scan proximally. Pay attention to the orientation of the probe so that it is revealing the short axis of the nerve.

The whole course of the LFCN, as well as its branches, is highly variable among individuals. A few anatomical variations that one should bear in mind in scanning the LFCN: it may course over or through the IL rather than under it, it may branch before crossing the IL in up to 28% of cases, and it may pass over or posterior the ASIS in 4–29%. Note that the nerve is subfascial and not subcutaneous.

If ultrasound cannot identify the LFCN, an injection of 5% dextrose can be used to dissect between the fascia lata and the sartorius muscle, decompressing the trapped nerve.

Literature Review

Grossman et al. classified MP as iatrogenic or idiopathic, which in turn may have sub-classification as mechanical or metabolic. Idiopathic mechanical factors can result in compression of the LFCN along its anatomical course. MP has been related to obesity (BMI $\geq$ 30), pregnancy, tight garments such as underwear and jeans, seat belts, military armor and police uniforms, prone position, direct trauma, muscle spasm, scoliosis, iliacus hematoma, and leg length changes. Certain sports such as gymnastics, baseball, soccer, bodybuilding, and strenuous exercise have higher incidences of MP. Metabolic factors include diabetes mellitus, alcoholism, and lead poisoning. It has also been reported as a post-surgical complication after spine surgery and hip joint replacement.

The incidence of MP in posterior spine surgery ranged between 12% and 24%. The presence of red flags such as weight loss and appetite change and acute onset of severe pain on pressure may suggest metastasis at the iliac crest or avulsion fracture of ASIS, respectively. In the situation of uncertainty, both electrophysiological tests and diagnostic nerve blocks can be useful. The limitation of nerve conduction test is that it evaluates mainly large myelinated axons. The test can be normal in patients whose condition principally affects the small myelinated A δ and C fibers.

The technique and importance of the application of ultrasound in order to perform the LFCN blockade has been well published. Validation studies demonstrated greater accuracy in identifying the LFCN with ultrasound in both cadavers and volunteers. Li et al. described the accuracy of identifying LFCN in a cadaveric study through landmark, and US was 1/19 and 16/19, respectively, and 0/20 and 16/20, respectively, in a healthy volunteer study. Nielsen et al. described a novel US-guided approach. Their technique focused on the fat-filled flat tunnel (FFFT), an area formed deep to the fascia lata between the sartorius and TFL. This approach significantly increased the chances of achieving more proximal blockade effects.

Tagliafico et al. described a series of 20 patients who underwent ultrasound-guided injections of local anesthetic and steroid for treatment of meralgia paresthetica. The authors reported a significant reduction in visual analog scale pain scores in all patients at 2 months after the procedure. However, relatively large volumes (9 mL) of injectate were used, and 4 of the 20 patients had required a repeat ultrasound-guided LFCN block procedure at 1 week.

Suggested Reading

Beresford HR. Meralgia paresthetica after seat-belt trauma. J Trauma. 1971;11(7):629–30.

Blake SM, Treble NJ. Meralgia paraesthetica--an addition to 'seatbelt syndrome'. Ann R Coll Surg Engl. 2004;86(6):W6–7.

Bodner G, Bernathova M, Galiano K, Putz D, Martinoli C, Felfernig M. Ultrasound of the lateral femoral cutaneous nerve: normal findings in a cadaver and in volunteers. Reg Anesth Pain Med. 2009;34(3):265–8.

Carai A, Fenu G, Sechi E, Crotti FM, Montella A. Anatomical variability of the lateral femoral cutaneous nerve: findings from a surgical series. Clin Anat. 2009;22(3):365–70.

Damarey B, Demondion X, Boutry N, Kim HJ, Wavreille G, Cotten A. Sonographic assessment of the lateral femoral cutaneous nerve. J Clin Ultrasound. 2009;37(2):89–95.

Dias Filho LC, Valença MM, Guimarães Filho FA, et al. Lateral femoral cutaneous neuralgia: an anatomical insight. Clin Anat. 2003;16(4):309–16.

Dibenedetto LM, Lei Q, Gilroy AM, Hermey DC, Marks SC, Page DW. Variations in the inferior pelvic pathway of the lateral femoral cutaneous nerve: implications for laparoscopic hernia repair. Clin Anat. 1996;9(4):232–6.

Fargo MV, Konitzer LN. Meralgia paresthetica due to body armor wear in U.S. soldiers serving in Iraq: a case report and review of the literature. Mil Med. 2007;172(6):663–5.

Goel A. Meralgia paresthetica secondary to limb length discrepancy: case report. Arch Phys Med Rehabil. 1999;80(3):348–9.

Grossman MG, Ducey SA, Nadler SS, et al. Meralgia paresthetica: diagnosis and treatment. J Am Acad Orthop Surg. 2001;9(5):336–44.

Gupta A, Muzumdar D, Ramani PS. Meralgia paraesthetica following lumbar spine surgery: a study in 110 consecutive surgically treated cases. Neurol India. 2004;52(1):64–6.

Haim A, Pritsch T, Ben-Galim P, et al. Meralgia paresthetica: a retrospective analysis of 79 patients evaluated and treated according to a standard algorithm. Acta Orthop. 2006;77(3):482–6.

Harney D, Patijn J. Meralgia paresthetica: diagnosis and management strategies. Pain Med. 2007;8(8):669–77.

Hui GKM, Peng PWH. Meralgia paresthetica- what an anesthesiologist needs to know. Reg Anesth Pain Med. 2011;36:156–61.

Jiang GX, Xu WD, Wang AH. Spinal stenosis with meralgia paraesthetica. J Bone Joint Surg Br. 1988;70(2):272–3.

Kho KH, Blijham PJ, Zwarts MJ. Meralgia paresthetica after strenuous exercise. Muscle Nerve. 2005;31(6):761–3.

Korkmaz N, Ozcakar L. Meralgia paresthetica in a policeman: the belt or the gun. Plast Reconstr Surg. 2004;114(4):1012–3.

Li J, Tang S, Lam D, et al. Novel utilization of fascial layer blocks in hip and knee procedures. Best Pract Res Clin Anaesthesiol. 2019;33(4):539–51. https://doi.org/10.1016/j.bpa.2019.07.010.

Macgregor J, Moncur JA. Meralgia paraesthetica-a sports lesion in girl gymnasts. Br J Sports Med. 1977;11(1):16–9.

Martinez-Salio A, Moreno-Ramos T, Diaz-Sanchez M, et al. Meralgia paraesthetica: a report on a series of 140 cases. Rev Neurol. 2009;49(8):405–8.

Mirovsky Y, Neuwirth M. Injuries to the lateral femoral cutaneous nerve during spine surgery. Spine (Phila Pa 1976). 2000;25(10):1266–9.

Mondelli M, Rossi S, Romano C. Body mass index in meralgia paresthetica: a case-control study. Acta Neurol Scand. 2007;116(2):118–23.

Moritz T, Prosch H, Berzaczy D, et al. Common anatomical variation in patients with idiopathic meralgia paresthetica: a high resolution ultrasound case-control study. Pain Physician. 2013;16(3):E287–93.

Moscona AR, Sekel R. Post-traumatic meralgia paresthetica--an unusual presentation. J Trauma. 1978;18(4):288.

Ng I, Vaghadia H, Choi PT, et al. Ultrasound imaging accurately identifies the lateral femoral cutaneous nerve. Anesth Analg. 2008;107(3):1070–4.

Nielsen TD, Moriggl B, Barckman J, et al. The lateral femoral cutaneous nerve: description of the sensory territory and a novel ultrasound-guided nerve block technique. Reg Anesth Pain Med. 2018;43(4):357–66.

Otoshi K, Itoh Y, Tsujino A, et al. Case report: meralgia paresthetica in a baseball pitcher. Clin Orthop Relat Res. 2008;466(9):2268–70.

Parisi TJ, Mandrekar J, Dyck PJ, et al. Meralgia paresthetica: relation to obesity, advanced age, and diabetes mellitus. Neurology. 2011;77(16):1538–42.

Park JW, Kim DH, Hwang M, et al. Meralgia paresthetica caused by hip-huggers in a patient with aberrant course of the lateral femoral cutaneous nerve. Muscle Nerve. 2007;35(5):678–80.

Sax TW, Rosenbaum RB. Neuromuscular disorders in pregnancy. Muscle Nerve. 2006;34(5):559–71.

Swezey E, Bordoni B. Anatomy, bony pelvis and lower limb, lateral femoral cutaneous nerve. [Updated 2021 Aug 11]. In: StatPearls [Internet]. Treasure Island (FL): StatPearls Publishing; 2022. Available from: https://www.ncbi.nlm.nih.gov/books/NBK532301/

Szewczyk J, Hoffmann M, Kabelis J. Meralgia paraesthetica in a bodybuilder. Sportverletz Sportschaden. 1994;8(1):43–5.

Ulkar B, Yildiz Y, Kunduracioglu B. Meralgia paresthetica: a long-standing performance-limiting cause of anterior thigh pain in a soccer player. Am J Sports Med. 2003;31(5):787–9.

van Slobbe AM, Bohnen AM, Bernsen RM, et al. Incidence rates and determinants in meralgia paresthetica in general practice. J Neurol. 2004;251(3):294–7.

Yang SH, Wu CC, Chen PQ. Postoperative meralgia paresthetica after posterior spine surgery: incidence, risk factors, and clinical outcomes. Spine (Phila Pa 1976). 2005;30(18):E547–50.

Yi TI, Yoon TH, Kim JS, et al. Femoral neuropathy and meralgia paresthetica secondary to an iliacus hematoma. Ann Rehabil Med. 2012;36(2):273–7.

Zhu J, Zhao Y, Liu F, Huang Y, Shao J, Hu B. Ultrasound of the lateral femoral cutaneous nerve in asymptomatic adults. BMC Musculoskelet Disord. 2012;22(13):227.

Obturator Nerve Block

58

Thomas Fichtner Bendtsen

Contents

General Consideration

All branches of the obturator nerve (ON) can be anesthetized in the thigh. The ON can be blocked by either a subpectineal approach or selective approaches to each of the anterior and posterior branches (Fig. 58.1). The ON can also be anesthetized as part of a lumbar plexus block, also known as a psoas compartment block. In that case, ON is anesthetized together with the femoral nerve, the lateral femoral cutaneous nerve, and the genitofemoral nerve. The lumbar plexus approach to obturator nerve block will be discussed in another chapter of this book.

A "fascia iliaca compartment block" (FICB) is an injection of local anesthetic into the compartment between the iliopsoas muscle and the transversalis fascia extending from the iliac crest to the lesser trochanter. It is a common assumption among regional anesthetists that a FICB anesthetizes the ON, as a short segment of this nerve runs through the fascia iliaca compartment on the posteromedial aspect of the psoas major muscle between the emergence of the ON from the psoas compartment and its entrance into the retroperitoneal compartment. However, even large volumes of local anesthetic injected using a suprainguinal FICB technique do not extend to the said posteromedial part of the fascia iliaca compartment and thus do not produce an obturator nerve block.

It is also assumed in the literature that injecting local anesthetic in the so-called iliopsoas compartment deep to the iliopsoas muscle (i.e., the iliopsoas plane block or the PENG block) would anesthetize the ON branches innervating the hip joint capsule and intra-articular joint structures. However, that is unlikely. The dense iliopsoas fascia is tightly adherent to the hip capsule from the inguinal ligament to the lesser trochanter, which effectively impedes spread of injectate from the iliopsoas compartment to the ON. Even a large injectate proximal to the inguinal ligament does not reach the location, where the obturator nerve exits the psoas compartment on the posteromedial aspect of the psoas major.

T. F. Bendtsen (✉)
Department of Anesthesiology, Aarhus University Hospital, Aarhus, Denmark
e-mail: tfb@dadlnet.dk

D. Jankovic, P. Peng (eds.), *Regional Nerve Blocks in Anesthesia and Pain Therapy*,
https://doi.org/10.1007/978-3-030-88727-8_58

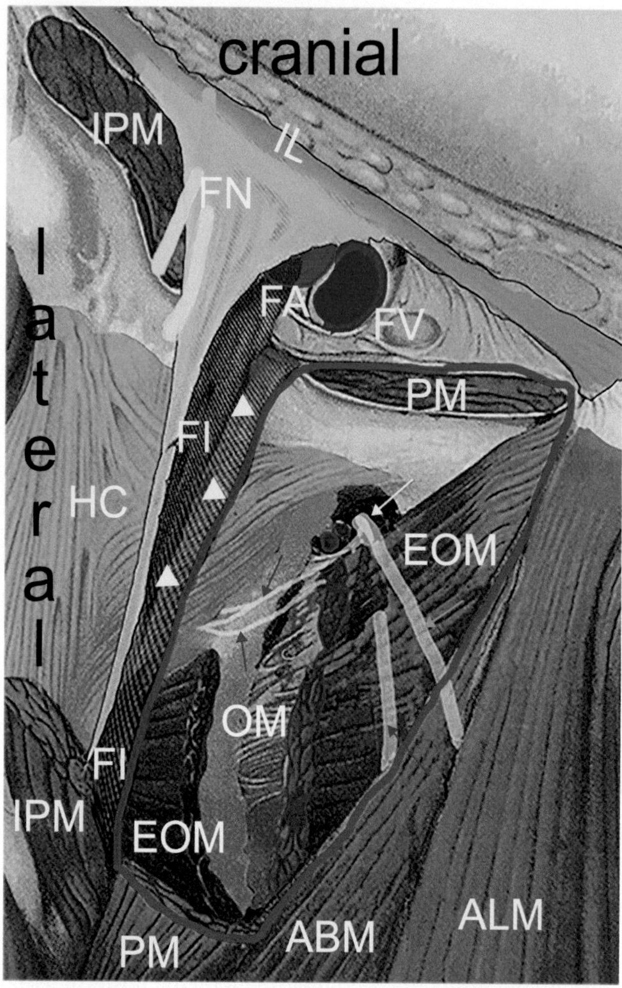

Fig. 58.1 Anatomy of the obturator nerve in the subinguinal region. The red "window" is made by resection of the pectineus muscle (PM). Part of the external obturator muscle (EOM) is also resected. This exposes the obturator nerve (ON), where it exits the obturator canal (white arrow). The anterior branch of the ON (green arrow) descends between the PM (resected) and EOM before it becomes sandwiched between the adductor longus muscle (ALM) and the adductor brevis muscle (ABM). The posterior branch (blue arrow) of the ON is seen to pierce the EOM before it descends posterior to the ABM. The hip articular branches (red arrows) deviate medially toward the acetabular notch at the exit of the ON from the obturator canal (white arrow). The PM is the "floor" of the vascular infra-inguinal compartment that contains the femoral artery (FA) and vein (FV), which are both resected. The lateral wall of the vascular compartment is the very dense fascia iliopsoica (FI). The entire FI is the "quiver" that contains the iliopsoas muscle (IPM) and the femoral nerve (FN) in the muscular infra-inguinal compartment. The FI is tightly adherent to the hip capsule (HC) from the inguinal ligament (IL) to the minor trochanter (not shown), and thus effectively obstructs any infra-inguinal spread of injectate from the muscular compartment (i.e., the "fascia iliaca compartment") to the vascular compartment and the subpectineal space that contains the ON. Printed at the courtesy of Thomas Bendtsen

Indications (Patient Selection)

A subpectineal ON block is indicated as a supplement to a femoral nerve block or a fascia iliaca compartment block for pain relief of hip fracture pain after arrival to the emergency ward prior to surgery. An obturator nerve block has no effect on pain after total hip replacement with a posterior surgical approach. Whether it relieves pain after an anterior approach is not known.

A subpectineal ON block can be indicated for suppression of adductor spasms due to the obturator reflex elicited by diathermy current during transurethral resection of urinary bladder tumors. In addition, a subpectineal ON block can be indicated for major knee surgery (total knee arthroplasty or anterior cruciate ligament repair) when distal approaches to ON contribution to posterior knee innervation (i.e., selective posterior obturator nerve block, popliteal plexus block, or infiltration between popliteal artery and capsule of the knee, also called iPACK) are not feasible. Finally, a subpectineal ON block is indicated for pain relief after amputation above the knee.

A selective posterior ON branch block can be indicated for pain relief after total knee arthroplasty and anterior cruciate ligament repair. However, it is not the first choice for anesthesia of the obturator innervation of the posterior part of the knee joint. A popliteal plexus block or an iPACK block would be preferable because of the motor-sparing effect and extended coverage to posterior innervation of the knee joint, including the other branches of ON and the proximal component of sciatic nerve. That said, the paralysis of the hip adductors with a subpectineal obturator nerve block or a selective posterior obturator nerve block does not impede ambulation critically after total knee arthroplasty.

A selective anterior obturator nerve block is only indicated in combination with a selective posterior obturator nerve block for amputation above the knee or suppression of adductor spasms in cases where such a combination is preferable to a subpectineal obturator nerve block. Of note, the distal dual block of the anterior and posterior branches is a more basic, easier to learn nerve block compared to the proximal subpectineal obturator nerve block. Thus, the combined distal approach is preferable compared to the proximal approach for nonexpert regional anesthetists.

Functional Anatomy

The obturator nerve originates from the lumbar L2–L4 ventral rami fusing in the psoas compartment between the anterior and posterior lamina of the psoas major muscle. It exits the psoas compartment at the posteromedial aspect of the psoas major muscle, where it crosses the so-called fascia iliaca compartment posterior to the internal iliac artery and vein. Subsequently, it enters the pelvic part of the retroperitoneal compartment. The obturator nerve exits the pelvis via the obturator canal, where it splits in an anterior and a posterior branch (Fig. 58.1).

First, the anterior branch is sandwiched between the obturator externus muscle posteriorly and the pectineus muscle anteriorly. It then descends between the adductor brevis and

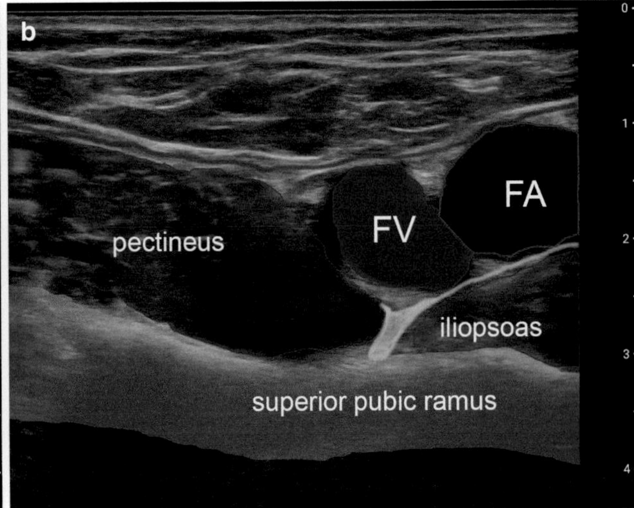

Fig. 58.2 The starting position. (**a**) Without labels. (**b**) With labels. The femoral artery (FA) and vein (FV) are tracked proximally with ultrasound until they are visualized anterior to the superior pubic ramus together with the pectineus muscle medially and the iliopsoas muscle laterally. This is the *starting position*. Fascia lata, pink. Iliopsoas fascia, cyan. Printed at the courtesy of Thomas Bendtsen

longus muscles (Fig. 58.1). It innervates the adductor longus and brevis muscles, the gracilis muscle, the hip joint, and occasionally a small and variable cutaneous area either in the popliteal fossa or the posteromedial aspect of the thigh. However, this cutaneous innervation has no relevance for pain after knee surgery. The hip articular branches (Fig. 58.1) from the obturator nerve depart immediately at the exit of the obturator canal between the pectineus and external obturator nerve.

The posterior branch often pierces the obturator externus muscle separate from the anterior branch (Fig. 58.1). The posterior branch descends between the adductor brevis and magnus muscles before it pierces the proximal part of the adductor magnus muscle. It emerges either on the anterior or the posterior aspect of the adductor magnus near the inferior tendinous margin of the muscle. The terminal posterior branch of the obturator nerve and a major branch from the tibial nerve are the main contributors to the dense popliteal plexus formed around the popliteal artery and vein and innervating the posterior part of the knee joint. In addition, the posterior branch innervates the obturator externus muscle and the proximal part of the adductor magnus muscle.

Techniques

The obturator nerve can be anesthetized selectively with a subpectineal approach. The anterior branch can be anesthetized selectively between the adductor longus and brevis muscles. The posterior branch can be anesthetized selectively between the adductor brevis and magnus muscles.

Generally, the patient is placed supine with the thigh slightly externally rotated. A high-frequency linear ultrasound transducer is placed in the inguinal crease, visualizing the femoral artery on top of the pectineus muscle anterior to the superior pubic ramus midway between the anterior superior iliac spine and the pubic symphysis. This is the *starting position* (Fig. 58.2).

Selective Obturator Nerve Block: Subpectineal Approach

The transducer is shifted distally from the starting position along the medial margin of the pectineus until the interfascial plane between the pectineus and obturator externus muscles is visualized inferomedial to the inferior border of the superior pubic ramus (Fig. 58.3). At this level, the adductor brevis emerges medially between the pectineus and external obturator muscles, and the adductor longus tendon is located medial to the pectineus and anterior to the adductor brevis muscle (Fig. 58.3). Oftentimes, a distal tilt of the transducer is required to obtain good visualization of the target interfascial plane. Usually, the ON branches can be visualized ultrasonographically. However, visualization of the target nerve branches is not required for successful nerve block, as this is a fascial plane block. Injection of 10 mL of local anesthetic into the target interfascial plane effectively spreads to the external orifice of the obturator canal and thus anesthetizes both the anterior and posterior branches of the obturator nerve, despite the fact that often the posterior branch intersects the target interfascial plane some distance from the anterior branch (Fig. 58.3).

Once the target interfascial plane is in the center of the monitor and the image depth, focus, and gain are optimized, a needle is inserted either in-plane or out-of-plane and care-

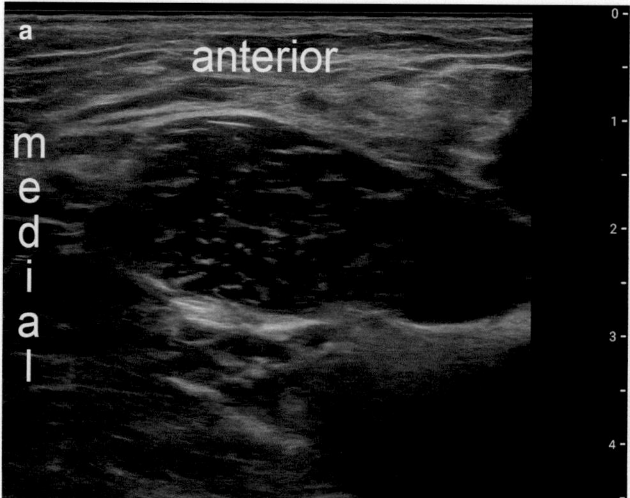

Fig. 58.3 The subpectineal obturator nerve block. (**a**) Without labels. (**b**) With labels. The ultrasound transducer is shifted distally from the starting position until the target interfascial plane between the pectineus and external obturator muscles become visible on the inferomedial side of the inferior border of the superior pubic ramus. The adductor longus muscle/tendon and the adductor brevis muscle are visible medially. The anterior branch of the obturator nerve (aON) is consistently visible in the target interfascial plane. Oftentimes, the posterior branch of the obturator nerve (pON) is separate from the aON and is seen in the external obturator muscle. Injection into the target interfascial plane is sufficient as the injectate spreads proximally to the external orifice of the obturator canal, thus anesthetizing the pON and the hip articular branches of the obturator nerve in addition to the aON. Target of injection, cyan asterisk. Femoral vein, FV. Fascia lata, pink. Printed at the courtesy of Thomas Bendtsen

fully advanced until the needle tip is located between the pectineus and obturator externus muscles. Typically, a palpable loss of resistance is felt when the needle tip enters the target interfascial plane between the two muscles. After careful aspiration to exclude intravascular needle tip placement, 10 mL of local anesthetic is injected while observing appropriate spread of the injectate between the pectineus and external obturator muscles. As the injectate effectively reaches the external orifice of the obturator canal, the hip branches are consistently anesthetized with this approach.

Selective Anterior and Posterior Obturator Nerve Branch Blocks

The transducer is shifted distally and medially from the starting position until the three adductor muscles (longus, brevis, and magnus) become clearly visible just medial to the pectineus muscle (Fig. 58.4). The anterior ON branch is located in the interfascial plane between the adductor longus muscle anteriorly and the adductor brevis muscle posteriorly (Fig. 58.4). The posterior ON branch is located in the interfascial plane between the adductor brevis muscle anteriorly and the adductor magnus muscle posteriorly (Fig. 58.4). The two ON branches are ultrasonographically visible as hyperechoic round or elliptical structures in cross section. Sonographic visibility of the target nerve branches is facilitated by shifting the transducer up and down in the proximal thigh while tracking the target nerves from an inter-adductor position to a position between the pectineus muscle and external obturator muscle and vice versa.

The needle is inserted either in-plane or out-of-plane and carefully advanced until the needle tip is located in the target interfascial plane. The two target planes can easily be injected with a single needle trajectory. Perineural injection of 5–10 mL of local anesthetic is carried out for each of the target ON branches. The nerve branches typically become distinctly visible after injection due to the contrast effect generated between the anechoic injectate and the hyperechoic target nerve branches.

Complications

1. Intravascular injection of local anesthetic
2. Hematoma due to injury of the great saphenous vein, femoral artery, or femoral vein

Practical Tips

The risk of intravascular injection of local anesthetic can be minimized by meticulous intermittent aspiration before and during injection of local anesthetic and real-time ultrasonographic observation of perineural spread of injectate. In addition, the transducer pressure should be released prior to injection in order to check for intravenous location of the needle tip with sonography. Furthermore, color or power

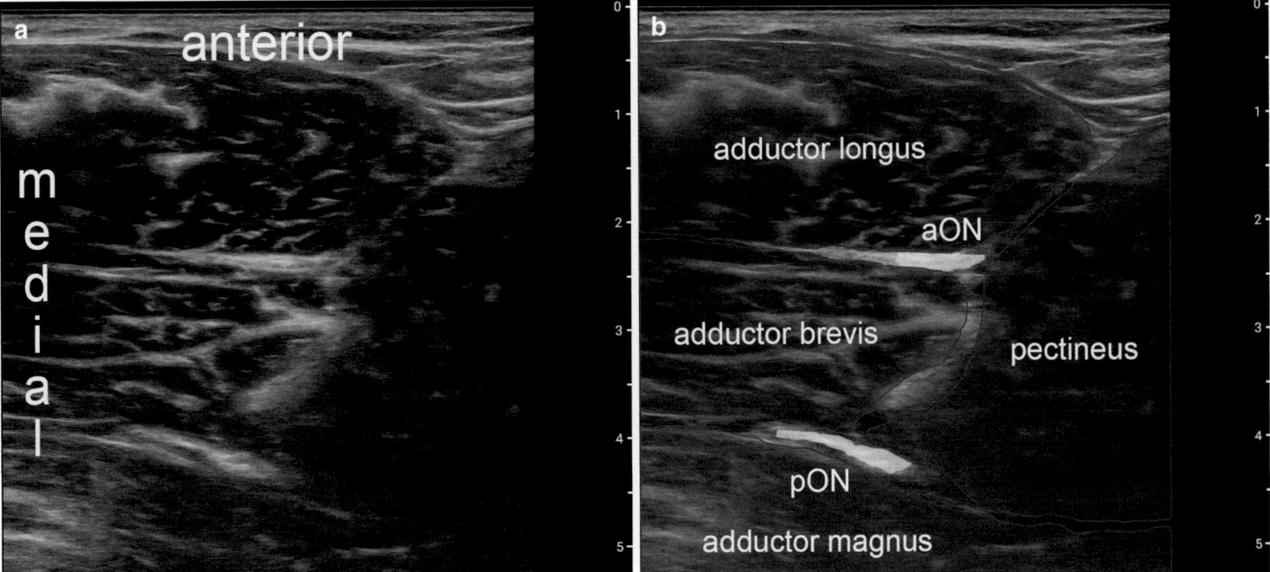

Fig. 58.4 Selective anterior and posterior obturator nerve block. (**a**) Without labels. (**b**) With labels. The transducer is shifted medial and distal from the starting position until the characteristic three-layered presentation of the adductor longus, brevis, and magnus muscles becomes visible medial to the pectineus muscle. The anterior obturator nerve (aON) is sandwiched between the adductors longus and brevis, while the posterior branch of the obturator nerve (pON) emerges between the adductor brevis and magnus muscles. Fascia lata, pink. Printed at the courtesy of Thomas Bendtsen

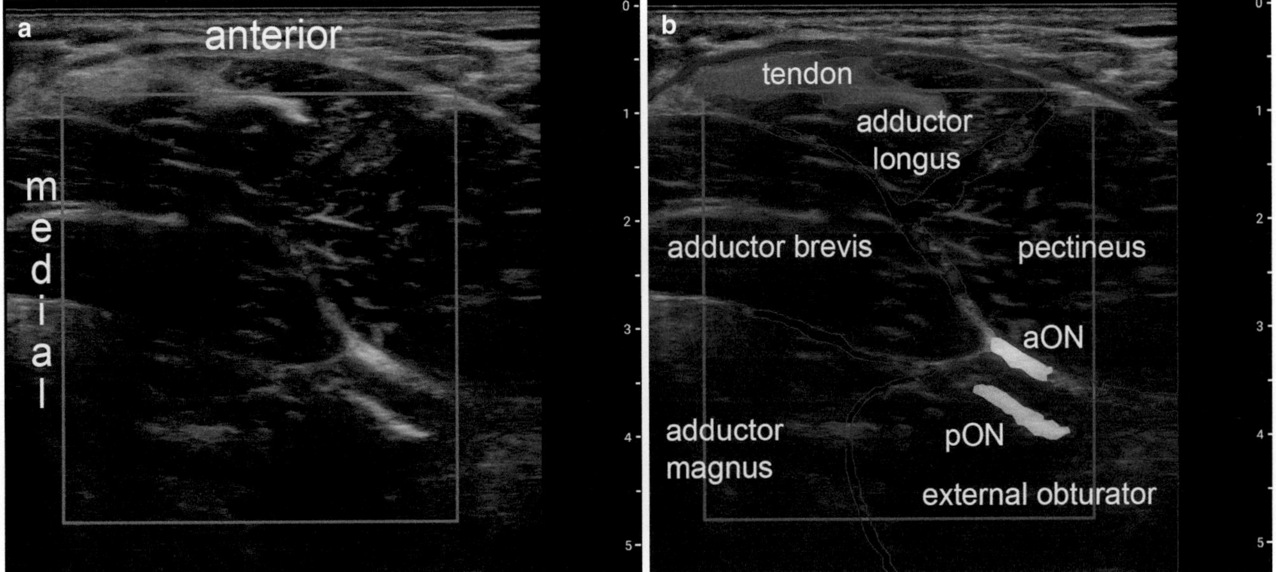

Fig. 58.5 Color Doppler for vascular visualization. (**a**) Without labels. (**b**) With labels. Color Doppler should always be applied to avoid a needle trajectory that intersects branches of the obturator artery and vein (red profiles) in addition to the great saphenous vein, the femoral artery, and the femoral vein. Anterior branch of the obturator nerve, aON. Posterior branch of the obturator nerve, pON. Fascia lata, pink. Printed at the courtesy of Thomas Bendtsen

Doppler should be applied prior to needle insertion and injection of local anesthetic to avoid vascular injury and intravascular injection (Fig. 58.5). Meticulous care is mandated in order to minimize the risk of accidental injury of the great saphenous vein or the femoral artery or femoral vein. The result of vascular injury can be a large hematoma in the thigh. Expert regional anesthetists with a preference for in-plane approach to the obturator nerve blocks should carry out a pre-scan meticulously identifying the great saphenous vein and the femoral artery and vein and plan the anticipated needle track in order to avoid these blood vessels.

Oftentimes, the tail of the transducer needs to be tilted distal in order to visualize the target interfascial plane between the pectineus muscle and the external obturator muscle with the subpectineal approach. An out-of-plane approach can make it a challenge to obtain intersection of the ultrasound beam and the needle when the needle is inserted distal to the transducer. In that case, appropriate ultrasonographic visualization of the needle tip in the target position can be facilitated by out-of-plane insertion of the needle proximal to the transducer.

Literature Review

The hip articular branches are effectively reached with a subpectineal obturator nerve block approach.

An obturator nerve block has no analgesic effect on pain after total hip replacement with a posterior approach. Probably because all the intra-articular nociceptors from the obturator nerve are excised.

A subinguinal obturator nerve block probably is effective as a supplement to a femoral nerve block or fascia iliaca compartment block for relieving pain due to hip fracture prior to surgery. However, no well-designed trials have assessed this.

MRI scans in a volunteer trial assessed the spread of 40 mL injectate after suprainguinal fascia iliaca compartment block. The authors concluded that the spread reached the ON. Unfortunately, this was a misinterpretation of the topography of the obturator nerve.

The posterior branch of the obturator nerve consistently contributes to the posterior innervation of the knee joint via the popliteal plexus. A supplementary infrainguinal, subpectineal obturator nerve block effectively relieves pain after total knee arthroplasty. However, in order to avoid hip adductor paralysis, it would probably be preferable to block the genicular innervation from the posterior branch of the obturator nerve with a more distal approach like the popliteal plexus block or the iPACK. In clinical practice, peripheral nerve blocks for pain relief after major knee surgery is practically always applied as a supplement to intraoperative local infiltration analgesia (LIA). However, LIA is most likely redundant with effective nerve blockade of the posterior innervation of the knee. Further clinical studies are required to clarify this.

The cutaneous obturator nerve innervation of the medial mid-thigh is small and highly variable when present, but the obturator nerve has no cutaneous innervation in more than 50% of human beings. The anteromedial cutaneous genicular innervation is practically always due to the medial femoral cutaneous nerve. Thus, the cutaneous obturator nerve innervation has no relevance for pain after knee surgery.

Suggested Reading

Bendtsen TF, Moriggl B, Chan V, Børglum. The optimal analgesic block for total knee arthroplasty. Reg Anesth Pain Med. 2016;41(6):711–9.

Bendtsen TF, Pedersen EM, Peng P. Course of the obturator nerve. Reg Anesth Pain Med. 2019;44(11):1039–40.

Bjørn S, Nielsen TD, Moriggl B, Hoermann R, Bendtsen TF. Anesthesia of the anterior femoral cutaneous nerves for total knee arthroplasty incision: randomized volunteer trial. Reg Anesth Pain Med. 2020;45(2):107–16.

Bouaziz H, Vial F, Jochum D, Macalou D, Heck M, Meuret P, Braun M, Laxenaire M. An evaluation of the cutaneous distribution after obturator nerve block. Anesth Analg. 2002;94(2):445–9.

Fonkoué L, Behets C, Kouassi JK, Covette M, Detrembleur C, Thienpont E, Cornu O. Distribution of sensory nerves supplying the knee joint capsule and implications for genicular blockade and radiofrequency ablation: an anatomical study. Anesth Pain Med. 2019;44(2):234–8.

Layera S, Aliste J, Bravo D, Saadawi M, Salinas FV, Tran Q. Motor-sparing nerve blocks for total knee replacement: a scoping review. J Clin Anesth. 2021;68:110076.

Nielsen TD, Moriggl B, Søballe K, Kolsen-Petersen JA, Børglum J, Bendtsen TF. A cadaveric study of ultrasound-guided subpectineal injectate spread around the obturator nerve and its hip articular branches. Reg Anesth Pain Med. 2017;42(3):357–61.

Nielsen ND, Madsen MN, Østergaard HK, Bjørn S, Pedersen EM, Nielsen TD, Søballe K, Børglum J, Bendtsen TF. An iliopsoas plane block does not cause motor blockade - a blinded randomized volunteer trial. Acta Anaesthesiol Scand. 2020;64:368–77.

Runge C, Børglum J, Jensen JM, Kobborg T, Pedersen A, Sandberg J, Mikkelsen LR, Vase M, Bendtsen TF. The analgesic effect of obturator nerve block added to a femoral triangle block after Total knee arthroplasty: a randomized controlled trial. Reg Anesth Pain Med. 2016;41(4):445–51.

Runge C, Moriggl B, Borglum J, Bendtsen TF. The spread of ultrasound-guided injectate from the adductor canal to the genicular branch of the posterior obturator nerve and the popliteal plexus a cadaveric study. Reg Anesth Pain Med. 2017;42(6):725–30.

Tran J, Giron Arango L, Peng P, Sinha SK, Agur A, Chan V. Evaluation of the iPACK block injectate spread: a cadaveric study. Reg Anesth Pain Med. 2019a;44(7):689–94.

Tran J, Peng PWH, Gofeld M, Chan V, Agur AMR. Anatomical study of the innervation of posterior knee joint capsule: implication for image-guided intervention. Reg Anesth Pain Med. 2019b;44(2):234–8.

Vermeylen K, Desmet M, Leunen I, Soetens F, Neyrinck A, Carens D, Caerts B, Seynaeve P, Hadzic A, Van de Velde M. Supra-inguinal injection for fascia iliaca compartment block results in more consistent spread towards the lumbar plexus than an infra-inguinal injection: a volunteer study. Reg Anesth Pain Med. 2019;44:483–91.

Proximal Nerve Block Approaches to the Sciatic Nerve

59

Reva Ramlogan, Jordan Zunder, and Colin J. L. McCartney

Contents

Introduction

This chapter presents two common approaches to ultrasound-guided sciatic nerve blockade, the subgluteal approach and the anterior approach. Patients having lower limb surgery, particularly orthopaedic surgery, are potential candidates for sciatic nerve blocks, for the provision of not only post-operative analgesia but also surgical anaesthesia.

Indication

The indications are listed in Table 59.1.

Anatomy of the Sciatic Nerve

The sciatic nerve (also known at the *ischiadic* nerve) originates from the convergence of the L4–S3 ventral rami of the lumbosacral plexus. It is both the widest and longest peripheral nerve in the body, measuring up to 2 cm at its proximal origin at the greater sciatic foramen and extending from the inferior aspect of the piriformis muscle to the superior aspect of the popliteal fossa. It is composed of a tibial component (formed from the anterior divisions of the ventral rami of the lumbosacral plexus) and a common peroneal component (formed from the posterior divisions of the ventral rami of the lumbosacral plexus). These components are bound together within the same connective tissue sheath and travel together as the sciatic nerve before dividing at the popliteal fossa into the terminal branches of the tibial nerve and common peroneal nerve.

At its origin at the greater sciatic foramen, the sciatic nerve is bordered anteriorly by the body of the ischium and posteriorly by the piriformis muscle, deep to gluteus maximus which forms the most dorsal structure overlying this space (Fig. 59.1). The sciatic nerve is quite superficial at the inferior border of the gluteus maximus muscle, and here it is amenable to peripheral nerve blockade via the subgluteal approach (Fig. 59.2). Medial to the sciatic nerve at this level are the inferior gluteal nerve, artery and veins, as well as the pudendal nerve, artery and veins. The sciatic nerve itself is the lateral-most structure as it exits the greater sciatic foramen. Here, it descends, running inferolaterally

R. Ramlogan · J. Zunder · C. J. L. McCartney (✉)
Department of Anesthesiology and Pain Medicine, The Ottawa Hospital, University of Ottawa, Ottawa, ON, Canada
e-mail: rramlogan@toh.ca; jzunder@toh.ca; cmccartney@toh.ca

D. Jankovic, P. Peng (eds.), *Regional Nerve Blocks in Anesthesia and Pain Therapy*,
https://doi.org/10.1007/978-3-030-88727-8_59

Table 59.1 Possible indications for subgluteal and anterior sciatic nerve blocks

SUBGLUTEAL APPROACH	ANTERIOR APPROACH
1. **Above-knee amputation in conjunction with femoral and obturator nerve blocks** (n.b. PFCN is blocked only 68% of the time)	1. **To avoid patient repositioning or when the patient is not able to reposition**
2. **Below-knee amputation in conjunction with femoral or saphenous nerve block**	2. **Below-knee amputation in conjunction with femoral or saphenous nerve block**
3. **Tibial, fibular or ankle surgery in conjunction with saphenous nerve block** (if procedure is on medial aspect)	3. **Tibial, fibular or ankle surgery in conjunction with saphenous nerve block** (if procedure is on medial aspect)
4. **If a popliteal approach to the sciatic nerve or a popliteal-fossa catheter is not feasible**	4. **If a popliteal approach to the sciatic nerve or a popliteal-fossa catheter is not feasible**
	5. **Possibly easier for catheter tip visualization when the longitudinal approach is used**

PFCN posterior femoral cutaneous nerve of the thigh

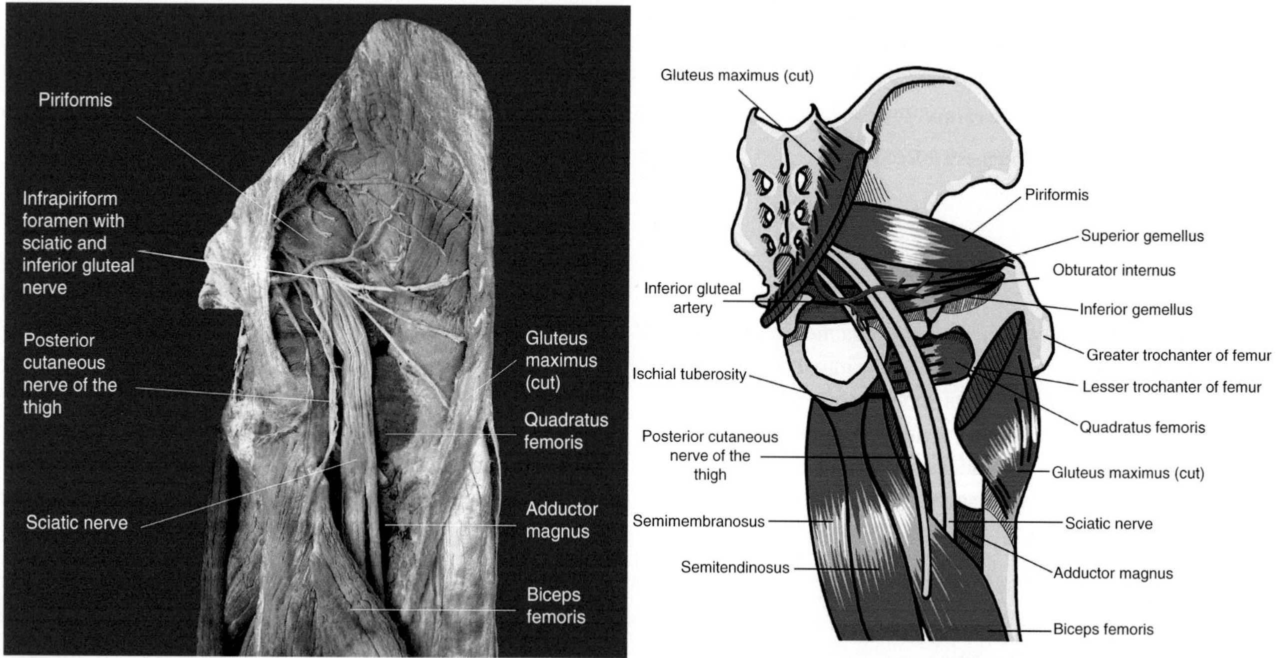

Fig. 59.1 Posterior muscle dissection of thigh showing the course of the sciatic nerve and its anatomic relations. Left. Cadaveric dissection. Reprinted with permission from Dr. Danilo Jankovic. Right. Schematic diagram

between the greater trochanter of the femur and the ischial tuberosity, bordered anteriorly by the superior and inferior gemelli, obturator internus, quadratus femoris and adductor magnus muscles and posteriorly by the long head of biceps femoris, before entering the posterior compartment of the thigh. As the sciatic nerve continues further distally, it becomes bordered anteriorly by the adductor magnus muscle and posteriorly by the muscles, which comprise the hamstrings (biceps femoris, semimembranosus and semitendinosus muscles). At this location, the sciatic nerve may be the target of peripheral nerve blockade via the anterior approach (Fig. 59.3).

The sciatic nerve and its two branches (the tibial and common peroneal nerves) supply all motor innervation to the posterior thigh, as well as the leg and foot muscles. It supplies cutaneous sensory innervation to the lower leg (except for the medial aspect) and is the origin of the articular sensory branches of the lower limb joints.

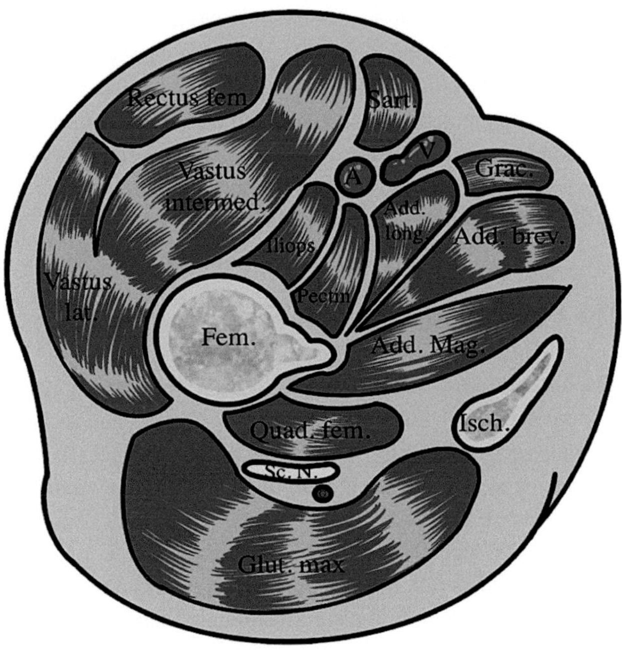

Fig. 59.2 Cross section of the thigh at the level of the posterior (subgluteal) approach to the sciatic nerve. *A* femoral artery, *V* femoral vein, *G* inferior gluteal nerve, *Sc. N* sciatic nerve, *Fem* femur, *isch* ischial tuberosity, *glut. max* gluteus maximus, *sart* sartorius, *grac* gracilis, *pectin* pectineus, *iliops* iliopsoas, *vastus lat* vastus lateralis, *vastus intermed* vastus intermedius, *rectus fem* rectus femoris, *add. long* adductor longus, *add. mag* adductor magnus, *quad fem* quadratus femoris, *add brev* adductor brevis

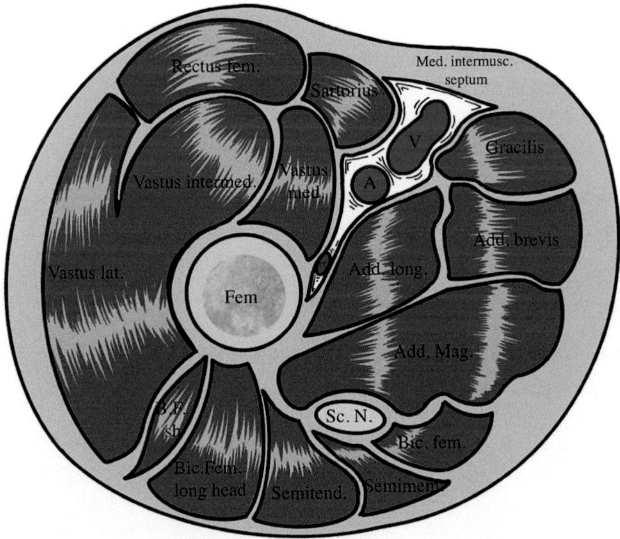

Fig. 59.3 Cross section of the thigh at the level of the anterior approach to the sciatic nerve. *A* femoral artery, *V* femoral vein, *PF* profunda femoris artery, *Fem* femur, *Sc. N* sciatic nerve, *med. Intermusc. septum* medial intermuscular septum of the thigh, *add. long* adductor longus, *add. mag* adductor magnus, *bic. fem.* biceps femoris, *semimem* semimembranosus, *semitend* semitendinosus, *bic. fem. long head* biceps femoris long head, *b.f. short head* biceps femoris short head, *vastus lat* vastus lateralis, *vastus intermed* vastus intermedius, *rectus fem* rectus femoris, *vastus med* vastus medialis

Techniques

The Ultrasound-Guided Subgluteal Approach

Because of the depth of the sciatic nerve, traditional approaches relying solely on surface landmarking and nerve stimulation are rarely performed. Furthermore, nerve stimulation of the sciatic nerve may not always produce a motor response. The ultrasound-guided subgluteal approach affords proximal blockade using traditional surface anatomy combined with visual reassurance that the block needle is at the appropriate depth and proximity to the sciatic nerve.

The term subgluteal should not be taken to mean the block is performed at the subgluteal *fold* but instead to the space or compartment between the gluteus maximus muscle and the quadratus femoris muscle. The subgluteal space is an intermuscular plane extending from the greater trochanter laterally to the ischial tuberosity medially. The amount of overlying adipose tissue decreases more distally; thus, better nerve visualization may be achieved within the distal portion of subgluteal compartment. At the level of these two bony landmarks, the sciatic nerve appears as an oval hyperechoic structure 1.5–2 cm wide and is situated closer to the ischial tuberosity, as opposed to equidistant between them, which was traditionally described.

Scanning Technique

The patient may be positioned prone, lateral or in the Sims position with the operative limb up. The Sims and lateral positions may stretch the gluteus maximus muscle when the hip is flexed, thereby making the sciatic nerve more superficial and echogenic. Standard monitors are applied and supplementary oxygen provided. As this is a fairly deep transmuscular block, sedation is recommended for patient comfort.

With the patient in the lateral or Sims position, the operator usually stands behind the patient (Fig. 59.4). Following skin preparation with chlorhexidine, a curvilinear low-frequency probe is prepared with a sterile probe cover. The greater trochanter and ischial tuberosity are palpated with the *needling hand*, and the scanning hand places the transducer transversely between the two bony landmarks, to obtain a short-axis view of the nerve. The image quality should be optimized for depth, gain and focus as required. The oval, hyperechoic, multi-fascicular sciatic nerve can be visualized within the subgluteal compartment, bordered by the hyperechoic epimysium of the gluteus maximus muscle dorsally, and the epimysium of the quadratus femoris ventrally.

Injection

Prior to needle insertion, colour should be applied to the overlying needle trajectory, to avoid the inferior gluteal artery and its branches (Fig. 59.5). Following skin and subcutaneous infiltration with lidocaine, an 80–100 mm block (depending on depth of the nerve) needle can be inserted in-plane or out-of-plane. Hydrolocation with small aliquots of 5% dextrose can be used to confirm needle tip location as the needle advances. This may be particularly useful in the out-of-plane approach. Some practitioners may find the out-of-plane approach easier for advancement of a catheter within the paraneurium.

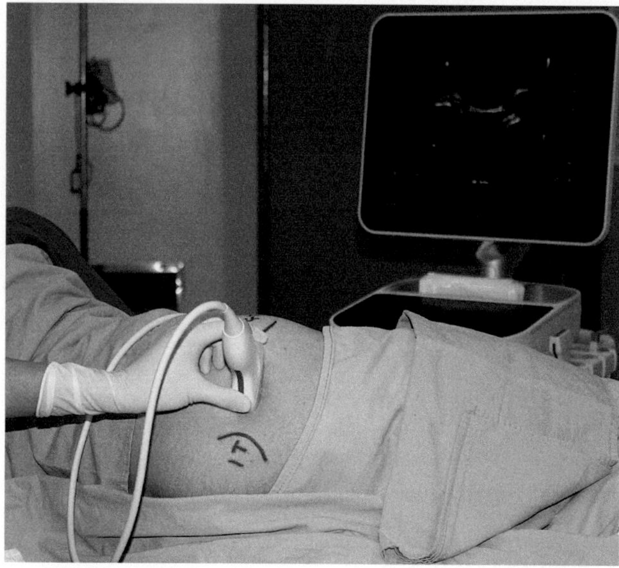

Fig. 59.4 Positioning for the subgluteal approach. The patient lies lateral with the operative side up; the hip and knee are flexed. The operator is positioned behind the patient. Note that the operator, the transducer and the ultrasound screen are all ergonomically aligned

Appropriate needle position can be confirmed with nerve stimulator or hydrolocation. After ensuring there is no expansion of nerve tissue with dextrose injection, the local anaesthetic is injected and the assistant should aspirate after every 5 ml to ensure the absence of blood. Relatively large volumes (20–40 mls) are required for surgical anaesthesia, due to the large circumference of the sciatic nerve.

The Ultrasound-Guided Anterior Approach

The anterior approach to the sciatic nerve may be warranted in patients who cannot turn laterally or prone due to body habitus or immobility factors such as external fixation devices. It is also advantageous from an efficiency perspective when a femoral or saphenous nerve block is also required, as repositioning for each block is not required. However, the depth to the sciatic nerve from the anterior thigh is greater than in the subgluteal approach and can vary considerably, depending on body habitus. Increasing depth makes needle visualization more challenging. Ota et al. examined the efficacy and procedure time for the ultrasound-guided anterior approach compared to the ultrasound-guided subgluteal approach. There was no difference in execution time or efficacy between the two approaches. The average depth of the sciatic nerve in the anterior approach was 6 cm, compared to 3.5 cm with the subgluteal approach. It should be noted, however, that the average BMI in both groups was approximately 23. Performing the block using either a short-axis or longitudinal view of the nerve in the proximal thigh has been described.

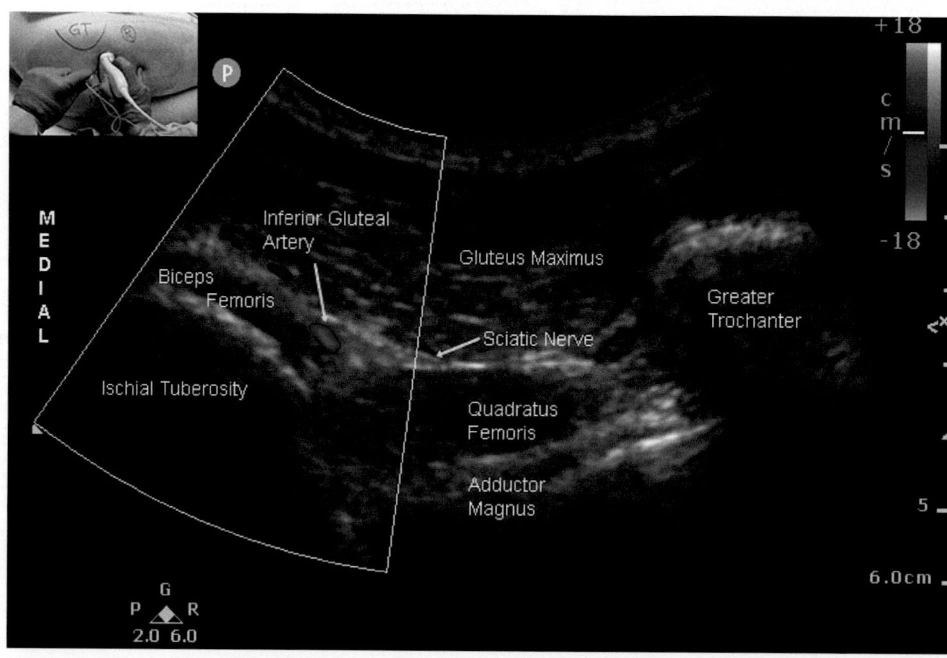

Fig. 59.5 In the subgluteal approach, the bony shadows of the greater trochanter (lateral) and the ischial tuberosity (medial) are easily identifiable. The sciatic nerve is a hyperechoic round/oval structure in the subgluteal space, between the gluteus maximus and the quadratus femoris. Colour Doppler identifies the inferior gluteal artery just medial to the sciatic nerve. Depth to the nerve is approximately 4 cm

As the sciatic travels caudally past the ischial tuberosity, it descends medial and parallel to the shaft of the femur, between the biceps femoris muscle posteriorly and the adductor magnus muscle anteriorly (Fig. 59.1). It is easier to perform the block distal to the lesser trochanter as this bony protuberance has been found to obscure the passage of the needle, unless the leg is internally rotated.

Scanning Technique

Standard monitors are applied and supplementary oxygen provided. As this is a deep transmuscular block, sedation is recommended for patient comfort. With the patient in the supine position, maintain the leg in neutral position, and prep with chlorhexidine from the inguinal crease to the distal thigh. The operator usually stands on the same side to be blocked.

A curvilinear low-frequency probe is prepared with a sterile probe cover. The additional use of nerve stimulation is advocated to due to the proximity of the branches from the femoral and obturator nerves, as well as for confirmation of needle tip position. Place the transducer transversely on the antero-medial thigh approximately one-third of the distance from the inguinal crease. This corresponds to a position overlying the sartorius and the adductor muscles (Fig. 59.6). The image quality should be optimized for depth, gain and focus as required. The oval, hyperechoic, multi-fascicular sciatic nerve can be visualized medial to the hypoechoic shadow of the femur. Appropriate transducer pressure, along with compression of the thigh with a hand under the hamstrings, may be required when visualization is challenging. Apply colour Doppler to visualize vessels, which may be in the path of the needle, such as the superficial femoral vessels, the profunda femoris vessels and their perforating muscle branches.

Injection

Either an in-plane or out-of-plane approach may be chosen. Even with an in-plane approach, the needle trajectory may be steep, making needle visualization challenging. Thus, hydrolocation with 5% dextrose and nerve stimulation are useful adjuncts. Because of challenges with both the nerve and needle visualization, some experts have proposed rotating the probe to view the sciatic in its longitudinal axis, thereby providing for a greater target. In this transducer orientation, the sciatic nerve appears as a hyperechoic cable-like structure (Fig. 59.7).

The needle may be inserted cephalad to caudad or vice versa. For a single-shot injection, there *may* be some advantage of injecting the local anaesthetic from caudad to cephalad, in order to obtain more proximal spread to potentially block the posterior cutaneous nerve of the thigh. Once a clear path is determined, the skin and subcutaneous tissue is infiltrated with lidocaine and an 80–120 mm block needle inserted. The nerve stimulator is turned on to 1–2 mA. Initially, there will be local muscle contractions of the thigh as the needle advances. Once the needle traverses the epimysium of the adductor magnus muscle, the muscle response will change to the foot due to stimulation of the sciatic nerve. Often, a fascial 'pop' can be ascertained. Ensure there is loss of motor response at ≤0.5 mA to avoid intra-neural injection,

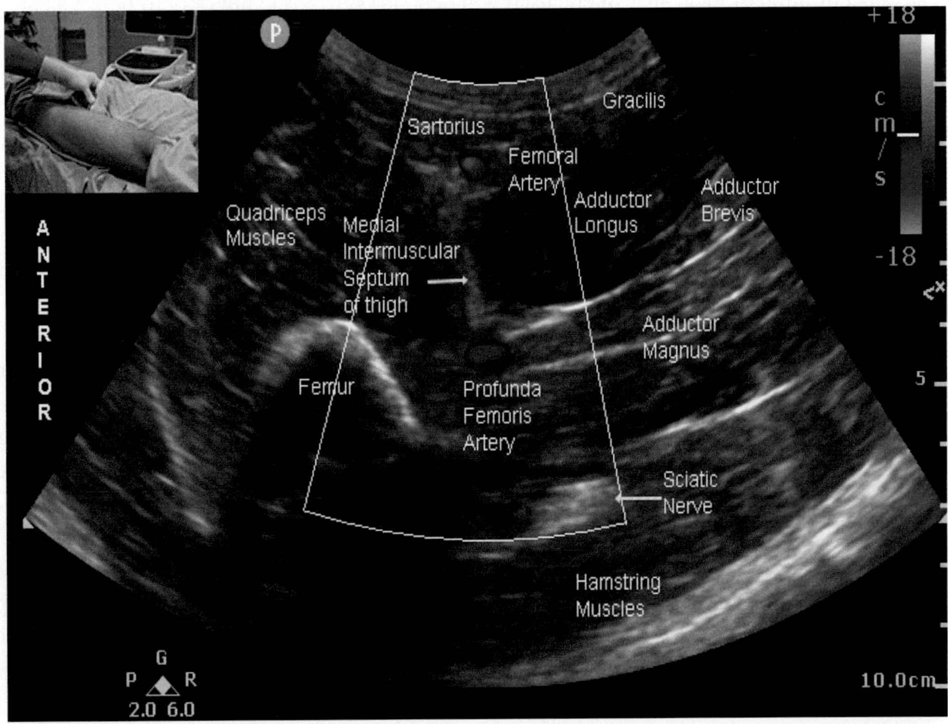

Fig. 59.6 In the anterior approach, the transducer is placed approximately 10 cm distal to the inguinal crease, on the anteromedial surface of the thigh. The sciatic nerve can be visualized as a hyperechoic oval shaped structure posteromedial to the femur, between the adductor magnus anteriorly and the biceps femoris (hamstring) muscles. Colour Doppler demonstrates the location of the femoral and profunda femoris vessels. Note the nerve is deeper in this approach, at approximately 6 cm

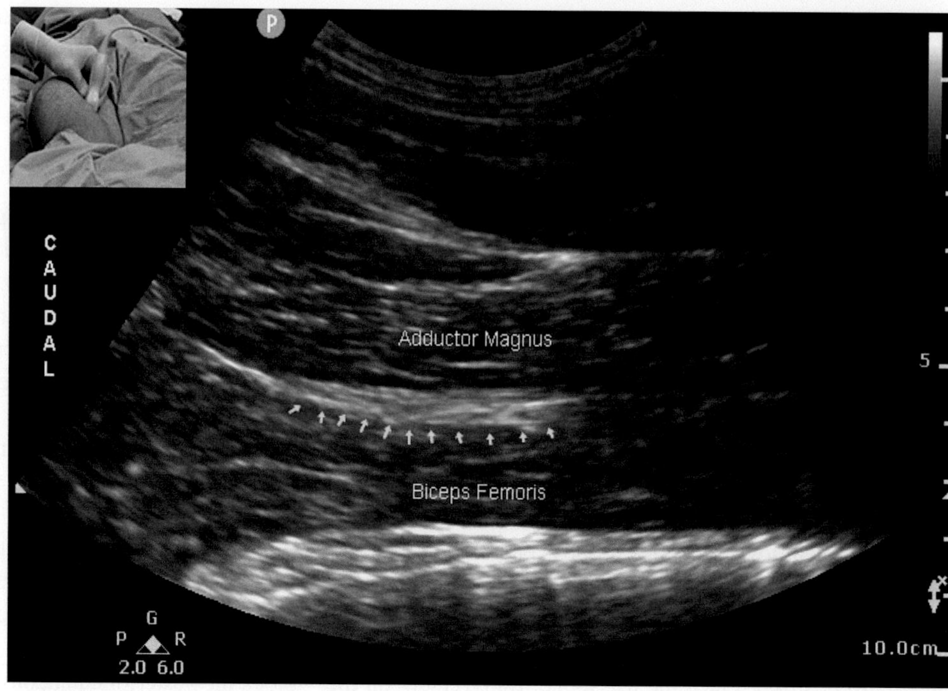

Fig. 59.7 A longitudinal view of the sciatic can be obtained by rotating the probe, once the image in Fig. 59.6 is achieved. Alternatively, one can palpate for the groove between the sartorius and the rectus femoris muscle and place the probe longitudinally. It may be necessary to slide the transducer lateral or medial to obtain the image of the sciatic nerve as a hyperechoic rope like structure (yellow arrows). The depth is approximately the same as in the transverse view (Fig. 59.6)

especially in the face of challenging needle tip visualization. On injection of local anaesthetic in the correct intermuscular plane, the nerve is displaced posteriorly and the adductor magnus elevates.

Local Anaesthetic Doses and Continuous Catheter Technique

The concentration of local anaesthetic used will depend on if surgical anaesthesia is required or just analgesia. In general, we use 0.5% ropivacaine with 2.5 mcg/ml epinephrine, as an intravascular marker, for surgical anaesthesia. Volumes of 30–40 mls are used depending on the patient's weight.

Inserting a catheter provides the benefit of extending post-operative analgesia. Post-operatively, we use 0.2% ropivacaine to provide analgesia. An electronic pump is used to deliver 5mls/hour with a patient bolus of 5mls every 30 minutes, as required.

There is no strong evidence to favour one catheter insertion technique over another in terms of long-axis versus short-axis view, with an in-plane versus out-of-plane needle approach. An in-plane approach with a shallow angle improves needle visibility. A long-axis view of the nerve with an in-plane view of the needle may allow for easier confirmation of the catheter in the correct plane. However, this technique may potentially take longer to perform due to challenges in maintaining the nerve, needle and catheter in view. Regardless of insertion technique, once the needle is in the correct position, a bolus of 5 mls of 5% dextrose solution can be used to dilate the space and make room for the catheter.

Literature Review

We have described two common methods of blocking the proximal sciatic nerve, but it should be noted that these are advanced blocks. The anterior approach may be challenging due not only to poor visualization of the nerve, as a result of anisotropy or its depth, but also because of the intervening blood vessels. New techniques and variations of previous techniques have been described to address these issues. Dolan described an approach using the same transducer position, but instead of inserting the needle adjacent to the transducer, the needle was inserted into the posterior-medial thigh at the level of the adductor magnus muscle. This insertion point places the needle perpendicular to the ultrasound beam, resulting in improved needle visualization and also avoiding neurovascular structures.

Recently, a lateral approach to the proximal sciatic nerve has been described in volunteers and cadavers. Nielsen et al. described placing the transducer 2–3 cm distal to the prominence of the greater trochanter, and posterior to the femur, in the transverse plane. At this level, the sciatic nerve is located in the intermuscular space between the gluteus maximus and the adductor magnus muscles. This approach appears promising as it avoids patient repositioning and major vascular structures. No clinical studies to evaluate the efficacy of either of these techniques have yet been performed.

Another lateral approach was recently investigated by Yoshida et al., to avoid patient repositioning and to improve blockade of the posterior femoral cutaneous nerve (PFCN). For above-the-knee amputations or for procedures requiring a thigh tourniquet, it may be necessary to block the PFCN, if the procedure is to be performed solely under peripheral nerve blockade. The PFCN (also known as the posterior cutaneous nerve of the thigh) supplies cutaneous innervation to the posterior thigh. It should be noted that this nerve diverges from the sciatic and becomes more superficial distal to the gluteus maximus muscle, and thus, it will not be blocked consistently when performing the subgluteal or anterior sciatic nerve block. The PFCN has previously been shown to be blocked about 68% of the time with the subgluteal approach but only 15% with the anterior approach. Yoshida et al. placed a curvilinear transducer at the most prominent level of the greater trochanter, to visualize both the greater trochanter and the ischial tuberosity. The transducer position was then translated cephalad or caudad to identify the origin of the biceps femoris on the ischium, and the sciatic nerve was blocked at this level. This lateral approach is more cephalad than Nielsen et al.'s but only successfully blocked the PFCN in 60% of cases.

As evidenced by recent studies and new block descriptions, blockade of the proximal sciatic nerve continues to be of practical clinical use and inspires investigators to develop methods to simply the technique.

Suggested Reading

Anderson T, Vilella R. Anatomy, bony pelvis and lower limb, posterior thigh. Treasure Island, FL: StatPearls Publishing; 2020. https://www.ncbi.nlm.nih.gov/books/NBK554598/. Accessed 3 December 2020

Chan VWS, Nova H, Abbas S, McCartney CJL, Perlas A, Quan Xu D. Ultrasound examination and localization of the sciatic nerve: a volunteer study. Anesthesiology. 2006;104(2):309–14. https://doi.org/10.1097/00000542-200602000-00017.

Dolan J. Ultrasound-guided anterior sciatic nerve block in the proximal thigh: an in-plane approach improving the needle view and respecting fascial planes. Br J Anaesth. 2013;110(2):319–20. https://doi.org/10.1093/bja/aes492.

Karmakar MK, Kwok WH, Ho AM, Tsang K, Chui PT, Gin T. Ultrasound-guided sciatic nerve block: description of a new approach at the subgluteal space. Br J Anaesth. 2007;98(3):390–5.

Koscielniak-Nielsen ZJ, Rasmussen H, Hesselbjerg L. Long-axis ultrasound imaging of the nerves and advancement of perineural catheters under direct vision: a preliminary report of four cases. Reg Anesth Pain Med. 2008;33(5):477–82. https://doi.org/10.1016/j.rapm.2008.02.009.

Moore KL, Agur AMR, Dalley AF. Clinically oriented anatomy. 8th ed. Wolters Kluwer; 2017.

Nielsen JK, Tranum-Jensen J, Bøgevig S. Proximal lateral approach to ultrasound-guided sciatic nerve block: a volunteer and cadaveric study. Reg Anesth Pain Med. 2019;44(7):715. https://doi.org/10.1136/rapm-2018-100203.

Ota J, Sakura S, Hara K, Saito Y. Ultrasound-guided anterior approach to sciatic nerve block: a comparison with the posterior approach. Anesth Analg. 2009;108(2):660–5.

Tran DQ, Salinas FV, Benzon HT, Neal JM. Lower extremity regional anesthesia: essentials of our current understanding. Reg Anesth Pain Med. 2019;44(2):143. https://doi.org/10.1136/rapm-2018-000019.

Tsui BCH, Özelsel TJ-P. Ultrasound-guided anterior sciatic nerve block using a longitudinal approach: "expanding the view". Reg Anesth Pain Med. 2008;33(3):275–6. https://doi.org/10.1016/j.rapm.2007.11.008.

Vloka JD, Hadžic A, April E, Thys DM. Anterior approach to the sciatic nerve block: the effects of leg rotation. Anesth Analg. 2001;92(2):460–2.

Wang A-Z, Gu L, Quan-Hong Z, Wen-Zong N, Wei J. Ultrasound-guided continuous femoral nerve block for analgesia after total knee arthroplasty: catheter perpendicular to the nerve versus catheter parallel to the nerve. Reg Anesth Pain Med. 2010;35(2):127–31.

Yoshida T, Nakamoto T, Hashimoto C, Aihara S, Nishimoto K, Kamibayashi T. An ultrasound-guided lateral approach for proximal sciatic nerve block: a randomized comparison with the anterior approach and a cadaveric evaluation. Reg Anesth Pain Med. 2018;43(7):712. https://doi.org/10.1097/AAP.0000000000000835.

Popliteal Sciatic Nerve Block

60

Amit Pawa and Ki Jinn Chin

Contents

A. Pawa
Department of Anaesthesia, Guy's and St Thomas' NHS Foundation Trust, London, UK

K. J. Chin (✉)
Department of Anesthesiology and Pain Medicine, Toronto Western Hospital, University of Toronto, Toronto, ON, Canada
e-mail: kijinn.chin@uhn.ca

D. Jankovic, P. Peng (eds.), *Regional Nerve Blocks in Anesthesia and Pain Therapy*,
https://doi.org/10.1007/978-3-030-88727-8_60

General Considerations

The popliteal sciatic nerve block is a well-established and popular technique of peripheral nerve blockade in the lower limb. It is a versatile block in that it may be performed in varying patient positions (prone, lateral, or supine), using different approaches (lateral-to-medial, posterior-to-anterior). The landmark-guided technique uses neurostimulation to locate the nerves and is both effective and easy to perform. The advent of ultrasound imaging though has both revolutionized our approach to the popliteal sciatic nerve block and enhanced our understanding of neural anatomy. In particular, the concept of a paraneural sheath in this region is now well-accepted and has changed the way we think about "intraneural" and "extraneural" injections.

Indications (Patient Selection)

- Anesthesia or analgesia of the lower limb below the knee, except the medial aspect of the calf/ankle/foot, which is supplied by the saphenous nerve
- Anesthesia or analgesia of the posterior aspect of the knee
- Notes
  - The primary advantage over a more proximal sciatic nerve block is preservation of the ability to flex at the knee, which allows more mobility, e.g., ambulation with crutches.
  - If immediate postoperative ambulation is anticipated, the patient will require a surgical boot or cast to overcome the issue of foot drop.
  - The popliteal block must be combined with a saphenous nerve block for complete sensory block of the lower leg and foot.
  - Additional provisions for anesthesia will have to be made if a thigh tourniquet is to be used during surgery, i.e., general anesthesia or neuraxial block.
  - Heel protection with soft padding during the duration of the block is essential to avoid the development of a pressure sore.

Contraindications

- Absolute
  - There are no absolute contraindications specific to this block. Generic contraindications such as patient refusal, allergy to local anesthetics, and local infection at the site of injection apply as usual.
- Relative
  - Preexisting neuropathy in the distribution of the sciatic nerve.
  - Traumatic injuries of the lower leg where there is a concern of compartment syndrome. This may be overcome by adequate postoperative monitoring for clinical features of compartment syndrome other than patient-reported pain.
  - Coagulation abnormalities are not a significant contraindication. The use of ultrasound should prevent vascular puncture. There are no major blood vessels in the immediate vicinity of the target nerves (the popliteal artery and vein are usually more than 2 cm anterior to the nerves at the level of injection) that are at risk during the landmark-guided approach. It can however be a deep block that traverses muscle (biceps femoris) when performed at the mid-thigh level.

Functional Anatomy

The sciatic nerve (L4, L5, S1–S3) is the largest nerve in the body and exits the pelvis as a structure consisting of two nerve bundles: the more medially placed tibial nerve and the common peroneal (fibular) nerve lying laterally. These two bundles are enclosed within a common paraneural sheath. At its origin, it is broad and flat, but as it passes peripherally, it becomes more rounded. The branching of this sciatic nerve bundle into the two separate nerves occurs at a variable location during its course in the posterior aspect of the thigh, but it has usually occurred within 8–10 cm of the popliteal crease.

The popliteal fossa is a closely packed compartment through which all of the nerves and vessels pass from the thigh to the leg posteriorly. The biceps femoris muscle forms the upper lateral border. The upper medial border is formed by the muscle of semimembranosus and by the tendon of the semitendinosus (*Anatomy* Fig. 60.1). Appearing from between the biceps femoris and semimembranosus are the two heads of gastrocnemius, which form the lower medial and lateral muscular borders of the fossa. Within the popliteal fossa are the popliteal artery (which terminates as the anterior and posterior tibial arteries), popliteal vein, and the tibial and common peroneal nerves (*Anatomy* Fig. 60.2).

Tibial Nerve

The tibial nerve is the larger of the two sciatic divisions, being almost twice as thick as the common peroneal (fibular) nerve. It traverses the popliteal fossa lying posterior and slightly lateral to the popliteal vessels.

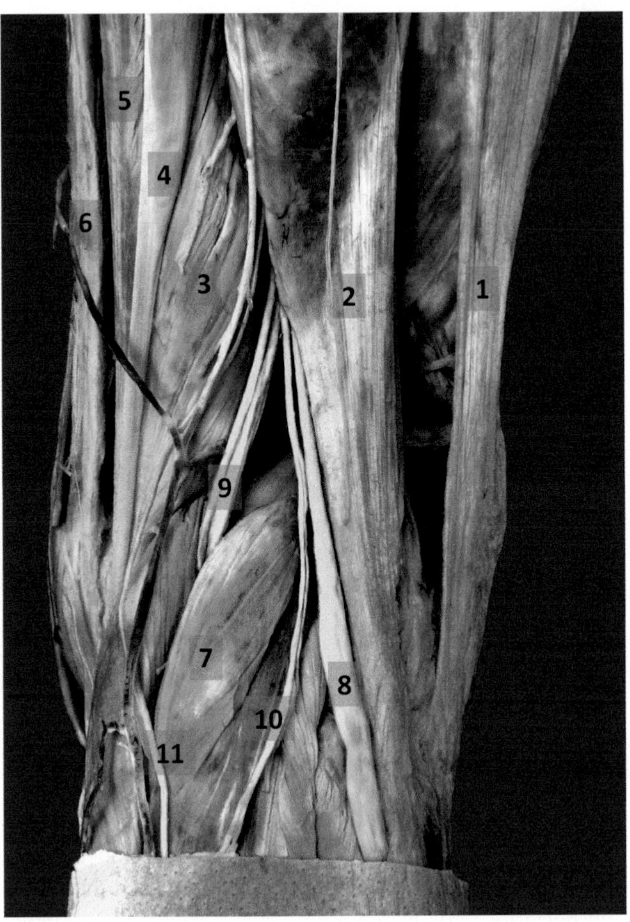

Fig. 60.1 Tibial and common peroneal (fibular) nerve in the popliteal area. (1) Iliotibial tract, (2) biceps femoris muscle, (3) semimembranosus muscle, (4) semitendinosus muscle, (5) gracilis muscle, (6) sartorius muscle, (7) gastrocnemius muscle, (8) common peroneal (fibular) nerve, (9) tibial nerve, (10) lateral sural cutaneous nerve (originates from peroneal nerve), (11) medial sural cutaneous nerve (originates from tibial nerve) (with permission from Danilo Jankovic)

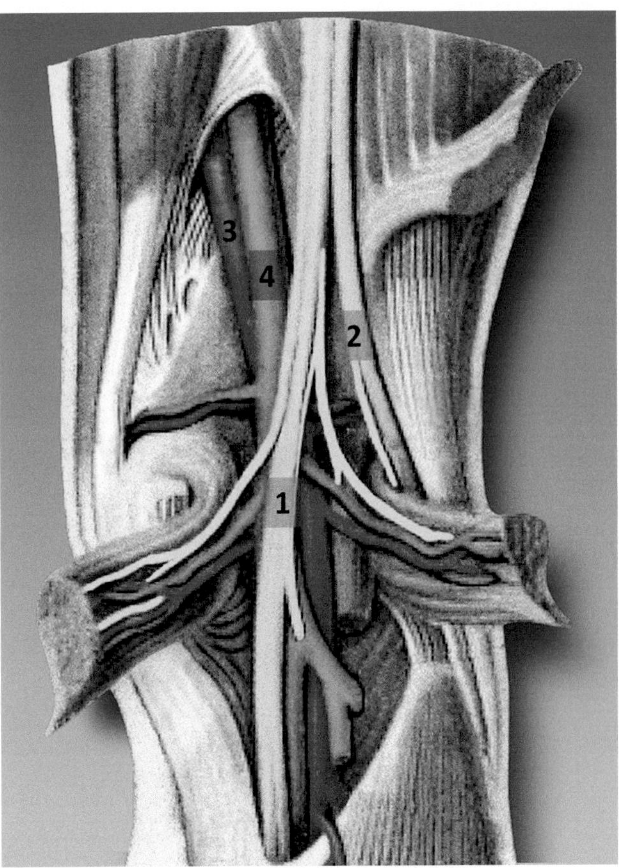

Fig. 60.2 Tibial and common peroneal (fibular) nerve in the popliteal fossa. (1) Tibial nerve, (2) common peroneal (fibular) nerve, (3) popliteal artery, (4) popliteal vein (with permission from Danilo Jankovic)

It then passes between the two heads of the gastrocnemius muscle to the upper edge of the soleus muscle, giving off the medial sural cutaneous nerve, which unites with the lateral sural cutaneous nerve (a branch of the common peroneal nerve) to form the sural nerve. The tibial nerve continues distally between the posterior tibial muscle and the soleus muscle and runs together with the posterior tibial artery through the calf musculature, between the medial malleolus and the calcaneus, and to the medial side of the foot joint (*Anatomy* Fig. 60.3). It divides into its two end branches, the medial and lateral plantar nerves, behind the medial malleolus. These pass under the flexor retinaculum to the sole of the foot and provide it with its sensory innervation.

Common Peroneal (Fibular) Nerve

After separating from the tibial nerve, the common peroneal (fibular) nerve runs along the medial edge of the biceps femoris muscle over the lateral head of the gastrocnemius muscle to the lateral angle of the popliteal fossa. At the neck of the fibula, it passes to the lateral surface of the bone. Before entering the peroneus longus muscle, which originates here, it divides into the superficial peroneal nerve (which is mainly sensory innervation of the foot) and the deep peroneal nerve (mainly motor innervation of the foot).

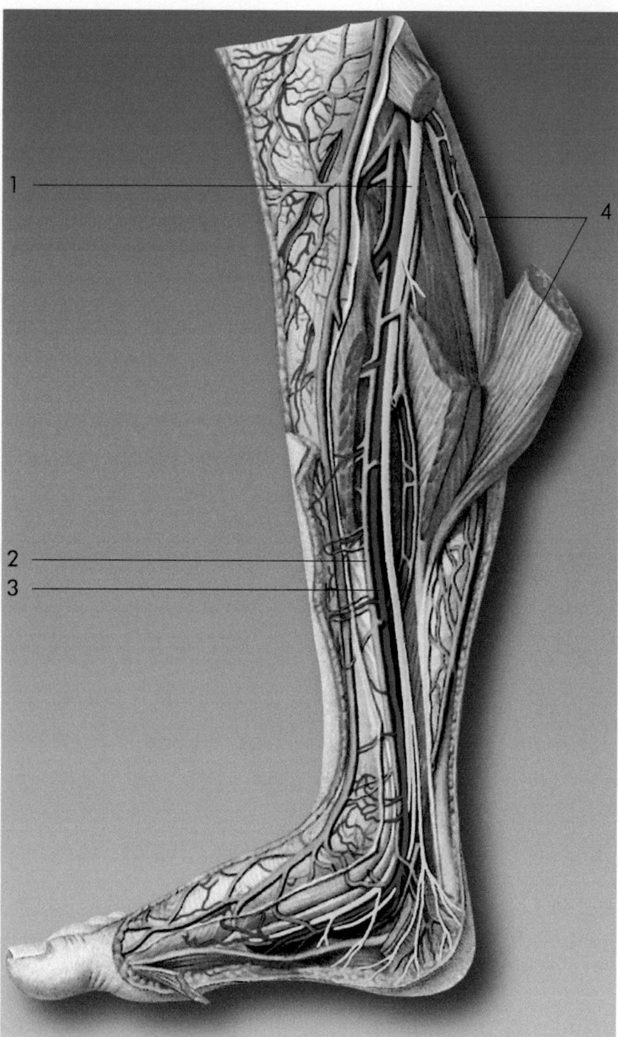

Fig. 60.3 The course of the tibial nerve through the leg and foot. It runs with the posterior tibial artery through the calf to lie behind the medial malleolus, where it divides into the medial and lateral plantar nerves. (1) Tibial nerve, (2) posterior tibial vein, (3) posterior tibial artery, (4) gastrocnemius muscle (with permission from Danilo Jankovic)

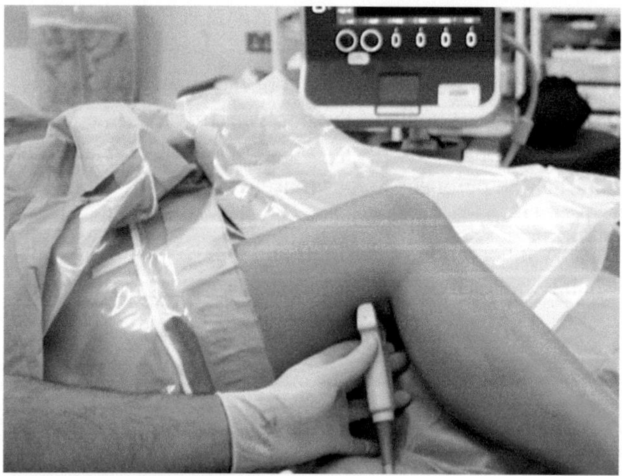

Fig. 60.4 Ultrasound probe position in the popliteal fossa with the patient in the supine position

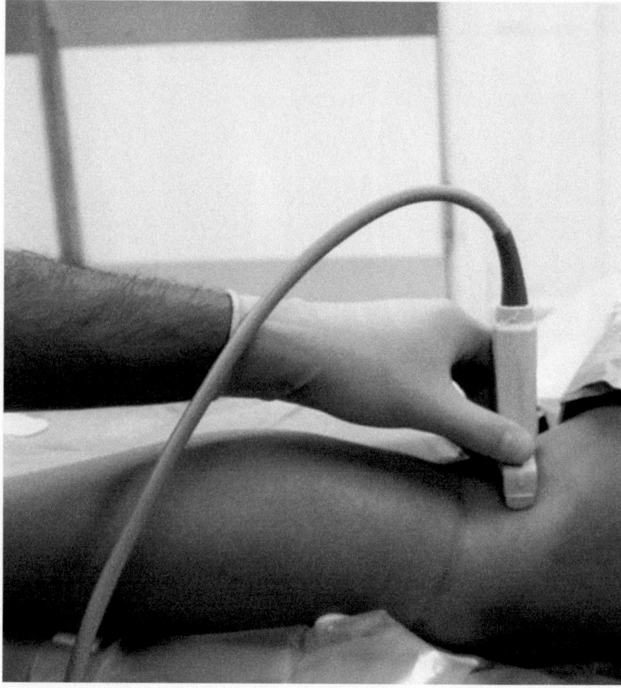

Fig. 60.5 Ultrasound probe position in the popliteal fossa with the patient in the prone position

Up to the point at which it divides, its small branches supply the short head of the biceps femoris muscle, the lateral and posterior parts of the joint capsule, and the tibiofibular joint.

The common peroneal nerve also gives off the lateral sural cutaneous nerve (*Anatomy* Fig. 60.1). The anterior branch of the lateral sural cutaneous nerve runs subcutaneously on the lateral surface of the lower leg, as far as the lateral malleolus, and supplies sensory innervation to the posterior and lateral aspects of the lower leg. Its posterior branch unites with the medial sural cutaneous nerve (branch of the tibial nerve) in the middle of the lower leg to form the sural nerve, although it can also occasionally continue as a separate branch as far as the lateral malleolus.

Sonoanatomy of the Sciatic Nerve in the Popliteal Fossa

The sciatic nerve is imaged by placing the ultrasound probe in a transverse orientation on the posterior aspect of the patient's leg, in the popliteal fossa (*Sonoanatomy* Figs. 60.4 and 60.5). It is recommended that a systematic scan be performed starting at the level of the popliteal skin crease (where structures are most superficial) and moving proximally or cephalad (the traceback approach). On the lateral aspect of the image, the muscle bulk is made up of biceps femoris and, medially, the

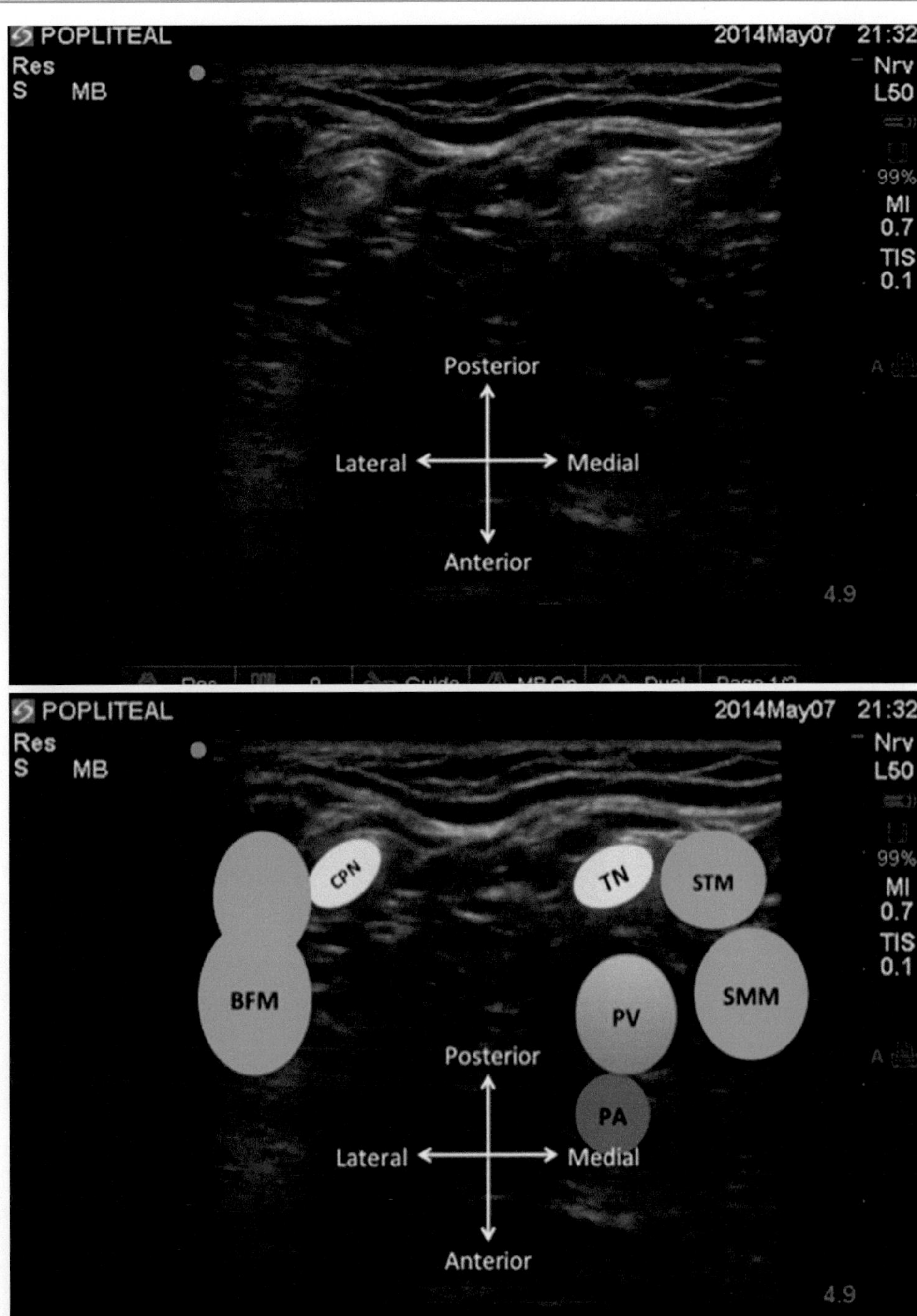

Fig. 60.6 Transverse view of the popliteal fossa and associated structures. The tibial nerve (TN) is located superficial to the popliteal artery (PA) and vein (PV). The common peroneal nerve (CPN) is visible lateral to the tibial nerve. *BFM* biceps femoris muscle, *STM* semimembranosus muscle, *SMM* semimembranosus muscle

muscles of semitendinosus and semimembranosus (*Sonoanatomy* Fig. 60.6). The popliteal vessels are identified as dark hypoechoic circular structures and can be distinguished by the fact that the artery is pulsatile, and the vein is compressible. Color Doppler can also be used for additional confirmation (*Sonoanatomy* Fig. 60.7). The hyperechoic tibial nerve is located superficial (posterior) to the popliteal vessels and is

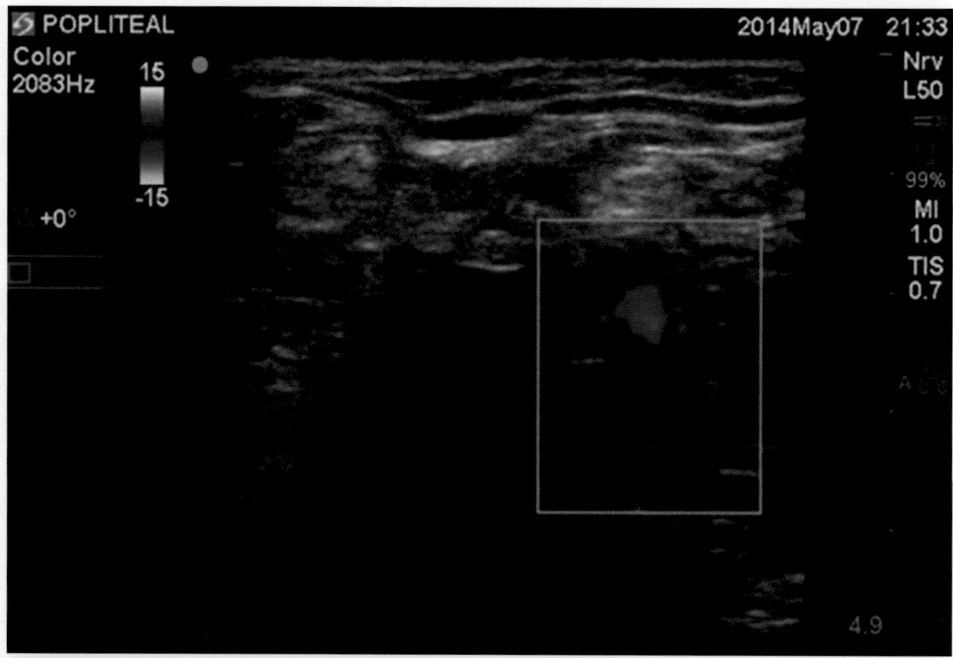

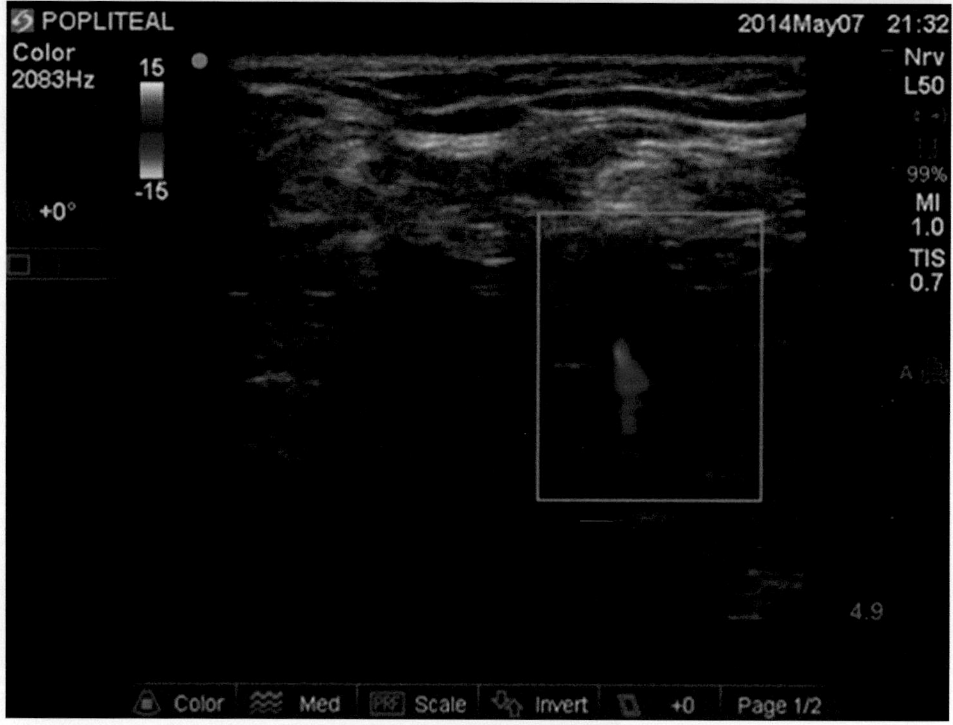

Fig. 60.7 Color Doppler may be used to help identify the popliteal vein (upper image) and artery (lower image)

most commonly lateral to the vein. As the probe is moved proximally, the smaller common peroneal (fibular) nerve will be seen to move from the lateral aspect of the thigh toward the midline to join the tibial nerve to form the sciatic nerve within a common (paraneural) sheath (*Sonoanatomy* Fig. 60.8).

Clinical Pearls for Optimal Imaging of the Popliteal Sciatic Nerve

- The neural structures are often more laterally positioned in the popliteal fossa than initially anticipated; bear this in mind with an initial probe placement.

- Use color Doppler to identify the popliteal vessels. Use minimal pressure initially to ensure that the popliteal vein is not occluded.
- The traceback method allows you to identify the point at which the common peroneal (fibular) nerve unites with the tibial nerve to form the common sciatic nerve. Blockade at this point is ideal.
- The tibial and common peroneal (fibular) nerves rarely lie in a parallel plane to the skin surface and are therefore usually poorly visible if the ultrasound probe is placed perpendicular to the skin surface. The probe will need to be tilted (often in a plantar direction) to a varying degree to increase the echogenicity and visibility of the nerves (a phenomenon known as anisotropy).

Landmark-Guided Popliteal Sciatic Nerve Block - Preparation

Required Supplies and Equipment

- Disinfectant solution and swabs for skin preparation
- Sterile gloves and drapes
- Short-beveled 22G block needle with extension tubing
  - 50–80 mm (posterior approach)
  - 80–100 mm needle (lateral approach)
- Local anesthetic of choice in 10 ml or 20 ml syringes
- Lidocaine 1–2% in 3 ml syringe with a 25–27G hypodermic needle for skin infiltration (at operator's discretion)
- Equipment and supplies for managing life-threatening acute complications, including intralipid for local anesthetic systemic toxicity
- Drugs for intravenous sedation during the block (at operator's discretion)

Preparation of Patient

- Obtain informed consent for the block.
- Explain expected clinical course including care of the insensate limb and managing the transition to systemic analgesia.
- Establish intravenous access, supplemental oxygen delivery, and standard monitors (ECG, noninvasive blood pressure, pulse oximetry).
- Perform a time-out to confirm patient identity and site and side of surgery.

Block Performance

There are two main landmark-guided approaches that may be used.

1. The posterior popliteal sciatic nerve block
2. The lateral popliteal sciatic nerve block

Landmark-Guided Popliteal Sciatic Nerve Block: Posterior Approach

Patient Position

- The patient is placed prone with little to no flexion at the knees and in a neutral position – internal or external rotation at the hips should be avoided. This is done by placing a small soft roll under the ankles or by allowing the feet to dangle off the foot of the bed.
- A right-handed operator should always stand on the left side of the patient, to allow use of the dominant hand for needling, and vice versa.

Surface Landmarks

- Different methods of determining the appropriate needle insertion point have been described (see Table 1 in Nader et al.), but all are based upon the principle of targeting the sciatic nerve in the mid-thigh, proximal to its bifurcation into tibial and peroneal nerves.
- The modified intertendinous approach (*LMG* Fig. 60.9)
  - Palpate the upper (cephalad) borders of the popliteal fossa, which are formed by the tendons and muscle bellies of the semimembranosus and semitendinosus (medial) and the biceps femoris (lateral). Identification of these landmarks can be facilitated by asking the patient to flex their knee against resistance.
  - Trace the borders to where they meet at the apex of the popliteal fossa—this is the site of needle insertion.
- Alternative method (*LMG* Fig. 60.9)
  - Draw a transverse line between the lateral and medial epicondyles of the femur and mark its midpoint.
  - From a point 1 cm lateral to the midpoint of this first line, draw a second line perpendicular to the first one, extending 5–7 cm in a cephalad direction—this is the site of needle insertion.

Needle Insertion and Injection Technique

- Disinfect the skin, drape the area appropriately, prime the block needle and tubing with local anesthetic solution, and attach a nerve stimulator at an initial current setting of 1–2 mA, a pulse duration of 0.1–0.3 msec, and a frequency of 1–2 Hz.
- Fixing the skin over the skin insertion point with the second and third fingers of the nondominant hand, insert a 50–80 mm block needle at a 45–60° angle in a cephalad

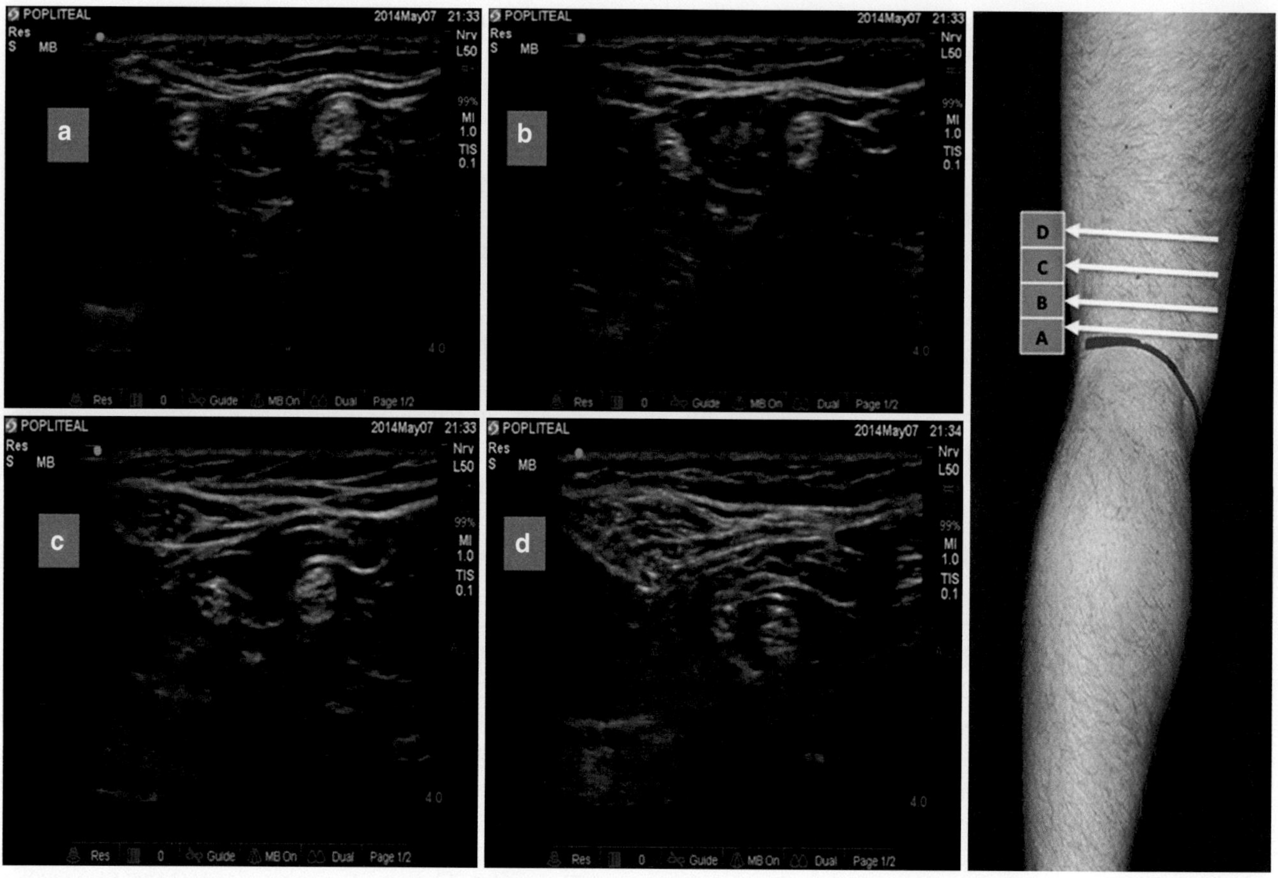

Fig. 60.8 Scanning the sciatic nerve in the popliteal fossa from distal to proximal (sequential images **a** to **d**) using the traceback method. The tibial (TN) and common peroneal (CPN) components of the sciatic nerve will be seen to approach each other and join within a common sheath

direction and parallel to the long axis of the leg (*LMG* Fig. 60.10).

- Advance the needle slowly and steadily until plantarflexion and inversion (tibial nerve – medial aspect of sciatic nerve) or dorsiflexion and eversion (peroneal nerve—lateral aspect) of the foot is obtained at a current threshold of 0.3–0.5 mA.
- Incremental injection of local anesthetic is performed with intermittent aspiration to exclude intravascular injection.
- If no motor response is obtained despite inserting the needle to its full depth, the needle should be withdrawn to the skin and redirected in a slightly medial or lateral direction.

Landmark-Guided Popliteal Sciatic Nerve Block: Lateral Approach

Patient Position

- The patient is placed supine; the knee may be slightly flexed by placing a soft roll underneath it.
- The operator stands on the side of the patient that is to be blocked.

Surface Landmarks (LMG Fig. 60.11)

- The groove between the lateral (posterior) edge of vastus lateralis and biceps femoris is identified; this can be accentuated by asking the patient to extend the knee against resistance.
- A point in the groove 7 cm proximal to the lateral femoral epicondyle is marked—this is the initial needle insertion point. Alternatively, a point 8 cm proximal to the popliteal crease in the groove can also be used.

Needle Insertion and Injection Technique

- Disinfect the skin, drape the area appropriately, prime the block needle and tubing with local anesthetic solution, and attach a nerve stimulator at an initial current setting of 1.5 mA, a pulse duration of 0.1–0.3 ms, and a frequency of 1–2 Hz.
- Fixing the skin over the skin insertion point with the second and third fingers of the nondominant hand, insert an 80–100 mm block needle perpendicular to the skin in the horizontal plane (*LMG* Fig. 60.12).

- Advance the needle slowly and steadily until the femur is contacted. The depth of insertion is noted – the sciatic nerve is expected to lie 1–2 cm deeper, posterior to the femur (*LMG* Fig. 60.13).
- The needle is then withdrawn to the skin and redirected approximately 30 degrees posteriorly (downwards) and advanced posterior to (under) the femur until plantarflexion and inversion (tibial nerve – medial aspect of sciatic nerve) or dorsiflexion and eversion (peroneal nerve – lateral aspect) of the foot is obtained at a current threshold of 0.2–0.5 mA.
- Biceps femoris twitches should not be accepted as they may represent local muscle stimulation. If the appropriate motor response is not obtained within 2 cm of cessation of the biceps femoris twitches, it is likely that the nerve has been missed, and the needle should be withdrawn and redirected at a shallower or steeper angle.
- Once an appropriate distal motor response has been obtained, incremental injection of local anesthetic is performed with intermittent aspiration to exclude intravascular injection.

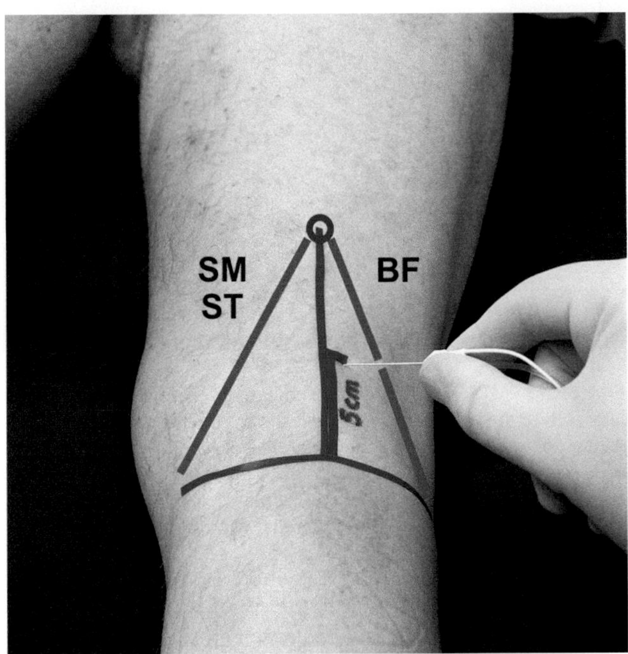

Fig. 60.9 Surface landmarks for the posterior approach to the popliteal nerve block. A transverse line between the lateral and medial epicondyles of the femur (corresponding approximately to the popliteal crease) is drawn block and its midpoint marked. The upper borders of the popliteal fossa, formed by semimembranosus (SM), semitendinosus (ST), and biceps femoris (BF) muscles, are palpated and marked. There are two possible insertion points: (1) at the apex of the popliteal fossa (the modified intertendinous approach) or (2) at a point 5–7 cm cephalad and 1 cm lateral to the midpoint of the transverse line between femoral epicondyles (with permission from Danilo Jankovic)

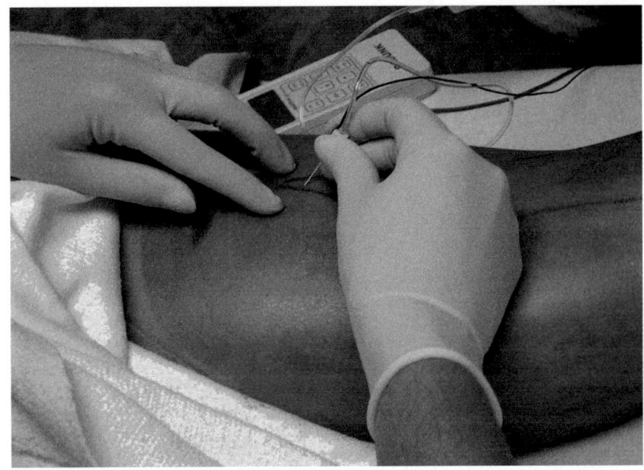

Fig. 60.10 Needle insertion in the surface landmark-guided posterior approach to the popliteal nerve block. The needle is advanced at 45–60° angle in a cephalad direction until an appropriate motor response is obtained at 0.3–0.5 mA

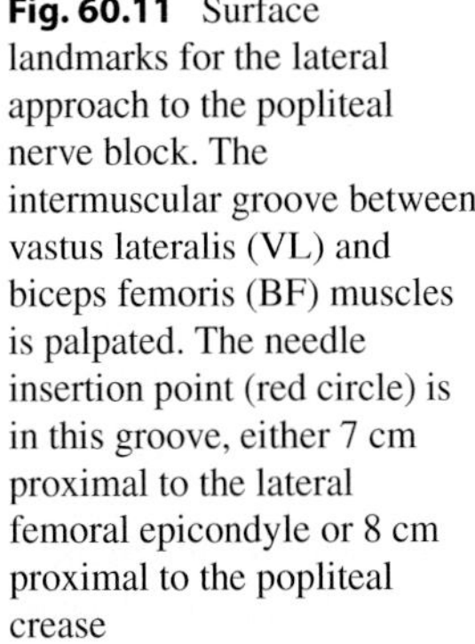

Fig. 60.11 Surface landmarks for the lateral approach to the popliteal nerve block. The intermuscular groove between vastus lateralis (VL) and biceps femoris (BF) muscles is palpated. The needle insertion point (red circle) is in this groove, either 7 cm proximal to the lateral femoral epicondyle or 8 cm proximal to the popliteal crease

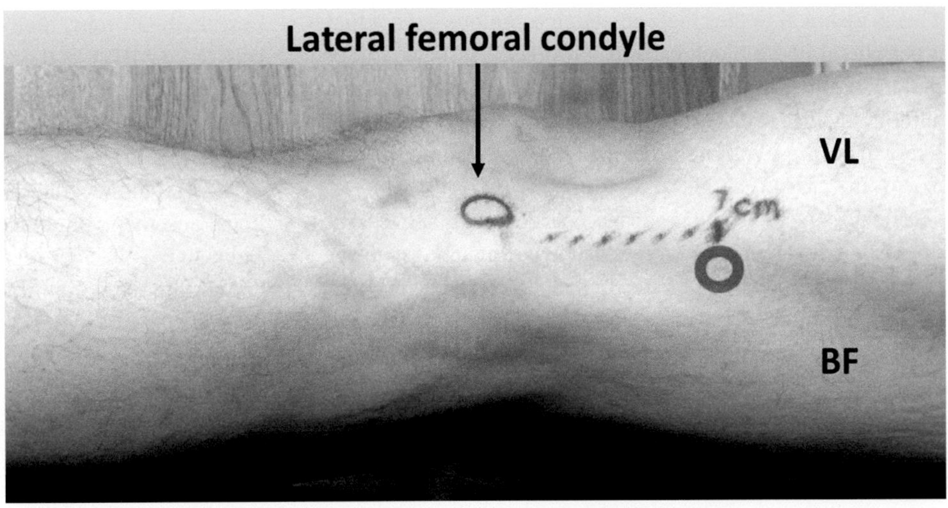

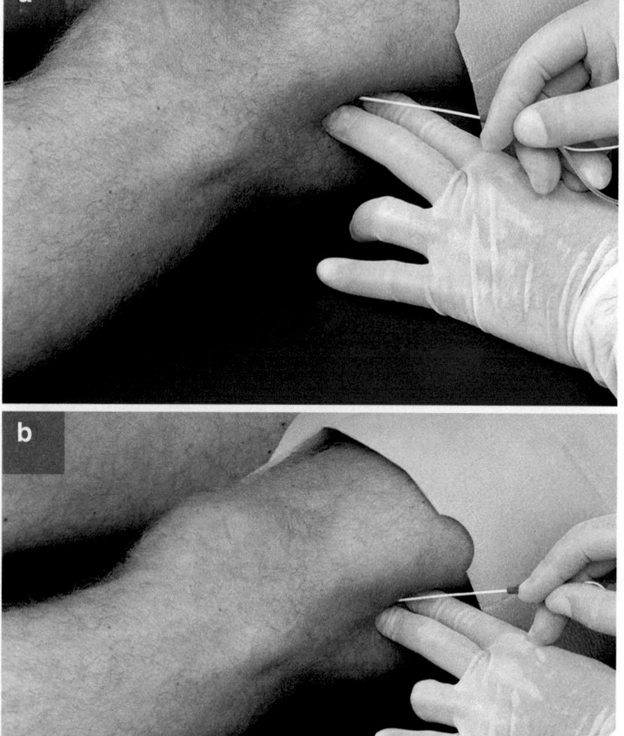

Fig. 60.12 Needle insertion in the surface landmark-guided lateral approach to the popliteal nerve block. (**a**) The needle is initially advanced perpendicular to the skin to contact the femur and the depth noted. (**b**) The needle is then withdrawn to the skin and redirected posteriorly under the femur until an appropriate motor response is obtained at 0.3–0.5 mA (with permission from Danilo Jankovic)

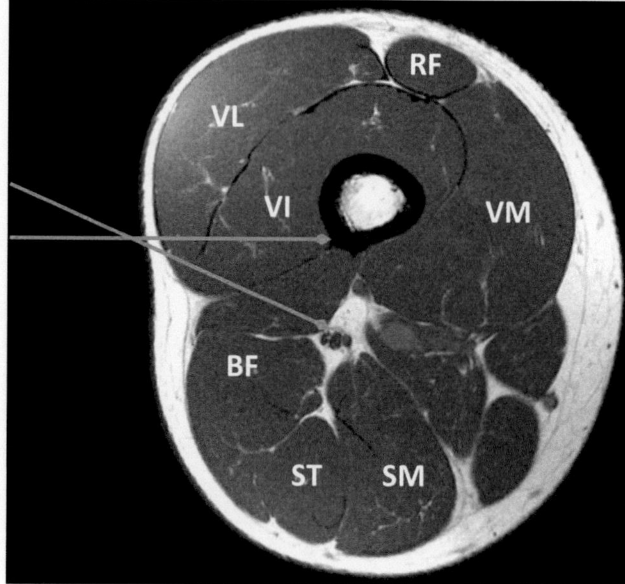

Fig. 60.13 MRI cross-section of the thigh indicating the lateral approach to the sciatic nerve. The needle is initially advanced perpendicular to the skin to contact the femur, before being redirected posteriorly at approximately 30° angle to reach the sciatic nerve. *BF* biceps femoris, *RF* rectus femoris, *SM* semimembranosus, *ST* semitendinosus, *VI* vastus intermedius, *VL* vastus lateralis, *VM* vastus medialis

Continuous Landmark-Guided Popliteal Sciatic Nerve Block Technique

This is identical to the single-injection technique except that a peripheral nerve block catheter kit is used instead. Either the posterior or lateral approach may be used, although the authors favor the posterior approach as the catheter is more likely to advance within the paraneural sheath along the long axis of the nerve.

The introducer needle is advanced as described above until the desired motor response is obtained. If a stimulating catheter is being used, 5–10 ml of 5% dextrose solution can be injected through the introducer needle to distend the paraneural sheath. This should also result in augmentation of the motor response. Injection of other solutions will abolish the motor response.

The catheter is then advanced 3–5 cm beyond the tip of the introducer needle, looking to maintain a motor response from the sciatic nerve at current thresholds of at least 0.2 mA and up to 0.8–1 mA. The needle is then withdrawn and the catheter fixed in place in the usual manner.

Ultrasound-Guided Popliteal Sciatic Nerve Block

Required Supplies and Equipment

- Disinfectant solution and swabs for skin preparation
- Sterile gloves, drapes, and ultrasound probe cover
- Linear 38–50 mm, high-frequency ultrasound probe (at least 7–13 MHz), and machine
- Nerve stimulator (at operator's discretion)
- Short-beveled 22G block needle with extension tubing
  - 50–80 mm (posterior approach)
  - 80–100 mm needle (lateral approach)
- Local anesthetic of choice in 10 ml or 20 ml syringes
- Lidocaine 1–2% in 3 ml syringe with a 25–27G hypodermic needle for skin infiltration (at operator's discretion)
- Equipment and supplies for managing life-threatening acute complications, including intralipid for local anesthetic systemic toxicity (LAST)
- Drugs for intravenous sedation during the block (at operator's discretion)

Preparation of Patient

- Obtain informed consent for the block.
- Explain expected clinical course including care of the insensate limb and managing the transition to systemic analgesia.
- Establish intravenous access, supplemental oxygen delivery, and monitoring (ECG, noninvasive blood pressure, pulse oximetry).
- Perform time-out to confirm patient identity and site and side of surgery.

Block Performance

Patient Position

The patient may be placed in 1 of 3 positions:

1. Prone position
2. Supine position
3. Lateral position

- The prone position is probably the most ergonomic one for the operator. The patient is placed prone with little to no flexion at the knees and in a neutral position—internal or external rotation at the hips should be avoided. This is done by placing a small soft roll under the ankles or by allowing the feet to dangle off the foot of the bed.
- The supine position is useful if there are hindrances to turning the patient prone (morbid obesity, leg in a plaster cast, etc.). To allow probe access to the popliteal fossa, the lower leg may be elevated by placing a roll or other support (e.g., a padded Mayo stand) underneath the calf. The leg may also be simply flexed at the knee, in which case access can be further improved by slight internal rotation at the hip.
- The lateral decubitus position is a third alternative to the prone and supine positions. The operative leg should be uppermost and extended at the knee, with padding (e.g., a small pillow) placed between the knees for comfort.
- Regardless of patient position, attention should be paid to ergonomics to ensure the operator, needle, and machine are aligned to minimize unnecessary movements during the procedure.

Probe Position and Image Optimization

- Place the probe in a transverse orientation above the popliteal crease to obtain a short-axis view of the popliteal fossa.
- Select appropriate depth of field (normally up to 5 cm), gain, and focus.
- Ensure the orientation marker is correctly positioned.
- Use the traceback method described previously to obtain a transverse, short-axis view of the sciatic nerve just distal to its bifurcation.
- Note that with the patient in the supine position, the ultrasound image and needle movements will appear inverted or "upside down" on the screen relative to the actual patient position. The orientation of the image on the screen can also be inverted using the machine settings to compensate for this, or the operator may choose to mentally compensate when redirecting the needle.

Needle Insertion and Injection Technique

- Disinfect the skin, drape the area appropriately, apply the cover to the ultrasound probe, prime the block needle and tubing with local anesthetic solution, and, if being used, attach a nerve stimulator at an initial current setting of 0.5–6 mA, a pulse duration 0.1–0.3 ms, and a frequency of 1–2 Hz.
- The needle can be inserted either in-plane or out-of-plane to the ultrasound probe and beam (see below).
- If a nerve stimulator is to be used, there should be no twitches elicited below 0.2 mA. This helps to exclude intraneural needle placement. It may not be necessary to reposition the needle just to obtain a minimum current threshold (<0.5 mA) if the injectate is clearly observed to spread within the paraneural sheath and around the nerves.
- The nerves should be carefully observed during injection to exclude intraneural injection, which is indicated by an increase in their cross-sectional area.

Out-of-Plane Needling Technique

- The out-of-plane approach may be used with the patient in either the prone or lateral position.
- Insert the needle perpendicular to the ultrasound probe and parallel to the long axis of the nerve (*USG* Fig. 60.14).
- The needle can be challenging to visualize with this technique, and at best, it will appear in short axis on the screen as a white dot (*USG* Fig. 60.15). However, progress of the needle tip can usually be easily tracked by tissue movement as it penetrates the various layers.
- Care must be taken to distinguish between the shaft and the tip of the needle. To aid needle-tip identification, small "side-to-side" or "jiggling" movements can be made and the resultant tissue movement observed to identify the tip.
- Small aliquots (0.5–1 ml) of fluid (5% dextrose if neurostimulation is being used as it preserves the motor response) can be injected to "hydrolocate" the tip of the needle.

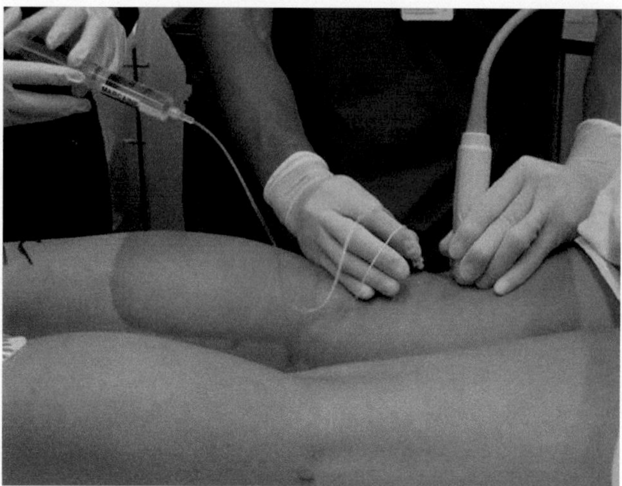

Fig. 60.14 Out-of-plane needle insertion in the popliteal nerve block with the patient in the prone position. As the needle is inserted progressively deeper, the probe must be scanned proximally to track the needle tip

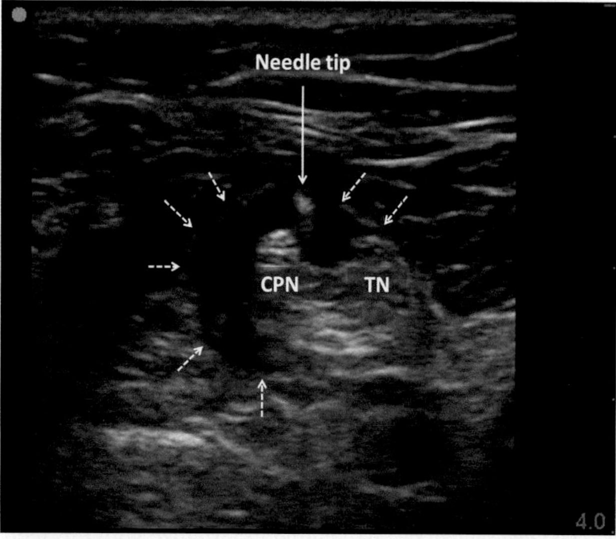

Fig. 60.15 Transverse short-axis view of the common peroneal nerve (CPN) and tibial nerve (TN) in the popliteal fossa. The needle has been inserted out-of-plane to the probe, and the tip is within the paraneural sheath (dashed arrows). Injected local anesthetic has distended the sheath and has begun to spread around the nerves, outlining them and increasing their visibility

- The aim is to place the needle tip within the paraneural sheath and between the tibial and common peroneal (fibular) nerves and to observe spread of local anesthetic within the sheath. Do not aim directly for the neural structures. Local anesthetic spread within the sheath should be observed (*USG* Fig. 60.15).

In-Plane Needling Technique

- The in-plane approach may be used with the patient in either the prone (*USG* Fig. 60.16), lateral, or supine (*USG* Fig. 60.17) position.
- The needle is inserted from the lateral aspect of the patient's thigh, either immediately adjacent to the probe (*USG* Fig. 60.16a) or in the intermuscular groove between biceps femoris and vastus lateralis (*USG* Fig. 60.16b). The second approach may allow better needle visualization as the shaft will be perpendicular to the ultrasound beam.
- It is essential to constantly visualize the tip of the needle as it advances, and small sliding movements of the probe should be made as needed to ensure needle-beam alignment.

- The aim is to place the needle tip within the paraneural sheath and between the tibial and common peroneal (fibular) nerves and to observe spread of local anesthetic

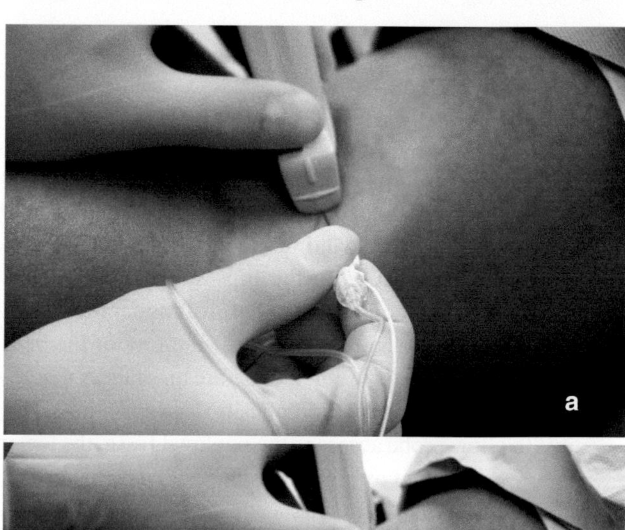

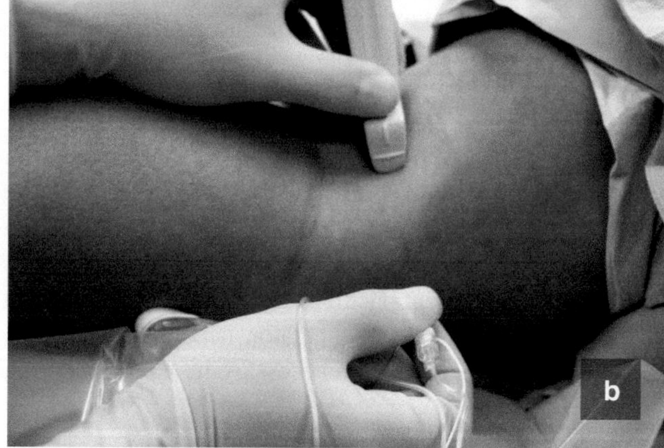

Fig. 60.16 In-plane needle insertion in the popliteal nerve block with the patient in prone position. The needle may be inserted (**a**) immediately adjacent to the probe or (**b**) in the intermuscular groove between vastus lateralis and biceps femoris. The second approach maximizes needle visibility as the shaft will be perpendicular to the ultrasound beam

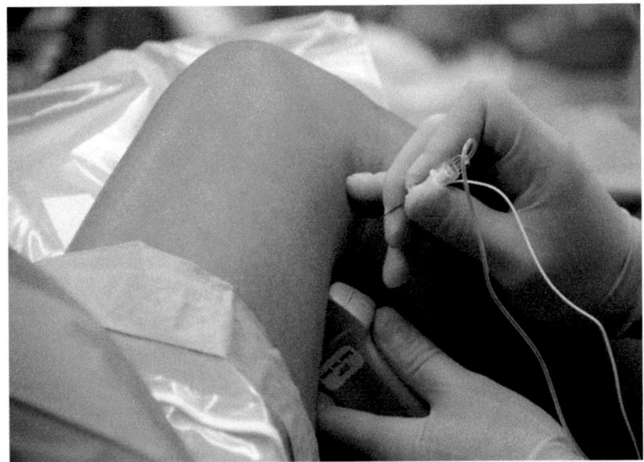

Fig. 60.17 In-plane needle insertion in the popliteal nerve block with the patient in the supine position. The knee has been flexed and rotated slightly inward to facilitate probe placement

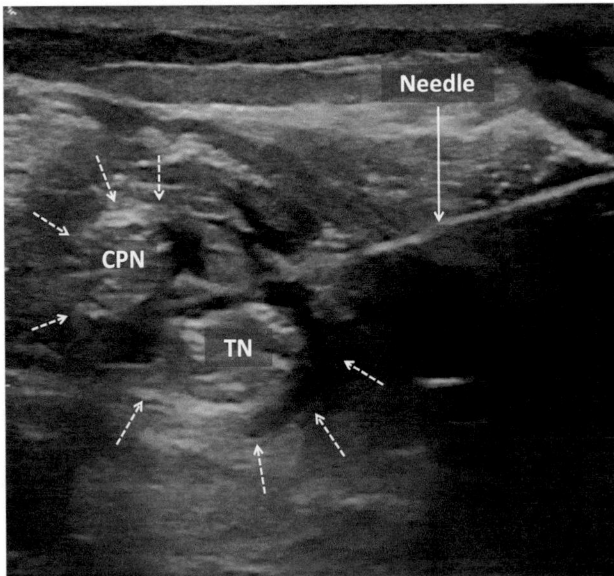

Fig. 60.18 Transverse short-axis view of the common peroneal nerve (CPN) and tibial nerve (TN) in the popliteal fossa. The needle has been inserted in-plane to the probe, and the tip is within the paraneural sheath (dashed arrows) and between the two nerves. Injected local anesthetic is spreading within the paraneural sheath and beginning to outline the nerves

within the sheath. Do not aim directly for the neural structures. Local anesthetic spread within the sheath should be observed (*USG* Fig. 60.18).

Continuous Ultrasound-Guided Popliteal Sciatic Nerve Block

There are three possible approaches for siting a catheter in the popliteal fossa under ultrasound guidance. These are:

1. Needle in-plane with the nerve viewed in the short axis
2. Needle out-of-plane with the nerve viewed in the short axis
3. Needle in-plane with the nerve viewed in the long axis

Even after considerable mastery of ultrasound-guided regional anesthesia, it is a challenge to maintain in-plane visualization of the needle, nerve, and catheter during the procedure, so the authors do not recommend using the third approach for catheter insertion.

Needle in-Plane with Nerve Viewed in Short Axis

This is identical to the single-injection in-plane technique except that a peripheral nerve block catheter kit is used instead. Either the posterior or lateral approach may be used.

The introducer needle is advanced as described above, and an initial bolus of either local anesthetic or 5% dextrose solution can be used to distend the paraneural sheath. The catheter is then advanced through the introducer needle no more than 2–3 cm beyond the tip. The introducer needle is then withdrawn. Local anesthetic injection is observed through the catheter under ultrasound guidance, and the catheter can then be withdrawn slightly if required to achieve the optimal position.

The catheter is fixed in place in the usual manner.

Needle Out-of-Plane with Nerve Viewed in Short Axis

This is identical to the single-injection out-of-plane technique except that a peripheral nerve block catheter kit is used instead. Either the posterior or lateral approach may be used, though technically, it may be easier to perform with the patient in the prone position. This is the authors' preferred technique as the catheter can be advanced further within the paraneural sheath along the long axis of the nerve, which reduces the risk of dislodgement.

The introducer needle is advanced as described above, and an initial bolus of either local anesthetic or 5% dextrose solution can be used to distend the paraneural sheath. The catheter is then advanced through the introducer needle 3–5 cm beyond the tip. Local anesthetic injection is observed through the catheter under ultrasound guidance to confirm optimal position. If necessary, in addition, a proximal scan should be able to confirm perineural catheter placement. The introducer needle is withdrawn, and the catheter is fixed in place in the usual manner.

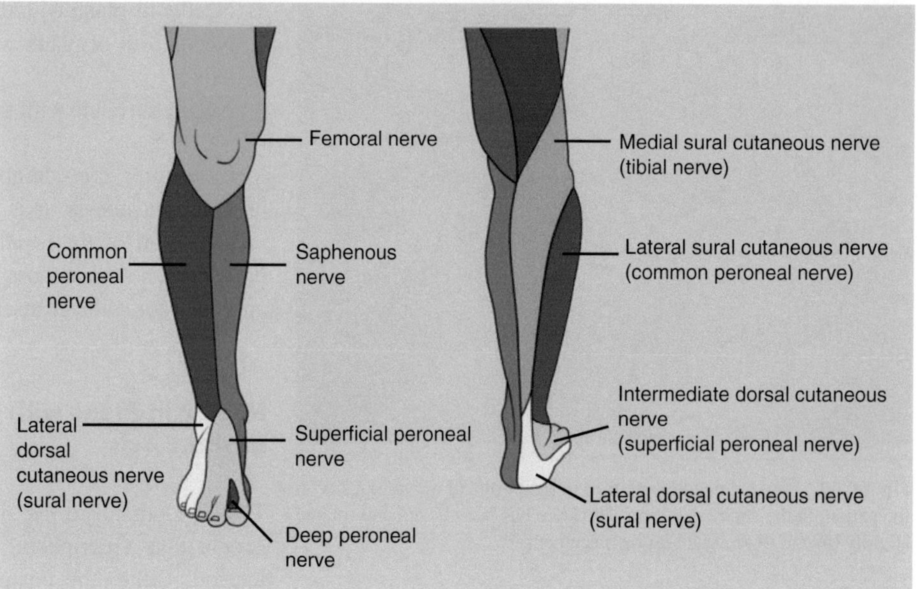

Fig. 60.19 Sensory innervation areas in the lower leg (reproduced with permission from Danilo Jankovic)

The areas of cutaneous innervation of the individual nerves discussed in this chapter are illustrated in Fig. 60.19.

Local Anesthetic Dosage

Single-Injection Block

- A volume of 30–40 ml (0.4–0.5 ml/kg) is generally recommended for the landmark-guided approach to popliteal nerve block.
- The choice of local anesthetic and concentration depends on the desired speed of onset and duration. Commonly used local anesthetics include the following:
  - A 1:1 mixture of an intermediate-acting local anesthetic (e.g., 2% mepivacaine or lidocaine) and a long-acting local anesthetic (e.g., 0.5% bupivacaine), which will have a faster onset than bupivacaine alone and a longer duration than lidocaine alone.
  - 0.25–0.5% bupivacaine.
  - 0.5–0.75% ropivacaine.
- Epinephrine may be added in a concentration of 2.5 mcg/ml as a marker of intravascular injection and to reduce systemic vascular absorption.

Continuous Popliteal Sciatic Nerve Block

- 0.2–0.4% ropivacaine at 4–8 ml/h.
- 0.125–0.25% bupivacaine at 4–8 ml/h.
- PCA boluses of 2–5 ml may be added if this function is available on the infusion pump.
- Both infusion rates and bolus volumes should be titrated to achieve the optimal balance between adequate analgesia and an excessively dense sensory and motor block.
- The current evidence indicates that both continuous infusion and programmed intermittent bolus regimens appear equally effective.

Complications

- Complications associated with popliteal nerve block are uncommon.
- Potential complications are similar to that of any peripheral nerve block and include:
  - Local bruising and pain at the site of needle insertion.
  - Hematoma formation.
  - Intravascular injection.
  - Local anesthetic systemic toxicity (LAST).
  - Neurologic injury and deficit.
- Patients should be counselled on appropriate care of the insensate limb, and, in particular, the heel should be protected against pressure injury.

Suggested Reading

Andersen HL, Andersen SL, Tranum-Jensen J. Injection inside the paraneural sheath of the sciatic nerve: direct comparison among ultrasound imaging, macroscopic anatomy, and histologic analysis. Reg Anesth Pain Med. 2012;37:410–4.

Edward Kim T, Howard SK, Funck N, Kyle Harrison T, Walters TL, Wagner MJ, Ganaway T, Mullens J, Lehnert B, Mariano ER. A randomized comparison of long-axis and short-axis imaging for in-plane ultrasound-guided popliteal-sciatic perineural catheter insertion. J Anesth. 2014; https://doi.org/10.1007/s00540-014-1832-8.

Franco CD. Connective tissues associated with peripheral nerves. Reg Anesth Pain Med. 2012;37:363–5.

Ilfeld BM, Loland VJ, Gerancher JC, Wadhwa AN, Renehan EM, Sessler DI, Shuster JJ, Theriaque DW, Maldonado RC, Mariano ER. PAINfRE investigators: the effects of varying local anesthetic concentration and volume on continuous popliteal sciatic nerve blocks: a dual-center, randomized, controlled study. Anesth Analg. 2008;107:701–7.

Ilfeld BM, Fredrickson MJ, Mariano ER. Ultrasound-guided perineural catheter insertion: three approaches but few illuminating data. Reg Anesth Pain Med. 2010;35:123–6.

Karmakar MK, Shariat AN, Pangthipampai P, Chen J. High-definition ultrasound imaging defines the paraneural sheath and the fascial compartments surrounding the sciatic nerve at the popliteal fossa. Reg Anesth Pain Med. 2013;38:447–51.

Nader A, Kendall MC, Candido KD, Benzon H, McCarthy RJ. A randomized comparison of a modified intertendinous and classic posterior approach to popliteal sciatic nerve block. Anesth Analg. 2009;108:359–63.

Paqueron X, Narchi P, Mazoit J-X, Singelyn F, Bénichou A, Macaire P. A randomized, observer-blinded determination of the median effective volume of local anesthetic required to anesthetize the sciatic nerve in the popliteal fossa for stimulating and nonstimulating perineural catheters. Reg Anesth Pain Med. 2009;34:290–5.

Perlas A, Wong P, Abdallah F, Hazrati L-N, Tse C, Chan V. Ultrasound-guided popliteal block through a common paraneural sheath versus conventional injection: a prospective, randomized, double-blind study. Reg Anesth Pain Med. 2013;38:218–25.

Sala-Blanch X, Vandepitte C, Laur JJ, Horan P, Xu D, Reina MA, Karmakar MK, Clark TB, Hadzic A. A practical review of perineural versus intraneural injections: a call for standard nomenclature. Int Anesthesiol Clin. 2011;49:1–12.

Short AJ, Ghosh M, Jin R, Chan VWS, Chin KJ. Intermittent bolus versus continuous infusion popliteal sciatic nerve block following major foot and ankle surgery: a prospective randomized comparison. Reg Anesth Pain Med. 2019;44:1053–8.

Taboada M, Rodríguez J, Valiño C, Carceller J, Bascuas B, Oliveira J, Alvarez J, Gude F, Atanassoff PG. What is the minimum effective volume of local anesthetic required for sciatic nerve blockade? A prospective, randomized comparison between a popliteal and a subgluteal approach. Anesth Analg. 2006;102:593–7.

Tsui BCH, Finucane BT. The importance of ultrasound landmarks: a "traceback" approach using the popliteal blood vessels for identification of the sciatic nerve. Reg Anesth Pain Med. 2006;31:481–2.

Femoral Triangle and Adductor Canal Blocks

61

Thomas Fichtner Bendtsen

Contents

General Consideration

A fast-track strategy for total knee replacement (TKR) focusing on early ambulation and minimum length of stay is facilitated by postsurgical pain management, including motor-sparing nerve blocks as an alternative to a femoral nerve block that impedes ambulation by generating paralysis of the quadriceps femoris muscles. The so-called adductor canal block in the midthigh has become an important component of this motor-sparing nerve block strategy. Most published trials assessing the effect of the midthigh 'adductor canal block' have—as a matter of fact—been carried out as a 'femoral triangle block'. More accurately, an injection adjacent to the femoral artery midway between the anterior superior iliac spine and the base of patella is anatomically a 'distal femoral triangle block'—not an 'adductor canal block'. Originally, almost 200 years ago, John Hunter localized the proximal end of the adductor canal anatomically correct as the middle of the thigh defined as the midpoint from the intersection point of the femoral artery and the inguinal crease to the most prominent point of the medial femoral epicondyle. The prevalent misnomer 'adductor canal block' appears to be due to a loss in translation of the historic meaning of 'middle of the thigh'. In this chapter, an 'adductor canal block' is referring to an injection of local anaesthetic around the femoral artery inside the anatomic adductor canal between the apex of the femoral triangle and the adductor hiatus. An injection of local anaesthetic proximal to the apex of the femoral triangle is referred to as a 'distal femoral triangle block'.

The common denominator of femoral triangle and adductor canal blocks is that the local anaesthetic is injected adjacent to the femoral artery. The anaesthetic effect of femoral triangle and adductor canal blocks depends on the level of injection along the femoral artery. It is clinically relevant to distinguish between (1) proximal femoral triangle block, (2) distal femoral triangle block, (3) proximal adductor canal block, and (4) distal adductor canal block (Fig. 61.1).

T. F. Bendtsen (✉)
Department of Anesthesiology, Aarhus University Hospital, Aarhus, Denmark
e-mail: tfb@dadlnet.dk

D. Jankovic, P. Peng (eds.), *Regional Nerve Blocks in Anesthesia and Pain Therapy*,
https://doi.org/10.1007/978-3-030-88727-8_61

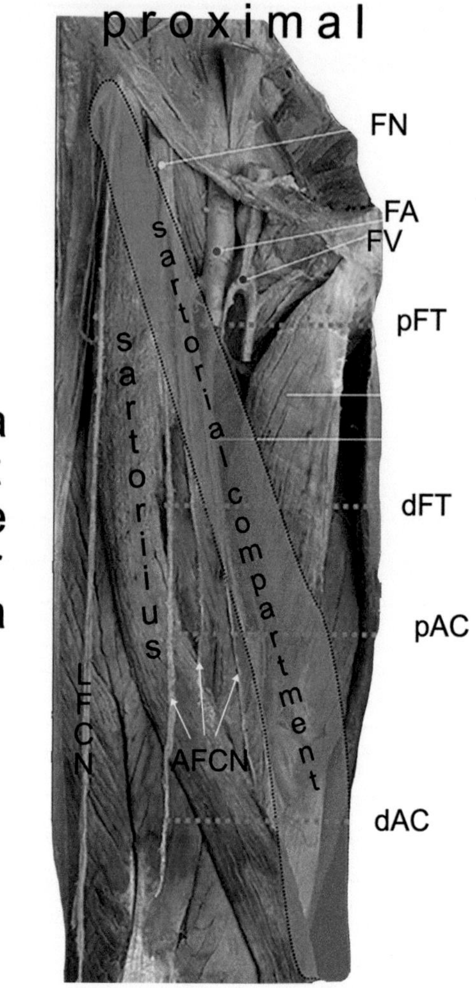

Fig. 61.1 The dissection shows the four levels of nerve blocks presented in this chapter: proximal femoral triangle (pFT), distal femoral triangle (dFT), proximal adductor canal (pAC), and distal adductor canal (dAC). The yellow 'sartorial compartment' indicates the in situ position of the holster of fascia lata containing the sartorius muscle (here drawn lateral). *FA* Femoral artery, *FV* femoral vein, *FN* femoral nerve, *LFCN*, lateral femoral cutaneous nerve, *AFCN* anterior femoral cutaneous nerves

Indications (Patient Selection)

Typically, TKR is performed by a midline skin incision followed by a medial parapatellar approach to access the knee joint.

In general, motor-sparing nerve block of femoral nerve terminals along the femoral artery in the femoral triangle or the adductor canal is used for pain relief after TKR performed with a medial approach as a supplement to intraoperative local infiltration analgesia (LIA).

A proximal femoral triangle block anaesthetizes the saphenous nerve, the nerve to vastus medialis (NVM), and the anterior femoral cutaneous nerves. A distal femoral triangle block (commonly known by the anatomic misnomer 'adductor canal block') anaesthetizes the saphenous nerve and the NVM. A proximal femoral triangle block provides a more effective analgesia after TKR compared to a distal femoral triangle block with a similar and moderate reduction of quadriceps femoris motor power. Thus, a proximal femoral triangle block should be the first choice for pain relief after TKR. Distal femoral triangle block should be the second choice, if the first choice is contraindicated.

A proximal adductor canal block only anaesthetizes the saphenous nerve as long as the local anaesthetic is contained in the lumen of the adductor canal. This nerve block is indicated for pain relief after hindfoot and ankle surgery but would only be the third choice for motor-sparing blockade of femoral nerve terminals innervating the anteromedial knee region. Probably the injectate sometimes spreads proximal to reach the NVM in the distal part of the femoral triangle or permeate the fascial layers separating the NVM from the lumen of the adductor canal. However, this cannot be assumed to be consistent in living human beings.

A distal adductor canal injection does not anaesthetize any femoral nerve branches. However, this block can be relevant for pain relief after knee surgery as the injectate spreads through the adductor hiatus into the popliteal fossa and anaesthetizes some of the major contributors to the popliteal plexus from the posterior branch of obturator nerve and the sciatic nerve, thereby presumed to provide analgesia of the posterior innervation of the knee. This could be an alternative to iPACK (infiltration between the popliteal artery and the capsule of the posterior knee).

Sometimes, TKR is carried out by a lateral parapatellar approach. In that case, the motor-sparing nerve block of femoral nerve terminals along the femoral artery in the femoral triangle or the adductor canal are not relevant, except that an injection in the distal adductor canal would still be a relevant alternative to iPACK.

Functional Anatomy

Motor-sparing nerve block of femoral nerve terminals innervating the anteromedial knee region is carried out by injecting local anaesthetic at various levels along the femoral artery in the femoral triangle or the adductor canal.

The 'femoral triangle' is a triangular groove in the anterior thigh. The base is the inguinal crease, and the apex is the intersection of the medial borders of the sartorius and adductor longus muscles. The femoral triangle is entirely roofed by the fascia lata (i.e. the deep fascia of the thigh). The sartorius muscle is a very special muscle as it is completely embedded in a duplication of the fascia lata. In this way, the sartorius muscle makes a 'half roof' of the femoral triangle.

The 'adductor canal' is a triangular vascular passageway from the apex of the femoral triangle to the popliteal fossa. It is the canal delimited by the fusion of the vastoadductor membrane with the epimysium of the medial vastus muscle and the adductor longus and magnus muscles. The distal opening of the adductor canal into the popliteal fossa is called the 'adductor hiatus'. It is the opening between the two tendons of the adductor magnus inserting on the linea aspera of the femur and the medial femoral epicondyle, respectively. The adductor magnus and longus muscles both insert on the linea aspera, and together they make the posteromedial wall of the adductor canal. The medial vastus muscle is also attached to the linea aspera and makes the anterolateral wall of the adductor canal. The vastoadductor membrane makes a dense anteromedial roof of the proximal superficial part of the adductor canal by fusing with the epimysium of the adductors and the medial vastus muscle. The distal part of the adductor canal is sandwiched between the adductor muscles posteriorly and the medial vastus muscle anteriorly.

The femoral artery descends from the base to the apex of the femoral triangle, where it dives into the adductor canal. From there, the femoral artery ends at the adductor hiatus, where it becomes the popliteal artery. The femoral nerve ramifies into numerous muscular and sensory terminal nerves at the level of the inguinal crease. These nerve terminals pass from the infrainguinal subcompartment of the fascia iliaca compartment into the femoral triangle, by piercing the dense iliopsoas fascia. The muscular nerve terminals innervating the quadriceps femoris muscles immediately deviate lateral away from the femoral artery—except the NVM. The femoral nerve terminals relevant for pain relief after anteromedial knee surgery are as follows: the infrapatellar branch of the saphenous nerve, the NVM, and the anterior femoral cutaneous nerves. They all have a relationship to the femoral artery that is relevant for regional anaesthesia of these nerves.

The sensory saphenous nerve and the mixed sensorimotor NVM originate from a common trunk of the femoral nerve and descend close together along the anterolateral side of the femoral artery throughout the femoral triangle from the base to the apex. At the apex, the saphenous nerve dives into the adductor canal, while the NVM deviates away from the femoral artery and continues inside its own fascial tunnel on top of the medial vastus muscle outside the adductor canal (Fig. 61.2). The NVM innervates this muscle and terminates as the superior medial genicular nerve, innervating the anteromedial aspect of the genicular retinaculum and the knee joint.

The saphenous nerve runs throughout the superficial proximal part of the adductor canal roofed by the vastoadductor membrane, where the adductor longus muscle makes the posterior wall. In this part of the canal, the saphenous nerve crosses obliquely anterior to the femoral artery from anterolateral to anteromedial. Approximately at the point where the posterior wall changes from the adductor longus to become the adductor magnus and the femoral artery dives into the deep distal part of the adductor canal towards the adductor hiatus, the saphenous nerve pierces the vastoadductor membrane and enters the subsartorial space between the vastoadductor membrane and the sartorius muscle. Here, it typically gives off an infrapatellar branch that emerges from the anterior border of the sartorius muscle tendon on the medial side of the knee. This branch innervates the skin and fascia, covering the inferior anteromedial part of the knee.

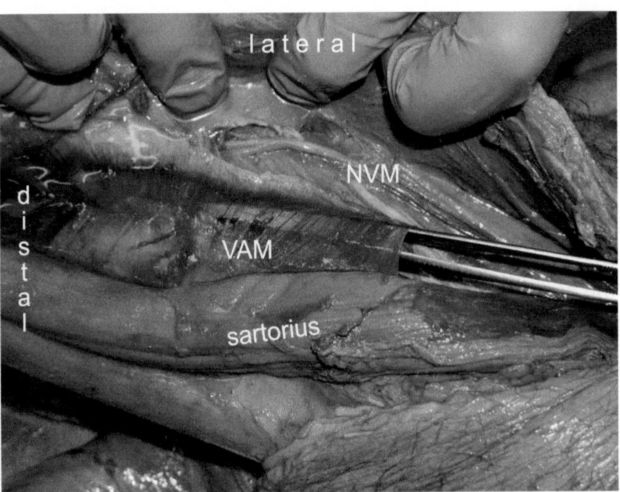

Fig. 61.2 The dissection shows how the nerve to the vastus medialis (NVM) deviates away from the saphenous nerve (position indicated by forceps) when reaching the proximal end of the AC, indicated by the sharp margin of the vastoadductor membrane (VAM). The sartorius muscle is lifted medial to expose the VAM. The methylene blue injected into the lumen of the adductor canal shows a patchy and inconsistent spread to the NVM by proximal spread as well as by permeating the fascial layers separating the adductor canal and the fascial tunnel containing the NVM. Whether this is similar in living human beings is not known. Reprinted with courtesy of Bernhard Moriggl and Thomas Fichtner Bendtsen

The anterior femoral cutaneous nerves comprise the intermediary and the medial femoral cutaneous nerves. They pierce the iliopsoas fascia just distal to the inguinal crease, and they make the most superficial layer of ramifications from the femoral nerve at this level. Typically, two intermediary femoral cutaneous nerves descend almost vertically across the sartorius muscle from the medial to the lateral border piercing the fascia lata in long 'flat fatty tunnels' before they become subcutaneous and innervate the skin and fascia of the distal half of the anterior thigh as far as the base of patella. The medial femoral cutaneous nerve descends approximately 10 cm along the lateral margin of the femoral artery before it crosses anterior to the artery and ramifies in anterior and posterior branches. The crossing is typically where the femoral artery dives deep to the medial border of the sartorius muscle. At a variable level, the anterior branches wind around the medial border or pierce the sartorius muscle and descend approximately vertically in 'tunnels' in the fascia lata across the sartorius. From there, these anterior branches emerge in the subcutaneous tissue when they cross the lateral border of the sartorius and continue across the medial vastus muscle as far as the anteromedial knee region. The posterior branches descend deep to the medial margin of the sartorius muscle, and the terminal branch emerges into the subcutaneous tissue approximately at the level of the proximal end of the adductor canal. The medial femoral cutaneous nerves innervate the skin and fascia lata in the anteromedial region between the territories innervated by the intermediary femoral cutaneous nerves and the infrapatellar branch of the saphenous nerve.

An injection into the most distal end of the adductor canal immediately proximal to the adductor hiatus does not anaesthetize any branches of the femoral nerve—except occasionally the saphenous nerve due to spread of injectate into the superficial proximal part of the adductor canal.

Techniques

Generally, the patient is placed supine with the thigh slightly externally rotated. The ultrasound transducer is placed on the anteromedial thigh approximately midway between the anterior superior iliac spine and the base of patella. The femoral artery is visualized deep to the sartorius muscle and aligned to the centre of the monitor by adjusting image depth and transducer position. Gain and focus point are adjusted as well. The transducer is shifted up and down along the femoral artery until the apex of the femoral triangle is identified as the intersection of the medial borders of the sartorius and adductor longus muscle (Fig. 61.3). This is the *reference point,* which is the interface between the femoral triangle proximally and the adductor canal distally.

Proximal Femoral Triangle Block

The high-frequency linear transducer is shifted proximally from the *reference point* along the femoral artery until the level where the artery is about to dive or has just dived deep to the medial margin of the sartorius muscle. This is typically approximately 10 cm distal to the inguinal crease (Fig. 61.4). At this level, the medial femoral cutaneous nerve has not yet crossed anterior to the femoral artery and is still located anterolateral to the femoral artery superficial to the saphenous and medial vastus nerves. Frequently, the latter two nerves are united in a common trunk at this level (Fig. 61.4).

The needle is inserted in-plane from the lateral end of the transducer with a trans-sartorial approach. It is mandatory to visualize and avoid piercing and injuring the intermediary femoral cutaneous nerves with this approach (Fig. 61.4). First, 5 mL of local anaesthetic is deposited anterolateral around the femoral artery in order to anaesthetize the medial femoral cutaneous nerve (Fig. 61.5). Second, the needle tip is redirected to a slightly deeper posterolateral position in relation to the femoral artery, and 10 mL of local anaesthetic is injected around the saphenous nerve and NVM (Fig. 61.5). Third, the needle is retracted, and the intermediary femoral

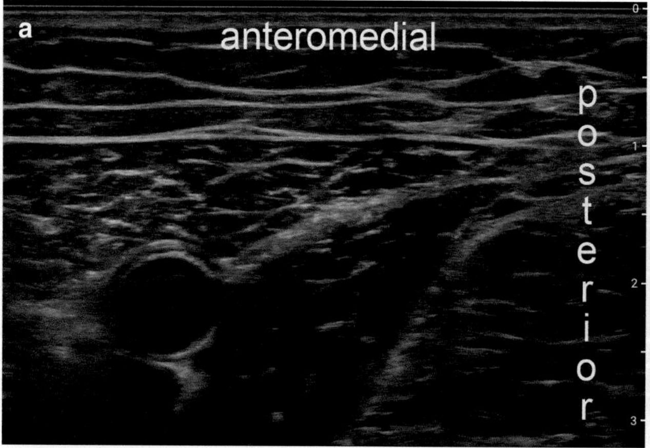

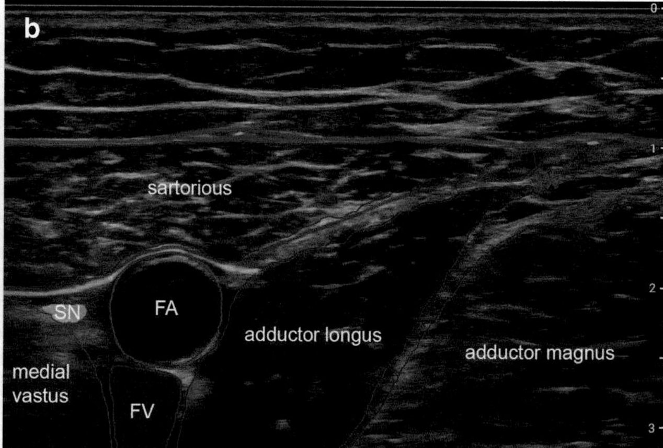

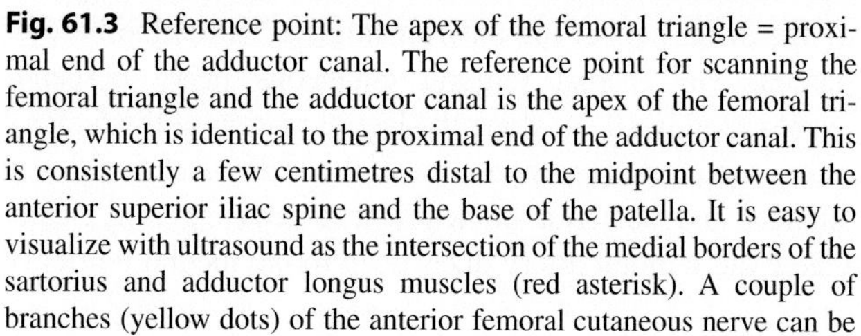

Fig. 61.3 Reference point: The apex of the femoral triangle = proximal end of the adductor canal. The reference point for scanning the femoral triangle and the adductor canal is the apex of the femoral triangle, which is identical to the proximal end of the adductor canal. This is consistently a few centimetres distal to the midpoint between the anterior superior iliac spine and the base of the patella. It is easy to visualize with ultrasound as the intersection of the medial borders of the sartorius and adductor longus muscles (red asterisk). A couple of branches (yellow dots) of the anterior femoral cutaneous nerve can be identified embedded in the layer of the fascia lata (pink) that is anterior to the sartorius muscle. Of note, the sartorius is enmeshed in a duplicature of the fascia lata. The dense vastoadductor membrane (cyan stripe) is the anteromedial roof the adductor canal. The proximal end of the membrane is at the apex of the femoral triangle. The ultrasound image (**a**) is shown with a graphical overlay in (**b**). *SN* saphenous nerve, *FA* femoral artery, *FV* femoral vein. Reprinted with courtesy of Thomas Fichtner Bendtsen

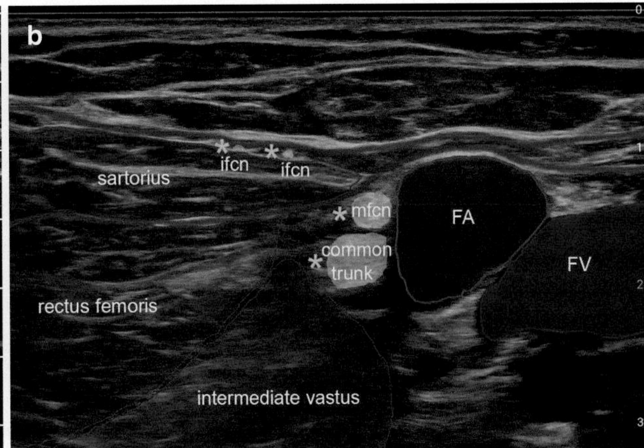

Fig. 61.4 The proximal femoral triangle block. The proximal femoral triangle block is carried out where the femoral artery (FA) is diving—or is about to dive—deep to the medial border of the sartorius muscle. This is typically approximately 10 cm distal to the intersection of the FA and the inguinal crease. At this level, the saphenous nerve and nerve to vastus medialis are frequently fused in a common trunk adjacent and lateral to the FA. The common trunk is located posterior to the medial femoral cutaneous nerve (MFCN) on the lateral side of the FA. This is just proximal to the level, where the MFCN crosses anterior to the FA and ramifies in anterior and posterior branches along the posteromedial border of the sartorius muscle. The intermediary femoral cutaneous nerves (ifcn) are located anterior to the sartorius muscle at this level. Four targets of injection are marked by cyan asterisks. They can be carried out by a single-needle insertion with redirections. The ultrasound image (**a**) is shown with a graphical overlay in (**b**). *FA* femoral artery, *FV* femoral vein. Reprinted with courtesy of Thomas Fichtner Bendtsen

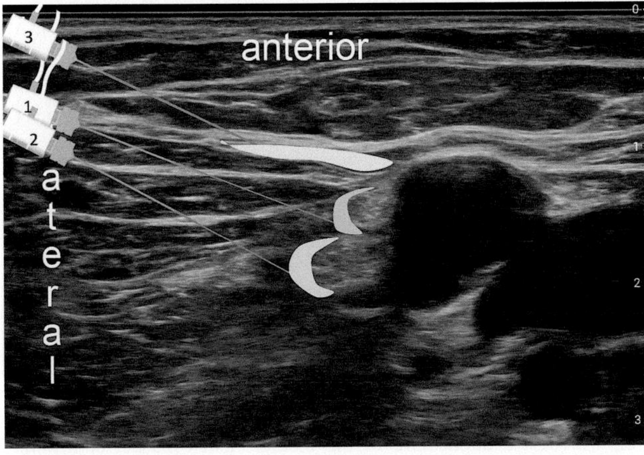

Fig. 61.5 Injections with the proximal femoral triangle block. Three injections are carried out: (1) 5 mL is injected (blue) around the medial femoral cutaneous nerve, (2) 10 mL is injected (orange) around the common trunk of the nerve to vastus medialis and the saphenous nerve located slightly deeper, and (3) 2–3 mL is injected (yellow) around the intermediary femoral cutaneous nerves inside their flat fatty tunnels in the fascia lata. Reprinted with courtesy of Thomas Fichtner Bendtsen

cutaneous nerves are anaesthetized inside their interfascial tunnels inside the deep fascia (i.e. fascia lata) or in the subcutaneous tissue by injecting 2–3 mL of local anaesthetic around each of the nerves (typically two) (Fig. 61.5).

Distal Femoral Triangle Block

The high-frequency linear transducer is shifted 3–5 cm proximal to the *reference point* along the femoral artery in order to secure anaesthesia of both the saphenous and the NVM.

The needle is inserted in-plane from the lateral end of the transducer and carefully advanced between the sartorius muscle and the medial vastus muscle. Optimally, the needle is advanced on the internal side of the sartorius epimysium, thereby avoiding painful and potentially harmful piercing of the branches of the medial vastus nerve that ramify in the interfascial plane between the sartorius and vastus medialis muscles (Fig. 61.6). In the awake patient, this approach is much less painful compared to a trans-sartorial approach. When the needle tip is close to the anterolateral aspect of the femoral artery, the epimysium is pierced, and the needle tip is located in the interfascial plane adjacent to the femoral artery containing the saphenous nerve and the main trunk of the NVM (Fig. 61.6). After meticulous check of no intravascular needle tip placement by aspiration, 10 mL of local anaesthetic is injected while observing perineural spread around the saphenous and NVM. In the case that the nerves are not visible, 20 mL of local anaesthetic should be injected adjacent to the femoral artery.

Proximal Adductor Canal Block

The high-frequency linear transducer is shifted 2–4 cm distal to the *reference point* along the femoral artery until the posterior wall of the adductor canal transitions from the adductor longus muscle to the adductor magnus muscle (Fig. 61.7). This is approximately where the saphenous nerve begins to emerge from the adductor canal by piercing the vastoadductor membrane. The needle is carefully advanced trans-sartorially in-plane from the lateral end of the ultrasound transducer, and 10 mL of local anaesthetic is injected around the femoral

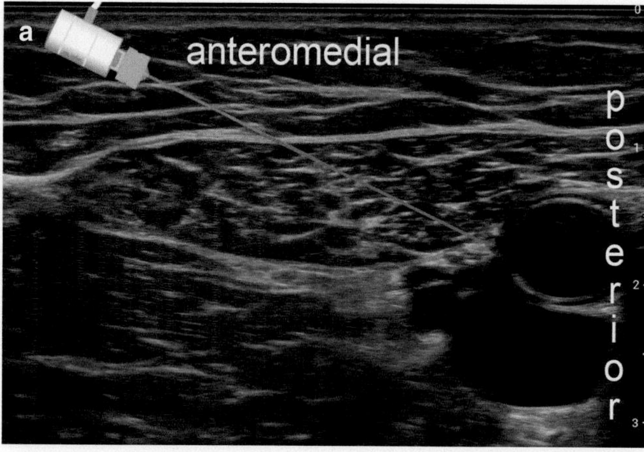

Fig. 61.6 The distal femoral triangle block. The distal femoral triangle block is carried out midway between the anterior superior iliac spine and the base of the patella. That is consistently 2–5 cm proximal to the proximal end of the true anatomical adductor canal. At this level, the saphenous nerve (SN) is adjacent to the femoral artery (FA) in the interfascial plane between the sartorius and medial vastus muscles. The medial vastus nerve (MVN) is localized slightly more anterolateral in the same interfascial plane. Typically, this block is performed as a fascial plane block by injecting adjacent to the FA. However, frequently the SN and the MVN are clearly visible with ultrasound and can be targeted by direct perineural injection. The targets of injection are marked by cyan asterisks. The ultrasound image (**a**) is shown with a graphical overlay in (**b**). *FA* femoral artery, *FV* femoral vein. Fascia lata, pink. Reprinted with courtesy of Thomas Fichtner Bendtsen

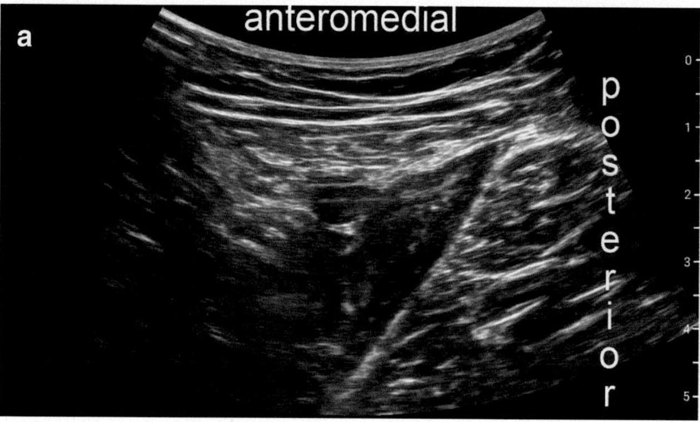

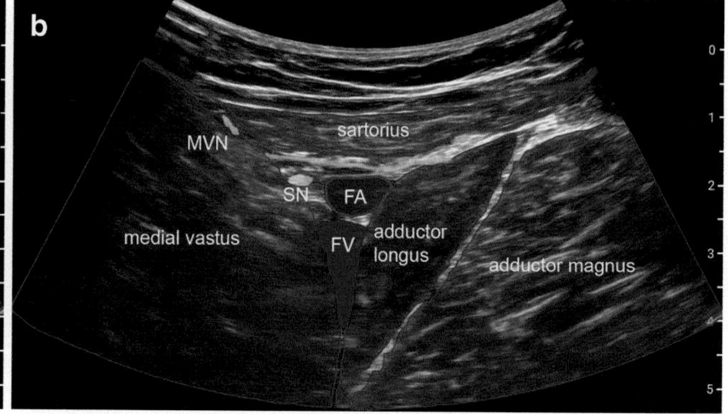

Fig. 61.7 The proximal adductor canal block. Only one nerve—the saphenous nerve—is consistently located in the proximal end of the adductor canal. The proximal part of the adductor canal is characterized by a posterior wall made by the adductor longus muscle. An injection into the proximal end of the adductor canal cannot be expected to anaesthetize the medial vastus nerve (MVN) as it is embedded in its own fascial tunnel, which is a duplicature of the medial vastus muscle epimysium. Vastoadductor membrane, cyan. Fascia lata, pink. The ultrasound image (**a**) is shown with a graphical overlay in (**b**). *FA* femoral artery, *FV* femoral vein. Reprinted with courtesy of Thomas Fichtner Bendtsen

artery. At this level, the saphenous nerve has shifted around the femoral artery and is typically localized antero-medial to the artery. On the ultrasound monitor, this appears as 'medial'.

Distal Adductor Canal Block

A curved-array transducer is placed in the distal anteromedial aspect of the thigh approximately 6 cm proximal to the base of patella, which is the typical location of the adductor hiatus. From this position, the transducer is shifted along the femoral artery until the femoral artery and vein are visualized, sandwiched between the medial vastus muscle and the adductor magnus in the deep distal part of the adductor canal (Fig. 61.8). The needle is advanced through the medial vastus muscle in-plane from the lateral end of the transducer until the needle tip is adjacent to the femoral artery inside the adductor canal. Ten to 15 mL of local anaesthetic is injected perivascularly in order to obtain spread of the injectate through the adductor hiatus to the posterior obturator nerve and tibial nerve main contributors to the popliteal plexus, innervating the posterior part of the knee and its capsule.

Complications

1. Intravascular injection of local anaesthetic
2. Injury of the anterior femoral cutaneous nerves
3. Injury of the NVM between the sartorius and medial vastus muscles

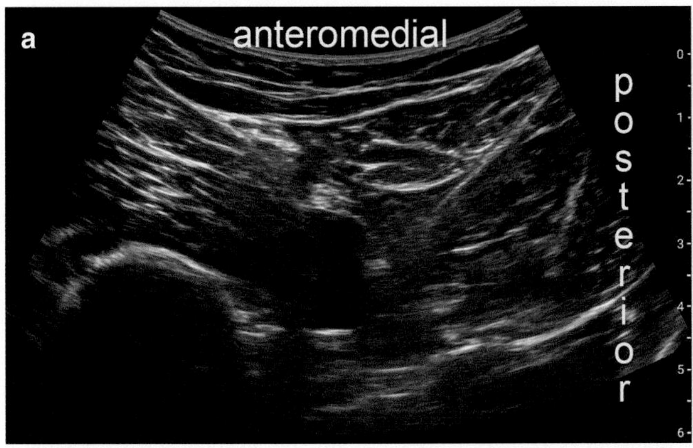

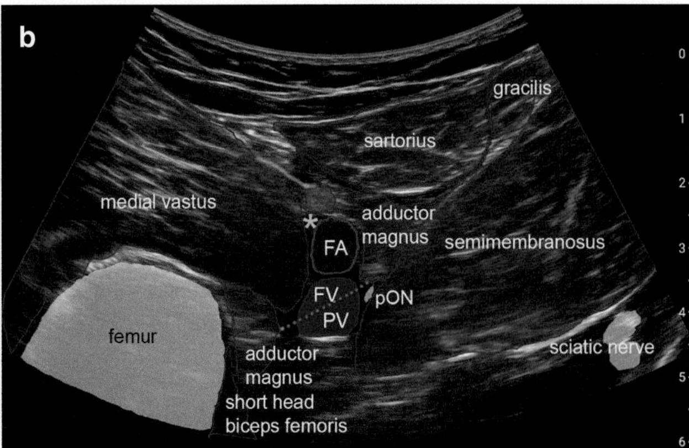

Fig. 61.8 Distal adductor canal block (popliteal plexus block). The distal end of the adductor canal is the adductor hiatus (dotted green line), which is the passage between the musculotendinous insertions (red asterisks) of the adductor magnus on the linea aspera and the medial epicondyle of the femur. This is where the femoral artery (FA) and vein (FV) become the popliteal artery and vein (PA and PV). The target of injection is marked by a cyan asterisk. The injectate spreads via the adductor hiatus into the popliteal fossa around the popliteal artery and PV. Thus, it anaesthetizes some of the main genicular branches from the posterior branch of the obturator nerve (pON) and the sciatic nerve to the popliteal plexus. The popliteal plexus winds around the popliteal artery and PV. At the level just proximal to the femoral epicondyles terminal nerve branches ramify from the popliteal plexus into the fatty connective tissue posterior to the knee joint capsule. These branches innervate the posterior part of the knee capsule. Vastoadductor membrane, cyan stripe. Fascia lata, pink. The ultrasound image (**a**) is shown with a graphical overlay in (**b**). Reprinted with courtesy of Thomas Fichtner Bendtsen

Practical Tips

The risk of intravascular injection of local anaesthetic can be minimized by (a) frequent intermittent aspiration during injection, (b) aborting injection if perineural injection is not sonographically visible, and (c) releasing the transducer pressure before injection in order to visualize accidental intravenous location of the needle tip.

The risk of injury of major cutaneous nerves should be minimized by visualizing these nerves prior to needle insertion (Figs. 61.3 and 61.5).

The risk of injury of the NVM between the sartorius and medial vastus muscles can be minimized by carefully advancing the needle on the inner side of the sartorial epimysium and by combining ultrasound with electrical nerve stimulation using an output of 0.2 mA.

Literature Review

The adductor canal was originally described by John Hunter 235 years ago. He wanted to ligate the femoral artery in the proximal end of the adductor canal and identified this point as midways from the intersection of the femoral artery and the groin to the medial side of the knee. This was also reported in older editions of Gray's anatomy. However, newer editions just state that the adductor canal is located in 'the middle of the thigh' with no reference. The originators of the so-called adductor canal block located the 'middle of the thigh' as the midpoint from the anterior superior iliac spine to the base of patella, thereby introducing an anatomical bias. Thus, what is widely known in the literature as 'adductor canal block' is in fact a distal femoral triangle block.

In an RCT, the proximal femoral triangle block has been compared to distal femoral triangle block and proximal adductor canal block. Unfortunately, the authors call the three blocks 'proximal, mid-, and distal adductor canal blocks', which contributes to the confusion about this topic in the literature. However, a proximal femoral triangle block reduces opioid consumption without reducing quadriceps strength after ACL repair compared to distal femoral triangle block and proximal adductor canal block.

In another RCT, proximal femoral triangle block is compared to distal femoral triangle block. Again, the authors confuse the femoral triangle with the adductor canal. The authors observed no difference between the groups concerning opioid consumption, pain, and ability to ambulate.

A recent volunteer study demonstrated that the cutaneous anteromedial knee innervation—including the area of surgical incision of total knee arthroplasty—is primarily due to the anterior femoral cutaneous nerves. However, no clinical studies have intentionally included nerve block of the anterior femoral cutaneous nerves when performing the proximal femoral triangle block. This volunteer study also compared the motor effect of proximal and distal femoral triangle blocks with 10 and 20 ml of local anaesthetic, respectively. No statistically significant intergroup difference was observed. That said, some volunteers had clinically significant quadriceps weakness in both groups.

Cadaveric studies show effective spread of injectate from the distal adductor canal to the popliteal fossa and the main contributors to the posterior knee innervation from the popliteal plexus. No comparative clinical studies of this mechanism have been carried out.

Suggested Reading

Abdallah FW, Mejia J, Prasad GA, Moga R, Chahal J, Theodoropulos J, Dwyer T, Brull R. Opioid- and motor-sparing with proximal, mid-, and distal locations for adductor canal block in anterior cruciate ligament reconstruction: a randomized clinical trial. Anesthesiology. 2019;131(3):619–29.

Bendtsen TF, Moriggl B, Chan V, Børglum. The optimal analgesic block for total knee arthroplasty. Reg Anesth Pain Med. 2016;41(6):711–9.

Bjørn S, Nielsen TD, Moriggl B, Hoermann R, Bendtsen TF. Anesthesia of the anterior femoral cutaneous nerves for total knee arthroplasty incision: randomized volunteer trial. Reg Anesth Pain Med. 2020;45(2):107–16.

Fonkoué L, Behets C, Kouassi JK, Covette M, Detrembleur C, Thienpont E, Cornu O. Distribution of sensory nerves supplying the knee joint capsule and implications for genicular blockade and radiofrequency ablation: an anatomical study. Anesth Pain Med. 2019;44(2):234–8.

Gray H. Anatomy - descriptive and surgical. London: Longmans, Green & Co; 1897.

Home E. An account of Mr. Hunter's method of performing the operation for the popliteal aneurism. Lond Med J. 1786;7(Pt 4):391–406.

Jæger P, Lund J, Jenstrup MT, Brøndum V, Dahl JB. Reply to Dr. Bendtsen. Reg Anesth Pain Med. 2014;39(3):254–5.

Layera S, Aliste J, Bravo D, Saadawi M, Salinas FV, Tran Q. Motor-sparing nerve blocks for total knee replacement: a scoping review. J Clin Anesth. 2021;68:110076.

Meier AW, Auyong DB, Yuan SC, Lin SE, Flaherty JM, Hanson NA. Comparison of continuous proximal versus distal adductor canal blocks for total knee arthroplasty: a randomized, double-blind, noninferiority trial. Reg Anesth Pain Med. 2018;43(1):36–42.

Runge C, Moriggl B, Borglum J, Bendtsen TF. The spread of ultrasound-guided injectate from the adductor canal to the genicular branch of the posterior obturator nerve and the popliteal plexus - a cadaveric study. Reg Anesth Pain Med. 2017;42(6):725–30.

Standring S, Gray H. Gray's anatomy: the anatomical basis of clinical practice. Edinburgh: Churchill Livingstone/Elsevier; 2008.

Tran J, Peng PWH, Gofeld M, Chan V, Agur AMR. Anatomical study of the innervation of posterior knee joint capsule: implication for image-guided intervention. Reg Anesth Pain Med. 2019;44(2):234–8.

Wong WY, Bjørn S, Strid JM, Børglum J, Bendtsen TF. Defining the location of the adductor canal using ultrasound. Reg Anesth Pain Med. 2017;42(2):241–5.

iPACK Block: Infiltration in the Interspace Between Popliteal Artery and Capsule of the Knee

62

James M. Jack, Maria Fernanda Rojas Gomez, and Vincent Chan

Contents

General Considerations

The iPACK block is a motor-sparing analgesic intervention that blocks the articular branches of the tibial, common peroneal and obturator nerves in the popliteal region.

J. M. Jack
Guy's and St Thomas' NHS Foundation Trust, London, UK
e-mail: James.jack@doctors.org.uk

M. F. Rojas Gomez
Cirulaser Andes Clinic, Bogota, Colombia

V. Chan (✉)
Department of Anesthesiology and Pain Medicine, Toronto Western Hospital, University of Toronto, Toronto, ON, Canada
e-mail: Vincent.Chan@uhn.ca

Indications (Patient Selection)

The iPACK block is indicated for patients undergoing total knee arthroplasty (TKA).

Functional Anatomy

Pain relief after TKA can be achieved by blocking the sensory innervation to the anterior and posterior compartments of the knee. Anterior knee joint innervation is complex and not yet fully elucidated (Fig. 62.1). Sensory innervation to the anteromedial compartment of the knee is supplied by the branches of the femoral nerve and either the anterior branch of the tibial nerve or directly from the sciatic nerve (SN). The anterolateral compartment is supplied by the branches of the femoral nerve, the common fibular nerve (CFN) or directly

D. Jankovic, P. Peng (eds.), *Regional Nerve Blocks in Anesthesia and Pain Therapy*,
https://doi.org/10.1007/978-3-030-88727-8_62

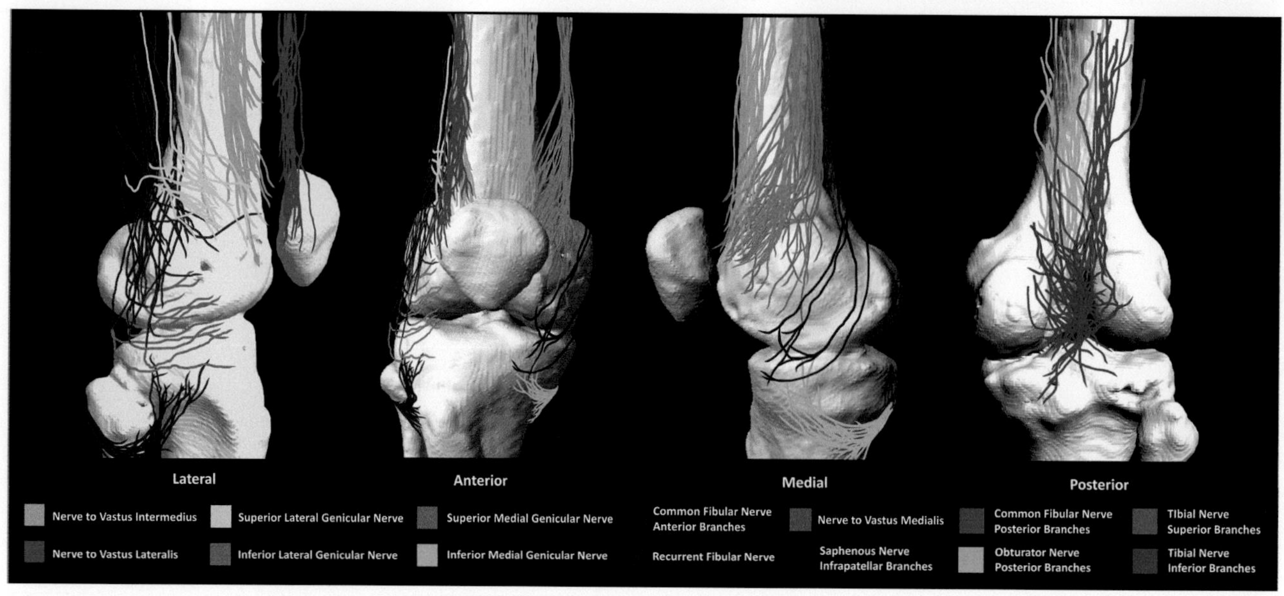

Fig. 62.1 Anterior knee joint innervation. Reprinted with permission from Philip Peng Educational Series

from the SN. Sensory innervation of the anterior knee compartment can also be divided into quadrants.

Collectively 10 nerves innervate four quadrants of the anterior knee joint capsule: superomedial and inferomedial (collectively known as the anteromedial component) and superolateral and inferolateral (collectively known as the anterolateral component). Nerve supply to four quadrants of the anterior knee joint is summarized in Fig. 62.2.

Furthermore, these nerves also innervate the following structures:

- Soft tissues—medial and lateral retinacula, patellar periosteum, infrapatellar fat pad, suprapatellar pouch and medial and lateral collateral ligaments
- Bony structures—the synovial surface of the lateral epicondyle of the femur, the periosteal anterior surface of the femur to the border of articular cartilage, the periosteal anterolateral surface of the tibia, tibial tuberosity and superior tibiofibular joint
- Vascular structures—blood vessels supplying the medial and lateral condyles of femur and tibia

Sensory innervation to the posterior knee compartment is supplied by the popliteal plexus (PP), which is derived principally from the tibial nerve (TN), and the posterior branch of the obturator nerve (ON) and, when present, either the posterior branch of the common peroneal nerve (CPN) or the SN (Fig. 62.3). The PP supplies the menisci, perimeniscular joint capsule, cruciate ligaments, infrapatellar fat pad and posterior part of the fibrous knee capsule. Posterior capsule innervation can be further divided into four quadrants—(1) superomedial quadrant innervated by the TN and posterior ON; (2) superolateral quadrant innervated by the TN and posterior CPN or posterior SN, when present; (3) inferomedial quadrant; and (4) inferolateral quadrant innervated by the TN.

Articular branches of the popliteal plexus travel through a tissue space between the popliteal artery and the posterior aspect of the distal femur (Fig. 62.4). This is the anatomic basis of the iPACK block injection.

Block Techniques

Anatomically, two iPACK block injection approaches have been described: (1) injection at the level of the distal femoral shaft and (2) injection more distally at the level of the intercondylar fossa just above the femoral condyles (Fig. 62.4). Both a high-frequency (8–12 MHz) linear transducer and a

Fig. 62.2 Innervation of the four quadrants of the anterior knee compartment. *SLGN* superior lateral genicular nerve, *NVILB* nerve to vastus intermedius lateral branch, *NVL* nerve to vastus lateralis, *CFNAB* common fibular nerve anterior branch, *RFN* recurrent fibular nerve, *ILGN* inferior lateral genicular nerve, *SMGN* superior medial genicular nerve, *NVIMB* nerve to vastus intermedius medial branch, *NVM* nerve to vastus medialis, *IMGN* inferior medial genicular nerves, *IPBSN* infrapatellar branch of saphenous nerve. Reprinted with permission from Philip Peng Educational Series

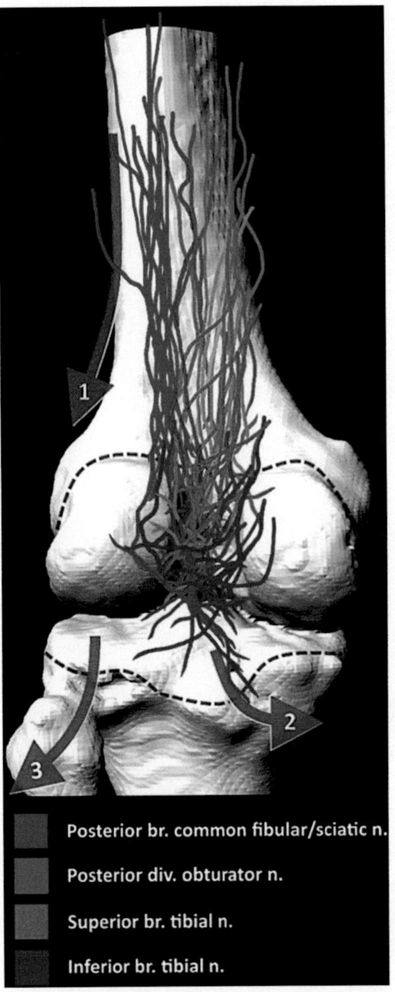

Fig. 62.3 Posterior view of the innervation of the knee. Arrows indicate course of the 1. superior lateral genicular nerve, 2. recurrent fibular nerve and 3. inferior medial genicular nerve. Reprinted with permission from Philip Peng Educational Series

low-frequency (2–5 MHz) curvilinear transducer may be employed. The latter offers a wider field of view, a deeper ultrasound penetration for patients with higher BMI and an easier needle visualization.

For each approach, a 22G 80 mm needle, preferably echogenic, is advanced in plane under ultrasound guidance in either a medial to lateral direction or a lateral to medial direction, with the patient lying in a variety of positions (supine, lateral or prone), as summarized in Table 62.1. At the level of the distal femoral shaft, a medial to lateral approach is often used with the patient in the supine position. At the intercondylar fossa level, a lateral to medial approach is often used with the patient lying lateral decubitus.

Blocking at the Level of the Intercondylar Fossa: Lateral to Medial Needling Approach

This is one of the most popular approaches with the patient lying lateral decubitus (Fig. 62.5). When administered at the intercondylar fossa level, an iPACK block injection can be performed using a lateral to medial needle approach after conduct of an isobaric spinal anaesthetic (hypobaric at body temperature) with the operative limb uppermost. However, a medial to lateral needle approach is preferred after conduct of hyperbaric spinal anaesthesia. With the patient in the lateral decubitus position, apply the transducer transversely just proximal to the popliteal crease (Fig. 62.6) to visualize the two femoral condyles (Fig. 62.6).

The transducer is then moved cephalad to visualize the intercondylar fossa, which is indicated by a continuous hyperechoic line joining two femoral condyles, with the popliteal artery and vein(s) posteriorly (Fig. 62.6). This is the level of injection.

We recommend sliding the transducer further cephalad to visualize the TN and CPN as they merge to form the SN. Knowing the location of the SN and its branches will help monitor for unintentional needle-nerve contact, during needle advancement, and potential local anaesthetic spread to the SN or CPN, resulting in foot-drop (Fig. 62.7). Then, move the transducer back to the level of injection after nerve visualization.

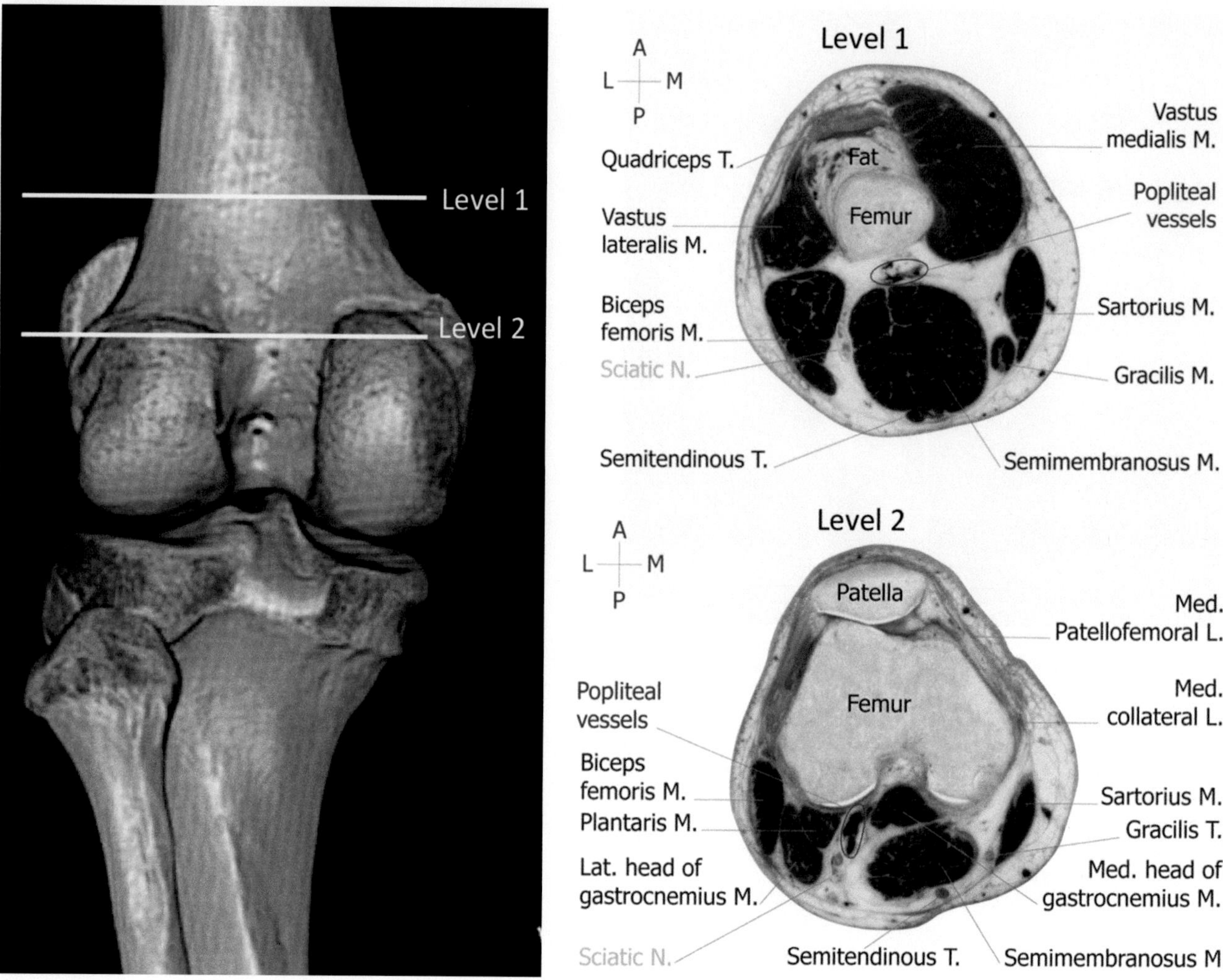

Fig. 62.4 Axial view of relevant anatomy at level of distal femoral shaft at two levels where iPACK is performed: 1 distal femoral shaft, 2. intercondylar fossa. Reprinted with permission from Dr. Maria Fernanda Rojas

Table 62.1 Patient position, transducer position and needle approach for iPACK

Level	Patient position	Transducer position	Needle approach
Distal femoral shaft	Supine	Medial thigh Posterior thigh	Medial to lateral Medial to lateral
	Prone	Posterior thigh	Medial to lateral Lateral to medial
Intercondylar fossa	Supine	Posterior thigh	Medial to lateral Lateral to medial
	Prone	Posterior thigh	Medial to lateral Lateral to medial
	Lateral decubitus	Posterior thigh	Medial to lateral Lateral to medial

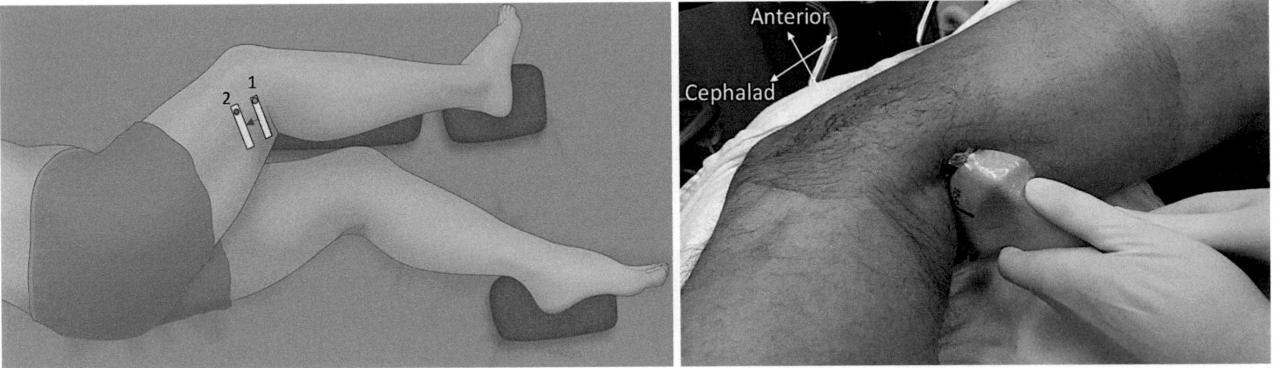

Fig. 62.5 Left. Schematic diagram of lateral decubitus position for lateral to medial intercondylar fossa approach. Transducer position is initially placed at 1 and then move to 2. Right. Initial position of transducer in lateral to medial intercondylar iPACK in a patient positioned lateral decubitus. Reprinted with permission from Dr. Maria Fernanda Rojas

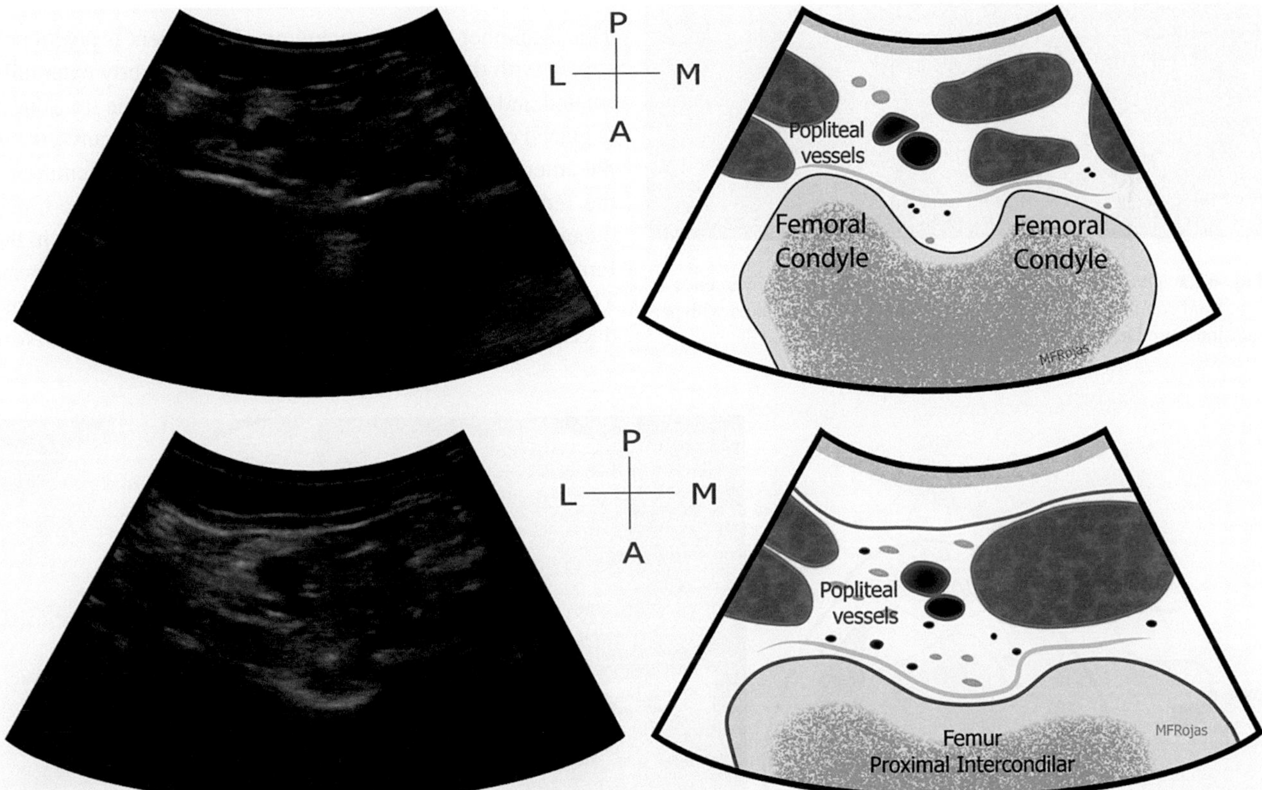

Fig. 62.6 The upper image corresponds to transducer position 1 in Fig. 62.5 at the level of femoral epicondyles with the transducer applied to posterior aspect of the knee. The lower image corresponds to transducer position 2 in Fig. 62.5 at the level of distal femoral shaft superior to the femoral condyles with the transducer applied to posterior aspect of the knee. Reprinted with permission from Dr. Maria Fernanda Rojas

Before needle insertion, the distance from the skin surface to the intercondylar fossa is measured using the on-screen calipers of the ultrasound device. This distance, usually 3–5 cm, equates to the needle insertion point distance from the transducer edge (Fig. 62.8). For the lateral to medial needle approach, the needle is inserted in plane at this distance, anterior to the tendon of long head of biceps femoris, parallel to the transducer (Fig. 62.8). Ensure the SN or its branches are not in the path of needle advancement. If visualization of needle advancement is difficult, then move the transducer laterally to meet the needle. Once the needle is visualized, the transducer is returned medially to the popliteal fossa whilst tracking needle advancement. The standard use of a curved transducer offers a wider field of view, allowing an earlier needle visualization.

Needle advancement is continuously monitored towards the interspace between the posterior aspect of the femur and the popliteal artery, ensuring the needle tip is far away from the CPN. Once the needle tip has reached 1–2 cm beyond the medial edge of the popliteal artery and negative aspiration is confirmed, local anaesthetic is injected slowly and incrementally. Local anaesthetic spread is monitored in real time for potential spread towards the CPN whilst withdrawing the needle (Fig. 62.9). Tissue expansion is usually seen superficial to the site of injection, towards the skin. A 10–20 mL bolus of a long-acting local anaesthetic solution (bupivacaine or ropivacaine 0.25–0.5% with epinephrine 1:200,000) is recommended. Injection may be performed continuously with the goal of depositing local anaesthetic at three sites: 1/3 medially, 1/3 underneath and 1/3 laterally to the artery whilst withdrawing the needle incrementally. Do not inject more than 2 cm lateral to the popliteal artery to minimize potential spread to the CPN. At this time, the optimum volume, concentration, needle tip location before injection and injection technique have not been determined.

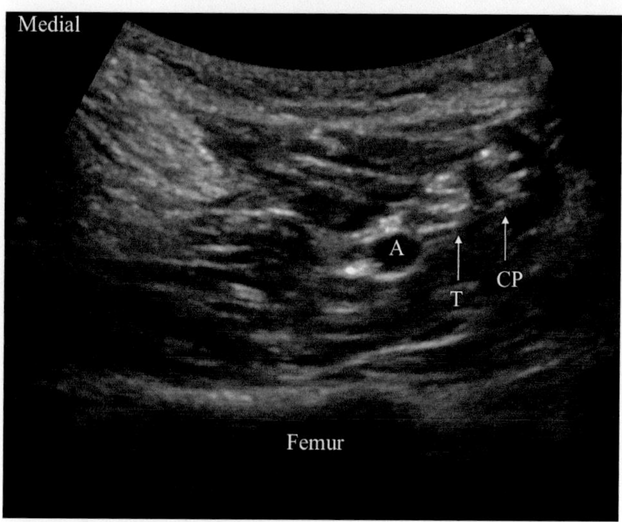

Fig. 62.7 Dynamic proximal scanning to visualize convergence of tibial and common peroneal nerves to sciatic nerve. Reprinted with permission from Dr. Maria Fernanda Rojas

Blocking at the Level of the Distal Femoral Shaft, Medial to Lateral Needling Approach

This is another common technique. The patient is positioned supine with the operative knee flexed and slightly externally rotated and the thigh supported (Fig. 62.10). The transducer is placed on the lower third of the medial thigh, transverse in the anterior to posterior direction, to visualize the femur and the femoral vessels in the cross section. Ensure the transducer is distal to the adductor hiatus through which the femoral artery passes through to become the popliteal artery. The main body of vastus medialis will be closest to the transducer, with the sartorius posterior to this superficially. Note

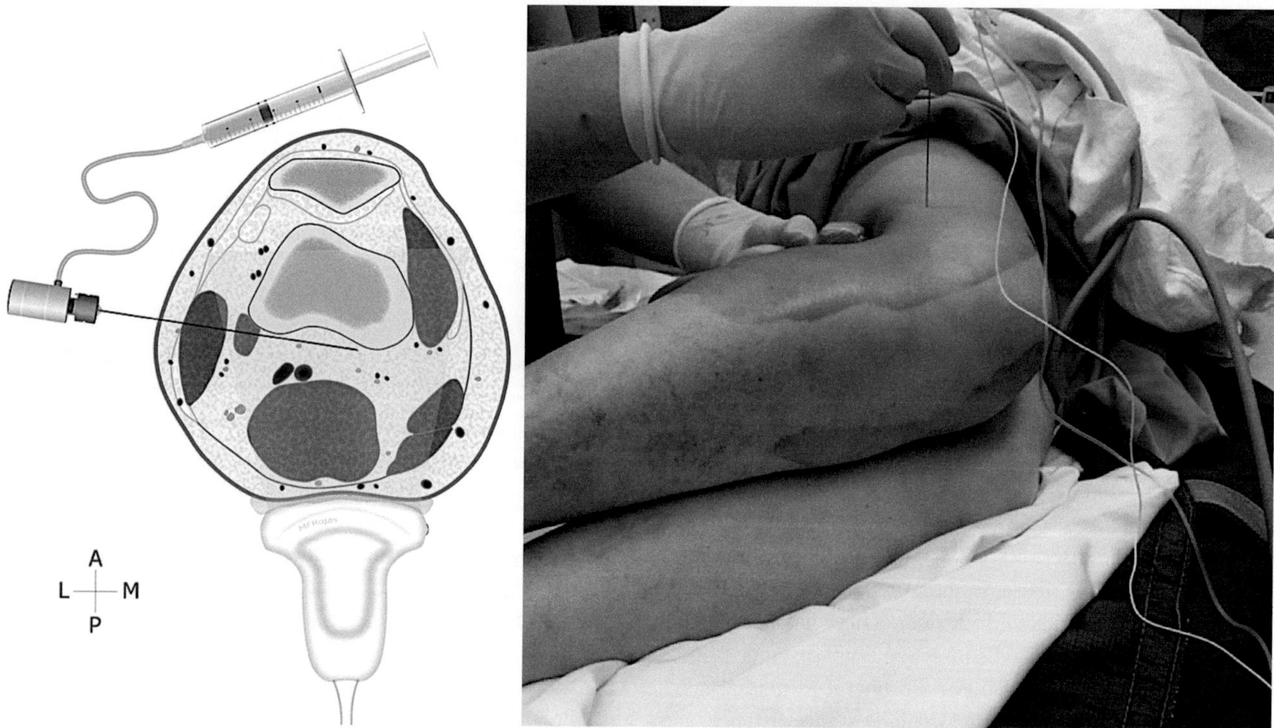

Fig. 62.8 Left. Insertion of needle in parallel to acoustic window of transducer at measured distance from skin at transducer edge to intercondylar fossa. Lateral movement of transducer to meet needle during advancement. Once the needle tip is visualized, return the transducer to the correct position. Reprinted with permission from Dr. Maria Fernanda Rojas

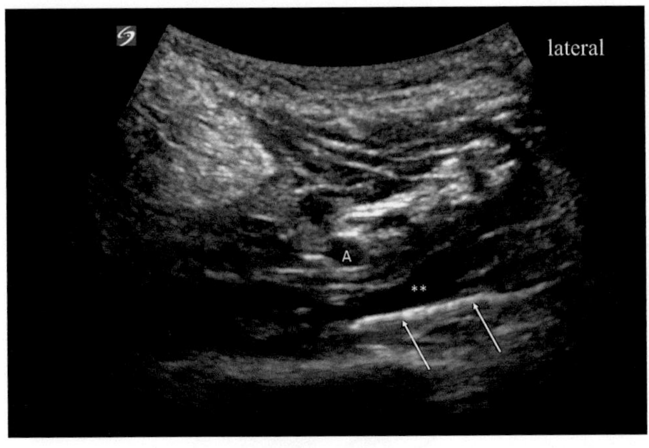

Fig. 62.9 Slow withdrawal of needle whilst injecting in real time to monitor for injectate spread to the common peroneal nerve. Arrows, the needle; A, popliteal artery; **, local anaesthetic

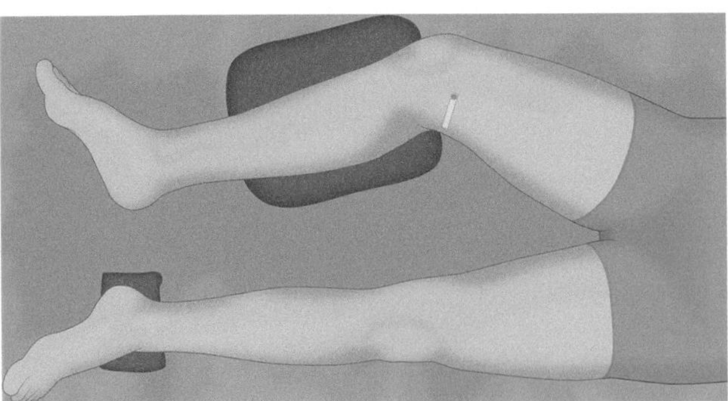

Fig. 62.10 Supine position with operative limb externally rotated, with slight knee flexion for medial to lateral approach iPACK (both variants). Reprinted with permission from Dr. Maria Fernanda Rojas

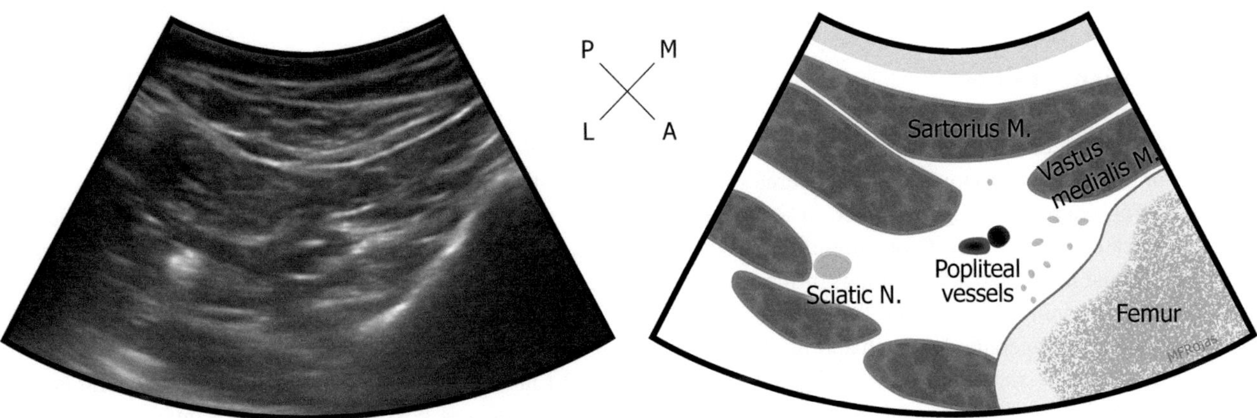

Fig. 62.11 Medial to lateral view at distal femoral shaft, with the femur at the edge of the transducer image. Reprinted with permission from Dr. Maria Fernanda Rojas

the hypoechoic femoral shaft with a curved hyperechoic bony outline (Fig. 62.11). Deep to the vastus medialis and posterior to the curved hypoechoic femoral shaft lie the femoral artery and vein, which may require colour Doppler to visualize. The SN is not seen in this view since it is located more laterally and posteriorly. The transducer is moved to visualize the femoral shaft at the edge of the screen, so that it does not obstruct needle advancement (Fig. 62.11).

The needle is inserted at the anterior end of the transducer in a medial to lateral trajectory and advanced in plane at a steep angle, penetrating the vastus medialis muscle (Fig. 62.12). The needle is advanced into the interspace until the needle tip has reached no more than 2 cm beyond the lateral border of the artery. The needle should be kept parallel to the acoustic shadow of the femur (Fig. 62.12). Starting in this position, after a negative aspiration, 10–20 mL of local anaesthetic is injected incrementally whilst withdrawing the needle until it is 1–2 cm medial to the popliteal artery.

Complications

Potential complications common to any regional technique include block failure, infection, vascular puncture and nerve injury. Specific complications include unintentional common peroneal nerve injury, due to needle trauma, and unintentional anaesthesia of the common peroneal nerve and its branches, resulting in foot drop.

Practical Tips

Optimal Needle Insertion Site

It is important to ensure there is an adequate space between the intercondylar fossa and popliteal artery for injection, ideally 1–2 cm.

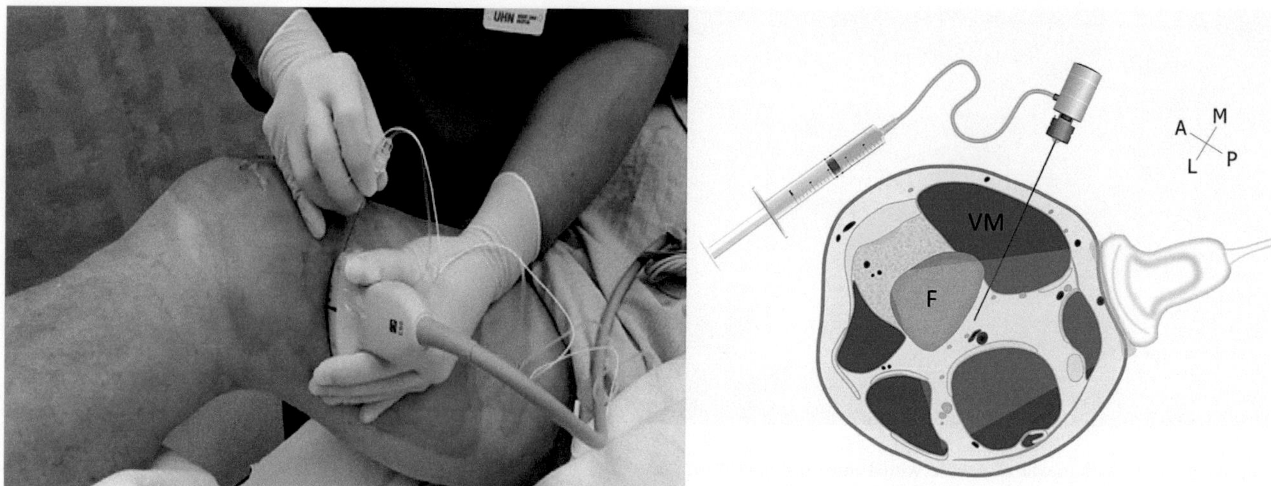

Fig. 62.12 Left. Needle insertion at the anterior end of the transducer in a medial to lateral trajectory. Right. Injection into the interspace with needle kept parallel to the acoustic shadow of the femur

Optimal Patient Position

This should be tailored in each clinical situation to maximize comfort for the patient, ergonomics for the operator and time efficiency. For example, when performed in a supine position, this block can be performed concurrently with adductor canal/saphenous nerve block, negating further prepping, draping and positioning (Fig. 62.12). This is often related to the preference of the operator. For each approach, the needle insertion points and site of injection are often the same regardless of patient position. The advantages and disadvantages of each block approach and its variant may not be fully appreciated at this time, pending further evaluation.

Optimal Needle Approach

This is not known at this time. Conceivably, the medial to lateral distal femoral shaft needle approach has the advantage of minimizing the chance of needle contact with SN. However, the disadvantages are as follows: (1) a challenging ultrasound view especially in patients with a large body habitus, (2) a steep needle to transducer angle which is required to reach the interspace between the popliteal vessels and the distal femoral shaft and (3) a higher chance of unintentional local anaesthetic spread to reach and block the CPN since the needle tip points laterally. This can be minimized by not advancing the needle more than 1–2 cm lateral to the popliteal artery.

On the other hand, the lateral to medial intercondylar fossa needle approach has the advantage of easy needle visualization, because the needle is inserted parallel to the acoustic window of the transducer at the same depth as the intended site of injection (Fig. 62.11). This ensures maximal needle distance from the CPN and optimal needle visualization. Whilst an oblique needle insertion from the lateral edge of the transducer is possible to reach the interspace, this needling technique may contact the CPN along the path of needle advancement, thus should be avoided.

Optimal Timing of iPACK Block

Performing iPACK block after spinal anaesthesia is a minor advantage, improving patient comfort.

Literature Review

Because the iPACK block is a relatively novel intervention, there is a lack of robust clinical data comparing different needle insertion techniques and clinical outcomes. The nee-

Table 62.2 Percentage staining of individual nerves with each technique

Anterior capsule	Technique		Posterior capsule	Technique	
Nerve	Proximal (%)	Distal (%)	Nerve	Proximal (%)	Distal (%)
Anterior branch CFN	71	100	Superior branch TN	75	85
Superior lateral genicular nerve	71	100	Inferior branch TN	29	42
Medial branch NVI	71	100	Posterior branch CFN	50	80
Superior medial genicular nerve	100	57	Genicular branch PON	100	100
Saphenous nerve	43	57			

dling techniques we described in this chapter are based on our own clinical experience at this time.

Cadaver Studies

A cadaveric dye study investigated spread of injectate following two variants of the medial to lateral iPACK needle approach: a proximal injection 1 finger breadth above the base of the patella and a distal injection at the superior border of the femoral condyles. Both injection techniques achieved similar mean area of injectate spread and nerves stained. Distal injection resulted in higher percentage capture of nerves supplying the posterior and anterolateral regions, whereas proximal injection had greater percentage capture of nerves supplying the anteromedial region of the knee.

Nerves most commonly stained by both injection techniques were the genicular branch of the ON, superior branch of TN, anterior branch of common peroneal nerve (innervating the anterior compartment) and the posterior branch of CPN (Table 62.2). Anterior capsule staining was noted, due to spread through the adductor hiatus.

Clinical Studies

We systematically reviewed the literature and identified six trials, one prospective non-inferiority trial, one prospective controlled trial and four retrospective studies investigating iPACK in total knee arthroplasty and one prospective randomized comparative trial, investigating the use of ACB and iPACK for knee pain secondary to osteoarthritis. The findings are summarized in (Table 62.3).

Four studies compared iPACK and ACB to ACB alone in TKA, all finding iPACK decreased pain scores, with the duration being 6–12 h. No study reported any difference in opioid consumption or length of stay. One study reported increased mobility and range of movement. These studies found iPACK provided a modest benefit or no benefit compared to ACB alone.

Five studies compared iPACK to periarticular infiltration (PAI). In those investigations, two studies found iPACK decreased pain scores both at rest and on ambulation for up to 5 days, one found non-inferiority and one found no difference. Two studies reported decreased opioid consumption, one found no difference and one increased. One study reported no difference in range of movement. iPACK was associated with a greater reduction in quadriceps strength on day 0 and lower timed up and go test scores on days 1 and 2, although it was associated with a significantly shorter length of stay, lower incidence of opioid-related side effects and higher patient satisfaction.

Three heterogeneous studies investigated iPACK with femoral nerve block. When compared to femoral nerve catheter, there was no difference in pain scores between femoral nerve block, femoral nerve catheter with iPACK and ACB with iPACK, although opioid consumption was significantly reduced with combined femoral nerve catheter and iPACK. Physical therapy performance was better on day 1 in ACB with iPACK, with a decreased length of stay. ACB with iPACK provided equivalent analgesia and improved physical therapy performance, allowing earlier hospital discharge. ACB and iPACK compared to femoral and sciatic blocks required less opioid after surgery, ambulated further on day 0 and had a significantly shorter length of stay. Adductor canal catheter plus iPACK compared to single-shot femoral nerve block with pericapsular liposomal bupivacaine resulted in lower opioid consumption, shorter length of stay and fewer opioid-related side effects.

In knee pain secondary to osteoarthritis, addition of iPACK to ACB resulted in significantly improved pain scores at all follow-up points and better functional outcome.

Table 62.3 Summary of published literature regarding iPACK

Study	Intervention	Pain score	Opioid consumption	Motor effect & ROM	LOS	Complications
Randomized controlled trials						
Kampitak et al. (2020)	Proximal iPACK block (iPACK1), distal iPACK block (iPACK2), or TNB, along with spinal anaesthesia, modified LIA, and CACB	Posterior knee pain score was significantly higher in the iPACK1 group than in other groups during the 24-h postoperative period ($P = 0.001$)	No significant difference in first-time morphine requirement or total intravenous opioid consumption between the groups	Significantly more CPN block in the TNB group vs. iPACK1 ($P = 0.001$) and iPACK2 ($P = 0.001$) groups. No difference between iPACK1 and iPACK2 groups. TN motor function better preserved with iPACK1 and iPACK2 groups than TNB group ($P < 0.001$) No difference in ROM, TUG and quadriceps muscle strength between groups	Hospital length of stay was significantly shorter in the iPACK2 group than that in the TNB group ($P = 0.016$), but no difference was observed between iPACK1 and iPACK2	No complications in any group
Kim et al. (2019)	iPACK + ACB + modified PAI or PAI	iPACK + ACB + modified PAI: lower NRS pain scores on ambulation POD 1 (difference in means [95% confidence interval], −3.3 [−4.0 to −2.7]; $P < 0.001$). Lower ambulatory NRS POD 0 (−3.5 [−4.3 to −2.7]; $P < 0.001$) and POD 2 (−1.0 [−1.9 to −0.1]; $P = 0.033$)	iPACK + ACB + modified PAI: lower opioid consumption PACU ($P = 0.005$), POD 0 ($P = 0.028$). Less IV opioids POD0 ($P = 0.001$), reduced need for IVPCA ($P = 0.037$).	iPACK + ACB + modified PAI: less pain interfering with walking reported POD 0 ($P = 0.001$) and POD 1 ($P < 0.001$)	No difference in LOS	iPACK + ACB + modified PAI: lower opioid-related side effects on POD 0 ($P = 0.039$) and POD 1 ($P = 0.048$)
Li et al. (2020)	Group A: ACB + iPACK + LFCNB, group B: ACB + iPACK, group C: ACB + LFCNB, group D: ACB	A, B and C: lower postoperative pain scores first 12 h at rest and first 8 h with activity than Group D ($P < 0.05$). Group A: longest analgesic duration (19.21 ± 3.22 h)	Group A (9.20 ± 7.52 mg) and Group B (10.8 ± 8.77 mg) had less morphine consumption for pain rescue compared with Group D (16.00 ± 7.82 mg) ($P < 0.05$) first 24 h. No difference in opioid consumption second and third 24 h. Total morphine consumption Group A (10.8 ± 10.85 mg) lower than Group C (18.40 ± 13.15 mg) ($P = 0.025$) and D (21.0 ± 12.16 mg) ($P = 0.01$). Analgesic durations groups A, B and C significantly longer than Group D ($P < 0.05$). Group A had lower morphine consumption than both Group C ($P < 0.05$) and Group D ($P < 0.01$)	No difference in mobility, quadriceps strength, TUG test and ROM	There was no significant difference among the groups ($P > 0.05$) in terms of the postoperative hospital stays	No difference

Ochroch et al. (2019)	ACB + iPACK or ACB + sham block	ACB + iPACK: lower incidence posterior knee pain at 6 h: 21.7% vs 45.8%, $P < 0.01$	No difference in opioid consumption	No difference in functional measures between groups	Not reported	Not reported
Patterson et al. (2020)	Continuous ACB + iPACK block or continuous ACB + sham subcutaneous saline injection	Continuous ACB + iPACK: lower pain scores in PACU at rest (average: 3 [2–5] vs. 5 [3–7], $P = 0.0122$, and worst: 5 [2–8] vs. 7 [5–8], $P = 0.0168$) No difference in the pain scores during physical therapy ($P = 0.2080$)	No difference in opioid consumption	No difference in walking distance	No difference in LOS	Not reported
Vichainarong et al. (2020)	iPACK + LIA + CACB or LIA + CACB	No differences in pain scores between the groups	No difference in opioid consumption first 24 h postoperatively	iPACK + LIA + CACB: Lower TUG test scores POD 1 and 2 ($P < 0.05$)	iPACK + LIA + CACB: Shorter LOS (60.4 ± 14.9 h vs. 51.4 ± 10.6 h $P = 0.007$)	No complications
Prospective randomized comparative study						
El-Emam et al. (2020)	Group I received ultrasound-guided ACB with 10 mL of 0.125 bupivacaine plus 40 mg methylprednisolone and Group II received ultrasound-guided ACB with 10 mL of 0.125 bupivacaine plus 40 mg methylprednisolone and i-PACK block for knee osteoarthritis	Significant lower value of visual analog and Western Ontario and McMaster Universities scores at all follow-up intervals compared to Group I		Better functional outcome		
Prospective non-inferiority trial						
Kertkiatkachorn et al. (2020)	Continuous ACB + iPACK or continuous ACB + PAI	ACB + iPACK: non-inferior to ACB + PAI @ 12 h: (0.9 (0.2) vs. 1.5 (0.3)) adjusted difference 95% confidence interval: −0.6 (−1.6, 0.4), $P = 0.266$ ACB + iPACK: lower VAS anterior knee pain score both at rest and on movement @ 24 h ($P < 0.05$) + Posterior knee pain score at rest 36 h-2 weeks after surgery ($P < 0.05$)	ACB + iPACK: higher cumulative IV morphine requirement at 12 h (0 [0, 2] vs 0 [0, 0] mg, $P = 0.004$), 24 h (2 [0, 4] vs 0 [0, 0] mg, $P = 0.002$) and 48 h (2 [0, 4] vs 0 [0, 0] mg, $P = 0.002$)	No differences in TUG test, knee ROM or quadriceps strength test. ACB + iPACK group: reduced quadriceps strength from baseline at both 0 ($P = 0.006$) and 45° ($P = 0.04$)	No difference in LOS	No difference in complications

(continued)

Table 62.3 (continued)

Study	Intervention	Pain score	Opioid consumption	Motor effect & ROM	LOS	Complications
Prospective controlled trial						
Sankineani et al. (2018)	iPACK + ACB vs ACB alone	iPACK + ACB: lower VAS scores up to POD 2: 2.55 ± 0.7274 vs. 3.4500 ± 0.67460, $P < 0.001$	Not reported	iPACK + ACB: increased mean ROM POD 2 (71.8° vs. 62.2°, $P < 0.05$). Increased ambulation distance: Increased ambulation distance day 3 (8.51 ± 1.85 m vs. 7.1333 ± 1.434 m, $P < 0.001$)	Not reported	Not reported
Retrospective study						
Eccles et al. (2019)	ACB + iPACK or FNB + Sciatic nerve block	Not reported	iPACK + ACB: less opioid POD 1 (mean, 15.7 vs. 24.0 morphine equivalents $P < 0.0001$) and at 2 weeks (mean, 6.2 vs. 9.3 morphine equivalents, $P = 0.025$)	iPACK + ACB: ambulated further on postoperative day 0 (mean 21.4 ft vs. 5.3 ft, $P < 0.001$)	iPACK + ACB: 62% patients discharged POD 1 vs. FNB + Sciatic: 14% ($P < 0.0001$). iPACK + ACB: shorter LOS (mean 1.48 days vs. 2.02 days, $P < 0.001$)	iPACK + ACB: higher proportion discharge POD 1 62% vs 14% ($P < 0.0001$, and shorter LOS (mean 1.48 days vs. 2.02 days, $P < 0.001$) than Fem + Sci group
Thobhani et al. (2017)	ACB + iPACK, FNC or FNC + iPACK	No differences in pain scores between the 3 groups	FNC + iPACK: reduced 48 h opioid consumption: 93 (72–124) mg vs FNC: 146 (98–164) mg, and ACB + iPACK: 150 (107–186) mg, $P = 0.0101$	ACB + iPACK: better distance travelled POD (1 42 (22–106) m) vs FNC: 20 (2–25) m & FNC + iPACK: 25 (9–35) m, $P < 0.0001$	ACB + iPACK: shorter LOS $P = 0.0024$. 100% patients discharged before POD 4	No complications in any group
Jung et al. (2020)	ACB + iPACK or ACB + PAI	iPACK with ACB: decreased rest pain at 45° flexion POD 1&2. Decreased rest pain POD 3, decreased pain at 45° flexion POD3-5	Significantly higher use of PCA on POD 1 in iPACK group. Significantly higher use of IVPCA dose in ACB+iPACK group (p=0.027).	Nil change reported	Not reported	Nil
Klement et al. (2019)	Continuous ACB + iPACK or FNB + liposomal bupivacaine PAI	ACB + iPACK: lower VAS POD 0 (3.8 ± 2.1 vs 4.5 ± 2.4, $P = 0.009$) and morning POD 1(3.7 ± 2.0 vs 4.8 ± 2.2, $P < 0.001$)	ACB + iPACK: less median opioid consumption (20.0 mg vs 44.1 mg, $P < 0.001$) than the FNB + LB-PAI group	ACB + iPACK: further median ambulation up to POD 1: (115 vs 34 ft, $P < 0.001$)	ACB + iPACK: shorter median length of stay (LOS, 2.0 vs 3.0, $P < 0.001$)	ACB + iPACK: fewer opioid-related adverse events (0.8 vs 5.5, $P = 0.045$), lower rate MUA (0.8% vs 6.2%, $P = 0.026$)

FNC femoral nerve catheter, *IVME* IV morphine equivalents, *IV* intravenous, *IVPCA* intravenous patient-controlled analgesia, *LFCNB* lateral femoral cutaneous nerve block, *OME* oral morphine equivalents, *PACU* postanaesthesia care unit, *PAI* periarticular infiltration, *ROM* range of movement, *TUG* Timed Up and Go

Suggested Reading

Eccles CJ, Swiergosz AM, Smith AF, Bhimani SJ, Smith LS, Malkani AL. Decreased opioid consumption and length of stay using an IPACK and adductor canal nerve block following total knee arthroplasty. J Knee Surg. 2019; https://doi.org/10.1055/s-0039-1700840.

El-Emam E-S, El motlb EAA. Ultrasound-guided adductor canal block versus combined adductor canal and infiltration between the popliteal artery and the posterior capsule of the knee block for osteoarthritis knee pain. Anesth Essays Res. 2020;14:127.

Gardner E. The innervation of the knee joint. Anat Rec. 1948;101:109–30.

Jung D-W, Shon W-Y, Seo S-S, Kim O-G, Lee I-S. Comparison of the postoperative analgesic effect for infiltration between the popliteal artery and the capsule of the posterior knee and that of periarticular multimodal drug injection in total knee arthroplasty: retrospective study in the immediate postoperative period. Knee Surg Relat Res. 2020;32:1.

Kampitak W, Tanavalee A, Ngarmukos S, Tantavisut S. Motor-sparing effect of iPACK (interspace between the popliteal artery and capsule of the posterior knee) block versus tibial nerve block after total knee arthroplasty: a randomized controlled trial. Reg Anesth Pain Med. 2020;45:267–76.

Kertkiatkachorn W, Kampitak W, Tanavalee A, Ngarmukos S. Adductor canal block combined with iPACK (interspace between the popliteal artery and the capsule of the posterior knee) block vs periarticular injection for analgesia after total knee arthroplasty: a randomized noninferiority trial. J Arthroplasty. 2020; https://doi.org/10.1016/j.arth.2020.06.086.

Kim DH, Beathe JC, Lin Y, et al. Addition of infiltration between the popliteal artery and the capsule of the posterior knee and adductor canal block to periarticular injection enhances postoperative pain control in total knee arthroplasty: a randomized controlled trial. Anesth Analg. 2019;129:526–35.

Klement MR, Bullock WM, Nickel BT, et al. Continuous adductor canal blockade facilitates increased home discharge and decreased opioid consumption after total knee arthroplasty. Knee. 2019;26:679–86.

Li D, Alqwbani M, Wang Q, Liao R, Yang J, Kang P. Efficacy of adductor canal block combined with additional analgesic methods for postoperative analgesia in total knee arthroplasty: a prospective, double-blind, randomized controlled study. J Arthroplasty. 2020; https://doi.org/10.1016/j.arth.2020.06.060.

Ochroch J, Qi V, Badiola I, et al. Analgesic efficacy of adding the IPACK block to a multimodal analgesia protocol for primary total knee arthroplasty. Region Anesth Pain Med. 2020;45(10):799–804. https://doi.org/10.1136/rapm-2020-101558.

Patterson ME, Vitter J, Bland K, Nossaman BD, Thomas LC, Chimento GF. The effect of the IPACK block on pain after primary TKA: a double-blinded, prospective, randomized trial. J Arthroplasty. 2020;35:S173–7.

Roberts SL, Stout A, Dreyfuss P. Review of knee joint innervation: implications for diagnostic blocks and radiofrequency ablation. Pain Med (Malden, MA). 2020;21:922–38.

Sankineani SR, Reddy ARC, Eachempati KK, Jangale A, Gurava Reddy AV. Comparison of adductor canal block and IPACK block (interspace between the popliteal artery and the capsule of the posterior knee) with adductor canal block alone after total knee arthroplasty: a prospective control trial on pain and knee function in immediate postoperative period. Eur J Orthop Surg Traumatol. 2018;28:1391–5.

Thobhani S, Scalercio L, Elliott CE, et al. Novel regional techniques for total knee arthroplasty promote reduced hospital length of stay: an analysis of 106 patients. Ochsner J. 2017;17:233–8.

Tran J, Peng PWH, Lam K, Baig E, Agur AMR, Gofeld M. Anatomical study of the innervation of anterior knee joint capsule: implication for image-guided intervention. Reg Anesth Pain Med. 2018;43:407–14.

Tran J, Peng PWH, Gofeld M, Chan V, Agur AMR. Anatomical study of the innervation of posterior knee joint capsule: implication for image-guided intervention. Reg Anesth Pain Med. 2019a;44:234–8.

Tran J, Giron Arango L, Peng P, Sinha SK, Agur A, Chan V. Evaluation of the iPACK block injectate spread: a cadaveric study. Reg Anesth Pain Med. 2019b;44:689–94.

Vichainarong C, Kampitak W, Tanavalee A, Ngarmukos S, Songborassamee N. Analgesic efficacy of infiltration between the popliteal artery and capsule of the knee (iPACK) block added to local infiltration analgesia and continuous adductor canal block after total knee arthroplasty: a randomized clinical trial. Region Anesth Pain Med. 2020;45(11):872–9. https://doi.org/10.1136/rapm-2020-10139.

Hip Joint and Trochanteric Bursa Injection

63

Piera Santullo and Agnes R. Stogicza

Contents

General Considerations

Pain related to hip is common and it affects 14% of people over 60 years old. The source of pain can originate from a wide array of pathologies in hip joint and surrounding tissues. Understanding the complexity of the anatomy in this region is crucial to formulate the differential diagnosis. Clinicians need to consider both local and distant osteoligamentous, tendinous, nervous, and muscular anatomy when examining patients with complaints related to the

P. Santullo (✉)
Department of Rehabilitation Medicine, Nottingham University Hospitals, Nottingham, UK

A. R. Stogicza
Department of Anesthesiology and Pain Medicine, Saint Magdolna Private Hospital, Budapest, Hungary

D. Jankovic, P. Peng (eds.), *Regional Nerve Blocks in Anesthesia and Pain Therapy*,
https://doi.org/10.1007/978-3-030-88727-8_63

posterior, lateral, or anterior hip. Moreover, myofascial pain is common and overlooked cause of pain.

Majority of anterior hip pain arises from the following conditions: hip osteoarthritis (OA), femoroacetabular impingement (FAI), acetabular labral tear, internal snapping hip, stress fracture, osteonecrosis of the femoral head, hip joint laxity, inguinal disruption, and neuropathy from femoral, obturator, ilioinguinal, and genitofemoral nerves.

Hip OA is very common over 60 years old, affecting 3–9% of the Western population and needs to be primarily considered. Acetabular labral tears must be excluded in a young patient with anterior hip pain. In individuals practicing sports requiring repetitive end-range hip motions, such as hockey, soccer, dance, and golf, FAI should be suspected as the differential diagnosis of anterior hip pain. Internal snapping hip can occur during the attrition of the iliopsoas tendon over the iliopubic eminence with hip movement. Neuropathy of the femoral, ilioinguinal, and genitofemoral nerves may cause anterior hip and thigh pain especially in patient with hip arthroplasty or inguinal hernia repair in the past history.

Intra-articular pathology often manifests as anterior hip/groin pain owing to the innervation of the hip capsule. The majority of the sensory innervation of the anterior hip is provided by the femoral and obturator nerves (Fig. 63.1). Therefore, most intra-articular conditions radiate to the anterior groin, whereas the majority of extra-articular conditions radiate to the lateral or posterior aspects of the hip.

Lateral hip pain is often due to chronic overuse. Gluteal and iliotibial tendinopathies are the most common causes of lateral hip pain. Other causes can be primary trochanteric bursitis that is not very common, external snapping hip where the iliotibial band or gluteus creates a snap during hip extension, lateral femoral cutaneous neuropathy, and iliohypogastric neuropathy.

In this chapter, we will focus on the injection techniques of two common hip conditions: hip osteoarthritis and greater trochanter pain syndrome.

Indication (Patient Selection)

Hip Joint Injection

Osteoarthritis is the main indication, and patients are selected when they had moderate to severe symptoms from the hip joint (pain localized at the inguinal region with hip flexion and internal rotation movements limited by pain) with imaging that confirms osteoarthritis and not responding to conservative measures.

Tears of the acetabular labrum can cause pain in the inguinal region, clicking and locking sensation, and stiffness. Diagnosis is often made with clinical history and MRI of the hip with contrast (although in some specialized center, they prefer MRI without arthrogam). Labral tear can lead to early osteoarthritis.

Gluteus Peritendinous or Trochanteric Bursa Injection

The main indication is greater trochanteric pain syndrome. This syndrome refers to the pain around the greater trochanter

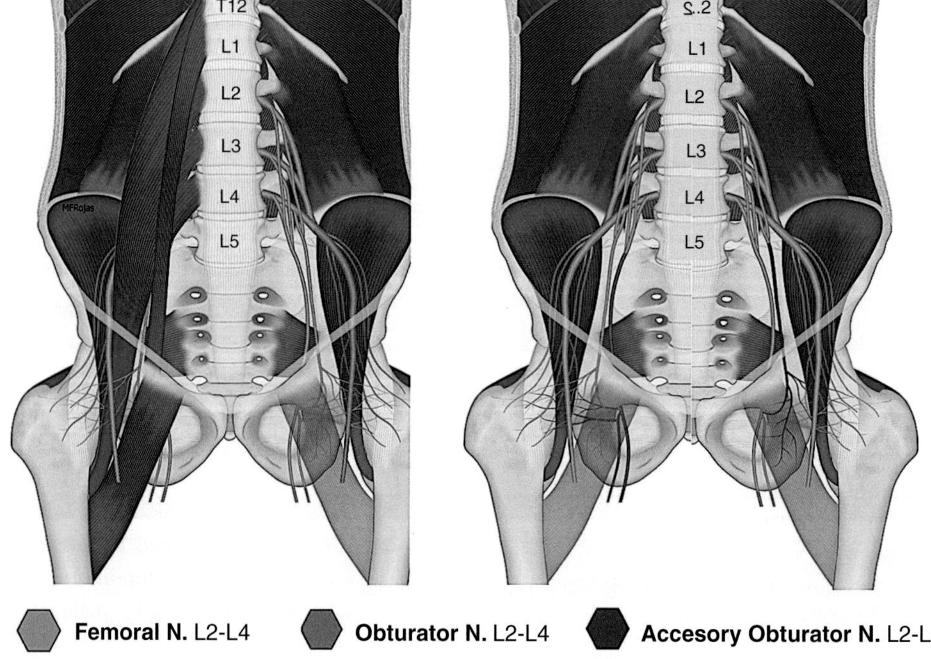

Fig. 63.1 Schematic diagram to show the articular branches to the anterior hip joint capsule. The femoral, obturator, and accessory obturator nerves are color coded. Reprinted with permission from Philip Peng Educational Series. The original artwork was created and modified with the permission from Dr. Maria Fernanda Rojas, Bucaramanga, Colombia

at the insertion of the gluteal tendons. It can radiate to the lateral thigh and to the knee. Aggravating factors are active abduction, climbing stairs, and lying on the side. It commonly accompanies sacroiliac joint pathologies. Special clinical signs include tenderness on palpation of the greater trochanter (jump sign), Trendelenburg sign, and pain on resisted hip abduction. Ultrasound or MRI may show tendinosis and calcification of the gluteal tendons, thickened iliotibial band, with or without trochanteric bursitis.

Functional Anatomy

The coxofemoral joint is an enarthrosis, a tight-fitting spheroidal joint that has three axes of freedom: a transverse plane for flexion-extension movements, a sagittal plane for abduction and adduction movements, and a vertical plane for external and internal rotation movements. It is composed of osseous, ligamentous, and muscular structures. The ilium, ischium, and pubis together with the acetabular labrum form the acetabular socket.

Caudal to the labrum, there is the capsule that inserts distally to the intertrochanteric region and posterior aspect of the femoral neck. The anterior capsule has two layers that are divided by the anterior recess of the joint space (Fig. 63.2). The articular surfaces are covered by hyaline cartilage arranged in a specific distribution to appropriately handle the forces placed across the hip joint. The acetabular labrum has been implicated as a cause of osteoarthritis of the hip. Absence of the labrum transfers the contact area of the femur-acetabular cartilage laterally toward the acetabular margin, with associated translational motion of the femoral head within the articulation, and significantly reduces resistance to distraction of the joint surfaces.

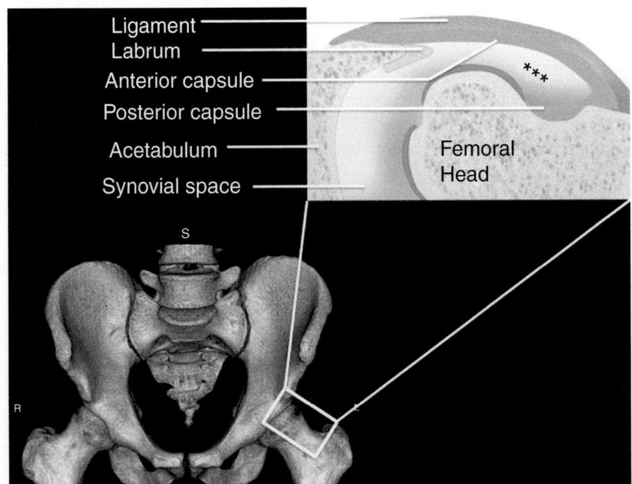

Fig. 63.2 Figure showing the anterior synovial recess (***). Under normal circumstances, the amount of synovial fluid in the recess is kept at a minimum. This figure showed a hip with effusion for demonstration. Reproduced with permission from Philip Peng Educational Series

Hip joint stability and capsular laxity are an important element to predict and prevent hip OA. The interlocking system formed by acetabulum and its labrum, capsule, ligaments, and muscles guarantee hip stability, together with gravity in the erect position. Any pathologic conditions (congenital, traumatic, or degenerative) that alter the biomechanics of the hip can predispose to the degeneration and osteoarthritis of hip.

Anteriorly, the hip is strengthened by two very strong periarticular ligaments: the iliofemoral ligament (ILF) and the pubofemoral (PF), and muscles play a less important role in providing stability. Posteriorly, the surrounding stabilizing structures are mainly muscles, and the only ligament is only the ischiofemoral (IsF). Adductor muscles run longitudinally and tend to dislocate the femoral head above the acetabulum. The transverse stability is guaranteed by coordinated and synchronized bilateral contraction of adductors and abductors muscles in double limb support. If one of these muscles are weak, it results in a tilt of the line joining the shoulders: Duchenne Trendelenburg's sign on single limb support. Hip instability can be secondary to traumatic and atraumatic causes. Traumatic origin can lead to ligamentous injury, bony injuries to the femoral head or acetabular wall, or shearing injuries to the articular cartilage with a compromise in the load-transferring ability of the joint. Atraumatic instability may be the result of repeated injury to the ligamentous capsule during activities that force the hip into abduction and external rotation. These positions increase the forces in the iliofemoral ligament, resulting in the development of capsular laxity and predisposing the acetabular labrum to injury. Once the static stabilizers of the hip including the capsule and labrum are compromised, there is an increased reliance on the dynamic stabilizers of the hip during activity, with the development of overuse syndromes and associated symptoms of the surrounding musculature and muscle attachments.

Anatomic alterations could also lead to early hip OA, including hip dysplasia, coxa vara, and coxa valga. In this context, the contact between the articular surfaces is concentrated on a small area of articular cartilage on the lateral aspect of the acetabulum leading to early hip osteoarthritis. The hypertrophy of the labrum can participate in providing load transfer. Coxa valga, in combination with insufficient acetabular coverage, creates a large contact force concentrated on a narrowband of articular surface on the lateral edge of the acetabulum, potentially leading to early symptomatic osteoarthritis. Coxa vara can lead to increased stress on the medial articular cartilage and medial migration of the femoral head, *leading to* cartilage breakdown.

Greater trochanteric pain syndrome is related to the tendonitis or tendinosis of the muscles in the lateral region of the hips that insert on the greater trochanter of the femur and consequential inflammation of the various trochanteric bursae.

The muscles that surround the hip joint in the lateral region are the gluteal muscles. These muscles extend the hip (maximus) and are responsible for abduction (minimus and medius), internal rotation (minimus), and external rotation (maximus). Tearing, strain, and degeneration of the gluteal muscles could lead to lateral hip pain. A good understanding of the anatomy of the hip can help GTPS diagnosis. The bony surface of the greater trochanter (GT) consists of four facets: anterior, lateral, superoposterior, and posterior (Fig. 63.3) The gluteus medius muscle attaches to the superoposterior and lateral facets. The gluteus minimus muscle attaches to the anterior facet. There are two layers of muscles in the lateral region: the superficial one that is formed by gluteus maximus and tensor fascia lata. In the superficial layer, there is the iliotibial (IT) tract that is part of the fascia lata commencing at the level of GT, passes along the posterolateral aspect of the thigh, and inserts in the Gerdy's tubercle of tibia. The deeper layer is formed by the "deltoid" of the hip, the gluteus medius and minimus. The gluteus medius muscle fans around the hip with anterior, medius, and posterior fibers.

There are three principal bursae in the lateral hip region: The trochanteric bursa covers the posterior facet of the GT, and it is located beneath the gluteus maximus muscle and iliotibial tract. It does not extend over the anterior border of the lateral facet. The subgluteus medius bursa is situated anterior to the apex of the GT (deep to the lateral part of the gluteus medius tendon) and proximal to its insertion, covering an area of the superior part of the lateral facet of the GT. The subgluteus minimus bursa lies beneath the gluteus minimus tendon, medial to its insertion, in the area of the anterior facet of the GT.

Technique

Hip intra-articular injection and trochanteric bursa injections are performed under sterile conditions, landmark-guided, ultrasound-guided, or fluoroscopy-guided. Before treatment, informed consent is required, and all advantages and disadvantages of the procedure are discussed with the patient. Use of anticoagulants and antiplatelets should be assessed according to the latest guidelines. Currently, percutaneous joint injections are considered low-risk procedures.

Intra-Articular Hip Joint Injection

The landmark-guided technique has shown to have an accuracy of 72%. However, the risk of piercing the femoral nerve with a blinded anterior approach was 27%, and the needles tips were in close proximity (<5 mm) to the femoral nerve in 60% of the punctures. Therefore, landmark-guided technique is not advocated in this chapter. In contrast, US- or fluoroscopy-guided techniques have shown to have an accuracy approaching 100%, significantly higher than landmark-guided technique.

Ultrasound-Guided Hip Joint Injection

Preparation

The needles used are 22–25-gauge 3.5–5-inch spinal needle, depending on the habitus of the patient. Low-frequency curvilinear probe (2–5 MHz) is used, but at times, linear high-frequency probe could also be used for patient with low body mass index. The patient is placed in supine position. The aim is the anterior recess at the anterior femur head-neck junction. The needle is introduced using caudal to cranial and lateral to medial approaches.

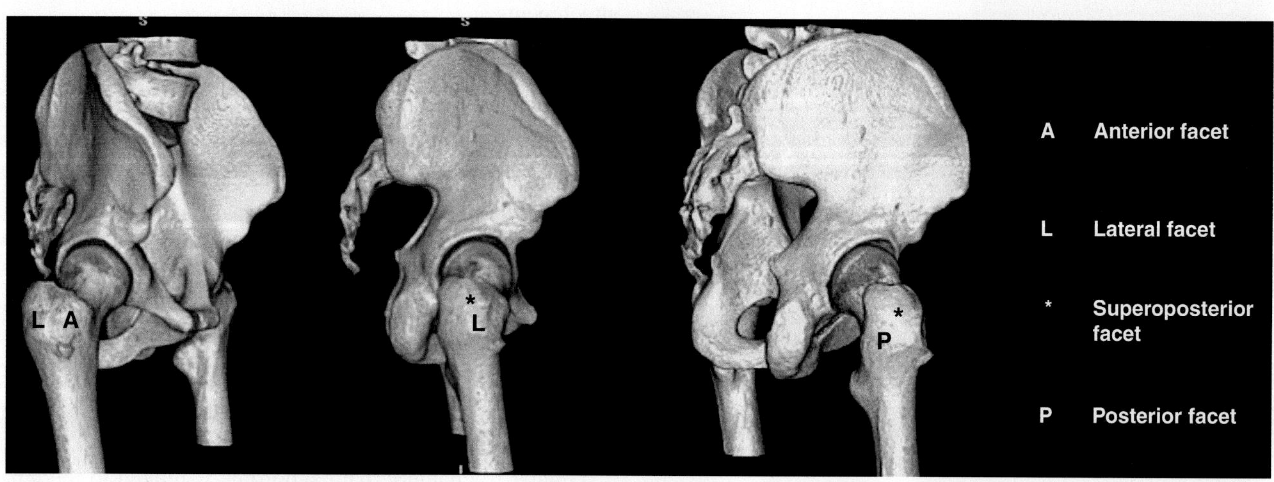

Fig. 63.3 Figure showing the four facets of greater trochanter. Reproduced with permission from Philip Peng Educational Series

Procedure

Step 1. Position the ultrasound probe in the short axis over the femoral shaft as shown on Fig. 63.4b. The femur diaphysis will appear as a rounded hyperechoic line.

Step 2. Slide the probe in cranial direction until hyperechoic shadow of the femur flattens to visualize the anterior trochanteric area (Fig. 63.4c).

Step 3. Rotate the probe perpendicularly to the inguinal line. The femoral head-neck junction should be directly visualized as well as the anterior recess (Fig. 63.4d). Color Doppler identifies the branches of the circumflex femoral artery, which should be avoided by slight manipulation of the probe (Fig. 63.4e). Insert the needle using in-plane technique as shown on (Fig. 63.4a–f) and aim to pierce the capsule of anterior recess and to touch the bone. In-plane technique is suggested to allow direct visualization of the length of the needle. This reduces the risk of neurovascular injuries and may also enhance precision needle placement.

Step 4. Color Doppler confirms capsular spread.

Technique: Fluoroscopy-Guided Hip Joint Injection

The positioning and the target are the same as that of ultrasound-guided procedure described above.

Procedure

Step 1. Take a posteroanterior view of the hip area, and identify the lateral aspect of the femoral head neck/neck junction. Palpate the femoral artery to ensure the neurovascular bundle is away from the needle trajectory.

Step 2. Following infiltration with local anesthetic, advance a 22-gauge 3.5-inch spinal needle under intermittent fluoroscopy in coaxial view until osseous contact is felt (Fig. 63.5a).

Step 3. Inject small volume test dose of anesthetic, and if low resistance is encountered, then administer the contrast dye to verify intracapsular needle location. The most classic dye pattern is the "ring of Saturn" pattern (Fig. 63.5b), with contrast pooling above the level of the zona orbicularis; otherwise, contrast will collect in the dependent portion of the capsule, extending inferiorly along the femoral neck. Inject medication after appropriate contrast spread.

Complications

The procedure is low risk, no devastating consequences should be expected. However, damage to the tissues in the vicinity can further worsen the patient's condition, so care must be taken during procedure.

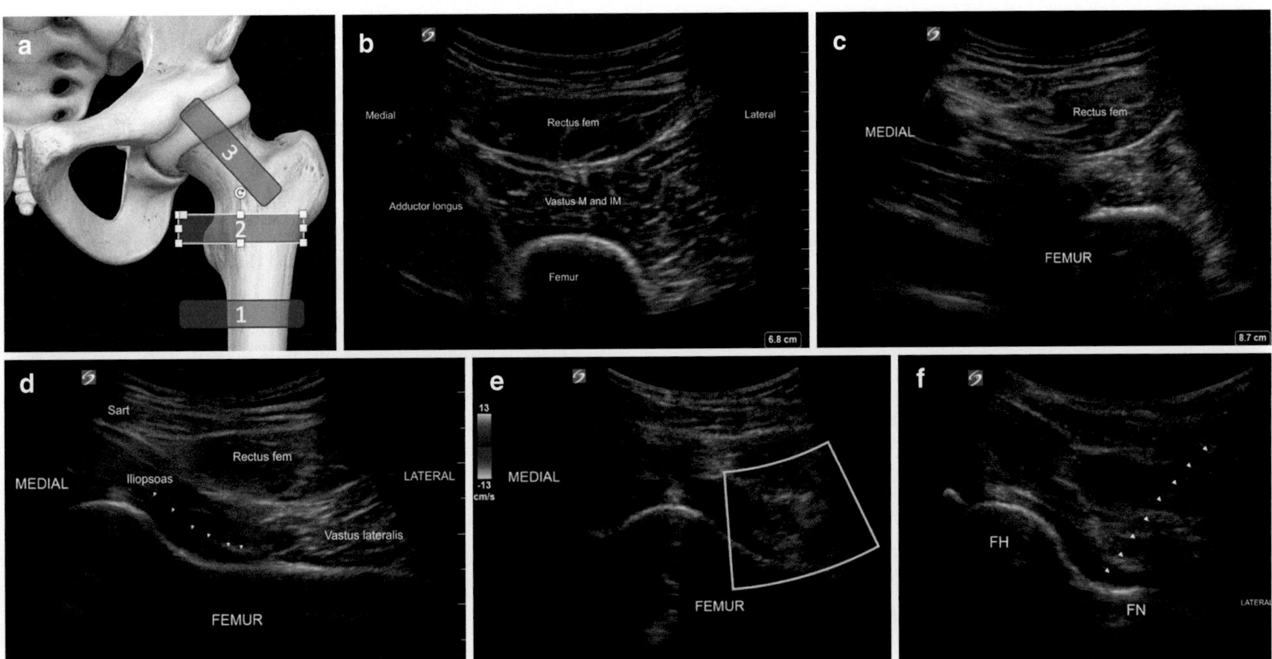

Fig. 63.4 Ultrasound probe position to identify anterior access to the hip joint (**a**). US probe placed on the femoral shaft (**b**) and then moved cephalad, until the flattening of the femur marks the anterior surface of the greater trochanter (GT) (**c**). The probe is rotated 45° in order to visualize femoral head and neck. Arrows mark the hip capsule/pubofemoral ligaments (**d**). Color doppler shows the ascending branch of the lateral femoral circumflex artery between iliopsoas and rectus femoris muscles (**e**). The needle reaches the junction of the femoral head and neck (**f**). Color doppler shows the injectate under the hip capsule. Reprinted with permission from Dr. Agnes Stogicza

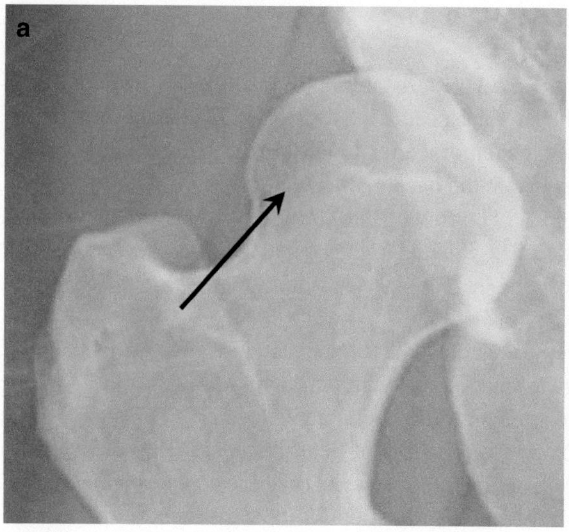

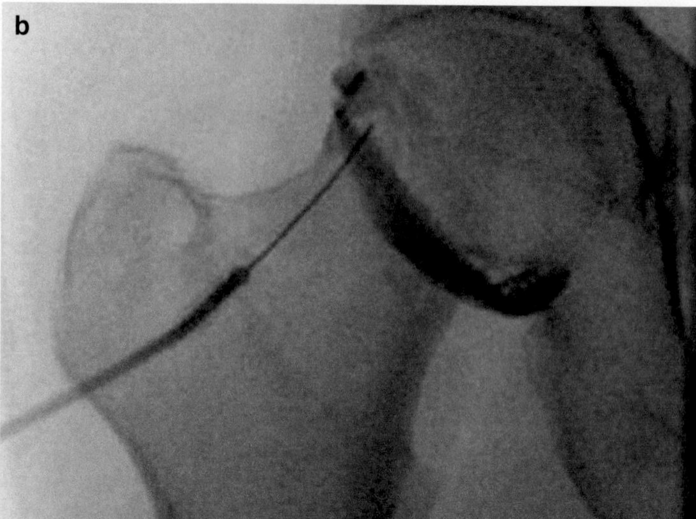

Fig. 63.5 Fluoroscopic hip injection. (**a**) AP image shows proposed needle placement in the lateral portion of the femoral head-neck junction. (**b**) Contrast confirms intra-articular needle position and outlines the zona orbicularis (ring of Saturn pattern). Reprinted with permission from Dr. Fabricio Assis

Injury to the labrum may increase pain and worsen OA. Injury to the psoas may result in psoas muscle hematoma or tendinopathy, leading to decreased hip flexion due to pain. Injury to femoral nerve injury can lead to permanent neuralgia or loss of function. If one is not cognizant of the femoral artery and vein or its branches in the needle trajectory, injury can lead to bleeding and hematoma. Septic arthritis may result if sterility is compromised. Infection rate of intra-articular steroid injection is very low (< 0.1%).

Pain and postinjection flare can occur especially after corticosteroid injection. Extra-articular injection can occur if there is no contact to the bone when injecting the medication or if the needle tip is not visualized, with possible decreased effect of the procedure.

Practical Tips

Keep a 2–3 cm distance between the needle and US probe to allow a shallow needle entry angle and facilitate good needle visualization.

Pay attention to patient feedback (injection of the labrum is very painful).

When using ultrasound guidance, always check for vascular structures in the needle trajectory before moving forward with an injection to prevent damage to the nerves and vessels and bleeding.

Switch on color Doppler to directly visualize the lateral circumflex femoral artery and smaller vessels. If the artery is within the trajectory, the probe is tilted laterally to establish another needle trajectory.

Literature Review

Intra-Articular Steroid for Hip Osteoarthritis

Intra-articular steroid injection is a very common procedure, and it is an also a recommended treatment in guidelines like the European League Against Rheumatism; the American College of Rheumatology, and Osteoarthritis Research Society International. However, literature reports very limited effect with short-term benefits and risks of osteoarthritis progression.

A systematic review that included five randomized controlled trials (RCTs) with less than 101 patients affected with OA showed that intra-articular steroid injection resulted in significant temporary short-term pain relief (less than a week) and transient improvement of function. It also demonstrated the safety of the procedure. It could not demonstrate any long-term improvement of this treatment compared to placebo.

Regarding the duration of effect of steroid intra-articular hip injections, a retrospective study that included 78 patients suggested that the steroid beneficial effect is not long term and that 49% of patients had to undergo hip surgery within 2 years. This was confirmed by another retrospective study of 44 patients that received steroid hip injection, in which 78% of patients had to have hip replacement. Moreover, literature shows that hip intra-articular steroid injection could accelerate cartilage loss and increase risk of periprosthetic joint infection.

Intra-Articular Hyaluronic Acid

A meta-analysis of six prospective RCTs demonstrated that intra-articular hip HA injection did not have significant effect on the reduction of pain and WOMAC compared to controls. Limitations to this study was related to RCTs eligibility criteria and the size of the comparative groups that was small.

A prospective study of 226 patients showed that patients with moderate grade of hip OA (Kellgren Lawrence stage 2) treated with intra-articular high-molecular-weight hyaluronic acid injection had significant improvement in terms of functional scores measured with WOMAC scale and Harris hip score. However, a multicenter double-blind randomized study with 357 patients did not demonstrate any difference between hyaluronic acid injection (hylan G-F20) and normal saline in terms of function improvement and pain reduction.

Intra-Articular Platelet-Rich Plasma (PRP) Injections for Hip Osteoarthritis

There are a number of meta-analyses investigating the effect of intra-articular PRP injection for the treatment of hip osteoarthritis. There is currently no evidence that intra-articular hip joint injections of PRP can lead to significant pain and function improvement compared to placebo.

Unfortunately, all of these studies included researches that investigated low-concentration PRP injections. In fact, all these studies gained between 4 and 20 mls of PRP from 8 to 150 mls of venous blood sample. Very low concentration of PRP has shown to be less effective than HA injections. Studies with high concentration of PRP reported better results for PRP treatment. Limitations of these meta-analysis is related to small sample sizes of RCTs considered.

The superiority of PRP compared to other intra-articular hip injections is still questionable.

Mesenchymal Stem Cell (MSC) Injections for Hip Osteoarthritis

Bone marrow-derived MSC is the common form of stem cell injection. Despite there is little evidence on the effectiveness of this treatment for hip osteoarthritis, it is a promising treatment option considering its effectiveness on knee osteoarthritis.

A meta-analysis collecting 12 trials of 608 patients showed evidence that MSC transplantation for the treatment of cartilage injury improves cartilage lesions, cartilage inflammatory symptoms, and the articular cartilage volume. This meta-analysis included studies that used stem cells of different type, and four kinds of mesenchymal stromal cells were applied in cartilage repair; bone marrow mesenchymal stromal cells were the most widely used. Recent systematic review showed encouraging results of bone marrow aspirate for the treatment of osteonecrosis of femoral head without causing serious adverse events.

A cohort study examined 18 patients with hip, knee, and ankle osteoarthritis treated with bone marrow (BM) MSC followed up over 30 months. All patients experienced a reduction in pain by VAS, reduced WOMAC, and increased physical function over the course of the study. No significant adverse events were observed beyond minor erythema. Of note, hip OA comprised a small fraction of cases in this study, making it difficult to generalize the findings to specifically hip OA.

A recent cohort study that included 19 patients and 25 joints showed encouraging results of BM MSC for the treatment of early hip osteoarthritis in terms of improving function, pain, and stiffness at 6 months from injection, and it demonstrated to be a safe procedure because of the lack of major complications. A case series showed encouraging results on the effectiveness of BM MSC in terms of reducing pain.

Prolotherapy for Hip Osteoarthritis

Prolotherapy refers to the injection of an irritant into a specific site with the main aim being pain relief via improving the biomechanical properties of the area. The mechanism is not completely understood, but increased cartilage and tenocyte growth has been observed, in vitro. The presence of a local irritant might attract inflammatory mediators and possibly stimulate the release of growth factors or act as a vascular sclerosant.

One RCT controlled study showed that pain reductions and functional improvement were statistically significant in the prolotherapy group for the treatment of osteoarthritis secondary to developmental dysplasia of the hip in comparison with the control (exercise group) group, starting from day 21 through the end of the trial. Prolotherapy was performed intra-articular and/or periarticular for hip dysplasia, Crowe type I and II. Periarticular injections performed were at the iliopsoas, gluteus medius/minimus, piriformis, and adductor tendons. Limitations of the study are its small sample size, relatively short follow-up period, and lack of a placebo control group.

Greater Trochanter Bursae Injection

This procedure can be performed using different guidance techniques: landmark-guided, ultrasound-guided and fluoroscopy-guided technique. The accuracy for landmark technique is 67% and can be improved to more than 90% with ultrasound guidance. Ultrasound guidance is highly recommended in the following situations: when the patient had a previous failed response to blinded injection but the clinical picture is compatible with greater trochanteric pain syndrome, when the greater trochanter cannot be palpated, when the previous imaging suggested the pathology is at the gluteus minimus, and when fenestration and PRP injection is planned.

Landmark-Guided Technique for Greater Trochanteric Bursae Injection

The patient is put on lateral decubitus with the injection site on the nondependent side and hip and knee bent.

Step 1. Mark the area of tenderness.

Step 2. Insert the needle perpendicular to skin at marked area.

Step 3. Once bony contact is encountered, the needle is withdrawn 3 mm, and 1 ml of medication is injected.

Ultrasound-Guided Greater Trochanteric Complex and Bursae Injection

The positioning is same as the landmark-guided injection.

Procedure Steps

Step 1. Palpate and visualize the greater trochanter GT (the bony prominence on the lateral aspect of the femur that looks like the apex of a tent). The anterior facet is where the gluteus minimus tendon inserts and the lateral facet where the gluteus medius tendon inserts (Fig. 63.6). The two facets are separated by a ridge. Both gluteus muscles are covered by the fascia lata, which is attached by the tensor fascia lata anteriorly and gluteus maximus posteriorly. The target is the bursa superficial to the gluteus medius and/or gluteus minimus tendon.

Step 2: For the trochanteric bursa superficial to the gluteus medius tendon, a 22G spinal needle is inserted in-plane from posterior to anterior direction. Upon hydrodissection, 5 mL of local anesthetic and steroid is injected.

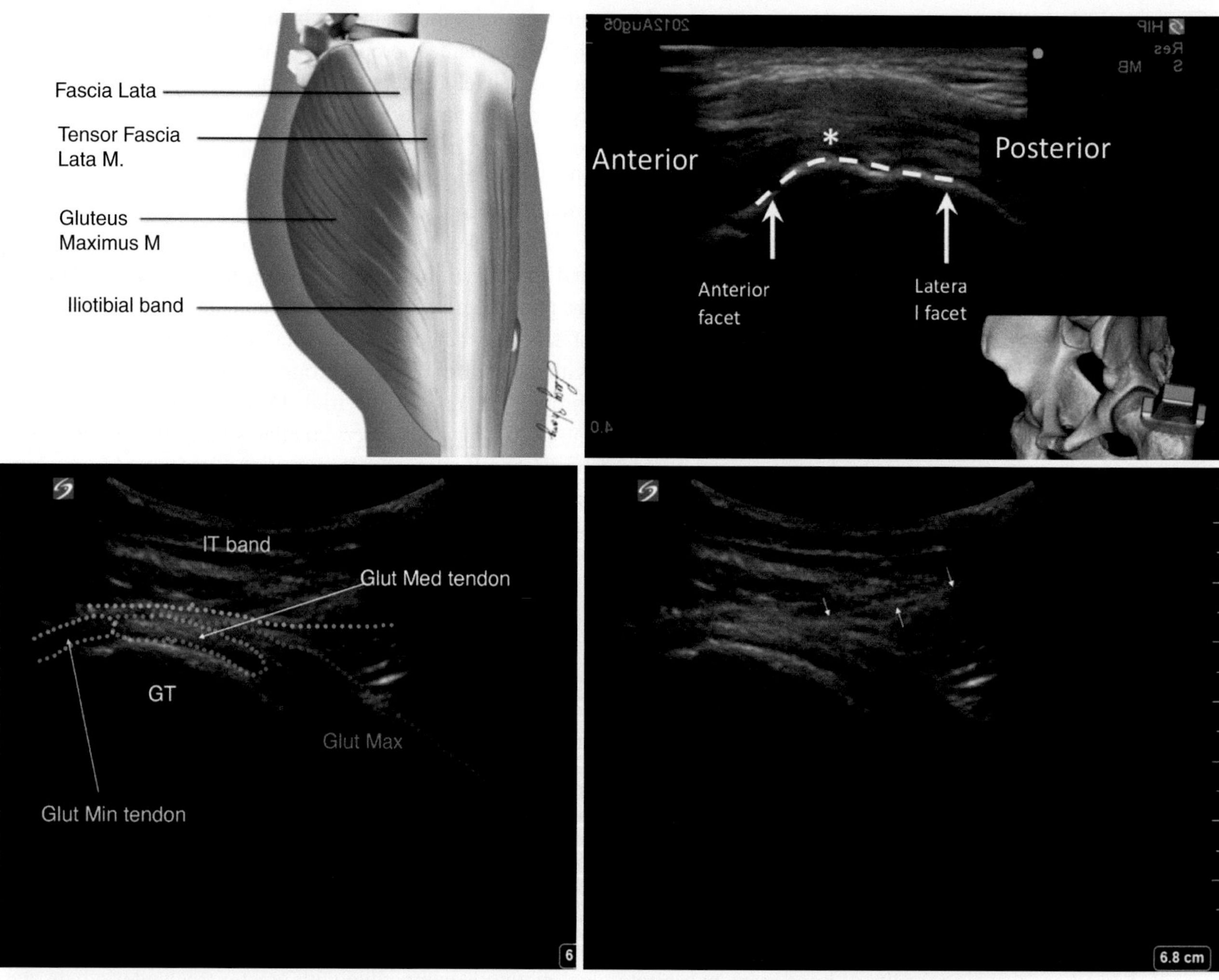

Fig. 63.6 Upper left. The most superficial layer is the tensor fascia lata (TFL) or the gluteus maximus (GMax). Upper right. When the ultrasound probe is placed at the greater trochanter as shown in the insert, the ridge (*) dividing the anterior and lateral facet is seen. Lower left. Different structures overlying the greater trochanter (GT) are shown: gluteus minimus (min) and medius (med) tendons, gluteus maximus (max) muscle, and iliotibial (IT) band. Lower right. Needle insertion (arrows) to the bursa superficial to the gluteus medius tendon. Reprinted with permission from Philip Peng Educational series and courtesy of Dr. Agnes Stogicza

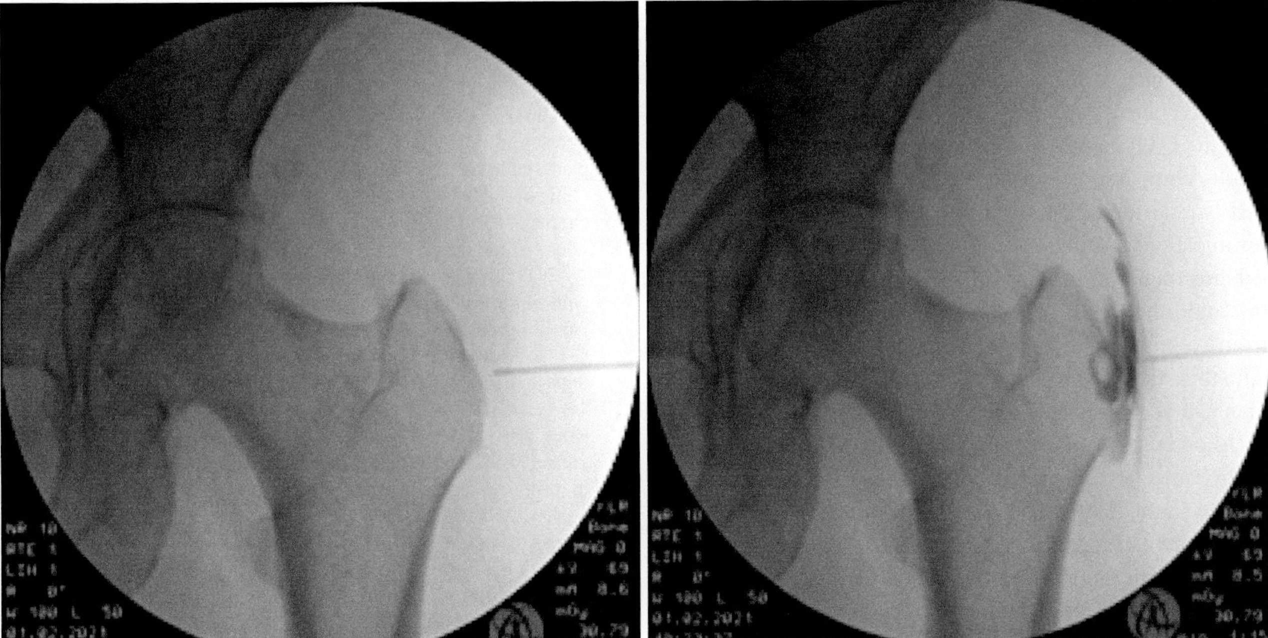

Fig. 63.7 Fluoroscopy-guided trochanteric bursa injection before and after contrast injection. Reprinted with permission from Dr. Fabricio Assis

Step 3: For the bursa superficial to the gluteus minimus tendon, the probe is slided anteriorly to the anterior facet, and the injection target is between the fascia lata and gluteus minimus tendon.

Fluoroscopy-Guided Greater Trochanteric Bursae Injection

The patient is placed in lateral decubitus position with the injection side up.

Procedure Steps

Step 1. Palpate the GT of interest and confirm the anterior and posterior side of the hip joint.

Step 2. Place a 22–25G spinal needle directly onto the GT in coaxial view (Fig. 63.7).

Step 3. Inject the contrast to confirm the pattern of spread.

Step 4. Inject medication.

Complications

Injury to gluteus tendon, with tendinopathy of gluteus medius or minimus, leads to worsening pain.

The most serious complication is infection.

If the injection contains steroid, there is the possibility of fat necrosis causing skin dimpling and skin discoloration.

Practical Tips (How to Improve the Success and Avoid Complications)

The procedure performance is usually not challenging, unless patient BMI is very high.

The success of this procedure lays in identifying the underlying biomechanical issues (often uneven pelvis, SI arthropathy) that led to the enthesopathy in the first place, as often these also require treatment for sustained relief.

If regenerative medicine (PRP, prolotherapy) is used, precise identification of the pathology (e.g., gluteus medius tendinopathy, calcification, etc.) and precise injection of it will improve outcomes. Important is to locate the area of tenderness and see whether there is tendonitis-tendinosis that will be proven triggering pain after the activation of the muscle involved.

Literature Review

Steroid for GTPS

Corticosteroid injections are commonly performed for GTPS because of their strong anti-inflammatory properties. There is strong evidence of benefit up to 3 months, with greatest effect at 6 weeks. However, the long-term benefits have not been shown. No significant difference in outcomes has been shown with or without image guidance.

PRP for GTPS

The evidence on the effectiveness of PRP for GTPS compared to control is limited. One study investigated the use of PRP in GTPS and demonstrated a longer-lasting clinical results compared to steroid treatment. In this study, 4 ml of PRP was gained from 40 ml blood. US guidance was used for injection. Limitation of this study was small sample size. Ribeiro found no benefit of PRP versus steroid in pain control and function. In this study, 4 mls of PRP was extracted from 25 mls of blood, and US guidance was used. The issue with this study was that the injectate had lower platelet count than had been indicated to be effective in other studies.

Another study did not show any evidence of effectiveness of PRP injection compared to placebo in a RCT double blind. In this study, 5 mls of PRP were injected from 54 mls of blood, and no imaging guidance was used.

In a fourth randomized controlled trial, it was compared the effect of a single ultrasound-guided injection of PRP into the deepest aspect of tendon abnormality with another group treated with repeated fenestration and found subsequent improvement over the next 3 months in both groups with no statistically significant difference between them. In this study, 10 ml of PRP were harvested from 60 mls of blood, and US guidance was used.

Conclusion

Pain arising from the hip joint and trochanteric bursae is very common, and it is a frequent cause of disability. First-line treatment for this pain is conservative management and physical therapy. Minimally invasive treatments might be required, aiming to relieve pain and to improve disability. Intra-articular steroids have shown to have limited effects, give temporary relief, and contribute to joint degeneration. Viscosupplementation with HA has shown some evidence to improve function for up to 6 months but has no disease-modifying effect. Regenerative medicine is the next frontier and shows very promising in terms of targeting the pathophysiology of inflammation and degenerative changes. Further large studies are needed to better demonstrate efficacy of techniques such as PRP, mesenchymal stem cells injections, and prolotherapy.

Suggested Reading

Athanasiou KA, Agarwal A, Dzida FJ. Comparative study of the intrinsic mechanical properties of the human acetabular and femoral head cartilage. J Orthop Res. 1994;12(3):340–9. https://doi.org/10.1002/jor.1100120306.

Battaglia M, Guaraldi F, Vannini F, Rossi G, Timoncini A, Buda R, Giannini S. Efficacy of ultrasound-guided intra-articular injections of platelet-rich plasma versus hyaluronic acid for hip osteoarthritis. Orthopedics. 2013;36(12):1501–8. https://doi.org/10.3928/01477447-20131120-13.

Begkas D, Chatzopoulos S-T, Touzopoulos P, Balanika A, Pastroudis A. Ultrasound-guided platelet-rich plasma application versus corticosteroid injections for the treatment of greater trochanteric pain syndrome: a prospective controlled randomized comparative clinical study. Cureus. 2020;12(1):1–9. https://doi.org/10.7759/cureus.6583.

Brander V, Skrepnik N, Petrella RJ, Jiang GL, Accomando B, Vardanyan A. Evaluating the use of intra-articular injections as a treatment for painful hip osteoarthritis: a randomized, double-blind, multicenter, parallel-group study comparing a single 6-ML injection of hylan G-F 20 with saline. Osteoarthr Cartil. 2019;27(1):59–70. https://doi.org/10.1016/j.joca.2018.08.018.

Brinks A, van Rijn RM, Willemsen SP, Bohnen AM, Verhaar JAN, Koes BW, Bierma-Zeinstra SMA. Corticosteroid injections for greater trochanteric pain syndrome: a randomized controlled trial in primary care. Ann Fam Med. 2011;9(3):226–34. https://doi.org/10.1370/afm.1232.

Chambers AW, Lacy KW, Liow MHL, Manalo JPM, Freiberg AA, Kwon YM. Multiple hip intra-articular steroid injections increase risk of periprosthetic joint infection compared with single injections. J Arthroplasty. 2017;32(6):1980–3. https://doi.org/10.1016/j.arth.2017.01.030.

Cohen SP, Strassels SA, Foster L, Marvel J, Williams K, Crooks M, Gross A, Kurihara C, Nguyen C, Williams N. Comparison of fluoroscopically guided and blind corticosteroid injections for greater trochanteric pain syndrome: multicentre randomised controlled trial. BMJ (Online). 2009;338(7701):986–8. https://doi.org/10.1136/bmj.b1088.

Coombes BK, Bisset L, Vicenzino B. Efficacy and safety of corticosteroid injections and other injections for management of tendinopathy: a systematic review of randomised controlled trials. Lancet. 2010;376(9754):1751–67. https://doi.org/10.1016/S0140-6736(10)61160-9.

Dallari D, Stagni C, Rani N, Sabbioni G, Pelotti P, Torricelli P, Tschon M, Giavaresi G. Ultrasound-guided injection of platelet-rich plasma and hyaluronic acid, separately and in combination, for hip osteoarthritis. Am J Sports Med. 2016;44(3):664–71. https://doi.org/10.1177/0363546515620383.

Darrow M, Shaw B, Darrow B, Wisz S. Short-term outcomes of treatment of hip osteoarthritis with 4 bone marrow concentrate injections: a case series. Clin Med Insight Case Rep. 2018;11:1179547618791574. https://doi.org/10.1177/1179547618791574.

Doria C, Mosele GR, Caggiari G, Puddu L, Ciurlia E. Treatment of early hip osteoarthritis: ultrasound-guided platelet rich plasma versus hyaluronic acid injections in a randomized clinical trial. Joints. 2017;5(3):152–5. https://doi.org/10.1055/s-0037-1605584.

Emadedin M, Liastani MG, Fazeli R, Mohseni F, Moghadasali R, Mardpour S, Hosseini SE, et al. Long-term follow-up of intra-articular injection of autologous mesenchymal stem cells in patients with knee, ankle, or hip osteoarthritis. Arch Iran Med. 2015;18(6):336–44.

Estrela GQ, Furtado R, Natour J, Narimatsu S, Rosenfeld A. Blinded vs ultrasound-guided corticosteroid injections for the treatment of the greater trochanteric pain syndrome (SDPT): a randomized controlled trial. Ann Rheum Dis. 2014;73(Suppl)

Ferguson SJ, Bryant JT, Ganz R, Ito K. The influence of the acetabular labrum on hip joint cartilage consolidation: a poroelastic finite element model. J Biomech. 2000;33(8):953–60. https://doi.org/10.1016/S0021-9290(00)00042-7.

Fernandes L, Hagen KB, Bijlsma JWJ, Andreassen O, Christensen P, Conaghan PG, Doherty M, et al. EULAR recommendations for the non-pharmacological core management of hip and knee osteoarthritis. Ann Rheum Dis. 2013;72(7):1125–35. https://doi.org/10.1136/annrheumdis-2012-202745.

Gazendam A, Ekhtiari S, Bozzo A, Phillips M, Bhandari M. Intra-articular saline injection as effective as corticosteroids, platelet-rich plasma and hyaluronic acid for hip osteoarthritis pain: a systematic review and network meta-analysis of randomised controlled trials. Br J Sports Med. 2020; https://doi.org/10.1136/bjsports-2020-102179.

Grumet RC, Frank RM, Slabaugh MA, Virkus WW, Bush-Joseph CA, Nho SJ. Lateral hip pain in an athletic population: differential diagnosis and treatment options. Sports Health. 2010;2(3):191–6. https://doi.org/10.1177/1941738110366829.

Gül D, Orsçelik A, Akpancar S. Treatment of osteoarthritis secondary to developmental dysplasia of the hip with prolotherapy injection versus a supervised progressive exercise control. Med Sci Monit. 2020;26:1–8. https://doi.org/10.12659/MSM.919166.

Hochberg MC, Altman RD, April KT, Benkhalti M, Guyatt G, McGowan J, Towheed T, Welch V, Wells G, Tugwell P. American college of rheumatology 2012 recommendations for the use of non-pharmacologic and pharmacologic therapies in osteoarthritis of the hand, hip, and knee. Arthritis Care Res. 2012;64(4):465–74. https://doi.org/10.1002/acr.21596.

Hoeber S, Aly AR, Ashworth N, Rajasekaran S. Ultrasound-guided hip joint injections are more accurate than landmark-guided injections: a systematic review and meta-analysis. Br J Sports Med. 2016;50(7):392–6. https://doi.org/10.1136/bjsports-2014-094570.

Jacobson JA, Yablon CM, Troy Henning P, Kazmers IS, Urquhart A, Hallstrom B, Bedi A, Parameswaran A. Greater trochanteric pain syndrome: percutaneous tendon fenestration versus platelet-rich plasma injection for treatment of gluteal tendinosis. J Ultrasound Med. 2016;35(11):2413–20. https://doi.org/10.7863/ultra.15.11046.

Jayaram P, Ikpeama U, Rothenberg JB, Malanga GA. Bone marrow–derived and adipose-derived mesenchymal stem cell therapy in primary knee osteoarthritis: a narrative review. PM R. 2019;11(2):177–91. https://doi.org/10.1016/j.pmrj.2018.06.019.

Lai WC, Arshi A, Wang D, Seeger LL, Motamedi K, Levine BD, Hame SL. Efficacy of intraarticular corticosteroid hip injections for osteoarthritis and subsequent surgery. Skelet Radiol. 2018;47(12):1635–40. https://doi.org/10.1007/s00256-018-3052-z.

Law L, Hunt CL, Van Wijnen AJ, Ahmad Nassr A, Larson N, Eldrige JS, Mauck WD, et al. Office-based mesenchymal stem cell therapy for the treatment of musculoskeletal disease: a systematic review of recent human studies. Pain Med (U S). 2019;20(8):1570–83. https://doi.org/10.1093/pm/pny256.

Leite VF, Amadera JED, Buehler AM. Viscosupplementation for hip osteoarthritis: a systematic review and meta-analysis of the efficacy on pain and disability, and the occurrence of adverse events. Arch Phys Med Rehabil. 2018;99(3):574–583.e1. https://doi.org/10.1016/j.apmr.2017.07.010.

McAlindon TE, LaValley MP, Harvey WF, Price LL, Driban JB, Zhang M, Ward RJ. Effect of intra-articular triamcinolone vs saline on knee cartilage volume and pain in patients with knee osteoarthritis a randomized clinical trial. JAMA. 2017;317(19):1967–75. https://doi.org/10.1001/jama.2017.5283.

McCabe PS, Maricar N, Parkes MJ, Felson DT, O'Neill TW. The efficacy of intra-articular steroids in hip osteoarthritis: a systematic review. Osteoarthr Cartil. 2016;24(9):1509–17. https://doi.org/10.1016/j.joca.2016.04.018.

Medina-Porqueres I, Ortega-Castillo M, Muriel-Garcia A. Effectiveness of platelet-rich plasma in the management of hip osteoarthritis: a systematic review and meta-analysis. Clin Rheumatol. 2020; https://doi.org/10.1007/s10067-020-05241-x.

Murphy NJ, Eyles JP, Hunter DJ. Hip osteoarthritis: etiopathogenesis and implications for management. Adv Ther. 2016;33(11):1921–46. https://doi.org/10.1007/s12325-016-0409-3.

Narouze S, Benzon HT, Provenzano D, Buvanendran A, De Andres J, Deer T, Rauck R, Huntoon MA. Interventional spine and pain procedures in patients on antiplatelet and anticoagulant medications (second edition): guidelines from the American Society of Regional Anesthesia and Pain Medicine, the European Society of Regional Anaesthesia and Pain Thera. Reg Anesth Pain Med. 2018;43:225–62. https://doi.org/10.1097/AAP.0000000000000700.

Peng PWH. Ultrasound-guided interventional procedures in pain medicine: a review of anatomy, sonoanatomy, and procedures. Part IV: hip. Reg Anesth Pain Med. 2013;38(4):264–73. https://doi.org/10.1097/AAP.0b013e318291c8ed.

Pogliacomi F, Schiavi P, Paraskevopoulos A, Leigheb M, Pedrazzini A, Ceccarelli F, Vaienti E. When is indicated viscosupplementation in hip osteoarthritis? Acta Biomed. 2019;90(11):67–74. https://doi.org/10.23750/abm.v90i1-S.8000.

Rabago D, Slattengren A, Zgierska A. Prolotherapy in primary care practice. Prim Care. 2010;37(1):65–80. https://doi.org/10.1016/j.pop.2009.09.013.

Raythatha M, Spitz D, Tang JY. Fluoroscopically-guided joint and bursa injection techniques: a comprehensive primer. Semin Roentgenol. 2019;54(2):124–48. https://doi.org/10.1053/j.ro.2018.09.002.

Reidy M, Cousins G, Finlayson D. Corticosteroid injection of the arthritic hip: what is the indication? Scott Med J. 2015;60(1):29–31. https://doi.org/10.1177/0036933014563237.

Ribeiro AG, Junior RW, Silva AR, Polesello GC, Guimarães RP. PRP in the treatment of trochanteric syndrome: a pilot study. Acta Ortop Bras. 2016;24(4):208–12. https://doi.org/10.1590/1413-785220162404159837.

Rodriguez-Fontan F, Piuzzi NS, Kraeutler MJ, Pascual-Garrido C. Early clinical outcomes of intra-articular injections of bone marrow aspirate concentrate for the treatment of early osteoarthritis of the hip and knee: a cohort study. PM and R. 2018;10(12):1353–9. https://doi.org/10.1016/j.pmrj.2018.05.016.

Sante LD, Villani C, Santilli V, Valeo M, Bologna E, Imparato L, Paoloni M, Iagnocco A. Intra-articular hyaluronic acid vs platelet-rich plasma in the treatment of hip osteoarthritis. Med Ultrason. 2016;18(4):463–8. https://doi.org/10.11152/mu-874.

Shah JP, Thaker N, Heimur J, Aredo JV, Sikdar S, Gerber L. Myofascial trigger points then and now: a historical and scientific perspective. PM and R. 2015;7(7):746–61. https://doi.org/10.1016/j.pmrj.2015.01.024.

Shbeeb MI, O'Duffy JD, Michet CJ Jr, O'Fallon WM, Matteson EL. Evaluation of glucocorticosteroid injection for the treatment of trochanteric bursitis. J Rheumatol. 1996;23:2104–6.

Shindle MK, Ranawat AS, Kelly BT. Diagnosis and management of traumatic and atraumatic hip instability in the athletic patient. Clin Sports Med. 2006;25(2):309–26. https://doi.org/10.1016/j.csm.2005.12.003.

Simeone FJ, Vicentini JRT, Bredella MA, Chang CY. Are patients more likely to have hip osteoarthritis progression and femoral head collapse after hip steroid/anesthetic injections? A retrospective observational study. Skelet Radiol. 2019;48(9):1417–26. https://doi.org/10.1007/s00256-019-03189-x.

Stephens MB, Beutler AI, O'Connor FG. Musculoskeletal injections: a review of the evidence. Am Fam Physician. 2008;78(8):971–6.

Thompson G, Pearson JF. No attributable effects of PRP on greater trochanteric pain syndrome. N Z Med J. 2019;132(1507):22–32.

Tibor LM, Sekiya JK. Differential diagnosis of pain around the hip joint. Arthroscopy. 2008;24(12):1407–21. https://doi.org/10.1016/j.arthro.2008.06.019.

Wu B, Li YM, Liu YC. Efficacy of intra-articular hyaluronic acid injections in hip osteoarthritis: a meta-analysis of randomized controlled trials. Oncotarget. 2017;8(49):86865–76. https://doi.org/10.18632/oncotarget.20995.

Xu S, Liu H, Xie Y, Sang L, Liu J, Chen B. Effect of mesenchymal stromal cells for articular cartilage degeneration treatment: a meta-analysis. Cytotherapy. 2015;17(10):1342–52. https://doi.org/10.1016/j.jcyt.2015.05.005.

Zhang W, Doherty M, Arden N, Bannwarth B, Bijlsma J, Gunther KP, Hauselmann HJ, et al. EULAR evidence based recommendations for the management of hip osteoarthritis: report of a task force of the EULAR Standing Committee for International Clinical Studies Including Therapeutics (ESCISIT). Ann Rheum Dis. 2005;64(5):669–81. https://doi.org/10.1136/ard.2004.028886.

Zhang W, Moskowitz RW, Nuki G, Abramson S, Altman RD, Arden N, Bierma-Zeinstra S, et al. OARSI recommendations for the management of hip and knee osteoarthritis, Part II: OARSI evidence-based, expert consensus guidelines. Osteoarthr Cartil. 2008;16(2):137–62. https://doi.org/10.1016/j.joca.2007.12.013.

Pericapsular Nerve Group Block and Ablation

64

Tony K. T. Ng, Laura Girón-Arango, and Philip Peng

Contents

General Consideration

Pain of hip origin can be in the form of acute (e.g., hip fracture) or chronic (e.g., hip osteoarthritis). From the literature, there are opportunities to improve the management of both the types of conditions.

Osteoarthritis (OA) of the hip is common with advancing age, and it is associated with pain, functional impairment, and instability. Investigators had examined the feasibility of ablation the articular branch network of hip joint by radiofrequency technique. However, the clinical results were mixed as there was no clear understanding of the course of articular branches to the hip joint.

Hip fracture is a condition found more frequently in the elderly population. An adequate pain control before surgery is a cornerstone in the management of these patients as suboptimal analgesia increases the risk of delirium and other morbidities. Regional anesthesia has become the preferred technique for pain relief in hip fracture patients as it provides an opioid-sparing analgesia with less side effects such as constipation, nausea, and altered mentation. The existing regional blocks are effective in controlling their pain at rest but not enough for movement-related pain.

Over the recent years, anatomical studies have brought greater understanding of the sensory innervation of the hip. The application of this new knowledge to sonoanatomy led to a novel technique, termed Pericapsular Nerve Group (PENG) block, which targets the sensory articular branches

T. K. T. Ng
Pain Management Unit, Department of Anaesthesia and Operating Theatre Services, Tuen Mun Hospital, Tuen Mun, Hong Kong

Department of Anaesthesiology, LKS Faculty of Medicine, The University of Hong Kong, Pok Fu Lam, Hong Kong

L. Girón-Arango
Department of Anesthesia, Hospital Pablo Tobón Uribe, Medellín, Colombia

P. Peng (✉)
Department of Anesthesia and Pain Medicine, Toronto Western Hospital, University of Toronto, Toronto, ON, Canada
e-mail: philip.peng@uhn.ca

D. Jankovic, P. Peng (eds.), *Regional Nerve Blocks in Anesthesia and Pain Therapy*,
https://doi.org/10.1007/978-3-030-88727-8_64

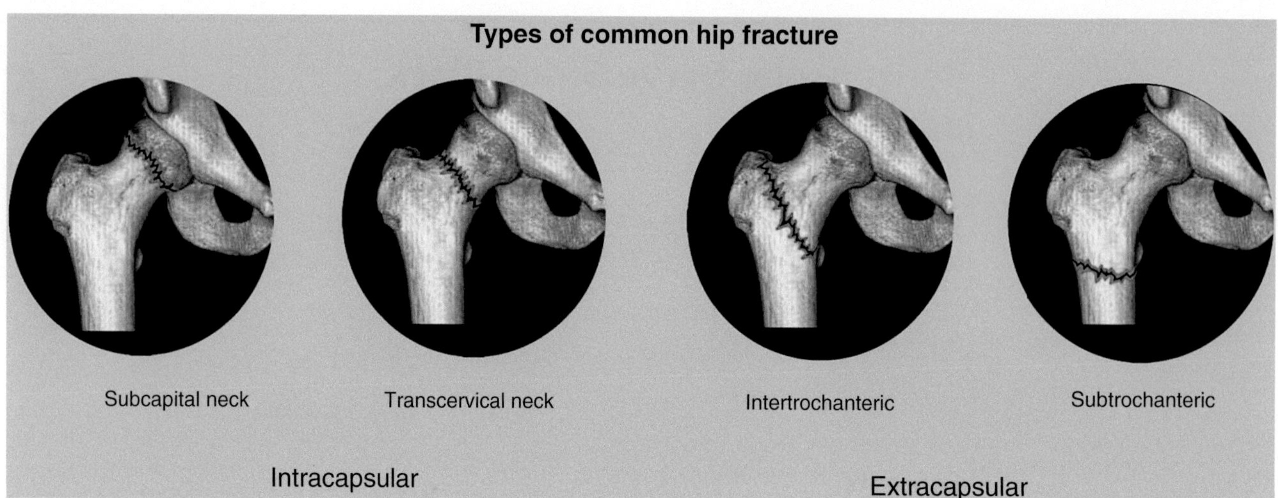

Fig. 64.1 Four common types of hip fracture. (Reprinted with permission from Philip Peng Educational Series)

of the hip providing analgesia without affecting the motor branches.

Patient Selection

In the peri-operative setting, this technique was initially described for hip fracture analgesia. There are different types of hip fractures (Fig. 64.1), and the PENG procedure is indicated for patient intracapsular and intertrochanteric fracture. Nevertheless, recent publications have described its use in other hip surgeries like hip arthroscopy and total hip replacement. It is important to point out that this technique is recommended primarily for analgesic purposes and not for surgical anesthesia as it covers only the articular branches of the hip without any cutaneous coverage. However, recent literature also showed promising result of applying this block to the post-operative pain control for both hip fracture surgery and hip arthroplasty.

For patients with chronic hip pain, the candidates for ablation described in the literature are patients with osteoarthritis. Other chronic hip pain conditions such as rheumatoid arthritis, avascular necrosis or post-infection destruction of the hip had not been well studied.

Anatomy

A review of the anatomy of the articular branches of hip joint in the last 200 years showed that 16 of 19 articles were published more than 50 years ago and only one article investigated the obturator articular branches with reference to discernable landmark by imaging equipment. Subsequently, a detailed anatomic dissection showed that the anterior hip capsule is consistently supplied by the articular branches from femoral, obturator, and accessory obturator (if present) nerves.

There are two types of articular branches from femoral nerve (L2, L3, and L4): high and low based on their origin superior or inferior to the inguinal ligament. The high branches emerge from the femoral nerve (FN) on the lateral border of this muscle at around the L4–L5 levels and travel intramuscularly through iliacus muscle. At the level of the inguinal ligament, up to 14 articular branches can be seen traveling between the anteroinferior iliac spine (AIIS) and iliopubic eminence (IPE) deep to the iliopsoas muscle and tendon, supplying all four quadrants of the anterior hip capsule (Fig. 64.2). Lower branches are less uncommon and are the exclusive supply from femoral nerve in only 1 in 13 cadavers. They perforated the iliopsoas to supply the anterior capsule directly or coursed inferiorly before recurring superiorly to innervate the capsule. The course of these lower branches cannot be related to the space between AIIS and IPE.

The accessory obturator nerve (AON)), if present, also originates in the lumbar plexus at the L2–L5 levels. This nerve descends as a single branch deep into the medial aspect of the psoas muscle and passes over the IPE before it enters the medial hip joint capsule (Fig. 64.2). The obturator nerve (ON) travels through the obturator foramen and divides into anterior and posterior divisions. It gives the articular branches either proximal or distal to the obturator foramen and travels across the inferomedial acetabulum (IMA) to supply the inferior half of the hip capsule (Fig. 64.2).

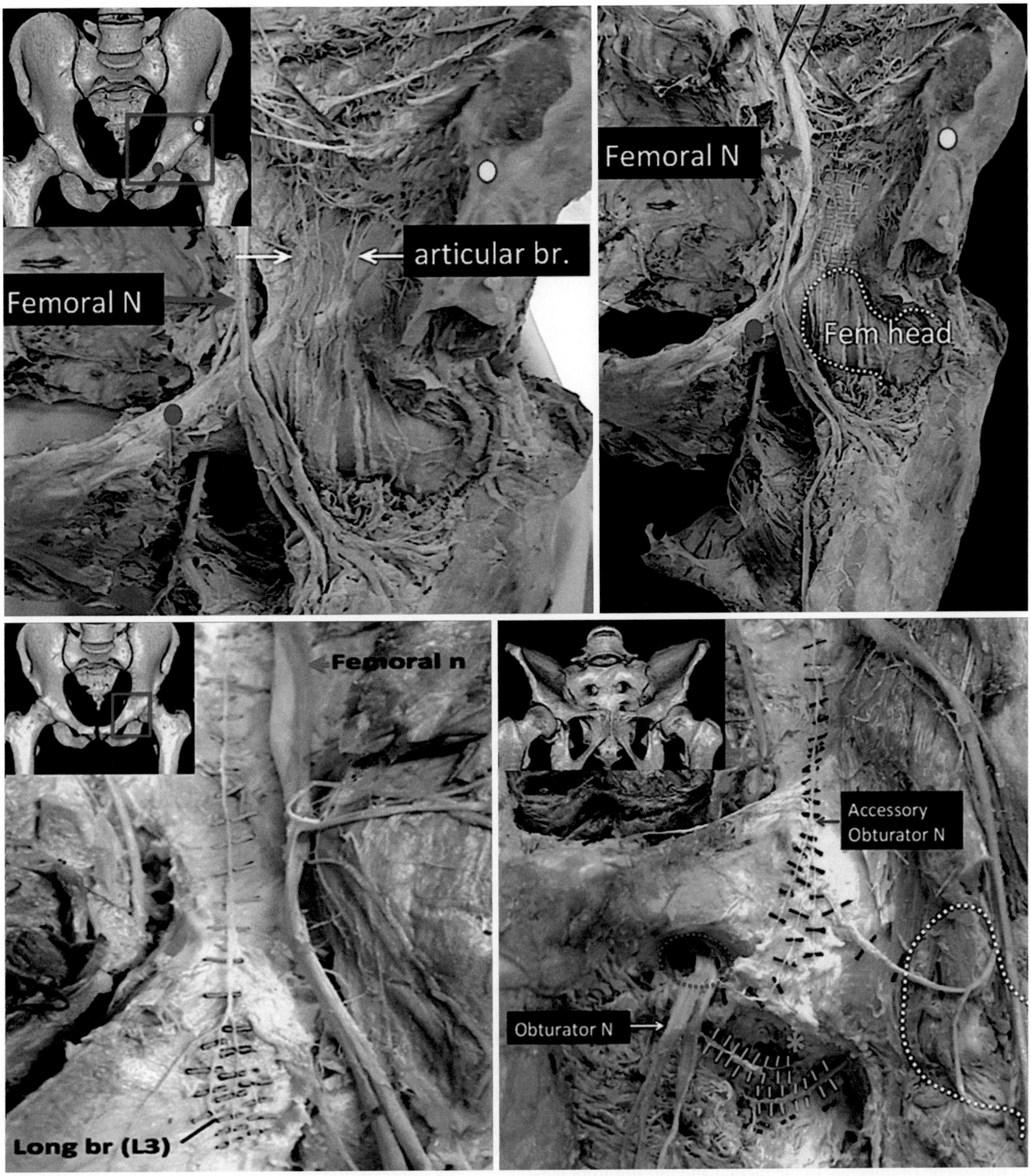

Fig. 64.2 Articular branches of the anterior hip capsule. Upper panel: Articular branches of femoral nerve (highlighted on the right with green sutures run between the anterior inferior iliac spine (yellow dot) and iliopubuc eminence (red dot). Lower left panel: Accessory obturator nerve runs over the iliopubic eminence. Lower right panel: The obturator nerve comes out from the obturator foramen (circle outlined by red dotted line) and divides into anterior and posterior divisions. The obturator nerve also sends articular branches coursing deep into the inferomedial acetabulum (*) toward the hip joint. In this figure, the accessory obturator can also be seen (highlighted by black suture). The locations of the dissections are all indicated with the insert in the left upper corner. (Reprinted with permission from Philip Peng Educational Series)

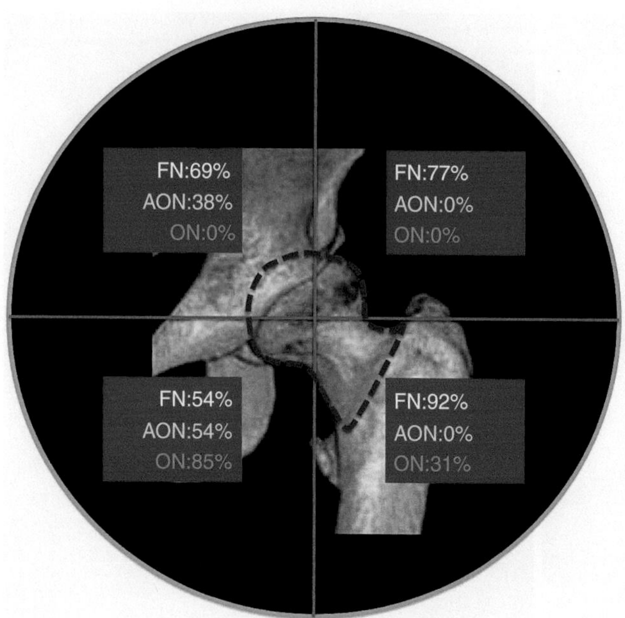

Fig. 64.3 The four quadrants of anterior hip capsule covered by femoral (FN), accessory obturator (AON), and obturator (ON) nerves. (Reprinted with permission from Philip Peng Educational Series)

The contribution of different articular branches to the anterior capsule varies (Fig. 64.3). The posterior aspect is supplied by the sacral plexus such as nerve to quadratus femoris, sciatic, and superior gluteal nerves. The highest concentration of nociceptive fibers is located in the anterior and superolateral hip capsule, and the posterior hip innervation is mainly comprised of mechanoreceptors and contains no nociceptive fibers. Thus, the main target to mitigate the pain from hip is the anterior articular branches.

Technique

The articular branches of FN and AON can be easily reached by directing the needle deep to the iliopsoas muscle between AIIS and IPE. The latter two landmarks can be easily visualized with ultrasound, and the IMA can be visualized by fluoroscopy as the "tear drop" or by ultrasound. A recent injection study showed that injection in the vicinity of the FN and AON articular branches between the AIIS and IPE resulted in the spread of injectate to the medial and inferior joint capsule, where the obturator nerve innervated. This pericapsular injection is the basis of the PENG block.

With the understanding of the innervation and the relationship of the articular branches to the bony landmark, the interventional procedure can be applied in four different settings:

1. Peri-operative block for hip fracture and hip arthroplasty
2. Diagnostic block for chronic hip pain
3. Chemical ablation for persistent hip pain
4. Radiofrequency ablation for chronic hip pain

Peri-operative Block for Hip Fracture and Arthroplasty

Scanning Technique

With the patient in supine and the leg in the neutral position, a low-frequency curved transducer (2–5 MHz) is used for scanning (use linear probe for patient with low BMI) after prepping the patient in sterile manner. The first landmark for scanning is the palpable anterior superior iliac spine (ASIS), which is a subcutaneous structure. From there, the probe is moved in caudal direction until the anterior inferior iliac spine (AIIS) is revealed. The AIIS can be found on the medial side of ASIS and is deeper in location. The probe is then rotated to align the AIIS with another bony landmark, the iliopubic eminence (IPE). A typical picture will show AIIS, IPE, psoas tendon and muscle, femoral neurovascular bundle superficial and medial to the iliopsoas (Fig. 64.4). The target is the fascial plane between the psoas muscle/tendon and the bone between AIIS and IPE.

Needle Insertion Approach

An 80- to 100-mm needle is inserted in plane in a lateral to medial direction toward the plane deep to the psoas muscle/tendon between AIIS and IPE. Hydrodissection should be used to identify the needle in the fascial plane instead of the intramuscular compartment in location. Having bony contact does not mean that the needle is on the bone (Fig. 64.5). It is recommended to use normal saline for hydrodissection instead of the local anesthetic as an intramuscular injection of the active solution could result in spread to the femoral nerve and cause quadriceps weakness. A successful injection will result in the spread of injectate between psoas and pubic bone (Fig. 64.5).

Alternatively, a catheter can be inserted in the pericapsular space as described above or iliopsoas plane (which is revealed by placing the probe in long axis to the femoral head and neck, and this plane is superficial to the iliofemoral ligament deep to the psoas). PENG catheter can be a useful option for preoperative analgesia of hip fracture when a few days to a week is required to optimize the patient comorbidities before hip surgery. The catheter tip is placed deep to the iliopsoas muscle at the midway between AIIS and IPE. The catheter can be left in situ during the surgery or be reinserted after the surgery.

Volume of the Local Anesthetic

Currently, there is no definite dose volume spread study to guide clinician the practice. However, Tran et al. investigated the spread and found that a volume of 10 mL was enough to cover the articular branches between AIIS and IPE, and therefore, this volume should be sufficient for neck of fracture femur. However, in patient with intertrochanteric fracture, a wider pericapsular spread including ON is important, and a volume of 20 mL is recommended based on those authors' recommendation. A volume higher than that is not

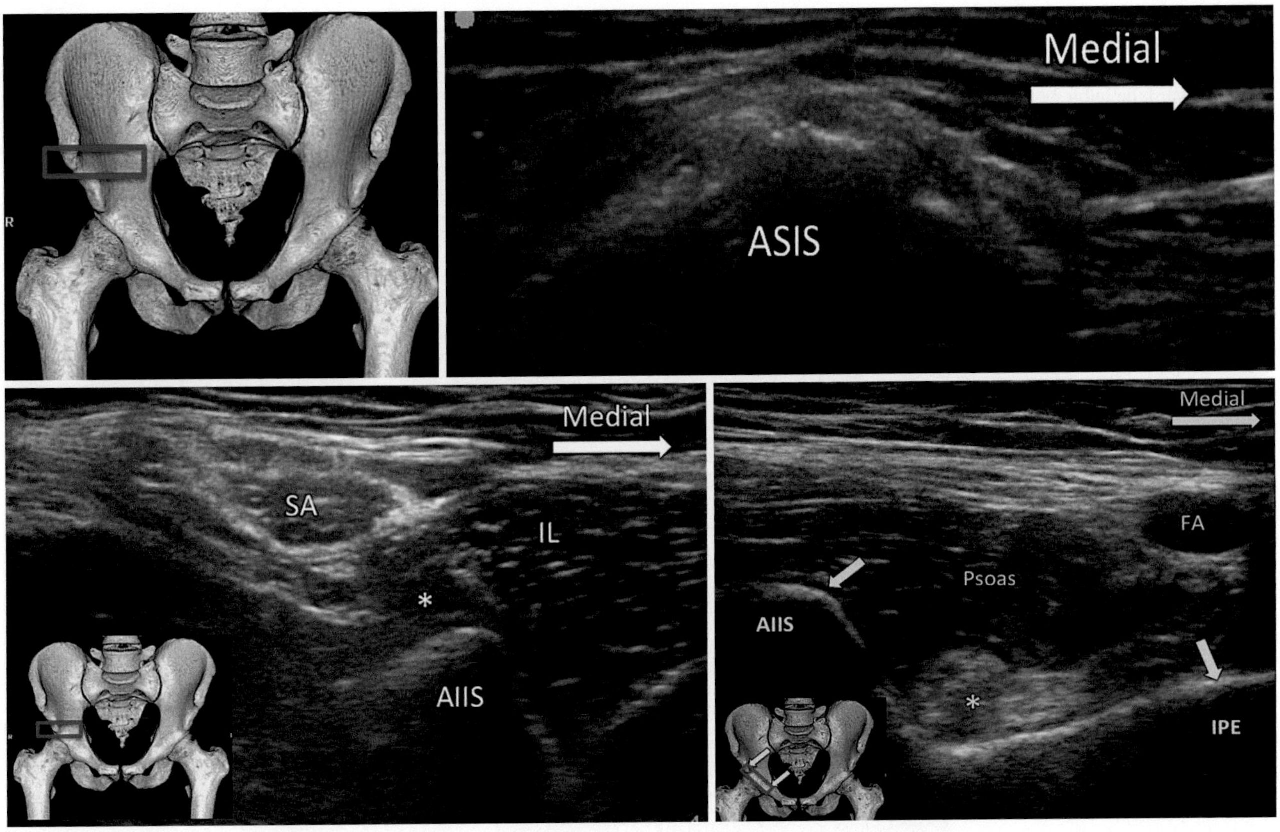

Fig. 64.4 Sonographic appearance of anterior hip. The probe position is indicated by the red box. The first scan is with the probe over the anterior superior iliac spine (ASIS). The probe is then slide in caudal direction to reveal the anterior inferior iliac spine (AIIS). At this space, the straight head of the rectus femoris (*) can be seen over the AIIS. From here, the probe is rotated to align the AIIS and iliopubic eminence (IPE) indicated by the arrows. *SA* sartorius. In this scan, the psoas muscle and tendon (*) are seen. *FA* femoral artery. (Reprinted with permission from Philip Peng Educational Series)

recommended as the injectate can spread lateral to the psoas muscle or in between the imperfect intermuscular fascia plane between pectineus and psoas to the femoral nerve superficial to the psoas-pectineus muscles.

After catheter insertion, Singh et al. published a case series that they injected a bolus dose of 20 mL 0.25% bupivacaine preoperatively, followed by keeping the PENG catheter postoperatively at 5 mL/h 0.25% bupivacaine for 48 h. The result was promising with a VAS range of 0–2 out of 10.

Diagnostic/Prognostic Block for Chronic Hip Pain

The rationale of a diagnostic or prognostic block is to determine whether the patient will benefit from a potential ablation procedure. The scanning and needle insertion technique is the same as described above. There are two differences. One is related to the volume which is typically 3–5 mL of long-acting local anesthetic such as 0.75–1% ropivacaine or 0.5% levobupivacaine or bupivacaine. Because of the small volume of injectate, the hydrodissection injectate of choice is normal saline. The other difference is the requirement of a separate injection for the articular branch of obturator nerve as the lower volume of injectate is unlikely to spread to the ON. The target is inferomedial acetabulum and can be visualized as a "tear drop" in X-ray (Fig. 64.6). However, a needle cannot be directed simply by fluoroscopic guidance as the femoral vessels and nerve overlay this structure (Fig. 64.6). Instead, the target can be approached by ultrasound guidance. This technique was suggested in one article but had not been validated. So at the present time, this ultrasound-guided technique is better reserved for experienced hand or used in adjunct with fluoroscopy guidance (Fig. 64.7).

For the scanning of the inferomedial acetabulum, the probe is first placed to reveal the superomedial acetabulum by aligning the acetabulum, femoral head and neck as shown in Fig. 64.7. The probe is then moved in the inferomedial direction until the disappearance of femoral head, which signifies the location of inferomedial acetabulum. A Doppler scan is advised at this stage to make sure there is no vessel in the trajectory of the needle insertion. If there is any vessel, the probe can be rotated slightly to a different plane to

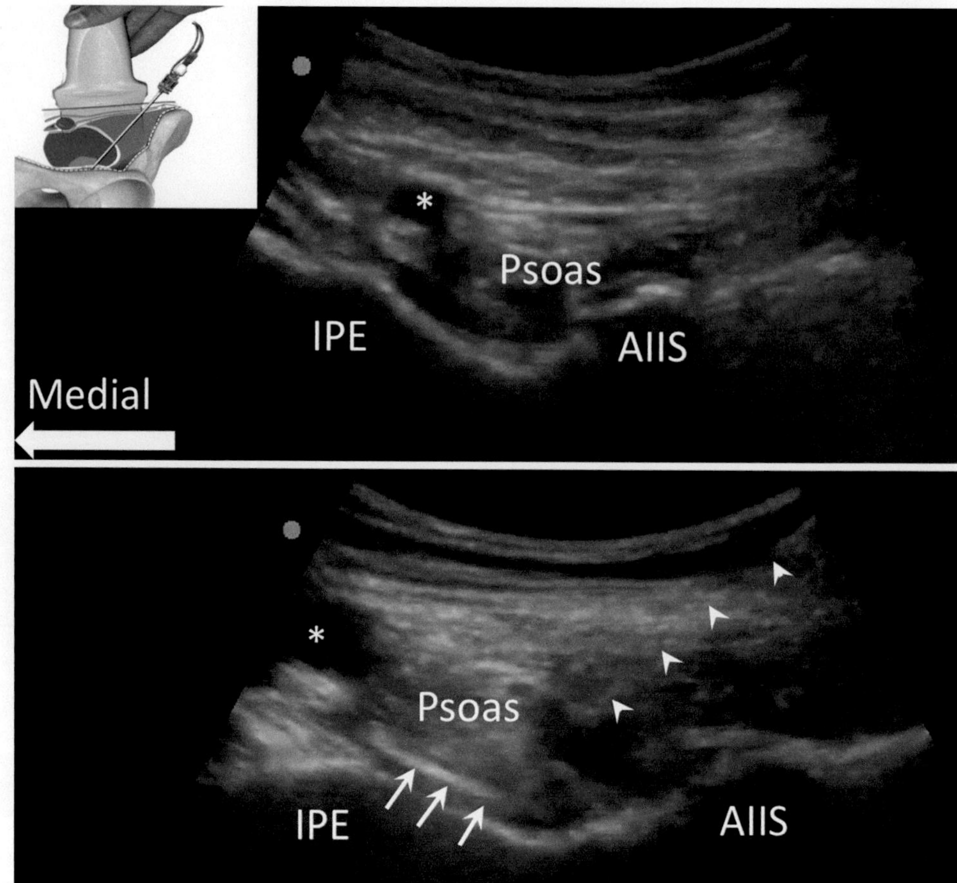

Fig. 64.5 Needle placement is performed by inserting the needle in-plane from lateral to medial toward the pubic bone between the anterior inferior iliac spine (AIIS) and iliopubic eminence (IPE). A successful injectate is indicated by the lifting of the psoas fascia (arrows). Femoral artery is indicated by *. The needle is indicated by the arrowheads. The optimal view for needle insertion should include the femoral artery as the femoral nerve is lateral to it and the needle trajectory should be away from the femoral nerve. (Reprinted with permission from Philip Peng Educational Series)

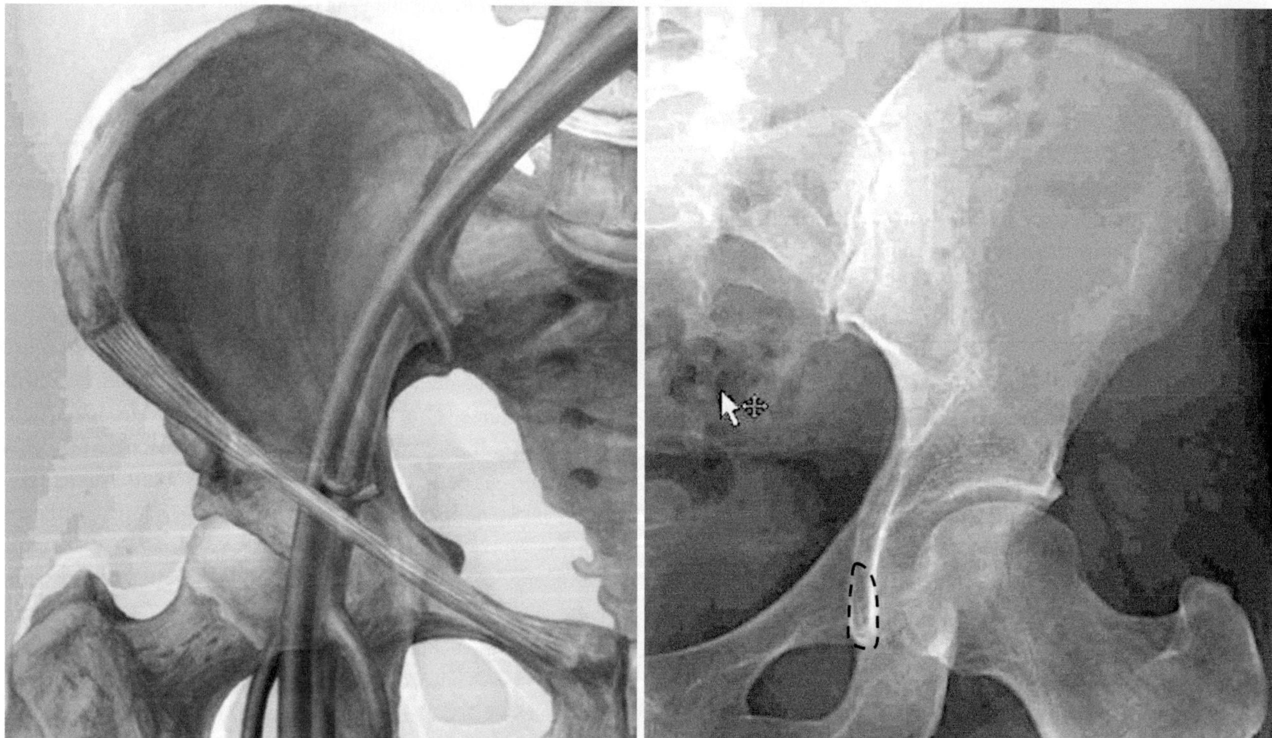

Fig. 64.6 Hybrid diagram to show the X-ray of the pelvis on the right side and pelvis bone on the left side. Note the inferomedial acetabulum (tear drop outlined by dotted line) is covered by femoral vessels. (Reprinted with permission from Philip Peng Educational Series)

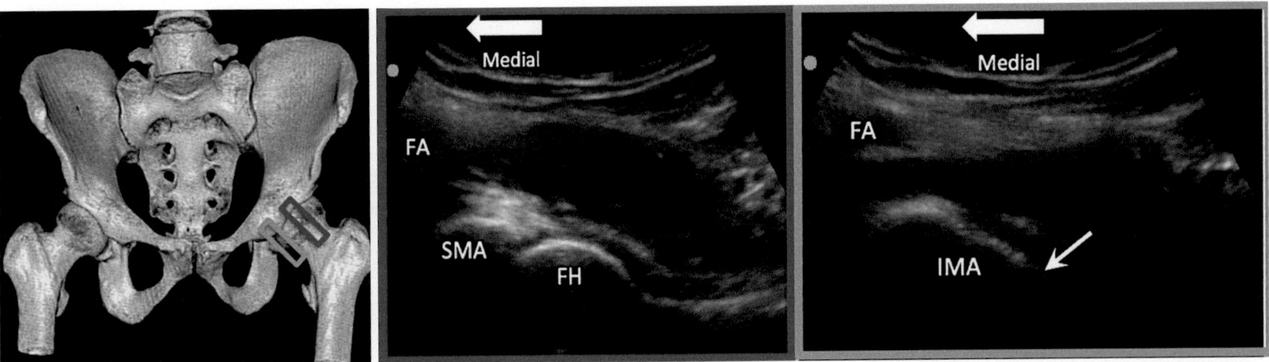

Fig. 64.7 Ultrasound scanning of the inferomedial acetabulum. The left figure shows the position of the ultrasound probes (red and green boxes). The corresponding images are shown in red and green boxes. *FA* femoral artery, *FH* femoral head, *SMA* superomedial acetabulum, *IMA* inferomedial acetabulum. (Reprinted with permission from Philip Peng Educational Series)

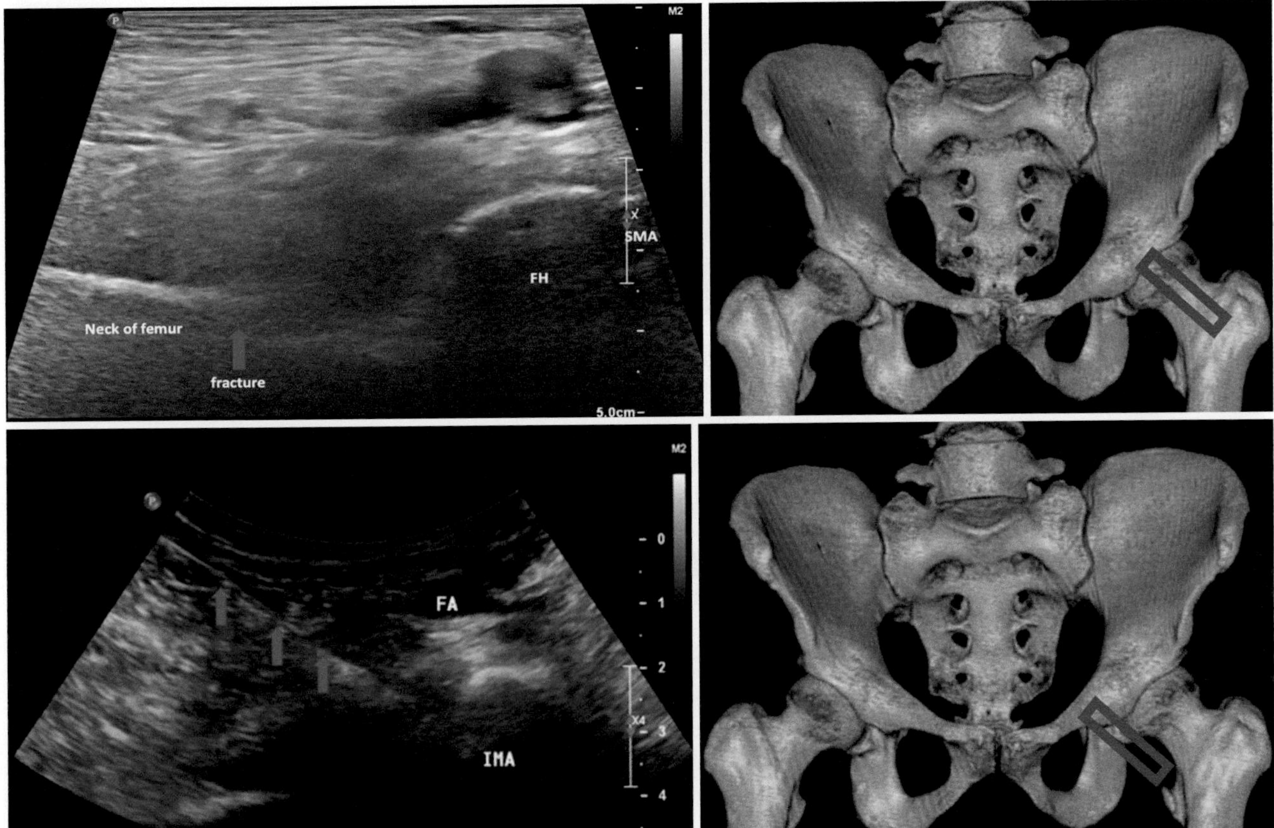

Fig. 64.8 Needle placement to the inferomedial acetabulum in a patient with hip fracture. *FA* femoral artery, *SMA* superomedial acetabulum, *IMA* inferomedial acetabulum. (Reprinted with permission from Philip Peng Educational Series)

avoid vessel puncture. A 22-gauge, 3.5-in. Quincke needle is inserted in-plane from laterally to medially until the needle tip is in contact with the inferomedial acetabulum Fig. 64.8, followed by injecting 1 mL of 0.5% levobupivacaine or 0.75–1% ropivacaine to the articular branch of obturator nerve.

Following the procedure, the patient is encouraged to ambulate afterwards. Pain reduction on ambulation is of paramount importance in this group of patients. A diagnostic/prognostic block is usually defined as positive if there is a reduction of ≥50% in pain intensity on walking for a relatively reasonable distance with respect to the patient's need.

However, for inoperable hip fracture or bone metastasis, the clinician can decide to waive the diagnostic block and go directly to the ablation. Alternatively, the needles are usually left in situ, and if the diagnostic block is positive, the needle

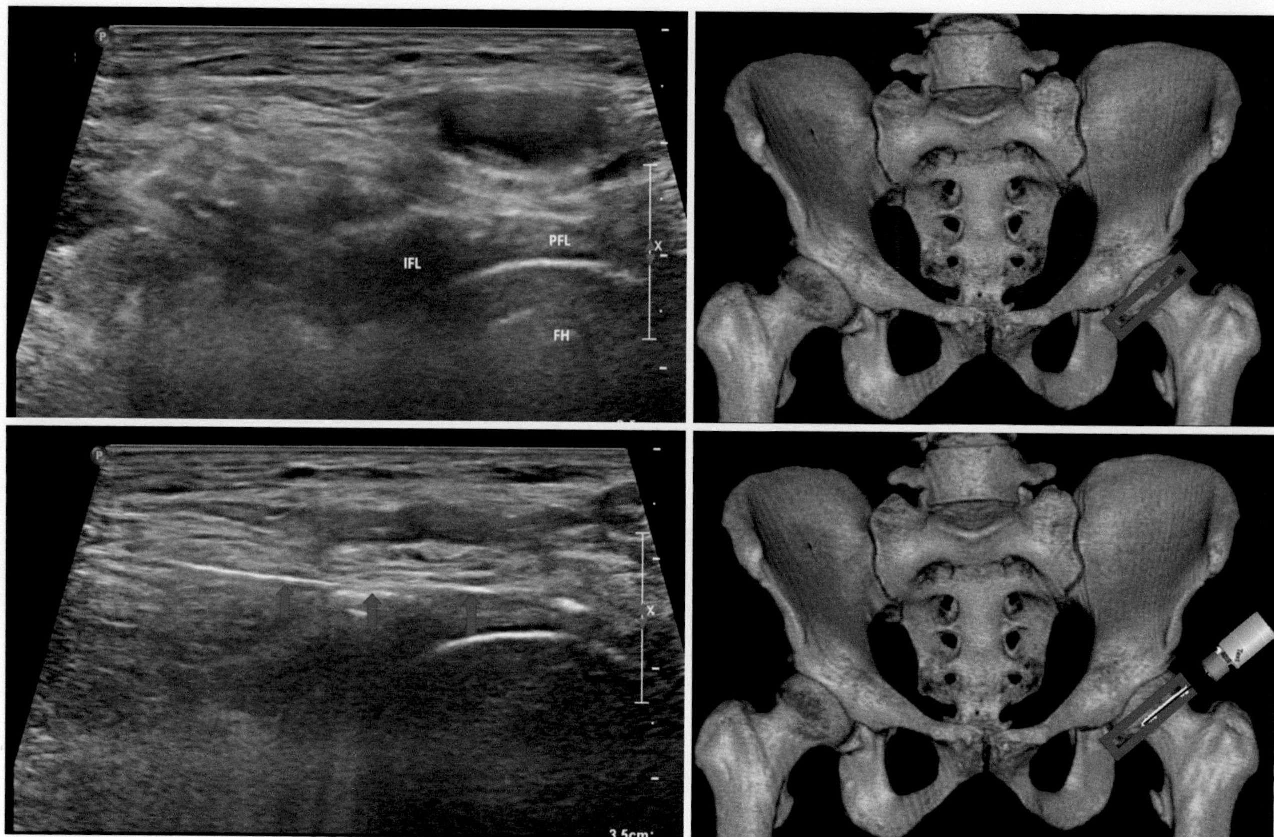

Fig. 64.9 Needle placement over the pubofemoral ligament (PFL) in a patient with hip fracture. *IFL* iliofemoral ligament, *FH* femoral head. (Reprinted with permission from Philip Peng Educational Series)

positions are reconfirmed before denervation (see "Chemical Ablation for Hip Pain" section). A diagnostic block is usually defined as positive if there is a reduction of ≥50% in pain intensity on hip flexion after injecting the local anesthetic for 10 min or more. The reason for this is to minimize the necessity for patients to come twice.

Chemical Ablation for Hip Pain

This procedure is mainly considered in the palliative setting, such as inoperable hip fracture, or bone metastasis to hip joint. Occasionally, this can also be considered in advanced hip osteoarthritis when there is any significant comorbidity, lack of radiofrequency equipment, or contraindication to radiofrequency ablation (internal pulse generator of stimulator in the vicinity). The neurolytic procedure is performed after a positive diagnostic block.

Scanning and Injection Technique

This technique involves a two-needle or three-needle insertion technique. For the articular branches of FN and AON, the first needle placement is the same as the perioperative block described above. The classical PENG approach of targeting the articular branches from FN and the AON between the AIIS and the IPE may potentially miss the low branches of FNAB (see "Anatomy" section). As such, in order to cover all the articular branches from FN, a second needle placed above the anterior iliofemoral and pubofemoral ligaments is recommended based on the experience from the Hong Kong group. The anterior iliofemoral ligament and the pubofemoral ligament can be easily identified by shifting the probe slightly caudally from the AIIS-IPE trough until the hip capsule is seen (Fig. 64.9). The Quincke needle is advanced until the needle tip is above the pubofemoral ligament deep to the femoral artery (Fig. 64.9). The third needle is placed at the inferomedial acetabulum described in the last section.

Chemical Agents and Volume

Both alcohol (100%) and phenol (6–10%) can be used. For the target between AIIS and IPE, or over the pubofemoral ligament, the authors usually put in 1.5 mL of long-acting local anesthetic first followed by 3.5 mL of neurolytic agent. If 100% alcohol is used, the final concentration will be 75%. An additional 1 mL of anesthetic was injected on removal of the needle to prevent the neurolytic agent from remaining in the soft tissue track. For the target in the inferomedial acetabulum, 0.5 mL of local anesthetic is administered first, then followed by another 1 mL of neurolytic agents. The lower the volume of local anesthetic is injected, the more burning discomfort the patient would experience upon absolute alcohol injection in an exchange of a higher final alcohol concentration. A final concentration of at least 50% alcohol is commonly believed to be the minimum for a long-lasting neurolytic effect.

The experience in Hong Kong where the chemical ablation is performed in patients with inoperable hip fracture is as follows. Upon reaching the target, either between the AIIS/IPE or over the pubofemoral ligament, 3–5 mL of long-acting local anesthetic (0.5–1% ropivacaine or 0.25–0.5% levobupivacaine) is administered. The needle is then kept in situ and the movement-related pain is tested after 10 min by gently flexing the hip. If there is a 50% reduction in the movement-related pain, 3–5 mL of the neurolytic agent (100% alcohol) is then administered. The denervation over the inferomedial acetabulum follows a similar sequence except that the total volume (local anesthetic and neurolytic agent 1:1 ratio) is limited to 2–3 mL. The reason of using a higher injectate volume in this group of patients is that the sonoanatomical image is often less optimal in the presence of hematoma or swollen soft tissues in the vicinity. A higher volume can improve the successful rate of neurolysis.

Radiofrequency (Thermal) Ablation

The advantage of chemical ablation is that the lesion size is dictated by the area of spread of the neurolytic agent. A volume of 2–3 mL can spread well along the space between AIIS and IPE. In contrast, the lesion size of a radiofrequency (RF) ablation is discrete and depends on the type of lesioning (conventional vs. cooled), configuration (monopolar, bipolar or strip), as well as other factors (adding hypertonic saline). The lesion size from the conventional RF ablation is unlikely to cover all the area between AIIS and IPE. The authors also prefer multi-tined needle (18G 100 mm with 5 mm active tip) because this needle will give the maximum lesion size with the trajectory of needle. The literature is scant in the RF ablation of the hip articular branches since the detailed description of the innervation of anterior hip capsule by Short et al. The following is based on the authors experience and preference.

Between the AIIS and IPE, a minimum of three needles are inserted, and the needles are quite often multi-tined (18G 10 cm with 5 mm active tip). The first needle is placed just medial to the AIIS. To have the needle lateral enough, the probe is tilted laterally to allow a more lateral placement of the needle (see "Practical Tips" section). The second needle is placed just medial to the first needle 1 cm apart. A bipolar lesion is created between these two needles. If the medially placed needle is not close to the IPE, a third needle placement is required to be at the IPE within 1 cm to the needle next to it. Depending on the size of the interval between AIIS and IPE, a fourth needle may be required with the distance in between the needle no more than 1 cm to create another bipolar lesion (Fig. 64.10).

For the articular branches of ON, the target size is small and a single needle (whether it is cooled RF system or multi-tined system) is usually sufficient. Using the scan technique described above, the author starts with needle insertion in-plane from lateral to medial. However, the clinician must scan the needle trajectory and the vicinity for any vessel. If necessary, the distal end of the probe can be rotated while keeping the inferomedial acetabulum in view. Once the needle makes a bony contact, the tip position is further fine-tuned under fluoroscopy. The main obturator trunk is closer to the medial half of the teardrop. Thus, the author prefers to put the needle on the lateral half of the teardrop. Sensory and motor test will add to the safety of the procedure (Fig. 64.11).

Complications

Complication from the Perioperative PENG Block

The complications are neurological complication from either direct needle injury or spread of local anesthetic.

An inadvertent femoral nerve block can cause an undesired quadriceps weakness. There are two plausible explanations for this phenomenon. First, instead of injecting local anesthetic deep to the fascia of the psoas muscle, there may have been intramuscular injection into the psoas, which subsequently spread to the FN. Alternatively, a medial placement of the needle closer to the pectineus or use of injectate volumes greater than 20 mL could result in anesthetic spread through the intermuscular plane between the pectineus and psoas, to capture the FN and resulting in the undesired motor block (Fig. 64.12). Additionally, high volume injectate may spread to the main trunk of the obturator nerve as it courses along the lateral wall within the pelvis.

Even though it has not been described in the literature, the injection point entry lies in close proximity to the LFCN, lateral to the ultrasound probe (Fig. 64.13). Therefore, it could be possible to cause an inadvertent puncture of the nerve. It is advised to look for the LFCN during the preliminary scanning, and if it is identified, try to avoid this structure in the needle trajectory. Alternatively, attention is paid to the local anesthetic infiltration of skin, and if the patient complains of paresthesia on the lateral aspect of the thigh, the needle needs to be relocated.

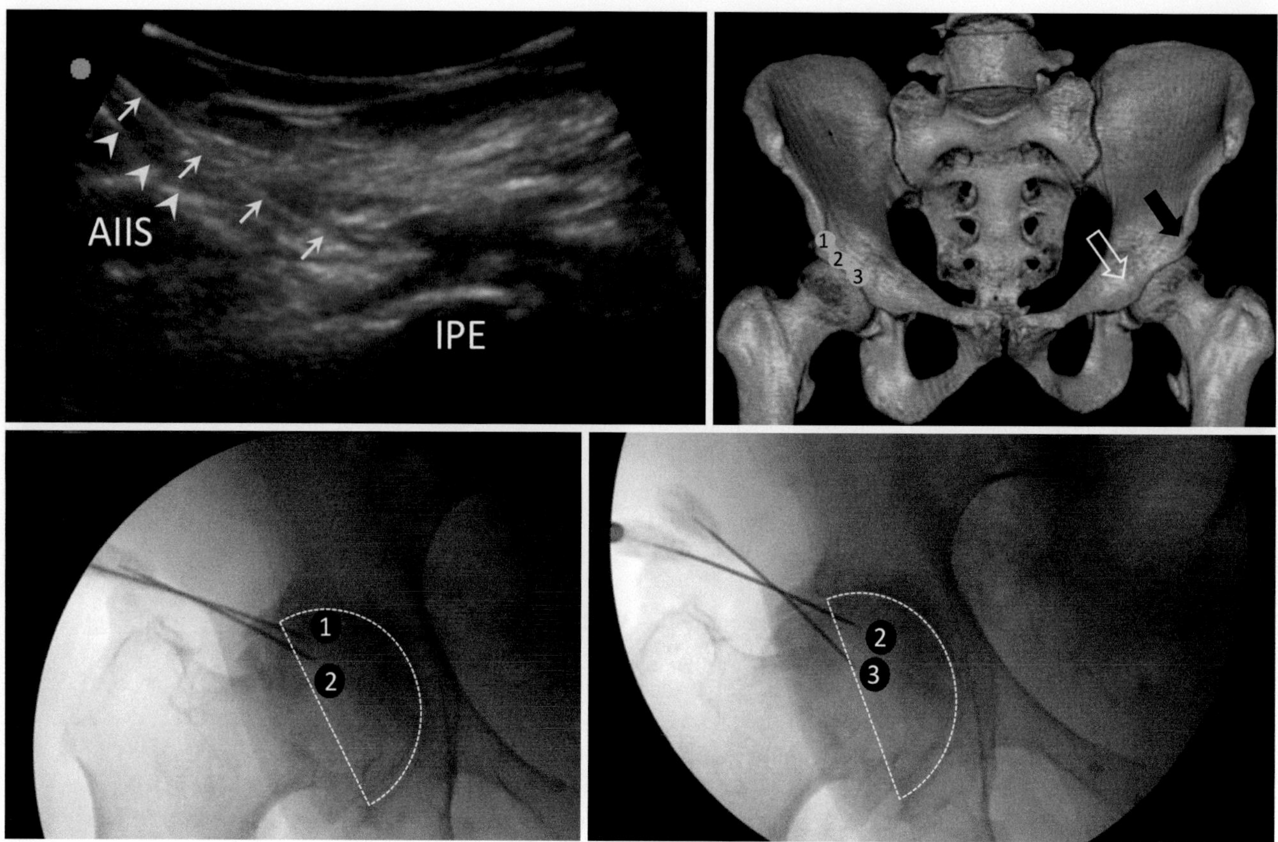

Fig. 64.10 Ultrasound and X-ray correlation of the placement of radiofrequency needles for ablation of femoral and accessory obturator nerves. Upper left: Two needles are inserted (one indicated by arrows and another by arrowheads) between the anterior inferior iliac spine (AIIS) and iliopubic eminence (IPE) in this sonogram. Upper right: Usually three needles are required to provide a palisade lesion between the anterior inferior iliac spine (AIIS) and iliopubic eminence (IPE), indicated by black bold arrow and white open arrow. Lower two figures are the X-ray showing the position of the three needles. The "cup" of acetabulum is shown by dotted line. (Reprinted with permission from Philip Peng Educational Series)

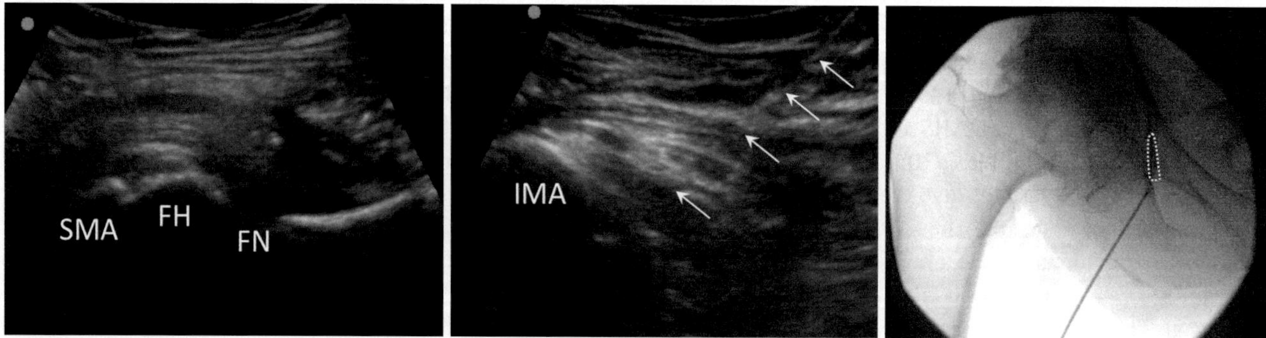

Fig. 64.11 Ultrasound and X-ray correlation of the radiofrequency needle inserted at the inferomedial acetabulum (IMA). The left figure shows the initial placement of probe to reveal the femoral head and neck (FH and FN, respectively). The radiofrequency needle is seen on the inferior aspect of the inferomedial acetabulum which is commonly called the tear drop (dotted line) in X-ray. (Reprinted with permission from Philip Peng Educational Series)

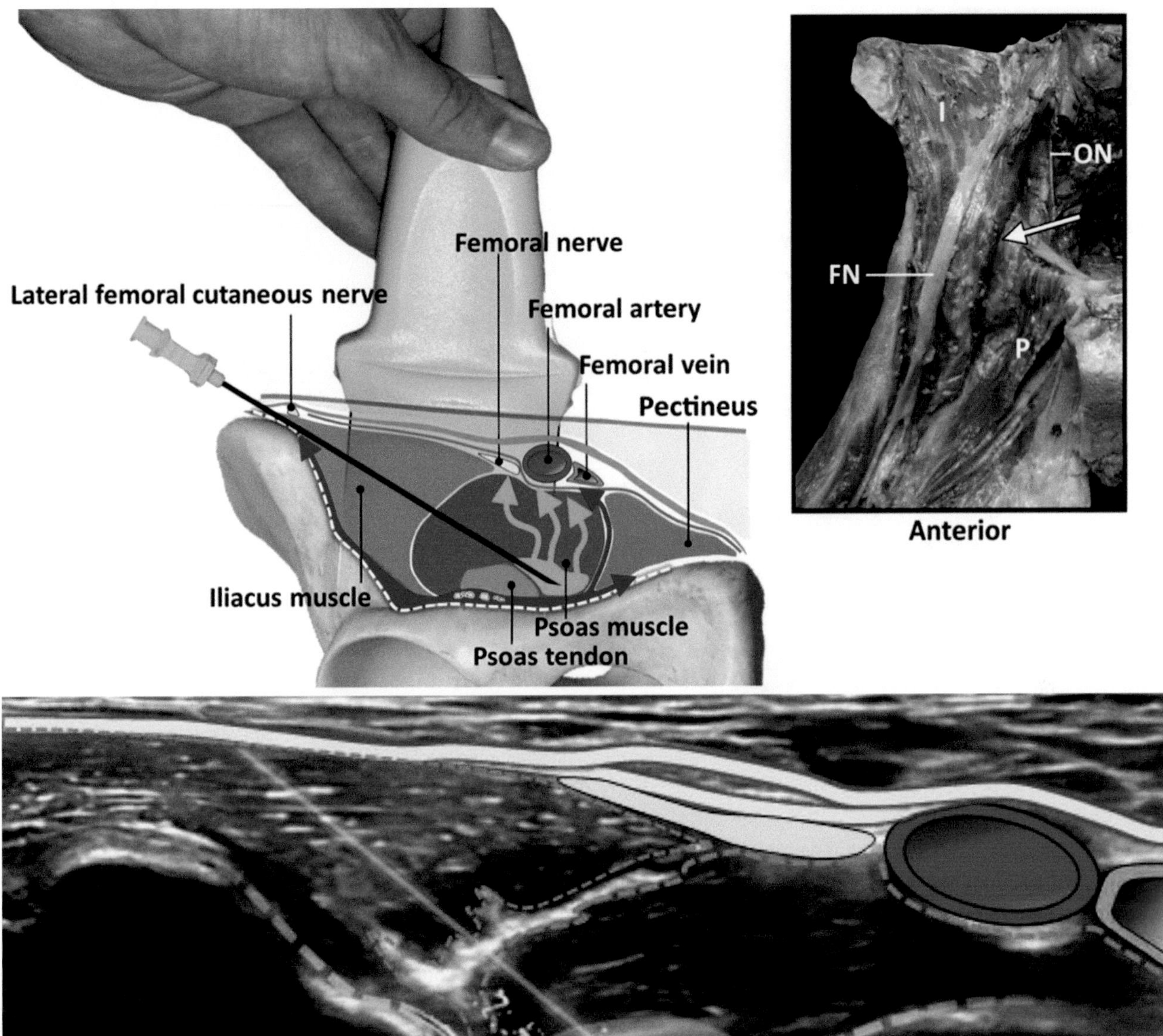

Fig. 64.12 The left upper figure shows possible route of spread to the surrounding nerve. Overzealous intramuscular spread is indicated by the green arrows which can spread to the femoral nerve. High volume of local anesthetic (blue arrows) can push the local anesthetic to the lateral femoral cutaneous nerve laterally, to the femoral nerve (FN) through the intermuscular septum between the psoas and pectineus (P), on to obturator nerve (ON) medially. The top right figure is the dissection showing the possibility of spread to the ON trunk. The lower figure shows the deposition of the local anesthetic in the sonogram. The schematic drawing was provided with the permission of Dr. Vicente Roques. (The whole figure was reprinted with permission from Philip Peng Educational Series)

Complication from the Diagnostic Block or Ablation

The complications can be categorized into procedure-related and medication-related.

For the medication-related complications, apart from the general risk of allergy and the local anesthetic toxicity, alcohol-related adverse effects have to be kept in mind. Of note, when a larger volume (>10 mL) of absolute alcohol is administered, patients are more susceptible to develop tachycardia and hypotension secondary to vasodilatation and its direct effect to the heart. The risk factors of such a complication include advanced frailty, low body weight (<50 kg), pre-procedural dehydration, and congestive heart failure. In case the risks of alcohol injection outweigh its benefits, thermal radiofrequency should be considered despite a more prolonged procedure.

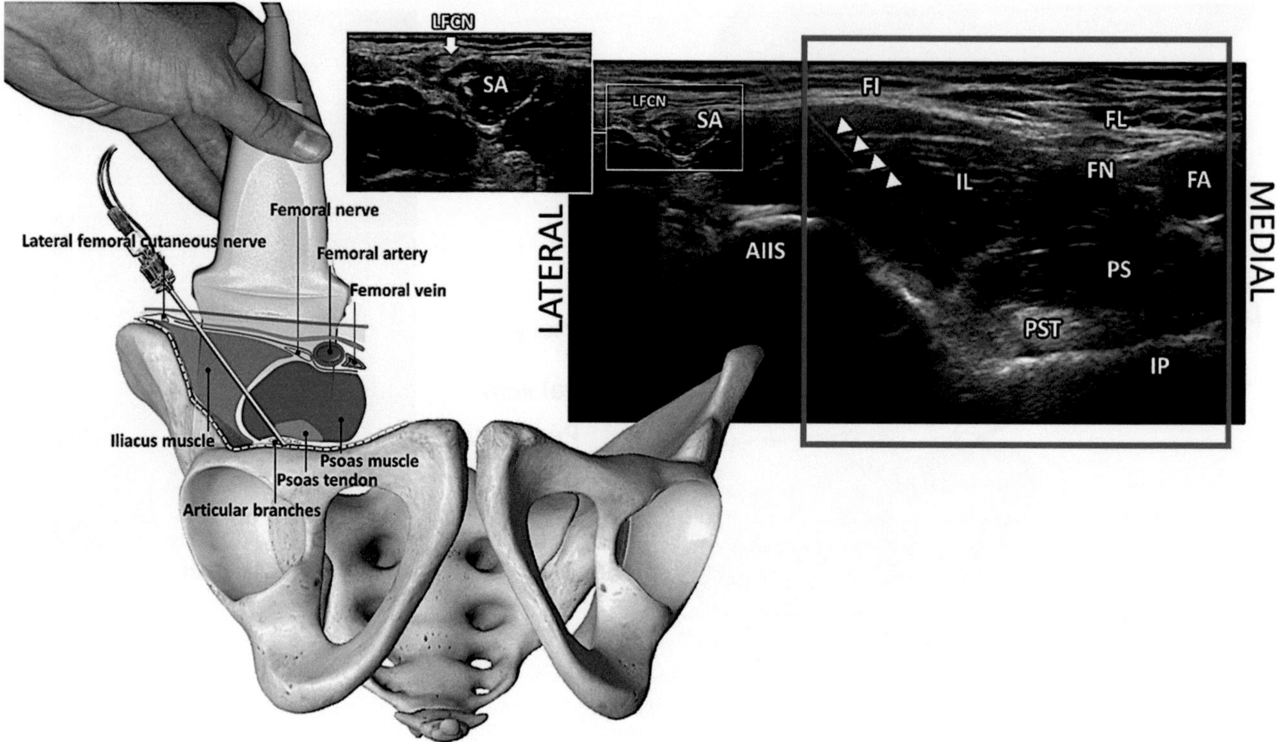

Fig. 64.13 Figure to show the possibility of direct needle trauma to the lateral femoral cutaneous nerve (LFCN), which is commonly outside the probe coverage but in the vicinity of the needle insertion site. *SA* sartorius, *FI* fascia iliacus, *FL* fascia lata, *AIIS* anterior inferior iliac spine, *IP* iliopubic eminence, *FN* femoral nerve, *FA* femoral artery, *PS* psoas, *PST* psoas tendon. (Reprinted with permission from Dr. Vicente Roques)

For the procedure-related complications, it is generally very safe when blocking the articular branches of FN and AON. However, the needle trajectory should avoid the femoral nerve and iliopsoas tendon. The former can be avoided if the clinician is cognizant about the location of the femoral nerve just lateral to the femoral artery. Concerning the needle placement of ON block, one should pay attention to the risk of puncturing the femoral artery and the posterior/acetabular branch of obturator vessels near the IMA. The needle tip should be well visualized when approaching the inferomedial acetabulum to avoid inadvertently puncturing the obturator membrane of obturator foramen, resulting in visceral (bladder) injury potentially. In addition, the patient may experience adductor weakness or numbness of the medial aspect of the thigh with local anesthetic injection because of the proximity of the inferomedial acetabulum to the obturator main trunk.

Practical Tips

1. Following the placement of the needle between the AIIS and IPE, if the injection is met with some resistance, one can adjust the needle depth as the needle tip may be subperiosteal or deep into the iliofemoral ligament. Withdrawing the needle slightly or change the direction of the needle bevel can change the injection resistance greatly. Alternatively, the needle does not puncture through the psoas fascia, and further "pushing" is hindered by the pubic bone (Fig. 64.14). In that case, performing rotating motions of the needle facilitates the piercing of the psoas fascia. A proper location of the needle should result in lifting of the psoas muscle. If an inadequate distribution toward the IPE is observed, the needle can be withdrawn and re-directed medially, followed by depositing a certain amount of local anesthetic at that level. This will help to block the AON more successfully, as its location is more medial.
2. When inserting the needle between the AIIS and IPE, the needle trajectory is between the straight head of rectus femoris and femoral nerve (Fig. 64.15). To avoid the injury to the femoral nerve, the range of needle trajectory can be widened by the lateral tilt of the probe (Fig. 64.15).
3. In patients with hip fracture, it is quite common to see a certain degree of external rotation of the hip. This posture, however, would lead to a lateral shift of the femoral vessels. As a result, the vessels often overlay the needle trajectory for the inferomedial acetabulum (Fig. 64.16). A solution to this technical challenge is to target the articular branches of ON in a sagittal plane. The key advantage of this approach is that the location of femoral vessels can be ignored.

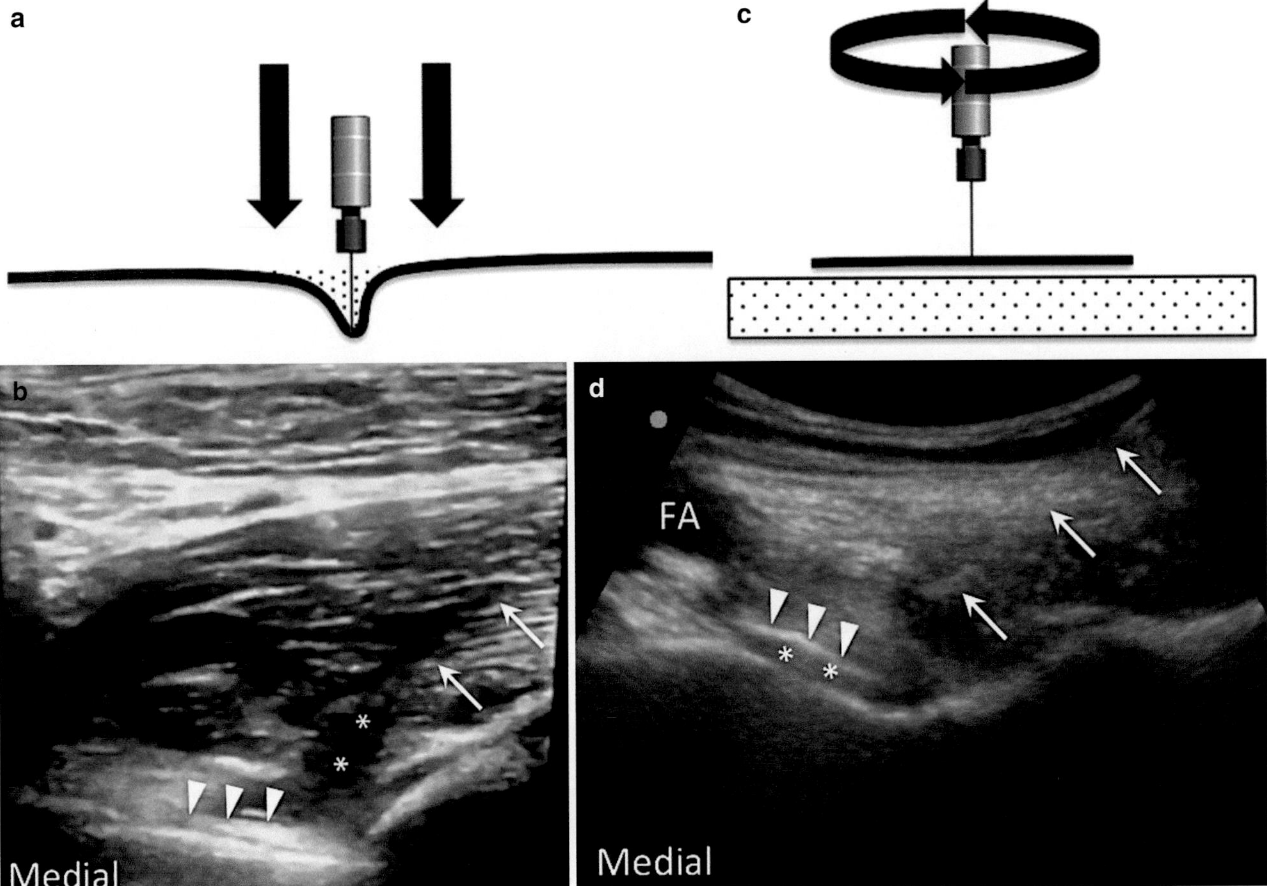

Fig. 64.14 (**a** and **c**) Schematic diagram to show that the needle pierces through fascia initially by indenting the fascia. However, when the fascia is supported by bone, as in the situation when psoas on pubis, the indentation may not happen. Having a bone contact does not imply the needle is on the bone. Injection in this circumstance will result in intramuscular spread (lower left figure, **b**). One tip is to rotate the needle to pierce the fascia, resulting in the lifting of the fascia (lower right figure, **d**). Arrows, needle; arrowheads, fascia; **, local anesthetic; *FA* femoral artery. (Reprinted with permission from Philip Peng Educational Series)

The IMA is first identified in the ordinary way as described above by either a linear probe or a curved probe (a linear probe is preferable for better image quality). The probe is then adjusted until the inferomedial acetabulum is in the middle of the image, followed by rotating the probe by approximately 60° (Fig. 64.16). In this scan, the pectineus, obturator externus, and the inferomedial acetabulum are revealed. Occasionally, the articular branches from the ON can be visualized in the wedge of the fascial plane between pectineus and obturator externus adjacent to the IMA (Fig. 64.16). Before any needle insertion, one should further tilt the probe medially toward the obturator foramen to locate the acetabular/posterior branch of obturator vessels. A 3.5-in. 22G Quincke needle is then inserted from caudal to cephalad in-plane until the needle tip reaches the wedge space containing the articular branches of ON. In case the wedge space cannot be clearly visualized, the needle tip would then be advanced until touching the bony surface of the IMA.

Literature Review

The main indication of PENG for the perioperative setting is for the control of hip pain from hip fracture. With the blockade of articular branches of the anterior hip capsule, it provides a dramatic reduction in movement-related pain without any motor blockade. However, it does not provide coverage for the incision. Investigators had explored the use of this outside hip fracture including hip arthroplasty, hip arthroscopy, and pelvic fracture. In 2021, there are 5 randomized trials supporting the use of the PENG block for the perioperative analgesia in both hip fracture surgery and total hip arthroplasty. Evidence is emerging to support the use of the PENG block for these settings.

For denervation of the articular branches, a recent narrative review captured 17 studies for radiofrequency denervation, and there are three further studies for chemical denervation. All are case series, and so far, there is no ran-

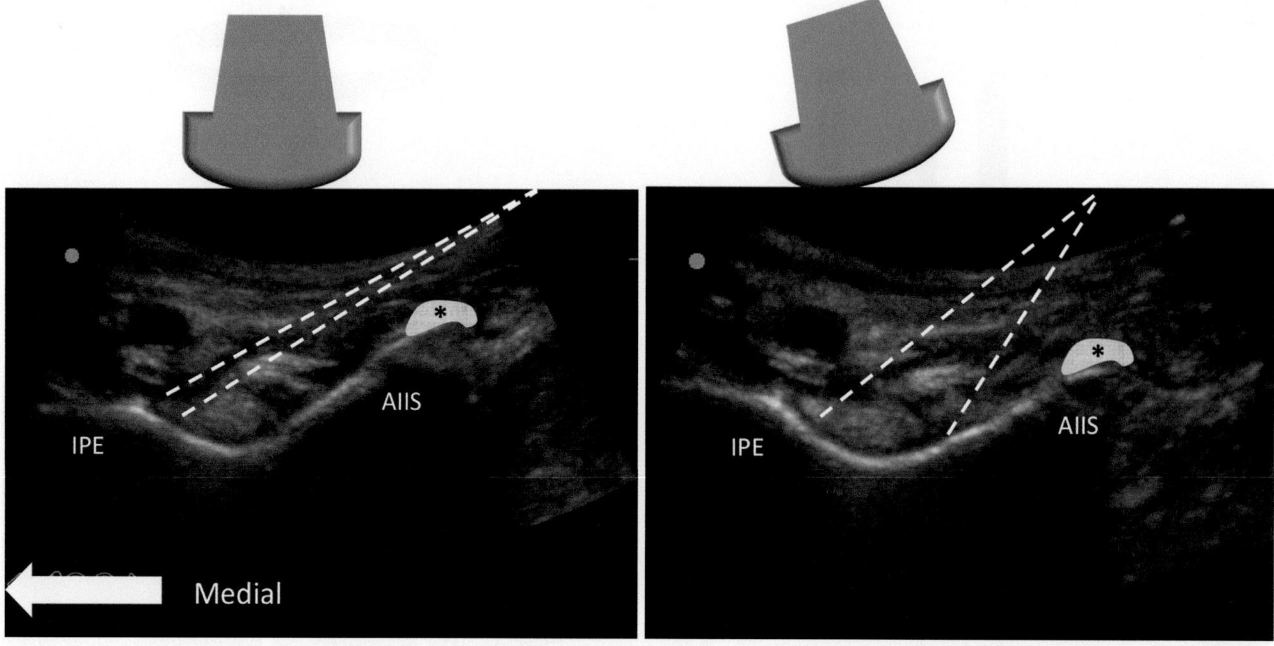

Fig. 64.15 Figure shows the effect of tilting the probe. Without tilting, the area of possible needle trajectory as highlighted by the dotted lines between the anterior inferior iliac spine (AIIS) and iliopubic eminence (IPE) is narrow. By tilting the probe, the area widens on the right figure. *, straight head of rectus femoris. (Reprinted with permission from Philip Peng Educational Series)

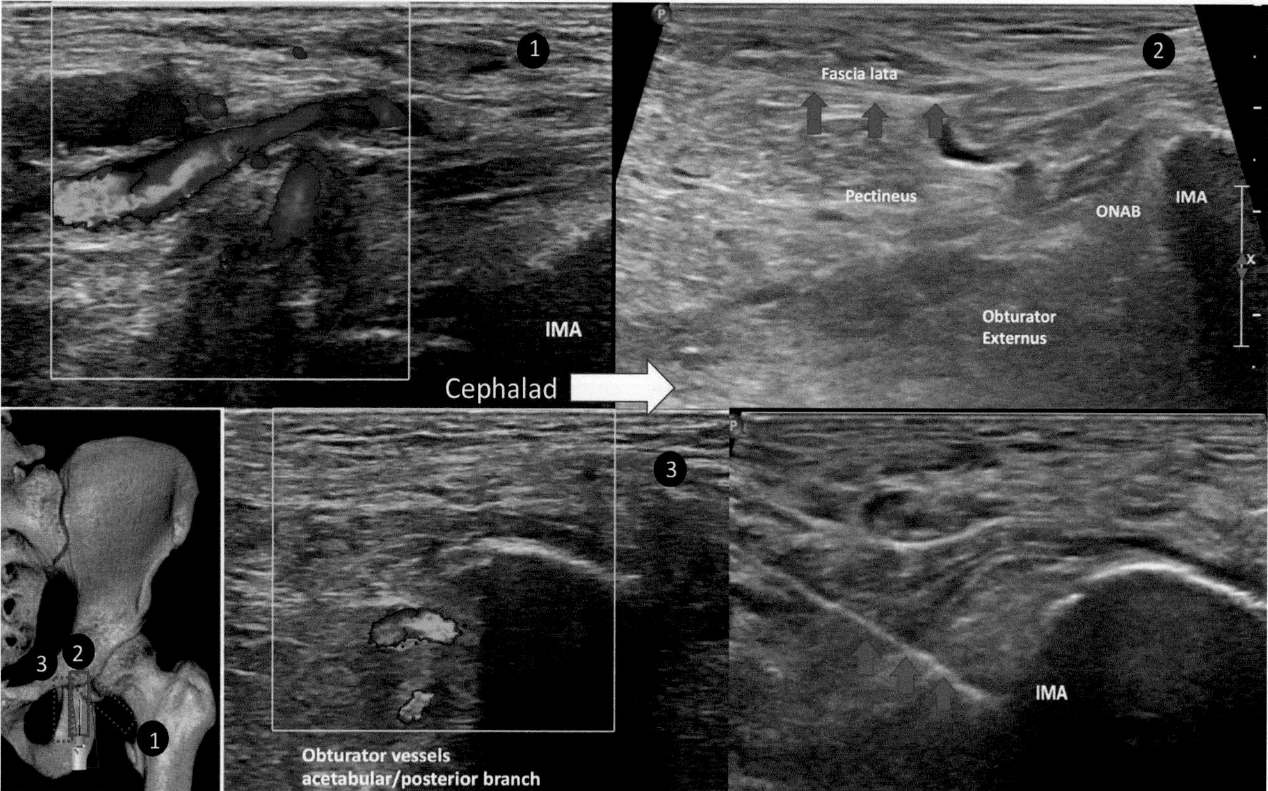

Fig. 64.16 The figure shows how rotation of the probe avoids the vessel in the needle trajectory. In probe position 1, the femoral artery is in the trajectory of the needle. 2. By rotating the probe, it establishes a trajectory without vessel in the needle trajectory. 3. Medial tilting of the probe may reveal the obturator vessels. By going back to position 2 and using Doppler to check the absence of vessel in the trajectory, the needle can be safely placed in the inferomedial acetabulum (IMA). ONAB obturator nerve articular branches. (Reprinted with permission from Philip Peng Educational Series)

domized controlled trial. In the most recent review of the radiofrequency ablation of hip, Kumar et al. demonstrated reductions in pain scores in all series, ranging from 30% to more than 90% at 8 days to 36 months after the procedures. There was evidence for an improvement in function and a lack of serious adverse events after RF treatments. They, however, reported attrition of analgesic benefits with time with an inability to reproduce the benefits with repeat procedures, whereas one publication reported almost complete absence of pain 24 months after the ablation.

From those radiofrequency studies, obturator nerve is the target in almost all studies. The landmark for those studies is the "teardrop" which is the inferomedial acetabulum revealed in the X-ray. However, this landmark is not directly approachable as the femoral artery and nerve overlay this landmark (Fig. 64.6). Ultrasound is useful in locating the inferomedial acetabulum and the vessels nearby while fluoroscopy is to confirm the final location. The landmark for femoral articular branches was not clear in those case series, and the upper outer quadrant of the acetabulum is the commonly described target. Since the detailed description of the anatomy of the articular branches of femoral and accessory obturator nerves, clinicians are now aware of the location between AIIS and IPE. As the location is wide, a logical approach to denervate those articular branches is by a palisade lesion as described above.

For chemical ablation, the initial description of a purely ultrasound-guided pericapsular alcohol neurolysis in a patient with inoperable hip fracture was from Sasaki et al. in early 2018. The procedure involved infiltrations of a high volume of the local anesthetic superficial to the pubofemoral and iliofemoral ligament over the hip capsule followed by the use of alcohol. With the recent understanding of the anatomy of the anterior capsule innervation, the use of chemical ablation with a much lower volume of injectate had been used in a case series of inoperable hip fractures and a patient with hip metastasis. Both phenol and alcohol have been described.

Suggested Reading

Barnett JJ, Peng J, Short A, Gofeld M, Peng PWH, Agur AR. Innervation of the anterior hip joint: a blast to the past (abstract). American Association of Clinical Anatomists Annual Meeting, Minneapolis, MN; 2017.

Bhatia A, Hoydonckx Y, Peng P, Cohen S. Radiofrequency procedures to relieve chronic hip pain: an evidence-based narrative review. Reg Anesth Pain Med. 2018;43:72–83.

Bijlsma JW, Berenbaum F, Lafeber FP. Osteoarthritis: an update with relevance for clinical practice. Lancet. 2011;377:2115–26.

Gardner E. The innervation of the hip joint. Anat Rec. 1948;101:353–71.

Gerhardt M, Johnson K, Atkinson R, et al. Characterisation and classification of the neural anatomy in the human hip joint. Hip Int. 2012;22:75–81.

Girón-Arango L, Peng PWH, Chin KJ, Brull R, Perlas A. Pericapsular nerve group (PENG) block for hip fracture. Reg Anesth Pain Med. 2018;43:859–63.

Giron-Arango L, Tran J, Peng P. Reply to Dr. Aydin et al. A novel indication of pericapsular nerve group (PENG) block: surgical anesthesia for vein ligation and stripping. J Cardiothorac Vasc Anesth. 2020;34:845–6.

Guay J, Parker MJ, Griffiths R, Kopp S. Peripheral nerve blocks for hip fractures. Cochrane Database Syst Rev. 2017;5:CD001159.

Kapural L. Cooled radiofrequency neurotomy of the articular sensory branches of the obturator and femoral nerves—combined approach using fluoroscopy and ultrasound guidance: technical report, and observational study on safety and efficacy. Pain Phys. 2018;21:279–84.

Kukreja P, Avila A, Northern T, et al. A retrospective case series of pericapsular nerve group (PENG) block for primary versus revision total hip arthroplasty analgesia. Cureus. 2020;12(5):e8200.

Kumar P, Hoydonckx Y, Bhatia A. A review of current denervation techniques for chronic hip pain: anatomical and technical considerations. Curr Pain Headache Rep. 2019;23:38.

Luftig J, Dreyfuss A, Mantuani D, et al. A new frontier in pelvic fracture pain control in the ED: Successful use of the pericapsular nerve group (PENG) block. Am J Emerg Med. https://doi.org/10.1016/j.ajem.2020.05.085.

Mysore K, Sancheti SA, Howells SR, Ballah EE, Sutton JL, Uppal V. Postoperative analgesia with pericapsular nerve group (PENG) block for primary total hip arthroplasty: a retrospective study. Can J Anaesth. 2020; https://doi.org/10.1007/s12630-020-01751-z.

Ng TKT, Chan WS, Peng PWH, et al. Chemical hip denervation for inoperable hip fracture. Anesth Analg. 2020;130:498–504.

Nielson ND, Madsen MN, Ostergaard HK, et al. An iliopsoas plane block does not cause motor blockade—a blinded randomized volunteer trial. Acta Anaesthesiol Scand. 2020;64:368–77.

Romero AR, Valdy GC, Lemus AJ. Ultrasound-guided pericapsular nerve group (PENG) hip joint phenol neurolysis for palliative pain. Can J Anesth. 2019;66:1270–1.

Sahoo RK, Jadon A, Sharma SK, Peng P. Pericapsular nerve group (PENG) block provides excellent analgesia in hip fractures and positioning for spinal anaesthesia: a prospective cohort study. Ind J Anesth. 2020;64:898–900.

Sandri M, Blasi A, De Blasi RA. PENG block and LIA as a possible anesthesia technique for total hip arthroplasty. J Anesth. 2020;34(3):472–5.

Sasaki S, Chan WS, Ng TKT, et al. Ultrasound-guided pericapsular hip joint alcohol neurolysis for the treatment of hip pain: a case report of a novel approach. A A Pract. 2018a;11:60–2.

Short AJ, Barnett JJG, Gofeld M, Baig E, Lam K, Agur AMR, Peng PWH. Anatomic study of innervation of the anterior hip capsule: implication for image guided intervention. Reg Anesth Pain Med. 2018;43:186–92.

Singh S, Singh S, Ahmed W. Continuous pericapsular nerve group block for hip surgery: a case series. A&A Pract. 2020;14:e01320.

Thallaj A. Combined PENG and LFCN blocks for postoperative analgesia in hip surgery—a case report. Saudi J Anaesth. 2019;13:381–3.

Tran J, Peng P, Agur A. Is pericapsular nerve group (PENG) block a true pericapsular block? Reg Anesth Pain Med. 2019:44–257.

Intra-Articular Knee Injection

65

Ning Nan Wang, Sofia Alejandra Velasco Figueroa, and Philip Peng

Contents

General Consideration

Osteoarthritis (OA) is a slowly progressive chronic disease that is characterized by a loss of joint cartilage. It represents a major disease burden worldwide, affecting 9.6% of men and 18.0% of women over 60 years of age. The lifetime risk of a single symptomatic knee OA is estimated at 44.7% (95% confidence interval [95% CI] 40.0–49.3%), and OA is only one of the many pathologies causing acute and chronic knee pain.

Knee pain can be classified into three categories: intra-articular, extra-articular, and the combination of both categories. A complete evaluation including history and physical examination, laboratory testing, and radiologic findings are mandatory for appropriate diagnosis and treatment. A multidisciplinary approach is often recommended. The first-line treatments include conservative management, such as physical therapy, rehabilitation, weight-loss, braces, acetaminophen, and nonsteroidal anti-inflammatory drugs (NSAIDs). Interventional approaches are often offered in conjunction or after failing conservative treatments.

Interventional knee procedures can be performed using image-guided or landmark techniques. The image-guided techniques include fluoroscopy, ultrasound, and magnetic resonance imaging (MRI). Image-guided techniques provide additional diagnostic value and improves the accuracy of the treatment over traditional landmark techniques. Ultrasound

N. N. Wang (✉)
Anesthesia Department, CIUSSS-du-Nord-de-l'Île-de-Montréal, Montreal, QC, Canada
e-mail: ning.n.wang@mail.mcgill.ca

S. A. Velasco Figueroa
Pain Management Department, Hospital Zambrano Hellion, TecSalud, San Pedro Garza Garcia, Nuevo Leon, Mexcio, USA
e-mail: sofia.velasco@ONE-Mail.on.ca

P. Peng
Department of Anesthesia and Pain Medicine, University of Toronto Toronto Western Hospital, Toronto, ON, Canada
e-mail: philip.peng@uhn.ca

D. Jankovic, P. Peng (eds.), *Regional Nerve Blocks in Anesthesia and Pain Therapy*,
https://doi.org/10.1007/978-3-030-88727-8_65

guidance allows a safe, radiation-free, accurate, and easy-to-perform bedside technique.

This chapter reviews the most common knee pathologies, indication, patient selection, functional anatomy, detailed explanation of the ultrasound-guided procedure, and its possible complication.

Indication and Patient Selection

Indication for ultrasound-guided knee intra-articular procedure include osteoarthritis, other types of arthritis, and knee joint aspiration.

Relative contraindications of intra-articular injection include active local and systemic infection, bleeding diathesis, known hypersensitivity to intra-articular agent, osteochondral or intra-articular fracture, prosthetic joint, recent injection with steroid in the same joint or other body parts, and inability to stay still during the procedure.

A complete evaluation including history and physical examination, laboratory testing, and radiologic findings are mandatory for appropriate diagnosis and treatment. A multidisciplinary approach is often recommended. A detailed discussion concerning the risks and benefits of the procedure should be carried out with the patient. Possible risks discussed include infection, bleeding, allergic reaction, transient increase in pain, focal fat necrosis, adverse reaction to injection of local anesthetic, and steroids. Short-term steroid risks include a temporary rise in blood sugar and blood pressure. Long-term steroid exposure is associated with an increased risk of myopathy, avascular necrosis, cataract, and osteoporosis.

Functional Anatomy of Knee Joints and Its Surrounding Tissue

The knee joint can be divided into three compartments: the patellofemoral, medial, and lateral tibiofemoral joints. As the medial tibiofemoral compartment receives the weight-bearing more than the other, the effect of OA is most prominent here. For the intra-articular compartment, there are two components: joint surface (articular cartilage and synovium), where the pathogenesis of OA takes place, and the stabilizing structures inside the joint (meniscus and cruciate ligaments). For the extra-articular structures, there are multiple bursae, ligaments, and tendons, which can contribute to pain symptomatology (Fig. 65.1). Thus, a clinician should be familiar with various components to decide whether the intra-articular (IA) injection is the options.

Technique of the Ultrasound Scan Intra-Articular Injection

The procedure is performed with the patient placed in a supine position with the knee slightly flexed and supported. Following sterile preparation, a high-frequency linear probe (6–13 Hz) is placed over the patella and quadriceps tendon. The target is suprapatellar recess (SPR), which is a recess that connects with the knee joint and is bounded by the suprapatellar and prefemoral fat pad (Fig. 65.2). The initial ultrasound probe position is in long axis to the femur just on the superior border of the patella (Fig. 65.3). This will reveal the SPR. When there is difficulty in visualizing the recess, applying pressure in the parapatellar space to squeeze the synovial fluid to the SPR may help when there is no large effusion.

Once the SPR is seen, the ultrasound probe is rotated 90° above the patella (Fig. 65.4). A 20- or 22-gauge needle is inserted from lateral to medial in-plane toward the SPR. Alternatively, the ultrasound probe is rotated 45° with the cephalad end directed to the lateral side (Fig. 65.5). The rotation of the probe is to avoid needle trauma to the quadriceps tendon.

Before injection, it is always advisable to aspirate the joint fluid as much as possible. Aspiration gives the patient with large effusion instantaneous relief due to the release of pressure. Once aspiration is attempt, 5 mL of mixture of steroid and local anesthetic or viscosupplement or platelet-rich supplement can be administered.

Practical Tips

In case of difficulty of in the visualization of SPR, two maneuvers can be used: to ask the patient to perform isometric contraction of the quadriceps or to apply pressure in the parapatellar space to squeeze the synovial fluid to the SPR.

Complications

Localized pain and swelling at the site of the injection is the most common side effect for intra-articular injections. Serious intra-articular knee injection complications are low, estimating to less than 1%. Rare but serious complications include localized pain or swelling at the site of injection, granulomatous inflammation of the synovium, nerve injury involving the saphenous nerve, aseptic acute arthritis, septic arthritis, and embolia cutis medicamentosa (Nicolau Syndrome).

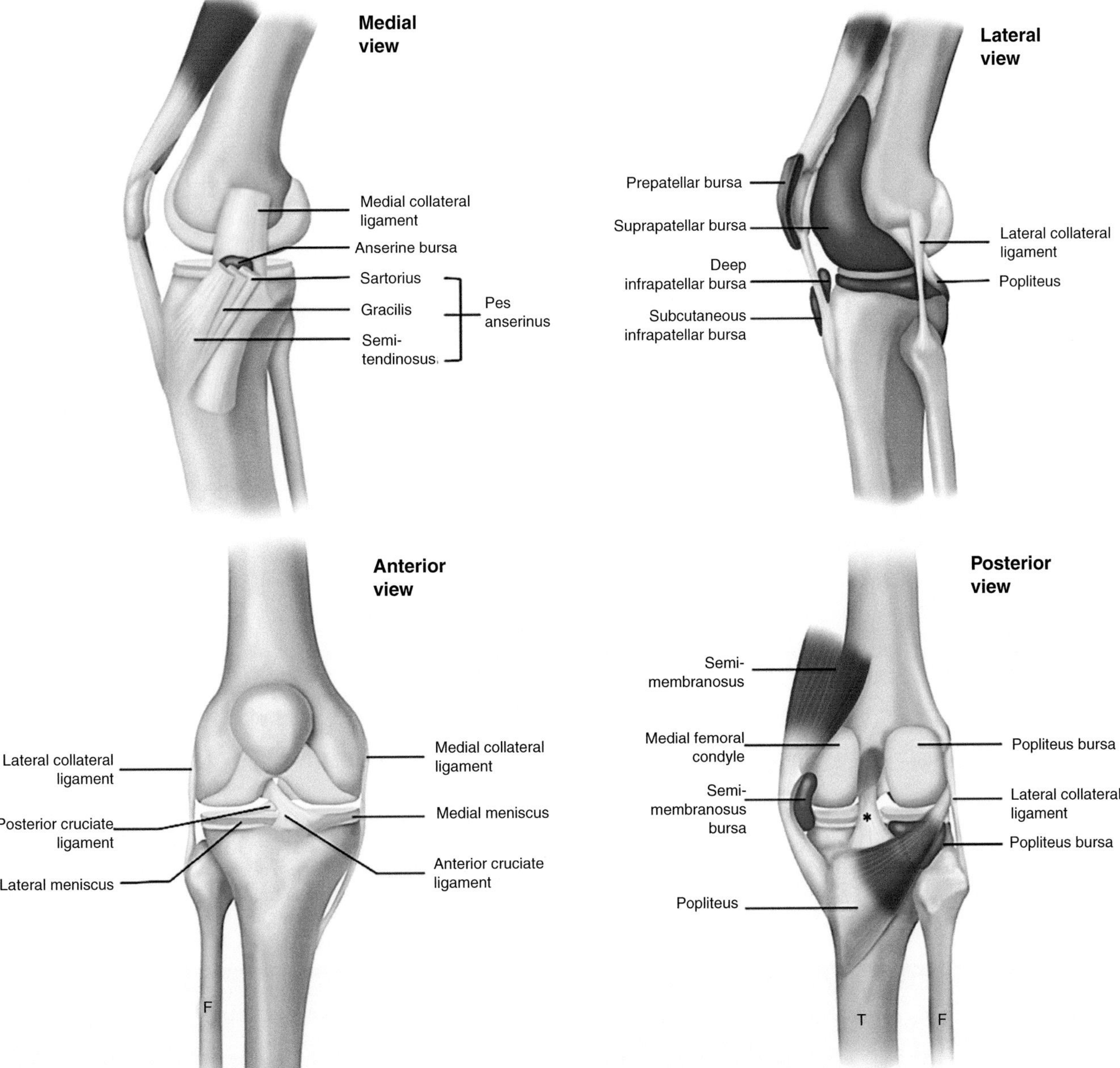

Fig. 65.1 Fours views (anterior, posterior, medial, and lateral) of the knee showed the ligaments and bursa. In the posterior view, the medial head of gastrocnemius was removed to reveal the intra-articular structures. F—fibula, T—tibia. Reproduced with permission from Philip Peng Educational Series

Specific adverse reactions after injections of intra-articular corticosteroids include accelerated osteoarthritis progression or rapid progressive OA, subchondral insufficiency fracture, osteonecrosis, and rapid joint destruction including bone loss.

Literature Review

Commonly used injection agents include corticosteroids, hyaluronic acid (HA), and platelet-rich plasma (PRP).

The Accuracy of Ultrasound-Guided Techniques Compared to Other Techniques

Interventional knee procedures can be performed using landmark or image-guidance (fluoroscopy or ultrasound) techniques. Current literature demonstrates that image guidance improved the accuracy of intra-articular injections of the knee (96.7% vs. 81.0%, $p < 0.001$). In contrast to fluoroscopy, ultrasound allows the procedure to be performed in office-based settings. The accuracies of landmark-based vs. ultrasound guidance techniques were also significantly

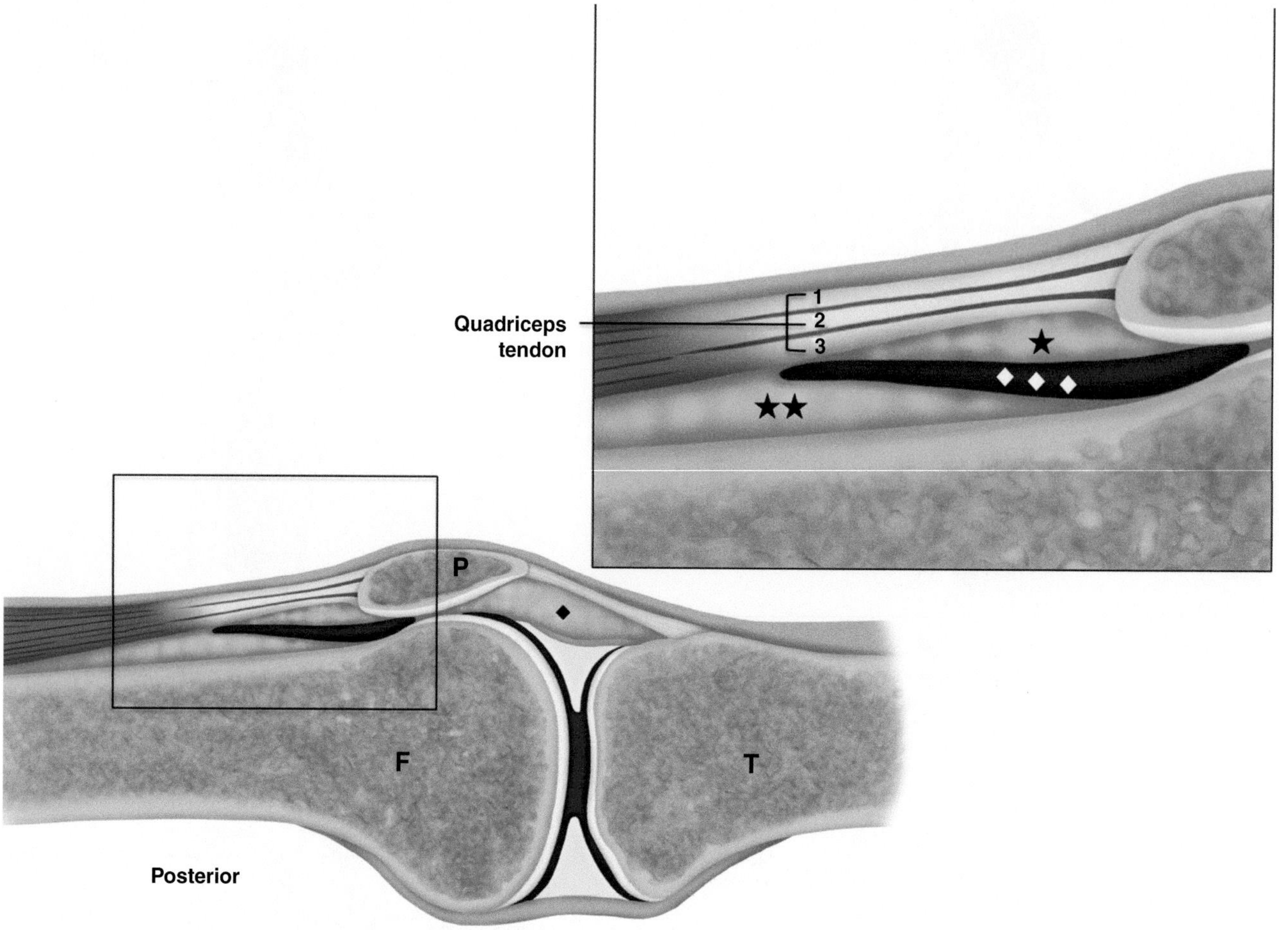

Fig. 65.2 Lateral view of the knee showed the details of the trilaminar nature of the quadriceps tendon. The insert on the right upper corner was the expanded view of the rectangle over the quadriceps tendon. P—patella, F—femur, T—tibia, ★★—prefemoral fat pad, ★—suprapatellar fat pad, ◆◆◆—suprapatellar recess, ◆—infrapatellar (Hoffa's) fat pad. Reproduced with permission from Philip Peng Educational Series

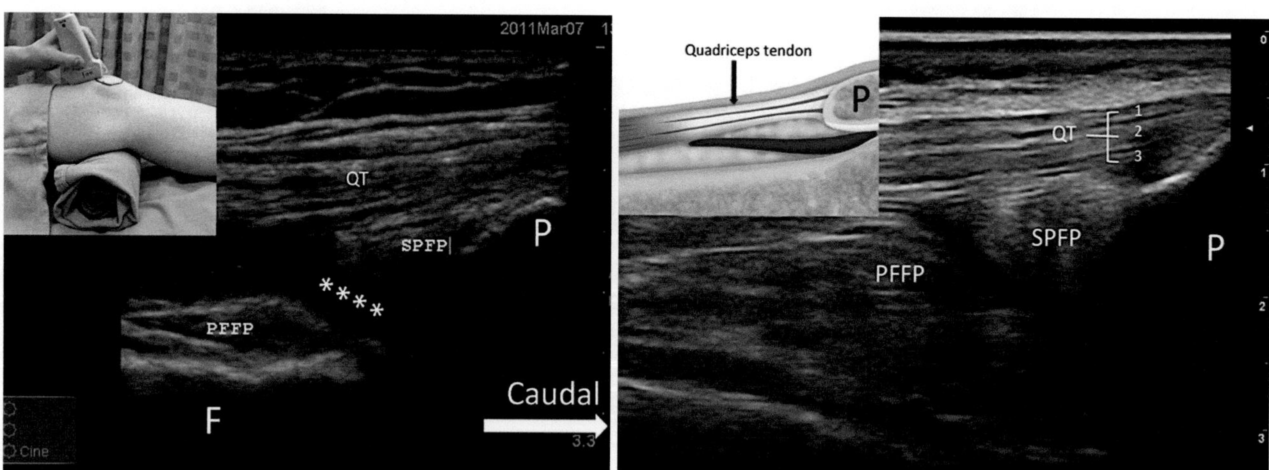

Fig. 65.3 Left. Sonogram of the suprapatellar view of a patient with knee effusion. Note the presence of effusion fluid filling the space between prefemoral fat pad and quadriceps tendon (QT). The insert showed the position of the patient and the ultrasound probe. Right. Sonogram of the details of quadriceps tendon. SPFP—suprapatellar fat pad; PFFP—prefemoral fat pad; P—patella; F—femur; ** indicates the suprapatellar recess. Reproduced with permission from Philip Peng Educational Series

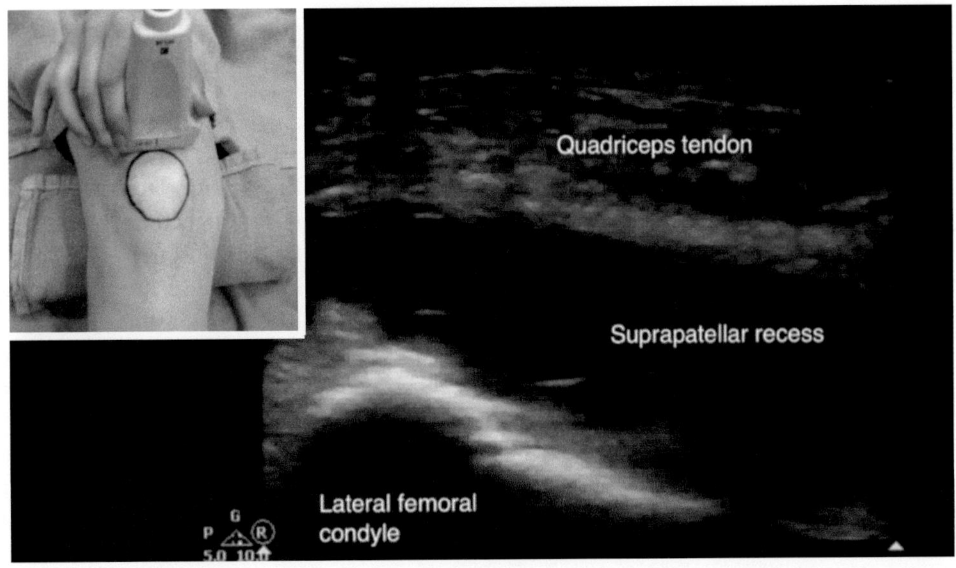

Fig. 65.4 Picture showed the rotation of the ultrasound probe upon visualization of the suprapatellar recess. The corresponding sonogram is shown on the right. Reproduced with permission from Philip Peng Educational Series

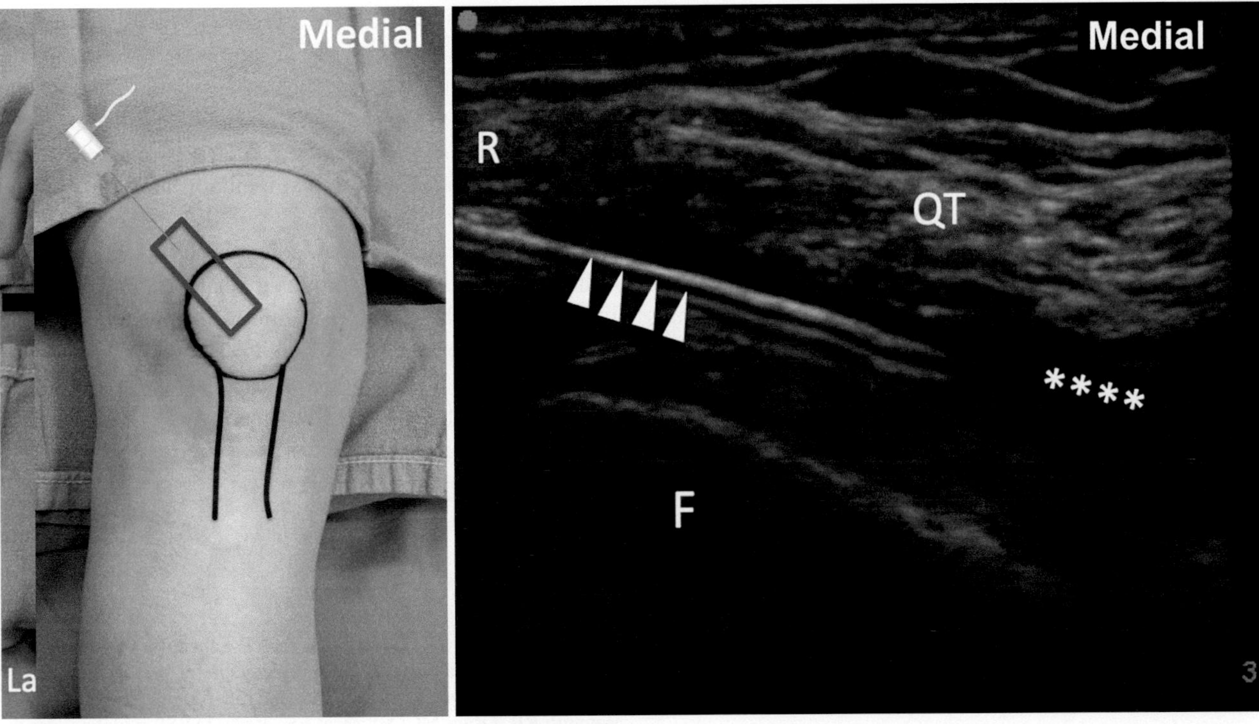

Fig. 65.5 Alternatively, the ultrasound is rotated 45° to the lateral side, and the needle is inserted in-plane from lateral to medial to avoid puncturing the quadriceps tendon. The needle is indicated by the arrowheads and the suprapatellar recess by asterisks (****). R—retinaculum; Q—quadriceps tendon, F—femur. Reproduced with permission from Philip Peng Educational Series

different, 77.8% and 95.8%, respectively. The experience of the injector was linked to improved accuracy for blinded though not image-guided technique.

Intra-Articular Corticosteroid Injections

Jüni et al. performed a systematic meta-analysis Cochrane database review to assess the efficacy in pain and quality of life associated with and the function and safety of intra-articular corticosteroid (IA-CS) injection when compared with sham injection or no treatment in patients with knee OA. A total of 27 RCTs with high heterogeneity demonstrated that IA-CS is more beneficial to placebo or no treatment group in pain reduction (SMD -0.40, 95% CI −0.58 to −0.22). The difference in visual analog score (VAS) for pain represents 1.0 cm on a 10 cm VAS scale between IA-CS and control group. The number needed to treat for an additional beneficial outcome (NNTB) of 8 (95% CI 6 to 13). A small improvement in the functional status in the WOMAC score (SMD −0.33, 95% CI −0.56 to −0.09) was also noted. This corresponded to a difference in functions scores of −0.7 units on a standardized WOMAC disability scale ranging from 0 to 10, which translates into an NNTB of 10 (95% CI 7 to 33). However, the overall quality of evidence was graded as low for all outcomes, because treatment effect estimates were inconsistent. The duration of beneficial effects is in the magnitude of weeks.

Although IA-CS showed improved analgesia in the meta-analysis, a few issues are highlighted here. The effect size of analgesia is small. There is no clinical meaningful functional improvement. This duration of effect is short, and repeated injection of IS-CS is associated with accelerated progression of OA. Possible corticosteroid-associated chondrotoxicity has been raised as a mechanism causing significantly greater cartilage volume loss when IA-CS compared with IA-saline.

Intra-Articular Hyaluronic Acid Injections

Hyaluronic acid is indicated for symptomatic OA without the complete collapse of the joint space. Multiple systematic review supported the analgesia efficacy of HA injection. The effect size is moderate and results in functional improvement. It is best for OA of early to moderate grades. The duration of relief is usually in terms of months (3–6 months). High molecular weight (>3000 kDA) demonstrated better efficacy and safety compared to mid molecular weight (1500kDA–3000 kDA) or low molecular weight (<1500 kDA).

He et al. compared the IA-HA and IA-CS injections' efficacy in pain relief in 12 RCTs. The IA-CS is more effective than IA-HA in short-term follow-up up to 1 month. However, the results at VAS or WOMAC is comparable at 3 months. By 6 months, IA-HA was more effective than IA-CS for pain relief.

Intra-Articular Plasma-Rich Platelet Injections

Intra-articular injections of plasma-rich platelet, PRP, is a subject of many controversies. PRP is obtained by centrifugation of autologous blood. It contains platelet growth factors and cytokines that are released during platelets' degranulation. PRP has anti-inflammatory and regenerative properties, including the potential to accelerate cartilage matrix synthesis, restrain synovial membrane inflammation, and promote cartilage healing.

Different meta-analysis reports various findings in terms of efficacy of PRP vs. HA or placebo. Limitations in the current literature concerning large heterogeneity of PRP preparation methods, resulting in different compositions of the PRP, make it difficult to assess its efficacy. Another concern is the high risk of bias among published studies. Four meta-analyses with knee OA patients demonstrated that PRP was somewhat superior to HA. Xu et al. analyzed a total of 10 RCTs, PRP showed no superiority over hyaluronic acid in well-designed double-blind trials, and beneficial effects of PRP in most trials probably resulted from insufficient blinding methods. Kanchanatawan et al. included a total of nine RCTs demonstrating a higher functional outcome in PRP vs. HA and placebo group at 1 year. Shen et al. confirm that PRP injection was more effective to reduce pain and improve self-report function than saline, HA, ozone, and corticosteroid injection. Filardo et al. reviewed 34 RCTs of PRP vs. placebo or other intra-articular treatments for knee osteoarthritis for pain and functional outcomes. PRP has limited short-term effects, no statistically significant difference compared to placebo at 6 months, but clinically significant at 12 months. Similar results are obtained for PRP vs. HA and PRP vs. steroids, statistically insignificant result at 1 and 3 months but clinically significant WOMAC score changes at 6- and 12-month intervals. Similarly, another meta-analysis by Dai et al. showed that PRP and HA had similar pain and functional outcomes at 6 months and superior outcomes at 12 months.

From this pile of data, a few points can be made. Compared with placebo, the PRP provided analgesia and function improvement. The duration of improvement tends to be longer in the range of 6 to 12 months. Therefore, when compared with HA, the analgesic efficacy is very similar in the first 6 months, but the PRP is superior than HA after that time frame. Leucocyte-poor is associated with better outcome than leucocyte-rich PRP.

Suggested Reading

Altman RD, Bedi A, Karlsson J, Sancheti P, Schemitsch E. Product differences in intra-articular hyaluronic acids for osteoarthritis of the knee. Am J Sports Med. 2016;44(8):2158–65.

Bannuru RR, Osani MC, Vaysbrot EE, et al. OARSI guidelines for the non-surgical management of knee, hip, and polyarticular osteoarthritis. Osteoarthr Cartil. 2019;27(11):1578–89.

Beissert S, Presser D, Rutter A, et al. Embolia cutis medicamentosa (Nicolau syndrome) after intra-articular injection. Hautarzt. 1999;50:21421–6.

Bone and Joint Canada. Osteoarthritis. 2014. http://boneandjointcanada.com/osteoarthritis/. Accessed 10 Oct 2020.

Boswell SG, Cole BJ, Sundman EA, et al. Platelet-rich plasma: a milieu of bioactive factors. Arthroscopy. 2012;28(3):429–39.

Campbell KA, Saltzman BM, Mascarenhas R, et al. Does intra-articular platelet-rich plasma injection provide clinically superior outcomes compared with other therapies in the treatment of knee osteoarthritis? A systematic review of overlapping meta-analyses. Arthroscopy. 2015;31(11):2213–21.

Charalambous CP, Tryfonidis M, Sadiq S, et al. Septic arthritis following intra-articular steroid injection of the knee–a survey of current practice regarding antiseptic technique used during intra-articular steroid injection of the knee. Clin Rheumatol. 2003;22:386–90.

Chen AL, Desai P, Adler EM, et al. Granulomatous inflammation after Hylan G-F 20 viscosupplementation of the knee: a report of six cases. J Bone Joint Surg (Am Vol). 2002;84-A(7):1142–7.

Cheng J, Abdi S. Complications of joint, tendon, and muscle injections. Tech Reg Anesth Pain Manag. 2007;11(3):141–7. https://doi.org/10.1053/j.trap.2007.05.006.

Concoff A, Sancheti P, Niazi F, Shaw P, Rosen J. The efficacy of multiple versus single hyaluronic acid injections: a systematic review and meta-analysis. BMC Musculoskelet Disord. 2017;18(1):542.

Dai WL, Zhou AG, Zhang H, et al. Efficacy of platelet-rich plasma in the treatment of knee osteoarthritis: a meta-analysis of randomized controlled trials. Arthroscopy. 2017;33(3):659–70.

Gregori D, Giacovelli G, Minto C, et al. Association of pharmacological treatments with long-term pain control in patients with knee osteoarthritis: a systematic review and meta-analysis. JAMA. 2018;320(24):2564–79.

He WW, Kuang MJ, Zhao J, et al. Efficacy and safety of intraarticular hyaluronic acid and corticosteroid for knee osteoarthritis: a meta-analysis. Int J Surg. 2017;39:95–103.

Huang Y, Liu X, Xu X, Liu J. Intra-articular injections of platelet-rich plasma, hyaluronic acid or corticosteroids for knee osteoarthritis: a prospective randomized controlled study. Orthopade. 2019;48(3):239–47.

Iizuka M, Yao R, Wainapel S. Saphenous nerve injury following medial knee joint injection: a case report. Arch Phys Med Rehabilit. 2005;86:2062–5.

Jevsevar DS. Treatment of osteoarthritis of the knee: evidence-based guideline, 2nd edition. J Am Acad Orthop Surg. 2013;21(9):571–6.

Jordan KM, Arden NK, Doherty M, et al. EULAR Recommendations 2003: an evidence-based approach to the management of knee osteoarthritis: Report of a Task Force of the Standing Committee for International Clinical Studies Including Therapeutic Trials (ESCISIT). Ann Rheum Dis. 2003;62(12):1145–55.

Jüni P, Hari R, Rutjes AWS, Fischer R, Silletta MG, Reichenbach S, da Costa BR. Intra-articular corticosteroid for knee osteoarthritis. Cochrane Database Syst Rev. 2015;(10):CD005328. https://doi.org/10.1002/14651858.CD005328.pub3.

Kanchanatawan W, Arirachakaran A, Chaijenkij K, et al. Short-term outcomes of platelet-rich plasma injection for treatment of osteoarthritis of the knee. Knee Surg Sports Traumatol Arthrosc. 2016;24(5):1665–77.

Kolasinski SL, Neogi T, Hochberg MC, et al. 2019 American College of Rheumatology/Arthritis Foundation guideline for the management of osteoarthritis of the hand, hip, and knee. Arthritis Care Res (Hoboken). 2020a;72(2):149–62.

Kolasinski SL, Neogi T, Hochberg MC, et al. 2019 American College of Rheumatology/Arthritis Foundation guideline for the management of osteoarthritis of the hand, hip, and knee. Arthritis Rheumatol. 2020b;72(2):220–33.

Kompel AJ, Roemer FW, Murakami AM, Diaz LE, Crema MD, Guermazi A. Intra-articular corticosteroid injections in the hip and knee: perhaps not as safe as we thought? Radiology. 2019 Dec;293(3):656–63. https://doi.org/10.1148/radiol.2019190341.

Law TY, Nguyen C, Frank RM, Rosas S, McCormick F. Current concepts on the use of corticosteroid injections for knee osteoarthritis. Phys Sportsmed. 2015;43(3):269–73.

Maricar N, Parkes MJ, Callaghan MJ, Felson DT, O'Neill TW. Where and how to inject the knee--a systematic review. Semin Arthritis Rheum. 2013;43(2):195–203. https://doi.org/10.1016/j.semarthrit.2013.04.010. Erratum in: Semin Arthritis Rheum. 2015;44(5):e18.

McAlindon TE, LaValley MP, Harvey WF, Price LL, Driban JB, Zhang M, Ward RJ. Effect of intra-articular triamcinolone vs saline on knee cartilage volume and pain in patients with knee osteoarthritis: a randomized clinical trial. JAMA. 2017;317(19):1967–75. https://doi.org/10.1001/jama.2017.5283.

Milano G, Deriu L, Sanna PE, et al. Repeated platelet concentrate injections enhance reparative response of microfractures in the treatment of chondral defects of the knee: an experimental study in an animal model. Arthroscopy. 2012;28(5):688–701.

Murphy L, Schwartz TA, Helmick CG, Renner JB, Tudor G, Koch G, Dragomir A, Kalsbeek WD, Luta G, Jordan JM. Lifetime risk of symptomatic knee osteoarthritis. Arthritis Rheum. 2008;59:1207–13. https://doi.org/10.1002/art.24021.

Nicholls M, Shaw P, Niazi F, Bhandari M, Bedi A. The impact of excluding patients with end-stage knee disease in intra-articular hyaluronic acid trials: a systematic review and meta-analysis. Adv Ther. 2019;36(1):147–61.

Papadopoulos PJ, Edison JD. The Clinical Picture - soft tissue atrophy after corticosteroid injection. Cleve Clin J Med. 2009;76:373–4.

Pendleton A, Arden N, Dougados M, et al. EULAR recommendations for the management of knee osteoarthritis: report of a task force of the Standing Committee for International Clinical Studies Including Therapeutic Trials (ESCISIT). Ann Rheum Dis. 2000;59(12):936–44.

Peng PWH, Shankar H. Ultrasound-guided interventional procedures in pain medicine: a review of anatomy, sonoanatomy, and procedures. Part V. Reg Anesth Pain Med. 2014;39:368–80.

Roos J, Epaulard O, Juvin R, et al. Acute pseudoseptic arthritis after intraarticular sodium hyaluronan. Joint Bone Spine. 2004;71:352–4.

Shen L, Yuan T, Chen S, et al. The temporal effect of platelet-rich plasma on pain and physical function in the treatment of knee osteoarthritis: systematic review and meta-analysis of randomized controlled trials. J Orthop Surg Res. 2017;12(1):16. https://doi.org/10.1186/s13018-017-0521-3.

Wehling P, Evans C, Wehling J, Maixner W. Effectiveness of intra-articular therapies in osteoarthritis: a literature review. Ther Adv Musculoskelet Dis. 2017;9(8):183–96. https://doi.org/10.1177/1759720X17712695.

Wernecke C, Braun HJ, Dragoo JL. The effect of intra-articular corticosteroids on articular cartilage: a systematic review. Orthop J Sports Med. 2015;3:2325967115581163.

Xu Z, Luo J, Huang X, et al. Efficacy of platelet-rich plasma in pain and self-report function in knee osteoarthritis: a best-evidence synthesis. Am J Phys Med Rehabil. 2017;96(11):793–800.

66 Knee Joint Denervation

Nimish Mittal, Michael Catapano, and Philip Peng

Contents

Background

Osteoarthritis (OA) of the knee joint is ranked as the 11th highest contributor to global disability, with the global age-standardized prevalence of 3.8%. Common conservative treatment options for knee OA treatment include oral analgesics, nonsteroidal anti-inflammatory drugs, intra-articular corticosteroid injections, and local anesthetic injections. All these modalities have shown poor long-term results, and their repeated usage is associated with significant adverse events. For this group of patients, the next option is usually knee arthroplasty.

Since the first publication of a randomized control trial (RCT) on the use of radiofrequency ablation (RFA) of genicular nerves with promising results, there is an emerging interest in applying RFA to manage knee OA. By December 2019, there are 33 case series and 13 randomized controlled trials published. The increase in clinical interest is also paralleled by an increase in the anatomic evaluation of the genicular nerve supplying the knee and the landmark validation studies for RFA.

N. Mittal (✉) · M. Catapano
Division of Physical Medicine and Rehabilitation, Department of Medicine, University of Toronto, Toronto, ON, Canada

Toronto Rehabilitation Institute, Toronto, ON, Canada
e-mail: Nimish.Mittal@uhn.ca; Michael.Catapano@uhn.ca

P. Peng
Department of Anesthesia and Pain Management, Toronto Western Hospital, University Health Network, Toronto, ON, Canada
e-mail: Philip.Peng@uhn.ca

D. Jankovic, P. Peng (eds.), *Regional Nerve Blocks in Anesthesia and Pain Therapy*,
https://doi.org/10.1007/978-3-030-88727-8_66

Indications (Patient Selection)

This procedure is offered to patients eligible for total knee arthroplasty, i.e., those who have moderate to severe symptomatic OA with grade II to IV Kellgren-Lawrence classification and are refractory to conservative treatment. The exception is that this modality is offered to patients who are at high risk for surgery or unwillingly to receive surgical options.

At present, there are two cohorts of patients that await more evidence for this procedure. One is the patient group with persistent knee pain following total knee arthroplasty. The other is to provide this preoperatively to facilitate postoperative rehabilitation and reduce the risk of persistent postsurgical pain.

Although the RFA provides pain relief for the patient with pain related to OA, patients with unstable knee joints will not benefit from this procedure, and the surgical option should be considered.

Anatomy

The first RCT on RFA adopted three different landmarks for the superomedial, inferomedial, and superolateral genicular nerves, although the anatomic basis for those landmarks has not been previously validated. Since the publication, a number of anatomy investigations were published trying to reconcile the findings. Those publications neither comprehensively investigate all the articular branches of the knee nor fully document the frequency of various articular branches. As a matter of fact, the article published by Gardner back in 1948 provided one of the most comprehensive accounts of all the articular supply to the knee. In 2018, Tran and colleagues published a comprehensive article detailing the course of all ten articular branches supplying the anterior knee capsule (Fig. 66.1). Their work outlined the courses of each branch and the relationship to the landmarks discernable to imaging modalities. The articular branches can be divided into four quadrants, as in Fig. 66.2.

Recently, some additional landmarks were suggested. However, the benefit of optimizing the outcome by adding further sites of ablation is still being investigated. Therefore, in this chapter, only the conventional landmarks for genicular nerve ablation are discussed. They are superomedial, superolateral, and inferomedial genicular nerves (SMGN, SLGN, IMGN, respectively).

Superomedial Genicular Nerve

The early literature described it as a branch of the tibial nerve. Recently, the investigators performed meticulous dissection and traced the nerve to the origin, and they revealed

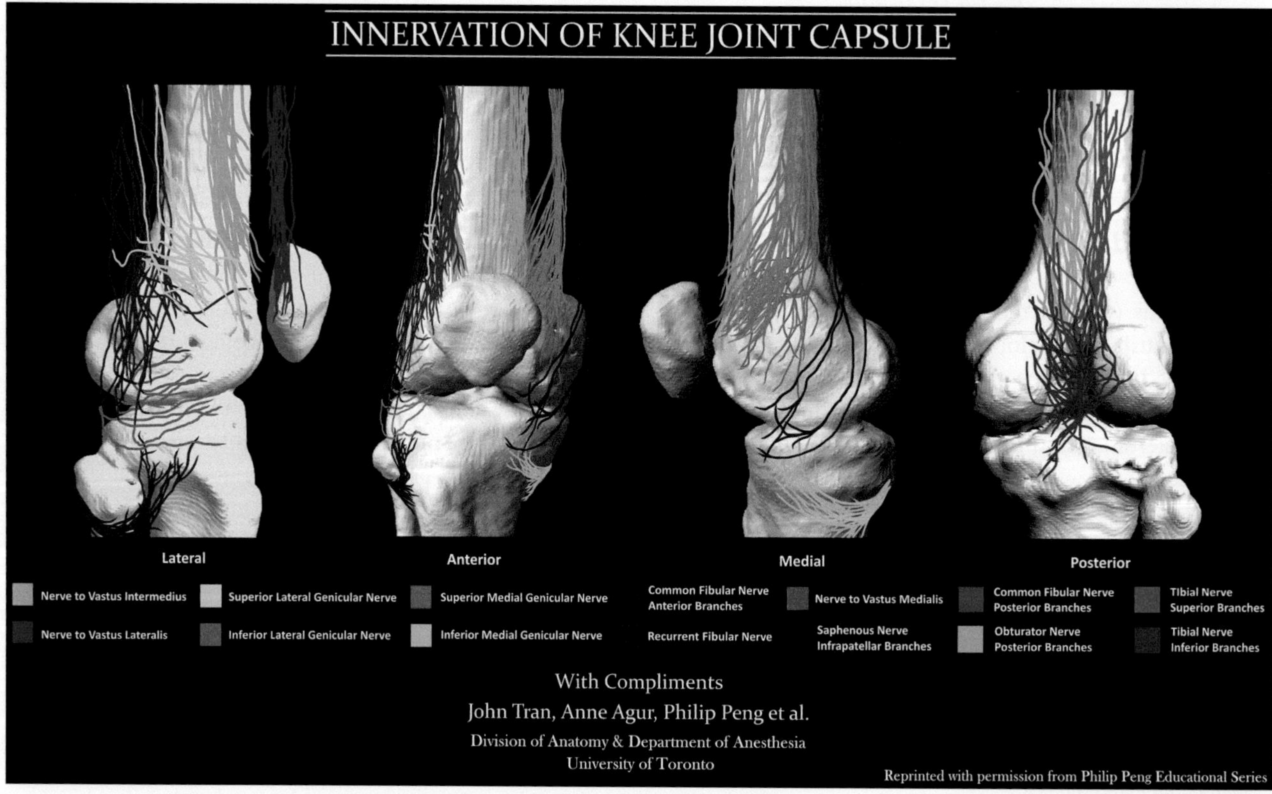

Fig. 66.1 Innervation of the joint capsule. Reprinted with permission from Philip Peng Educational Series

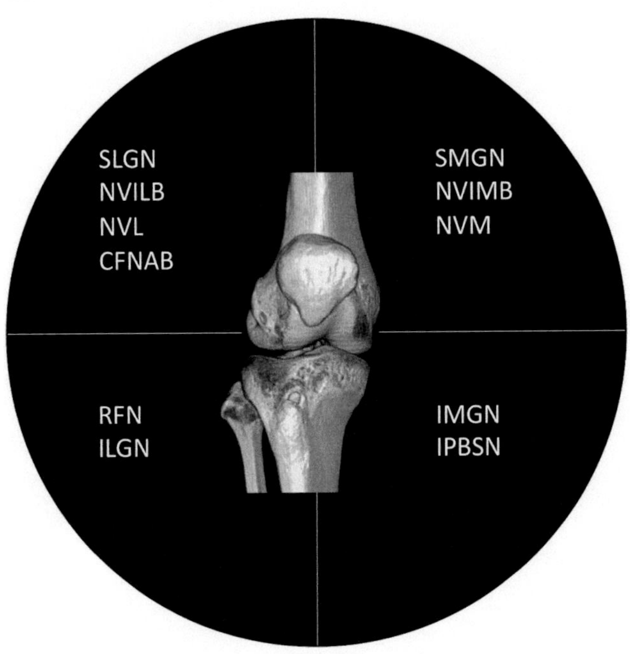

Fig. 66.2 The articular branches in four quadrants of the knee. *SMGN* superomedial genicular nerve, *NVIMB* nerve to vastus intermedius medial branch, *NVM* nerve to vastus medialis, *IMGN* inferomedial genicular nerve, *IPBSN* infrapatellar branch of saphenous nerve, *SLGN* superolateral genicular nerve, *NVILB* nerve to vastus intermedius lateral branch, *NVL* nerve to vastus lateralis, *CFNAB* common fibular nerve anterior branch, *RFN* recurrent fibular nerve, *ILGN* inferolateral genicular nerve. Reprinted with permission from Philip Peng Educational Series

that the SMGN is a terminal branch of the nerve to vastus medialis (NVM) originating from the femoral nerve. The SMGN runs by the posteromedial surface of the vastus medialis and descends along the adductor magnus tendon (Fig. 66.3). From there, the SMGN gives off articular branches proximal and distal to the adductor tubercle innervating the superomedial knee joint capsule and medial femoral condyle.

The landmark of SGMN can be either at or just inferior to the adductor tubercle (distal branches) or the junction of the femoral shaft and medial femoral condyle (proximal branch). The latter is the basis for the conventional landmark, and the former is the proposed new landmark in a recent anatomic article (Fig. 66.3).

Superolateral Genicular Nerve

The SLGN is a branch of the sciatic nerve (SCN) that runs deep to the biceps femoris tendon and courses toward the posterosuperior angle of the lateral femoral condyle. It shares a common trunk with articular branches of the common fibular nerve (CFN) and coursed along the posterolateral aspect of the femur. Here, the nerve joins the superior lateral genicular artery, which gives the nerve the original name. Tran et al. reported that the SLGN originated from the SCN in 5 out of 15 specimens and from an articular nerve of the CFN in the remaining 10 specimens (Fig. 66.1). When originating from the SCN, the SLGN descends to the level of the superior border of the lateral femoral condyle to accompany the superior lateral genicular artery (SLGA). The landmark to locate both the SLGN and SLGA is the junction of the femoral shaft and lateral femoral condyle (Fig. 66.4).

Inferior Medial Genicular Nerve

The origin of the IMGN was described coming from the tibial nerve by Gardner and Tran et al. but from the SCN by Fonkoue et al. Regardless of its origin, the IMGN courses deep to the medial collateral ligament accompanied by the inferior medial genicular artery to supply to anterior knee joint capsule (Fig. 66.1). The landmark for the IMGN is the junction between epiphysis and diaphysis deep to the medial collateral ligament.

Nerve to Vastus Intermedius

Although it is not described in any of the current landmarks, the course of the nerve to vastus intermedius (NVI) is well misunderstood in the literature and bears some importance in the current landmark. Most of the literature described the course of the articular branches of the NVI deep to the vastus intermedius muscle along the anterior/anteromedial aspect of the femur. Tran et al. found consistently in all their specimens that the NVI gives distinct medial and lateral articular branches, instead of a single branch. These branches coursed along the anteromedial and anterolateral aspect of the distal femur, deep to the vastus intermedius, to supply the suprapatellar bursa (anterior divisions of those branches) and superomedial/superolateral knee joint capsule (a posterior division of those branches) (Figs. 66.3 and 66.4). This pattern was consistent with the illustration of articular branches of NVI by Gardner. The posterior division of both medial and lateral articular branches is in the vicinity of the convention landmark for RF ablation.

Technique

Both ultrasound and fluoroscopy guidance techniques have been described for both diagnostic and ablation. A randomized trial comparing the genicular nerve injection did not find a difference in the outcome. Both techniques will be discussed.

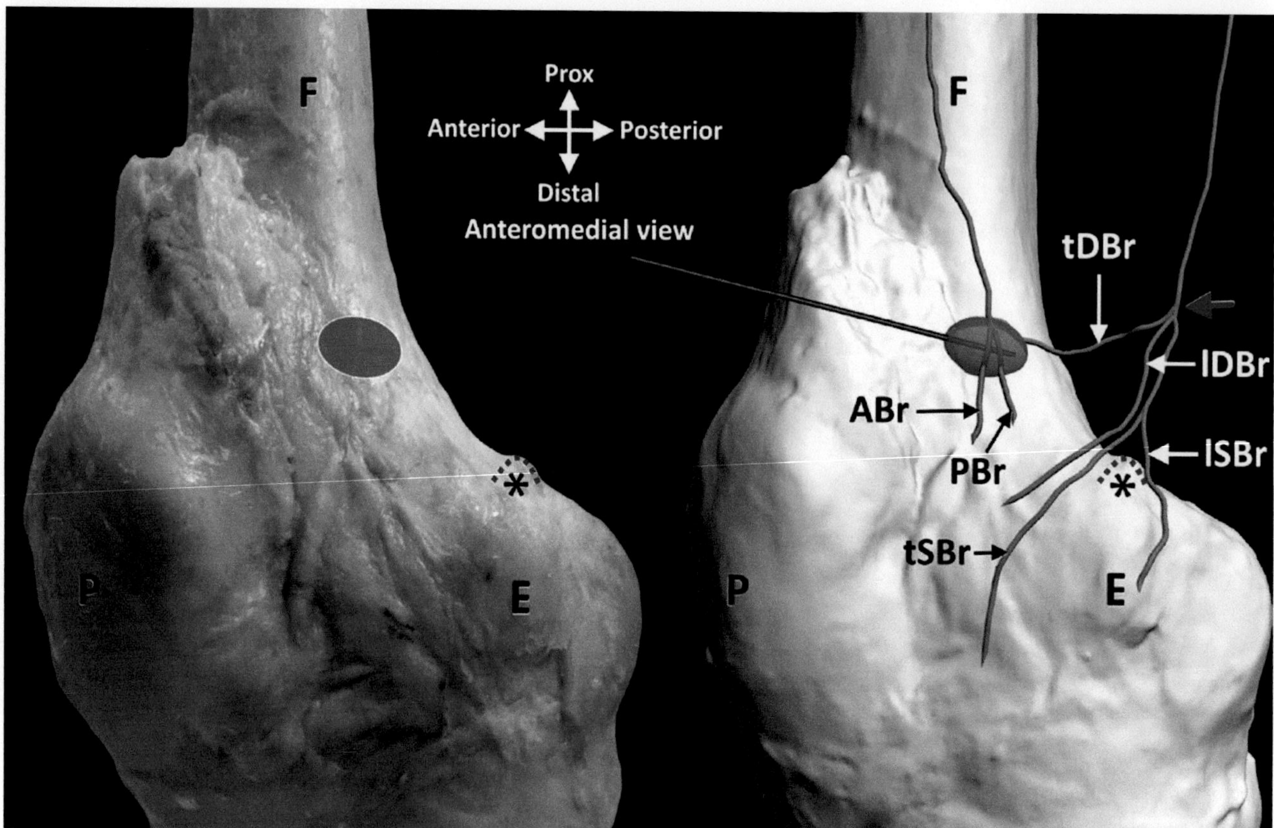

Fig. 66.3 Left: Skeletonized specimen with intact joint capsule showing simulated lesion (red) relative to shaft of femur F, E, adductor tubercle (*), and patella (P). Right: 3D model showing articular branches and simulated lesion relative to reconstructed bony landmarks. Lesion captures tDBr of SMGN (orange), ABr and PBr of the medial nerve to the vastus intermedius (green). Branches not captured include lDBr, tSBr, and lSBr of SMGN. Blue dashed line: outline of the adductor tubercle. *3D* three-dimensional, *ABr* anterior branch, *DBr* deep branch, *E* medial epicondyle, *F* femur, *lDBr* longitudinal deep branch, *lSBr* longitudinal superficial branch, *PBr* posterior branch, *SBr* superficial branch, *SMGN* superior medial genicular nerve, *tDBr* transverse deep branch, *tSBr* transverse superficial branch. Reprinted with permission from Philip Peng Educational Series

Fluoroscopy Guidance

The patient is put in the supine position and has a bolster or pillow to keep the knee in flexion.

For the superomedial and superolateral genicular nerve, the target is the junction between epiphysis and diaphysis in anteroposterior view and midpoint between anterior and posterior cortex in the lateral view (Fig. 66.5). The key is to have the needle on around the bone; otherwise, it may be in the muscle. For the inferomedial genicular nerve, the target is the junction between epiphysis and diaphysis deep to the medial collateral ligament (Fig. 66.5).

For the diagnostic block, a 22G 3.5-inch spinal needle is used. Upon close to the periosteum, which is sensitive to pain, the needle gently makes contact with the bone. The position is then checked with a lateral view. Following confirmation of the position, 1.5 mL of 0.25–0.5% bupivacaine is administered to the superomedial and superolateral targets and 1 mL to the inferomedial target.

For RFA, the targets are the same. The systems quite often described in the literature are either a cooled RF system or a regular RF system with single needle placement. The parameter for a cooled RF system is usually set at temperature 60 °C for 150 s, with the heat generated in the tissue approximating 77 to 80 °C. For the regular thermal RF system, various systems have been used and described in the literature, and the parameter is generally set at 80–82 °C for 120 s.

Given the variable course of superomedial genicular nerve, and most of the disease burden is on the medial aspect of the knee, the authors incorporated a palisade lesion in the superomedial area (Fig. 66.6). The first needle is inserted in the classical target for the superomedial genicular nerve. Two additional needles are inserted: one cephalad and anterior and another caudal and posterior to the first needle (Fig. 66.6). This palisade lesion creates a strip interrupting virtually all articular branches approaching the anterior joint capsule in the superomedial quadrant. This modification is based on the authors' preference and no literature investigating this ablation configuration so far.

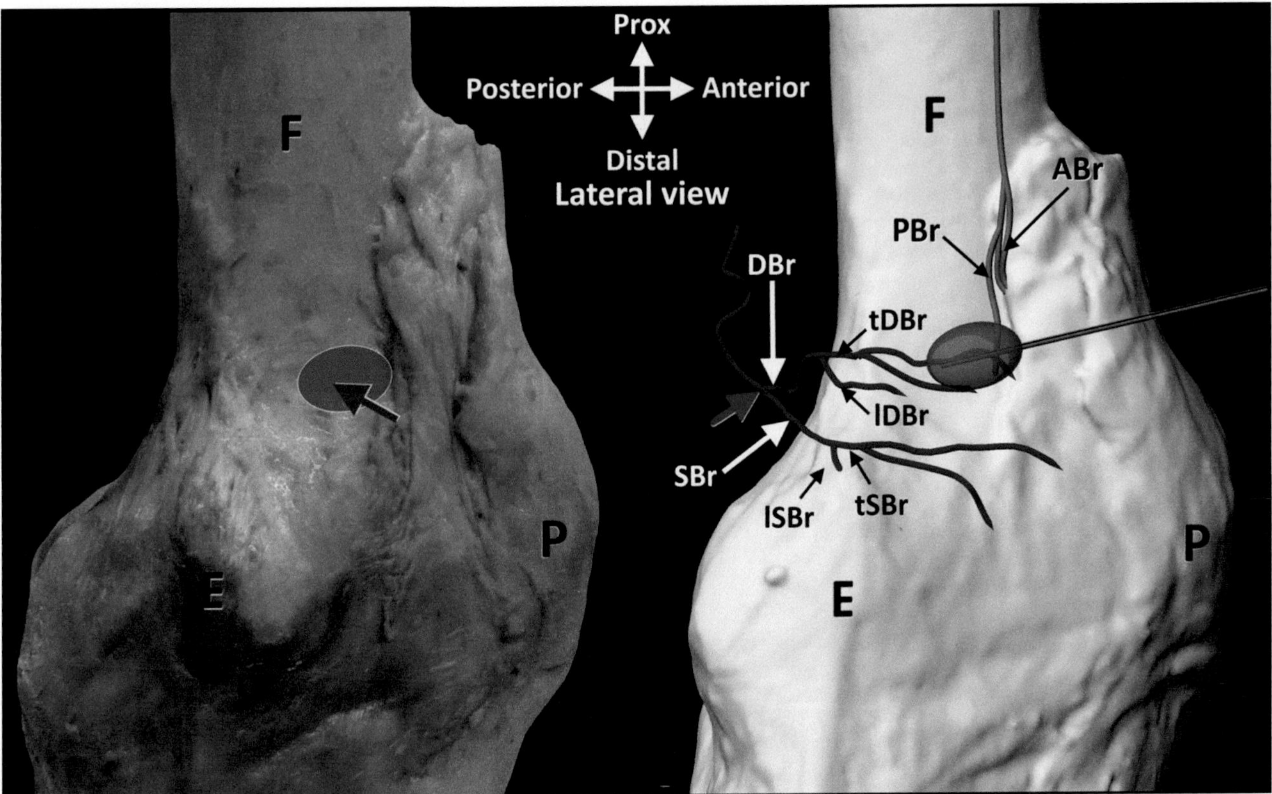

Fig. 66.4 Left: Skeletonized specimen with intact joint capsule showing simulated lesion (red) relative to shaft of F, E, and P. Right: 3D model showing articular branches and simulated lesion relative to reconstructed bony landmarks. Lesion captures the tDBr of the SLGN (purple) and PBr of the lateral nerve to the vastus intermedius (green). Branches not captured include lDBr, tSBr, and lSBr of SLGN. Blue arrow: origin of DBr of SLGN. *3D* three-dimensional, *ABr* anterior branch of lateral nerve to vastus intermedius, *DBr* deep branch, *E* lateral epicondyle, *F* femur, *lDBr* longitudinal deep branch, *lSBr* longitudinal superficial branch, *P* patella, *PBr* posterior branch, *SBr* superficial branch, *SLGN* superolateral genicular nerve, *tDBr* transverse deep branch, *tSBr* transverse superficial branch. Reprinted with permission from Philip Peng Educational Series

Ultrasound Guidance

The easy access to an ultrasound machine in pain clinics makes it an appealing method for a diagnostic block. Since no sedation is required, the diagnostic block can be performed in the clinic. A high-frequency probe (6–15 MHz) is used unless inpatient with a very high body mass index.

For diagnostic block, the patient is placed in a supine position, and the authors' preferred position is to have the leg in the figure-of-four position with the hip externally rotated. After the usual prepping and draping, the ultrasound probe is placed along the long axis of the femur in a strict coronal plane simulating the X-ray beam in obtaining a lateral view. The first target will be the SMGN. The medial condyle and femoral shaft can be revealed as well as the fascia expansion deep to the vastus medialis (Fig. 66.7). The target is the junction between epiphysis and diaphysis as in the fluoroscopy-guided technique. The target's depth is measured, and the probe is turned 90° to keep the bone shadow at the same depth. A 22G 3.5-inch spinal needle is inserted in-plane in the anterior-posterior direction to reach the target. The volume and dose of the injectate are the same as the fluoroscopy-guided procedure.

With the patient in the same position, the probe is placed over the medial aspect of the tibiofemoral joint. From there, the probe is moved in the caudal direction keeping in the long axis of the tibia until the IMGN and vessel are seen deep to the medial collateral ligament (Fig. 66.8). The depth of the target is measured, and the probe is turned 90°, keeping the target at the same depth. The needle insertion method and the dose of injectate are the same as the fluoroscopy-guided method.

Upon finishing the SMGN and IMGN, the patient is asked to turn on the side so that the lateral side of the knee is on the non-dependent side. The probe is placed along the long axis of the femur to reveal the epiphysis and diaphysis. The target is the fascia expansion deep to the vastus lateralis/intermedius. Again, the depth of the target is measured,

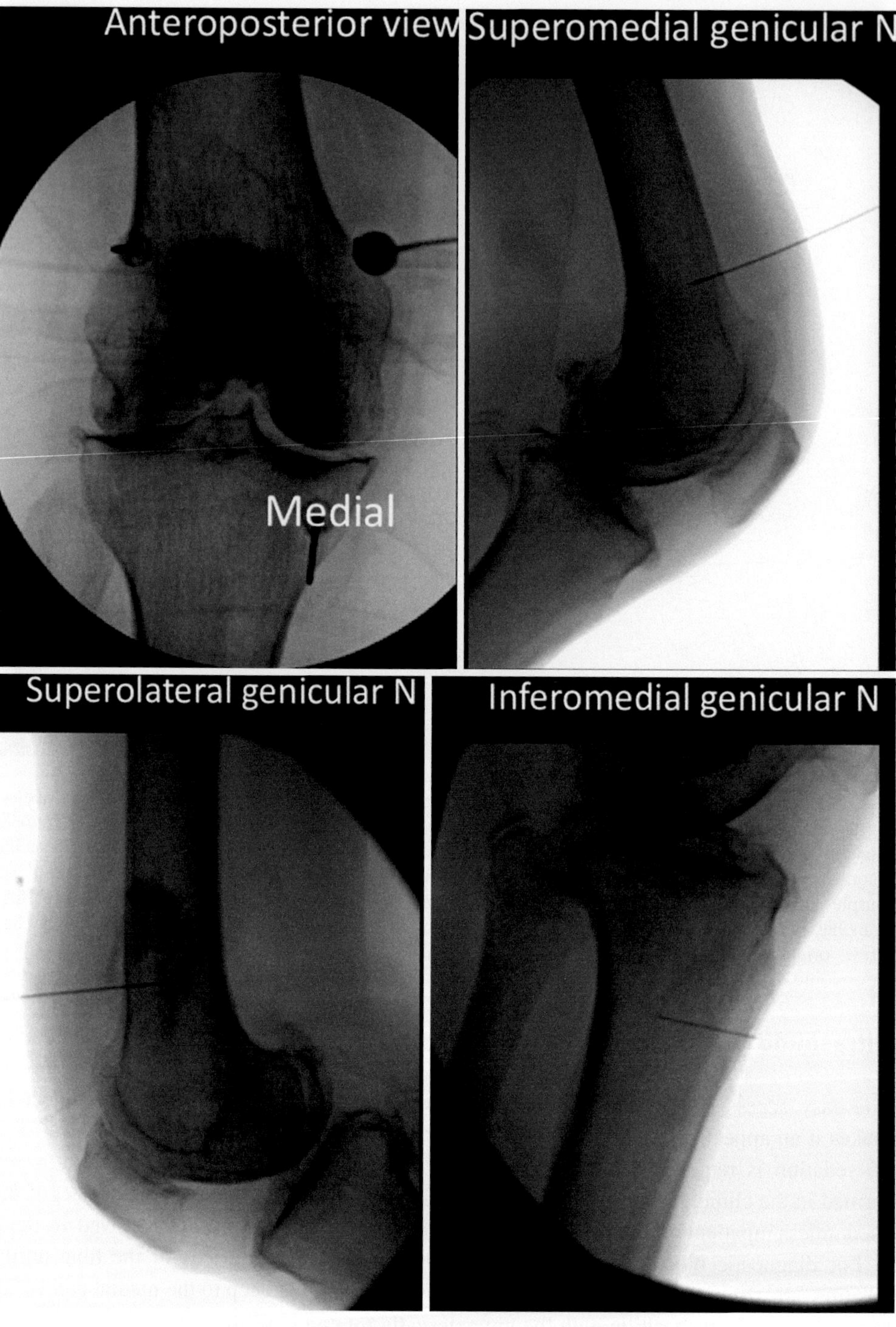

Fig. 66.5 Fluoroscopic images of the classical targets for radiofrequency ablation. Reprinted with permission from Philip Peng Educational Series

and the probe is turned 900 to keep the target at the same depth. The needle insertion method and the dose of the injectate are the same as that of the fluoroscopy-guided method.

It is important to note that the target is the fascia expansion at the junction of epiphysis and diaphysis in all three landmarks. The vessels in those areas are not necessarily detectable in the ultrasound scan or the genicular arteries. Sometimes, more than one vessel is discovered, and therefore, the authors do not recommend the routine use of the vessel as the landmark in the ultrasound method.

For the RFA procedure, the authors suggest following two principles to guide the RF needle to the target similar to that in the fluoroscopic method. First, the probe's orientation should be in a strict coronal plane simulating the X-ray beam in taking the lateral view. Second, the clinician should understand the sonographic "signature" of the lower end of the femur. These two technical components allow the clini-

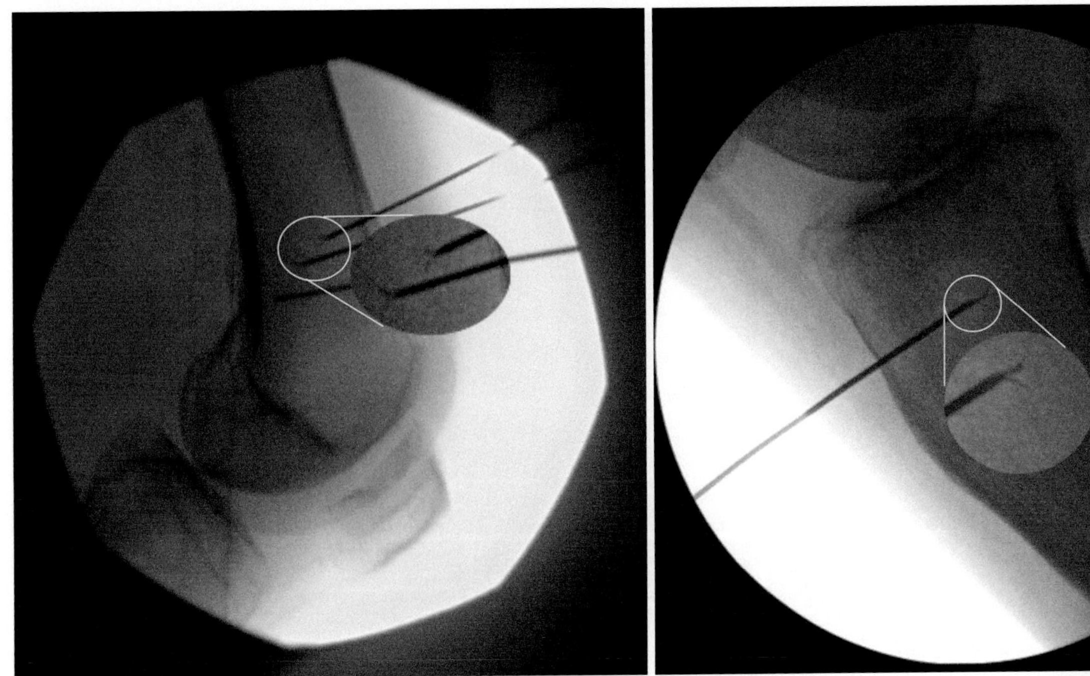

Fig. 66.6 Palisade lesion of superomedial (left) and inferomedial (right) genicular nerve with three needles. A zoom image from the white circle showed the tine of the radiofrequency needle. Reprinted with permission from Philip Peng Educational Series

cian to place the needle at the bony target under ultrasound guidance.

Complications

Hematoma formation, hemarthrosis, pseudoaneurysm, infection, sepsis, chondrolysis, osteonecrosis of the patella, and skin burns have been reported.

Practical Tips

When the needle tip is in contact with the bone, it does not necessarily mean that the tip is on the bone. It may be still in the muscle and results in inadvertent intramuscular injection and thus false-negative diagnostic test. This can be avoided simply by gently rotating the needle and piercing through the muscle fascia. With the use of ultrasound, the spread of injectate can be seen deep to the muscle in real time. Alternatively, injection of contrast under fluoroscopy can confirm the location of the tip.

The needle placement for genicular nerves lies adjacent to the genicular artery as it is challenging to visualize the nerve itself. Although the literature has identified the genicular nerves travel adjacent to the artery, it may not be accurate in all the cases and could lead to the procedure's failure. The clinician can rely on the fascia expansion and the bony contour signature of the femur to guide the needle to the target with ultrasound.

After blood is seen coming out of the needle after inserting a large-bore RF cannula, it is best to leave the needle and proceed with RFA as the heat can stimulate the coagulation and stop the bleeding.

Review of Literature

Since the first randomized trial on genicular nerve radiofrequency ablation, there has been outpouring interest culminating in over 35 clinical studies and 15 randomized controlled trials that are all of moderate to high methodological quality.

The clinical efficacy of genicular RFA is best exemplified with the largest double-blind, randomized control trial of cooled RFA (CRFA) compared to intra-articular steroid (IAS) in 151 patients with symptomatic knee OA (KL grade 2–4). Despite having similar pre-intervention numeric pain rating scores, the mean knee pain score was less in the CRFA group than in the IAS group at every follow-up interval, including 1, 3, and 6 months post-intervention. Mean improvement at 1 month in the CFRA group at 1 and 6 months was 4.2 and 4.9 points, respectively, on a 10-point NRS scale compared to 3.3 and 1.3 in the IAS group. Similarly, at 6 months, 74% and 22% in the CRFA group met successful outcome criteria (>50% reduction in NRS score)

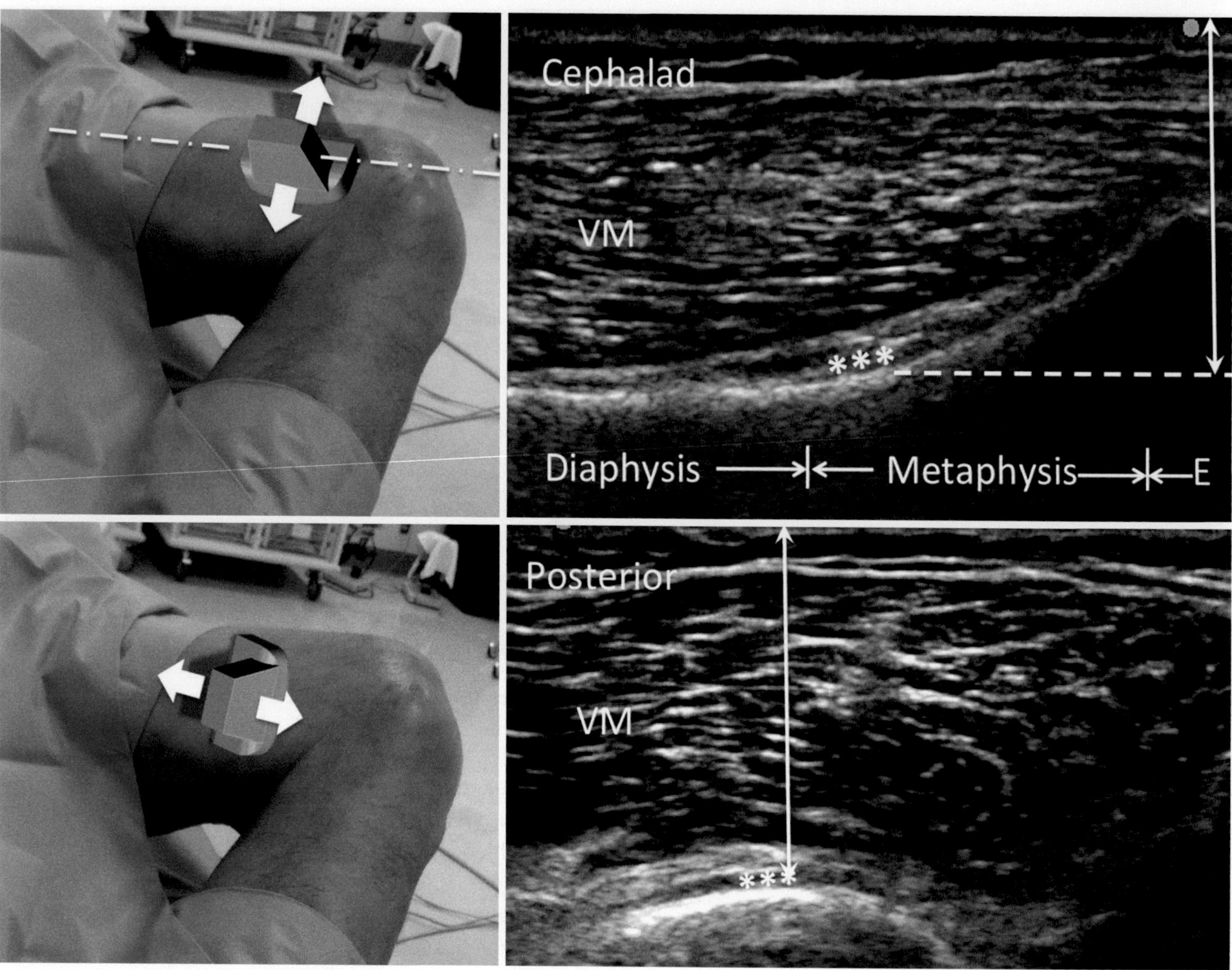

Fig. 66.7 Ultrasound imaging technique and the corresponding sonographic image of the superomedial knee. Upper left panel: The ultrasound probe was placed along the long axis of femur between the diaphysis and epiphysis. Upper right panel: A fascia expansion (***) deep to the vastus medial (VM) could be seen. E, epiphysis. Lower left panel: The ultrasound probe was then turned 90 °C to obtain a short axis view of the femur. Move or align the probe in the cephalad-caudal direction until the target of the same depth as the long axis view is obtained. It is important that the probe should not be tilted but aligned in cephalad-caudal direction. When the appropriate depth was found, the same fascia expansion (***) could be located. Reprinted with permission from Philip Peng Educational Series

and 100% pain relief, respectively, compared to only 26% and 4% in the IAS group. Similarly, functional outcome demonstrated clinically and statistically significant improvements in the CRFA group compared to the IAS group.

Multiple systematic reviews and meta-analyses have supported the clinical efficacy of genicular RFA. Genicular RFA has demonstrated >50% pain relief in 194/296 patients (65.5%) at 6 months when combining all available comparative studies or a pooled mean difference in the VAS of 4 (from 0 to 10) when combining only ultrasound-guided RFA studies. Similarly, 27/28 (96%) comparative studies demonstrated enhanced functionality from baseline up until 6 months in those undergoing RFA or a pooled mean difference in the WOMAC scores of 23 points when combining only ultrasound-guided RFA studies.

The large majority of randomized controlled trials have final follow-ups at the 6-month post-intervention period; however, long-term follow-up studies of these large, randomized trials have demonstrated sustained pain relief and improved function up to 24 months post-intervention. At 18 and 24 months post-intervention, there was a demonstration of a significant decrease in NRS pain scores from 6.6 ± 1.6 at baseline to 3.1 2.7(n = 25) and 3.6 2.8 (n = 18) at 18 and 24 months, respectively, with 12/25 subjects reporting ≥50% pain relief at 18 months and 11/18 demonstrating ≥50% pain relief at 24 months from the baseline. Similarly, there was a demonstration of prolonged functional improvement as measured by the Oxford Knee Score, with an overall mean change from baseline of 26.0 ± 9.6 points (MCID = 5) at 18 months and 29.9 ± 10.4 points at 24 months.

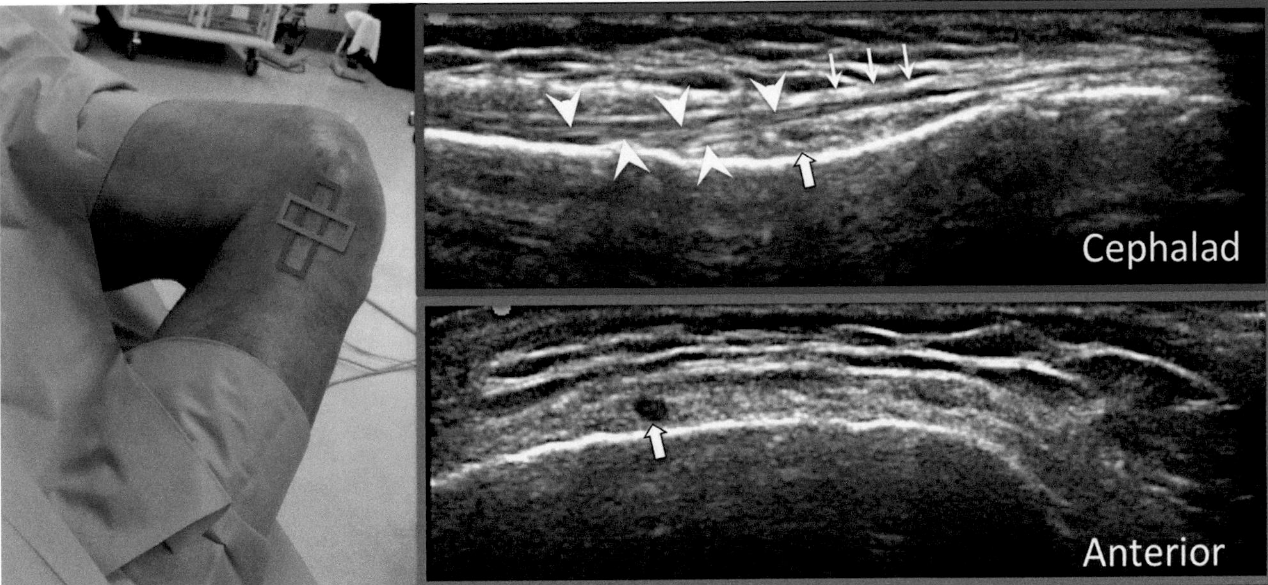

Fig. 66.8 Left panel: The two positions of the ultrasound probe just distal to the epiphysis of the tibia. Right upper panel in red rectangle: The ultrasound probe was in long axis of the tibia. The inferior medial genicular nerve (IMGN) and vessel (bold arrow) are deep to the medial collateral ligament (arrowheads), which is deep to the crural fascia (arrows). Mark the depth of the bone hyperechoic shadow deep to the IMGN. Right lower panel in green rectangle: The ultrasound was rotated 90 °C and aligned in the cephalad-caudal direction so that the hyperechoic bone shadow is at the same depth as the previous scan. The neurovascular bundle (bold arrow) was seen again. Reprinted with permission from Philip Peng Educational Series

While the evidence supports the use of RFA in patients with chronic knee pain due to osteoarthritis in the native knee, this procedure has not shown expected benefits in some scenarios: preoperative for those undergoing TKA or in those with persistent chronic TKA pain. A single-center sham-controlled prospective trial that assessed the efficacy of preoperative knee RF done 2–6 weeks prior to total knee arthroplasty reported a lack of benefit in terms of postoperative pain, consumption of analgesics including opioid medications, and functional recovery. The authors proposed a 26% non-responder rate of this procedure and is probably explained by the variable course of genicular nerves and co-presence of central sensitization with chronic advanced knee osteoarthritis. Similarly, RFA of the knee joint has not been rigorously tested in subacute and chronic persistent knee pains post arthroplasty.

A retrospective comparative study of ultrasound-guided knee RFA in chronic pains secondary to TKA or advanced knee OA (KL grade III–IV) in 23 patients reported comparable benefits (67% in the TKA group and 88% in knee OA group of >50% improvement in VAS pain scores) in both groups at 3 months. A few isolated case reports of knee RF in acute posttraumatic pains and acute postoperative TKA pains have been published, although the clinical efficacy in these conditions remains to be established.

Comparison with Other Treatment Groups

Eight studies have compared genicular nerve radiofrequency ablation to standard injection therapies, including corticosteroid injection, ozone injection, HA injection, platelet-rich plasma (PRP) with sodium hyaluronate injection, solely sodium hydrate injection and IA prolotherapy with erythropoietin and dextrose injection.

All randomized controlled trials of RFA compared to corticosteroid injection have demonstrated significant improvements at all follow-ups for pain reduction; however, only 2/3 of studies have demonstrated significant improvements in functional scores. Similarly, to corticosteroid, RFA has demonstrated improvements in pain and functional scores when compared to PRP and hyaluronic acid in a randomized fashion, with the RFA group demonstrating significant improvements in VAS and WOMAC function scores.

Unfortunately, compared to nontraditional intra-articular injections, including erythropoietin plus dextrose injection and ozone injection, RFA has not demonstrated significant benefits. The significance of these randomized control trials, despite being of moderate quality, necessitates further investigation due to the infrequent utilization of these intra-articular therapies for knee osteoarthritis.

Comparative Efficacy of Ultrasound Vs Fluoroscopy-Guided RFA Techniques

Both fluoroscopy and ultrasound have been used as imaging modalities for guiding the needle to the target position. Knee RFA was initially performed using a fluoroscopy-guided approach. Later, ultrasound (US) was suggested as an alternate radiation-free office-based technique. Several studies, both cadaveric and clinical, on the US-based approach for knee RFA asserted the adjacent location of genicular arteries as a surrogate marker for localizing genicular nerves to yield better outcomes. Yet, subsequent cadaveric studies investigating the relationship of genicular nerves and arteries did not find this assumption to be true. Clinically, a couple of RCTs have compared the efficacy of pain relief in US and RFA techniques and reported similar outcomes with both techniques. Each technique offers a unique set of advantages. Fluoroscopy guidance can easily identify the nerve targets as they run adjacent to the periosteum and offer better needle visualization regardless of tissue depth and needle gauze. In contrast, ultrasound guidance offers the benefit of an office-based cheaper alternative with no radiation exposure and improved safety due to better visualization of adjacent soft tissue structures. The choice of technique should be based on the availability of setup and individual experience and comfort with the imaging modalities.

Complications/Adverse Events

The majority of publications regarding genicular nerve RFA have not demonstrated any significant adverse events related to the procedure. With the significant increase in the procedure rate of genicular nerve RFA, there have been reports of rare, however significant, safety concerns. Transient hypoesthesia numbness and periosteal touch allodynia were reported in few studies and significantly improved within a few weeks after the procedure. Rare complications include vascular injury of the knee, including large subcutaneous bleeding, ecchymosis, hematoma formation, skin burns, hemarthrosis, pes anserine tendon damage, septic arthritis, or pseudoaneurysm; also, osteonecrosis of the patella has been described in the literature. Direct comparison of fluoroscopy and US-guided knee RFA was done in two studies and did not report any adverse effects.

Several clinicians argue Charcot's neuropathy is a possible catastrophic side effect of knee joint nerve ablation. Nevertheless, Charcot's neuropathy has never been reported as a complication post knee RFA, even in the studies with relatively more prolonged follow-up duration. The reasons for the non-occurrence of Charcot's neuropathy are twofold. First, the nerve supply of the joint is partially preserved with knee RFA as the articular sensory branches to the posterior joint are spared. Second, Charcot neuropathy develops in systemic conditions with inflammatory mediators that disrupt the homeostasis of bone mineralization, causing osteolysis. Due to the rarity of these adverse events and no description in large cohort studies, it is unknown what the true prevalence of these adverse events are, nor the procedural aspects that may increase or decrease the risk of these events.

Disclosure Statement We declare that we have no conflicts of interest in the authorship or publication of this contribution.

Suggested Reading

Choi WJ, Hwang SJ, Song JG, et al. Radiofrequency treatment relieves chronic knee osteoarthritis pain: a double-blind randomized controlled trial. Pain. 2011;152:481–7.

Davis T, Loudermilk E, DePalma M, et al. Prospective, multicenter, randomized, crossover clinical trial comparing the safety and effectiveness of cooled radiofrequency ablation with corticosteroid injection in the management of knee pain from osteoarthritis. Reg Anesth Pain Med. 2018;43(1):84–91.

Fonkoué L, Behets C, Kouassi JK, et al. Distribution of sensory nerves supplying the knee joint capsule and implications for genicular blockade and radiofrequency ablation: an anatomical study. Surg Radiol Anat. 2019;41:1461–71.

Fonkoue L, Behets CW, Steyaert A, et al. Accuracy of fluoroscopic-guided genicular nerve blockade: a need for revisiting anatomical landmarks. Reg Anesth Pain Med. 2019; https://doi.org/10.1136/rapm-2019-100451.

Gardner E. The innervation of the shoulder joint. Anat Rec. 1948;102:1–18.

Hunter C, Davis T, Loudermilk E, Kapural L, DePalma M. Cooled radiofrequency ablation treatment of the genicular nerves in the treatment of osteoarthritic knee pain: 18- and 24-month results. Pain Pract. 2020;20:238–46.

Kim DH, Lee MS, Lee S, Yoon SH, Shin JW, Choi SS. A prospective randomized comparison of the efficacy of ultrasound- vs fluoroscopy-guided genicular nerve block for chronic knee osteoarthritis. Pain Physician. 2019;22(2):139–46.

Park MR, Kim D, Rhyu IJ, et al. An anatomical neurovascular study for procedures targeting peri-articular nerves in patients with anterior knee pain. Knee. 2020;27(5):1577–84.

Tran J, Peng PWH, Lam K, Baig E, Agur AMR, Gofeld M. Anatomical study of the innervation of anterior knee joint capsule: implication for image-guided intervention. Reg Anesth Pain Med. 2018;43:407–14.

Tran J, Peng P, Agur A. Evaluation of nerve capture using classical landmarks for genicular nerve radiofrequency ablation: 3D cadaveric study. Reg Anesth Pain Med. 2020;45:898–906.

Walega D, McCormick Z, Manning D, Avram M. Radiofrequency ablation of genicular nerves prior to total knee replacement has no effect on postoperative pain outcomes: a prospective randomized sham-controlled trial with 6-month follow-up. Reg Anesth Pain Med. 2019; https://doi.org/10.1136/rapm-2018-100094.

Ankle Nerve Block

67

Philip Peng

Contents

Introduction

Ankle block provides excellent anesthesia to surgery in the foot especially forefoot. Conventionally, the procedure is performed with landmark guidance, but application of ultrasound guidance is gaining popularity. Without relying on field infiltration as in landmark-guided procedure, ultrasound-guided injection reduces the discomfort association with ankle block and improves the success rates. It affects the motor function minimally as mainly the intrinsic muscles of foot are blocked. The use of long-acting local anesthetic allows prolonged postoperative analgesia.

In addition, foot and ankle injury can result in neuropathic pain, and a series of injection can provide a window period for rehabilitation.

Indication (Patient Selection)

1. Surgical anesthesia and analgesia for foot distal to the malleoli, especially in the forefoot, including hallux valgus repair surgery, forefoot arthroplasty, reconstruction, osteotomy, and amputation.
2. Perineural injections around the foot and ankle nerves may be offered as diagnostic or therapeutic procedures for patients with neuropathic pain, particularly in the context of peripheral nerve injury or entrapment.

P. Peng (✉)
Department of Anesthesia and Pain Medicine, University of Toronto, Toronto Western Hospital, Toronto, ON, Canada
e-mail: philip.peng@uhn.ca

D. Jankovic, P. Peng (eds.), *Regional Nerve Blocks in Anesthesia and Pain Therapy*,
https://doi.org/10.1007/978-3-030-88727-8_67

Contraindication

1. In surgery when surgeons require long duration of tourniquet
2. Patients with difficult landmarks: severe edema, multiple scar, and peripheral vascular disease
3. Local infection at the site of injection

Anatomy

Tibial Nerve

The tibial nerve (TN) in the ankle region is the direct continuation of the tibial nerve distal to the bifurcation of the sciatic nerve in the popliteal fossa. The nerve descends through the calf sandwiched between gastrocnemius/soleus and the deep flexors. It reaches the distal lower leg posterior to the medial malleolus running deep to the flexor retinaculum and is usually posterior to the artery. It gives off medial calcaneal branches to the heel and divides into its two end branches, the medial and lateral plantar nerves, which pass to the sole of the foot and provide it with its sensory supply (Figs. 67.1 and 67.2).

Superficial Peroneal (Fibular) Nerve

This nerve arises from the common peroneal (fibular) nerve, runs through the peroneus longus muscle, and extends between the peroneus longus and brevis muscles. In the distal half of the leg, the nerve is sandwiched between peroneus brevis and extensor digitorum longus (EDL) in the intermuscular septum that separates the anterior and lateral compartments of the leg and gradually ascends into a superficial location before eventually piercing the crural fascia (Fig. 67.3). Subcutaneously, or still at the subfascial level, it divides into the thicker medial dorsal cutaneous nerve and the smaller intermediate dorsal cutaneous nerve, providing the sensory supply for the skin on the back of the foot and the toes (Fig. 67.4).

Deep Peroneal (Fibular) Nerve

This nerve runs between the tibialis anterior muscle and the extensor hallucis longus (EHL) muscle in the direction of the ankle, where it divides into a medial and a lateral end branch. The medial end branch continues in the same direction as the nerve trunk and passes with the dorsalis pedis artery to the first interosseous space, crossing under the tendon of the extensor hallucis brevis muscle to the distal end of the inter-

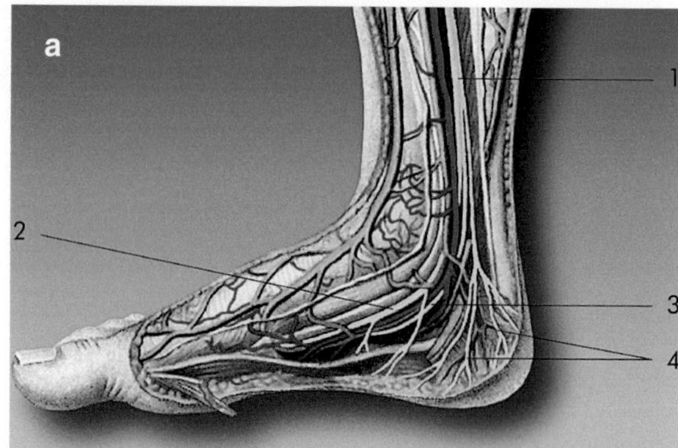

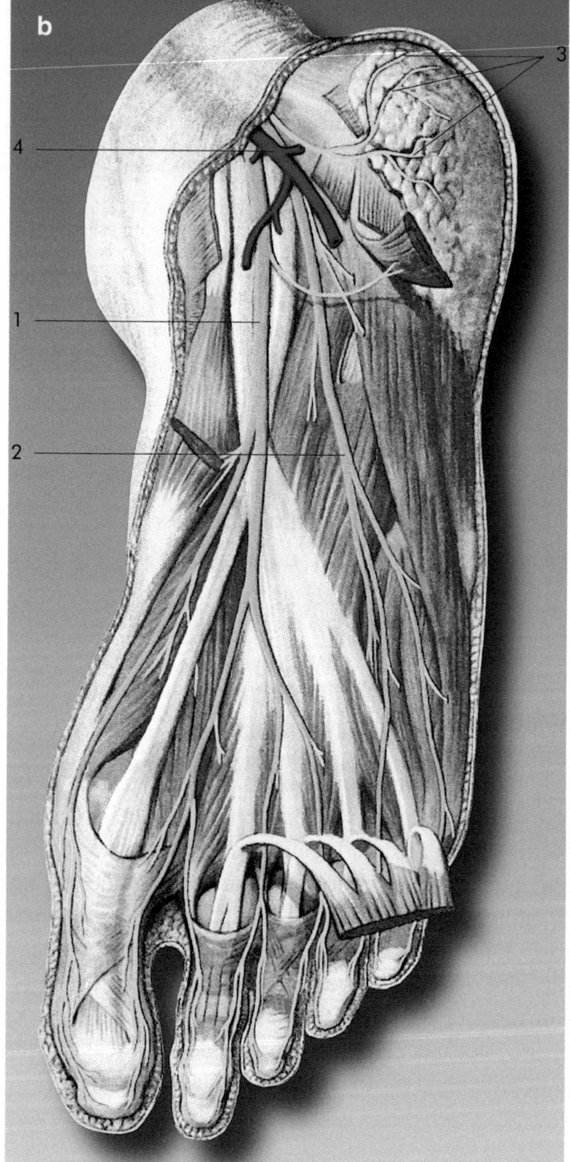

Fig. 67.1 (**a**) Tibial nerve. (1) Tibial nerve, (2) medial plantar nerve, (3) lateral plantar nerve, (4) calcaneal branches. Reprinted with permission from Danilo Jankovic. (**b**) Tibial nerve – sole of the foot. (1) Medial plantar nerve, (2) lateral plantar nerve, (3) medial calcaneal branches, (4) posterior tibial artery. Reprinted with permission from Danilo Jankovic

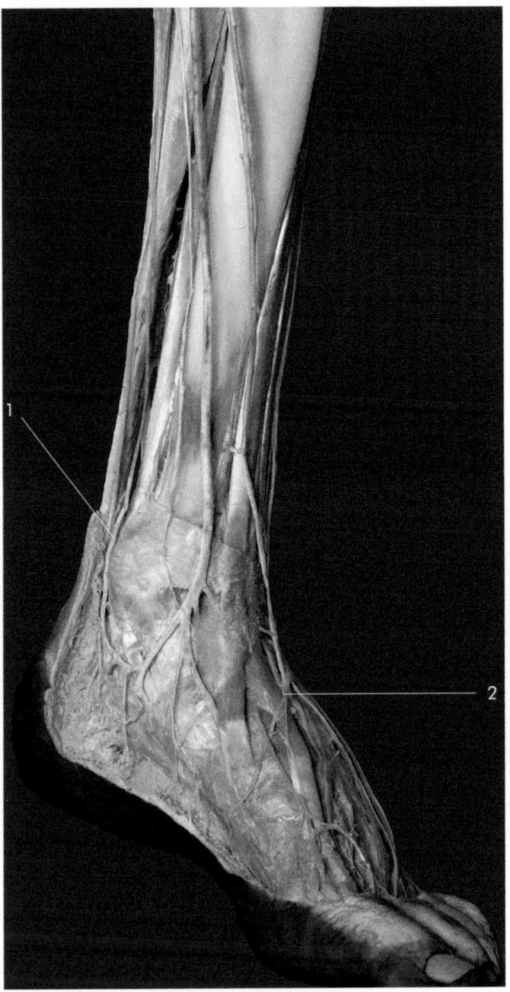

Fig. 67.2 Dissection of the medial ankle. (1) Tibial nerve, (2) deep peroneal nerve. Reprinted with permission from Danilo Jankovic

osseous space (Fig. 67.2 and 67.4). Here it joins with a strand of the superficial peroneal nerve (SPN) and divides into the end branches for the facing sides of the dorsal surfaces of the first and second toes. The lateral end branch turns laterally and supplies the extensor digitorum brevis muscle, sending off three interosseous nerves.

Sural Nerve

The medial sural cutaneous nerve arises in the proximal part of the popliteal fossa, runs down between the two heads of the gastrocnemius muscle, and joins the peroneal communicating branch (lateral sural nerve) to form the sural nerve. Accompanied by the small saphenous vein, the sural nerve runs behind the lateral malleolus and is contained within the same superficial fascial sheath. It passes as the lateral dorsal cutaneous nerve along the lateral side of the foot, where it gives off a connecting branch to the intermediate dorsal cutaneous nerve and ends as the dorsalis digiti minimi nerve on the lateral edge of the dorsum of the small toe (Fig. 67.4). Behind the lateral malleolus, it sends off branches (the lateral calcaneal branches) to the skin there and at the heel. The branches for the lateral side of the ankle, for the anterior capsular wall, and for the tarsal sinus originate proximal to the malleolus.

Saphenous Nerve

Below the knee, it runs along the tibial surface close to the great saphenous vein. Its relationship to the saphenous vein is inconstant, and the nerve may be either posterior or anterior to the vein. A common fascia has been described that envelops both the vein and the nerve in the distal third of the calf. At the level of the lower leg, the saphenous nerve courses along the medial side of and anterior to the medial malleolus and sends off branches to the skin of the medial side of the foot. It usually ends in the metatarsal area, without reaching the big toe (Fig. 67.4).

Technique

Ultrasound-Guided Approach

Preparation for the Block

Before performing the procedure, full prior information for the patient is mandatory. Since the location of nerves is superficial, a 30 mm 25-G needle should be sufficient. The procedure is performed with sterile technique. A high-frequency linear ultrasound probe is used. Local anesthetic involved long-acting drugs 0.5–0.75% ropivacaine, 0.25–0.5% bupivacaine, or combined lidocaine 2% lidocaine/0.5% bupivacaine 1:1 ratio.

Sonoanatomy and Injection Technique

Tibial Nerve

The patient is in the supine position with hip in external rotation, so that the medial side of ankle is facing upward. The ultrasound probe is placed in a transverse orientation just proximal to the prominence of the medial malleolus. The main landmark is the posterior tibial artery and is usually accompanied by two venae comitantes. The tibial nerve is a round hyperechoic structure usually posterior to the artery and rests on the fascia of flexor hallucis longus (FHL). By extending and flexing the big toe, the tibial nerve can be seen moving up and down, a maneuver to help identify the tibial nerve (Fig. 67.5).

Both in-plane and out-of-plane needle approach to the nerve are feasible. The nerve lies within a fascial sheath, and

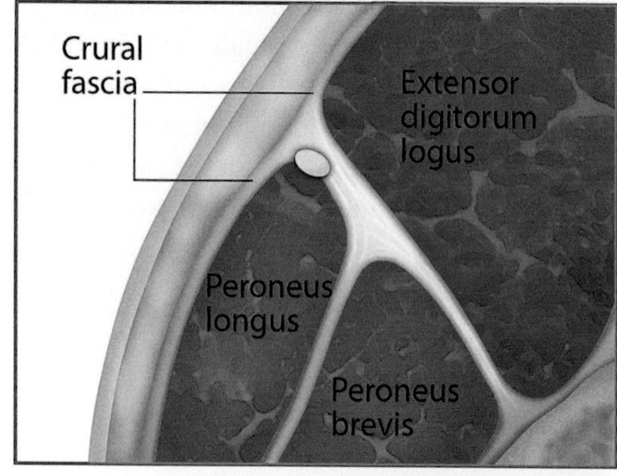

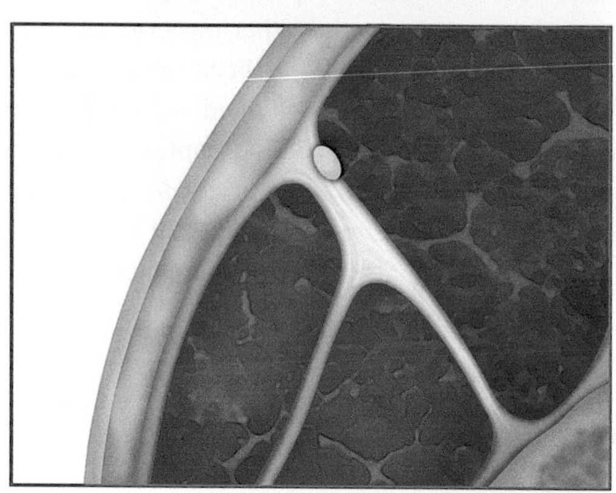

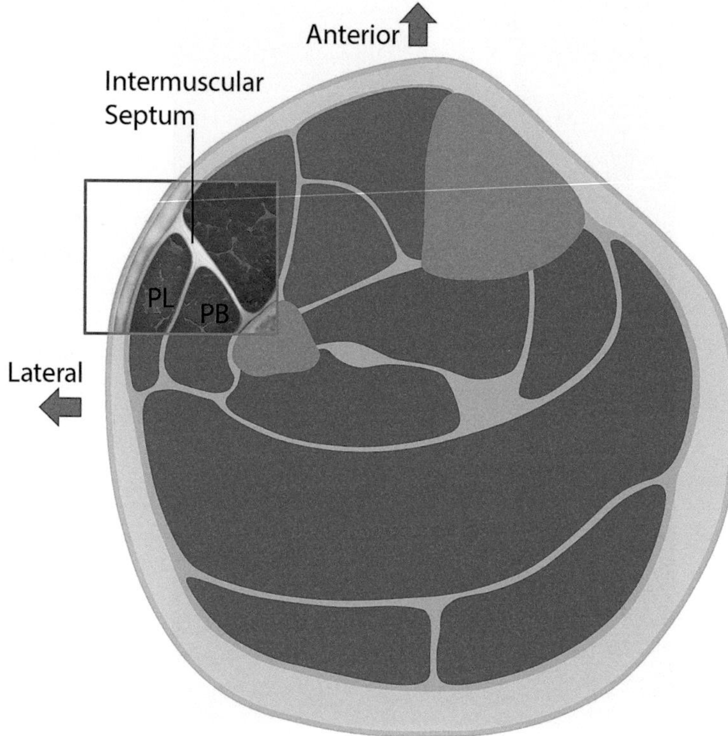

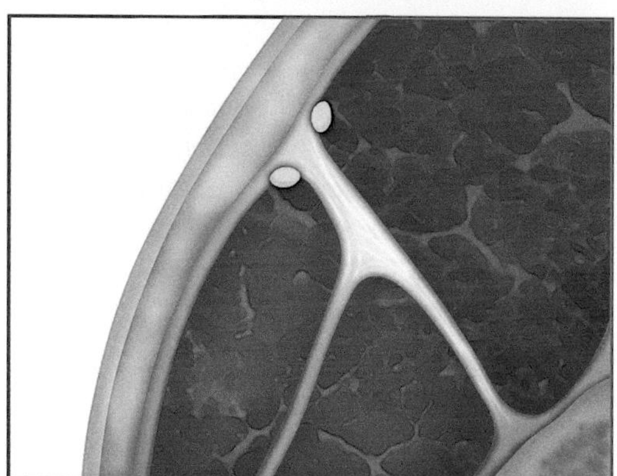

Fig. 67.3 Variation of superficial peroneal nerve in the mid leg. Reprinted with permission from Philip Peng Educational Series

injecting the local anesthetic within this sheath will produce a characteristic circumferential spread of local anesthetic around the nerve. The author prefers out-of-plane and directs the needle into the space behind the nerve formed between the flexor retinaculum and fascia of flexor hallucis longus (Fig. 67.6). 8 to 10 mL of local anesthetic is sufficient to produce a good block.

Saphenous Nerve

The position is the same as that for tibial nerve scanning. The probe is placed gently just proximal to the medial malleolus in the approximate location of the greater saphenous vein. The vein is the primary landmark. The saphenous nerve, which is a small hyperechoic structure, is not always clearly visible and does not have a constant relationship to the vein. However, the saphenous vein indicates the plane where the saphenous nerve is (Fig. 67.7).

For injection, the vein is the primary landmark, and light pressure from the ultrasound probe should be applied. The target is the plane around the vein, and the needle can be inserted in-plane or out-of-plane. The volume of local anesthetic is 3–5 mL.

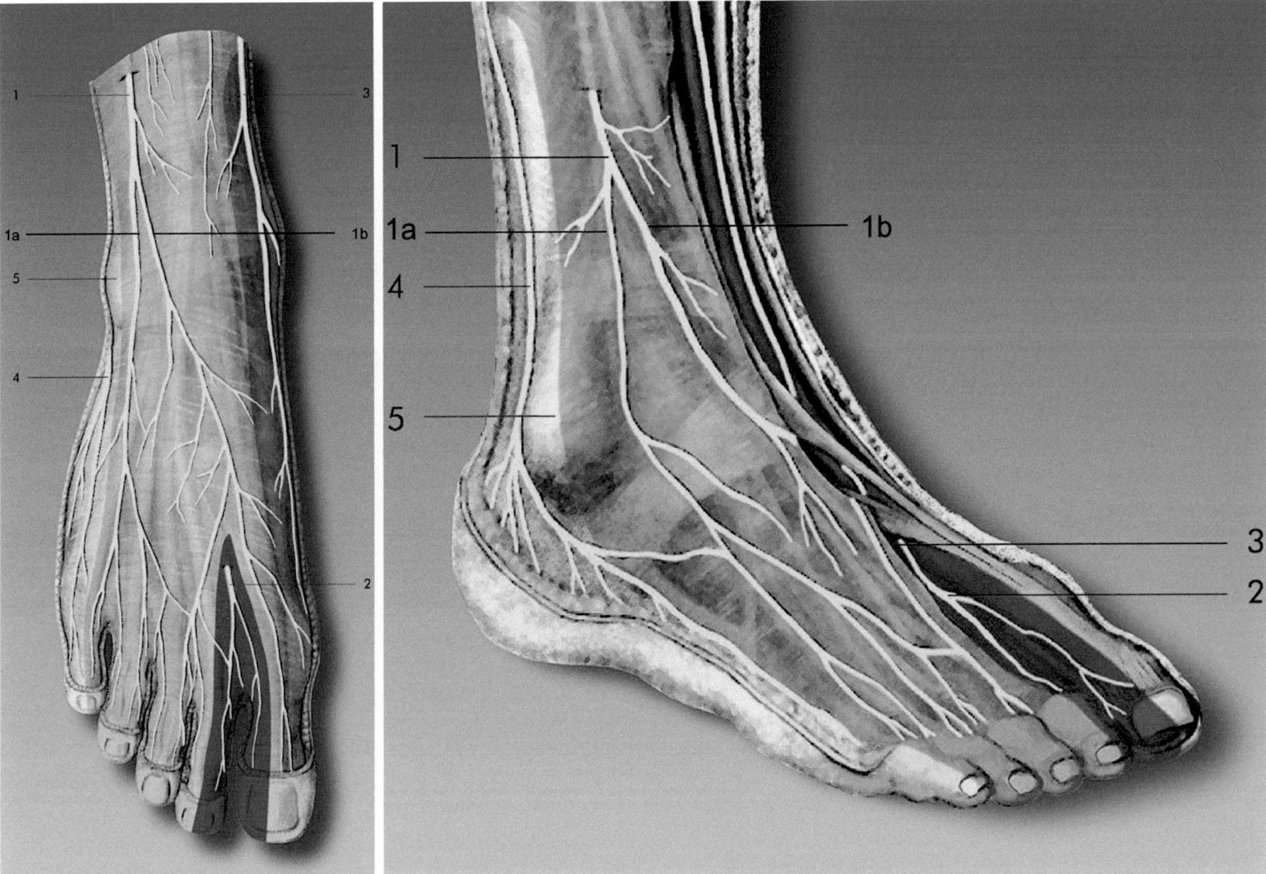

Fig. 67.4 Cutaneous innervation of the foot. Left. Anterior view. (1) Superficial peroneal (fibular) nerve, (1a) medial dorsal cutaneous nerve, (1b) intermediate dorsal cutaneous nerve, (2) deep peroneal (fibular) nerve, (3) saphenous nerve, (4) sural nerve, (5) lateral malleolus. Right. Lateral view. (1) Superficial peroneal (fibular) nerve, (1a) medial dorsal cutaneous nerve, (1b) intermediate dorsal cutaneous nerve, (2) deep peroneal (fibular) nerve, (3) dorsalis pedis artery, (4) lateral dorsal cutaneous nerve (sural nerve), (5) lateral malleolus. Reprinted with permission from Danilo Jankovic

Deep Peroneal (Fibular) Nerve

The patient is placed in supine position with the leg in a neutral position. Place the probe in a transverse orientation on the anterior surface of the ankle at the intermalleolar line (that is proximal to the ankle joint). The landmark is the anterior tibial/dorsalis pedis artery, which is usually deep to the extensor hallucis longus. The deep peroneal nerve (DPN) is sometimes, but not always, visible as a small hyperechoic structure lateral to the artery in the same tissue plane. It is not essential to visualize the nerve to perform this block; the main reason to visualize it is so as to avoid inadvertently piercing it with the block needle (Fig. 67.8).

It is not essential to visualize the nerve to perform this block. An in-plane or out-of-plane needle approach may be used, although out-of-plane allows a more direct needle entry for a superficial nerve. The needle tip should be directed to either side of the artery, and local anesthetic should be injected to distend the plane in which the artery lies. 3 mL of local anesthetic is sufficient for a good block.

Superficial Peroneal (Fibular) Nerve

With the patient in the supine position, the knee is flexed and the hip rotated inward, to make the lateral aspect of the leg accessible. Alternatively, the patient is put in the lateral position with the procedure side on the non-dependent side. The probe is placed in a transverse orientation on the lateral aspect of the mid-leg above the subcutaneous part of the fibula (Fig. 67.9). The superficial peroneal nerve is visible as a small triangular hyperechoic structure in the intermuscular septum between the peroneus brevis and extensor digitorum longus muscles just deep to the crural fascia. Its identity can be confirmed by sliding the probe distally and observing the nerve rise through the crural fascia to eventually lie above it in a superficial location.

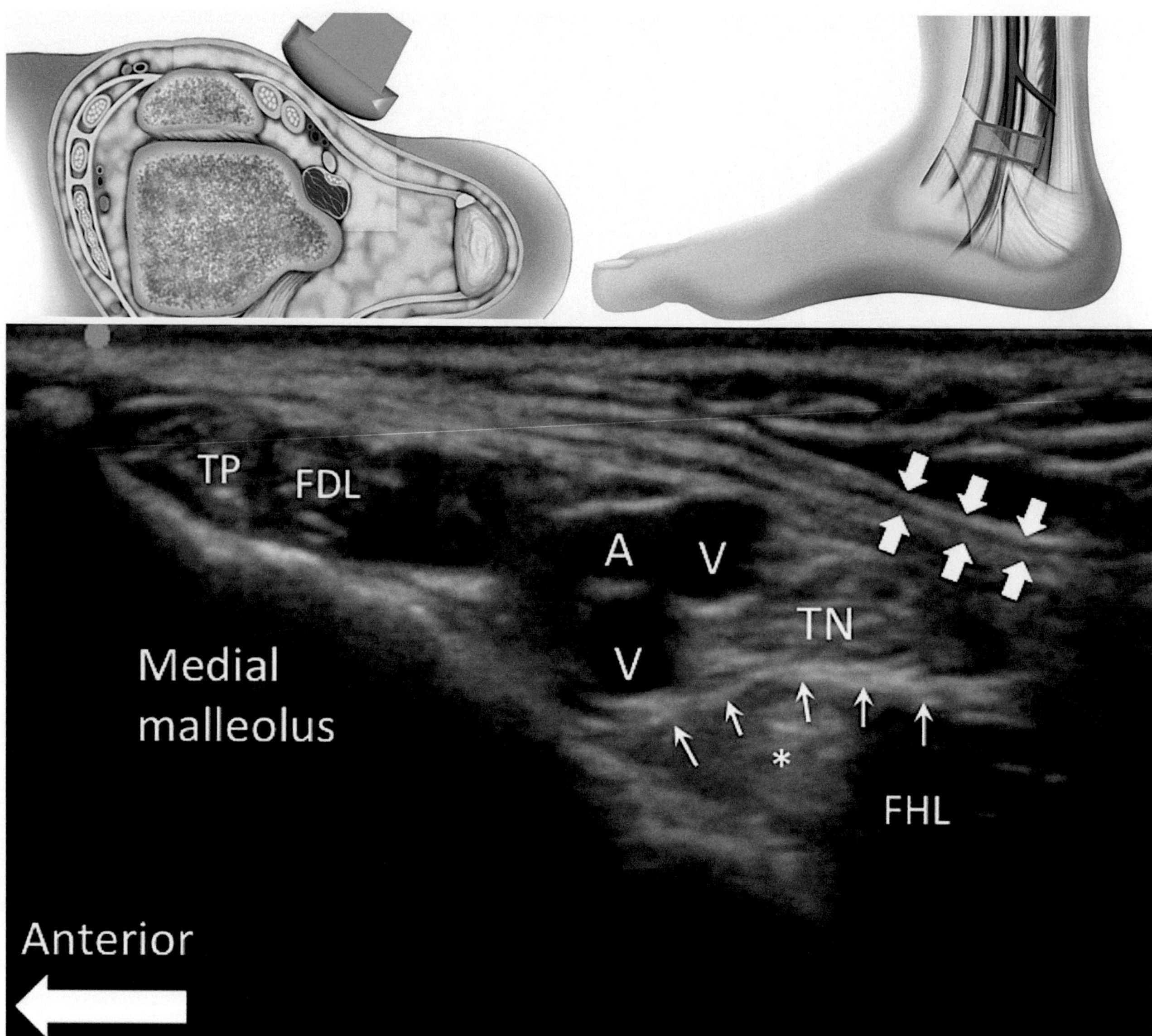

Fig. 67.5 Sonography of the tibial nerve at the level of medial malleolus. The ultrasound probe position is shown on the top left and right. The flexor retinaculum is indicated by the block arrows. From anterior to posterior, the structures are tibialis posterior tendon (TP), flexor digitorum longus tendon and muscle (FDL), posterior tibial artery (A) and veins (V), tibial nerve (TN), and flexor hallucis longus (FHL). Please note that the tibial nerve is usually seen resting on the fascia overlying FHL (line arrows). The tendon of the FHL (*) is deep to the fascia and should not be mistaken as the tibial nerve. Reproduced with permission from Philip Peng Educational Series

The nerve can be blocked where it lies above the crural fascia using either an in-plane or out-of-plane approach. In-plane approach is preferred as it allows easier entry into the narrow fascial plane. 5 mL of local anesthetic should be sufficient to establish a good block.

Sural Nerve

The patient is placed in lateral position with the knee flexed. The probe is placed in a transverse orientation across the groove between the lower fibula and Achilles tendon with minimal pressure to avoid compression of the lesser saphenous vein. Both the vein and the nerve are contained with the fascial plane between the peroneus tendon and Achilles tendon (Fig. 67.10). The sural nerve is a small hyperechoic round structure lying adjacent to the lesser saphenous vein in the same fascial subcutaneous plane.

The target is the fascia expansion between the between the fibula and Achilles tendon. If the nerve is not visible, local anesthetic may be injected around the vein. The nerve may be approached using an in-plane or out-of-plane technique, taking care not to pierce the nerve itself. 3 to 4 mL of local anesthetic is injected in the fascial plane of the nerve.

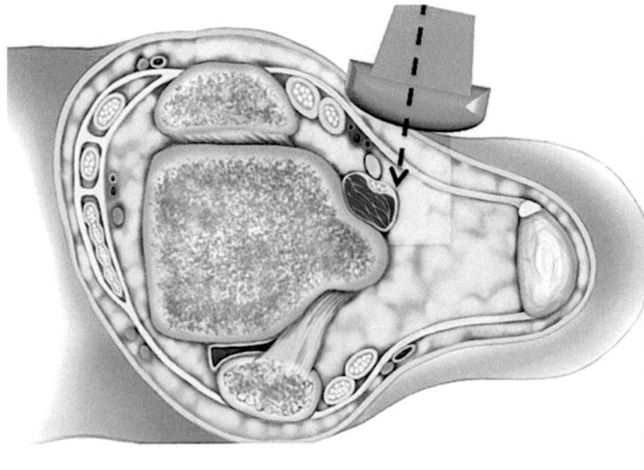

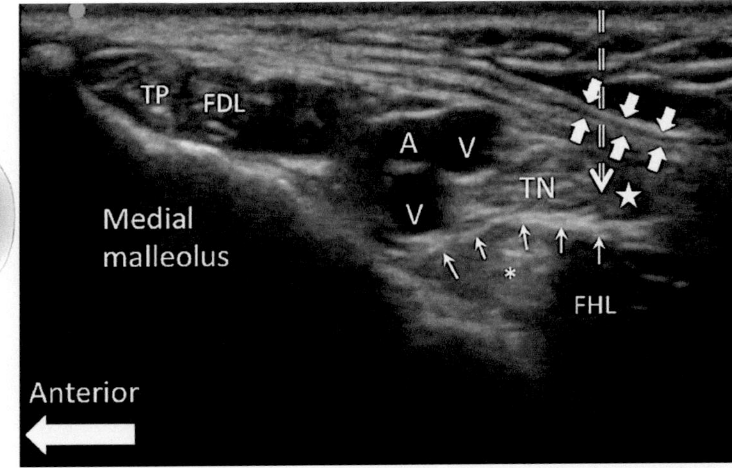

Fig. 67.6 Out-of-plane needle insertion for tibial nerve. The probe and needle insertion are shown in the left diagram. The trajectory of the needle is shown with dotted arrow to the target (star) formed between the flexor retinaculum and fascia over the flexor hallucis longus. Reproduced with permission from Philip Peng Educational Series

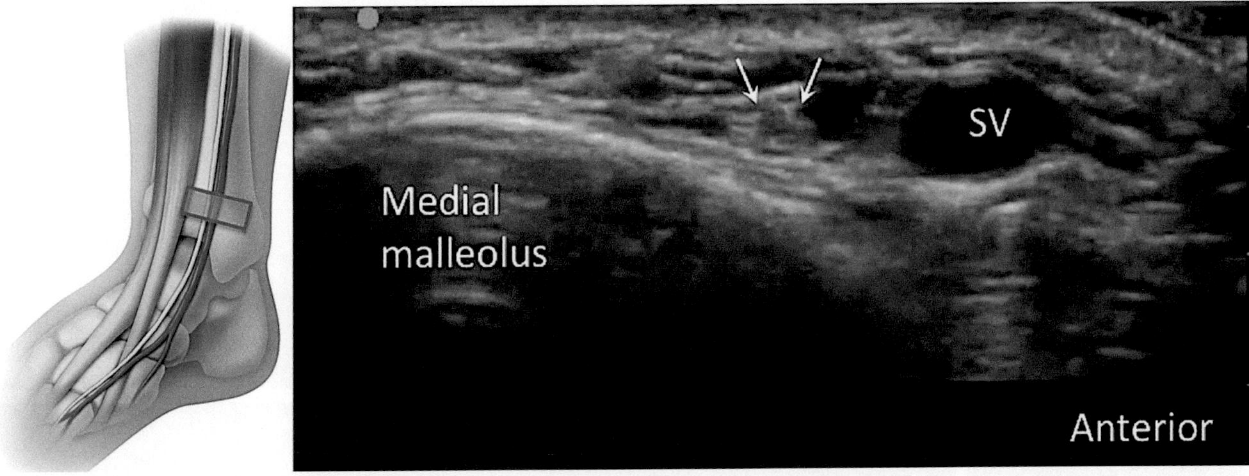

Fig. 67.7 Sonography of the saphenous nerve (line arrows). It lies within the same fascia plane with the greater saphenous vein. The ultrasound position is shown in the left diagram. Reproduced with permission from Philip Peng Educational Series

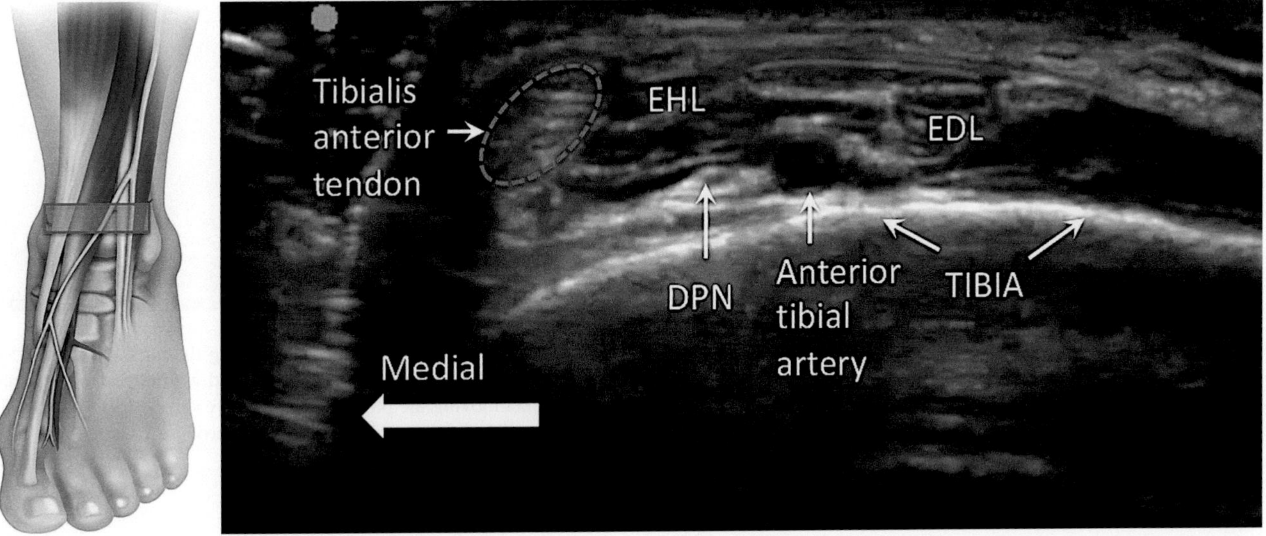

Fig. 67.8 Sonography of deep peroneal (fibula) nerve (DPN) at the low tibia area. The nerve is seen lateral to the anterior tibial (dorsalis pedis) artery which is deep to the extensor hallucis longus (EHL) and extensor digitorum longus (EDL). The ultrasound position is shown in the left diagram. Reproduced with permission from Philip Peng Educational Series

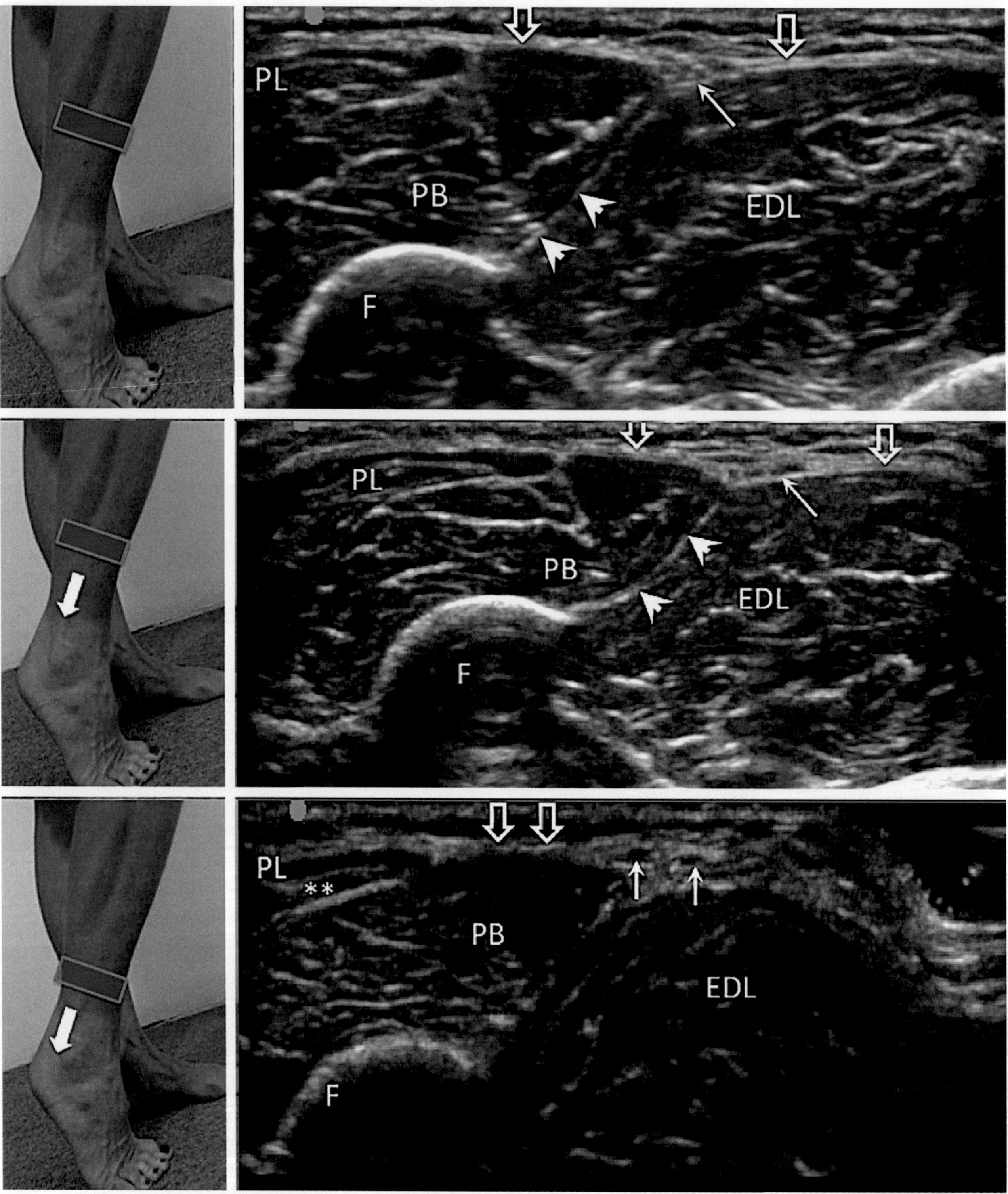

Fig. 67.9 Sonography of the superficial peroneal (fibula) nerve (SPN) at three different levels in the distal third of the leg. Upper panel at the level where the fibula (F) is covered by s longus (PB and PL), the SPN (line arrows) is seen in the intermuscular septum (arrowheads) between peroneus brevis and extensor digitorum longus (EDL) deep to the crural fascia (bold arrows). Middle panel advancing the ultrasound probe in the distal direction reveals the SPN embedded within the crural fascia. Lower panel moving the probe further distally shows the SPN superficial to the crural fascia. ** PL tendon. Reproduced with permission from Philip Peng Educational Series

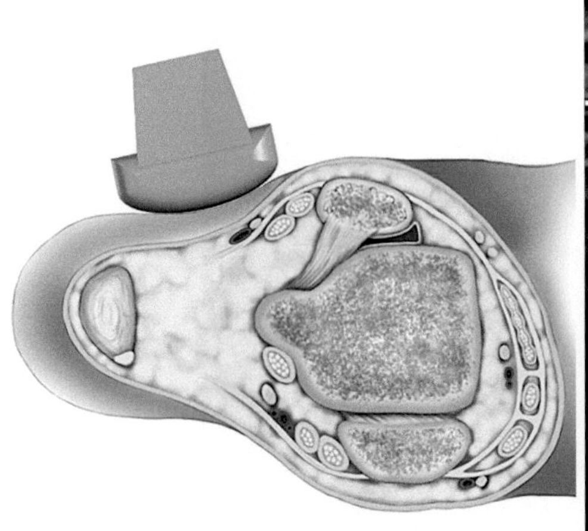

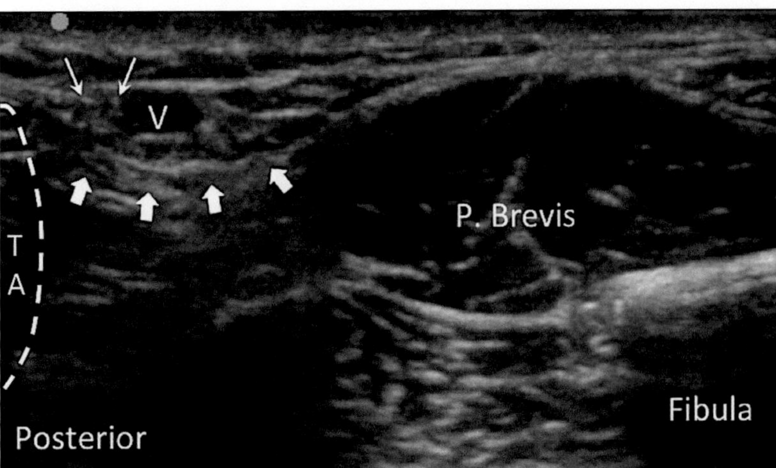

Fig. 67.10 Sonography of the sural nerve (indicated by line arrows). It is accompanied by the lesser saphenous vein, and both are located within the fascia plane (block arrows) between the peroneus brevis muscle and tendon Achilles (TA). The ultrasound position is shown in the left diagram. Reproduced with permission from Philip Peng Educational Series

Landmark-Guided Technique

Care must be taken to avoid nerve injury, as paresthesia is not available as a warning sign here.

Tibial Nerve

Patient is placed in prone, with a pillow under the ankle (or the patient may be seated or supine with the hip and knee externally rotated). The landmarks are medial malleolus and posterior tibial artery.

Lateral to the palpated pulse of the posterior tibial artery, a fine 25-G needle, 30 mm long, is introduced at a right angle to the posterior side of the tibia and just posterior to the posterior tibial artery. After paresthesia is elicited and after a negative aspiration test, 5 mL of local anesthetic is injected. If paresthesia cannot be elicited, then after reaching the posterior tibia, the needle is withdrawn for about 1 cm, and 5–10 mL of local anesthetic is injected (Figs. 67.1, 67.11, and 67.12).

Another technique is to carry out perpendicular puncture of the skin at the level of the medial malleolus, dorsal, and then ventral to the posterior tibial artery and to distribute the total dose of local anesthetic in two equal halves on each side.

Deep Peroneal Nerve

The patient is either placed in supine or sitting position, and the landmarks are the dorsalis pedis artery and proximal back of the foot.

A fine 25-G injection needle, 30 mm long, is introduced perpendicular to the skin surface; 5 mL of the local anesthetic is injected on each side, first lateral to the artery and then medial to it (Figs. 67.4 and 67.13).

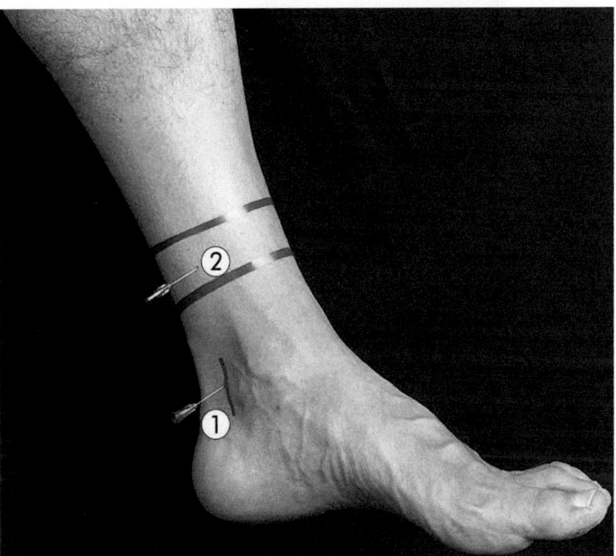

Fig. 67.11 Tibial nerve (1) (red needle) and posterior tibial artery (red), (2) saphenous nerve (black needle). Reprinted with permission from Danilo Jankovic

Sural Nerve and Superficial Peroneal Nerve

The patient is placed in supine or sitting position, and the landmark is lateral malleolus. About 10 cm above the lateral malleolus, parallel to the upper ankle, fan-shaped subcutaneous infiltration of the Achilles tendon is carried out as far as the edge of the tibia, using about 10 mL of local anesthetic (Figs. 67.4, 67.12 and 67.14).

Saphenous Nerve

The patient is placed in supine or sitting position, and the landmark is medial malleolus. About 10 cm above the medial malleolus, 5–10 mL of local anesthetic is injected subcutane-

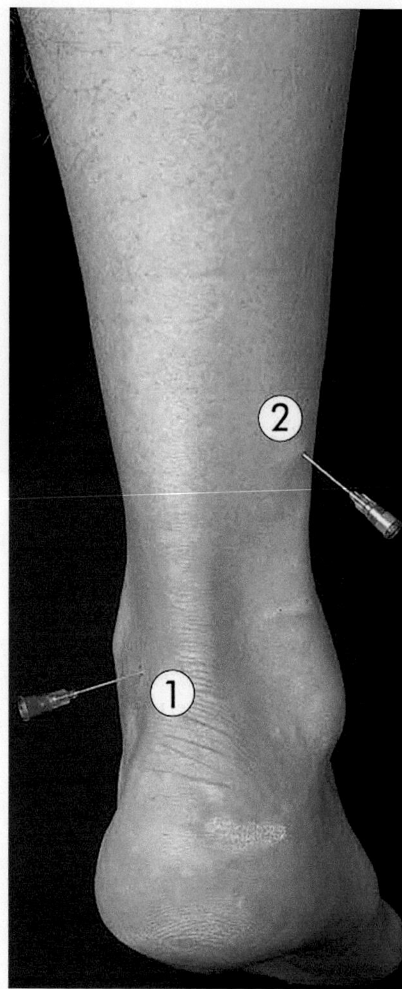

Fig. 67.12 Tibial nerve (1) (red needle) and (2) sural nerve (green needle). Reprinted with permission from Danilo Jankovic

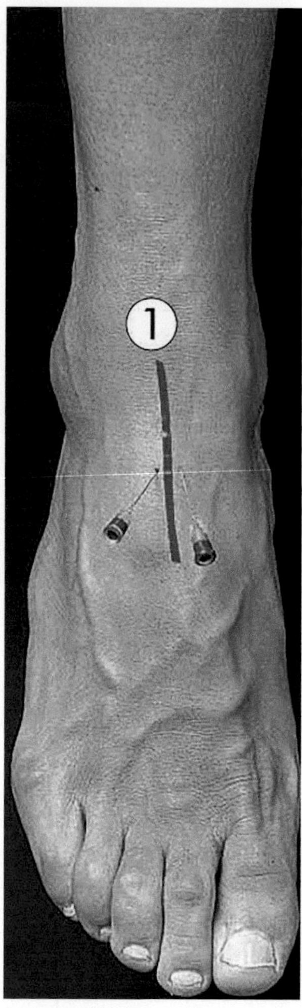

Fig. 67.13 Deep peroneal (fibular) nerve. (1) Dorsalis pedis artery. Reprinted with permission from Danilo Jankovic

ously around the long saphenous vein and, in a fan-shaped fashion, in a mediolateral direction (Fig. 67.11). The cutaneous innervation areas of the individual nerves are shown in Fig. 67.15.

Practical Tips

When performing the ankle block, always consider performing blockade of tibial nerve first as it is the biggest nerve and requires longer time for the onset of full block.

When scanning the block of superficial peroneal nerve, start from high when the nerve is deep to the crural fascia, and observe the movement of the nerve emerging superficial to the crural fascia. The nerve in the latter site may be difficult to see because it is smaller and hypoechoic.

Both deep peroneal and saphenous nerves may be difficult to visualize. However, pay attention to the fascial plane that defines the vessel, and deposit the local anesthetic within that plane.

For sural nerve, it is consistently found within the fascial expansion between the peroneus and Achilles tendons.

Literature Review

Hallux valgus repair or bunion surgery is a commonly performed foot surgery and is associated with moderate to severe pain. Ankle nerve block is commonly performed for this procedure. A recent systematic review using the PROcedure SPECific Postoperative Pain ManagemenT (PROSPECT) methodology showed that a few interventions improved postoperative pain control, including the use of pharmacologic measures: paracetamol, nonsteroidal anti-inflammatory drugs, or cyclooxygenase-2 selective inhibitors, or systemic steroids. They also found that ankle

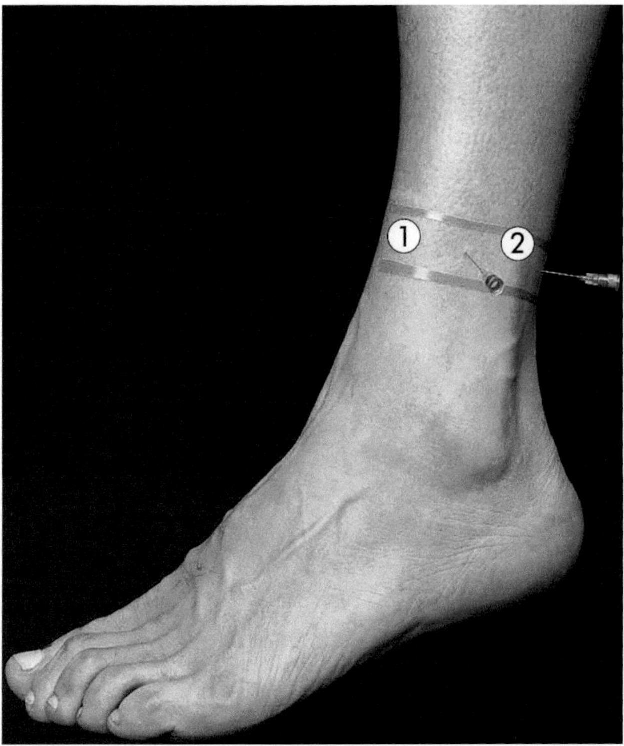

Fig. 67.14 (1) Superficial peroneal (fibular) nerve (blue needle) and (2) sural nerve (green needle). Reprinted with permission from Danilo Jankovic

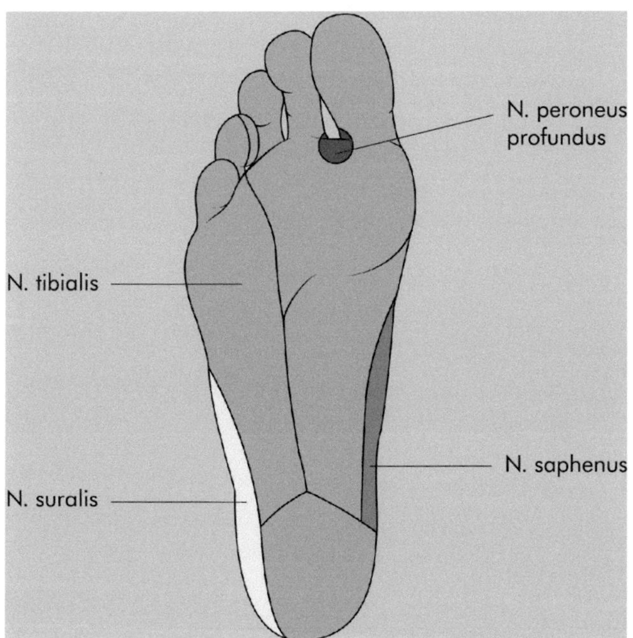

Fig. 67.15 Cutaneous innervation areas in the region of the sole of the foot. Reprinted with permission from Danilo Jankovic

block and local anesthetic wound infiltration also improved postoperative pain.

Ankle nerve block was originally described by Braun, Pauchet, and Sourdat back in 1914. The procedure typically involved blocking all five ankle nerves with landmark guidance. Since the first description of ultrasound-guided ankle nerve block by Fredrickson in 2009, a few randomized trials examined the accuracy and superiority of the use of ultrasound guidance. These studies supported the improved success rates in tibial nerve and sural nerve with ultrasound guidance. However, the success rates were equivalent for the deep peroneal nerve. Some investigators questioned the necessity of blocking saphenous nerve in bunion surgery as they showed that the saphenous nerve did not supply beyond the first tarsometatarsal joint in 97% of the patients, and for the rest of the patients, the surgical anesthesia was simply supplemented by local infiltration. For the superficial peroneal nerve, the anatomy can be complicated, and the sonoanatomy was recently described and had been discussed in detail in this chapter. A large retrospective review by Chin et al. concluded that US-guided ankle blocks (primarily involving US-guided tibial and deep peroneal nerve blocks) resulted in statistically and clinically significant higher success rates and less conversion to unplanned general anesthesia. The use of US and the total amount of local anesthetic were the only two variables predictive of a successful surgical block.

Suggested Reading

Antonakakis JG, Scalzo DC, Jorgenson AS, Figg KK, Ting P, Zuo Z, Sites BD. Ultrasound does not improve the success rate of a deep peroneal nerve block at the ankle. Reg Anesth Pain Med. 2010;35:217–21.

Canella C, Demondion X, Guillin R, Boutry N, Peltier J, Cotten A. Anatomic study of the superficial peroneal nerve using sonography. AJR Am J Roentgenol. 2009;193:174–9.

Chin KJ. Ultrasound visualization of the superficial peroneal nerve in the mid-calf. Anesthesiology. 2013;118(4):956–65.

Chin KJ, Wong NW, Macfarlane AJ, Chan VW. Ultrasound-guided versus anatomic landmark-guided ankle blocks: a 6-year retrospective review. Reg Anesth Pain Med. 2011;36(6):611–8.

Fredrickson MJ, White R, Danesh-Clough TK. Low-volume ultrasound-guided nerve block provides inferior postoperative analgesia compared to a higher-volume landmark technique. Reg Anesth Pain Med. 2011;36:393–8.

Hoerster W. Blockaden peripherer Nerven im Bereich des Kniegelenkes; Blockaden im Bereich des Fußgelenkes. In: Hoerster W, Kreuscher H, Niesel HC, editors. Regionalanaesthesie. Fischer Verlag Stuttgart; 1981. p. 124–399.

Husni A, Chin KJ. Ankle. In: Peng PWH, editor. Ultrasound for pain medicine intervention. A practical guide. Volume 1. Peripheral structures. Philip Peng educational series. 1st ed. iBook, CA: Apple Inc.; 2013. p. 74–88.

Jankovic D. Blocking peripheral nerves in the ankle joint region. In: Jankovic D, editor. Regional nerve blocks & infiltration therapy. Textbook and color atlas. 3rd ed. Blackwell; 2004. p. 254–8.

Kofoed H. Peripheral nerve blocks at the knee and ankle in operations for common foot disorders. Clin Orthop. 1982;168:97–101.

Lopez AM, Sala-Blanch X, Magaldi M, Poggio D, Asuncion J, Franco CD. Ultrasound-guided ankle block for forefoot surgery: the contribution of the saphenous nerve. Reg Anesth Pain Med. 2012;37:554–7.

Redborg KE, Antonakakis JG, Beach ML, Chinn CD, Sites BD. Ultrasound improves the success rate of a tibial nerve block at the ankle. Reg Anesth Pain Med. 2009a;34:256–60.

Redborg KE, Sites BD, Chinn CD, Gallagher JD, Ball PA, Antonakakis JG, Beach ML. Ultrasound improves the success rate of a sural nerve block at the ankle. Reg Anesth Pain Med. 2009b;34:24–8.

Snaith R, Dolan J. Ultrasound-guided superficial peroneal nerve block for foot surgery. AJR Am J Roentgenol. 2010;194:W538; author reply W42.

Ankle Joint Injection

68

Philip Peng

Contents

General Consideration

Foot and ankle pain is a common complaint in the primary care practice. The prevalence of ankle pain is estimated as 11.7% in the community setting and symptomatic ankle osteoarthritis proven by radiographic imaging 3.4%. Tibiotalar and subtalar osteoarthritis are the two common causes of foot and ankle pain, and trauma is a common etiology for the joint arthritis.

Indications and Contraindications

The main indication is osteoarthritis, especially post-traumatic. Arthrosis of the ankle joint is rare in the absence of a causative factor (e.g., fracture, instability, or posture-related joint strain). The patient reports local pain and swelling in the ankle region. The examination reveals capsular-pattern movement restriction, with plantar flexion more severely restricted than dorsal flexion. Contraindications are similar to other joint injections, such as infection in the skin around the joint area and in patients who are taking anticoagulants.

Anatomy

The bones of the foot are divided into the tarsus, metatarsus, and toes (Fig. 68.1a, b). The tarsus consists of seven bones (tarsal bones): the talus, calcaneus, navicular, and cuboid bones and three cuneiform bones. The metatarsus consists of the five metatarsal bones. The toes are formed by the phalanges. A distinction is made in the foot joints between the upper ankle joint (the talocrural joint) and the lower ankle joint (subtalar and talocalcaneonavicular joints) (Fig. 68.2).

The joint surfaces of the talocrural joint are formed by the malleolar mortise (mortise joint) at the trochlea of the talus, with its superior facet and medial and lateral malleolar facets. The ligaments of the upper ankle joint are the medial collateral ligament (deltoid ligament), anterior talofibular ligament, posterior talofibular ligament, and calcaneofibular ligament (Figs. 68.3 and 68.4a, b).

P. Peng (✉)
Department of Anesthesia and Pain Medicine, University of Toronto, Toronto Western Hospital, Toronto, ON, Canada
e-mail: philip.peng@uhn.ca

D. Jankovic, P. Peng (eds.), *Regional Nerve Blocks in Anesthesia and Pain Therapy*,
https://doi.org/10.1007/978-3-030-88727-8_68

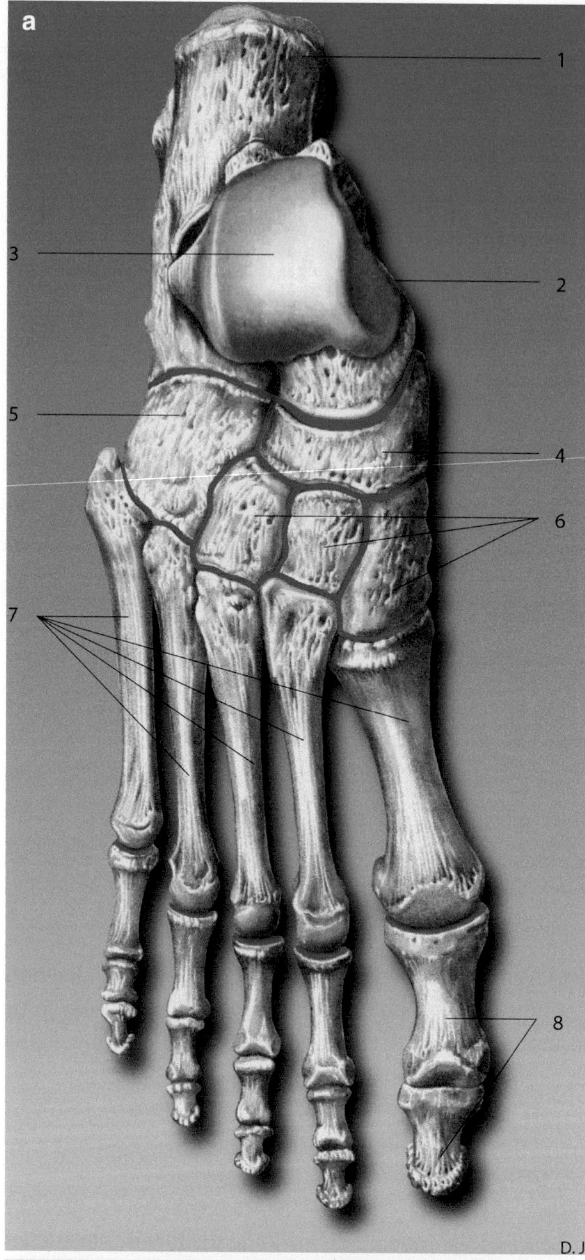

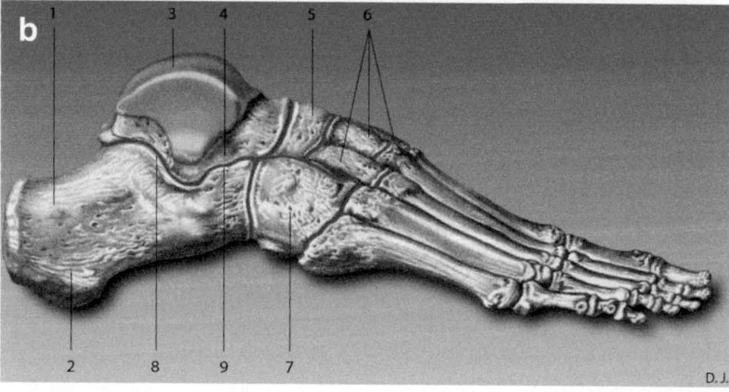

Fig. 68.1 (**a**) Foot skeleton. Dorsal view. (1) Calcaneus, (2) talus, (3) Trochlea tali, (4) navicular bone, (5) cuboid bone, (6) cuneiform bone, (7) metatarsal bones, (8) phalanges. Reproduced with permission from Danilo Jankovic. (**b**) Foot skeleton. Lateral view. (1) Calcaneus, (2) tuber calcaneus, (3) talus, (4) sinus tarsi, (5) navicular bone, (6) cuneiform bones, (7) cuboid bone, (8) subtalar joint, (9) talocalcaneonavicular joint. Reproduced with permission from Danilo Jankovic

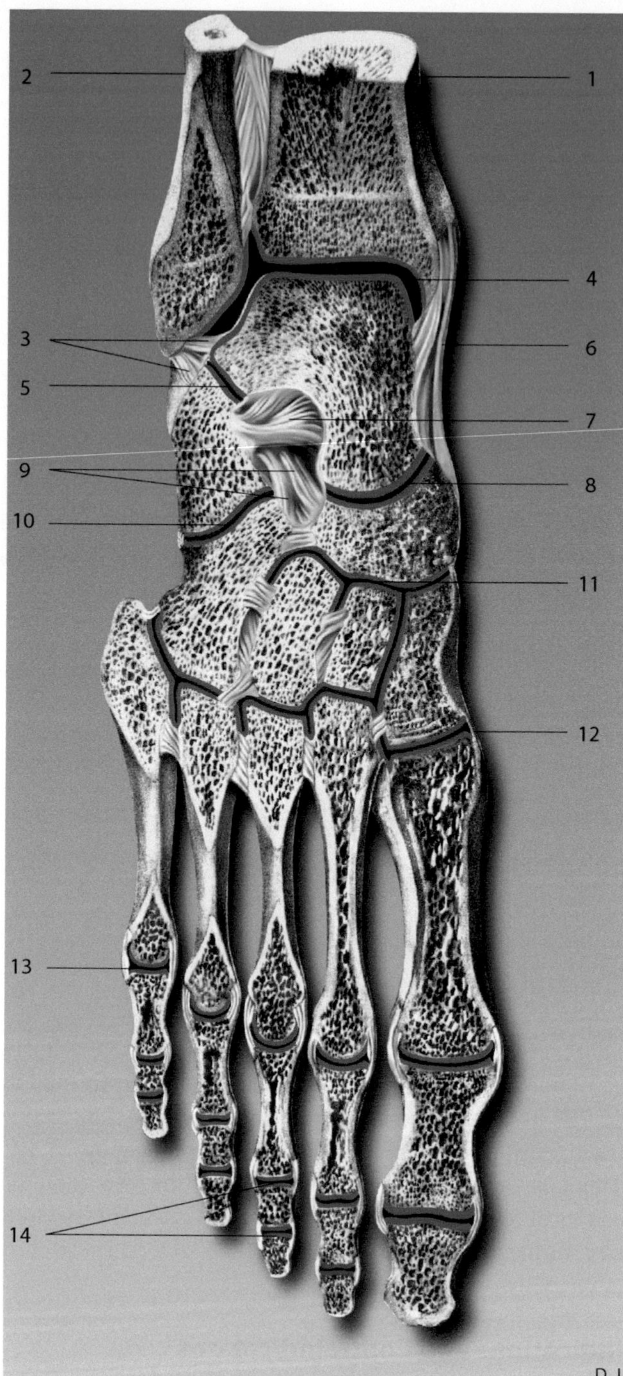

Fig. 68.2 (1) Tibia, (2) Fibula, (3) posterior talofibular ligament, (4) talocrural joint, (5) subtalar joint, (6) deltoid ligament, (7) talocalcaneus ligament, (8) talonavicular ligament, (9) bifurcated ligament, (10) calcaneocuboid ligament, (11) cuneonavicular ligament, (12) tarsometatarsal ligament, (13) metatarsophalangeal ligament, (14) articulationes digiti. Reproduced with permission from Danilo Jankovic

The lower ankle joint consists of two separate joints—the subtalar joint, which forms the posterior part of the lower ankle joint, and the talocalcaneonavicular joint, which forms the anterior part of it. These two separate joints act together. The joint surfaces in the subtalar joint are formed by the talus and calcaneus (Figs. 68.3 and 68.4a, b).

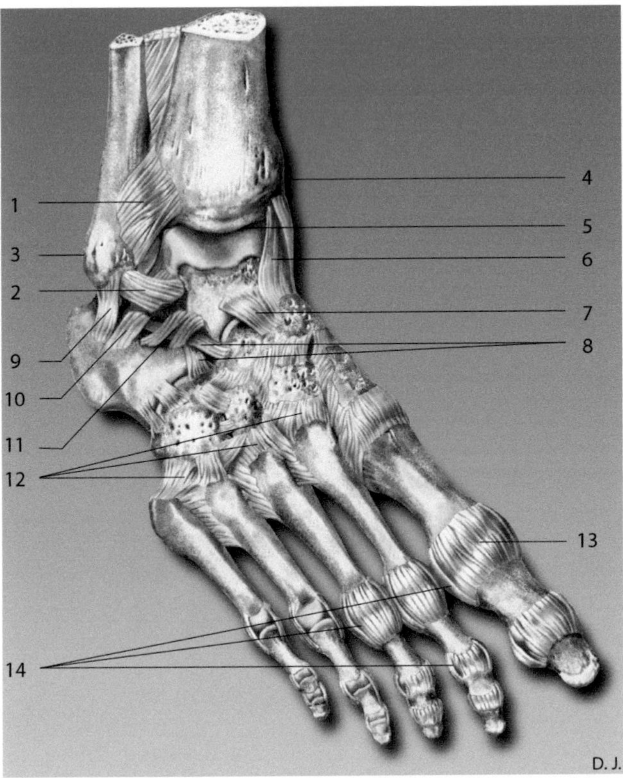

Fig. 68.3 Foot joints. Lateral view. (1) Anterior tibiofibular joint, (2) anterior talofibular ligament, (3) lateral malleolus, (4) medial malleolus, (5) talocrural joint, (6) deltoid ligament (medial collateral ligament), (7) talonavicular ligament, (8) bifurcated ligament, (9) calcaneofibular ligament, (10) talocalcanean ligament, (11) interosseous talocalcanean ligament, (12) dorsal tarsometatarsal ligaments, (13) articular capsule, (14) collateral ligaments. Reproduced with permission from Danilo Jankovic

The vascular supply to the ankle is from branches of the posterior tibial artery (the medial and lateral plantar arteries) and from the anterior tibial artery (the dorsalis pedis artery). The ankle is innervated from the tibial nerve (lateral and medial plantar nerves and calcaneal branches) and from the deep fibular (peroneal) nerve (Fig. 68.5a–c).

Technique

Tibiotalar or Talocrural Joint Injection

For tibiotalar or talocrural joint, the target is the anterior tibiotalar recess between the tibialis anterior tendon and medial malleolus (Fig. 68.6). The patient is placed in supine position with the knee flexed 90 degrees and the foot flat on the table or in semi-recumbent with the ankle in a plantar-flexed position. A linear (8–12 MHz) ultrasound probe is placed over the tibialis anterior tendon first. The fat pad in the anterior recess of the tibiotalar joint is revealed (Fig. 68.7).

Both in-plane and out-of-plane techniques have been described. For out-of-plane technique, ultrasound probe is placed over the tibialis anterior tendon, and a 1.5-inch 25G needle is inserted medial to the tibialis anterior tendon into the anterior recess. The injectate should be seen spread deep to the fat fad. In the presence of joint effusion, one should consider a larger-gauge needle for aspiration. A total volume of 3–5 mL of injectate is sufficient, either a mixture of local anesthetic with steroid (2% lidocaine and 40 mg Depo-Medrol) or a commercially available hyaluronic acid solution (Fig. 68.8). For in-plane technique, the ultrasound probe is first placed over the tibialis anterior tendon first. The probe is then moved slightly in medial direction to reveal the anterior joint recess. A 3.5-inch 22G needle is inserted in-plane deep to the fat pad (Fig. 68.9).

Subtalar Joint

For subtalar joint, the joint space can be revealed with either medial or lateral approach. The author-preferred approach is the lateral approach. The patient is placed in lateral position (injection side as non-dependent side), and a small pillow is placed on the medial aspect of ankle. A linear (8–12 MHz) ultrasound probe is placed anterior to lateral malleolus right on sinus tarsi (Fig. 68.10). The probe is then moved and tilted in posterior direction to reveal the subtalar joint (Fig. 68.11).

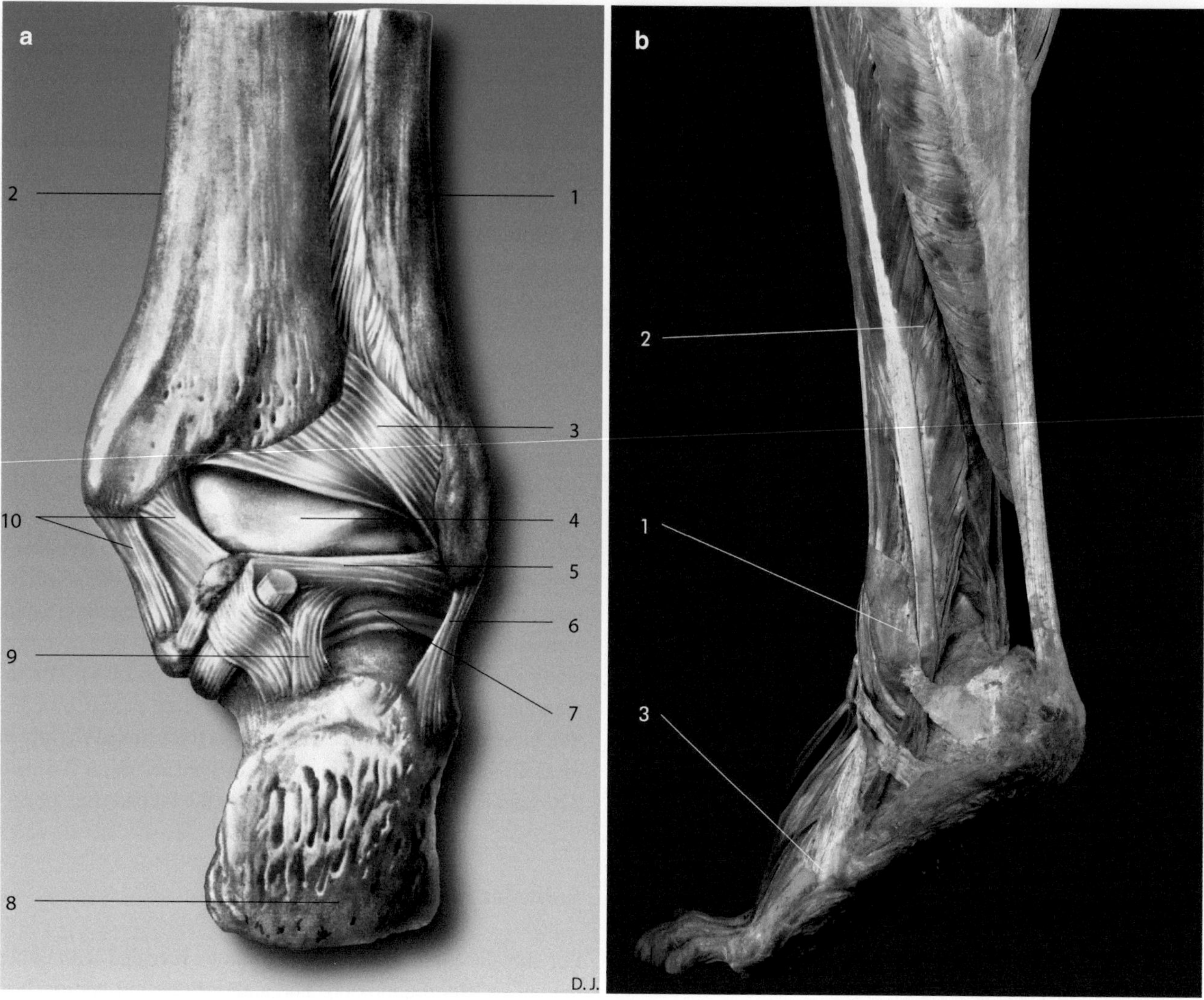

Fig. 68.4 (**a**) A Foot joints. Dorsal view. (1) Fibula, (2) tibia, (3) posterior tibiofibular ligament, (4) talus, (5) posterior talofibular ligament, (6) calcaneofibular ligament, (7) subtalar joint, (8) calcaneus,(9) posterior talocalcaneal joint, (10) deltoid ligament, Reproduced with permission from Danilo Jankovic. (**b**) Ankle joint. Lateral view. (1) Lateral malleolus, (2) peroneal muscles, (3) tuberosity of the metatarsal bone with tendon of the peroneus brevis and tertius muscle. Reproduced with permission from Danilo Jankovic

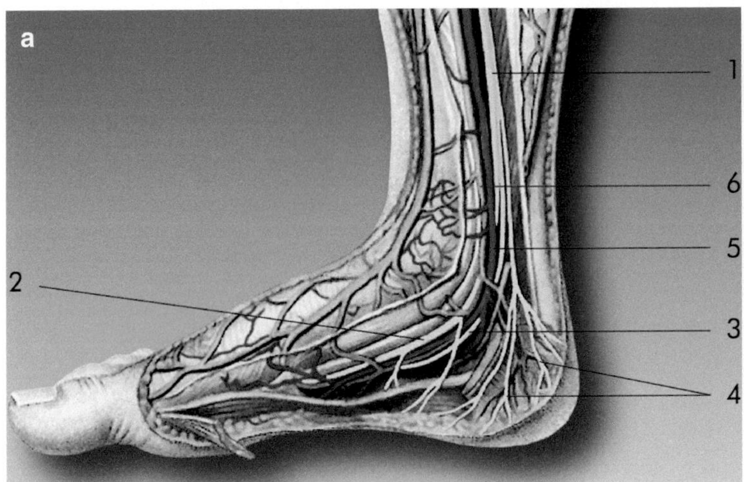

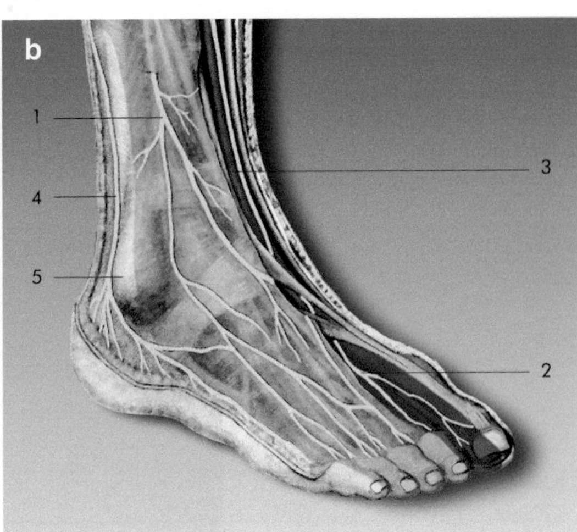

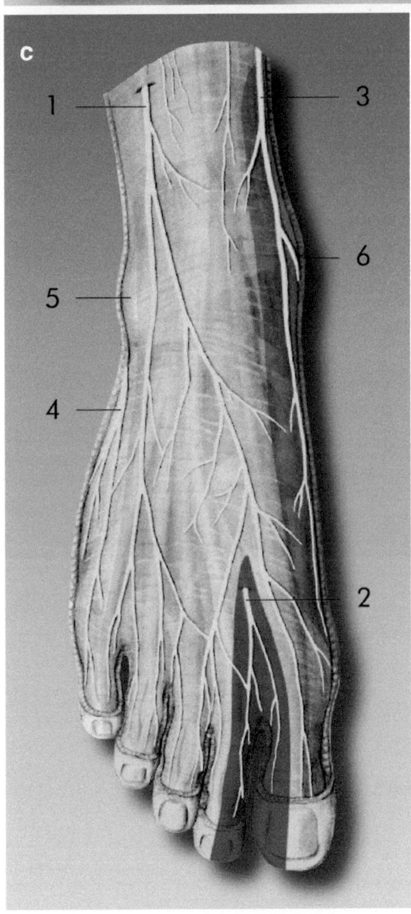

Fig. 68.5 (**a**) Foot. Vascular supply and Innervation. (1) Tibial nerve, (2) medial plantar nerve, (3) lateral plantar nerve, (4) calcaneal branches, (5) posterior tibial artery, (6) posterior tibial vein. Reproduced with permission from Danilo Jankovic. (**b**) Cutaneous innervation areas of the back of the foot. Lateral view. (1) Superficial peroneal (fibular) nerve, (2) deep peroneal (fibular) nerve, (3) anterior tibial artery, (4) sural nerve, (5) lateral malleolus. Reproduced with permission from Danilo Jankovic. (**c**) Cutaneous innervation areas in the region of the back of the foot (from the front). Superficial peroneal (fibular) nerve, (2) deep peroneal (fibular) nerve, (3) saphenous nerve, (4) sural nerve, (5) lateral malleolus, (6) medial malleolus. Reproduced with permission from Danilo Jankovic

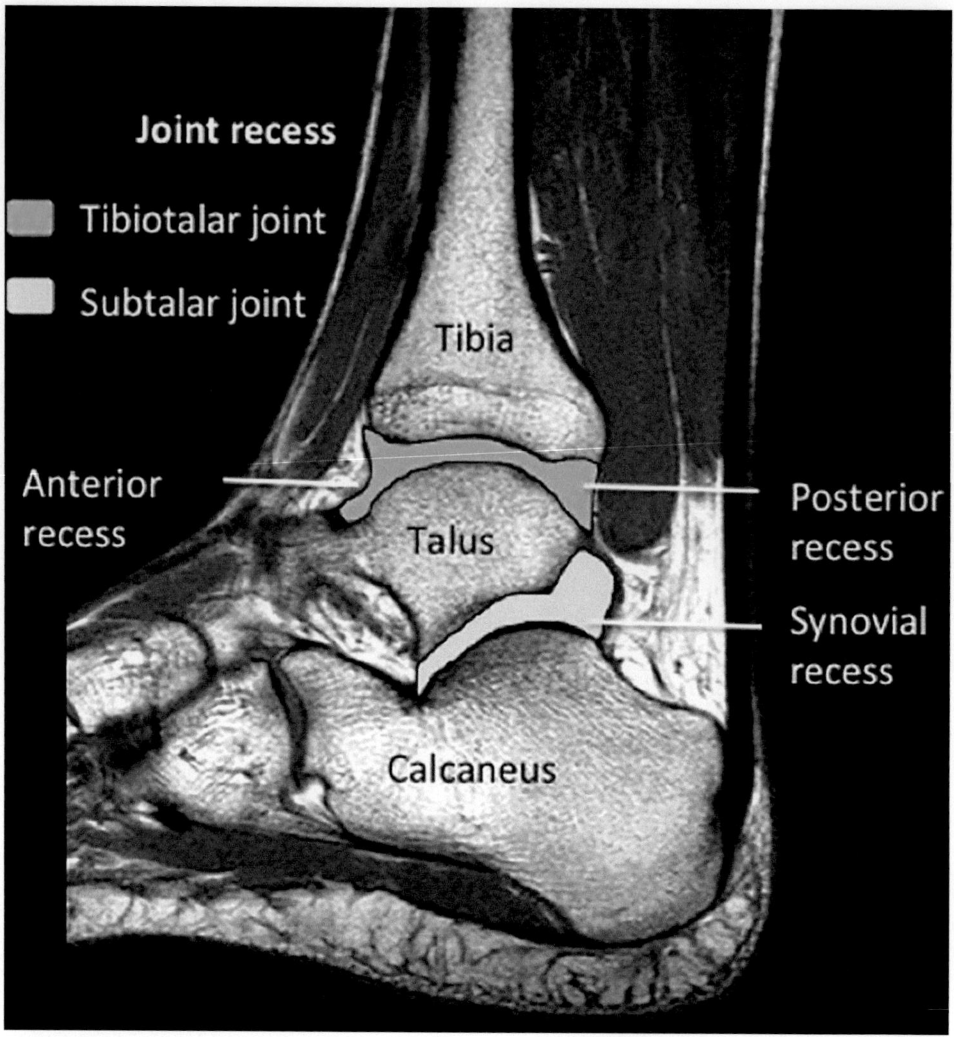

Fig. 68.6 Joint recess for tibiotalar joint and subtalar joint. Reproduced with permission from Philip Peng Educational Series

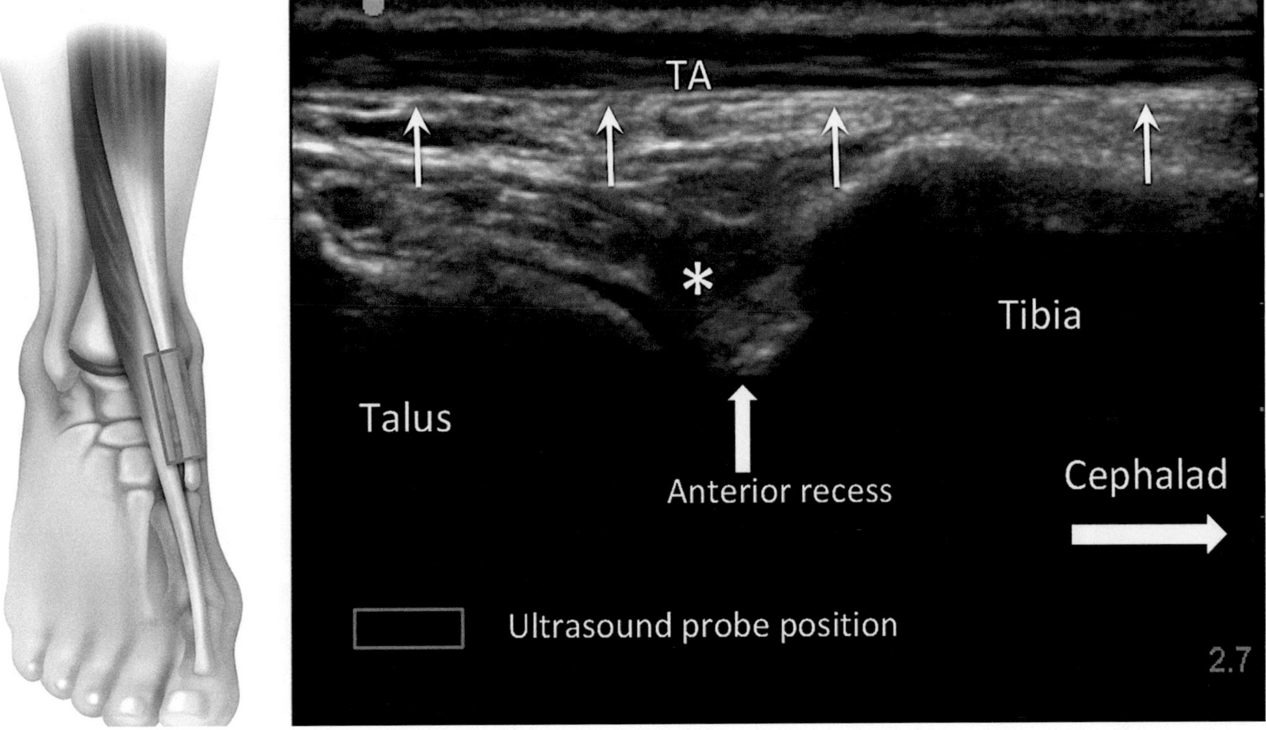

Fig. 68.7 Sonogram of the anterior aspect of tibiotalar joint. The inserts on the left side show the position of the ultrasound probe (orange rectangle). Reproduced with permission from Philip Peng Educational Series

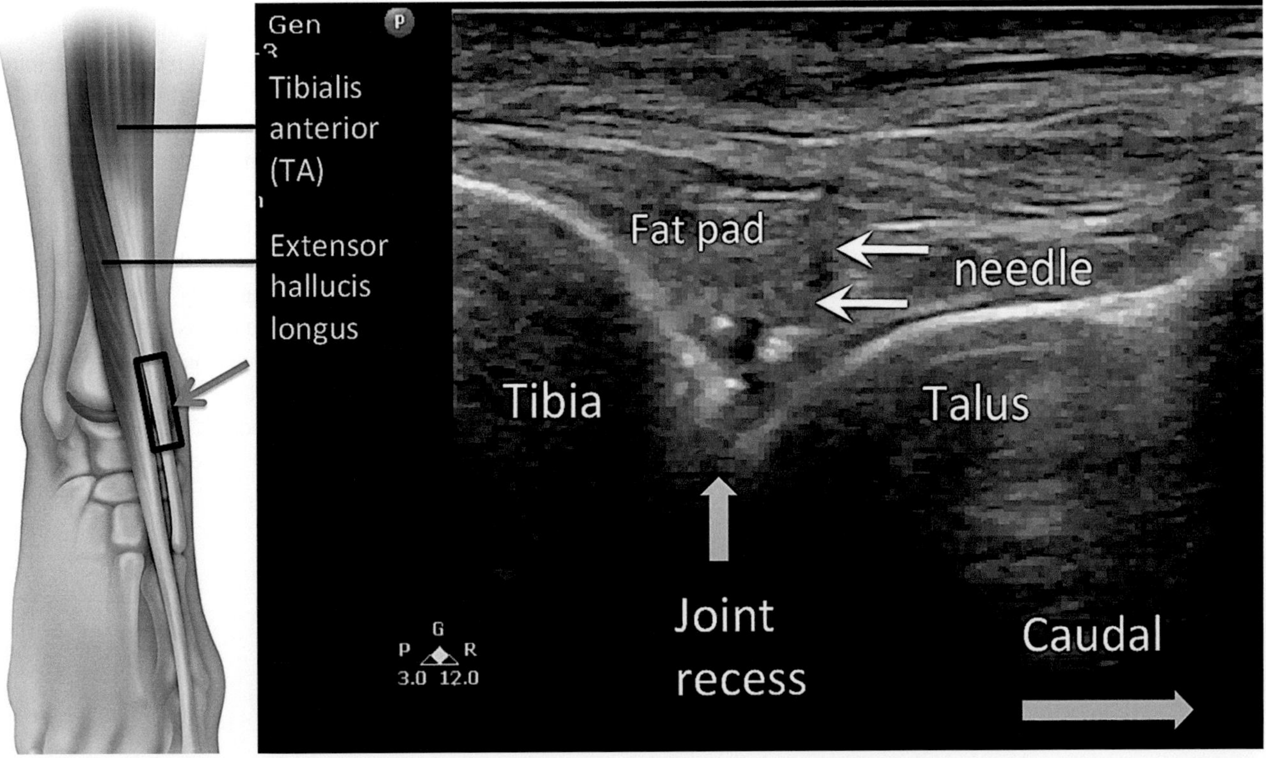

Fig. 68.8 Sonogram shows out-of-plane needle insertion for tibiotalar joint. The line arrows indicate the needle path. The insert shows the anatomy and the ultrasound probe position. Reproduced with permission from Philip Peng Educational Series

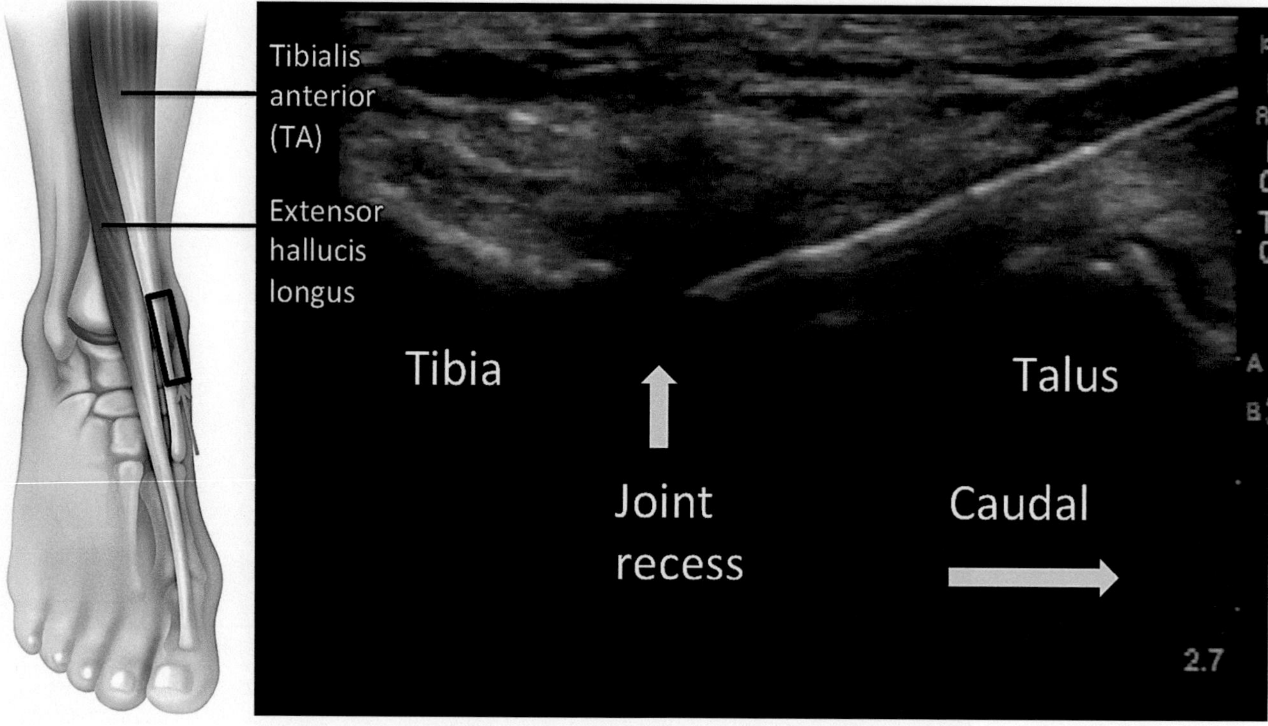

Fig. 68.9 Sonogram shows in-plane needle insertion for tibiotalar joint. The insert shows the anatomy and the ultrasound probe position. Reproduced with permission from Philip Peng Educational Series

Once the subtalar joint is visualized, a 1.5-inch 25G needle is inserted out-of-plane from posterior to anterior direction (Fig. 68.12). A total volume of 1–2 mL of either a mixture of local anesthetic with steroid (2% lidocaine and 20 mg Depo-Medrol) or a commercially available hyaluronic acid solution is sufficient.

Complications

- Infection (prophylaxis: extremely strict asepsis).
- Injury to cartilage or bone.
- A temporary increase in pain may occur in approximately 25% of patients (who should be informed about this).
- Hematoma formation.

Practical Tips

Upon injection into the tibiotalar joint, the injectate should be seen deep to the fat pad. If not, the needle tip is not in the joint.

When performing out-of-plane injection for tibiotalar joint, the needle advancement may be stopped by the initial bony contact. A simple jiggling movement of the needle allows the needle to be advanced deeper into the joint.

For a small subtalar joint which is very superficial, one of the tricks is to allow easy insertion of the needle initially under the probe (the needle orientation is almost tangential to the skin). To facilitate this, a generous amount of gel is placed under the probe. With this arrangement, the needle can be moved until it is seen right over the joint entrance. Once it is over the entrance, the needle is then pulled back so that the tip is directed into the joint space.

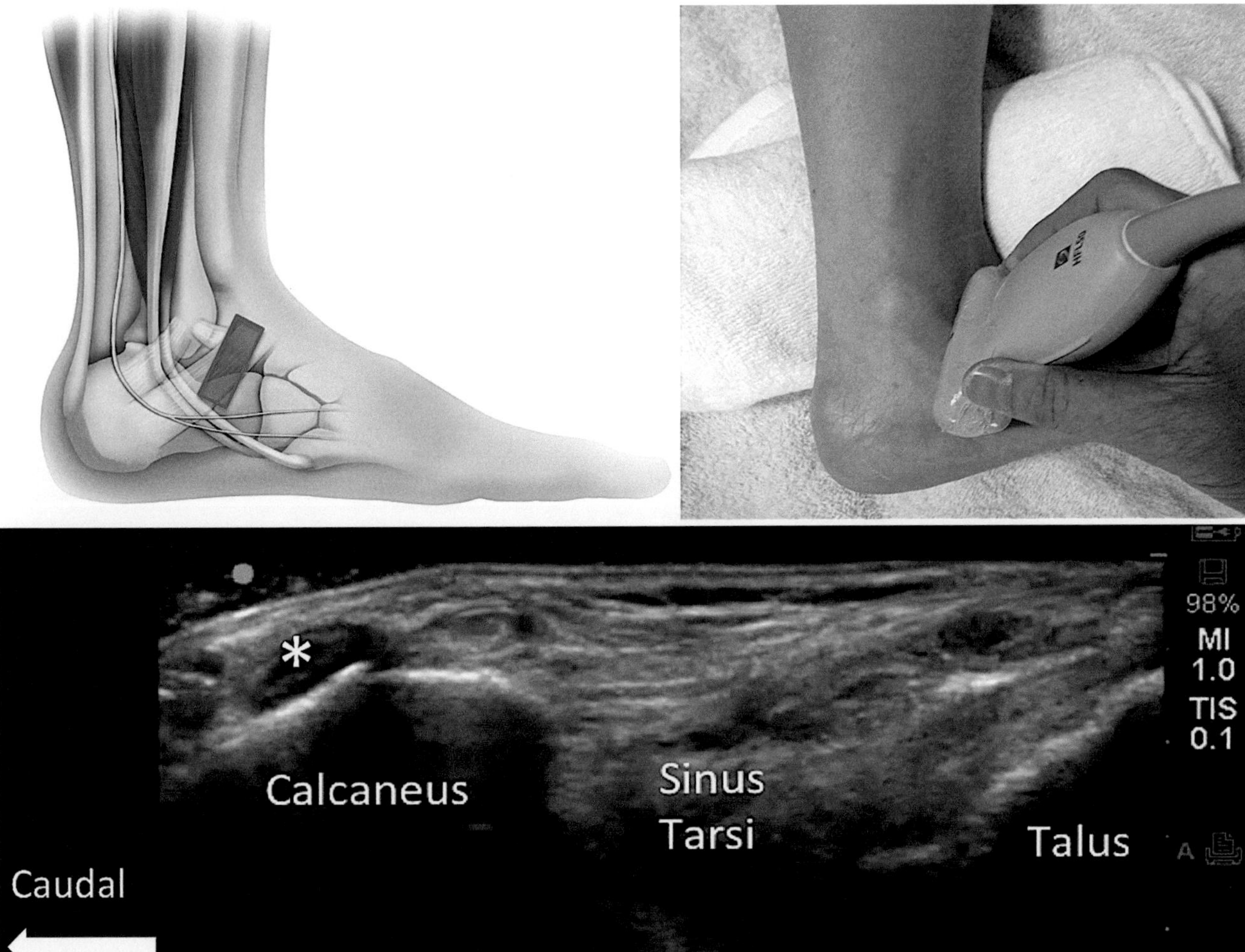

Fig. 68.10 Top two figures showed the position of the foot and probe. A small towel roll is placed on the medial aspect of the ankle to allow inversion of the joint. The lower figure is the sonogram of sinus tarsi. * The peroneus tendon. Reproduced with permission from Philip Peng Educational Series

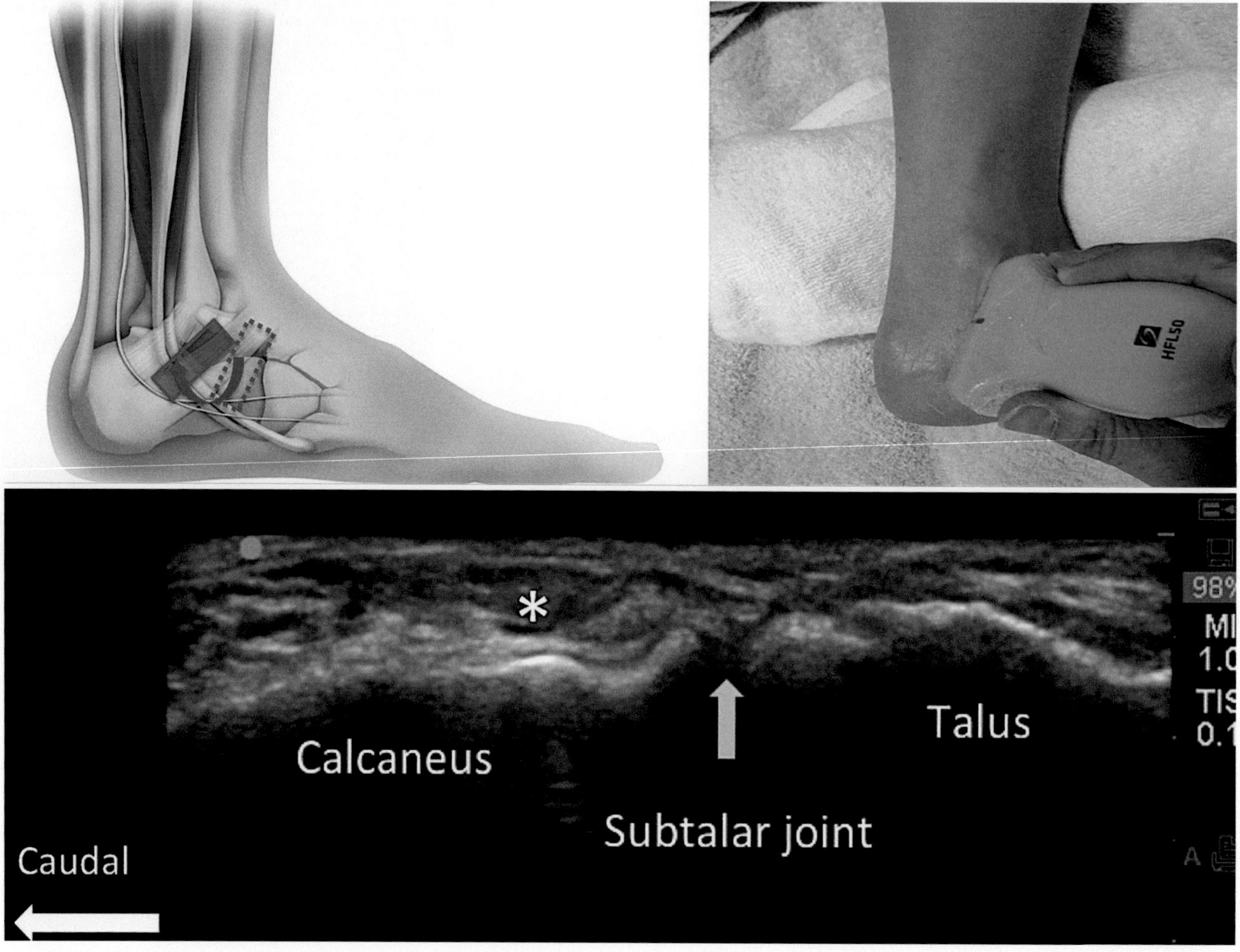

Fig. 68.11 Sonogram of the lateral aspect of posterior subtalar joint. The top two figures showed the position of the ultrasound probe. The probe position is similar to that of sinus tarsi but moved and tilted toward the lateral malleolus. * The peroneus tendon. Reproduced with permission from Philip Peng Educational Series

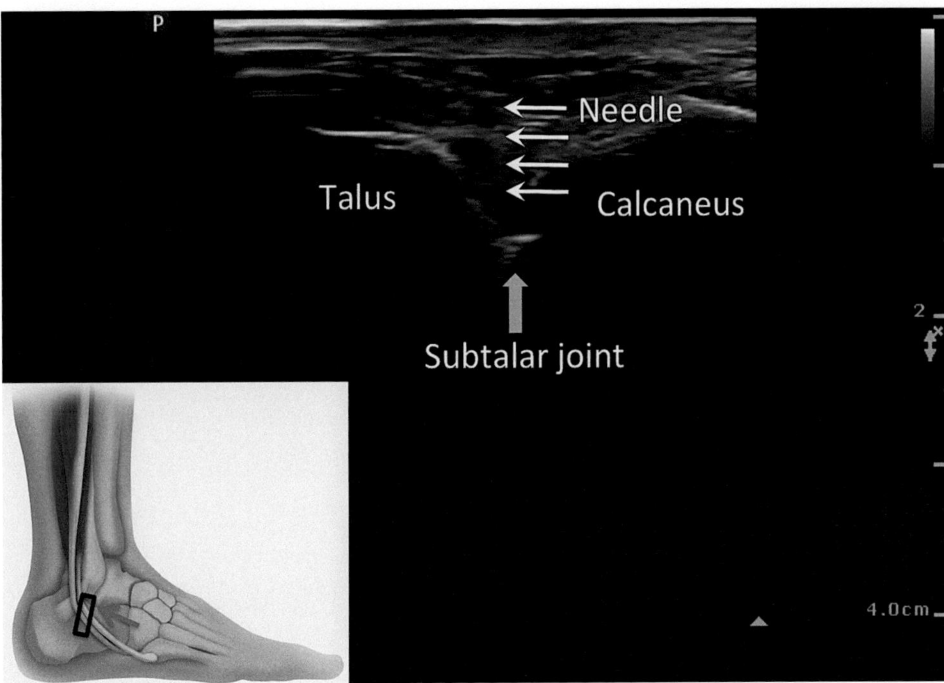

Fig. 68.12 Sonogram shows out-of-plane needle insertion for subtalar joint. The insert shows the anatomy and the ultrasound probe position. The line arrows indicate the needle path. Reproduced with permission from Philip Peng Educational Series

Literature

Ultrasound guidance is a validated technique for tibiotalar and subtalar joint injections. Studies have shown 100% accuracy rates when ultrasound guidance is used for tibiotalar joint injections. Accuracy rates for subtalar joint injections also approach 100%. Due to the anatomy of the subtalar joint, extravasation of the injectate to surrounding structures occurs in approximately 20% of injections. Rates of extravasation to areas such as the subtalar joint and peroneal tendons are similar between ultrasound and other injection techniques such as fluoroscopy and anatomic guidance. Foot and ankle joint injections with local anesthetic and steroid can be valuable for diagnostic purposes. Literature generally supports the correlation between response to local anesthetic and steroid and good surgical outcome. From a therapeutic standpoint, a limited number of studies demonstrate short-term benefit with foot and ankle injections with local anesthetic and steroid. Viscosupplementation is another viable option for ankle joint injections. A recent meta-analysis concluded that viscosupplementation for ankle arthritis can significantly reduce pain and is likely superior to reference therapy; however, the number of studies is limited. Larger good quality randomized studies are required to assess longer-term efficacy of foot and ankle injections.

Suggested Reading

Chang KV, Hsiao MY, Chen WS, Wang TG, Chien KL. Effectiveness of intra-articular hyaluronic acid for ankle osteoarthritis treatment: a systematic review and meta-analysis. Arch Phys Med Rehabil. 2013;94:951–60.

Cunnington J, Marshall N, Hide G, Bracewell C, Isaacs J, Platt P, Kane D. A randomized, double-blind, controlled study of ultrasound-guided corticosteroid injection into the joint of patients with inflammatory arthritis. Arthritis Rheum. 2010;62(7):1862–9.

Gilliland CA, Salazar LD, Borchers JR. Ultrasound versus anatomic guidance for intra-articular and periarticular injection: a systematic review. Phys Sportsmed. 2011;39:121–13.

Khosla S, Thiele R, Baumhauer JF. Ultrasound guidance for intra-articular injections of the foot and ankle. Foot Ankle Int. 2009;30:886–90.

Khoury NJ, el-Khoury GY, Saltzman CL, Brandser EA. Intraarticular foot and ankle injections to identify source of pain before arthrodesis. AJR Am J Roentgenol. 1996;167:669–73.

Lucas PE, Hurwitz SR, Kaplan PA, Dussault RG, Maurer EJ. Fluoroscopically guided injections into the foot and ankle: localization of the source of pain as a guide to treatment—prospective study. Radiology. 1997;204:411–5.

Newman JS. Diagnostic and therapeutic injections of the foot and ankle. Semin Roentgenol. 2004;39:85–94.

Papaliodis DN, Vanushkina MA, Richardson NG, DiPreta JA. The foot and ankle examination. Med Clin North Am. 2014;98:181–204.

Reach JS, Easley ME, Chuckpaiwong B, Nunley JA 2nd. Accuracy of ultrasound guided injections in the foot and ankle. Foot Ankle Int. 2009;30:239–42.

Smith J, Finnoff JT, Henning PT, Turner NS. Accuracy of sonographically guided posterior subtalar joint injections: comparison of 3 techniques. J Ultrasound Med. 2009;28:1549–57.

Smith J, Maida E, Murthy NS, Kissin EY, Jacobson JA. Sonographically guided posterior subtalar joint injections via the sinus tarsi approach. J Ultrasound Med. 2015;34:83–93.

Soneji N, Peng P. Ultrasound-guided interventional procedures in pain medicine: a review of anatomy, sonoanaotmy and procedures. Part VI: ankle joint. Reg Anesth Pain Med. 2016;41:99–116.

Thomas MJ, Roddy E, Zhang W, Menz HB, Hannan MT, Peat GM. The population prevalence of foot and ankle pain in middle and old age: a systematic review. Pain. 2011;152:2870–80.

Ward ST, Williams PL, Purkayastha S. Intra-articular corticosteroid injections in the foot and ankle: a prospective 1-year follow-up investigation. J Foot Ankle Surg. 2008;47:138–44.

Wisniewski SJ, Smith J, Patterson DG, Carmichael SW, Pawlina W. Ultrasound-guided versus nonguided tibiotalar joint and sinus tarsi injections: a cadaveric study. PM R. 2010;2:277–81.

MTP Joint and Morton's Neuroma

69

David A. Spinner and Erica R. Eldon

Contents

First Metatarsophalangeal Joint (MTPJ)

General Consideration

The first metatarsophalangeal joint (MTPJ) is a common source of medial forefoot pain. Differential diagnosis includes arthritis (osteoarthritis, rheumatoid, and psoriatic), gout (podagra), MTP joint sprain (turf toe) in athletes, sesamoiditis, fracture, infection, and EHL tendon rupture. The diagnosis is clinical and based largely on history and physical exam. When comorbidities such as diabetes are present, infection and osteomyelitis should be ruled out with imaging. Conservative management includes rest, ice, compression, elevation (RICE), activity modification, and in some cases immobilization. When pain persists despite conservative management, ultrasound-guided injection into the MTP joint with corticosteroids or hyaluronic acid can provide symptom relief and has been shown to be both practical and accurate.

D. A. Spinner (✉)
Rehabilitation and Human Performance, Mount Sinai, New York, NY, USA
e-mail: David.spinner@mountsinai.org

E. R. Eldon
Rehabilitation and Human Performance, Icahn School of Medicine at Mount Sinai, New York, NY, USA
e-mail: erica.eldon@mountsinai.org

Indication

Persistent pain in the area of the MTP joint despite conservative management and negative evaluation of other etiologies.

Functional Anatomy

The first MTP joint is a synovial joint comprised of the first metatarsal proximally, the proximal phalanx of the

D. Jankovic, P. Peng (eds.), *Regional Nerve Blocks in Anesthesia and Pain Therapy*,
https://doi.org/10.1007/978-3-030-88727-8_69

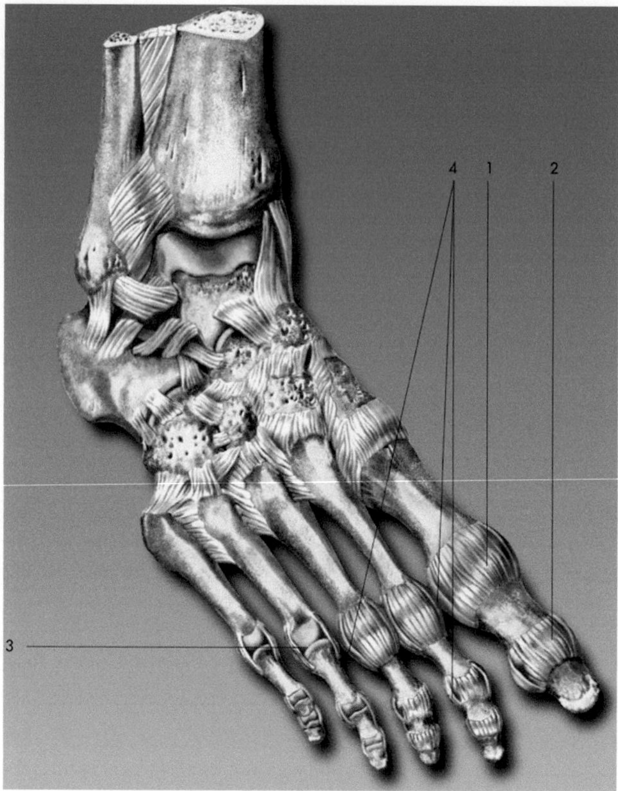

Fig. 69.1 (1) Joint capsule of the metatarsophalangeal joint, (2) capsule of interphalangeal joint of the first digit, (3) metatarsophalangeal joint, (4) collateral ligaments. Reproduced with permission from Dr. Danilo Jankovic

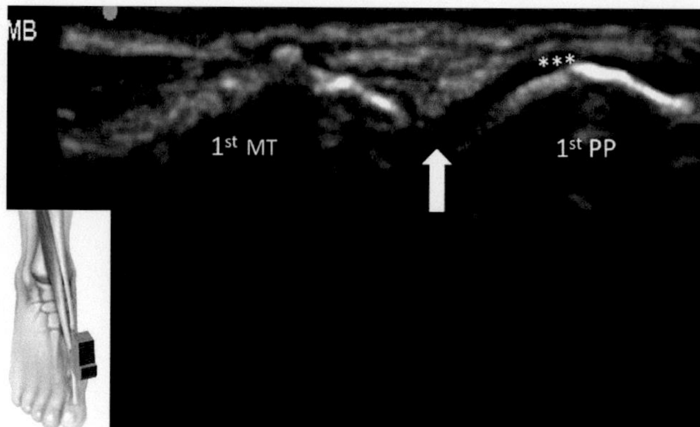

Fig. 69.2 Sonography of the long-axis view of the first metatarsophalangeal joint (MTPJ). The ultrasound probe position was indicated in the insert in the left lower corner. The MTPJ was indicated by the bold arrow. first PP first proximal phalanx; first MT first metatarsal; ** metatarsophalangeal joint recess. Reproduced with permission from Philip Peng Educational Series

hallux distally, and two sesamoids (medial and lateral) that are located within the fibrous plantar pad. Medial collateral and lateral collateral ligaments reinforce the joint capsule (Fig. 69.1). The extensor hallucis longus tendon makes up the dorsal aspect of the joint, inserts onto the base of the proximal phalanx, and contributes to extensor motion of the MTP joint. The proper digital nerves and arteries run along the medial and lateral aspects of the joint.

Technique

Preparation

To prepare for the procedure, an ultrasound machine with a small footprint linear array "hockey stick" transducer (18 MHz) or medium frequency linear array transducer is needed. In addition, the equipment required for the procedure are 22G–25G 1.5-inch needle, 1–3 mL local anesthetic, and 0.5 mL corticosteroid.

With patient supine and leg flexed so the foot rests flat on the table with the forefoot hanging over the edge, use the small footprint linear array transducer, and place the probe in the sagittal plane over the EHL tendon as it crosses the MTP joint. The MTP joint can be readily identified (Fig. 69.2).

Injection: In-Plane Gel-Standoff Approach

Use copious sterile gel between the transducer and the skin to allow for gel standoff technique (Fig. 69.3). Identify the proximal phalanx, metatarsal, and EHL tendon. Traction and flexion of the proximal phalanx will open up the dorsal MTP joint space. Move the probe just medially off the EHL tendon, and center the joint space in view. Advance the needle through the gel parallel to the transducer using the in-plane approach, from distal to proximal, and enter the skin just distal to the joint using a superficial angle (Fig. 69.3). When the needle tip is visualized directly in the joint capsule, before reaching the metatarsal, inject 0.5 mL of corticosteroid under direct visualization.

Injection: Short-Axis Out-of-Plane Approach

With patient supine and leg flexed so the foot rests flat on the table. A small footprint linear array transducer is placed in the sagittal plane across the MTP joint. Use a small quantity of sterile gel. Identify the two ends of the joint articulation. Line a small needle up in the center of the probe at a 45–75° angle directed toward the center of the joint. Once under the joint capsule, the needle does not needle to be advanced further. The needle will appear as a hyperechoic dot.

Complications

Careful to avoid extravasation of steroids into the surrounding soft tissue. Too much volume will pressurize the joint and cause more pain.

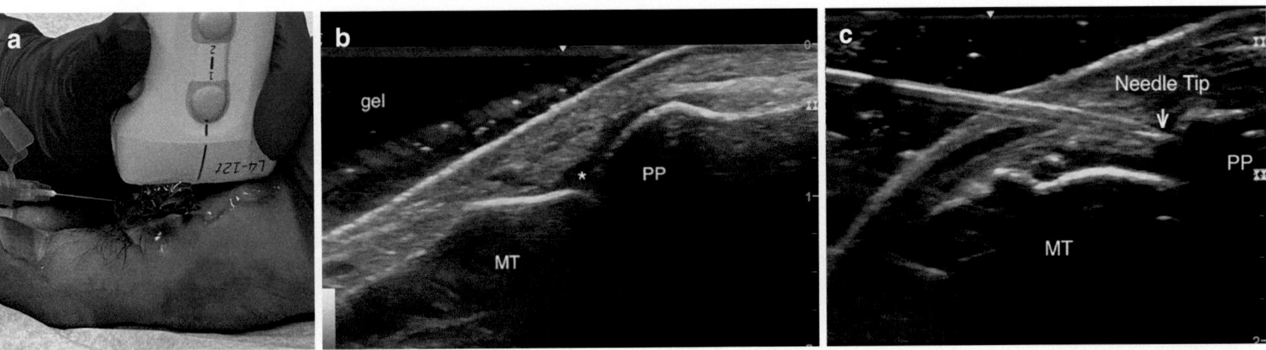

Fig. 69.3 (**a**) Probe placement over the MTP joint with in-plane gel standoff injection technique. (**b**) Long-axis view of MTP joint. (**c**) Needle placement in joint capsule. *MT* metatarsal, *PP* proximal phalanx, * joint capsule and needle target

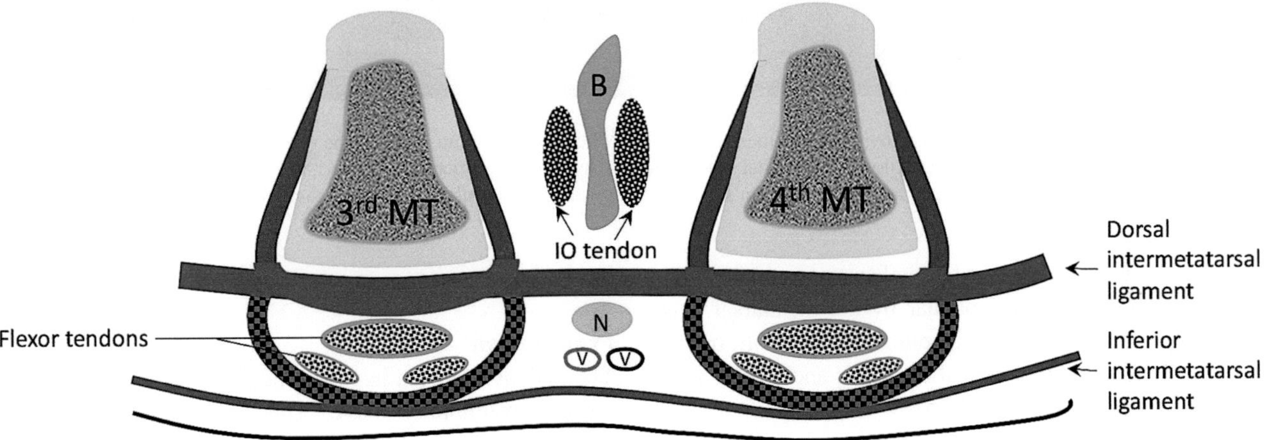

Fig. 69.4 Schematic diagram of the cross-section view of the metatarsophalangeal joint. IO tendon-interosseous tendon, MT metatarsal bone, N digital nerve, V vessels, B- synovial intermetatarsal bursa. Reprinted with permission from Philip Peng Educational Series

Practical Tips

Use the small footprint and high-frequency linear array transducer for better visualization for superficial structures. Gentle traction and flexion of the proximal phalanx open the dorsal joint space.

Literature Review

Palpation-guided MTP joint aspiration has been shown to be inaccurate, while ultrasound-guided joint aspiration has 97% accuracy and 100% accuracy for MTP joint injection. In addition to injection with corticosteroids, an increase in the use of viscosupplementation and biologic injectables has contributed to reports of platelet-rich plasma (PRP) and autologous conditioned plasma (ACP) for the treatment of orthopedic conditions, including MTP joint pain due to turf toe in athletes. However, literature review is currently limited to case reports.

Morton's Neuroma

General

Morton's neuroma (MN), also known as interdigital neuroma or interdigital nerve compression syndrome, is a common source of forefoot pain. Pain is commonly described as gradual onset of shooting pain and/or paresthesias in the digits, cramping, and a sensation of walking on a lump in the forefoot that progressively worsens and is relieved with removal of shoes and with massage. Morton's neuroma is a misnomer since it is not a true neuroma. Compression of the digital branch of the medial plantar nerve, most commonly distal to the deep transverse metatarsal ligament in the third web space, followed by the second web space, leads to non-neoplastic enlargement of the nerve, axonal degeneration, edema, and fibrous proliferation in the endoneurium (Fig. 69.4). MN is caused by nerve entrapment or trauma. Provocative tests include Mulder's sign, where medial to lateral compression of the forefoot with simultaneous dorsal to

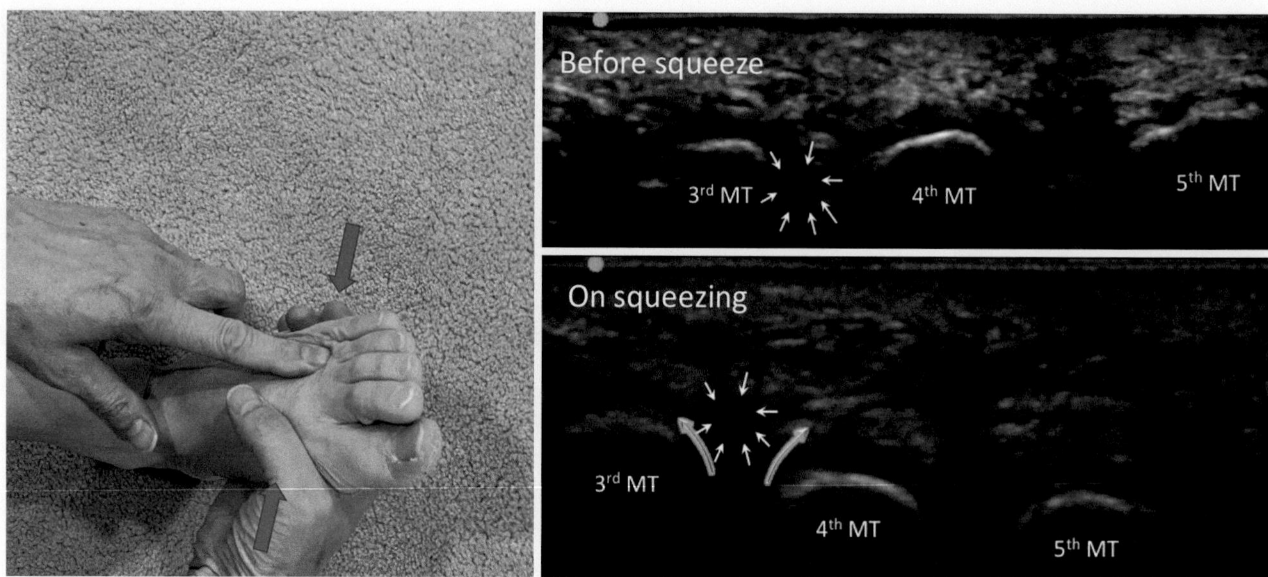

Fig. 69.5 Mulder sign. This is performed by squeezing the metatarsals together while applying pressure from the dorsal interdigital space. The right panel shows the sonographic appearance of the Morton's neuroma when applying ultrasound on the plantar side. The neuroma appears as a hypoechoic structure (arrows). MT metatarsal. Reprinted with permission from Philip Peng Educational Series

plantar pressure over the third digital space results in a click as the neuroma is pushed plantar by the metatarsal heads (Fig. 69.5). Ultrasound visualization of the neuroma can assist in confirming the clinical diagnosis and is 91% sensitive and 100% specific (Fig. 69.5).

Indications

Corticosteroid injection, alcohol ablation, cryoablation, or radiofrequency ablation (RFA) of MN should be considered in patients who have confirmed Morton's neuroma based on history, physical exam, and diagnostic studies, who have failed conservative therapy. Conservative therapy includes wearing footwear with a wide toe box and use of tarsal pads.

Functional Anatomy

MN is most commonly found in the third interdigital web space distal to the deep or inferior transverse metatarsal ligament (Fig. 69.4). There is a communicating branch of the lateral plantar nerve that joins the third common digital branch of the medial plantar nerve as it enters the third web space where it divides into the proper digital branches. There are small digital arteries within each web space.

Technique

Preparation

The patient is placed in supine position with the leg resting on the examination table. The following equipment is required: high-frequency linear array transducer, 25G 1.5-inch needle, 2–4 mL local anesthetic, 0.5 mL corticosteroid, or 0.5–1 mL alcohol for neurolysis (50–70% alcohol mixed with local anesthetic).

Ultrasound-Guided Injection

A medium-frequency linear transducer is placed on the plantar side of the foot over the metatarsophalangeal joint (Fig. 69.6). The depth of the metatarsal and proximal phalanx is measured. The probe is moved laterally to the interdigital space, and the neuroma should be revealed at the similar depth. The neuroma appears as a non-compressible hypoechoic mass. If the hypoechoic mass is compressible, it is likely to be a bursa.

A 25-gauge 1.5-inch needle is inserted in the interdigital space (Fig. 69.6) in plane toward the neuroma. If a perineural injection is planned, the needle is placed outside the neuroma with the injectate deposited in the perineural space (usually 2–3 mL). The location applies to the technique for cryoanalgesia. If the intention is chemical ablation, the needle is directed inside the neuroma, and a volume of 0.5 mL

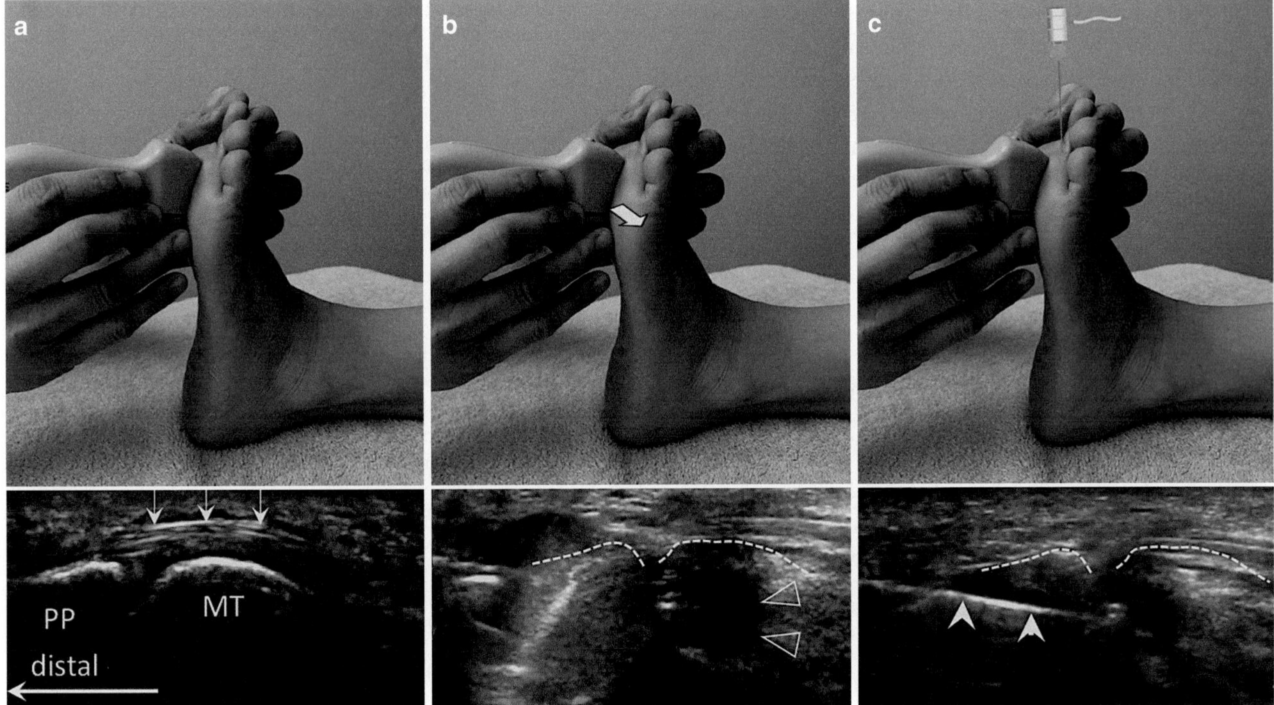

Fig. 69.6 (**a**) Placement of the ultrasound probe over the metatarsophalangeal joint of the third digit with corresponding sonography below. MT-metatarsal, PP-proximal phalanx, arrows-flexor tendons. (**b**) Moving the probe to the interdigital space between third and fourth digit revealed the corresponding sonography below. The corresponding outline of adjacent phalange and metatarsal was illustrated with dotted lines. The Morton neuroma appears as a hypoechoic mass indicated by bold arrows. (**c**) The figure shows the needle insertion in the interdigital space in-plane, and the corresponding sonography below shows the needle (arrowheads) inserted into the neuroma for neurolysis. Reprinted with permission from Philip Peng Educational Series

of injectate is administered (Fig. 69.6). Extreme care is important to avoid the spread of the chemical outside of neuroma and spillage toward the flexor tendon, which will cause severe pain after the procedure.

Ultrasound-Guided Radiofrequency Ablation

The procedure will require a wider sterile field with proper prepping (chlorhexidine) and draping. Sterile ultrasound gel and a 22G 5 cm RFA needle with a 10 mm electrode active tip will also be required.

The technique is similar to the one described above. Following a subcutaneous wheal of local anesthetic at the skin entry site, the needle is advanced to the neuroma, and local anesthetic is administered around the neuroma. After local anesthetic has taken effect, advance the sterile RFA needle through the wheal until the needle tip is centered within the hypoechoic lesion. Remove the stylet and insert the RFA wire. According to Masal et al., a protocol of continuous RF with one cycle of 90 s and probe temperature of 85 °C (impedance 95–210 mΩ) resulted in reduction of pain intensity within 1 week with symptoms stabilization that lasted up to 1 year.

Complications

Keep the needle tip within view to verify correct placement and depth. Advancing the needle too deep can perforate the plantar aspect of the forefoot.

Practical Tips

Doppler will assist in identifying vasculature. Power Doppler may assist in differentiating between inflamed symptomatic and asymptomatic neuromas.

Literature Review

While MN is a nerve entrapment syndrome, forefoot postural overload is a contributing factor and may result in other overlapping forefoot pain pathologies such as hallux valgus, MTP joint capsulitis, and hammer toe. Thorough evaluation and accurate diagnosis are critical to successful outcomes. Some authors recommend confirmation of the diagnosis and localization with MRI in addition to ultrasound. 20% alcohol solution is the minimum concentration to achieve successful neural inhibition, with several studies preferring a 50% solution, and a recent study recommending increased volume and concentration, 2.5 mL of 70% alcohol, yielded an 82% success rate defined as pain-free daily life at the 5-year mark.

Suggested Reading

Adams WR. Morton's neuroma. Clin Podiatr Med Surg. 2010;27(4):535–45.

Balint PV, Kane D, Hunter J, McInnes IB, Field M, Sturrock RD. Ultrasound guided versus conventional joint and soft tissue fluid aspiration in rheumatology practice: a pilot study. J Rheumatol. 2002;29(10):2209–13.

Honvo G, Reginster J-Y, Rannou F, Rygaert X, Geerinck A, Rabenda V, et al. Safety of intra-articular hyaluronic acid injections in osteoarthritis: outcomes of a systematic review and meta-analysis. Drugs Aging. 2019;36(1):101–27.

Kawalec JS. Mechanical testing of foot and ankle implants. In: Friis E, editor. Mechanical testing of orthopaedic implants. Woodhead Publishing; 2017. p. 231–53.

Lu VM, Puffer RC, Everson MC, Gilder HE, Burks SS, Spinner RJ. Treating Morton's neuroma by injection, neurolysis, or neurectomy: a systematic review and meta-analysis of pain and satisfaction outcomes. Acta Neurochir. 2020; https://doi.org/10.1007/s00701-020-04241-9.

Manadan AM, Mushtaq S, Block JA. Radiocarpal and first metatarsophalangeal intraarticular injection site confirmation with fluoroscopy and review of accuracy of intraarticular injections. Am J Ther. 2015;22(1):11–3.

Mares AV, Schreiter R, van Eck CF, Blanc R, Musahl V. Management of athletic turf toe using biologics. Oper Tech Orthop. 2016;26(2):117–21.

Masala S, Cuzzolino A, Morini M, Raguso M, Fiori R. Ultrasound-guided percutaneous radiofrequency for the treatment of Morton's neuroma. Cardiovasc Intervent Radiol. 2018;41(1):137–44.

Morgan P, Monaghan W, Richards S. A systematic review of ultrasound-guided and non–ultrasound-guided therapeutic injections to treat Morton's neuroma. J Am Podiatr Med Assoc. 2014;104(4):337–48.

Pabinger C, Malaj I, Lothaller H, Samaila E, Magnan B. Improved injection technique of ethanol for Morton's neuroma. Foot Ankle Int. 2020;41(5):590–5.

Pasquali C, Vulcano E, Novario R, Varotto D, Montoli C, Volpe A. Ultrasound-guided alcohol injection for Morton's neuroma. Foot Ankle Int. 2015;36(1):55–9.

Perini L, Perini C, Tagliapietra M, Varotto D, Valcarenghi A, Postorino A, et al. Percutaneous alcohol injection under sonographic guidance in Morton's neuroma: follow-up in 220 treated lesions. Radiol Med. 2016;121(7):597–604.

Sahler CS, Spinner DA, Kirschner JS. Ultrasound-guided first metatarsophalangeal joint injections: description of an in-plane, gel standoff technique in a cadaveric study Foot Ankle Spec. 2013. https://journals-sagepub-com.eresources.mssm.edu/doi/10.1177/1938640013493465.

Spinner DA, Mazzola AJ. General principle of musculoskeletal scanning and intervention. In: Peng P, Finlayson R, Lee SH, Bhatia A, editors. Ultrasound for interventional pain management: an illustrated procedural guide. Cham: Springer; 2020. p. 207–12. https://doi.org/10.1007/978-3-030-18371-4_18.

Vadada K, Chang RG, Sahler C, Kirschner JS. Foot and ankle. In: Spinner DA, Kirschner JS, Herrera JE, editors. Atlas of ultrasound guided musculoskeletal injections. New York, NY: Springer; 2014. p. 69–88. (Musculoskeletal Medicine). https://doi.org/10.1007/978-1-4614-8936-8_7.

70 Landmark-Guided Technique for Regional Anesthesia of the Lower Limb

Danilo Jankovic and Battista Borghi

Contents

D. Jankovic (✉)
Pain Management Centre DGS – Cologne – Huerth, Cologne-Hürth, Germany
e-mail: danilo@jankovic1.de

B. Borghi
Anesthesia Research Unit, Instituti Orthopedici Rizzoli, Bologna, Italy
e-mail: battista.borghi@ior.it

D. Jankovic, P. Peng (eds.), *Regional Nerve Blocks in Anesthesia and Pain Therapy*,
https://doi.org/10.1007/978-3-030-88727-8_70

General Consideration

In no anatomic site outside the neuraxis are the lower extremity plexuses as compactly packaged as are the nerves to the upper extremity in the brachial plexus. When considering lower extremity innervation, it is essential to understand that two major nerve plexuses innervate the lower extremity: the lumbar plexus and the lumbosacral plexus. The concept of a regional anesthesia technique that provides neural blockade of the entirety of the lumbar plexus, a lumbar plexus block, dates back nearly 50 years. Winnie proposed that a large volume of local anesthetic injected in the femoral nerve sheath could spread proximally to produce blockade of the obturator, lateral femoral cutaneous, as well as femoral nerve. Later work would show that, in fact, this rarely succeeded and typically only blocked the femoral and femoral lateral cutaneous nerves. Since Winnie's original descriptions of the approach to the lumbar plexus, there have been several alternative descriptions.

In 1976, Chayen et al. described a posterior lumbar plexus block, or "psoas compartment block," which proved to be a more reliable realization of that goal of blocking the whole of the lumbar plexus with a single injection.

Functional Anatomy of the Lumbar Plexus, Sacral Plexus, and Coccygeal Plexus

These plexuses, closely related to one another, are formed by the ventral branches of the lumbar, sacral, and coccygeal spinal nerves (Figs. 70.1, 70.2, 70.3, 70.4, and 70.5).

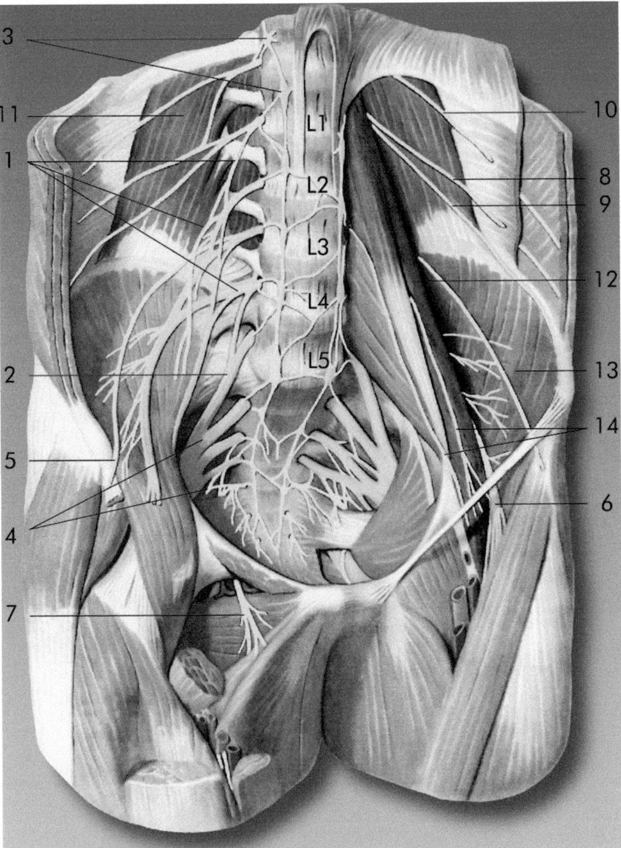

Fig. 70.1 Anatomy: lumbar plexus, sacral plexus, and coccygeal plexus. *(1)* Lumbar plexus, *(2)* lumbosacral trunk, *(3)* sympathetic trunk, *(4)* sacral plexus, *(5)* lateral femoral cutaneous nerve, *(6)* femoral nerve, *(7)* obturator nerve, *(8)* iliohypogastric nerve, *(9)* ilioinguinal nerve, *(10)* subcostal nerve, *(11)* quadratus lumborum muscle, *(12)* psoas major muscle, *(13)* iliacus muscle, *(14)* genitofemoral nerve. (Reproduced with permission from Danilo Jankovic)

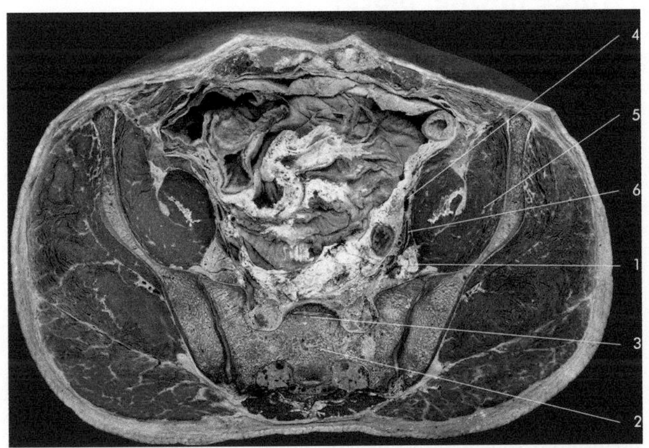

Fig. 70.2 Lumbar plexus. Transversal dissection. *(1)* Lumbar plexus, *(2)* os sacrum, *(3)* intervertebral disc, *(4)* left external iliac artery, *(5)* iliopsoas muscle, *(6)* left external iliac vein. (Reproduced with permission from Danilo Jankovic)

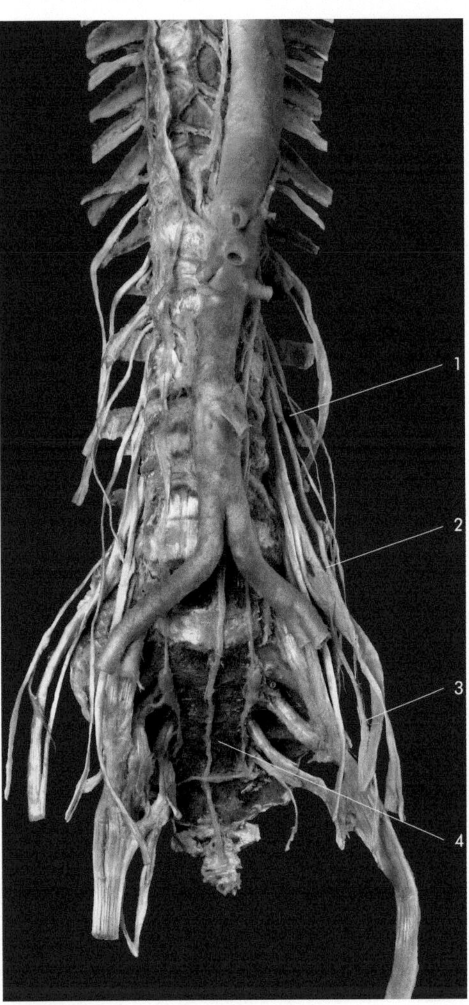

Fig. 70.3 Lumbosacral plexus. Ventral view. *(1)* Lumbar plexus, *(2)* lumbosacral trunk, *(3)* sacral plexus, *(4)* medial sacral artery: left and right side – sympathetic trunk. (Reproduced with permission from Danilo Jankovic)

The lumbar plexus lies in front of the transverse processes of the lumbar vertebrae. It mainly arises from the ventral branches, the first three lumbar nerves, most of the fourth lumbar nerve, and the twelfth thoracic nerve (subcostal nerve).

The most important branches of the plexus are located in a fascial compartment that is enclosed ("sandwiched") by the quadratus lumborum, psoas major, and iliacus muscles. The first lumbar nerve, which contains a branch from the twelfth thoracic nerve, divides into an upper branch (iliohypogastric nerve and ilioinguinal nerve) and a lower branch (genitofemoral nerve). Most of the second, third, and parts of the fourth lumbar nerves form ventral branches, from which the femoral nerve and obturator nerve branch off. The lateral femoral cutaneous nerve is formed from fibers of the ventral branches of L2. The caudal parts of the ventral branches of L4 and L5 combine to form the lumbosacral trunk. Together with the ventral branches of the first three sacral nerves and the upper part of the ventral branch of the fourth sacral nerve, the lum-

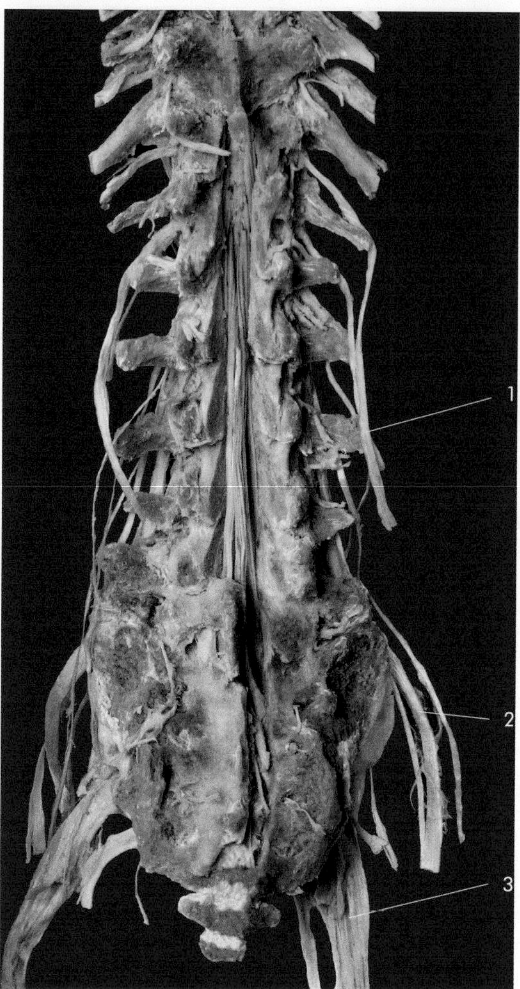

Fig. 70.4 Lumbosacral plexus. Dorsal view. *(1)* lumbar plexus, *(2)* lumbosacral plexus, *(3)* sacral plexus. (Reproduced with permission from Danilo Jankovic)

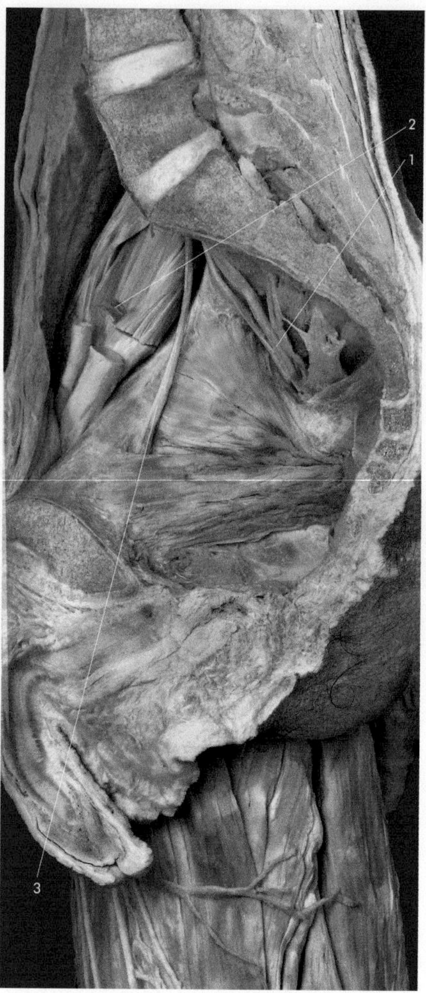

Fig. 70.5 Anatomy. Medial sagittal dissection. *(1)* Lumbosacral plexus, *(2)* iliopsoas muscle with femoral nerve, *(3)* obturator nerve. (Reproduced with permission from Danilo Jankovic)

bosacral trunk forms the sacral plexus, the largest branch of which is the sciatic nerve. The lumbar plexus is also connected with the lumbar part of the sympathetic nervous system via two or three long communicating branches.

The thickness of the ventral branches of the lumbar nerves increases markedly from the first to the fifth nerve (L1 has a diameter of ca. 2.5 mm, L2 is already ca. 4 mm, L3 and L4 are ca. 6 mm, and L5 is as large as 7 mm). The coccygeal plexus arises from the lower part of the ventral branches of the fourth and fifth sacral nerves, as well as the coccygeal nerves.

Lumbar Plexus Blocks

Two techniques are described that belong to the standard methods for blocking the lumbar plexus:

1. The caudal (ventral) psoas compartment block ("three in-one" inguinal femoral paravascular block)
2. The cranial (dorsal) psoas compartment block

Inguinal Femoral Paravascular Nerve Block ("Three-in-One" Block)

General Consideration

The concept underlying lumbar plexus blocks is that the course of the neural network from the transverse processes to the inguinal ligament lies within a perivascular and perineural space. Like the epidural space, this space limits the spread of the local anesthetic and conducts it to the various nerves.

The initial description of the three-in-one block (an infero-antero approach to the femoral, lateral femoral cutaneous, and obturator nerves) was published by Winnie et al. in 1973 involving a small number of patients. The authors postulated that a block of the entire lumbar plexus can be accomplished by a single perivascular injection slightly distal to the inguinal ligament. Consequently, a single injection should result in anesthesia of the femoral, the lateral femoral cutaneous, and obturator nerves (Figs. 70.6, 70.7, and 70.8). Winnie et al. suggested that the underlying mechanism of

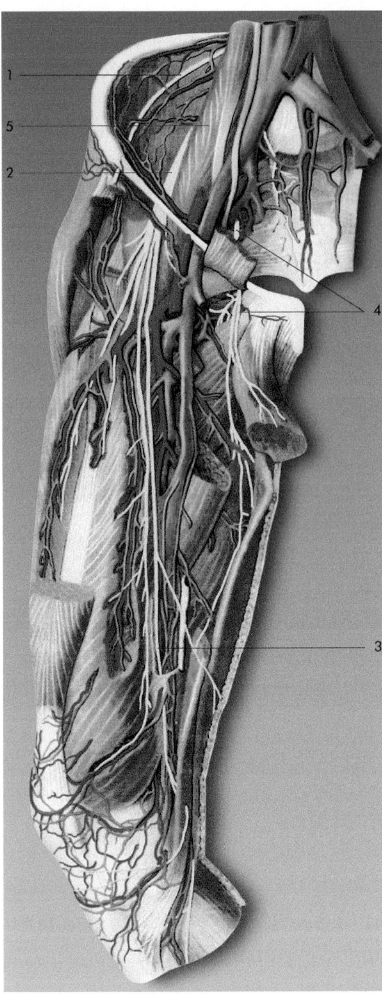

Fig. 70.6 Anatomy: femoral nerve, lateral femoral cutaneous nerve, and obturator nerve. *(1)* Lateral femoral cutaneous nerve, *(2)* femoral nerve, *(3)* saphenous nerve, *(4)* obturator nerve, *(5)* psoas major muscle. (Reproduced with permission from Danilo Jankovic)

this regional anesthetic technique should be a cephalad distribution of the local anesthetic along the fascial layer. Within the connective tissue and neural sheath, the concentration and volume of the local anesthetic determine the extent of the block's spread. This hypothesis, however, was never confirmed clinically. Moreover, an MRI study clarified the spread of local anesthetic after an inguinal injection of local anesthetic lateral to the femoral artery and concluded that the distribution of local anesthetic follows a lateral and slightly medial direction, but never a cephalad direction. One of the main proposed advantages of the three-in-one block was the ability to achieve block of the obturator nerve using this approach. In clinical practice, however, the obturator nerve (posterior branch) has never been shown to be anesthetized effectively using this approach. Capdevila et al. reported that the local anesthetic used in three-in-one block spreads under the iliac fascia, but rarely to the lumbar plexus. Both techniques resulted in poor blocks of the obturator nerve.

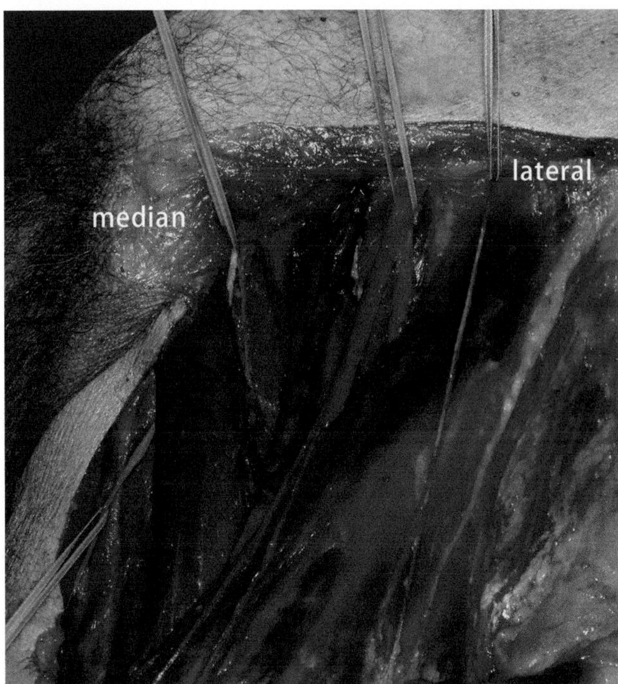

Fig. 70.7 *(1)* Femoral nerve *(yellow)*, (2) lateral cutaneous femoral nerve *(blue)*, obturator nerve *(green)*. In clinical practice, the obturator nerve (posterior branch) has never been shown to be anesthetized effectively. (Reproduced with permission from Danilo Jankovic)

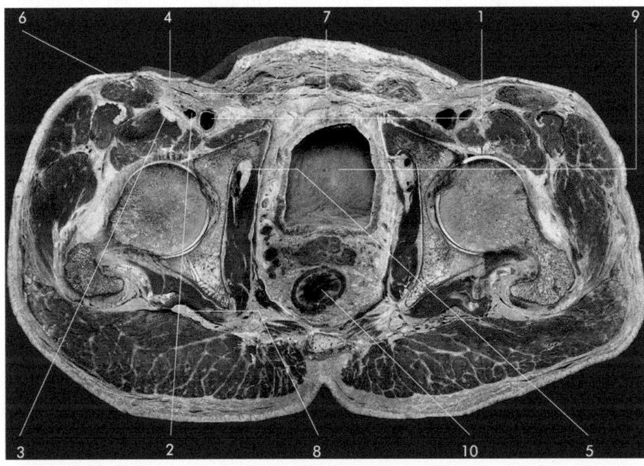

Fig. 70.8 Transversal dissection. *(1)* Femoral vein, *(2)* femoral artery, *(3)* femoral nerve, *(4)* lateral cutaneous femoral nerve, *(5)* obturator nerve with vasa obturatoria, *(6)* sartorius muscle, *(7)* fascia lata, *(8)* sciatic nerve, *(9)* vesica urinaria, *(10)* rectum. (Reproduced with permission from Danilo Jankovic)

Functional Anatomy

The *femoral nerve* divides slightly distal to the inguinal ligament in several branches, which is the rationale for the nerve block needle to be inserted close to the distal ligament when performing the three-in-one block. The femoral nerve supplies motor branches to the quadriceps femoris, sartorius, and pectineus muscles, and its sensory branch (saphenous nerve) innervates the anterior-medial side of the lower leg down to the medial ankle. Both the obturator nerve and the lateral femoral cutaneous nerve divide at variable levels from the femoral nerve (Figs.70.6, 70.7, and 70.8). The *lateral femoral cutaneous nerve* arises from the ventral branches of the L2 and L3 spinal nerves, passing lateral to the psoas muscle and then to the iliacus muscle.

Covered by the iliac fascia, it then runs to the region of the anterior superior iliac spine. It passes under the inguinal ligament and under the deep circumflex iliac artery and enters the thigh, where it lies under the superficial sheet of the fascia and divides into a thicker descending branch and a smaller posterior branch, which penetrate the fascia separately. The posterior branch runs posteriorly over the tensor fascia lata muscle and reaches the gluteal region. The anterior branch runs 3–5 cm below the inguinal ligament and then downward along the anterior surface of the vastus lateralis muscle as far as the lateral knee area, where it sends off lateral branches (Figs. 70.6, 70.7, and 70.8). The *obturator nerve* arises from the ventral branches of the L2–L4 spinal nerves. The trunk runs downward along the medial edge of the psoas muscle, passing behind the common iliac vessels to reach the pelvis and the obturator canal. Within the canal, it divides into its two end branches – the anterior and posterior branches. It provides the motor supply for the obturator externus muscle and the adductors of the thigh, sends off branches to the hip and knee joints and to the femur, and provides the sensory supply for a highly variable cutaneous area on the inside of the thigh and lower leg (Figs. 70.6, 70.7, and 70.8).

Indications

Surgical

- Superficial surgical interventions in the innervated area: wound care, skin grafts, and muscle biopsies.
- Analgesia for positioning for neuraxial block anesthesia in femoral neck fractures.
- Performing surgical interventions in the area of the lower extremity in ischemia or tourniquet, in combination with sciatic nerve block. Larger volumes of local anesthetic have to be used here (toxicity!).
- Outpatient procedures.

Therapeutic

- Postoperative pain therapy (e.g., after femoral neck, femoral shaft, tibial and patellar fractures, knee joint operations)
- Post-traumatic pain
- Postoperative neurolysis or nerve reimplantations for better innervation
- Early mobilization after hip or knee joint operations
- Arterial occlusive disease and poor perfusion in the lower extremities
- Complex regional pain syndrome (CRPS) types I and II
- Post-amputation pain
- Edema in the leg after radiotherapy
- Diabetic polyneuropathy
- Knee joint arthritis
- Elimination of adductor spasm in paraplegic patients

Block Series

A series of six to eight blocks is recommended. When there is evidence of improvement in the symptoms, additional blocks can also be carried out.

Prophylactic

- Postoperative analgesia
- Prophylaxis against post-amputation pain
- Prophylaxis against complex regional pain syndrome (CRPS)

Contraindications

Specific

- Infections (e.g., osteomyelitis, pyoderma) or malignant diseases in the inguinal region
- Local hematoma
- Anticoagulant treatment (see Chap. 1)
- Distorted anatomy (due to prior surgical interventions or trauma to the inguinal and thigh region)

Relative

The decision should be taken after carefully weighing up the risks and benefits:

- Hemorrhagic diathesis
- Stable central nervous system disorders
- Local nerve injury (when it is difficult to determine whether the cause is surgical or anesthetic)
- Contralateral nerve paresis
- Patients with a femoral bypass

Procedure

This block should be carried out by experienced anesthetists, or under their supervision. Full information for the patient is mandatory.

Preparations

Check that the emergency equipment is complete and in working order: sterile precautions, intravenous access, ECG monitoring, pulse oximetry, intubation kit, ventilation facilities, emergency medication.

Materials

Fine 26 G needle, 25 mm long, for local anesthesia. Peripheral nerve stimulator

Single-Shot Technique

50 (80)-mm-long atraumatic 22 G (15°) short-bevel insulated stimulating needle with injection lead ("immobile needle")

Continuous Technique

[1]Peripheral nerve stimulator

Catheter kit (including a 50–80 mm 18 G (15°) stimulating needle and catheter 0.45 × 0.85 × 400 mm, or Tuohy set, 52 (102)-mm-long 18 G Tuohy needle with catheter)

Syringes: 2 and 20 mL

Local anesthetics, disinfectant, swabs, compresses, sterile gloves, and drape

Patient Positioning

Supine, with the thigh slightly abducted. The patient's ipsilateral hand lies under the head. The person carrying out the injection must stand on the side being blocked.

Landmarks

The femoral artery is palpated 1–2 cm distal to the inguinal ligament. It is held between the spread index and middle finger. The injection point lies about 1.5–2 cm laterally.
Skin prep, subcutaneous local anesthesia, sterile drapes; draw up local anesthetic into 20 mL syringes, check patency of injection needles and functioning of nerve stimulator, and attach electrodes.
Preliminary puncture with a large needle or stylet.

> The quadriceps femoris muscle and the patella must be observed throughout the procedure.

[1]<Footnote ID="Fn1"><Para ID="Par53">If technical difficulties arise, the catheter and Tuohy needle must always be removed simultaneously. A catheter must never be removed through the Tuohy needle (as the catheter may shear!).</Para></Footnote>

Technique

Single-Injection Technique

1. The injection is carried out in a cranial direction at an angle of about 30–40° to the skin surface, almost parallel to the course of the femoral artery. Stimulation current of 1–2 mA at 2 Hz is selected with a stimulus duration of 0.1 ms (Fig. 70.9). Usually, the nerve is at the depth of 12± 4 mm.
2. The needle is advanced until contractions of the quadriceps femoris muscle and patellar movements become visible ("dancing patella"). Contractions of the sartorius muscle alone suggest incorrect positioning and are inadequate (Fig. 70.10).
3. Do not advance the needle further! The stimulation current is reduced to 0.2–0.3 mA. Slight twitching suggests that the stimulation needle is in the immediate vicinity of the nerve.
4. Aspiration test.
5. Test dose of 3 mL local anesthetic (e.g., 1% prilocaine). During the injection, the twitching slowly disappears.
6. Incremental injection of a local anesthetic (injection-aspiration after each 3–4 mL).
7. After the injection, compression massage of the injection area is carried out and then flexing of the thigh for about 1 min (Fig. 70.11).
8. Careful cardiovascular monitoring.

> During the injection, distal compression should be applied with the finger to support proximal spread of the local anesthetic.

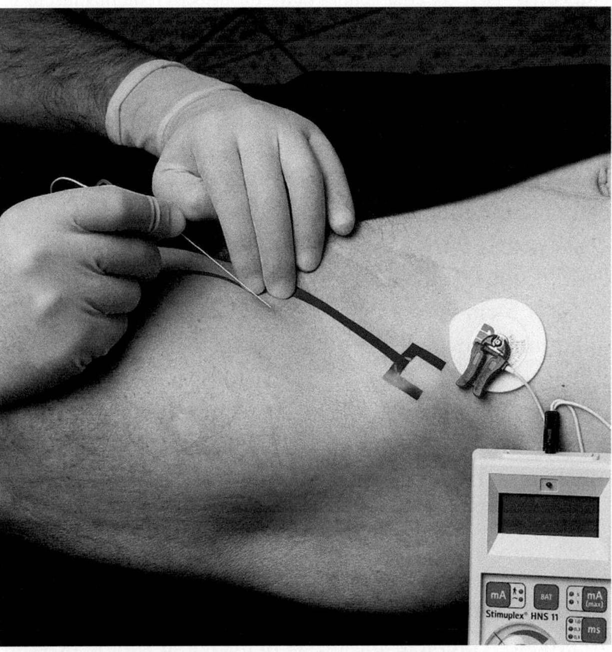

Fig. 70.9 Injection. Cranial direction, at an angle of about 30–40° to the skin surface. (Reproduced with permission from Danilo Jankovic)

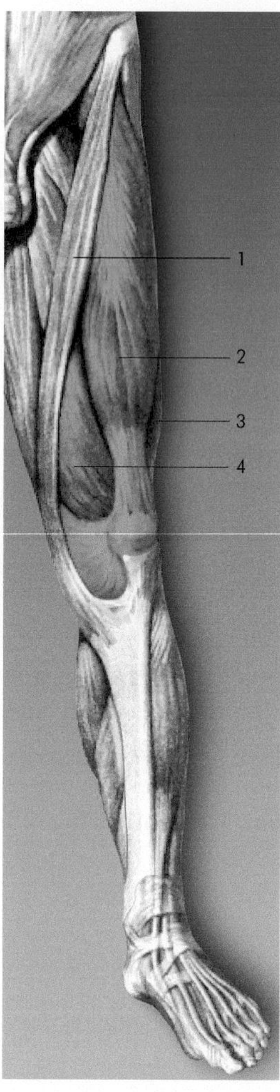

Fig. 70.10 Note the contractions of the quadriceps femoris muscle and patellar movements. *(1)* Sartorius muscle, *(2)* rectus femoris muscle, *(3)* vastus lateralis muscle, *(4)* vastus medialis muscle. (Reproduced with permission from Danilo Jankovic)

Continuous Technique

Either non-stimulating (conventional) or stimulating catheters can be used. The site is located in the same way as described for the unilateral technique. The injection is carried out about 2–2.5 cm below the inguinal ligament and 1–1.5 cm lateral to the femoral artery and in a cranial direction at an angle of about 30–40°. Using the Seldinger technique, the catheter is advanced at least 10 cm deep into the fascial compartment. An aspiration test, administration of a test dose, fixation of the catheter, and placement of a bacterial filter then follow. After aspirating again, the local anesthetic is given on an incremental basis.

Distribution of Anesthesia

To produce complete anesthesia in the leg, it should be combined with a sciatic nerve block (Figs.70.12 and 70.13).

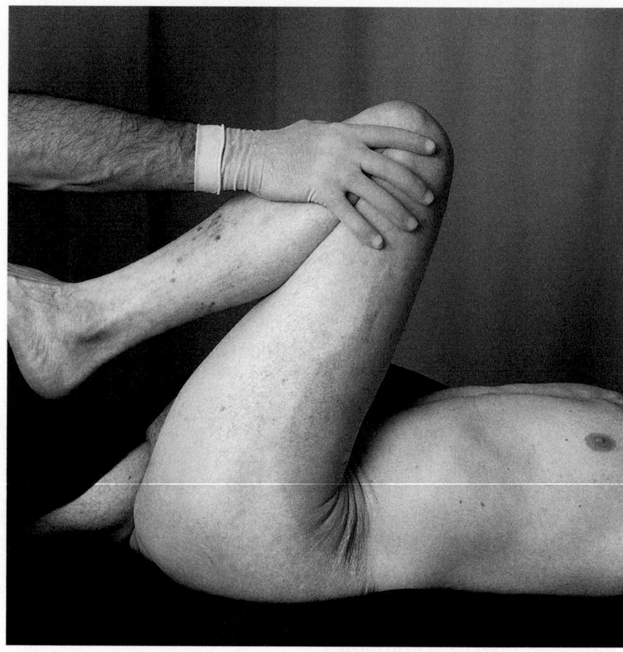

Fig. 70.11 After the injection: flexing the thigh for about 1 min. (Reproduced with permission from Danilo Jankovic)

Dosage

Surgical

- 15–20 mL—single-injection femoral nerve block
- 40–50 mL local anesthetic—e.g., 0.5–0.75% ropivacaine, 0.5% bupivacaine (0.5% levobupivacaine), 1% prilocaine, and 1% mepivacaine

A combination of local anesthetics with longer-term and medium-term effect has proved particularly valuable for surgical indications—e.g., 1% prilocaine (20 mL) + 0.5–0.75% ropivacaine (20 mL) or 1% prilocaine (20 mL) + 0.25–0.5% bupivacaine (0.25–0.5% levobupivacaine, 20 mL).

Therapeutic

10–15 mL local anesthetic – e.g., 0.2–0.375% ropivacaine, 0.125–0.25% bupivacaine (0.125–0.25% levobupivacaine)

Important Notes for Outpatients

Long-lasting block can occur (even after administration of low-dose local anesthetics—e.g., 0.125% bupivacaine or 0.2% ropivacaine). The blocked leg can give way even 10–18 h after the injection. The patient must therefore use walking aids during this period. The same rules apply to the treatment of post-amputation pain. During the period of effect of the local anesthetic, the patient should not wear a prosthesis.

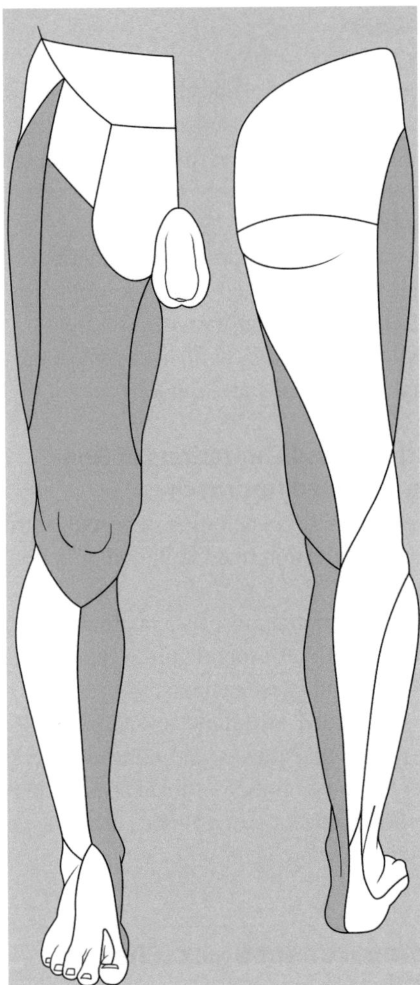

Fig. 70.12 The neural areas most frequently blocked after administration of a "three-in-one" block. (Reproduced with permission from Danilo Jankovic)

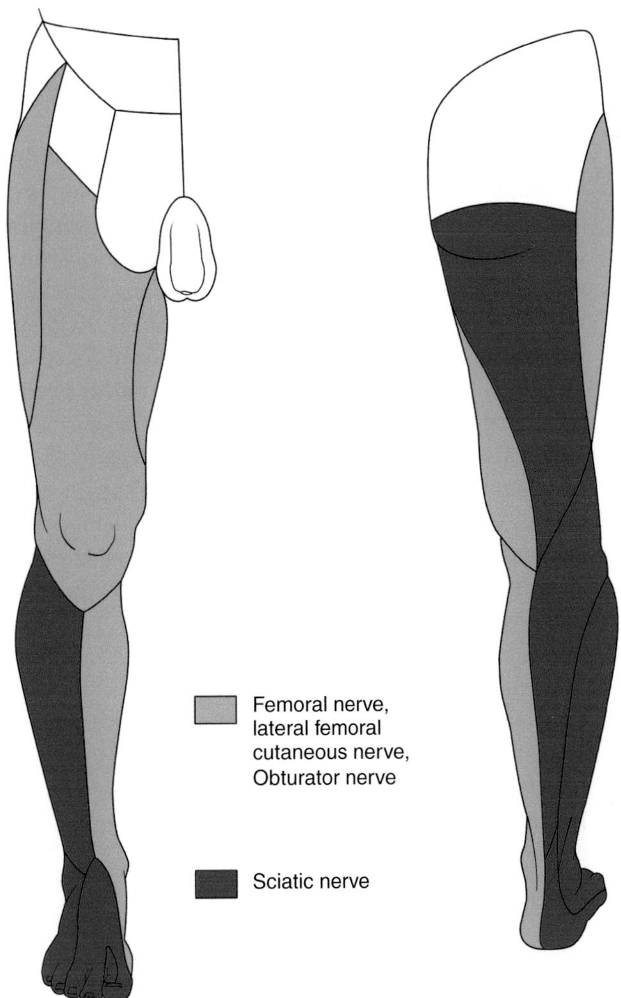

Fig. 70.13 Comparison of the innervation areas of the femoral nerve, lateral femoral cutaneous nerve, and obturator nerve *(blue)* with the innervation area of the sciatic nerve *(red)*. (Reproduced with permission from Danilo Jankovic)

A record must be kept of patient information and consent.

Continuous Technique

Test dose: 3–5 mL 1% prilocaine (1% mepivacaine)

Bolus administration: 30 mL 0.5–0.75% ropivacaine or 0.25–0.5% bupivacaine

Maintenance Dose

Intermittent Administration

15–20 mL of local anesthetic every 4–6 h (0.5–0.75% ropivacaine or 0.25–0.5% bupivacaine) after a prior test dose

Reduction of the dose and/or adjustment of the interval, depending on the clinical picture

Continuous Infusion

Infusion of the local anesthetic via the catheter should be started 30–60 minutes after the bolus dose. A test dose is obligatory.

Ropivacaine: 0.2–0.375%	6–14 mL/h
	(max. 37.5 mg/h)
Levobupivacaine: 0.125–0.25%	8–15 mL/h
Bupivacaine: 0.125%	10–14 mL/h
Bupivacaine: 0.25%	8–10 mL/h

If necessary, the infusion can be supplemented with bolus doses of 5–10 mL 0.5–0.75% ropivacaine (0.25–0.5% bupivacaine or 0.25% levobupivacaine).

Individual adjustment of the dosage and period of treatment is essential.

Complications

1. Nerve injuries (see Chap. 4, Complications of Regional Anesthesia).

   Traumatic nerve injury is a rare complication of this technique. It can occur as a result of the use of sharp needles (due to nerve puncture), intraneural or microvascular injury (hematoma and its sequelae), prolonged ischemia, as well as toxic effects of intraneurally injected local anesthetic (see Chap. 4, Complications of Regional Anesthesia). Probable effects of intraneural injection include a transient neurological deficit (unexpectedly prolonged block, lasting up to 10 days). A suspicion of intraneural needle positioning arises if there is strong twitching even at low levels of stimulation current (e.g., 0.2 mA) and if there is no cessation of the twitching after administration of the test dose. The local anesthetic may also be difficult to inject. Correction of the needle position is essential.
2. Intravascular injection (see Chap. 5, Local Anesthetic Systemic Toxicity).
3. CNS intoxication (see Chap. 5, Local Anesthetic Systemic Toxicity).
4. Infection in the injection area (continuous techniques).
5. Hematoma formation (note the obligatory prophylactic compression).

Practical Tips

- Use a strict aseptic technique.
- The femoral artery is palpated 1–2 cm distal to the inguinal ligament. The injection point lies about 1.5–2 cm laterally.
- Keep the palpating finger in the same position throughout the procedure.
- When the femoral artery or vein is punctured, the procedure should be stopped and firm, constant pressure applied over the femoral artery for 5 min before proceeding with the blockade.
- The needle should never be redirected medially. Redirections should all be made more lateral.
- Avoid stimulation at <0.2 mA and advance needle slowly.
- Do not inject when the patient complains of pain or when high resistance is present.

Advantages

- Suitable for postoperative or post-traumatic analgesia and for therapeutic blocks
- Suitable for patients in whom a unilateral block is desired – particularly in outpatient procedures

Disadvantages

- Success is unpredictable.
- Larger amounts of local anesthetic are necessary (particularly if the sciatic nerve is also being blocked).
- The likelihood of systemic toxicity is increased.
- Longer-onset times have to be expected (surgical indications).
- Despite larger amounts of local anesthetic, not all nerves in the plexus are blocked (e.g., the obturator nerve and lateral femoral cutaneous nerve).
- For surgical procedures with ischemia or a tourniquet, neuraxial anesthesia is preferable.

Disadvantages and Limitations of Non-ultrasound-Guided Approaches

- Higher potential for penetration of vascular structures and intravascular injection (the likelihood of systemic toxicity is increased).
- Palpating the femoral pulse as a landmark for the block is not required with ultrasound guidance, a process that can be challenging in obese patients.
- Ultrasound-guided technique allows multiple injections around the lumbar plexus and can be successfully performed with lower dosage of local anesthetic solution.
- Distribution of the local anesthetic cannot be visualized to assure adequate spread around the lumbar plexus.

Psoas Compartment Block (Chayen Approach)

General Consideration

Since the initial description of the posterior lumbar plexus block (Chayen 1976), a number of variations of the technique have been described. Most of these differ from the original technique of Chayen et al. in only minor detail and are related to the distance of the needle insertion point from midline or the lumbar level at which the block is performed. The psoas compartment block is an advanced nerve block technique. Because the placement of the needle is in the deep muscles, the potential for systemic toxicity is greater than it is with more superficial techniques. The proximity of the lumbar nerve roots to the epidural space also carries a risk of epidural spread of the local anesthetic. For these reasons, care should be taken when selecting the type, volume, and concentration of local anesthetic, particularly in elderly, frail, or obese patients. When combined with a sciatic nerve block, anesthesia of the entire leg can be achieved. Because of the complexity of the technique, potential for complications, and existence of simpler alternatives (e.g., fascia iliaca or femoral blocks), the benefits of lumbar plexus blocks should always be weighed against the risks.

Functional Anatomy

The psoas compartment block represents a cranial and dorsal paravertebral access route to the lumbar plexus. The concept is to block the closely juxtaposed branches of the lumbar plexus and parts of the sacral plexus by injecting local anesthetic through a high access route to the plexus (L4–L5) (see above, lumbar plexus anatomy). When the quality of the block is good, the area of distribution is comparable with that of the "three-in-one" block (see "three-in-one" femoral nerve block, Figs. 70.12 and 70.13). The most important branches of the plexus are located in a fascial compartment that is enclosed ("sandwiched") by the quadratus lumborum, psoas major, and iliacus muscles (Figs. 70.14 and 70.15). The following nerves are affected: lateral femoral cutaneous nerve, femoral nerve, genitofemoral nerve, obturator nerve, and parts of the sciatic and posterior femoral cutaneous nerve. A combination of this block with block of the sciatic nerve is necessary to achieve complete anesthesia of the lower extremity.

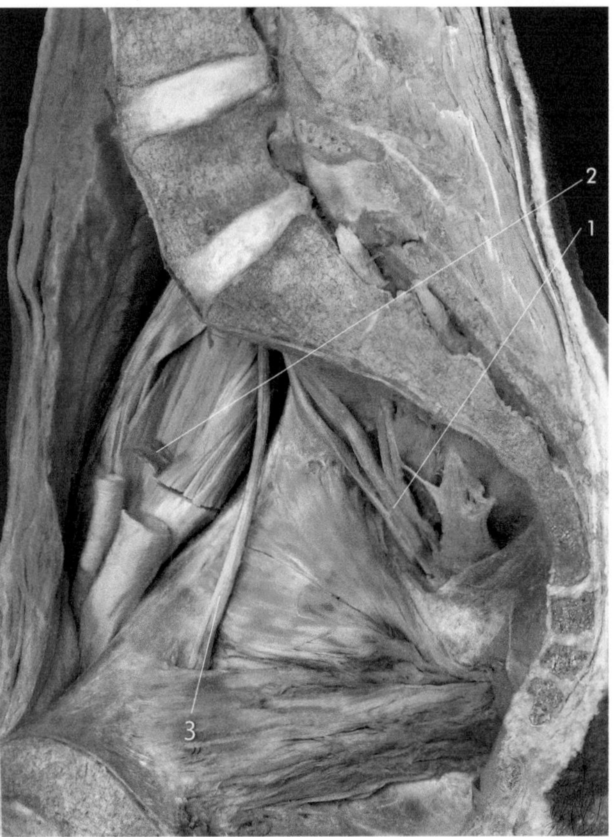

Fig. 70.15 Lumbosacral plexus. Median sagittal dissection. *(1)* Lumbosacral plexus at the level of L5–S3 segment, *(2)* iliopsoas muscle with femoral nerve, *(3)* obturator nerve. (Reproduced with permission from Danilo Jankovic)

Indications

Surgical

- As a continuous or single-shot block for all surgical procedures in the region of the lower extremity, but in combination with a block of the sciatic nerve. A need for larger volumes of local anesthetics must be expected (toxicity!).
- Outpatient procedures.

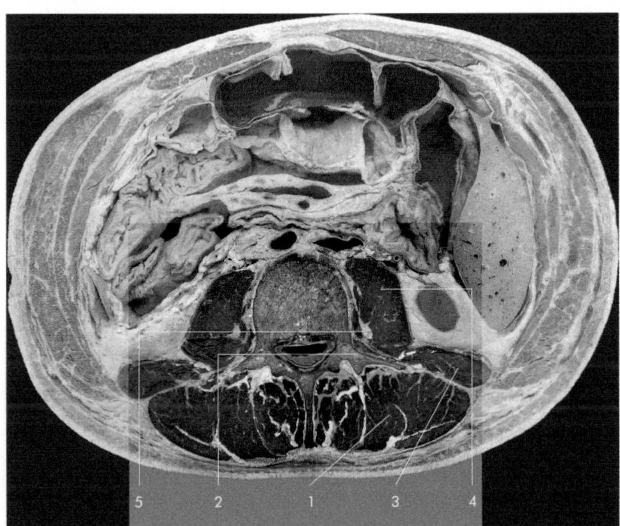

Fig. 70.14 Anatomy. Transversal dissection on the level of the L3/L4. *(1)* Erector spinae muscle, *(2)* transverse process, *(3)* quadratus lumborum muscle, *(4)* psoas major muscle, *(5)* lumbar plexus. (Reproduced with permission from Danilo Jankovic)

Therapeutic

- Postoperative and post-traumatic pain therapy
- Early mobilization after hip and knee operations
- Arterial occlusive disease and poor perfusion of the lower extremities
- Complex regional pain syndrome (CRPS), types I and II
- Post-surgical neurolysis or nerve reimplantations for better innervation
- Edema after radiotherapy
- Post-amputation pain
- Diabetic polyneuropathy
- Tumors and metastases in the hip joint and pelvis

Block Series

A series of six to eight blocks is recommended. When there is evidence of improvement in the symptoms, additional blocks can also be carried out.

Prophylactic

- Postoperative analgesia
- Prophylaxis against post-amputation pain
- Prophylaxis against development of complex regional pain syndrome

Contraindications

Specific

- Infection or hematoma in the injection area
- Anticoagulant treatment (see Chap. 1)
- Lesion in the nerves to be stimulated distal to the injection site

Relative

The decision should be taken after carefully weighing up the risks and benefits:

- Hemorrhagic diathesis
- Stable systemic neurological diseases
- Local nerve injury (when there is doubt whether the fault lies with the surgeon or anesthesiologist)
- Contralateral nerve paresis

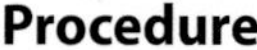

Procedure

This block should be carried out by experienced anesthetists, or under their supervision. Full information for the patient is mandatory.

Preparations

Check that the emergency equipment is complete and in working order: sterile precautions, intravenous access, ECG monitoring, pulse oximetry, intubation kit, ventilation facilities, and emergency medication.

Materials

Fine 26 G needle, 25 mm long, for local anesthesia

Electrostimulation Technique

- Peripheral nerve stimulator
- 120-mm-long short bevel insulated atraumatic 22 G needle (15°) with injection lead ("immobile needle")

Continuous Technique

[2]Tuohy set: 1.3 × 102 (152)-mm-long 18 G Tuohy insulated needle with catheter, or 18 G (15°) insulated stimulating needle (1.3 × 110 mm with catheter)

Syringes: 2 and 20 mL

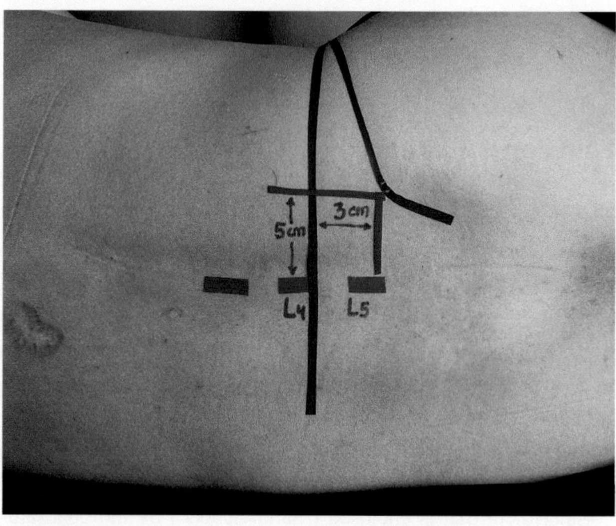

Fig. 70.16 Location. (Reproduced with permission from Danilo Jankovic)

Local anesthetics, disinfectant, swabs, compresses, sterile gloves, and drape

Patient Positioning

Lateral decubitus or sitting, as in the position for neuraxial anesthesia; legs drawn up, with the leg being blocked on top

Landmarks

The iliac crest and the midline of the spinous process are located. From the intersection between these (L4 spinous process), a line is drawn 3 cm caudally, and from the end of it, another line is drawn 5 cm laterally as far as the medial edge of the iliac crest and marked as the injection point (Fig. 70.16).

Skin prep, local anesthesia, sterile draping, drawing up the local anesthetic into 20 mL syringes, checking the patency of the injection needle and functioning of the nerve stimulator, and attaching the electrodes

Preliminary puncture with a large needle or stylet

> The quadriceps femoris muscle must be observed throughout the procedure.

Technique

Single-Injection Technique

1. The palpating hand should be firmly pressed and anchored against the paraspinal muscles to facilitate needle insertion and redirection of the needle when necessary.

[2]<Footnote ID="Fn2"><Para ID="Par159">If technical difficulties arise, the catheter and Tuohy puncture needles are always removed simultaneously. A catheter must never be withdrawn through a Tuohy puncture needle that remains in place (because of catheter shearing).</Para></Footnote>

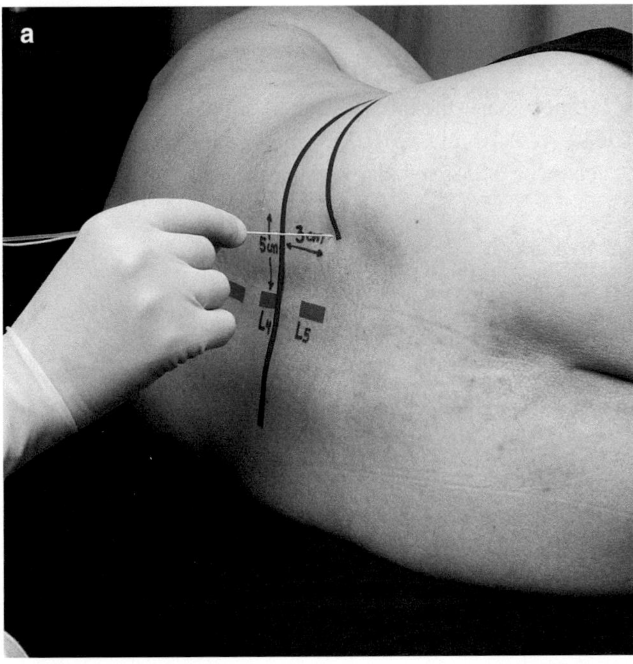

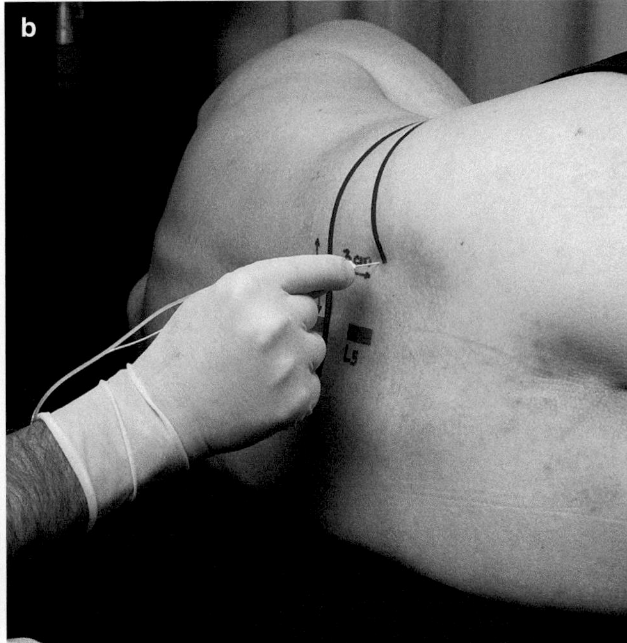

Fig. 70.17 (**a**) The injection needle is introduced perpendicular to the skin surface until bone contact is made with the transverse process of L5 (Reproduced with permission from Danilo Jankovic). (**b**) The injection needle is advanced until contractions of the quadriceps femoris muscle become visible. (Reproduced with permission from Danilo Jankovic)

2. Introduce an electrostimulation needle perpendicular to the skin surface until bone contact is made with the transverse process of L5 (Figs. 70.17a and 70.18).

   The location of the transverse process is very important. The lumbar plexus is situated at the depth of 8.35 cm in average in males (6.1–10.1 cm) and 7.1 cm in average in females (5.7–9.3 cm). The distance from the skin to the transverse process is variable and depends from the anatomy. The distance between transverse process and lumbar plexus is relatively constant (app. 2 cm).

   It is then withdrawn slightly and advanced further cranially, past the transverse process (Figs. 70.17b and 70.18). Stimulation current of 1.5 mA at 2 Hz is selected with a stimulus duration of 0.1 ms.
3. Advance the needle further until contractions of the quadriceps femoris muscle become visible (usually at the depth of 6–8 cm).
4. Reduce the stimulation current to 0.5–1.0 mA. If contractions of the muscle are still visible at this level of current, the needle is in the correct position.
5. Aspiration test.
6. Test dose of 3–5 mL of a local anesthetic.
7. Incremental injection of a local anesthetic (injection-aspiration after each 3–4 mL).
8. Careful cardiovascular monitoring.

Continuous Technique

The needle is attached to the nerve stimulator and to a syringe with local anesthetic.

A Tuohy, continuous block needle is inserted at the perpendicular angle to the skin and advanced until the quadriceps twitch response is obtained at 0.5–1.0 mA current. At this point, after aspiration test and injection of test dose, the initial volume of local anesthetic is injected (e.g., 15–25 mL), and the catheter is advanced ca. 8–10 cm beyond the needle tip into the fascial compartment. The needle is then withdrawn back to the skin level, while the catheter is simultaneously advanced. The opening of the needle should be oriented cephalad before threading the catheter. This method prevents inadvertent removal of the catheter and intravascular and intrathecal placement by negative aspiration test.

Dosage

Surgical

40–50 mL local anesthetic—e.g., 1% prilocaine (20–30 mL) + 0.5–0.75% ropivacaine (20 mL); 1% prilocaine (20–30 mL) + 0.25–0.5% bupivacaine (0.25–0.5% levobupivacaine; 20 mL)

Therapeutic

10–20 mL local anesthetic—e.g., 0.2–0.375% ropivacaine, 0.125–0.25% bupivacaine (0.125–0.25% levobupivacaine)

> Important notes for outpatients (see "three-in-one" block)

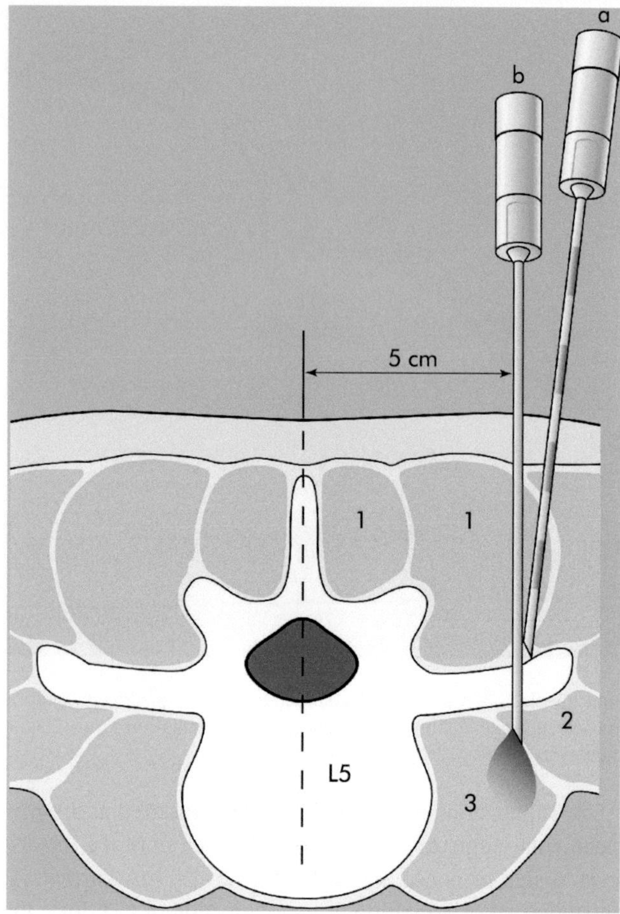

Fig. 70.18 Diagram: *(a)* contact with the transverse process of L5; *(b)* the needle is advanced past the transverse process until contractions of the quadriceps femoris muscle become visible. *(1)* Erector spinae muscle, *(2)* quadratus lumborum muscle, *(3)* psoas muscle. (Reproduced with permission from Danilo Jankovic)

Continuous Technique

Test dose: 3–5 mL 1% prilocaine (1% mepivacaine)

Bolus administration: 30 mL

0.5–0.75% ropivacaine or 0.25–0.5% bupivacaine

Maintenance Dose

Intermittent administration

15–20 mL of local anesthetic every 4–6 h (0.5–0.75% ropivacaine or 0.25–0.5% bupivacaine) after a prior test dose

Reduction of the dose and/or adjustment of the interval, depending on the clinical picture

Continuous Infusion

Infusion of the local anesthetic via the catheter should be started 30–60 min after the bolus dose. A test dose is obligatory.

Ropivacaine: 0.2–0.375%	6–14 mL/h
	(max. 37.5 mg/h)
Levobupivacaine: 0.125–0.25%	8–15 mL/h
Bupivacaine: 0.125%	10–14 mL/h
Bupivacaine: 0.25%	8–10 mL/h

If necessary, the infusion can be supplemented with bolus doses of 5–10 mL 0.5–0.75% ropivacaine (0.25–0.5% bupivacaine or 0.25% levobupivacaine).

> Individual adjustment of the dosage and period of treatment is essential.

Complications

1. Nerve injury (see Chap. 4, Complications of Regional Anesthesia)
2. Intravascular injection
3. Local anesthetic systemic toxicity (see Chap. 5)
4. Subarachnoid or epidural injection with the potential risk of high neuraxial anesthesia (see Chap. 42, Neuraxial Anesthesia)
5. Hypotension
6. Iliopsoas or renal hematoma formation
7. Pneumatocele
8. Intra-abdominal injuries
9. Post-injection pain due to spasm in the lumbar paravertebral musculature

Practical Tips

- Use a strict aseptic technique.
- Visible or palpable twitches of the quadriceps muscle at 0.5 to 1.0 mA.
- Deep needle insertion should be avoided (puncture of the vena cava or aorta).
- Large volumes of long-acting anesthetic should be avoided in older and frail patients. Consider using a less toxic local anesthetic (e.g., prilocaine) or mixtures of two local anesthetics (e.g., prilocaine, mepivacaine, or lidocaine with ropivacaine) to decrease the total dose of more toxic, long-acting local anesthetics.
- Careful and frequent aspiration should be performed during injection.
- Avoid fast, forceful injection of local anesthetic. Forceful injections carry a greater risk of systemic toxicity and epidural spread.
- Do not inject when the patient complains of pain or when high resistance is present.

Advantages

- Better block quality in comparison with the “three-in-one” block.

- Suitable for patients in whom a unilateral block is desired, particularly in outpatient procedures.
- The method is suitable for postoperative and post-traumatic analgesia and for therapeutic blocks.

Disadvantages

- Success of the block is unpredictable.
- Larger quantities of local anesthetic are needed (particularly if the sciatic nerve is also being anesthetized).
- There is an increased likelihood of systemic toxicity (because the placement of the needle is in the deep muscles, the potential for systemic toxicity is greater than it is with more superficial techniques).
- The proximity of the lumbar nerve roots to the epidural space also carries risk of the epidural spread of the local anesthetics.
- Slower onset must be expected (surgical indications).
- For surgical procedures with ischemia or tourniquet, neuraxial anesthesia is preferable.

Proximal Sciatic Nerve Block Traditional Techniques

1. Classic dorsal transgluteal technique (Labat technique)
2. Subgluteal technique
3. Proximal thigh (anterior technique)

General Consideration

The sciatic nerve is the workhorse of the lower extremity, suppling the vast majority of the motor and sensory function to the lower limb. It supplies motor function to the posterior thigh and all muscles below the knee. Sensory function is provided to the posterior thigh, posterior knee joint, and everything below the knee except a narrow band on the medial lower leg. This area is supplied by the saphenous nerve, which is derived from the lumbar plexus. The posterior approach to sciatic nerve block has wide clinical applicability for surgery and pain management and is one of the more commonly used techniques in regional anesthesia for lower extremity. This block is relatively easy to perform and associated with a high success rate. It is particularly suited for surgery on the knee, calf, Achilles tendon, ankle, and foot. It provides complete anesthesia of the leg below the knee with the exception of the medial strip of skin, which is innervated by the saphenous nerve. When combined with femoral nerve or lumbar plexus block, anesthesia of the entire lower extremity can be achieved.

Functional Anatomy

The sciatic nerve arises from the ventral branches of the spinal nerves from L4 to S3. Exiting from the pelvic cavity at the lower edge of the piriformis muscle (in about 2% of individuals, the nerve pierces the piriformis) (Fig. 70.19a, b), its 16–20-mm-thick trunk runs between the ischial tuberosity and the greater trochanter; turns downward over the gemelli, the obturator internus tendon, and the quadratus femoris, which separate it from the hip joint; and leaves the buttock to enter the thigh beneath the lower border of the gluteus maximus (Figs. 70.19a, b and 70.20).

Distal to this, the nerve lies on the posterior surface of the adductor magnus muscle, where it is covered by the flexor muscle originating from the ischial tuberosity and thus extends as far as the popliteal fossa (Figs. 70.19a and 70.20). Here it lies slightly laterally and above the popliteal vein and artery, with thick popliteal fascia overlying it. At the proximal end of the popliteal fossa, the nerve usually divides into the thicker tibial nerve, which continues the trunk and the smaller common peroneal (fibular) nerve (Fig. 70.19a).

The sensory branches of the nerve innervate the dorsal thigh, the dorsolateral lower leg, and lateral half of the foot, the hip and knee joint, as well as the femur.

Its muscular branches are responsible for supplying the biceps femoris, semimembranosus, semitendinosus, and adductor magnus muscles.

Classic Dorsal Transgluteal Technique (Labat Technique)

General Considerations

The classic transgluteal approach of sciatic nerve block was first described in anesthesia literature in 1923 by Gaston Labat in his book, *Regional Anesthesia: Its Technic and Clinical Application*. Alon Winnie modified the Labet approach in 1975. The transgluteal approach to sciatic nerve block has wide clinical applicability for surgery and pain management of the lower extremity. This block is relatively easy to perform and associated with a high success rate.

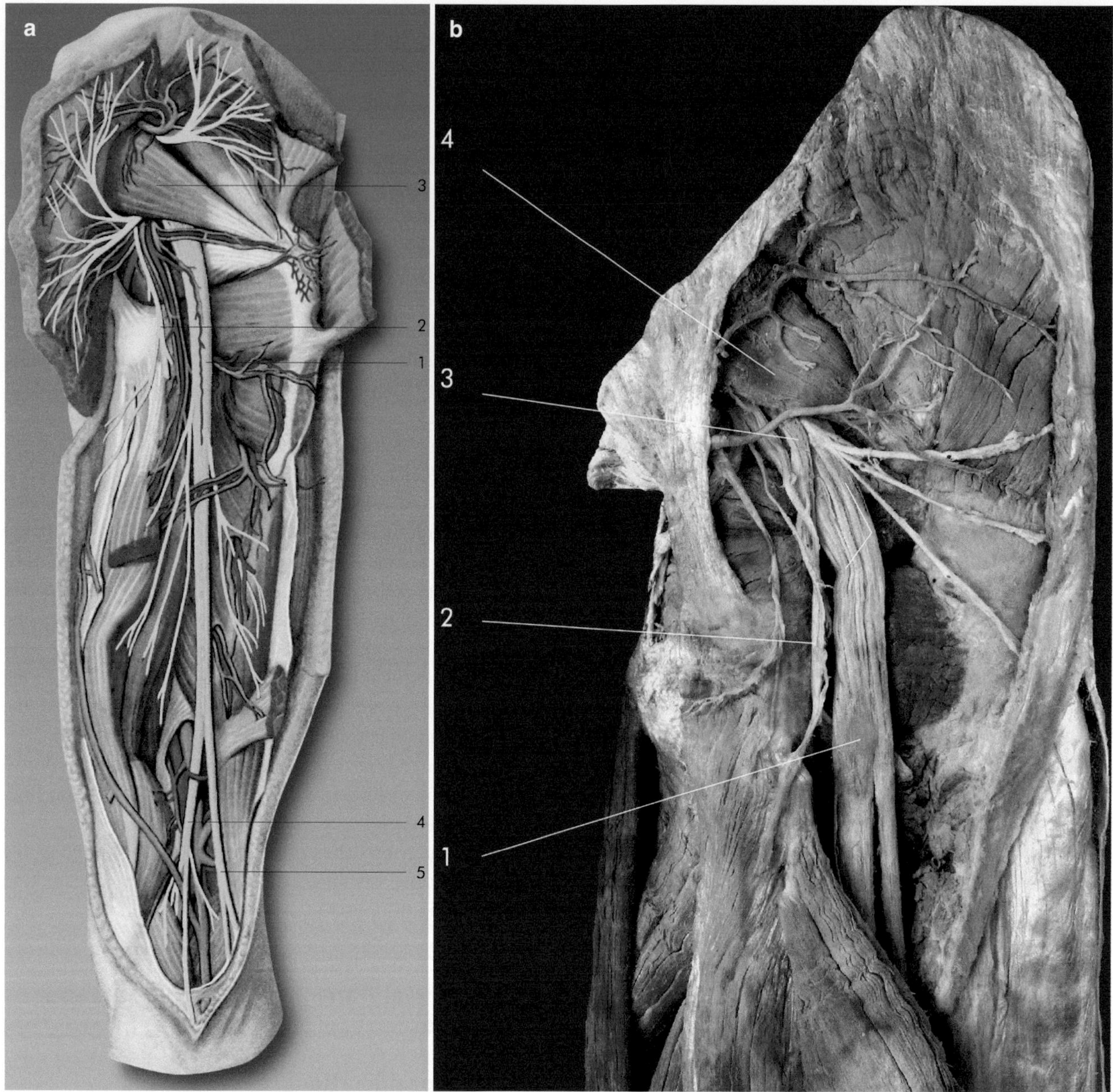

Fig. 70.19 (**a**) Anatomy of the sciatic nerve. *(1)* Sciatic nerve, *(2)* posterior femoral cutaneous nerve, *(3)* piriformis muscle, *(4)* tibial nerve, *(5)* common peroneal (fibular) nerve. (Reproduced with permission from Danilo Jankovic). (**b**) *(1)* Sciatic nerve, *(2)* posterior cutaneus femoris nerve, *(3)* infrapiriform foramen with sciatic nerve and gluteal inferior nerve, *(4)* piriformis muscle. (Reproduced with permission from Danilo Jankovic)

Functional Anatomy

(See above)

Indications

Surgical

- Superficial procedures in the innervated area.
- Carrying out surgical procedures in the region of the lower extremity under tourniquet, but in combination with a block of the lumbar plexus ("three-in-one" block or dorsal psoas compartment block). A need for larger volumes of local anesthetics must be expected (toxicity!).

Therapeutic

An isolated block of the sciatic nerve is rarely indicated. A combination with block of the lumbar plexus or femoral nerve is recommended.

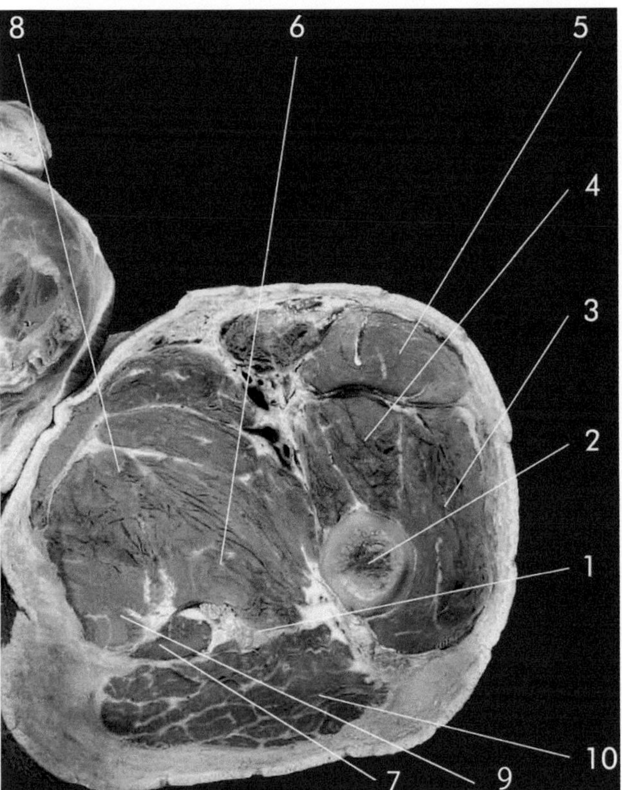

Fig. 70.20 Transversal dissection. *(1)* Sciatic nerve, *(2)* femur, *(3)* vastus lateralis muscle *(4)* vastus intermedius muscle, *(5)* rectus femoris muscle, *(6)* semimembranosus muscle, *(7)* semitendinosus muscle, *(8)* adductor brevis muscle, *(9)* adductor magnus muscle, *(10)* gluteus maximus muscle. (Reproduced with permission from Danilo Jankovic)

Block Series

A series of six to eight blocks is recommended. When there is evidence of improvement in the symptoms, additional blocks can also be carried out.

Contraindications

Specific

- Infection or hematoma in the injection area
- Anticoagulant treatment (see Chap. 1)
- Lesion in the nerves to be blocked distal to the injection site

Relative

The decision should be taken after carefully weighing up the risks and benefits:

- Hemorrhagic diathesis
- Stable central nervous system diseases
- Local nerve injury

Procedure

This block should be carried out by experienced anesthetists, or under their supervision. Full prior information for the patient is mandatory.

Preparations

Check that the emergency equipment is complete and in working order: sterile precautions, intravenous access, ECG monitoring, pulse oximetry, intubation kit, ventilation facilities, and emergency medication.

Materials

Peripheral nerve stimulator

Single-Shot Technique

Fine 26 G needle, 25 mm long, for local anesthesia 80–100 mm long (120–150 mm for ventral access), short-bevel insulated stimulating atraumatic 22 G needle (15°) with injection lead ("immobile needle")

Continuous Technique

Tuohy set: 102-mm-long 18 G Tuohy needle with catheter

Catheter kit: 18 G needle (80–110 mm, 15°) with catheter

Syringes: 2, 10, and 20 mL

Local anesthetics, disinfectant, swabs, compresses, sterile gloves, and drape

Patient Positioning (Fig. 70.21a)

Lateral decubitus, with the leg being blocked on top (Sims position). The upper leg is bent at the hip and knee joints, and the upper knee lies on the table. The lower leg is straight.

Landmarks (Fig. 70.21b)

The important landmarks are the greater trochanter and posterior superior iliac spine (and/or sacral hiatus). From the midpoint of the connecting line, a line is drawn medially, and the injection point is marked at 5 cm (Labat line). To check this, another line connecting the greater trochanter and the sacral hiatus is bisected (Winnie line). The two points should coincide.

Procedure

Skin prep, local anesthesia, sterile draping, drawing up local anesthetic into a 20 mL syringe, checking patency of the injection needle and correct functioning of the nerve stimulator, and attaching the electrodes

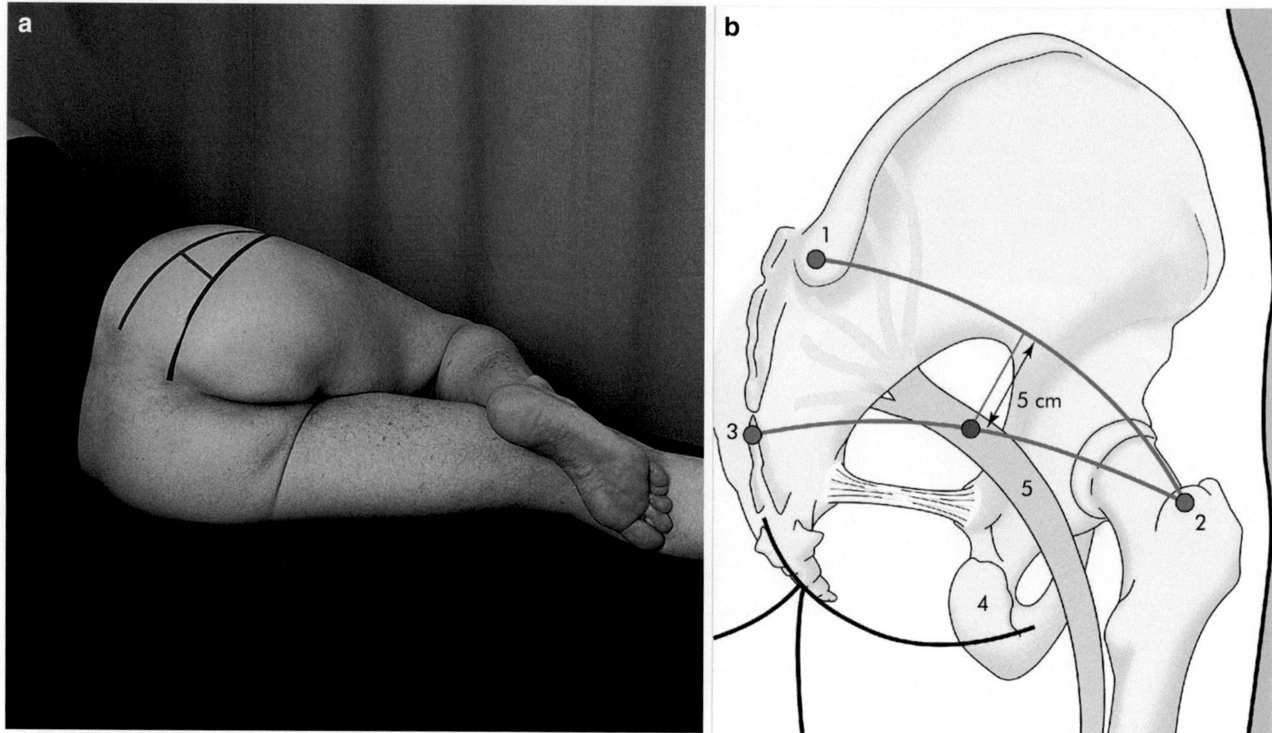

Fig. 70.21 (**a**) Classic dorsal transgluteal technique (positioning) (Reproduced with permission from Danilo Jankovic). (**b**) Landmarks. *(1)* Posterior superior iliac spine, *(2)* greater trochanter, *(3)* sacral hiatus, *(4)* ischial tuberosity, *(5)* sciatic nerve. (Reproduced with permission from Danilo Jankovic)

Preliminary puncture with a large needle or stylet

> During the procedure, the biceps femoris, semimembranosus, and semitendinosus muscles and the foot must be observed.

Injection Technique

1. The injection needle is introduced perpendicular to the skin surface (Fig. 70.22). Stimulation current of 1 mA at 2 Hz is selected with a stimulus duration of 0.1 ms.
2. After about 1–4 cm, there should be direct stimulation of the gluteus maximus muscle.
3. At a depth of about 5 cm, contractions of the biceps femoris, semimembranosus, and semitendinosus muscles are produced (Fig. 70.23).
4. After the needle is advanced further, at a depth of about 6–8 cm, there is plantar and dorsal flexion of the foot as a response to the stimulus from the tibial or peroneal part of the sciatic nerve.
5. Do not advance the needle any further.
6. The stimulation current is reduced to 0.3 mA. Slight twitching suggests that the needle is positioned in the immediate vicinity of the nerve.
7. Aspiration test.

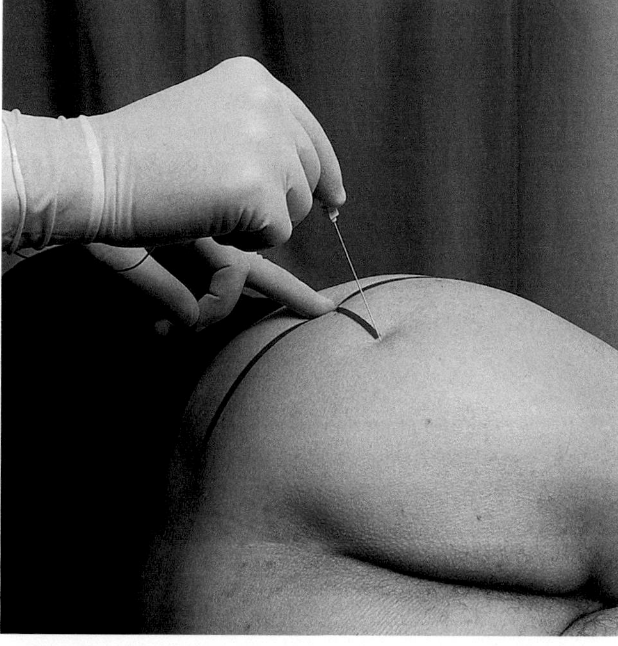

Fig. 70.22 The injection needle is introduced perpendicular to the skin surface. (Reproduced with permission from Danilo Jankovic)

8. Test dose of 3 mL local anesthetic (e.g., 1% lidocaine, mepivacaine, or prilocaine). During the injection, the twitching should slowly disappear.

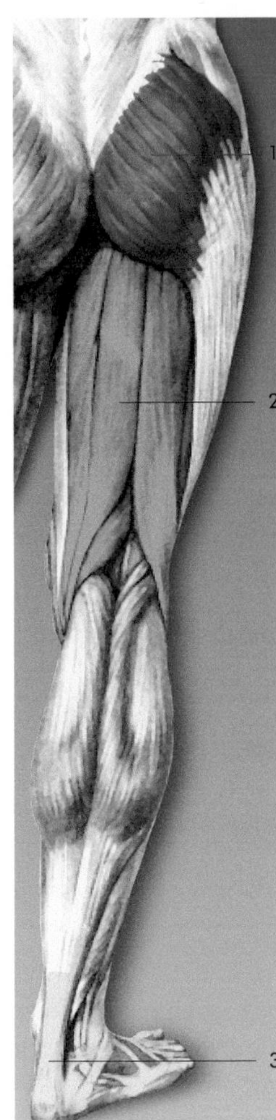

Fig. 70.23 Sequence of muscle contractions. *(1)* Gluteus maximus muscle, *(2)* semitendinosus muscle, semimembranosus muscle, biceps femoris muscle, *(3)* plantar/dorsal flexion of the foot. (Reproduced with permission from Danilo Jankovic)

9. Incremental injection of a local anesthetic (injection-aspiration after each 3–4 mL).
10. Careful cardiovascular monitoring.

The area of anesthesia is shown in Fig. 70.24.

Problem Situations

- Bone contact at a depth of 8 cm without visible twitching. The injection needle should be withdrawn, and the direction should be altered laterally.
- Intraneural positioning:

The following signs suggest intraneural positioning of the injection needle:

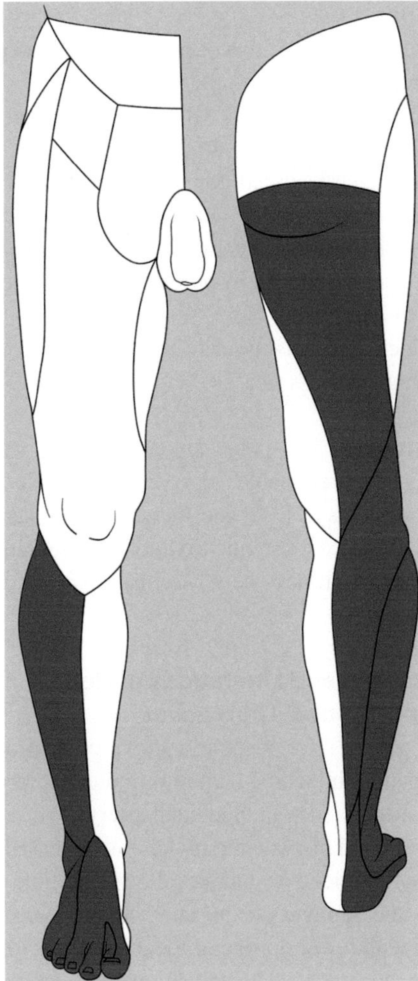

Fig. 70.24 Cutaneous innervated area of the sciatic nerve. (Reproduced with permission from Danilo Jankovic)

- Strong twitching (even at a stimulant current of 0.2 mA).
- No disappearance of the twitching during injection of a test dose.
- High resistance and severe pain during the injection.
- The injection must be stopped immediately and the needle must be withdrawn.

Continuous Technique

The injection is carried out as in the single-shot technique.

An 18-G Tuohy needle 102 mm long or a short bevel stimulating atraumatic needle 110 mm long is usually used as stimulation needles. After correct stimulation and aspiration, a test dose is injected. The catheter is then advanced ca. 3 cm beyond the end of the container, and the stimulation needle is slowly withdrawn while the thumb and index finger of the left hand simultaneously hold the catheter at the injection site. A bacterial filter is then placed, and the catheter is fixed with a skin suture and dressing.

Advantages

- Suitable for postoperative or post-traumatic analgesia and for therapeutic blocks.
- Suitable for patients in whom a unilateral block is desired—particularly in outpatient procedures.
- It is particularly suited for surgery on the knee, calf, Achilles tendon, ankle, and foot. It is most often combined with femoral, lateral femoral cutaneous, and/or obturator nerve blocks to produce surgical anesthesia of the lower leg.
- This block is relatively easy to perform and associated with a high success rate.

Disadvantages

- Success is unpredictable.
- Larger amounts of local anesthetic are necessary.
- The likelihood of systemic toxicity is increased.
- Longer-onset times have to be expected (surgical indications).

Disadvantages and Limitations of Non-ultrasound-Guided Approaches

- Higher potential for penetration of vascular structures and intravascular injection (superior gluteal artery, inferior gluteal artery and vein, pudendal artery).
- The likelihood of systemic toxicity is increased.
- Ultrasound-guided technique allows multiple injections around the lumbar plexus and can be successful performed with lower dosage of local anesthetic solution.
- The use of ultrasound visualization decreases need for the geometry and measurements that are required for the classic landmark-based approaches (particularly important in obese patients).
- Distribution of the local anesthetic cannot be visualized to assure adequate spread around the sciatic nerve.

Sciatic Nerve Block (Subgluteal Approach: Di Benedetto-Borghi)

General Consideration

The subgluteal block of the sciatic nerve has the advantage over the classic posterior transgluteal technique in that it is less stressful to the patient during the procedure, as the sciatic nerve has a more superficial course in the subgluteal region than in the gluteal region. The reduced patient discomfort during block placement is probably related to the shallower depth at which the sciatic nerve is identified, because proper sciatic stimulation was elicited at 4–5 cm as compared with 6.7 cm in classic Labat approach. The reduced depth at which the sciatic nerve can be reached with the subgluteal approach could be helpful particularly in obese patients. In fact, the increased amount of adipose tissue in the gluteal region usually makes it quite difficult and unpredictable to identify the sciatic nerve with needles of normal length if the classic posterior approach is used. This access route also makes it easier to place and fix a catheter for postoperative analgesia.

Functional Anatomy

(See above; transgluteal approach)

Indications

(See above; transgluteal approach)

Contraindications

(See above; transgluteal approach)

Procedure

This block should be carried out by experienced anesthetists or under their supervision. Full prior information for the patient is mandatory.

Preparations

Check that the emergency equipment is complete and in working order: sterile precautions, intravenous access, ECG monitoring, pulse oximetry, intubation kit, ventilation facilities, and emergency medication.

Skin prep, local anesthesia, sterile draping, drawing up local anesthetic, checking the patency of the injection needle and correct functioning of the nerve stimulator, and attaching the electrodes

Materials

(See above, transgluteal approach)

Patient Positioning

Lateral decubitus, with the leg being blocked on top (Sims position; see transgluteal approach (Fig. 70.21a)

Landmarks

From the midpoint of a line connecting the greater trochanter and the ischial tuberosity, a second line is drawn to the upper edge of the popliteal fossa (known as the "sciatic line"). The injection site is located ca. 3–4 cm caudal to this (Fig. 70.25). If the patient is lying in the Sims position, for easier guidance, one can palpate a groove along this line between the semitendinosus muscle and the biceps femoris muscle.

> In this technique, the distance between the skin and the sciatic nerve is shorter (4.7 cm) than in Labat's classic transgluteal access route (6.7 cm).

Technique

Preliminary puncture with a large needle or stylet.
An injection needle ca. 50 (80) mm long is introduced perpendicular to the skin (Fig. 70.26a). Stimulation current is applied at 1–1.5 mA at 2 Hz with a stimulus duration 0.1 ms. At a depth of ca. 4 cm, plantar flexion and dorsiflexion of the foot occur in response to the stimulation of the tibial or peroneal parts of the sciatic nerve. The needle should not be advanced any further. The stimulation current is reduced to 0.3 mA. Slight twitching indicates that the stimulation needle is located in the immediate vicinity of the nerve. After an aspiration test, a test dose (e.g., 3 mL 1% prilocaine) is injected, and incremental injection of the local anesthetic follows.

> During the procedure, the biceps femoris, semimembranosus, and semitendinosus muscles and the foot must be observed.

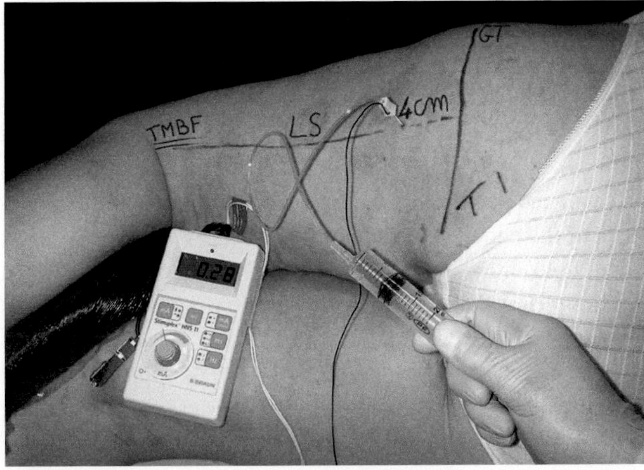

Fig. 70.25 Subgluteal approach. Landmarks. *GT* greater trochanter, *TI* ischial tuberosity, *LS* sciatic line, *TMBF* tendon of the biceps femoris muscle. (Reproduced with permission from Battista Borghi)

Continuous Technique

After skin prep, an adhesive sterile transparent drape with a hole is applied.

Materials

Tuohy continuous set—52 (102)-mm-long 18-G Tuohy needle with a catheter—or catheter kit, 18-G- short-bevel insulated atraumatic needle 80–110 mm (15°) long with a catheter

Technique

The injection is carried out as in the single-shot technique. After injection of 5 mL 0.9% saline, the catheter is introduced through the already positioned needle. The catheter is advanced ca. 3–4 cm beyond the end of the needle or cannula (Fig. 70.26b). After removal of the needle or cannula, fixing of the catheter and placement of a bacterial filter (Fig. 70.26c), after careful aspiration, and injection of a test dose, bolus administration of the local anesthetic is carried out.

Dosage

Surgical

30–40 mL local anesthetic—e.g., 0.5–0.75% ropivacaine, 0.5% bupivacaine (0.5% levobupivacaine), 1% prilocaine, 1% mepivacaine.

A combination of long-duration and medium-duration local anesthetics has proved particularly useful for surgical indications.

Continuous Administration

0.2–0.375% ropivacaine

5–15 mL/h (max. 37.5 mg/h)

Alternatively, as a bolus dose: 0.2–0.375% ropivacaine, 10–30 mL

Patient-controlled analgesia (PCA): baseline rate of 4 mL/h 0.4% ropivacaine, 0.25% levobupivacaine, 0.25% bupivacaine

Bolus dose of 2 mL

Lockout time 10 min

Therapeutic

10–20 mL local anesthetic – e.g., 0.2–0.375% ropivacaine, 0.125–0.25% bupivacaine

Cutaneous innervated area of the sciatic nerve (see Fig. 70.24)

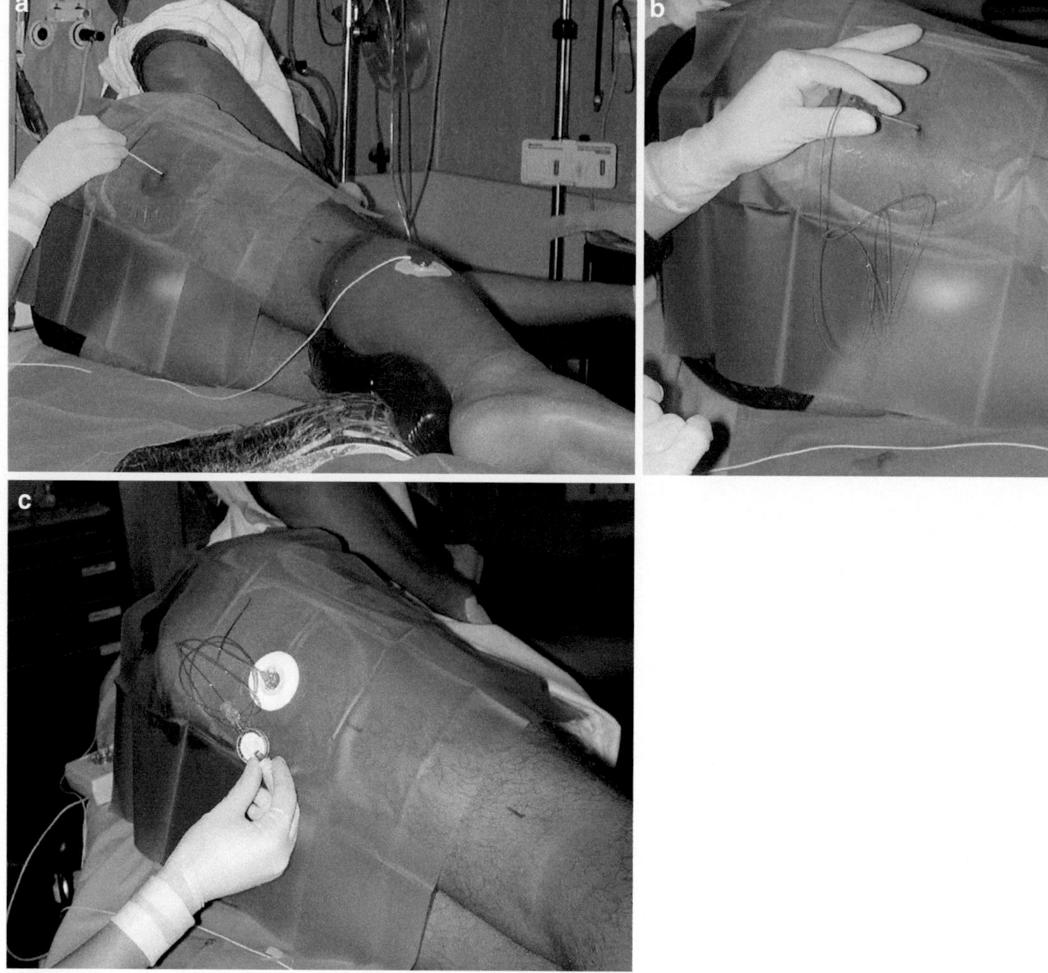

Fig. 70.26 (**a**) Introducing the needle. (Reproduced with permission from Battista Borghi.) (**b**) Introducing the catheter. (Reproduced with permission from Battista Borghi.) (**c**) Fixing the catheter and placing a bacterial filter. (Reproduced with permission from Battista Borghi)

Complications

(See above, transgluteal technique)

Complications are rare, but possible:

1. Nerve injury
2. Intravascular injection
3. CNS toxicity
4. Infection in the area of the injection
5. Hematoma formation

Advantages and Disadvantages

(See above: transgluteal technique)

Sciatic Nerve Block (Anterior Approach)

General Consideration

Among the various approaches to perform regional nerve blocks on the sciatic nerve, the anterior approach is considered to be the most difficult. This approach to sciatic nerve block is an advanced nerve block technique. It requires minimal movement of the patient, a benefit in trauma cases, when movement may be severely limited or painful. When combined with a femoral nerve block, the anterior sciatic nerve block provides complete anesthesia of the lower extremity. Beck was the first to describe the anterior approach in 1963. His approach located the sciatic nerve near the lesser trochanter using the anatomic landmarks of the anterior superior iliac spine, lateral border of the pubic symphysis, and the greater trochanter. In 1999, Chelly and Delaunay described a new anterior approach to the sciatic nerve without using the greater trochanter as a landmark (line between the inferior border of the anterior iliac spine and the superior angle of the pubic tubercle).

Functional Anatomy (Fig. 70.28a, b)

The sciatic nerve, terminal branch of the sacral plexus that exits the pelvis through the greater sciatic foramen, has initially a curved route before becoming more or less parallel to the femoral shaft at the thigh. In this technique, the sciatic nerve is blocked while posterior and medial to the lesser trochanter, or to the femoral shaft immediately distal to the lesser trochanter. Anatomic variations are common, and the nerve may be more or less medial to the femur. The landmarks described by Beck aim at locating the lesser trochanter based on the position of the greater trochanter, which is palpated at the lateral aspect of the upper thigh.

Indications

- For patients who cannot be repositioned into the lateral decubitus position (Sims position). It requires minimal movement of the patient, a benefit in trauma cases, when movement may be severely limited or painful (see transgluteal approach).

Contraindications

- This block is relatively contraindicated in patients who had vascular surgery in the groin area (as ultrasound is not used).
- Coagulopathic patients (see Chap. 1).

Patient Positioning

A supine position that is comfortable for the patient, with slight outward rotation of the leg being blocked.

Landmarks

Important landmarks are the anterior superior iliac spine, pubic tubercle, and greater trochanter. Two lines are drawn for orientation:

- A line connecting the anterior superior iliac spine with the pubic tubercle, which is marked into thirds
- A second line parallel to the first, from the greater trochanter across the thigh

A perpendicular line is drawn from the intersection of the medial and central third of the upper inguinal ligament line to the parallel line and marked as the injection point (Figs. 70.27a, b and 70.28a, b).

Technique

A 22 G (15°) short-bevel insulated stimulating atraumatic needle 120–150 mm long, with an injection lead, is advanced perpendicular to the skin until bone contact is made with the femur. The needle is then withdrawn slightly and introduced about 5 cm deeper, past the medial border of the femur.

During the anterior approach to sciatic nerve block, the needle traverses between the sartorius and rectus femoris and through the iliopsoas, pectineus, adductor longus, brevis, and magnus muscles before reaching the sciatic nerve (Fig. 70.28b). The correct needle position is confirmed when paresthesias or twitches are produced during electrostimulation. After aspiration and administration of a test dose, incremental injection of a local anesthetic is carried out.

Problem Situations and Practical Tips

- Contractions of the quadriceps femoris muscle and patelar movements become visible (needle position is too superficial – stimulation of the branches of the femoral nerve) (Fig. 70.28a). Continue advancing the needle.
- Local twitch at the femoral crease area (stimulation of iliopsoas or pectineus muscles—too cephalad insertion of the needle (Fig. 70.28b)).
- The needle is placed deep (12–15 cm), but twitches were not elicited, and bone is not contacted (too medial insertion of the needle). Withdraw the needle and redirect it slight laterally.
- Bone contact is frequently encountered during needle advancement (usually the lesser trochanter). Withdraw the needle back to the subcutaneous tissue, and rotate the foot inward. Eventually, reinsert the needle 1–2 cm medial to initial insertion.

Complications

1. Hematoma formation (avoid multiple needle insertions). Note the obligatory prophylactic compression.
2. Infection in the injection area (continuous techniques).
3. Intravascular injection (avoid medial placement of the needle- femoral artery and vein-) (Fig. 70.28a) (see Chap. 5).
4. Local anesthetic systemic toxicity (see Chap. 5).

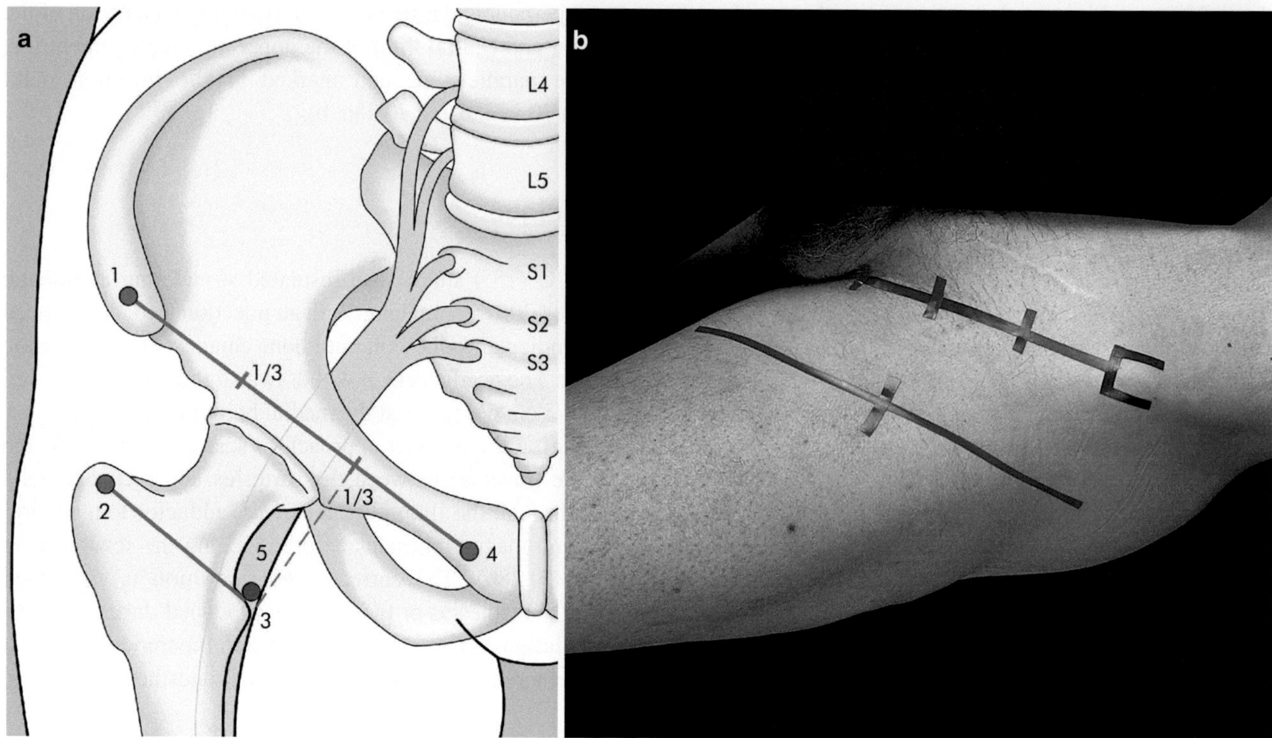

Fig. 70.27 (**a**) Anterior approach. Location (diagram). *(1)* Anterior superior iliac spine, *(2)* greater trochanter, *(3)* injection site, *(4)* pubic tubercle, *(5)* sciatic nerve. (Reproduced with permission from Danilo Jankovic.) (**b**) Location (in patient). (Reproduced with permission from Danilo Jankovic)

5. Nerve injuries (see Chap. 4, Complications of Regional Anesthesia).

   Traumatic nerve injury is a rare complication of this technique. It can occur as a result of the use of sharp needles (due to nerve puncture), intraneural or microvascular injury (hematoma and its sequelae), prolonged ischemia, as well as toxic effects of intraneurally injected local anesthetic. Probable effects of intraneural injection include a transient neurological deficit (unexpectedly prolonged block, lasting up to 10 days). A suspicion of intraneural needle positioning arises if there is strong twitching even at low levels of stimulation current (e.g., 0.2 mA) and if there is no cessation of the twitching after administration of the test dose. The local anesthetic may also be difficult to inject. Correction of the needle position is essential.
6. Tourniquet damage (avoid the use of a tourniquet if possible).

Important Notes for Outpatients

Long-lasting block can occur (even after administration of low-dose local anesthetics—e.g., 0.125% bupivacaine or 0.2% ropivacaine). The blocked leg can give way even 10–18 h after the injection. The patient must therefore use walking aids during this period. The same rules apply to the treatment of postamputation pain. During the period of effect of the local anesthetic, the patient should not wear a prosthesis.

A record must be kept of patient information and consent.

Advantages

- The use of this block is reserved for patients who cannot be repositioned into the lateral position needed for posterior approach.

Disadvantages

- The needle crosses more tissue and muscle planes. Thus, the procedure might be more painful for the patient (Fig. 70.28b).
- The block is more distal, and there is a risk of not blocking the posterior cutaneous nerve of the thigh, with consequently no anesthesia of the posterior aspect of the thigh. A thigh tourniquet would then be poorly tolerated.
- The superficial and deep femoral vessels, as well as branches of the femoral nerve, lie anterior and medial to

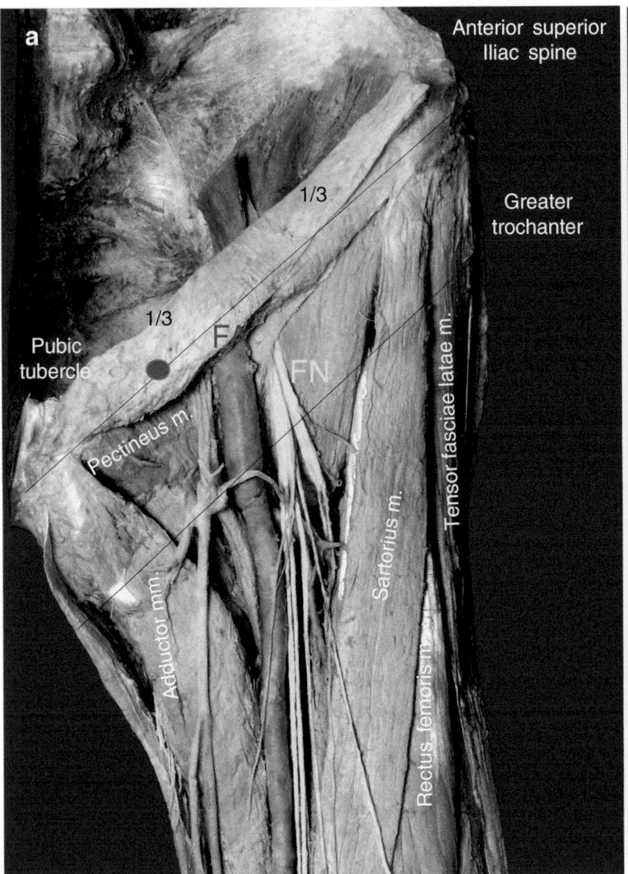

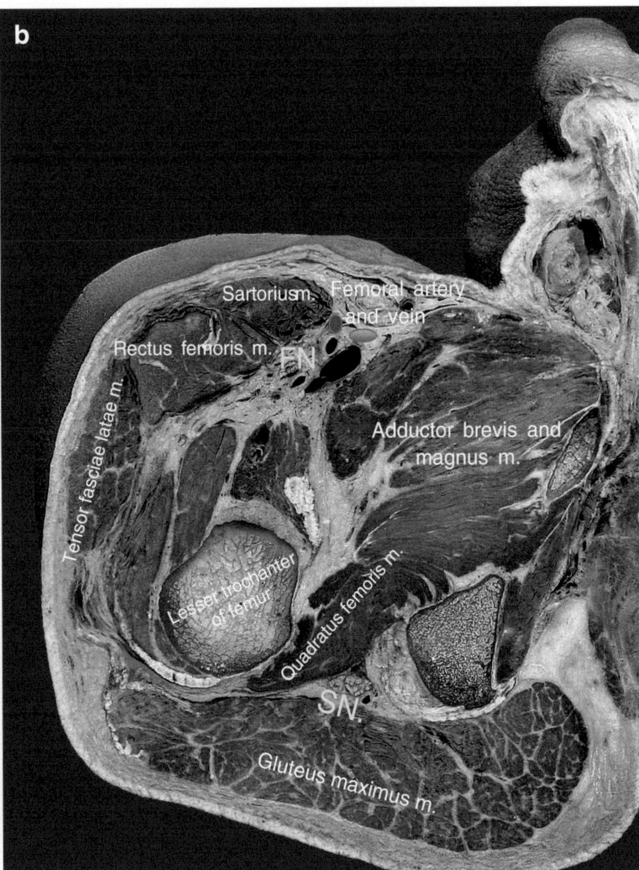

Fig. 70.28 (**a**) Anatomic preparation. Anterior approach. Location. FA femoral artery, FN femoral nerve. (Reproduced with permission from Danilo Jankovic.) (**b**) Transversal dissection: the needle traverses between the sartorius and rectus femoris and through the iliopsoas, pectineus, adductor longus, brevis, and magnus muscles before reaching the sciatic nerve. *FN* femoral nerve, *SN* sciatic nerve. (Reproduced with permission from Danilo Jankovic)

the femoral shaft, and there is a theoretical risk of injuring them during the block performance.

- This technique is not ideal for catheter insertion because of the deep location and perpendicular angle of insertion.
- Because of the large size of the sciatic nerve, 25–40 min may be necessary for full blockade.

Popliteal Sciatic Nerve Block

See Chap. 60 Popliteal Sciatic Nerve Block.

Suggested Reading

Functional Anatomy of the Lumbar Plexus, Sacral Plexus and Coccygeal Plexus

Farny J, Drolet P, Girard M. Anatomy of the posterior approach to the lumbar plexus block. Can J Anesth. 1994;41:480–5.

Gosling JA, Harris PF, Whitmore I, Willan PLT. Fotoatlas Anatomie. Urban & Fischer; 2005. p. 225–43.

Hanna M, Peat SJ, D'Costa F. Lumbar plexus block: an anatomical study. Anesthesia. 1993;48:675–8.

Jankovic D. Anatomie des plexus lumbalis, sacralis und coccygeus. In: Jankovic D, editor. Regional blockade and infiltrationstherapie. 4th ed. ABW-Berlin; 2007. p. 316–8.

Kirchmair L, Entner T, Wissel J, et al. A study of the paravertebral anatomy for ultrasound guided posterior lumbar plexus block. Anesth Analg. 2001;93:477–8.

Netter FH. Nervous system. Part 1. Anatomy and physiology. The Ciba Collection of Medical Illustrations. Ciba 1991. Plates 1–16.

Rohen J, Yokochi C, Lütjen-Drecoll E. Anatomie des Menschen. Fotografischer Atlas. Schattauer; 2002. p. 456–70.

Thiel W. Photographischer Atlas der Praktischen Anatomie, vol. 208-27. Springer; 2003. p. 246–60.

Inguinal Femoral Nerve Block ("Three-in-One" Block)

Berkowitz A, Rosenberg H. Femoral block with mepivacaine for muscle biopsy in malignant hyperthermia patients. Anesthesiology. 1985;62:651–2.

Capdevila X, Biboulet P, Bouregba M, et al. Comparison of the three-in-one and fascia iliaca compartment blocks in adults: clinical and radiographic analysis. Anesth Analg. 1998;86:1039–44.

Capdevila X, Biboulet P, Morau D, Bernard N, Deschodt J, Lopez S, d'Athis F. Continuous three-in-one block for postoperative pain after lower limb orthopaedic surgery: where do the catheters go? Anesth Analg. 2002;94:1001–6.

Cauhepe C, Oliver M, Colombani R, et al. The "3-in-1" block: myth or reality? Ann Fr Anesth Reanim. 1989;8:376–8.

Elmas C, Atanassoff P. Combined inguinal paravascular (3 in 1) and sciatic nerve blocks for lower limb surgery. Reg Anesth. 1993;18:88–92.

Frerk CM. Palsy after femoral nerve block. Anaesthesia. 1988;43:167–8.

Hirst GC, Lang SA, Dust WN, Cassidy D, Yip RW. Femoral nerve block. Single injection versus continuous infusion for total knee arthroplasty. Reg Anesth. 1996;21(4):292–7.

Lang S, Yip R, Chang P, Gerard M. The femoral 3-in-1 block revisited. J Clin Anesth. 1993;5:292–6.

Lang S. Electromyographic comparison of obturator nerve block to 3-in-1 block. Anesth Analg. 1996;83:436–7.

Lynch J. Prolonged motor weakness after femoral nerve block with bupivacaine 0,5%. Anaesthesia. 1990;45:421.

Marhofer P, Nasel C, Sitzwohl C, Karpal S. Magnetic resonance imaging of the distribution of local anesthetic during the three-in-one block. Anesth Analg. 2000;90:119–24.

Misra U, Pridie AK, McClymont C, Bower S. Plasma concentrations of bupivacaine following combined sciatic and femoral 3 in 1 nerve blocks in open knee surgery. Br J Anaesth. 1991;66:310–3.

Ringrase NH, Cross MJ. Femoral nerve block in knee joint surgery. Am J Sports Med. 1984;12:398–402.

Ritter J. Femoral nerve "sheath" for inguinal paravascular lumbar plexus block is not found in human cadavers. J Clin Anesth. 1995;7:470–3.

Rooks M, Fleming LL. Evaluation of acute knee injuries with sciatic femoral nerve blocks. Clin Orthop. 1983;179:185–8.

Rosenblatt R. Continuous femoral anesthesia for lower extremity surgery. Anesth Analg. 1980;59:631.

Singelyn F, Vanderelst P, Gouverneur J. Extended femoral nerve sheath block after total hip arthroplasty: continuous versus patient-controlled techniques. Anesth Analg. 2001;92:455–9.

Singelyn FJ, Gouverneur JM. The continuous "3-in-1" block as post-operative pain treatment after hip, femoral shaft or knee surgery: a large scale study of efficacy and side effects. Anesthesiology. 1994;81:1064.

Winnie AP, Ramamurthy S, Durani Z. The inguinal paravascular technic of lumbar plexus anesthesia: the "3-in-1" the inguinal paravascular block. Anesth Analg. 1973;52:989–96.

Winnie A. Regional anesthesia. Surg Clin North Am. 1975;55:861–92.

Winnie A, Ramamurthy S, Durrani Z, Radonjic R. Plexus blocks for lower extremity surgery. Anesthesiol Rev. 1974;1:11–6.

Psoas Compartment Block (Cheyen Approach)

Aida S, Takahashi H, Shimoji K. Renal subcapsular hematoma after lumbar plexus block. Anestesiology. 1996;84:452–5.

Aveline C, Bonnet F. Delayed retroperitoneal hematoma after failed lumbar plexus block. Br. J Anesth. 2004;93:589–91.

Blumenthal S, Ekatodramis G, Borgeat A. Ropivacaine plasma concentrations are similar during continuous lumbar plexus blockade using two techniques: pharmacokinetics or pharmacodynamics? Can J Anesth. 2004;51:851.

Bogoch ER, Hence M, Mackenzie T, et al. Lumbar paravertebral nerve block in the management of pain after total hip and knee arthroplasty: a randomize controlled trial. J Arthroplast. 2002;17:398–401.

Capdevila X, Macaire P, Dadure C, Choquet O, Biboulet P, Ryckwaert YD, D'Athis F. Continuous psoas compartment block for postoperative analgesia after total hip arthroplasty: new landmarks, technical guidelines and clinical evaluation. Anesth Analg. 2002;94:1606–13.

Chayen D, Nathan H, Clayen M. The psoas compartment block. Anesthesiology. 1976;45:95–9.

Chelly JE, Casati A, Al-Samsam T, et al. Continuous lumbar plexus block for acute postoperative pain management after open reduction and internal fixation of acetabular fractures. J Orthop Trauma. 2003;17:362–7.

Gentilli M, Aveline C, Bonnet F. Total spinal anesthesia after posterior lumbar plexus block. Ann Fr Anesth Reanim. 1998;17:740–2.

Huet O, Eyrolle LJ, Mazoit JX, et al. Cardiac arrest after injection of ropivacaine for posterior lumbar plexus blockade. Anesthesiology. 2003;99:1451–3.

Hsy DT. Delayed retroperitoneal hematoma after failed lumbar plexus block. Br J Anesth. 2005;93:589–91.

Indelli PF, Grant SA, Nielsen K, et al. Regional anesthesia in hip surgery. Clin Orthop Relat Res. 2005;441:250–5.

Litz RJ, Vicent O, Wiessner D, et al. Misplacement of a psoas compartment catheter in the subarachoidal space. Reg Anesth Pain Med. 2004;29:60–4.

Mannion S, Barrett J, Kelly D, et al. A description of the spread of injectate after psoas compartment block using magnetic resonance imaging. Reg Anesth Pain Med. 2005;30:567–71.

Pham-Dang C, Beaumont S, Floch H, et al. Acute toxic accident following lumbar plexus block with bupivacaine. Ann Fr Anesth Reanim. 2000;19:356–9.

Reddy MB. Pneumocoele following psoas compartment block. Anesthesia. 2002;57:938–9.

Robards C, Hadzic A. Lumbar plexus block. In: Hadzic: textbook of regional anesthesia and acute pain management. Mc Graw Hill; 2007. p. 481–8.

Proximal Sciatic Nerve Block-Traditional Techniques

Beck GP. Anterior approach to sciatic nerve block. Anesthesiology. 1963;24:222–4.

Ben-David B, Schmalenberger K, Chelly JE. Analgesia after total knee arthroplasty: is continuous sciatic blockade needed in addition to continuous femoral blockade? Anesth Analg. 2004;98(3):747–9.

di Benedetto P, Bertini L, Casati A, Borghi B, et al. A new posterior approach to the sciatic nerve block. A prospective, randomized comparison with the classical posterior approach. Anesth Analg. 2001;93:1040–4.

di Benedetto P, Casati A, Bertini L. Continuous subgluteal sciatic nerve block after orthopedic foot and ankle surgery: comparison of two infusion techniques. Reg Anesth Pain Med. 2002;27(2):168–72.

Bertini L, Casati A, Borghi B, et al. A new posterior approach to the sciatic nerve block. A prospective, randomized comparison with the classical posterior approach. Anesth Analg. 2001;93:1040–4.

Bridenbaugh PO, Wedel DJ. The lower extremity: somatic blockade. In: Cousins MJ, Bridenbaugh DL, editors. Neural blockade in clinical anesthesia and management of pain. 3rd ed. Lippincott-Raven; 1998. p. 375–94.

Candido KD, Sukhani R, McCarthy RJ. Posterior approach to the sciatic nerve: can "common sense" replace science and logic? Anesthesiology. 2003;99(5):1237–8.

Capdevilla X, Ponrouch M, Choquet O. Continuous peripheral nerve blocks in clinical practice. Curr Opin Anaesthesiol. 2008;21(5):619–23.

Casati A, et al. Using stimulating catheters for continuous sciatic nerve block shortens onset time of surgical block and minimizes postoperative consumption of pain medication after halux valgus repair as compared with conventional nonstimulating catheters. Anesth Analg. 2005;101(4):1192–7.

Casati A, et al. A double-blinded, randomized comparison of either 0.5% levobupivacaine or 0.5% ropivacaine for sciatic nerve block. Anesth Analg. 2002;94(4):987–90.

Casati A, et al. Levobupivacaine 0.2% or 0.125% for continuous sciatic nerve block: a prospective, randomized, double-blind comparison with 0.2% ropivacaine. Anesth Analg. 2004;99(3):919–23.

Chely JE, Delaunay L. A new anterior approach to the sciatic nerve block. Anesthesiology. 1999;91:1655–60.

Farny J, Girard M, Drolet P. Posterior approach to the lumbar plexus combined with a sciatic nerve block using lidocaine. Can J Anesth. 1994;41(6):486–91.

Fournier R, et al. Levobupivacaine 0.5% provides longer analgesia after sciatic nerve block using Labat approach then the same dose of ropivacaine in foot and ankle surgery. Anesth Analg. 2010;110(5):1486–9.

Grabtree EC, et al. A method to estimate the depth of the sciatic nerve during subgluteal block by using thigh diameter as a guide. Reg Anesth Pain Med. 2006;31(4):358–62.

Hadzic A. Peripheral nerve blocks. Sciatic Block Mc Graw Hill; 2012. p. 229–48.

Jankovic D. Sciatic nerve block. In: Jankovic D, editor. Regional nerve blocks & infiltration therapy. Textbook and color atlas. Blackwell; 2004. p. 230–7.

Kilpatrick AW, Coventry DM, Todd JG. A comparison of two approaches to sciatic nerve block. Anesthesia. 1992;47(2):155–7.

Latzke D, et al. Minimal local anesthetic volumes for sciatic nerve block: evaluation of ED 99 in volunteers. Br J Anaesth. 2010;104(2):239–44.

Mansour NY, Bennetts FE. An observational study of combined continuous lumbar plexus and single –shot sciatic nerve blocks for post-knee surgery analgesia. Reg Anesth. 1996;21:287–91.

Misra U, Pridie AK, McClymont C, et al. Plasma concentrations of bupivacaine following combined sciatic and femoral 3in1 nerve blocks in open knee surgery. Br J Anesth. 1991;66:310–3.

Smith BE, Sggins D. Low volume, high concentration block of the sciatic nerve. Anaesthesia. 1988;43:8–11.

Tran D, Clemente A, Finlayson RJ. A review of approaches and techniques for lower extremity nerve blocks. Can J Anesth. 2007;54(11):922–34.

Wiegel M, Reske A, Hennebach R, et al. Anterior sciatic nerve block-new landmarks and clinical experience. Acta Anaesthesiol Scand. 2005;49:552–7.

Winnie AP. Regional anesthesia. Surg Clin North Am. 1975;55:861–92.

Part VIII

Neuromodulation Therapy

Ultrasound-Guided Peripheral Nerve Stimulation

71

Alexander Sable-Smith and Einar Ottestad

Contents

General Consideration

Electrical stimulation has been used for centuries to relieve pain since the serendipitous discovery, described in 15 AD by the Roman physician Scribonius, that contact with an electric fish relieved gout pain. In the late nineteenth and early twentieth centuries, compact devices capable of transcutaneous electrical nerve stimulation were developed and marketed to consumers as a treatment for pain and other maladies, though without any scientific substantiation of these claims. Modern neuromodulation was born in the late 1960s after Melzack and Wall postulated the mechanism by which electrical stimulation can produce analgesia, known as the gate control theory. This theory was substantiated in a case series of peripheral nerve stimulation used to diminish pain. Peripheral nerve stimulation (PNS) was followed soon by the first reports of dorsal column stimulation by Shealy. Miniaturization of batteries and electrical leads, along with widespread adoption of fluoroscopy, transformed dorsal column stimulation from an open neurosurgical procedure to one that could be performed percutaneously by anesthesiologists who were already adept in percutaneous epidural access techniques. Peripheral nerve stimulation, however, remained the purview of surgeons, whose skills were necessary to meticulously expose peripheral nerves and attach cuff-like electrodes. Just as fluoroscopy transformed dorsal column stimulation, widespread adoption of ultrasound proved transformative for the field of peripheral neuromodulation. Ultrasound allowed clinicians to easily identify peripheral nerve targets for percutaneous intervention. Dorsal column stimulation systems with implantable pulse generators (IPGs) were re-purposed for peripheral use. More recently, PNS systems consisting of small monopolar or multipolar leads with external power sources have been developed.

A. Sable-Smith · E. Ottestad (✉)
Anesthesiology, Perioperative and Pain Medicine, Stanford University School of Medicine, Stanford, CA, USA
e-mail: ottestad@stanford.edu

D. Jankovic, P. Peng (eds.), *Regional Nerve Blocks in Anesthesia and Pain Therapy*,
https://doi.org/10.1007/978-3-030-88727-8_71

Presently, commercially available peripheral nerve stimulators are designed for either temporary or permanent implantation. Temporary stimulators (Fig. 71.1a) intended for 60-day use are implanted percutaneously with the monopolar lead adjacent to the target nerve. The lead exits the skin where it is secured under an occlusive adhesive dressing and connected externally to a pulse generator. Systems designed for permanent implantation are similarly placed; however, the tail end of the lead is either tunneled subcutaneously where it either functions as a receiver for an external pulse transmitter (EPT) (Fig. 71.1b) or connects to a miniature IPG (Fig. 71.1c).

Peripheral nerve stimulation is indicated for chronic, intractable pain of peripheral nerve origin, primarily mononeuropathies. Prototypical conditions include mononeuropathies such as CRPS type II (causalgia) or phantom

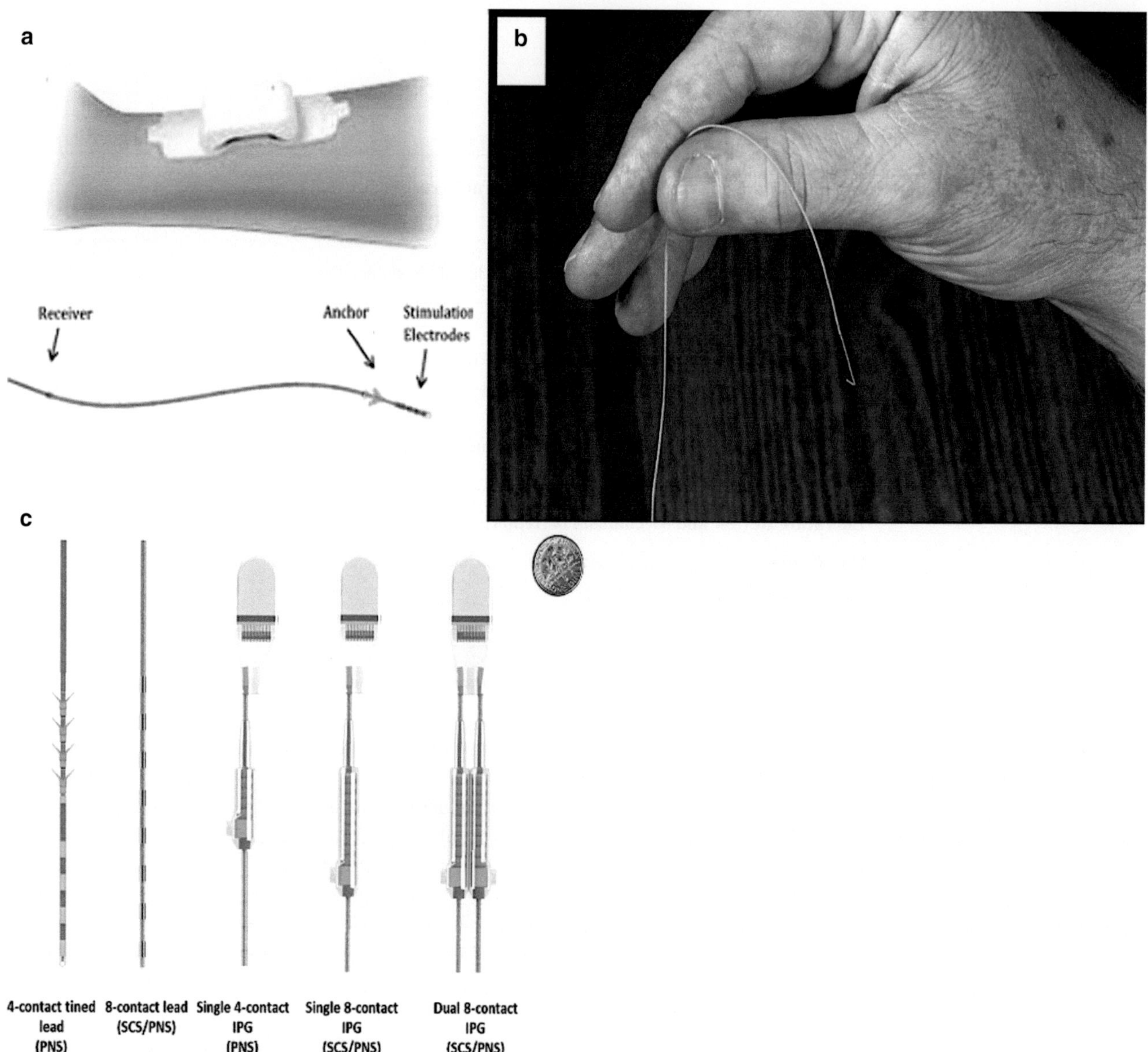

Fig. 71.1 This figure depicts examples of commercially available peripheral nerve stimulator systems including (**a**) permanent implantable monopolar lead with a disposable adhesive external pulse transmitter worn on the skin overlying the implanted lead; (**b**) temporary monopolar coiled lead which exits the body and connects to a pulse generator; and (**c**) permanent multipolar lead with implantable pulse generator, with a dime for size reference. The system pictured here is designed for both peripheral nerve (PNS) and spinal cord stimulation (SCS)

limb pain following amputation. However, there is evidence that PNS can provide analgesia for painful conditions with a predominant somatic origin, such as hemiplegic shoulder pain after stroke and for postoperative analgesia of the shoulder and knee. Generally, the pain being treated should be confined to the distribution of the sensory innervation of the target nerve. It is postulated that PNS has beneficial and durable effects on neuroplasticity in the central nervous system, which has led to applications for pain that is not primarily neuropathic in nature such as low back pain, and even non-painful symptoms such as overactive bladder.

Though many peripheral nerves can be targeted using multi-modal imaging for guidance, in this chapter, we will describe ultrasound-guided approaches for two targets, one in the upper extremity (suprascapular nerve for shoulder pain) and one in the lower (posterior tibial nerve for foot pain), as illustrative examples.

Indications and Patient Selection for Peripheral Nerve Stimulation

General patient selection involves a thorough history and physical exam to identify the origins of pain and identify medical and psychosocial factors that may influence the efficacy of PNS systems. Patients must have the capacity to make an informed decision to undergo the procedure and plan appropriately for the use of the device. The implanting clinician must consider the visualization of the target nerve and surrounding landmarks, lead trajectory, and tunneling site as well as ergonomics of the use of the power source or charger. Leads should not be placed across joints in order to minimize chances that everyday movement causes lead fracture or migration. Need for future magnetic resonance imaging should also be considered, and manufacturer-specific MRI recommendations should be followed. Patients who have other implanted electronic devices or metallic devices should not have PNS systems implanted in the immediate area of the other device.

Suprascapular Nerve

Stimulation of the suprascapular nerve is indicated for patients with chronic pain arising from the glenohumeral joint, particularly the superior-posterior aspect of the joint which is primarily innervated by this nerve. Conditions include glenohumeral arthritis and chronic supraspinatus tendinopathy. Pain originating from more anterior structures such as the acromioclavicular joint and biceps tendon may not benefit as much from this procedure.

Tibial Nerve

Stimulation of the tibial nerve is indicated for pain of the sole of the foot, including painful peripheral neuropathy, chronic pain following podiatric surgery, or other chronic pain following foot injury.

Stimulation of the Suprascapular Nerve for Chronic Shoulder Pain

Functional Anatomy

The suprascapular nerve arises from the superior cord of the brachial plexus, with contributions from primarily the C5 and C6 nerve roots, but with contributions from C4 in some cases. From the brachial plexus, it courses posteriorly with the suprascapular artery through the suprascapular notch to the supraspinatus fossa where it runs deep to the supraspinatus muscle. The nerve continues inferiorly through the spinoglenoid notch to the infraspinatus fossa. Medial projections innervate the supraspinatus and infraspinatus muscles. Laterally, the nerve sends sensory branches to the shoulder joint, primarily the superior and posterior aspects. Blockade of the suprascapular nerve with local anesthetic is used to control acute and chronic shoulder pain of numerous etiologies, while radiofrequency neuromodulation has demonstrated sustained pain relief for up to 6 months.

Technique

Positioning and Scanning

The patient is placed prone or sitting so that the posterior and superior portions of the shoulder are exposed. A high-frequency linear transducer is oriented in a coronal plane over the supraspinatus fossa (Fig. 71.2). From superficial to deep, the trapezius muscle, supraspinatus muscle, and supraspinatus fossa can be identified. The transducer is then moved slightly anteriorly to identify the suprascapular notch, which will appear as an indentation or divot in the supraspinatus fossa covered by the transverse scapular ligament (Figs. 71.3 and 71.4). The suprascapular nerve and vessels travel from an anterior to posterior direction through this notch. The artery can be seen in the notch but has a variable course and is not always immediately near the nerve.

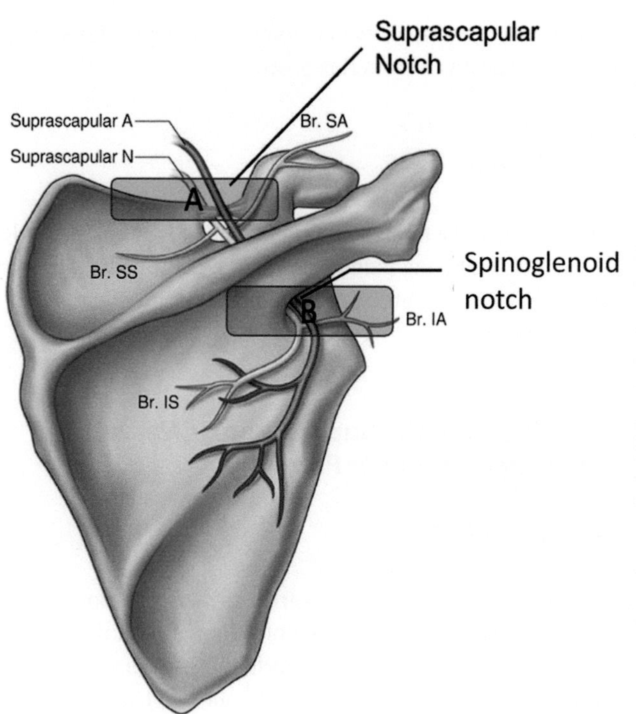

Fig. 71.2 Approximate scanning position and lead placement technique for stimulation of the suprascapular nerve. Position A demonstrates position for placement perpendicular to the nerve at the suprascapular notch. Position B demonstrates placement parallel to the nerve at the spinoglenoid notch. Reprinted with permission from the Philip Peng Educational Series, with modification by Einar Ottestad and Alexander Sable-Smith

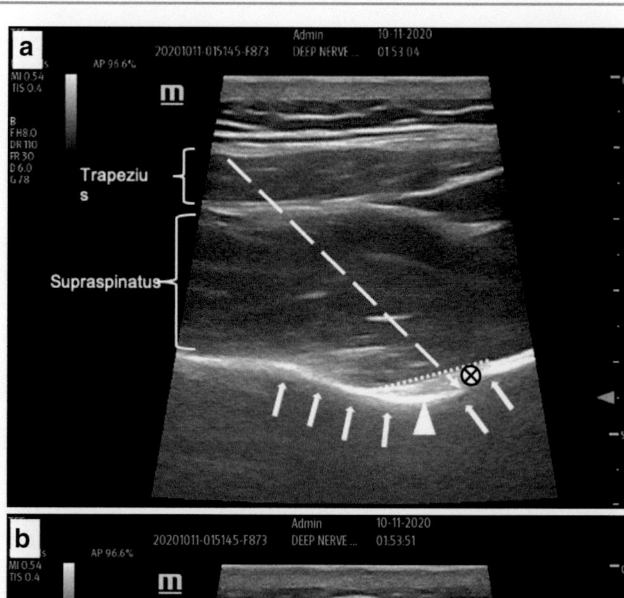

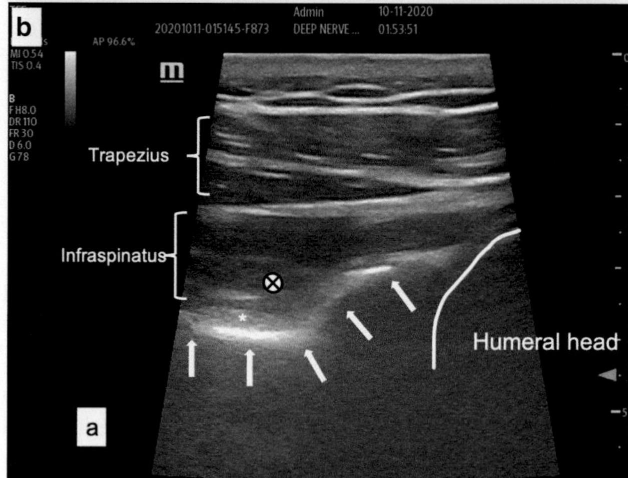

Fig. 71.3 (**a**) Ultrasound image of the suprascapular nerve (arrowhead) at the suprascapular notch (outlined with bold arrows). The suprascapular nerve lies deep to the transverse scapular ligament (dotted line). Dashed arrow indicates the approximate trajectory of the lead introducer. Final lead position deep to the ligament is similar whether the lead is inserted perpendicular to the nerve (arrowhead on dashed arrow) or inserted parallel to the nerve (circle with X) at the spinoglenoid notch as seen in 3b and then advanced superiorly under the scapular spine. (**b**) Ultrasound image of the suprascapular nerve (*) at the spinoglenoid notch (bold arrows). Approximate lead placement parallel to the nerve, out-of-plane approach with lead viewed in cross-section (circle with X) as it is advanced superiorly under the scapular spine. The final lead position is represented with the "circle with X" in Fig. 71.3a. Reprinted with permission Einar Ottestad and Alexander Sable-Smith

Lead Placement

A lead can be placed either perpendicular or parallel to the suprascapular nerve, though in either case, the tip of the lead rests in a similar location, illustrated in Fig. 71.4.

Perpendicular Approach

Lead placement is a sterile procedure and should be performed in the appropriate setting. Administration of preoperative antibiotics is at the discretion of the implanting clinician but is generally recommended for all implantable neuromodulation devices. Once the target is identified, the skin and tissues along the needle trajectory are anesthetized, with care not to anesthetize the target nerve, as sensory testing is required. The lead-introducer apparatus (manufacturer specific) is then advanced to the target medially to laterally using an in-plane approach. At this point, sensory and motor stimulation is performed to confirm pleasant paresthesia is in the appropriate distribution in conjunction with an absence of uncomfortable motor stimulation. The introducer apparatus is removed. In the case of temporary PNS systems, the lead exit site is secured with topical skin glue and a sterile occlusive dressing applied. In the case of a fully implantable

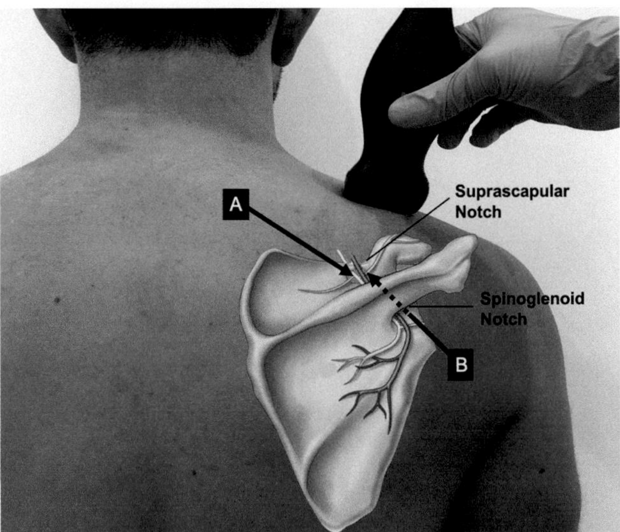

Fig. 71.4 Lead insertion trajectories perpendicular to the nerve at the suprascapular notch (**A**) and parallel to the nerve at the spinoglenoid notch (**B**). Dotted line indicates the portion of the lead which is deep to the scapular spine. Reprinted with permission from Einar Ottestad and Alex Sable-Smith

system, the tail end of the lead is tunneled under the skin. Depending on the system, at this point, the tail end remains subcutaneously where it will receive charge from an external power transmitter or it is directly connected to a tiny IPG. For the shoulder joint especially, it is best to orient the lead so that the external power source can be placed using the contralateral hand without discomfort. If patients have difficulty crossing the contralateral arm to the PNS site, they must have somebody at home who can help them place and remove the external power source.

Parallel Approach

The probe is placed caudad to the scapular spine to identify the spinoglenoid notch medial to the humeral head and glenoid fossa. Place the "valley" of the fossa in the middle of the ultrasound view, and choose a needle entry position 4–5 cm caudad of the center of the US probe for needle insertion. Figure 71.4 demonstrates an out-of-plane technique walking the needle down toward the spinoglenoid notch. Using both in-plane and out-of-plane techniques will help guide the needle to the scapula. Upon touching bone, the needle is directed slightly lateral and superficial through the spinoglenoid notch, so that it slides under the scapular spine and into the supraspinatus fossa, approaching the suprascapular notch. Final adjustments are made once the lead is in the suprascapular notch parallel with the nerve using the suprascapular notch view. Whether the lead is place perpendicular or parallel to the nerve, the final position of the tip of the lead is roughly the same.

Stimulation of the Posterior Tibial Nerve for Foot Pain

Functional Anatomy

The tibial nerve receives innervation from the L4–S3 nerve roots and arises from the sciatic nerve as it bifurcates in the superior aspect of the popliteal fossa. The nerve passes through the popliteal fossa and travels in the posterior compartment of the leg where it supplies the muscles responsible for ankle flexion and inversion as well as toe flexion. The nerve courses posterior to the medial malleolus through the tarsal tunnel (Fig. 71.5) and then bifurcates into the three sensory nerves that innervate the sole of the foot, the medial (L4–L5) and lateral (S1–S2) plantar nerves, and medial calcaneal branch. The medial calcaneal branch usually branches proximal to the tarsal tunnel. The lateral calcaneal branches of the sural nerve (which receives contributions more proximally from the tibial and common peroneal nerves) also innervate the skin of the heel. The posterior tibial nerve is an appropriate target for PNS (usually placed proximal to the tarsal tunnel) for patients experiencing neuropathic pain of the plantar aspect of the foot. Stimulation of this nerve has been shown to reduce neuropathic pain in the foot, including painful diabetic peripheral neuropathy, in the foot in our experience, as well as in open-label studies. The tibial nerve is also the main target for PNS treatment of overactive bladder and fecal incontinence.

Technique

Positioning and Scanning

The posterior-medial aspect of the calf is best exposed with the patient in the prone position with the ankle inverted or supine with the lower extremity externally rotated. The posterior tibial nerve is traditionally identified in the tarsal tunnel, where it travels posterior to the medial malleolus and deep to the flexor retinaculum. It can be identified by placing a high-frequency linear probe in a transverse orientation between the medial malleolus and the calcaneus. Adjacent structures are the posterior tibial artery and vein and tendons of the tibialis posterior, flexor digitorum, and flexor hallicus longus (Fig. 71.5). Using dynamic scanning, the nerve is traced proximally with the neurovascular bundle. It will be deep to the thin gastrocnemius muscle and soleus muscle tendons (Achilles tendon) and superficial to the flexor digitorum longus, flexor hallicus longus, and tibialis posterior. More proximally, the soleus muscle belly will be superficial to the nerve.

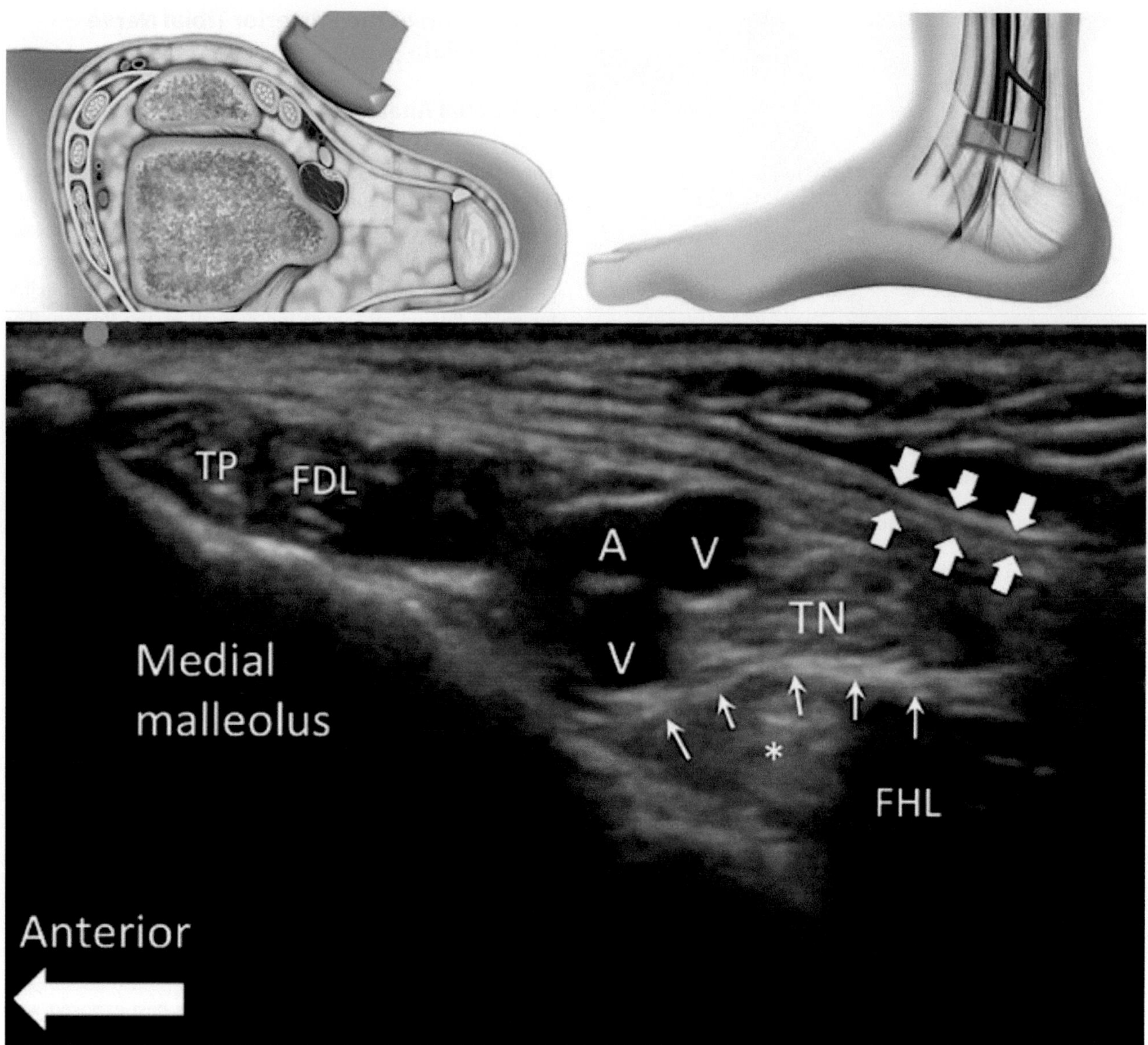

Fig. 71.5 Sonoanatomy of the tibial nerve. *TP* Tibialis posterior tendon, *FDL* flexor digitorum longus tendon, *bold arrows* flexor retinaculum, *A* posterior tibial artery, *V* posterior tibial vein, *TN* tibial nerve. Moving the great toe can bring the flexor hallucis longus (FHL) tendon (*) and overlying fascia (line arrows) into view. Reprinted with permission from the Philip Peng Educational Series

Lead Placement

Lead placement is a sterile procedure and should be performed in the appropriate setting. Administration of preoperative antibiotics is at the discretion of the implanting clinician but is generally recommended for all implantable neuromodulation devices. The lead can be placed parallel or perpendicular to the nerve, though we prefer a parallel approach, which allows a longer "runway" of tissue to hold the lead in place. Once the target is identified, the lead is inserted in a proximal-to-distal approach in the supine (Fig. 71.6) or prone (Fig. 71.7) position. The exact approach depends on the ergonomics of where the external pulse transmitter will be worn and whether or not a portion of the lead will be buried. The skin and tissues along the needle trajectory are anesthetized, with care not to anesthetize the target nerve, as sensory testing is required. The lead-introducer apparatus (manufacturer specific) is then advanced using either an in-plane or out-of-plane technique to the target site. At this point, sensory and motor stimulation is performed to confirm pleasant paresthesia is in the appropriate distribution in conjunction with an absence of uncomfortable motor stimulation. The introducer apparatus is removed. In the case of temporary PNS systems, the lead exit site is secured with topical skin glue and a sterile occlusive dressing applied. In the case of a fully implantable system, the tail end of

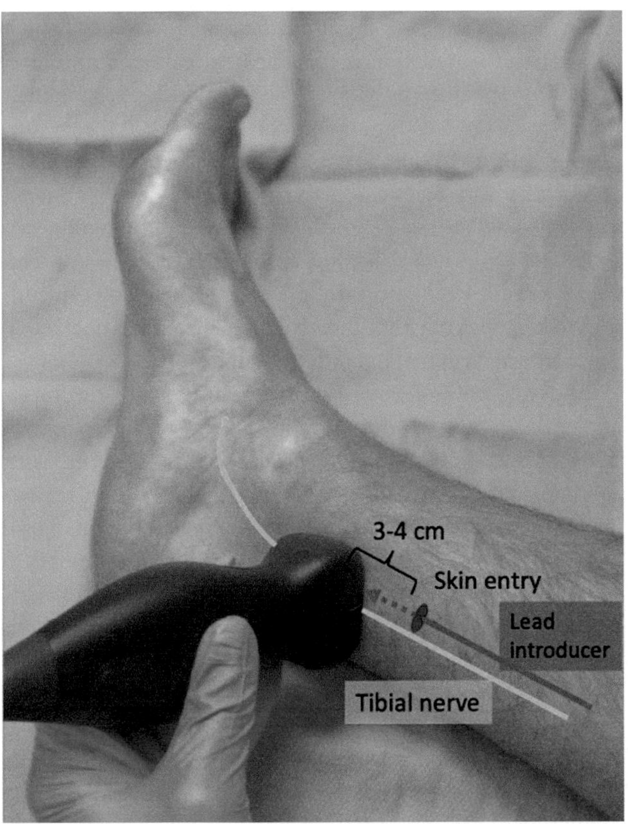

Fig. 71.6 Schematic of lead insertion parallel to the nerve in an out-of-plane approach with the patient positioned supine with the lower extremity externally rotated. Reprinted with permission from Alexander Sable-Smith

the lead is tunneled under the skin. Depending on the system, at this point, the tail end remains subcutaneously where it will receive charge from an external power transmitter or it is directly connected to a tiny IPG. In the case of temporary PNS systems, the lead exit site is secured with topical skin glue, and a sterile occlusive dressing is applied.

Complications of Peripheral Nerve Stimulation

Transient, superficial skin irritation, redness, and pruritus at the implantation site or adhesive site is the most commonly reported adverse reaction in studies of modern percutaneous lead systems. Lead fracture is another complication that implanters should discuss with PNS candidates. In a study of a 60-day temporary PNS system, the distal lead fracture rate at removal was 15%, though the authors report no sequelae of retained lead fragments in 10 months' follow-up after lead removal, and the fragments were designated as MR conditional. A stronger version of the lead should ameliorate this risk. Risk of lead infection is very low and estimated to be 0.03 and 0.83 infections per 1000 indwelling days for coiled and non-coiled leads, respectively. Lead migration is another potential complication of implantation, especially when spinal cord leads are repurposed for peripheral use. The prevalence of lead migration with modern percutaneous systems which have anchor barbs is not reported.

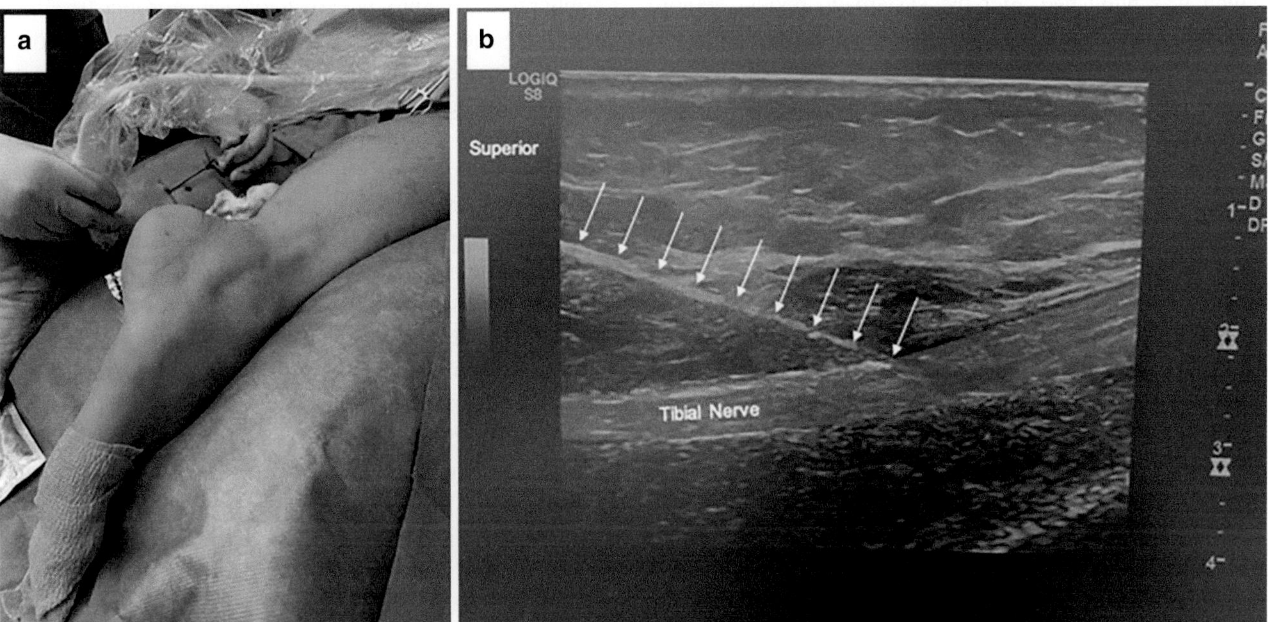

Fig. 71.7 (**a**) Intraoperative photo showing lead insertion parallel to the nerve in an out-of-plane approach with the patient positioned prone. (**b**) An ultrasound image of the lead introducer after the probe was rotated 90 °. Reprinted with permission from Einar Ottestad

Practical Tips

- PNS systems require daily attention from patients. Select patients who have the necessary support to use their devices.
- Pre-procedure planning is key. Consider your approach, lead exit site (temporary systems), and implantation sites.
  - Consider ergonomics of applying and removing adhesive external pulse generators, and optimize position to account for clothing and daily activity.
  - Don't cross major joints with leads to reduce rate of lead fracture and migration.
  - The patient can trial wearing the battery to evaluate ergonomics and ensure no allergies to adhesive.
- Temporary PNS systems need 3–4 cm of lead buried in muscle and subcutaneous tissues to prevent migration.
- Presence of an implant may affect the patient's ability to get an MRI. MRI compatibility varies by manufacturer.

Literature Review and Mechanism of Action

Peripheral nerve stimulation has been shown to be beneficial in randomized controlled trials for chronic pain conditions including headache (targeting the occipital nerve and sphenopalatine ganglion), post-stroke shoulder pain (targeting the axillary nerve), neuropathic pain of the legs or trunk with a variety of targets, low back pain (multifidus stimulation), and chronic pelvic pain (targeting the tibial nerve) as detailed in a recent systematic review. A randomized controlled trial which was published after the systematic review demonstrates long-term efficacy for post-amputation pain. There is heterogeneity in the primary outcomes reported in these studies (pain reduction on visual analog scale, 30% and 50% responder rates) and secondary outcomes (psychosocial measures, medication use, disability, etc.). Limitations of the body of evidence as a whole include a relatively small number of trials with variable follow-up periods, heterogeneity of nerve targets, potential bias introduced by industry funding, and challenges with reliable blinding and inconsistent use of sham control procedures. Nonetheless, the available research provides moderate- to-high-quality evidence that peripheral nerve stimulation is a promising treatment for chronic pain, a common and impactful condition with a paucity of safe and effective treatments. Beyond randomized controlled trials, there is an abundance of published case reports and series describing benefit of peripheral nerve stimulation in peripheral nerve targets head to toe.

Numerous mechanisms are thought to be responsible for pain relief achieved by peripheral nerve stimulation. The prevailing explanation for the immediate analgesic mechanism of electrical stimulation is the so-called gate control theory originally described by Melzack and Wall in 1965. As applied to peripheral nerve stimulation, the gate control theory suggests an electrical field is applied in the periphery at parameters such that it selectively activates large, highly myelinated, low-threshold A-beta sensory axons in the peripheral nerve. In the dorsal horn of the spinal cord, input from these A-beta fibers activates inhibitory interneurons which subsequently inhibit signals from high-threshold A-delta and C-fiber axons that carry nociceptive input to the spinal cord.

The gate control theory provides an explanation for the analgesia produced during application of the stimulus, whether that stimulus is an electrical field or a parent gently rubbing an injured area of a child. However, clinical evidence in peripheral nerve stimulation shows that analgesia can persist for at least 10 months after the stimulus is removed. The processes that underlie this sustained benefit are complex and not completely understood. Experimental models suggest molecular and cellular changes at the peripheral and spinal levels that alter the process of peripheral and central sensitization. Peripheral electrical stimulation has been shown to induce local antinociceptive changes such as modulation of the sympathetic nervous system and downregulation of pro-inflammatory cytokines and prostaglandins in the periphery and CSF. In the spinal cord, experimental evidence implicates modulation of the endogenous opioid system, as well as changes in serotonin, GABA, and glutamate receptors. Peripheral nerve injury and peripheral nerve stimulation have implications at the cortical level as well. Peripheral nerve injury is known to have neuroplastic effects on sensory and motor cortical organization, and the cortical changes may be partially responsible for maintaining pain. Flor and colleagues demonstrated that deafferentation after upper extremity limb amputation led to cortical changes such that the area for the lip invaded the cortex once devoted to the upper limb. Furthermore, greater plastic changes correlated with increased phantom limb pain. Subsequently, the same researchers demonstrated that sensory discrimination training led to reversal for cortical plastic changes and decreases in phantom limb pain. It has been hypothesized that peripheral nerve stimulation can lead to long-term pain relief (even after stimulation is removed) by helping restore normal cortical organization, analogous to the effect of rehabilitative strategies such as mirror therapy and desensitization therapy. If substantiated by additional evidence, PNS may be thought of as more than just a treatment for peripheral mononeuropathies, but rather a means to influence the central nervous system though peripheral channels and thus augment and expedite recovery from painful conditions.

Conclusions

The field of peripheral nerve stimulation is still in its infancy and already shows tremendous promise. Technological advances and additional miniaturization will likely make implantation safer and less burdensome to the patient. PNS systems are already under investigation for applications beyond chronic pain, including perioperative analgesia. Additional research will enrich our understanding of the mechanisms of analgesia in PNS and help physicians select the patients likely to benefit from PNS with increasing precision.

Suggested Reading

Chakravarthy KV, Xing F, Bruno K, et al. A review of spinal and peripheral neuromodulation and neuroinflammation: lessons learned thus far and future prospects of biotype development. Neuromodulation. 2019;22:235–43. https://doi.org/10.1111/ner.12859.

Dabby R, Sadeh M, Goldberg I, Finkelshtein V. Electrical stimulation of the posterior tibial nerve reduces neuropathic pain in patients with polyneuropathy. J Pain Res. 2017;10:2717–23. https://doi.org/10.2147/JPR.S137420.

Deer T, Pope J, Benyamin R, et al. Prospective, multicenter, randomized, double-blinded, partial crossover study to assess the safety and efficacy of the novel neuromodulation system in the treatment of patients with chronic pain of peripheral nerve origin. Neuromodulation. 2016;19:91–100. https://doi.org/10.1111/ner.12381.

Deer TR, Provenzano DA, Hanes M, et al. The neurostimulation appropriateness consensus committee (NACC) recommendations for infection prevention and management. Neuromodulation. 2017;20:31–50. https://doi.org/10.1111/ner.12565.

Deer TR, Esposito MF, McRoberts WP, et al. A systematic literature review of peripheral nerve stimulation therapies for the treatment of pain. Pain Med. 2020;21:1590–603. https://doi.org/10.1093/pm/pnaa030.

Flor H, Elbert T, Knecht S, et al. Phantom-limb pain as a perceptual correlate of cortical reorganization following arm amputation. Nature. 1995;375:482–4. https://doi.org/10.1038/375482a0.

Flor H, Denke C, Schaefer M, Grüsser S. Effect of sensory discrimination training on cortical reorganisation and phantom limb pain. Lancet Lond Engl. 2001;357:1763–4. https://doi.org/10.1016/S0140-6736(00)04890-X.

Gildenberg PL. History of electrical neuromodulation for chronic pain. Pain Med. 2006;7:S7–S13. https://doi.org/10.1111/j.1526-4637.2006.00118.x.

Gilmore CA, Ilfeld BM, Rosenow JM, et al. Percutaneous 60-day peripheral nerve stimulation implant provides sustained relief of chronic pain following amputation: 12-month follow-up of a randomized, double-blind, placebo-controlled trial. Reg Anesth Pain Med. 2019a; https://doi.org/10.1136/rapm-2019-100937.

Gilmore C, Ilfeld B, Rosenow J, et al. Percutaneous peripheral nerve stimulation for the treatment of chronic neuropathic postamputation pain: a multicenter, randomized, placebo-controlled trial. Reg Anesth Pain Med. 2019b;44:637–45. https://doi.org/10.1136/rapm-2018-100109.

Gilmore CA, Kapural L, McGee MJ, Boggs JW. Percutaneous peripheral nerve stimulation for chronic low back pain: prospective case series with 1 year of sustained relief following short-term implant. Pain Pract. 2020;20:310–20. https://doi.org/10.1111/papr.12856.

Gofeld M, Restrepo-Garces CE, Theodore BR, Faclier G. Pulsed radiofrequency of suprascapular nerve for chronic shoulder pain: a randomized double-blind active placebo-controlled study. Pain Pract. 2013;13:96–103. https://doi.org/10.1111/j.1533-2500.2012.00560.x.

Ilfeld BM, Gilmore CA, Grant SA, et al. Ultrasound-guided percutaneous peripheral nerve stimulation for analgesia following total knee arthroplasty: a prospective feasibility study. J Orthop Surg. 2017a;12:4. https://doi.org/10.1186/s13018-016-0506-7.

Ilfeld BM, Gabriel RA, Saulino MF, et al. Infection rates of electrical leads used for percutaneous neurostimulation of the peripheral nervous system. Pain Pract Off J World Inst Pain. 2017b;17:753–62. https://doi.org/10.1111/papr.12523.

Ilfeld BM, Finneran JJ, Gabriel RA, et al. Ultrasound-guided percutaneous peripheral nerve stimulation: neuromodulation of the suprascapular nerve and brachial plexus for postoperative analgesia following ambulatory rotator cuff repair. A proof-of-concept study. Reg Anesth Pain Med. 2019a; https://doi.org/10.1136/rapm-2018-100121.

Ilfeld BM, Said ET, Finneran JJ, et al. Ultrasound-guided percutaneous peripheral nerve stimulation: neuromodulation of the femoral nerve for postoperative analgesia following ambulatory anterior cruciate ligament reconstruction: a proof of concept study. Neuromodulation. 2019b;22:621–9. https://doi.org/10.1111/ner.12851.

Jiang JF, Leung AK, Pettitt-Schieber B, et al. Efficacy of percutaneous tibial nerve stimulation for overactive bladder in women and men at a safety net hospital. J Urol. 2020;203:385–91. https://doi.org/10.1097/JU.0000000000000539.

Lin T, Gargya A, Singh H, et al. Mechanism of peripheral nerve stimulation in chronic pain. Pain Med. 2020;21:S6–S12. https://doi.org/10.1093/pm/pnaa164.

Melzack R, Wall PD. Pain mechanisms: a new theory. Science. 1965;150:971–9. https://doi.org/10.1126/science.150.3699.971.

Moseley GL, Flor H. Targeting cortical representations in the treatment of chronic pain: a review. Neurorehabil Neural Repair. 2012;26:646–52. https://doi.org/10.1177/1545968311433209.

Ottestad E, Orlovich DS. History of peripheral nerve stimulation-update for the twenty-first century. Pain Med. 2020;21:S3–5. https://doi.org/10.1093/pm/pnaa165.

Shealy CN, Mortimer JT, Reswick JB. Electrical inhibition of pain by stimulation of the dorsal columns: preliminary clinical report. Anesth Analg. 1967;46:489–91.

Shin C, Lee S-E, Yu K-H, et al. Spinal root origins and innervations of the suprascapular nerve. Surg Radiol Anat. 2010;32:235–8. https://doi.org/10.1007/s00276-009-0597-5.

Sokal P, Harat M, Zieliński P, Kierońska S. Tibial nerve stimulation with a miniature, wireless stimulator in chronic peripheral neuropathic pain. J Pain Res. 2017;10:613–9. https://doi.org/10.2147/JPR.S128861.

Wall PD, Sweet WH. Temporary abolition of pain in man. Science. 1967;155:108–9. https://doi.org/10.1126/science.155.3758.108.

Wang M, Jian Z, Ma Y, et al. Percutaneous tibial nerve stimulation for overactive bladder syndrome: a systematic review and meta-analysis. Int Urogynecology J. 2020; https://doi.org/10.1007/s00192-020-04429-8.

Wilson RD, Gunzler DD, Bennett ME, Chae J. Peripheral nerve stimulation compared with usual care for pain relief of hemiplegic shoulder pain: a randomized controlled trial. Am J Phys Med Rehabil. 2014;93:17–28. https://doi.org/10.1097/PHM.0000000000000011.

Spinal Cord Stimulation

72

Leonardo Kapural and James Deering

Contents

Introduction

Spinal cord stimulation (SCS) has been used for several decades and just recently has been considered a superior treatment for patients with chronic, intractable pain. Currently, about 34,000 patients worldwide receive a spinal cord stimulator annually for any chronic pain. Spinal cord stimulation (SCS) leads are placed in the epidural space to deliver electrical stimulation to the dorsal columns of the spinal cord. Successful pain relief generally requires activation of dorsal column fibers that innervate the patient's painful area.

Historically, using traditional low-frequency (40–90 Hz) stimulation, the patient feels paresthesia located over the painful area and pain relief due to spinal and supraspinal mechanisms. However, only about 30–50% of patients respond to conventional low-frequency SCS therapy. Recent advances in SCS therapies are improving SCS outcomes. For example, continuous stimulation at a higher frequency (10 kHz) was shown to provide superior pain relief for low back and leg pain compared to traditional lower SCS stimulation frequencies. Additionally, prior studies have indicated that 1 kHz continuous stimulation or 500 Hz burst patterns of stimulation may provide an additional pain relieving benefit while reducing the stimulation energy required. More recently, both closed-loop and differential target multiplex types of SCS demonstrated, in well-conducted randomized controlled trials (RCTs), comparable outcomes to 10 kHz SCS in optimizing the overall outcomes of this therapy.

Mechanisms of Action

Traditionally, low-frequency, traditional type of SCS was thought to provide long-term pain relief by the activation of the gate control mechanisms, conductance blockade of the spinothalamic tracts, blockade of supraspinal sympathetic

L. Kapural (✉) · J. Deering
Carolinas Pain Institute and Chronic Pain Research Institute, Winston-Salem, NC, USA

D. Jankovic, P. Peng (eds.), *Regional Nerve Blocks in Anesthesia and Pain Therapy*,
https://doi.org/10.1007/978-3-030-88727-8_72

mechanisms, and activation or release of neuromodulators. When SCS is active, unmyelinated afferent fibers (A delta and C) are inhibited by the electrical stimulation of non-nociceptive, myelinated afferent fibers. Conductance blockade of the spinothalamic tract is accomplished by depression of the spinothalamic tract cells by SCS during thoracic or cervical stimulation of the ipsilateral dorsal columns. Such inhibition of actual transmission of electrochemical information can be accomplished anywhere along the spinothalamic tract. Blockade of supraspinal sympathetic mechanisms results in an increase of the peripheral blood flow in the skin which remains after the transection of the dorsal roots and after spinal cord section rostrally to the stimulating electrode. There is also transitory inhibition of sympathetic vasoconstriction documented in studies conducted in the early 1990s. Activation and release of neuromodulators included an induction of GABA release in the dorsal horn, glycine release in the extracellular space of the spinal cord, and reduction of glutamate and aspartate release in the dorsal horn.

Measured effects of SCS to heart function include reduction of intrinsic cardiac nervous system activity and preemptive suppression of marked increase in cardiac NSA following local occlusion of coronary blood flow which may inhibit local heart circuits and decrease frequency of arrhythmias in the ischemic heart. We do know that SCS has no effects on coronary blood flow during ischemic conditions, left ventricular function, or left ventricular blood flow distribution. However, positive and anti-ischemic effects include decrease of myocyte oxygen demand, significant increase of pacing tolerance, decreased ST segment depression, and improved myocardial lactate metabolism, which in turn results in pain relief and improvement in exercise tolerance.

SCS improves ischemic extremity pain providing vasodilator effect via peripheral release of calcitonin gene-related peptide (CGRP), prostacyclin release, and neuronal release of nitric oxide. During SCS, there is a decreased sensitivity to vasoconstrictive sympathetic stimuli mainly by suppression of efferent sympathetic activity. Such effect is inhibited after complete surgical sympathectomy and blockade of nicotinic transmission in the ganglia or postganglionic $[\text{alpha}]_1$ adrenoceptors. It has been determined that an increase in skin blood flow during SCS correlates with resulting pain relief, increase in transcutaneous partial oxygen pressure, and increased pulse-wave amplitude.

Other possible mechanisms of SCS were proposed recently when very specific types of SCS waveform are used, different than traditional low-frequency type of SCS. For example, recruitment of the dorsal horn with activation of inhibitory neurons was a proposed additional mechanism of action seen with 10 kHz. This is independent of any effect that SCS may produce on the dorsal columns. Such effect results in additional pain relief, not exhibited greatly when low frequencies (1–1200 Hz) of SCS were used.

Recently, much work was done on neuromodulation, mainly SCS, involving glial cells in addition to neurons. These cells (microglia, astrocytes, and oligodendrocytes) are abundant in the spinal cord and carry ratio of about 12:1 to neurons in the gray matter and 20:1 in the white matter. While glial cells support normal brain function by cleaning damaged areas and regulating neurotransmitters, in chronic disease conditions, they can become "activated" and contribute to a pathological state, such as chronic pain. Glial cells respond to electrical field application by depolarizing, releasing neurotransmitters, and communicating with each other. Differential target multiplex (DTM) type of SCS is directed toward modulation of glial cell response. In an acute neuropathic pain model in rodents and mammals, DTM type of SCS provided superior thermal and mechanical hypersensitivity suppression compared to low and high (1000 Hz) type of SCS. During DTM SCS in an animal model of neuropathic pain, gene expression is better restored toward the baseline, non-pain state, when compared to low- and high-frequency SCS, including the genes related to neuroinflammation.

Finally, a recent development in spinal cord stimulation waveform optimization is a closed-loop stimulation. During closed-loop stimulation, data regarding the spinal cord response to stimulation, measured as evoked compound action potentials (ECAPs), is recorded in real time. This allows the spinal cord stimulator system to adjust its stimulation parameters to maintain ideal therapeutic response.

Spinal Cord Stimulator Trial Technique

As opposed to any other interventional therapy for control of chronic pain, patients can undergo temporary SCS trial. Time interval of SCS trial may vary between 3 and 30 days (in the United States, most frequently 7–10 days). Based on NACC guidelines, patients who have been identified by the physician as potential SCS candidates should be screened for risk factors that may predispose them to complications from SCS, referred for psychological evaluation to rule out any prohibitive psychological disorders that may hinder successful response to neuromodulation, and thorough history and physical examination must be performed. Vital questions for the SCS candidate include whether or not they are anticoagulated, have a history of poorly controlled diabetes, are current smokers, or have a history of surgical site infection/poor wound healing. If the patient is anticoagulated, American Society of Regional Anesthesia and Pain Medicine (ASRA) guidelines should be strictly adhered to in order to minimize the risk of catastrophic epidural hematoma formation or any other bleeding. Attention should be given to the patient's body habitus, as increase in body mass index may affect procedural technique and predispose the patient to postoperative infection. Spine imaging should be carefully reviewed in order to rule out structural instability that would warrant surgical attention, as well as central canal stenosis that may preclude the safe insertion of SCS leads.

The patient is brought to the fluoroscopy suite and positioned prone with adequate padding under the abdomen to minimize lumbar lordosis. Weight-based antibiotics are administered 30–90 minutes prior to epidural space access. Sterility should be maintained while prepping and draping the patient. If sedation is required, it should be minimal in order to facilitate patient-physician communication throughout the procedure. AP fluoroscopy is centered over the intended epidural entry point, most commonly L2–L3 to T12–L1 for thoracolumbar SCS (back and leg pain). The image is optimized with fine oblique adjustments to center the spinous processes between the pedicles and cephalad or caudal tilt to square the endplates of the vertebral body at the intended level of epidural entry (Fig. 72.1).

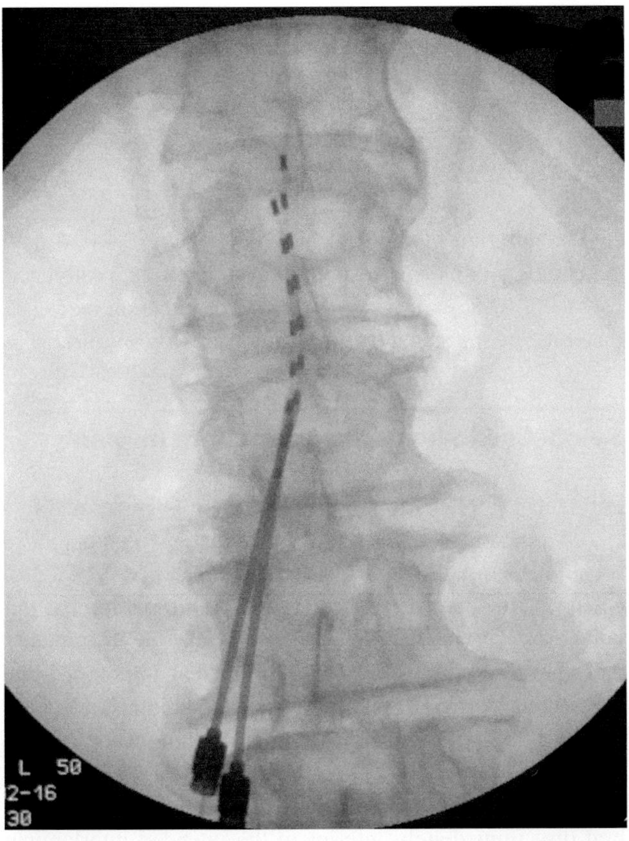

Fig. 72.1 Anterior-posterior fluoroscopic view of an entry point to the lumbar epidural space. Notice that both Tuohy needles are placed next to each other within the same lumbar interspace. Final advancement of the needles was achieved in lateral view (see Fig. 72.2a) and after the confirmation of an epidural space, and leads accessed epidural space in lateral view, further advancement of the leads is commenced in anterior-posterior fluoroscopic view as shown in Fig. 72.2b

Once the optimal AP image has been obtained, needle entry point must be determined. The goal is to enter the epidural space at a relatively flat angle of 30–45°. Individual patient body habitus greatly impacts the proper skin insertion point. The greater the amount of subcutaneous tissue, the further the skin entry point will be from the intended interlaminar target. In a patient of average BMI, local anesthetic is injected in the skin overlying the medial border of the pedicle one level caudad to the interlaminar epidural target. Deep local anesthetic infiltration may be achieved using a spinal needle along the intended trajectory. Next, the 14-gauge Tuohy needle is directed toward the midline of the intended interlaminar space. Note that the necessary length of the Tuohy needle may vary based on point of skin entry.

Utilizing frequent AP fluoroscopy, contact should be made with the cephalad aspect of the lamina immediately below the intended epidural target. This serves as a depth gauge and minimizes the risk of inadvertent entry into the epidural or intrathecal space. Once contact has been made, a lateral fluoroscopic image is obtained.

The angle of approach is further reduced, and the Tuohy needle is advanced anteriorly toward the epidural space. As the needle approaches the base of the spinous processes under lateral fluoroscopy, a loss of resistance technique is utilized to safely identify the epidural space. Once loss of resistance is obtained, the SCS lead is slowly advanced into the epidural space. A lateral image is obtained to confirm the lead is positioned posteriorly in the spinal column (Fig. 72.2a, b).

The lead is advanced superiorly through the epidural space under continuous fluoroscopic guidance to the desired vertebral level. This target varies based on the diagnosis being treated and various device manufacturer recommendations.

Once the first lead has been advanced to the intended target site, attention is directed to the placement of the second Tuohy needle. This can be inserted ipsilateral to the first needle at the same interlaminar level, at the level above or the level below the insertion site of the first needle. It may also be inserted from the contralateral side aiming toward the intended interlaminar entry point. After entering the epidural space, the second lead is advanced alongside the first lead until it reaches its target vertebral level (Fig. 72.3).

After satisfactory lead location has been established, the Tuohy needles are removed with intermittent fluoroscopy to ensure they do not advance or withdraw during needle movement. Once the needles are removed, the leads are secured in a fashion that suits the physician's preference. This may include suturing in place using manufacturer provided anchoring devices, suturing to the lead itself, securing it using Steri-Strip, and dressing only or tunneling leads for possible prolonged trials (Fig. 72.4).

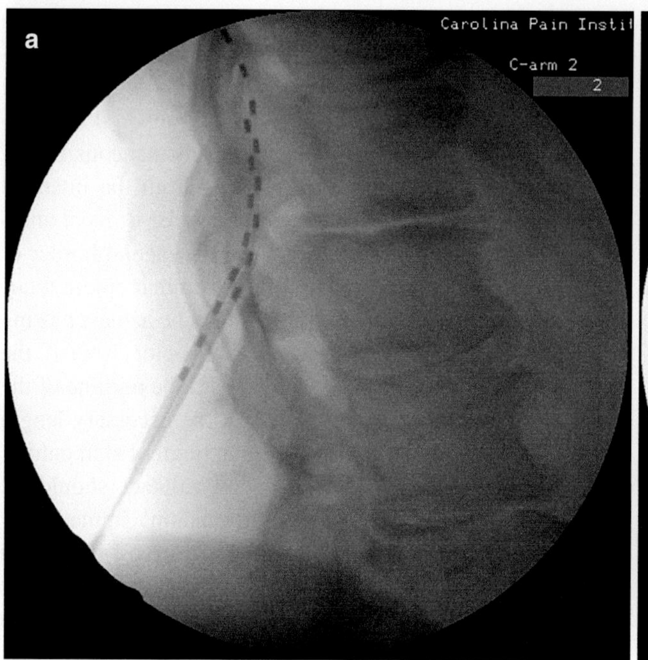

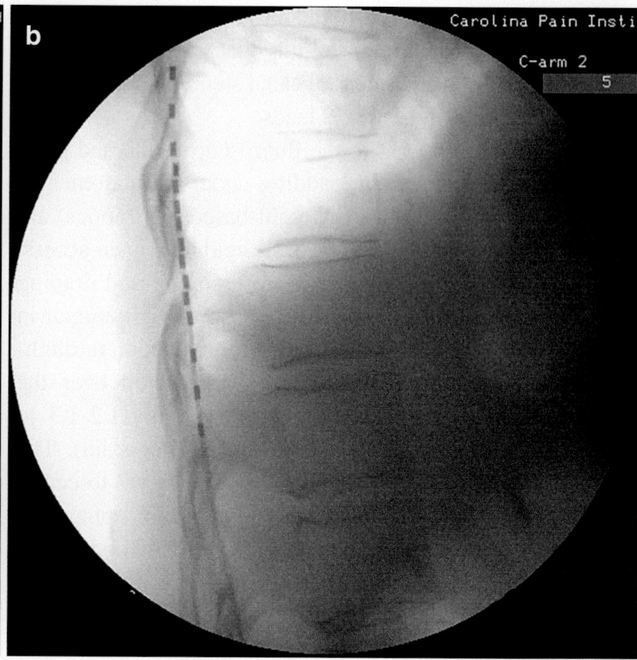

Fig. 72.2 Lateral fluoroscopic views during Tuohy needle and lead insertion in the epidural space. (**a**) Needle insertion level, typically upper lumbar, for the lead placement that would be used for back and leg chronic pain. Notice that both needles are inserted at the same ligamentum flavum level and leads with eight contacts each were just confirmed to be positioned in the posterior epidural space. (**b**) A final position of two 8-contact leads in the posterior epidural space. In this example, leads were stacked from the top of T8 vertebral body to mid vertebral body of T11

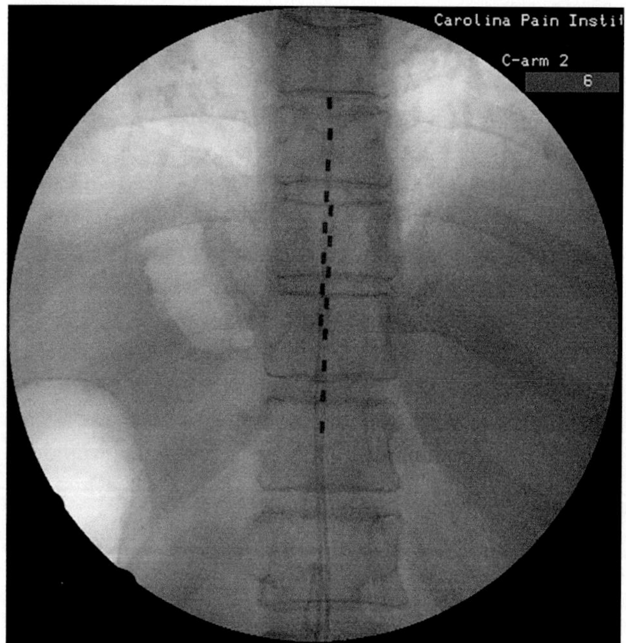

Fig. 72.3 Final positioning of two Octrode leads in the anterior-posterior view. One lead reached top of T8 vertebral body, the other one top of T9

The duration of the trial may range from 3 to 10 days depending on patient response and physician preference. Beyond a 10-day trial period, the risk of infection increases, but could be mitigated by tunneling leads (Fig. 72.3b).

Spinal Cord Stimulator Permanent Implant

Permanent implantation of a SCS system is performed in a sterile operating room setting. The patient is positioned prone in a similar fashion as described for the SCS trial procedure, with adequate padding to reduce normal lumbar lordosis (or cervical lordosis for cervical SCS implant). Anesthesia is administered and the patient is prepped and draped in a sterile fashion. Intravenous antibiotics have been administered within 1 h of incision. AP fluoroscopy is utilized to identify the intended interlaminar target. A vertical incision site is marked starting at the level of the intervertebral disc immediately inferior to the intended interlaminar insertion site and extending inferiorly 3 to 4 cm.

The skin and subcutaneous tissue is anesthetized with 1% lidocaine containing 1:200,000 epinephrine. A vertical incision is made using a scalpel blade. Careful dissection is per-

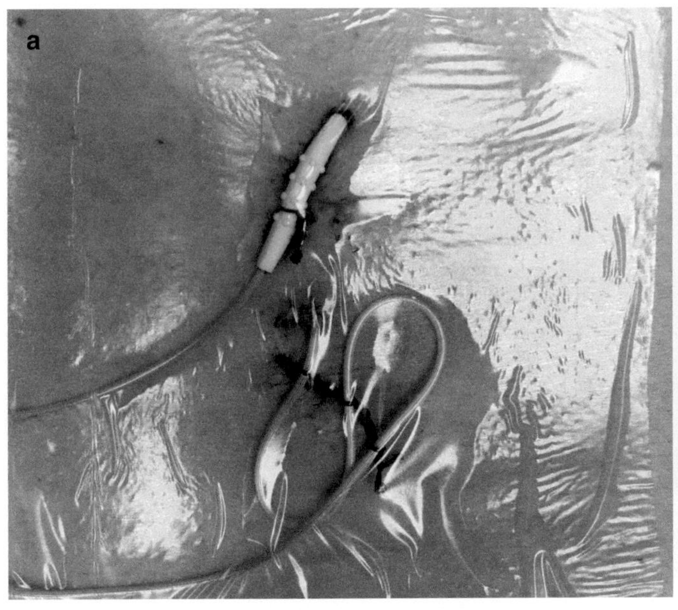

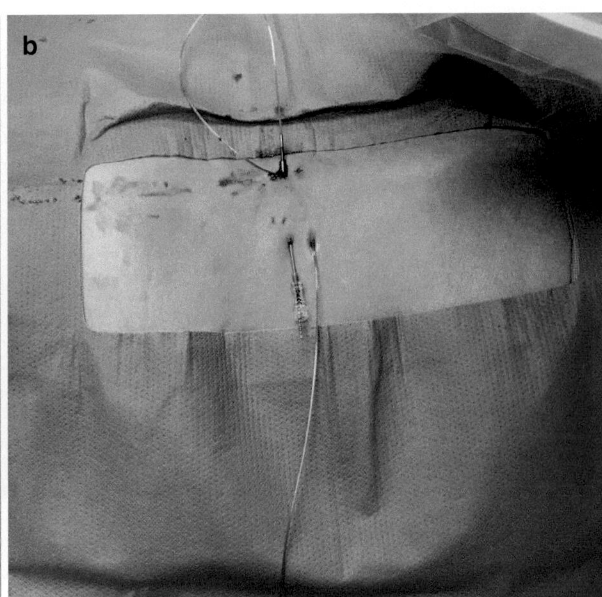

Fig. 72.4 Photographs of various externalized lead skin anchoring techniques at the conclusion of lead placement. (**a**) Examples of industry-offered anchor secured to the skin (left) vs directly tied lead in number-eight-shape form to prevent migration. (**b**) Two epidural leads tunneled about 4–5 cm under the skin for possible prolonged trial. Notice that second epidural needle is inserted in a small stab wound to facilitate tunneling

formed, assisted by electrocautery to achieve hemostasis, until the fascia overlying the spinous processes/supraspinous ligament is exposed. A Weitlaner retractor may assist during the dissection as well as Tuohy needle placement.

Next, the first epidural needle is inserted lateral to the palpable spinous processes at a 30–45° angle, directed toward the midline of the target interlaminar space. This insertion site should be within the superior one third of the incision in order to allow adequate space below for the insertion of the second needle. Contact may be made with the lamina just caudad to the intended interlaminar space in order to gauge depth. The needle is further advanced utilizing lateral fluoroscopy and a loss of resistance technique until the epidural space is reached. The stimulator lead is then advanced through the needle into the epidural space, which is confirmed by posterior location of the lead on lateral fluoroscopy. The lead is then advanced under continuous AP fluoroscopy to the intended vertebral level. Next the second epidural needle is placed either ipsilateral and inferior to the first needle or on the contralateral side (Fig. 72.5). Proper entry into the epidural space is confirmed as described for the first needle, and the second lead is advanced in parallel to the first lead.

The epidural needles are removed leaving the leads in place. The leads are then secured to the underlying fascia using the SCS manufacturer provided anchoring devices and non-absorbable suture (Fig. 72.6). A final fluoroscopy image is captured to ensure no lead migration occurred with needle removal and anchoring of the leads.

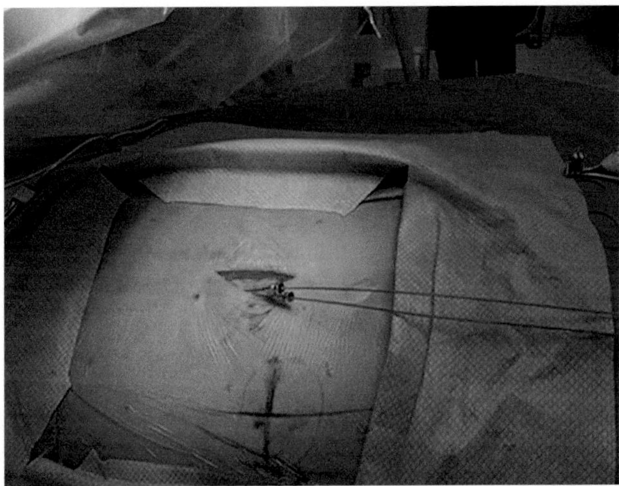

Fig. 72.5 Tuohy needles and epidural lead placement during the percutaneous SCS system implantation. Two needles in final position, inserted ipsilaterally and vertical to one another, with SCS leads advanced through those needles

It is essential to discuss IPG location with the patient prior to implantation. It is vital to examine the potential site of implantation while the patient is in the sitting position, paying attention to the location of the iliac crest, the inferior aspect of the ribs, as well as the level at which the patient's belt-line typically lies to avoid postoperative discomfort. The desired site is marked preoperatively before proceeding to the operating room.

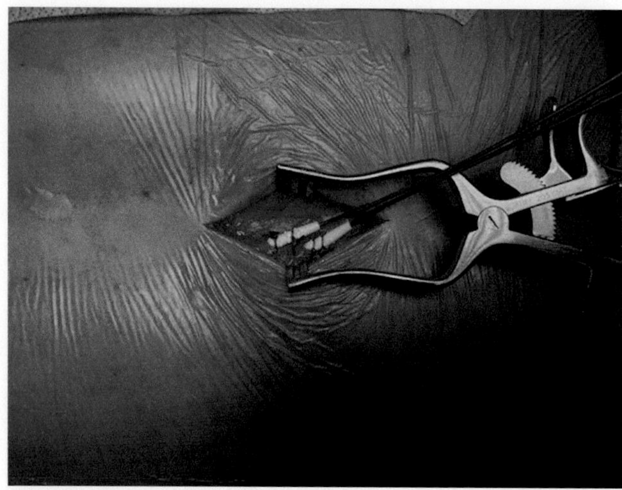
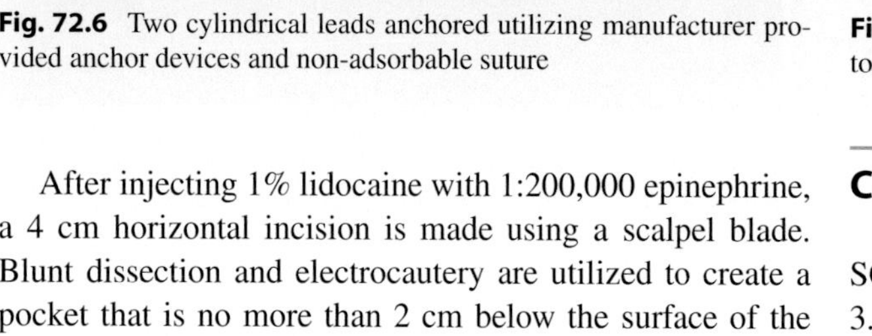

Fig. 72.6 Two cylindrical leads anchored utilizing manufacturer provided anchor devices and non-adsorbable suture

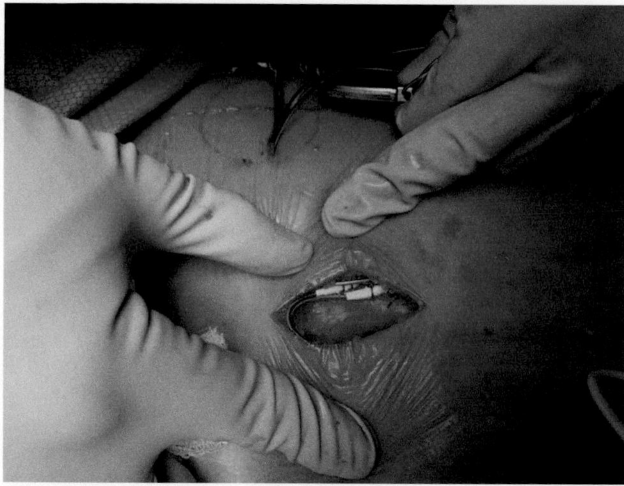

Fig. 72.7 Retention loop created within the midline incision intended to decrease/prevent incidence of lead migration

After injecting 1% lidocaine with 1:200,000 epinephrine, a 4 cm horizontal incision is made using a scalpel blade. Blunt dissection and electrocautery are utilized to create a pocket that is no more than 2 cm below the surface of the skin. This ensures the ability to effectively charge the device. A sizer may be utilized to check that the pocket size will fit the IPG.

Once the pocket has been created and hemostasis has been achieved, the leads must be tunneled from the midline incision to the pocket. The tunneling device may be bent slightly to ensure the ability to remain superficial while tunneling. It is inserted through the tissue at the inferior aspect of the midline incision and directed toward the IPG pocket. Care should be taken to palpate the tip of the tunneler as it is advanced to prevent deep penetration. Once the tunneler emerges in the IPG pocket site, the two SCS leads are fed into the tunneling device until they are visualized on the IPG pocket side of the tunnel. Enough lead may be left within the midline incision to create a retention loop in order to reduce the risk of lead migration (Fig. 72.7). The sheath is then pulled through the tunnel and removed through the IPG pocket incision.

Next, the electrodes are cleaned with a wet and dry Raytec and inserted into the IPG. An impedance check is performed, and the leads are locked into place.

Copious irrigation of both incisions is performed prior to closure. The excess length of SCS lead is looped behind the IPG as it is placed inside the pocket. Non-absorbable suture is utilized to secure the IPG within the pocket. The wounds are closed in a layered fashion using simple interrupted absorbable suture. The skin is closed using a running absorbable suture or staples.

Complications

SCS device-related infection rate has been estimated to be 3.11% based on a logistic regression (n = 6615) over a 12-month postoperative period. It is most commonly seen at the IPG pocket site. Lead migration has been reported as a possible complication of SCS, occurring at a rate of approximately 2.1–12% of implants depending on the reference source. Pocket site discomfort has also been noted with some frequency. Other less common complications that have been described include electrode fracture, IPG failure, and CSF leak following dural puncture, among others.

Clinical Outcomes

Traditional 0–1200 Hz

Traditional SCS has been demonstrated to be a superior treatment option for patients suffering from failed back surgery syndrome when compared to conventional medical management or reoperation. In addition to traditional SCS being more efficacious in improving pain scores and quality of life, it was also found to be less costly than long-term medical management or reoperation for failed back surgery syndrome. Low-frequency SCS has traditionally been reliant on paresthesia coverage overlapping the distribution of a patient's pain. However, some studies have demonstrated superior response to sub-perception stimulation at less than 1200 Hz when compared to traditional tonic stimulation. A multicenter, prospective, randomized controlled trial that enrolled 70 subjects and randomized to either receive supra-perception or sub-perception stimulation at less than 1200 Hz demonstrated non-inferiority to subthreshold stimulation. 39% of subjects with sub-perception settings and 29% with supra-perception settings had a greater than or equal to 50% reduction in their overall pain scores at 3 months post-activation as compared with baseline. Notably, there has been evidence to suggest the contrary that there is no significant difference between patient response to sub-perception versus supra-perception. Attempts have been made to elucidate the exact threshold frequency of stimulation at which patients have an improved response. In a prospective RCT, mean low back pain VAS scores were compared in patients suffering from failed back surgery syndrome who were treated with either sham stimulation, 1200, 3030, or 5882 Hz. There was no significant difference found between the sham stimulation group, 1200 Hz, and 3030 Hz groups. Patients in the 5882 Hz group did experience a greater reduction in VAS score. The overall trend in study results appears to be in favor of higher-frequency stimulation. However, the exact stimulation frequency threshold in which the greatest results are obtained has yet to be determined.

Burst

Burst stimulation is another recently studied waveform with significant evidence to support its use. A "burst" is characterized by a five-pulse train with internal frequency of 500 Hz delivered at 40 Hz utilizing a passive recharge pattern and waveform. It was first described by De Ridder et al. in 2013. This early study examined 15 patients that were randomized to placebo, tonic, or burst stimulation groups. Patients receiving burst SCS experienced improvement in back, limb, and general limb pain VAS scores by 51%, 53%, and 55%, respectively, whereas the tonic SCS group and placebo group experienced 30%, 52%, and 31% and 18.9%, 11.7%, and 10.9% improvement, respectively. Deer et al. conducted a large RCT (SUNBURST) in which 100 patients were randomized to receive traditional or burst stimulation for 12 weeks. At the conclusion of the 12-week period, the patients were then crossed over to comparing stimulation group 12 additional weeks. Burst stimulation was found to be superior to traditional tonic stimulation, with slightly better average pain scores ($P < 0.017$). Of note, at 1 year post-implant, 68.2% of patients preferred burst stimulation.

10 kHz

There is substantial, Level 1 evidence to support the efficacy and durability of high-frequency (10 kHz) SCS for treating back and leg pain and superiority of high-frequency stimulation to traditional stimulation. In a large prospective randomized controlled trial published in 2015 (SENZA-RCT), the response rates of 171 patients who were implanted with either a 10 kHz or traditional low-frequency 2–1200 Hz SCS system to treat back and leg pain were compared. At 12 months post-implant, both groups had sustained response, but the 10 kHz therapy provided in 80% of patients more than 50% of pain relief, versus less than 50% responders in the traditional SCS group. Mean back pain was reduced from VAS of 7.4 ± 1.2 to 2.5 (67% decrease) in the 10 kHz group versus being reduced from 7.8 ± 1.2 to 4.3 (44% decrease) in the traditional SCS group. These results were noted to be durable through a 24-month follow-up, with 76.5% ongoing responder rate in the 10 kHz SCS group versus 49.2% responder rate in the traditional SCS group. Evidence for the efficacy of 10 kHz SCS has been further substantiated by two large randomized prospective studies on chronic nonsurgical back pain patient population and those with neuropathic pain in peripheral neuropathy in diabetes. Both studies substantiated superiority of 10 kHz SCS to conventional medical management in control of chronic pain with consistent responder rate exceeding 80% of treated patients. This therapy is currently the only SCS modality supported by three large prospective RCTs. Furthermore, a recent elegant retrospective study measured 10 kHz SCS's ability as rescue therapy in patients who were previously implanted and failed conventional, low-frequency SCS systems. Out of 105 patients analyzed, 81% of patients experienced greater than 50% pain relief after transitioning from the traditional (less than 1200 Hz) to 10 kHz SCS.

Closed Loop

Levi et al. conducted a multicenter, double-blind, parallel-arm, RCT which enrolled 134 patients. The participants were randomized to the control group which received fixed output, open-loop stimulation or the experimental group which received ECAP-controlled closed-loop spinal cord stimulation. The primary outcome measure was the percentage of patients that obtained greater than 50% pain relief in the back and legs at 3 and 12 months. The closed-loop group had 82.3% responder rate at 3 months, and 83.1% at 12 months, compared to the open-loop group, which had a 60.3% and 61% responder rate at 3 and 12 months, respectively (20). Closed-loop SCS stimulation is not currently available for commercial use, but preliminary data shows promising results for sustained and even improved response rates over time.

Conclusions

Spinal cord stimulation for control of chronic pain recently became the fastest advancing therapy in the area of neuromodulation. The main reason is an introduction of novel waveforms in SCS therapy providing better long-term outcomes than long-standing traditional 0–1200 Hz SCS. Closed-loop, 10 kHz, and differential target multiplex therapies for the first time in well-conducted RCTs demonstrated in more than 80% of patients 50% or more pain relief and very few procedural or long-term complications of therapy. There is a strong interest and much ongoing basic science and clinical research exploring novel approaches and waveforms to simplify techniques of electrical stimulation and improve the outcomes. Currently, the future of SCS for control of chronic pain looks bright and very promising.

Suggested Reading

Al-Kaisy A, Palmisani S, Pang D, Sanderson K, Wesley S, Tan Y, McCammon S, Trescott A. Prospective, randomized, sham-control, double blind, crossover trial of subthreshold spinal cord stimulation at various kilohertz frequencies in subjects suffering from failed back surgery syndrome (SCS frequency study). Neuromodulation. 2018 Jul;21(5):457–65.

Bendel MA, O'Brien T, Hoelzer BC, Deer TR, Pittelkow TP, Costandi S, Walega DR, Azer G, Hayek SM, Wang Z, Eldrige JS, Qu W, Rosenow JM, Falowski SM, Neuman SA, Moeschler SM, Wassef C, Kim C, Niazi T, Saifullah T, Yee B, Kim C, Oryhan CL, Warren DT, Lerman I, Mora R, Hanes M, Simopoulos T, Sharma S, Gilligan C, Grace W, Ade T, Mekhail NA, Hunter JP, Choi D, Choi DY. Spinal cord stimulator related infections: findings from a multicenter retrospective analysis of 2737 implants. Neuromodulation. 2017;20(6):553–7.

Bendersky D, Yampolsky C. Is spinal cord stimulation safe? A review of its complications. World Neurosurg. 2014;82(6):1359–68.

Benyamin R, Galan V, Hatheway J, Kim P, Choi D, Falowski S, Calodney A, Sweet J, Yu C, Kapural L, Provenzano D. Options: a prospective, open-label study of high-dose spinal cord stimulation in patients with chronic Back and leg pain. Pain Physician. 2020;23(1):87–98.

Broseta J, Barberá J, de Vera JA, Barcia-Salorio JL, Garcia-March G, González-Darder J, Rovaina F, Joanes V. Spinal cord stimulation in peripheral arterial disease. A cooperative study. J Neurosurg. 1986;64(1):71–80.

Cedeno DL, Vera-Portocarrero L, Goodman Keiser M, et al. Translational comparison of rodent and sheep models of continuous spinal cord stimulation. Poster Presentation at International Society, Sydney, Australia, May 27–30, 2019.

Cedeño DL, Smith WJ, Kelley CA, Vallejo R. Spinal cord stimulation using differential target multiplexed programming modulates neural cell-specific transcriptomes in an animal model of neuropathic pain. Mol Pain. 2020;16:1744806920964360.

Chakravarthy K, Kent AR, Raza A, Xing F, Kinfe TM. Burst spinal cord stimulation: review of preclinical studies and comments on clinical outcomes. Neuromodulation. 2018;21(5):431–9.

Chakravarthy K, Fishman MA, Zuidema X, Hunter CW, Levy R. Mechanism of action in burst spinal cord stimulation: review and recent advances. Pain Med. 2019;20(Suppl 1):S13–22. https://doi.org/10.1093/pm/pnz073.

Croom JE, Foreman RD, Chandler MJ, Koss MC, Barron KW. Role of nitric oxide in cutaneous blood flow increases in the rat hindpaw during dorsal column stimulation. Neurosurgery. 1997;40(3):565–70; discussion 571. https://doi.org/10.1097/00006123-199703000-00027.

Cui JG, O'Connor WT, Ungerstedt U, Linderoth B, Meyerson BA. Spinal cord stimulation attenuates augmented dorsal horn release of excitatory amino acids in mononeuropathy via a GABAergic mechanism. Pain. 1997;73(1):87–95.

De Ridder D, Plazier M, Kamerling N, et al. Burst spinal cord stimulation for limb and back pain. World Neurosurg. 2013;80(5):642–9.

Deer TR, Lamer TJ, Pope JE, et al. The neurostimulation appropriateness consensus committee (NACC) safety guidelines for the reduction of severe neurological injury. Neuromodulation. 2017;20:13–30.

Deer T, Slavin KV, Amirdelfan K, North RB, Burton AW, Yearwood TL, Tavel E, Staats P, Falowski S, Pope J, Justiz R, Fabi AY, Taghva A, Paicius R, Houden T, Wilson D. Success using neuromodulation with BURST (SUNBURST) study: results from a prospective, randomized controlled trial using a novel burst waveform. Neuromodulation. 2018a Jan;21(1):56–66.

Deer T, Slavin KV, Amirdelfan K, et al. Success using neuromodulation with BURST (SUNBURST) study: results from a prospective, randomized controlled trial using a novel burst waveform. Neuromodulation. 2018b;21(1):56–66.

Falowski SM, Provenzano DA, Xia Y, Doth AH. Spinal cord stimulation infection rate and risk factors: results from a United States payer database. Neuromodulation. 2019 Feb;22(2):179–89.

Fishman M, Cordner H, Justiz R, et al. 12 month results from multicenter randomized controlled trial comparing DTM SCS and traditional SCS in subjects with chronic intractable back and leg pain. In: 2021 North American Neuromodulation Society annual meeting abstracts.

Foreman RD, Linderoth B. Neural mechanisms of spinal cord stimulation. Int Rev. Neurobiol. 2012;107:87–119.

Foreman RD, Linderoth B, Ardell JL, et al. Modulation of intrinsic cardiac neurons by SCS: implications for its therapeutic use in angina pectoris. Cardiovasc Res. 2000;47:367–75.

Gazelka HM, Freeman ED, Hooten WM, Eldrige JS, Hoelzer BC, Mauck WD, Moeschler SM, Pingree MJ, Rho RH, Lamer TJ. Incidence of clinically significant percutaneous spinal cord stimulator lead migration. Neuromodulation. 2015;18(2):123–5. discussion 125

Grider J. Effectiveness of spinal cord stimulation in chronic spinal pain: a systematic review. Pain Physician. 2016;19:E33–54.

Kapural L, Yu C, Doust MW, et al. Novel 10-kHz high-frequency therapy (HF10 therapy) is superior to traditional low-frequency spinal cord stimulation for the treatment of chronic back and leg pain: the SENZARCT randomized controlled trial. Anesthesiology. 2015;123:851–60.

Kapural L, Yu C, Doust MW, et al. Comparison of 10-kHz high frequency and traditional low-frequency spinal cord stimulation for the treatment of chronic back and leg pain: 24-month results froma multicenter, randomized, controlled pivotal trial. Neurosurgery. 2016;79:667.

Kapural L, Sayed D, Kim B, Harstroem C, Deering J. Retrospective assessment of salvage to 10 kHz spinal cord stimulation (SCS) in patients who failed traditional SCS therapy: RESCUE study. J Pain Res. 2020;10(13):2861–7.

Kapural L, Jameson J, Patel M, et al. Spinal cord stimulation at 10 kHz for non-surgical refractory back pain: multicenter RCT primary endpoint results. In: NANS 2021 annual meeting abstracts.

Kingma JG Jr, Linderoth B, Ardell JL, Armour JA, DeJongste MJ, Foreman RD. Neuromodulation therapy does not influence blood flow distribution or left-ventricular dynamics during acute myocardial ischemia. Auton Neurosci. 2001;91(1–2):47–54.

Kumar K, Taylor RS, Jacques L, et al. Spinal cord stimulation versus conventional medical management for neuropathic pain: a multicentre randomised controlled trial in patients with failed back surgery syndrome. Pain. 2007;132(1–2):179–88.

Lee KY, Bae C, Lee D, Kagan Z, Bradley K, Chung JM, La JH. Low-intensity, Kilohertz Frequency spinal cord stimulation differently affects excitatory and inhibitory neurons in the rodent superficial dorsal horn. Neuroscience. 2020;21(428):132–9.

Linderoth B, Fedorcsak I, Meyerson BA. Peripheral vasodilatation after spinal cord stimulation: animal studies of putative effector mechanisms. Neurosurgery. 1991a;28(2):187–95.

Linderoth B, Gunasekera L, Meyerson BA. Effects of sympathectomy on skin and muscle microcirculation during dorsal column stimulation: animal studies. Neurosurgery. 1991b;28(2):187–95.

Linderoth B, Herregodts P, Meyerson BA. Sympathetic mediation of peripheral vasodilation induced by spinal cord stimulation: animal studies of the role of cholinergic and adrenergic receptor subtypes. Neurosurgery. 1994;35(4):711–9.

Mannheimer C, Eliasson T, Andersson B, Bergh CH, Augustinsson LE, Emanuelsson H, Waagstein F. Effects of spinal cord stimulation in angina pectoris induced by pacing and possible mechanisms of action. BMJ. 1993;307(6902):477–80.

Mekhail N, Mehanny D, Armanyous S, Saweris Y, Costandi S. The impact of obesity on the effectiveness of spinal cord stimulation in chronic spine-related pain patients. Spine J. 2019;19(3):476–86.

Mekhail N, Levy RM, Deer TR, Kapural L, Li S, Amirdelfan K, Hunter CW, Rosen SM, Costandi SJ, Falowski SM, Burgher AH, Pope JE, Gilmore CA, Qureshi FA, Staats PS, Scowcroft J, Carlson J, Kim CK, Yang MI, Stauss T, Poree L. Evoke Study Group. Long-term safety and efficacy of closed-loop spinal cord stimulation to treat chronic back and leg pain (Evoke): a double-blind, randomized, controlled trial. Lancet Neurol. 2020;19(2):123–34.

Narouze S, Benzon HT, Provenzano D, et al. Interventional spine and pain procedures in patients on antiplatelet and anticoagulant medications (Second Edition): guidelines from the American Society of Regional Anesthesia and Pain Medicine, the European Society of Regional Anaesthesia and Pain Therapy, the American Academy of Pain Medicine, the International Neuromodulation Society, the North American Neuromodulation Society, and the World Institute of Pain. Reg Anesth Pain Med. 2018;43(3):225–62.

North RB, Kidd DH, Farrokhi F, Piantadosi SA. Spinal cord stimulation versus repeated lumbosacral spine surgery for chronic pain: a randomized, controlled trial. Neurosurgery. 2005;56(1):98–106. Discussion 7.

North RB, Kidd D, Shipley J, Taylor RS. Spinal cord stimulation versus reoperation for failed back surgery syndrome: a cost effectiveness and cost utility analysis based on a randomized, controlled trial. Neurosurgery. 2007;61(2):361–8. Discussion 368–9.

North J, Hong SJ, Young Cho P. Clinical outcomes of 1 kHz subperception spinal cord stimulation in implanted patients with failed paresthesia-based stimulation: results of a prospective randomized controlled trial. Neuromodulation. 2016;19(7):731–7.

North R, Desai MJ, Vangeneugden J, Raftopoulos C, Van Havenbergh T, Deruytter M, Remacle JM, Shipley J, Tan Y, Johnson MJ, Van den Abeele C, Rigoard P, PROMISE Study Group. Postoperative infections associated with prolonged spinal cord stimulation trial duration (PROMISE RCT). Neuromodulation. 2020;23(5):620–5.

Parker J, Karantonis DM, Single PS, et al. Compound action potentials recorded in the human spinal cord during neurostimulation for pain relief. Pain. 2012;153:593–601.

Peterson E, Stauss TG, Scowcroft JA, et al. 10 kHz spinal cord stimulation for treatment of painful diabetic neuropathy - a multicenter randomized controlled trial. In: 2021 annual North American Neuromodulation Society abstracts; late-breaking abstract 4.

Ruiz-Sauri A, Orduña-Valls JM, Blasco-Serra A, et al. Glia to neuron ratio in the posterior aspect of the human spinal cord at thoracic segments relevant to spinal cord stimulation. J Anat. 2019;235(5):997–1006.

Shamji MF, Westwick HJ, Heary RF. Complications related to the use of spinal cord stimulation for managing persistent postoperative neuropathic pain after lumbar spinal surgery. Neurosurg Focus. 2015;39(4):E15.

Simpson RK Jr, Robertson CS, Goodman JC, Halter JA. Recovery of amino acid neurotransmitters from the spinal cord during posterior epidural stimulation: a preliminary study. J Am Paraplegia Soc. 1991;14(1):3–8.

Southerland EM, Milhorn DM, Foreman RD, et al. Preemptive, but not reactive, SCS mitigates transient ischemia-induced myocardial infarction via cardiac adrenergic neurons. Am J Physiolol Heart Circ Physiol. 2007;292:H311–7.

Stiller CO, Cui JG, O'Connor WT, Brodin E, Meyerson BA, Linderoth B. Release of gamma-aminobutyric acid in the dorsal horn and suppression of tactile allodynia by spinal cord stimulation in mononeuropathic rats. Neurosurgery. 1996;39(2):367–74.

Tanaka S, Barron KW, Chandler MJ, Linderoth B, Foreman RD. Low intensity spinal cord stimulation may induce cutaneous vasodilation via CGRP release. Brain Res. 2001;896(1–2):183–7. https://doi.org/10.1016/s0006-8993(01)02144-8.

Valejo R, Bradley K, Kapural L. Spinal cord stimulation in chronic pain: mode of action. Spine (Phila Pa 1976). 2017;42(Suppl 14):S53–60.

Vallejo R, Kelley C, Smith WJ, et al. Cell-specific targeting in neural tissue using Differential Target Multiplexed (DTM) SCS. Poster presentation at the American Society for Regional Anesthesiology (ASRA) conference; Nov 2019.

Targeted Intrathecal Drug Delivery as Pain Therapy

73

Salim M. Hayek and Melinda M. Lawrence

Contents

Introduction

Unlike electric-based forms of neuromodulation, targeted intrathecal drug delivery (TIDD) is centered on pharmacodynamic interactions of spinally administered agents with target receptors in the central nervous system (CNS). An intrathecal drug delivery system (IDDS) consists of an intrathecally placed catheter attached to a drug delivery pump (Fig. 73.1). TIDD has demonstrated benefits over oral analgesics in the treatment of chronic intractable pain as it depos-

S. M. Hayek (✉) · M. M. Lawrence
Department of Anesthesiology, Division of Pain Medicine, University Hospitals Cleveland Medical Center, Cleveland, OH, USA
e-mail: salim.hayek@uhhospitals.org; melinda.lawrence@uhhospitals.org

D. Jankovic, P. Peng (eds.), *Regional Nerve Blocks in Anesthesia and Pain Therapy*, https://doi.org/10.1007/978-3-030-88727-8_73

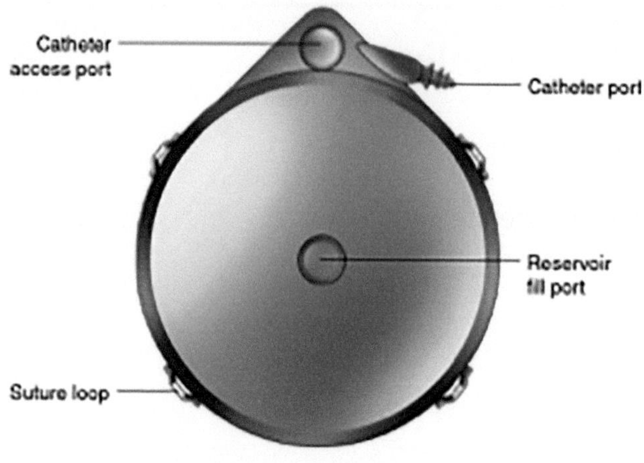

Fig. 73.1 Different component of an intrathecal pump

its medications directly at their site of action bypassing hepatic first-pass metabolism and the blood-brain barrier. Hence, neuromodulating substances that do not cross the blood-brain barrier—and would otherwise not reach their targets via systemic administration—are delivered to the CNS. TIDD also improves the efficiency of transfer of other centrally acting medications, thus allowing the use of miniscule amounts intrathecally compared to systemic administration, often resulting in less adverse effects and better pain control in comparison to other routes of medication delivery. The advantages of TIDD in managing chronic pain may have become even more relevant recently given the opioid abuse epidemic in the United States.

Whereas a number of intrathecal (IT) agents are used in TIDD as standard of care, only two—morphine and ziconotide—have been approved for intrathecal monotherapy of chronic pain by the US Food and Drug Administration (FDA). The Polyanalgesic Consensus Conference (PACC) panel provides periodic consensus guidelines regarding the efficacy and safety of TIDD. It also postulates hierarchical lines of care in the choice of intrathecal agents, with the 2017 PACC guidelines taking into consideration disease state and patient factors in the medication selection process. While intrathecal monotherapy is recommended first and occasionally used, off-label combination TIDD therapy is the norm in the management of chronic pain, driven mostly by insufficient pain relief with monotherapy. Thus, there remains a need for novel, safe, and more effective intrathecal agents for the management of chronic pain. To that end, a number of potential substances have been explored for TIDD using animal experiments, and some are currently undergoing preliminary safety clinical trials.

The goal of this chapter is to provide an overview on intrathecal targeted drug delivery including combination therapy for the management of chronic pain.

Patient Selection

Patient selection is arguably the most important factor for successful outcomes with TIDD. TIDD has been utilized in a wide range of chronic pain disorders, and it is routinely used for patients with cancer or chronic noncancer pain. For a number of years, the generalized prerequisites for an appropriate patient selection for TIDD were considered to include failure to achieve adequate pain control with more conservative measures (medication, therapy, and interventions), inability to tolerate systemic pain medication or presence of intolerable side effects, presence of objective pathology, and lack of untreated psychological disorder or presence of an unfavorable psychological disorder (personality disorder). More recent research has brought attention to other important factors in patient selection including patient demographics and medical history, pain characteristics, and concurrent use of opioids.

In terms of patient demographics, an important factor to consider is age. Prior studies have revealed that younger subjects have a faster pace of opioid tolerance and higher opioid dose escalation than older subjects taking oral opioids for chronic noncancer pain. Similar results have also been seen in the pain literature on TIDD.

Location of pain (diffuse vs. localized) and type of pain (nociceptive vs. neuropathic) are also factors to take into account when evaluating a patient for possible TIDD. In the 2017 version of the PACC guidelines, the authors not only considered type of pain but also took into consideration the location of pain for the first time in making recommendations for treatment. In general, patients who have localized pain are thought to have better results with TIDD than patients with diffuse and widespread pain. CSF dynamics and the physicochemical properties of intrathecal agents generally allow better responses when targeting areas very close to the tip of the intrathecal catheter rather than treating the whole spine or multiple far away segments. Limitation of drug spread may be especially evident when using hydrophobic drugs like fentanyl or bupivacaine. These important drug properties and CSF dynamics will be discussed more in depth later in the chapter but are important factors to consider in patient selection. The use of TIDD for nociceptive, neuropathic, or mixed pain have all been described in the literature. In general, there is not a lot of evidence to support specific intrathecal medications in the treatment of neuropathic pain, moderate effect for ziconotide in spinal cord injury patients, and little evidence that opioids are more or less effective in neuropathic versus nociceptive pain. Certainly further research is necessary to determine which medications may best serve the treatment of particular pain types.

Trialing

The trialing period is a critical precursor to the implant and a necessary evaluation for both the patient and the provider to assess if the therapy is appropriate and efficacious. Each trial may be individually tailored based on the type of trial (single shot, infusion), medications selected for intrathecal infusion, and location or level in the spine targeted. Though there are many trialing techniques, a continuous infusion catheter in the intrathecal space is thought to be the "gold standard" for trialing as it most closely mimics the permanent implant. Even though the continuous infusion is thought to be the "gold standard," there is limited evidence to support this technique as superior. It is also difficult to mimic the trial exactly as most externalized pumps deliver much higher rates or volumes of drug as compared to fully implanted IDDS pumps. High infusion rates can result in wider and deeper spinal spread and may explain better relief with the temporary infusion trial on occasion than a permanent implant. The technique for implantation of the targeted intrathecal drug delivery system is summarized in Figs. 73.2 and 73.3.

Intrathecal Drug Delivery Targets

Except for local anesthetics, pharmacologic targets for intrathecal analgesic drug delivery reside in superficial layers of the dorsal horn of the spinal cord. While dorsal root ganglia house the cell bodies of the primary nociceptive afferent neurons, these consistently synapse with second-order neurons in the superficial laminae of the dorsal horn. Hence, peripheral nociceptive input is encoded at the level of the spinal dorsal horn. The spinal dorsal horn is the first CNS relay station whereby the pain signal is modulated. This critical relay area involves not only ascending afferent signal input but also local neuronal and non-neuronal modulation as well as descending supraspinal (bulbospinal) effects. Non-neuronal modulation involves spinal cord glial cells, which outnumber neurons by as much as 7:1 and play a key role in chronic pain

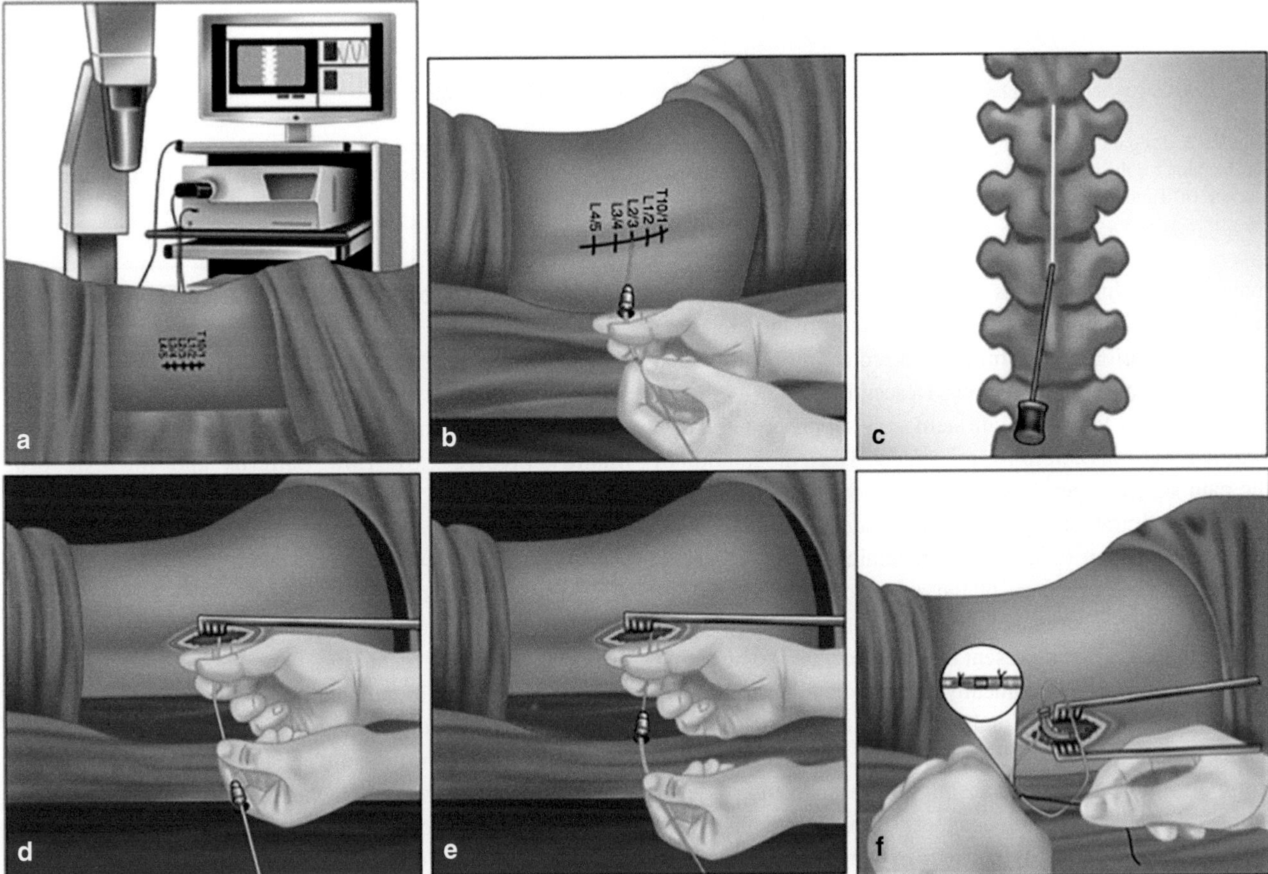

Fig. 73.2 Preparation of the catheter site. (**a**) Mark the spine level with the fluoroscopy. (**b**) Percutaneous insertion of the needle and catheter in the intrathecal space. (**c**) Monitor the location and tip of the catheter with the fluoroscopy. (**d**) and (**e**) Incision of skin and removal of needle. (**f**) Insertion of anchor to secure the catheter

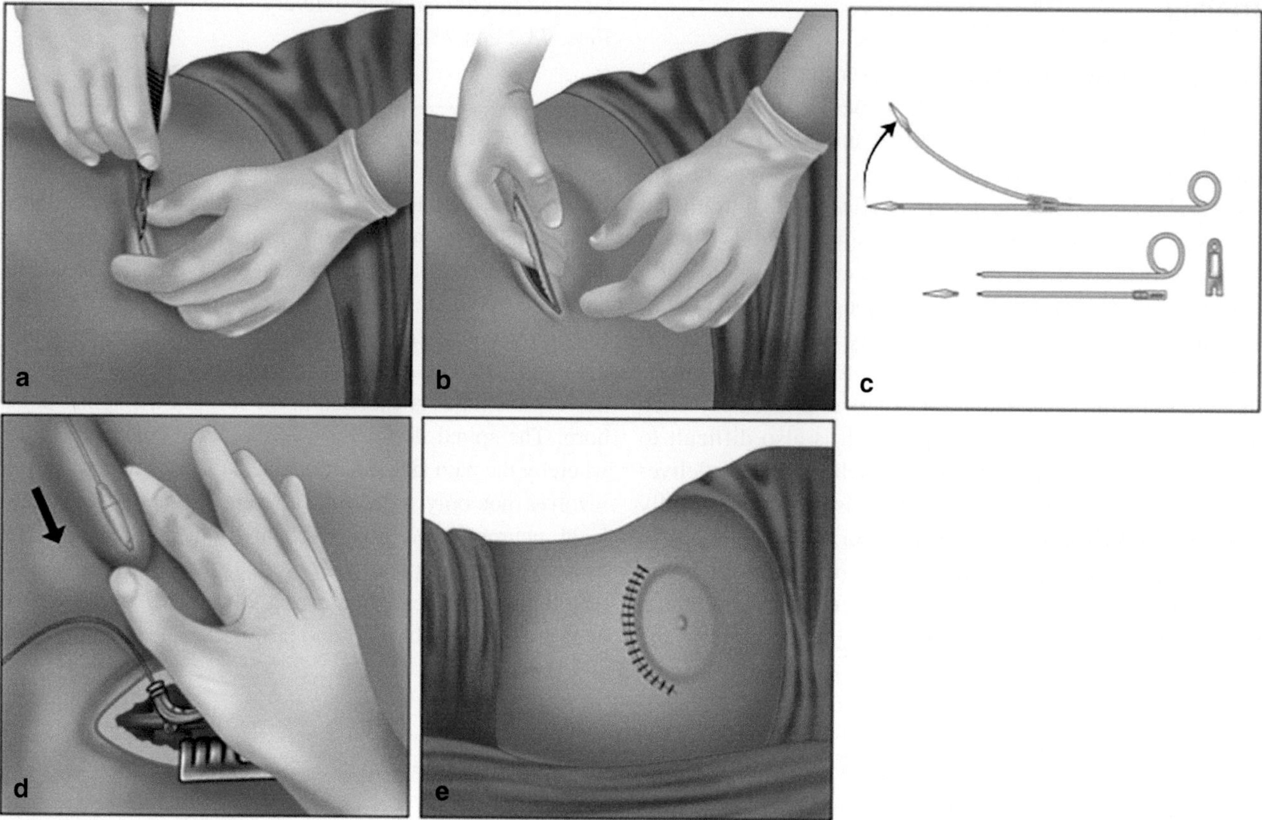

Fig. 73.3 Preparation of pump and connection to the spinal catheter. (**a**) Incision for the pump pocket. (**b**) blunt dissection for the creation of pocket. (**c**) Tunneling device; bend to conform to anatomy. (**d**) Creation of a tunnel from between abdominal incision and posterior pocket where the spinal catheter was inserted. (**e**) Closure of the incisions

maintenance. Interneurons in the superficial dorsal horn, which may be inhibitory or excitatory, modify the incoming information prior to transmission to projection neurons that relay the signals to brain regions. Descending control of nociception, mostly from the brain stem, may suppress or enhance neuronal transmission to rostral centers. Thus, modulation of the pain signal at the dorsal horn alters the supraspinal pain experience. Intrathecal opioids, ziconotide, alpha-2 agonists, and baclofen exert their effects predominantly at superficial layers of the dorsal horn of the spinal cord, at a depth of 1–2 mm from the surface of the cord.

Local anesthetics represent the one exception to targeting the dorsal horn among clinically used medications in IDDSs. Bupivacaine is the predominant local anesthetic used in TIDD and, similar to all local anesthetics, exerts its effects by interrupting neuronal transmission through blockade of voltage-dependent sodium channels. Bupivacaine has a sensory to motor differential blockade making it preferable over most other local anesthetics. While sodium channels are ubiquitously distributed along neuronal fibers, they are more readily blocked intrathecally along the thin nerve rootlets that merge into the dorsal horn (fila radicularia)—as opposed to the thicker spinal cord.

Determinants of Intrathecal Drug Delivery

Intrathecal targeted drug delivery depends on a number of parameters that govern pharmacokinetic drug distribution within the cerebrospinal fluid (CSF). These predominantly involve CSF flow patterns and intrinsic drug properties.

CSF Flow Dynamics

Modern imaging techniques and animal models have debunked the traditional bulk flow theory for CSF flow. Indeed, CSF is no longer believed to circulate throughout the neuraxis between the cranium and the caudal canal in a cyclical recurring fashion but has been rather shown to oscillate locally in a rostro-caudad pattern with an amplitude around 1 cm. The models for the CSF flow emphasize pulsatile flow with oscillatory bidirectional craniocaudal CSF movement. These described CSF pulsations have been validated with CINE-MRI.

The major determinants of the pulsatile flow of the CSF in the spinal column are arterial pulsations and the changes in intrathoracic pressures associated with respiration. Cardiac and respiratory cycle pulsations are measurable in the spinal canal; and regional changes are associated with segmental differences in the arterial and venous supplies and posture. As a result of arterial pulsation, there is cranial CSF flow in diastole and caudad flow during systole in the cervical and cervicothoracic regions. In the lower thoracic spine, respiratory influence is the predominant factor affecting flow. During deep inspiration, CSF moves cephalad, while exhalation moves CSF caudad, and CSF mean flow is augmented post-Valsalva maneuver.

Intrathecal drug delivery is also determined by factors other than CSF dynamics including drug dose, drug volume, certain intrinsic drug properties, and the rate of administration. When considering these factors and drug properties, lipid solubility may be the most important factor for targeting drug delivery to its site of action. When intrathecal medications are infused into the CSF, the drug then diffuses through the pia mater and into the target sites in lamina II of the dorsal horn of the spinal cord. Morphine, a hydrophilic drug with low lipophilicity is more likely to penetrate deeper into the spinal cord and spread more widely throughout the CSF. A hydrophobic, high-lipophilicity drug like fentanyl is more likely to rapidly diffuse into the fat-rich epidural space and from there cleared into the systemic circulation. Hydrophobic drugs are quickly cleared from the CSF through small vessels after uptake into epidural fat.

Rate of administration and drug volume also contribute to the drug distribution in the CSF. Much of the literature in the past has been based on spinal anesthesia which may be difficult to directly apply to chronic infusions of intrathecal medication which utilize low flow rates and drug volumes. The most commonly utilized permanently implanted intrathecal infusion devices for chronic pain infuse at no more than 0.01–0.02 mL/min (at maximal rate) typically utilizing a continuous infusion with a peristaltic pump or small 2–3 μL boluses with a valve gated pump. In general, boluses and larger volumes of drug can allow for drug to spread further, while low-rate continuous infusions allow for drug to stay closer to the catheter tip. Due to these determinants and known CSF dynamics that result in localized spread of drug, it is important to have the intrathecal catheter tip appropriately placed adjacent to the dorsal horn targeting the spinal segment that causes the patient's pain when using common agents such as opioids, alpha-2 agonists, and ziconotide. Some biological agents may target the dorsal root ganglion cell which is a target that lives distal to the dural cuff formed by the meninges. Since the dorsal root ganglion lies outside of the dural cuff and blood-brain barrier, mobilization of drug from the CSF to the DRG is currently a barrier for intrathecally administered agents, including adenoviruses.

Intrathecal Medications

Opioids

While a number of agents are used clinically in TIDD, opioids remain the most commonly used medications. When administered neuraxially, opioids have a primary site of action on the mu opioid receptors in the lamina II in the dorsal horn of the spinal cord. Although morphine (Infumorph) is the only FDA-approved intrathecal opioid for the treatment of chronic pain, many opioids are commonly used for the treatment of chronic pain. The most recent Polyanalgesic Consensus Conference (PACC) guidelines outline the appropriate use of commonly used IT opioids such as morphine, fentanyl, hydromorphone, and sufentanil. The guidelines have changed over the years but currently break down their recommendations for cancer and noncancer pain that is either localized or diffuse. PACC recommends the FDA-approved IT opioid morphine as first-line therapy in all treatment groups. Drugs with lower lipophilicity are typically recommended higher in the algorithms when treating diffuse pain whether it is cancer or noncancer-related due to the ability for wider spread in the CSF and deeper penetration into the gray matter, while drugs with higher lipophilicity like fentanyl are higher in the algorithm when treating localized pain due to known intrinsic drug properties previously reviewed.

Low-Dose Opioid TIDD

Historically, IT therapy was often considered to be a chronic pain treatment for cancer patients and highly opioid tolerant patients. Findings of better TIDD outcomes in opioid-naïve patients or those on low doses of systemic opioids prior to IDDS implant have led to the use of low-opioid dosing TIDD. Over the last decade, there has been more research evaluating the efficacy and usefulness of IT "microdosing." The concept of "microdosing," better referred to as low-opioid dosing, involves weaning a patient off systemic opioids prior to trialing or implanting an IDDS and then utilizing low-dose IT opioid. There have been several low-opioid dosing methods described in the literature, but there is no specific method or limit that has been defined. Limiting the amount of intrathecal opioid may be beneficial in decreasing opioid tolerance, opioid hyperalgesia, and risk of catheter-tip granuloma and limiting adverse effects from opioid administration. Although there is some evidence to support low-dose TIDD, further research including prospective randomized control trials is needed.

Opioid Adverse Effects and Complications

Drug-related adverse effects for opioids include respiratory depression, peripheral edema, hormonal changes, tolerance, opioid-induced hyperalgesia, constipation, pruritus, and granuloma formation.

One complication that is unique to chronic intrathecal opiate drug delivery is granuloma formation. A granuloma is a sterile fibrotic mass found at the tip of an IT catheter. Granuloma formation has been associated with the use of high-dose opiates in the intrathecal space. Intrathecal catheter tip granuloma (ICTG) formation is most commonly associated with high-dose morphine but has also been reported with hydromorphone. In general, it is thought that higher-dose and higher-concentration IT opioids are associated with increased likelihood for granuloma formation. Veizi et al. reported four cases of ICTG formation in patients receiving relatively low-dose hydromorphone (160–360 mcg/day, 0.75–1.0 mg/mL). Outside of unusual and excessively high doses, fentanyl has not been associated with granuloma formation and may be a useful option in properly selected patients. To minimize the chance of developing a granuloma, one should use the lowest effective dose of opioid and the lowest concentration of opioid.

Combination of Opioids with Bupivacaine

Opioid dose escalation is an unfortunate accompaniment of opioid TIDD and may predispose to higher risks of complications, including granuloma formation, lower extremity edema, and potential opioid-induced hyperalgesia. Although monotherapy with the FDA-approved/on-label intrathecal agents morphine and ziconotide is recommended as first line (1A) by the PACC guidelines, off-label use prevails. Inadequate analgesia with opioid monotherapy has given rise to combination therapy with bupivacaine being the most common used adjuvant in conjunction with opioids. Bupivacaine in combination with intrathecal opioids is a 2017 PACC guidelines line 1B treatment in the management of cancer and noncancer pain. Bupivacaine when combined with opioids at initiation of TIDD may help in limiting IT opioid dose escalation. In a retrospective study examining patients with chronic noncancer pain treated with TIDD, patients receiving combination of opioids with bupivacaine from the outset of TIDD experienced a blunted rise in opioid dose escalation (185 ± 85%) vs. those who only had opioids (535 ± 180%). The use of bupivacaine in combination with hydromorphone in 57 patients with refractory low back pain in the setting of previous lumbar spine surgery resulted in significant and sustained analgesic response over a 2-year follow-up period. The same center examined the intrathecal trialing of patients with persistent pain who have had previous spine surgeries and received a combination therapy of hydromorphone with bupivacaine. These patients were trialed overnight using a continuous catheter intrathecal infusion with an external pump. The success rate at trial was 87% (54/62 patients proceeded to implant). No demographic factors, including pre-trial daily morphine equivalent requirements, were found to be predictive for success or failure of trial. However, similar to other studies, higher pre-trial opioid requirements were associated with higher opioid requirements at trial and after implant.

Given risk of ICTG with hydromorphone, the same group transitioned to the use of fentanyl in combination with bupivacaine, even though fentanyl may have less than optimal pharmacokinetic characteristics. They compared effectiveness of hydromorphone/bupivacaine in 30 consecutive patients with lumbar post-laminectomy syndrome and low back pain to 28 similar consecutive patients who received fentanyl/bupivacaine. Both patient groups were followed for at least 2 years, with the fentanyl cohort being the more recent. The fentanyl cohort had lower pre-implant opioid dosage consistent with the shift in practice toward low-opioid dosing, but other demographic parameters were similar. Given lower starting systemic opioid doses, the fentanyl cohort had a lower rate of opioid dose escalation. However, both groups had similar reductions in pain scores over the 2-year follow-up period suggesting that fentanyl/bupivacaine is an effective combination that may be safer. Of note, a small case series from the same group reported on the effectiveness of intrathecal fentanyl in resolving intrathecal hydromorphone- or morphine-induced peripheral edema.

Ziconotide

Ziconotide (Prialt) is a synthetic form of a 25-amino acid peptide that was originally isolated from the venom of a marine snail (*Conus magus*). Ziconotide selectively blocks the presynaptic N-type calcium channels in the dorsal horn of the spinal cord which then impedes pain signal transmission by inhibiting the release of calcitonin gene-related peptide, glutamate, and substance P. Although ziconotide has been shown to be safe and efficacious in the treatment of intractable pain, studies have shown significantly more adverse effects than placebo (11.6–30.6% for ziconotide and 2–10% for placebo). Reported adverse effects include psychiatric disturbances, dizziness, nystagmus, somnolence, confusion, memory impairment, myopathy, nausea, and abnormal gait.

Ziconotide is the only non-opioid IT medication that is FDA approved for the treatment of chronic pain. The PACC guidelines consider ziconotide as a first-line monotherapy (1A) treatment for diffuse or localized chronic noncancer and cancer pain. Although not FDA approved for combination therapy, ziconotide is recommended to be used in combination by PACC and often used with other agents in clinical practice. Despite its common use in combination, there is little evidence to support its use in that capacity. One retrospective review of 15 chronic noncancer patients who had suboptimal pain control were trialed with intrathecal ziconotide as a second-line agent (add-on) to their existing IT infusions (either hydromorphone/bupivacaine or fentanyl/bupivacaine). Eleven patients were deemed to have a successful trial of ziconotide which was then added in combination with existing IT medications. Seven patients discontinued ziconotide treatment due to adverse effects, while only four patients were able to continue with ziconotide as an add-on through the end of the study (24 months). Five out of seven patients who had the ziconotide removed due to adverse effects also did not see improvement in pain, while two did see improvement. A study by Deer et al. using combination therapy with ziconotide showed early improvement in pain scores at 3 months which was similar to the aforementioned study by Hayek et al. After the initial 3 months however, patients failed to show ongoing improvement in pain scores while developing more adverse effects that led to attrition.

Ziconotide Stability

Stability is a concern whenever two or more chemicals are mixed together as chemical interactions can occur and physical and/or chemical changes may lead to a variation in therapeutic properties and undesirable side effects. The stability of the ziconotide peptide has been studied alone and in combination. Proteins and peptides are known to be highly sensitive to hydrolysis and oxidation which may lead to chemical instability and impact the overall efficacy of a treatment. The primary mechanism of ziconotide degradation is oxidation which occurs when oxygen dissolved in water reacts with the methionine bonds in the peptide. The literature has shown that opioids can speed up the degradation of ziconotide and interfere with its stability. As a monotherapy, the ziconotide peptide has been shown to be more stable. Ziconotide stability as a monotherapy was 90% at 60 days, while stability was reduced when combined with opioids (90% at 8 days down to 75% at 17 days). There are larger declines in ziconotide concentrations (more instability) when more dilute concentrations of ziconotide are used. Dupoiron et al. found a nearly linear decline in the concentration of ziconotide admixed in vitro with morphine, bupivacaine, and clonidine. Additionally, temperature plays a role in the degradation of ziconotide. When ziconotide in admixtures is stored in syringes at 5 °C, there is no degradation which is particularly important when considering storage and transport of medication. Finally, due to degradation of ziconotide, there may be decreases in clinical effectiveness in patients whose pumps are refilled at longer intervals. Decline in ziconotide concentrations should be taken into account when considering refill frequency. In general, studies have found that other intrathecal admixtures and single agents are stable.

Alpha-2 Agonists

Clonidine is a selective alpha-2 adrenergic agonist that can be used intrathecally for the treatment of chronic pain. Clonidine inhibits the nociceptive impulses at the dorsal spinal cord by activating pre- and post-junctional alpha-2 adrenoceptors. Clonidine has also been shown to inhibit the neuroimmune activation associated with neuropathic pain states, specifically by inhibiting the activation glial cells that contribute to enhanced pain states through the release of proinflammatory cytokines.

Intrathecal clonidine is not recommended for use as a single agent to treat chronic pain. Clonidine is recommended for use with opioids, ziconotide, and local anesthetics or in combination with two or more of the aforementioned IT agents. Clonidine can potentiate the effect of opioids as alpha-2 agonist, and opioids are known to have a synergistic relationship. Analgesia with clonidine is dose dependent when utilized in the spinal space, and in some cases, the side effects associated with clonidine may limit its use. While pain relief may be better with higher dosing, the observed cardiovascular effects with intrathecal clonidine are more prevalent at lower dosing and stabilize as dosing increases. Adverse effects may include bradycardia, confusion, dizziness, dry mouth, hypotension, nausea, orthostasis, sedation, depression, night terrors, and insomnia. Another concern with clonidine is that with abrupt discontinuation, rebound hypertension can occur. The potential for rebound hypertension can make it challenging to down titrate clonidine, especially when used in combination.

Future of Intrathecal Therapy: Agents and Applications

The treatment of pain is ever evolving, and the future of IT pain treatment will involve novel agents and applications. Targeted use of novel intrathecal toxins may have specific advantages, and the most promising toxin for TIDD is resiniferatoxin.

Resiniferatoxin (RTX)

RTX seems to be a promising drug on the horizon for the treatment of pain and for use in the IT space. RTX is a naturally occurring plant molecule that is found in a cactus-like plant native to Morocco that is named *Euphorbia resinifera*. This drug molecule is the most potent among all known endogenous and synthetic agonists of the transient receptor potential vanilloid 1 (TRPV1) receptor, also well known as the capsaicin receptor. TRPV1 channels are found on the endings of the small high threshold primary nociceptive afferents and when activated will lead to stimulation, then desensitization, and loss of nerve terminal activities. RTX causes cytotoxicity and death only of those sensory nociceptive neurons that express the TRPV1 ion channel leading to selective targeting and permanent deletion of the TRPV1 expressing C-fiber neuronal cell bodies in the dorsal root ganglia. RTX has been found to exhibit anti-hyperalgesic effects in canine models.

RTX may prove to be a versatile agent for the treatment of a wide variety of pain problems as it has been studied for use in acute and chronic pain settings, and it may be administered both peripherally and centrally to the intrathecal space. One major advantage of RTX is that it is selective for a subpopulation of the nociceptive primary afferent fibers. Consequently, the sensations of pressure, vibration, proprioceptive, and cold temperature are left intact. Preclinical studies also showed long-lasting, selective analgesia, but the drug did not affect motor activity, coordination, or mechanosensitivity. There is also an important difference in route of administration and the effects on the neurons. Animals studies showed that after using RTX peripherally (subcutaneous, perineural, topical), the peripheral sensitivity returns to baseline unlike with intrathecal use. The intrathecal route of administration leads to a permanent failure of conduction, without regeneration, between TRPV1-expressing neurons and the spinal cord. A recent study using a swine model ($n = 12$) was performed to test whether the contrast injected during a transforaminal or intralaminar epidural procedure would reliably predict the extent of resiniferatoxin-mediated nociceptive neurolysis. In all animals, there was unilateral spread of contrast but bilateral neurolysis of spinal nociceptive afferents. This study suggests that the true neuroanatomical range of a new drug delivered to the dorsal epidural space cannot absolutely be predicted by intraprocedural imaging of contrast. Another potential role for targeting TRPV1 is that activated TRPV1 forms a pore that can pass local anesthetics (e.g., QX314), which cannot normally enter the axon. Further studies are needed to determine how RTX may be employed in TIDD in the future.

Non-traditional Applications: Facial Pain and Hypertension

Facial Pain

The treatment of refractory facial and head pain using IT therapy has been described in the pain literature. Using a high cervical IT catheter may be a viable option for the treatment of facial pain due to the fact that the more inferior portion of the trigeminal nucleus is located mainly in the C1 and C2 segments of the spinal cord and possibly even lower in the cervical spine.

Hayek et al. described the first case of the successful management of corneal neuropathic pain with an intrathecal drug delivery system. In this case, a fentanyl/bupivacaine infusion was used to target the nerves that supply the cornea by utilizing a catheter placed at the C1 level. The cornea itself has a very high neuronal density that is 300–600 times that of the skin with unmyelinated sensory fibers that transmit nociceptive input by way of the ciliary nerves to the ophthalmic branch of the trigeminal nerve. These nociceptive afferents from the cornea travel via the ophthalmic division of the trigeminal nerve along the descending spinal trigeminal tract. These nerves and synapse travel through the caudal portion of the trigeminal nucleus. TIDD with a high intrathecal cervical catheter may be able to target these low-lying nerve pathways that were causing the refractory eye or facial pain. This type of intrathecal therapy targeting the high cervical area could be utilized for many other refractory facial pain conditions, especially when the trigeminal system is involved. Further prospective studies would be needed to characterize the long-term benefits and specific disease state applications.

Hypertension

A recent retrospective review of 82 patients with an IDDS for chronic noncancer pain in an academic medical center looked at the effect of long-term intrathecal bupivacaine on blood pressure. In this novel study, the patients were found to have significant decreases in systolic blood pressure and mean arterial pressure at follow-up intervals (1 week, 1 month, 3 months, 1 year) relative to their baseline pressures prior to implant. Despite the change in systolic and mean pressures, there was no significant change in diastolic blood pressure throughout the study. Prior to this study, there were no studies regarding the long-term effects of intrathecal bupivacaine on blood pressure. Local anesthetics in the acute setting often cause hypotension, and it is thought to be related to sympathetic blockade. In this study, the decrease in systolic blood pressure was thought to reflect a partial sympathetic blockade by bupivacaine in the lower thoracic spinal levels as there was no change in heart rate that may be seen in the upper thoracic areas. Decreases in systolic and mean pressures were seen in patients who had a diagnosis of hypertension and those who did not—suggesting an effect on preganglionic sympathetic fibers. This effect on blood pressure certainly is interesting as the change in systolic pressure was equal to or greater than the effect seen with prescription antihypertensives. Larger, prospective randomized studies examining the effect of bupivacaine on blood pressure as well as other intrathecal medications with antihypertensive effects like an intrathecal alpha-2 agonist (clonidine) also warrant further studies.

Conclusions

Targeted intrathecal drug delivery is an important therapy in the armamentarium of the pain physician. Understanding CSF flow dynamics, intrathecal medication pharmacokinetics, and device capabilities coupled with sound patient selection and technical performance of the procedure can result in very favorable outcomes for an otherwise refractory chronic pain population. Additionally, novel agents and indications may be on the horizon.

Suggested Reading

Alperin N, Vikingstad EM, Gomez-Anson B, Levin DN. Hemodynamically independent analysis of cerebrospinal fluid and brain motion observed with dynamic phase contrast MRI. Magn Reson Med. 1996;35(5):741–54.

Bahney J, von Bartheld CS. The cellular composition and glia-neuron ratio in the spinal cord of a human and a nonhuman primate: comparison with other species and brain regions. Anat Rec (Hoboken). 2018;301(4):697–710.

Bates BD, Mitchell K, Keller JM, Chan CC, Swaim WD, Yaskovich R, et al. Prolonged analgesic response of cornea to topical resiniferatoxin, a potent TRPV1 agonist. Pain. 2010;149(3):522–8.

Battal B, Kocaoglu M, Bulakbasi N, Husmen G, Tuba Sanal H, Tayfun C. Cerebrospinal fluid flow imaging by using phase-contrast MR technique. Br J Radiol. 2011;84(1004):758–65.

Bernards CM. Cerebrospinal fluid and spinal cord distribution of baclofen and bupivacaine during slow intrathecal infusion in pigs. Anesthesiology. 2006;105(1):169–78.

Bert RJ, Hayek SM, Yaksh TL. Modeling spinal intrathecal drug distribution: the challenge of defining and predicting cerebrospinal fluid dynamics. Anesth Analg. 2017;124(5):1403–6.

Bevacqua BK, Fattouh M, Backonja M. Depression, night terrors, and insomnia associated with long-term intrathecal clonidine therapy. Pain Pract. 2007;7(1):36–8.

Bhadelia RA, Madan N, Zhao Y, Wagshul ME, Heilman C, Butler JP, et al. Physiology-based MR imaging assessment of CSF flow at the foramen magnum with a Valsalva maneuver. AJNR Am J Neuroradiol. 2013;34(9):1857–62.

Binshtok AM, Bean BP, Woolf CJ. Inhibition of nociceptors by TRPV1-mediated entry of impermeant sodium channel blockers. Nature. 2007;449(7162):607–10.

Boswell MV, Iacono RP, Guthkelch AN. Sites of action of subarachnoid lidocaine and tetracaine: observations with evoked potential monitoring during spinal cord stimulator implantation. Reg Anesth. 1992;17(1):37–42.

Brinzeu A, Berthiller J, Caillet JB, Staquet H, Mertens P. Ziconotide for spinal cord injury-related pain. Eur J Pain. 2019;23(9):1688–700.

Brown J, Klapow J, Doleys D, Lowery D, Tutak U. Disease-specific and generic health outcomes: a model for the evaluation of long-term intrathecal opioid therapy in noncancer low back pain patients. Clin J Pain. 1999;15(2):122–31.

Brown DC, Iadarola MJ, Perkowski SZ, Erin H, Shofer F, Laszlo KJ, et al. Physiologic and antinociceptive effects of intrathecal resiniferatoxin in a canine bone cancer model. Anesthesiology. 2005;103(5):1052–9.

Brown DC, Agnello K, Iadarola MJ. Intrathecal resiniferatoxin in a dog model: efficacy in bone cancer pain. Pain. 2015;156(6):1018–24.

Buntin-Mushock C, Phillip L, Moriyama K, Palmer PP. Age-dependent opioid escalation in chronic pain patients. Anesth Analg. 2005;100(6):1740–5.

Burton AW, Deer TR, Wallace MS, Rauck RL, Grigsby E. Considerations and methodology for trialing ziconotide. Pain Physician. 2010;13(1):23–33.

Capogna G, Celleno D, Zangrillo A, Costantino P, Foresta S. Addition of clonidine to epidural morphine enhances postoperative analgesia after cesarean delivery. Reg Anesth. 1995;20(1):57–61.

Covino BG. Pharmacology of local anaesthetic agents. Br J Anaesth. 1986;58(7):701–16.

De Conno F, Caraceni A, Martini C, Spoldi E, Salvetti M, Ventafridda V. Hyperalgesia and myoclonus with intrathecal infusion of high-dose morphine. Pain. 1991;47(3):337–9.

Deer TR, Kim C, Bowman R, Tolentino D, Stewart C, Tolentino W. Intrathecal ziconotide and opioid combination therapy for noncancer pain: an observational study. Pain Physician. 2009;12(4):E291–6.

Deer TR, Prager J, Levy R, Rathmell J, Buchser E, Burton A, et al. Polyanalgesic Consensus Conference--2012: consensus on diagnosis, detection, and treatment of catheter-tip granulomas (inflammatory masses). Neuromodulation. 2012;15(5):483–95. discussion 96

Deer TR, Pope JE, Hayek SM, Bux A, Buchser E, Eldabe S, et al. The polyanalgesic consensus conference (PACC): recommendations on intrathecal drug infusion systems best practices and guidelines. Neuromodulation. 2017;20(2):96–132.

Deer TR, Pope JE, Hanes MC, McDowell GC. Intrathecal therapy for chronic pain: a review of morphine and ziconotide as firstline options. Pain Med. 2019;20(4):784–98.

Dominguez E, Sahinler B, Bassam D, Day M, Lou L, Racz G, et al. Predictive value of intrathecal narcotic trials for long-term therapy with implantable drug administration systems in chronic non-cancer pain patients. Pain Pract. 2002;2(4):315–25.

Dupoiron D, Richard H, Chabert-Desnot V, Devys C, Leynia P, Boisdron-Celle M. In vitro stability of low-concentration ziconotide alone or in admixtures in intrathecal pumps. Neuromodulation. 2014;17(5):472–82. discussion 82

Eisenach JC, Hood DD, Curry R. Intrathecal, but not intravenous, clonidine reduces experimental thermal or capsaicin-induced pain and hyperalgesia in normal volunteers. Anesth Analg. 1998;87(3):591–6.

Feng X, Zhang F, Dong R, Li W, Liu J, Zhao X, et al. Intrathecal administration of clonidine attenuates spinal neuroimmune activation in a rat model of neuropathic pain with existing hyperalgesia. Eur J Pharmacol. 2009;614(1–3):38–43.

Filos KS, Goudas LC, Patroni O, Polyzou V. Hemodynamic and analgesic profile after intrathecal clonidine in humans. A dose-response study. Anesthesiology. 1994;81(3):591–601. Discussion 27A–28A.

Fitzgibbon D, Rapp S, Butler S, Terman G, Dolack G, DuPen S, et al. Rebound hypertension and withdrawal associated with discontinuation of an infusion of epidural clonidine. Anesthesiology. 1996;84(3):729–31.

Flack SH, Anderson CM, Bernards C. Morphine distribution in the spinal cord after chronic infusion in pigs. Anesth Analg. 2011;112(2):460–4.

Friese S, Hamhaber U, Erb M, Kueker W, Klose U. The influence of pulse and respiration on spinal cerebrospinal fluid pulsation. Investig Radiol. 2004;39(2):120–30.

Galica RJ, Hayek SM, Veizi E, McEwan MT, Katta S, Ali O, et al. Intrathecal trialing of continuous infusion combination therapy with hydromorphone and bupivacaine in failed back surgery patients. Neuromodulation. 2018;21(7):648–54.

Gikic M, Di Paolo ER, Pannatier A, Cotting J. Evaluation of physicochemical incompatibilities during parenteral drug administration in a paediatric intensive care unit. Pharm World Sci. 2000;22(3):88–91.

Gissen AJ, Covino BG, Gregus J. Differential sensitivity of fast and slow fibers in mammalian nerve. III. Effect of etidocaine and bupivacaine on fast/slow fibers. Anesth Analg. 1982;61(7):570–5.

Grider JS, Harned ME, Etscheidt MA. Patient selection and outcomes using a low-dose intrathecal opioid trialing method for chronic nonmalignant pain. Pain Physician. 2011;14(4):343–51.

Guevara-Lopez U, Aldrete JA, Covarrubias-Gomez A, Hernandez-Pando RE, Lopez-Munoz FJ. Absence of histological changes after the administration of a continuous intrathecal clonidine in Wistar rats. Pain Pract. 2009;9(2):122–9.

Hamza M, Doleys D, Wells M, Weisbein J, Hoff J, Martin M, et al. Prospective study of 3-year follow-up of low-dose intrathecal opioids in the management of chronic nonmalignant pain. Pain Med. 2012;13(10):1304–13.

Hao JX, Yu W, Xu XJ, Wiesenfeld-Hallin Z. Effects of intrathecal vs. systemic clonidine in treating chronic allodynia-like response in spinally injured rats. Brain Res. 1996;736(1–2):28–34.

Hassenbusch SJ, Portenoy RK. Current practices in intraspinal therapy--a survey of clinical trends and decision making. J Pain Symptom Manag. 2000;20(2):S4–11.

Hayek SM, Hanes MC. Intrathecal therapy for chronic pain: current trends and future needs. Curr Pain Headache Rep. 2014;18(1):388.

Hayek SM, Joseph PN, Mekhail NA. Pharmacology of intrathecally administered agents for treatment of spasticity and pain. In: Seminars in pain medicine. Elsevier; 2003. p. 238–53.

Hayek SM, Veizi IE, Narouze SN, Mekhail N. Age-dependent intrathecal opioid escalation in chronic noncancer pain patients. Pain Med. 2011;12(8):1179–89.

Hayek SM, Veizi E, Hanes M. Intrathecal hydromorphone and bupivacaine combination therapy for post-laminectomy syndrome optimized with patient-activated bolus device. Pain Med. 2015a;17(3):561–71.

Hayek SM, Hanes MC, Wang C, Veizi IE. Ziconotide combination intrathecal therapy for noncancer pain is limited secondary to delayed adverse effects: a case series with a 24-month follow-up. Neuromodulation. 2015b;18(5):397–403.

Hayek SM, Sweet JA, Miller JP, Sayegh RR. Successful management of corneal neuropathic pain with intrathecal targeted drug delivery. Pain Med. 2016;17(7):1302–7.

Hayek SM, McEwan MT, Veizi E, Roh J, Ali O, Katta S, et al. Effect of long-term intrathecal bupivacaine infusion on blood pressure. Neuromodulation. 2019;22(7):811–7.

Heinricher MM, Tavares I, Leith JL, Lumb BM. Descending control of nociception: specificity, recruitment and plasticity. Brain Res Rev. 2009;60(1):214–25.

Henry-Feugeas MC, Idy-Peretti I, Baledent O, Poncelet-Didon A, Zannoli G, Bittoun J, et al. Origin of subarachnoid cerebrospinal fluid pulsations: a phase-contrast MR analysis. Magn Reson Imaging. 2000;18(4):387–95.

Hildebrand KR, Elsberry DD, Deer TR. Stability, compatibility, and safety of intrathecal bupivacaine administered chronically via an implantable delivery system. Clin J Pain. 2001a;17(3):239–44.

Hildebrand KR, Elsberry DE, Anderson VC. Stability and compatibility of hydromorphone hydrochloride in an implantable infusion system. J Pain Symptom Manag. 2001b;22(6):1042–7.

Hildebrand KR, Elsberry DD, Hassenbusch SJ. Stability and compatibility of morphine-clonidine admixtures in an implantable infusion system. J Pain Symptom Manag. 2003;25(5):464–71.

Iadarola MJ, Gonnella GL. Resiniferatoxin for pain treatment: an interventional approach to personalized pain medicine. Open Pain J. 2013;6:95–107.

Iadarola MJ, Mannes AJ. The vanilloid agonist resiniferatoxin for interventional-based pain control. Curr Top Med Chem. 2011;11(17):2171–9.

Jain KK. An evaluation of intrathecal ziconotide for the treatment of chronic pain. Expert Opin Investig Drugs. 2000;9(10):2403–10.

Karai L, Brown DC, Mannes AJ, Connelly ST, Brown J, Gandal M, et al. Deletion of vanilloid receptor 1-expressing primary afferent neurons for pain control. J Clin Invest. 2004;113(9):1344–52.

Kerr FW. Evidence for a peripheral etiology of trigeminal neuralgia. J Neurosurg. 1967;26(1):Suppl:168-74.

Kerr FW, Olafson RA. Trigeminal and cervical volleys. Convergence on single units in the spinal gray at C-1 and C-2. Arch Neurol. 1961;5:171–8.

Krames ES. Intraspinal opioid therapy for chronic nonmalignant pain: current practice and clinical guidelines. J Pain Symptom Manag. 1996;11(6):333–52.

Kroin JS. Intrathecal drug administration. Present use and future trends. Clin Pharmacokinet. 1992;22(5):319–26.

McCarthy TJ. Chemical incompatibility of parenteral drug admixtures. S Afr Med J. 1974;48(46):1951–3.

McGivern JG. Ziconotide: a review of its pharmacology and use in the treatment of pain. Neuropsychiatr Dis Treat. 2007;3(1):69–85.

Mogensen T, Eliasen K, Ejlersen E, Vegger P, Nielsen IK, Kehlet H. Epidural clonidine enhances postoperative analgesia from a combined low-dose epidural bupivacaine and morphine regimen. Anesth Analg. 1992;75(4):607–10.

Neubert JK, Karai L, Jun JH, Kim HS, Olah Z, Iadarola MJ. Peripherally induced resiniferatoxin analgesia. Pain. 2003;104(1–2):219–28.

Newton DW. Physicochemical determinants of incompatibility and instability in injectable drug solutions and admixtures. Am J Hosp Pharm. 1978;35(10):1213–22.

Paice JA, Penn RD, Shott S. Intraspinal morphine for chronic pain: a retrospective, multicenter study. J Pain Symptom Manag. 1996;11(2):71–80.

Pollay M. The function and structure of the cerebrospinal fluid outflow system. Cerebrospinal Fluid Res. 2010;7:9.

Rauck RL, Cherry D, Boyer MF, Kosek P, Dunn J, Alo K. Long-term intrathecal opioid therapy with a patient-activated, implanted delivery system for the treatment of refractory cancer pain. J Pain. 2003;4(8):441–7.

Rauck RL, Wallace MS, Leong MS, Minehart M, Webster LR, Charapata SG, et al. A randomized, double-blind, placebo-controlled study of intrathecal ziconotide in adults with severe chronic pain. J Pain Symptom Manag. 2006;31(5):393–406.

Rauck RL, Wallace MS, Burton AW, Kapural L, North JM. Intrathecal ziconotide for neuropathic pain: a review. Pain Pract. 2009;9(5):327–37.

Reina MA, Villanueva MC, Maches F, Carrera A, Lopez A, De Andres JA. The ultrastructure of the human spinal nerve root cuff in the lumbar spine. Anesth Analg. 2008;106(1):339–44.

Rudd RA, Seth P, David F, Scholl L. Increases in drug and opioid-involved overdose deaths - United States, 2010-2015. MMWR Morb Mortal Wkly Rep. 2016;65(50–51):1445–52.

Saulino M. Successful reduction of neuropathic pain associated with spinal cord injury via of a combination of intrathecal hydromorphone and ziconotide: a case report. Spinal Cord. 2007;45(11):749–52.

Schmidtko A, Lotsch J, Freynhagen R, Geisslinger G. Ziconotide for treatment of severe chronic pain. Lancet. 2010;375(9725):1569–77.

Shields D, Montenegro R, Ragusa M. Chemical stability of admixtures combining ziconotide with morphine or hydromorphone during simulated intrathecal administration. Neuromodulation. 2005;8(4):257–63.

Shields DE, Liu W, Gunning K, Montenegro R. Statistical evaluation of the chemical stability of ziconotide solutions during simulated intrathecal administration. J Pain Symptom Manag. 2008;36(1):e4–6.

Siddall PJ, Molloy AR, Walker S, Mather LE, Rutkowski SB, Cousins MJ. The efficacy of intrathecal morphine and clonidine in the treatment of pain after spinal cord injury. Anesth Analg. 2000;91(6):1493–8.

Singla A, Stojanovic MP, Chen L, Mao J. A differential diagnosis of hyperalgesia, toxicity, and withdrawal from intrathecal morphine infusion. Anesth Analg. 2007;105(6):1816–9.

Sites BD, Beach M, Biggs R, Rohan C, Wiley C, Rassias A, et al. Intrathecal clonidine added to a bupivacaine-morphine spinal anesthetic improves postoperative analgesia for total knee arthroplasty. Anesth Analg. 2003;96(4):1083–8.

Southwell DG, Osorio JA, Liverman CS, Friedman LM, Naidu RK, Poree LR, et al. Intrathecal catheter-associated inflammatory mass in a neurofibromatosis type-1 patient receiving fentanyl and bupivacaine. Surg Neurol Int. 2017;8:159.

Staats PS, Yearwood T, Charapata SG, Presley RW, Wallace MS, Byas-Smith M, et al. Intrathecal ziconotide in the treatment of refractory pain in patients with cancer or AIDS: a randomized controlled trial. JAMA. 2004;291(1):63–70.

Tangen KM, Hsu Y, Zhu DC, Linninger AA. CNS wide simulation of flow resistance and drug transport due to spinal microanatomy. J Biomech. 2015;48(10):2144–54.

Tangen KM, Leval R, Mehta AI, Linninger AA. Computational and in vitro experimental investigation of intrathecal drug distribution: parametric study of the effect of injection volume, cerebrospinal fluid pulsatility, and drug uptake. Anesth Analg. 2017;124(5):1686–96.

Taren JA, Kahn EA. Anatomic pathways related to pain in face and neck. J Neurosurg. 1962;19:116–21.

Todd AJ. Neuronal circuitry for pain processing in the dorsal horn. Nat Rev. Neurosci. 2010;11(12):823–36.

Tonra JR, Mendell LM. Rabbit IgG distribution in skin, spinal cord and DRG following systemic injection in rat. J Neuroimmunol. 1997;80(1–2):97–105.

Ummenhofer WC, Arends RH, Shen DD, Bernards CM. Comparative spinal distribution and clearance kinetics of intrathecally administered morphine, fentanyl, alfentanil, and sufentanil. Anesthesiology. 2000;92(3):739–53.

Unger MD, Pleticha J, Steinauer J, Kanwar R, Diehn F, LaVallee KT, et al. Unilateral epidural targeting of resiniferatoxin induces bilateral neurolysis of spinal nociceptive afferents. Pain Med. 2019;20(5):897–906.

Veizi IE, Hayek SM, Narouze S, Pope JE, Mekhail N. Combination of intrathecal opioids with bupivacaine attenuates opioid dose escalation in chronic noncancer pain patients. Pain Med. 2011;12(10):1481–9.

Veizi IE, Hayek SM, Hanes M, Galica R, Katta S, Yaksh T. Primary hydromorphone-related intrathecal catheter tip granulomas: is there a role for dose and concentration? Neuromodulation. 2016;19(7):760–9.

Veizi E, Tornero-Bold M, Hayek SM. Resolution of intrathecal hydromorphone or morphine-induced peripheral edema by opioid rotation to fentanyl: a case series. Pain Pract. 2016c;16(6):E94–8.

Wallace MS, Charapata SG, Fisher R, Byas-Smith M, Staats PS, Mayo M, et al. Intrathecal ziconotide in the treatment of chronic nonmalignant pain: a randomized, double-blind, placebo-controlled clinical trial. Neuromodulation. 2006;9(2):75–86.

Wallace MS, Rauck R, Fisher R, Charapata SG, Ellis D, Dissanayake S. Intrathecal ziconotide for severe chronic pain: safety and tolerability results of an open-label, long-term trial. Anesth Analg. 2008a;106(2):628–37.

Wallace MS, Kosek PS, Staats P, Fisher R, Schultz DM, Leong M. Phase II, open-label, multicenter study of combined intrathecal morphine and ziconotide: addition of ziconotide in patients receiving intrathecal morphine for severe chronic pain. Pain Med. 2008b;9(3):271–81.

Wang Y, Mitchell J, Moriyama K, Kim KJ, Sharma M, Xie GX, et al. Age-dependent morphine tolerance development in the rat. Anesth Analg. 2005;100(6):1733–9.

Weaver T, Wells M, Roediger M, Stromberg K. Medtronic 2013 product performance report. 2013. https://www.medtronic.com/wcm/groups/mdtcom_sg/@mdt/@corp/documents/documents/annual_report_2013pdf. p 1–151.

Webster LR, Fisher R, Charapata S, Wallace MS. Long-term intrathecal ziconotide for chronic pain: an open-label study. J Pain Symptom Manag. 2009;37(3):363–72.

Wilkes DM, Orillosa SJ, Hustak EC, Williams CG, Doulatram GR, Solanki DR, et al. Efficacy, safety, and feasibility of the morphine microdose method in community-based clinics. Pain Med. 2018;19(9):1782–9.

Wu J, Kraja AT, Oberman A, Lewis CE, Ellison RC, Arnett DK, et al. A summary of the effects of antihypertensive medications on measured blood pressure. Am J Hypertens. 2005;18(7):935–42.

Yaksh TL, Wilson PR, Kaiko RF, Inturrisi CE. Analgesia produced by a spinal action of morphine and effects upon parturition in the rat. Anesthesiology. 1979;51(5):386–92.

Yaksh TL, Rathbun M, Jage J, Mirzai T, Grafe M, Hiles RA. Pharmacology and toxicology of chronically infused epidural clonidine HCl in dogs. Fundam Appl Toxicol. 1994;23(3):319–35.

Yaksh TL, Fisher CJ, Hockman TM, Wiese AJ. Current and future issues in the development of spinal agents for the management of pain. Curr Neuropharmacol. 2017;15(2):232–59.

Yamada S. Cerebrospinal fluid physiology: visualization of cerebrospinal fluid dynamics using the magnetic resonance imaging Time-Spatial Inversion Pulse method. Croat Med J. 2014;55(4):337–46.

Yamada S, Miyazaki M, Yamashita Y, Ouyang C, Yui M, Nakahashi M, et al. Influence of respiration on cerebrospinal fluid movement using magnetic resonance spin labeling. Fluids Barriers CNS. 2013;10(1):36.

Zacest AC, Carlson JD, Nemecek A, Burchiel KJ. Surgical management of spinal catheter granulomas: operative nuances and review of the surgical literature. Neurosurgery. 2009;65(6):1161–4. Discussion 4–5.

Part IX

Regional Anesthesia for Children

Pediatric Regional Anesthesia for the Upper Limb

74

Farrukh Munshey and Ban C. H. Tsui

Contents

F. Munshey
Department of Anesthesiology and Pain Medicine, University of Toronto, Toronto, ON, Canada

Department of Anesthesia and Pain Medicine, The Hospital for Sick Children, Toronto, ON, Canada
e-mail: farrukh.munshey@sickkids.ca

B. C. H. Tsui (✉)
Department of Anesthesiology Perioperative, and Pain Medicine, Lucille Packard Children's Hospital, Stanford, CA, USA
e-mail: bantsui@stanford.edu

D. Jankovic, P. Peng (eds.), *Regional Nerve Blocks in Anesthesia and Pain Therapy*,
https://doi.org/10.1007/978-3-030-88727-8_74

Interscalene Nerve Block

General Considerations

A well-studied peripheral nerve block that is relatively easy to perform and has a low risk of complications. The interscalene nerve block should be avoided in children with limited respiratory reserve as blockade of the phrenic nerve can significantly impair diaphragmatic muscle use for ventilation. The ulnar nerve is often inconsistently blocked with this technique.

Indication

Suitable for analgesia and surgical anesthesia for shoulder surgery, proximal humerus, and arm. Distal arm procedures will likely require supplementation with ulnar nerve blockade.

Functional Anatomy

After leaving the intervertebral foramina, the roots of the brachial plexus travel between the anterior and middle scalene muscles at the level of the cricoid cartilage (C6). The carotid artery and internal jugular vein will appear more medially, and the sternocleidomastoid muscle lies more super-medially. The interscalene nerve block is performed at this anatomical location at the level of the roots and proximal trunks of the brachial plexus (Fig. 74.1).

Technique

The patient is placed with the head turned approximately 45° away from the side to be blocked with a rolled towel placed underneath the shoulders. The skin is cleaned with antiseptic solution. If ultrasound guidance is used, prepare the probe surface by applying a sterile adhesive dressing. A 50 mm, 22G–25G insulated short-beveled needle is used. Recommended local anesthetics are 0.125–0.25% bupivacaine or 0.1–0.2% ropivacaine. Using 0.25% bupivacaine at 0.2–0.3 mL/kg is a reasonable option for this block. The duration of sensory block averages 15 ± 4.5 h, independent of the type and concentration of the local anesthetic used. Epinephrine 1:200,000 may be added to detect intravascular injection.

Nerve Stimulation

The point of needle insertion is at the level of cricoid cartilage (C6) within the interscalene groove (Fig. 74.2). The interscalene groove is located between the anterior and middle scalene muscles posterior to the lateral border of sternocleidomastoid muscle (SCM), approximately slightly above the point where the sternal and clavicular heads of the SCM

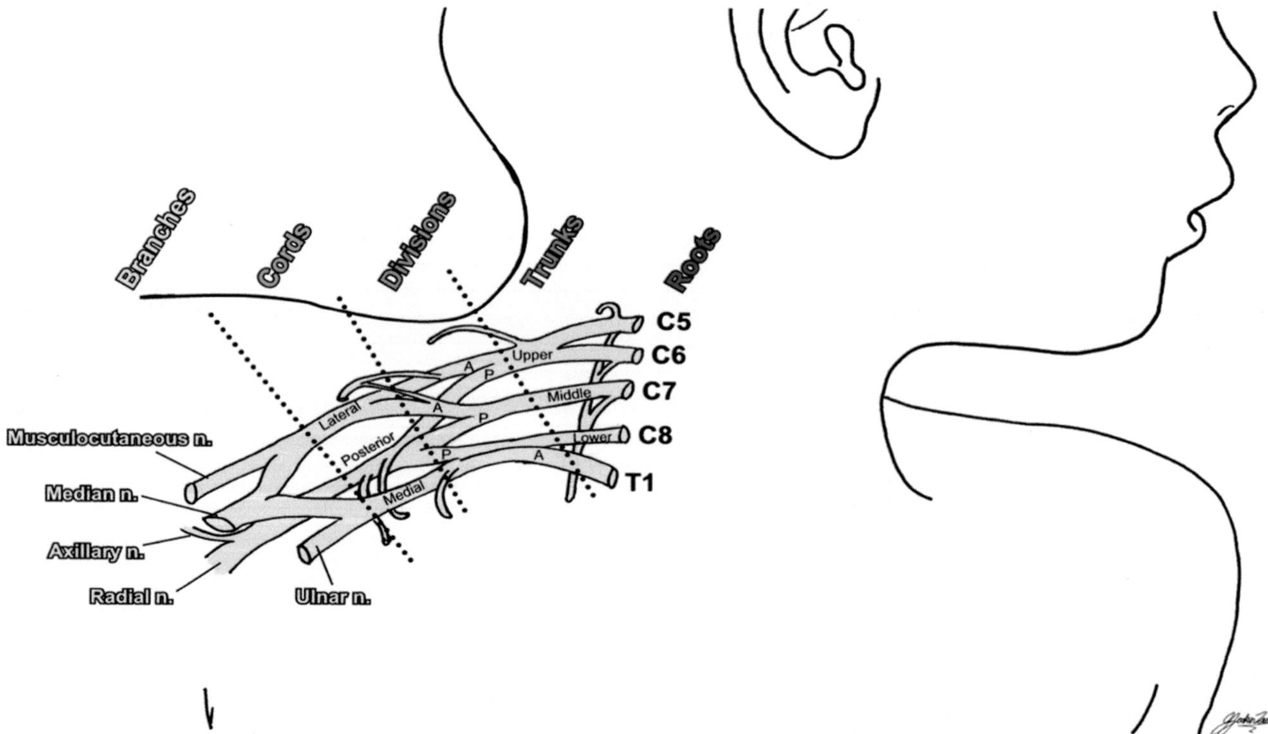

Fig. 74.1 Anatomy of the brachial plexus. *A* anterior divisions, *P* posterior divisions

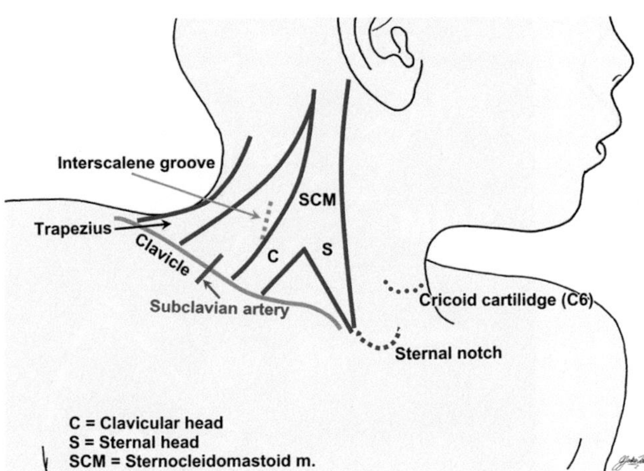

Fig. 74.2 Patient positioning and surface landmarks for interscalene brachial plexus block

separate. The line between the point of needle insertion and the cricoid cartilage should cross the Chassaignac's tubercle (anterior tubercle of the transverse process of the C6 vertebra), which can be felt easily. The needle is inserted at 60° to the skin and directed medially, posteriorly, and caudally to prevent inadvertent puncture of the vertebral artery or epidural/intrathecal space. The initial current is set at 0.8–1.0 mA (2 Hz, 100–300 μs) and then gradually reduced to a threshold current of 0.2–0.4 mA (0.1–0.2 msec) after eliciting appropriate motor responses. Response at a current >0.4 mA indicates that the needle is too far away from the plexus; a current ≤0.2 mA signifies intraneural placement.

Ultrasound-Guided

A high-frequency (13–6 MHz) linear transducer probe is suitable for this block. As shown in Fig. 74.3, the probe is placed on the neck in an axial oblique view at the level of the cricoid cartilage (C6). The anechoic great vessels (common carotid artery and internal jugular vein) and the overlying triangular-shaped sternocleidomastoid muscle are identified first. If necessary, color Doppler can be used to locate the vessels. Move the probe proximally and distally to identify the roots/trunks of the brachial plexus (commonly seen as three round- or oval-shaped hypoechoic structures) in the interscalene groove between the anterior and middle scalene muscles. Occasionally, the vertebral artery can be seen deep to the plexus and anterior to the C6 transverse process. Extra caution should be exercised not to confuse the artery with a nerve and inject into it. Visualization of the neural structures can be difficult in small children, so a "traceback" approach is recommended (Fig. 74.4). In the traceback approach, the probe is placed in a coronal oblique plane at the upper border of the clavicle. The brachial plexus at this point appears as "a bunch of grapes," superolateral to the subclavian artery. The plexus is then traced back to the interscalene region by scanning in a cephalad direction. The needle is inserted either in-plane or out-of-plane, although the in-plane approach is preferred to ensure visualization of the needle, thereby minimizing the risk of complications. For the in-plane approach, the needle is inserted in a lateral-to-medial fashion into the interscalene groove. When using the out-of-plane approach, the plexus is centered in the middle of the screen, and the needle is inserted cranial to the probe at the midline. Direct the needle tip, which appears as bright dot on the screen, in a "walk-down" manner in proximity to the nerves. Nerve structures can be confirmed by nerve stimulation. A test dose with D5W is useful to visualize the spread and confirm nerve localization. After negative aspiration for blood or CSF, local anesthetic is deposited to achieve good spread surrounding the nerves within the interscalene groove. The depth should be less than 1–2 cm, even in teenage adolescents.

Complications

Phrenic nerve block, vertebral artery puncture and injection, epidural or intrathecal injection, Horner's syndrome, recurrent laryngeal nerve blockade, and hematoma formation in the neck due to arterial or venous puncture, block failure, infection, and local anesthetic systemic toxicity (LAST) are possible, but rare, complications.

Practical Tips

- The nerve roots lie anterior to the transverse process.
- If a trapezius muscle twitch is encountered with nerve stimulation, withdraw and angle needle more anteriorly.
- If the carotid artery is punctured, remove needle, and apply pressure. Subsequent attempt should direct needle more posteriorly.

Literature Review

The interscalene nerve block for shoulder surgery in the pediatric population has shown superior postoperative analgesia and minimized inpatient hospital admissions in a retrospective cohort. Case reports of children with acute respiratory tract infections and acute hepatitis needing emergency shoulder surgery have successfully reported on the use of an interscalene nerve block to provide surgical anesthesia while avoiding a general anesthetic.

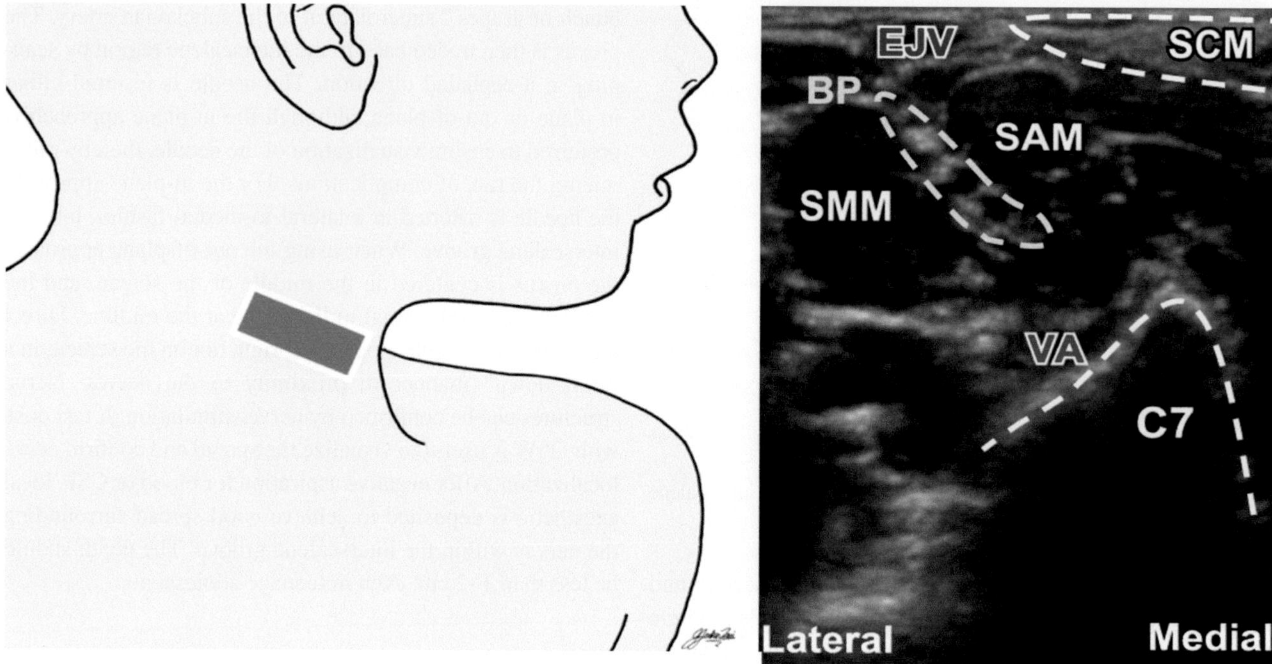

Fig. 74.3 Ultrasound image of the brachial plexus at the interscalene groove. *EJV* external jugular vein, *SCM* sternocleidomastoid muscle, *SAM* scalenus anterior muscle, *SMM* scalenus medius muscle, *VA* vertebral artery, *BP* brachial plexus, *C7* C7 vertebra

Supraclavicular Nerve Block

General Considerations

A well-studied peripheral nerve block that is relatively easy to perform and has a low risk of complications. The supraclavicular nerve block is less likely to cause phrenic nerve blockade compared to the interscalene nerve block. Given the proximity of the location of blockade to the pleura, the risk of pneumothorax is present.

Indication

Provides reliable anesthesia and analgesia for surgeries distal to the shoulder involving the entire upper extremity, elbow, forearm, and hand.

Functional Anatomy

The trunks continue to travel between the anterior and middle scalene muscles until they reach the level of the first rib which lies anterior. Superior and posterior to the subclavian artery, the upper, middle, and lower trunks conform tightly and are the ideal location for the supraclavicular nerve block. With the use of ultrasound, the rib and pleura can be seen slightly deeper to the subclavian artery.

Technique

The head of the patient is turned to the contralateral side. The arm is placed on the side, and the shoulder is pushed backward on to the mattress and down toward the feet. The skin is cleaned with antiseptic solution. If the ultrasound approach is used, prepare the probe surface by applying a sterile adhesive dressing.

A 50 mm, 21G–23G insulated needle is used. Depth of insertion is related to the age and weight of the patient in a nonlinear manner. For a 10 kg child, the depth of insertion is about 10 mm. For every 10 kg increase in weight, the depth of insertion increases 3 mm until the child reaches 50 kg. After that, advance 1 mm for every 10 kg increase in weight. The maximum depth should not exceed 35 mm. The required depth of penetration is usually less than 1 cm for children and 1–2 cm for teenagers.

Recommended local anesthetics are 0.25–0.5% bupivacaine, 0.2% ropivacaine, or 2% lidocaine. Blockade at this level can be achieved with volumes as low as 0.15–0.2 mL/kg.

Nerve Stimulation

The needle insertion point is located 1 cm above the midpoint of the clavicle posterolateral to the subclavian artery (Fig. 74.5). The subclavian artery pulsation serves as the landmark for localization of the plexus. The current is initially set at 0.8 mA (2 Hz, 100–300 μs) and then gradually reduced to a threshold current of 0.2–0.4 mA (0.1–0.2 m)

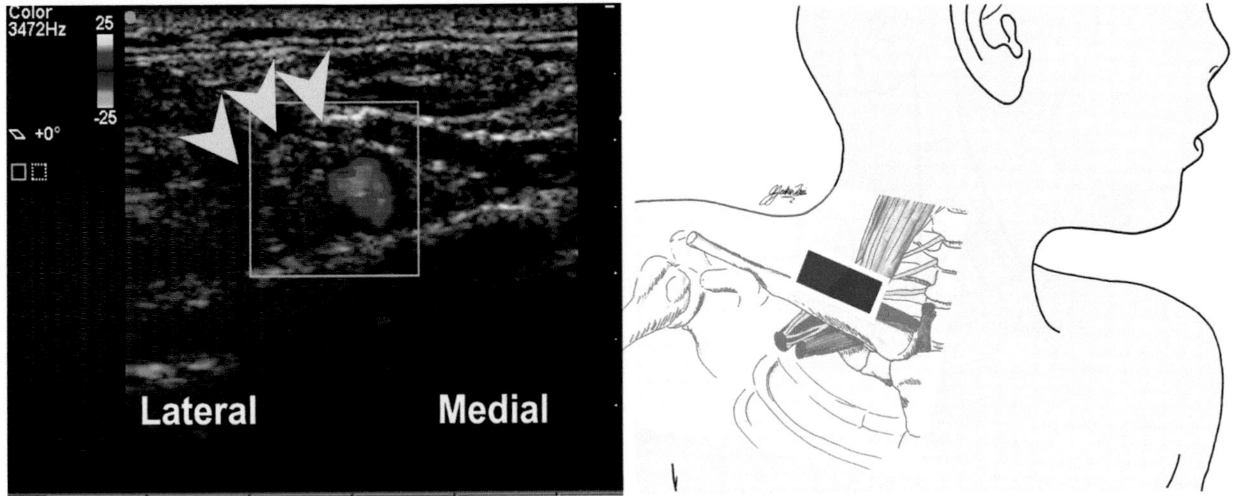

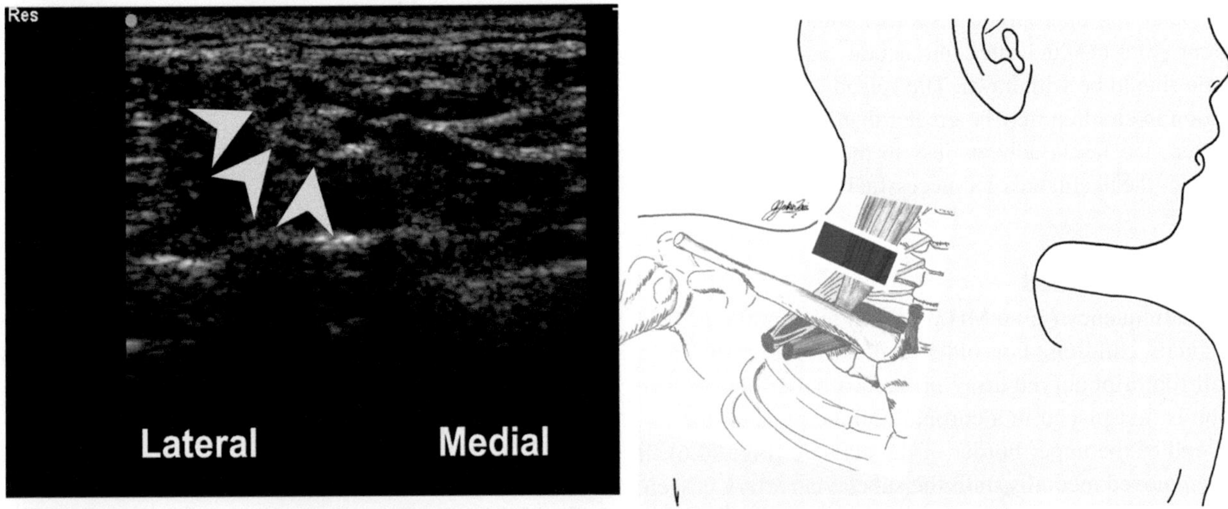

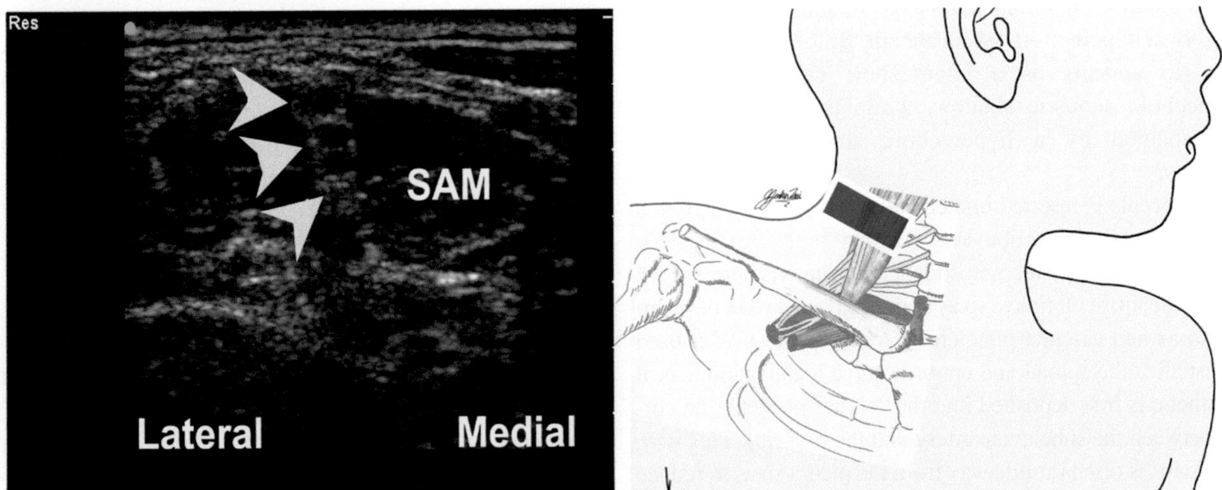

Fig. 74.4 Ultrasound traceback approach for interscalene block. *SAM* scalenus anterior muscle; arrowheads show location of brachial plexus

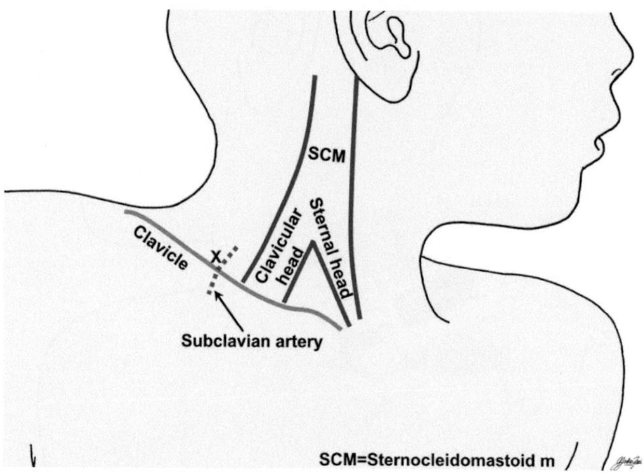

Fig. 74.5 Patient positioning and surface landmarks for supraclavicular brachial plexus block

after obtaining appropriate response. Motor response at a current ≤0.2 mA indicates intraneural placement, and the needle should be withdrawn. The spread of local anesthetic solution in children may be greater than for adults since, in children, the fascia adheres less to the nerve trunks. This increases the likelihood of a successful block with any motor response.

Ultrasound-Guided

A high-frequency (13–6 MHz) hockey stick probe is ideal for small children. For older and/or obese children, a small footprint curved array probe is a better option. The probe is first placed in a coronal oblique plane at the lateral end of the upper border of the clavicle (Fig. 74.6). It is then moved medially until the subclavian artery is seen. The subclavian artery is anechoic, hypodense, pulsatile, and round; its identity can be confirmed by color Doppler. The plexus is located superior and lateral to the artery above the first rib and appears as a "bunch of grapes" outlined by a hyperechoic fascia sheath. Below the artery, the first rib appears as a hyperechoic structure with a hypoechoic acoustic shadow, while the lung pleura is accompanied by a hyperechoic shadow due to air artifacts.

The needle is inserted immediately above the clavicle in a lateral-to-medial direction at a shallow angle. An in-plane approach is strongly recommended, to ensure visualization of the needle tip, at all times, so as to minimize the risks of pneumothorax and vascular puncture. A test dose of D5W is used to visualize the spread and confirm nerve localization. Local anesthetic is first deposited into the "corner pocket" (the corner between the subclavian artery and the first rib). This way, the plexus is often raised away from the pleura so as to reduce the chance of pleural puncture upon subsequent injection. The needle may then be repositioned to achieve good local anesthetic spread around the nerves within the fascia.

Complications

Pneumothorax, phrenic nerve block, subclavian artery puncture and injection, epidural or intrathecal injection, Horner's syndrome, recurrent laryngeal nerve blockade, and hematoma formation in the neck due to arterial or venous puncture, block failure, infection, and local anesthetic systemic toxicity (LAST) are possible, but rare, complications.

Practical Tips

- The use of Doppler to identify vascular structures (i.e., suprascapular artery and transverse cervical artery) in the vicinity of the brachial plexus at this location is recommended.
- If a pneumothorax occurs, the clinical presentation is often delayed as opposed to immediate.

Literature Review

The use of single shot and continuous infusion supraclavicular nerve blocks in children have been reported for both sole surgical anesthesia and postoperative analgesia of upper extremity orthopedic surgery.

Infraclavicular Nerve Block

General Considerations

A well-studied brachial plexus block that is moderately challenging to perform given the depth of the brachial plexus divisions at this location. The risk of complications is low, and this block is preferable in children with respiratory compromise who are dependent on diaphragmatic muscle use for respiration.

Indication

This block is indicated for surgery on the upper arm, elbow, forearm, and hand. Continuous infusion of local anesthetic via an infraclavicular catheter provides excellent postoperative analgesia for major upper limb surgery and is preferred over supraclavicular and axillary catheters because of ease of placement and securement.

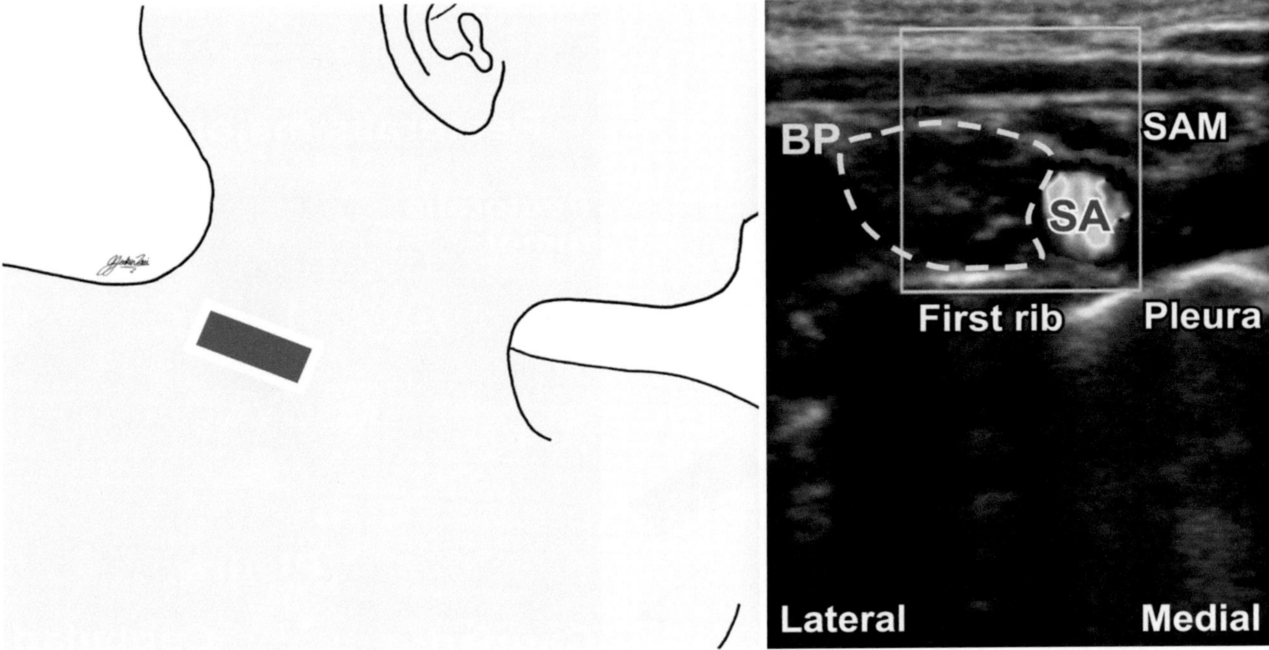

Fig. 74.6 Ultrasound image of the brachial plexus at the supraclavicular level. *BP* brachial plexus, *SAM* scalenus anterior muscle, *SA* subclavian artery

Functional Anatomy

As the trunks of the brachial plexus pass over the lateral border of the first rib heading toward the axilla, they become anterior and posterior divisions. In the infraclavicular region, near the lateral chest wall, the infraclavicular plexus block is performed to anesthetize the lateral, medial, and posterior cords that surround the axillary artery. The pectoralis major and minor muscles lie superficial to the cords, while the axillary vein is deep to the cords.

Technique

A pillow is placed underneath the patient's shoulder. The elbow is flexed with the hand resting on the abdomen or with the arm resting at the side. Alternatively, the arm can be abducted and externally rotated with the elbow flexed. This maneuver has the advantage of stretching the cords and bringing them closer to the surface, enhancing the ultrasonographic appearance as well as facilitating local anesthetic spread. The skin is cleaned with antiseptic solution. If ultrasound guidance is used, prepare the probe surface by applying a sterile adhesive dressing.

A 50 mm, 21G–24G needle is commonly used for this block. An insulated needle should be chosen if nerve stimulation is used. The depth of penetration is usually within 2–3 cm at a lateral location inferior to the coracoid process. Recommended local anesthetic doses are 0.5 mL/kg of 0.2–0.5% ropivacaine or 0.25–0.5% bupivacaine. Concentrations may need to be reduced in small children to obtain a volume of at least 5 mL for this block.

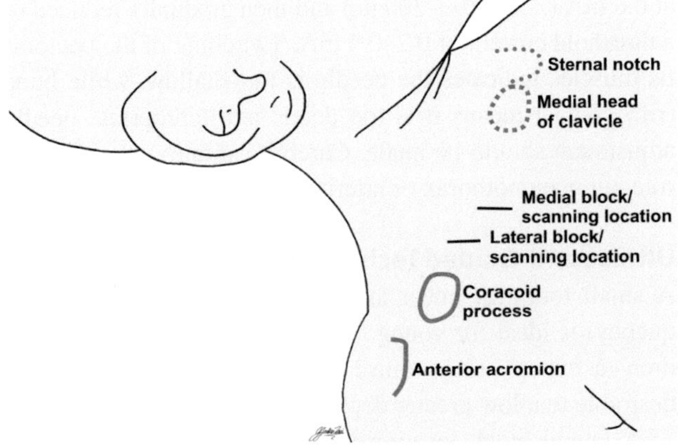

Fig. 74.7 Patient positioning and surface landmarks for infraclavicular brachial plexus block

Nerve Stimulation Technique

A lateral approach is recommended, where the point of needle insertion is approximately 0.5–1 cm inferior and slightly medial to the coracoid process (Fig. 74.7). At this point, the pleura is further away so the risk of pneumothorax is lower compared to a more medial injection site. The needle is advanced in a vertical direction until distal motor response (hand or wrist flexion) is obtained. The current is initially set

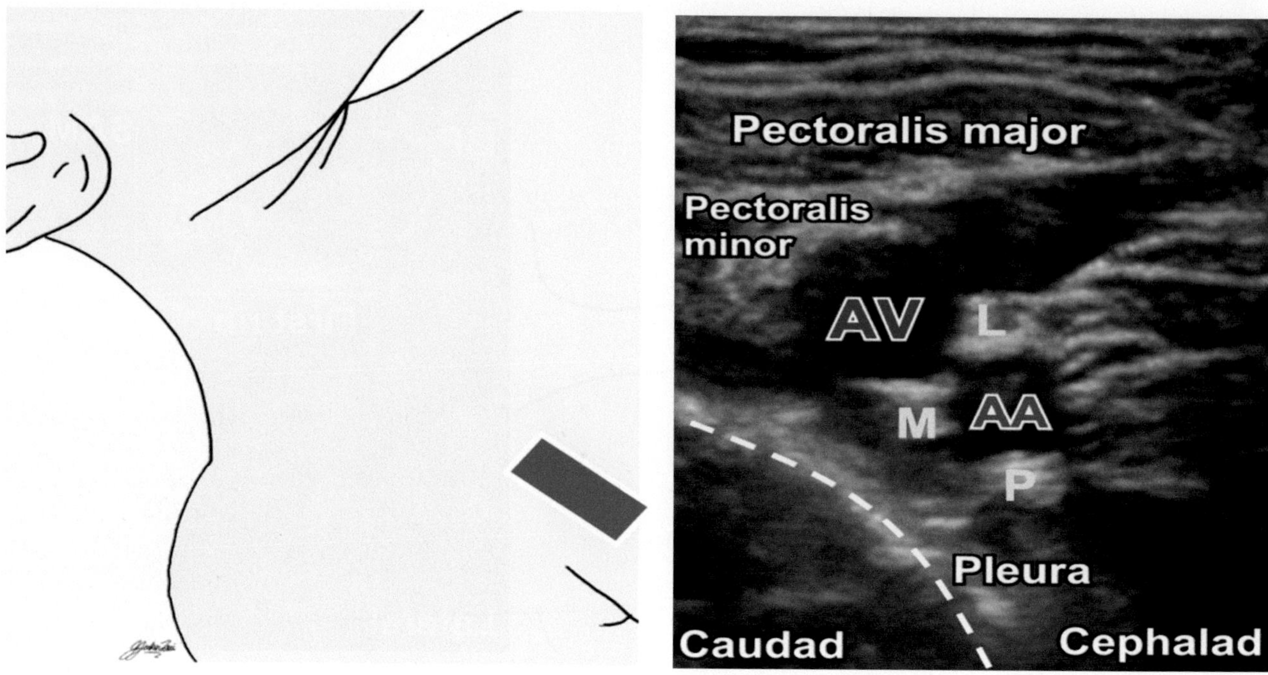

Fig. 74.8 Ultrasound image of the brachial plexus at the infraclavicular level at a lateral scanning location. *AV* axillary vein, *AA* axillary artery, *L* lateral cord, *M* medial cord, *P* posterior cord

at 0.8 mA (2 Hz, 100–300 μs) and then gradually reduced to a threshold current of 0.2–0.4 mA. Twitching of the pectoralis muscles indicates the needle is too shallow, while bone (rib) contact means it is too deep, and appropriate needle adjustment should be made. Careful aspiration is crucial to rule out pneumothorax or arterial/venous puncture.

Ultrasound-Guided Technique

A small footprint linear array transducer (13–6 MHz frequency) is ideal for young children. In older or larger children, a curved array transducer (5–2 MHz frequency) is desirable to allow greater depth of penetration.

A lateral block location is recommended. The probe is placed in a parasagittal plane below and slightly medial to the coracoid process. Scan medially and laterally to locate the axillary neurovascular bundle, which sits underneath the pectoralis major and minor muscles (Fig. 74.8). The axillary artery can be identified as a round- or oval-shaped pulsatile structure. The axillary vein is almost always medial and caudad to the artery and is irregularly shaped. Color Doppler can be used to identify the vessel in cases of doubt. At this point, the cords, which are seen as hyperechoic oval structures, can be found posterolateral to the artery. The medial cord may be difficult to identify because it may be hidden between the axillary artery and vein and can be posterior or even slightly cephalad to the artery.

If a medial approach is to be used, the probe is positioned at the midpoint of the line between the anterior acromion and jugular notch. It is important to maintain the pleura and needle in view at all times during the time of needle insertion. The pleura usually appears as a hypoechoic cavity outlined by a hyperechoic line and is often located proximal to the vessels and plexus (Fig. 74.9).

Both in-plane and out-of-plane approaches can be used for this block. The in-plane approach is strongly recommended, especially when a more medial block location is chosen, because it allows visualization of the needle tip and shaft, thereby minimizing the risk of pleural puncture. The needle is inserted at the cephalad end of the probe at a 45–60° angle to the skin and advanced caudally. The needle is then directed to the posterior cord, and local anesthetic is deposited around it. This often results in a "U-shaped" spread around the artery and hence complete blockade of the plexus. If the spread is deemed inadequate, a further dose of local anesthetic is deposited as the needle is withdrawn to the lateral cord position. Another injection between the artery and the vein may be needed to ensure blockade of the medial cord. Nerve stimulation offers additional confirmation of the neural structure and is recommended. A test dose of D5W prior to injection of local anesthetic can visualize spread and confirm nerve localization.

Occasionally, the out-of-plane approach is required when there is not enough space for the in-plane needle insertion between the probe and the clavicle, especially in very small children. This approach also has the advantage of a reduced length of needle path for better patient comfort if the block is to be performed on a conscious child. A 45°-angled needle insertion is used so that the distances between the needle

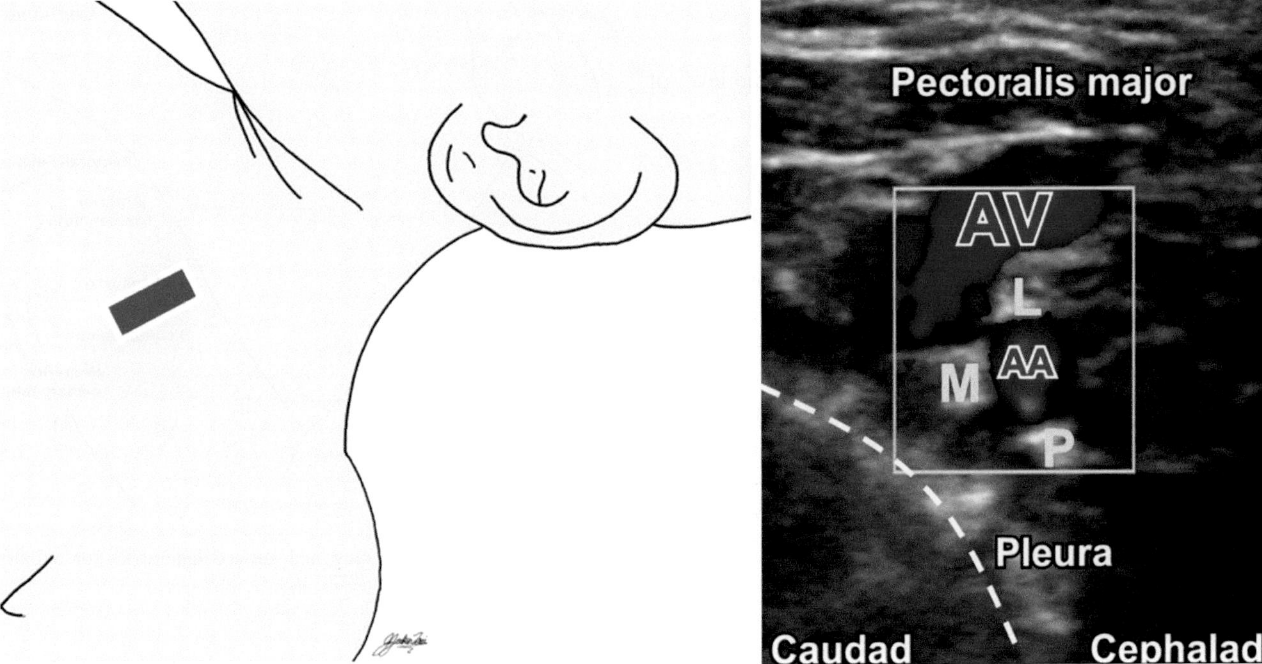

Fig. 74.9 Ultrasound image of the brachial plexus at the infraclavicular level at a medial scanning location. *AV* axillary vein, *AA* axillary artery, *L* lateral cord, *M* medial cord, *P* posterior cord

insertion point, probe, and brachial plexus are equal (i.e., forming a right-angled triangle). The needle then "walks down" to reach the posterior cord while the needle tip is being tracked.

Complications

Axillary artery puncture and injection, hematoma formation in the neck due to arterial or venous puncture, block failure, infection, local anesthetic systemic toxicity (LAST), and pneumothorax are possible, but rare, complications.

Practical Tips

- Common causes of pneumothorax with the infraclavicular nerve block can occur with medial insertion of needle, excessive medial redirection of needle, and deep needle placement.
- The ultrasound probe should be placed medial to the coracoid process, an easy-to-palpate bony landmark.
- The lateral cord is cephalad, posterior cord is posterior, and medial cord is caudad to the axillary artery.

Literature Review

The infraclavicular brachial plexus has been reported in children requiring upper extremity forearm and elbow surgery. Relative to the supraclavicular nerve block, it is reported as having a slightly higher incidence of arterial puncture and lower risk of pneumothorax and requiring longer to perform. The duration of motor block and analgesia with the two techniques is similar. Continuous infraclavicular catheter placement in children has been described with good success.

Axillary Nerve Block

General Considerations

Prior to routine use of ultrasound, the axillary nerve block was the most commonly performed brachial plexus block in children given the low risk of complications. Though quite consistent in its sensory and motor blockade, limitations of arm positioning in a sedated child who is in pain and sparing of the musculocutaneous nerve make it less ideal.

Indication

Elbow, forearm, wrist, and hand surgery below the level of the antecubital fossa.

Functional Anatomy

At the apex of the axilla, the axillary artery continues its trajectory along with three of the terminal branches of the brachial plexus: the ulnar, median, and radial nerves. The other two terminal branches (axillary and musculocutaneous) arise earlier in the brachial plexus and follow a different trajectory such that they are not within the neurovascular sheath of the axillary artery.

Technique

The arm of the patient is abducted 70–80° and externally rotated. The skin is cleaned with antiseptic solution. If ultrasound is used, prepare the probe surface by applying a sterile adhesive dressing.

A 50 mm, 22–24G insulated needle is typically used. The recommended dose of local anesthetic for an ultrasound-guided technique is 0.2–0.3 mL/kg of 0.25–0.5% bupivacaine, ropivacaine, or levobupivacaine and 0.5–1.0 mL for the musculocutaneous nerve. Higher volumes are needed if nerve stimulation is used.

Nerve Stimulation Technique

The axillary artery is first palpated at the apex of axilla. The needle is introduced at an approximately 45° angle to the skin at the upper edge of the axillary artery, pointing cephalad toward the midpoint of clavicle (Fig. 74.10). Advance the needle until a "pop" or "give" is felt as the needle enters the neurovascular sheath. Pulsations in the needle indicate that the needle tip is in immediate vicinity of the artery. An initial current is applied at 0.8 mA (2 Hz, 100 μs) and then gradually reduced to a threshold current of 0.4 mA (0.1 ms) after obtaining a distal motor response in the hand, wrist, or forearm. Local anesthetic is deposited after careful aspiration to rule out any intra-arterial/intravenous placement. A second injection can be made at the lower edge of the artery in a similar fashion ("two-puncture technique").

To block the musculocutaneous nerve, direct the needle (using the same needle insertion site) toward the belly of the coracobrachialis muscle, and inject local anesthetic. Elbow flexion can be elicited if nerve simulation is used.

If a tourniquet is required for the surgery, the intercostobrachial nerve should be blocked; this can be done by subcutaneous injection of local anesthetic across the medial surface of the upper arm.

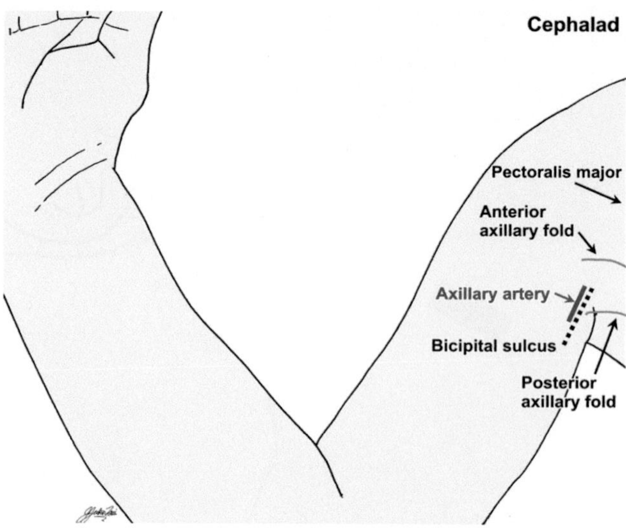

Fig. 74.10 Patient positioning and surface landmarks for axillary block of the brachial plexus

Ultrasound-Guided Technique

A high-frequency (13–6 MHz) linear probe is suitable for this block. In small children, a small footprint ("hockey stick") probe is desirable. The probe is placed in a transverse plane along the axillary crease and scanned as proximally as possible to obtain the best transverse view of the neurovascular bundle surrounded by the biceps brachii, coracobrachialis, and triceps muscles. The anechoic axillary artery can be identified as pulsatile circular structure, while the anechoic axillary vein(s) is/are irregular in shape, compressible, and usually more superficial. The nerves, which appear as round- or oval-shaped structures with a honeycomb-like appearance, are situated around the artery (Fig. 74.11). The median nerve can be found between the artery and biceps brachii muscle and is located superficial to the artery. The ulnar nerve lies between the artery and the triceps muscle and is also superficial to the artery. The radial nerve is deep to the artery at the midline and can sometimes be difficult to locate. The musculocutaneous nerve, whose appearance can vary from round or oval to flat, can usually be found in the plane between the biceps and the coracobrachialis muscles. If necessary, each of these terminal branches can be traced distally for confirmation. The use of nerve stimulation can also help identify individual nerves according to the corresponding motor responses.

The needle is inserted either in-plane or out-of-plane in relation to the probe. Commonly, multiple injections and needle redirections are required to ensure circumferential spread of local anesthetic around each individual nerve. For the in-plane approach, the needle is inserted at an acute angle (20–30°) to the skin in a superior-to-inferior direction in parallel to the long axis of the probe. The needle is initially directed underneath the artery to reach the radial nerve. It is

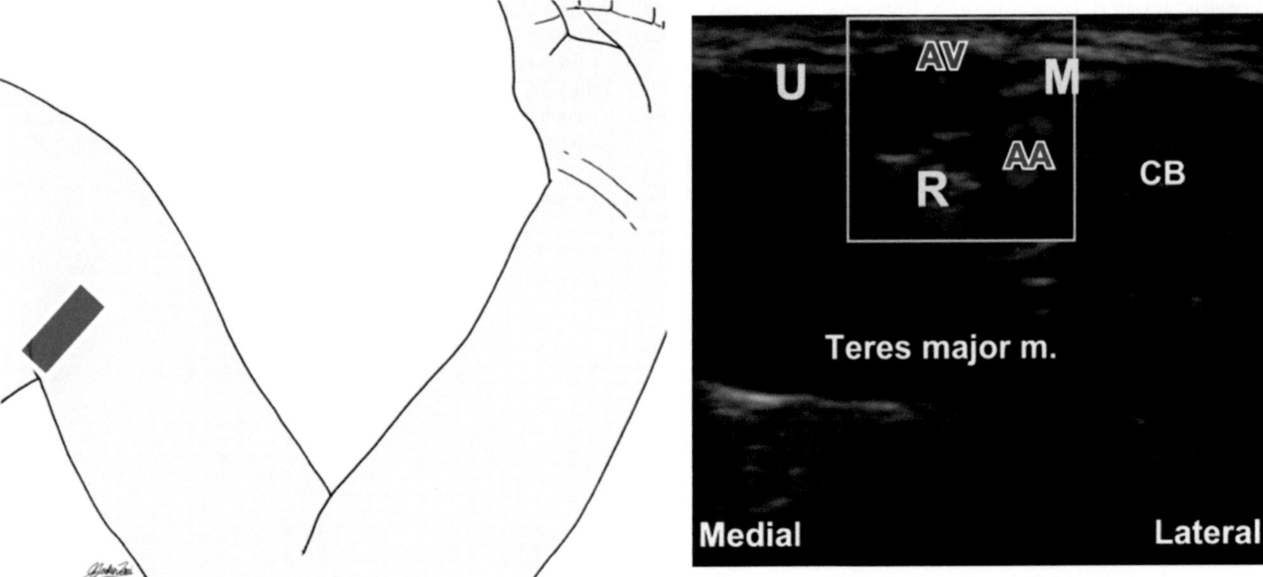

Fig. 74.11 Ultrasound image of the brachial plexus at the axilla. *AV* axillary vein, *AA* axillary artery, *CB* coracobrachialis, *U* ulnar nerve, *R* radial nerve, *M* median nerve

recommended to block the radial nerve first to minimize image distortion from the spread of local anesthetic. After that, the needle is withdrawn and redirected to deposit local anesthetic around the ulnar and the median nerves. A test dose with D5W is useful to visualize the spread and confirm nerve localization prior to injection of local anesthetic. If an out-of-plane approach is used, the needle is inserted approximately 1 cm away from the midpoint of the probe at a 30–45° angle from the skin to reach the nerves.

Complications

Axillary artery puncture and injection, hematoma formation, block failure, infection, and local anesthetic systemic toxicity (LAST) are possible, but rare, complications.

Practical Tips

- Procedures of the forearm require musculocutaneous nerve block supplementation.
- Though the exact orientation of the nerves vary, in general, the median nerve may be identified lateral and superficial to the axillary artery, the ulnar nerve is typically medial and superficial to the artery, and the radial nerve location is posterior to the artery.
- Make sure to identify the axillary vein medial to the axillary artery as it can be easily compressed and potentially serve as a location for intravascular injection.

Literature Review

Unlike in adults, where multiple injections during performance of an axillary nerve block may improve quality of sensory and motor blockade, in children, a single injection is sufficient.

Distal Nerve Blocks of the Upper Extremity

The terminal nerves of the upper extremity including the median, ulnar, and radial nerve can be blocked with local anesthetic either individually or in combination. Though the technique is well described and reported in the adult literature, utility of distal nerve blocks of the upper extremity has not been reported. Further, in common pediatric anesthesia practice, these blocks are rarely performed by the anesthesiologist. As such, the reader is directed to the "Regional Anesthesia for the Upper Limb in Adults" chapter for further description of these blocks.

Suggested Reading

Altinay M, Turk HS, Ediz N, Talmac MA, Oba S. Our ultrasound guided brachial plexus block experiences for upper extremity surgeries in pediatric patients. Sisli Etfal Hastan Tip Bul. 2020;54(2):231–5.

Aminian DM, Bhalla T, Sprague K, et al. A retrospective review of interscalene nerve blockade for shoulder surgery in the pediatric population. Anaesth Pain Intens Care. 2014;18(4):345–9.

Carre P, Joly A, Cluzel Field B, et al. Axillary block in children: single or multiple injection? Paediatr Anaesth. 2000;10(1):35–9.

Ergönenç T, Can H, Gökhan Beyaz S. Ultrasound-guided interscalene brachial plexus block in a child with acute upper respiratory infection: a case report. Anaesthesist. 2017;66(10):782–5.

Lee JH, Kim YR, Yu HK, et al. Ultrasound-guided interscalene brachial plexus block in a pediatric patient with acute hepatitis – a case report. Korean J Anesthesiol. 2012;62(6):568–70.

Pande R, Pande M, Bhadani U, et al. Supraclavicular brachial plexus block as a sole anesthetic technique in children: an analysis of 200 cases. Anaesthesia. 2000;55:798–810.

Ponde VC. Continuous infraclavicular brachial plexus block: a modified technique to better secure catheter position in infants and children. Anesth Analg. 2008;106(1):94–6.

Yang CW, Cho CK, Kwon HU, Roh JY, Heo YM, Ahn SM. Ultrasound-guided supraclavicular brachial plexus block in pediatric patients -a report of four cases. Korean J Anesthesiol. 2010;59(Suppl):S90–4.

Pediatric Regional Anesthesia for the Lower Limb

75

Farrukh Munshey and Ban C. H. Tsui

Contents

F. Munshey
Department of Anesthesiology and Pain Medicine, University of Toronto, Toronto, ON, Canada

Department of Anesthesia and Pain Medicine, The Hospital for Sick Children, Toronto, ON, Canada
e-mail: farrukh.munshey@sickkids.ca

B. C. H. Tsui (✉)
Department of Anesthesiology Perioperative, and Pain Medicine, Stanford, CA, USA

Lucille Packard Children's Hospital, Palo Alto, CA, USA
e-mail: bantsui@stanford.edu

D. Jankovic, P. Peng (eds.), *Regional Nerve Blocks in Anesthesia and Pain Therapy*,
https://doi.org/10.1007/978-3-030-88727-8_75

Femoral Nerve Block

General Considerations

A well-studied peripheral nerve block that is relatively easy to perform, provides consistent results, and has a low risk of complications.

Indication

Suitable for surgery involving the anterior aspect of the thigh and medial part of the leg below the knee. The femoral nerve block (FNB) can be used for femur fractures, quadriceps tendon injury, knee ligament injury, knee arthroscopy, and anterior thigh wound injuries requiring exploration and washout. For surgeries on the lower leg and ankle, a FNB can supplement a sciatic nerve block to provide complete analgesia of the lower leg.

Functional Anatomy

The largest branch of the lumbar plexus, this mixed nerve arises from the anterior rami of L2–L4. It descends through the psoas major muscle, emerging inferiorly from its lateral border. Continuing its descent, the femoral nerve lies between the lateral border of psoas major and the anterior surface of the iliacus muscle. Deep to the fascia iliaca and lateral to the femoral artery, the nerve passes posterior to the inguinal ligament and enters the anterior compartment of the thigh. Cutaneous branches supply the skin of the anterior thigh (medial and intermediate cutaneous nerves) and the skin of the medial leg (saphenous). The motor branches innervate the iliacus, pectineus, sartorius, rectus femoris, vastus medialis, vastus intermedius, and vastus lateralis muscles. Articular branches supply the hip and knee joints.

Technique

With the patient supine, the leg is externally rotated. The skin is cleaned with antiseptic solution. If ultrasound is used, prepare the probe surface by applying a sterile adhesive dressing. A 50 mm, 22G short-beveled needle is used for children under 40 kg (use a 22G, 80 mm needle for children >40 kg). An insulated needle should be chosen if nerve stimulation is used. Commonly recommended local anesthetic doses are 0.2–0.5 mL/kg of 0.25% bupivacaine or 0.2% ropivacaine without exceeding the toxic dose limits (2.5 mg/kg for bupivacaine and 3 mg/kg for ropivacaine without epinephrine).

Nerve Stimulation

The point of needle insertion is approximately 0.5–1 cm lateral to the femoral artery at the inguinal crease (which is about 0.5–1 cm below the inguinal ligament) (Fig. 75.1). This insertion point may vary according to the age and

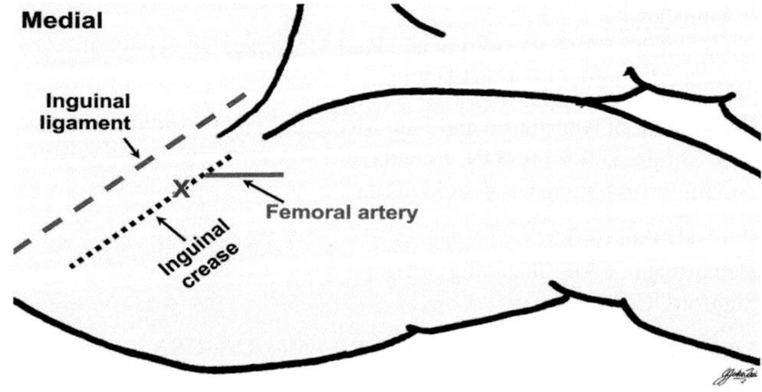

Fig. 75.1 Surface anatomy and landmarks for femoral nerve block

weight of the child. The needle is inserted at 30–45° to the skin, directed cephalad and medial. Advance the needle until "patellar twists" (contraction of quadriceps femoris muscle) are obtained. The current is initially set at 0.8–1 mA (1 Hz, 0.1–0.2 msec) and then gradually reduced to a threshold current of 0.5 mA. Currents less than 0.3 mA indicate intraneural placement, and the needle should be withdrawn slightly. As the needle is advanced, two "pops" or "gives" can be felt as the needle passes through the fascia lata and fascia iliaca, respectively. Local anesthetic is injected after the second "pop" following negative aspiration. Depending on the age and size of the patient, the depth of insertion is usually around 0.5–1 cm.

Ultrasound-Guided

A high-frequency (13–6 MHz) linear probe is suitable for this block. In infants, a small footprint ("hockey stick") probe is desirable. The probe is placed in a transverse plane along the inguinal crease to obtain a transverse view of the femoral artery and the vein (Fig. 75.2). The nerve, which often appears oval or triangular shaped, is located lateral to the femoral artery and just underneath the hyperechoic fascia iliaca. The femoral artery is anechoic, circular, and pulsatile, whereas the femoral vein is more irregular in shape, compressible, and located medial to the artery. The femoral nerve is usually found lateral to the artery.

Both in-plane and out-of-plane techniques can be used. For the in-plane approach, the needle is inserted at the lateral edge of the probe and angled medially to reach the nerve. Two "pops" or "gives" are felt as the needle penetrates the fascia lata and fascia iliaca. When using the out-of-plane approach, the nerve is centered in the middle of the screen, and the needle is inserted at 0.5–1 cm away from the midpoint of the caudad edge of the probe at 45°to the skin. The needle then "walks down" to reach the nerve while maintaining the needle tip in view. A test dose of D5W can visualize spread and confirm nerve localization prior to injection of local anesthetic.

Complications

Block failure, vascular puncture, hematoma, nerve injury, infection, and local anesthetic systemic toxicity (LAST) are possible, but rare, complications.

Practical Tips

If localization of the nerve with ultrasound is difficult, scan distally to look for the profunda femoris artery, and trace it proximally to the point where it joins the femoral artery.

- If the artery or vein is accidentally punctured, apply pressure to the site for 1–2mins prior to re-attempting.
- If it is hard to injection, stop injecting, and redirect needle to avoid possible intraneural injection.
- Similarly, during needle stimulation technique, currents less than 0.3 mA indicate intraneural placement, and the needle should be withdrawn slightly.

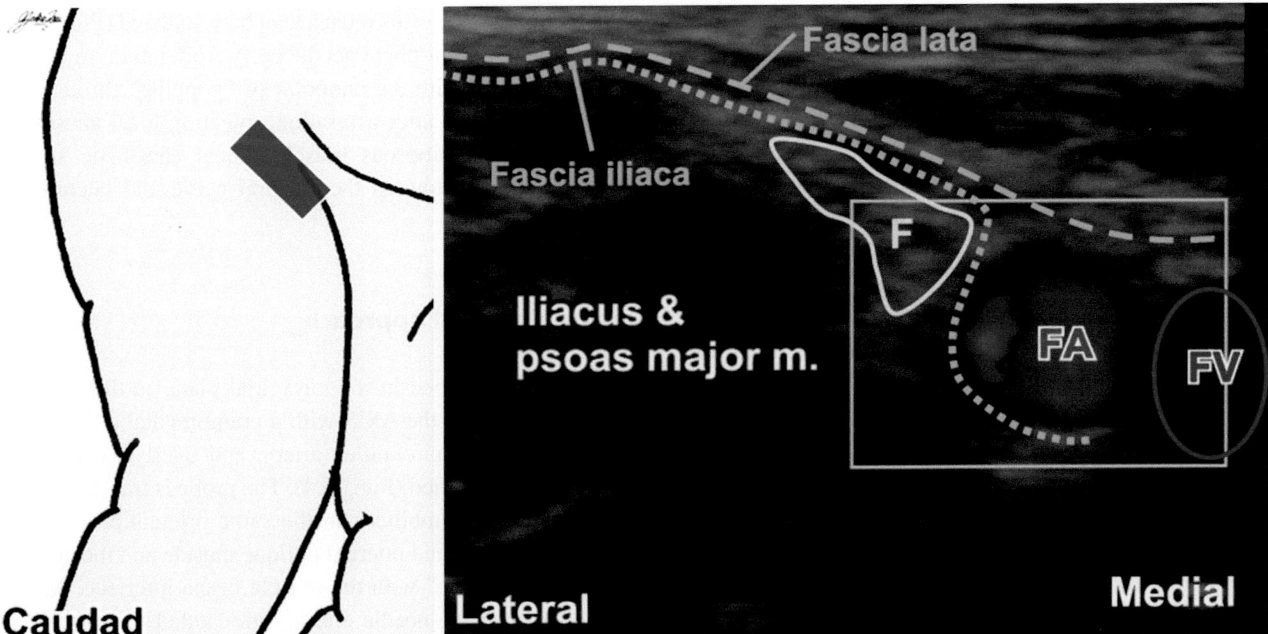

Fig. 75.2 Ultrasound image of major anatomical structures surrounding the femoral nerve. *F* Femoral nerve, *FA* femoral artery, *FV* femoral vein

Literature Review

In emergency departments, FNB have been used to provide longer-lasting analgesia in comparison to intravenous morphine for cases of hip fractures, femur fractures, patellar injuries, and anterior thigh wounds. For knee arthroscopy, FNBs reduced the amount of general anesthetics and opioid analgesics needed intraoperatively as well as the level of postoperative pain and consumption of analgesics postoperatively. A retrospective review showed in pediatric arthroscopic knee surgery, FNBs shortened hospital stay, reduced opioid requirements, and decreased postoperative pain scores. For anterior cruciate ligament repairs, FNBs lowered postoperative admission rates.

Fascia Iliaca Block

General Considerations

A well-known fascial plane block that is safe and easy to perform with the benefits of anesthetizing primarily the lateral cutaneous femoral nerve along with consistent spread to the femoral nerve and inconsistent obturator nerve coverage.

Indications

Useful in pediatric hip surgery, analgesia for proximal femoral fracture and lower limb surgeries with proximal lateral incisions.

Functional Anatomy

The fascia iliaca compartment is a potential space with the anterior border being the posterior surface of the fascia iliaca and the posterior border consisting of the anterior surface of the iliacus muscle and the psoas major muscle. The vertebral column marks the medial border. Cranio-laterally, the border is the inner lip of the iliac crest, and cranio-medially, the border is continuous with the space between the quadratus lumborum muscle and its fascia. This compartment allows deposition of local anesthetic of sufficient volumes spread to the lateral femoral cutaneous, femoral, and, potentially, the obturator nerve.

The lateral femoral cutaneous nerve is a pure sensory nerve which innervates the lateral thigh up to the knee. It arises from the anterior divisions of the L2 and L3 roots. After emerging from the lateral border of the psoas muscle, the nerve runs obliquely toward the anterior superior iliac spine (ASIS) beneath the fascia iliaca. It then passes underneath the inguinal ligament at a point approximately one fingerbreadth medial to the ASIS and then enters the thigh deep to the fascia lata, where it divides into anterior and posterior branches to supply the skin of the lateral thigh.

Technique

With the patient supine, the leg is slightly abducted. The skin is cleaned with antiseptic solution. If ultrasound is used, prepare the probe surface by applying a sterile adhesive dressing. A 50 mm, 22G short-beveled needle is used for children under 40 kg (use a 22G, 80 mm needle for children >40 kg). As the LFCN is a sensory nerve, nerve stimulation is not used. Commonly recommended local anesthetic doses are 0.5–1.0 mL/kg of 0.25% bupivacaine or 0.2% ropivacaine without exceeding the toxic dose limits (2.5 mg/kg for bupivacaine and 3 mg/kg for ropivacaine without epinephrine).

Ultrasound-Guided

A high-frequency (13–6 MHz) linear probe is suitable for this block. In infants, a small footprint ("hockey stick") probe is desirable.

Infra-Inguinal Approach

The probe is placed in a transverse plane along the inguinal crease between the pubic symphysis and ASIS. The femoral nerve, iliopsoas muscle, and fascia iliaca are identified (Fig. 75.2). The transducer is moved laterally toward the ASIS until the sartorius muscle can be visualized (Fig. 75.3). At this location, in-plane needle entry from lateral to medial is commenced with the endpoint of "popping" through the fascia iliaca and, after aspiration, injecting local anesthetic just above the iliopsoas muscle. Local anesthetic should spread medially toward the femoral nerve and laterally to cover the LFCN.

Supra-Inguinal Approach

The probe is placed in a parasagittal plane in the inguinal crease, medial to the ASIS with a craniomedial oblique tilt. The ASIS, deep circumflex artery, and overlying iliopsoas muscle are identified (Fig. 75.4). The probe is translated caudad toward the umbilicus in the same orientation until the sartorius muscle and internal oblique muscle and the appearance of a "bowtie" with the muscle fascia interface. At this location, in-plane needle entry from caudad to cephalad is commenced with the endpoint of "popping" through the fascia iliaca, and after aspiration, local anesthetic is injected

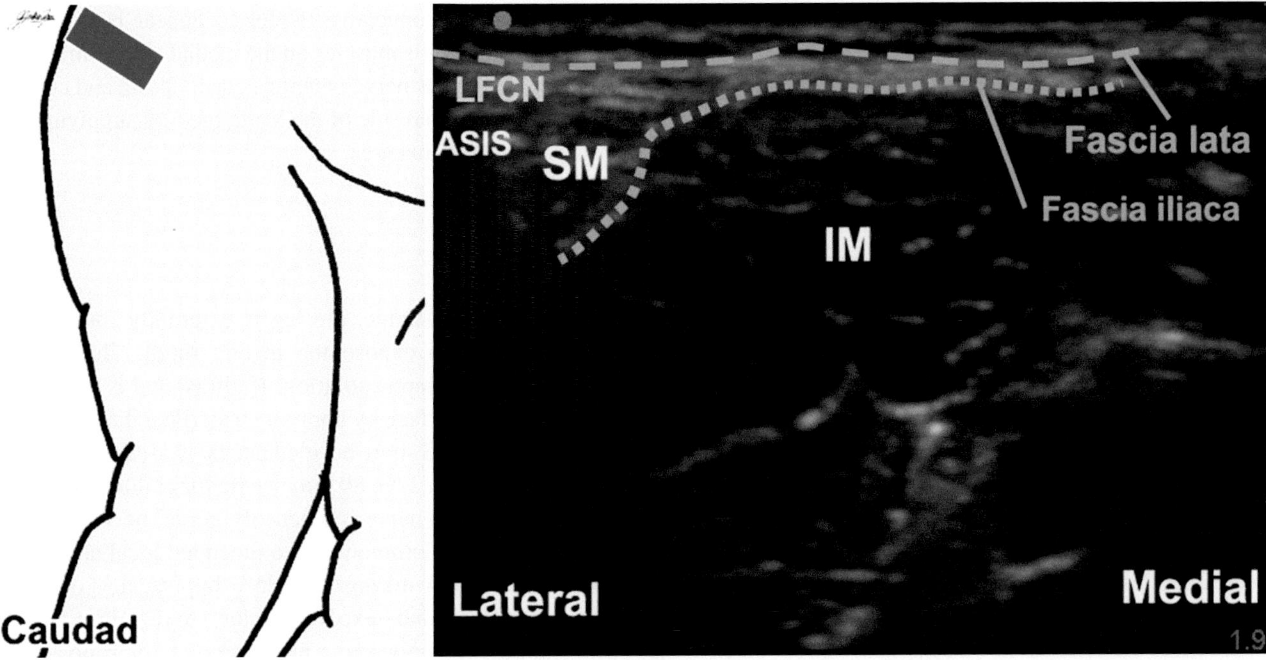

Fig. 75.3 Infra-inguinal fascia iliaca block. Ultrasound image of the lateral femoral cutaneous nerve (LFCN) between the fascia lata and fascia iliaca. *ASIS* Anterior superior iliac spine, *SM* sartorius muscle, *IM* iliacus muscle

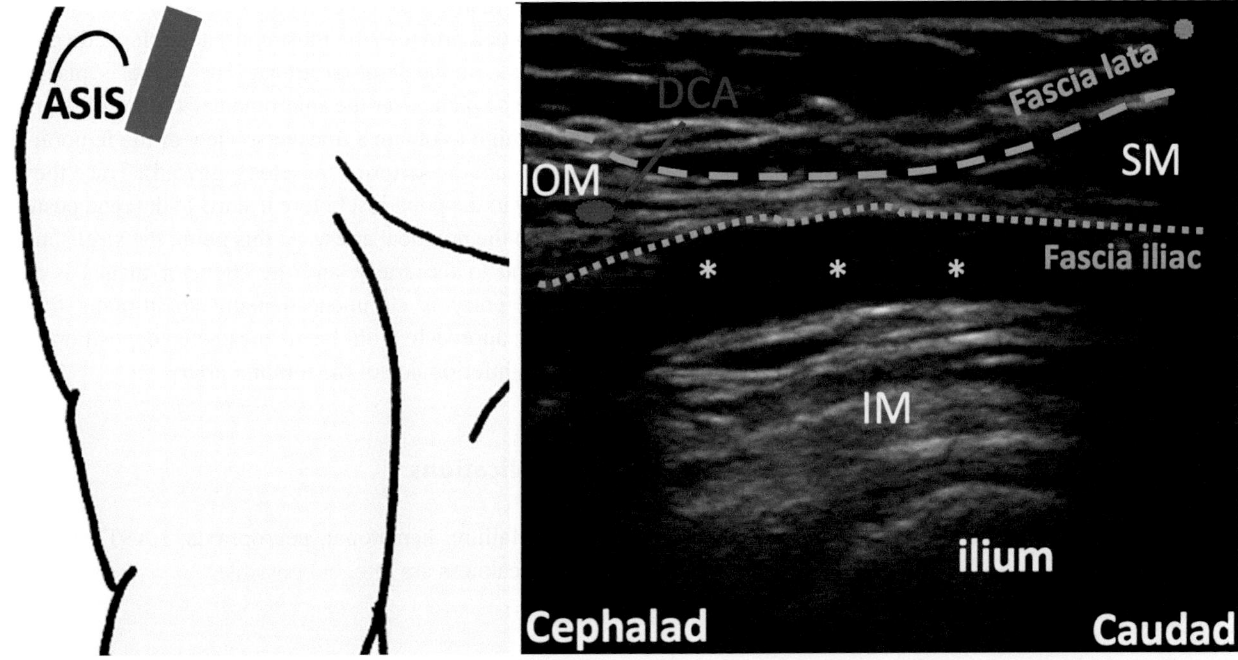

Fig. 75.4 Supra-inguinal fascia iliaca nerve block. *ASIS* Anterior superior iliac spine, *SM* sartorius muscle, *IM* iliacus muscle, *IOM* internal oblique muscle, *DCA* deep circumflex artery. *** Local anesthetic

above the iliopsoas muscle. Given the more proximal deposition of local anesthetic, this approach may more consistently anesthetize the LFCN and femoral nerve and possibly anesthetize the obturator nerve, thus providing superior analgesia after hip surgery.

Complications

Block failure, hematoma, neuropraxia, LAST, quadriceps weakness, perforation of peritoneal cavity, and bladder puncture are rare, but possible, complications.

Practical Tips

- If the femoral artery is seen in the supra-inguinal approach, translate probe superior-laterally.
- Deep circumflex artery is always superficial to the fascia iliaca and can be used as a landmark. Upward movement of the artery upon injection with a supra-inguinal approach is a positive sign.
- Hydro-dissection of the fascia iliaca from the iliopsoas muscle further helps spread of local anesthetic. Fascia iliaca block is a fascial plane block and requires adequate volume for spread.

Literature Review

In emergency departments, FIB have shown improved pain scores and less use of systemic opioids for femur fractures. For hip arthroscopy and hip osteotomy, the supra-inguinal approach to the FIB has shown consistent sensory block in the FN and LFCN among adolescents and improved pain scores. In burn patients needing lateral thigh skin grafting, FIB improved the postoperative pediatric patient pain experience when compared to local anesthetic infiltration at the site. Finally, in adolescent children having thigh surgery, FIB reduced emergence agitation and pain scores when compared to those patients who received intravenous opioids alone.

Adductor Canal Block

General Considerations

A well-described sensory nerve block of the saphenous nerve performed at the level of the mid-thigh which provides an alternative to a femoral nerve block with motor-sparing properties. The saphenous nerve can be blocked more distally using alternative approaches (subsartorius, infra-patellar), but these will not be discussed.

Indications

Procedures involving the medial aspect of the lower leg, knee, and foot.

Functional Anatomy

The terminal branch of the femoral nerve, this sensory nerve accompanies the femoral artery through the adductor canal in the mid- to lower thigh and subsequently penetrates directly through connective tissues to appear between the sartorius and gracilis muscles on the medial side of the knee. Here the saphenous nerve penetrates deep fascia and continues down the medial side of the leg to the foot supplying the overlying skin in that area.

Technique

With the patient supine, the leg is externally rotated and slightly flexed to expose the medial thigh. The skin is cleaned with antiseptic solution. If ultrasound is used, prepare the probe surface by applying a sterile adhesive dressing. A 50 mm, 22G short-beveled needle is used for children under 40 kg (use a 22G, 80 mm needle for children >40 kg). As the saphenous nerve is a sensory nerve, nerve stimulation is not used. Commonly recommended local anesthetic doses are 0.2–0.4 mL/kg of 0.25% bupivacaine or 0.2% ropivacaine without exceeding the toxic dose limits (2.5 mg/kg for bupivacaine and 3 mg/kg for ropivacaine without epinephrine).

Ultrasound-Guided

Though many approaches have been described, an adductor canal block provides the most consistent blockade given the landmark of the femoral artery. The probe is placed in a transverse plane over the anteromedial surface of the mid- to lower thigh to obtain a transverse view of the femoral artery underneath the sartorius muscle (Fig. 75.5). Trace the artery distally to the point just before it starts to descend posteriorly to form the popliteal artery. At this point, the vastus medialis is lateral to the artery, and the adductor magus is medial. Needle entry is commenced using an in-plane lateral to medial approach with local anesthetic deposition on the medial-inferior side of the femoral artery.

Complications

Block failure, hematoma, neuropraxia, LAST, and quadriceps weakness are rare, but possible.

Practical Tips

- The saphenous nerve will not always be visualized under ultrasound guidance, especially in obese patients. In such situations, injection beside the femoral artery in the plane between the sartorius and vastus medialis muscle is sufficient.
- The more proximal the site of blockade, the higher the likelihood of proximal muscle weakness.

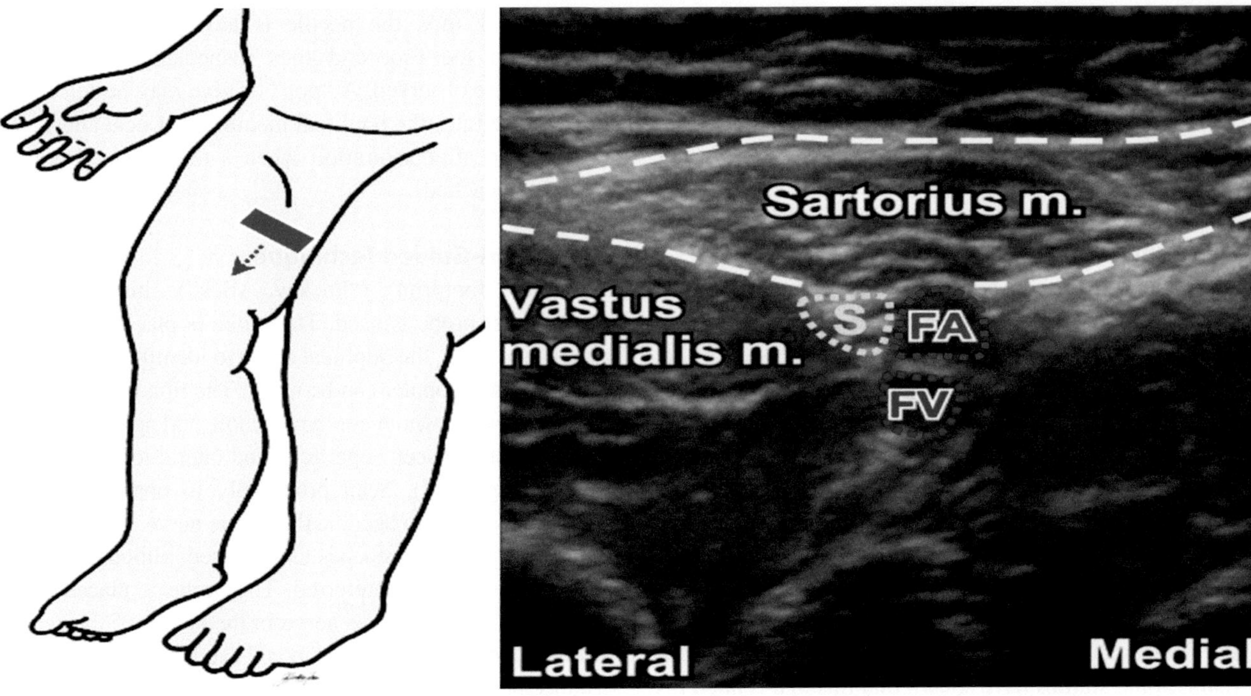

Fig. 75.5 Ultrasound image showing the saphenous nerve in the adductor canal. Often, the probe is moved distally until the femoral artery is further away from the nerve. *S* Saphenous nerve, *FA* femoral artery, *FV* femoral vein

Literature Review

Single-shot ACB for patellar dislocation surgery showed low pain scores and minimal postoperative opioid use in a case series of patients.

Popliteal Nerve Block

General Considerations

A commonly performed block used to anesthetize the posterior leg covering the branch point of one of the major nerves of the lower limb, the sciatic nerve. The sciatic nerve can be blocked using several different approaches (anterior, posterior gluteal, subgluteal) at different locations. We will however, focus, only on the popliteal nerve block approach to the sciatic nerve.

Indications

Foot and ankle surgery, below-knee procedures, distal femur procedures with involvement of the posterior compartment. Often done in combination with a saphenous nerve block to provide complicate anesthesia of the lower limb.

Functional Anatomy

The sciatic nerve is the largest peripheral nerve in the body. Derived from the L4–S3 roots, it exits the pelvis along with the posterior cutaneous nerve of the thigh via the greater sciatic foramen underneath the piriformis. It then passes midway between the greater trochanter of the femur and ischial tuberosity and descends along the back of the thigh. Proximally, the nerve lies deep to the gluteus maximus, after which it lies underneath the long head of the biceps femoris muscle. In the distal thigh, the nerve divides into the tibial nerve medially and common peroneal nerve laterally. The sciatic nerve supplies the posterior aspect of the thigh, the hamstring muscles, the entire lower leg (except the territory supplied by the saphenous nerve), as well as the hip and knee joints.

Technique

The nerve is blocked at a superficial level in the popliteal fossa just before the bifurcation. This is the most commonly, performed approach to the sciatic block for surgery on the lower leg and foot. The child lies in the lateral or prone position with the knee extended. It can also be performed in the supine position with the knee slightly bent and elevated. The foot is kept off the bed if nerve stimulation is used. The skin is cleaned with antiseptic solution. Prepare the ultrasound probe surface by applying a sterile adhesive dressing. A 50 mm, 22–25G short-beveled block needle is used. Recommended local anesthetic doses are 0.25–0.5 mL/kg (without exceeding the toxic dose limit) of 0.2% ropivacaine, 0.25% bupivacaine, or 0.25% levobupivacaine.

Nerve Stimulation Technique

The popliteal fossa is bordered superolaterally by the biceps femoris, superomedially by the semimembranosus and semitendinosus, and inferiorly by the medial and lateral heads of the gastrocnemius (Fig. 75.6). It is divided by the popliteal crease in the middle, creating the superior and inferior triangles of popliteal fossa. The sciatic nerve runs lateral and superficial to the popliteal vessels and then branches into tibial nerve (medially) and common peroneal nerve (laterally) near the upper apex of the fossa. According to an age-related formula,(Chen et al., 2015) the nerve bifurcates at a mean distance of 4.1 cm ± 0.8 cm in children under 8 years and at 5.8 cm ± 1.3 cm in children older than 8 years. Some studies have shown that this age-related distance is not consistent and found wide variability in the location of the bifurcation point.(Dadure et al., 2006) Thus, the use of nerve stimulation together with ultrasound guidance is recommended to obtain a higher success rate of blocking the sciatic nerve before it divides or blocking the individual nerves distal to the bifurcation. The point of needle insertion is midpoint between the semimembranosus and semitendinosus tendons and the biceps femoris tendon in the superior popliteal triangle, immediately lateral to the popliteal pulse, with the distance from the popliteal cease according to the weight of the child: 1 cm if <10 kg, 2 cm if 10–20 kg, etc.(Jan van Geffen et al., 2007) Introduce the needle at 45° to the skin, pointing cephalad. With an initial current of 1 mA, the needle is advanced slowly until twitches in the foot and toes (especially tibial nerve response) are observed. A "pop" or give may be felt as the needle penetrates the popliteal membrane. Local anesthetic is deposited after aspiration when a threshold current of 0.4 mA is reached.

Ultrasound-Guided Technique

A small footprint ("hockey stick") high-frequency (13–6 MHz) probe is used. The probe is placed in a transverse plane along the popliteal cease to identify the popliteal vessels (color Doppler can be used). The tibial and common peroneal nerves, which are hyperechoic and appear round or oval, are usually seen superficial and lateral to the popliteal vessels (Fig. 75.7). Scan proximally to observe the two nerves converging to become the sciatic nerve. Both in-plane and out-of-plane approaches can be used, although the out-of-plane approach is preferred. The probe is placed at the bifurcation point with the nerve in the center of the screen. Insert the needle 45° to the skin and caudal to the probe. The distance between the probe and insertion point should be the same as the distance between the nerve and skin surface; the needle can then be "walked down" to reach the nerve while keeping the needle tip in view. Local anesthetic is deposited after negative aspiration. For optimal blockade, aim for a circumferential spread around both branches of the sciatic nerve.

Complications

Block failure, hematoma, neuropraxia, local anesthetic systemic toxicity (LAST), and quadriceps weakness are rare, but possible, complications.

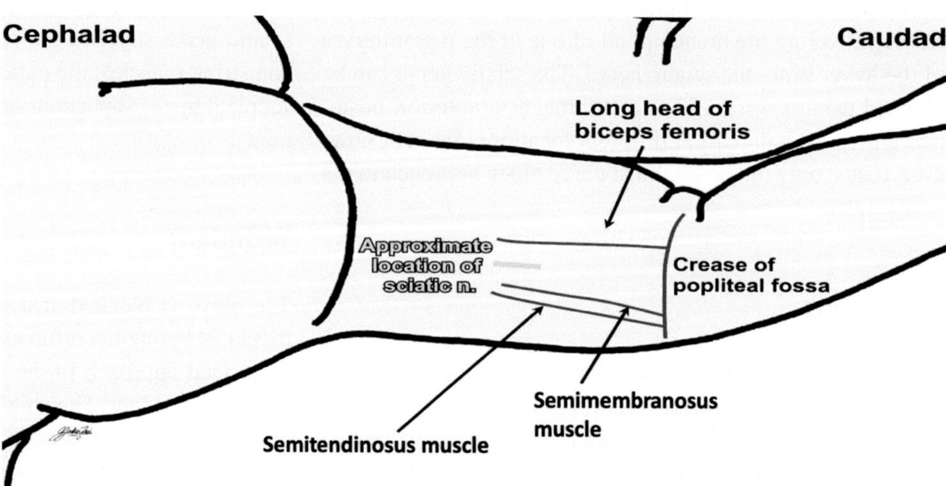

Fig. 75.6 Surface anatomy of the popliteal fossa

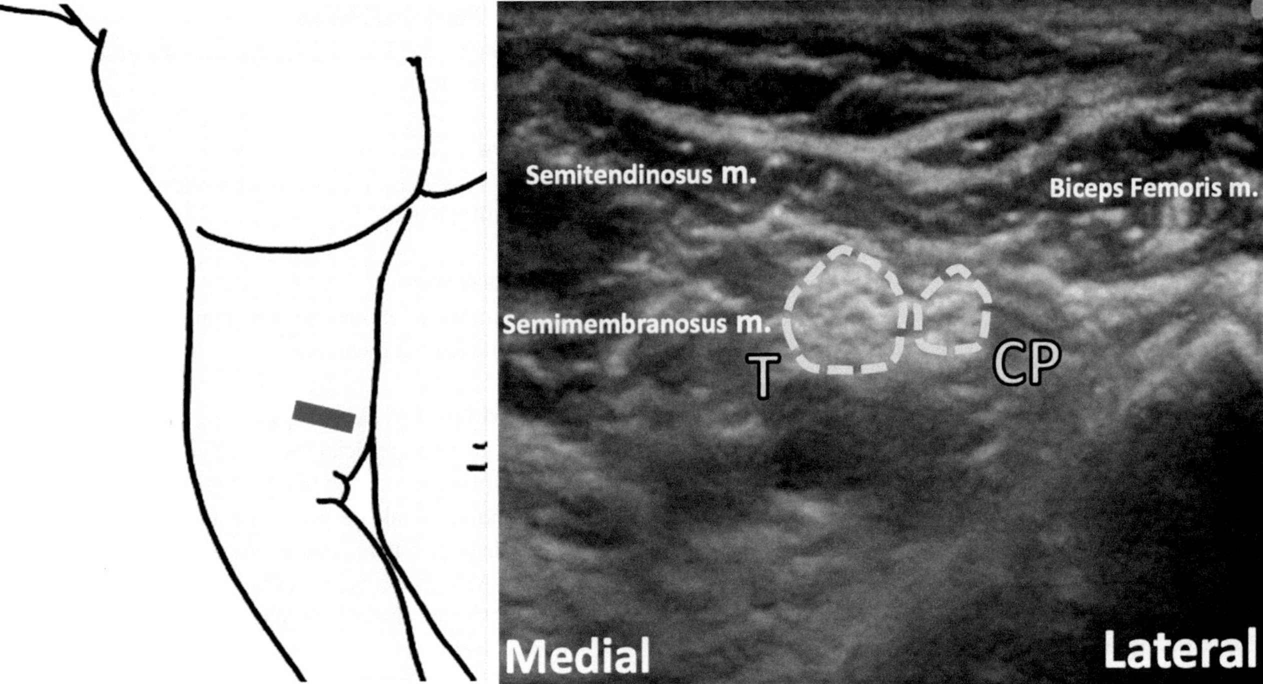

Fig. 75.7 Ultrasound image of the popliteal sciatic nerve block location. T, Tibial nerve; CP, common peroneal nerve

Practical Tips

- The popliteal artery and vein should always be below the sciatic nerve and its branches.
- Considerable transducer pressure is required to elucidate the echogenic nerve structure of the sciatic nerve and its branches.
- In the lateral approach, ensure needle entry is at least 2–3 cm away from the transducer to improve needle visualization without need for extensive angulation of the needle.

Literature Review

In children ages 1–12 years undergoing podiatric surgery, a continuous sciatic nerve block provided equivalent postoperative analgesia to a continuous epidural block with less urinary retention, nausea, and vomiting. In case reports of children aged 3 and 12 yrs., a continuous sciatic nerve block provided excellent analgesia for Lisfranc midfoot amputation and revision of a lower limb amputation stump.

Ankle Block

General Considerations

A commonly performed sensory and motor block of the five nerves supplying the foot.

Indications

Can be used for foot and toe surgery.

Functional Anatomy

Five nerves supply the foot: the posterior tibial, deep peroneal, superficial peroneal, sural, and saphenous nerves. The first four are derived from the sciatic nerve, while the saphenous is from the femoral nerve. The posterior tibial nerve is responsible for plantarflexion and cutaneous sensation of the sole of the foot. The deep peroneal nerve is responsible for ankle and toe extension and cutaneous sensation of the web space between the first and second toes. The other three nerves are mainly sensory: the superficial peroneal nerve innervates the dorsum of the foot (except the area supplied by the deep peroneal), the sural innervates the heel and lateral malleolus, and the saphenous innervates the anteromedial aspect.

Technique

The foot is raised and supported on a pillow. The skin is cleaned with antiseptic solution. If ultrasound is used, prepare the probe surface by applying a sterile adhesive dressing.

A 50 mm, 25–27G short-beveled or hypodermic needle is suitable for these blocks. Recommended local anesthetic doses are 0.1 mL/kg of 0.25% bupivacaine or 0.2% ropivacaine (a volume of 1–3 mL is usually adequate for each block). Epinephrine should not be added because of the presence of end arteries.

Nerve Stimulation Technique

Among the five nerves that supply the foot, only the posterior tibial and deep peroneal have motor fibers. Since the others are sensory, nerve stimulation is not necessary.

Posterior Tibial Nerve

The needle is inserted immediately posterior to the posterior tibial pulse, which is about midway between the medial malleolus and the medial border of the Achilles tendon (Fig. 75.8). With an initial current of 0.8 mA (2 Hz, 0.1–0.3 msec), the needle is advanced until plantarflexion of the toes is observed. Local anesthetic is injected after aspiration when a threshold current of 0.4 mA is reached.

Deep Peroneal Nerve

The needle is inserted perpendicular to the skin with a slight anterior tilt at the mid-foot, lateral to the extensor hallucis longus tendon and immediately lateral to the anterior tibial pulse (Fig. 75.9). Observe for toe extension upon nerve stimulation. Local anesthetic is deposited when twitches are seen at a current of 0.4 mA.

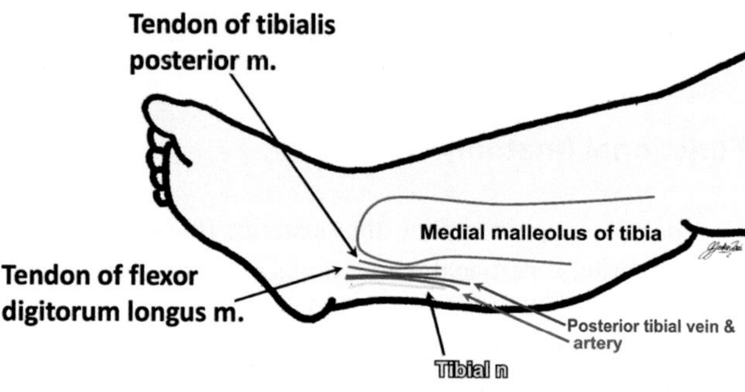

Fig. 75.8 Surface anatomy and landmarks for posterior tibial nerve block

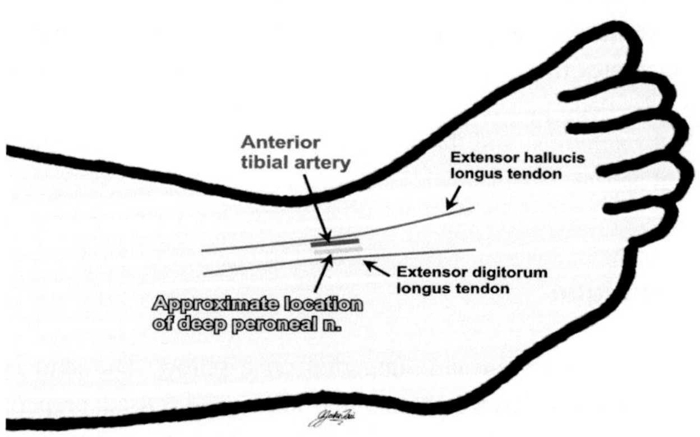

Fig. 75.9 Surface anatomy and landmarks for deep peroneal nerve block

Superficial Peroneal Nerve

Local anesthetic is infiltrated subcutaneously along the line between the malleoli.

Sural Nerve

The needle is inserted midway between the lateral malleolus and the Achilles tendon.

Saphenous Nerve

Local anesthetic is infiltrated subcutaneously above and anterior to the medial malleolus.

Ultrasound-Guided Technique

While the more superficial nerves (superficial peroneal, sural, and saphenous) can be blocked reliably using the landmark technique, blockade of the deeper nerves (posterior tibial and deep peroneal) can be facilitated by the use of ultrasound. A high-frequency (13–6 MHz) small footprint "hockey stick" transducer is preferred.

Posterior Tibial Nerve

The probe is placed in a transverse plane posterior to medial malleolus to locate the posterior tibial artery (color Doppler can be used). The nerve, which is round or oval with a honeycomb appearance, is found posterior and deep to the artery (Fig. 75.10). Local anesthetic is deposited at the point beforc it divides into the medial and lateral plantar nerves.

Deep Peroneal Nerve

The probe is placed in a transverse plane on the dorsum of the foot along the line between the malleoli to locate the deep peroneal artery (color Doppler can be used). The nerve, which is small and may be difficult to visualize, is found lateral to the artery (Fig. 75.11).

Although both in-plane and out-of-plane techniques can be used for these blocks, the out-of-plane approach is often easier due to the limited space at the ankle. A "donut sign" upon injection of local anesthetic indicates good circumferential spread around the nerve.

Complications

Block failure, hematoma, neuropraxia, local anesthetic systemic toxicity (LAST), and foot drop (weakness) are rare, but possible, complications.

Practical Tips

– There is variant anatomy of the nerves, and on occasion individual nerves are difficult to identify on ultrasound.

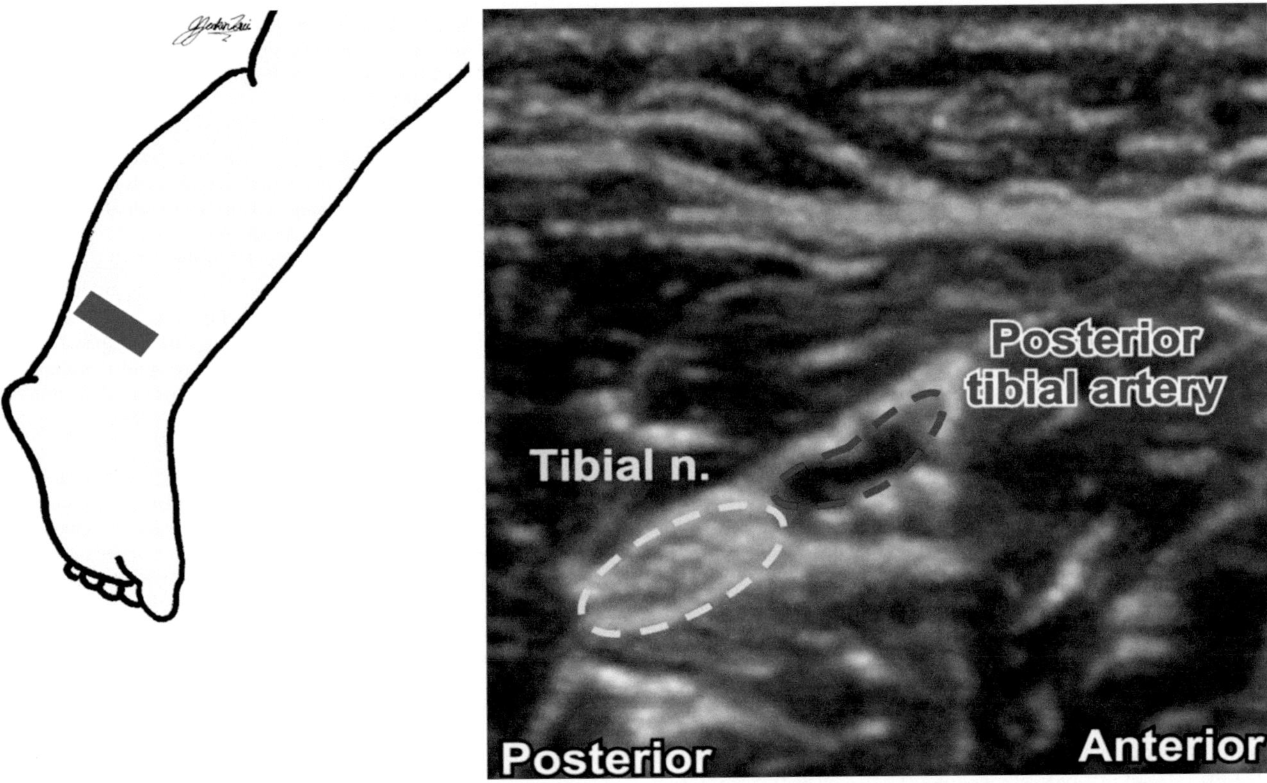

Fig. 75.10 Ultrasound image of major anatomical structures surrounding the tibial nerve

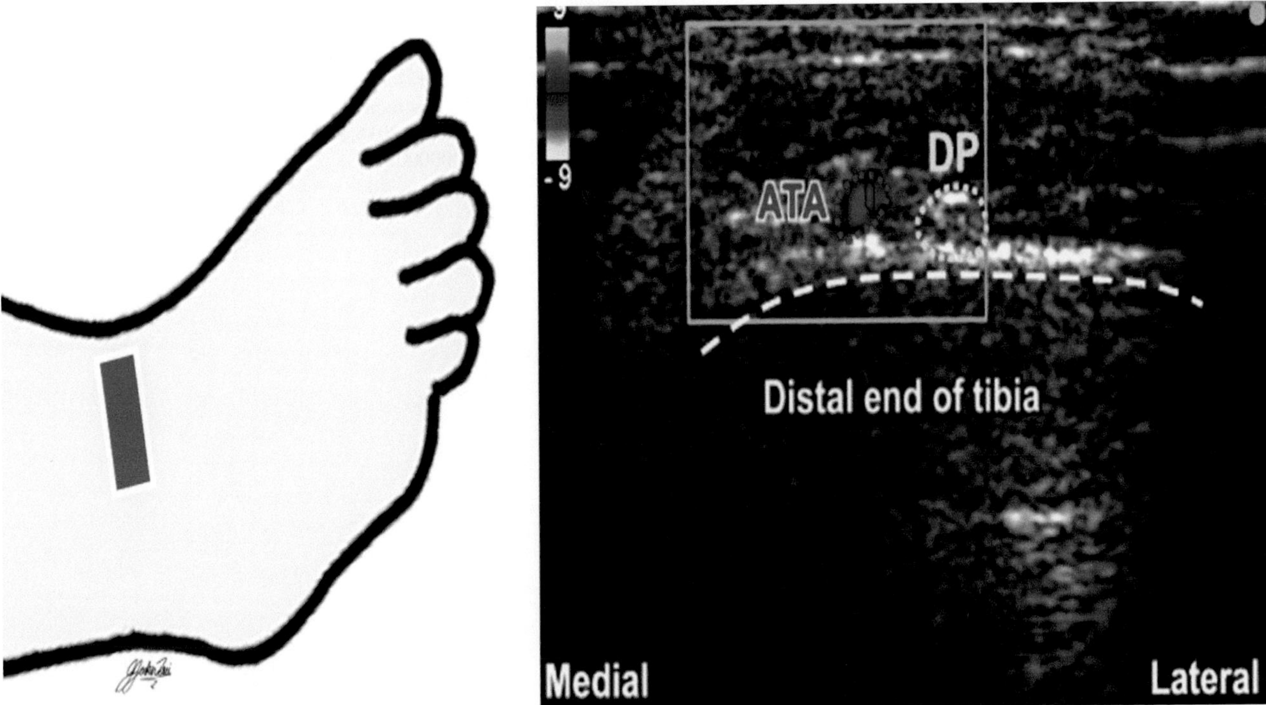

Fig. 75.11 Ultrasound image of major anatomical structures surrounding the deep peroneal nerve. *ATA* Anterior tibial artery, *DP* deep peroneal nerve

- Minimal volume is needed to block the nerves given the superficial nature of the nerve and the proximity of injection.
- Ensure adequate soak time, and a supplementary proximal block may be needed if tourniquet is used.

Literature Review

Though extensively reported in the adult literature, no reports of use of ankle block have been reported in children.

Miscellaneous Blocks

Additional peripheral nerve blocks of the lower extremity have been well described in the adult literature including the lateral femoral cutaneous, obturator, saphenous, and sciatic nerve blocks with different approaches (posterior gluteal, infragluteal/subgluteal, anterior). Since there is a limited of distinct literature with new information and approaches in pediatric surrounding such blocks, as such, we have chosen to not include them in this chapter. The reader is directed to the "Regional Anesthesia for the Lower Limb in Adults" chapter for further description of these blocks and approaches.

Suggested Reading

Baker MD, Gullett JP. Ultrasound-guided femoral nerve blocks. Pediatr Emerg Care. 2015;31:864–8.

Chen JY, Li N, Xu YQ. Single shot Adductor Canal block for postoperative analgesia of pediatric patellar dislocation: a case-series report. Medicine (Baltimore). 2015;94(48):e2217. https://doi.org/10.1097/MD.0000000000002217.

Dadure C, Bringuier S, Nicolas F, et al. Continuous epidural block versus continuous popliteal nerve block for postoperative pain relief after major podiatric surgery in children: a prospective, comparative randomized study. Anesth Analg. 2006;102(3):744–9. https://doi.org/10.1213/01.ane.0000195439.54650.dc.

Eastburn E, Hernandez MA, Boretsky K. Technical success of the ultrasound-guided supra-inguinal fascia iliaca compartment block in older children and adolescents for hip arthroscopy. Paediatr Anaesth. 2017;27(11):1120–4. https://doi.org/10.1111/pan.13227.

Jan van Geffen G, Bruhn J, Gielen M. Ultrasound-guided continuous sciatic nerve blocks in two children with venous malformations in the lower limb. Can J Anesth. 2007;54(11):952–3. http://dx.doi.org.myaccess.library.utoronto.ca/10.1007/BF03026804

Kim HS, Kim CS, Kim SD, Lee JR. Fascia iliaca compartment block reduces emergence agitation by providing effective analgesic properties in children. J Clin Anesth. 2011;23(2):119–23. https://doi.org/10.1016/j.jclinane.2010.08.007.

Marinković D, Simin J, Drasković B, Kvrgić I, Pandurov M. Efficiency of ultrasound guided lower limb peripheral nerve blocks in perioperative pain management for knee arthroscopy in children. A randomized study. Med Pregl. 2016;69(1–2):5–10.

Neubrand TL, Roswell K, Deakyne S, Kocher K, Wathen J. Fascia iliaca compartment nerve block versus systemic pain control for acute femur fractures in the pediatric emergency department. Pediatr Emerg Care. 2014;30(7):469–73. https://doi.org/10.1097/PEC.0000000000000163.

Schloss B, Bhalla T, Klingele K, Phillips D, Prestwich B, Tobias J. A retrospective review of femoral nerve block for postoperative analgesia after knee surgery in the pediatric population. J Pediatr Orthop. 2014;34(4):459–61.

Shank ES, Martyn JA, Donelan MB, Perrone A, Firth PG, Driscoll DN. Ultrasound-guided regional anesthesia for pediatric burn reconstructive surgery: a prospective study. J Burn Care Res. 2016;37(3):e213–7. https://doi.org/10.1097/BCR.0000000000000174.

Pediatric Nerve Block: Trunk and Neuraxial

76

Stephanie Pan, Sara S. K. Cheung, and Ban C. H. Tsui

Contents

Backgrounds

Although the early days of regional anesthesia focused on spinal cord analgesia, pediatric anesthesiologists have continually sought to decrease the devastating risks associated with neuraxial techniques including hematoma, infection, and paralysis. The logical alternative target was the peripheral nerve or nerve plexus that would give rise to techniques such as the paravertebral, intercostal, and ilioinguinal and iliohypogastric nerve blocks.

Prior to the advent of ultrasound imaging, these blocks were performed using anatomical landmark techniques and had their share of associated complications such as pneumothorax, peritoneal and bowel puncture, and local anesthetic systemic toxicity. Nerve stimulation techniques improved our ability to locate specific nerves and to deposit local anesthetics closer to the target nerves. However, the incidence of persistent paresthesias and failed blocks was still high. When two-dimensional ultrasound imaging for regional anesthesia was first described by Kapral in 1994, these peripheral nerve

S. Pan · B. C. H. Tsui (✉)
Department of Anesthesiology, Perioperative and Pain Medicine, Stanford University School of Medicine, Stanford, CA, USA

Lucile Packard Children's Hospital, Palo Alto, CA, USA
e-mail: sjpan@stanford.edu; bantsui@stanford.edu

S. S. K. Cheung
University of Alberta, Edmonton, AB, Canada

Department of Anaesthesia, Pamela Youde Nethersole Eastern Hospital, Hong Kong, Hong Kong

D. Jankovic, P. Peng (eds.), *Regional Nerve Blocks in Anesthesia and Pain Therapy*,
https://doi.org/10.1007/978-3-030-88727-8_76

blocks could finally be visualized albeit with often grainy images compared to current standards.

But as ultrasound technology and image quality improved, there was a shift in regional anesthesia from targeting specific nerve(s) to depositing local anesthetic in interfascial planes where the nerves travel through (e.g., transversus abdominis plane (TAP) block). What if analgesia could be achieved without targeting individual nerves or nerve plexuses? And so began the explosion of interfascial plane blocks including the pectoralis blocks, the serratus anterior plane block, the quadratus lumborum blocks, and the erector spinae plane block. These new interfascial plane blocks aim to increase the safety and efficiency of regional anesthesia. Whether they hold equivalent analgesic efficacy as their older counterparts remains to be studied and seen.

It is important to understand the advantages and disadvantages of each interfascial plane block (Table 76.1), perineural nerve block (Table 76.2), and central neuraxial block (Table 76.3) to optimize their use in various analgesic applications. Understandably, interfascial plane blocks have gained popularity due to their ease of placement and potential opioid-sparing properties. However, they tend to be only effective at blunting somatic pain and do not provide a reliable dense surgical and sympathetic block.

Table 76.1 Interfascial plane blocks

Regional technique	Advantages	Disadvantages	Physiologic effects	Catheter placement
Erector spinae plane (ESP) block	• Potentially opioid-sparing • Less invasive compared to neuraxial and paravertebral techniques • Theoretically lower risk of hematoma and other major complications	• Effectiveness not well studied • Higher risk of muscle spasm • Large studies are lacking	Somatic blockade, possible sympathetic blockade	Well suited
Pectoralis (PECS) 1 and 2 block	• Opioid-sparing • Theoretically lower risk of hematoma and other major complications	• Effectiveness not well studied • Large doses of local anesthetic needed for analgesic effect	Somatic blockade only	Poorly suited
Serratus anterior plane (SAP) block	• Potentially opioid-sparing • Theoretically lower risk of hematoma and other major complications	• Effectiveness not well studied • Large doses of local anesthetic needed for analgesic effect	Somatic blockade only	Poorly suited
Transversus thoracic muscle plane (TTMP) block	• Theoretically lower risk of hematoma and other major complications, excluding pneumothorax	• Effectiveness not well studied • Risk of pneumothorax • Risk of local anesthetic toxicity	Somatic blockade only	Poorly suited
Parasternal (intercostal) block	• Opioid-sparing • May facilitate early extubation • Theoretically lower risk of hematoma and other major complications	• Effectiveness not well studied	Somatic blockade only	Poorly suited
Quadratus lumborum (QL) block	• Opioid-sparing • May facilitate early extubation • Theoretically lower risk of hematoma and other major complications	• Effectiveness not well studied • Large doses of local anesthetic needed for analgesic effect • Risk of bowel and/or renal puncture	Somatic and visceral blockade	Well suited
Transversus abdominis plane (TAP) block	• Theoretically lower risk of hematoma and other major complications	• Effectiveness not well studied • Large doses of local anesthetic needed for analgesic effect • Risk of bowel puncture	Somatic blockade only	Poorly suited
Rectus sheath block	• Theoretically lower risk of hematoma and other major complications	• Effectiveness not well studied • Large doses of local anesthetic needed for analgesic effect • Risk of bowel puncture	Somatic blockade only	Poorly suited

Table 76.2 Peripheral nerve blocks

Regional technique	Advantages	Disadvantages	Physiologic effects	Catheter placement
Paravertebral block	• Equivalent analgesia to neuraxial anesthesia • Lower incidence of minor complications compared to neuraxial techniques • Improved safety profile with ultrasound guidance	• Risk of hematoma • Risk of pneumothorax • Risk of epidural migration	Somatic and sympathetic blockade	Well suited
Lumbar plexus block	• Opioid-sparing • Provides effective hip analgesia	• Deep block • Risk of hematoma	Somatic blockade only	Well suited
Intercostal nerve block	• Potentially opioid-sparing	• Effectiveness not well studied • Risk of pneumothorax • Risk of local anesthetic toxicity • Large doses of local anesthetic needed for analgesic effect	Somatic blockade only	Poorly suited
Ilioinguinal and iliohypogastric nerve block	• Opioid-sparing • Theoretically lower risk of hematoma and other major complications	• Risk of bowel puncture	Somatic blockade only	Poorly suited

Table 76.3 Central neuraxial blocks

Regional technique	Advantages	Disadvantages	Physiologic effects	Catheter placement
Epidural anesthesia	• Well-studied • Proven efficacy • Reduced risk of myocardial infarction, respiratory depression, atrial arrhythmia • Reduced mortality	• Risk of hematoma, potentially exacerbated by cardiopulmonary bypass OR • Risk of dural puncture	Somatic and sympathetic blockade	Well suited
Caudal anesthesia	• May facilitate early extubation in pediatric patients • Decreased stress response to surgery	• Risk of hematoma • Risk of dural puncture • Commonly, only used in pediatric patients	Somatic and sympathetic blockade	Well suited
Spinal anesthesia	• Well-studied • Proven efficacy • Decreased stress response to surgery	• Risk of hematoma, potentially exacerbated by cardiopulmonary bypass • Risk of postdural puncture headache	Somatic and sympathetic blockade	Well suited

Interfascial Plane Blocks

Erector Spinae Plane (ESP) Block

General Considerations

The erector spinae plane (ESP) block is a newer interfascial plane block developed as an alternative to the paravertebral nerve block and neuraxial techniques. Its mechanism of analgesia is believed to involve the dorsal and ventral rami of the spinal nerves at the level of injection with spread to adjacent cephalad and caudal vertebral levels. Its attraction is partly spurred by its superficial clear ultrasonographic targets and ease of performance for both single injection and catheter placement. The ESP block carries a lower risk of complications given its distance away from neuraxial structures, major blood vessels, and pleura, its highly compressible location, and its use of the transverse process as an osseous backstop. Although large studies directly comparing the ESP block to its counterparts are lacking, early data has shown significant opioid-sparing effects in several different surgeries that highlight the potential versatility of the ESP block.

Indications

The erector spinae plane block was first described in 2016 for the management of thoracic neuropathic pain caused by metastatic disease of the ribs and rib fractures. Multiple applications of ESP blocks have since been reported for acute postoperative pain management in patients undergoing procedures including thoracic surgeries, cardiac surgeries with and without cardiopulmonary bypass, breast surgeries, abdominal surgeries, spine fusions, and hip reconstructions.

Functional Anatomy

The erector spinae plane is a fascial plane located between the anterior aspect of the erector spinae muscle group and the posterior aspect of the transverse process. This fascial plane extends along the length of the erector spinae muscle group from the spinous processes of T1 and the cervical vertebrae to the medial crest of the sacrum on both sides of the vertebral column. The mechanism of analgesia of the ESP block is believed to involve the ventral and dorsal rami of the spinal nerves closest to the level of local anesthetic injection with lateral spread to the intercostal spaces. Some cadaver dye studies have shown inconsistent spread of local anesthetic to the paravertebral and epidural spaces.

Technique

Patient Positioning, Preparation, Equipment, and Dosage

The child can be in the prone or lateral decubitus position if under general anesthesia or heavy sedation. Alternatively, the child can be in the sitting position under minimal sedation with the back assuming a kyphotic posture. Standard patient monitoring should be in place, including continuous ECG monitoring, pulse oximetry, and blood pressure measurement. The skin is cleaned with antiseptic solution.

A 50 or 100 mm insulated needle (21–22 G for single injection, 18 G for catheter placement) is commonly used depending on the depth of the transverse process from the skin. Choices of local anesthetic include 0.125–0.25% bupivacaine, 0.2–0.5% ropivacaine, or 0.125–0.5% lidocaine. A volume of 3.5 mL is needed to cover one thoracic vertebral level in an adult, while a volume of 5 mL is needed to cover one lumbar vertebral level. The volume of injectate needed to cover one vertebral level in a child is unknown.

Landmark Technique

Like the landmark technique for the paravertebral block, palpate and mark the targeted spinous process for the chosen thoracic or lumbar level to ensure appropriate analgesia to cover surgical incision. Mark the adjacent spinous processes as well. Next, locate and mark the transverse processes which are 1–2.5 cm lateral to the spinous processes, depending on the child's age (see equation for paravertebral block). In the thoracic region, the transverse processes are generally located at one intervertebral space higher than the corresponding spinous process because of the inferior angulation of the spinous processes. In the lumbar region, the transverse processes are located lateral to the corresponding spinous process.

The needle is inserted perpendicularly to the skin to contact the transverse process. Once contact with the transverse process is made, there is no need to redirect the needle. The local anesthetic can be injected after aspiration. If resistance on initial injection is observed, withdraw the needle very slightly. Note that withdrawing the needle too much can result in an intramuscular injection rather than an injection within the erector spinae fascia. Thus, the use of ultrasound is recommended for guidance and confirmation.

Nerve Stimulation Technique

Nerve stimulation for the ESP block has not been reported.

Ultrasound-Guided Technique

A high-frequency (13–6 MHz) linear probe (Fig. 76.1) is used in smaller children, while a curvilinear transducer (8–3 MHz) is used in larger children. Both "offline" and real-time scanning can be used although real-time scanning is recommended. The "offline" approach has been described and involves performing a pre-procedural scan to locate the point of needle insertion and depth of the transverse process. The real-time approach involves performing needle insertion under real-time ultrasound guidance.

The probe is placed in the cephalocaudal orientation over the midline of the back at the desired thoracic or lumbar level. Slide the probe laterally until the transverse process is visible. For the thoracic region, the transverse processes appear as superficial rectangular structures with hyperechoic outlines and acoustic shadowing, as compared to the overlapping diagonal lines of the lamina and deeper smooth arcs of the ribs. The pleura appears as a hyperechoic line between the acoustic shadowing of osseous structures.

The needle can be inserted superior or inferior to the probe using an in-plane approach in a cephalad to caudal direction or caudal to cephalad direction, respectively. The bevel of the needle should point posteriorly. Once the tip of the needle is below the erector spinae muscle, even touching the transverse process, a small bolus of saline should be given through the needle to confirm the correct interfascial plane. If resistance is observed, withdraw the needle slightly away from the transverse process while remaining underneath the erector spinae muscle. The erector spinae muscle should be visualized separating from the transverse process with minimal injection pressures. Once confirmation of the correct interfascial plane is achieved, inject the local anesthetic after aspiration. The ultrasound probe can slide in a cephalad or caudad direction from the needle insertion site to ensure appropriate spread along the erector spinae fascial plane.

Complications

Given that an ESP block is less difficult to perform than a paravertebral or epidural technique due to its more superficial target, the ESP block has fewer complications and contraindi-

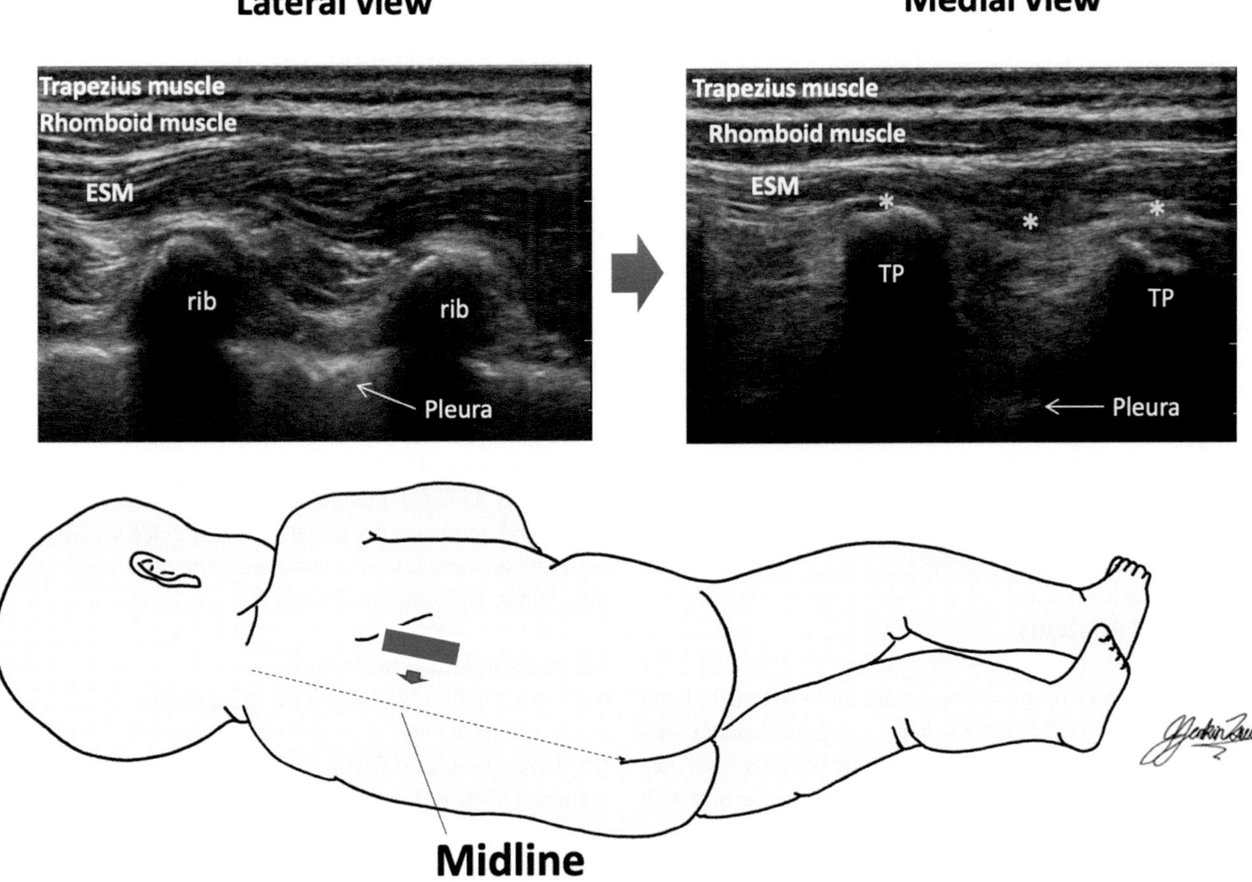

Fig. 76.1 Ultrasound images of longitudinal views of the back, scanning from lateral to medial at T4–T5. (*Left*) intercostal view (*right*) erector spinae plane (ESP) view. *ESP* erector spinae muscle, *TP* transverse process, * ESP fascial plane

cations. The ESP block can be performed without ultrasound guidance, but the use of ultrasound allows for more accurate visualization of the transverse process and spread of the local anesthetic anterior to the erector spinae muscles while minimizing inadvertent puncture of the pleura, neuraxial structures, and retroperitoneal organs. Sterile technique should be used to minimize any risk of infection. And although located in a compressible location, caution should be used when placing any ESP block in patients with a history of anticoagulation to avoid hematomas.

Practical Tips

The ESP block can be used for both unilateral and bilateral surgical procedures. Like the paravertebral block, the ESP block can be performed at the thoracic levels for thoracic and abdominal surgeries and at the lumbar levels for lower extremity procedures. A catheter can be placed in the open interfascial space created by the local anesthetic. Placement of an ESP catheter is relatively easy and smooth as compared to the placement of a paravertebral catheter. If resistance is felt on placement of the ESP catheter, remove the catheter from the needle, and re-confirm the location of the needle tip by ultrasound. It may be helpful to withdraw the needle slightly away from the transverse process and inject a small bolus of saline to create a more open interfascial plane before re-attempting catheter insertion. Avoid maneuvering the needle with the catheter through the needle tip as this can cause shearing and compromise of the catheter integrity.

Literature Review

The ESP block has shown great promise in its ability to provide postoperative analgesia and reduce postoperative complications in cardiac, thoracic, and abdominal surgeries, particularly in the early postoperative period. However, there remains a lack of large-sized randomized control trials directly comparing the ESP block to alternative blocks such as neuraxial and paravertebral blocks.

Pectoralis (PECS 1 and 2) Block

General Considerations

The pectoralis (PECS) 1 and 2 blocks are part of a series of newer interfascial anterior chest wall blocks that avoid the need for significant positioning of the patient to provide analgesia. The safety of the PECS block relies on its superficial targets that have clear anatomical delineations and the location of the ribs that provide a backstop against pleural puncture. Although small branches of the thoracoacromial artery can be found, the location of the PECS block allows for easy compressibility against the formation of any hematomas. The ability to perform the PECS 1 and 2 block safely and easily with one needle insertion has led to its popularity.

Indications

In addition to breast surgery, the PECS 1 and 2 blocks are also used for pacemaker and implantable cardioverter defibrillator (ICD) implantation, transapical transcatheter aortic valve implantation, minimally invasive mitral valve repair, port placement and removal, postherpetic neuralgia in the thoracic region, midshaft and distal clavicle surgery, and proximal anterior humeral surgery.

Functional Anatomy

The pectoralis 1 (PECS 1) block was first described in 2011 for breast surgery by providing analgesia to the medial and lateral pectoral nerves between the pectoralis major and minor muscles. Because analgesic sparing was observed during breast expander and subpectoral prosthesis insertion with the PECS 1 block, the pectoralis 2 (PECS 2) block was used to supplement the long thoracic, intercostobrachial, and III to VI intercostal nerves between the pectoralis minor and serratus anterior muscles.

Technique

Patient Positioning, Preparation, Equipment, and Dosage

The child is placed in the supine position with the arm slightly abducted. Standard patient monitoring should be in place, including continuous ECG monitoring, pulse oximetry, and blood pressure measurement. The skin is cleaned with antiseptic solution.

A 50 mm, 22G short-beveled needle is used. Recommended local anesthetic doses are 0.5 mL/kg of 0.25% bupivacaine or 0.2% ropivacaine on each side (up to a maximum of 3 mg/kg in total).

Landmark Technique

The PECS 1 and 2 blocks are typically performed under ultrasound guidance to target the two interfascial planes between the three layers of muscles: pectoralis major, pectoralis minor, and serratus anterior.

Nerve Stimulation Technique

Nerve stimulation is not used for these blocks.

Ultrasound-Guided Technique

A linear (13–6 MHz) probe (Fig. 76.2) is placed in the deltopectoral groove below the clavicle (the similar location for performing an infraclavicular nerve block). Once the subclavian vessels are identified, identify the second rib in this view. Slide the probe inferolaterally to the level of the third

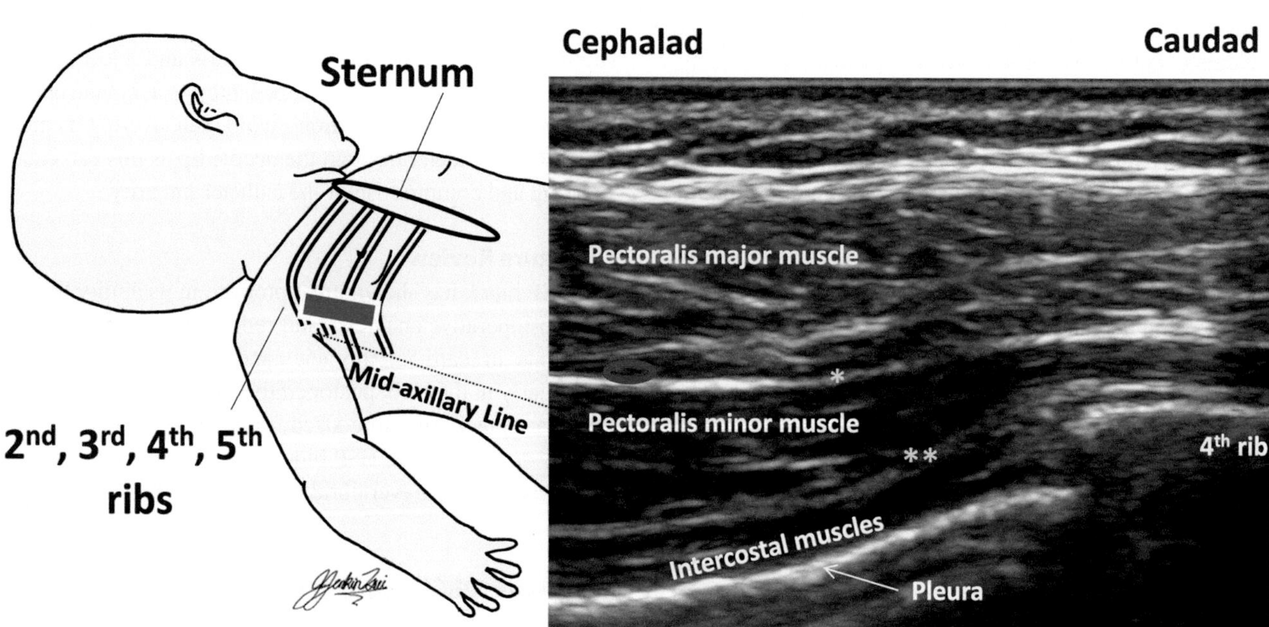

Fig. 76.2 Ultrasound image of pectoralis blocks (PECS1) and (PECS2) with longitudinal view at T4. *O* Thoracoacromial artery; * PECS1 block; ** PECS2 block

and fourth ribs. The serratus anterior muscle appears as a very thin band of muscle overlying the ribs with the pectoralis minor muscle lying on top of the serratus anterior muscle and tapering caudally. The pectoralis major muscle is located above the pectoralis minor muscle. Branches of the thoracoacromial artery can be found between the pectoralis major and minor muscles. Care should be taken to avoid these branches in the needle trajectory.

The in-plane approach is typically used with the needle inserted in a cephalad to caudad direction. The PECS 2 block is performed first to avoid any accidental injection of air that could decrease visualization of deeper structures. To perform the PECS 2 block, the needle tip is placed in between the pectoralis minor and serratus anterior muscles. If the plane between these two muscles is difficult to visualize, the needle can target the fascial plane between the fourth rib and the muscle on top. Ensure that the spread of the local anesthetic is not intramuscular. Once the PECS 2 block is complete, slowly withdraw the needle to perform the PECS 1 block where the local anesthetic is injected in between the pectoralis major and pectoralis minor muscles.

Complications

Potential complications include infection, pneumothorax, hematoma, winging of the scapula from blockade of the long thoracic nerve, and local anesthetic toxicity.

Practical Tips

Although the out-of-plane approach can be performed, good technique must be used to avoid causing a pneumothorax. Catheters can be placed for PECS blocks. However, the location of PECS catheters can be in the surgical field thus necessitating their placement after surgical closure.

Literature Review

The PECS block has shown to reduce postoperative pain intensity and opioid consumption in the first 24 h in breast surgery when compared to systemic analgesia alone. However, there remains a lack of large-sized randomized control trials directly comparing the PECS block to neuraxial techniques and other chest wall blocks.

Serratus Anterior Plane (SAP) Block

General Considerations

The serratus anterior plane (SAP) block falls into the family of new interfascial anterior chest wall blocks that include the PECS 1 and 2 blocks. It offers analgesia that supplements the lateral and posterior areas spared by the PECS 1 and 2 blocks. The safety profile of the SAP block is similar to the PECS 1 and 2 blocks given its superficial target and osseous backstop.

Indications

The serratus anterior plane block was first described in 2013 to provide improved analgesia to the lateral thorax after breast surgery. Since its introduction, the SAP block has been applied to breast surgery, thoracotomy and thoracoscopic surgeries, chest tube placement, and rib fracture pain.

Functional Anatomy

The SAP block covers the anterior, lateral, and posterior chest wall from T2 to T9 but spares the mid-chest. It blocks the lateral cutaneous branches of the intercostal nerves as well as the long thoracic nerve and the thoracodorsal nerve, which lie on top of the serratus anterior muscle.

Technique

Patient Positioning, Preparation, Equipment, and Dosage

The child can be placed in either the supine or lateral position to gain exposure to the fifth rib along the mid-axillary line. Standard patient monitoring should be in place, including continuous ECG monitoring, pulse oximetry, and blood pressure measurement. The skin is cleaned with antiseptic solution.

A 25 or 50 mm, 22G short-beveled needle is used depending on the size of the child. Although recommended local anesthetic doses are 0.5 mL/kg of 0.25% bupivacaine or 0.2% ropivacaine for each side (up to a maximum of 3 mg/kg total), the spread of this fascial plane block is volume dependent. In adults, achieving a spread from T1 to T8 requires 40 ml of local anesthetic volume. The ideal volume to achieve the same spread has not been explored in children.

Landmark Technique

Count the number of ribs along the anterior aspect of the chest until the fifth rib is located. Palpate the fifth rib more laterally to the mid-axillary line. The fifth rib is kept in place by the proceduralist's index and middle finger along the cephalad and caudal aspects of the fifth rib. The needle is inserted perpendicularly to the skin between the proceduralist's index and middle finger to contact the fifth rib. The local anesthetic can be injected after aspiration. If resistance on initial injection is observed, withdraw the needle very slightly. A small volume of local anesthetic can be reserved at the end of the nerve block to be injected while the needle is slowly withdrawn, but this is not required to achieve an optimal block.

Nerve Stimulation Technique

Nerve stimulation is not used for this block.

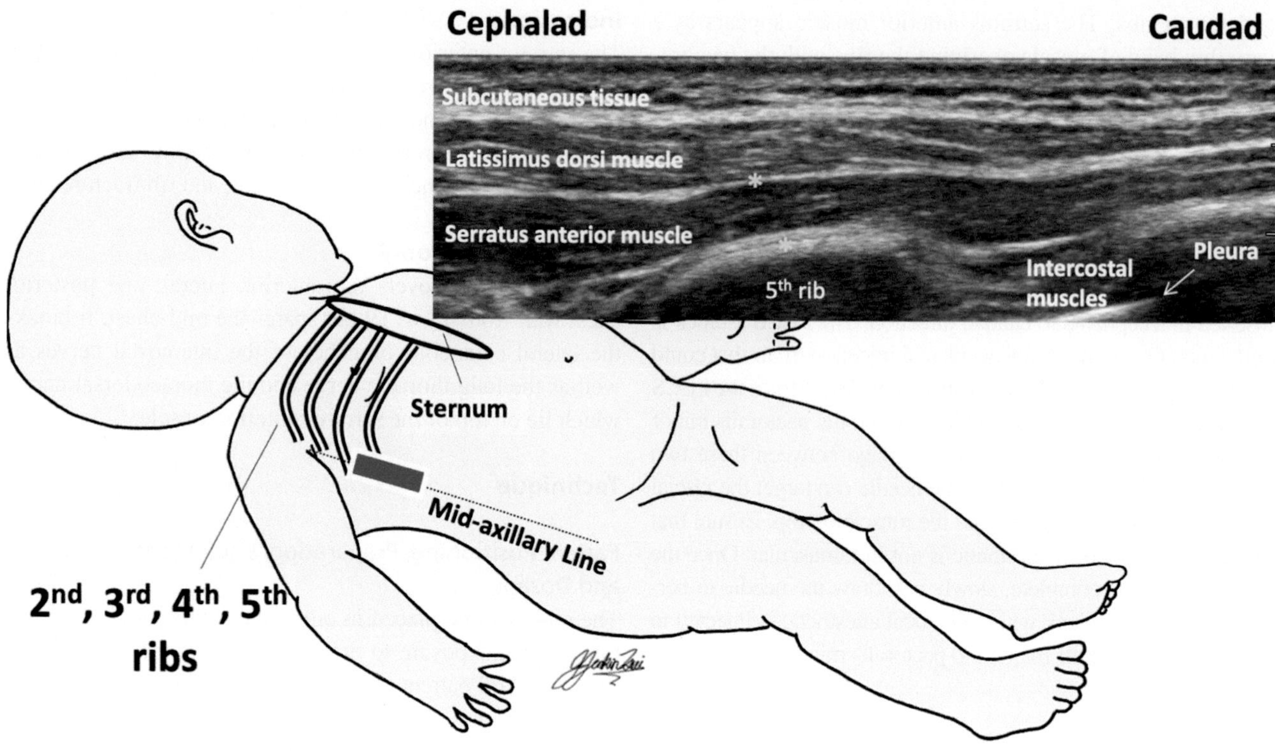

Fig. 76.3 Ultrasound image of mid-axillary longitudinal view of serratus anterior plane (SAP block) at T5 level

Ultrasound-Guided Technique

Using a linear (13–6 MHz) probe (Fig. 76.3), start at the midclavicular line just below the clavicle. Count the ribs by slowly sliding the probe in a caudal and lateral direction until the fourth and fifth ribs are identified in the mid-axillary line. At this location, the latissimus dorsi muscle can be seen superficial to the serratus anterior muscle which overlies the ribs. The pleura can be seen in between each rib shadow.

The thoracodorsal artery can occasionally be seen in the plane above the serratus anterior muscle. Applying color Doppler ultrasound can increase the safety of the intended needle trajectory.

The in-plane approach is usually performed by advancing the needle in a cephalad to caudal direction. The ideal point of injection can be superficial to the serratus anterior muscle (between the latissimus dorsi and the serratus anterior muscles) or deep to the serratus anterior muscle (between the serratus anterior muscle and the rib). After negative aspiration, inject the local anesthetic. If both the superficial and deep approaches are performed, always perform the deeper injection first to avoid any accidental injection of air that could decrease visualization of deeper structures.

Complications

Potential complications include infection, pneumothorax, hematoma, winging of the scapula from blockade of the long thoracic nerve, and local anesthetic toxicity.

Practical Tips

If interfascial spread along the superficial plane (between the latissimus dorsi and serratus anterior muscles) is challenging to achieve, target the deeper plane instead between the serratus anterior muscle and the rib. Analgesic efficacy appears to be similar for both planes. Catheters can be placed for SAP blocks but are difficult to maintain with a high risk of dislodgment. The location of the SAP catheter can be in the surgical field thus necessitating its placement after surgical closure. PECS 1 and 2 and SAP can be performed as a single pass (Fig. 76.4).

Literature Review

The SAP block has shown to reduce postoperative pain intensity and opioid consumption in the first 24 hours in thoracic surgery when compared to systemic analgesia alone. However, there remains a lack of large-sized randomized controlled trials directly comparing the SAP block to neuraxial techniques and other chest wall blocks.

Transversus Thoracic Muscle Plane (TTMP) Block

General Considerations

The transversus thoracic muscle plane (TTMP) block falls into the family of new interfascial anterior chest wall blocks

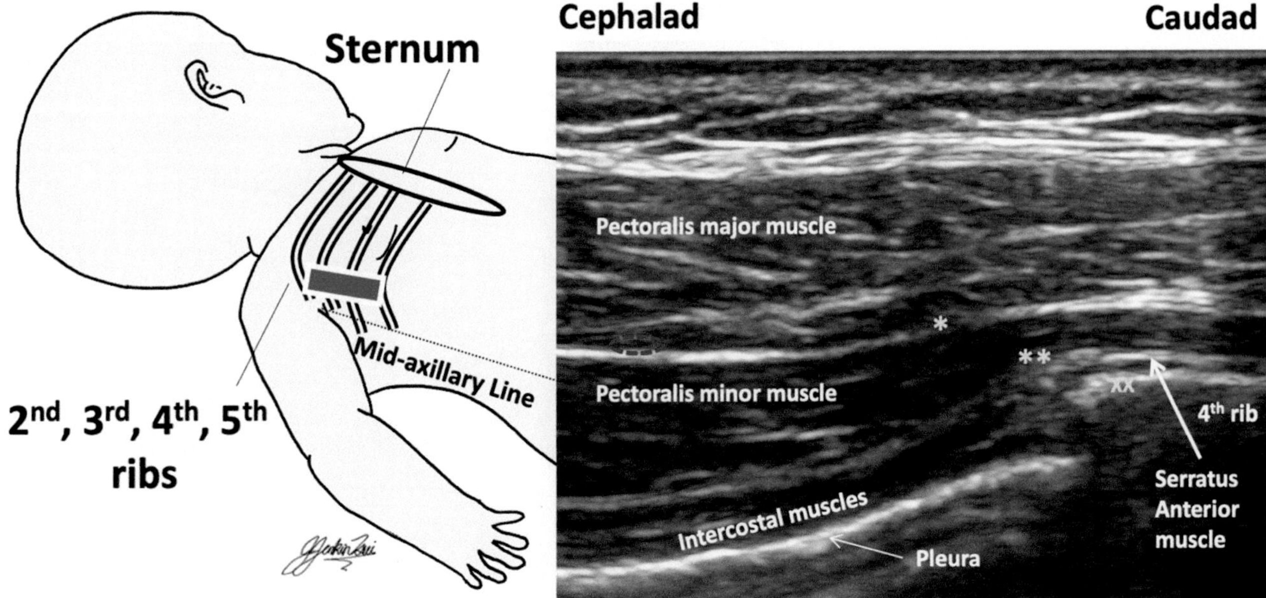

Fig. 76.4 Ultrasound image of pectoralis (PECS1 and 2) and serratus anterior plane (SAP) blocks with longitudinal view at T4. *O* Thoracoacromial artery; * PECS1 block; ** PECS2 block. XX, SAP

that also includes the SAP and PECS 1 and 2 blocks. It offers analgesia that supplements anteromedial chest wall areas spared by the PECS 1 and 2 blocks. Unlike the SAP and PECS blocks, the TTMP block can be slightly more challenging to perform given the smaller sizes of the transversus thoracic and internal intercostal muscles and their proximity to the pleura without any osseous backstop. Thus needle technique must be optimized to perform the TTMP block in a pediatric patient.

Indications

The TTMP block was first described in 2015 to supplement medial chest analgesia after pectoralis (PECS) block. Reported analgesic use has included median sternotomy, breast surgery, implantable cardioverter-defibrillator (ICD) placement, and pericardiocentesis. There has also been a case report of a combined TTMP block with bilateral PEC 2 blocks for bilateral breast cancer resection without the use of general anesthesia.

Functional Anatomy

The TTMP block targets the fascial plane between the transversus thoracic muscle and the internal intercostal muscle, just lateral to the sternum, at the level between the fourth and fifth ribs. Anatomic studies demonstrate sensory block of the anterior branches of the second to sixth intercostal nerves from a single injection point. The TTMP block therefore provides analgesia to the internal mammary region.

Technique

Patient Positioning, Preparation, Equipment, and Dosage

The child is placed in the supine position. Standard patient monitoring should be in place, including continuous ECG monitoring, pulse oximetry, and blood pressure measurement. The skin is cleaned with antiseptic solution.

A 25 or 50 mm, 22G short-beveled needle is used depending on the size of the child. Recommended local anesthetic doses are 0.5 mL/kg of 0.25% bupivacaine or 0.2% ropivacaine on each side (up to a maximum of 3 mg/kg).

Landmark Technique

The TTMP block is typically performed under ultrasound guidance to target the interfascial planes between the transversus thoracic and the internal intercostal muscles while avoiding pleural puncture.

Nerve Stimulation Technique

Nerve stimulation is not used for this block.

Ultrasound-Guided Technique

Using a high-frequency linear (13–6 MHz) probe in the sagittal plane next to the sternum (Fig. 76.5), count the ribs by slowly sliding the probe in a caudal direction until the fourth and fifth ribs are identified. Although both the sagittal (Fig. 76.5) and transverse approaches (Fig. 76.6) can be used to perform the TTMP block, the sagittal approach is recommended for greater local anesthetic spread.

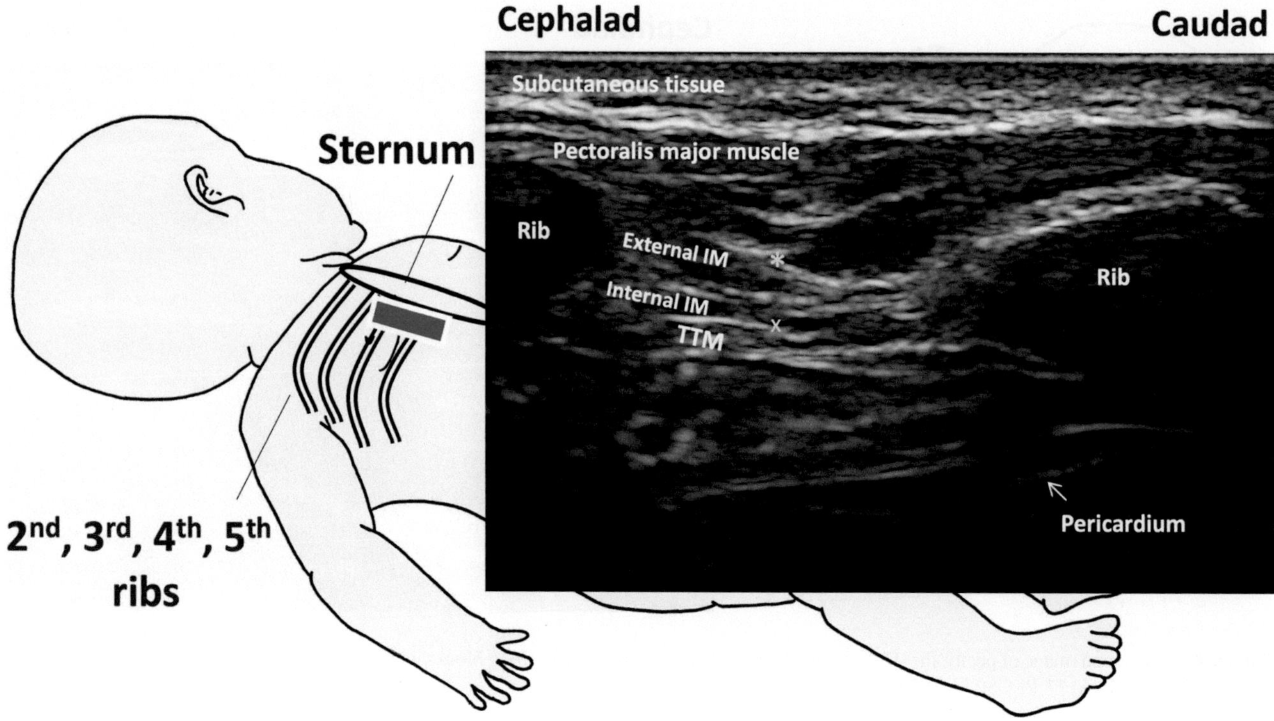

Fig. 76.5 Sagittal ultrasound view of the transversus thoracic muscle plane (TTMP) block next to sternum at T4 and T5 level

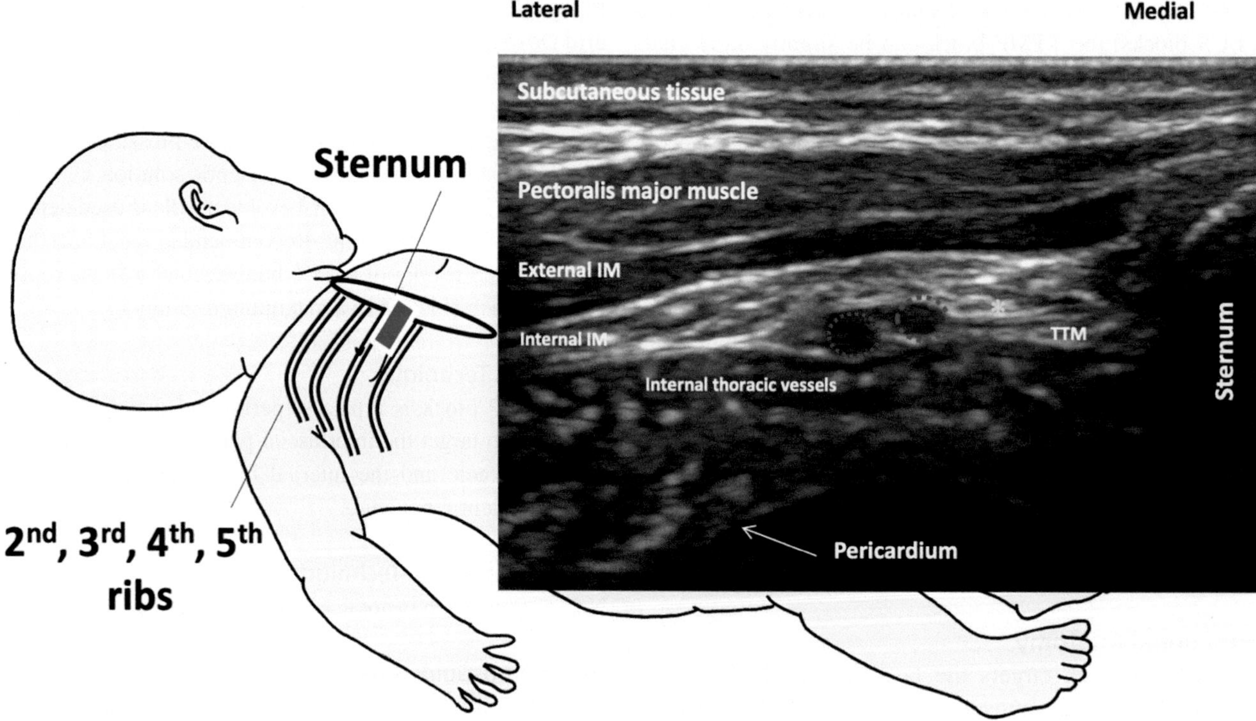

Fig. 76.6 Transverse ultrasound view of the transversus thoracic muscle plane (TTMP) block next to sternum at T4 and T5 level. *O* Internal thoracic vessels

To perform the sagittal approach, identify the transversus thoracic and the internal intercostal muscles. The pleura can be seen in between each rib shadow. Insert the needle in-plane from a cephalad to caudal direction such that the ideal point of injection is in between the transversus thoracic and the internal intercostal muscles. After negative aspiration, inject the local anesthetic.

To perform the transverse approach, identify the fourth and fifth ribs along the sternum as before. Rotate the probe 90°, and identify the transversus thoracic and the internal intercostal muscles. Insert the needle in-plane from a lateral to medial direction. The ideal point of injection is in between the transversus thoracic and the internal intercostal muscles. After negative aspiration, inject the local anesthetic.

Complications

Potential complications include infection, pneumothorax, hematoma, local anesthetic toxicity, and puncture of the internal thoracic artery (also known as the internal mammary artery).

Practical Tips

Catheters can be placed for TTMP block but are difficult to maintain with a high risk of dislodgment or migration outside of the interfascial plane. The location of the TTMP catheter(s) is typically in the surgical field thus necessitating placement after surgical closure.

Literature Review

Although various case reports have described postoperative analgesia with TTMPBs after cardiac and breast surgery in adults and children, there have been no large, reproducible studies examining its efficacy.

Parasternal Intercostal Nerve Block

General Considerations

The parasternal intercostal nerve block (or parasternal block) was first introduced in 2016 in response to the technical challenges associated with placement of the transversus thoracic muscle plane (TTMP) block. These challenges include difficult visualization and differentiation of the transversus thoracic muscle by ultrasound given its small size and the need for excellent needling technique to avoid puncture of the pleura and internal thoracic artery. The parasternal nerve block instead targets the more superficial interfascial layer between the larger pectoral major and external intercostal muscles (Fig. 76.5).

There are similarities between the parasternal block to the subpectoral interfascial plane (SIP) block and the pectointercostal fascial block (PIFB). All three blocks target the same fascial plane between the pectoral major and external intercostal muscles. Their subtle difference lies in the distance away from the sternum.

Indications

The parasternal block has been used for sternotomy pain after cardiac surgery, sternal fractures, medial anterior chest pain following breast surgery, and minimally invasive thoracotomy.

Functional Anatomy

Parasternal nerve blocks target the anterior and posterior intercostal nerves. Thus, the parasternal nerve block provides analgesia to the internal mammary area.

Technique

Patient Positioning, Preparation, Equipment, and Dosage

The child is placed in the supine position. Standard patient monitoring should be in place, including continuous ECG monitoring, pulse oximetry, and blood pressure measurement. The skin is cleaned with antiseptic solution.

A 25 or 50 mm, 22G short-beveled needle is used depending on the size of the child. Recommended local anesthetic doses are 0.5 mL/kg of 0.25% bupivacaine or 0.2% ropivacaine on each side (up to a maximum of 3 mg/kg).

Landmark Technique

The parasternal block is typically performed under ultrasound guidance to target the interfascial planes between the pectoral major and external intercostal muscles while avoiding pleural puncture.

Nerve Stimulation Technique

Nerve stimulation is not used for this block.

Ultrasound-Guided Technique

Place a high-frequency linear (13–6 MHz) probe in the sagittal plane between the sternum and midclavicular line. Count the ribs by slowly sliding the probe (Fig. 76.5) in a caudal direction until the third, fourth, and fifth ribs are identified.

Identify the pectoral major and external intercostal muscles. The pleura can be seen in between each rib shadow. Insert the needle in-plane from a cephalad to caudal direction such that the ideal point of injection is in between the pectoral major and external intercostal muscles. After negative aspiration, inject the local anesthetic.

Complications

Potential complications include infection, pneumothorax, hematoma, and local anesthetic toxicity.

Practical Tips

Catheters can be placed for parasternal blocks but are difficult to maintain with a high risk of dislodgment. The location of the parasternal catheter can be in the surgical field thus necessitating its placement after surgical closure.

Literature Review

In randomized studies in both adult and pediatric patients undergoing cardiac surgery, the use of parasternal blocks decreased morphine consumption after surgery and reduced mean extubation times. However, there remains a lack of large-sized randomized control trials directly comparing the parasternal block to neuraxial techniques and other chest wall blocks.

Transversus Abdominis Plane (TAP) Block

General Considerations

The transversus abdominis plane (TAP) block has become a commonly used regional block technique, as an alternative to epidural, for intraoperative and postoperative analgesia for abdominal surgery. Its use in children has gained popularity in recent years with the use of ultrasound. However, because of the lack of visceral pain blockade and limited fascial spread, newer techniques (e.g., quadratus lumborum (QL) block which will be described in the next section) have also been developed for improved analgesic effect.

Indications

This block is commonly indicated in abdominal and pelvic surgery for intraoperative and postoperative pain control. It is useful as an alternative to epidural analgesia in children who have contraindications to a neuraxial block. Since blockade of the L1 nerve can be achieved, it may also be used as a substitute for ilioinguinal and iliohypogastric block. Like rectus sheath block, this block can only cover somatic pain.

Functional Anatomy

The anterior abdominal wall is innervated by the ventral divisions of the lower seven intercostal nerves (T6–T12) and the L1 nerve. These nerves lie in the transversus abdominis plane (TAP) – the fascial plane between the internal oblique and transversus abdominis muscles. The nerves give rise to lateral cutaneous branches, which supply the anterolateral torso, near the mid-axillary line. They then terminate as anterior cutaneous branches which supply the anterior torso. Deposition of local anesthetic in this plane results in unilateral blockade of the skin, muscle, and parietal peritoneum of the anterior abdominal wall. In order for this block to provide the best coverage especially for non-midline incision, it is important to perform the block as laterally as possible to cover the lateral cutaneous branches. One should be reminded that conventional TAP blocks provide analgesia from T10 to L1, which is good for lower abdominal surgery. For upper abdominal incisions involving T6 to T10, subcostal TAP blocks should be used instead.

Technique

Patient Positioning, Preparation, Equipment, and Dosage

This block should be performed with the child under general anesthesia or deep sedation. The child is positioned either in the supine (lateral approach) or lateral decubitus position (posterior approach), although a more posterior approach gives better results. The skin is cleaned with antiseptic solution.

A 50 mm, 22G short-beveled needle is used. Choices of local anesthetic include 0.2% ropivacaine or 0.25% bupivacaine. A volume of 0.2–0.3 mL/kg of local anesthetic is recommended on each side (up to a maximum of 3 mg/kg). It is important to have adequate volume to promote spread for this block.

Landmark Technique

The needle insertion point is at the triangle of Petit – an area at the lateral abdominal wall bounded anteriorly by the external oblique, posteriorly by the latissimus dorsi, and inferiorly by the iliac crest. In this triangle, the internal oblique muscle forms the floor of this triangle, so it is the only area of the abdominal wall where this muscle can be localized directly. The needle is inserted perpendicularly to the skin at the point just anterior to the attachment of the latissimus dorsi to the external lip of the iliac crest. The needle is then walked off the iliac crest when the needle contacts the bone. As the needle penetrates the internal oblique muscle to enter the TAP, a "pop" or give is felt. After negative aspiration, local anesthetic is injected. The block is repeated on the other side for a midline or transverse incision.

Ultrasound-Guided Technique

On the mid-axillary line, a high-frequency (13–6 MHz) linear probe is placed transversely between the costal margin and the iliac crest. The three muscle layers separated by the hyperechoic fascia are seen: external oblique, internal oblique, and transversus abdominis (Fig. 76.7). The internal oblique is the widest muscle layer, and it lies laterally to rectus abdominis on the same plane. The transversus abdominis is the thinnest muscle layer and is generally more hypoechoic. It continues and goes underneath the rectus muscle near the costal margin. Underneath the transversalis fascia deep to the transversus abdominis, the peritoneum and bowel are seen. Occasionally, a curved probe is used for obese patients.

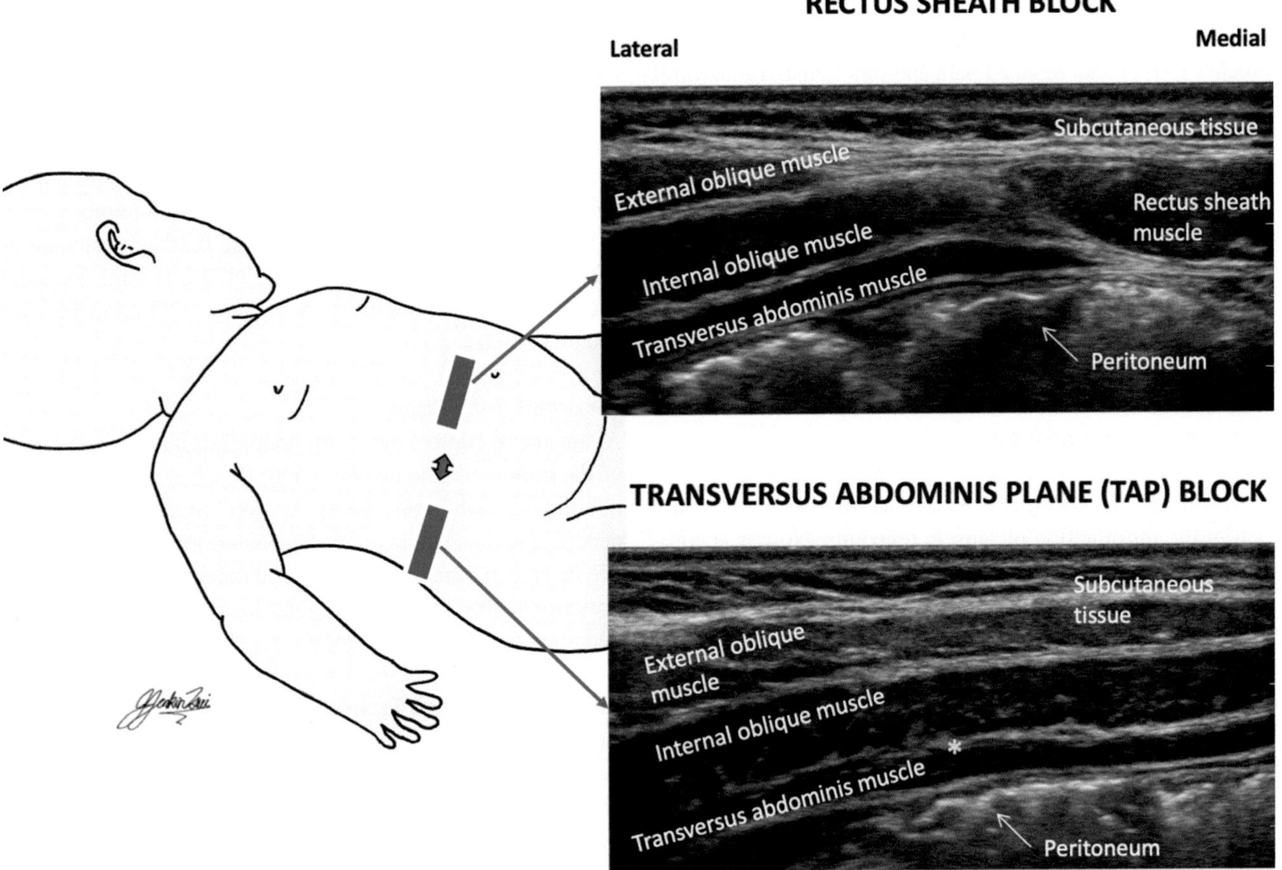

Fig. 76.7 Ultrasound images of the abdominal muscles. (*Upper*) rectus sheath. (*Lower*) * transversus abdominis plane

Both in-plane and out-of-plane approaches can be used. With an in-plane approach, the needle can be introduced either in a medial-to-lateral or lateral-to-medial direction to reach the TAP. A medial-to-lateral approach is preferred because the needle can be directed more posteriorly for block placement. Two "pops" or gives can sometimes be felt as the needle passes through the fascial planes between the external oblique and internal oblique muscles, as well as between the internal oblique and transversus abdominis muscles. Hydrodissection can be used to visualize spread and confirm needle tip position. Local anesthetic is deposited after negative aspiration. Hydrodissection and local anesthetic is seen to open the fascial plane and spread along TAP. For an out-of-plane approach, the needle is introduced at the cephalad edge of the probe and directed caudally. With the needle tip in view, the needle then "walks down" to reach the TAP.

For the subcostal TAP block, the probe is placed obliquely along the costal margin where the same three muscle layers as before can be seen. The needle is introduced in-plane to reach the fascial plane between the transversus abdominis and the internal oblique muscles.

Complications

Specific complications of this block include hematoma, local anesthetic toxicity, and inadvertent peritoneal puncture resulting in trauma to the abdominal viscera.

Practical Tips

Cadaver studies have found that the triangle of Petit varies largely in position and size. Palpation of the triangle of Petit in an anesthetized child can be difficult, especially if the child is obese. An ultrasound-guided approach is therefore recommended.

For a large abdominal incision which involves both the upper and lower abdomen, bilateral dual TAP blocks (two lateral/posterior TAP blocks, two subcostal TAP blocks) or an alternative block approach may be required to ensure complete analgesic coverage.

To prolong the analgesic effect, continuous TAP blocks can be achieved by the use of TAP catheters (one on each side) with either intermittent boluses or continuous infusion of local anesthetic.

Literature Review

A systematic review showed that together with rectus sheath blocks, TAP blocks reduced pain and opioid use for abdominal operations in children.

A multicenter observational study showed that the overall and specific complication rate of TAP blocks in children was very low (0.1% and 0.05%, respectively). In addition, complications were very minor and did not require any interventions.

Rectus Sheath Block

General Considerations

The rectus sheath block was first described in 1899 and was used initially for abdominal wall relaxation for laparotomy before the introduction of muscle relaxants. Now it is commonly used in the pediatric population as postoperative pain relief for umbilical and midline surgery.

Indications

This block is most commonly indicated for midline abdominal incisions (e.g., epigastric and umbilical hernia repair). However, one should be reminded that only somatic pain is covered with this block.

Functional Anatomy

The rectus abdominis is a pair of oval-shaped muscles running vertically on each side on the anterior abdominal wall. It is enveloped by the rectus sheath, which is formed by the aponeuroses of the three abdominal muscles – external oblique, internal oblique, and transversus abdominis. The left and right rectus sheaths join at the linea alba in the midline. Above the arcuate line (which is located roughly one-third the distance from the umbilicus to the pubic crest), the rectus muscles sit on the posterior rectus sheath derived from the aponeurosis of internal oblique and transversus abdominis. Below the arcuate line, the posterior rectus sheath terminates, and all three aponeuroses pass superficial to the rectus muscles, so the rectus muscles are sitting directly on the fascia transversalis. The anterior abdominal wall is innervated by the lower seven intercostal nerves (T6–T12) and the L1 nerve. Running in the plane between the internal oblique and transversus abdominis muscles, the nerves course anteriorly and pierce the posterior rectus sheath at the posterolateral edge, penetrate through the rectus abdominis muscle, and then exit anteriorly to supply the skin. A para-umbilical block can be produced if local anesthetic is placed between the rectus muscle and the posterior rectus sheath bilaterally.

Technique

Patient Positioning, Preparation, Equipment, and Dosage

This block should be performed with the child under general anesthesia or deep sedation. With the child in the supine position, the skin is cleaned with antiseptic solution.

Choices of local anesthetic include 0.2% ropivacaine or 0.25–0.5% bupivacaine. A volume of 0.2–0.3 mL/kg local anesthetic is recommended. A 50 mm, 22G short-beveled needle is used.

Landmark Technique

At the lateral edge of the rectus abdominis muscle at the level of the umbilicus, the needle is introduced at 60° to the skin, pointing medially (Fig. 76.8). A "pop" or give is felt as the needle is advanced and pierces the anterior rectus sheath. The needle is then advanced further until the firm resistance of the posterior rectus sheath is felt, and local anesthetic is deposited after aspiration. The block is repeated on the other side.

Ultrasound-Guided Technique

At one side on the anterior abdominal wall, place a high-frequency (13–6 MHz) linear probe in a transverse plane above the umbilicus to scan for the three muscle layers: external oblique, internal oblique, and transversus abdominis (Figs. 76.7 and 76.8). Identify the oval-shaped rectus abdominis muscle which lies medial to the internal oblique on the same plane. At this level (i.e., above the arcuate line), the posterior rectus sheaths can be seen, and it appears as a hyperechoic double line just posterior to the rectus muscle. The superior and inferior epigastric vessels which run through the rectus muscle may be seen on color Doppler. The target site for local anesthetic is the plane between the rectus muscle and the posterior rectus sheath.

The needle is inserted in-plane (in either a lateral-to-medial direction or mediatl-to-lateral direction) and directed to the plane between the rectus muscle and the posterior rectus sheath. The needle tip position in the fascial plane can be confirmed using hydrodissection. Local anesthetic is deposited after negative aspiration.

Complications

Specific complications include peritoneal puncture and puncture of the epigastric vessels causing hematoma.

Practical Tips

To achieve optimal blockade, the block can be performed at the upper and lower ends of the incision bilaterally (i.e., a total of four blocks).

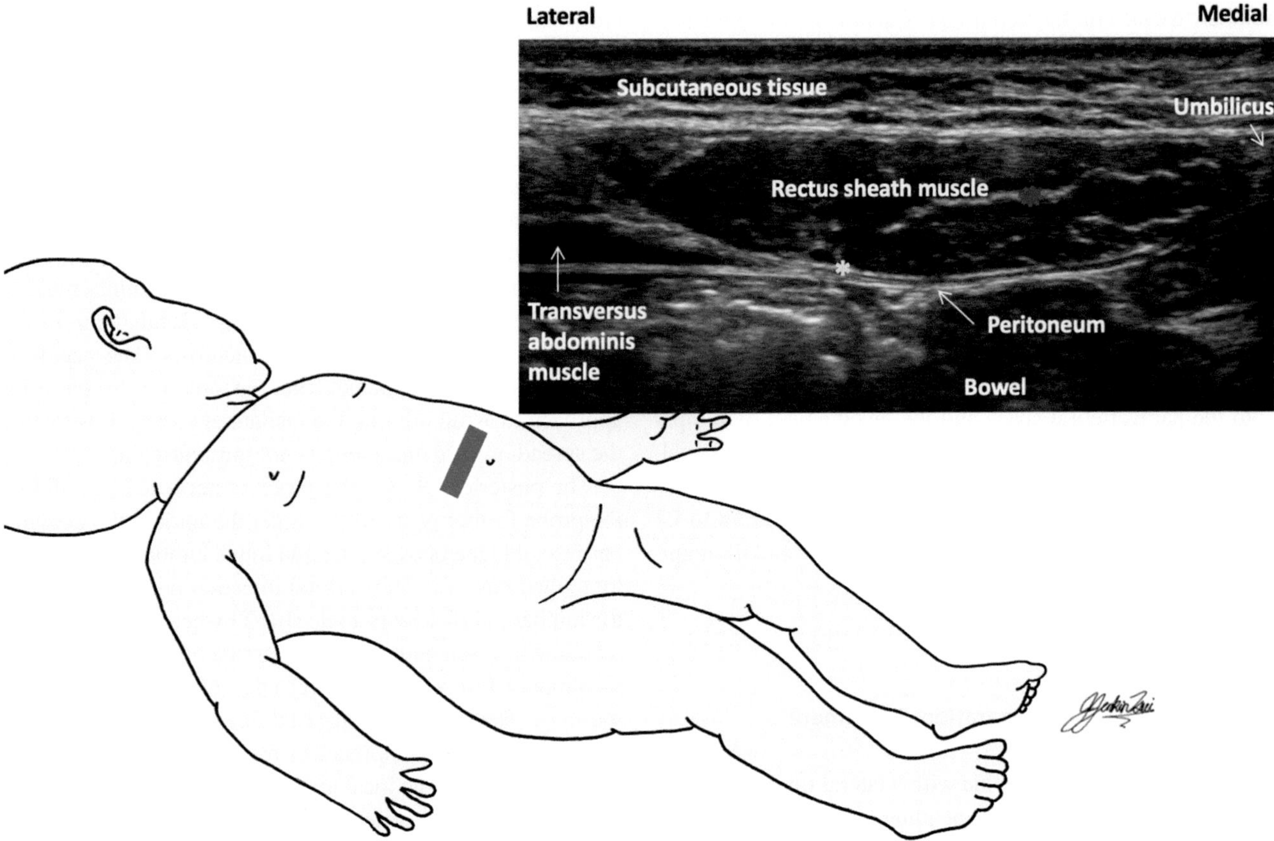

Fig. 76.8 Ultrasound image of the abdominal wall and rectus sheath. *O* epigastric vessel, * target for rectus sheath block

Although the depth of the posterior sheath is usually less than 1 cm, there is poor correlation between the depth of the posterior sheath and the age, weight, or height in children. The use of ultrasound for this block is recommended to avoid complications.

In up to 30% of the population, the anterior cutaneous branches are formed before the rectus sheath and so do not penetrate the posterior sheath. This results in incomplete block despite correct placement of local anesthetic.

Literature Review

Several studies had demonstrated that ultrasound-guided rectus sheath blocks provided more effective analgesia than local anesthetic wound infiltration for umbilical hernia repairs in children. A catheter can be placed to prolong analgesic effect. Regimens with intermittent boluses are shown to be more effective than those containing only continuous infusion.

Quadratus Lumborum (QL) Block

General Considerations

The quadratus lumborum (QL) block is a more posterior and lateral version of the transversus abdominus plane (TAP) block without the technical difficulties of a paravertebral or neuraxial technique. Because the local anesthetic placed with a QL block spreads toward the paravertebral space, the QL block offers somatic as well as visceral analgesia. Although there are three major types of QL blocks (not including the intramuscular psoas muscle injection variation), there have been no large studies directly comparing the efficacy of each of the three major QL blocks in efficacy and superiority for different surgeries.

Indications

The QL block has been used for mid-to-lower abdominal surgeries, Cesarean section, gynecologic surgeries, urologic surgeries, renal transplant, and orthopedic surgeries involving the proximal anterior and lateral femur. Like the TAP block, the QL block can be used as an alternative block when a neuraxial technique is contraindicated. The QL block can also be used as an alternative for the following: rectus sheath block, TAP block, ilioinguinal and iliohypogastric nerve block, paravertebral block, ESP block, fascia iliaca block, and femoral nerve block (for proximal hip and femur surgeries to limit quadriceps weakness).

Functional Anatomy

The quadratus lumborum block was first reported in 2007 as a posterior variation of the TAP block targeting the thoracolumbar fascia. The thoracolumbar fascia (TLF) is an extension of the abdominal wall muscle fascia. Composed of three layers (anterior, middle, and posterior), the TLF extends from the thoracic spine to the lumbar spine in a craniocaudal direction. The anterior TLF lies anterior to the quadratus lumborum and psoas muscles. The middle TLF runs between the quadratus lumborum and erector spinae muscles. And the posterior TLF encloses the erector spinae muscles. The QL block provides analgesia through the spread of local anesthetic to the paravertebral space through the thoracolumbar fascia which contains mechanoreceptors, nocicepters, and sympathetic fibers. Local anesthetic spread from the TLF into the paravertebral space and the involvement of sympathetic fibers in the TLF are thought to provide visceral analgesia that is not seen in the TAP block. Cadaver and in vivo studies have shown dermatomal spread to include T8 to L1 with consistent coverage of the iliohypogastric and ilioinguinal nerves.

Technique

Patient Positioning, Preparation, Equipment, and Dosage

The child can be either supine with a lateral tilt (also known as a "hip bump") or lateral depending on the proceduralist's preference and planned needle trajectory. The lateral position facilitates a more posterior needle approach. Standard patient monitoring should be in place, including continuous ECG monitoring, pulse oximetry, and blood pressure measurement. The skin is cleaned with antiseptic solution.

A 50–100 mm, 22G short-beveled needle is used. Recommended local anesthetic doses are 0.5 mL/kg of 0.25% bupivacaine or 0.2% ropivacaine on each side (up to a maximum of 3 mg/kg).

Landmark Technique

The QL block is typically performed under ultrasound guidance to target the thoracolumbar fascia around the quadratus lumborum muscle while minimizing potential injury to the ipsilateral kidney, peritoneum, and bowel.

Nerve Stimulation Technique

Nerve stimulation is not used for these blocks.

Ultrasound-Guided Technique (Fig. 76.9)

A linear (13–6 MHz) probe is used for babies and younger children, while a curvilinear (8–3 MHz) probe is used for larger children and teenagers. The probe is placed in a transverse plane on the mid-axillary line, between the costal margin and the iliac crest to visualize the three muscle layers for the TAP block. Slide the probe posteriorly above the iliac crest until the tapering of the transversus abdominis can be seen and the quadratus lumborum muscle comes into view.

There are three different approaches to the QL block based on the anatomical location of the needle tip in relation to the quadratus lumborum muscle and the TLF: lateral QL (QL1), posterior QL (QL2), and anterior QL (QL3).

The lateral QL or QL1 block is performed by targeting the lateral border of the quadratus lumborum muscle and the tapering aponeurosis of the transversus abdominis muscle. Tilting the probe caudally can improve visualization of the tapered end of the transversus aponeurosis. The needle is typically inserted in-plane from an anterior to posterior approach to avoid injuring the ipsilateral kidney. Ensure that the spread of local anesthetic is not intramuscular.

The posterior QL or QL2 block is performed by sliding the probe further posterior to target the middle thoracolumbar fascial plane between the quadratus lumborum and erector spinae muscles. The optimal injection point is known as the lumbar interfascial triangle (LIFT) where the middle thoracolumbar fascia joins the deep lamina of the posterior thoracolumbar fascia at the lateral edge of the erector spinae muscles. The needle is inserted in-plane either from an anterior-to-posterior approach or from a posterior-to-anterior approach. Ideally, the local anesthetic should spread posteriorly toward the paravertebral space.

The anterior QL or QL3 block is performed by targeting the anterior thoracolumbar fascial plane between the quadratus lumborum and psoas muscles. The needle is typically inserted in-plane from posterior-to-anterior to minimize the travel distance of the needle.

Complications

There are few contraindications to performing the QL block. Unintentional puncture of the peritoneum, bowel, or kidney should not occur with careful needle visualization under ultrasound guidance. Caution should be used in the case of anticoagulation as the presence of the fourth lumbar artery in the thoracolumbar fascia can cause large hematomas. Quadriceps weakness can be seen when the QL3 block is performed due to local anesthetic spread from the thoracolumbar fascia to the fascia iliaca.

Practical Tips

Catheters can be placed for all approaches of the QL block. If the location of the QL catheter is in the surgical field, place the catheters after surgical closure.

Literature Review

The QL block has been shown to reduce pain intensity and opioid consumption in the early postoperative period in Cesarean delivery and renal surgery when compared to sys-

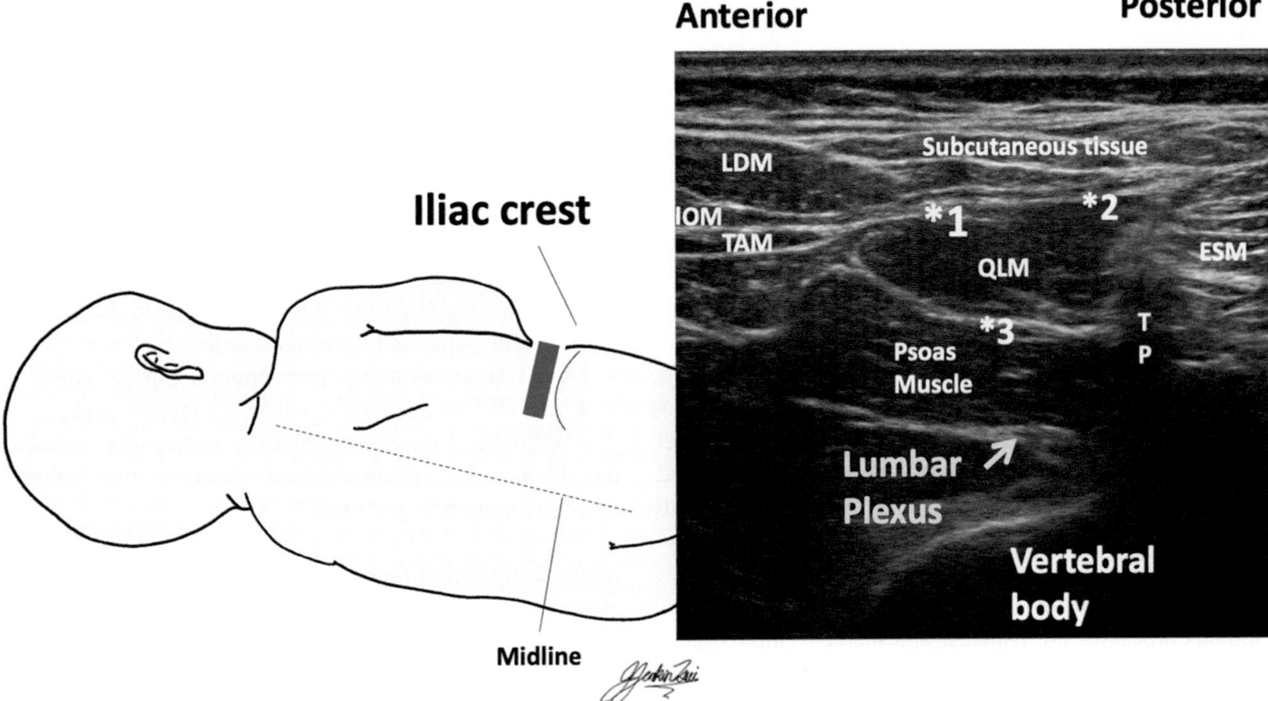

Fig. 76.9 Ultrasound image of the quadratus lumborum (QL) blocks. ESM, erector spinae muscles; *1 Lateral QL (QL1); *2 posterior QL (QL2); and *3 anterior QL (QL3) blocks

temic analgesia alone. The same evidence for other surgeries is limited. Although a meta-analysis of QL blocks compared to TAP blocks showed less opioid consumption with QL blocks after abdominal surgery, there remains a lack of large-sized randomized controlled trials directly comparing the different QL blocks to each other as well as to neuraxial, paravertebral, and ESP techniques for different surgical applications.

Peripherial Nerve Blocks

Paravertebral Block

General Considerations

The paravertebral block has become an increasingly popular alternative to epidural analgesia. It can produce somatic and visceral pain relief with fewer side effects on hemodynamics, urinary retention, neurological injuries, etc. The safety of this block is further improved with the use of ultrasound.

Indications

Common indications for thoracic paravertebral blocks include breast surgery, abdominal surgery, thoracotomy, and pain management for rib fractures. Bilateral blocks have also been used for sternotomy pain, cardiac surgery, and chest wall correction surgery (e.g., Nuss procedure). Lumbar paravertebral blocks are less frequently performed but have been reported in inguinal herniorrhaphy and lower limb surgeries.

Functional Anatomy

The paravertebral space is a wedge-shaped area located on either side of the vertebral column which contains the spinal nerves as they exit the intervertebral foramina. After exiting the foramen, the spinal nerve divides into ventral and dorsal rami. The dorsal ramus supplies the paravertebral muscles and skin of the back, while the ventral ramus forms the intercostal nerve which supplies the trunk in the thoracic region (or in the lumbar region, the lumbar plexus which supplies the lower extremity). The paravertebral space is bounded medially by the vertebral body, intervertebral disc and foramen, and spinous processes; anterolaterally by the parietal pleura in the thoracic region and psoas muscle in the lumbar region; and posteriorly by the anterior surface of transverse process and superior costotransverse ligament. The space communicates medially with the epidural space and, in the thoracic region, laterally with the intercostal space. When local anesthetic is deposited into this space, the ipsilateral spinal nerves can be anesthetized, producing ipsilateral somatic and sympathetic blockade similar to a "unilateral epidural." Blockade of several thoracic segments is possible due to contiguous spread to the vertebral levels above and below. Occasionally true epidural spread occurs due to the extension of the dural cuff.

Technique

Patient Positioning, Preparation, Equipment, and Dosage

This block should be performed with the child under general anesthesia or deep sedation. The child is placed in the prone or lateral decubitus position with the back assuming a kyphotic posture. The skin is cleaned with antiseptic solution.

Choices of local anesthetic include 0.125–0.25% bupivacaine. To achieve a vertical spread of 4–5 vertebral levels, a volume of 0.5 mL/kg with or without epinephrine (up to 15–20 mL on each side without exceeding the toxic dose) is required. If blocks are performed individually at each level, a smaller volume of 0.1 mL/kg (up to 5 ml) should be used. A 50–100 mm, 21-22G short-beveled needle is commonly used.

Landmark Technique

Spinous processes are palpated and marked. Surface landmarks are identified and can be correlated to various vertebral levels: the tip of the scapula (T7), the most prominent spinous process (C7), the intercristal line (L4) (L5/S1 for younger children), and the line between two posterior superior iliac spines (PSIS) (S1). In adults, the transverse processes are then marked at 1–2.5 cm lateral to the spinous processes. The distance of the needle insertion point lateral to the spinous process can be estimated based on the child's age using the equation below.

- Spinous process to space distance (mm) = 0.12 x body weight (kg) + 10.2
- Alternatively: 13.56 + 0.33 × age (years) + 0.06 x weight (kg) + 0.47 × gender (female = 0, male = 1) [6]

Unlike in the lumbar region where the transverse processes are located lateral to the corresponding spinous process, the transverse processes in the thoracic region are generally located at one intervertebral space higher than the corresponding spinous process because of the inferior angulation of the spinous processes.

The needle is inserted perpendicularly to the skin and advanced until contact is made with the transverse process. The needle is then redirected 10° superiorly or inferiorly to walk off the transverse process. Inferior redirection is preferred to minimize risk of vascular and nerve injury. Upon redirection, the needle is advanced deeper (up to a maximum of 1 cm) until a "give" can be felt as the needle punctures the costotransverse ligament. If an epidural set is used, a loss of resistance to air or saline can be elicited but an 18- or lower-gauge needle must be used. Alternatively, a "hanging drop" test can be used to verify that the tip of the needle is not intrapleural or in the lung if the patient is spontaneously breathing and cooperative. To perform the "hanging drop" test, place a drop of saline or local anesthetic at the top of the needle or the end of extension tubing connected to the needle with the opening aimed upwards. The patient is asked to take in a deep breath. If the drop is sucked into the needle on inspiration, this is considered a positive test and the needle should be repositioned. If the drop is not affected by inspiration, then the needle tip is not intrathoracic. Keep in mind that the "hanging drop" test cannot be performed while the patient is intubated and on positive pressure ventilation. A third method is to calculate the depth of the paravertebral space, which has been found to correlate with the patient's body weight using the following formula:

- Depth from skin to paravertebral space (mm) = 17.49 – 0.35 × age (years) + 0.55 × weight (kg) [6]

The lumbar paravertebral block is technically similar to the thoracic paravertebral block. However, the "hanging drop" test cannot be performed.

Nerve Stimulation Technique

Nerve stimulation is not a common technique used for paravertebral block placement. After the needle is inserted, a current of 1.5–3 mA is applied. The needle is advanced slowly, and appropriate motor responses (twitches in ipsilateral thoracic/abdominal wall for thoracic paravertebral block or twitches in the ipsilateral quadriceps muscle for lumbar paravertebral block) are observed while the current is decreased gradually. When a threshold current of 0.4–0.6 mA is reached, local anesthetic is injected after negative aspiration. If bilateral motor responses are obtained, it may signify intrathecal/subdural or epidural placement (with higher threshold currents) and thus the needle should be withdrawn.

Ultrasound-Guided Technique

A high-frequency (13–6 MHz) linear probe is used for in smaller children, while a curvilinear transducer (8–3 MHz) is used in larger children. The paravertebral space can be appreciated in the transverse and parasagittal views.

Transverse scan: With the probe in the transverse plane in the midline, the spinous process and laminae (with hyperechoic outline and acoustic shadowing) are identified. The transverse process can be located laterally. In the thoracic region, lateral to the transverse process is the hyperechoic pleura (Fig. 76.10). Needle placement should be in-plane under ultrasound guidance from a lateral to medial direction. The needle tip should not be advanced past the lateral edge of the transverse process as visualization of structures deep to the transverse process are hidden by acoustic shadowing. Advancing the needle tip past the lateral edge of the transverse process can lead to increased risk of dural puncture. The paravertebral block in the transverse scan is often easier to navigate in smaller children than in the parasagittal scan due to the narrow space between transverse processes and the steep needle angle required in the parasagittal scan. The

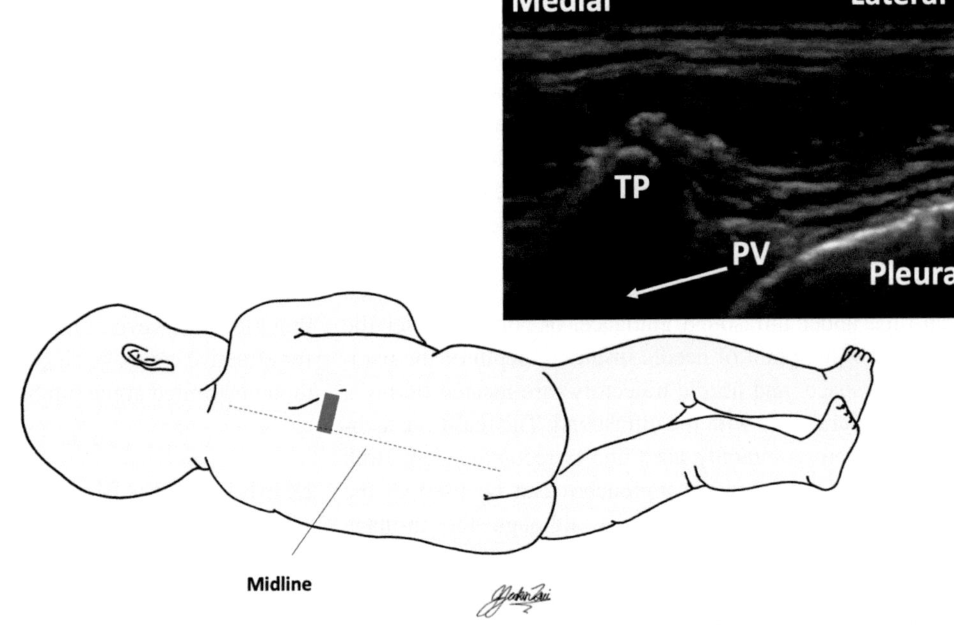

Fig. 76.10 Ultrasound image of transverse view of paravertebral block at T8–T9. *TP* transverse process, *P* Pleura, *PV* paravertebral block

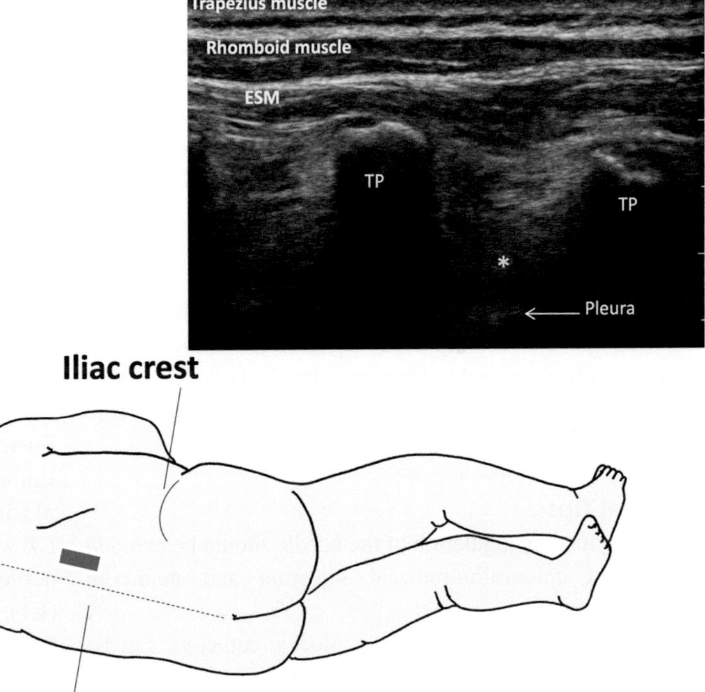

Fig. 76.11 Ultrasound image of parasagittal view of the paravertebral block at T8–T9. *ESM* erector spinae muscles, *TP* transverse process, * paravertebral space

transverse scan also allows for a greater length of catheter to be tunneled in the body to decrease the risk of accidental catheter dislodgment.

Parasagittal scan: The probe is placed longitudinally along the midline to locate the spinous processes. As the probe is moved laterally, the lamina, articular processes, and transverse processes (and then ribs in the thoracic region) can be located accordingly. In the thoracic region, the ribs often have a roundish hyperechoic outline with acoustic shadowing, whereas the transverse processes appear as tall rectangles (see the ESP block section). The pleura is seen as a deep hyperechoic line between the ribs/transverse processes (Fig. 76.11). The lamina appears as a sawtooth pattern with diagonal hyperechoic lines.

In the thoracic region, the paravertebral space can be found deep to the transverse processes between the intercostal muscle and parietal pleura. Occasionally, the superior costotransverse ligament (which forms the posterior border of the paravertebral space and is continuous with the internal intercostal membrane laterally) can be seen between two transverse processes. In the lumbar region, the lumbar plexus lies in the "psoas compartment" inside the psoas major muscles.

The block can be performed either with the needle inserted real-time under ultrasound guidance, or "offline" after the landmarks (the point of needle insertion, depth of the paravertebral space, and needle trajectory) are located during a pre-procedural scan with the ultrasound. The real-time technique is more commonly used and is recommended. Both in-plane and out-of-plane approaches can be used in the transverse and parasagittal scans although the in-plane approach is preferred for higher block accuracy. Local anesthetic is deposited into the paravertebral space after negative aspiration for blood or air. For thoracic paravertebral blocks placed under real-time ultrasound guidance, the pleura will appear to be downwardly displaced upon injection of the hypoechoic local anesthetic. If pleural depression is not clearly seen, the "hanging drop" test used in the landmark based technique can also be used as confirmation. In addition, vertical spread to adjacent levels can be seen on ultrasound imaging. For lumbar paravertebral blocks, the injectate is seen posterior to the psoas.

Complications

Potential serious complications may occur including unintentional epidural or intrathecal injection (resulting in total spinal anesthesia, postdural puncture headache, etc.), vascular puncture, systemic toxicity, and, in the case of thoracic blocks, pneumothorax.

Practical Tips

Excessive medial angulation of the needle should be avoided to prevent epidural/intrathecal injection and neuraxial complications.

In addition to single-injection blocks, catheters can be placed to provide analgesia by continuous infusion.

Literature Review

Compared to epidural or caudal epidural analgesia, paravertebral blocks demonstrate comparable analgesia with fewer side effects in the pediatric population. Paravertebral blocks also have superior analgesia over ilioinguinal blocks in children undergoing inguinal hernia repair, although paravertebral blocks, in theory, are more invasive.

The use of ultrasound can improve the accuracy of needle placement with visualization of local anesthetic spread while at the same time minimizing inadvertent puncture of pleura or neuraxial structures. Therefore, ultrasound-guided paravertebral blocks should be considered whenever possible.

The thoracic paravertebral block can be performed as a single injection with a larger volume of local anesthetic or as multiple injections of smaller volumes of local anesthetic. The dermatomal spread and duration of analgesia are not significantly different between the two methods of injection although the single-injection technique takes less time to perform and hence may be preferred. For lumbar paravertebral block, however, injection at each level is recommended for effective coverage since the vertical spread of local anesthetic is limited at the lumbar level.

Lumbar Plexus Block

General Considerations

The lumbar plexus block is also known as the psoas compartment block or the posterior lumbar plexus block. It is a deep regional technique that blocks the lumbar plexus as it runs within the psoas major muscle. The deep location of the lumbar plexus in adults often makes ultrasound visualization and performance of this block difficult. In children, the lumbar plexus is more superficially located facilitating clearer ultrasound visualization and easier block placement.

Indications

The lumbar plexus block can be used for surgery in the distribution of the lumbar plexus (e.g., groin, anterolateral and medial thigh, knee, medial part of the lower leg). When combined with a sciatic nerve block, the entire leg can be anesthetized.

Functional Anatomy

Embedded in the substance of the psoas muscle, the lumbar plexus is formed by the ventral rami of the lumbar roots L1–L4 with contributions from T12. The following individual nerves arise from the plexus: ilioinguinal and iliohypogastric (L1), genitofemoral (L1 and L2), lateral femoral cutaneous (L2 and L3), obturator (anterior divisions of L2, L3, and L4), and femoral (posterior divisions of L2, L3, and L4).

The psoas muscle can be divided into posterior and anterior sections. The anterior section originates from the anterolateral surface of the lumbar vertebrae while the posterior section originates from the anterior aspect of the lumbar transverse processes. The lumbar plexus lies between the two sections of the psoas muscle in a compartment known as the psoas compartment. The psoas compartment is bordered medially by the psoas major muscle fiber insertions (which insert onto the bodies of the lumbar vertebrae), posteriorly by the lumbar transverse processes, and anteriorly by the fascia iliaca.

Technique

The lumbar plexus block is traditionally performed using of anatomical landmarks and the plexus is located using either loss of resistance, paresthesia, or nerve stimulation. Recently there has been increasing evidence supporting the use of ultrasound for placement of this block. The relevant anatomy can be identified easily in children, and the location and depth of bony and muscular landmarks can be obtained. Insertion of the needle under real-time ultrasound guidance can improve the block's success rate and minimize needle-related complications.

Patient Positioning, Preparation, Equipment, and Dosage

This block should be performed with the child under general anesthesia or deep sedation. The child is placed in the lateral decubitus position (the side to be blocked facing upwards) with the hips and knees flexed. The skin is cleaned with antiseptic solution.

Choices of local anesthetic include 0.2% ropivacaine or 0.25% bupivacaine. A volume of 0.2–0.5 mL/kg (without exceeding the toxic limit) of local anesthetic is recommended. A 50–100 mm, 21-22G short-beveled needle is used. A nerve stimulator should be available with the ground electrode attached to the child's body surface if nerve stimulation technique is used.

Nerve Stimulation Technique

In Winnie's approach (Fig. 76.12), the needle is inserted perpendicularly to the skin at the intersection of the intercristal line (the line joining the upper borders of the iliac crests) and a line parallel to the midline and crossing the ipsilateral posterior superior iliac spine (PSIS). With the initial current at 1–2 mA (2 Hz), the needle is then advanced slowly until twitches of the quadriceps muscle are observed at a threshold current of 0.5 mA. A loss of resistance may be felt as the needle enters the psoas compartment. Local anesthetic is injected after negative aspiration. For children aged 3–12 years old, the skin-to-plexus distance correlates with weight and ranges from 1.24 mm/kg to 1.74 mm/kg.

Ultrasound-Guided Technique

Ultrasound scanning of the lumbar plexus can occur in the transverse or sagittal axis. For the sagittal scan in small children, a 13–6 MHz linear probe is placed longitudinally just lateral to the midline (in older children, a curvilinear probe with a frequency of 5–2 MHz should be used). After the sacrum is identified, the probe is moved cephalad to locate the L4/L5 and L3/L4 interspaces (Fig. 76.13).

Deep to the erector spinae muscle, the psoas muscle can be seen between the transverse processes. The plexus is located within the posterior third of the psoas.

For the transverse scan (Fig. 76.14), the probe is rotated 90° from sagittal view and placed along the intercristal line just above the iliac crest with a medial direction. In this view, the erector spinae muscle (superficial to the lamina and transverse process; lateral to the spinous process), and the quadratus lumborum muscle (lateral to the transverse process and deep to the erector spinae muscle) can be seen. Deep to the quadratus lumborum muscle is the psoas muscle, which appears slightly hypoechoic with multiple hyperechogenic striations (i.e., a "starry night" appearance). The lumbar plexus is located within the muscle belly as a hyperechoic structure.

In older children, it may be necessary to switch between the transverse and sagittal views to survey the area because the plexus may be difficult to visualize due to the greater depth and poorer differentiation between muscle and nerves. Occasionally, the more superficial L3/L4 interspace can be used for better resolution. Note that the lower pole of the kidney is usually found at L2/L3 level in adolescents and can reach as low as L4/L5 in young children.

The block can be performed either with the needle inserted real time under ultrasound guidance, or "offline" after the landmarks are located with the ultrasound. To perform the lumbar plexus block using a sagittal view with real-time ultrasound guidance, the needle can be inserted either from a

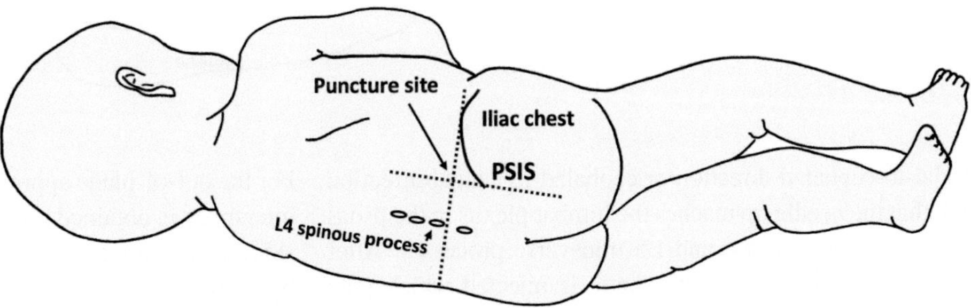

Fig. 76.12 Surface anatomy for lumbar plexus block. *PSIS* posterior superior iliac spine

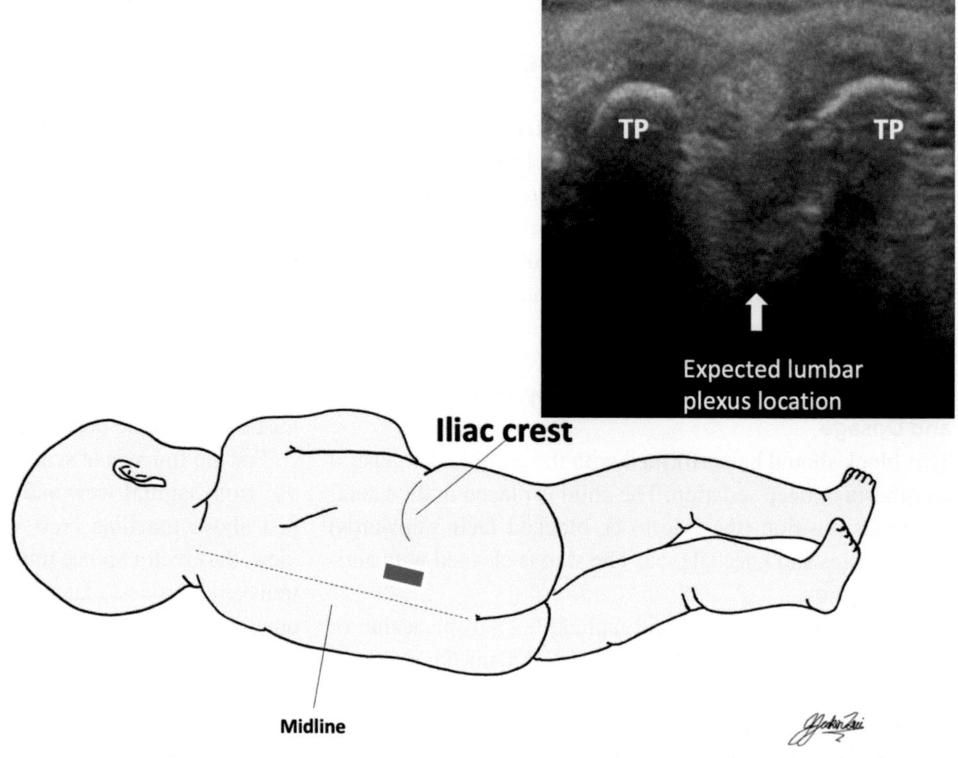

Fig. 76.13 Longitudinal ultrasound image of lumbar plexus at L3 and L4 transverse processes

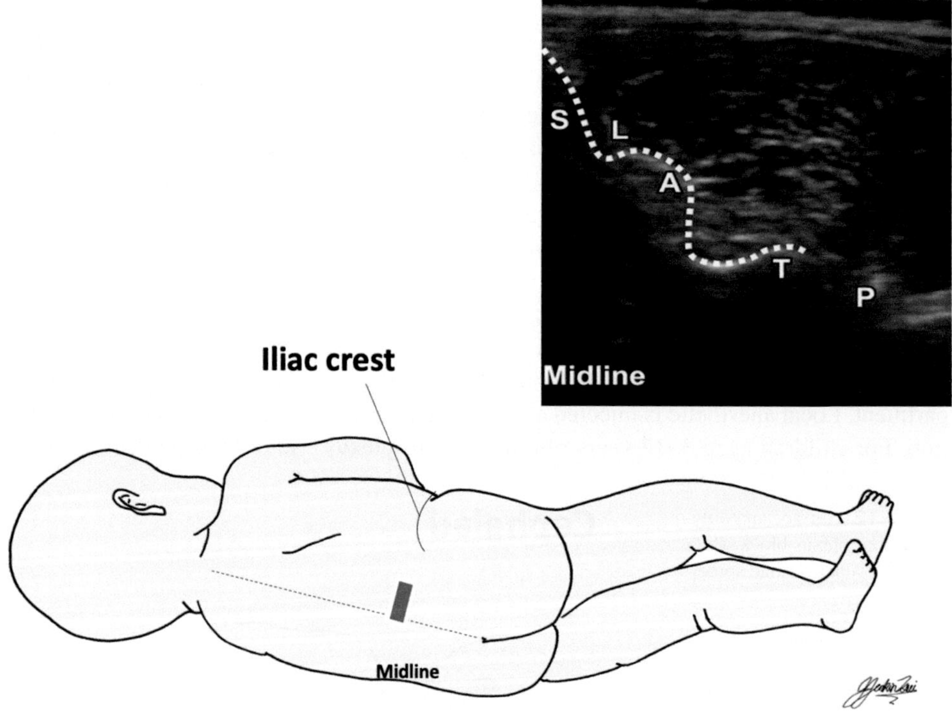

Fig. 76.14 Ultrasound image of major anatomical structures in the lumbar plexus. *S* spinous process, *L* lamina, *A* articular process, *T* transverse process, *P* psoas muscle

caudal-to-cephalad direction or cephalad-to-caudal direction such that the needle tip reaches the lumbar plexus in the psoas muscle between the L4 and L5 transverse processes. After negative aspiration, local anesthetic is injected which may create a "flow-like" pattern within the psoas compartment. For the out-of-plane approach, a transverse view of the L4/L5 interspace is obtained. The needle is introduced at 45–60° to skin, 1 cm from the caudad end of the probe. With the needle tip in view, walk the needle down to reach the plexus. The plexus is then confirmed using nerve stimulation.

To perform the lumbar plexus block using a transverse view with real-time ultrasound guidance, the probe is placed parallel to the intercristal line just above the iliac crest to visualize the abdominal wall muscles (Fig. 76.9). The probe is moved posteriorly with a medial angulation until the quadratus lumborum muscle is seen. From here, a "shamrock" pattern can be visualized: the L4 transverse process can be viewed as the stem of the shamrock, while the erector spinae, quadratus lumborum, and psoas muscles are the three leaves, arranged in a posterior-anterior direction. The lumbar plexus may be seen as a hyperechoic structure in the posterior aspect of the psoas. The probe is then tilted caudally until the L4 transverse process disappears, and the needle is introduced just lateral from the midline and advanced in a posterior-anterior direction under real-time ultrasound guidance to reach the plexus. Because the ultrasound beam is perpendicular to the needle, needle visualization should be excellent.

Complications

The lumbar plexus block is an advanced level block. Potential serious complications include retroperitoneal hematoma, injury to retroperitoneal structures (e.g., kidney, major vessels), systemic toxicity, and unintentional epidural or intrathecal injection. The use of this block should be well justified and is contraindicated in coagulopathic patients, especially when simpler and safer alternatives are present.

Practical Tips

Directing the needle medially may result in unintentional epidural/intrathecal injection.

Surveying the area with color Doppler decreases the chance of unrecognized inadvertent intravascular puncture or injection during block placement as the area is supplied by lumbar arteries and veins.

A combined approach with nerve stimulation and ultrasound guidance can improve accuracy and safety.

A catheter can be placed for continuous infusion of a local anesthetic for postoperative pain management in children undergoing hip, femur, and knee surgery.

Literature Review

The lumbar plexus block causes less hypotension with better postoperative analgesia in adults compared with spinal and general anesthesia. Large-sized randomized controlled trials to compare this block with other analgesic modalities in pediatrics are lacking.

Intercostal Block

General Considerations

The intercostal nerve block is a relatively simple and straightforward block. It blocks the intercostal nerve, producing a unilateral dermatomal band of analgesia for the vertebral level at which the block is performed. This block had been shown to produce effective analgesia with improved respiratory function in patients. However, for a large incision or multiple rib fractures, several intercostal blocks are required which may greatly increase the chance of pneumothorax and local anesthetic systemic toxicity, making the intercostal block less desirable compared with paravertebral or epidural blocks in such situations.

Indications

Common indications for the intercostal block include pain management for rib fractures, thoracotomy, breast surgery, pectus excavatum repair, hepatobiliary and gastric surgery, as well as minor procedures such as chest tube placement.

Functional Anatomy

The thoracic spinal nerves emerge from the intervertebral foramina and divide into the dorsal rami (which supply the paravertebral region) and ventral rami (which gives rise to the intercostal nerves). There are 11 pairs of intercostal nerves (T1–T11) and one pair of subcostal nerves (T12). Near the angle of rib, the intercostal nerve pierces the intercostal membrane to travel between the innermost and internal intercostal muscles. At the mid-axillary line, the intercostal nerve then gives rise to the lateral cutaneous branch, which innervates the lateral trunk, and terminates as the anterior cutaneous branch, which innervates the anterior trunk. Because the lateral cutaneous branch arises near the mid-axillary line, the intercostal nerve block should be performed posterior to the mid-axillary line (most commonly at the angle of the rib or at the posterior axillary line).

There are also variations among these intercostal nerves. The first thoracic nerve (T1) does not divide into lateral or anterior branches. It joins the C8 cervical nerve to form the brachial plexus. The lateral cutaneous branch of the second thoracic nerve (T2) (and some fibers of the third thoracic nerve (T3)) forms the intercostobrachial nerve which supplies the axilla and medial side of the arm. The lateral cutaneous branch of the subcostal nerve (T12) also does not divide. It joins the L1 lumbar nerve to form the iliohypogastric, ilioinguinal, and genitofemoral nerves.

The upper intercostal nerves (T2–T6) supply the thoracic wall, while the lower intercostal and subcostal nerves (T7–T12) supply the abdominal wall. Within the intercostal space, the intercostal nerve travels in the costal groove underneath the intercostal vein and artery.

Technique

Patient Positioning, Preparation, Equipment, and Dosage

The intercostal block should be performed with the child under general anesthesia or deep sedation. The child is placed in the lateral decubitus position (for unilateral blocks) or prone position (for bilateral blocks). The arm(s) are extended forward so that the scapula(e) are displaced laterally away from midline. The skin is cleaned with antiseptic solution.

Depending on the required duration of action, choices of local anesthetic include 0.25–1% lidocaine, 0.125–0.25% bupivacaine, or 0.1–0.5% ropivacaine. A volume of 0.5–1 mL of local anesthetic is usually adequate for each level. For small children, solutions using lower concentrations should be used to avoid overdose. Alternatively, epinephrine 1:400,000 (with a maximum dose of 4 μg/kg) can be added to decrease systemic absorption. A 50 mm, 22–24G short-beveled needle, attached to extension tubing to minimize movement of the needle upon respiration, is used.

Landmark Technique

The point of needle insertion is at the inferior border of the rib at the posterior axillary line, which runs midway between the mid-axillary line and the spinous processes (Fig. 76.15). With the fingers of one hand retracting the skin up and over the rib, the needle is inserted at a 20° cephalad angle with the bevel facing cephalad. The needle is advanced slowly until it makes contact with the bone and then redirected off the inferior border of the rib while applying a constant pressure to the syringe. A sudden loss of resistance can be felt when the needle enters the intercostal space. After careful aspiration for blood and air, local anesthetic is injected. Blockade of two dermatomes above and two dermatomes below the level of incision are usually needed for effective analgesia.

Ultrasound-Guided Technique

A high-frequency (13–6 MHz) linear probe is placed in a coronal plane along the posterior axillary line to obtain a longitudinal view of two ribs (Fig. 76.16). The ribs are characterized by hyperechoic outlines with acoustic shadowing. The intercostal muscle layers and the pleura can be found between the ribs (the pleura is distinguished by its sliding movement with respiration). Using color Doppler, the intercostal vessels can be found between the internal and innermost intercostal muscles. The intercostal nerve may be seen next to the vessels in this plane.

The in-plane approach is commonly adopted. The needle is inserted at the inferior end of the probe and directed cephalad to reach the inferior border of the rib. The tip of the needle is placed in the plane between the internal and innermost intercostal muscles where the nerve lies. However, the innermost intercostal muscle is not always clearly visualized with ultrasound. In this scenario, the goal is to inject local anesthetic just beneath the internal intercostal muscle to avoid pleural puncture. Thus, the internal intercostal muscle is the more important sonographic landmark. Hydrodissection can be used to confirm needle tip position. After negative aspiration, local anesthetic injection will cause the fascial plane to expand and push the pleura deeper.

Complications

Complications include pneumothorax, hematoma, nerve damage, and epidural spread. Total spinal anesthesia has been reported. If multiple blocks are performed, systemic absorption can be significant resulting in local anesthetic systemic toxicity.

Practical Tips

Because of the overlapping innervation from adjacent intercostal nerves, performing additional intercostal blocks one level above and one level below the site of the surgical incision or fracture is recommended.

Blockade of the T1 to T7 intercostal nerves may be technically challenging because of the scapulae. A thoracic paravertebral block can be considered instead.

A catheter can be placed to prolong the analgesic effect of the intercostal block but there is a high risk of dislodgment.

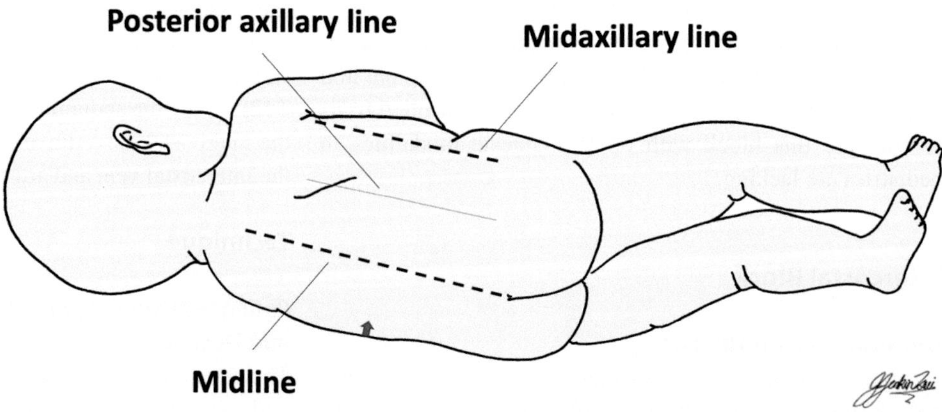

Fig. 76.15 Surface anatomy for intercostal nerve block (posterior approach)

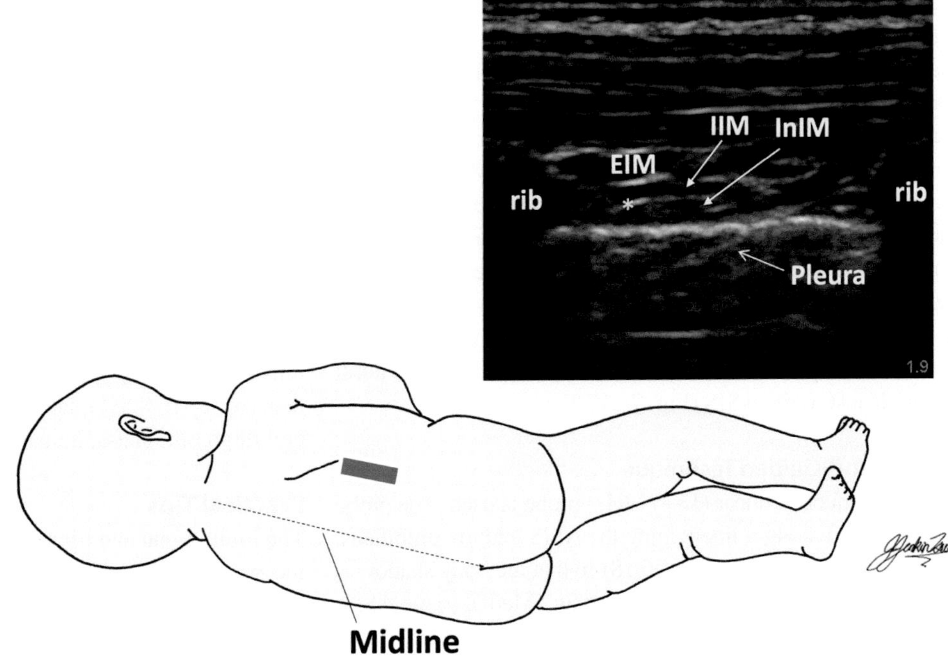

Fig. 76.16 Longitudinal ultrasound image of the intercostal space. *EIM* external intercostal muscle, *IIM* internal intercostal muscle, *InIM* innermost intercostal muscle, * injection site

Literature Review

Newer blocks such as the serratus anterior plane block and the PECS II block have been shown to be equally efficacious in post-thoracotomy pain management in children, compared with intercostal nerve blocks, with the additional benefits of being longer-lasting and easier to perform. Overall, there is a paucity of large-scale studies comparing the intercostal block to other analgesic modalities in children.

Ilioinguinal and Iliohypogastric Nerve Blocks

General Considerations

Ilioinguinal and iliohypogastric nerve blocks are one of the most commonly performed regional nerve blocks in pediatrics. They produce excellent postoperative analgesia, reduce the use of high-dose opioids, and facilitate early discharge of patients undergoing inguinal and lower abdominal wall surgeries. The use of ultrasound makes these blocks more accurate and safer.

Indications

Indications for the ilioinguinal and iliohypogastric blocks include procedures involving the inguinal region and lower abdominal wall (e.g., inguinal herniorrhaphy, orchidopexy, hydrocele repair). The two nerves can also be blocked by the use of a TAP or QL block.

Functional Anatomy

The ilioinguinal and iliohypogastric nerves are branches of the ventral division of the L1 nerve root (with contributions from T12 via the subcostal nerve). Superior and medial to the anterior superior iliac spine (ASIS), the nerves pierce the transversus abdominis to run in the transversus abdominis plane between the transversus abdominis and internal oblique muscles. The iliohypogastric nerve divides into a lateral cutaneous branch and an anterior branch, both of which pierce the internal and external oblique muscles. The lateral cutaneous branch supplies the gluteal region, while the anterior branch supplies the skin above the inguinal ligament and the suprapubic area. The ilioinguinal nerve, which has no lateral branch, travels anteroinferiorly and pierces the internal and external oblique muscles to enter the inguinal canal to supply the upper medial thigh, root of the penis, and scrotum in males (or labium majus and mons pubis in females).

Technique

Patient Positioning, Preparation, Equipment, and Dosage

This block should be performed under general anesthesia or deep sedation. The child is placed in a supine position. The skin is cleaned with antiseptic solution.

Choices of local anesthetic include 0.25%–0.5% bupivacaine and 0.2–0.5% ropivacaine. A volume of 0.3 mL/kg (or 0.2 mL/kg into each fascial plane if the nerves are not visible) is recommended. A 50 mm, 22G short-beveled needle is used.

Landmark Technique

One approach is to insert the needle about 0.5–2 cm medial and 0.5–2 cm below the ASIS. After the needle is introduced perpendicularly to the skin, it is advanced slowly until two fascial clicks or losses of resistance are felt as the needle passes through the external and internal oblique muscles (although often, only one fascial click is felt). Local anesthetic is injected after the first click (between the external and internal oblique) and the second click (between the internal oblique and transversus abdominis) after negative aspiration. Local anesthetic is deposited from cephalad to caudad in a fan-like pattern. Another 0.5–1 mL is injected subcutaneously upon withdrawal of the needle. Another approach is to draw a line from the ASIS to the umbilicus and divide the line into thirds. The needle should be inserted at the lateral third closest to the ASIS (Fig. 76.17).

Ultrasound-Guided Technique

A high-frequency linear (13–6 MHz) probe is used. The probe is positioned along a line joining the ASIS and the umbilicus, just medial to the ASIS (Fig. 76.18) so that the bony shadow is seen on one side of the ultrasound image. Medial to the ASIS, the external oblique, internal oblique, and transversus abdominis muscles are identified. The peritoneum and the bowel can be seen underneath the transversus abdominis. The ilioinguinal and iliohypogastric nerves can be seen lying side-by-side as two small hyperechoic ovals in the fascial plane between the internal oblique and transversus abdominis. Occasionally, the two nerves may pierce the internal oblique muscle layer at the ASIS level and travel more superficially between the internal and external oblique muscles. The deep circumflex iliac artery is often found adjacaent to the nerves and can be identified using color Doppler.

The in-plane approach is typically used with the needle inserted in a medial-to-lateral direction at the medial end of the probe and directed laterally at a shallow angle to avoid inadvertent bowel puncture. The needle is targeted to the plane where the nerves are seen. Hydrodissection can be used to confirm needle position. If the nerves are not well visualized, a fascial block can be performed by placing local anesthetic between the internal oblique and transversus abdominis muscles.

If the out-of-plane approach is used, the needle is inserted at 45° to the skin at the same distance as the depth of the nerves and "walked down" to reach the nerves while keeping the needle tip in view. After negative aspiration, local anesthetic is deposited.

Complications

Special complications related to this block include transient femoral nerve palsy with quadriceps weakness (with an incidence of up to 8.8%), lateral cutaneous nerve block with lateral thigh numbness, hematoma, and trauma to the bowel.

Practical Tips

The ilioinguinal and iliohypogastric blocks cannot be used as the sole anesthetic for inguinal hernia repair due to additional innervation supplied by the genitofemoral nerve and contralateral branches of the ilioinguinal and iliohypogastric nerves. Visceral pain is also not blocked, thus the spermatic cord and sac (peritoneum) are not anesthetized.

The T11 and T12 intercostal nerves also supply sensation to the inferior abdominal wall. It is important to block these nerves as well for inguinal hernia repair.

Literature Review

These blocks have been shown to significantly reduce pain associated with inguinal hernia repair.

The ultrasound-guided approach has been shown to produce higher success rates, better analgesia with smaller volumes of local anesthesia, and decreased complication rates.

Depending on the age and size of the child, the needle insertion point to ASIS varies. In a study involving 50 children of mean age 3.3 years and mean weight 13 kg, the mean distance from the ilioinguinal nerve to the ASIS was 6.7 mm.

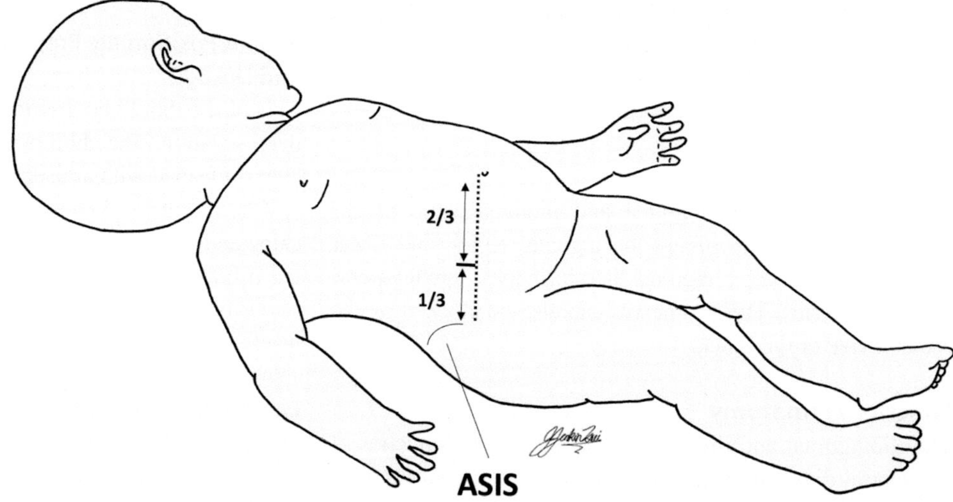

Fig. 76.17 Surface anatomy for ilioinguinal nerve block. *ASIS* anterior superior iliac spine

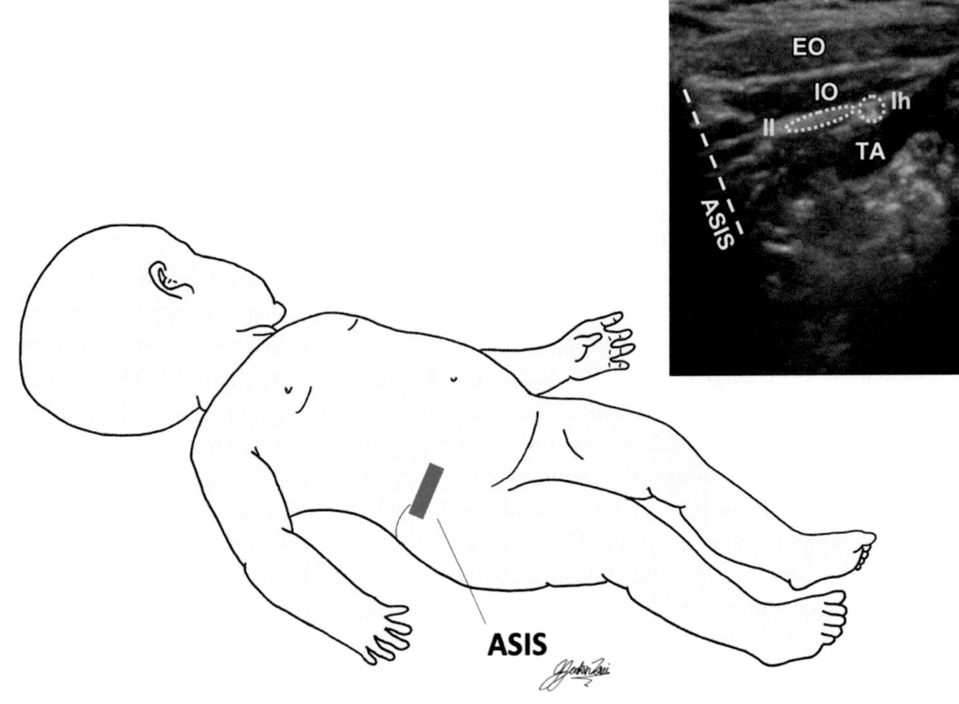

Fig. 76.18 Ultrasound images of the ilioinguinal and iliohypogastric nerves and major landmarks. *EO* External oblique, *IO* internal oblique, *TA* transversus abdominis muscle; *Il* ilioinguinal nerve, *Ih* iliohypogastric nerve, *ASIS* anterior superior iliac spine

Neuraxial Blocks

Epidural Anesthesia

Epidural analgesia is an effective treatment modality for postoperative pain. The epidural space can be approached at the thoracic, lumbar, or caudal level. Although both the single-injection and continuous catheter techniques can be used, the continuous catheter technique has the advantage of offering prolonged postoperative analgesia.

Lumbar and Thoracic Epidural Anesthesia

General Considerations

Placement of epidural catheters via the direct approach can be technically difficult for many reasons. Firstly, landmarks and the distance between tissue planes are small. Secondly, the ability to detect intrathecal or subdural placement is challenging (especially without fluoroscopy) as the procedure is often performed under general anesthesia or heavy sedation. Thirdly, despite the use of ultrasound sonographic visibility of the epidural space decreases for children over 1 year old. An alternative to the direct approach is to insert an epidural catheter at the lumbar or caudal level and thread it to the desired level. However, catheter advancement becomes more difficult in children over 1 year old because of the lumbar curvature.

Indications and Contraindications

Common indications for thoracic and lumbar epidurals include major surgeries involving the thorax, abdomen, pelvis, and unilateral or bilateral lower extremities.

Contraindications of epidural insertion include patient/parental refusal, coagulopathy, local infection or septicemia, uncorrected hypovolemia, and raised intracranial pressure.

Functional Anatomy

The spine anatomy in children is different from adults in many ways. In younger children, the conus medullaris ends at a lower level (L3 in neonates, L2–L3 in infants, L1–L2 in 1-year-olds) compared to adults (L1–L2). Similarly, the dural sac terminates at a more caudal position in neonates and infants (S3) compared to adults (S1). In neonates and infants, the spinous processes may be palpated as two bony structures because of incomplete fusion of the neural arches. Because the epidural space is loosely packed, an epidural catheter can be easily threaded cranially from the lumbar or caudal approaches to the thoracic level. The epidural block also has a faster onset in children as a result of the easier spread.

Technique

Patient Positioning, Preparation, Equipment, and Dosage

This block can be performed with the child under general anesthesia or deep sedation. The child is placed in the lateral decubitus position with the spine assuming a kyphotic posture. Alternatively, if the child is awake and cooperative, a sitting position can be adopted. The skin is cleaned with antiseptic solution and covered with sterile drapes. Sterile adhesive dressing is applied to the probe surface if an ultrasound technique is planned. The size of the Tuohy needle, catheter, and syringe are chosen according to the size of the child. A 50 mm, 19-20G Tuohy needle may be used for small infants while an 100 mm, 18G needle is more suitable for larger children. A nerve stimulator should be available if the epidural stimulation test is used (described later).

A loading dose of 0.3 mL/kg 0.1–0.2% ropivacaine or 0.125–0.25% bupivacaine/levobupivacaine is recommended for thoracic epidural and 0.5 mL/kg for lumbar epidural. This is followed by an infusion. A commonly used regimen is 0.2–0.25 mg/kg/hour for children 4 months or less due to decreased protein binding and alpha-1 glycoprotein levels in the setting of immature hepatic clearance while an infusion rate of 0.5 mg/kg/hour is more appropriate for children older than 4 months. The amount of volume is commonly a limiting factor when dosing epidurals in children. If epidural spread is a concern, the local anesthetic can be switched from ropivacaine or bupivacaine to chloroprocaine for both the loading dose and continuous infusion. Commonly used adjuvants include clonidine, dexmedetomidine, morphine, and ketamine. Table 76.4 contains a list of commonly used neuraxial adjuvants.

Table 76.4 Commonly used neuraxial adjuvants

Adjuvants	Dose
Clonidine	1 μg/kg
Dexmedetomidine	1 μg/kg
Morphine	10 μg/kg
Ketamine	0.5 mg/kg

Landmark Technique

The spinous processes are palpated along the midline. The relevant intervertebral space can be identified by the use of surface bony landmarks. For example, the most prominent cervical spinous process corresponds to the C7 vertebra, the inferior tip of the scapula corresponds to the T7 vertebra, the intercristal line intersects with the L4 vertebra in older children, and the line between two posterior superior iliac spines (PSIS) intersects with the S1 vertebra.

Both midline and paramedian approaches can be used. The paramedian approach is performed for thoracic epidurals since the midline approach requires an acute insertion angle due to the angle of the spines. In young children, however, the thoracic spinous processes are more horizontal, so the midline approach is still preferred for thoracic epidural placement because it is easier to master. If a paramedian approach is used, insert the Tuohy needle 1–2 finger breadths (patient's finger breadths) lateral to the cranial aspect of the spinous process and perpendicularly to the skin. The needle is advanced until contact is made with the lamina and then angled 15° medially. From there, the needle is redirected cephalad and "walked off" the lamina slowly into the intervertebral foramen while using a loss of resistance (LOR) to identify the epidural space. For lumbar epidurals, the midline approach is typically used. The needle is inserted between the two spinous processes and directed cephalad. It is then advanced slowly into the epidural space until loss of resistance is achieved. Although both saline and air can be used for the LOR test, saline is recommended over air to avoid the risk of air embolism and to give a more defined loss of resistance to the operator. If air has to be used in neonates and infants, the volume of air should be limited to 1 ml. In infants, identification of the epidural space by LOR is more difficult because the ligamentum flavum is softer so the characteristic "give" is less obvious. The hanging drop technique can be used, but it is less accurate in sedated patients in a lateral position. Alternatively, epidural placement can be confirmed by the electrical epidural stimulation test. For epidurals with a midline approach, the depth of epidural space from the skin can be estimated using the following formulae (although the most accurate assessment is still by the use of an ultrasound):

Rough estimate: Depth (mm) = 1 mm/kg total body weight

Depth (cm) = 1 + (0.15 × age in years)

Depth (cm) = 0.8 + (0.05 × weight in kg)

After negative aspiration for blood and cerebrospinal fluid, a test dose of 1.5% lidocaine with 1:200,000 epinephrine (0.1 mL/kg, max of 3 mL for thoracic epidurals, max of 5 mL for lumbar epidurals) should be administered. Blood pressure (an increase of SBP $\geq$ 15 mmHg, heart rate (an increase of $\geq$ 20 beats per minute), and ECG changes (>25% increase in T-wave amplitude, is the most specific) should be observed to exclude intravascular injection. Be mindful that while a positive result is always reassuring, a negative result does not rule out intravascular placement because the hemodynamic effects of epinephrine can be affected by many factors. Therefore, it is recommended that injection of local anesthetic should be performed slowly in small aliquots with intermittent aspiration.

Epidural Stimulation Test and ECG Monitoring Technique

The epidural stimulation test (Tsui test) is a simple test that is based on the current versus nerve-distance relationship. It is used to confirm correct positioning of an epidural catheter and exclude intrathecal, subdural, and intravascular catheter placement. It allows guidance of catheters (inserted via the lumbar or caudal route) to an appropriate position within two segmental levels. The test can also be applied to epidural needles to confirm correct needle placement. The Tsui test has a positive predictive value of 80–100%.

An epidural stimulating catheter is used to perform the Tsui test. An adapter is attached to the connector of the epidural stimulating catheter, and then the adaptor and catheter are filled with normal saline to enhance conduction. The cathode lead of the nerve stimulator is attached to the metal hub of the adapter, while the grounding anode is attached to the child's body surface (upper limbs for lumbar epidurals and lower limbs for thoracic). The nerve stimulator is initially set to a frequency of 2 Hz and a pulse width of 0.2 msec. The current is increased slowly up to 10 mA for lumbar and caudal catheters and 17 mA for thoracic catheters. By applying current to the catheter, motor responses of the corresponding segment are observed upon a current of 1–10 mA (or 17 mA for thoracic level). Presence of a motor response indicates that the epidural catheter tip is within 1–2 cm from the desired nerve roots and confirms epidural placement. If twitches are present with a current of <1 mA, the tip is either is abutting a nerve root or is in the intrathecal or subdural space. Normally the threshold current increases after a test dose of local anesthetic. Intravascular injection should be suspected if the threshold current remains the same after injection of the test dose. The location of the motor responses (upper limbs, trunk, or lower limbs) also represents the segmental level of the catheter tip. Table 76.5 shows the interpretations of various responses to the test.

In the ECG monitoring technique, a reference ECG waveform is obtained by placing the right-arm ECG lead at the target segmental level on the child's back (with the left-leg and left-arm leads at the standard positions). The lead is then attached to the metal hub of the electrode adaptor to obtain the epidural ECG waveform. If the catheter tip is within two vertebral spaces of the target segmental level, the amplitudes of the two waveforms will be similar. This technique is useful to confirm catheter tip position in paralyzed patients or when a local anesthetic has already been given via the epidural catheter. However, it cannot detect intrathecal or intravascular catheter placement.

Table 76.5 Motor responses and threshold currents with different catheter locations during epidural stimulation test

Catheter location	Threshold current	Motor responses
Epidural	1–10 mA (or 17 mA for thoracic level)	Unilateral or bilateral
Subcutaneous	N/A	No motor response
Subdural	<1 mA	Bilateral (many segments)
Subarachnoid	<1 mA	Unilateral or bilateral
Against nerve root	<1 mA	Unilateral
Non-intravascular	Threshold current increase upon local anesthetic injection	Unilateral or bilateral
Intravascular	No change in threshold current upon local anesthetic injection	Unilateral or bilateral

Ultrasound-Guided Technique

In neonates and infants, the largely cartilaginous posterior vertebral column allows neuraxial structures to be well visualized with the ultrasound beam. The visibility, however, decreases in children over 1 year old. The use of ultrasound allows for the evaluation of the location, depth, and needle trajectory to guide epidural placement. This reduces the number of puncture attempts with the possibility of improving safety. It also allows for confirmation of the catheter position and local anesthetic spread.

A high-frequency (13–6 MHz) linear probe is used. Occasionally, a low-frequency (5–2 MHz) curvilinear probe is required for deeper ultrasound visualization in older children. The lower lumbar region has the largest acoustic windows compared to the high lumbar or thoracic regions. The spine can be flexed to open the acoustic window for better visualization of the neuraxial structures. Common scan views are:

- Transverse view (Fig. 76.19): The probe is placed transversely over the spinous process. In the thoracic region, it may be necessary to tilt the probe cephalad because of the inferior inclination of the spinous process. In this view, the spinous process and lamina appear as an inverted "V" with hypoechoic shadows. In young children, circular hyperechoic lines are seen which represent the ligamentum flavum and the dura, although the ligamentum flavum may not be visible in some cases. Inside the spinal canal, the cauda equina fibers appear as hyperechoic dots surrounded by the anechoic cerebrospinal fluid. In the thoracic region, the oval hypoechoic spinal cord with a hyperechoic center (which represents the invaginated median sulcus) may be seen.
- Paramedian longitudinal view (Fig. 76.20): This view provides the best acoustic window and visibility of the dura. The probe is placed in a longitudinal direction slightly lateral to the midline and tilted medially to visualize the laminae (seen as slanted hyperechoic lines with acoustic shadows) with the intervertebral spaces in between. Within the intervertebral spaces, the hyperechoic ligamentum flavum and dura can be seen on either side of an anechoic CSF (or hypoechoic spinal cord in the thoracic region). Again, the dura is usually more visible than the ligamentum flavum. The cauda equine appears as a fibrillar structure at the lumbar level.
- Midline longitudinal scan (Fig. 76.21): The probe is placed in a longitudinal direction directly over the midline. Spinous processes are seen with interspinous spaces. The use of this view is limited in older children especially in the

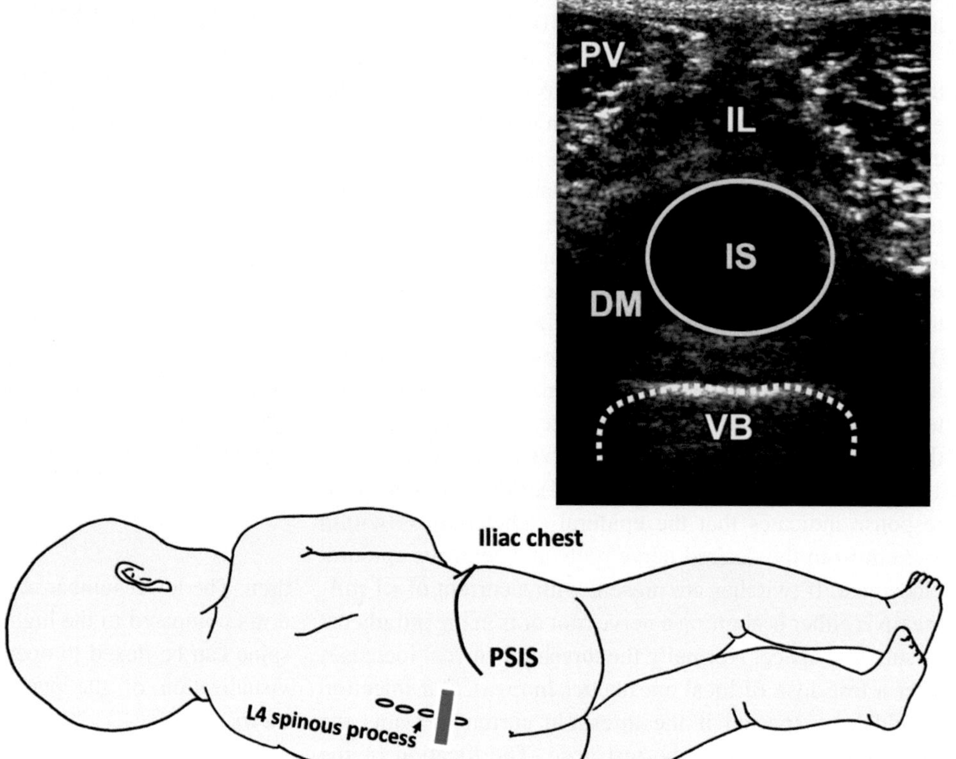

Fig. 76.19 Sonographic appearance of the transverse view of lumbar spine in a 10-year-old. *PV* paravertebral muscles, *IL* intraspinous ligament, *IS* intrathecal space, *DM* dura mater, *VB* vertebral body, *L* lamina

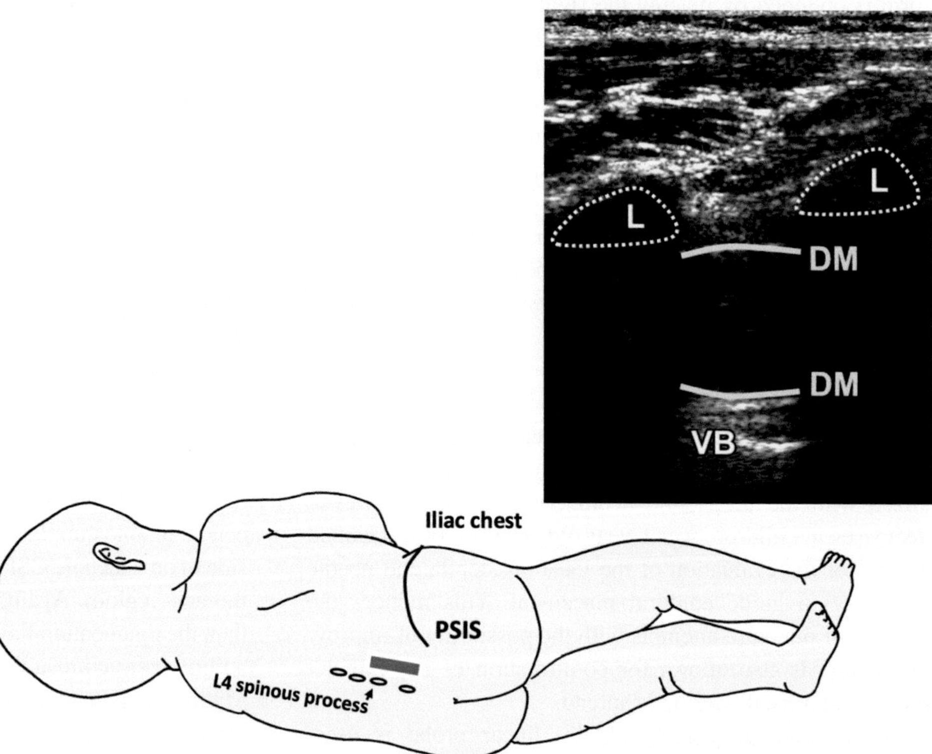

Fig. 76.20 Sonographic appearance of the paramedian longitudinal view of lumbar spine in a 10-year-old. *DM* dura mater, *VB* vertebral body, *L* lamina

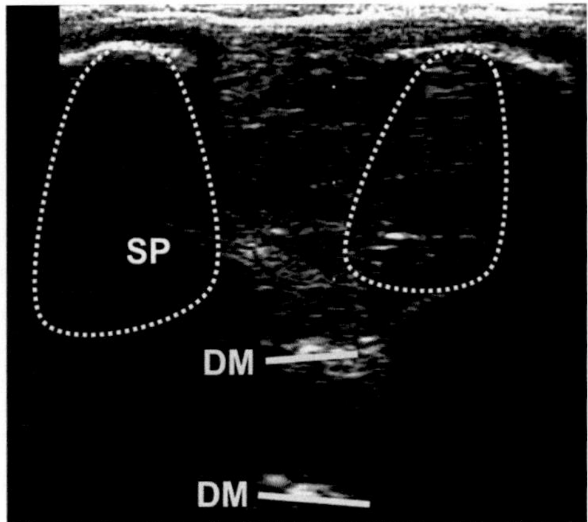

Fig. 76.21 Sonographic appearance of the midline longitudinal view of lumbar spine in a 10-year-old.; *DM* dura mater, *SP* spinal process

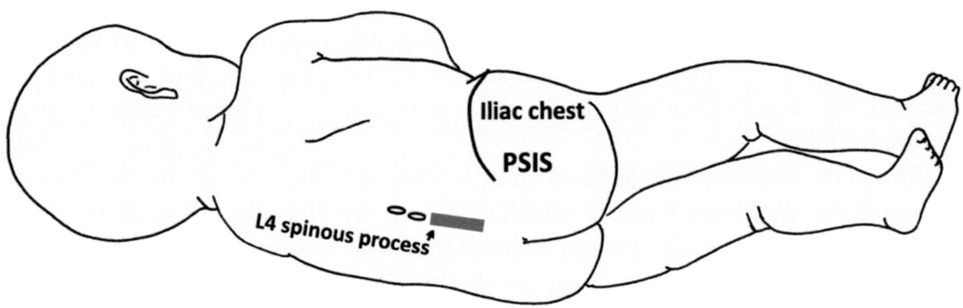

thoracic region because the long spinous processes obscure the acoustic window through the interspinous spaces.

Both "offline" (pre-procedural) scanning and real-time approaches can be used, although the latter may be most suitable in infants. For the real-time approach, the probe is placed in the longitudinal paramedian plane by an assistant. The needle is introduced at the midline. The needle is then advanced and is seen piercing through the ligamentum flavum into the epidural space under real-time ultrasound guidance, while at the same time loss of resistance is used. Once loss of resistance is achieved, the injection of saline should result in dural movement and widening of the epidural space. The epidural catheter can then be threaded into the epidural space. The tip of the catheter may be identified directly on ultrasound or indirectly by dural movement and local anesthetic spread.

For "offline" (pre-procedural) scanning, both the paramedian longitudinal view and the transverse view are used to survey the neuraxial anatomy and assess the location and the depth of the epidural space to provide guidance on the insertion point and needle trajectory prior to needling. The depth of epidural space is measured as the distance between the skin and the space between the ligamentum flavum and dura if both lines are seen, or the distance between the skin and dorsal side of the dura if only the dura is seen. Imaging studies have shown that the epidural space in neonates and infants is less than 2 mm wide.

Complications

Complications include nausea and vomiting, pruritus, post-dural puncture headache, urinary retention, neurological injury, paralysis, epidural hematoma, infection (cutaneous or neuraxial), catheter-related issues (e.g., kinking, occlusion, dislodgement), respiratory depression or apnea, high block or total spinal block, and local anesthetic toxicity.

Practical Tips

Although ultrasound imaging allows for real-time needle guidance into the epidural space, the simultaneous use of loss of resistance is still necessary because the differentiation between the needle tip and needle shaft can be difficult as the needle (midline) and probe (paramedian) are out of plane to the ultrasound beams. Alternatively, a true in-plane technique can be used with both the needle and the probe in the paramedian longitudinal planes, but its use in children is still under investigated.

Literature Review

A recent Cochrane review of 33 randomized controlled trials suggested that ultrasound guidance for regional blockade in children increased the block duration and decreased the risk of failed block and pain scores at 1 hour after surgery. There was no significant difference in the risk of minor complications.

Caudal Epidural Anesthesia

General Considerations

Caudal epidural blockade is one of the most widely used techniques of regional anesthesia in children. Single-injection caudal blocks are commonly performed to anesthetize the lumbar and sacral regions for urogenital and lower limb surgery. The analgesic effect can be prolonged with the use of a catheter. Under ultrasound guidance or the use of an epidural stimulation test, the caudal approach also allows for lumbar and thoracic epidural catheterization, which can be used as a safer alternative to a direct thoracic and lumbar epidural placement.

Indications and Contraindications

Caudal epidural bocks are commonly indicated in surgeries below the umbilicus (e.g., inguinal hernia repair), urogenital and anal surgery (e.g., circumcision, anal atresia repair), as well as lower limb surgery.

Apart from the contraindications listed under lumbar and thoracic epidural anesthesia, specific contraindications to caudal block include pilonidal cyst and spinal dysraphism such as tethered cord syndrome.

Functional Anatomy

The sacrum is a wedge-shaped bone with a base that connects with the fifth lumbar vertebra and an apex that articulates with the coccyx. In children, the five sacral vertebrae are incompletely ossified, so the sacral intervertebral spaces can be palpated. The dorsal surface is convex with a midline median crest. The sacral hiatus, which is a fissure created by the incomplete fusion of the fifth sacral vertebral laminae, marks the caudal opening of the sacral canal and serves as the accesspoint to the caudal epidural space. The sacrococcygeal membrane or ligament, which is made of tough fibrous tissue, covers the sacral hiatus.

Technique

Patient Positioning, Preparation, Equipment, and Dosage

The caudal block can be performed with the child under general anesthesia or deep sedation. The child is placed in the lateral decubitus position with the spine assuming a kyphotic posture (note that a prone position can be a more amenable position for catheter placement to the thoracic or lumbar levels). The skin is cleaned with antiseptic solution and covered with sterile drapes. Sterile adhesive dressing is applied to the probe surface if an ultrasound technique is planned. For a single-injection block, a 20G needle is used for older children (greater than 10 kg), whereas a 22G is used for children weighing 10 kg or less. A Tuohy or Crawford needle is chosen if a catheter technique is planned. If epidural stimulation is used, an insulated needle and a nerve stimulator are required. The nerve stimulator should be set to a low frequency (1–2 Hz) with a pulse width of 0.1–0.2 ms.

Choices of local anesthetic include 0.1–0.2% ropivacaine or 0.125–0.25% bupivacaine. For single injections, the recommended volume is 1 mL/kg of either 0.2% ropivacaine or 0.25% bupivacaine for coverage to the umbilicus. For coverage to the xyphoid, 1.2 mL/kg of either 0.2% ropivacaine or 0.25% bupivacaine should be used. For continuous infusions via a caudal catheter, the dosage and rate are similar to lumbar and thoracic epidurals.

Landmark Technique

The sacral hiatus can be located by drawing a line between the bilateral posterior superior iliac spines (PSIS), known as Tuffier's line, to form the base of an equilateral triangle where the apex is the sacral hiatus. Another way to locate the sacral hiatus is to first palpate for the coccyx. From the coccyx, the bilateral sacral cornua can be palpated by moving the hand in a cephalad direction. At the midpoint between the sacral cornua is the sacral hiatus which forms as a slight depression. Once the sacral hiatus is identified, the needle is introduced into the sacral hiatus at a 45 degree angle until a characteristic "pop" is felt as the needle is advanced through the sacrococcygeal membrane. The angle of the needle is then reduced to 20–30 degrees and the needle is advanced for a few more millimeters. Local anesthetic is injected after negative aspiration. Avoid advancing the needle too much as the dural sac ends as low as S3 in neonates and infants and excessive advancement will result in dural puncture.

Ultrasound-Guided Technique

A high-frequency (13–6 MHz) small footprint linear ("hockey stick") probe is used. A larger footprint linear probe is needed in older children. Common scan views are:

- Transverse view (Fig. 76.22): The probe is placed transversely at the S5 level. The sacral cornua appear as two hyperechoic humps. Two hyperechoic lines are seen between the cornua which represent the sacrococcygeal membrane (upper line) and the dorsal side of the pelvic surface of the sacrum (bottom line). The sacral hiatus lies between these two lines and is hypoechoic.
- Longitudinal view (Fig. 76.23): The probe is placed longitudinally at the midline between the two sacral cornua. The sacrococcygeal membrane appears as a thick hyperechoic bank sloping caudally. The hyperechoic dorsal surface of the sacrum can be found cephalad to the membrane, while the dorsal side of the pelvic surface of sacrum lies at the bottom. The sacral hiatus is identified as a hypoechogenic space between the sacrococcygeal membrane and sacral bone.

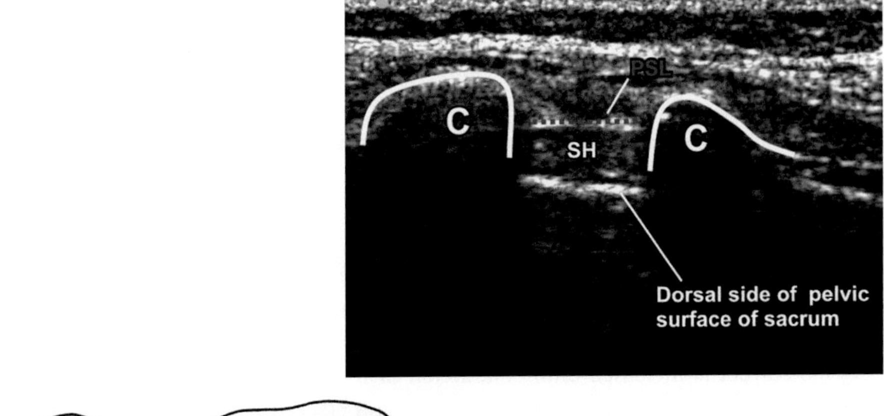

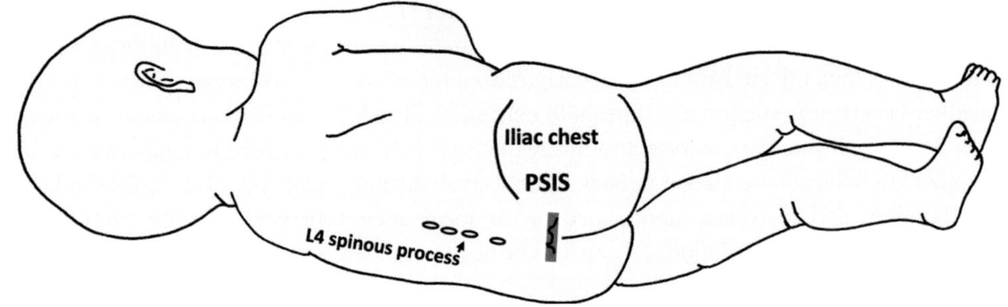

Fig. 76.22 Sonographic appearance of the transverse view of sacral region. *C* sacral cornu, *SH* sacral hiatus, *PSL* posterior sacrococcygeal ligament

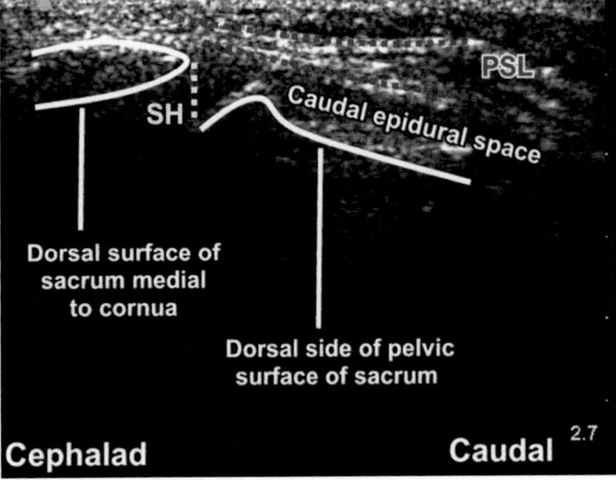

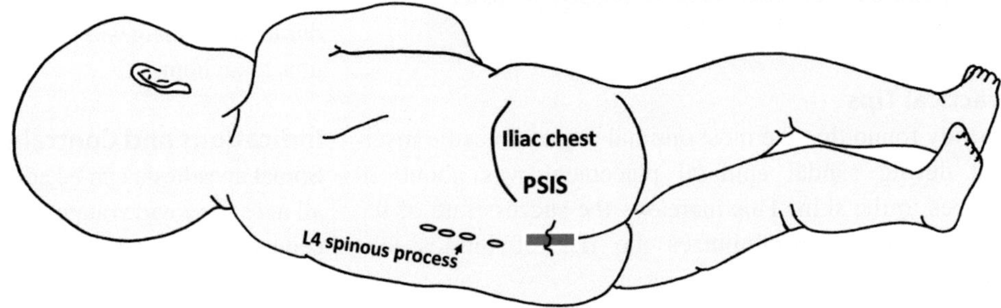

Fig. 76.23 Sonographic appearance of the longitudinal view of sacral region. *SH* sacral hiatus, *PSL* posterior sacrococcygeal ligament

After the sacrococcygeal anatomy is identified with the transverse view, the needle is inserted at the sacral hiatus. The probe is then rotated 90° to obtain a longitudinal view, and the needle is advanced in-plane toward the sacrococcygeal membrane and is seen piercing into the caudal epidural space (a characteristic "pop" is felt as the sacrococcygeal membrane is punctured). Switching back to the transverse view, the needle is seen as a dot on the screen between the sacrococcygeal membrane and the dorsal side of the pelvic surface of sacrum. A test dose with epinephrine can help rule out intravascular injection. Local anesthetic injected will be seen as an expansion of hypoechogenicity that causes movement of the dura.

To guide an epidural catheter through the caudal route, the probe is placed longitudinally over the lumbar or thoracic spine to capture the catheter during its advancement. In older children, however, the paramedian longitudinal view is needed because of the ossification of the spine. If the catheter cannot be seen directly, look for surrogate markers such as the movement of the dura and fluid expansion of the epidural space after saline injection.

Epidural Stimulation Technique

The epidural stimulation technique can be used to confirmed caudal needle placement. After a distinct "pop" is felt with the insulated needle indicating entry into the caudal epidural space, the current is increased until contraction of the anal sphincter (S2–S4) is seen. For correct caudal epidural placement, the threshold current should be within 1–10 mA. Local anesthetic is then injected after negative aspiration. Incorrect needle placement is suggested if threshold current is <1 mA or > 8 mA or if there are incorrect motor responses such as localized twitches in the gluteal or back muscles, subcutaneous bulging, and resistance upon injection of local anesthetic. The epidural stimulation test can also be used to guide a caudal epidural catheter to the lumbar or thoracic level within two segmental levels. Corresponding motor responses are observed which indicate the location of the catheter tip (see a more detailed description under lumbar and thoracic epidurals).

Although promising, the clinical value of the epidural stimulation test for caudal epidural placement has not been extensively studied. It may be more valuable as a supplementary test to other means such as ultrasound. There are other tests that can be used to confirm epidural placement. Verification by epidurogram is the gold standard but involves exposure to radiation and contrast agents. Acoustic tests such as the "whoosh" and "swoosh" tests can be used; however, their sensitivities and specificities are inferior to those of ultrasonography. The use of Doppler imaging has been reported, but more data is needed to determine its merits.

Practical Tips

A study found that the most optimal angle of needle insertion during caudal epidural placement was about 20 degrees to the skin. This increases the success rate of the caudal block and minimizes the risk of intraosseous injection.

Cephalad advancement of a caudal catheter becomes increasingly difficult in children over 1 year old due to development of the lumbar lordosis. If resistance is encountered while threading the catheter to a thoracic or lumbar level, injecting a small amount of normal saline through the catheter or flexing and extending the child's spine may help. If the problem still cannot be solved, the position of the catheter should be checked.

Complications

Complications of caudal epidurals are similar to those of lumbar and thoracic epidurals. Rectal puncture and sacral osteomyelitis have been reported with caudal epidural insertion. Local anesthetic toxicity can also result from intraosseous injection.

Literature Review

Large-scale prospective studies evaluating the superiority of ultrasound to landmark-based techniques in caudal blocks for children are lacking. However, the advantages of visualizing the sacral structures with the ability to confirm local anesthetic spread makes ultrasound an attractive option, especially in children with difficult anatomy.

Although lumbar and caudal epidural blocks produce superior analgesia for lower limb surgery, current literature still recommends the use of peripheral nerve blocks whenever possible (unless bilateral or multiple nerve blocks are needed and the toxic dose of local anesthetic may be exceeded) because peripheral nerve blocks produce equally effective analgesia with less complications.

Spinal Anesthesia

General Considerations

Spinal anesthesia in pediatrics is used primarily to avoid complications and risks associated with general anesthesia. It is generally performed in neonates or infants, especially preterm babies with a history of apnea, bradycardia, and/or chronic lung disease who have high risk of developing postoperative apnea or bradycardia if they receive a general anesthetic. In addition, there are concerns about the unknown neurotoxic effects of general anesthetic on the brains of preterm infants. Compared to adults, spinal blockade in children usually produces greater hemodynamic stability although the duration of analgesia is significantly shorter, about 30 minutes to an hour.

Indications and Contraindications

Spinal anesthesia can be administered to pediatric patients of all ages for a wide range of short (<90 minutes) surgical procedures, including lower abdominal (e.g., inguinal hernia repair), urologic, and lower extremity surgery. It has also been used for postoperative pain control in children undergoing cardiac surgery.

Absolute contraindications include patient/parental refusal, coagulopathy, local or systemic infection, hypovolemia, increased intracranial pressure, spinal abnormalities, degeneration or demyelinating diseases affecting the central nervous system, and presence of ventriculoperitoneal shunts or intrathecal catheters.

Functional Anatomy

The subarachnoid space is much shallower in children. At birth, the depth to the subarachnoid space is only 10–15 mm. This increases to 20, 25, and > 30 mm at 3, 5, and 10 years old, respectively. The cerebrospinal fluid volume is greater in infants compared to adults (4 mL/kg vs. 2 mL/kg), with a greater proportion in the spinal canal. Therefore, higher doses of local anesthetics are required for spinal anesthetics in infants, and duration of action is shorter.

As mentioned in the previous section, the spinal cord terminates at a lower position in neonates and infants; hence, the procedure should not be performed at a level higher than L4–L5 interspace to prevent spinal injuries. The spinous processes may be felt as two bony structures in neonates and infants because of incomplete fusion of the neural arches. The intercristal line crosses the L5–S1 interspace in neonates and infants and L4–L5 interspace in children older than 1 year old.

Technique

Patient Positioning, Preparation, Equipment, and Dosage

The skin puncture site can be topicalized by EMLA (eutectic mixture local anesthetic) cream (2.5% lidocaine and 2.5% prilocaine) 30 minutes to 1 hour before the procedure. This helps minimize discomfort and facilitate smooth performance of the procedure. Alternatively, an inhalational anesthetic or intravenous sedation can be given for the procedure, but caution is needed in preterm babies who are at risk of apnea.

With the help of a trained assistant, the child is placed either in the lateral decubitus or sitting position. In either position, the child is flexed at the knees and hips to open the spine for spinal insertion. Avoid excessive neck flexion which may compromise the airway. The skin is then cleaned with antiseptic solution and covered with sterile drapes. Sterile adhesive dressing is applied to the probe surface if an ultrasound technique is planned. A short 25–27G styletted spinal needle is used. An introducer is usually not necessary in neonates and younger infants.

Recommended choices of local anesthetic include isobaric or hyperbaric bupivacaine, levobupivacaine, tetracaine, and ropivacaine. A dose of 0.5–1.0 mg/kg of bupivacaine 0.5% or ropivacaine 0.5% is generally used in children less than 10 kg, with a dose towards the higher end of the range for smaller infants. In our experience, a dose of 1 mg/kg (= 0.2 mL/kg) preservative-free plain bupivacaine 0.5% will provide 60 minutes of surgical anesthesia for inguinal hernia repair. Adjuvants can also be added intrathecally to prolong the block duration (see Table 76.5). A 1 ml syringe can be used for injection of drugs.

Landmark Technique (Fig. 76.24)

Under aseptic technique, palpate the iliac crests and identify the intercristal line, which crosses the L5–S1 interspace in neonates and infants (or L4–L5 interspace in children older than 1 year old). Next, feel for the midline with spinous processes (two bony structures may be felt in neonates and infants). In neonates and infants, the block should be performed at either the L4–L5 or L5–S1 interspaces.

If the skin has not been topicalized with EMLA cream, infiltrate the skin with 1% lidocaine using a 27–30G needle. A midline approach is preferred. The needle is inserted perpendicular to the skin and advanced slowly into the subarachnoid space. The classic "pop" experienced upon puncturing the dura may be absent since the ligamentum flavum is soft in children. Remove the stylet to look for cerebrospinal fluid (CSF) flow. After ensuring that the CSF flow is smooth and without blood, inject the local anesthetic slowly (e.g., over a 15–20-second period).

To minimize development of high block, avoid the barbotage method during injection of the local anesthetic. Also, avoid elevating the patient's legs or trunk after the block has been administered. If a rapidly rising block level is observed, place the child in a reverse Trendelenburg position to avoid further cranial spread of the local anesthetic.

Ultrasound-Guided Technique

A high-frequency (13–6 MHz) linear probe is used. Occasionally, a low-frequency (5–2 MHz) curvilinear probe

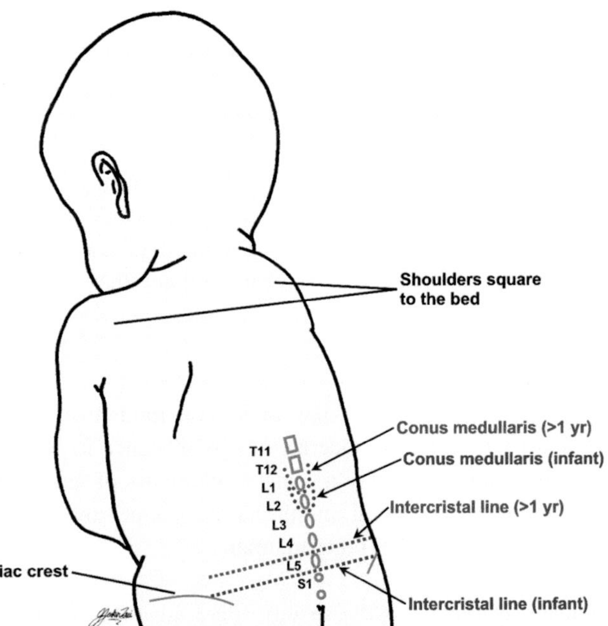

Fig. 76.24 Surface landmarks for spinal anesthesia. Positions of the conus medullaris and intercristal line are shown for infants less than 1 year old (blue) and children over 1 year old (red)

is required in adolescents for better penetration. As mentioned earlier, the sonographic visibility is best in infants and neonates and declines with increasing age.

Overall, there is limited literature concerning the use of ultrasound for spinal anesthesia in children. Theoretically, ultrasound can be used as an "offline" (pre-procedural) scanning technique to evaluate the relevant lumbar and sacral levels, the level of the conus medullaris, and the depth to subarachnoid space. Injection of local anesthetic with the use of real-time color Doppler may allow for confirmation of the intrathecal injection. Similar to epidurals, both the transverse and longitudinal views can be used.

Complications

Common complications include difficult spinal requiring multiple attempts, block failure requiring conversion to general anesthetic, and premature wearing off of the spinal block. Less common complications include postdural puncture headache, bleeding or hematoma, infection, allergic reaction, local anesthetic toxicity, and neurological injury or paralysis. Occasionally, bradycardia and high block are observed. Methemoglobinemia is a risk with the use of tetracaine and prilocaine.

Practical Tips

Assessment of a spinal block can be difficult in young and/or sedated children. Objective assessments utilizing the Bromage scale or cold stimulus can be used.

To avoid the devastating consequences of an epidural hematoma, a pre-procedural coagulation panel can be obtained, especially in former preterm infants in which coagulopathy is common and difficult to detect solely by clinical history. Test results should be compared to the age-specific ranges.

A single-shot spinal block usually has an approximate duration of 90 minutes. If the surgery is anticipated to be longer than 1 hour, spinal anesthesia alone may not be sufficient. Supplementary sedation or general anesthesia may be needed.

Literature Review

In a recent Cochrane review of several randomized controlled trials, there is moderate-quality evidence to suggest that the administration of a spinal (without use of sedatives) in preference to general anesthesia may reduce the risk of postoperative apnea in preterm infants.

Acknowledgments This chapter was written using Dr. Tsui's textbook, *Ultrasound and Nerve Stimulation-Guidance in Pediatric Regional Anesthesia* as a template. The authors thank Jenkin Tsui for providing original artwork for the figures.

Suggested Reading

Jankovic D, Wells C. Regional nerve blocks: textbook and color atlas. 2nd ed. Wiley; 2001.

Peutrell JM, Mather SJ. Regional anesthesia for babies and children. Oxford University Press; 1997.

Saint-Maurice C, Schulte SO, Armitage E, editors. Regional Anaesthesia in children. Mediglobe: Appleton & Lange; 1990.

Tsui BC. Atlas of ultrasound and nerve stimulation-guided regional anesthesia. Springer; 2007.

Erector Spinae Plane (ESP) Block

Adhikary SD, Bernard S, Lopez H, Chin KJ. Erector spinae plane block versus retrolaminar block: a magnetic resonance imaging and anatomical study. Reg Anesth Pain Med. 2018;43:756–62.

Almeida CR, Oliveira AR, Cunha P. Continuous bilateral erector of spine plane block at T8 for extensive lumbar spine fusion surgery: case report. Pain Pract. 2019;19(5):536–40.

Bonvicini D, Tagliapietra L, Giacomazzi A, Pizzirani E. Bilateral ultrasound-guided erector spinae plane blocks in breast cancer and reconstruction surgery. J Clin Anesth. 2018;44:3–4.

Cai Q, Liu GQ, Huang LS, Yang ZX, Gao ML, Jing R, Liu Z, Pan LH. Effects of erector spinae plane block on postoperative pain and side-effects in adult patients underwent surgery: a systematic review and meta-analysis of randomized controlled trials. Int J Surg. 2020;80:107–16.

Chin KJ, Adhikary S, Sarwani N, Forero M. The analgesic efficacy of pre-operative bilateral erector spinae plane (ESP) blocks in patients having ventral hernia repair. Anaesthesia. 2017;72(4):452–60.

Chin KJ, Lewis S. Opioid-free analgesia for posterior spinal fusion surgery using erector spinae plane (ESP) blocks in a multimodal anesthetic regimen. Spine (Phila Pa 1976). 2019;44(6):E379–83.

Chin KJ, Malhas L, Perlas A. The erector spinae plane block provides visceral abdominal analgesia in bariatric surgery: a report of 3 cases. Reg Anesth Pain Med. 2017;42(3):372–6.

De Cassai A, Andreatta G, Bonvicini D, Boscolo A, Munari M, Navalesi P. Injectate spread in ESP block: a review of anatomical investigations. J Clin Anesth. 2020;61:109669.

De Cassai A, Bonvicini D, Correale C, Sandei L, Tulgar S, Tonetti T. Erector spinae plane block: a systematic qualitative review. Minerva Anestesiol. 2019;85(3):308–19.

Elkoundi A, Bentalha A, Kettani SEE, Mosadik A, Koraichi AE. Erector spinae plane block for pediatric hip surgery -a case report. Korean J Anesthesiol. 2019;72(1):68–71.

Forero M, Adhikary SD, Lopez H, Tsui C, Chin KJ. The erector spinae plane block: a novel analgesic technique in thoracic neuropathic pain. Reg Anesth Pain Med. 2016;41(5):621–7.

Gürkan Y, Aksu C, Kuş A, Yörükoğlu UH, Kılıç CT. Ultrasound guided erector spinae plane block reduces postoperative opioid consumption following breast surgery: a randomized controlled study. J Clin Anesth. 2018;50:65–8.

Ivanusic J, Konishi Y, Barrington MJ. A cadaveric study investigating the mechanism of action of erector spinae blockade. Reg Anesth Pain Med. 2018;43(6):567–71.

Luis-Navarro JC, Seda-Guzmán M, Luis-Moreno C, Chin KJ. Erector spinae plane block in abdominal surgery: case series. Indian J Anaesth. 2018;62(7):549–54.

Macaire P, Ho N, Nguyen T, et al. Ultrasound-guided continuous thoracic erector spinae plane block within an enhanced recovery program is associated with decreased opioid consumption and improved patient postoperative rehabilitation after open cardiac surgery-a patient-matched, controlled before-and-after study. J Cardiothorac Vasc Anesth. 2019;33(6):1659–67.

Nagaraja PS, Ragavendran S, Singh NG, Asai O, Bhavya G, Manjunath N, Rajesh K. Comparison of continuous thoracic epidural analgesia with bilateral erector spinae plane block for perioperative pain management in cardiac surgery. Ann Card Anaesth. 2018;21(3):323–7.

Raft J, Chin KJ, Belanger ME, et al. Continuous erector spinae plane block for thoracotomy analgesia after epidural failure. J Clin Anesth. 2019;54:132–3.

Vidal E, Giménez H, Forero M, Fajardo M. Erector spinae plane block: a cadaver study to determine its mechanism of action. Rev Esp Anestesiol Reanim. 2018;65:514–9.

Yoshizaki M, Murata H, Ogami-Takamura K, Hara T. Bilateral erector spinae plane block using a programmed intermittent bolus technique for pain management after Nuss procedure. J Clin Anesth. 2019;57:51–2.

Pectoralis (PECS 1 & 2) Block

Blanco R. The 'pecs block': a novel technique for providing analgesia after breast surgery. Anaesthesia. 2011;66(9):847–8.

Blanco R, Fajardo M, Parras MT. Ultrasound description of pecs II (modified pecs I): a novel approach to breast surgery. Rev Esp Anestesiol Reanim. 2012;59(9):470–5.

Blanco R, Parras T, McDonnell JG, Prats-Galino A. Serratus plane block: a novel ultrasound-guided thoracic wall nerve block. Anaesthesia. 2013;68:1107–13.

Bossolasco M, Fenoglio LM. Yet another PECS usage: a continuous PECS block for anterior shoulder surgery. J Anaesthesiol Clin Pharmacol. 2018;34(4):569–70.

Hussain N, Brull R, McCartney CJL, Wong P, Kumar N, Essandoh M, Sawyer T, Sullivan T, Abdallah FW. Pectoralis-II myofascial block and analgesia in breast cancer surgery: a systematic review and meta-analysis. Anesthesiology. 2019;131(3):630–48.

Kim YD, Park SJ, Shim J, Kim H. Clinical usefulness of pectoral nerve block for the management of zoster-associated pain: case reports and technical description. J Anesth. 2016;30(6):1074–7.

Kulhari S, Bharti N, Bala I, Arora S, Singh G. Efficacy of pectoral nerve block versus thoracic paravertebral block for postoperative analgesia after radical mastectomy: a randomized controlled trial. Br J Anaesth. 2016;117(3):382–6.

Munshey F, Ramamurthi RJ, Tsui B. Early experience with PECS 1 block for port-a-Cath insertion or removal in children at a single institution. J Clin Anesth. 2018;49:63–4.

Schuitemaker RJB, Sala-Blanch X, Rodriguez-Pérez CL, Mayoral RJT, López-Pantaleon LA, Sánchez-Cohen AP. The PECS II block as a major analgesic component for clavicle operations: a description of 7 case reports. Rev Esp Anestesiol Reanim. 2018;65(1):53–8.

Shakuo T, Kakumoto S, Kuribayashi J, Oe K, Seo K. Continuous PECS II block for postoperative analgesia in patients undergoing transapical transcatheter aortic valve implantation. JA Clin Rep. 2017;3(1):65.

Yalamuri S, Klinger RY, Bullock WM, Glower DD, Bottiger BA, Gadsden JC. Pectoral fascial (PECS) I and II blocks as rescue analgesia in a patient undergoing minimally invasive cardiac surgery. Reg Anesth Pain Med. 2017;42(6):764–6.

Serratus Anterior Plane (Sap) Block

Biswas A, Castanov V, Li Z, Perlas A, Kruisselbrink R, Agur A, Chan V. Serratus plane block: a cadaveric study to evaluate optimal Injectate spread. Reg Anesth Pain Med. 2018;43(8):854–8.

Jack JM, McLellan E, Versyck B, Englesakis MF, Chin KJ. The role of serratus anterior plane and pectoral nerves blocks in cardiac surgery, thoracic surgery and trauma: a qualitative systematic review. Anaesthesia. 2020;75(10):1372–85.

Kunhabdulla NP, Agarwal A, Gaur A, Gautam SK, Gupta R, Agarwal A. Serratus anterior plane block for multiple rib fractures. Pain Physician. 2014;17:E553–5.

Kunigo T, Murouchi T, Yamamoto S, Yamakage M. Injection volume and anesthetic effect in serratus plane block. Reg Anesth Pain Med. 2017;42(6):737–40.

Liu X, Song T, Xu HY, Chen X, Yin P, Zhang J. The serratus anterior plane block for analgesia after thoracic surgery: a meta-analysis of randomized controlled trails. Medicine (Baltimore). 2020;99(21):e20286.

Madabushi R, Tewari S, Gautam SK, Agarwal A, Agarwal A. Serratus anterior plane block: a new analgesic technique for post-thoracotomy pain. Pain Physician. 2015;18:E421–4.

Moon S, Lee J, Kim H, Kim J, Kim J, Kim S. Comparison of the intraoperative analgesic efficacy between ultrasound-guided deep and superficial serratus anterior plane block during video-assisted thoracoscopic lobectomy: a prospective randomized clinical trial. Medicine (Baltimore). 2020;99(47):e23214.

Ohgoshi Y, Yokozuka M, Terajima K. Serratus-intercostal plane block for breast surgery. Masui Jpn J Anesthesiol. 2015;64:610–4.

Zhang X, Zhang C, Zhou X, Chen W, Li J, Wang H, Liu J. Analgesic effectiveness of perioperative ultrasound-guided serratus anterior plane block combined with general anesthesia in patients undergoing video-assisted Thoracoscopic surgery: a systematic review and meta-analysis. Pain Med. 2020;21(10):2412–22.

Transversus Thoracic Muscle Plane (TTMP) Block

Fujii S, Bairagi R, Roche M, Zhou JR. Transversus Thoracis muscle plane block. Biomed Res Int. 2019;2019:1716365.

Nakanishi T, Yoshimura M, Toriumi T. Pectoral nerve II block, transversus thoracic muscle plane block, and dexmedetomidine for breast surgery in a patient with achondroplasia: a case report. JA Clin Rep. 2019;5(1):47.

Ueshima H, Hara E, Marui T, Otake H. The ultrasound-guided transversus thoracic muscle plane block is effective for the median sternotomy. J Clin Anesth. 2016;29:83.

Ueshima H, Hiroshi O. Clinical experiences of ultrasound-guided transversus thoracic muscle plane block for children. J Clin Anesth. 2017a;40:23.

Ueshima H, Hiroshi O. Comparison of spread of transversus thoracic plane block by sagittal and transverse approach in a clinical setting. J Clin Anesth. 2017b;43:4–5.

Ueshima H, Kitamura A. Blocking of multiple anterior branches of intercostal nerves (Th2-6) using a transversus thoracic muscle plane block. Reg Anesth Pain Med. 2015a;40(4):388.

Ueshima H, Kitamura A. Clinical experiences of ultrasound-guided transversus thoracic muscle plane block: a clinical experience. J Clin Anesth. 2015b;27(5):428–9.

Ueshima H, Otake H. Ultrasound-guided transversus thoracic muscle plane block: complication in 299 consecutive cases. J Clin Anesth. 2017a;41:60.

Ueshima H, Otake H. Continuous transversus thoracic muscle plane block is effective for the median sternotomy. J Clin Anesth. 2017b;37:174.

Ueshima H, Takeda Y, Ishikawa S, Otake H. Ultrasound-guided transversus thoracic muscle plane block: a cadaveric study of the spread of injectate. J Clin Anesth. 2015;27:696.

Parasternal Intercostal Nerve Block

Chaudhary V, Chauhan S, Choudhury M, et al. Parasternal intercostal block with ropivacaine for postoperative analgesia in pediatric patients undergoing cardiac surgery: a double-blind, randomized, controlled study. J Cardiothorac Vasc Anesth. 2012;26:439–42.

Ellouze O, Missaoui A, Berthoud V, Bouhemad B, Guinot PG. Parasternal pectoral block for right anterior minimally invasive thoracotomy in cardiac surgery. J Cardiothorac Vasc Anesth. 2020;34(2):450–3.

McDonald SB, Jacobsohn E, Kopacz DJ, et al. Parasternal block and local anesthetic infiltration with levobupivacaine after cardiac surgery with desflurane: the effect on postoperative pain, pulmonary function, and tracheal extubation times. Anesth Analg. 2005;100:25–32.

Ohgoshi Y, Ino K, Matsukawa M. Ultrasound-guided parasternal intercostal nerve block. J Anesth. 2016;30(5):916.

Piraccini E, Biondi G, Corso RM, Maitan S. The use of rhomboid intercostal block, parasternal block and erector spinae plane block for breast surgery. J Clin Anesth. 2020;59:10.

Piraccini E, Calli M, Corso RM, Maitan S. Pectointercostal fascial block (PIFB) and parasternal block (PSB): two names for the same block? J Clin Anesth. 2019;58:130.

Raza I, Narayanan M, Venkataraju A, Ciocarlan A. Bilateral subpectoral interfascial plane catheters for analgesia for sternal fractures: a case report. Reg Anesth Pain Med. 2016;41:607–9.

Transversus Abdominis Plane (TAP) Block

Borglum J, et al. Ultrasound-guided bilateral dual transversus abdominis plane block: a new four-point approach. Acta Anaesthesiol Scand. 2011;55(6):658–63.

Carney J, et al. Ipsilateral transversus abdominis plane block provides effective analgesia after appendectomy in children: a randomized controlled trial. Anesth Analg. 2010 Oct;111(4):998–1003.

Hamill JK, et al. Rectus sheath and transversus abdominis plane blocks in children: a systemic review and meta-analysis of randomized trials. Paediatric Anaesth. 2016;26(4):363–71.

Hebbard P, et al. Subcostal transversus abdominis plane block under ultrasound guidance. Anesth Analg. 2008;106(2):674–5.

Jankovic ZB, et al. An anatomical study of the transversus abdominis plane block: location of the lumbar triangle of petit and adjacent nerves. Anesth Analg. 2009;109:981–5.

Laghari ZA, Harmon D. Ultrasound-guided transabdominus plane block. J Clin Anesth. 2008;20:156–8.

Long JB, et al. Transversus abdominis plane block in children: a multicenter safety analysis of 1994 cases from the PRAN (pediatric regional anesthesia network) database. Anesth Analg. 2014;119(2):395–9.

Rafi AN. Abdominal field block: a new approach via the lumbar triangle. Anaesthesia. 2001;56:1024–6.

Rectus Sheath Block

Dingeman RS, et al. Ultrasonography-guided bilateral rectus sheath block vs local anesthetic infiltration after pediatric umbilical hernia repair: a prospective randomized clinical trial. JAMA Surg. 2013;148(8):707–13.

Flack SH, et al. Ultrasound-guided rectus sheath block or wound infiltration in children: a randomized blinded study of analgesia and bupivacaine absorption. Paediatr Anaesth. 2014;24(9):968–73.

Gurnaney HG, et al. Prospective randomized observer-blinded study comparing the analgesic efficacy of ultrasound-guided rectus sheath block and local anaesthetic infiltration for umbilical hernia repair. Br J Anaesth. 2011;107(5):790–5.

de Jose MB, Gotzens V, Mabrok M. Ultrasound-guided umbilical nerve block in children: a brief description of a new approach. PaediatrAnaesth. 2007;17:44–50.

Purdy M, et al. A prospective, randomized, open label, controlled study investigating the efficiency and safety of 3 different methods of rectus sheath block analgesia following midline laparotomy. Medicine. 2018;97:e9968.

Skinner AV, et al. Rectus sheath block: successful use in the chronic pain management of pediatric abdominal wall pain. Paediatr Anaesth. 2007;17:1203–11.

Willschke H, Bosenberg A, Marhofer P, Johnston S, Kettner SC, Wanzel O, Kapral S. Ultrasonography-guided rectus sheath block in paediatric anaesthesia--a new approach to an old technique. BrJ Anaesth. 2006;97:244–9.

Quadratus Lumborum (QL) Block

Blanco R. TAP block under ultrasound guidance: the description of a 'non-pop-technique'. Reg Anaesth Pain Med. 2007;32(Suppl 1):130.

Blanco R, Ansari T, Riad W, Shetty N. Quadratus Lumborum block versus transversus abdominis plane block for postoperative pain after cesarean delivery: a randomized controlled trial. Reg Anesth Pain Med. 2016;41(6):757–62.

Carline L, McLeod GA, Lamb C. A cadaver study comparing spread of dye and nerve involvement after three different quadratus lumborum blocks. Br J Anaesth. 2016;117:387–94.

Elsharkawy H, El-Boghdadly K, Kolli S, Esa WAS, DeGrande S, Soliman LM, Drake RL. Injectate spread following anterior sub-costal and posterior approaches to the quadratus lumborum block: a comparative cadaveric study. Eur J Anaesthesiol. 2017;34(9):587–95.

Hernandez MA, Vecchione T, Boretsky K. Dermatomal spread following posterior transversus abdominis plane block in pediatric patients: our initial experience. Paediatr Anaesth. 2017;27(3):300–4.

Ishio J, Komasawa N, Kido H, Minami T. Evaluation of ultrasound-guided posterior quadratus lumborum block for postoperative analgesia after laparoscopic gynecologic surgery. J Clin Anesth. 2017;41:1–4.

Jin Z, Liu J, Li R, Gan TJ, He Y, Lin J. Single injection quadratus Lumborum block for postoperative analgesia in adult surgical population: a systematic review and meta-analysis. J Clin Anesth. 2020;62:109715.

Liu X, Song T, Chen X, Zhang J, Shan C, Chang L, Xu H. Quadratus lumborum block versus transversus abdominis plane block for postoperative analgesia in patients undergoing abdominal surgeries: a systematic review and meta-analysis of randomized controlled trials. BMC Anesthesiol. 2020a;20(1):53.

Liu X, Song T, Chen X, Zhang J, Shan C, Chang L, Xu H. Quadratus lumborum block versus transversus abdominis plane block for postoperative analgesia in patients undergoing abdominal surgeries: a systematic review and meta-analysis of randomized controlled trials. BMC Anesthesiol. 2020b;20(1):53.

Öksüz G, Bilal B, Gürkan Y, Urfalioğlu A, Arslan M, Gişi G, Öksüz H. Quadratus Lumborum block versus transversus abdominis plane block in children undergoing low abdominal surgery: a randomized controlled trial. Reg Anesth Pain Med. 2017;42(5):674–9.

Parras T, Blanco R. Randomised trial comparing the transversus abdominis plane block posterior approach or quadratus lumborum block type I with femoral block for postoperative analgesia in femoral neck fracture, both ultrasound-guided. Rev Esp Anestesiol Reanim. 2016;63:141–8.

Sato M. Ultrasound-guided quadratus lumborum block compared to caudal ropivacaine/morphine in children undergoing surgery for vesicoureteric reflex. Paediatr Anaesth. 2019;29(7):738–43.

Sindwani G, Sahu S, Suri A, Sureka S, Thomas M. Efficacy of ultrasound guided quadratus lumborum block as postoperative analgesia in renal transplantation recipients: a randomised double blind clinical study. Indian J Anaesth. 2020;64(7):605–10.

Ueshima H, Yoshiyama S, Otake H. The ultrasound-guided continuous transmuscular quadratus lumborum block is an effective analgesia for total hip arthroplasty. J Clin Anesth. 2016;31:35.

Visoiu M, Pan S. Quadratus lumborum blocks: two cases of associated hematoma. Paediatr Anaesth. 2019;29(3):286–8.

Yousef NK. Quadratus Lumborum block versus transversus abdominis plane block in patients undergoing Total abdominal hysterectomy: a randomized prospective controlled trial. Anesth Essays Res. 2018;12(3):742–7.

Paravertebral Block

Ben-Ari A, et al. Ultrasound-guided paravertebral block using an intercostal approach. Anesth Analg. 2009;109:1691–4.

Conacher ID. Resin injection of thoracic paravertebral spaces. Br J Anaesth. 1988;61:657–61.

Jiashan Q, et al. A prospective randomized observer-blinded study to assess postoperative analgesia provided by an ultrasound-guided bilateral thoracic paravertebral block for children undergoing the Nuss procedure. Reg Anesth Pain Med. 2014;39(3):208–13.

Karmakar MK. Thoracic paravertebral block. Anesthesiology. 2001;95:771–80.

Krediet AC, et al. Different approaches to ultrasound-guided thoracic paravertebral block: an illustrated review. Anesthesiology Aug. 2015;123:459–74.

Yoo SH, Lee DH, Moon DE, Song HK, Jang Y, Kim JB. Anatomical investigations for appropriate needle positioning for thoracic paravertebral blockade in children. J Int Med Res. 2012;40(6):2370–2380.

Lonnqvist PA. Continuous paravertebral block in children. Initial Exp Anaesthesia. 1992;47:607–9.

Luyet C, et al. The location of paravertebral catheters placed using the landmark technique. Anaesthesia. 2012;67:1321–6.

Narasimhan P, et al. Comparison of caudal epidural block with paravertebral block for renal surgeries in pediatric patients: a prospective randomize, blinded clinical trial. J Clin Anesth. 2019 Feb;52:105–10.

Page EA, et al. Paravertebral block in paediatric abdominal surgery – a systematic review and meta-analysis of randomized trials. Br J Anaesth. 2017;118(2):159–66.

Purcell-Jones G, et al. Paravertebral somatic nerve block: a clinical, radiographic, and computed tomographic study in chronic pain patients. Anesth Analg. 1989;68:32–9.

Shibata Y, et al. Ultrasound-guided intercostal approach to thoracic paravertebral block. Anesth Analg. 2009;109:996–7.

Uppal V, et al. Single-injection versus multiple-injection technique of ultrasound-guided paravertebral blocks: a randomized controlled study comparing dermatomal spread. Reg Anesth Pain Med. 2017;42:575–81.

Xie J, et al. Comparison of regional analgesia techniques for pleurodesis pain in pediatric patients. Paediatr Anaesth. 2020;30(10):1102–8.

Yoo SH, et al. Anatomical investigations for appropriate needle positioning for thoracic paravertebral blockade in children. J Int Med Res. 2012;40(6):2370–80.

Lumbar Plexus Block

Chayen D, Nathan H, Chayen M. The psoas compartment block. Anesthesiology. 1976;45:95–9.

De Visme V, et al. Combined lumbar and sacral plexus block compared with plain bupivacaine spinal anesthesia for hip fractures in the elderly. Reg Anesth Pain Med. 2000;25:158–62.

Ganidagli S, et al. The comparison of two lower extremity block techniques combined with sciatic block: 3-in-1 femoral block vs psoas compartment block. Int J Clin Pract. 2005;59:771–6.

Jankowski CJ, et al. A comparison of psoas compartment block and spinal and general anesthesia for outpatient knee arthroscopy. Anesth Analg. 2003;97:1003–9.

Karmakar MK, Ho AM, Li X, et al. Ultrasound-guided lumbar plexus block through the acoustic window of the lumbar ultrasound trident. Br J Anaesth. 2008;100:533–7.

Kirchmair L, Enna B, Marhofer P, Kapral S. The right thing in the right place: lumbar plexus block in children. Anesthesiology. 2005;102:865–6.

Kirchmair L, Enna B, Mitterschiffthaler G, Moriggl B, Greher M, Marhofer P, Kapral S, Gassner I. Lumbar plexus in children. A sonographic study and its relevance to pediatric regional anesthesia. Anesthesiology. 2004a;101:445–50.

Kirchmair L, Entner T, Kapral S, Mitterschiffhaler G. Ultrasound guidance for the psoas compartment block: an imaging study. Anesth Analg. 2002;94:706–10.

Kirchmair L, et al. Lumbar plexus in children. A sonographic study and its relevance to pediatric regional anesthesia. Anesthesiology. 2004b;101(2):445–50.

Morimoto M, Kim JT, Popovic J, et al. Ultrasound-guided lumbar plexus block for open reduction and internal fixation of hip fracture. Pain Prac. 2006;6(2):124–6.

Nielsen MV, et al. Superiority of ultrasound-guided shamrock lumbar plexus block. Minerva Anestesiol. 2018;84(1):115–21.

Sato M, et al. Ultrasound-guided lumbar plexus block using three different techniques: a comparison of ultrasound image quality. J Anesth. 2018;32(5):694–701.

Sauter AR, Ullensvang K, Bendtsen TF, Borglum J. The "shamrock method" a new and promising technique for ultrasound guided lumbar plexus block. Br J Anaesth 2013. http://bja.oxfordjournals.org/forum/topic/brjana_el%3B9814. Accessed 15 March 2015.

Strid JMC, et al. Ultrasound-guided lumbar plexus block in volunteers; a randomized controlled trial. Br J Anaesth. 2017;118(3):430–8.

Winnie AP, Ramamurthy S, Durrani Z. The inguinal paravascular technic of lumbar plexus anesthesia: the "3-in-1 block". Anesth Analg. 1973;52:989–96.

Intercostal Block

Karmakar MK, et al. Acute pain management of patients with multiple fractured ribs. J Trauma. 2003;54:612–5.

Kaushal B, et al. Comparison of the efficacy of ultrasound-guided serratus anterior plane block, pectoral nerves II block, and intercostal nerve block for the management of postoperative thoracotomy pain after pediatric cardiac surgery. J Cardiothoracic and Vascular Anesth. 2019;33(2):418–25.

Kopacz DJ, et al. Intercostal blocks for thoracic and abdominal surgery. Tech Reg Anesth Pain Manage. 1998;2:25–9.

Lukosiene L, et al. Single shot intercostal block for pain management in pediatric patients undergoing the Nuss procedure: a double-blind, randomized, controlled study. J Pediatric Surgery. 2014;49(12):1753–7.

Luo M, et al. Comparison of ultrasonography-guided bilateral intercostal nerve blocks and conventional patient-controlled intravenous analgesia for pain control after the Nuss procedure in children. The Clinical J of Pain. 2017;33(7):604–10.

Schlatter MG, et al. Progressive reduction of hospital length of stay following minimally invasive repair of pectus excavatum: a retrospective comparison of three analgesia modalities, the role of addressing patient anxiety, and reframing patient expectations. J Pediatric Surgery. 2019;54(4):663–9.

Strombskag KE, et al. Continuous intercostals and interpleural nerve blockades. Tech Reg Anesth Pain Manage. 1998;2:79–89.

Vlassakov K, et al. A prospective, randomized comparison of ultrasonographic visualization of proximal intercostal block vs paravertebral block. BMC Anesthesiol. 2020;20(1):13.

Ilioinguinal and Iliohypogastric Nerve Blocks

Ghani KR, et al. Transient femoral nerve palsy following Ilio-inguinal nerve blockade for day case inguinal hernia repair. J R Coll Surg Edinb. 2002;47:626–9.

Lipp AK, et al. Leg weakness is a complication of Ilio-inguinal nerve block in children. Br J Anaesth. 2004;92(2):273–4.

van Schoor AN, Boon JM, Bosenberg AT, Abrahams PH, Meiring JH. Anatomical considerations of the pediatric ilioinguinal/iliohypogastric nerve block. PaediatrAnaesth. 2005;15:371–7.

Van Schoor AN, Bosman MC, Bosenberg AT. Revisiting the anatomy of the ilioinguinal/iliohypogastric nerve block. Paediatr Anaesth. 2013 May;23(5):390–4.

Wanzel O, Coz SG, Sitzwohl C, Kapral S. Ultrasonography for ilioinguinal/iliohypogastric nerve blocks in children. Br J Anaesth. 2005;95(2):226–30.

Willschke H, Marhofer P, Bosenberg A, Johnston S, Wanzel O, Cox SG, Sitzwohl C, Kapral S. Ultrasonography for ilioinguinal/ iliohypogastric nerve blocks in children. Br J Anaesth. 2005;95(2):226–30.

Epidural Anaesthesia

Byun S, Pather N. Pediatric regional anesthesia: a review of the relevance of surface anatomy and landmarks used for peripheral nerve blockades in infants and children. Clin Anat. 2019;32(6):803–23.

Ecoffey C, et al. Epidemiology and morbidity of regional anesthesia in children: a follow-up one-year prospective survey of the French-language society of pediatric anesthesiologists (ADARPEF). Paediatr Anaesth. 2010;20:1061–9.

Guay J, et al. The use of ultrasound guidance for perioperative neuraxial and peripheral nerve blocks in children: a Cochrane review. Anesth Analg. 2017 Mar;124(3):948–58.

Gunter JB, et al. Thoracic epidural anesthesia via the caudal approach in children. Anesthesiology. 1992;76(6):935–8.

Gupta A, et al. Evolving pediatric epidural practice: an institution's clinical experience over 20 years – a retrospective observational cohort study. Paediatr Anesth. 2019;1:25–33.

Hasan MA, et al. Depth of epidural space in children. Anaesthesia. 2007;49(12):1085–7.

Karmakar MK, Li X, Ho AMH, Kwok WH, Chui PT. Real-time ultrasound-guided paramedian epidural access: evaluation of a novel in-plane technique. Br J Anaesth. 2009;102(6):845–54.

Kesler H, Dias MS, Kalapos P. Termination of the normal conus medullaris in children: a whole-spine magnetic resonance imaging study. NeurosurgFocus. 2007;23:E7.

Kil HK, et al. Prepuncture ultrasound-measured distance: an accurate reflection of epidural depth in infants and small children. Reg Anesth Pain Med. 2007;32:102–6.

Lonnqvist PA, et al. The European Society of Regional Anesthesia and Pain Therapy and the American Society of Regional Anesthesia and Pain Medicine joint committee practice advisory on controversial topics in pediatric regional anesthesia I and II: what do they tell us? Curr Opin in Anesth. 2017;30(5):613–20.

Marhofer P, et al. Pilot study of neuraxial imaging by ultrasound in infants and children. Pediatr Anesth. 2005;15:671–6.

Oberndorfer U, et al. Ultrasonographic guidance for sciatic and femoral nerve blocks in children. Br J Anaesth. 2007;98:797–801.

Rapp HJ, et al. Ultrasound-guided epidural catheter insertion in children. Anesth Analg. 2005;101:333–9.

Taenzer AH, et al. Asleep versus awake: does it matter?: pediatric regional block complications by patient state: a report from the pediatric regional anesthesia network. Reg Anesth Pain Med. 2014;39(4):279–83.

Tsui BC. Thoracic epidural catheter placement in infants via the caudal approach under electrocardiographic guidance: simplification of the original technique. Anesth Analg. 2004;98:273.

Tsui BC, Gupta S, Finucane B. Confirmation of epidural catheter placement using nerve stimulation. Can J Anesth. 1998;45:640–4.

Tsui BC, Wagner A, Cave D, Seal R. Threshold current for an insulated epidural needle in pediatric patients. Anesth Analg. 2004;99:694–6.

Tsui BCH, Suresh S. Ultrasound imaging for regional anesthesia in infants, children, and adolescents: a review of current literature and its application in the practice of neuraxial blocks. Anesthesiology. 2010;112:719–28.

Walker BJ, et al. Complications in pediatric regional anesthesia: an analysis of more than 100,000 blocks from the pediatric regional anesthesia network. Anesthesiology. 2018;129:721–32.

Caudal Epidural Anesthesia

Bachman SA, et al. Thoracic caudal epidural catheter localization using ultrasound guidance. Paediatr Anaesth. 2020;30(2):194–5.

Bromage PR. A comparison of the hydrochloride and carbon dioxide salts of lidocaine and prilocaine in epidural analgesia. Acta Anaesthesiol Scand Suppl. 1965;16:55–69.

Lewis MP, Thomas P, Wilson LF, Mulholland RC. The 'whoosh' test. A clinical test to confirm correct needle placement in caudal epidural injections. Anaesthesia. 1992;47:57–8.

Orme RM, Berg SJ. The 'swoosh' test-an evaluation of a modified 'whoosh' test in children. Br J Anaesth. 2003;90:62–5.

Park JH, et al. Determination of the optimal angle for needle insertion during caudal block in children using ultrasound imaging. Anesthesia. 2006;61:946–9.

Ponde VC, et al. Does ultrasound guidance add accuracy to continuous caudal-epidural catheter placements in neonates and infants? Paediatr Anaesth. 2017;27(10):1010–4.

Raghunathan K, et al. Determining the accuracy of caudal needle placement in children: a comparison of the swoosh test and ultrasonography. Pediatr Anesth. 2008;18:606–12.

Roberts SA, et al. Ultrasound assessment of caudal catheter position in infants. Pediatr Anesth. 2005;15:429–32.

Tsui B, Leipoldt C, Desai S. Color flow Doppler ultrasonography can distinguish caudal epidural injection from intrathecal injection. Anesth Analg. 2013;116:1376–9.

Tsui BC, Tarkkila P, Gupta S, Kearney R. Confirmation of caudal needle placement using nerve stimulation. Anesthesiology. 1999;91:374–8.

Tsui BC, Wagner AM, Cunningham K, Perry S, Desai S, Seal R. Can continuous low current electrical stimulation distinguish insulated needle position in the epidural and intrathecal spaces in pediatric patients? Paediatr Anaesth. 2005;15:959–63.

Wiegele M, Marhofer P, Lonnqvist PA. Caudal epidural blocks in paediatric patients: a review and practical considerations. Br J Anaesth. 2019 Apr;122(4):509–17.

Wiegele M, Marhofer P, Lonnqvist PA. Caudal epidural blocks in paediatric patients: a review and practical considerations. Br J Anaesth. 2019;122(4):509–17.

Spinal Anesthesia

Arthurs OJ, Murray M, Zubier M, Tooley J, Kelsall W. Ultrasonographic determination of neonatal spinal canal depth. ArchDisChild Fetal Neonatal Ed. 2008;93:F451–4.

Bonadio WA, Smith DS, Metrou M, Dewitz B. Estimating lumbar-puncture depth in children. N Engl J Med. 1988;319:952–3.

Cote CJ, Lerman J, Todres ID. A practice of anesthesia for infants and children. Philadelphia: Saunders Elsevier; 2009. p. 877.

De Saint BL, Simon L, Laplace C, Egu JF, Hamza J. Preoperative coagulation tests in former preterm infants undergoing spinal anaesthesia. Paediatr.Anaesth. 2002;12:304–7.

Hammer GB, et al. Postoperative analgesia after spinal blockade in infants and children undergoing cardiac surgery. Anesth Analg. 2005;100:1283–8.

Jones LJ, et al. Regional (spinal, epidural, caudal) versus general anaesthesia in preterm infants undergoing inguinal herniorrhaphy in early infancy. Cochrane Database Syst Rev. 2015;6:CD003669.

Kachko L, et al. Spinal anesthesia in neonates and infants - a single-center experience of 505 cases. Paediatr Anaesth. 2007;17(7):647–53.

Lopez T, et al. Spinal anesthesia in pediatric patients. Minerva Anestesiol. 2012;78(1):78–87.

Puncuh F, et al. Use of spinal anaesthesia in paediatric patients: a single Centre experience with 1132 cases. Paediatr Anaesth. 2004;13:564–7.

Shenkman Z, Rathaus V, Jedeikin R, Konen O, Hoppenstein D, Snyder M, Freud E. The distance from the skin to the subarachnoid space can be predicted in premature and former-premature infants. Can J Anaesth. 2004;51:160–2.

Shenkman Z, et al. Hemodynamic changes during spinal anesthesia in premature infants with congenital heart disease undergoing inguinal hernia correction. Paediatr Anaesth. 2012;22(9):865–70.

Suresh S, et al. The European Society of Regional Anaesthesia and Pain Therapy/American Society of Regional Anesthesia and Pain Medicine recommendations on local anesthetics and adjuvants dosage in pediatric regional anesthesia. Reg Anesth Pain Med. 2018;43(2):211–6.

Tobias JD. Spinal anaesthesia in infants and children. Paediatr Anaesth. 2000;10:5–16.

Whitaker EE, et al. Spinal anesthesia for pediatric urological surgery: reducing the theoretic neurotoxic effects of general anesthesia. J Pediatr Urol. 2017;13(4):396–400.

Correction to: Celiac Plexus Block

Arash Yousefi, Neal Rakesh, Amitabh Gulati,
and Sushma Bhatnagar

Correction to chapter 44 in:
D. Jankovic, P. Peng (eds.), *Regional Nerve Blocks in Anesthesia and Pain Therapy*,
https://doi.org/10.1007/978-3-030-88727-8_44

The original version of this chapter was inadvertently published with incorrect authorship. The first author Arash Yousefi's name was not included. The authorship has been updated with this erratum, and the correct authorship reads as:

Arash Yousefi, Neal Rakesh, Amitabh Gulati, and Sushma Bhatnagar

The updated version of this chapter can be found at https://doi.org/10.1007/978-3-030-88727-8_44

D. Jankovic, P. Peng (eds.), *Regional Nerve Blocks in Anesthesia and Pain Therapy*,
https://doi.org/10.1007/978-3-030-88727-8_77

Index

D. Jankovic, P. Peng (eds.), *Regional Nerve Blocks in Anesthesia and Pain Therapy*,
https://doi.org/10.1007/978-3-030-88727-8

M

Q

R

Printed by Printforce, the Netherlands